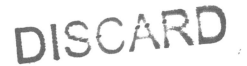

Clinical Infectious Disease

This is a clinically oriented, user-friendly text on infectious disease. Written to address the needs of both general internists and infectious disease specialists, this book focuses on the diagnostic protocols and treatment strategies with which physicians must be familiar when managing infectious disease patients.

The orientation of the volume is multi-faceted: in addition to the traditional organization of organ system and pathogen-related information, this text includes specific sections on the susceptible host (with individual chapters on the diabetic, the elderly, the injection drug user, and the neonate), travel-related infections, nosocomial infections, infections related to surgery and trauma, and bioterrorism.

Informative algorithms, tables, and high-quality color photographs supplement many of the chapters. Moreover, the size of this book places it between the available encyclopedic tomes and the small pocket guides, making it a comprehensive but convenient and practical reference for the practicing clinician.

David Schlossberg, MD, FACP, is Professor of Medicine at Temple University School of Medicine in Philadelphia; Adjunct Professor of Medicine, University of Pennsylvania School of Medicine; and Medical Director of the Tuberculosis Control Program for the Philadelphia Department of Public Health. He is a Fellow of the American College of Physicians and a Fellow of the Infectious Diseases Society of America. In addition to winning numerous teaching awards, he has been invited to lecture throughout the United States and East Asia. He is a reviewer for a number of medical journals, including the *New England Journal of Medicine*, *Clinical Infectious Diseases*, the *Annals of Internal Medicine*, the *Journal of Infectious Disease*, and the *Journal of the American Medical Association*.

Clinical Infectious Disease

Edited by

David Schlossberg

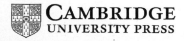

CAMBRIDGE UNIVERSITY PRESS
Cambridge, New York, Melbourne, Madrid, Cape Town, Singapore, São Paulo, Delhi

Cambridge University Press
32 Avenue of the Americas, New York, NY 10013-2473, USA

www.cambridge.org
Information on this title: www.cambridge.org/9780521871129

First published 2008

Printed in Hong Kong by Golden Cup

A catalog record for this publication is available from the British Library.

Library of Congress Cataloging in Publication Data

Clinical infectious disease/edited by David Schlossberg.
    p. ; cm
Includes bibliographical references and index.
ISBN 978-0-521-87112-9 (hardback)
1. Communicable diseases.   I. Schlossberg David.   II. Title.
[DNLM: 1. Communicable Diseases. WC 100 C6416 2008]
RC111.C562   2008
616.9–dc22   2007050649

ISBN 978-0-521-87112-9 hardback

This book is dedicated to Dr. Bennett Lorber – physician, teacher, musician, artist, raconteur, colleague, and valued friend.

"and gladly wolde he lerne and gladly teche."
– Chaucer, Canterbury Tales

Contents

Part V. Clinical Syndromes – Respiratory Tract

Part VI. Clinical Syndromes – Heart and Blood Vessels

Part VII. Clinical Syndromes – Gastrointestinal Tract, Liver, and Abdomen

Part VIII. Clinical Syndromes – Genitourinary Tract

[†] Deceased

[†] Deceased

Preface

David Schlossberg, MD, FACP

Our goal with *Clinical Infectious Disease* is to provide to physicians a complete and user-friendly guide to both the diagnosis and treatment of infectious diseases.

The book is divided into 10 sections. First, clinical presentation by organ system provides a traditional anatomic orientation, although within this section additional chapters are devoted to particularly challenging entities that are often difficult to research, such as infectious thyroiditis, deep neck infection, periocular infection, lymphadenopathy, mediastinitis, pacemaker infection, sexually transmitted enteric infection, bursitis, polyarthritis, psoas abscess, splenic abscess, spinal epidural abscess, cerebrospinal shunt infection, myelitis and peripheral neuropathy, and prion disease.

The second section, "The Susceptible Host," includes individual chapters on a variety of immunocompromised states, including diabetes, transplantation, neutropenia, dialysis, pregnancy, and asplenia. Subsequent entire sections are devoted to HIV, nosocomial infection, surgery and trauma, prophylaxis, travel and recreation, and bioterrorism.

Organism-specific chapters follow, with separate chapters dedicated to individual bacteria, viruses, fungi, parasites, and other pathogens, and then a major section on antimicrobial therapy comprises chapters on principles of antibiotic therapy, antifungal therapy, antiviral therapy, and hypersensitivity to antibiotics. A final chapter lists antimicrobial agents in tabular form, providing a convenient reference for dosage, side effects, cost, pregnancy class, effect of food, and dose adjustment for renal dysfunction. All chapters include suggested readings.

We hope this text provides a practical, clinically oriented, and convenient resource for the diagnosis and treatment of infectious disease.

I am enormously grateful for the vision, talent, and dedication of the staff at Cambridge University Press, particularly publishing director Marc Strauss and editorial assistant Carlos Aguirre. I also thank Jennifer Bossert and Barbara Walthall for their valuable contributions and guidance.

Contributors

Judith A. Aberg, MD, FIDSA
Department of Medicine (Infectious
  Diseases and Immunology)
New York University School of Medicine,
  New York, New York
100. Prophylaxis of Opportunistic
  Infections in HIV Infection

Elias Abrutyn, MD[†]
Division of Infectious Diseases
Drexel University College of Medicine,
  Philadelphia, Pennsylvania
64. Urinary Tract Infection

David W. K. Acheson, MD
U.S. Food and Drug Administration.
Rockville, Maryland
129. Campylobacter, 153. Shigella

Elisabeth E. Adderson, MD
Department of Infectious Diseases
St. Jude Children's Research Hospital,
  Departments of Molecular Sciences and
  Pediatrics
University of Tennessee Health Sciences
  Center, Memphis, Tennessee
81. Cerebrospinal Fluid Shunt Infections

Adaora A. Adimora, MD, MPH
Division of Infectious Diseases,
  Department of Medicine
University of North Carolina
  School of Medicine, Chapel Hill,
  North Carolina
161. Syphilis and Other Treponematoses

N. Franklin Adkinson, Jr., MD
Professor of Medicine
Johns Hopkins Asthma and Allergy Center
Division of Allergy and Clinical
  Immunology
The Johns Hopkins School of Medicine,
  Baltimore, Maryland
206. Hypersensitivity to Antibiotics

Timothy R. Aksamit, MD, FCCP
Division of Pulmonary and Critical Care
  Medicine and Internal Medicine
Mayo Clinic, Rochester, Minnesota
156. Nontuberculous Mycobacteria

Daniel M. Albert, MD, MS
Department of Ophthalmology and
  Visual Sciences
University of Wisconsin School of Medicine
  and Public Health, Madison, Wisconsin
14. Retinitis

Phillip B. Amidon, MD, FACP
Liver and Digestive Disease Section
Maine General Medical Center,
  Waterville, Maine
57. Whipple's Disease and Sprue

Vincent T. Andriole, MD
Emeritus Professor of Medicine
Yale University School of Medicine,
  New Haven, Connecticut
66. Focal Renal Infections and Papillary
  Necrosis

Donald Armstrong, MD
Member Emeritus
Memorial Sloan-Kettering Cancer Center,
  New York, New York
85. Infections in Patients with Neoplastic
  Disease

Andrew W. Artenstein, MD, FACP, FIDSA
Physician in Chief, Department of Medicine
Director, Center for Biofeedback and
  Emerging Pathogens
Memorial Hospital of Rhode Island
Associate Professor of Medical and
  Community Health
The Warren Alpert School Medical School
  of Brown University
Providence, Rhode Island
120. Bioterrorism

[†] Deceased

Stephen Ash, MB, BS, FRCP
Infection and Immunity Unit
Ealing Hospital, London, UK
22. Deep Soft-Tissue Infections: Necrotizing
   Fasciitis and Gas Gangrene

Aristides P. Assimacopoulos, MD, FIDSA
Department of Internal Medicine
University of South Dakota, Sanford School
   of Medicine, Vermillion, South Dakota
18. Staphylococcal and Streptococcal Toxic
   Shock and Kawasaki Syndromes

Alfred E. Bacon III, MD, FACP
Clinical Assistant Professor of Medicine
Jefferson Medical College, Philadelphia,
   Pennsylvania
Section of Infectious Disease
Christiana Care Health System,
   Newark, Delaware
167. Chlamydia Psittaci (Psittacosis)

Johan S. Bakken, MD, PhD
St. Luke's Infectious Disease Associates,
   Duluth, Minnesota
169. Ehrlichiosis and Anaplasmosis

Robert S. Baltimore, MD
Professor, Departments of Pediatrics and
   Epidemiology and Public Health
Division of Infectious Diseases
Yale University School of Medicine
   New Haven, Connecticut
92. Neonatal Infection

**Jamie S. Barkin, MD, MACG, FACP,
   AGAF, FASGE**
Professor of Medicine University of Miami,
   Miller School of Medicine
Chief, Division of Gastroenterology
Mt. Sinai Medical Center, Miami, Florida
46. Infectious Complications of Acute
   Pancreatitis

John G. Bartlett, MD
Division of Infectious Diseases,
   Department of Medicine
The Johns Hopkins School of Medicine,
   Baltimore, Maryland
50. Antibiotic-Associated Diarrhea

Jules Baum, MD
Department of Ophthalmology
Tufts University School of Medicine, Boston,
   Massachusetts
12. Keratitis

Stephen G. Baum, MD
Senior Associate Dean for Students
Albert Einstein College of Medicine
Bronx, New York
5. Infectious Thyroiditis

Daniel G. Bausch, MD, MPH&TM
Department of Tropical Medicine
Tulane School of Public Health and Tropical
   Medicine, New Orleans, Louisiana
192. Viral Hemorrhagic Fevers

Susan E. Beekmann, RN, MPH
Coordinator, Emerging Infections
   Network Program
Department of Internal Medicine
University of Iowa, Iowa City, Iowa
40. Vascular Infection

Irmgard Behlau, MD
Instructor, Medicine and Ophthalmology
Harvard Medical School
Massachusetts Eye and Ear Infirmary,
The Schepens Eye Research Institute,
   Boston, Massachusetts
Infectious Diseases Division, Mt. Auburn
   Hospital, Cambridge, Massachusetts
29. Croup, Supraglottitis, and Laryngitis

Elise M. Beltrami, MD, MPH
Division of Healthcare Quality Promotion
Center for Infectious Diseases
Centers for Disease Control and Prevention,
   Atlanta, Georgia
102. Percutaneous Injury: Risks and
   Management

Joseph R. Berger, MD
Instructor, Harvard Medical School,
   Boston, Massachusetts
Infectious Disease Service/Opthalmology,
   Massachusettes Eye and Ear Infirmary
   (Harvard), Boston, Massachusetts
The Schepens Eye Reasearch Institute,
   Boston, Massachusetts
Infectious Diseases Division, Mount
   Auburn Hospital (Harvard), Cambridge,
   Massachusetts

Newton-Wellesley Hospital, Tufts/Harvard, Newton, Massachusetts
Department of Neurology, University of Kentucky Medical Center, Lexington, Kentucky
80. Progressive Multifocal Leukoencephalopathy

Anitra S. Birnbaum, MD
Department of Medicine
Sinai Hospital of Baltimore, Baltimore, Maryland
10. Deep Neck Infections

Charles D. Bluestone, MD
Division of Pediatric Otolaryngology
Children's Hospital of Pittsburgh, Pittsburgh, Pennsylvania
7. Sinusitis

Joseph A. Bocchini, Jr., MD
Department of Pediatrics
Louisiana State University Health Sciences Center–Shreveport, Shreveport, Louisiana
127. Moraxella (Branhamella) Catarrhalis

Andrea K. Boggild, MSc, MD, DTMH
Division of Infectious Diseases, Department of Laboratory Medicine and Pathobiology
University of Toronto, Toronto, Ontario, Canada
118. Recreational Water Exposure

Charlotte E. Bolton, MD
Department of Respiratory Medicine
Wales College of Medicine, Cardiff University, Wales, UK
35. Empyema and Bronchopleural Fistula

Fouad Bou Harb, MD
Member of Infectious Disease Society of America
Member of American Academy of HIV Medicine, Bellerose, New York
96. HIV Infection: Initial Evaluation and Monitoring

Suzanne F. Bradley, MD
Professor of Internal Medicine
Division of Infectious Diseases and Geriatric Medicine
University of Michigan Medical School, GRECC, VA Ann Arbor Healthcare System Ann Arbor, Michigan
149. Staphylococcus

David M. Brett-Major, MD
Department of Internal Medicine, Division of Infectious Diseases
National Naval Medical Center, Bethesda, Maryland
26. Mycetoma (Madura Foot)

Roy D. Brod, MD
Department of Opthalmology
Hershey Medical Center
Pennsylvania State School of Medicine, Hershey, Pennsylvania
15. Endophthalmitis

Itzhak Brook, MD, MSc
Professor of Pediatrics
Department of Pediatrics
Georgetown University School of Medicine, Washington, D.C.
4. Pharyngotonsillitis

Arthur E. Brown, MD
Infectious Disease Service
Memorial Sloan-Kettering Cancer Center, New York, New York
103. Hospital-Acquired Fever

Steven C. Buckingham, MD
Department of Pediatrics
University of Tennessee Health Science Center, Memphis, Tennessee
117. Tick-Borne Disease

Stefan Bughi, MD
Assistant Professor of Clinical Medicine
Division of Endocrinology, Keck School of Medicine
University of Southern California, Los Angeles, California
88. Diabetes and Infection

Joseph J. Burrascano, MD
Internal Medicine
Southampton Hospital, Southampton,
   New York
163. Relapsing Fever

Michael Cappello, MD
Professor of Pediatrics, Microbial
   Pathogenesis, and Epidemiology and
   Public Health
Yale University School of Medicine,
   New Haven, Connecticut
37. Acute Pericarditis

Denise M. Cardo, MD
Director, Division of Healthcare Quality
   Promotion
National Center for Infectious Diseases
Centers for Disease Control and Prevention,
   Atlanta, Georgia
102. Percutaneous Injury: Risks and
   Management

Jeanne Carey, MD
Department of Medicine, Division of
   Infectious Diseases
Beth Israel Medical Center, New York,
   New York
5. Infectious Thyroiditis

Christopher F. Carpenter, MD
Department of Medicine, Division of
   Infections Diseases
William Beaumont Hospital, Royal Oak,
   Michigan
170. Candidiasis

Carlos Carrillo, MD, MSc
Instituto de Medicina Tropical Alexander
   von Humboldt Universidad Peruana
   Cayetano Heredia, Lima, Peru
Departamento de Enfermedades
   Transmisibles, Hospital Nacional
   Cayetano Heredia, Lima, Peru
128. Brucellosis

Gulfem E. Celik, MD
Associate Professor, Department of Allergy
Ankara University School of Medicine,
   Ankara, Turkey
206. Hypersensitivity to Antibiotics

Tempe K. Chen, MD
Department of Pediatrics, Division of
   Infectious Diseases
David Geffen School of Medicine at the
   University of California, Los Angeles,
   Los Angeles, California
199. Human Babesiosis

Sanford Chodosh, MD, FCCP
Boston University School of Medicine
   (retired), Boston, Massachusetts
28. Acute and Chronic Bronchitis

Mashiul H. Chowdhury, MD
Department of Medicine, Division of
   Infectious Disease
Drexel University College of Medicine,
   Philadelphia, Pennsylvania
36. Endocarditis of Natural and Prosthetic
   Valves: Treatment and Prophylaxis

Vivian H. Chu, MD, MHS
Department of Medicine, Division of
   Infectious Diseases and International
   Health
Duke University Medical Center, Durham,
   North Carolina
135. HACEK

L. W. Preston Church, MD
Department of Medicine, Division of
   Infectious Diseases
Medical University of South Carolina
Ralph H. Johnson Veterans Affairs Medical
   Center, Charleston, South Carolina
132. Enterobacteriaceae

Clay J. Cockerell, MD
Department of Dermatology, Division of
   Dermatopathology
University of Texas Southwestern Medical
   Center at Dallas, Dallas, Texas
140. Leprosy

Carlo Contoreggi, MD
Clinical Director, National Institute on
   Drug Abuse
National Institutes of Health Clinical Center,
   Baltimore, Maryland
89. Infectious Complications in the Injection
   Drug User

Roberto Baun Corales, DO
Community Health Network, Rochester,
New York
159. Miscellaneous Gram-Positive
Organisms

Kent Crossley, MD
Division of Infectious Diseases and
International Medicine
University of Minnesota Medical School,
Minneapolis, Minnesota
91. Infections in the Elderly

Burke A. Cunha, MD, MACP
Infectious Disease Division
Winthrop-University Hospital, Mineola,
New York
Department of Medicine
SUNY School of Medicine, Stony Brook,
New York
1. Fever of Unknown Origin, 32.
Nosocomial Pneumonia

John S. Czachor, MD, FACP
Division of Infectious Diseases
Wright State University Boonshoft School
of Medicine, Dayton, Ohio
203. Principles of Antibiotic Therapy

Titus L. Daniels, MD
Assistant Professor of Medicine
Division of Infectious Diseases
Vanderbilt University School of Medicine,
Associate Hospital Epidemiologist
Nashville, Tennessee
146. Pseudomonas, Stenotrophomonas,
and Burkholderia

Scott F. Davies, MD
Department of Medicine
University of Minnesota Medical School
Hennepin County Medical Center,
Minneapolis, Minnesota
172. Zygomycosis (Mucormycosis)

Charles Davis, MD
Associate Professor of Medicine
Institute of Human Virology
Division of Infectious Diseases
University of Maryland School of Medicine,
Baltimore, Maryland
141. Meningococcus and Miscellaneous
Neisseriae

Anastácio de Queiroz Sousa, MD
Department of Clinical Medicine and
Director, São José Hospital for Infectious
Diseases, Federal University of Ceará,
Fortaleza, Brazil
200. Trypanosomiases and Leishmaniases

Jorgelina de Sanctis, MD
Department of Medicine, Division of
Infection Disease
William Beaumont Hospital, Royal Oak,
Michigan
170. Candidiasis

E. Patchen Dellinger, MD
Division of General Surgery
University of Washington School of
Medicine, Seattle, Washington
107. Postoperative Wound Infections

Carmen E. DeMarco, MD
Department of Medicine, Division of
Infectious Diseases
Wayne State University School of Medicine,
Detroit, Michigan
2. Sepsis and Septic Shock

Louise M. Dembry, MD, MS, MBA
Section of Infectious Diseases, Department
of Medicine
Yale University School of Medicine,
New Haven, Connecticut
66. Focal Renal Infections and Papillary
Necrosis

Stanley C. Deresinski, MD
Division of Infectious Diseases,
Department of Medicine
Stanford University School of Medicine,
Stanford, California
Santa Clara Valley Medical Center,
San Jose, California
177. Coccidioidomycosis

Lisa L. Dever, MD
Division of Infectious Diseases,
Department of Medicine
New Jersey Medical School, Newark,
New Jersey
34. Lung Abscess

Catherine Diamond, MD, MPH
Division of Infectious Diseases
University of California, Irvine School of
Medicine, Orange, California
38. Myocarditis

Gordon Dickinson, MD
Department of Medicine, Division of
Infectious Diseases
Miller School of Medicine, University of
Miami, Coral Gables, Florida
109. Infected Implants

Mark J. DiNubile, MD
Medical Communications Department
Merck Research Laboratories, North Wales,
Pennsylvania
77. Spinal Epidural Abscess: Diagnosis
and Management

J. Stephen Dumler, MD
Division of Medical Microbiology,
Department of Pathology
The Johns Hopkins School of Medicine,
Baltimore, Maryland
169. Ehrlichiosis and Anaplasmosis

Herbert L. DuPont, MD
University of Texas Health Sciences Center
at Houston
School of Public Health, Center for
Infectious Diseases
St. Luke's Episcopal Hospital and Baylor
College of Medicine, Houston, Texas
119. Travelers' Diarrhea

Marlene L. Durand, MD
Assistant Professor of Medicine, Division of
Infectious Diseases
Massachusetts General Hospital, Boston,
Massachusetts
16. Periocular Infections

Asim K. Dutt, MD
Chief, Medical Service (retired)
Alvin C. York Veterans Administration
Medical Center, Murfreesboro, Tennessee
Professor and Vice Chairman (retired)
Department of Medicine
Meharry Medical College, Nashville,
Tennessee
155. Tuberculosis

N. Cary Engleberg, MD
Division of Infectious Diseases, Departments
of Internal Medicine, Microbiology, and
Immunology
University of Michigan Medical School,
Ann Arbor, Michigan
3. Chronic Fatigue Syndrome

Lawrence J. Eron, MD
Department of Medicine
John Burns School of Medicine, University
of Hawaii, Honolulu, Hawaii
188. Papillomavirus

Janine Evans, MD
Associate Professor of Medicine
Department of Internal Medicine
Yale University School of Medicine,
New Haven, Connecticut
162. Lyme Disease

Matthew E. Falagas, MD, MSc, DSc
Adjunct Associate Professor of Medicine
Tufts University School of Medicine, Boston,
Massachusetts
Director, Alfa Institute of Biomedical
Sciences, Athens, Greece
58. Urethritis and Dysuria

Sebastian Faro, MD
Clinical Professor of Obstetrics and
Gynecology
The University of Texas Health Sciences
Center at Houston, Houston, Texas
59. Vaginitis and Cervicitis

Michael J. G. Farthing, MD, FRCP
Medicine
St George's University of London,
London, UK
201. Intestinal Protozoa

Henry M. Feder, Jr., MD
Department of Pediatrics
University of Connecticut Health Center,
Farmington, Connecticut
19. Classic Viral Exanthems

Thomas Fekete, MD, FACP
Infectious Disease Section
Temple University School of Medicine,
Philadelphia, Pennsylvania
60. Epididymo-Orchitis

Thomas M. File, Jr., MD, MACP, FCCP
Professor, Internal Medicine
Head, Infectious Disease Section
Northeastern Ohio Universities College
    of Medicine, Rootstown, Ohio
Chief, Infectious Disease Service, Summa
    Health System, Akron, Ohio
30. Atypical Pneumonia

Sydney M. Finegold, MD
Infectious Diseases Section
VA Medical Center, West Los Angeles
Department of Microbiology, Immunology
    and Molecular Genetics
David Geffen School of Medicine,
    University of California at Los Angeles,
    Los Angeles, California
122. Anaerobic Infections

Neil Fishman, MD
Director, Antimicrobial Management
    Program
Hospital of the University of
    Pennsylanvia
Associate Professor of Medicine
University of Pennsylvania School
    of Medicine, Philadelphia,
    Pennsylvania
187. Influenza

Thomas A. Fleisher, MD
Chief, Laboratory of Medicine
National Institutes of Health,
    Bethesda, Maryland
83. Evaluation of Suspected
    Immunodeficiency

Harry W. Flynn, Jr., MD
Department of Ophthalmology
University of Miami Miller School of
    Medicine
Bascom Palmer Eye Institute, Miami,
    Florida
15. Endophthalmitis

Patricia M. Flynn, MD
Department of Infectious Diseases
St. Jude Children's Research Hospital,
    Memphis, Tennessee
81. Cerebrospinal Fluid
    Shunt Infections

Joshua Forman, MD
Senior Fellow, Division of
    Gastorenterology and Hepatology
Department of Medicine
University of Maryland School
    of Medicine, Baltimore, Maryland
47. Esophageal Infections

**Michelle E. Freshman, MPH, MSN,
    APRN, BC**
Nurse Practitioner/Ambulatory Services
    Coordinator
Newton-Wellesley Hospital, Newton,
    Massachusetts
43. Chronic Hepatitis

Gerald Friedland, MD
Professor of Medicine and Epidemiology
    and Public Health
Director, Yale University School of Medicine,
    AIDS Program Section of Infectious
    Diseases, Department of Internal
    Medicine, New Haven, Connecticut
27. Fever and Lymphadenopathy

Harvey M. Friedman, MD
Professor of Medicine
Chief of Infectious Disease
University of Pennsylvania, School of
    Medicine, Philadelphia, Pennsylvania
187. Influenza

Lawrence S. Friedman, MD
Professor of Medicine, Harvard Medical
    School, Boston, Massachusettes
Professor of Medicine, Tufts University
    School of Medicine, Boston,
    Massachusetts
Chair, Department of Medicine,
    Newton-Wellesley Hospital, Newton,
    Massachusetts
Assistant Chief of Medicine, Massachusetts
    General Hospital, Boston, Massachusetts
43. Chronic Hepatitis

Patrick G. Gallagher, MD
Professor, Department of Pediatrics,
    Division of Perinatal Medicine
Yale University School of Medicine,
    New Haven, Connecticut
92. Neonatal Infection

Leanne Gasink, MD, MSCE
Instructor in Medicine, Division
of Infectious Diseases
Associate Hospital Epidemiologist,
Hospital of the University of
Pennsylvania, Philadelphia,
Pennsylvania
187. Influenza

Dany Ghannam, MD
Department of Anesthesia
Stanford University School of Medicine,
Stanford, California
105. Intravascular Catheter-Related
Infections

George S. Ghneim, DVM, MPVM, PhD
RTI International, Research Triangle Park,
North Carolina
116. Systemic Infection from Animals

Aaron E. Glatt, MD, FACP, FIDSA, FSHEA
President and Chief Executive Officer
Professor of Clinical Medicine
New Island Hospital, Bethpage, New York
96. HIV Infection: Initial Evaluation and
Monitoring

Richard A. Gleckman, MD[†]
Medicine
Mt. Sinai Medical Center, New York,
New York
203. Principles of Antibiotic Therapy

Marshall J. Glesby, MD, PhD
Department of Medicine
Weill Cornell Medical College, New York,
New York
99. Differential Diagnosis and
Management of Opportunistic
Infections Complicating
HIV Infection

Roderick Go, MD
Department of Internal Medicine
SUNY School of Medicine at Stony Brook,
Stony Brook, New York
197. Toxoplasma

Matthew Bidwell Goetz, MD
Chief, Infectious Diseases,
Veterans Administration Greater Los
Angeles Healthcare System, Los Angeles,
California
Professor of Clinical Medicine, David
Geffen School of Medicine, University of
California, Los Angeles, California
33. Aspiration Pneumonia

Mitchell Goldman, MD
Associate Professor of Medicine, Indiana
University School of Medicine,
Indianapolis, Indiana
175. Histoplasmosis

Ellie J. C. Goldstein, MD
Director, R.M. Alden Research Laboratory
Clinical Professor of Medicine, David
Geffen School of Medicine, University
of California, Los Angeles, Los Angeles,
California
23. Human and Animal Bites

Eduardo Gotuzzo, MD, FACP
Principal Professor of Medicine
Universidad Peruana Cayetano Heredia
Alexander von Humboldt Instituto de
Medicina Tropical
Lima, Peru
128. Brucellosis

Jeremy D. Gradon, MD
Department of Medicine, Division of
Infectious Disease
Sinai Hospital of Baltimore, Baltimore,
Maryland
10. Deep Neck Infections

David Y. Graham, MD
Department of Medicine, Section of
Gastroenterology and Hepatology
Michael E. DeBakey VA Medical Center and
Baylor College of Medicine, Houston, Texas
136. Helicobacter Pylori

Elizabeth Graham, FRCP, DO, FRCO
Medical Eye Unit
St. Thomas' Hospital, London, UK
13. Iritis

[†] Deceased

Jennifer Rubin Grandis, MD, FACS
Department of Otolaryngology
University of Pittsburgh School of Medicine,
  Pittsburgh, Pennsylvania
8. Dental Infection and Its Consequences

Jane M. Grant-Kels, MD
Dermatology Residency Program, Residency
  Director
University of Connecticut School of
  Medicine, Farmington, Connecticut
19. Classic Viral Exanthems

Ruth M. Greenblatt, MD
Departments of Clinical Pharmacy,
  Medicine, and Epidemiology
University of California, San Francisco
  Schools of Pharmacy and Medicine, San
  Francisco, California
186. Human Herpesviruses 6, 7, and 8

Ronald A. Greenfield, MD
Department of Internal Medicine, Section of
  Infectious Disease
University of Oklahoma College of
  Medicine, Oklahoma City, Oklahoma
173. Sporotrichosis

Donald L. Greer, PhD
Professor Emeritus
Department of Dermatology
Louisiana State University Health Sciences
  Center, New Orleans, Louisiana
179. Miscellaneous Fungi and Algae

David W. Gregory, MD
Associate Professor of Medicine, Emeritus
Division of Infectious Diseases
Vanderbilt University School of Medicine,
  Nashville, Tennessee
146. Pseudomonas, Stenotrophomonas,
  and Burkholderia

David E. Griffith, MD
Professor of Medicine
The University of Texas Health Sciences
  Center, Tyler, Texas
156. Nontuberculous Mycobacteria

Ray Y. Hachem, MD
Department of Infectious Diseases,
  Infection Control and Employee Health
University of Texas M.D. Anderson Cancer
  Center, Houston, Texas
9. Infection of the Salivary and Lacrimal
  Glands

Sohail G. Haddad, MD
Department of Infectious Diseases
Cleveland Clinic Foundation, Cleveland,
  Ohio
159. Miscellaneous Gram-Positive
  Organisms

Lisa Haglund, MD, FACP
Division of Infectious Diseases
University of Cincinnati College of
  Medicine, Cincinnati, Ohio
143. Nocardia

Margaret R. Hammerschlag, MD
Professor of Pediatrics and Medicine
Director, Division of Pediatric Infectious
  Diseases
SUNY Downstate Medical Center, Brooklyn,
  New York
166. Chlamydia Pneumoniae

W. Lee Hand, MD
Department of Internal Medicine,
  Division of Infectious Diseases
Texas Tech University School of Medicine,
  El Paso, Texas
134. Erysipelothrix

Shahbaz Hasan, MD
Infectious Care
Presbyterian Hospital of Dallas, Dallas,
  Texas
67. Infection of Native and Prosthetic Joints

Rodrigo Hasbun, MD
Infectious Diseases Section
Tulane University School of Medicine, New
  Orleans, Louisiana
78. Myelitis and Peripheral Neuropathy

Bridget Hathaway, MD
Department of Otolaryngology
University of Pittsburgh School of Medicine,
  Pittsburgh, Pennsylvania
8. Dental Infection and
  Its Consequences

Arash Heidari, MD
Assistant Clinical Professor of Medicine,
  Department of Medicine, Division of
  Infectious Diseases
David Geffen School of Medicine,
  University of California, Los Angeles,
Kern Medical Center, Bakersfield,
  California
33. Aspiration Pneumonia

David K. Henderson, MD
Associate Professor, Department of
  Psychiatry
Harvard Medical School, Boston,
  Massachusetts
40. Vascular Infection

H. Franklin Herlong, MD
Division of Hepatology, Department of
  Medicine
The Johns Hopkins University School of
  Medicine, Baltimore, Maryland
45. Pyogenic Liver Abscess

Lisa S. Hodges, MD
Department of Pediatrics
Louisiana State University Health Sciences
  Center–Shreveport, Shreveport, Louisiana
127. Moraxella (Branhamella) Catarrhalis

Craig J. Hoesley, MD
Associate Professor of Medicine
University of Alabama at Birmingham,
  Birmingham, Alabama
124. Bartonellosis (Carrión's Disease)

Charles H. Hoke, Jr., MD, FIDSA
Military Infectious Disease Research
  Program
U.S. Army Medical Research and
  Materiel Command, Fort Detrick,
  Maryland
181. Dengue and Dengue-Like Illness

Paul D. Holtom, MD
Associate Professor of Medicine and
  Orthopaedics
Keck School of Medicine, University
  of Southern California, Los Angeles,
  California
168. Rickettsial Infections

Richard B. Hornick, MD
Clinical Professor of Medicine, University
  of Florida, Florida State University, and
  University of Central Florida
Orlando Regional Healthcare, Orlando,
  Florida
154. Tularemia

Thomas R. Howdieshell, MD, FACS, FCCP
Department of Surgery, Trauma/Surgical
  Critical Care
University of New Mexico School of
  Medicine, Albuquerque, New Mexico
55. Splenic Abscess

Ping-I Hsu, MD
Division of Gastroenterology,
  Department of Internal Medicine
Kaoshiung Veterans General Hospital
National Yang-Ming University,
  Kaohsiung, Taiwan
136. Helicobacter Pylori

Robert Huang, MD, DTM&H
Division of Infectious Diseases,
  Department of Medicine
University of California, San Diego School
  of Medicine, San Diego, California
202. Extraintestinal Amebic Infection

Walter T. Hughes, MD
Department of Infectious Diseases
St. Jude Children's Research Hospital,
  Memphis, Tennessee
178. Pneumocystis Pneumonia

Thomas L. Husted, MD
Department of Surgery
University of Cincinnati College of
  Medicine, Cincinnati, Ohio
112. Surgical Prophylaxis

Christopher D. Huston, MD
Assistant Professor, Departments of
  Medicine, Microbiology and Molecular
  Genetics
University of Vermont College of Medicine,
  Burlington, Vermont
164. Leptospirosis

Newton E. Hyslop, Jr., MD
Professor of Medicine Emeritus
Infectious Diseases Section
Tulane University School of Medicine, New
  Orleans, Louisiana
78. Myelitis and Peripheral Neuropathy

Michelle J. Iandiorio, MD
Division of Infectious Disease, Department
  of Medicine
University of New Mexico School of
  Medicine, Albuquerque, New Mexico
184. Hantavirus Cardiopulmonary
  Syndrome in the Americas

David N. Irani, MD
Department of Neurology
University of Michigan Medical School,
  Ann Arbor, Michigan
75. Acute Viral Encephalitis

Raul E. Isturiz, MD, FACP
Departamento de Medicina
Centro Medico de Caracas, Caracas,
  Venezuela
Centro Medico Docente La Trinidad,
  Caracas, Venezuela
93. Pregnancy and the Puerperium:
  Infectious Risks

William R. Jarvis, MD
President, Jason and Jarvis, Hilton Head
  Island, South Carolina
104. Transfusion-Related Infection

Selma M. B. Jeronimo, MD, PhD
Department of Biochemistry
Bioscience Center Universidade Federal
  do Rio grande do Norte, Rio Grande do
  Norte, Brazil
200. Trypanosomiases and Leishmaniases

Caroline C. Johnson, MD
Philadelphia Department of Public Health
  Philadelphia, Pennsylvania
151. Viridans Streptococci

Jonas T. Johnson, MD
Department of Otolaryngology
University of Pittsburgh School of Medicine,
  Pittsburgh, Pennsylvania
8. Dental Infection and Its Consequences

Richard T. Johnson, MD
Department of Neurology
The Johns Hopkins School of Medicine,
  Baltimore, Maryland
82. Prion Diseases

Royce H. Johnson, MD, FACP
KMC Department of Medicine
UCLA David Geffen School of Medicine,
  Los Angeles, California
158. Yersinia

Ronald N. Jones, MD
JMI Laboratories, North Liberty, Iowa
133. Enterococcus

Elaine C. Jong, MD, FIDSA
Department of Medicine
University of Washington School of
  Medicine, Seattle, Washington
113. Immunizations

Harmit Kalia, DO
Division of Gastroenterology
New Jersey Medical School, Newark,
  New Jersey
42. Acute Viral Hepatitis

Niranjan Kanesa-thasan, MD, MTMH
Early Development, Novartis Vaccines and
  Diagnostics, Cambridge, Massachusetts
181. Dengue and Dengue-Like Illness

Ravi Karra, MD, MHS
Clinical Fellow, Harvard Medical School
Department of Medicine, Brigham and
  Women's Hospital
Boston, Massachusetts
39. Mediastinitis

Keith S. Kaye, MD, MPH
Department of Medicine, Division of
  Infectious Diseases and International
  Health
Duke University School of Medicine,
  Durham, North Carolina
39. Mediastinitis

Paul Kelly, MD, FRCP
Barts and The London, Queen Mary's
  School of Medicine and Dentistry,
  University of London, London, UK
201. Intestinal Protozoa

Michael Kessler, Pharm D
Cooper University Hospital, Camden,
New Jersey
207. Antimicrobial Agent Tables

Jay S. Keystone, MD, MSc. (CTM), FRCPC
Tropical Disease Unit, Toronto General
Hospital
University of Toronto, Toronto, Ontario,
Canada
114. Advice for Travelers, 193. Intestinal
Roundworms, 198. Malaria: Treatment
and Prophylaxis

David W. Kimberlin, MD
Division of Pediatric Infectious
Diseases
University of Alabama at Birmingham
School of Medicine, Birmingham,
Alabama
185. Herpes Simplex Viruses 1 and 2

Evelyn K. Koestenblatt, MS
Department of Dermatology
St. Luke's/Roosevelt Hospital Center,
New York, New York
25. Superficial Fungal Diseases of the
Hair, Skin, and Nails

James R. Korndorffer, Jr., MD, FACS
Associate Professor of Surgery
Tulane University School
of Medicine, New Orleans, Louisiana
53. Diverticulitis

Phyllis E. Kozarsky, MD
Professor of Medicine and Infectious
Diseases, Travelers' Health and Tropical
Medicine Section
Emory University School of Medicine,
Atlanta, Georgia
114. Advice for Travelers,
198. Malaria: Treatment and Prophylaxis

Peter J. Krause, MD
Professor of Pediatrics
University of Connecticut School of
Medicine, Farmington, Connecticut
Director of Infectious Disease
Connecticut Children's Medical Center,
Hartford, Connecticut
199. Human Babesiosis

William L. Krinsky, MD, PhD
Division of Entomology
Peabody Museum of Natural History,
Yale University, New Haven, Connecticut
24. Lice, Scabies, and Myiasis

Amol D. Kulkarni, MD
Department of Ophthalmology and
Visual Sciences
University of Wisconsin School of
Medicine and Public Health, Madison,
Wisconsin
14. Retinitis

Sampath Kumar, MD
Department of Infectious Diseases,
RML Specialty Hospital, Hinsdale, Illinois
160. Miscellaneous Gram-Negative
Organisms

Alvaro Lapitz, MD
Assistant Clinical Professor of Medicine
Indiana University School of Medicine,
Indianapolis, Indiana
175. Histoplasmosis

Fiona Larsen, MBChB, FRACP
Department of Dermatology, Division
of Dermatopathology
University of Texas Southwestern Medical
Center at Dallas, Dallas, Texas
140. Leprosy

William J. Ledger, MD, FACOG
Weill Cornell Medical College
New York Presbyterian Hospital,
New York, New York
63. Pelvic Inflammatory Disease

Matthew E. Levison, MD
Adjunct Professor of Medicine, Department
of Medicine
Drexel University College of Medicine
Professor
Drexel University School of Public Health,
Philadelphia, Pennsylvania
56. Peritonitis

Stuart M. Levitz, MD
Division of Infectious Diseases and
Immunology
University of Massachusetts Medical School,
Worcester, Massachusetts
171. Aspergillosis

Daniel P. Lew, MD
Department of Medicine
University of Geneva, Switzerland
69. Acute and Chronic Osteomyelitis

Neil S. Lipman, VMD
Professor of Veterinary Medicine in
    Pathology and Laboratory Medicine,
    Research Animal Resource Center
Weill Cornell Medical College
    New York, New York
147. Rat-Bite Fevers

Pamela A. Lipsett, MD, FACS, FCCM
Professor of Surgery, Anesthesia, Critical
    Care, and Nursing
Program Director, General Surgery and
    Surgical Critical Care
The Johns Hopkins School of Medicine,
    Baltimore, Maryland
72. Psoas Abscess

Gustine Liu-Young, MD
Department of Internal Medicine,
    Division of Infectious Disease
Yale University School of Medicine,
    New Haven, Connecticut
27. Fever and Lymphadenopathy

Sarah S. Long, MD
Professor of Pediatrics
Drexel University College of Medicine,
    Philadelphia, Pennsylvania
126. Bordetella

Bennett Lorber, MD
Thomas M. Durant Professor of Medicine
    and Professor of Microbiology and
    Immunology
Temple University School of Medicine,
    Philadelphia, Pennsylvania
142. Listeria

Benjamin J. Luft, MD
Department of Medicine
SUNY School of Medicine at Stony Brook,
    Stony Brook, New York
197. Toxoplasma

Larry I. Lutwick, MD
Director, Infectious Diseases
VA New York Harbor Health Care System,
    Brooklyn, New York (Brooklyn Campus)
95. Overwhelming Postsplenectomy
    Infection

Rodger D. MacArthur, MD
Department of Medicine, Division of
    Infectious Diseases
Wayne State University School of Medicine,
    Detroit, Michigan
2. Sepsis and Septic Shock

Karl Madaras-Kelly, PharmD
Department of Pharmacy Practice
College of Pharmacy, Idaho State
    University, Boise, Idaho
150. Streptococcus Groups A, B, C,
    D, and G

Joanne T. Maffei, MD
Associate Professor, Department of
    Medicine, Section of Infectious Diseases/
    HIV
Louisiana State University Health Sciences
    Center, New Orleans, Louisiana
20. Skin Ulcer and Pyoderma

Rafael Gerardo Magaña, MD
Department of Surgery
New York-Presbyterian/Weill Cornell
    Medical College, New York, New York
110. Infection in the Burn-Injured Patient

James H. Maguire, MD
Department of Epidemiology and
    Preventive Medicine
University of Maryland School of Medicine,
    Baltimore, Maryland
195. Schistosomes and Other Trematodes

Francis S. Mah, MD
Department of Ophthalmology
University of Pittsburgh School
    of Medicine, Pittsburgh, Pennsylvania
12. Keratitis

Anita Mahadevan, MBBS, MD
Department of Neuropathology
National Institute of Mental Health and
    Neurosciences, Bangalore, India
190. Rabies

Mark A. Malangoni, MD
Department of Surgery
Case Western Reserve University School
    of Medicine, Cleveland, Ohio
108. Trauma-Related Infection

Stephen E. Malawista, MD
Department of Internal Medicine
Yale University School of Medicine,
  New Haven, Connecticut
162. Lyme Disease

Peter Mariuz, MD
Associate Professor in Medicine
Department of Medicine
University of Rochester, School of Medicine
  and Dentistry, Rochester, New York
94. Dialysis-Related Infection

Thomas J. Marrie, MD, FRCP(C)
Department of Medicine
University of Alberta, Edmonton, Alberta,
  Canada
139. Legionellosis

Paul Martin, MD
Professor of Medicine
Chief, Division of Hepatology, Schiff Liver
  Institute, University of Miami Miller
  School of Medicine, Miami, Florida
42. Acute Viral Hepatitis

Rebecca Edge Martin, MD
Division of Infectious Diseases,
  Department of Medicine, Central
  Arkansas Veterans' Healthcare
  System
University of Arkansas for Medical
  Sciences, Little Rock, Arkansas
31. Community-Acquired Pneumonia

Richard A. Martinello, MD
Assistant Professor, Departments of
  Medicine and Pediatrics, Infectious
  Diseases
Yale University School of Medicine and
  VA Connecticut Healthcare System,
  New Haven, Connecticut
37. Acute Pericarditis

Omar Massoud, MD, PhD
Hepatology, Milwaukee, Wisconsin
79. Reye's Syndrome

John E. McGowan, Jr., MD
Department of Epidemiology
Rollins School of Public Health, Emory
  University, Atlanta, Georgia
101. Prevention of Nosocomial Infection
  in Staff and Patients

J. Anthony Mebane, MD
Division of Infectious Diseases
VA Medical Center, Boise, Idaho
150. Streptococcus Groups A, B, C, D, and G

Jeffery L. Meier, MD
Department of Internal Medicine
University of Iowa Carver College of
  Medicine
Iowa City Veterans Affairs Medical Center
  Iowa City, Iowa
180. Cytomegalovirus, 183. Epstein–
  Barr Virus and Other Causes of the
  Mononucleosis Syndrome

Gregory Mertz, MD
Division of Infectious Diseases,
  Department of Medicine
University of New Mexico School of
  Medicine, Albuquerque, New Mexico
184. Hantavirus Cardiopulmonary
  Syndrome in the Americas

Burt R. Meyers, MD
Clinical Professor Medicine
Division of Infectious Diseases,
  Department of Medicine
Mt. Sinai School of Medicine,
  New York, New York
74. Aseptic Meningitis Syndrome

Laurence F. Mirels, MD
Division of Infectious Diseases, Department
  of Medicine, Santa Clara Valley Medical
  Center, San Jose, California
Stanford University, School of Medicine,
  Stanford, California
177. Coccidioidomycosis

Thomas A. Moore, MD, FACP
Clinical Professor and Associate
  Program Director
Department of Internal Medicine
University of Kansas School of Medicine,
  Wichita, Kansas
194. Tissue Nematodes

Douglas R. Morgan, MD, MPH
Division of Digestive Diseases, School of
  Medicine
University of North Carolina School,
  Chapel Hill, North Carolina
48. Gastroenteritis

Maurice A. Mufson, MD, MACP
Department of Medicine
Joan C. Edwards School of Medicine,
    Marshall University, Huntington,
    West Virginia
145. Pneumococcus

Jorge Murillo, MD
Infectious Diseases and Internal Medicine,
    Miami, Florida
93. Pregnancy and the Puerperium:
    Infectious Risks

Robert L. Murphy, MD
Department of Infectious Disease
Northwestern University Feinberg School
    of Medicine, Chicago, Illinois
86. Corticosteroids, Cytotoxic Agents,
    and Infection

Timothy F. Murphy, MD
Distinguished Professor of Medicine and
    Microbiology
Chief, Infectious Diseases, University at
    Buffalo, State University of New York,
    Buffalo, New York
138. Haemophilus

Avindra Nath, MD
Department of Neurology
The Johns Hopkins School of Medicine,
    Baltimore, Maryland
190. Rabies

Dionissios Neofytos, MD
Department of Medicine,
Division of Infectious Diseases
Jefferson Medical College of Thomas
    Jefferson University, Philadelphia,
    Pennsylvania
97. HIV-1 Infection: Antiretroviral
    Therapy

Ronald Lee Nichols, MD, MS, FACS
William Henderson Professor of Surgery
    Emeritus, Professor of Microbiology
    and Immunology
Department of Surgery
Tulane University School of Medicine,
    New Orleans, Louisiana
53. Diverticulitis

Lindsay E. Nicolle, MD, FRCPS
Professor, Departments of Internal
    Medicine and Medical Microbiology
University of Manitoba, Winnipeg,
    Manitoba, Canada
106. Infections Associated with
    Urinary Catheters

Deborah J. Nicolls, MD
Department of Medicine, Division
    of Infectious Diseases
Emory University School of Medicine,
    Atlanta, Georgia
198. Malaria: Treatment and Prophylaxis

Ahmad R. Nusair, MD
Department of Internal Medicine,
    Infectious Disease Division
Marshall University School of Medicine,
    Huntington, West Virginia
90. Infections in the Alcoholic

Judith A. O'Donnell, MD
Division of Infectious Diseases
Drexel University College of Medicine,
    Philadelphia, Pennsylvania
64. Urinary Tract Infection

Anthony Ogedegbe, MD
Department of Medicine
Weill Cornell Medical College,
    New York, New York
99. Differential Diagnosis and Management
    of Opportunistic Infections Complicating
    HIV Infection

Todd D. Otteson, MD
Division of Pediatric Otolaryngology
Children's Hospital of Pittsburgh,
    Pittsburgh, Pennsylvania
7. Sinusitis

Robert L. Owen, MD
Gastroenterology Section IICI
Department of Veteran Affairs Medical
    Center, San Francisco, California
48. Gastroenteritis

Michael N. Oxman, MD
Department of Medicine, Division of
    Infectious Diseases
University of California, San Diego School
    of Medicine, La Jolla, California
182. Enteroviruses

Brandon Palermo, MD, MPH
Temple University School of Medicine,
  Philadelphia, Pennsylvania
60. Epididymo-Orchitis

George A. Pankey, MD, MACP
Director, Infectious Disease Research
Ochsner Clinic Foundation, New Orleans,
  Louisiana
179. Miscellaneous Fungi and Algae

Monica Panwar, MD, MACP
Fellow in Infectious Diseases
Ochsner Clinic Foundation, New Orleans,
  Louisiana
95. Overwhelming Postsplenectomy
  Infection

Georgios Pappas, MD
Institute of Continuing Medical Education
  of Ioannina, Ioannina, Greece
58. Urethritis and Dysuria

Peter G. Pappas, MD
Department of Medicine, Division of
  Infectious Diseases
University of Alabama School of Medicine,
  Birmingham, Alabama
176. Blastomycosis

Richard H. Parker, MD
Section of Infectious Diseases
Providence Hospital, Washington, D.C.
68. Bursitis

Eleni Patrozou, MD
Division of Infectious Diseases
The Warren Alpert Medical School of Brown
  University School, Providence, Rhode
  Island
120. Bioterrorism

Thomas F. Patterson, MD
Department of Medicine, Division of
  Infectious Diseases
University of Texas Health Science Center
  at San Antonio, San Antonio, Texas
204. Antifungal Therapy

Andrew T. Pavia, MD
Professor of Pediatrics and Medicine
University of Utah School of Medicine,
  Salt Lake City, Utah
49. Food Poisoning

Zbigniew S. Pawlowski, MD, DTMH
Professor Emeritus of Parasitic and
  Tropical Diseases
Poznan University of Medical Sciences,
  Poznan, Poland
196. Tapeworms (Cestodes)

Carlos V. Paya, MD, PhD
Department of Infectious Diseases
Mayo Clinic, Rochester, Minnesota
87. Infections in Transplant Patients

Richard D. Pearson, MD
Departments of Medicine and Pathology
Division of Infectious Diseases and
  International Health
University of Virginia Health System,
  Charlottesville, Virginia
200. Trypanosomiases and Leishmaniases

Stephen I. Pelton, MD
Professor of Pediatrics and Epidemiology
Boston University Schools of Medicine and
  Public Health
Chief, Section of Pediatric Infectious
  Diseases
Boston Medical Center, Boston,
  Massachusetts
6. Otitis Media and Externa

Rosalie Pepe, MD
Department of Infectious Diseases
 Cooper University Hospital, Camden,
  New Jersey
207. Antimicrobial Agent Tables

Kristine M. Peterson, MD
Assistant Professor of Medicine
Division of Infectious Diseases and
  International Health
University of Virginia Health System,
  Charlottesville, Virginia
76. Intracranial Suppuration

Robert S. Pinals, MD
Department of Medicine
Robert Wood Johnson Medical School,
  University of Medicine and Dentistry of
  New Jersey, New Brunswick, New Jersey
70. Polyarthritis and Fever

Roger J. Pomerantz, MD, FACP
Tibotec
Yardley, Pennsylvania
205. Antiviral Therapy

William G. Powderly, MD
School of Medicine and Medical Science
University College, Dublin, Dublin,
    Ireland
174. Cryptococcus

Laurel C. Preheim, MD
Department of Medicine, Division of
    Infectious Diseases
Creighton University School of Medicine
University of Nebraska College of Medicine,
    VA Medical Center, Omaha, Nebraska
90. Infections in the Alcoholic

Thomas C. Quinn, MD, FACP
Division of Infectious Disease
The Johns Hopkins School of
    Medicine, Baltimore, Maryland
51. Sexually Transmitted Enteric
    Infections

Richard Quintiliani, Jr., MD
Director, Hartford Hospital Clinical
    Research Center, Hartford, Connecticut
130. Clostridia

Richard Quintiliani, Sr., MD, FACP
Medicine and Pharmacology
University of Connecticut School of
    Medicine, Farmington, Connecticut
130. Clostridia

Issam Raad, MD, FACP
Department of Infectious Diseases,
    Infection Control and Employee Health
University of Texas M. D. Anderson
    Cancer Center, Houston, Texas
9. Infection of the Salivary and Lacrimal
    Glands, 105. Intravascular Catheter-
    Related Infections

Sanjay Ram, MD
Division of Infectious Diseases and
    Immunology
University of Massachusetts Medical
    School, Worcester, Massachusetts
171. Aspergillosis

Carlos R. Ramírez-Ramírez, MD
Department of Medicine
University of Puerto Rico, School of
    Medicine, San Juan, Puerto Rico
131. Corynebacteria

Carlos H. Ramírez-Ronda, MD, MACP
Department of Medicine
University of Puerto Rico School of
    Medicine, San Juan, Puerto Rico
131. Corynebacteria

Jean-Pierre Raufman, MD
Professor of Medicine
Head, Division of Gastroenterology
    and Hepatology, Department
    of Medicine
University of Maryland School of
    Medicine, Baltimore, Maryland
47. Esophageal Infections

Raymund R. Razonable, MD
Division of Infectious Diseases,
    Department of Medicine
Mayo Clinic, Rochester, Minnesota
87. Infections in Transplant Patients

S. Frank Redo, MD[†]
Chief of Pediatric Surgery,
    Department of Surgery
New York Presbyterian Hospital,
    Weill Cornell Medical Center,
    New York, New York
52. Acute Appendicitis

Sharon Reed, MD
Pathology and Medicine, Division of
    Infectious Diseases
School of Medicine, University
    of California, San Diego, San Diego,
    California
202. Extraintestinal Amebic Infection

Robert V. Rege, MD
Department of Surgery
University of Texas Southwestern
    Medical Center at Dallas, Dallas, Texas
44. Biliary Infection: Cholecystitis and
    Cholangitis

[†] Deceased

Michael F. Rein, MD
Jordan Professor of Epidemiology in
    Medicine, Division of Infectious Diseases
    and International Health
University of Virginia Health System,
    Charlottesville, Virginia
137. Gonococcus: Neisseria Gonorrhoeae

Bruce S. Ribner, MD, MPH
Department of Medicine, Division of
    Infectious Diseases
Emory University School of Medicine,
    Atlanta, Georgia
148. Salmonella

Stacey A. Rizza, MD
Division of Infectious Diseases
Mayo Clinic, Rochester, Minnesota
41. Pacemaker, Defibrillator, and VAD
    Infections

Allan Ronald, OC, MD, FRCPC, MACP
Distinguished Emeritus Professor
University of Manitoba, Winnipeg,
    Manitoba, Canada
61. Genital Ulcer Adenopathy Syndrome

Isabella Rosa-Cunha, MD
Department of Medicine, Division of
    Infectious Diseases
Miller School of Medicine, University
    of Miami, Coral Gables, Florida
109. Infected Implants

Virginia R. Roth, MD
Associate Professor of Medicine,
    University of Ottawa
Director, Infection Prevention and Central
    Program, the Ottawa Hospital
Ottawa, Ontario, Canada
104. Transfusion-Related Infection

Nadine G. Rouphael, MD
Division of Infectious Diseases
Department of Medicine
Emory University School of Medicine,
    Atlanta, Georgia
111. Nonsurgical Antimicrobial
    Prophylaxis

Thomas A. Russo, MD, CM
Professor of Medicine and
    Mircrobiology
Departments of Medicine and Microbiology,
    Division of Infectious Diseases
University at Buffalo
Veterans Administration Western New York
    Health Care System
Buffalo, New York
121. Actinomycosis

William A. Rutala, MD, MPH
Division of Infectious Diseases,
    Department of Medicine
University of North Carolina at Chapel Hill,
    Chapel Hill, North Carolina
116. Systemic Infection from Animals

Mandi P. Sachdeva, MD
Department of Dermatology
Cleveland Clinic, Cleveland, Ohio
21. Cellulitis and Erysipelas

Amar Safdar, MD, FACP
Associate Professor of Medicine,
M. D. Anderson Cancer Center,
    Houston, Texas
85. Infections in Patients with Neoplastic
    Disease

Mirella Salvatore, MD
Division of Infectious Diseases,
    Department of Medicine
Mt. Sinai School of Medicine, New York,
    New York
74. Aseptic Meningitis Syndrome

Rafik Samuel, MD
Division of Infectious Diseases
Temple University School of Medicine,
    Philadelphia, Pennsylvania
84. Infections in the Neutropenic Patient

Naveed Saqib, MD
Department of Surgery
University of New Mexico School of
    Medicine, Albuquerque, New Mexico
55. Splenic Abscess

Divya Sareen, MD
Division of Infectious Disease
Cooper University Hospital, Camden,
    New Jersey
207. Antimicrobial Agent Tables

George A. Sarosi, MD, MACP
Professor of Medicine
Indiana University School of Medicine,
  Indianapolis, Indiana
175. Histoplasmosis

Nicoline Schiess, PhD
Department of Neurology
The Johns Hopkins School of Medicine,
  Baltimore, Maryland
190. Rabies

Patrick M. Schlievert, PhD
Department of Microbiology
University of Minnesota Medical School,
  Minneapolis, Minnesota
18. Staphylococcal and Streptococcal Toxic
  Shock and Kawasaki Syndromes

David Schlossberg, MD, FACP
Medical Director, Tuberculosis Control
  Program, Philadelphia Department of
  Public Health
Professor of Medicine, Temple University
  School of Medicine
Adjunct Professor of Medicine, University of
  Pennsylvania School of Medicine
Philadelphia, Pennsylvania
207. Antimicrobial Agent Tables

Steven K. Schmitt, MD
Department of Infectious Diseases
Cleveland Clinic Foundation, Cleveland,
  Ohio
159. Miscellaneous Gram-Positive
  Organisms

John Schmittner, MD, DHHS
National Institutes of Health, National
  Institute on Drug Abuse, Baltimore,
  Maryland
89. Infectious Complications in the
  Injection Drug User

William A. Schwartzman, MD
Associate Clinical Professor
David Geffen School of Medicine, University
  of California, Los Angeles
Division of Infectious Diseases, VA West
  Los Angeles Health Care Center,
  Los Angeles, California
125. Cat Scratch Disease and Other
  Bartonella Infections

John W. Sensakovic, MD
Infectious Disease
St. Michael's Medical Center, Newark,
  New Jersey
17. Fever and Rash

Susan K. Seo, MD
Antibiotic Management Program
Infectious Disease Service
Memorial Sloan-Kettering Cancer Center,
  New York, New York
103. Hospital-Acquired Fever

Daniel J. Sexton, MD
Department of Medicine, Division of
  Infectious Diseases and International
  Health
Duke University Medical Center, Durham,
  North Carolina
135. HACEK

Dennis J. Shale, MD
Department of Respiratory Medicine
Wales College of Medicine, Cardiff
  University, Wales, UK
35. Empyema and Bronchopleural Fistula

Susarla K. Shankar, MD
Department of Neuropathology
National Institute of Mental Health and
  Neurosciences, Bangalore, India
190. Rabies

Sylvia J. Shaw, MD
Assistant Professor of Clinical Medicine
Division of Endocrinology, Keck School
  of Medicine, University of Southern
  California, Los Angeles, California
88. Diabetes and Infection

Samuel A. Shelburne III, MD
Department of Infectious Diseases
Baylor College of Medicine, Houston, Texas
98. Immune Reconstitution Inflammatory
  Syndrome

Kamaljit Singh, MD
Department of Infectious Diseases
Rush University Medical Center, Chicago,
  Illinois
160. Miscellaneous Gram-Negative
  Organisms

Upinder Singh, MD
Department of Internal Medicine
Stanford University School of Medicine,
    Stanford, California
71. Infectious Polymyositis

Linda A. Slavoski, MD
Doctor of Infectious Disease Medicine
    and Internal Medicine
Wilkes Barre, Pennsylvania
56. Peritonitis

James W. Smith, MD
Clinical Professor of Internal Medicine
Infectious Diseases Division
University of Texas Southwestern
    Medical School, Dallas, Texas
67. Infection of Native and
    Prosthetic Joints

Leon G. Smith, MD
Chairman, Department of Medicine,
    St. Michael's Medical Center, Newark,
    New Jersey
Chairman, Department of Medicine,
    Seton Hall University School
    of Graduate Medical Education
Professor of Preventative Medicine,
    New Jersey Medical School,
    New Brunswick, New Jersey
17. Fever and Rash

Jack D. Sobel, MD
Division of Infectious Diseases
Wayne State University School
    of Medicine, Detroit, Michigan
65. Candiduria

Paola R. Solari, MD
Department of Medicine, Division
    of Infectious Disease
Drexel University College of Medicine,
    Philadelphia, Pennsylvania
36. Endocarditis of Natural and Prosthetic
    Valves: Treatment and Prophylaxis

Joseph S. Solomkin, MD
Department of Surgery, Division
    of Trauma and Critical Care
University of Cincinnati College of
    Medicine, Cincinnati, Ohio
112. Surgical Prophylaxis

Kathleen E. Squires, MD
Department of Medicine
Division of Infectious Diseases
Jefferson Medical College of Thomas
    Jefferson University, Philadelphia,
    Pennsylvania
97. HIV-1 Infection: Antiretroviral Therapy

Barbara W. Stechenberg, MD
Department of Pediatrics, Division of
    Pediatric Infectious Diseases,
(Tufts University School of Medicine
    Baystate Children's Hospital,)
    Springfield, Massachusetts
152. Poststreptococcal Immunologic
    Complications

James M. Steckelberg, MD
Division of Infectious Diseases
Mayo Clinic, Rochester, Minnesota
41. Pacemaker, Defibrillator, and VAD
    Infections

Roy T. Steigbigel, MD
Division of Infectious Disease
University at Stony Brook, Stony Brook,
    New York
94. Dialysis-Related Infection

James P. Steinberg, MD
Department of Medicine
Emory University School of Medicine,
    Atlanta, Georgia
111. Nonsurgical Antimicrobial Prophylaxis

David S. Stephens, MD
Professor of Medicine and Microbiology
    and Immunology
Director, Division of Infectious Disease,
    Department of Medicine
Emory University School of Medicine,
    Atlanta, Georgia
144. Pasteurella Multocida

Dennis L. Stevens, MD, PhD
Professor of Medicine, Division of
    Infectious Diseases
University of Washington School of
    Medicine, Seattle, Washington
Chief Infectious Disease Section, Veterans
    Affairs Medical Center, Boise, Idaho
150. Streptococcus Groups A, B, C, D,
    and G

Nimalie D. Stone, MD
Division of Infectious Diseases
Emory University School of Medicine,
    Atlanta, Georgia
101. Prevention of Nosocomial Infection
    in Staff and Patients

J. B. Stricker, DO
Fred Hutchinson Cancer Research Center,
    Seattle, Washington
140. Leprosy

Kathryn N. Suh, MD, FRCPC
Medicine and Pediatrics
University of Ottawa, Ontario, Canada
193. Intestinal Roundworms

Babafemi O. Taiwo, MD
Division of Infectious Diseases
Northwestern University Feinberg School
    of Medicine, Chicago, Illinois
86. Corticosteroids, Cytotoxic Agents, and
    Infection

Naasha J. Talati, MD
Division of Infectious Diseases
Emory University School of Medicine,
    Atlanta, Georgia
144. Pasteurella Multocida

Jeremiah G. Tilles, MD
Pacific AIDS Education and Training Center
University of California, Irvine School
    of Medicine, Irvine, California
38. Myocarditis

Frank L. Tomaka, MD
Tibotec
Yardley, Pennsylvania
205. Antiviral Therapy

Kenneth J. Tomecki, MD
Department of Dermatology
Cleveland Clinic, Cleveland, Ohio
21. Cellulitis and Erysipelas

Edmund C. Tramont, MD, MACP
Associate Director, Special Projects
Division of Clinical Research
National Institute of Allergy and Infectious
    Diseases, National Institutes of Health,
    Bethesda, Maryland
141. Meningococcus and Miscellaneous
    Neisseriae

Donald D. Trunkey, MD
Professor of Surgery
Oregon Health and Science University,
    Portland, Oregon
54. Abdominal Abscess

Elmer Y. Tu, MD
Director, Cornea and External Disease
    Service
Associate Professor Clinical Ophthalmology
Department of Ophthalmology and
    Visual Sciences
University of Illinois at Chicago College
    of Medicine, Chicago, Illinois
11. Conjunctivitis

Allan R. Tunkel, MD, PhD
Chair, Department of Medicine
Monmouth Medical Center, Long Branch,
    New Jersey
Professor of Medicine, Drexel University
    College of Medicine, Philadelphia,
    Pennsylvania
73. Bacterial Meningitis

Arlo Upton, MBChB, FRACP
Department of Microbiology
Auckland City Hospital, Auckland,
    New Zealand
140. Leprosy

Rajiv R. Varma, MD
Division of Gastroenterology and
    Hepatology
Medical College of Wisconsin,
    Milwaukee, Wisconsin
79. Reye's Syndrome

Boris Velimirovic, MD
World Health Organization
Pan American Health Organization
Washington, D. C.
123. Anthrax and Other Bacillus Species

Anita Venkataramana, MBBS
Department of Neurology
The Johns Hopkins School of Medicine,
    Baltimore, Maryland
190. Rabies

Karen J. Vigil, MD
Infectious Disease
University of Texas–Houston, School
    of Medicine, Houston, Texas
119. Travelers' Diarrhea

Duc J. Vugia, MD, MPH
Infectious Diseases Branch
California Department of Public Health,
    Richmond, California
157. Vibrios

Kenneth F. Wagner, DO, FIDSA
Consultant, Infectious Diseases and
    Tropical Medicine
Islamorada, Florida
26. Mycetoma (Madura Foot)

Ken B. Waites, MD
Department of Pathology, Division of
    Laboratory Medicine
University of Alabama at Birmingham
    School of Medicine, Birmingham,
    Alabama
165. Mycoplasma

Francis A. Waldvogel, MD
Department of Medicine
University of Geneva, Switzerland
69. Acute and Chronic Osteomyelitis

David J. Weber, MD, MPH
Departments of Medicine, Pediatrics, and
    Epidemiology
University of North Carolina Schools
    of Medicine and Public Health, Chapel
    Hill, North Carolina
116. Systemic Infection from Animals

Amy Wecker, MD
Fellow in Infectious Diseases
State University of New York, Downstate
    Medical Center, Brooklyn, New York
95. Overwhelming Postsplenectomy
    Infection

Jeffrey M. Weinberg, MD
Director, Clinical Research Center
Department of Dermatology
St. Luke's - Roosevelt Hospital Center, Beth
    Israel Medical Center,
Assistant Clinical Professor of Dermatology,
    Columbia University College of
    Physicians and Surgeons, New York,
    New York
25. Superficial Fungal Diseases of the Hair,
    Skin, and Nails

Richard J. Whitley, MD
Department of Medicine
University of Alabama at Birmingham
    School of Medicine, Birmingham,
    Alabama
185. Herpes Simplex Viruses 1 and 2

Nathan P. Wiederhold, PharmD
College of Pharmacy
The University of Texas at Austin, Austin,
    Texas
 204. Antifungal Therapy

Mary Elizabeth Wilson, MD, FACP, FIDSA
Associate Professor of Population and
    International Health
Harvard School of Public Health, Boston,
    Massachusetts
118. Recreational Water Exposure

Brian Wispelwey, MD
Division of Infectious Diseases and
    International Health
University of Virginia Health System,
    Charlottesville, Virginia
76. Intracranial Suppuration

Martin S. Wolfe, MD
Travelers' Medical Service of Washington
George Washington School of Medicine and
    Health Sciences, Washington, D. C.
115. Fever in the Returning Traveler

Daniel Wolfson, MD
Administrative Gastroenterology Fellow
University of Miami, Miller School of
    Medicine, Miami, Florida
46. Infectious Complications of Acute
    Pancreatitis

Henry M. Wu, MD
Division of Infectious Disease
Drexel University College of Medicine,
    Philadelphia, Pennsylvania
64. Urinary Tract Infection

Neal S. Young, MD
Hematology Branch,
National Heart Lung and Blood Institute,
    National Institutes of Health, Bethesda,
    Maryland
189. Acute and Chronic Parvovirus
    Infection

Souad Youssef, MD
Department of Infectious Diseases
Infection Control and Employee Health
University of Texas M. D. Anderson Cancer
  Center, Houston, Texas
9. Infection of the Salivary and Lacrimal
  Glands

Roger W. Yurt, MD
New York Presbyterian Hospital,
  New York, New York
110. Infection in the Burn-Injured Patient

Sarah S. Zaher, MD
Division of Medicine
Imperial College London, London, UK
13. Iritis

John A. Zaia, MD
Division of Virology
Beckman Research Institute of City of
  Hope, Duarte, California
191. Varicella-Zoster Virus

Jonathan M. Zenilman, MD
Chief, Division of Infectious Diseases
Johns Hopkins Bayview Medical Center,
  Baltimore, Maryland
62. Prostatitis

PART I

Clinical Syndromes – General

1. Fever of Unkown Origin

Burke A. Cunha

OVERVIEW

Fever of unknown origin (FUO) describes prolonged undiagnosed fevers. In 1961, Petersdorf introduced a standard definition of FUO; his criteria included fevers of temperature >101°F that lasted ≥3 weeks that remained undiagnosed after 1 week of intensive, in-hospital diagnostic testing. This classical definition of FUO still applies today but with one modification. Because of advanced imaging techniques available on an outpatient basis, the intensive diagnostic workup may be conducted in the outpatient setting. The causes of FUO include a wide variety of infectious and noninfectious disorders capable of eliciting fever. By definition, acute febrile disorders are not included in the definition and, even if diagnosed, should not be termed FUOs. Prolonged, difficult-to-diagnose fevers may be due to infection, malignancy, rheumatic diseases, or a variety of other miscellaneous causes.

CAUSES OF FEVER OF UNKNOWN ORIGIN

The types of disorders that are associated with prolonged fevers have remained relatively constant over time, but the relative proportion of different disease categories has changed over the years. In Petersdorf's initial description, infectious diseases constituted the largest single category of disorders causing FUO. Decades later, in reevaluating the distribution of FUO causes, Petersdorf noted that malignancies had exceeded infectious diseases as the most important singular cause of FUO. Recently, in some series, the distribution has changed again, which reflects the demographics of the population being studied. For example, a recent study of FUOs indicates a majority of patients had unexplained fevers due to noninfectious, inflammatory conditions (ie, predominantly rheumatic disorders). Therefore, the relative distribution of disorders presenting as FUO depends on a variety of factors, including the patient's age, geographical location, and underlying host immune defects. Some authors have even further broken down FUOs into those occurring in specific subpopulations (ie, HIV, returning travelers, nosocomial FUOs, etc). Although the differential diagnosis in each subcategory reflects a preponderance of diseases that are specific to age, region, or host defense defects, the overall causes of FUOs in each subpopulation remain essentially the same (Table 1.1).

DIAGNOSTIC APPROACH

Because the appropriateness of any therapy is based on a correct diagnosis, the main focus of the proper approach to the FUO patient is diagnostic rather than therapeutic. The diagnostic workup of the FUO patient should take into account the frequency of distribution of disorders, noninfectious as well as infectious, that relates to the patient's age, geography, and host defense status. The diagnostic workup should further be refined and focused based on the presence of signs, symptoms, and laboratory abnormalities, which can either eliminate diagnostic categories or suggest a particular diagnosis. Nonspecific laboratory tests are often overlooked as potential clues in the FUO workup. Nonspecific laboratory tests are, by definition, nonspecific but, particularly when taken together, should suggest a particular diagnosis and prompt specific diagnostic testing. Importantly, the diagnostic workup should not be shot-gun, including diagnostic testing for every conceivable cause of FUO. Diagnostic testing should be focused and appropriate to the patient's age and geographical location and based particularly on the findings/absence of findings on physical examination and pertinent aspects of the patient's history.

NONSPECIFIC LABORATORY TEST CLUES

Nonspecific laboratory clues are also important in further focusing the diagnostic workup. There are certain radiologic/laboratory investigations that are generally useful when no particular cause of FUO is apparent from the initial diagnostic history, physical, and workup. In addition to basic laboratory tests, computer tomography/magnetic resonance imaging (CT/MRI) scans of the chest, abdomen, and pelvis are high-yield diagnostic tests. Gallium or indium scanning also may localize otherwise

Table 1.1 Diseases Causing Classical Fever of Unknown Origin

Type of Disorder	Common	Uncommon	Rare
Malignancy	Lymphoma Hypernephromas	Preleukemias Hepatomas Myeloproliferative disorder (MPDs) Pancreatic carcinoma Metastases to liver	Atrial myxomas CNS tumors Multiple myeloma Colon carcinoma
Infections	Miliary TB Extrapulmonary TB (Renal TB, TB meningitis) Intraabdominal/pelvic abscesses SBE Typhoid fever malaria	CMV Toxoplasma gondii Salmonella enteric fevers Intra/perinephric abscess Splenic abscess Cat scratch fever EBV	Periapical dental abscesses Chronic sinusitis Subacute vertebral osteomyelitis Listerial Yersinia Brucellosis Relapsing fever Rat bite fever Chronic Q fever HIV Leptospirosis Histoplasmosis Coccidioidomycosis LGV Whipple's disease Relapsing mastoiditis Leishmaniasis (Kala-azar)
Rheumatologic	Still's disease (adult JRA) Polymyalgia rheumatica/ temporal arteritis	PAN Rheumatoid arthritis (elderly)	SLE Takayasu's arteritis Kikuchi's disease Felty's syndrome Pseudogout (CPPD) Behçet's disease FMF
Miscellaneous causes	Drug fever Cirrhosis	Granulomatous hepatitis Regional enteritis Subacute thyroiditis	Fabray's disease Hyperthyroidism Pheochromocytomas Addison's disease Cyclic neutropenia Pulmonary emboli (multiple, Hypothalamic dysfunction Factitious fever Pseudolymphomas Hyper IgD syndrome

Abbreviations: CNS = central nervous system; TB = tuberculosis; SBE = subacute bacterial endocarditis; CMV = cytomegalovirus; HIV = human immunodeficiency virus; EBV = Epstein-Barr virus; LGV = lymphogranuloma venereum; JRA = juvenile rheumatoid arthritis; PAN = polyarteritis nodosa; SLE = systemic lupus erythematosus; FMF = familial Mediterranean fever.
Adapted from: Cunha BA. Fever of unknown origin (FUO). In: Gorbach SL, Bartlett JB, Blacklow NR, eds. *Infectious Diseases in Medicine and Surgery*. 3rd ed. Philadelphia, PA: WB Saunders, 2004:1568–1577.
Adapted from: Cunha BA. Overview. In: Cunha BA, ed. *Fever of Unknown Origin*. New York, NY: Informa Healthcare; 2007.

unsuspected areas of inflammation, infection, or malignancy. Other nonspecific tests are helpful in suggesting or eliminating particular diagnostic categories as well as refining the diagnostic workup, for example, serum ferritin levels, serum protein electrophoresis (SPEP), febrile agglutinins. The SPEP is useful and important, not only for detecting monoclonal gammopathies but also in the differential diagnosis of FUO in demonstrating a polyclonal gammopathy. Polyclonal gammopathy in SPEP in a patient with a heart murmur, signs of endocarditis, and negative blood cultures should suggest the possibility of atrial myxoma rather than culture-negative endocarditis. Perhaps the most underutilized laboratory test in the FUO workup is serum ferritin determinations. Highly elevated serum ferritin levels most frequently suggest a neoplasm/myeloproliferative disorder. However, elevated serum ferritins levels are also present in flares of systemic lupus erythematosus (SLE) or

Table 1.2 FUO: Initial Laboratory Tests

For all FUO categories
- CBC
- ESR
- LFTs
- Chest x-ray
- UA
- Routine blood cultures
- Imaging studies-chest (if abnormal CXR) abdominal/pelvic CT/MRI

CBC[a]
- Leukocytosis → neoplastic and infectious disease panels[a]
- Leukopenia → neoplastic, infectious, and RD panel[a]
- Anemia → neoplastic, infectious, and RD panel[a]
- Myelocytes/metamyelocytes → neoplastic panel[a]
- Lymphocytosis → neoplastic and infectious panels
- Lymphopenia → neoplastic, infectious, and RD panel[a]
- Atypical lymphocytes
- Eosinophilia → neoplastic, RD, and infectious panels[a]
- Basophilia → neoplastic panel[a]
- Thrombocytosis → neoplastic, infectious disease, and RD panels[a]
- Thrombocytopenia → neoplastic, infectious disease, and RD panels[a]

ESR
- Highly elevated → neoplastic, infectious, and RD panels[a]

LFTs
- ↑ SGOT/SGPT → infectious and RD panel[a]
- ↑ Alk. phosphatases → neoplastic and RD panels[a]

Chest x-ray
- Any lung parenchymal abnormality/adenopathy/pleural effusion → neoplastic, infectious and RD panels[a]

[a] See Table 1.3.
Abbreviations: CBC = complete blood count; CXR= chest X-ray; CT= Computer tomagraphy; ESR = erythrocyte sedimentation rate; LFTs = liver function tests; MRI= Magnnetic Resonance Imaging; UA = urine analysis; RD = rheumatic disease; SGOT/SGPT = serum glutamic-oxaloacetic transaminase/serum glutamic pyruvate transaminase.
Adapted from Cunha BA. A focused diagnostic approach. In: Cunha BA, ed. *Fever of Unknown Origin*. New York, NY: Informa Healthcare; 2007.

adult Still's disease (juvenile rheumatoid arthritis) or temporal arteritis. Elevated ferritin level also has important exclusionary value as a nonspecific test in FUO patients. For example, the likelihood of a patient having a malignancy is greatly decreased if the patient has a normal serum ferritin level. The diagnostic workup should be focused and guided by findings and laboratory abnormalities as they become apparent after the initial diagnostic workup (Tables 1.2–1.4).

THERAPEUTIC APPROACH

Empiric therapy of FUOs is rarely justified. Fever, per se, should not be treated, as it eliminates an important sign that may be helpful diagnostically. The only rational antipyretic intervention that may be employed in a patient with FUO is the use of the Naprosyn test (naproxen 375 mg orally every 12 hours for 3 days) for *diagnostic*, not therapeutic, purposes. In FUO patients where the differential diagnosis is between malignancy and infection, the Naprosyn test has important diagnostic implications. The Naprosyn test is positive when the patient's temperature dramatically decreases during the test period. Little or no decrease in the patient's temperature indicates an infectious disorder, whereas a prompt/dramatic decrease in the febrile response indicates a malignancy.

Table 1.3 FUO: Laboratory Clues

Leukopenia	Atypical Lymphocytosis	ESR (>100 mm/hr)
Miliary TB	EBV	Adult JRA
Brucellosis	CMV	PMR/TA
SLE	Brucellosis	Hypernephroma
Lymphomas	Toxoplasmosis	SBE
Pre-leukemias	Drug fever	Drug fever
Typhoid fever	**Thrombocytosis**	Carcinomas
Kikuchi's disease	MPDs	Lymphomas
Monocytosis	TB	MPDs
TB	Carcinomas	Abscesses
PAN	Lymphomas	Subacute osteomyelitis
TA	Sarcoidosis	LORA
CMV	Vasculitis	Hyper IgD syndrome
Sarcoidosis	Temporal arteritis	**SPEP**
Brucellosis	Subacute osteomyelitis	Polyclonal gammopathy
SBE	Hypernephroma	Atrial myxoma
SLE	**Thrombocytopenia**	Alcoholic cirrhosis
Lymphomas	Leukemias	Sarcoidosis
Carcinomas	Lymphomas	PAN
Regional enteritis (Crohn's disease)	MPDs	HIV
MPDs	EBV infectious mono	Takayasu's arteritis
Eosinophilia	Drug fever	↑ α_1/α_2 globulin
Trichinosis	Vasculitis	Lymphoma
Lymphomas	SLE	SLE
Drug fever	**Rheumatoid Factor**	↑ gammaglobulin spike
Addison's disease	SBE	Multiple myeloma
PAN	Chronic active hepatitis	Schnitzler's syndrome
Hypersensitivity vasculitis	Malaria	Hyper Ig D syndrome
Hypernephroma	Hypersensitivity vasculitis	**Increased Serum**
MPDs	LORA	**Transaminases**
Basophilia	**Alkaline Phosphatase**	EBV mononucleosis
Carcinomas	Hepatoma	CMV
Lymphomas	Miliary TB	Q fever
Pre-leukemia (AML)	Lymphomas	Drug fever
MPDs	EBV	Leptospirosis
Lymphocytosis	CMV	Toxoplasmosis
TB	Adult JRA	Brucellosis
EBV	Subacute thyroiditis	Kikuchi's diseases
CMV	TA	**Abnormal Renal Tests**
Toxoplasmosis	Hypernephroma	SBE
Non-Hodgkin's lymphoma	PAN	Renal TB
Lymphocytopenia	Liver metastases	PAN
Whipple's disease	Granulomatous hepatitis	Leptospirosis
Miliary TB	**Serum Ferritin**	Brucellosis
SLE	Malignancies	Lymphomas
Lymphomas	SLE	SLE
Multiple myeloma	TA	Hypernephroma
	LORA	MPDs
	Adult JRA	

Abbreviations: CMV = cytomegalovirus; EBV = Epstein-Barr virus; ESR = erythrocyte sedimentation rate; PAN = periarteritis nodosa; SBE = subacute bacterial endocarditis; SLE = systemic lupus erythematosus; TB = tuberculosis; MPDs = myeloproliferative disorders; LORA = late onset rheumatoid arthritis.
Adapted from Cunha BA. Nonspecific tests in the diagnosis of fever of unknown origin. In: Cunha BA, ed. *Fever of Unknown Origin*. New York, NY: Informa Healthcare; 2007.

The patient's temperature as well as the pulse response has important diagnostic implications, which is another reason antipyretic therapy should be used only under unusual circumstances.

Among the infectious diseases, empiric therapy of presumed culture-negative endocarditis and presumed miliary TB are two of the few exceptions to blindly treating patients with prolonged undiagnosed fevers. With rheumatic diseases, empiric therapy of polymyalgia rheumatica with low-dose prednisone (ie, 5–10 mg orally per day) is important diagnostically. The main difficulty in FUO is to arrive at a correct diagnosis.

Table 1.4 FUO Infectious Panel/Neoplastic Panel/Rheumatic Panel

FUO Infectious Panel	FUO Neoplasic Panel	FUO Rheumatic Panel
Blood Tests		

• Special blood cultures (↑ CO_2/6 weeks
• Q fever serology
• Brucella serology
• Bartonella serology
• Salmonella serology
• Viral serologies
  EBV
  CMV
  HHV-6
	• Ferritin
	• SPEP
		• ANA RF
		• Ds DNA
		• SPEP
		• Ferritin
		• CPK
		• ACE

Radiologic Tests		
• CT/MRI abdomen/pelvis[a] • Gallium scan • Panorex film of jaws (if all else negative)	• CT/MRI abdomen/pelvis[a] • Gallium scan	• Head/chest CT/MRI • Low dose steroids (prednisone 10 mg/day if PMR likely)
Other Tests		
• Naprosyn test • Anergy panel/PPD	• Naprosyn test • BM biopsy (if myelophthistic anemia/abnormal RBCs/WBCs) • TTE (if heart murmur with negative blood cultures)	• Temporal artery biopsy (if ESR >100, without alternate diagnosis)

[a] Chest/head CT/MRI (if infectious etiology suspected in head/chest).
Abbreviations: EBV = Epstein-Barr virus; CMV = cytomegalovirus; HHV-6 = human herpes virus-6; CPK = creatinine phosphokinase; SPEP = serum protein electrophoresis; ACE = angiotensin converting enzyme.
Adapted from Cunha BA. A focused diagnostic approach. In: Cunha BA, ed. *Fever of Unknown Origin*. New York, NY: Informa Healthcare; 2007.

Table 1.5 Therapy in Fever of Unknown Origin

Empiric Therapy	Disorder
Infectious diseases	• Culture negative subacute bacterial endocarditis • Miliary TB
Rheumatic diseases	• Polymyalgia rheumatica (PMR) • Temporal arteritis (TA)
Specific Therapy	**Disorder**
Infectious diseases	• All treatable with effective antibiotics
Rheumatic diseases	• All treatable with effective therapies
Neoplastic diseases	• All treatable with effective therapies

Abbreviations: TB = tuberculosis; TA = temporal arteritis; PMR = polymyalgia rheumatica.

Empiric antimicrobial therapy of a patient with an FUO should be reserved for unusual circumstances, when a therapeutic intervention with an antimicrobial may be of critical importance (eg, culture-negative endocarditis) and may be lifesaving (eg, miliary tuberculosis [TB]). There is a place for specific therapy of FUO once the diagnosis has been determined. Clearly, patients with treatable malignant disorders should receive appropriate antineoplastic therapies/interventions, those with rheumatic diseases should receive steroids/immunosuppressives as appropriate for the disorder and the severity of the illness, and infectious disorders should be treated if therapy is available against the etiologic agent (Table 1.5).

Fever of Unknown Origin

SUGGESTED READING

Brusch JL, Weinstein L. Fever of unknown origin. *Med Clin North Am*. 1988;72:1247–1261.

Chang JC, Gross HM. Utility of naproxen in the differential diagnosis of fever of undetermined origin in patients with cancer. *Am J Med*. 1984;76:597.

Cunha BA. Fever of unknown origin. *Infect Dis Clin North Am*. 1996;10:111–128.

Cunha BA. Fever of unknown origin. In: Gorbach SL, Bartlett JG, Blacklow NR, eds. *Infectious Diseases*. 3rd ed. New York, NY: Lippincott Williams & Wilkins; 2004:1568–1577.

Cunha BA. Nonspecific tests in infectious diseases. In: Gorbach SL, Bartlett JG, Blacklow NR, eds. *Infectious Diseases*. 3rd ed. New York, NY: Lippincott Williams & Wilkins; 2004:158–166.

Cunha BA. FUO due to adult juvenile rheumatoid arthritis (adult onset Still's disease): the diagnostic significance of double quotidian fevers and elevated serum ferritin levels. *Heart Lung*. 2004;33;417–421.

Cunha BA, Mohan S, Parchuri S. Fever of unknown origin: chronic lymphatic leukemia versus lymphoma (Richter's transformation). *Heart Lung*. 2005;34:437–441.

Cunha BA, Hamid N, Krol V, Eisenstein L. Fever of unknown origin due to preleukemia/myelodysplastic syndrome: the diagnostic importance of monocytosis with elevated serum ferritin levels. *Heart Lung*. 2006;35:277–282.

Cunha BA, ed. *Fever of Unknown Origin (FUO)*. New York, NY: Informa Healthcare; 2007.

Cunha BA, Fever of unknown origin (FUO): diagnostic serum ferritin levels. *Scand J Infect Dis*. 2007: 39:651–652.

Kazanjian PH. Fever of unknown origin: review of 86 patients treated in community hospitals. *Clin Infect Dis*. 1992;15:968–973.

Knockaert DC, Vanneste LJ, Vanneste SB, Bobbaers HJ. Fever of unknown origin in the 1980s: an update of the diagnostic spectrum. *Arch Intern Med*. 1992;152:51–55.

Knockaert DC, Vanneste LJ, Bobbears HJ. Fever of unknown origin in elderly patients. *J Am Geriatr Soc*. 1993;41:1187–1192.

Krol V, Cunha BA. Diagnostic significance of serum ferritin levels in infectious and noninfectious diseases. *Infect Dis Pract*. 2003;27:196–197.

Petersdorf RG, Beeson PB. Fever of unexplained origin: reports on 100 cases. *Medicine (Baltimore)*. 1961;40:1–30.

Remé P, Cunha BA. Indocin and the Naprosyn test in fever of unknown origin (FUO). *Infect Dis Pract*. 2000;24:32.

Weinstein L. Clinically benign fever of unknown origin: a personal retrospective. *Rev Infect Dis*. 1985:7:692–699.

Zenone T. Fever of unknown origin in adults: evaluation of 144 cases in a non-university hospital. *Scand J Infect Dis*. 2006:38:632–638.

8

Clinical Syndromes – General

2. Sepsis and Septic Shock

Carmen E. DeMarco and Rodger D. MacArthur

DEFINITIONS

Sepsis is a complex syndrome comprising a constellation of systemic symptoms and signs in response to infection, including inflammatory, pro-coagulant, and immunosuppressive events. Septic shock occurs when there is significant hypotension in the presence of sepsis. The definitions and diagnostic criteria for sepsis and related conditions were developed in 1991 at a consensus conference sponsored jointly by the American College of Chest Physicians and the Society for Critical Care Medicine and reviewed by the 2001 International Sepsis Definitions Conference (sponsored by the Society of Critical Care Medicine, European Society of Critical Care Medicine, American College of Chest Physicians, American Thoracic Society, and the Surgical Infections Society). Apart from expanding the list of signs and symptoms of sepsis to reflect clinical bedside experience, the definitions remained unchanged. The sepsis-related terminology and definitions are presented in Table 2.1; the diagnostic criteria for sepsis presented in Table 2.2 have been updated by the Conference to include a variety of signs of systemic inflammation in response to infection. This international group proposed a classification scheme for sepsis that stratifies patients based on their predisposing conditions, the nature and extent of the insult (infection), the host response, and the degree of concomitant organ dysfunction (acronym PIRO). This concept will have to be further tested and refined before it can be routinely applied in clinical practice.

EPIDEMIOLOGY

The incidences of sepsis, severe sepsis, and septic shock are probably underestimated because most of the available estimates are based on hospital discharge diagnoses. A recent review by Martin et al. found that the incidence of sepsis increased fourfold from 1979 to 2000 to 240 cases per 100 000 population per year (approximately 750 000 cases/year). In-hospital mortality rates in patients with a sepsis-related diagnosis remain high, with estimates between 18 and 70%, depending on the severity. Approximately 150 000 persons die annually in Europe from severe sepsis and more than 200 000 die annually in the United States. Certain populations such as the elderly, neutropenic patients, and infants (especially low-birth-weight newborns) have higher attack and mortality rates. The incidence of sepsis is higher in men and nonwhite persons, as compared with women and white persons, respectively, for unclear reasons.

PATHOGENESIS

The clinical manifestations of the sepsis syndrome are caused by the body's immune, inflammatory, and coagulation responses to toxins and other components of microorganisms. For example, infusion of endotoxin into humans is sufficient to initiate the cascade of inflammatory mediators seen in sepsis. Endotoxin is the lipoidal acylated glucosamine disaccharide core of the cell wall of many aerobic gram-negative bacteria. This moiety, known as *lipid A,* is highly conserved among the Enterobacteriaceae and, to a lesser extent, among the Pseudomonaceae. Anaerobic gram-negative bacteria, such as *Bacteroides fragilis,* lack *lipid A,* perhaps explaining why sepsis is not commonly seen when infection is caused solely by this anaerobe.

Once a pathogenic microorganism invades a host barrier, these highly conserved microbial cell wall molecules, usually lipids or sugars, are sensed by the local defense cells (eg, tissue macrophages, mast cells, dendritic cells) expressing specific host proteins on their surface, such as CD14 and toll-like receptors (TLRs). The bacterial peptidoglycan of gram-positive bacteria is recognized by TLR2 and the lipopolysaccharide of gram-negative bacteria is recognized by TLR4. The activation of the TLR receptors initiates intracellular signaling pathways that lead to the production of cytokines and immunomodulatory molecules that mediate the inflammatory response and contribute to the clinical manifestations of sepsis.

Table 2.1 Sepsis-Related Terminology and Definitions

Infection	A pathological process caused by invasion of normally sterile host tissue by pathogenic or potentially pathogenic microorganisms
Bacteremia	The presence of viable bacteria in the blood
SIRS	The systemic inflammatory response to a wide range of infectious and noninfectious conditions. Currently used criteria include 2 or more of the following: temperature >38°C or ≤36°C; heart rate >90 beats/min; respiratory rate >20 breaths/min, or $Paco_2$ ≤32 mm Hg; WBC >12 000 cells/mm^3 or ≤4000 cells/mm^3, or ≤10% immature (band) forms
Sepsis	The clinical syndrome defined by the presence of both infection and a systemic inflammatory response
Severe sepsis	Sepsis complicated by organ dysfunction, hypotension, or signs of hypoperfusion (eg, lactic acidosis, renal failure, altered mental status, and acute respiratory failure)
Septic shock	Sepsis accompanied by acute circulatory failure, characterized by persistent arterial hypotension that, despite adequate fluid resuscitation, requires pressor therapy
MODS	Multiple organ dysfunction syndrome; the presence of altered organ function in an acutely ill patient such that homeostasis cannot be maintained without intervention; primary multiple organ dysfunction syndrome is the direct result of a well-defined insult in which organ dysfunction occurs early and can be directly attributable to the insult itself; secondary multiple organ dysfunction syndrome develops as a consequence of a host response and is identified in the context of SIRS

Abbreviations: SIRS = systemic inflammatory response syndrome; MODS = multiple organ dysfunction syndrome; WBC= white blood cells.

Tumor necrosis factor-α (TNF-α); interleukin (IL)-1β, IL-10, IL-12, and other interleukins; interferon-γ; and several colony-stimulating factors are produced rapidly (minutes to hours) after the interaction of monocytes and macrophages with the microbial molecules. Although the effects of TNF-α appear to be central to the pathophysiology of sepsis, many other immune modulators interact with TNF-α, host defense mechanisms, and bacterial pathogens in complex ways.

The sepsis cascade can be simplified by dividing it into at least five components with feedback loops among them. The process starts with the release of intracellular or extracellular bacterial activators, such as lipid A in gram-negative sepsis and peptidoglycan, teichoic acid, or toxic shock toxin-1 (TSST-1) in gram-positive sepsis. The second event is the activation of macrophages by the bacterial products. This activation leads to the third component of sepsis, which consists of the release of highly active molecules (eg, cytokines) that have many potent biologic effects. The most important and best studied cytokine is TNF-α; IL-1β is another cytokine that is released early in the sepsis cascade, with effects similar to those of TNF-α. The release of TNF-α and IL-1β leads to the fourth component in the sepsis cascade, which includes the release of stress hormones, other cytokines (eg,

IL-2, IL-6, IL-8, IL-10), and other inflammatory mediators of sepsis (eg, nitric oxide released by activated endothelial cells, the lipooxygenase and cyclooxygenase metabolites, platelet activation factor, interferon γ, adhesion molecules in neutrophils and endothelial cells). All of these immune modulators interact in a complex fashion to effect, in the fifth stage, the various observable changes to multiple organ systems (eg, vascular endothelium, myocardial cells, pulmonary alveolar cells, liver cells). The result is the clinical picture of sepsis and the development of multiorgan system failure. Table 2.3 lists some of the important biologic effects of the mediators involved in the sepsis syndrome with the ensuing clinical manifestations.

There are several points to be made based on our understanding of sepsis: (1) it is essential to contain and eliminate the infection source with all possible measures (eg, antibiotics, surgical or needle drainage of pus); (2) after the sepsis cascade has been activated, the clinical outcome of the patient may depend not only on effective antiinfective therapy but also on the ability to control the vigorous inflammatory response that led to the manifestations of sepsis; (3) elevations of many of the cytokines have been correlated with poor outcome among persons with sepsis. Greatly elevated levels of the inflammatory mediator IL-6, in particular,

Table 2.2 Diagnostic Criteria for Sepsis

Infection (documented or suspected) *and* some of the following parameters must be present:	
General appearance	Altered mental status
Vital signs	Core temperature >38° C (100.4°F) or ≤36°C (96.8°F) Heart rate >90 beats/min or >2 SD above the normal value for age Tachypnea
Laboratory parameters	Hyperglycemia (plasma glucose >110 mg/dL or 7.7 mM/L) in the absence of diabetes White blood cells >12 000 cells/mm^3 or ≤4000 cells/mm^3 or >10% immature (band) forms
Hemodynamic parameters	Arterial hypotension (SBP ≤90 mm Hg, MAP ≤70 mm Hg, or an SBP decrease of >40 mm Hg in adults or >2 SD below normal for age) Mixed venous oxygen saturation >70%[a] Cardiac index >3.5 L/min/m^2 BSA Significant edema or positive fluid balance (>20 mL/kg over 24 h)
Organ dysfunction parameters	Arterial hypoxemia (PaO$_2$/FIO$_2$ ≤300) Acute oliguria (urine output ≤0.5 mL/kg/h or 45 mmol/L for at least 2 h) Creatinine increase ≥0.5 mg/dL Coagulation abnormalities (INR >1.5 or aPTT >60s) Ileus (absent bowel sounds) Thrombocytopenia (platelet count ≤100 000/mm^3) Hyperbilirubinemia (plasma total bilirubin >4 mg/dL or 70 mmol/L)
Tissue perfusion parameters	Hyperlactatemia (>3 mmol/L) Decreased capillary refill or mottling

Abbreviations: SBP = systolic blood pressure; MAP = mean arterial pressure; SD = standard deviation; BSA = body surface area; INR = international normalized ratio; aPTT = activated partial thromboplastin time.
[a] Normal values in children and newborns are 75%–80%, therefore this criterion should not be used as a sign of sepsis in this population.

have been shown in multiple studies to be correlated with decreased likelihood of survival.

The first biologic treatment for sepsis, activated protein C, was approved by the U.S. Food and Drug Administration (FDA) in 2001. More recently, the administration of systemic hydrocortisone has been shown to decrease mortality in adults with relative adrenal insufficiency in one randomized clinical trial. However, in a retrospective cohort study in critically ill pediatric patients with severe sepsis, steroids were not found to improve outcome and their use was associated with increased mortality. In addition, the diagnosis of adrenal insufficiency in patients with sepsis is challenging. For instance, patients with sepsis and low serum albumin levels may have low total serum cortisol levels but normal or increased free serum cortisol levels. Therefore, at this time, corticosteroids in patients with sepsis should be used only with extreme caution, if at all.

Multiple large, well-controlled trials have failed to demonstrate any efficacy of monoclonal antibodies directed against lipid A, other components of the gram-negative bacterial cell wall, and TNF-α. However, a large prospective, randomized, double-blind, placebo-controlled, multiple-center clinical trial published in 2004 showed that afelimomab (an anti-TNF F(ab')2 monoclonal antibody fragment) resulted in a significant reduction in TNF and IL-6 levels and a more rapid improvement in organ failure scores compared with placebo with an adjusted reduction in the risk of death of 5.8% ($P = .041$) and a corresponding reduction of relative risk of death of 11.9% at 28 days. Nevertheless, this monoclonal antibody has not been developed further for clinical use, perhaps because of the relatively modest effects on survival (especially when compared to activated protein C).

Etiology

Historically, antibiotic recommendations for therapy of sepsis and septic shock were based primarily on coverage of gram-negative organisms. However, sepsis caused by gram-positive organisms is clinically identical to sepsis caused by gram-negative organisms and, since 1987, gram-positive pathogens have become the predominant pathogens. In most clinical series 30%–50% of the cases are caused

Table 2.3 Selected Biologic and Clinical Manifestations Seen in Sepsis Syndrome

Mediator	Selected Biologic Manifestations	Selected Clinical Manifestations
Endotoxin	Activation of macrophages Release of TNF-α Release of IL-1β	Clinical effect is mediated by the release of TNF-α and the other mediators
TNF-α	↑ IL-1β ↑ IL-6 ↑ IL-8 ↑ Nitric oxide (NO) ↑ Myocardial depressant factor Activate arachidonic metabolism PMN activation	Fever ↑ Catabolic state Microthrombi Mental status changes ↑ Cortisol level
IL-1β	Virtually identical to TNF-α effects, except less effect on PMN function and chemotaxis	Same as TNF-α
Nitric oxide	↓ Myocardial performance ↓ Vascular smooth muscle tone High levels suppress TH1 T-cell function	↓ Tissue oxygen supply Hypotension Ileus and abdominal distension Hypoxemia from increased shunting
Thromboxanes	Platelet and PMN aggregation Increased PMN adhesiveness Vasoconstriction of regional blood vessels Enhanced capillary permeability Increased airway resistance	Regional hypoperfusion ARDS Pulmonary shunting Edema Wheezing
Prostaglandins	Vasodilation (PGI$_2$, PGE$_1$) Vasoconstriction (PGF$_2$) Antiaggregatory effects on platelets Enhanced capillary permeability	Hypotension ↑ Systemic and pulmonary shunting Arterial hypoxemia ↑ Edema

Abbreviations: ARDS = acute respiratory distress syndrome; PMN = polymorphonuclear cell; TNF = tumor necrosis factor.

by *Staphylococcus aureus*, coagulase-negative staphylococci, and enterococci. *Escherichia coli* has remained the most common gram-negative pathogen isolated in nosocomial infections and *Staphylococcus epidermidis* has become the most common cause of nosocomial bacteremias, followed by *Staphylococcus aureus*, enterococci, and *Candida* species. Infections caused by vancomycin-resistant enterococci (VRE), particularly *Enterococcus faecium*, and non-*albicans Candida* species have become increasingly common in the past several years. Gram-negative bacteria such as *Pseudomonas aeruginosa, Enterobacter* species, and *Acinetobacter* species also are increasingly likely to be resistant to multiple antibiotics.

Diagnosis

The diagnosis of sepsis should be considered when a patient displays symptoms and signs of systemic inflammation in response to infection (see Table 2.2). Unfortunately, there are no bedside tests currently available to differentiate quickly and reliably infectious causes of systemic inflammatory response syndrome

(SIRS) from noninfectious causes. The 2001 International Sepsis Definitions Conference emphasized the nonspecificity of these symptoms and signs, while recognizing the importance of bedside clinical diagnosis. Therefore the diagnosis of sepsis is based on the presence of infection and some of the criteria listed in Table 2.2. The mortality from septic shock or sepsis with multiple organ dysfunction syndrome (MODS) is between 25% and 45%. Consequently, prompt empiric administration of antibiotics is appropriate in most situations. However, every attempt should be made to determine the source, microbiology, and pathophysiology of the infection because this knowledge will guide the optimal management. Often, various underlying risk factors predispose individuals to infection with specific organisms. Some of these conditions and associated pathogens are listed in Table 2.4.

A thorough history and physical examination are crucial in the diagnosis of sepsis; their importance cannot be overemphasized. Multiple cultures from multiple sites need to be obtained when infection is suspected.

Table 2.4 Special Circumstances in Septic Patients

Circumstance	Possible Pathogens
Splenectomy (traumatic or functional)	Encapsulated organisms: *Streptococcus pneumoniae*, *Haemophilus influenzae*, and *Neisseria meningitidis*
Neutropenia (≤500 neutrophils/µL)	Gram-negatives, including *Pseudomonas aeruginosa*; gram-positives, including *Staphylococcus aureus*; fungi, especially *Candida* species
Hypogammaglobulinemia (eg, CLL)	*Streptococcus pneumoniae, Escherichia coli*
Burns	MRSA, *Pseudomonas aeruginosa*, resistant gram-negatives, *Candida* species
AIDS	*Pseudomonas aeruginosa* (if neutropenic), *Salmonella* species, *Staphylococcus aureus, Pneumocystis jirovecii* (pneumonia)
Intravascular devices	*Staphylococcus aureus, Staphylococcus epidermidis*
Nosocomial infections	MRSA, *Staphylococcus epidermidis, Enterococcus* species, resistant gram-negatives, *Candida* species

Abbreviations: CLL = chronic lymphocytic leukemia; AIDS = acquired immunodeficiency syndrome; MRSA = methicillin-resistant *Staphylococcus aureus*.

All culture material needs to be delivered promptly to the microbiology laboratory. Gram stains should be made and read as soon as possible on all specimens submitted for culture. Ideally, cultures should be obtained before initiation of antibiotics. However, the administration of antibiotics should not be delayed for patients who are clinically or hemodynamically unstable.

Two sets of blood cultures, drawn from different sites, should be obtained from all patients suspected of being septic. Each blood culture consists of one aerobic and one anaerobic bottle. Typically, at least 10 mL of blood needs to be injected into each bottle to increase the likelihood of culturing pathogens. If an indwelling venous or arterial catheter is present, it is important to obtain additional cultures through each port of the device.

Sputum for culture can be spontaneously expectorated, induced with 3% saline, or obtained by nasotracheal, endotracheal, or transtracheal techniques. Specimens should have fewer than 25 squamous epithelial cells per low-power (100×) microscopic field to decrease the chance that the specimen is contaminated with upper airway flora.

Urine should be obtained for culture when possible. Clean-catch or straight-catheterization specimens are preferred. Urine that has been present in a closed collection system for more than 1 hour should not be sent for culture. If necessary, urine can be obtained directly from the catheter tubing or bladder (suprapubic aspiration) using a syringe and a small-gauge needle. It is important to remember that many bacteriuric patients, especially those with indwelling urinary catheters, may be septic from another source. Although the presence of more than 100 000 bacteria/mL of urine cultured suggests infection, this criterion has been validated only for ambulatory young adults with gram-negative bacillary organisms.

Cultures from other sites should be obtained if clinically indicated. Computer tomography (CT) scans of the abdomen can reveal previously overlooked fluid collections that may be accessible by needle aspiration. Certain infections prevalent in intravenous drug users, such as epidural abscesses and psoas muscle abscesses, may be diagnosed by magnetic resonance imaging (MRI). Patients with diarrhea should have stool sent for a cytotoxic assay for *Clostridium difficile* toxin A and B. Ultrasonography is useful for detecting ascites and biliary, hepatic, and pancreatic pathologic conditions. A portable (bedside) ultrasound can be obtained for critically ill patients who are too unstable to be transported to the radiology department. A lumbar puncture for cell count, protein, glucose, bacterial antigens, Gram stain, and culture should be performed on any septic patient with unexplained altered mentation.

Treatment of Sepsis

Consensus guidelines for the management of sepsis were published in 2004. The concept of early goal-directed therapy (EGDT) was initially introduced as a quality initiative and later validated in studies, emphasizing a timely and coordinated approach to sepsis management and showing a significant mortality benefit when hemodynamic optimization was provided within the first few hours of disease presentation. During the first critical 6 hours of presentation, aggressive correction of hemodynamic abnormalities and organ dysfunction is pursued to correct the global tissue hypoxia that can lead to more severe stages of sepsis. This approach has been shown to improve outcomes and decrease health-care resource utilization.

ANTIMICROBIAL THERAPY: SELECTION AND DURATION

Antibiotics form the cornerstone of therapy for sepsis. Studies by MacArthur et al., among others, have shown that outcome is improved in septic patients if the diagnosis is suspected early and appropriate antibiotics are started without delay. A recently published retrospective cohort study by Kumar et al. showed that administration of effective antimicrobials within the first hour of hypotension was associated with increased survival to hospital discharge in adults with septic shock; each hour of delay beyond the initial 6 hours following the onset of hypotension was associated with an average decrease in survival of 7.6%. In addition, appropriate surgical intervention ("surgical source control") often is as important as the choice of antibiotics.

Our suggestions for empiric antibiotic therapy are outlined in Figure 2.1 and Table 2.5. A few principles are worth emphasizing: (1) Antipseudomonal agents should be used for empirical therapy for nosocomial infection and (2) antibiotic dosages should be optimized for the site of infection, usually requiring the highest allowable dosage adjusted for organ dysfunction. Intravenously administered antibiotics often result in higher serum and tissue levels than orally administered antibiotics. The oral route of antibiotic administration should not be used for persons in whom gut absorption is compromised (eg, mucositis and severe colitis). (3) Community-acquired infections are likely to be caused by organisms different from those encountered in the hospital. For example, *Pseudomonas aeruginosa* is unlikely to

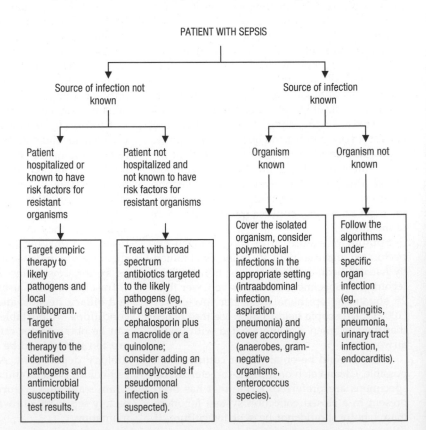

Figure 2.1 Algorithm for antibiotic coverage in patients with sepsis.

Table 2.5 Recommended Initial[a] Antibiotic Regimens for Septic Patients with Normal Renal Function

Clinical Situation	Regimen
Empiric coverage (includes antipseudomonal drugs)	Either imipenem[b] 0.5 g IV q6h, or meropenem 1g IV q8h or piperacillin-tazobactam 3.375 g IV q4h with or without an aminoglycoside (eg, tobramycin[c, d] 5 mg/kg IV q24h)
Community-acquired pneumonia[e]	Ceftriaxone 1 g IV q24h plus azithromycin 500 mg IV or PO q24h or a fluoroquinolone (eg, levofloxacin 500 mg IV or PO qd)
Community-acquired urosepsis	Ciprofloxacin 400 mg IV q12h with or without ampicillin 2 g IV
Meningitis	Vancomycin 25 mg/kg q12h plus ceftriaxone 2 g q24h. Add ampicillin 2 g IV q4h if *Listeria* is a likely pathogen (eg, elderly, neonates, immunosuppressed)
Nosocomial infections *or* Neutropenia[f]	Piperacillin-tazobactam[g] 3.375 g IV q4–6h or ceftazidime 2 g IV q8h or cefepime 1–2 g IV q8h or imipenem 0.5 g IV q6h with or without an aminoglycoside (eg, tobramycin[c, d] 5 mg/kg IV q24h)
HIV+ with pneumonia[h]	Trimethoprim-sulfamethoxazole, 5 mg/kg IV q6h or pentamidine 4 mg/kg IV q24h, either with ceftriaxone 1 g IV q12h and with or without azithromycin 500 mg IV or PO q24h. When treating for *Pneumocystis* pneumonia add prednisone (or equivalent) 40 mg PO q12h for room air PaO2 ≤ 70 mmHg or alveolar-arterial gradient >35 mmHg

Abbreviation: HIV = human immunodeficiency virus.
[a] Antibiotics should be adjusted according to the microbiologic results.
[b] Imipenem dosage should be adjusted according to weight, age, and creatinine clearance.
[c] Amikacin at 15 to 20 mg/kg/day can be substituted for tobramycin at institutions with significant bacterial resistance to tobramycin.
[d] Aminoglycosides should be used in patients with hemodynamic instability because of their rapid killing of bacteria and broad spectrum of activity against aerobic gram-negative organisms. Single daily dosing is recommended when feasible.
[e] Vancomycin 25 mg/kg q12h may be substituted for ceftriaxone for beta-lactam allergic patients with *Streptococcus pneumoniae* or *Staphylococcus aureus* or if the infection is caused by resistant organisms.
[f] Antipseudomonal agents are recommended for empiric therapy of sepsis in neutropenic patients. Meropenem may be substituted for Imipenem, particularly in the elderly, patients with renal failure, patients with seizure disorders or patients with central nervous system infections.
[g] Must dose every 4 h if covering *Pseudomonas aeruginosa* infection.
[h] Use the above recommendations for HIV-positive patients with CD4+ cell counts ≤200 cell/mm[3] when *Pneumocystis* is a likely pathogen; otherwise, cover the same as in community-acquired pneumonia without HIV. If Gram stain reveals gram-negative rods, antibiotics appropriate for *Pseudomonas aeruginosa* must be added.

be encountered in community-acquired infections; with few exceptions (eg, intravenous drug users), antipseudomonal coverage is not warranted routinely. However, *Streptococcus pneumoniae* is one of the most common causes of community-acquired sepsis. This organism needs to be covered adequately, something that may not be accomplished with the use of many of the antipseudomonal antibiotics currently available; (4) aminoglycosides offer rapid killing of gram-negative aerobic bacteria in a dose-dependent fashion, whereas toxicity depends on the time that serum levels are above the toxicity threshold. The risk of nephrotoxicity and ototoxicity, the poor penetration of aminoglycosides into abscesses and lung parenchyma, and the lack of data to indicate that the addition of aminoglycosides affects the

outcome in septic patients call for judicious use of aminoglycosides. Our current suggestions for the use of aminoglycosides are as follows: (1) large single daily doses (eg, 5 mg/kg of tobramycin daily) in patients who are hemodynamically unstable, (2) small doses (eg, 1 to 1.5 mg/kg of tobramycin every 8 hours) when used for synergy against streptococcal and enterococcal infections, (3) use aminoglycosides only in the first few days to provide empriric coverage for aerobic gram-negative bacteria. Important potential advantages of combination therapy over monotherapy include a higher probability that the infecting pathogen will be covered by at least one of the antimicrobials, a potential synergistic effect, and possible suppression of emergence of resistant subpopulations of bacteria.

Table 2.6 Factors That May Affect the Choice of Antibiotics in Sepsis

Factor Affecting the Choice of Antibiotic	Appropriate Antibiotic Choice	Less Favorable Antibiotic Choice
Antibiotic Penetration into Infected Site		
Pyelonephritis	Ciprofloxacin	Moxifloxacin
Biliary infection	Ciprofloxacin, moxifloxacin	Penicillin
Pneumonia	Ceftriaxone, quinolones	
Central nervous system infection	Meropenem, third-generation cephalosporins	Daptomycin Imipenem, quinolones
Underlying Medical Problems that Affect Antibiotic Metabolism or Safety		
Renal dysfunction	Meropenem	Imipenem, trimethoprim-sulfametoxazole
Seizure disorder		Imipenem
Identification of the Organism		
Enterobacter species	Carbapenems, trimethoprim-sulfametoxazole	Cephalosporins, penicillins
Staphylococcus aureus	Nafcillin (MSSA), Vancomycin (MRSA)	Quinolones
Enterococci	Ampicillin, piperacillin, imipenem, vancomycin, daptomycin, linezolid	Quinolones, cephalosporins, trimethoprim-sulfametoxazole
Allergies		
	Use a different class of antibiotic if the allergy is significant	Avoid the offending agent
Hemodynamically Unstable Patient		
	Use bactericidal agent; consider aminoglycosides	Avoid bacteriostatic agents

The choice of the specific antibiotic agents depends on multiple factors. Table 2.6 lists some of the factors that affect the choice of antibiotics beyond what is outlined in the Figure 2.1 algorithm and in Table 2.5. For instance, the carbapenemens (eg, imipenem or meropenem) and trimethoprim/sulfamethoxasole are preferred over the cephalosporins and extended-spectrum penicillins for the treatment of infections caused by *Enterobacter* species, due to the potential for the *Enterobacter* species to become constitutive producers of beta-lactamase.

In recent years an increase in the incidence of nosocomial beta-lactam-resistant gram-positive organisms has been reported, and community-acquired methicillin-resistant *Staphylococcus aureus* (MRSA) infections also are on the rise. Although the routine empiric use of vancomycin is not advocated because of concerns about the emergence of VRE infections, the treating physician should be aware of the patterns of antimicrobial resistance in the community when selecting an empiric regimen; an antibiotic with activity against MRSA (such as vancomycin, linezolid, or daptomycin) should be empirically initiated if this pathogen is prevalent (>10%–20% of all *Staphylococcus aureus* isolates) in the community.

Fungi account for 5% of all cases of severe sepsis or septic shock; therefore routine use of antifungal therapy also is not recommended in patients with sepsis, unless the patient is at high risk (eg, neutropenic or post bone marrow transplant). In these high-risk patients, delaying administration of antifungal therapy until fungal blood cultures are reported as positive should be avoided due to the associated increase in mortality rates. The presence of macronodular skin lesions shown on biopsy to be consistent with candidal infection or the presence of Candidal endophthalmitis is synonymous with dissemination. Because only a fraction of patients with systemic candidiasis will have positive blood cultures, a number of schemes have been developed to stratify the risk for systemic fungal infection in hospitalized patients. In general, when *Candida* species are isolated from three or more nonblood sites, the risk of subsequent infection of the blood by these fungi increases. Determining when to initiate therapy in such situations typically depends on evaluating the total clinical picture. In any case, the efficacy of the azole antifungals (eg, fluconazole), with their associated favorable toxicity profiles, has made the empiric use of antifungal therapy much more acceptable. However, a nonazole antifungal (eg, caspofungin, micafungin) may be advisable initially at institutions with high rates of azole resistance.

The duration of antibiotic therapy depends on the clinical response and, occasionally, the infecting pathogen. A "typical" course of antibiotics is given for 7 to 14 days. A good rule of thumb is to administer the antibiotics for 3 days beyond the point at which the patient becomes afebrile or has normalization of laboratory values. There are some important exceptions: (1) neutropenic patients (absolute neutrophil count ≤500 cells/mm^3) should receive 14 days of antibiotic therapy. The therapeutic approach is a compromise between stopping antibiotics shortly after the patient becomes afebrile and continuing the antibiotics for the entire duration of neutropenia. If a previously febrile neutropenic patient becomes afebrile and is no longer neutropenic, a shorter course of antibiotic therapy can be considered. (2) Patients with *Staphylococcus aureus* pneumonia or bacteremia should receive at least 14 days of antibiotics. Many infectious disease practitioners recommend 4 weeks or more of antistaphylococcal antibiotic therapy if bacteremia with *Staphylococcus aureus* is prolonged (ie, persists for >48 hours). In general, if a patient has responded rapidly to antibiotics, the last several days of therapy can be given via the oral route. (3) Patients with *Pneumocystis jirovecii* pneumonia should receive 21 days of therapy.

Antibiotic decisions should be reevaluated at least daily. Changes need to be considered as culture and sensitivity results become available or as the clinical course dictates. In addition, a patient who has not responded to therapy or who has relapsed after an initial improvement needs to be reevaluated thoroughly. Additional diagnostic studies may be indicated, and repeat cultures should be obtained to search for new or resistant pathogens. If the clinical syndrome is determined to be noninfectious, antibiotics should be stopped promptly.

The persistently febrile neutropenic patient represents an especially challenging problem. Antifungal therapy should be started if fever persists despite broad-spectrum antibiotic coverage for more than 5 to 7 days. A number of amphotericin B lipid formulations are now available that may decrease the number and severity of side effects compared to non-liposomal amphotericin B preparations. In addition, fluconazole has been shown to be at least as good as amphotericin B in multiple clinical situations. The recent introduction of the echinocandins (eg, caspofungin and micafungin) offers additional options for antifungal therapy in both neutropenic and nonneutropenic patients. Although the optimal duration of antifungal therapy is unknown, it probably is prudent to continue antifungal therapy as long as neutropenia exists. For therapy of microbiologically documented *Candida* infection, fluconazole is the drug of choice for infections due to *Candida albicans*, *Candida tropicalis*, or *Candida parapsilosis*. When infections are caused by the more frequently azole-resistant *Candida glabrata* or by *Candida krusei*, caspofungin or the lipid formulations of amphotericin B deoxycholate should be used.

Poor decisions about antibiotic use have immediate and future negative consequences. Long-term antibiotic use will not protect patients from infection; rather, patients will become infected with resistant organisms. The best practical way to avoid widespread resistance problems is to continuously reevaluate the need for antibiotic therapy and to deescalate therapy when microbial susceptibility panels become available. In addition, side effects, such as rashes and *Clostrida difficile* diarrhea, are much more common after long courses of multiple antibiotics.

SUPPORTIVE THERAPY

Sepsis is a systemic disease, and proper management requires diligent and prompt attention to resuscitation and supportive care, particularly in the presence of multiorgan dysfunction. There has been considerable controversy about the extent to which organ perfusion is to be optimized. Our recommendation is to aim to achieve normal perfusion parameters. Supernormal perfusion is not warranted and may be harmful. Crystalloids should be administered to maintain central venous pressure (CVP) at 8 to 12 mm Hg; vasopressors should be added if mean arterial pressure is less than 65 mm Hg. It also has been suggested that the manner in which organ failure is managed could affect the outcome and that supportive therapy may have a negative or a positive effect on the process of sepsis. For example, there is evidence that the approach used to mechanically ventilate patients with acute respiratory distress syndrome (ARDS) may affect outcome, and strategies to minimize oxygen demand should be considered (eg, analgesia, sedation, intubation, and mechanical ventilation). If myocardial dysfunction is identified, inotropic therapy should be instituted after volume repletion.

Strict glucose control with levels below 150 mg/dL should be implemented immediately after initial stabilization, because it has been shown to reduce morbidity and mortality rate (4.6 vs 8% in controls) in patients with an ICU stay of longer than 5 days.

Other supportive therapies recommended in septic patients are as follows: (1) deep-vein thrombosis prophylaxis with low-dose un-fractionated heparin or low-molecular-weight heparin or graduated compression devices if heparin is contraindicated and (2) stress ulcer prophylaxis should be given to all patients with severe sepsis using histamine-2 receptor antagonists that are more effective than sucral-fate in decreasing bleeding risk and transfusion requirements. Proton pump inhibitors may be used as well, although they have not been directly compared with histamine-2 receptor antagonists.

Table 2.7 describes some of the current recommendations regarding supportive care in patients with sepsis.

Adjunctive Therapies

Protein C has been studied as an endog-enous anticoagulant with profibrinolytic and antiinflammatory properties. The mul-ticenter, randomized controlled PROWESS study (Recombinant Human Activated Protein C Worldwide Evaluation in Severe Sepsis) showed that administration of recombinant-activated protein within 24 hours after the cri-teria for sepsis were met was associated with a reduction in the relative risk of death of 19% and a reduction in the absolute risk of death of 6% compared with placebo, whereas the risk of bleeding increased (3.5 vs 2%, $P = .06$). Carefully selected patients with severe sepsis and more than one organ dysfunction and/or an APACHE II (Acute Physiology and Chronic Health Evaluation) score greater than 25 could benefit from this novel therapy.

Corticosteroids have well-known antiinflam-matory and hemodynamic effects, therefore their use in sepsis has been studied extensively. Based on well-conducted studies, at the cur-rent time the use of steroids is recommended in proven or suspected meningitis of any eti-ology in children and adults, severe typhoid fever, late acute respiratory distress syndrome, *Pneumocystis jirovecii* pneumonia in patients

Table 2.7 General Principles in the Management of Sepsis

1. Control the infection.
   - Provide appropriate antibiotics (see Tables 2.5 and 2.6 and Figure 2.1)
   - Initiate surgical or invasive management of the infection if appropriate (drain any abscess, correct a perforated viscus, remove infected device if appropriate)

2. Optimize tissue perfusion and oxygenation.
   - Optimize arterial oxygen saturation
   - Optimize fluid status (crystalloids are preferred)
   - Optimize cardiac output and oxygen delivery (note that supernormal values have not been proven to be beneficial and may be harmful)
   - Transfuse blood only if patient is symptomatic and hemoglobin is ≤7 g/dL.

3. Consider active nutritional support.
   - If the patient has malnutrition or is expected to be without nutrition for more than 3 days
   - Gut feeding is preferable to parenteral feeding

4. Optimally manage organ failure.
   - Implementing strict glucose control
   - Use PEEP and low tidal volume in the management of ARDS complicating sepsis
   - Norepinephrine may improve visceral perfusion
   - Consider the use of gastric tonometry to evaluate visceral organ perfusion

5. Prevent nosocomial complications.
   - Prevention of line infections and nosocomial pneumonia (semirecumbent positioning)
   - DVT prophylaxis
   - Stress ulcer prophylaxis
   - Judicious use of antibiotics to avoid nosocomial infections by resistant organisms

Abbreviations: ARDS = acute respiratory distress syndrome; DVT= deep venous thrombosis; PEEP= positive and expiratory pressure.

with acquired immunodeficiency syndrome, and in patients with documented adrenal insufficiency. In patients with septic shock and relative adrenal insufficiency (diagnosed as failure to increase serum cortisol level above 9 µg/dL after administration of 250 µg of adre-nocorticotropin), one multicenter randomized controlled trial demonstrated a 10% absolute reduction in 28-day mortality rate in patients receiving corticosteroids. As recommended by the Surviving Sepsis Guidelines, intrave-nous corticosteroids (hydrocortisone 200–300 mg/day for 7 days in 3 or 4 divided doses or by continuous infusion) are recommended in patients with septic shock who, despite ad-equate fluid replacement, require vasopressor therapy to maintain adequate blood pressure. However, as discussed in the pathogenesis sec-tion, the use of corticosteroids in this setting remains controversial; they should be used only with extreme caution, if at all. High doses of corticosteroids (>300 mg/day) should not be used in severe sepsis or septic shock unless warranted by other medical conditions.

Conclusions

The sepsis syndrome is incredibly complex, involving many mediators that we are just starting to appreciate. Better identification of the subset of patients likely to benefit from modulation of these mediators is necessary, as are rapid diagnostic assays for endotoxin, TNF, and various cytokines. For now, we must continue with our attempts to improve patient survival by aggressively diagnosing the cause of sepsis and promptly treating the manifestations of the syndrome with antibiotics, source control, and supportive/adjunctive therapy.

SUGGESTED READING

Bernard GR, Vincent J-L, Laterre P-F, et al. Efficacy and safety of recombinant human activated protein C for severe sepsis. *N Engl J Med*. 2001;344:699–709.

Dellinger RP, Carlet JM, Masur H, et al. Surviving Sepsis Campaign guidelines for management of severe sepsis and septic shock. *Crit Care Med*. 2004;32:858–873. [Errata, *Crit Care Med*. 2004;32:1448, 2169–2170.]

Kumar A, Roberts D, Wood KE, et al. Duration of hypotension before initiation of effective antimicrobial therapy is the critical determinant of survival in human septic shock. *Crit Care Med*. 2006;34(6):1589–1596.

Levy MM, Fink MP, Marchall JC, et al. 2001 SCCM/ESICM/ACCP/ATS/SIS International Sepsis Definitions Conference. *Intensive Care Med*. 2003;29:530–538.

MacArthur RD, Miller M, Albertson T, et al. Adequacy of early empiric antibiotic treatment and survival in severe sepsis: experience from the MONARCS trial. *Clin Infect Dis*. 2004;38:284–288.

Martin GS, Mannino DM, Eaton S, et al. The epidemiology of sepsis in the United States from 1979 through 2000. *N Engl J Med*. 2003;348:1546–1554.

Munford RS. Sepsis, severe sepsis and septic shock. In Mandell GL, Bennett JE, Dolin R, eds. *Principles and Practice of Infectious Diseases*. 6th ed. Philadelphia: Churchill Livingstone, 2005.

Otero RM, Nguyen HB, Huang DT, et al. Early goal-directed therapy in severe sepsis and septic shock revisited. Concepts, controversies, and contemporary findings. *Chest*. 2006;130(5):1579–1595.

Panacek EA, Marshall JC, Albertson TE, et al. Efficacy and safety of the monoclonal anti-tumor necrosis factor antibody F(ab')2 fragment afelimomab in patients with severe sepsis and elevated interleukin-6 levels. *Crit Care Med*. 2004;32(11):2173–2182.

Russell JA. Management of sepsis. *N Engl J Med*. 2006;355:1699–1713.

3. Chronic Fatigue Syndrome

N. Cary Engleberg

INTRODUCTION: NATURE OF THE SYNDROME

Chronic fatigue syndrome (CFS) is a syndrome of subjective complaints, most prominently featuring profound and prolonged physical exhaustion. Many experts suggest that this syndrome is the late-20th-century formulation of an illness that has been described under various designations in medical literature for centuries, such as *febricula* ("little fevers") in the 18th century, *neurasthenia* in the 19th century, and *myalgic encephalomyelitis* (ME), in Great Britain and Canada, or *chronic fatigue and immune dysfunction syndrome* (CFIDS), in the United States, during the late 20th century. The designation *chronic fatigue syndrome* was adopted by the Centers for Disease Control and Prevention (CD) and the National Institutes of Health (NIH) because this name does not assume a direct role for infection, inflammation, or immune system dysfunction in the genesis of the symptoms. Indeed, an abundance of research has failed to attribute the syndrome to any specific infection or immunologic disturbance. Nevertheless, CFS concerns infectious disease physicians because it is frequently recognized as a sequel of infection, ie, as postviral or postinfectious fatigue.

The association of chronic fatigue and infection was first studied systematically in a study of chronic brucellosis. In a 1951 study, Wesley Spink found that 20% of patients with serologic evidence of brucellosis went on to develop persistent fatigue, muscle weakness, myalgia, mental confusion, and depression without evidence of ongoing infection with *Brucella*. He suggested that the symptoms of chronic brucellosis depended on both a previous *Brucella* infection and a psychological predisposition. Evidence for this theory was provided by investigators from John Hopkins during the Asian influenza pandemic of 1957–1958. During that epidemic season, these investigators conducted a retrospective cohort analysis of military personnel and their dependents who had completed the Minnesota Multiphasic Personality Inventory (MMPI) prior to the epidemic. Prolonged convalescence after influenza was associated with

unfavorable scores on certain subscales of the test. Moreover, the MMPI profiles of subjects with prolonged postinfluenza symptoms were nearly identical to MMPI profiles of patients with chronic brucellosis. This observation implies that the persistent fatigue and associated symptoms may reflect a programmed response to a variety of different infections in predisposed subjects.

Acute mononucleosis has also long been recognized as a precipitant of prolonged postinfectious fatigue. Consequently, when two large studies in 1985 reported an association between chronic fatigue and elevated titers of Epstein-Barr virus (EBV) antibodies, EBV became a leading candidate as the etiologic agent, and chronic mononucleosis became a popular designation for fatigue syndrome. As with other attempts to link CFS to a specific infectious agent, the association between active EBV and CFS was not confirmed by subsequent virological studies. EBV infection is now best understood as one more of the infectious precipitants of the syndrome rather than as a chronic infectious agent that is directly causative of the persistent symptoms. A similar role has also been assigned to enteroviruses, cytomegalovirus, Ross River virus, parvovirus, and human herpesvirus 6, *Borrelia burgdorferi*, Q fever, and *Candida albicans*, to name a few of the most cited potential etiologic candidates. The notion that CFS is a direct consequence of chronic active infection with any of these agents is not supported by existing evidence. Studies are either inconclusive or definitively negative. Making a distinction between infection as an acute precipitant and as a chronic persistent cause of the syndrome is critical. It explains why attempts to treat the syndrome with antibiotics, antivirals, and antifungals have been uniformly disappointing.

In the absence of a simple etiology or a uniformly applicable diagnostic test for CFS, the NIH and the CDC sponsored a series of conferences between 1985 and 1994 to develop a consensus definition of the syndrome. This definition was intended to serve as a single standard for epidemiologic, pathophysiologic, clinical, and therapeutic studies in the future. Because fatigue is one of the most common complaints encountered in general medicine, the definition was formulated to exclude patients with trivial or medically explainable fatigue states and to capture those with illnesses that most experts recognize as being characteristic of the syndrome. The 1994 definition of the syndrome (see Table 3.1) has been consistently applied in most studies undertaken during the past decade, and it is used by many practitioners as criteria for clinical diagnosis in individual patients. However, there are inescapable problems with both specificity and sensitivity of a case definition of this kind. Because the syndrome consists of nonspecific, subjective symptoms, the case definition requires a minimal number of these symptoms. If the definition requires too few nonspecific symptoms, it will capture a collection of fatiguing disorders with more than one etiology and/or pathophysiology, a situation that will confound the interpretation of research findings. Alternatively, as the number of symptoms required for defining CFS increases, the definition captures an increasing proportion of patients with somatization disorders. Clinicians who use the case definition for clinical diagnosis of individual patients face an additional potential problem. The case definition may formally exclude patients whose illness closely resembles that of the defined cases and who may suffer the same pathophysiology. The authors of the CFS criteria recognized this problem and stipulated that fatigue lasting 6 months but not associated with the required number of associated symptoms should be designated as idiopathic chronic fatigue. In reality, many of those who fall into this category and those with CFS as defined in Table 3.1 may have the same disorder. Thus, rigid application of the CFS criteria in medical practice (eg, requiring 6 symptomatic months) may exclude patients who might profit from an early, appropriate intervention.

EPIDEMIOLOGY

Idiopathic chronic fatigue is very common (5%–10% of patients in general medical practice), but very few (≤1%) can be diagnosed with chronic fatigue syndrome using the 1994 criteria. The U.S. national prevalence of chronic fatigue syndrome was estimated by the CDC through a network of physicians in four American cities. The prevalence ranged from 3 to 11 per 100 000 population, and the gender and age distribution were similar in all four sites. Most patients were female (7:1) in the fourth and fifth decades

of life. Estimates from clinic-based studies in Australia and the United Kingdom yield similar results. However, a population-based survey in San Francisco and other community-based studies elsewhere suggest a prevalence of about 0.2%, with a greater proportion of males, ethnic minorities, and those of lower socioeconomic classes. The discrepancy between community- and clinic-based studies is attributable to the greater utilization of clinical services by middle- and upper-class women. It belies the notion of a "yuppie flu," a pejorative term applied to this disorder in the past.

Illnesses consistent with CFS also occasionally occur in epidemic fashion. In some instances, the outbreaks may be associated with an infectious event; however, in others, the distribution of illness among the populations at risk clearly does not resemble the spread of an infection. Examples of the latter type include the large hospital-based outbreaks in Los Angeles, California, and London, UK, that affected the hospital professional staff but not the hospitalized patients or nonprofessional staff.

PATHOPHYSIOLOGY

Research on the pathophysiology of CFS has been complicated by the definitional problems described above; most importantly by the problem of selecting a homogenous group of subjects for study who have symptoms that are attributable to the same cause or causes. Many patients have an acute onset of the syndrome. A small proportion can be traced to a diagnosed infectious disease; more often this is presumed based on the history but cannot be confirmed. CFS may also follow other physically and psychologically stressful events, such as surgeries, accidents, deaths, and divorces. Many patients have an insidious onset with no definite precipitating event. Regardless of the onset, the majority of patients have past or current psychiatric disorders, but a large minority has no active or past psychiatric symptoms.

Numerous infections have been associated with CFS, but evidence that the syndrome is not likely associated with any specific infectious agent is of three main types. First, there is no single infectious agent that is detectable in all cases of CFS; the disorder may occur even in the absence of the most common cosmopolitan agents, such as EBV. Second, the development of the same syndrome occurs during convalescence after infections with nonoverlapping geographical distribution (eg, Ross River virus, Q fever, or Lyme disease). Third, attempts to treat

Table 3.1 Case Definition of Chronic Fatigue Syndrome (Fukuda et al., 1994)

Clinically evaluated, unexplained chronic fatigue for more than 6 months' duration, which is not lifelong or the result of ongoing exertion and is not substantially alleviated by rest. The fatigue is associated with a significant reduction in occupational, educational, social, or personal activities.

PLUS
Four or more of the following concurrent symptoms:
   Impaired memory or concentration
   Sore throat
   Tender cervical or axillary lymph nodes
   Muscle pain
   Generalized or migratory arthralgia
   New headaches
   Nonrestorative sleep
   Prolonged postexertional malaise

CFS with anti-infectives have been uniformly disappointing. It may be true that only a specific type of infection with prolonged duration or severity is necessary to precipitate CFS. Indeed, patients seen in general practice for common, simple infections do not have an increased frequency of prolonged fatigue relative to patients seen for other medical problems. However, postinfectious cases and those with no apparent precipitant are clinically indistinguishable with respect to symptoms and psychosocial features once the defining criteria are met. These observations lead to the conclusion that the syndrome is a nonspecific sequel to a variety of infections or other precipitants. Whether patients who have CFS will reactivate latent viruses more frequently than well individuals is an unsettled issue, but no correlation between viral reactivation (eg, EBV) and the expression of symptoms has been demonstrated.

Apart from infections, disruptions in various biologic systems associated with CFS have been proposed as inciting or perpetuating factors. These include subtle alterations in immunologic, neuroendocrine, and neuropsychological function. The most consistent immune alterations include increased numbers of T lymphocytes expressing activation markers, eg, the CD45RA differentiation marker and a reduction in the natural killer cell function and number of CD16-positive lymphocytes. The clinical relevance of these changes is unclear, because similar differences occur in monozygotic twin pairs that are discordant for CFS, and changes in lymphocyte number and function do not necessarily correlate with changes in clinical status. Attempts to correlate cytokine levels with the presence or severity of CFS have been inconsistent. However, interferons are known to activate expression of the enzyme 2′,5′-oligoadenylate synthetase. This enzyme generates 2′,5′-adenylate oligonucleotides that bind to and activate RNAse L, leading to the cytoplasmic degradation of viral and other RNAs. CFS is associated with increased levels of 2′,5′A oligonucleotides, RNAse L activity, and the expression of a low-molecular-weight RNAse L molecule. The pathophysiologic significance of this phenomenon is uncertain, but measurement of this pathway has been suggested as a potential biologic marker for CFS.

The hypothesis that the central nervous system is the principle site of the pathophysiology in CFS has gained support in recent years. This hypothesis is bolstered by presence of neuropsychological symptoms in the active syndrome, the observation of prior or preexisting psychiatric disorders in a large proportion of patients, and subtle alterations of hormones regulated at the hypothalamic level. Previous or concurrent depression is frequently present in CFS. When patients in general practice are evaluated for "viral" illnesses, the psychiatric morbidity and the patients belief structure concerning the illness are better predictors of subsequent chronic fatigue than the severity of symptoms at the time of presentation. More objective evidence of central nervous system involvement includes the observed disruption of the hypothalamic-pituitary-adrenal (HPA) axis. As a group, patients with CFS appear to have lower HPA axis activity than age- and gender-matched controls. Most evidence points to the hypothalamus as the affected element of the axis; however, it is not known whether this defect is primary or secondary to inactivity, sleep disruption, or continuing stress accompanying CFS. Nevertheless, the decreased HPA activity in CFS contrasts with the increased activity of the HPA axis observed in patients with major depressive disorder. It is more consistent with findings in posttraumatic stress disorder (PTSD), suggesting that CFS may represent a dysfunctional capacity to respond to both physical and psychological stress, either acquired or genetic or both.

Some evidence for a genetic predisposition to CFS has been generated by studying the occurrence of the disorder in twin pairs. Studies in the United States, Australia, and Great Britain have shown an increased frequency of concordance in monozygotic, rather than dizygotic, twins. This observation and the other findings mentioned above suggest a particular pathophysiologic theory of CFS. The syndrome is a complex and multifactorial process. There is a predisposition to the disorder involving genetic or environmental predispositions or both. In the presence of an acute provocation, such as an infection, the stress response system fails and results in both the production and perpetuation of subjective symptoms (ie, fatigue, pain, disrupted sleep, poor cognition) and detectable immune alterations.

DIAGNOSIS

Chronic fatigue syndrome is a clinical diagnosis that depends almost entirely on the history and the patient's report of symptoms. There are no characteristics clinical signs. There are no laboratory tests that can be used with any reliability to rule in or rule out the diagnosis. The purpose of the physical examination and basic laboratory testing is to confirm that there is not another medically definable condition that may be causing the symptoms. In the absence of any confounding medical conditions, the diagnosis of CFS may be guided by the published consensus criteria. For reasons explained above, the clinician need not apply these criteria stringently for individual patients.

The illness occasionally develops in the aftermath of an infection, such as infectious mononucleosis or influenza, or some other physically stressful event, such as surgery or trauma. In postinfectious fatigue, the chronic symptoms may appear to be an extension of the inciting infection. Most often, there is no identifiable precipitating event, and the same flulike symptoms develop gradually. They include sore throat, low-grade fever, tender cervical lymphadenopathy, generalized myalgia or arthralgia, headache, sleep disturbances, and a perception of impaired cognition. Objective physical findings accompanying these symptoms (eg, pharyngeal erythema or exudate, fever greater than 100.5°F, muscle weakness, signs of arthritis, or enlarged lymph nodes) are rare. The presence of any of these signs should raise suspicion of an alternative diagnosis.

The cardinal symptom of the syndrome is, of course, persistent and disabling fatigue, and the fatigue has several characteristic qualities. Most importantly, it is unrelenting and of long duration (>6 months according to the CDC/NIH criteria in Table 3.1). It is generally not improved by rest but typically worsens after physical exertion. Postexertional malaise may persist for hours to days after even a modest expenditure of effort. Many patients perceive that they have a limited allotment of energy to expend each day, and once it is used, they cannot function.

Most patients describe impaired concentration and poor short-term memory. Standard neuropsychological testing typically shows no evidence of an organic syndrome and need not be ordered unless there is objective evidence for cognitive or memory deficit on physical examination. This problem may be the most alarming for the patient who fears a loss of intellectual function; however, such patients can be reassured that the "mental fog" that they experience will lift as the physical symptoms improve.

Most patients will also report either insomnia or excessive sleep. A thorough sleep history is important, because many primary sleep disorders present with chronic fatigue as the chief complaint. If there is a suspicion of sleep apnea or a nocturnal movement disorder, a formal polysomnography is indicated. Similarly, many patients will have symptoms of depression or anxiety. The clinician must determine whether these symptoms are reactive, and part of the CFS syndrome, or primary, accounting for all of the patient's symptoms. If all of the symptoms can be attributed to an episode of major depression or anxiety, then CFS should not be diagnosed.

A laboratory evaluation should be performed for the purpose of ruling out unrecognized medical conditions. All patients should have a complete blood count with differential count, a serum chemistry profile, urinalysis, and thyroid function testing. Additional testing may be ordered to rule out other specific medical conditions if the history or physical examination is suggestive. However, certain laboratory tests may be nonspecifically abnormal in patient with CFS. For example, 15% to 54% of patients may have a low-titer antinuclear antibody test. This is usually nonspecific, and anti-DNA antibodies and antibodies to extractable nuclear antigens are typically absent. Patients with CFS are more likely than healthy controls to have small areas of increased single intensity by brain MRI. These are usually nonspecific and easily distinguished from plaques of demyelinating disease. Urinary free cortisol levels may be relatively low in CFS, but this finding is not reliable enough to be of any diagnostic value. Hormonal testing, other than thyroid-stimulating hormone, should be ordered only when a particular disorder is suspected. Similarly, measurement of the 2′,5′-oligoadenylate synthetase pathway can be ordered from some commercial laboratories. Although opinions differ about the value of these tests, this author finds them insufficiently sensitive and specific to be useful.

CFS often overlaps or coexists with other common idiopathic disorders. Patients with CFS may also meet diagnostic criteria for fibromyalgia, irritable bowel syndrome, interstitial cystitis, premenstrual syndrome, migraine, restless leg syndrome, neurally mediated hypotension or postural orthostatic tachycardia, atypical depression, or spastic dysphonia. The pathophysiologic relationship between these entities and CFS is unclear, but it is important to identify these coexisting disorders, because they often respond to treatments that are not necessarily appropriate for use in CFS alone.

TREATMENT

Guiding Principles

At present, the pathophysiology of CFS is not sufficiently understood to inform specific therapy. Consequently, specific medical or psychiatric therapy is indicated only when there is an alternate or coexisting diagnosis. There is no rationale for treating infectious agents unless there is clear evidence of an active infection that is producing symptoms. Antivirals and other anti-infective agents are not of value in treating the symptoms of CFS because known infectious agents are not typically perpetuating factors in the syndrome.

In the absence of specific therapy for CFS, treatment should be focused on the remediation of symptoms, nonpharmacologic interventions, and physical rehabilitation. There are only a few treatment modalities that can be recommended based on consistent efficacy demonstrated in well-designed, controlled studies (Table 3.2). Many other treatments have less evidence-based support because controlled

Table 3.2 Treatments for Chronic Fatigue Syndrome

Therapies supported by several randomized controlled trials	Graded exercise program Cognitive behavioral therapy
Empiric, symptomatic treatments	Nonnarcotic pain relievers Antidepressants Sleep hygiene Sleep aids
Controversial treatments not supported by a consensus of experimental data and not recommended	Anti-infectives Hydrocortisone Galantamine Fludrocortisone DHEA IV immunoglobulin Interferons Nutritional supplements and vitamins Restrictive diets

treatment trials have not been done or have produced inconsistent results. Conclusions of conflicting studies may differ because of differences in treatment protocols, criteria for patient selection, and disability and duration of illness at the time of recruitment. Because the evidence-based information is inconclusive, clinicians must use their own judgment when using empiric, symptomatic therapies based on the patient's complaints and their own comfort when prescribing the medications. Several other treatments have been proposed, but a preponderance of studies suggests that they are unhelpful or potentially harmful (Table 3.2). Clinicians should also be aware that there is typically a robust placebo effect in trials with CFS patients; therefore, treatment trials that lack appropriate control groups should be considered uninterpretable.

When initiating treatment of any CFS patient, it is useful to objectify the symptoms as much as possible. Patients should be asked to rate their symptoms and to keep personal logs so that their response to any treatment can be assessed. This approach is consistent with the principles of one of the known effective treatments, cognitive-behavioral therapy (see below). Therapeutic interventions should be initiated sequentially so that their positive and negative effects can be assessed. In addition, it is especially important to ask the patient about the use of unconventional or alternative therapies, because many patients may resort to using these products in addition to whatever is prescribed. Polypharmacy, including alternative treatments, may confuse the patient's ability to assess their response to any particular treatment that may be prescribed. In general, the empiric use of allopathic medications and the patient's experimentation with alternative therapies should both be guided by concerns for safety and cost, and empiric trials of treatment should be undertaken systematically in a manner that allows the patient and the doctor to assess the value of the intervention.

Therapies with Demonstrated Efficacy

Several studies using disparate groups of patients have demonstrated that graded aerobic exercise is helpful in reducing the symptoms of CFS. A program of exercise tailored to the individual patient's tolerance should be a part of any treatment effort. The form of exercise should be quantifiable (eg, distance walked, time on an exercise machine, and laps swimming) so that it can be reliably reproduced day to day. Adherence to such a program usually requires substantial reinforcement by the physician, especially among patients who experience serious postexertional fatigue. As a rule-of-thumb, patients should be counseled to exercise daily up to, but not beyond, a level that will not interfere with their ability to repeat the same amount of exercise the following day. Gradual increases in the amount of exercise, over weeks or months, is usually tolerated and leads to overall improvement. In contrast, there is no evidence to support the prescription of bed rest and some suggestion that continuous inactivity may both reinforce illness behavior and lead to complicating myofascial pain syndromes.

Cognitive-behavioral therapy (CBT) is helpful for symptom control in a variety of organic diseases, so it is not surprising to find that it is also of benefit in CFS. CBT involves a restructuring of the patient's beliefs about the illness and encourages objective assessment of the symptoms and disabilities. CBT programs for CFS patients are not universally available; however, the physician can integrate some of the principles of CBT into routine medical care. Educating the patient about the causes and manifestations of CFS is critical, particularly when there are misconceptions that may lead to counterproductive behaviors. Having the patient objectify their symptoms and identify factors that exacerbate or relieve them may also be helpful in management (see above). A rational and sympathetic approach to the patient is essential. Challenging the reality of symptoms or attributing them some other cause (eg, depression in the absence of standard criteria) is distinctly unhelpful because these ideas will not

be consistent with the patient's own experience and beliefs. Similarly, classical insight-oriented psychotherapy is not indicated in most cases of CFS and should be reserved for those patients who have significant, continuing emotional stress at home or work.

Empiric Treatment of Symptoms

Certain medications may be useful for symptomatic therapy in selected patients. Nonnarcotic pain relievers for myalgia, arthralgia, or headache may be helpful. Some combination of nonsteroidal anti-inflammatory medications, acetaminophen, and tramadol may improve symptoms in some patients with prominent pain symptoms.

Although studies conflict on the value of antidepressant therapy for all CFS patients, there are two rationales for considering their use in selected patients: (1) certain antidepressants are generally considered effective symptomatic treatment (eg, for mood disturbances, anxiety, insomnia, pain, and poor concentration) and (2) CFS and fibromyalgia frequently coexist or have substantial symptom overlap, and a benefit of tricyclic antidepressants and similar medications has been demonstrated in fibromyalgia. It should be noted that studies that show benefit of these agents in CFS generally report relief of the associated symptoms noted above rather than the cardinal symptom—fatigue. Therefore, a particular antidepressant may be favored for a given patient depending on the intensity of these symptoms. The remarkable safety profile of antidepressants makes them a reasonable choice for an empiric trial.

Many CFS patients also suffer from sleep disturbances. Pharmacologic sleep aids (eg, eszopiclone, zolpidem, and clonazepam) may be helpful but have the potential risk of creating dependency. Various antidepressants (eg, low-dose trazadone or amitriptyline) may also be useful for this purpose and better suited for long-term use. Melatonin is a popular over-the-counter sleep remedy, but CFS patients have normal levels and timing of endogenous melatonin secretion. Nevertheless, a trial of high-dose melatonin improved CFS symptoms in patients with delayed melatonin secretion; however, the trial used historical controls and must be interpreted with caution.

Perhaps as important as pharmacologic agents is some attention to sleep hygiene. All patients should be instructed to keep regular sleep hours. Patients who are sleeping excessively should be encouraged to reduce their hours of sleep gradually. Those with insomnia should be encouraged to reduce daytime napping to less than 1 hour a day to avoid further disruption of nighttime sleep architecture.

Some therapies have been evaluated in only a single positive study, so it is difficult to determine where they may fit into a therapeutic regimen. These include magnesium sulfate, methylphenidate, and massage therapy.

Controversial or Contraindicated Therapies

Several specific therapies for CFS have been tried based on a particular pathophysiologic hypothesis. Up to the present, none of these therapies has been shown to have meaningful benefit. As noted in the pathophysiology section above, a carefully conducted trial of anti-herpesvirus therapy with acyclovir to test the hypothesis that EBV replication is associated with ongoing symptoms failed to show any benefit. Similarly, a randomized therapeutic trial of oral nystatin was conducted to assess the effect on CFS-like symptoms in patients who claimed to have yeast hypersensitivity. The only benefit was a slight reduction in *Candida vaginitis* in the treatment group.

The finding of depressed HPA-axis activity prompted a trial of low-dose hydrocortisone and subsequently a trial of galantamine (to stimulate HPA axis activity centrally). Investigators judged that the bone mineral loss and prolonged suppression of the HPA axis that resulted from hydrocortisone therapy was not justified by the minimal benefit gained by treatment. The study of galantamine showed no substantial benefit. Another neuroendocrine hypothesis involves the hormone dihydroepiandosterone (DHEA). DHEA supplementation in CFS has reportedly improved fatigue and other symptoms in patients with depressed levels of this enzyme at baseline; however, there has been no controlled trial of this treatment, and it should be regarded skeptically. A study connecting neurally mediated hypotension (diagnosed by a 45-minute tilt table protocol) with CFS prompted therapeutic trials of volume expansion with fludrocortisone. Two independent studies showed no significant benefit of this approach.

Using a model of immune dysfunction as a key factor in the production of CFS symptoms, immune modulation with immunoglobulins, and interferons has been studied. These therapies are extremely costly and inconvenient, so the benefit should outweigh these negative factors. In fact, the preponderance of evidence shows no benefit associated with the use of intravenous immunoglobulin, and studies with interferon are contradictory. Other therapies that have been ineffective or conflicted in randomized controlled trials include the thiamine precursor, sulbutiamine, growth hormone, homeopathic preparations, and essential fatty acids.

Occasionally, patients report relief of symptoms with specialized dietary alterations. A common example is the restrictive diet recommended to reduce intestinal "yeast." There is no experimental evidence to support these diet therapies in CFS, and highly restrictive diets may impair nutrition and general health. Trials of nutritional supplements (eg, vitamins and liver extract) have also been discouraging. Two small trials of activated NADH showed some benefit, but both can be criticized on methodological grounds, and the conclusions have not yet been replicated in a larger study.

Physicians should be aware that there is a lucrative Internet market catering to desperate patients with CFS whose primary care physicians are dismissive. Most of the on-line sales involve unproven supplements and remedies. Many are very expensive (such as replacement of all amalgam dental fillings) and some may be hazardous (such as various hormones and ephedra). Some patients with CFS are motivated to take risks and to spend abundantly from their personal resources to achieve relief from their suffering. Sympathetic physicians should attempt to guide patients through this "medicine show" and to protect them from financial exploitation or harm.

SUMMARY

CFS may occur spontaneously or as a result of an acute stressor, such as an infection. However, there is no evidence that a chronic infection is the cause of the chronic symptoms. Diagnostic criteria have been established by expert consensus in an attempt to standardize research on this disorder, but these criteria may not capture all patients with the variations of this condition that are encountered in clinical practice. Diagnosis based on the patient's subjective report; physical examination and laboratory tests are useful only to rule out confounding medical conditions. Medical treatments directed at specific symptoms may be helpful, but their effectiveness should be assessed in individual patients to justify ongoing therapy. Treatments based on a pathophysiologic hypothesis of the disorder have been uniformly disappointing.

Consequently, the most important elements of care include (1) educating the patient with restructuring of beliefs and perceptions of the illness, (2) initiating a graded exercise program, (3) evaluating symptomatic treatments, and (4) protecting the patient from physical or financial harm associated with unproven therapies.

SUGGESTED READING

Afari N, Buchwald D. Chronic fatigue syndrome: a review. *Am J Psychiatr*. 2003; 160:221–236.

Edmonds M, McGuire H, Price J. *Exercise Therapy for Chronic Fatigue Syndrome (Review)*. The Cochrane Library; 2007. Issue 1.

Fukuda K, Straus S, Hickie I, et al. The chronic fatigue syndrome: a comprehensive approach to its definition and study. International Chronic Fatigue Syndrome Study Group. *Ann Int Med*. 1994;121:953–959.

Imboden JB, Canter A, Cluff LE. Convalescence from influenza. A study of the psychological and clinical determinants. *Arch Int Med*. 1961;108:393–399.

Price JR, Couper J. *Cognitive Behavioral Therapy for Chronic Fatigue Syndrome in Adults (Review)*. The Cochrane Library; 2007. Issue 1.

Straus SE. Pharmacotherapy of chronic fatigue syndrome; another gallant attempt. *JAMA*. 2004; 292:1234–1235.

Stulemeijer M, de Jong LWAM, Fiselier TJW, et al. Cognitive behaviour therapy for adolescents with chronic fatigue syndrome: randomised controlled trial. *Br Med J*. 2005; 330;14–19.

Vercoulen J, Swanink C, Zitman F, et al. Randomised, double-blind, placebo-controlled study of fluoxetine in chronic fatigue syndrome. *Lancet*. 1996;347: 858–861.

Whiting P, Bagnall AM, Sowden AJ, et al. Interventions for the treatment and management of chronic fatigue syndrome: a systematic review. *JAMA*. 2001;286: 1360–1368.

PART II

Clinical Syndromes –
Head and Neck

4. Pharyngotonsillitis

Itzhak Brook

Pharyngotonsillitis (PT) is characterized by the presence of increased redness and finding of an exudate, ulceration, or a membrane covering the tonsils. Because the pharynx is served by lymphoid tissues of the Waldeyer ring, an infection can spread to include various parts of the ring such as the nasopharynx, uvula, soft palate, tonsils, adenoids, and the cervical lymph glands. Based on the extent of the infection, the infection can be described as pharyngitis, tonsillitis, tonsillopharyngitis, or nasopharyngitis. The duration of any of these illnesses can be acute, subacute, chronic, or recurrent.

ETIOLOGY

The diagnosis of PT generally requires the consideration of group A β-hemolytic streptococci (GABHS) infection. However, numerous other bacteria, viruses, and other infections and noninfectious causes should be considered. Recognition of the cause and choice of appropriate therapy are of utmost importance in assuring rapid recovery and preventing complications.

Table 4.1 lists the different causative agents and their characteristic clinical features. The occurrence of a certain etiological agent depends on numerous variables that include environmental conditions (season, geographical location, exposure) and individual variables (age, host resistance, and immunity). The most prevalent agents accounting for PT are GABHS, adenovirus, influenza virus, parainfluenza virus, Epstein–Barr virus (EBV), and enterovirus. However, the exact etiology is generally not determined and the role of some potential pathogens is not certain.

Recent studies suggested that interactions between various organisms, including GABHS, other aerobic and anaerobic bacteria, and viruses, may occur during PT. Some of these interactions may be synergistic (ie, between EBV and anaerobic bacteria), thus enhancing the virulence of some pathogens, whereas others may be antagonistic (ie, between GABHS and certain "interfering" α-hemolytic streptococci). Furthermore, β lactamase-producing bacteria (BLPB) can protect themselves as well as other bacteria from β-lactam antibiotics.

Aerobic Bacteria

Because of the potential of serious suppurative and nonsuppurative sequellae, GABHS are the best known cause of sore throat. Occasionally groups B, C, and G β-hemolytic streptococci are responsible. The clinical presentation of PT due to all types of streptococci is generally identical and is characterized by exudation, palatal petechiae, follicles, tender cervical adenitis, and scarlet fever rash. What are generally absent are the classical signs of viral infections such as cough, rhinitis, conjunctivitis, and diarrhea.

GABHS PT should be suspected in the presence of abrupt onset of fever in a child older than 2 years (with or without "sore throat"), higher temperature, ill appearance, headache, neck muscle pain, tenderness, abdominal pain, nausea, or vomiting, flushed cheeks, circumoral pallor, palatal "petechiae" and semicircular red marks, early strawberry tongue or scarlatinaform rash, a history of exposure to the organism, winter season, and the presence of a peculiar, sour-sweet, yeasty breath odor.

The isolation rate of GABHS varies with patient age, with the highest prevalence in school years. The isolation rate of non-GABHS is higher in adults than in children.

There was a marked decrease in the incidence of acute rheumatic fever in the United States over the past 4 decades that is correlated with the replacement of rheumatogenic types by nonrheumatogenic types. However, streptococcal tonsillitis is still a potential serious illness because rheumatic fever still occurs, and GABHS is manifesting increased virulence. More cases of sepsis, pneumonia, and toxic shock syndrome due to streptococci have been observed in the past decade. Streptococci can be involved in suppurative complications of tonsillitis such as peritonsillar and retropharyngeal abscesses.

Streptococcus pneumoniae can also be involved in PT that can either subside or spread to other sites. *Corynebacterium diphtheria* can cause a

Table 4.1 Infectious Agents of Pharyngotonsillitis

I. Bacteria	Clinical Lesions	Clinical Frequency
Aerobic		
Groups A, B, C, and G streptococci	F, Er, Ex, P	A
Streptococcus pneumoniae	E	C
Staphylococcus aureus	F, ER, Ex	C
Neisseria gonorrhoeae	Er, Ex	C
Neisseria meningitidis	Er, Ex	C
Corynebacerium diphtheriae	Er, Ex	C
Corynebacterium hemolyticum	Er, Ex	C
Arcanobacterium hemolyticum	Er, Ex	C
Bordetella pertussis	Er, Er	C
Haemophilus influenzae	Er, Ex	C
Haemophilus parainfluenzae	Er, Ex	C
Salmonella typhi	Er	C
Francisella tularensis	Er, Ex	C
Yersinia pseudotuberculosis	Er	C
Treponema pallidum	F, Er	C
Mycobacterium spp.	Er	C
Anaerobic		
Peptostreptococcus spp.	Er, E	C
Actinomyces spp.	Er, U	C
Pigmented *Prevotella* and *Porphyromonas* spp.	Er, Ex, U	B
Bacteroides spp.	Er, Ex, U	C
II. Mycoplasma		
Mycoplasma pneumoniae	F, Er, Ex	B
Mycoplasma hominis	Er, ex	C
III. Viruses and Chlamydia		
Adenovirus	F, Er, Ex	A
Enteroviruses (Polio, Echo, Coxsackie)	Er, Ex, U	A
Parainfluenzae 1–4	Er	A
Epstein-Barr	F, Er, Ex	B
Herpes hominis	Er, Ex, U	C
Respiratory syncytial	Er	C

III. Viruses and Chlamydia (continued)	Clinical Lesions	Clinical Frequency
Influenzae A and *B*	Er	A
Cytomegalovirus	Er	C
Reovirus	Er	C
Measles	Er, P	C
Rubella	P	C
Rhinovirus	Er	C
Chlamydia trachomitis		
IV. Fungi		
Candida spp.	Er, Ex	B
V. Parasites		
Toxoplasma gondi	Er	C
VI. Rickettsia		
Coxiella burnetii	Er	C

Abbreviations: Clinical lesions: F = Follicular, Er = Erythematous, Ex = Exudative, U = Ulcerative, P = Petechial; Frequency: A = most frequent (more than 66% of cases), B = frequent (between 66% and 33% of cases), C = uncommon (less than 33% of cases).

bull neck, as can *Corynebacterium hemolyticum*, and both can cause an early exudative PT with grayish-green thick membrane that may be difficult to dislodge and often leaves a bleeding surface when torn off. The infection can spread to the throat, palate, and larynx. *Corynebacterium hemolyticum* produces a lethal systemic exotoxin. *Arcanobacterium hemolyticum* incidence of causing PT is 2.5% to 10%, and occurs mostly in 15- to 18-year-old individuals, and about half of the patients have a scarlatiniform rash.

Neisseria gonorrheae is common in homosexual males and can be detected in adolescents with pharyngitis. The infection is often asymptomatic but can exhibit ulcerative or exudative pharyngitis, may result in bacteremia, and can persist after treatment. *Neisseria meningitidis* can cause symptomatic or asymptomatic PT that can be a prodrome for septicemia or meningitis.

Nontypable *Haemophilus influenzae* and *Haemophilus parainfluenzae* can be recovered from inflamed tonsils. These organisms can cause invasive disease in infants and elderly persons, as well as acute epiglotitis, otitis media, and sinusitis.

Staphylococcus aureus in PT is often recovered from chronically inflamed tonsils and

peritonsillar abscesses. It can produce the enzyme β-lactamase that may interfere with the eradication of GABHS. High tissue concentration of *Haemophilus influenzae*, *S. aureus*, and GABHS correlates with clinical parameters of recurrent infection and hyperplasia of the tonsils.

Rare causes of PT are *Francisella tularemia*, *Treponema pallidum*, *Mycobacterium* spp., and *Toxoplasma gondii*.

Anaerobic Bacteria

The anaerobic species that have been implicated in PT are *Actinomyces* spp., *Fusobacterium* spp., and pigmented *Prevotella* and *Porphyromonas* spp.

The role of anaerobes is supported by their predominance in tonsillar or retropharyngeal abscesses and Vincent's angina (*Fusobacterium* spp. and Spirochetes). Furthermore, patients with non GABHS tonsillitis as well as infectious mononucleosis respond to antibiotics directed only against anaerobes (metronidazole), and elevated serum levels of antibodies to *Prevotella intermedia* and *Fusobacterium nucleatum* were found in patients with recurrent non-GABHS tonsillitis and peritonsillar cellulitus and abscess.

Mycoplasma

Mycoplasma pneumoniae and *Mycoplasma hominis* can cause PT usually as a manifestation of a generalized infection. The prevalence of Mycoplasma infection increases with age.

Viruses and Chlamydia

Viral PT is generally characterized by the absence of an exudate, the presence of ulcerative lesions, minor nontender adenopathy, enanthems, cough, rhinitis, hoarseness, conjunctivitis, or diarrhea. The viruses known to cause PT are adenovirus (concomitant conjunctivitis), coxsackie A virus, parainfluenza virus, enteroviruses (pharyngeal vesicles or ulcers, vesicles on palms and soles in summer), Epstein-Barr virus (exudative pharyngitis, liver and spleen enlargement, cervical adenopathy), herpes simplex (anterior oral and lip lesions, fever), respiratory syncytial virus, rubeola (oral erythema and Koplik spots prior to exanthema) and cytomegalovirus. *Chlamydia pneumoniae* may cause PT, often accompanying pneumonia or bronchitis.

CLINICAL FINDINGS

Pharyngotonsillitis has generally a sudden onset, with fever and sore throat, nausea, vomiting, headache, and rarely abdominal pain. At an early stage redness of throat and tonsils is observed, and the cervical lymph glands become enlarged. The clinical manifestations may vary by causative agent (see above and also Table 4.1) but are rarely specific. Erythema is common to most agents; however, the occurrence of ulceration, petechiae, exudation, or follicles varies. The common features are exudative pharyngitis in GABHS infection, ulcerative lesions in enteroviruses, and membranous pharyngitis in *C. diphtheriae*. Petechiae can often be seen in GABHS, Epstein-Barr, measles, and rubella viruses infections.

Viral disease is generally self-limited, lasts 4 to 10 days, and is generally associated with the presence of nasal secretions. Bacterial illness lasts longer if untreated. The most unique features of anaerobic tonsillitis or PT are enlargement and ulceration of the tonsils associated with fetid or foul odor and the presence of fusiform bacilli, spirochetes, and other organisms on Gram stain.

DIAGNOSIS

Throat culture obtained by throat swab of both tonsillar surfaces and the posterior pharyngeal wall, plated on sheep blood agar media is the standard. Incubation in anaerobic condition and use of selective media can increase the recovery rate of GABHS. A single throat culture has the sensitivity of 90% to 95% in detection of GABHS in the pharynx. False-negative results can occur in patients who received antibiotics. Throat cultures that generally identify GABHS by direct growth may take 24 to 48 hours. Reexamination of plates at 48 hours is advisable. The use of bacitracin disk provides presumptive identification. Attempts to identify β hemolytic streptococci, other than group A, may be worthwhile in older individuals. Commercial kits containing group specific antisera are available for identifying the specific streptococcal group.

Rapid methods for detection of GABHS that take 10 to 60 minutes are available. They are more expensive than the routine culture but allow for rapid administration of therapy and reduction of morbidity. Antigen tests depend on the detection of the surface Lancefield group A carbohydrate. Newer tests use nucleic acid (DNA) probes and polymerase chain reaction (PCR) with greater sensitivity and identify more pathogenic serotypes of GABHS. Early kits showed low sensitivity, but the current ones have 85% to 90% sensitivity but are still associated with 5% to 15% false-negative results. It is therefore recommended that a bacterial culture be performed in instances where the rapid streptococcal test is negative.

More than 10 colonies of GABHS per plate are considered to represent a true infection rather than colonization. However, using the number of colonies of GABHS in the plate as an indicator for the presence of true infection is difficult to implement, as there is overlap between carriers and infected individuals. A rise in antistreptolysin O titer (ASO) streptococcal antibodies titer after 3 to 6 weeks can provide retrospective evidence for GABHS infection and assist in differentiating between the carrier state and infection.

Other pathogens should be identified in specific situations, when no GAHBS is found or when a search of other organisms is warranted. Because many of the other potential pathogens are part of the normal pharyngeal flora, interpretation of these data can be difficult. Attempts to identify corynebacteria should be made whenever a membrane is present in the throat. Cultures should be obtained from beneath the membrane, using special moisture-reducing transport media. A Loeffler slant, a tellurite plate, and a blood agar plate should be inoculated. Identification by fluorescent antibody technique is possible. Viral cultures, or

Table 4.2 Oral Antibiotics for 10-Day Course of Treatment of Acute GABHS Pharyngotonsillitis

Generic Name	Dosage (in mg)		
	Pediatric (mg/kg/d)	Adult	Frequency
Penicillin-V	25–50	250	q6–8 h
Amoxicillin	40	250	q8 h
Cephalexin[a]	25–50	250	q6–8 h
Cefadroxyl[a]	30	1000	q12 h
Cefaclor[a]	40	250	q8 h
Cefuroxime-axetil[a]	30	250	q12 h
Cefpodoxime-proxetil[a]	30	500	q12 h
Cefdinir[a,d]	7 mg 14 mg	300 600	q12 h q 24 h
Cefprozil[a]	30	250	q12 h
Cefditoren	NA	200	q12 h
Azithromycin[d]	12	250[c]	q24 h
Clarithromycin	7.5	250	q12 h
Cefixime	8	400	q24 h
Ceftibuten	9	400	q24 h
Erythromycin estolate	40	250	q8–12 h
Amoxicillin-calvulanate[b]	45	875	q12 h
Clindamycin[b]	20–30	150	q6–8 h

Abbreviations: NA = not approved for children younger than 12 years.
[a] Effective also against aerobic β-lactamase-producing bacteria (BLPB).
[b] Effective also against aerobic and anaerobic BLPB.
[c] First day dose is 500 mg.
[d] Duration of therapy 5 days.

rapid tests for some viruses (ie, respiratory syncytial virus) are available. A heterophile slide test or other rapid tests for infectious mononucleosis can also provide a specific diagnosis.

THERAPY

Many antibiotics are available for the treatment of PT caused by GABHS. However, the recommended optimal treatment for GABHS infection is penicillin administered three times a day for 10 days (Table 4.2). Oral penicillin-VK is used more often than intramuscular (IM) benzathine penicillin-G. However, IM penicillin can be given as initial therapy in those who cannot tolerate oral medication or to ensure compliance. An alternative medication is amoxicillin, which is as active against GABHS, but its absorption is more reliable, blood levels are higher, plasma half-life is longer, and protein binding is lower, giving it theoretical advantages. Furthermore, oral amoxicillin has better compliance (better taste). Amoxicillin should not be used, however, in patients suspected of infectious mononucleosis, where it can produce a skin rash.

The frequently reported inability of penicillin to eradicate GABHS from patients with PT despite its excellent in vitro efficacy is of concern. Although about half of the patients who harbor GABHS following therapy may be carriers, the rest may still show signs of infection and represent true clinical failure. Recent studies have shown that the recommended

Table 4.3 Oral Antimicrobials in Treatment of GABHS Tonsillitis

Acute	Recurrent/Chronic	Carrier State
Penicillin (amoxicillin)	Clindamycin, amoxicillin-clavulanate	Clindamycin
Cephalosporins[b]	Metronidazole plus macrolide	Penicillin plus rifampin
Clindamycin	Penicillin plus rifampin	
Amoxicillin-clavulanate		
Macrolides[a]		

[a] GABHS may be resistant.
[b] All generations.
Remark: For dosages and length of therapy see Table 4.2.

doses of either oral penicillin V or intramuscular (IM) penicillin failed to eradicate GABHS in acute-onset pharyngitis in 35% patients treated with oral penicillin V and 37% of those treated with IM penicillin.

Penicillin failure in eradicating GABHS tonsillitis has several explanations (Table 4.4). These include noncompliance with 10-day course of therapy, carrier state, reinfection from another person or object, and penicillin tolerance. Some postulate that bacterial interactions between GABHS and members of the pharyngotonsillar bacterial flora can explain these failures. These explanations include the "shielding" of GABHS from penicillins by BLPB that colonize the pharynx and tonsils, the absence of normal flora organisms that interfere with the growth of GABHS, and the coaggregation between *Moraxella catarrhalis* and GABHS. Repeated penicillin administration can induce many of these changes. It can result in a shift in the oral microflora with selection of β-lactamase-producing strains of *S. aureus, Haemophilus* spp., *Moraxella catarrhalis, Fusobacterium* spp., pigmented *Prevotella* and *Porphyromonas spp.*, and *Bacteroides* spp.

It is possible that BLPB can protect the GABHS from penicillin by inactivating the antibiotic. Such organisms in a localized soft-tissue infection may degrade penicillin in the area of the infection, protecting not only themselves but also penicillin-susceptible pathogens such as GABHS. Thus, penicillin therapy directed against a susceptible pathogen can be rendered ineffective. An increase in in vitro resistance of GABHS to penicillin was observed when GABHS was inoculated with *S. aureus, Haemophilus* spp., and pigmented *Prevotella* and *Porphyromonas*

Table 4.4 Possible Reasons for Antibiotic Failure or Relapse in GABHS Tonsillitis

Bacterial Interactions
- The presence of β-lactamase-producing organisms that "protects" GABHS from penicillins
- Co-aggregation between GABHS and *Moraxella catarrhalis*
- Absence of members of the oral bacterial flora capable of interfering with the growth of GABHS (through production of bacteriocins and/or competition on nutrients)

Internalization of GABHS (survives within epithelial cells escaping eradication by penicillins)

Resistance (ie, erythromycin) or tolerance (ie, penicillin) to the antibiotic used

Inappropriate dose, duration of therapy, or choice of antibiotic

Poor compliance with taking medication

Reacquisition of GABHS from a contact or an object (ie, toothbrush, dental retainer, or dental braces)

Carrier state, not disease

spp. *Bacteroides* spp. protected a penicillin-sensitive GABHS from penicillin therapy in mice. Both clindamycin and the combination of penicillin and clavulanic acid (a β-lactamase inhibitor), which are active against both GABHS and *Bacteroides*, eradicated the infection.

Penicillin therapy can also reduce the number of aerobic and anaerobic bacteria that can interfere with the growth of GABHS. The oropharyngeal flora of over 85% of individuals who are not tonsillitis prone contains numerous types of organisms that are capable of interfering with the in vitro growth of potential pathogens. In contrast, only 25 to 30% of children who suffer from recurrent tonsillitis harbor interfering organisms.

Acute Pharyngotonsillitis

Even though antibiotics other than penicillin were found to be more effective in the bacteriological and clinical cure of GABHS PT, penicillin is still recommended by some guidelines as the antibiotic of choice. The antibiotics found to be more effective included cephalosporins, lincomycin, clindamycin, macrolides, and amoxicillin-clavulanate. Some of these agents were more effective than penicillin in acute (cephalosporins, macrolides) and others in recurrent (lincomycin, clindamycin, and amoxicillin-clavulanate) GABHS PT.

There are patients where more effective antimicrobials that are less likely to fail to eradicate GABHS should be considered. Individual medical, economical, and social issues should be considered in each patient prior to selecting an antimicrobial for the treatment of GABHS PT (Table 4.5). These include the existence of a high probability for the presence in the pharyngotonsillar area of BLPB and the absence of interfering organisms, the recent failure of penicillin therapy, or a history of recurrent GABHS PT.

The macrolides are also an alternative choice in therapy of PT. Compliance with the newer macrolides (clarithromycin and azithromycin) is better compared with erythromycin, because of their longer half-life and reduced adverse gastrointestinal side effects. However, the increased use of macrolides for the treatment of various respiratory and other infections has been associated with increased GABHS resistance to these agents. Resistance of GABHS to macrolides has reached 70% in Finland, Italy, Japan, and Turkey. Of concern is the recent significant increase of such resistance in the United States that reached 48% in specific populations. The current resistance of GABHS to macrolides in the United States is 5% to 16%. It is therefore advisable to avoid the routine use of macrolides for GABHS PT and save these agents for those patients who are type I penicillin allergic.

The success rate of treatment of acute GABHS tonsillitis was consistently found to be higher with cephalosporins than with penicillin. The cephalosporins' increased efficacy may be due to their activity against aerobic BLPB such as *S. aureus*, *Haemophilus* spp., and *M. cattarrhalis*. Another possible reason is that the nonpathogenic interfering aerobic and anaerobic bacteria that compete with GABHS,

Table 4.5 Indications for the Use of Antimicrobials Other Than a Penicillin for GABHS Tonsillitis

Presence of β-lactamase-producing bacteria (recent antibiotic exposure, winter, region)
Absence of "interfering flora" (recent antibiotic therapy)
Recurrent GABHS tonsillitis
Past failures to eradicate GABHS
High failures of penicillins in the community
Comorbidities
When failure is a medical, economical, or social hardship
Penicillin allergy (non-type I)

and help to eliminate them, are less susceptible to cephalosporins than to penicillin. These organisms are therefore more likely to survive cephalosporin therapy.

The length of therapy of acute tonsillitis with medication other than penicillin has not been determined by large comparative controlled studies. However, certain new agents have been administered in shorter courses of 5 or more days (Table 4.2). Early initiation of antimicrobial therapy results in faster resolution of signs and symptoms. However, spontaneous disappearance of fever and other symptoms generally occurs within 3 to 4 days, even without antimicrobials. Furthermore, acute rheumatic fever can be prevented even when therapy is postponed up to 9 days.

Prevention of recurrent tonsillitis due to GABHS by prophylactic administration of daily oral or monthly benzathine penicillin should be attempted in patients who suffered from rheumatic fever. American Heart Committee guidelines on the prevention of rheumatic fever should be followed, and if any family members are carrying GABHS, the disease should be eradicated and the carrier state monitored.

When *C. diphtheriae* infection is suspected, erythromycin is the drug of choice, and penicillin or rifampin are alternatives. Supportive therapy of PT includes antipyretics and analgesics, such as aspirin or acetaminophen, and attention to proper hydration.

Recurrent and Chronic Pharyngotonsillitis

Penicillin failure in treatment of recurrent and chronic tonsillitis is even higher than the failure of therapy of acute infection. Several clinical studies demonstrated the superiority of lincomycin, clindamycin, and amoxicillin-clavulanic acid over penicillin. These antimicrobial agents are effective against aerobic as well as anaerobic BLPB and GABHS in eradicating recurrent tonsillar infection. However, no studies showed them to be superior to penicillin in treatment of acute tonsillitis. Other drugs that may also be effective in the therapy of recurrent or chronic tonsillitis are penicillin plus rifampin and a macrolide (eg, erythromycin) plus metronidazole (see Table 4.3). Referral of a patient for tonsillectomy should be considered only after these medical therapeutic modalities have failed.

SUGGESTED READING

Bisno AL, Gerber MA, Gwaltney JM Jr, Kaplan EL, Schwartz RH. Diagnosis and management of group A streptococcal pharyngitis: a practice guideline. Infectious Diseases Society of America. *Clin Infect Dis.* 1997;25:574–583.

Brook I. The role of anaerobic bacteria in tonsillitis. *Int J Pediatr Otorhinolaryngol.* 2005;69:9–19.

Brook I. The role of bacterial interference in otitis, sinusitis and tonsillitis. *Otolaryngol Head Neck Surg.* 2005;133:139–146.

Brook I, Gober AE. Persistence of group A beta-hemolytic streptococci in toothbrushes and removable orthodontic appliances following treatment of pharyngotonsillitis. *Arch Otolaryngol Head Neck Surg.* 1998;124:993–995.

Dajani AS, Taubert KA, Wilson W, et al. Prevention of bacterial endocarditis: recommendation by the American Heart Association. *Clin Infect Dis.* 1997;25:1448-58.

Kaplan EL, Johnson DR Unexplained reduced microbiological efficacy of intramuscular benzathine penicillin G and of oral penicillin V in eradication of group A streptococci from children with acute pharyngitis. *Pediatrics.* 2001;108:1180–1186.

Lindroos R. Bacteriology of the tonsil core in recurrent tonsillitis and tonsillar hyperplasia–a short review. *Acta Otolaryngol Suppl.* 2000;543:206–208.

Nouri S, Newburger JW, Hutto C, Pallasch TJ, Gage TW, Levison ME, Peter G, Zuccaro G Jr. Prevention of bacterial endocarditis: recommendations by the American Heart Association. *Clin Infect Dis.* 1997;25:1448–1458.

Richter SS, Heilmann KP, Beekmann SE, Miller NJ, Miller AL, Rice CL, Doern CD, Reid SD, Doern GV. Macrolide-resistant *Streptococcus pyogenes* in the United States, 2002–2003. *Clin Infect Dis.* 2005; 41:599–608.

Shulman ST, Stollerman G, Beall B, Dale JB, Tanz RR. Temporal changes in streptococcal M protein types and the near-disappearance of acute rheumatic fever in the United States. *Clin Infect Dis.* 2006;42:441–447.

5. Infectious Thyroiditis

Jeanne Carey and Stephen G. Baum

INTRODUCTION

Acute suppurative thyroiditis (AST) is a rare but potentially life-threatening infection. AST is usually bacterial in etiology, although fungal, parasitic, and mycobacterial organisms have also been documented causes. The routes of infection are predominantly hematogenous or lymphatic; however, thyroid infections may also be the result of direct spread from an adjacent deep fascial space infection, an infected thyroglossal fistula, or anterior perforation of the esophagus. Thus, infectious thyroiditis may either occur as a local infection or as part of a disseminated systemic infection. Because prognosis is dependent on prompt diagnosis and treatment, it is important to differentiate AST from the noninfectious inflammatory conditions of the thyroid and other inflammations in the neck that it may closely resemble.

PATHOGENESIS

The thyroid gland is rarely infected, and several protective factors have been postulated to explain why the gland is relatively resistant to infection. First, there is a rich blood supply to and extensive lymphatic drainage from the thyroid. Second, the high iodine content of the gland may be bactericidal; however, there are no data to show that the concentration of iodine present in the thyroid would be enough to inhibit the growth of microorganisms. Third, in addition to being surrounded by a complete fibrous capsule, the thyroid is separated from the other structures of the neck by fascial planes.

Primary infections of the thyroid are most likely to occur in individuals with preexisting thyroid disease or with certain congenital anomalies. Goiters, Hashimoto's thyroiditis, or thyroid cancer have been present in up to two-thirds of women and one-half of men with infectious thyroiditis. With respect to congenital anomalies, which are associated with AST more frequently in children than in adults, transmission of infective organisms via a pyriform sinus fistula is the most common direct route of thyroid infection (Figure 5.1). Episodes of AST are often preceded by an upper respiratory infection or another factor (eg, injury or obstruction of the fistula by food or foreign bodies) that may induce inflammation of the fistula and thus facilitate transmission of pathogens to the thyroid. Particularly in children, the left lobe is more commonly involved, reflecting the observation that pyriform sinus fistulae predominantly occur on the left.

Infected embryonic cysts of the third and fourth branchial pouches have also been identified as causes of AST. Infectious organisms may also spread directly to the thyroid via a patent thyroglossal duct fistula (Figure 5.2). AST may be caused by spread of microbes from adjacent sites of infection, such as the oropharynx and middle ear, although this occurs infrequently, presumably because the thyroid is encapsulated within its fibrous sheath. Perforation of the esophagus may also result in direct spread of infection to the thyroid gland.

Bacterial AST may also result from trauma to the anterior neck. One of us (SGB) has seen a single case of direct spread of infection to the thyroid from a neck wound. The patient was a mechanic who scraped his anterior neck while working on his back underneath an automobile. The wound appeared superficial, but infection spread to the thyroid with abscess formation. The offending organism was a staphylococcus. Even fine-needle aspiration (FNA) of thyroid nodules has resulted in thyroid infection.

Immunosuppressed patients, such as those with human immunodeficiency virus (HIV) infection or acquired immunodeficiency syndrome (AIDS) or hematologic malignancies, as well as patients with autoimmune diseases or organ transplants treated with immunosuppressive agents, are at risk for suppurative thyroiditis, which can occur as part of a disseminated infectious process. These infections arise when pathogens reach the thyroid hematogenously or through the lymphatic system.

MICROBIOLOGY

Gram-positive organisms are the most common etiologic pathogens in AST, although a wide

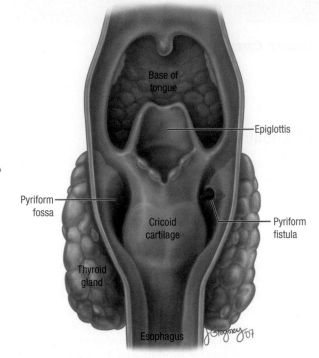

Figure 5.1 Anatomy of the thyroid gland and oropharynx, demonstrating the relationship to a pyriform fistula, anterior view.

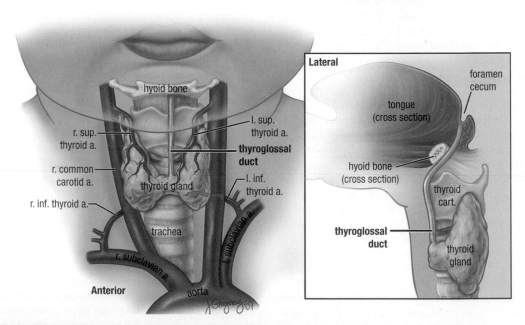

Figure 5.2 Anatomy of the thyroid gland and neck. A thyroglossal duct fistula is shown in frontal and lateral views.

variety of bacteria have been isolated as causative agents in case reports (Table 5.1). In a review of 224 cases of thyroid infections reported between 1900 and 1980, staphylococci, found in 23 of 66 (35%) of culture-positive specimens, were the most frequently identified organisms;

Staphylococcus aureus was the predominant species. *Streptococcus pyogenes*, presumably acquired after a recent pharyngeal infection or colonization, *Streptococcus pneumoniae*, and other streptococci were also commonly recovered. In a subsequent review of an additional

Table 5.1 Microbiology of Infectious Thyroiditis

Nonimmunocompromised Host
Staphylococcus aureus
Staphylococcus epidermidis
Streptococcus pyogenes
Other streptococcal species
Klebsiella species, especially in diabetic patients
Other Enterobacteriaceae
Anaerobic oral flora (foul smell on needle aspiration may give hint of this)

Other Gram-negative bacteria
    free-living in water
    secondary to upper respiratory tract infection

Mycobacterium tuberculosis
Mycobacterium bovis
Actinomyces species
Immunocompromised Host
Mycobacterium avium-intracellulare
Nocardia species
Pneumocystis jiroveci
Modified from Shah and Baum, 2000.

191 cases of AST reported between 1980 and 1997, in which 130 microorganisms were isolated, Yu et al. found that the most common bacterial isolates were gram-positive aerobes (39%), gram-negative aerobes (25%), and anaerobes (12%, mostly in mixed culture).

The true involvement of anaerobic bacteria in AST is unknown because past studies have not used uniform methods for the recovery of anaerobes. Because anaerobes are more difficult to isolate, it is possible that culture-negative cases of AST may represent purely anaerobic or mixed infections, an important consideration when choosing empiric therapy for AST.

The bacterial pathogens implicated in AST in children are similar to those found in adults. *S. aureus*, *S. pyogenes*, *Staphylococcus epidermidis*, and *Streptococcus pneumoniae* are the most commonly isolated organisms in pediatric cases of AST.

Following bacteria, fungi are the second most common microorganisms to infect the thyroid, representing 15% of cases of AST in the review by Yu and colleagues. Fungal thyroiditis most commonly occurs in immunocompromised patients, such as those with leukemia, lymphoma, and autoimmune diseases and in organ-transplant patients on immunosuppressive therapy. In a review of 41 fungal thyroiditis cases published between 1970 and 2005, Goldani et al. found that *Aspergillus* species (spp.) were the most commonly reported cause of fungal thyroid infection. Thyroid involvement by *Aspergillus* spp. was found at autopsy as part of disseminated aspergillosis in 13 (62%) of 21 patients, most of whom lacked clinical manifestations and laboratory evidence of thyroid dysfunction. After *Aspergillus* spp., *Candida* spp. were the second most common cause; other fungal etiologies reported include *Cryptococcus neoformans*, *Coccidioides immitis*, *Histoplasma capsulatum*, and *Pseudallescheria boydii*.

Pneumocytis jiroveci (then called *Pneumocytis carinii*), now classified as a fungus, was not included in the review by Goldani et al.; however, *P. jiroveci* has been found to cause of thyroid infections, almost exclusively in patients with AIDS. Yu et al. identified *P. jiroveci* as the causative agent in 16 of 19 cases of fungal thyroiditis in their literature review.

Mycobacterium tuberculosis as well as atypical mycobacteria have been described as causes of thyroid infection. Thyroidal tuberculosis occurs in the setting of miliary or disseminated disease. Disseminated *Mycobacterium avian-intracellulare* infection in AIDS patients has resulted in thyroidal infection. In their literature review, Yu et al. found that mycobacterial organisms were isolated in 12 of 130 (9%) cases of culture-positive AST. Unlike patients with pyogenic bacterial AST, those with mycobacterial thyroiditis are typically symptomatic for months and are much less likely to experience pain, tenderness, and fever.

Involvement of the thyroid gland by parasites is extremely rare and typically occurs in the setting of disseminated disease. In the United States, only nine cases of echinococcal (tapeworm) thyroiditis have been reported. These patients had chronic symptoms (1.5 to 35 years in duration), were generally diagnosed as having goiters, and were discovered to have thyroidal echinococcosis at the time of surgery. *Strongyloides stercoralis*, which is endemic in the southeastern United States and tropical climates, has been reported as a cause of thyroid infection only in the setting of disseminated disease in immunocompromised patients.

Viral infection causing thyroiditis has never been definitively proven. In postmortem studies of patients with AIDS, cytomegalovirus (CMV) inclusions have been found in thyroid tissue in association with disseminated CMV infection. However, symptomatic thyroiditis due to CMV has not been reported in these patients.

CLINICAL MANIFESTATIONS

The symptoms and signs of AST may be indistinguishable from those of a variety of both infectious and noninfectious inflammatory conditions of the anterior neck. Most patients with AST present with fever, pain and a tender, firm swelling in the anterior aspect of the neck that moves on swallowing and develops over days to a few weeks. In this clinical scenario, the differential diagnosis includes such entities as subacute thyroiditis, Grave's disease, thyroid cancer, hemorrhage into the thyroid, cervical lymphadenitis, and cellulitis (Table 5.2).

Other typical signs and symptoms of AST include dysphagia, dysphonia (both of which have been attributed to compression of local structures, including the recurrent laryngeal nerve), and concurrent pharyngitis. On examination the thyroid is tender with warmth and erythema of the overlying skin and, in the case of abscess formation, fluctuance. Suppurative areas may include one lobe, both lobes, or only the isthmus of the gland. Because a firm nodule may progress to become fluctuant over the course of 1 to 3 days, repeated physical examinations are advisable.

Children with AST present similarly; however, there are a few noteworthy differences. The left lobe of the thyroid gland is more frequently involved in pediatric cases, because pyriform fossa fistulae are predominantly observed on the left. Neonates and infants are more likely than adults to present with stridor and respiratory distress from tracheal compression by an enlarged thyroid gland.

Suppurative thyroiditis that occurs as part of a disseminated infectious process differs from locally spread bacterial thyroiditis in several important ways. First, suppurative thyroiditis due to a systemic infection often occurs in the absence of any clinical manifestations of thyroiditis. Second, the etiologic organisms are typically opportunistic pathogens, such as fungi, *P. jiroveci*, and mycobacteria, which tend to present with a chronic, insidious course. Finally, in contrast to bacterial thyroiditis, preexisting thyroid disease is not a significant risk factor for suppurative thyroiditis that occurs as part of a disseminated infection; rather, patients who are immunocompromised are those who are at particular risk for the latter type of infectious thyroiditis.

Table 5.2 Causes of Painful Anterior Neck Mass

Thyroid-related
Subacute, nonsuppurative thyroid inflammation (Hashimoto's thyroiditis)
Grave's disease
Thyroid cancer, with or without hemorrhage
Hemorrhage into the thyroid secondary to trauma
Radiation damage to thyroid
Acute suppurative thyroiditis
Nonthyroid-related
Cervical lymphadenitis due to infection or malignancy
Cellulitis
Infections of thyroglossal duct remnant, branchial cleft cyst, or cystic hygroma
Modified from Shah and Baum, 2000.

DIAGNOSIS

Leukocytosis and an elevated erythrocyte sedimentation rate and C-reactive protein level are nonspecific, but are commonly seen in AST. Although thyroid function test results are within normal limits in the majority of patients with AST, destruction of glandular tissue with release of preformed thyroid hormone into the circulation can lead to transient thyrotoxicosis. Hypothyroidism has also been reported. Although most patients with bacterial AST are euthyroid, Yu et al. found that those with fungal infections were often hypothyroid (63%) and that half of patients with mycobacterial infections were hyperthyroid.

Imaging studies help to differentiate AST from other causes of anterior neck pain and fever (Table 5.2). Plain neck radiography may reveal tracheal deviation or soft-tissue gas formation, indicative of infection with anaerobic gas-forming organisms, such as *Clostridium* spp. Magnetic resonance imaging (MRI), computed tomography (CT), and ultrasonography often reveal unilobular thyroidal swelling and are extremely useful in the identification of parathyroidal abscesses and spread of infection to contiguous structures (Figure 5.3). Radioactive-iodine scans characteristically demonstrate an area of diminished or absent tracer uptake (a "cold" area) localized to the infected lobe or region of the gland.

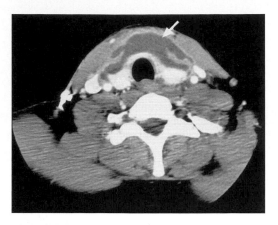

Figure 5.3 Computed tomographic scan of neck with contrast showing an abscess of the left lobe of the thyroid gland (arrow). Published in Jacobs A, David-Alexandre CG, Gradon JD. Thyroid abscess due to *Acinetobacter calcoaceticus*: case report and review of the causes of and current management strategies for thyroid abscesses. *South Med J.* 2003;96:300–7.

The most useful test in AST is FNA, which will frequently be diagnostic. FNA is especially helpful when there is no associated bacteremia or fungemia and when the patient's tenderness is limited to a localized area. Specimens for cytology, Gram stain, and aerobic and anaerobic cultures should be obtained. In the appropriate clinical setting, mycobacterial and fungal cultures as well as special stains for *P. jiroveci* and acid-fast bacilli should also be performed.

MANAGEMENT

Antimicrobial treatment must be targeted at the underlying etiology of AST. In cases of bacterial AST high-dose parenteral antibiotics should be started promptly, as early treatment may prevent complications such as bacteremia and abscess formation. Given the great variety of bacterial species that can cause AST, broad-spectrum antibiotics should be administered while cultures are pending.

In adults, because *S. aureus* and streptococci are the most common causative pathogens, empiric therapy should cover gram-positive cocci. An antistaphylococcal β-lactam (eg, nafcillin and cefazolin) combined with an aminoglycoside (eg, gentamicin) or monotherapy with a third-generation cephalosporin are appropriate initial regimens. Until culture results are available, patients who are penicillin-allergic or who may be at risk for infection with methicillin-resistant *S. aureus* (MRSA) should receive vancomycin. Because oral anaerobes may be involved in AST, antibiotic regimens for most patients should also include anaerobic coverage (eg, clindamycin or β-lactam/β-lactamase inhibitor).

In pediatric or recurrent cases of AST, it is particularly important to cover oral anaerobes, which are commonly involved in these infections. Empiric antibiotic therapy for children with AST should also provide adequate coverage for *S. aureus* and *S. pyogenes*.

If clinical examination or radiographic findings are consistent with an abscess or gas formation, surgical drainage is indicated. If an infection persists despite antibiotic treatment (eg, continued leukocytosis and fever, progressive local inflammation) or involves extensive necrosis, lobectomy may be required.

Patients with AST should be evaluated for the presence of predisposing conditions. Any preexisting thyroid pathology that is discovered, such as a goiter or adenoma, should be treated. Because a pyriform sinus fistula is the most common route of infection in bacterial AST, most patients with their first episode and all patients with recurrent episodes should undergo a barium swallow, CT scan, or MRI of the neck to exclude the presence of a communicating fistula. Because the tract may be obscured by inflammatory material during an acute phase of infection, imaging studies may not reveal a fistula until after the completion of antibiotic therapy. Surgical excision of such fistulae is necessary to prevent recurrent infections.

With appropriate treatment the prognosis of AST is excellent and the vast majority of patients recover completely. Rarely, however, episodes of AST are followed by hypothyroidism, which is almost always transient, vocal cord paralysis, and recurrent infection. As a result of severe, diffuse inflammation and necrosis of the gland, some patients may develop transient or prolonged hypothyroidism requiring L-thyroxine replacement therapy. Management of AST also includes diagnosing and treating any pre-existing thyroid pathology, such as a goiter or adenoma, which may have served as a predisposing condition.

Suppurative thyroiditis due to pathogens other than bacteria generally occurs in the setting of a disseminated infection, most commonly in immunocompromised hosts. In such cases, systemic therapy for the underlying disease (eg, fungal infection, mycobacterial infection) usually results in treatment of the thyroiditis.

CONCLUSION

Acute suppurative thyroiditis is a rare disease, but one that carries considerable morbidity unless promptly treated. Modern imaging techniques are very useful in demonstrating a focus of infection in the thyroid. This infection can occur as a result of systemic infection, in which case hematogenous or lymphatic spread settles in the thyroid. It can also be a result of direct spread from a surface wound or through local invasion from infected congenital anomalies of the neck. In view of the multiplicity and variability of the potential pathogens and their antimicrobial sensitivities, every attempt should be made to identify the offending pathogen. In the case of systemic infections (eg, bacteremias, fungemias, and disseminated tuberculosis), cultures of blood and other infected sites may be sufficient to establish the etiology. When AST is the single site of infection, prompt FNA should be used to identify the organism and dictate appropriate therapy.

SUGGESTED READING

Berger SA, Zonszein J, Villamena P, Mittman N. Infectious diseases of the thyroid gland. *Rev Infect Dis*. 1983;5:108–122.

Brook I. Microbiology and management of acute suppurative thyroiditis in children. *Int J Pediatr Otorhinolaryngol*. 2003;67: 447–451.

Chi H, Lee YJ, Chiu NC, Huang FY, Huang CY, Lee KS, Shih SL, Shih BF. Acute suppurative thyroiditis in children. *Pediatr Infect Dis J*. 2002;21:384–387.

Farwell AP. Subacute thyroiditis and acute infectious thyroiditis. In: Braverman LE, Utiger RD, eds. *Werner & Ingbar's the Thyroid: A Fundamental and Clinical Text*. 9th ed. Philadelphia: Lippincott Williams & Wilkins; 2005:536–547.

Goldani LZ, Zavascki AP, Maia AL. Fungal thyroiditis: an overview. *Mycopathologia*. 2006;161:129–139.

Jacobs A, David-Alexandre CG, Gradon JD. Thyroid abscess due to *Acinetobacter calcoaceticus*: case report and review of the causes of and current management strategies for thyroid abscesses. *South Med J*. 2003;96:300–307.

Miyauchi A, Matsuzuka F, Kuma K, Takai S. Piriform sinus fistula: an underlying abnormality common in patients with acute suppurative thyroiditis. *World J Surg*. 1990;14:400–405.

Nishihara E, Miyauchi A, Matsuzuka F, Sasaki I, Ohye H, Kubota S, Fukata S. Amino N, Kuma K. Acute suppurative thyroiditis after fine-needle aspiration causing thyrotoxicosis. *Thyroid*. 2005;15:1183–1187.

Shah SS, Baum SG. Diagnosis and management of infectious thyroiditis. *Curr Infect Dis Rep*. 2000;2:147–153.

Yu EH, Ko WC, Chuang YC, Wu TJ. Suppurative *Acinetobacter baumanii* thyroiditis with bacteremic pneumonia: case report and review. *Clin Infect Dis*. 1998;27:1286–1290.

6. Otitis Media and Externa

Stephen I. Pelton

INTRODUCTION

The last three decades have seen an expansion in the number of children treated with antibiotics for acute otitis media (AOM) both as a result of the failure to differentiate AOM from otitis media with effusion (OME) and true increases in the frequency of disease most likely associated with the changing nature of day-care attendance. This increased use of antibiotics has, in part, provided the selective pressure to promote the emergence of resistance among the three major otopathogens, *Streptococcus pneumoniae*, nontypable *Haemophilus influenzae*, and *Moraxella catharalis*. Although briefly halted in association with the introduction of pneumococcal conjugate vaccine, resistance has once again begun to increase among isolates of *Streptococcus pneumoniae* with multidrug-resistant serotype 19A emerging as a significant cause of treatment failure. These events warrant a re-evaluation of the diagnosis and treatment of AOM, with an emphasis on distinguishing acute disease from OME and selection of antimicrobial therapy that results in sterilization of the middle ear fluid.

DIAGNOSIS

The American Academy of Pediatrics (AAP) guidelines, published in 2003, codify principles for improving the diagnosis of AOM. Criteria that distinguish AOM from OME were established (Figure 6.1) to promote the judicious use of antimicrobial therapy in otitis media. The AAP guidelines require the presence of middle ear effusion as detected by physical exam or tympanometry as a critical criterion. In addition to middle ear fluid, the diagnosis requires new onset of signs and symptoms such as earache, ear tugging, or a bulging tympanic membrane. Specific ear findings, such as earache or ear tugging, increase the likelihood of bacterial AOM to greater than 85%. In contrast, among children with only nonspecific symptoms such as fever and irritability, bacterial pathogens are found at tympanocentesis in only 50% of cases. When it is less likely that bacterial otitis media is present, it is less likely the child will benefit from antimicrobial therapy as nonbacterial AOM is cured or improved in over 96% of cases with only supportive therapy.

Clinical symptoms and signs may suggest a specific otopathogen as pneumococcal disease is associated with higher fever and greater pain; however, the overlap in signs and symptoms is sufficiently large that clinical differentiation is not possible. The one clinical finding that is consistently associated with a specific pathogen is conjunctivitis with nontypeable Haemophilus influenzae (NTHi).

MICROBIOLOGY OF AOM IN THE ERA OF UNIVERSAL IMMUNIZATION WITH PCV7

The pathogenesis of AOM clearly establishes that nasopharyngeal otopathogens ascend the Eustachian tube into the middle ear where they elicit an inflammatory response resulting in the accumulation of exudate within the middle ear with resulting changes in the tympanic membrane and clinical symptomatology. The point is that, although tympanocentesis is necessary to define the etiology of a specific episode, the spectrum of otopathogens colonizing the nasopharynx will define the microbiology of AOM. Lacking recent studies of tympanocentesis in unselected U.S. children, the current microbiology of AOM can be deduced from studies of nasopharyngeal colonization (NP) and the results of tympanocentesis studies performed on children with persistent or recurrent AOM.

Immunization with PCV7 prevents not only pneumococcal invasive disease due to one of the 7 vaccine serotypes (4, 6B, 9V, 14, 18C, 19F, and 23F) but also new acquisitions of NP carriage of these serotypes. Clinical trials of PCV7 for prevention of otitis media in Finnish children establish a nearly 60% efficacy against vaccine serotypes. The FinOM study also demonstrates protection against several cross-reacting pneumococcal serotypes (isolates of *Streptococcus pneumoniae* (SP) that share the same serogroup designation but are of a different serotype) such as 6A. The overall reduction in pneumococcal otitis was only 34% as an increase in episodes

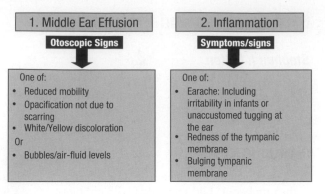

Figure 6.1 Acute otitis media.

1. Middle Ear Effusion
Otoscopic Signs

One of:
• Reduced mobility
• Opacification not due to scarring
• White/Yellow discoloration
Or
• Bubbles/air-fluid levels

2. Inflammation
Symptoms/signs

One of:
• Earache: Including irritability in infants or unaccustomed tugging at the ear
• Redness of the tympanic membrane
• Bulging tympanic membrane

Table 6.1 Distribution by Serotype Grouping of 87 Middle Ear Isolates of *Streptococcus pneumoniae* Resistant to Amoxicillin

	Amosicillin Resistant	
SP Serotype	No.	(%)
Vaccine ST	76	(87.4)
Vaccine Related	9	(10.3)
Non-Vaccine ST	2	(2.3)
Total	87	(100)
Adapted from Joloba, ML. *C/D* 2001		

due to non-vaccine serotypes of SP was observed providing initial evidence that "replacement" disease (that due to nonvaccine serotypes or alternative otopathogens) was significant.

Initially replacement of disease due to vaccine serotype (VST) with nonvaccine serotype (NVST) reduced episodes of AOM due to penicillin nonsusceptible pneumococci. This was a result of the clustering of resistance among a limited number of pneumococcal serotypes, primarily the vaccine serotypes. In one collection of 500 middle ear isolates, 87% of isolates with reduced susceptibility to amoxicillin were vaccine serotypes (Table 6.1). The evidence in support of a transition in pathogens (from VST to NVST) comes from the increased prevalence of NP carriage of NVST, the reported reduction in treatment failures following amoxicillin, and the predominance of *Haemophilus influenzae* rather than penicillin-resistant SP in middle ear cultures of children failing amoxicillin.

Recent studies of NP colonization in children with AOM compared with studies performed prior to the introduction of PCV7 demonstrate increased rates of carriage of *Moraxella catarrhalis* and nontypable *Haemophilus influenzae*, as well as diminished colonization with vaccine serotype pneumococci. Replacing the vaccine serotypes are nonvaccine serotypes, dominated

by serotypes 19A and 6A. Specifically, serotype 19A has become the most commonly recovered pneumococcal serotype in studies of NP colonization and a frequent cause of treatment failure in children with acute AOM.

TREATMENT

Concerns about the escalation of resistance among otopathogens have resulted in a reevaluation of the role of antibiotics in the treatment of AOM. In part this reflects the experience in the Netherlands, where otitis media guidelines recommend antimicrobial therapy to children less than 6 months of age and those who do not respond to supportive therapy. Multiple questions must be addressed to formulate a strategy for treatment of AOM. (1) Do children treated with antimicrobial therapy improve more quickly than those assigned to analgesia alone? (2) Does persistence of bacterial infection within the middle ear correlate with persistence of clinical signs or symptoms? (3) Is the risk of recurrence greater in children who are not initially treated with antimicrobial therapy? (4) Does amoxicillin remain the initial drug of choice when the decision to use antimicrobial therapy has been made?

Do children treated with antimicrobial therapy improve more quickly than those assigned to analgesia alone?

The availability of antimicrobial therapy for the treatment of AOM has resulted in a dramatic decline in suppurative complications, specifically mastoiditis, over the past five decades. Similarly, in special populations such as Native Americans and Eskimo children, the prevalence of otorrhea has declined in association with both the introduction of antimicrobial therapy for AOM and the improvement in public health and socioeconomic conditions. Today, AOM resolves in the majority of children without complications with or without antimicrobial therapy.

The observation that 20% to 30% of episodes are culture negative at the time of diagnosis and do not benefit from antimicrobial therapy and that a proportion of children with acute bacterial otitis spontaneously clear the pathogen (approximately 15% of those with pneumococcal disease, 40% of those due to NTHi, and 75% of those with AOM due to *M. catarrhalis*) had led some experts to suggest that symptomatic therapy should be the initial approach to children with AOM. However, therapeutic trials that include a placebo arm consistently report excess failure rates in children who receive only symptomatic treatment. Historically, Engelhard and associates reported greater than 70% failure in children with AOM who received myringotomy alone. Kaleida and colleagues observed a 2-fold higher failure rate among children with temperature greater than 103°F treated with myringotomy plus placebo compared with antibiotics (23.5% vs 11.5%). They also observed approximately 2-fold greater failure rate in children with nonsevere episodes who were treated with placebo compared with those who received amoxicillin (7.7% vs 3.9%). These studies appeared to establish the role of antimicrobial therapy in the treatment of AOM.

More recently, Little and coworkers compared the outcome of AOM in children initially treated with amoxicillin and in those given a prescription to be filled only if symptoms persisted for 72 hours. Children treated with antibiotics improved more quickly. McCormick and colleagues evaluated "watchful waiting" as a strategy for children with perceived nonsevere AOM. Increased treatment failures and persistent symptoms were observed in children, especially those younger than 2 years old, assigned to the delayed antibiotic treatment group. Although delayed resolution was observed in the cohort assigned to watchful waiting, parent satisfaction was not different among the early treatment and the initial observation groups. More mild adverse events as well as the emergence of multidrug resistance among isolates of SP in the nasopharynx occurred in the early treatment group.

Does persistence of bacterial infection within the middle ear correlate with persistence of clinical signs or symptoms?

The outcome measure selected is critical for determining the impact of antimicrobial treatment on the course of AOM. If outcome parameters such as resolution of signs and symptoms by day 7 to 10, or persistence of middle ear fluid at day 14 or 28 are selected, no differences between antimicrobial treatment and watchful waiting strategies can be consistently established. Effective antimicrobial therapy sterilizes the middle ear, resulting in a more rapid resolution of clinical signs (bulging and erythema) and symptoms (fever, earache, irritability). Therefore, evaluating outcomes within the first 3 to 5 days is necessary to demonstrate improved outcomes in antibiotic-treated cohorts as well as between antibiotic regimens.

Both Dagan and Carlin observed greater improvement in signs and symptoms in children with bacterial AOM when the middle ear fluid was sterilized by days 4 to 6 compared to children who had persistent middle ear infection further providing evidence of improved outcome with effective antimicrobial therapy. Figure 6.2 details the changes in clinical symptom score in children with effective antimicrobial therapy and sterilization of the middle ear compared to those with ineffective antimicrobial therapy and persistence of middle ear infection. The results also demonstrate that most children with persistent middle infection have decreased symptoms at days 4–6 compared to initial presentation.

Is the risk of recurrence greater in children who are not initially treated with antimicrobial therapy?

Only recently has an association between sterilization of the middle ear at days 4 to 6 and the risk of recurrence been suggested. In a recent study, Leibovitz reported that patients with clinical improvement or cure on days 4–6 but culture-positive MEF had an increased rate of recurrent AOM compared to those with culture-negative MEF and clinical improvement or cure (54/133 [35%] vs 126/476 [27%]; $P = .035$) (Figure 6.3). Forty one (76%) of the 54 culture-positive patients with clinical improvement or cure on days 4–6 underwent tympanocentesis at the time of recurrence and 29 were culture positive. Molecular analysis of the otopathogens isolated at recurrence and those identified on days 4–6 found concordance in 66% of patients. This study demonstrated that patients with persistence of MEF pathogens after 4–6 days of antibiotic therapy and clinical improvement or cure had a higher rate of recurrent AOM compared with those who achieved culture-negative status on days 4–6 of treatment. These observations emphasize the benefit of bacteriologic eradication in AOM.

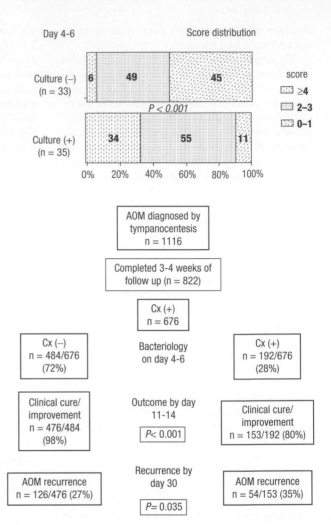

Figure 6.2 Symptoms score in children with AOM.

Figure 6.3 Association between eradication of ME pathogens during Rx.

Does amoxicillin remain the initial drug of choice when the decision to use antimicrobial therapy has been made?

The selection of antimicrobial therapy should be based on knowledge of the microbiology of AOM, pharmacodynamic principles, and clinical trials using both clinical and microbiologic outcomes. Eighteen antibiotics are currently approved by the U.S. Food and Drug Administration (FDA) for treatment of AOM; however, the emergence of otopathogens with reduced susceptibility to β-lactam antibiotics (*S. pneumoniae* and NTHi) has limited the efficacy of some antimicrobial. In the majority of cases of AOM, the specific pathogen is unknown, and presumptive therapy is based on the potential pathogens and their in vitro susceptibility. The proportion of isolates of NTHi producing β-lactamase has slowly risen to 40% over a 25-year period. A very limited number of β-lactamase-producing, amoxicillin-clavulanate-resistant isolates have also been reported in the United States, although these isolates are most common in Japan. The recent emergence of nonvaccine serotypes of pneumococci with reduced susceptibility to β-lactam agents as well as macrolides and trimethoprim-sulfamethoxazole must also be considered in selection of antimicrobial therapy. Because there are no clinical differences between cases with resistant and susceptible pathogens, epidemiologic risk features must be assessed and tympanocentesis employed when a specific microbiologic etiology is needed.

Children with infrequent episodes of OM, without recent antimicrobial therapy, without conjunctivitis, older than 2 years, or not in day care are at low risk for middle ear disease due to drug-resistant *Streptococcus pneumoniae* (DRSP) or β-lactamase-producing NTHi. For these children the AAP guidelines recommend amoxicillin at 90 mg/kg/day administered twice daily for initial therapy in most when the decision to treat has been reached (Table 6.2).

Table 6.2 AAP/AAFP Recommended Antibacterial Agents

Temperature ≥ 39°C and/or Severe Earache	At Diagnosis for Patients Being Initially Treated with Antibacterial Agents or Clinically Defined Treatment Failure at 48–72 Hours After Initial Managment with Observation	
	Recommended	Alternative for Penicillin Allergy
No	Amoxicillin 80–90 mg/Kg/day	Non-type I: Cefdinir Cefuroxime Cefpodoxime Type I: Azithromycin Clarithromycin
Yes	Amoxicillin-clavulanate 90/6.4 mg/Kg/day	Ceftriaxone 1 or 3 days
AAP/AAFP Clinical Practice Guideline: Diagnosis and Management of Acute Otitis Media 2004.		

Table 6.3 AAP/AAFP Recommended Antibacterial Agents

Temperature ≥ 39°C and/or Severe Earache	Clinically Defined Treatment Failure At 48–72 Hours After Initial Management with Antibacterial Agents	
	Recommended	Alternative for Penicillin Allergy
No	Amoxicillin-clavulanate 90/6.4 mg/Kg/day	Non-type I: Ceftriaxone 3 days Type I: Clindamycin
Yes	Ceftriaxone 3 days	Tympanocentesis Clindamycin
AAP/AAFP Clinical Practice Guideline: Diagnosis and Management of Acute Otitis Media 2004.		

Children with risk features such as recent antimicrobial therapy or conjunctivitis are at higher risk for disease due to DRSP or β-lactamase-producing NTHi. In these children only oral high dose amoxicillin and intramuscular ceftriaxone achieve middle ear concentrations high enough to exceed the MIC of all SP that are intermediately sensitive to penicillin and many, but not all, highly resistant strains as well as for strains of NTHi that do not produce β-lactamases. Cefuroxime axetil, cefprozil, and cefpodoxime represent alternatives to high-dose amoxicillin; however, each achieves sufficient middle ear concentration to be effective against only approximately 50% of SP isolates that are intermediately susceptible to penicillin. Also, cefprozil has limited activity against NTHi (Table 6.3). Macrolide are very effective when fully susceptible isolates of SP are present. Because amoxicillin clavulanate resists destruction by the β-lactamase, it effectively eradicates middle ear infection-caused NTHi. Although the AAP guidelines recommend the consideration of amoxicillin clavulanate as initial therapy only for children with severe disease, the increasing prevalence of AOM due to NTHi warrants consideration for broader use of amoxicillin clavulanate as first-line therapy in selected children.

Initial therapy for the child with type I allergy to penicillin (urticaria, laryngeal spasm, wheezing, or anaphylaxis) is limited. Alternatives to

Table 6.4 Treatment of Otalgia

Modality	Comments
Acetaminophen, Ibuprofen	• Effective analgesia for mild to moderate pain • Readily available • Mainstay of pain management for AOM
Home remedies: (no controlled studies that directly address effectiveness) Distraction External application of heat or cold Oil	• May have limited effectiveness
Topical agents: Benzocaline (Auralgan®, Americaine Otic®) Naturopathic agents (Otikon Otic Solution®)	• Additional, but brief, benefit over acetaminophen in patients > 5 years of age • Comparable to ametocain/phenazone drops (Anaesthetic®) in patients > 6 years of age
Homeopathic agents	• No controlled studies that directly address pain
Narcotic analgesia with codeine or analogs	• Effective for moderate or severe pain • Requires prescription • Risk of respiratory depression • Altered mental status • GI upset and constipation
Tympanostomy/myringotomy (EBOM 227–240)	• Requires skill and entails potential risk

β-lactams are limited by substantial resistance among otopathogens. Macrolides, including azithromycin and clarithromycin, are active against most pneumococcal isolates; however, up to 40% of SP have minimal inhibitory concentration (MIC) that are too high for these agents to be effective in some communities. Resistance to trimethoprim sulfamethoxazole among SP and NTHi also is frequent. The AAP guidelines acknowledge the potential limitations of these alternative agents but recommend their use as best alternative.

In 2003, β-lactamase-producing NTHi emerged as the most common pathogen in children failing initial therapy with amoxicillin. As detailed above, this resulted from the decline in disease due to multidrug-resistant SP (MIC > 2.0 ug/mL to amoxicillin) and replacement with susceptible nonvaccine serotypes reducing the likelihood that SP would be the cause of treatment failure. In these children, amoxicillin-resistant, β-lactamase-producing NTHi were identified in more than 50% of episodes. In 2006, DRSP, most often serotype 19A, in conjunction with the continued presence of β-lactamase-producing NTHi are equally likely to be recovered by tympanocentesis in children failing amoxicillin. For these children, a three-dose regimen of ceftriaxone (50 mg/kg/day) has demonstrated efficacy. Anecdotal data support the efficacy for clindamycin and linezolid against DRSP; however, neither is active against

Haemophilus influenza. High-dose amoxicillin in combination with cefixime or ceftibuten and standard-dose amoxicillin in combination with amoxicillin-clavulanate is also appropriate. Clinical studies of quinolones (specifically gatifloxacin and levofloxacin) demonstrate rapid sterilization and clinical resolution of middle ear infection due to both SP and NTHi. Currently, quinolones are not licensed for use in children for the treatment of AOM.

The AAP guidelines emphasize that watchful waiting includes providing analgesia for children suffering from AOM. A limited number of studies suggest that ibuprofen or acetaminophen is effective. Topical agents such as auralgen also may offer temporary symptomatic relief. For children with severe pain, myringotomy is an effective method to attain relief (Table 6.4).

PREVENTION OF RECURRENT ACUTE OTITIS MEDIA

Decreasing the burden of AOM has potential implications for decreasing acute febrile illness in children and associated discomfort, reducing health care costs and surgical procedures, and preventing the language and cognitive delays that occur in some children with recurrent AOM and prolonged conductive hearing loss. Middle ear disease has been identified as the most common reason for ambulatory health care visits. Paradise and colleagues reported that more than 45% of urban children in the first year of life, and 30% in the second year, spend at least 3 months of each year with middle ear effusion and 10% of children spent more 50% of each year with middle ear effusions.

Prevention of recurrent AOM can be achieved by preventing nasopharyngeal colonization with otopathogens, preventing viral respiratory infection, or providing specific antibacterial immunity. Insertion of tympanostomy tubes does not reduce the frequency of acute episodes substantially; however, the presence of such tubes shortens the duration of middle ear effusion. Antimicrobial prophylaxis lowers the frequency of colonization with respiratory otopathogens and decreases the number of acute episodes. Mandel and colleagues found a decrease in acute episodes from 1.04 per child per year in the placebo group to 0.28 in group receiving prophylactic amoxicillin. The reduction in acute episodes was accompanied by a reduction in episodes of OME. The greatest benefit occurs in otitis-prone children who have multiple episodes per year and in whom the problem does not resolve with increasing age. Chemoprophylaxis offers short-term benefits only. Most otitis-prone children continue to have recurrent episodes once prophylaxis is discontinued, until their immune systems and Eustachian tube function have matured.

The pathogenesis of AOM involves co-infection with respiratory viruses in more than 85% of episodes. Immunization with influenza vaccine reduces febrile AOM as well as in myringotomy and insertion of tympanostomy tubes over a winter season. Annual immunization is recommended for children with risk factors for recurrent OM, such as attendance at out-of-home child care, family history of recurrent AOM, or early onset of disease. Unfortunately, prevention strategies for other respiratory tract viruses such as respiratory syncytial virus have not demonstrated consistent protection against AOM.

Two 7-valent pneumococcal conjugate vaccines (PCV$_{CRM}$ and PCV$_{OMP}$), administered at 2, 4, and 6 months with a booster at 12 to 15 months of either 7-valent PCV or 23-valent pneumococcal polysaccharide vaccine have been shown to reduce AOM due to vaccine serotypes of S. pneumoniae by approximately 60%, and all episodes of pneumococcal otitis media by one-third. However, the overall reduction in clinical episodes of AOM was more modest (6% to 10%). A critical concern in the studies was the small increase in episodes of AOM due to nonvaccine serotypes and NTHi. Postmarketing studies

have confirmed an increase in the proportion of AOM due nonvaccine serotypes of SP. Follow up of the original clinical trials of PCV7 in both the Northern California Kaiser Permanente cohort and the FinOM cohort have identified significant reductions in tympanostomy tube insertions in the children immunized in infancy with PCV7. Studies of PCV7 in the child with frequent recurrences of otitis media has failed to demonstrate a significant reduction in recurrent episodes. Veenhoven observed that disease due to vaccine serotypes of SP was a small proportion of overall episodes and reducing these episodes had no impact on total recurrences.

COMPLICATIONS OF ACUTE OTITIS MEDIA

Perforation of the tympanic membrane is the most common complication of AOM and occurs most frequently in younger children. Certain ethnic groups, such as Alaska Eskimos and Native Americans, have a higher rate of spontaneous perforation with AOM. Differentiation between AOM with perforation and acute otitis externa can be difficult. In general, the history of increasing pain with relief when otorrhea occurs is found with AOM, whereas increasing pain without relief in the face of otorrhea is seen with otitis external. The microbiology of AOM in children with acute perforation reports a greater proportion of episodes due to Group A Streptococcus (GAS) and S. aureus. However, S. pneumoniae, NTHi, and M. catarrhalis remain predominant. The natural history of AOM with perforation is usually complete resolution with healing of the tympanic membrane. A small proportion of patients can have persistent dry perforation or experience chronic suppurative otitis media (persisting for more than 6 to 12 weeks). Streptococcus pneumoniae and NTHi are the most common pathogens in infants and toddlers where as Staphylococcus aureas and Pseudomonas aeruginosa are frequent pathogens in older children and during the summer months. An increasing proportion of the S. aureus isolates, even those acquired in the community, are resistant to methicillin. Amoxicillin is generally effective for the therapy of acute otorrhea through a tympanostomy tube and results in rapid clearing of bacterial pathogens and a resolution of otorrhea. Alternatively to oral antimicrobial therapy is topical otic suspensions, either ofloxacin or ciprofloxacin. Both quinolones are active against pseudomonas and quinolone susceptible staphylococci. When methicillin-resistant S. aureas (MRSA) is the pathogen standard therapy, oral amoxicillin or topical quinolone preparations have been ineffective. Resoluton of otorrhea with topical vancomycin (25 mg/mL) drops or the use of trimethoprin-sulfamethoxazole orally in combination with gentamicin otic has been reported. Caution with both of these regimens is necessary as safety has not been established.

Facial palsy as a complication of AOM has become less prominent with the routine use of antibiotic therapy. Facial weakness and earache are the predominant symptoms. Management with antimicrobial agents and myringotomy (with or without tube insertion) is usually sufficient to achieve complete resolution.

The incidence of mastoiditis has decreased dramatically with the routine use of antimicrobial therapy. However, it remains the most common suppurative complication of AOM. Although the potential for reemergence of mastoiditis when antimicrobial agents are withheld for AOM has been a concern, there is little convincing data available that this scenario is occurring. The management of acute mastoiditis depends on assessment of disease status. *Acute mastoiditis with periostitis* results from an obstruction of the connection between the middle ear and mastoid space (aditus ad antrum). Postauricular erythema, tenderness, and edema are the clinical manifestations. AOM is often but not universally present. *S. pneumoniae*, GAS, and NTHi are most common but *Pseudomonas aeruginosa* was found in 29% and *S. epidermidis* in 31% of cases in one large series. *Pseudomonas* and *Staphylococcus* should be suspected when a history of otorrhea precedes development of acute mastoiditis.

Labyrinthitis develops when AOM spreads (through the round window) into the cochlear space. The process may be suppurative or serous (due to toxins). The onset of labyrinthitis is often sudden, with vertigo and hearing loss being characteristic. Acute surgical intervention (myringotomy with tube insertion) with antimicrobial therapy is the treatment of choice. Additional rare complications of AOM are brain abscess, lateral sinus thrombosis, and otic hydrocephaly.

OTITIS EXTERNA

Acute otitis externa (AOE) is primarily a pediatric disease occurring most frequently in children 6 to 12 years of age. The disease results from a disruption of integrity of the ear canal and the normal self-cleaning process of epithelial migration toward the external

os. Swimming, local trauma, accumulation of debris from dermatologic conditions, or the wearing of hearing aids are predisposing factors. The early manifestations are itching, pain, and erythema of the canal but the disease can progress with severe swelling and obstruction of the external canal or extension to the bony external canal or even the base of the skull in the elderly or in patients with comorbidity (see discussion of malignant external otitis in Chapter 146, Pseudomonas, Stenotrophomonas and Burkholderia).

Early in the course, minimal, odorless secretions and erythema of the external canal in association with mild pain and pruritis are present. As the disease progresses, erythema increases and edema of the canal becomes manifest. Seropurulent secretions may be present and acute pain is elicited by movement of the auricle or direct pressure on the tragus. Severe disease is noted by edema of the canal wall obstructing the lumen, intense pain, and extension to cervical adenitis or auricular cellulitis.

The diagnosis of AOE requires rapid onset of symptoms over several days with evidence of inflammation of the external ear canal manifest by otalgia, itching, tenderness of the tragus or pinna and/or diffuse erythema. Systemic manifestations such as cervical adenitis or cellulitis of the pinna may be present. Distinguishing AOE from AOM is critical as the therapy is markedly different. Identification of complications that may be manifest by facial paralysis, vertigo, or meningeal signs or cranial nerve palsy or the presence of granulation tissue at the junction of the boney and cartilaginous portions of the canal is critical. A furuncle may be observed in the external canal. Often referred to as localized otitis externa, this represents an infected hair follicle in the outer third of the external canal. History is helpful in discriminating AOE from AOM. Often the pain in AOE is progressive where in AOM the pain will usually abruptly improve when perforation occurs. The tympanic membrane in both AOM and AOE is frequently erythematous but in AOE pneumatic otoscopy reveals normal motility. Otomycosis may manifest as thick otorrhea, white debris with hyphae in the canal (*Candida*), or a white plug with dark debris (*Aspergillus niger*).

Topical therapy is the initial choice for diffuse, uncomplicated AOE as there is no need to systemic antimicrobials unless there are comorbid conditions that are associated with disease complications, progression to cellulitis of the pinna or adenitis, or topical therapy is contraindicated. AOE is primarily a bacterial disease with *Pseudomonas aeruginosa* the dominant pathogen followed by *S. aureus*. Fungal infection is uncommon except in those who have failed initial topical therapy. Mild disease can be treated with 2% acetic acid with or without a steroid. Compliance may be poor as acetic acid is irritating and frequently causes stinging when administered topically to inflamed skin. Topical antimicrobial preparations contain an aminoglycoside, polymixin B, or a quinolone with or without a steroid are effective. These topicals achieve local tissue concentrations 1000-fold that of systemic administration and standard antimicrobial resistant profiles may not correlate with success. No significant difference in clinical outcome have been established for antiseptic vs antimicrobial preparations, for quinolone vs nonquinolone formulations, or for steroid-antimicrobial preparations compared to antimicrobials alone. However, when a perforation of the timpanic membrane (TM) is suspected, a tympanostomy tube is in place, or the TM has not visualized, only quinolone formulations are approved for use when a nonintact TM is present. All show benefit compared to placebo and all result in cure in most patients by 7 to 10 days. Critical for topical therapy to be successful is the delivery. Self-administration is difficult and often unsuccessful. Ototopical formulations should be administered with the patient lying on his/her side. The canal should be filled and, if necessary, the pinna pulled forward and back to assist filling. Some clinicians use aural lavage for removal of debris either initially or, if necessary, repeatedly. Pain may limit the ability to perform aural lavage or suction. If edema is present, a wick of either compressed cellulose or ribbon gauze will enable complete delivery of the ototopical agent. Once the edema resolves, the wick may be removed and therapy continued to complete 7 to 10 days. Adverse events with topical therapy are not common; however, sensitization especially to those formulations that contain neomycin can occur. If signs and symptoms fail to improve, systemic antimicrobial therapy should be added based on the results of susceptibility testing of external ear canal culture.

Fungal disease, most commonly *Candida* or *Aspergillus*, is most often found in patients failing initial topical therapy and should be suspected in that situation. Two approaches have been used successfully: ketoconozole cream can be applied to the external canal directly once with follow-up examination in 5 to 7 days and repeat application if needed or cresylate otic is applied three times a day. Both treatments achieve greater than 80% cure rates. Most recently, community-acquired methicillin-resistant *S. aureus* (CaMRSA) has emerged as an increasing cause of AOE. Treatments used successfully in the treatment of MRSA otitis externa were aural toilet and fucidic acid-betamathasone 0.5%. Most CaMRSA are susceptible to quinolones and it would be expected that ofloxacin or ciprofloxacin formulations should be effective.

Pain management is an integral part of treatment of AEO. Nonsteroidal anti-inflammatory agents and benzocaine otic have been used successfully to manage the discomfort of AOE.

In children with recurrent otitis externa, strategies such as the use of acidifying ear drops before or after swimming, the use of a hair dryer to dry the ear canal after swimming or bathing, or the use of ear plugs while swimming have all been used successfully.

SUGGESTED READING

American Academy of Pediatrics. Subcommittee on management of acute otitis media: diagnosis and management of acute otitis media. *Pediatrics.* 2004;113:1451–1465.

Arguedas A, Dagan R, Pichichero M, et al. An open-label, double tympanocentesis study of levofloxacin therapy in children with, or at high risk for, recurrent or persistent acute otitis media. *Pediatr Infect Dis J.* 2006;25(12):1102–1109.

Carlin SA, Marchant CD, Shurin PA, et al. Host factors and early therapeutic response in acute otitis media. *J Pediatr* (1991 Feb) 118(2):178-83.

Dagan R, Leibovitz E, Greenberg D, et al. Early eradication of pathogens from middle ear fluid during antibiotic treatment of acute otitis media is associated with improved clinical outcome. *Pediatr Infect Dis J.* 1998;17:776–782.

Del Mar C, Glasziou P, Hayem M. Are antibiotics indicated as initial treatment for children with acute otitis media? A meta-analysis. *Br Med J.* 1997;314:1526–1529.

Dowell SF, Marcy SM, Phillips WR, et al. Otitis media—principles of judicious use of antimicrobial agents. *Pediatrics.* 1998;101:165–171.

Eskola J, Kilpi T, Palmu A, et al. Efficacy of a pneumococcal conjugate vaccine against acute otitis media. *N Engl J Med.* 2001;344(6):403–409.

Leibovitz E. *The challenge of recalcitrant acute otitis media: Pathogens, resistance, and treatment strategy. PIDJ,* in press.

Lieberthal AS. Acute otitis media guidelines: review and update. *Curr Allergy Asthma Rep*. 2006;6(4):334–341.

Mandel EM, Casselbrant ML, Rockette HE, et al. Efficacy of antimicrobial prophylaxis for recurrent middle ear effusion. *Pediatr Infect Dis J* (1996 Dec) 15(12):1074-82.

McCormick DP, Chonmaitree T, Pittman C, et al. Nonsevere acute otitis media: a clinical trial comparing outcomes of watchful waiting versus immediate antibiotic treatment. Pediatrics. 2005;115(6):1455–1465.

Paradise JL, et al. Otitis media in 2253 Pittsburgh-Area infants: Prevalence and risk factors during the first two years of life. *Pediatrics* 1997: 1997;99:318-333.

Rosenfeld RM, Kay D. Natural history of untreated otitis media. In: Rosenfeld RM, Bluestone CD, eds. *Evidence-Based Otitis Media*. 2nd ed. Hamilton, ON, Canada: BC Decker Inc; 2003:180–198.

Segal N, Leibovitz E, Dagan R, et al. Acute otitis media—diagnosis and treatment in the era of antibiotic resistant organisms: updated clinical practice guidelines. *Int J Pediatr Otorhinolaryngol*. 2005;69(10):1311–1319.

Rosenfeld RM, Brown L, Cannon CR, et al. Clinical practice guideline: acute otitis externa. *Otolaryngol Head Neck Surg*. 2006;134: S4–S23.

Veenhoven R, Bogaert D, Uiterwaal C, et al. Effect of conjugate pneumococcal vaccine followed by polysaccharide pneumococcal vaccine on recurrent acute otitis media: a randomised study. *Lancet* (2003 Jun 28) 361(9376):2189-95.

7. Sinusitis

Charles D. Bluestone and Todd D. Otteson

Sinusitis is one of the most commonly diagnosed ailments in clinical practice, yet criteria for its diagnosis may be variable and a standard treatment protocol is nonexistent. The majority of patients with acute sinusitis improve without any therapy or with over-the-counter remedies. The temptation to treat an upper respiratory infection with antimicrobials should be avoided, especially in light of increasing bacterial resistance profiles. An understanding of the anatomy, pathophysiology with predisposing factors, and common microbiology helps drive therapeutic decision making.

SINUS ANATOMY

The paranasal sinuses consist of paired maxillary, ethmoid, sphenoid, and frontal sinuses. The maxillary and ethmoid sinuses are present at birth and fully pneumatize during childhood. The paired sphenoid and frontal sinuses appear in childhood and continue to pneumatize into early adulthood in some cases. The maxillary, anterior ethmoid, and frontal sinuses drain into the osteomeatal complex (OMC). The OMC is a functional physiological unit comprising the ethmoid infundibulum, middle meatus, and surrounding structures. The OMC and its patency are the keys to normal sinus drainage and the maintenance of physiologic mucociliary clearance.

PATHOPHYSIOLOGY

Any anatomic anomaly, environmental exposure, or disease process, acute or chronic, that prevents the normal mucociliary clearance either by functional obstruction or by thickening of nasal secretions may result in pathogen overgrowth and sinusitis. Typically these processes or exposures affect not only the paranasal sinus mucosa but also the intranasal mucosa, prompting use of the term rhinosinusitis. Table 7.1 outlines specific conditions that precipitate obstruction of the OMC, entities that cause thickened secretions, and diseases that involve dysfunction of mucosal cilia.

Rarely, direct inoculation of bacteria into the sinus via spread of odontogenic infection or during swimming or diving may cause acute sinusitis as well.

The bacteriology of sinusitis has been well documented in a number of studies using a variety of means for gathering specimens for culture. The results have been consistent for decades, with the most common organisms isolated in acute sinusitis being *Streptococcus pneumoniae, Haemophilus influenzae,* and *Moraxella catarrhalis.* Individual resistance to antibiotics either by β-lactamase production or by some other means has increased. The spectrum of organisms widens in chronic sinusitis to include anaerobic bacteria, *Staphylococcus aureus,* and gram-negative organisms, particularly *Pseudomonas aeruginosa.* Much research has been dedicated recently to the role of biofilm formation in the pathophysiology of chronic rhinosinusitis. A biofilm is a complex polysaccharide matrix synthesized by bacteria that is protective of bacterial colonies and renders them somewhat resistant to antibiotic therapy. *Pseudomonas aeruginosa* is a known biofilm former in patients with chronic rhinosinusitis.

DIAGNOSIS

Diagnosis of sinusitis is based on a complete history and a meticulous physical examination with radiographic support in certain cases. The physical examination consists of anterior rhinoscopy before and after topical decongestion. Any purulent drainage or edema in the area of the middle meatus should be documented as well as the general appearance of the nasal mucosa. Nasal endoscopy allows a more detailed examination of the nasal cavity. Palpation of the paranasal sinuses may elicit focal tenderness. Transillumination of the sinuses may be helpful in adults if the exam is normal or completely absent but is not reliable in children.

Distinguishing between bacterial sinusitis and viral upper respiratory infection may often be difficult but is important in planning a treatment strategy. A set of standardized definitions

Table 7.1 Conditions Precipitating Sinusitis

OMC Obstruction
Concha bullosa
Mucosal edema secondary to rhinitis
Nasal foreign body
Nasal septal deviation
Nasogastric/nasotracheal tubes Polyps
Secretion Thickness
Allergic rhinitis
Cystic fibrosis
Viral URI
Ciliary Dysfunction
Ciliary dyskinesia
Viral URI

for rhinosinusitis based on symptom profile and duration is well accepted. Symptoms are described as major or minor and include facial pain, nasal obstruction, nasal discharge/post-nasal drip, hyposmia/anosmia, purulence on examination (major), and headache, halitosis, dental pain, fatigue, and ear pain/pressure (minor). Rhinosinusitis is acute when symptoms last 4 weeks or less, subacute when symptoms are present for 4 to 12 weeks, and chronic for symptoms present longer than 12 weeks. Recurrent acute rhinosinusitis occurs in patients with four or more episodes per year with disease-free intervals in between. An acute exacerbation of chronic sinusitis is defined as a sudden worsening of symptoms with return to baseline after treatment.

Plain films add little to the diagnosis of sinusitis, especially if sinuses other than the maxillary sinuses are involved. If the clinical situation warrants it, the suspicion of sinusitis is confirmed by computed tomography (CT), which can demonstrate characteristic changes in the paranasal sinuses and especially the OMC. The best time to obtain a CT scan is at the end of a treatment course when the patient is not acutely ill. The CT scan is crucial if any surgical intervention is required. Figure 7.1A shows the paired maxillary sinuses (M) with some dependent fluid in the right maxillary sinus. Note also the right nasal septal deviation. Figure 7.1B shows the ethmoid

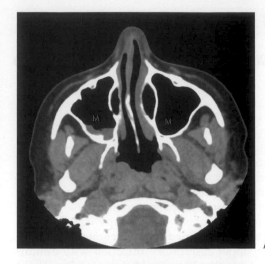

A

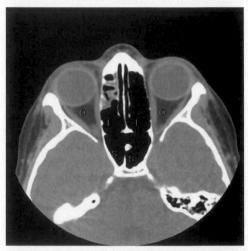

B

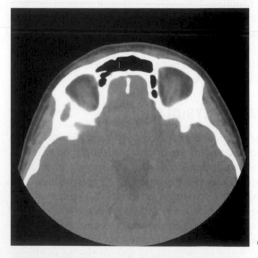

C

Figure 7.1 (A) Paired maxillary sinuses (M) with dependent fluid in the right maxillary sinus. (B) Ethmoid sinuses (E) with some right anterior ethmoid opacification and Orbit (O). (C) Frontal sinus (F).

sinuses (E) with some right anterior ethmoid opacification. Note also the proximity of the ethmoid sinuses to the orbit (O); the lamina papyracea is a layer of thin bone separating these structures. The sphenoid sinuses posteriorly are also present in this image. Figure 7.1C shows the frontal sinus (F).

TREATMENT

The treatment of acute sinusitis involves appropriate antibiotic therapy and should improve the patency of the sinus ostia. Topical decongestants, such as oxymetazolone, may alleviate nasal obstruction and decrease nasal mucosal edema but they can only be used for a short time. Systemic decongestants and mucolytics may assist with clearance of secretions.

Ideal antimicrobial therapy eliminates the common bacteria that cause acute sinusitis with as narrow a spectrum as possible. Current antibiotic treatment recommendations for acute bacterial rhinosinusitis as outlined by the Sinus and Allergy Health Partnership are stratified depending on disease severity and usage of recent antibiotics. First-line treatment for mild disease is with amoxicillin or amoxicillin-clavulanate unless the patient has had an antibiotic course within the past 4 to 6 weeks; in this case, first-line treatment includes fluoroquinolones or high-dose amoxicillin–clavulanate. For penicillin-allergic patients, macrolides are generally recommended as the first-line antimicrobial followed by fluoroquinolones or rifampin+clindamycin. Treatment failure after 72 hours may require directed cultures and treatment with a broader spectrum second-line agent.

Treatment of chronic sinusitis is aimed at both alleviation of symptoms and diminishing sinus inflammation. Irrigation of the nasal cavity with normal saline as well as treatment with topical nasal steroids, systemic antihistamines, systemic decongestants, and any additional allergy therapy should be attempted. Longer-term antimicrobial therapy lasting 4 weeks with a second-line antibiotic may improve symptoms when shorter courses have failed.

If patients with either chronic sinusitis or recurrent acute sinusitis fail to respond to these medical measures, consultation with an otolaryngologist should be considered. Investigation into the etiology of the inflammation causing rhinosinusitis, including any anatomic or physiologic source, should be undertaken. When maximal medical therapy has failed to resolve the rhinosinusitis, surgical management of the disease must be entertained. The goal of surgical intervention is to restore sinus drainage while preserving as much paranasal sinus and nasal mucosa as possible. This principle is especially crucial for surgery directed at the OMC. Postoperative patient satisfaction scores are generally high.

COMPLICATIONS

Complications of sinusitis are almost exclusively a phenomenon of acute sinusitis and generally involve spread of infection from the affected sinus to adjacent structures. Acute infection of the ethmoid sinuses may spread to become an orbital infection that may range from preseptal cellulitis to orbital cellulitis to subperiosteal orbital abscess to orbital abscess with possible spread to become cavernous sinus thrombosis. Infection involving the frontal sinus may precipitate meningitis or even intracranial abscess. Regardless of the location, therapy involves intravenous antibiotic therapy and may also include surgical drainage of the affected sinus or sinuses.

FUNGAL SINUSITIS

Fungal sinusitis describes a spectrum of diseases with treatment depending on the individual disease entity. The most severe and the rarest manifestation is invasive fungal sinusitis, which typically occurs in patients with immunodeficiency for any reason, including uncontrolled diabetes mellitus and patients taking immunosuppressive medications after transplant or hematologic malignancy. Treatment in these cases involves intravenous antifungal medications that may be quite toxic. Aggressive surgical debridement of necrotic tissue is required. Reversal of the immunosuppression is advised if possible. A less aggressive form of chronic invasive fungal sinusitis has been described in immunocompetent patients.

Allergic fungal sinusitis is characterized by an allergic inflammation of the sinonasal mucosa caused by colonizing fungi within the sinuses. Tissue samples of such sinonasal mucosa show no mucosal invasion. The abundant allergic response of the mucosa to the adjacent fungal elements is immunoglobulin E- (IgE) mediated inflammation. The production of thick, tenuous, allergic mucin is pathognomonic of allergic fungal sinusitis. Histological examination of the mucosa reveals chronic inflammation with an overabundance of eosinophils. A similar examination of the allergic mucin demonstrates fungal hyphae characteristic of the species involved and Charcot-Leyden crystals. Treatment consists of conservative surgical debridement, either topical or systemic antifungal therapy, and topical or systemic steroids depending on the clinical situation.

A fungal ball, or mycetoma, typically involves a single sinus, is not considered invasive, and may masquerade as chronic sinusitis. Treatment is surgical, addressing only the sinus(es) in question with no subsequent medical therapy required.

SUGGESTED READING

Anon JB, Jacobs MR, Poole MC, et al. Antimicrobial treatment guidelines for acute bacterial rhinosinusitis. *Otolaryngol Head Neck Surg.* 2004;130(Suppl 1):1–45.

Benninger MS, Ferguson BJ, Hadley JA, et al. Adult chronic rhinosinusitis definitions, diagnosis, epidemiology, and pathophysiology. *Otolaryngol Head Neck Surg.* 2003;129(Suppl 3):1–32.

Bent JP III, Kuhn FA. Diagnosis of allergic fungal sinusitis. *Otolaryngol Head Neck Surg.* 1994;111:580–588.

Cryer J, Schipor I, Perloff J, et al. Evidence of bacterial biofilms in human chronic rhinosinusitis. *ORL J Otorhinolaryngol Relat Spe* 2004;66(3):155–158.

Lanza, DC, Kennedy DW. Adult rhinosinusitis defined. *Otolaryngol Head Neck Surg.* 1997; 117:S1–S7.

Marple BF, Brunto S, Ferguson BJ. Acute bacterial rhinosinusitis: a review of U.S. treatment guidelines. *Otolaryngol Head Neck Surg.* 2006;135:341–348.

8. Dental Infection and Its Consequences

Bridget Hathaway, Jennifer Rubin Grandis, and Jonas T. Johnson

ANATOMY

It is helpful when discussing the manifestations and treatment of odontogenic infections to have an understanding of the fascial spaces surrounding maxillomandibular dentition (Figure 8.1). Although both maxillary and mandibular teeth can become infected, infections of mandibular dentition are more common. Anatomic spaces involved by maxillary infections include the canine and buccal spaces, with the orbit and cavernous sinus less commonly affected. If untreated, odontogenic infections tend to erode through the thinnest, closest cortical plate. The thinner bone in the maxilla is on the labial-buccal side, the palatal cortex being thicker. The canine space is that region between the anterior surface of the maxilla and the levator labii superioris (Figure 8.2). Infection of this fascial space usually results from maxillary canine tooth infection. The buccal space is located between the buccinator muscle and the skin and superficial fascia. Infections of this space usually result from maxillary molar processes with the premolars as the rare culprits. Orbital cellulitis or cavernous sinus thrombosis are unusual but serious manifestations of maxillary infection. Under such circumstances, the infection most likely spreads both by direct extension as well as hematogenously.

In the mandible, the thinnest region is on the lingual aspect around the molars and the buccal aspect anteriorly. The primary mandibular spaces include the submental, sublingual, and submandibular fascial spaces. The submental space is that area between the anterior belly of the digastric muscle, the mylohyoid muscle, and the skin. Infection here usually results from the mandibular incisors (Figure 8.3). Medially, the sublingual and submandibular spaces are typically affected by the mandibular molars. Whether the infection is in the sublingual or submandibular space is determined by the relationship between the area of perforation and the mylohyoid attachment. Specifically, if the apex of the offending tooth is superior to that of the mylohyoid (eg, premolars, first molar, and occasionally second molar), the sublingual space is affected; if the infection is inferior (eg, third molar and occasionally second molar), the submandibular space is involved. Multiple fascial spaces can be infected simultaneously. For example, the sublingual space lies between the oral mucosa and the mylohyoid and communicates along the posterior bounder of the mylohyoid muscle with the submandibular space. When infection involves the primary mandibular spaces bilaterally it is known as Ludwig's angina.

Odontogenic infection can extend beyond the mandibular spaces to the neck to involve the cervical fascial spaces. The secondary mandibular spaces include the pterygomandibular, masseteric, and temporal spaces. These fascial spaces become infected as the result of secondary spread from more anterior spaces, including the buccal, sublingual, and submandibular spaces. The pterygomandibular space lies between the medial aspect of the mandible and the medial pterygoid muscle. The masseteric space is that area between the lateral mandible and the masseter muscle, and the temporal space is superior and posterior to the pterygomandibular and masseteric spaces. Infection of these areas almost uniformly produces trismus resulting from inflammation of the muscles of mastication.

Infection in these spaces may progress to the deep neck spaces, which include the lateral pharyngeal (parapharyngeal) space, the retropharyngeal space, and the prevertebral space. Infections of these spaces are discussed in detail in Chapter 10, Deep Neck Infections. One should keep in mind, however, that up to 30% of deep neck infections may result from odontogenic processes. These so-called deep neck infections may spread distally into the mediastinum.

PATHOPHYSIOLOGY

Odontogenic infections and their complications may be encountered by any clinician who treats diseases of the mouth and throat. Most infections are minor and self-limited, confined to the offending tooth and its apex. Under certain circumstances, however, the infectious process

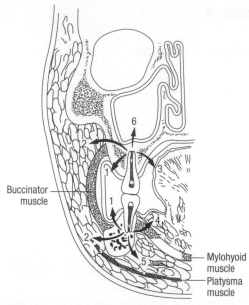

Figure 8.1 An odontogenic infection can express itself after erosion through jaw bone, depending on the thickness of the overlying bone and the nature of the surrounding soft tissues. This illustration displays six possible locations: (1) vestibular abscess, (2) buccal space, (3) palatal abscess, (4) sublingual space, (5) submandibular space, and (6) maxillary sinus. Cummings: *Otolaryngology: Head & Neck Surgery, 4th ed.*, Copyright © 2005 Mosby, Inc.

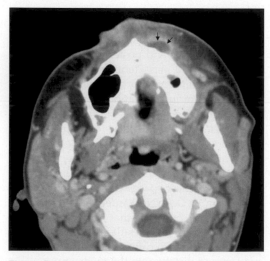

Figure 8.2 CT image demonstrating an abscess of the canine space (black arrows).

may break through the bony, muscular, fascial, and mucosal barriers and spread to contiguous spaces, resulting in soft-tissue infections.

Typically, infections originate within the dental pulp, periodontal tissue, or pericoronal tissue from a carious tooth. This results in

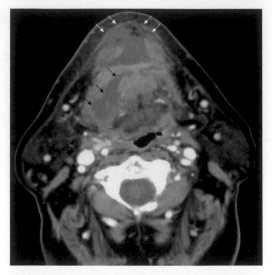

Figure 8.3 CT image demonstrating an abscess of the floor of mouth (black arrows) and submental space (white arrows).

bacterial invasion and a local inflammatory response, which includes vasodilation and edema leading to increased pressure, which exacerbates the pain and decreases the blood supply. This sequence of events serves only to further the periapical necrosis, with subsequent bacterial invasion into bone and erosion of the bony cortex into surrounding soft tissues. The spreading infection can result in a chronic sinus tract or, under the appropriate circumstances (eg, perforation of the cortical bone above the muscular attachment), a fascial space collection. (Alternatively, infections involving the maxillary dentition may spread to involve the maxillary sinus and present as unilateral maxillary sinusitis.)

The microbiology of odontogenic infection reflects the normal endogenous oral flora. A large number of bacteria are contained in the mouth, particularly around the dental crevices. These bacteria are primarily anaerobic although gram-positive aerobic organisms (primarily *Streptococci*) are found as well. Infections that result from the spread of these organisms into surrounding soft-tissue spaces are often polymicrobial (eg, more than one organism may be cultured). Anaerobes causing odontogenic infections generally consist of gram-positive anaerobic cocci (GPAC) and gram-negative anaerobic rods. Traditionally, most GPAC were included in the genus *Peptostreptococcus* with *Peptostreptococcus micros* being the most prevalent in odontogenic infections. Recently *P. micros* was reclassified as *Micromonas micros*. The anaerobic gram-negative rods are comprised of *Bacteroides* and *Fusobacterium* species. Reclassification of the *Bacteroides* species has resulted in the genera *Prevotella* (moderately sacchyarolytic) and *Porphyromonas* (asaccharolytic). DNA analysis has allowed for the identification of *Tannerella forsythensis* (formerly *Bacteroides forsythus*) as another potentially important anaerobic pathogen.

DIAGNOSIS

Odontogenic infections commonly present with pain and swelling around the infected tooth. As the infection progresses, a sinus tract may develop as detected by drainage and usually decreased discomfort. If the infection spreads into the surrounding soft tissues and fascial spaces, the signs and symptoms may become systemic and include fever, leukocytosis, and dehydration. It should be noted that with the spread of the infection, local signs and symptoms of odontogenic infection may diminish and the origin of the space infection may seem remote or obscure.

Signs and symptoms of fascial space involvement include swelling of the region (eg, face and lateral neck), trismus, dysphagia, and airway compromise. To assess the airway for impending compromise, one should note tongue mobility, floor-of-mouth edema, uvular deviation, and lateral pharyngeal swelling. The presentation of infection of the floor of the mouth, or Ludwig's angina, deserves special mention. Patients may develop this widespread fascial space infection as a result of second or third molar infection or widespread periodontal disease. Cellulitis of the floor of mouth rapidly becomes a spreading, gangrenous process producing elevation and displacement of the tongue and brawny induration of the entire submandibular region. Airway compromise can occur precipitously (Table 8.1), hence appropriate precautions should be undertaken.

Information regarding the causative dentition as well as the extent of infection may be gained through radiographic evaluation. A panoramic radiograph (panorex) of the maxilla and mandible is useful to examine the bone morphology and presence of impacted teeth or caries. When there is clinical suspicion of infection extending to the soft tissues of the the head and neck, computed tomography (CT) or magnetic resonance imaging (MRI) is warranted. CT with contrast is generally considered to be the first-line imaging modality given its lower cost, greater availability, and

Table 8.1 Emergency Considerations

Presence of subcutaneous air Consider necrotizing fasciitis
Ludwig's angina – progressive severe soft-tissue edema Consider tracheotomy

patient tolerance relative to MRI. However, in a prospective study of 47 patients, Muñoz et al. concluded that MRI was superior to CT in the initial evaluation of odontogenic infections in terms of anatomic discrimination, lesion conspicuity, and extension of the processes. MRI was also more precise in identifying the number of spaces involved. However, CT is more sensitive in detecting intralesional gas. It is yet unclear whether these advantages of MRI translate into improved patient outcomes to warrant its routine use in this setting.

THERAPY

Initial evaluation should seek to determine the site and nature of the infectious process. In the presence of palpable fluctuance on physical exam or radiographic evidence of abscess, treatment is surgical drainage.

It is often not difficult to obtain material for Gram stain and culture. One approach is needle aspiration. However, precautions should be taken to obtain the material in a sterile fashion, process it under anaerobic conditions, and make an effort to evaluate the Gram stain before starting antibiotics. The administration of antibiotics is necessary under most circumstances to control the infection. Antibiotics should be administered before surgical drainage or if the process is determined to be in the cellulitic phase. The choice of antimicrobial agent(s) sometimes must be made empirically. In addition, the general condition of the host (eg, dehydration, predisposing conditions such as diabetes mellitus and immunocompromise) must be taken into consideration when devising a treatment plan. The presence of palpable subcutaneous air or air on radiographs is an indication of infection by gas-forming organisms and is a hallmark of necrotizing fasciitis, a surgical emergency.

Choosing an effective antibiotic for an odontogenic infection depends on the ability of the clinician to correctly predict the offending organism(s). As noted, these infections are nearly always polymicrobial and caused by endogenous oral cavity flora. Monotherapy is generally preferable because of the reduced cost, fewer potential side effects, and greater ease of administration. The antibiotic should have activity against oral anaerobes and *Streptococci*.

Penicillin G, once a first choice for odontogenic infection, is rarely used for serious infection because of the rising incidence of penicillin-resistant *Streptococci* in the community as well as the frequency of β-lactamase–producing *Bacteroides* species (estimated to be greater than 30%). Amoxicillin or amoxicillin/clavulanate is acceptable first line agents for the treatment of early or mild odontogenic infections. Clindamycin is an effective alternative for penicillin-allergic patients. Much has been written about metronidazole in the treatment of odontogenic infections. One must keep in mind, however, that although effective against oral anaerobes, this agent has no activity against aerobic organisms and must be used in combination with another antimicrobial. If one chooses a cephalosporin, it should be noted that the higher "generations" tend to sacrifice gram-positive aerobic activity for gram-negative efficacy. First-generation agents, such as cefazolin and cefoxitin, are likely more effective than other, broader-spectrum drugs.

A recent study by Salinas et al. of antibiotic susceptibility of bacteria causing odontogenic infections found high susceptibility for amoxicillin, amoxicillin/clavulanate, linezolid, and clindamycin. Conversely, a relatively high proportion of bacteria cultured were resistant to metronidazole, erythromycin, and azithromycin. Antibiotics should be administered parenterally for severe infections and in the perioperative period (eg, 24 to 48 hours). Once the drainage catheters are removed and the patient is ready for discharge, the oral route of administration is adequate. Decisions regarding the duration of antimicrobial administration are made empirically, but a 2-week course usually is adequate.

Evacuation of the purulent collection is the standard of care for odontogenic infections. If the process is cellulitis that has not proceeded to abscess, administration of antibiotics may result in resolution. However, the patient must be followed closely and surgery undertaken if abscess ensues. Surgery may entail a minor procedure, such as drainage of a periapical abscess, or extensive debridements of adjacent fascial compartments in the case of necrotizing fasciitis.

The route of drainage should be evaluated on an individual basis. General principles to be followed include stabilization of the airway, protection of vital structures, adequate visualization at the time of drainage, copious irrigation of the abscess cavity with antibiotic-containing solution, and postoperative drainage of the wound. Canine and isolated sublingual space infections can usually be drained transorally. Buccal space infections can be drained transorally or extraorally with care taken to identify Stenson's duct and the buccal branch of the facial nerve. The submental space is best approached extraorally via an incision that parallels the inferior border of the mandibular symphysis. Buccal, submandibular, masseteric, pterygomandibular, and sublingual spaces can all be drained extraorally via a horizontal incision parallel to the inferior angle of the mandible.

Drainage catheters are generally used when a transcutaneous route is used and should be left in place until wound drainage has essentially ceased (≤10 mL in 24 hours). In our experience, the catheters do not serve as a route for infection (ie, to draw bacteria inward). In all cases, special attention should be paid to the status of the airway. Ideally, a team of clinicians with expertise in difficult airway management is involved. In Ludwig's angina, urgent tracheotomy is usually required. Other, less rapidly progressing, maxillomandibular space infections can usually be managed with careful endotracheal intubation. If the airway compromise continues in the postoperative period, the patient should remain intubated or an elective tracheotomy should be performed.

If necrotizing fasciitis is diagnosed based on identification of subcutaneous air or recognition of tissue necrosis at the time of drainage, the wound must be opened widely, necrotic tissue debrided, and the wound packed open for observation and potential further debridement. Hyperbaric oxygen administration may be beneficial in this circumstance.

The successful treatment of these infections depends on a combination of accurate diagnosis and institution of appropriate therapy in a timely fashion. Adjunctive laboratory and radiographic tests may confirm the diagnosis and help plan the drainage procedure, but a thorough history and physical examination often provides the clinician with sufficient information.

SUGGESTED READING

Bridgeman A, Weisenfeld D, Newland S. Anatomical considerations in the diagnosis and management of acute maxillofacial bacterial infections. *Aust Dent J.* 1996;41:238.

Flynn TR, Shanti RM, Levi MH, et al. Severe odontogenic infections, Part 1: Prospective report. *J Oral Maxillofac Surg.* 2006;64:1093–1103.

Flynn TR, Shanti RM, Hayes C. Severe odontogenic infections, Part 2: Prospective outcomes study. *J Oral Maxillofac Surg.* 2006;64:1104–1113.

Gill Y, Scully C. Orofacial odontogenic infections: review of microbiology and current treatment. *Oral Surg Oral Med Oral Pathol.* 1990;70:155.

Krishnan V, Johnson JV, Helfrick JF. Management of maxillofacial infections: a review of 50 cases. *J Oral Maxillofac Surg.* 1993;51:868.

Langford FP, Moon RE, Stolp BW, et al. Treatment of cervical necrotizing fasciitis with hyperbaric oxygen therapy. *Otolaryngol Head Neck Surg.* 1995;112:274.

Stefanopoulos PK, Kolokotronis AE. The clinical significance of anaerobic bacteria in acute orofacial odontogenic infections. *Oral Surg Oral Med Oral Pathol Oral Radiol Endod.* 2004;98:398–408.

Munõz A, Castillo M, Melchor MA, et al. Acute neck infections: prospective comparison between CT and MRI in 47 patients. *J Comput Assist Tomogr.* 2001;25(5):733–741.

Brescó-Salinas, Costa-Riu N, Berini-Aytés, L., et al. Antibiotic susceptibility of the bacteria causing odontogenic infections. *Oral Surg.* 2006;11:E70.

9. Infection of the Salivary and Lacrimal Glands

Souad Youssef, Ray Y. Hachem, and Issam Raad

Sialadenitis is infection of the salivary glands. This is a relatively common disease. Sialadenitis can be acute, subacute, or chronic in nature and can be of bacterial or viral origin. Bacterial infections may reach the salivary gland tissue mostly via the ductal system, whereas viral infections invade the salivary glands via the bloodstream. The incidence of bacterial sialadenitis is in direct relation to factors such as old age, nutritional and health status, trauma, anatomic abnormalities, and use of drugs that decrease the salivary flow. There are several etiological predisposing local and systemic generalized factors that play an important role in the development and course of sialadenitis (Table 9.1).

ACUTE BACTERIAL SIALADENITIS

Acute bacterial sialadenitis is also known as suppurative sialadenitis and mainly affects the parotid and submandibular glands. Sialadenitis of the intraoral and sublingual glands is very rare. This may be due to the fact that the serous saliva produced by the parotid gland has less bacteriostatic activity or may result from a secretory disorder that changes the amount and chemical composition of saliva, including most of the protein, mucins, and electrolytes. Primary acute bacterial parotitis (ABP) has been reported mainly in elderly patients suffering from dehydration, malnutrition, Sjogren's disease, poor oral hygiene, ductal obstructions due to sialolithiasis, tumor or foreign bodies, chronic tonsillitis, dental infection, neoplasm of the oral cavity, liver cirrhosis, or diabetes mellitus. The use of antisialanogic drugs, including antidepressants, anticholinergics, and diuretics, has been associated with acute bacterial sialadenitis. Studies have shown that bacteria can infect the parotid gland through ascending transmission through Stensen's duct or through bacteremia.

Acute postoperative parotitis as a special type of acute purulent parotitis is observed particularly after major abdominal surgery and accompanied by large fluid loss and reduction of salivary secretions. United States President James A. Garfield sustained an abdominal gunshot wound and subsequently died of complications of suppurative parotitis. A recent report has shown an association between neurosurgical procedures in sitting positions and acute parotitis.

Bahar et al. reported five cases of post fine-needle aspiration parotitis. All patients had Wharton's tumor as their underlying disease. Acute sialadenitis has been reported after intravascular iodinated radiocontrast agents. Neonatal suppurative sialadenitis is an uncommon infection in the neonatal period. Risk factors include prematurity, decreased saliva production related to prolonged orogastric or nasogastric feeds, dehydration, sialolith, anatomical abnormalities of Wharton's duct.

Pathogenic organisms are mostly *Staphylococcus aureus* followed by group A strep, particularly *viridans*, strict anaerobes such as *Fusobacterium nucleatum, Prevotella,* and *Porphyromonas. Peptostreptococcus anaerobius* may also play a major role. Brook reported that 43% of his patients with sialadenitis were related to strict anaerobes, and 57% to mixed aerobes and anaerobes organisms. Recent reports have shown an increasing incidence of gram-negative rods, especially in seriously ill patients who tend to be colonized by these bacteria. Less frequently isolated organisms included Arachnia, *Haemophilus influenza, Klebsiella pneumoniae, Salmonella* spp., *Pseudomonas aeruginosa, Treponema pallidum,* cat scratch bacillus, *Eikenella corrodens, Actinomyces israelii,* and *Actinomyces eriksonii.*

Clinically, the patient with parotitis experiences an intense radiating pain in the affected side of the face. It is usually unilateral. General malaise and fever with erythema and swelling are common (Figure 9.1). Some patients complain of limited movement of the mandible and difficulty in swallowing. Stenson's duct orifice appears red with expression of pus on palpation. In some cases disturbance of the facial nerve may be noticed. Sometimes a toxic state of mental obtundation occurs. In this situation aggressive treatment is required because the mortality is high.

The diagnosis of parotitis is based on the clinical presentation, Gram stain, and culture

Table 9.1 Etiological Classification of Sialadenitis

Acute Bacterial Sialadenitis
Acute purulent parotitis
Acute postoperative parotitis
Acute bacterial submandibular sialadenitis
Chronic Bacterial Sialadenitis
Chronic recurrent parotitis
Chronic sclerosing sialadenitis of submandibular gland
Obstructive sialadenitis
Viral Sialadenitis
Parotitis epidemica (Mumps)
Cytomegalovirus infection (salivary gland viral disease)
Other types (Coxsacki virus, infectious mononucleosis, measles, EMC virus, ECHO virus)
Granulomatous Sialadenitis
Giant cell sialadenitis
Tuberculosis

of the purulent material from Stensen's duct. Laboratory findings commonly include marked leukocytosis with left shift, elevated sedimentation rate and serum amylase. A plain film of the parotid gland may be useful to detect stones; however, this is not a common situation in parotitis. The use of sialography is discouraged because of the often painful swelling and the risk of ductal rupture. Computed tomography (CT) scanning often is the radiologic evaluation of choice because it shows evidence of a suppurative process in the gland parenchyma. Ultrasonography may also be helpful in demonstrating the presence of calculus.

The differential diagnosis of an enlarged parotid mass should include viral parotitis, cystic fibrosis, collagen vascular diseases, alcoholism, chronic recurrent parotitis, sarcoidosis, sialolithiasis, and neoplasms.

Treatment of ABP consists of elimination of the cause, such as a mucous plug, by using adequate hydration to increase the salivary flow and the use of systemic antibiotics that cover gram-positive cocci, spirochetes, and mouth anaerobes, awaiting the results of Gram stain and cultures. In cases involving abscess formation, incision and drainage are highly indicated. Drainage is done by surgical exposure of the gland and penetration of the capsule by blunt probing. Most of the time a semisynthetic antistaphylococcal penicillin such as nafcillin is adequate as initial empiric treatment.

First-generation cephalosporins are good alternatives as well as the addition of quinolones and third-generation cephalosporins, especially in the seriously ill hospitalized patient in whom infection with gram-negative rods is increasing (Table 9.2). Vancomycin should be considered in the setting where methicillin-resistant *Staphylococcus aureus* (MRSA) is predominant. The literature supports the use of antibiotics for 10 to 14 days.

Adjuvant treatment should include optimal oral hygiene, nutritional support, warm compress, discontinuation of anticholinergic drugs that reduce salivary flow or increase the viscosity of the saliva, and use of sialagogic agents such as lemon juice. Irradiation of the glands is no longer recommended. Needle aspiration of the gland is not indicated, because it is a blind procedure that endangers the facial nerve and does not provide adequate drainage. Surgical intervention is indicated in the following circumstances: lack of improvement after 3 to 5 days of antibiotic therapy, facial nerve or other vital organ involvement, and abscess formation. A follow-up CT scan or sialogram is recommended after resolution of the infection

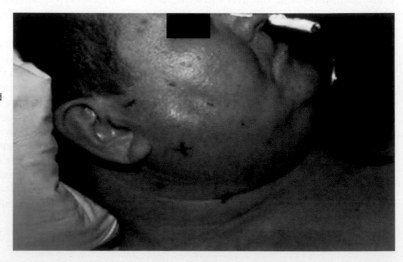

Figure 9.1 Staphylococcal parotitis in a post-operative patient. The enlarged parotid is outlined by ink marks with an X in the center. Note the characteristic diffuse enlargement of the gland, earlobe elevation and obliterated mandible landmarks. (Courtesy of David Schlossberg, MD.)

Table 9.2 Treatment of Sialadenitis

	Antibiotic Treatment	**Surgical Treatment**
Acute bacterial sialadenitis	Susceptible gm+ : penicillinase-resistant penicillin or first-generation cephalosporin Resistant Gm+ (MRSA, *S. pneumoniae*): vancomycin Gm- : third-generation cephalosporin, quinolone Anaerobes: flagyl or clindamycin	Parotid drainage may be needed; silolithectomy in submandibular infection
Chronic bacterial sialadenitis	Same as above	Gland extirpation usually required
Viral sialadenitis	None; symptomatic treatment	None
Granulomatous sialadenitis	Director to specific cause	Rarely needed

Abbreviations: Gm+ = gram positive; Gm- = gram negative; MRSA = multiresistant *Staphylococcus aureus*.

to treat the underlying disease such as calculi or stricture so recurrent parotitis may be prevented.

Acute bacterial submandibular sialadenitis (ABSS), unlike ABP, is very frequently associated with obstruction of Wharton's duct by stones or structures. Predisposition to stone formation in the submandibular gland is due to the alkalinity, calcium concentrations in and its secretions, and to anatomic factors such as the length and tortuosity of Wharton's duct. Medical treatment is the same as for ABP. If ductal calculi are present, excision is the only effective treatment. This can be done by ductal dilatation or sialolithotomy, depending on the location. Repeated ductal stone formation may cause chronic submandibular infection, in which case surgical excision of the gland is indicated.

Subacute necrotizing sialadenitis (SANS) has been recently described as an inflammatory disease of unknown origin. It usually affects the palatal salivary glands. Clinically the patient presents with pain or swelling or both. The main etiological factor seems to be infarction of the salivary gland by ischemic injury as a result of surgery or trauma. Nevertheless, it remains possible that SANS is part of necrotizing sialometaplasia.

Chronic Bacterial Sialadenitis

Chronic bacterial sialadenitis is also known as recurrent bacterial sialadenitis. It involves the parotid or submandibular glands. Chronic (adult) parotitis can follow a subclinical course. The infection usually occurs via the excretory duct. Inflammation of the oral mucosa and a decreased salivary flow may lead to an ascending or retrograde infection in the major sali-

vary glands. This chronic infection sometimes is associated with Sjogren's disease in which case manifestations xerostonia and systemic autoimmune disease are present. Chronic juvenile recurrent parotitis is a combination of a congenital malformation of a portion of the salivary ducts and infections ascending from the mouth following dehydration in children. Boys are more often affected than girls. The clinical course is characterized by recurrent episodes of acute sialadenitis of either the parotid or submandibular glands. Although the inflammation may occur bilaterally, the symptoms of a painful swelling are often unilateral. In cases involving swelling in the parotid glands area, salivary gland neoplasm should be considered, as well as sialadenonis and lymphadenopathies that may be caused by a variety of diseases such as catscratch disease, toxoplasmosis, and neoplasm. As in acute parotitis, microbiological culturing of the saliva is recommended. Several studies have identified *Streptococcus viridans* as the most common causative organism followed by *S. aureus, Streptococcus pneumoniae*, and mixed aerobic-anaerobe oral flora. Involvement of a specific microorganism, such as *Mycobacterium tuberculosis* and actinomycosis, is quite rare.

Sialography, which involves the retrograde injection of a radio-opaque dye into the main excretory duct, is the most important tool in establishing a diagnosis of chronic parotitis. In addition to plain radiographs, CT sialography may provide additional and more detailed information. Scintigraphy is considered to be a useful diagnostic aid in chronic recurrent parotitis, especially in patients in whom sialography cannot be performed. Ultrasound examination is not very useful in detecting chronic inflammation. Laboratory data commonly show a persistent elevation of the erythrocyte sedimentation rate. Histologically, in chronic parotitis the parenchymal structures may largely be replaced by fibrosis and fat. The ducts are often dilated and surrounded by a dense lymphocytic infiltrate. Initial treatment should be conservative; patients with chronic parotitis should be instructed to carefully massage the involved gland in a dorsoventral direction four to six times a day and to eat sour foods to stimulate parotic secretion. Systemic antibiotic irrigation and proper oral hygiene have been advocated as effective treatment. In spite of medical treatment some cases require surgical management. Submandibular sialadenitis usually presents earlier, is secondary to calculi and requires early intervention. Parotidectomy with facial nerve dissection is preferred.

Chronic Sclerosing Sialadenitis

Chronic sclerosing sialadenitis of the submandibular gland, also known as Kuttner's tumor (KT), is a chronic inflammatory process that produces a firm, sometimes painful, swelling in the submandibular area that is difficult to distinguish from tumor. Submandibular glands are the most involved, but involvement of other major and minor salivary glands has been reported.

In 29% to 83% of cases, it is associated with sialolithiasis and is most commonly seen in the elderly. Actually, it is unclear whether sialolithiasis is the cause or the result of KT. It affects males more often than females. Proposed etiologies include fibrotic immune process or secretory dysfunction with ductal inspissation, duct abnormalities, and infectious agents. Histologically, it is characterized by periductal sclerosis, dense lymphocyte infiltration, lymphoid follicle formation, acinar atrophy, and fibrosis. It is a benign disease, and no additional treatment is warranted.

Obstructive Sialadenitis

Obstructive sialadenitis is the most common type of sialadenitis. Thirty-seven percent of cases are localized in the submandibular gland, 30% in the salivary glands and 20% in the parotid gland. The remaining 13% are in the sublingual glands. There are two distinguishing factors that play a role in the pathogenesis of obstructive sialadenitis. One is a mechanical obstruction, including salivary cyst and tumor or lesion of the oral mucosa. The other is a disturbance of the secretory changes in electrolyte concentration, leading to the development of a viscous secretory product.

If a salivary calculus is not removed, the secretory congestion leads to an inflammatory reaction in the salivary gland tissue. Histologically, this is characterized by periductal lymphocyte infiltration, intralobular fibrosis, and parenchymal loss with functional loss of the gland. One possible mediator of this inflammatory process is the transforming growth factor-β. Transforming growth factor has a physiologic role in wound healing and tissue repair. However, overproduction of this cytokine can lead to excessive deposition of scar tissue and fibrosis.

Sialography is widely used to diagnose obstructive sialadenitis, but the etiology can be still unknown for about half of the patients. Recent reports highlighted the importance of sialoendoscopy for the diagnosis and treatment of sialolithiasis.

Viral Sialadenitis

Viral infection of the salivary glands is a frequent condition mainly affecting the parotid glands. Mumps, a paramyxo virus, is by far the most common virus producing clinically significant parotitis. This disease is contagious and is transmitted by droplets of saliva. Mumps is predominantly a childhood disease and is more common in boys than in girls. Young adults may also be affected and have a more aggressive clinical course. Mumps is often preceded by a viral infection in the oral cavity or the nose, leading to viremia and hematogenous infections of the salivary glands. Apart from the major salivary glands, the testes, meninges, pancreas, and mammary glands may become involved. The incubation period is approximately 3 weeks, followed by 1 to 2 days of fever, chills, headache, and jaw pain on chewing. After that comes rapid and painful swelling of the parotid gland. The submandibular glands may additionally become involved. In 30% to 40% of infected patients no clinical symptoms have been noticed. The virus can be isolated from the saliva during the first week of the clinical manifestation of the disease. During this period, leukopenia with relative lymphocytosis and elevation of serum analyses is observed. Serological diagnosis can be made using a complement-binding reaction, or a 4-fold increase in antibody titer, usually at the end of the second week. Apart from vaccination, no effective treatment for mumps is available. Cytomegalovirus (CMV) sialadenitis is rare and usually presents as painful salivary gland and swelling. The diagnosis is usually based on an elevated complement fixation titer of antibodies to CMV, a positive CMV titer, and detection of CMV in the salivary gland. Other viruses that produce sialadenitis are coxsackievirus, infectious mononucleosis, measles, echovirus, influenza A, parainfluenza, human immuno-deficiency virus, lymphocytic choriomeningitis virus, adenovirus, human herpes virus 6, parvo-virus B19, and Epstein-Barr virus. Most of these viral infections have a self-limiting condition, which produces lifelong immunocity. Chronic hepatitis C virus (HCV) infection has been associated with mild lymphocytic sialadenitis.

Granulomatous Sialadenitis

A rare condition, granulomatous sialadenitis is most often secondary to regional lymph node involvement rather than involvement of the gland parenchyma itself. Granulomatous giant cell sialadenitis is localized mostly in the sub-mandibular gland. The inflammatory reaction is caused by obstruction of the ducts and develop-ment of granulomas with multinuclear foreign body giant cells. Tuberculosis is the most com-mon type of granuloma and starts mostly from the parotid and submandibular lymphnodes. Clinically there is a firm, nontender swelling of the gland resembling tumor more than parotitis. Most patients have simultaneous pulmonary tuberculosis. The diagnosis may be established by acid-fast bacilli (AFB) smear and culture of the salivary gland drainage if present. Tissue biopsy with culture may be necessary to make the diagnosis.

Treatment, as in other forms of extrapul-monary tuberculosis, consists of a three- to four-drug regimen that usually includes isoniazid, rifampin, ethambutol, and pyra-zinamide. The duration of therapy depends on the clinical response but usually is 6 to 9 months. Surgical excision of salivary tissue is rarely needed. A typical *Mycobacterium* infec-tion most often affects children and usually presents as a facial or cervical mass that may drain spontaneously. As in tuberculosis, the diagnosis is based on AFB smears and cultures. Chemotherapy should be based on the kind of atypical *Mycobacterium* isolated and the sus-ceptibility pattern. Actinomycosis is usually caused by *Actinomyces israelii*, which can be part of the oral flora, particularly in patients with dental caries. It may present as acute supportive parotitis or have a more chronic course. The diagnosis is based on smears and cultures of draining material or tissue biopsy. Surgical drainage and high dose of penicillin for a prolonged period are indicated.

Other agents that have been reported to cause granulomatous sialadenitis are syphilis, tularemia, toxoplasmosis, cat scratch dis-ease, blastomycosis, and coccidiomycosis. Xantogranulomatous sialadenitis of parotid gland presenting as B-cell lymphoma has also been reported. Other noninfectious etiologies include sarcoidosis, Wegener's granulomatosis, or Crohn's disease.

Lacrimal System Infection

Infection of the lacrimal system includes three types: (1) canaliculitis, (2) dacryocystitis, and (3) dacryoadenitis.

Canaliculitis is inflammation of the cana-liculi that leads to obstruction of the lumen. It presents clinically as conjunctivitis, itching, burning sensation, mild to severe swelling of the canaliculus, and mucopurulent discharge from the punctum and is associated with exces-sive tears. *Staphylococcus* and *Actinomycosis* species and *Arachnia propionica* are commonly implicated. Other organisms less frequently causing canaliculitis include *Fusobacterium, Enterobacter cloacae, Lactococcus lactis, Eikenella corrodens,* nocardia, *Candida al-bicans,* and *Aspergillus.* Viruses like herpes also can be involved.

The diagnosis is based on isolation of the organism from the lacrimal passage and fluo-rescein to see the patency of the duct lumen. Treatment consists of topical antibiotics. Eye drops, penicillin, or macrolides may be used (Table 9.3). For others, canaliculotomy is the main mode of therapy to prevent recurrence.

Dacryocystitis is a common infection of the lacrimal sac. It can be either an acute or chronic infection. Dacryocystitis often occurs in children as a complication of congenital or acquired no-solacrimal proximal or distal duct obstruction of the drainage system. In the neonate period it is often due to dacryocele and presented as duct cyst. In older infants and children, nasolacrimal duct obstruction may occur as a consequence of ethmoidal sinusitis or facial fracture. Also it is common in adults over 40 with obstruction at the opening of the nasolacrimal duct into to inferior meatus being the most common risk factor. Clinically, it presents with epiphora (ie, excessive tearing), and an acute onset of suppuration at the level of the medial epican-thus can be associated with cellulitis of the tissue surrounding the lacrimal sac. The most

Table 9.3 Treatment of Lacrimal System Infection

	Antibiotic Treatment	Surgical Treatment
Canaliculits	Topical antibiotic drop plus antibiotic irrigation of canaliculi (pen G) plus intravenous/oral pen V or macrolides	Canaliculotomy
Acute dacrocystitis		
Neonatal (duct cyst)	Topical antibiotic drops or IV plus oral cephalosporin antibiotic	Duct probing nasal endoscopy
Preseptal cellulitis	IV antibiotics	Duct probing
Trauma	IV antibiotics	Dacryocystorhicostomy nasolacrimal intubation
Chronic dacryocystitis	IV antibiotics	Endoscopic intranasal, dacryocystorhinostomy
Acute dacryoadenitis	Systemic antibiotic	Incision and drainage if spontaneous resolution does not occur
Chronic dacryoadenitis	Directed toward specific cause	Rarely required

common organisms isolated in the acute stage are *S. aureus*, including methicillin-resistant *S. aureus*, *S. pneumoniae*, gram-negative rods (*P. aerugenosa*, *Haemophilus influenza*) and rarely *Stenotrophonomas maltophilia* in which setting quinolones are recommended for the treatment of chronic dacryocystitis. Other rare etiologies of dacryocystitis include mucocutaneous leishmaniasis, *Proteus mirabilis*, *Haemophilus parainfluenza*, *Peptostreptococcus*, *Propionibacterium*, *Prevotella*, *Fusobacterium*, and *Curvularia*. Acute dacryocystitis may lead to orbital cellulitis, abscess, or fistula.

The diagnosis can be made by culture, radiographically by dacryocystography, CT, or scintillography. Treatment consists of hot compresses applied to the affected area and systemic antibiotics based on Gram stain and culture results. Surgical intervention is indicated for abscess or when the symptoms do not resolve with medical therapy (Table 9.3). Recently the holmium:YAG laser has been used to decrease the risk of hemorrhage associated with traditional surgery. (See also Chapter 16, Periocular Infections.)

DACRYOADENITIS

Dacryoadenitis is inflammation of the lacrimal gland. It is usually present as localized tenderness and swelling of the eyelid. Acute bacterial infections can be due to pyogenic bacteria, such as *S. aureus* and streptococci. Viral infections with mumps and infectious mononucleosis are most often implicated as causes. The most common causes of acute dacryoadenitis are inflammation and infections. Chronic infection of the lacrimal gland can be associated with various infectious and noninfectious causes. Tuberculosis, syphilis, leprosy, and schistosomiasis, Epstein-Barr virus, *Brucella melitensis*, herpes simplex virus, and varicella-zoster virus have been also reported. It has also been associated with *Acanthameoba keratitis*, Wegener's granulomatosis, sarcoidosis, and Sweet's syndrome.

Clinically, patients with acute dacryoadenitis complain of severe pain in the lacrimal gland region, edema, and redness and swelling, whereas in chronic dacryoadenitis only minimal eyelid edema and mild tenderness can be observed. Management of dacryoadenitis includes symptomatic treatment with local hot compresses or systemic antibiotics in case of bacterial cause. The standard treatment for acute idiopathic inflammatory dacryoadenitis is oral corticosteroids. Others report the benefit of intralesional steroid injection.

If symptoms persist, irradiation or cyclosporine may be an option. Surgical drainage is necessary in case of abscess formation.

SUGGESTED READING

Baddini-Caramelli C, Matayoshi S. Chronic dacrocystitis in American mucocutaneous leishmaniasis. *Ophthal Plas Reconstr Surg.* 2001;17:48–52.

Batsakis JG. Granulomatous sialadenitis. *Ann Otol Rhinol Laryngol*. 1991;100:166–169.

Brook I. Acute Bacterial suppurative parotitis: microbiology and management. *J Craniofac Surg*. 2003;14:37–40.

Campolattaro BN, Lueder GT, Tychsen L. Spectrum of pediatric dacryocystitis: medical and surgical management of 54 cases. *J Pediatr Ophthalmol Strabismus*. 1997; 34:143–153.

Goldberg MH. Infections of the salivary glands. In: Topazian RG, Goldberg MH, eds. *Oral and Maxillofacial Infection*. Philadelphia, PA: WB Saunders; 1994:320.

Johnson A. Inflammatory conditions of the major salivary glands. *Ear Nose Throat*. 1989; 68:94–102.

Kitagawa S, Zen Y. Abundant IgG4-positive plasma cell infiltration characterizes chronic sclerosing sialadenitis. *Am J Surg Pathol*. 2005;29:783–791.

Medinam J. Hepatitis C virus-related extra-hepatic disease-aetiopathogenesis and management. *Aliment Pharmacol Ther*. 2004;20:129–141.

Newel FW. The lacrimal system. In: Newell FW, ed. *Ophthalmology: Principles and Concepts*. St. Louis, MO: Mosby; 1992:246.

Raad II, Sabbagh MF, Caranasos GJ. Acute bacterial sialadenitis: a study of 29 cases and review. *Rev Infect Dis*. 1990;12: 591–601.

Seifert G. Aetological and histological classification of sialadenitis. *Pathologica*. 1997; 89:7–17

10. Deep Neck Infections

Anitra S. Birnbaum and Jeremy D. Gradon

INTRODUCTION

Infections of the various deep spaces of the neck are uncommon. However, when they do occur, they are often life threatening, and even stable-appearing patients are at grave risk for sudden clinical decompensation. This degree of clinical severity is related to both the anatomic nature of the space (Figure 10.1) involved with numerous adjacent critical organs and structures being present as well as the nature of the hosts themselves. Patients with such infections are frequently diabetic or immune-compromised in some other way often having a history of injection drug use, neutropenia, or steroid use. There is often a dental source of these infections, and underlying poor dentition is commonly encountered. On rare occasions, deep neck space infection may complicate head and neck cancers or residual dentiginous cysts or lateral cleft. An example of a deep neck infection of the lateral pharyngeal space in a human immunodeficiency virus (HIV)-infected patient is shown in Figure 10.2. *Nocardia asteroides* grew from the deep neck cultures.

These infections are usually polymicrobial, reflecting the oral cavity source of most of these infections. When associated with injection drug use, community-acquired methicillin-resistant *Staphylococcus aureus* (MRSA) is the most likely organism to be encountered. The microbiology of these infections is shown in Table 10.1.

Relevant Anatomy of the Deep Neck Spaces

The deep neck spaces are bound by a variety of anatomic landmarks and are anatomically distinct. However, all have the potential for communicating with each other, and thus infection may spread from one region to another during the course of the illness. It is important to delineate the various spaces clinically and radiologically so that appropriate management can be provided. The main spaces are as follows:

- The submandibular space (composed of two spaces separated by the mylohyoid muscle: the sublingual space, which is superior, and the submaxillary space, which is inferior).
- The lateral pharyngeal spaces (anterior and posterior)
- The retropharyngeal spaces (including the retropharynx, the prevertebral space, and the "danger space").

Radiologic Testing in Deep Neck Infections

Computed tomography (CT) and magnetic resonance imaging (MRI) are both critical

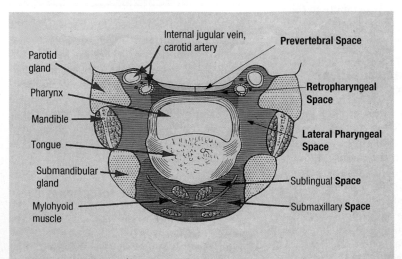

Figure 10.1 Oblique section of top of neck. Note contiguity of spaces and resultant potential for spread. Adapted with permission from Hollingshead WH. *Anatomy for Surgeons. Vol.1: The Head and Neck*. 2nd ed. New York, NY: Harper & Row; 1968.

Table 10.1 Pathogens Enountered in Deep Neck Space Infections

Common
Viridans and other streptococci
Staphylococcus aureus (including MRSA)
Prevotella, Fusobacterium, Bacteroides, Porphyromonas
Rare
Moraxella
Haemophilus species
Pseudomonas species
Actinomyces species

Table 10.2 Management of Deep Neck Space Infections

NEVER LEAVE THE PATIENT UNATTENDED out of a monitored unit
Protect the airway–experienced otolaryngology evaluation is essential
CT or MRI of mouth, neck, mediastinum to evaluate for drainable collections, airway compression, vascular complications, or mediastinal involvement
Dentist/oral surgery evaluation for a (removable) dental source of infection
Correct underlying medical issues—Maximize glycemic control, correct neutropenia, taper steroids (if feasible), etc.

Table 10.3 Antibiotic Therapy[a]

Nonimmune Compromised Host[b]
Penicillin G 3 million units IV q4h plus IV metronidazole 500 mg q6h
or
Ampicillin-sulbactam 3 g IV q6h (+/– gentamicin 1.5 mg/kg q8H IV)
or
Clindamycin 600 mg IV q8h plus moxifloxacin 400 mg IV q24h
Immune Compromised Host[b]
Imipenem-cilastatin 500 mg IV q6h plus vancomycin 1 g IV q12h
or
Piperacillin-tazobactam 4.5 g IV q6h plus vancomycin 1 g IV q12h

[a] These antibiotic recommendations are only examples of appropriate regimens. Multiple other combinations of antibiotics providing polymicrobial coverage for both aerobes and anaerobes are appropriate as well.
[b] In the setting of injection drug use, HIV infection or the recent use of antibiotics (within ≤3 months) would add anti-MRSA coverage with vancomycin, daptomycin, or linezolid.

diagnostic tools for deep neck space infections. However, it must be appreciated that these patients are critically ill and are at risk for acute airway obstruction at any time early in their clinical course. Thus, appropriately trained personnel must accompany these patients when they go for such scans. Equipment must be brought along that allows for immediate securing of the airway should sudden airway failure develop in (or on the way to) the radiology department.

Submandibular Space Infections ("Ludwig's Angina")

This bilateral infection of the submandibular space most commonly arises from the posterior two molar teeth. The infection is most commonly found in patients with diabetes, neutropenia, or lupus. It has a rapid onset with fever, mouth pain, and drooling of oral secretions. It spreads to cause woody induration of the submandibular space and stiff neck. Because the tongue may be displaced upward and backward, acute airway obstruction may develop. Tracheal compression due to surrounding edema is another cause of airway failure in this infection. Management is outlined in Tables 10.2 and 10.3 and complications in Table 10.4.

Lateral Pharyngeal Space Infections (Anterior and Posterior)

These are most common forms of deep neck space infection. Infections of the lateral pharyngeal spaces can result from preexisting submandibular space infections or may develop secondary to dental, salivary gland, lymph node, or retropharyngeal space infections. Injection drug use, with the patient attempting to access deep neck (jugular) veins with nonsterile needles is the most common cause of lateral pharyngeal space infections in inner-city hospitals (Figure 10.3).

Patients present with fever, neck pain, and rigors. If the anterior portion of the lateral pharyngeal space is involved, then trismus may develop. This may mimic the cephalic form of tetanus. However, posterior lateral pharyngeal space infection is not associated with either trismus or visible neck swelling. Management is outlined in Table 10.2 and 10.3 and complications in Table 10.4.

Retropharyngeal Space Infections

THE RETROPHARYNGEAL SPACE
Patients present with fever, sore throat, dysphagia, systemic toxicity, and neck stiffness. Inspection of the retropharynx will

Table 10.4 Complications of Deep Neck Space Infections

Submandibular Space Infection
Acute airway obstruction
Aspiration pneumonia
Tongue necrosis
Carotid artery erosion
Jugular vein thrombosis
Spread to the lateral pharyngeal space
Anterior Lateral Pharyngeal Space
Spread of infection to the parotid gland
Posterior Lateral Pharyngeal Space
Carotid artery erosion
Suppurative jugular vein thrombosis
Cranial nerve palsies (IX–XII)
Retropharyngeal Space
Respiratory distress
Spread to cervical vertebrae
Danger Space
Spread of infection to mediastinum
Spread of infection to the pleural space
Prevertebral Space
Spread of infection along the length of the vertebral column
Lemierre's Syndrome
Jugular venous thrombosis
Septic pulmonary emboli
Empyema
Septic arthritis

frequently demonstrate bulging or swelling of the retropharyngeal soft tissues. On occasion, the lesion may penetrate the posterior pharynx and pus may be visible on the intraoral portion of the retropharynx. Infection occurs as a complication of local pharyngeal infection or may be due to hematogenous seeding from a distal site. On occasion, the infection may be due to spread from acute cervical vertebral osteomyelitis, or follow penetrating trauma to the area. The differential diagnosis is shown in Table 10.5.

THE "DANGER SPACE"

The "danger space" is an anatomical potential space that connects the deep neck spaces with the mediastinum. Access to the mediastinum is via the pretracheal fascia to the parietal pericardium and posterior mediastinum via the "danger space" from the retropharynx. As a result of this connection, acute bacterial mediastinitis, a justly feared complication, may develop as a consequence of deep neck space infection. Conversely, postoperative mediastinal infections may track up this space to the retropharynx and present as an apparent primary neck infection.

THE PREVERTEBRAL SPACE

This fascial plane runs from the base of the skull to the coccyx along the anterior borders of the vertebrae. Thus, infection may spread from the retropharyngeal space to the whole length of the vertebral column. Management is outlined in Tables 10.2 and 10.3 and complications in Table 10.4.

LEMIERRE'S SYNDROME

Lemierre's syndrome is an eponym describing internal jugular vein septic thrombophlebitis. It is the most common vascular complication

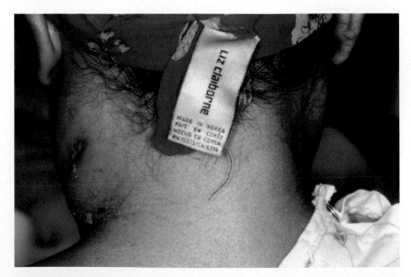

Figure 10.2 Recurring deep neck abscess of lateral pharyngeal space caused by Nocardia asteroides in an HIV-infected patient with CD4 count of 86/mm3.

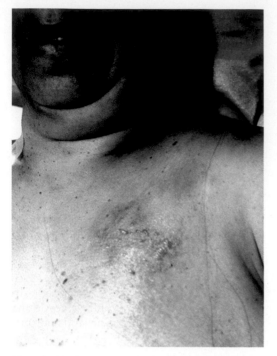

Figure 10.3 Group A streptococcal necrotizing fasciitis of the neck and anterior chest wall: preoperative photo, taken before wide surgical debridement was performed.

Table 10.5 Differential Diagnosis of Retropharyngeal Space Infections

Bacterial meningitis
Cervical vertebral osteomyelitis
Potts disease
Calcific tendonitis of the neck muscles
Inflammatory tumor / neoplasm
Mediastinal infection with spread via the "danger space'

Table 10.6 Management of Lemierre's Syndrome

IV Antibiotics (as shown in Table 10.3)
Drainage of metastatic abscesses (other than septic pulmonary emboli)
Rarely: ligation and resection of involved jugular vein (for unrelenting sepsis)
No clear role for anticoagulation

of parapharyngeal space infection. The most commonly encountered cause is the anaerobe *Fusobacterium necrophorum*. Other causative bacteria include *Bacteroides*, MRSA, anaerobic streptococci, and other assorted mouth flora.

The infection is classically preceded by a sore throat, following which the patients develop fever, systemic toxicity, and tenderness to palpation along the angle of the jaw and sternocleidomastoid muscle. Trismus is not present. As a result of the endovascular infection, bacteremia develops with associated septic pulmonary emboli, empyema formation, and septic arthritis. Lemierre's syndrome can also develop as a complication of attempts to access the jugular vein either for IV line placement or for purposes of injection drug use. The management of Lemierre's syndrome is outlined in Table 10.6.

CAROTID ARTERY EROSION

This may occur as a complication of almost any deep neck space infection. Initially, this entity may be difficult to recognize due the tight fascia binding the carotid artery. Once a false aneurysm has developed the patient may start to develop "herald bleeding" from the nose, mouth, or ears. Once major bleeding occurs death is common. Treatment involves urgent vascular surgery, and the risk of stroke is high.

SUGGESTED READING

Huang TT, Tseng FY, Liu TC, et al. Deep neck infection in diabetic patients: Comparison of clinical picture and outcomes with non-diabetic patients. *Head Neck Surg.* 2005;32: 943–947.

Huang TT, Tseng FY, Yeh TH, et al. Factors affecting the bacteriology of deep neck infection: a retrospective study of 128 patients. *Acta Oto-Laryngol.* 2006;126:396–401.

Ridder GJ, Technau-Ihling K, Sander A, et al. Spectrum and management of deep neck space infections: An eight year experience of 234 cases. *Otolaryngol Head Neck Surg.* 2005;133:709–714.

Wang CP, Ko JY, Lou PJ. Deep neck infection as the main initial presentation of primary head and neck cancer. *J Laryngol Otol.* 2006;120:305–309.

PART III

Clinical Syndromes – Eye

11. Conjunctivitis

Elmer Y. Tu

Conjunctivitis is a nonspecific term used to describe inflammation of the ocular surface and conjunctiva from either infectious or noninfectious causes. Infectious conjunctivitis is most commonly due to exogenous inoculation of the mucous membranes lining the surface of the eye and eyelid, resulting in an activation of a local inflammatory response. The vast majority of cases are acute but may also present as chronic or recurrent. Although most cases of acute infectious conjunctivitis are self-limited and result in few long-term sequelae, appropriate evaluation and therapy are indicated with specific presentations.

CLINICAL FEATURES

The hallmark of conjunctivitis is injection or hyperemia of the conjunctival vessels, resulting in a red eye as well as tearing and/or mucopurulent discharge. Conjunctivitis may also result in complaints of irritation, foreign body sensation, mattering or crusting of the eyelids, and mild visual blurring primarily due to alterations of the tear layer. The local inflammatory response may manifest as conjunctival lymphoid follicles or vascular papillae, eyelid edema, and/or preauricular adenopathy. Complaints of severe eye pain, photophobia, significant visual loss, or referred pain should alert the examiner to the possibility of other, more ominous, etiologies. Similarly, loss of normal corneal clarity either diffuse or focal, proptosis, pupillary abnormalities, conjunctival scarring, or restriction of eye movement is criteria for a detailed ophthalmic evaluation (Table 11.1).

ETIOLOGY

Numerous studies have demonstrated that, regardless of the etiology, acute conjunctivitis follows a benign course and results in few sequelae even without specific antibiotic therapy. Because characteristic signs and symptoms can distinguish bacterial and viral syndromes, the diagnosis of conjunctivitis is based largely on clinical history and examination. Cultures are normally reserved for neonatal or hyperacute conjunctivitis or in patients with a course greater than 2 to 3 weeks, classified as chronic conjunctivitis. A history of contact with other patients with conjunctivitis, bilateral involvement, or exposure to groups of children is associated with the more contagious viral agents. Signs of preauricular lymph node swelling (with the exception of hyperacute conjunctivitis), a follicular palpebral conjunctival reaction and clear discharge or copious tearing are also more consistent with acute viral conjunctivitis. A papillary conjunctival reaction, mucopurulent discharge, and the lack of local lymph node swelling is more suggestive of bacterial conjunctivitis. When indicated, diagnostic workup consists of conjunctival swabs for Gram and other histologic stains as well as culture.

VIRAL CONJUNCTIVITIS

Acute conjunctivitis, defined as less than 2 to 3 weeks duration, is most commonly viral, especially in adults. Adenovirus is a commonly identified pathogen in outbreaks of acute viral conjunctivitis. Although usually associated with types 8 and 19, epidemic keratoconjunctivitis (EKC) has been associated with several other serotypes and is highly contagious, spread by direct contact from hand to eye. In addition to the classic signs of viral conjunctivitis, patients with EKC may develop an immune keratitis consisting of corneal subepithelial infiltrates approximately 2 or 3 weeks after the onset of the conjunctivitis. The corneal inflammation results in complaints of foreign body sensation, photophobia, and, possibly, decreased vision sometimes lasting days to months. Pharyngoconjunctivitis has a similar ocular presentation but is associated with serotypes 3 and 7 and includes fever and pharyngitis. Viral cultures are reserved for tracking large outbreaks because results usually are available after symptoms have subsided. The recent introduction of an in-office, rapid, reproducible adenovirus antigen screening test should prove to be of more clinical utility. The virus may remain viable on surfaces for many days to weeks, making control of outbreaks

Table 11.1 Red Eye: Differential Features

	Conjunctivitis			Keratitis		Iritis	Glaucoma (Acute)
	Bacterial	**Viral**	**Allergic**	**Bacterial**	**Viral**		
Blurred vision	0	0	0	+++	0 to ++	+ to ++	++ to +++
Pain	0	0	0	++	0 to +	++	++ to +++
Photophobia	0	0	0	++	++	+++	+ to ++
Discharge	Purulent + to +++	Watery + to ++	White, ropy +	Purulent +++	Watery +	0	0
Injection	+++	++	+	+++	+	0 to + (limbal)	+ to ++ (limbal)
Corneal haze	0	0	0	+++	+ to ++	0	+ to +++
Ciliary flush	0	0	0	+++	+	+++ to +++	+ to ++
Pupil	Normal	Normal	Normal	Normal or miotic (iritis)	Normal	Miotic	Mid-dilated Nonreactive
Pressure	Normal	Normal	Normal	Normal	Normal	Normal, low or high	High
Preauricular nodes	Rare	Usual	0	0	0	0	0
Smear	Bacteria PMNs	Lymphs	Eosinophil	Bacteria PMNs	0	0	0
Therapy	Antibiotics	Nonspecific	Nonspecific	Antibiotics	Antivirals (if herpes)	Cycloplegia Topical steroids	Medical or surgical

+, Mild; ++, moderate; +++, severe; *PMNs*, polymorphonucleocytes.

problematic. True EKC may remain highly transmissible from patient to patient for 2 weeks or more, and, therefore, requires strict hygiene instruction as well as isolation precautions, especially during the phase of copious discharge. Acute hemorrhagic conjunctivitis associated with enterovirus 70 and coxsackievirus A24 is a highly transmissible follicular conjunctivitis with preauricular adenopathy with the added feature of subconjunctival hemorrhages (Figure 11.1). Currently available topical antivirals are not efficacious in any of these entities, making primary treatment supportive with topical lubricants, cool compresses, and topical nonsteroidal anti-inflammatory drugs (NSAIDs). Topical corticosteroids have been used cautiously in patients with debilitating symptoms of EKC-related keratitis, but their use is controversial.

Either herpes simplex type 1 or 2 may result in a primary follicular conjunctivitis seen in children and young adults. Primary conjunctivitis is normally unilateral with a

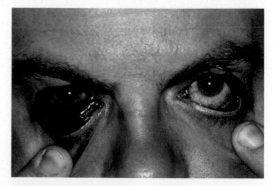

Figure 11.1 Self-limited acute hemorrhagic conjunctivitis.

palpable preauricular lymph node associated with a classic vesicular eyelid or periorbital eruption (Figure 11.2). Systemic antivirals are indicated for primary infection. Because vision-threatening sequelae are associated with corneal involvement, topical trifluridine 1% 5 to 9 times per day may also be added to either treat or reduce the risk of herpes simplex virus (HSV)

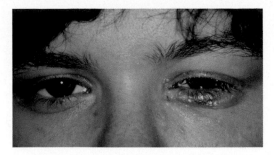

Figure 11.2 Primary herpes simplex blepharitis and conjunctivitis.

keratitis by shortening the duration of the HSV conjunctivitis. Recurrence is common.

Chronic viral conjunctivitis may be associated with *molluscum contagiosum*, usually seen in children. The chronic follicular conjunctivitis is caused by viral shedding into the eye from an eyelid or periorbital molluscum, characteristically a pearly white nodule with an umbilicated center (Figure 11.3). These lesions are typically small and multiple and spread by direct contact. Immunocompromised individuals may present with much larger lesions. Treatment of the molluscum lesion by incision and curettage of its center or excision is curative of the conjunctivitis.

BACTERIAL CONJUNCTIVITIS

Most bacterial conjunctivitis is self-limited, has low morbidity, and responds well to most available topical broad spectrum antibiotics, obviating the need for microbiologic identification. Definitive evaluation and specific treatment is, however, required in hyperacute conjunctivitis, a rapidly progressive, purulent, destructive infection, and neonatal conjunctivitis to avoid local and systemic complications more common to these two entities.

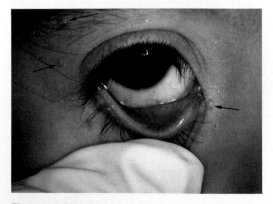

Figure 11.3 *Molluscum contagiosum* chronic follicular conjunctivitis.

HYPERACUTE CONJUNCTIVITIS

Hyperacute conjunctivitis is usually associated with *Neisseria* species, most commonly *Neisseria gonorrhoeae* in newborns and young sexually active adults. A copious, rapidly accumulating mucopurulent discharge, intense redness, and periorbital swelling are characteristic of hyperacute conjunctivitis. It is one of the few acute bacterial conjunctivitides that develops a preauricular lymphadenopathy. Rapid corneal and conjunctival penetration can result in severe corneal ulceration and ocular destruction if left untreated. It is considered a true ocular emergency. This potential for ocular complications and systemic infection with *N. gonorrhoeae* necessitates microbiologic identification as well as systemic antibiotic therapy (see Table 11.2). Local sterile saline lavage can be symptomatically helpful. Because of a significant incidence of co-infection, systemic therapy directed against Chlamydia infection is recommended in these cases (see below). Less commonly, *N. meningitides* may result in hyperacute conjunctivitis in a similar, but muted, presentation. The infection may be a primary conjunctivitis but is more likely secondary to systemic meningococcemia, requiring aggressive systemic therapy to prevent systemic complications.

NEONATAL CONJUNCTIVITIS

Conjunctivitis occurring within the first month of life is termed neonatal conjunctivitis and is either nosocomial or contracted during passage through the birth canal. The pathogens most commonly identified include *Chlamydia trachomatis* (30–50%), *Staphylococcus aureus*, and *N. gonorrhoeae*, with *Streptococcus pneumoniae*, *Haemophilus* spp., and *Pseudomonas* also identified. Prophylaxis with a single topical application of antibiotic within the hour of delivery has drastically reduced the incidence of neonatal conjunctivitis. The original solution of 1% silver nitrate (*Crede prophylaxis*) has been largely supplanted by topical erythromycin 0.5% or tetracycline 1% ointment both for better coverage for Chlamydia and a lower incidence of toxicity. Signs and symptoms are not helpful in discerning between these infections, necessitating microbiologic identification to direct appropriate therapy.

Infection with *N. gonorrhoeae* causes hyperacute conjunctivitis 1 to 13 days after birth and constitutes an ocular emergency. Clinical signs, symptoms, and treatment are similar to

Table 11.2 Systemic Treatment of Gonococcal Conjunctivitis

Adults	Dosage
Ceftriaxone (Drug of Choice)	1 g IM, single dose
Ciprofloxacin	500 mg PO, single dose
Ofloxacin	400 mg PO, single dose
Spectinomycin	2 g IM, single dose
Children (≤ 45 kg)	**Dosage**
Ceftriaxone	125 mg IM, single dose
Spectinomycin	40 mg/kg IM (max=adult dosage), single dose
Neonates	**Dosage**
Ceftriaxone	25–50 mg/kg IV or IM (max=125 mg), single dose

those seen in adults as described above. The proper use of neonatal prophylaxis reduces the incidence of gonococcal conjunctivitis to less than 2% in infected children born to infected mothers.

Neonatal inclusion conjunctivitis is caused by *C. trachomatis* and presents 5 to 14 days after birth. Signs may include lid swelling, redness, water, or mucopurulent discharge. In some cases a pseudomembrane may occur. Diagnostic workup is detailed below. Ocular infection can be associated with pneumonia and/or otitis media in up to 50% of patients, necessitating both topical and systemic therapy consisting of oral erythromycin or erythromycin ethylsuccinate 50 mg/kg/day in 4 divided doses.

Most other bacterial infections will respond to a topical broad spectrum antibiotic such as erythromycin, sulfacetamide, aminoglycoside, or fluoroquinolone.

HSV may also result in ophthalmia neonatorum either as an isolated conjunctivitis/keratitis or as part of a serious systemic neonatal infection. Prophylaxis of the mother with acyclovir or valacyclovir has been shown to reduce viral shedding during delivery. This combined with Cesarean section, in the presence of active genital herpes, has reduced the incidence of HSV neonatal infection. Transmission may, however, still occur in asymptomatic individuals and should be considered in the differential of neonatal conjunctivitis. Classic vesicular lesions are usually noted on the eyelid with a concomitant follicular conjunctivitis. Dendritic lesions of the cornea indicate HSV keratitis with the potential for loss of vision secondary to corneal scarring. Intraocular involvement may lead to more serious ocular damage. Although HSV type 2 is more common, HSV type 1 has also been isolated. Superficial scraping for smear and culture are helpful but not integral to diagnosis. Treatment includes systemic antivirals as well as topical trifluridine 1% 9 times per day. Other forms of neonatal viral conjunctivitis are otherwise uncommon.

ACUTE BACTERIAL CONJUNCTIVITIS

Overall, the majority of acute conjunctivitis is viral, except in the pediatric population where more bacterial pathogens are seen. Clinical features include a mild to moderate mucopurulent discharge, a papillary conjunctival inflammatory response, injection (hyperemia), and initial unilaterality. With few exceptions (see hyperacute conjunctivitis, chlamydia in this chapter), routine bacterial conjunctivitis does not result in preauricular adenopathy. Cultures and smears are not normally performed in its management, but, in prospective series, gram-positive bacteria, *S. pneumoniae*, *Streptococcus viridans*, *S. aureus*, and *Haemophilus* predominate. Gram-negative bacteria are seen less frequently. *S. pneumoniae* may cause a bilateral conjunctivitis with characteristic small petechial hemorrhages of the conjunctiva. Seen more commonly in children, *Haemophilus* may cause discoloration of the involved eyelid described as "violaceous" and create significant upper eyelid edema resulting in a characteristic S-shaped upper eyelid.

Treatment of acute bacterial conjunctivitis with any of number of broad spectrum topical antibiotics will achieve local concentrations that can easily overcome even mild to moderate resistance. The average duration of untreated acute bacterial conjunctivitis is 2 to 7 days. Topical antibiotics have been shown to shorten the overall course when administered early in the course of infection and to improve clinical and microbiologic signs of disease. Addition of antibiotics later in the course after day 4 is of limited benefit. Broad spectrum antibiotics are administered 4 to 6 times daily for 5 to 7 days (see Table 11.3). In adults presenting with conjunctivitis, it has been suggested that a delay in treatment for 3 to 4 days, instituted only with a lack of resolution, would significantly reduce the unnecessary use of topical antibiotics in viral or self-limited bacterial cases with no significant impact on overall outcome. Although unnecessary, the use of antibiotic–steroid combinations (Table 11.3) may speed symptomatic

Clinical Syndromes – Eye

Table 11.3 Common Topical Ophthalmic Antibiotics and Steroid Forms

Antibiotic	Common Brand Names	Form	Steroid-Containing Combination Product Brand Name
Sulfacetamide	Bleph-10	Drop/ointment	Blephamide, vasocidin
Erythromycin	Generic	Ointment	None
Bacitracin	Generic	Ointment	None
Bacitracin-polymyxin B	Polysporin	Ointment	
Polymyxin B-trimethorprim	Polytrim	Drop	None
Neomycin-polymyxin B		Drop/ointment	Maxitrol, cortisporin
Tetracycline-polymyxin B	Terramycin	Ointment	None
Gentamicin	Garamycin	Drop/ointment	Pred-G
Tobramycin	Tobrex	Drop/ointment	Tobradex, Zylet
Ciprofloxacin	Ciloxan	Drop/ointment	None
Ofloxacin	Ocuflox	Drop	None
Levofloxacin	Quixin	Drop	None
Gatifloxacin	Zymar	Drop	None
Moxifloxacin	Vigamox	Drop	None

relief but may potentiate serious masquerading conditions and should, therefore, be used with caution if the diagnosis is in question. Because of a relationship between *Haemophilus* conjunctivitis and acute otitis media or other involvement, the addition of appropriate systemic antibiotics is strongly considered, especially if systemic signs are present.

CHRONIC BACTERIAL ONJUNCTIVITIS

Conjunctivitis persisting for greater than 2 weeks is considered chronic and requires more detailed ophthalmic examination as well as Gram and Giemsa staining and culture. Chronic or recrudescent bacterial conjunctivitis may persist because of characteristics of the causative organism or a persistent local or external reservoir of the organism not exposed to normal ocular surface defense mechanisms. Although contaminated prosthetic devices such as contact lenses may be a source for pathogen reintroduction, the most common reservoir is the eyelids in the form of blepharitis, dacryocystitis, or, rarely, dacryoadenitis.

Blepharitis, or eyelid margin inflammation, is most commonly associated with chronic colonization by *S. aureus* or epidermidis and is characterized by eyelash debris, eyelid margin thickening, and telangiectasias (Figure 11.4). Angular blepharitis refers to infection of the lateral canthus causing inflammation and irritation of the eyelid skin and is associated with *Moraxella lacunata*. Seen more commonly in alcoholics and immunocompromised individuals, it may also result in conjunctivitis and keratitis. Swabs for Gram stain demonstrate the classic "double boxcar" gram-negative organisms. A concomitant conjunctivitis may accompany any form of blepharitis. Signs and symptoms are similar to other forms of bacterial conjunctivitis and respond to lid hygiene and topical antibiotic ointment such as erythromycin, bacitracin, or sulfacetamide at bedtime.

CHLAMYDIA CONJUNCTIVITIS

Serotypes A to C are associated with trachoma, a follicular bacterial conjunctivitis that because of its chronicity results in scarring of the superior tarsus. These cicatricial changes may lead to entropion and trichiasis, inward turning eyelashes, resulting in chronic corneal trauma and scarring. Seen primarily in endemic areas of the developing world, it is one of the most common causes of blindness. Diagnostic workup consists of

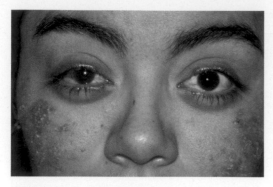

Figure 11.4 *S. aureus*-related chronic blepharoconjunctivitis.

Table 11.4 Causes of Parinaud's Oculoglandular Syndrome

Disease	Agents
Cat scratch disease	*Bartonella henselae*
Tularemia	*Francisella tularensis*
Sporotrichosis	*Sporotrichum schenckii*
Tuberculosis	*Mycobacterium tuberculosis*
Syphilis	*Treponema pallidum*
Coccidioidomycosis	*Coccidioides immitis*
Paracoccidioidomycosis	*Paracoccidioidomycosis brasiliensis*
Actinomycosis	*Actinomyces israelii, A. propionicus*
Blastomycosis	*Blastomyces dermatitidis*
Infectious mononucleosis	Epstein-Barr virus
Mumps	Paramyxovirus
Pasteurellosis	*Pasteurella multocida (septica)*
Yersinia infection	*Yersinia pseudotuberculosis*
	Yersinia enterocolitica
Glanders	*Burkholderia mallei*
Chancroid	*Haemophilus ducreyi*
Lymphogranuloma venereum (LGV)	Chlamydial LGV agent L, L_2, L_3
Rickettsiosis (Mediterranean spotted fever)	*Rickettsia conorii*
Listerellosis	*Listeria monocytogenes*
Ophthalmia nodosa (Non-infectious)	Lepidoptera (caterpillars) Tarantula hairs

conjunctival swabs/scrapings for culture or direct immunofluorescence. Courses of systemic erythromycin, doxycycline 100 mg twice daily for 7 days or a single 1-g oral dose of azithromycin are effective and curative, but because of its endemic nature, whole community programs are required to prevent recurrent reinfection. Alternatives include erythromycin, ofloxacin, and levofloxacin.

Adult inclusion conjunctivitis is also caused by *C. trachomatis* (serotypes D through K). The conjunctivitis is concurrent with, but may occur independent of, active genital infection. Transmission to the eye is by direct contact with contaminated secretions. Nonspecific symptoms of tearing, foreign body sensation, photophobia, and eyelid edema are presenting complaints. Chlamydia causes a follicular conjunctivitis with preauricular lymphadenopathy, but unlike trachoma, the lower eyelid is normally more involved. As in trachoma, systemic azithromycin or doxycycline is effective but also requires appropriate evaluation and treatment of sexual contacts.

MISCELLANEOUS CAUSES

In addition to *Neisseria* sp. and *Chlamydiae* sp., several other forms of conjunctivitis may be related to systemic infection. Parinaud's oculoglandular syndrome is the association of a follicular conjunctivitis, conjunctival granuloma, and an ipsilateral lymphadenopathy. Cat scratch disease caused by *Bartonella henselae* is the most common cause of Parinaud's and is transmitted by contact with an infected cat. The conjunctival granuloma may be single or multiple and is surrounded by intense inflammation accompanied by ipsilateral head, neck, or axillary lymphadenopathy. Other causes of Parinaud's include tularemia, sporotrichosis, tuberculosis, syphilis, and coccidioidomycosis

(Table 11.4). Evaluation should include a detailed history of exposures and appropriate serologic tests and systemic cultures. Treatment is directed toward the underlying process.

Chronic use of any topical ophthalmic medication may result in ocular medicamentosa. Signs and symptoms include tearing, redness, photophobia, and irritation, masquerading as an infectious conjunctivitis. Although it is most commonly associated with over-the-counter vasoconstrictors, it is also seen with topical antibiotics and may cause a self-perpetuating conjunctivitis until discontinued. Other etiologies should be considered in chronic conjunctivitis, including neoplasm, allergy, toxicity, autoimmune disease, and unusual pathogens.

SUGGESTED READING

American Academy of Ophthalmology. *Conjunctivitis, Preferred Practice Pattern*. San Francisco, CA: American Academy of Ophthalmology; 2003.

Buznach N, Dagan R, Greenberg D. Clinical and bacterial characteristics of acute bacterial conjunctivitis in children in the antibiotic resistance era. *Pediatr Infect Dis J*. 2005;24:823–828.

Mah FS. New antibiotics for bacterial infections. *Ophthalmol Clin North Am*. 2003;16:11–27.

Rubenstein JB. Disorders of the conjunctiva and limbus. In: Yanoff M, ed. *Ophthalmology*. Philadelphia, PA: Mosby; 1999:5.1.2–5.1.11.

Sambursky R, Tauber S, Schirra F, Kozich K, Davidson R, Cohen EJ. The RPS adeno detector for diagnosing adenoviral conjunctivitis. *Ophthalmology*. 2006;113:1758–1764.

Sheikh A, Hurwitz B. Antibiotics versus placebo for acute bacterial conjunctivitis. *Cochrane Database Syst Rev*. 2006:CD001211.

Tarabishy AB, Hall GS, Procop GW, Jeng BH. Bacterial culture isolates from hospitalized pediatric patients with conjunctivitis. *Am J Ophthalmol*. 2006;142:678–680.

12. Keratitis

Francis S. Mah and Jules Baum

Keratitis can lead to severe visual disability and requires prompt diagnosis and treatment. Sequelae can vary in severity from corneal scarring to perforation, endophthalmitis, and loss of the eye. Although the corneal surface is awash with microorganisms of the normal flora, an intact corneal epithelium and ocular defense mechanism serve to prevent infection in the normal eye. Although some organisms such as *Neisseria gonorrhoeae, Neisseria meningitides, Corynebacterium diptheriae, Listeria,* and *Shigella* can penetrate an intact epithelium, all others require damage to the epithelial layer to invade the cornea. Several risk factors predispose the cornea to infection. Dry eyes from Sjogren syndrome, Stevens-Johnson syndrome, or vitamin A deficiency can result in bacterial keratitis. Prolonged corneal exposure from ectropion, lagophthalmos or proptosis can lead to secondary infection. Entropion and trichiaisis resulting in epithelial defects put the cornea at risk. Neurotrophic keratopathy from cranial neuropathy, prior herpes simplex, or zoster infections predispose to secondary infections. Some systemic conditions such as chronic alcoholism, severe malnutrition, immunosuppressive drug use, immunodeficiency syndromes, and malignancy can impair immune defenses and allow infection by unusual organisms. Prior ocular surgery such as penetrating keratoplasty or refractive procedures are also risk factors. Trauma is a common predisposing factor of bacterial keratitis, especially for patients at the extremes of age and in developing countries. Injury to the corneal surface and stroma allows invasion of normal flora as well as organisms harbored by foreign bodies.

Contact lens wear is an established risk factor for bacterial keratitis. All types of contact lenses have been linked to infection, with extended-wear soft lenses conferring greater risk than daily wear hard or soft lenses. Corneal changes from contact lens use include an induced hypoxic and hypercapnic state promoting epithelial cell derangement and allowing bacterial invasion. Contact lenses also induce dry eye and corneal hypesthesia. Overnight rigid gas-permeable lens use for orthokeratology has also been associated with bacterial keratitis.

Although there are geographic variations in the order of incidence, the most common pathogenic organisms associated with bacterial keratitis include *Staphylococcus* species, *Streptococcus* species, *Pseudomonas aeruginosa*, and enteric gram-negative rods. A 5-year review of bacterial keratitis isolates from Pittsburgh showed a change in distribution with a decrease in gram-positive organisms, whereas gram-negative isolates remained stable (Figure 12.1). In South Florida, an increase in gram-positive isolates with a decrease in gram-negative isolates over a 30-year period has been reported. A similar trend has also been reported in North China. *Pseudomonas aeruginosa* is commonly associated with contact lens–related bacterial keratitis, causing up to two-thirds of cases, although a decline in the frequency of *P. aeruginosa* isolates in these patients has been noted. Nontuberculous mycobacteria is being reported with increasing frequency as a cause of infectious keratitis after laser in situ keratomileusis. Although the reported incidence of infection after LASIK is low, this condition is a management challenge requiring proper diagnosis and treatment. Bacterial colonization of the eyelid and conjunctiva is normal and helps reduce opportunities for pathogenic strains from gaining a foothold. Host defense mechanisms can be overcome, however, and lead to serious ocular morbidity if not treated properly. Although the clinical manifestations of corneal infections may be characteristic of certain pathogens, further laboratory evaluation with cultures and antibiotic susceptibility testing provide a definitive diagnosis and more focused treatment after empirical therapy has been initiated.

CLINICAL FEATURES

The presenting symptoms, clinical history, and exam findings may suggest an infectious keratitis but are not diagnostic for a particular organism. The presenting signs of bacterial keratitis vary depending on the virulence of the organism, duration of infection, structural status of the cornea, and host inflammatory response.

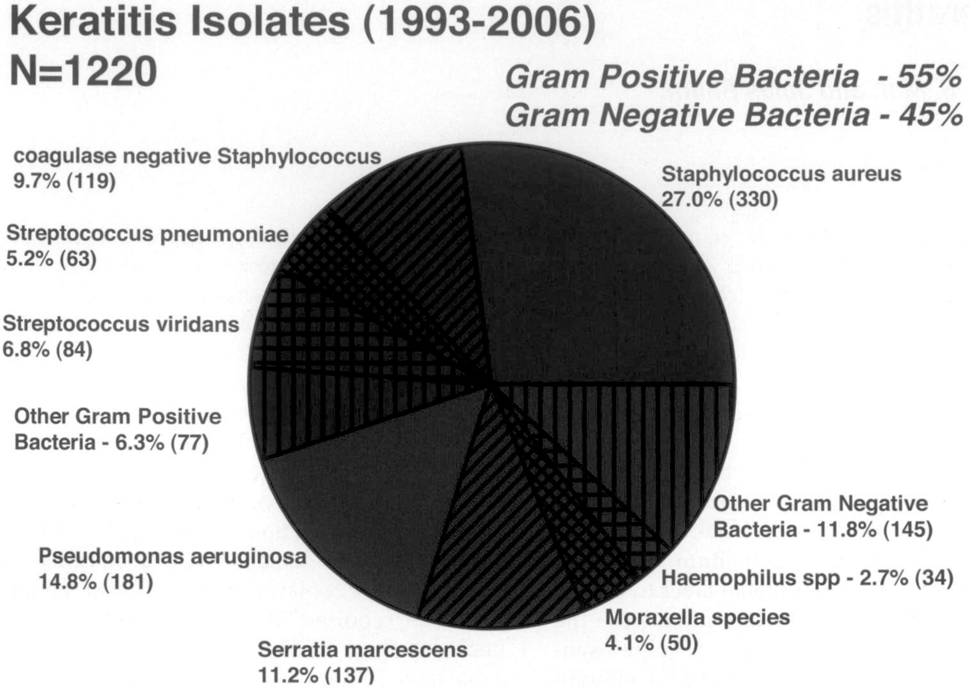

Keratitis Isolates (1993-2006)
N=1220

Gram Positive Bacteria - 55%
Gram Negative Bacteria - 45%

coagulase negative Staphylococcus
9.7% (119)

Staphylococcus aureus
27.0% (330)

Streptococcus pneumoniae
5.2% (63)

Streptococcus viridans
6.8% (84)

Other Gram Positive
Bacteria - 6.3% (77)

Other Gram Negative
Bacteria - 11.8% (145)

Pseudomonas aeruginosa
14.8% (181)

Haemophilus spp - 2.7% (34)

Moraxella species
4.1% (50)

Serratia marcescens
11.2% (137)

Figure 12.1 Keratitis isolates(1993–2006).

Common presenting symptoms include pain, decreased vision, tearing, and photophobia. Eyelid edema, conjunctival hyperemia with a papillary reaction, and chemosis are typical findings. A corneal epithelial defect with adherent mucopurulent exudate and underlying stromal infiltrate is a hallmark sign for infectious keratitis (Figure 12.2). Multiple focal infiltrates can be seen with contact lens use or with polymicrobial infections. Migration of inflammatory cells causes a diffuse cellular infiltration adjacent to and within the ulcerated stroma. An anterior chamber reaction can range from mild cells and flare to a marked hypopyon (Figure 12.3). A cornea damaged from prior disease can present with less distinct signs and symptoms. Preexisting corneal scars, epitheliopathy, or inflammation confuse the picture as does prior use of antibiotics and corticosteroids. On examination, all ocular abnormalities should be documented in detail to help track the clinical course on subsequent visits. Repeat measurements of the size of the epithelial defect, the depth of the stromal infiltrate, and the severity of inflammation can be used to assess the effectiveness of treatment.

Nontuberculous mycobacterial keratitis has been reported with increasing frequency after laser in situ keratomileusis including several clusters of cases. In two recent

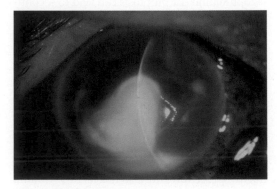

Figure 12.2 Infectious keratitis.

reviews of post-LASIK corneal infections, *Mycobacterium* represented the most common etiologic organism. The isolated subtypes include the fast-growing *Mycobacterium chelonae, Mycobacterium abscessus, Mycobacterium fortuitum,* and *Mycobacterium mucogenicum,* as well as the slow-growing *Mycobacterium szulgai.* Nontuberculous keratitis after LASIK is characterized by a delayed onset with an indolent course. Time of onset from fast-growing organisms averaged 3.4 weeks after the procedure, whereas the slow-growing *M. szulgai* can present 6 to 24 weeks after surgery. Symptoms can range from a mild foreign body sensation to pain, redness, photophobia, and decreased

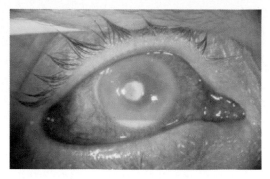

Figure 12.3 Hypopyon.

vision. The infiltrate, which can be multiple, begins in the interface and spreads to adjacent stroma of the flap and stromal bed. Anterior perforation through the flap can occur with progression of infection. The location can be central, paracentral, or peripheral. In addition to a focal infiltrate, a cracked windshield appearance of infectious crystalline keratopathy has been reported (Figures 12.4A and B).

DIAGNOSTIC TECHNIQUES

Routine culture of corneal infections is not the usual practice in the community. A small peripheral ulcer may be treated empirically, but a large, purulent, central ulcer that extends to the middle to deep stroma should be cultured. In addition, ulcers that are clinically suspicious for fungal, mycobacterial, or amebic infections or are unresponsive to initial broad spectrum antibiotics warrant cultures. Topical anesthesia with proparacaine hydrochloride is preferred because it has less antibacterial properties than other topical anesthetics. A sterile platinum spatula is used to scrape the leading edge as well as the base of the ulcer while carefully avoiding contamination from the lids and lashes. Organisms such as *Streptococcus pneumoniae* are

more readily recovered from the ulcer edge, whereas other organisms such as *Moraxella* are characteristically recovered from the base. The scrapings are inoculated onto solid media (blood, chocolate, mannitol, Sabouraud's agar) by streaking a row of Cs. New material is recovered for each row. Scrapings are also placed on microscope slides and stained as above. Special stains include Ziehl-Neelsen acid-fast stain for *Mycobacterium*, *Actinomyces*, and *Nocardia*. Acridine orange is a fluorescent dye that may be helpful in identifying bacteria when yields are low, but this stain does not yield classification information that Gram stain provides.

In cases of deep stromal suppuration that is not readily accessible or a progressive microbial keratitis unresponsive to therapy, a corneal biopsy may be warranted. A round 2-mm to 3-mm sterile disposable skin trephine is used to incise the anterior corneal stroma, and lamellar dissection is performed with a surgical blade. The specimen is then ground in a mortar with trypticase soy broth and plated on media.

TREATMENT
Routes of Administration

The topical application of drugs with eyedrops is the preferred method of treatment of bacterial keratitis. Increased drug penetration can be achieved by higher concentrations, more frequent applications, and by the typical presence of an epithelial defect. Fortified antibiotics are made by mixing the powdered drug or diluting the parenteral form with artificial tears or balanced salt solution. These freshly prepared solutions remain stable for up to a week without significant loss of activity. Although ointments prolong corneal contact time and lubricate the ocular surface, peak corneal concentrations may be limited when compared with

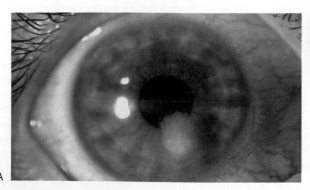
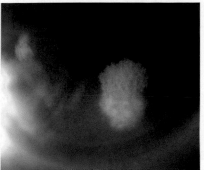

A   B

Figures 12.4A and 12.4B Infectious crystalline keratopathy.

solutions. They also retard antibiotic absorption delivered in eyedrop form. Ointments can be used as adjunctive therapy at bedtime in less severe cases.

Subconjunctival injections may not have a therapeutic advantage over topical solutions. However, they may be indicated in certain clinical situations such as imminent perforation or spread of infection to adjacent sclera, especially when patient compliance is an issue. Soft contact lenses and collagen shields can act as drug delivery devices and aid in sustaining high corneal drug levels. These "bandage" contact lenses may also provide structural support to promote reepithelialization. Systemic therapy is indicated for gonococcal infections as well as for young children with severe *H. influenzae* or *P. aeruginosa* keratitis. Systemic antibiotics are also indicated for perforations and scleral involvement.

Empiric Therapy

Because bacterial keratitis can rapidly progress and threaten vision, treatment should begin when an infectious process is suspected. Topical broad spectrum antibiotics are initially used and later modified according to culture results, antibiotic susceptibilities, and clinical response. For severe cases, combination therapy with fortified β-lactam (cefazolin 50 mg/mL) and aminoglycoside (tobramycin or gentamicin 14 mg/mL) (Figure 12.5) provides adequate coverage of both gram-positive and -negative organisms that cause bacterial keratitis.

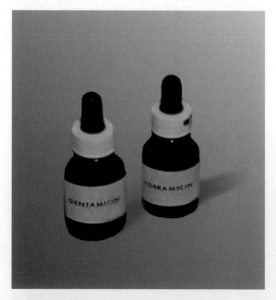

Figure 12.5 Topical aminoglycosides are combined with β-lactam therapy.

Vancomycin (50 mg/mL) can be substituted for cefazolin in cases of penicillin allergy or resistance to *Enterococcus* and *Staphylococcus* species. Some prefer to commence treatment with vanomycin instead of cefazolin. A loading dose is achieved with a drop every 5 minutes for five applications. Antibiotic is then continued every 30 minutes to 1 hour around the clock.

Single-agent therapy with fluoroquinolones has been shown to be as effective as combination therapy in treating bacterial keratitis. The widespread use of the second (ciprofloxacin and ofloxacin) and third (levofloxacin) generation fluoroquinolones has, however, led to the emergence of resistance in several bacterial species, including *Staphylococcus aureus* and *Pseudomonas aeruginosa*. The fourth-generation fluoroquinolones, gatifloxacin and moxifloxacin have been developed in response to this increasing resistance. They require two mutations to establish resistance and, therefore, are more effective against gram-positive organisms that already have a single mutation and are resistant to older generation fluoroquinolones.

A favorable response to empiric therapy merits continuing the treatment plan. Positive signs of clinical improvement include decreased pain and discharge, consolidation of the stromal infiltrate, decreased anterior chamber reaction, and corneal reepithelialization. Culture and antibiotic susceptibility results can be used to focus therapy against the offending organism or to discontinue unnecessary drugs. Clinical improvement may not be seen during the first 2 days due to increased inflammation and suppuration from bacterial exotoxins. Toxicity from topical medications can also mask changes. A lack of improvement or clinical worsening after 48 hours may warrant repeat cultures, although concomitant antibiotic therapy will decrease yields. Topical therapy can be tapered as the clinical picture improves.

Management of nontuberculous mycobacterial keratitis after LASIK can be challenging and requires aggressive treatment. The flap should be lifted for smears and culture as well as for soaking of the stromal bed and flap with antibiotics. Fortified amikacin, clarithromycin, and azithromycin are the drugs of choice. Fourth-generation fluoroquinolones have also been shown to be effective against mycobacterial keratitis. Combination therapy is recommended due to emergence of resistance on monotherapy. Lack of clinical improvement warrants repeat culture and tailoring of antibiotics accordingly. Flap amputation may also be necessary to allow increased antibiotic penetration.

Adjunctive Therapy

Bacterial keratitis is often associated with severe pain. Pain control with analgesics may provide not only comfort but also better compliance with the difficult regimen of around-the-clock topical drop instillation. Cycloplegic agents should also be used to decrease discomfort from ciliary spasm and to prevent synechiae formation. Cyanoacrylate glue can be used to reinforce an area of corneal thinning, a descemetocele, or a small perforation. A "bandage" contact lens is placed after the glue hardens. This procedure allows for further treatment of the infection and inflammation while postponing surgery. A corneal patch graft is an alternative for small perforations, whereas larger necrotic perforations require a therapeutic penetrating keratoplasty. Maximal topical antibiotic therapy as well as systemic antibiotics are given preoperatively.

Corticosteroids may play a role in treating bacterial keratitis with its potential for reducing the host inflammatory response and resultant corneal scarring. Adverse effects of corticosteroids include inhibition of corneal wound healing, promotion of stromal thinning and perforation, potentiation of microbial replication, and recrudescence of infection, secondary glaucoma, and cataract formation. Despite its theoretical advantages, studies have not shown a consistent or significant beneficial effect of corticosteroids on clinical outcome. Prior use of corticosteroids in eyes with preexisting corneal disease increased the risk of ulcerative keratitis. Worsening or recrudescence of *Pseudomonas* keratitis has been reported after the addition of topical steroids. Guidelines regarding the optimal use of corticosteroids are lacking; however, certain recommendations have been proposed: (1) Steroids should not be used initially or if the infection is improving, (2) steroids should be used after several days of antibiotics if there is persistent inflammation, (3) continue use of concomitant antibiotics, and (4) steroids should not be used if there is significant corneal thinning.

Acanthameba keratitis is a rare opportunistic infection that affects approximately 1.2 to 3.0 cases per million. Acanthamebae are ubiquitous protozoa that exist in two forms: trophozoites (the active form) and cysts (the inactive form). Under unfavorable conditions, trophozoites transform into cysts that are resistant to extremes of temperature, pH, and desiccation. Cysts are notoriously difficult to kill, and this is one reason why this infection is so difficult to eradicate. Indeed, only one class of medications, the biguanides, has cystocidal activity.

The initial report of Acanthameba keratitis was in 1975 in a patient who sustained eye trauma outdoors. This was followed by an epidemic of infection in soft contact lens wearers in the late 1980s, largely attributed to homemade saline. In addition to all types of contact lenses, additional risk factors include ocular trauma, corneal transplantation, and exposure to infected lake water, sea water, or hot tubs. Recently, an alarming increase in the rate of Acanthameba keratitis has been observed prompting the Centers for Disease Control and Prevention (CDC) to investigate possible etiologies.

Acanthameba infection presents with similar nonspecific symptoms as bacterial keratitis. Pain that is out of proportion to clinical findings is classic but not universal. Early corneal infection manifests as epithelial involvement, including elevated epithelial lines that may appear as dendritic, punctuate epithelial erosions, microcysts, and epithelial haze (Figure 12.6). Stromal findings, which occur later in the infection, include single or multiple stromal infiltrates and nummular keratitis. Ring infiltrates or satellite lesions usually suggest advanced disease (Figure 12.7). Tropism of

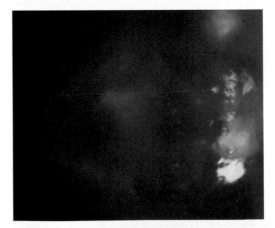

Figure 12.6 Epithelial haze.

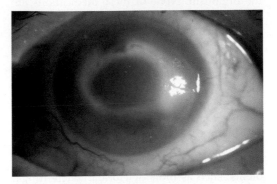

Figure 12.7 Ring infiltrates.

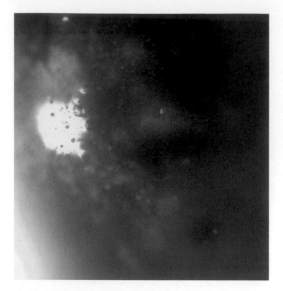

Figure 12.8 Radial keratoneuritis.

the Acanthameba organism for corneal nerves causes radial keratoneuritis, the reason for the extreme pain (Figure 12.8).

Diagnosis is typically delayed for a number of reasons. Early infections are commonly treated as bacterial keratitis, especially because many practitioners rely on empiric treatment with broad-spectrum topical fluoroquinolones. Early disease is commonly misdiagnosed as herpes simplex, whereas later disease can be confused with fungal keratitis. The delay in diagnosis makes it more difficult to treat because the infection is then more deeply seated.

Treatment of Acanthameba keratitis is long, involves toxic medications, and may be unsuccessful in curing the infection if the infection involves the posterior cornea. A combination of topical antiamebic agents, including biguanides (eg, PHMB and chlorhexidine), diamides (eg, propamidine), and aminoglycosides (eg, neomycin) are typically used. Of these, only the biguanides are active against the cystic form of the organism. None of these medications are available commercially in the United States and they must be compounded by a specialty pharmacy before use. Medications must be used for months, starting with hourly dosages and tapering off as the clinical situation improves. The use of steroids is controversial. It clearly improves patient comfort but may potentiate the infection.

In temperate climates, fungal keratitis is an uncommon infection. Fungal infections of the cornea are more common in hot, humid environments, such as India or Florida, where fungal keratitis accounts for 60% and 16% of all cornea

infections, respectively. Fungi are ubiquitous in the environment and can be broadly divided into yeast (*Candida* species) and molds (filamentous fungi, eg, *Fusarium* and *Aspergillus*). Although the ocular surface is continuously exposed to fungus, keratitis can occur only when the organism gains access to the corneal stroma through a break in the epithelial barrier, which is the most important defense mechanism against all forms of infections keratitis. By far the most important risk factor for fungal keratitis is ocular trauma, especially when the trauma involves contact with soil or vegetable matter. Other risk factors include ocular surface disease such as neurotrophic keratitis and prior use of steroids. Patients with atopic disease, immunocompromised patients or those hospitalized in intensive care units are at increased risk for fungal keratitis. Although contact lens wear has not been considered a major risk factor for fungal keratitis, a cluster of *Fusarium* keratitis cases in otherwise healthy soft-contact lens wearers was noted throughout the world in 2006 (Figure 12.9). The CDC report suggests patient noncompliance with recommended cleaning regimens especially associated with the contact lens cleaning solution Renu with MoistureLoc, which was withdrawn from the market in April 2006.

Clinical signs of fungal infection include nonspecific signs of any corneal infection. Specific clinical features that should raise suspicion include infiltrates with indistinct or "feathery" edges, multifocal infiltrates, satellite lesions, immune rings, and endothelial plaques (Figure 12.10). The patient history is an important clue to the diagnosis as patients typically have a history of outdoor trauma and a waxing and waning course of symptoms and signs that have been unresponsive to management. Early diagnosis is critical for successful treatment because fungi can penetrate intact Descemet's membrane and cause endolphthalmitis. Fungal

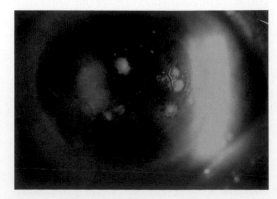

Figure 12.9 Fungal keratitis.

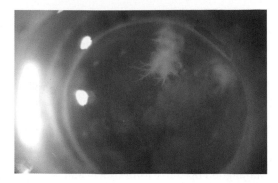

Figure 12.10 Fungal keratitis endothelial plaques.

keratitis is also difficult to diagnose because it is uncommon and the organism can be difficult to capture and culture if it has spread deep into the cornea. Culture and vital staining is key to diagnosis.

Treatment of fungal keratitis is difficult because currently available antifungal medications have limited efficacy and poor penetration into the cornea. The most widely used topical antifungal medications are the polyenes, amphotericin B, and natamycin. Natamycin is the only commercially available antifungal topical medication. Azole compounds have been used topically (clotrimazole and miconazole) and systemically (ketaconazole, fluconazole, itraconazole, and voriconazole). Voriconazole is particularly promising both topically and systemically. In addition to natamycin, these agents must be compounded from an IV formulation to be used topically. Treatment of fungal keratitis is prolonged and often lasts for months. The use of a topical steroid is contraindicated because it can worsen disease and interferes with the efficacy of certain antifungal agents.

SUGGESTED READING

Abshire R, et al. Topical antibacterial therapy for mycobacterial keratitis: potential for surgical prophylaxis and treatment. *Clin Ther*. 2004;26(2):191–196.

Alexandrakis G, et al. Corneal biopsy in the management of progressive microbial keratitis. *Am J Ophthalmol*. 2000;129(5):571–576.

Alexandrakis G, Alfonso EC, Miller D. Shifting trends in bacterial keratitis in south Florida and emerging resistance to fluoroquinolones. *Ophthalmology*. 2000;107(8):1497–1502.

Alfonso E, et al. Ulcerative keratitis associated with contact lens wear. *Am J Ophthalmol*. 1986;101(4):429–433.

Alfonso EC, et al. Fungal infections. In: *Smolin and Thoft's The Cornea: Scientific Foundations & Clinical Practice*. 4th ed. Philadelphia, PA: Lippincott, Williams & Wilkins; 2005.

Alfonso EC, et al. Insurgence of Fusarium keratitis associated with contact lens wear. *Arch Ophthalmol*. 2006;124:941–947.

Aliprandis E, et al. Comparative efficacy of topical moxifloxacin versus ciprofloxacin and vancomycin in the treatment of P. aeruginosa and ciprofloxacin-resistant MRSA keratitis in rabbits. *Cornea*. 2005;24(2):201–205.

Badenoch PR, Coster DJ. Antimicrobial activity of topical anaesthetic preparations. *Br J Ophthalmol*. 1982;66(6):364–367.

Baum J, Barza M. Topical vs subconjunctival treatment of bacterial corneal ulcers. *Ophthalmology*. 1983;90(2):162–168.

Bourcier T, et al. Bacterial keratitis: predisposing factors, clinical and microbiological review of 300 cases. *Br J Ophthalmol*. 2003;87(7):834–838.

Burns RP. Pseudomonas aeruginosa keratitis: mixed infections of the eye. *Am J Ophthalmol*. 1969;67(2):257–262.

Chandra NS, et al. Cluster of Mycobacterium chelonae keratitis cases following laser in-situ keratomileusis. *Am J Ophthalmol*. 2001;132(6):819–830.

Chang MA, Jain S, Azar DT. Infections following laser in situ keratomileusis: an integration of the published literature. *Surv Ophthalmol*. 2004;49(3):269–280.

Charukamnoetkanok P, Pineda R II. Controversies in management of bacterial keratitis. *Int Ophthalmol Clin*. 2005;45(4):199–210.

Chaudhry NA, et al. Emerging ciprofloxacin-resistant Pseudomonas aeruginosa. *Am J Ophthalmol*. 1999;128(4):509–510.

Cohen EJ, et al. Corneal ulcers associated with cosmetic extended wear soft contact lenses. *Ophthalmology*. 1987;94(2):109–114.

Cohen EJ, et al. Trends in contact lens-associated corneal ulcers. *Cornea*. 1996; 15(6): 566–570.

Dajcs JJ, et al. Effectiveness of ciprofloxacin, levofloxacin, or moxifloxacin for treatment of experimental Staphylococcus aureus keratitis. *Antimicrob Agents Chemother*. 2004; 48(6):1948–1952.

Dixon JM, et al. Complications associated with the wearing of contact lenses. *JAMA*. 1966; 195(11):901–903.

Driebe WT Jr. Present status of contact lens-induced corneal infections. *Ophthalmol Clin North Am*. 2003;16(3):485–494, viii.

Forster RK Conrad Berens lecture: the management of infectious keratitis as we approach the 21st century. *CLAO J.* 1998;24 (3):175–180.

Freitas D, et al. An outbreak of Mycobacterium chelonae infection after LASIK. *Ophthalmology.* 2003;110(2):276–285.

Fulcher SF, et al. Delayed-onset mycobacterial keratitis after LASIK. *Cornea.* 2002; 21(6):546–554.

Garg P, Sharma S, Rao GN. Ciprofloxacin-resistant Pseudomonas keratitis. *Ophthalmology.* 1999;106(7):1319–1323.

Goldstein MH, Kowalski RP, Gordon YJ. Emerging fluoroquinolone resistance in bacterial keratitis: a 5-year review. *Ophthalmology.*1999;106(7):1313–1318.

Harbin T. Recurrence of a corneal Pseudomonas infection after topical steroid therapy: report of a case. *Am J Ophthalmol.* 1964;58:670–674.

Holmes GP, et al. A cluster of cases of Mycobacterium szulgai keratitis that occurred after laser-assisted in situ keratomileusis. *Clin Infect Dis.* 2002;34(8):1039–1046.

Hsiao CH, et al. Infectious keratitis related to overnight orthokeratology. *Cornea.* 2005;24 (7):783–788.

Hyndiuk RA, et al. Comparison of ciprofloxacin ophthalmic solution 0.3% to fortified tobramycin-cefazolin in treating bacterial corneal ulcers. Ciprofloxacin Bacterial Keratitis Study Group. *Ophthalmology.* 1996;103 (11):1854–1862.

Hyon JY, et al. Comparative efficacy of topical gatifloxacin with ciprofloxacin, amikacin, and clarithromycin in the treatment of experimental Mycobacterium chelonae keratitis. *Arch Ophthalmol.* 2004;122(8):1166–1169.

John T, Velotta E. Nontuberculous (atypical) mycobacterial keratitis after LASIK: current status and clinical implications. *Cornea.* 2005.24(3):245–255.

Kalayci D, et al. Penetration of topical ciprofloxacin by presoaked medicated soft contact lenses. *CLAO J.* 1999;25(3):182–184.

Karp CL, et al. Infectious keratitis after LASIK. *Ophthalmology.* 2003;110(3):503–510.

Keay L, et al. Microbial keratitis predisposing factors and morbidity. *Ophthalmology.* 2006:113(1):109–116.

Kowalski RP, et al. Gatifloxacin and moxifloxacin: an in vitro susceptibility comparison to levofloxacin, ciprofloxacin, and ofloxacin using bacterial keratitis isolates. *Am J Ophthalmol.* 2003;136(3):500–505.

Laspina F, et al. Epidemiological characteristics of microbiological results on patients with infectious corneal ulcers: a 13-year survey in Paraguay. *Graefes Arch Clin Exp Ophthalmol.* 2004;242(3):204–209.

Liesegang TJ. Contact lens-related microbial keratitis: part I: epidemiology. *Cornea.* 1997;16(2):125–131.

Liesegang TJ. Contact lens-related microbial keratitis: part II: pathophysiology. *Cornea.* 1997;16(3):265–173.

Mah-Sadorra JH, et al. Trends in contact lens-related corneal ulcers. *Cornea.* 2005;24(1):51–58.

Marangon FB, et al. Ciprofloxacin and levofloxacin resistance among methicillin-sensitive Staphylococcus aureus isolates from keratitis and conjunctivitis. *Am J Ophthalmol.* 2004;137(3):453–438.

McDonnell PJ, et al. Community care of corneal ulcers. *Am J Ophthalmol.* 1992;114(5):531–538.

O'Brien TP et al. Efficacy of ofloxacin vs cefazolin and tobramycin in the therapy for bacterial keratitis: report from the Bacterial Keratitis Study Research Group. *Arch Ophthalmol.* 1995;113(10):1257–1265.

O'Brien TP. Bacterial keratitis. In: Foster CS, Azar DT, Dohlman CH, eds. *Smolin and Thoft's The Cornea,* Philadelphia, PA: Lippincott William & Wilkins; 2005;235–288.

Parmar P, et al. Comparison of topical gatifloxacin 0.3% and ciprofloxacin 0.3% for the treatment of bacterial keratitis. *Am J Ophthalmol.* 2006a;141(2):282–286.

Parmar P, et al. Microbial keratitis at extremes of age. *Cornea.* 2006b;25(2):153–158.

Radford CF, et al. Acanthamoeba keratitis: multicentre survey in England 1992–1996, National Acanthamoeba Keratitis Study Group. *Br J Ophthal.* 1998;82:1387–1392.

Sampath R, Ridgway AE, Leatherbarrow B. Bacterial keratitis following excimer laser photorefractive keratectomy: a case report. *Eye.* 1994;8(4):481–482.

Schein OD, et al. The incidence of microbial keratitis among wearers of a 30-day silicone hydrogel extended-wear contact lens. *Ophthalmology.* 2005;112(12):2172–2179.

Siganos CS, Solomon A, Frucht-Pery J. Microbial findings in suture erosion after penetrating keratoplasty. *Ophthalmology.* 1997;104(3):513–516.

Solomon R, et al. Infectious keratitis after laser in situ keratomileusis: results of an ASCRS survey. *J Cataract Refract Surg.* 2003;29(10):2001–2006.

Stern GA, Buttross M. Use of corticosteroids in combination with antimicrobial drugs in the treatment of infectious corneal disease. *Ophthalmology*. 1991;98(6):847–853.

Sun X, et al. Distribution and shifting trends of bacterial keratitis in north China (1989-98). *Br J Ophthalmol*. 2004;88(2):165–166.

Tauber J, Jehan F. Parasitic keratitis and conjunctivitis. In: *Smolin and Thoft's The Cornea: Scientific Foundations & Clinical Practice*. 4th ed. Philadelphia, PA: Lippincott, Williams & Wilkins; 2005:427–430.

Thebpatiphat N, et al. Acanthamoeba at Wills eye hospital: a parasite on the rise. *Invest Ophthalmol Vis Sci*. 2006:47:E–3568.

The Ofloxacin Study Group. Ofloxacin monotherapy for the primary treatment of microbial keratitis: a double-masked, randomized, controlled trial with conventional dual therapy. *Ophthalmology*. 1997;104(11): 1902–1909.

Umapathy T, et al. Non-tuberculous mycobacteria related infectious crystalline keratopathy. *Br J Ophthalmol*. 2005;89(10): 1374–1375.

Wilhelmus KR. Indecision about corticosteroids for bacterial keratitis: an evidence-based update. *Ophthalmology*. 2002;109(5): 835–842.

Willoughby CE, Batterbury M, Kaye SB. Collagen corneal shields. *Surv Ophthalmol*. 2002;47(2):174–182.

13. Iritis

Sarah S. Zaher and Elizabeth Graham

The uveal tract is a continuous vascular structure consisting of the iris, ciliary body, and choroid. It is convenient to subdivide inflammation of the uveal tract into anterior uveitis (iritis and iridocyclitis) and posterior uveitis (choroiditis and choroidoretinitis). This chapter relates to anterior uveitis or, more simply, iritis; for the related entity chorioretinitis please also see Chapter 14, Retinitis.

Exogenous iritis may follow injury or surgery to the eye or may have a local intraocular cause, which usually is obvious from history or examination. Endogenous iritis may be regarded as a symptom of some widespread infection or multisystem disorder.

Iritis may be the presenting feature of a systemic infection or merely "another organ" involved by an already diagnosed infection. However, the ocular fluids are relatively easily obtained and their analysis can prove very useful when specific diagnosis of the offending organism has proved elusive.

In the clinical setting iritis may be part of an acute or chronic systemic infection or be an immune response to a preceding systemic infection. The presentation of the iritis depends on both the immunity of the patient as well as the nature and the virulence of the organism. On occasions the iritis is the only sign of the infection which is entirely localized to the eye.

PRESENTATION OF IRITIS

Anterior uveitis, or iritis, may have an acute explosive or chronic insidious onset. Acute iritis is characterized by abrupt onset of pain, photophobia, and blurring of vision. All these symptoms are exacerbated by close work. There may be circumcorneal injection, which should not be confused with conjunctivitis. The eye is not sticky. There is a ciliary flush, but the pupil may not be stuck down and can react briskly. Inflammatory cells (keratic precipitates) are seen on the back of the cornea. These may be called granulomatous when they appear round, waxy, and yellow and nongranulomatous when they look finer and have a whiter appearance. Granulomatous keratic precipitates are classically seen in the granulomatous diseases, eg, tuberculosis or sarcoidosis, but by no means exclusively in these diseases so although the distinction has some value it must not carry too much weight when the cause of uveitis is being considered. In severe cases a hypopyon is present. This is a collection of inflammatory cells within the anterior chamber that due to their large number settle and form a visible line within the eye in the anterior chamber.

Chronic anterior uveitis has an insidious onset. The pupil is often small and reacts poorly to light or accommodation. It may be irregular due to adhesions between the iris and the lens called posterior synechiae. The patient may have had previous attacks and be able to anticipate a recurrence.

When the inflammation also involves the posterior segment of the eye, cells are seen in the vitreous cavity (vitritis) causing the patient to complain of floaters and, if involvement of the retina and optic nerve occurs, macular edema or disk edema develop. Macular edema produces reduction of central acuity, but disk edema may not be associated with signs of an optic neuropathy (reduced acuity, reduced color vision, visual field defect, and afferent papillary defect) unless there is additional infiltration or vascular involvement.

Ophthalmologists are extremely fortunate, as they are able to directly view all the structures of the eye and different patterns of ocular inflammation can lead them to the most likely underlying diagnosis, although obviously the systemic features are also vital to the process of reaching the correct diagnosis. Although ocular fluids are readily accessible, only miniscule amounts are available and therefore it is important to have a list of diagnostic probabilities in order of clinical likelihood to present to the microbiologist to maximize diagnostic yield. An ophthalmic opinion must always be sought in patients who are thought to have iritis, as an essential part of the examination is to dilate the pupil and examine the fundus where signs are often diagnostic. This chapter will consider those infections that can present with an isolated iritis without involvement of the retina or choroids, at least initially.

INFECTIONS PRESENTING WITH ACUTE ANTERIOR UVEITIS

Secondary Syphilis

This sexually transmitted infection commonly presents to the ophthalmologist. Patients develop a red eye and blurred vision a few weeks after the nonspecific illness often associated with a skin rash. A nonspecific panuveitis is present with granulomatous or nongranulomatous keratic precipitates. The vitritis may be associated with striking shiny retrohyaloid keratic precipitates. The optic disk is frequently swollen and despite good visual acuity and color vision an afferent pupillary defect may be noted. Diffuse retinal pigment epithelial abnormality can occur, and fluorescein angiography may highlight a pathognomonic picture of capillary leakage.

The diagnosis is made with routine serology, and this can be applied to ocular fluids. Treatment is with penicillin and systemic steroids to prevent the Herxheimer reaction and local steroids to treat the intraocular inflammation. Ocular prognosis is excellent. Patients should be jointly managed with genitourinary physicians to arrange antibiotic therapy, contact tracing, and screening for intercurrent infections.

Lyme Disease

This is a spirochaetal infection that results from tick-borne transmission of *Borrelia burgdorferi*. The disease is endemic where deer abound, such as Long Island Sound in the United States and the New Forest in the United Kingdom. Three stages of Lyme disease have been described: stage I, characterized by erythema chronicum migrans and flulike symptoms; stage II, characterized by dermatologic, ophthalmologic, neurologic, and cardiac disorders; and stage III, characterized by arthritis, a multiple sclerosis-like syndrome, psychiatric disorders, and a chronic fatigue syndrome. The ophthalmic disease may present with a nonspecific panuveitis and a special vitritis termed *spiderweb*, but more commonly there are neurophthalmological features that point to the diagnosis. These include oculomotor palsies and disk swelling associated with raised intracranial pressure. Therapy with penicillin or tetracycline hastens the resolution of stage I symptoms. Treatment

duration normally ranges between 10 days and 3 weeks. Tetracycline or doxycycline appears to be more effective than penicillin in preventing the development of late Lyme disease.

Cat Scratch

Bartonella is responsible for this condition where the eye often bears the brunt of the infection and the insult from the cat appears relatively minor. The patient develops a mild yet acute panuveitis, but the cardinal feature is a neuroretinitis with the characterisitic fundal appearance of a massively swollen optic disk and a macular star. The diagnosis is confirmed by serology, and conservative, symptomatic treatment is recommended for the majority of patients with mild or moderate cat scratch disease. For those with severe disease, antibiotic therapy is advised with the literature reporting good response to gentamicin and ciprofloxacin. The visual prognosis is good, although a minority of patients have permanent visual loss due to macular pathology.

HERPES VIRUSES

Herpes simplex is an important cause of keratitis and active corneal disease is frequently associated with anterior uveitis, which may be complicated by raised intraocular pressure. The diagnosis can be confirmed by polymerase chain reaction (PCR) of an aqueous sample. Treatment consists of local antiviral agents and mydriatics in addition to local steroids as long as these are covered with the antiviral agent.

Herpes zoster ophthalmicus results from involvement of the ophthalmic branch of the trigeminal nerve. Jonathan Hutchinson observed that vesicles on the tip of the nose indicated involvement of the nasociliary branch, and this correlated with the presence of intraocular inflammation that is a combination of a keratitis and anterior uveitis (Figure 13.1). This is usually mild but when associated with a vasculitis the results can be devastating and result in a blind and phthisical eye. Treatment is with local and systemic antiviral agents and local steroids and mydriatics as required. Frequent sequelae of even mild intraocular inflammation are iris atrophy, producing photophobia, and raised intraocular pressure.

ACUTE RETINAL NECROSIS

This is an ophthalmological syndrome characterized by anterior uveitis often associated with

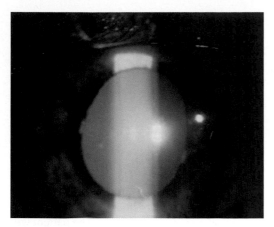

Figure 13.1 Irregular pupil and iris atrophy in a patient who has had herpes zoster anterior uveitis.

waxy, hexagonal, or spindly keratic precipitates, vitritis, and a necrotizing retinitis associated with predominantly retinal arteriolar sheathing that may lead to retinal ischaemia and then secondary neovascularization.

The particular pattern of both the anterior uveitis and the retinal findings are both extremely characteristic. This syndrome can be caused by either herpes simplex when the patients have often suffered with either recurrent cold sores or encephalitis in the past or herpes zoster when the patients are often older and apparently otherwise healthy. However, occasionally the syndrome can accompany active chickenpox or shingles. The patients present with a red eye due to the anterior uveitis. It is a situation when it is vital that the fundus is examined after pupil dilatation on presentation; otherwise, the diagnostic retinal signs may be missed as visual prognosis is poor and probably the only thing that improves it is early diagnosis and therefore treatment. The viral etiology is confirmed by PCR of the vitreous, and treatment is with systemic antivirals (usually given initially as intravenous acyclovir for 10 days and then oral preparation for 3 months) to prevent involvement of the other eye.

METASTATIC ENDOPHTHALMITIS

This is the term given to infection occurring in the eye secondary to systemic sepsis. These patients occasionally present to the ophthalmologist with a short history of a progressively painful red eye associated with rapidly deteriorating vision often with a story of no improvement following treatment with local steroids and mydriatics. Clues that should arouse suspicion of the underlying diagnosis for the ophthalmologist are the sudden presentation of a unilateral uveitis in an elderly patient who has never had uveitis before, particularly if diabetic. Pathogenic organisms range from meningococcus in children to *Staphylococcus*, *Escherichia coli*, *Streptococcus*, or *Klebsiella*; *Candida* is a potential pathogen in intravenous drug abusers and patients requiring intravenous treatment who are often in intensive care units. The most distinctive feature of the uveitis is that it is extremely severe, with the presence of a hypopyon, and often a view of the fundus is impossible (Figure 13.2).

The diagnosis is established by culture of any affected organ, eg, blood, skin, urine, and aqueous. Treatment is with systemic antibiotics and intracameral antibiotics, but visual prognosis is poor, at least in part because of a directly toxic affect of the bacteria on the retina. This condition not only has a terrible visual prognosis but also carries a systemic mortality and hence early diagnosis by the ophthalmologist is important. Unfortunately that is not always the case, and the average time between presentation and diagnosis is approximately 14 days.

PARAINFECTIOUS UVEITIS

An acute anterior uveitis may accompany or immediately follow certain viral infections, eg, adenovirus, influenza, mumps, and measles, and also *Campylobacter* infection, *Streptococcus*, or *Mycoplasma*. The uveitis is usually nongranulomatous and not associated with ocular complications and resolves quickly with local steroid and mydriatic.

INFECTIONS PRESENTING WITH CHRONIC UVEITIS
Tuberculosis

The most common ocular presentation of tuberculosis is anterior uveitis or choroiditis. The anterior uveitis is characteristically granulomatous often associated with posterior synechiae and cataract due to its chronicity. The incidence of uveitis in patients with active systemic tuberculosis is low, and a common scenario is the patient who presents with a chronic granulomatous uveitis, with no other systemic features of tuberculosis but a positive Mantoux test and a history of recent possible exposure. Diagnosis based on detection of mycobacterial DNA through PCR is becoming the method of choice, although further investigations are

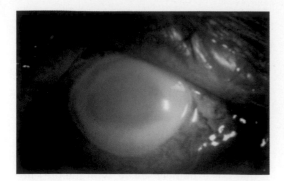

Figure 13.2 Severe anterior uveitis in a patient with klebsiella liver abscess and septicemia.

needed to determine the sensitivity and specificity of PCR and ELISA testing for tuberculosis in ocular tissues. Patients are usually treated with local steroids and mydriatics and a course of antituberculous therapy, usually in association with systemic steroids. Left untreated the inflammation can spread slowly to the ciliary body and sclera and eventually produce a panophthalmitis with consequent blindness. Patients with known tuberculosis may present with cold abscesses in the retina or choroidal tubercles depending on their immune response to the bacterium.

Brucellosis

Brucella is a very rare cause of uveitis and is a diagnosis that above all will never be made unless it is thought of. The bacterium infects the genitourinary tract of animals such as sheep and cows. Humans become infected by direct contact or by airborne spread after exposure to infected animals or contaminated meat or dairy products. Hence, countryfolk, farmers, and abattoir workers are particularly at risk of infection.

The pattern of uveitis that develops is indistinguishable from that of tuberculosis, producing a chronic granulomatous uveitis in the front and the back of the eye. There are several methods to make the diagnosis, including isolations of brucella from blood, body fluids, and bone marrow; agglutination test; and PCR. The standard treatment for brucellosis is a combination of doxycycline with rifampicin or gentamicin.

Leprosy

Leprosy affects 10 to 12 million people worldwide and around 5% of these are blind as the organism M. Leprae has a tropism for body parts with low temperature, including the eye. Intraocular inflammation more commonly occurs in lepromatous leprosy. Direct bacterial invasion of the external eye results in keratitis, scleritis, and iritis, and destruction of the autonomic nerve fibers result in a pinpoint pupil and a low grade iritis. Current treatment of leprosy involves use of three dugs: rifampicin, clofazimine, and dapsone.

Whipple's Disease

Whipple's disease is a rare cause of a chronic uveitis. The characterisitics of the uveitis are rather nonspecific and indolent. The patient will present with a very chronic nongranulomatous anterior uveitis as well as a persistent vitritis and little or no response to local or systemic steroids. Specific ocular features that can alert the ophthalmologist to the bizarre diagnosis are diffuse leakage from retinal capillaries on fluorescein angiography and subtle sheathing of both retinal arterioles and venules but not associated with capillary closure.

The diagnosis is confirmed on jejunal biopsy and treatment is with a long course of antibiotics. Unfortunately, the ocular inflammation can remain persistent.

UVEITIS IN PATIENTS WITH HUMAN IMMUNODEFICIENCY VIRUS OR IATROGENIC IMMUNOSUPPRESSION

Patients infected with HIV can present with a nongranulomatous uveitis as part of a seroconversion illness or merely associated with a high viral load, although in the latter circumstance the inflammation is predominantly in the vitreous.

These patients are particularly susceptible to some of the infections already discussed, particularly syphilis, tuberculosis, and herpes zoster, and the clinical manifestations may be altered by the additional immunosuppression so confirmation of the offending organism is always recommended. It is interesting that the presence of the HIV virus alone is not a risk factor for candida endophthalmitis and that for the eye to be involved additional intravenous access must be present.

Cytomegalovirus retinitis (CMVR) is seen in patients with a low CD4 count but is rarely associated with a significant uveitis, emphasizing the effectiveness of immune suppression that the HIV virus can produce. This is in contrast to the clinical presentation of patients who are iatrogenically immunosuppressed and develop

CMVR where a florid anterior uveitis with substantial keratic precipitates is seen and often a vitritis so severe that it precludes a good view of the fundus. Treatment of CMVR is with the appropriate antiviral agent, usually ganciclovir or foscarnet, but also restoration of the patients' immune response, either with antiretroviral therapy or reduction of immunosuppressive therapy.

SUGGESTED READING

Biswas J, Narain S, et al. Pattern of uveitis in a referral uveitis clinic in India. *Int Ophthalmol.* 1996-1997;20(4):223–228.

Corapi KM, White IM, et al. Strategies for primary and secondary prevention of Lyme disease. *Nat Clin Pract Rheumatol.* 2007;3(1):20–25.

Deriban G, Marth T. Current concepts of immunopathogenesis, diagnosis and therapy in Whipples disease. *Curr Med Chem.* 2006;13(24):2921–2926.

Donahue SP, et al. Intraocular candidaemia. *Ophthalmology.* 1994;101(7):1302–1309.

Doris JP, Saha K, et al. Ocular syphilis: the new epidemic. *Eye.* 2006; 20:703–705.

Goodwin SD, Sproat TT, Russell WL. Management of Lyme disease. *Clin Pharm.* 1990;9(3):192–205.

Jackson TL, Eykyn SJ, et al. Endogenous bacterial endophthalmitis: a 17-year prospective series and review of 267 reported cases. *Surv Ophthalmol.* 2003;48(4):403–423.

Kurup SK, Chan CC. Mycobacterium related ocular inflammatory disease: diagnosis and management. *Am Acad Med Singapore.* 2006;35:203–209.

Margileth AM. Antibiotic therapy for cat-scratch disease: clinical study of therapeutic outcome in 268 patients and review of the literature. *Pediatr Infect Dis J.* 1992;11(6):474–478.

Sakran W, Chazan B, et al. Brucellosis: clinical presentation, diagnosis, complications and therapeutic options.

Shaw IN, Christian M, et al. Effectiveness of multidrug therapy in multibacillary leprosy: a long term follow up of 34 multibacillary leprosy patients treated with multidrug regimens till skin smear negativity. *Lepr Rev.* 2003;74(2):141–147.

Thompson MJ, Albert DM. Ocular tuberculosis. *Arch Ophthalmol.* 2005;123:844–849.

14. Retinitis

Daniel M. Albert and Amol D. Kulkarni

CYTOMEGALOVIRUS RETINITIS

Cytomegalovirus (CMV) retinitis is the most common and clinically significant opportunistic ocular infection seen in immunocompromised patients, including those with acquired immune deficiency syndrome (AIDS). With the extensive use of highly active antiretroviral therapy (HAART) in human immunodeficiency virus (HIV)-positive patients, there has been a tremendous decrease in the incidence of CMV retinitis in these patients (23 per 10 000 HIV/ AIDS cases in the pre-HAART era to 8 per 10 000 HIV/AIDS cases in the post-HAART era).

The presentation of CMV retinitis may be unilateral or bilateral. The onset is insidious, and symptoms may include blurred vision, floaters, visual field defects, or other nonspecific visual complaints. Clinically, the various types of active chorioretinal lesions include (1) hemorrhagic pattern showing confluent area of full-thickness retinal necrosis with a yellow-white granular appearance and associated retinal hemorrhages, which has been referred to as a "pizza-pie" appearance (Figure 14.1); (2) "brush fire" pattern showing rapidly spreading zone of retinal necrosis with yellow-white margin; and (3) granular pattern showing areas of retinal atrophy amid white granular punctate lesions. In all of these, vitreous inflammation is minimal or absent. Visual loss may be profound if the macula or optic nerve (Figure 14.2) is involved. Without treatment, CMV retinitis will become bilateral in 80% of cases and eventually will result in blindness from retinal atrophy, retinal detachment, or optic nerve involvement.

In patients known to have HIV or to be immunosuppressed, the diagnosis of CMV retinitis is based on clinical examination and confirmed by positive blood cultures for CMV. In individuals not known to be HIV positive, the diagnosis is suspected based on clinical appearance, and an investigation of immune status is essential.

In an effort to halt its progression and improve visual outcome, CMV retinitis requires treatment with one of five currently available virostatic agents: ganciclovir, valganciclovir,

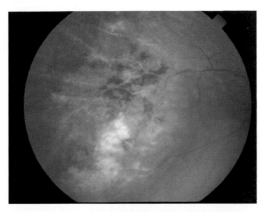

Figure 14.1 Photo of the peripheral fundus showing a yellow-white granular appearing area of retinal necrosis associated with retinal hemorrhages ("pizza-pie appearance"), representing an active chorioretinal lesion due to CMV retinitis.

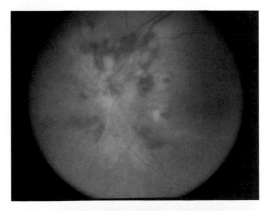

Figure 14.2 Fundus photo of the posterior pole showing swelling of the optic nerve head with peripapillary retinal necrosis and retinal hemorrhages, suggestive of optic nerve involvement with CMV retinitis.

foscarnet, cidofovir, and fomivirsen (Table 14.1). The choice of the antiviral agent and its route of delivery should be based on the location and extent of the infection, potential side effects, and the effectiveness of prior treatments.

Ganciclovir, an inhibitor of CMV DNA polymerase, may be administered intravenously, orally, or intravitreally. Intravenous (IV) ganciclovir should be used as induction therapy for 14 to 21 days, followed by maintenance

Table 14.1: Therapy for Retinitis

	Agent	Regimen	Side Effects
CMV retinitis	Ganciclovir	Induction of 5 mg/kg IV q12h for 14 to 21 days, then 5 mg/kg/d IV 7 d/wk or 6 mg/kg 5 d/wk 1000 mg PO three times daily as maintenance therapy	Granulocytopenia Thrombocytopenia Anemia
	Valaganciclovir	Induction dose of 900 mg twice daily PO for 14 to 21 days and maintenance dose of 900 mg once daily PO	Granulocytopenia Anemia
	Foscarnet	Induction of 60 mg/kg IV q8h for 14 to 21 days, then 90 to 120 mg/kg/d IV	Nephrotoxicity Electrolyte imbalance Seizures/headache
	Cidofovir	Induction of 3 to 5 mg/kg IV once per week for 2 weeks, then 3 mg/kg IV every 2 weeks as maintenance	Nephrotoxicity Neutropenia Uveitis
	Fomivirsen	Induction of 330-μg intravitreal injection weekly for 2 weeks, then 330-μg intravitreal injection every 4 weeks as maintenance	Uveitis Rise of intraocular pressure Visual field disturbance Retinal pigment epitheliopathy Bull's eye maculopathy
Ocular toxoplasmosis	Pyrimethamine	75 mg PO, then 25 mg PO daily for 4 to 6 weeks	Anemia Thrombocytopenia Leukopenia
	Sulfadiazine	2 g PO, then 1 g PO four times daily for 4 to 6 weeks	Stevens-Johnson syndrome Hypersensitivity reaction Crystalluria
	Clindamycin	300 mg PO four times daily for 4 to 6 weeks	Diarrhea Pseudomembranous colitis
Acute retinal necrosis	Acyclovir	500 mg/m^2 IV q8h for 7 to 10 days, then 800 mg PO five times daily for 6 to 12 weeks	Localized phlebitis Elevated serum creatinine

Abbreviations: CMV = cytomegalovirus; IV = intravenously; PO = orally.

therapy by either an IV or oral route. Because ganciclovir is virostatic, maintenance therapy is required indefinitely. The full dosage of ganciclovir cannot be tolerated and requires reduction in patients with impaired renal function. The most common side effect of ganciclovir is neutropenia, which arises in 20% to 40% of patients and is reversible on discontinuation of the drug. Because ganciclovir and zidovudine may result in granulocytopenia, the concomitant use of these two agents may result in pronounced bone marrow suppression.

The use of a sustained-release ganciclovir implant placed directly into the vitreous cavity of the eye protects against reactivation of CMV retinitis for up to 7 months. The intravitreal implant reduces intraocular recurrence of CMV retinitis and systemic side effects of ganciclovir, but it is not protective against involvement of the fellow eye or systemic CMV infection. Adverse effects associated with the ganciclovir implant include decreased vision in the postoperative period and an increased risk of retinal detachment.

Valganciclovir is a prodrug of ganciclovir and has good penetration into the vitreous cavity after oral administration. A positive response equivalent to ganciclovir given intravenously has been demonstrated with the use of oral induction therapy with valganciclovir. The adverse effects of the two drugs are similar.

Foscarnet, an inhibitor of DNA polymerase and reverse transcriptase, is administered intravenously for 14 to 21 days as induction therapy, followed by maintenance therapy indefinitely. The most common side effect of foscarnet is nephrotoxicity, which occurs in 25% of patients and is reversible with early cessation of the drug. Because foscarnet undergoes renal elimination and is nephrotoxic, careful monitoring of renal function is necessary. However, it is effective in the treatment of ganciclovir-resistant retinitis.

Cidofovir acts by inhibiting CMV DNA polymerase. It does not require virus-dependent phosphorylation for activation. The advantage of cidofovir over ganciclovir and foscarnet is that it requires less frequent IV administration: once weekly as induction for 2 weeks and once every 2 weeks for maintenance therapy thereafter. Nephrotoxicity is the most common dose-limiting side effect, which may be reduced with the concurrent administration of oral probenecid and IV hydration.

Fomivirsen, the newest agent available for the treatment of CMV retinitis, acts by interfering with CMV mRNA encoding. The mode of administration is intravitreal injection, and it is being used for CMV retinitis that is resistant to other antiviral agents. The various ocular toxic effects include uveitis, retinal pigment epitheliopathy, and bull's eye maculopathy.

The initial response to antiviral therapy usually occurs 1 to 2 weeks after the initiation of the induction regimen and is evident by termination of the growth of the retinal lesions and gradual atrophy of the involved retina. Ophthalmologists should examine patients' fundi every 2 to 3 weeks to monitor the effectiveness of the antiviral therapy. Recurrence of CMV retinitis occurs in 30% to 50% of patients receiving maintenance doses of systemic antiviral therapy. The treatment of recurring CMV retinitis is reinduction for 2 weeks followed by indefinite maintenance therapy. In the era of HAART therapy, HIV-positive patients with CMV retinitis having a sustained CD4$^+$ T-cell count greater than 100 cells/mL for 3 to 6 months can terminate maintenance therapy. However, maintenance therapy needs to be restarted if the immune status is compromised (CD4$^+$ T-cell count 50-100 cells/mL). Furthermore, these patients should undergo 3 to 6 monthly ophthalmic screenings, depending on the immune status.

The various surgical treatments that have been used in the management of CMV retinitis include laser photocoagulation and vitrectomy. Prophylactic laser photocoagulation surrounding areas of retinal necrosis has been shown to reduce the rate of retinal detachments. When retinal detachments develop, the standard approach for repair is vitrectomy surgery with silicone oil instillation.

OCULAR TOXOPLASMOSIS

Ocular toxoplasmosis, which accounts for 30% to 50% of all cases of posterior uveitis, is caused by the obligate intracellular parasite *Toxoplasma gondii*. Infection may be congenital through transplacental transmission or acquired through contact with cat excreta or by ingestion of oocysts from undercooked meat. Most cases of ocular toxoplasmosis occur as a result of reactivation of congenital ocular lesions.

Symptoms of active infection include blurred vision and vitreous floaters. Most commonly, ocular toxoplasmosis presents as a white-yellow area of focal necrotizing retinitis adjacent to an old atrophic chorioretinal scar (Figure 14.3). Vitreous inflammation typically is present over the area of active retinitis, and granulomatous iridocyclitis or optic nerve swelling may be present. The various complications associated with larger lesions include rhegmatogenous or exudative retinal detachment, macular edema, retinal vessel occlusions, subretinal neovascularization, and epiretinal membranes.

Not all active retinal lesions require treatment when present in immunocompetent

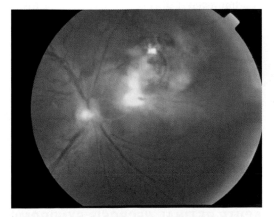

Figure 14.3 Fundus photo of the posterior pole showing an excavated atrophic chorioretinal scar and overlying epiretinal membrane in the macula consistent with resolved focal necrotizing chorioretinitis secondary to toxoplasmosis.

individuals. Small peripheral lesions, which often are self-limited and not visually threatening, can be observed. Without treatment, active lesions generally heal in 2 to 4 months. Medical therapy is indicated when the toxoplasma lesions involve or threaten the macula or optic nerve or when visually disabling vitreous inflammation is present.

The goal of treatment for ocular toxoplasmosis is to halt the infectious process and reduce scarring of the retina and vitreous. Traditional therapy consists of the concurrent use of two folate antagonists: sulfadiazine and pyrimethamine. Sulfadiazine is administered as a loading dose of 2 g orally, followed by 1 g four times daily for 4 to 6 weeks. Pyrimethamine is given as a loading dose of 75 mg followed by 25 mg orally per day for a similar duration. Pyrimethamine requires weekly complete blood counts and may be administered with leucovorin calcium, 5 mg orally twice weekly, to reduce the incidence of bone marrow suppression. Clindamycin, 300 mg orally four times daily for 4 to 6 weeks, has been suggested in combination with sulfadiazine and pyrimethamine for severe ocular toxoplasmosis infections. It has been shown to have high intraocular penetration and is also active against the cyst form. The other antibiotics that have been used include atovaquone, azithromycin, spiramycin, and tetracyclines.

Systemic corticosteroids should be administered when inflammation from the active toxoplasmosis lesions threaten the macula or optic nerve and when severe vitreous inflammation is present. Corticosteroids should never be used in the treatment of ocular toxoplasmosis without the concurrent use of antibiotic agents. Prednisone at a dosage of 60 to 80 mg/d is administered during the first week of treatment and rapidly tapered based on clinical response and patient tolerance.

The various regimens widely used for treatment of toxoplasmosis are as follows: (1) triple therapy consisting of pyrimethamine, sulfadiazine, and prednisone and (2) quadruple therapy consisting of pyrimethamine, sulfadiazine, clindamycin, and prednisone. A maintenance therapy with pyrimethamine/sulfadiazine is useful in severely immunocompromised patients. In the event of retinal detachment or vitreous opacification, vitrectomy surgery is performed.

ACUTE RETINAL NECROSIS SYNDROME

Acute retinal necrosis (ARN) is a necrotizing retinitis associated with infection by the varicella-zoster virus (VZV) or, less commonly,

the herpes simplex virus (HSV) types 1 and 2. Although initially described only in immunocompetent patients, recent cases have been reported in immunosuppressed individuals, including those with AIDS.

Clinically, ARN presents as patchy or confluent areas of white retinal necrosis in the far periphery (Figure 14.4), which may spread to the posterior pole rapidly within days. In addition, moderate to severe vitritis and occlusive retinal vasculitis (arteritis and phlebitis) are seen. Anterior uveitis, ischemic vasculopathy involving the optic nerve, and macular edema may be associated findings. The active phase of inflammation generally lasts several weeks and is followed by a convalescent phase. As many as 52% of patients with ARN may develop retinal breaks and subsequent rhegmatogenous retinal detachments. Retinal detachments may occur from 9 days to 5 months after the onset of retinitis.

The onset of ARN typically is unilateral, although bilateral involvement may occur in up to 30% of patients within several weeks of onset. The diagnosis of ARN is made based on the clinical findings, and polymerase chain reaction (PCR) analysis of vitreous samples for viral DNA is helpful in confirming the clinical impression.

The current standard of care for ARN includes IV acyclovir (1500 mg/m^2) administered in three divided doses daily for 7 to 10 days followed by oral acyclovir 800 mg five times daily for 4 to 6 weeks. The antiviral therapy is useful to suppress unilateral disease and reduce the risk of involvement of the fellow eye. The oral prodrugs valacyclovir and famciclovir, which have higher bioavailability than oral acyclovir, may be also considered. Systemic

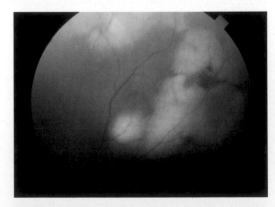

Figure 14.4 Photo of the peripheral fundus showing confluent white areas of retinal necrosis with occlusive retinal vasculitis and retinal hemorrhages, suggestive of acute retinal necrosis.

and periocular corticosteroids may be administered to reduce the tissue damage caused by the necrotizing intraocular inflammation but must be concomitant with antiviral therapy. A thorough search for retinal breaks is essential in the first 6 months, and prophylactic laser barrier photocoagulation should be performed within 3 weeks of onset of symptoms or at the earliest time possible. The barrier laser treatment consists of the application of confluent rows of argon laser burns posterior to the area of retinal necrosis and around retinal breaks. In spite of the intensive antiviral and anti-inflammatory therapy, visual impairment may occur due to vitreous hemorrhage secondary to retinal neovascularization or retinal detachment. In patients with vitreous hemorrhage or retinal detachment, vitreoretinal surgery with or without silicone oil tamponade has been shown to be of benefit.

SUGGESTED READING

Blumenkranz MS, et al. Treatment of acute retinal necrosis syndrome with intravenous acyclovir. *Ophthalmology* 1986;93:296–300.

Duker JS, Blumenkranz MS. Diagnosis and management of acute retinal necrosis syndrome. *Survey Ophthalmol.* 1991;35:327–343..

Hardy W. Management strategies for patients with cytomegalovirus retinitis. *J Acquir Immune Defic Syndr* 1997;14:S7–S14.

Jabs DA, Enger C, Bartlett JG. Cytomegalovirus retinitis and acquired immunodeficiency syndrome. *Arch Ophthalmol.* 1989;107:75–80.

Koo L, Young LH. Management of ocular toxoplasmosis. *Int Ophthalmol Clin.* 2006;46:183–193.

Lakhanpal V, Schocket SS, Nirankari VS. Clindamycin in the treatment of toxoplasmic retinochoroiditis. *Am J Ophthalmol.* 1983;95:605–613.

Lau CH, Missotten T, Salzmann J, Lightman SL. Acute retinal necrosis features, management, and outcomes. *Ophthalmology,* 2007;114(4):756–762.

Tamesis RR, Foster CS. Toxoplasmosis. In: Albert DM, Jakobiec FA, eds. *Principles and Practice of Ophthalmology,* vol 2. Philadelphia, PA: WB Saunders; 1994.

Wiegand TW, Young LH. Cytomegalovirus retinitis. *Int Ophthalmol Clin.* 2006;46(2):91–110.

Roy D. Brod and Harry W. Flynn, Jr.

INTRODUCTION

Endophthalmitis is a vision-threatening inflammation of the inner eye fluids and tissues. Infectious endophthalmitis results from either exogenous or endogenous entry of microbes into the eye. In reported clinical series, exogenous endophthalmitis is much more common than endogenous (or metastatic) endophthalmitis. By far, the most common cause of exogenous infection is intraocular surgery. Because cataract surgery is the most frequently performed type of intraocular surgery, it accounts for the greatest number of exogenous endophthalmitis cases. Exogenous endophthalmitis can also occur after other types of intraocular surgery, including secondary lens implantation, glaucoma filtering surgery, vitrectomy surgery, and corneal transplantation. Organisms may also enter the eye during penetrating trauma, intraocular injection of medication, and contiguous spread into the eye from an infected corneal ulcer. Gram-positive bacteria are the most common cause of exogenous endophthalmitis.

INCIDENCE

Postoperative endophthalmitis cases from the University of Miami (Bascom Palmer Eye Institute) over a 5-year period (January 2000 to December 2004) demonstrated the incidence of nosocomial endophthalmitis after cataract surgery to be 0.04%. Endophthalmitis occurs after penetrating trauma in 3% to 30% of patients depending on the nature of the injury. The rate of development of *Candida* endogenous endophthalmitis in patients with documented candidemia has been reported to range from 2.8% to 45%.

CLINICAL FEATURES

Endophthalmitis can be classified into the following general categories: (1) acute-onset postoperative endophthalmitis, (2) delayed-onset postoperative endophthalmitis, (3) conjunctival filtering bleb associated endophthalmitis, (4) posttraumatic endophthalmitis, (5) endogenous

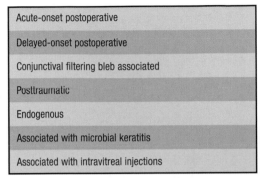

Table 15.1 Endophthalmitis Categories

| Acute-onset postoperative |
| Delayed-onset postoperative |
| Conjunctival filtering bleb associated |
| Posttraumatic |
| Endogenous |
| Associated with microbial keratitis |
| Associated with intravitreal injections |

endophthalmitis (metastatic), (6) endophthalmitis associated with microbial keratitis (corneal ulcer), and (7) endophthalmitis associated with intravitreal injections (Table 15.1). Each category has characteristic clinical features and often-predictable causative organisms.

Most cases of acute-onset endophthalmitis postcataract surgery present within 2 weeks of intraocular surgery (Figure 15.1). Symptoms may start as early as 12 hours after the surgery. The classic symptoms include visual loss and ocular pain in 75% of cases. The loss of vision is typically profound and is reduced out of proportion to the usual postoperative course. The presenting signs often include lid edema, conjunctival injection and swelling, conjunctival discharge, corneal edema, anterior chamber inflammation, fibrin formation, and vitreous inflammatory response. In most cases, a layer of inflammatory cells (hypopyon) can be visualized in the inferior portion of the anterior chamber (Figure 15.2). Redness and purulent discharge from the conjunctiva and lid margins are also commonly seen. A severe intraocular inflammatory response will often obscure a view of the posterior pole and may cause loss of the red reflex. In these cases echographic exam of the eye may be useful in ruling out posterior segment complications, such as retinal detachment and retained lens fragments.

In the Endophthalmitis Vitrectomy Study (EVS), the coagulase-negative staphylococci

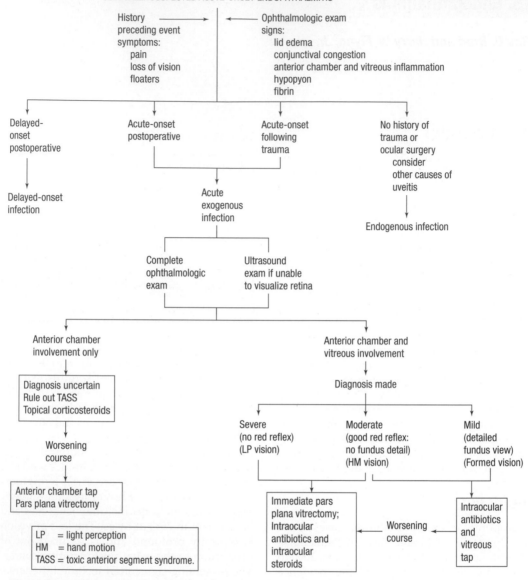

CLINICALLY SUSPECTED ACUTE-ONSET ENDOPHTHALMITIS

History
preceding event
symptoms:
   pain
   loss of vision
   floaters

Ophthalmologic exam
signs:
   lid edema
   conjunctival congestion
   anterior chamber and vitreous inflammation
   hypopyon
   fibrin

Delayed-onset postoperative

Acute-onset postoperative

Acute-onset following trauma

No history of trauma or ocular surgery
   consider other causes of uveitis

Delayed-onset infection

Acute exogenous infection

Endogenous infection

Complete ophthalmologic exam

Ultrasound exam if unable to visualize retina

Anterior chamber involvement only

Anterior chamber and vitreous involvement

Diagnosis made

Diagnosis uncertain
Rule out TASS
Topical corticosteroids

Severe
(no red reflex)
(LP vision)

Moderate
(good red reflex:
no fundus detail)
(HM vision)

Mild
(detailed
fundus view)
(Formed vision)

Worsening course

Anterior chamber tap
Pars plana vitrectomy

Immediate pars plana vitrectomy;
Intraocular antibiotics and intraocular steroids

Worsening course

Intraocular antibiotics and vitreous tap

LP   = light perception
HM = hand motion
TASS = toxic anterior segment syndrome.

Figure 15.1 Algorithm for management of acute-onset endophthalmitis.

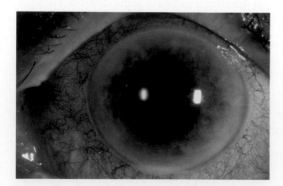

Figure 15.2 Hypoyon (layering of WBCs in the anterior chamber) in an eye with acute postcataract surgery endophthalmitis.

were the most commonly cultured organisms (68%) of the patients with confirmed growth. Other gram-positive organisms were cultured in 22% of patients and included *Streptococcus* and *Staphylococcus aureus*. Gram-negative organisms were isolated in 6% of the cases in the EVS and more than one species was confirmed in 4% of the cases. Fortunately, the coagulase-negative staphylococci are one of the least virulent causes of acute onset postoperative endophthalmitis. *Staphylococcus aureus*, *Streptococcus* species, and the gram-negative organisms usually produce a more rapidly progressive and fulminant inflammation often leading to severe vision loss.

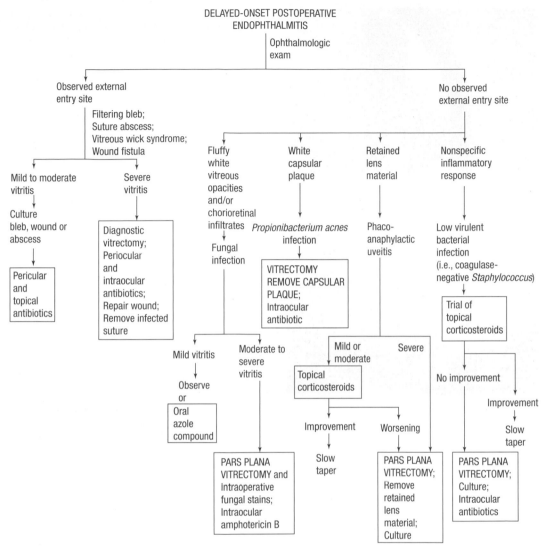

Figure 15.3 Algorithm for management of delayed-onset endophthalmitis.

Another subgroup of post cataract surgery endophthalmitis is the delayed-onset category (Figure 15.3). These patients present 6 weeks or more after cataract surgery with a slowly progressive, often milder, inflammatory response. The inflammation can be isolated to the anterior segment or involve both the anterior segment and vitreous. The intraocular inflammation may respond initially to topical steroid therapy but usually recurs as the topical steroids are tapered. A common cause of delayed-onset postoperative endophthalmitis is *Propionibacterium acnes*. This is a ubiquitous, gram-positive, nonspore-forming pleomorphic bacillus. Clinical features of intraocular infections caused by this organism include granulomatous inflammation with large keratitic precipitates (clumps of inflammatory cells)

on the corneal endothelium. A characteristic diagnostic feature is the presence of white intracapsular plaque, which has been shown to be composed of organisms mixed with residual lens cortex (Figure 15.4). Because *P. acnes* is a slow-growing anaerobic organism, it is important for the microbiology laboratory to be instructed to keep these anaerobic cultures for at least 2 weeks. Other organisms responsible for delayed-onset postoperative endophthalmitis include *Candida, Staphylococcus epidermidis*, and *Corynebacterium* species.

Delayed-onset endophthalmitis associated with conjunctival filtering blebs may present months or years after glaucoma filtering surgery. The organisms enter the eye directly through the thin wall of the conjunctival bleb, which may contain purulent material

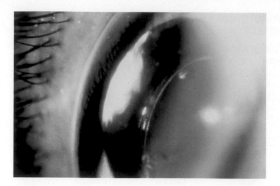

Figure 15.4 White capsular plaque in a patient with *Propionibacterium acnes* endophthalmitis.

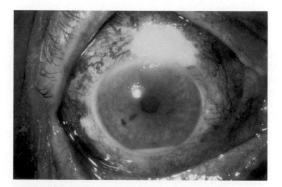

Figure 15.5 Purulent material in a filtering bleb in an eye with endophthalmitis 6 months following glaucoma filtering surgery.

(Figure 15.5). The presenting symptoms and signs are similar to acute-onset postoperative endophthalmitis. Streptococcal species are the most common organisms isolated. *Haemophilus influenza* is also a common cause of this category of endophthalmitis. Because these organisms are more virulent than those causing acute-onset postoperative endophthalmitis, the visual outcomes are generally worse. Optic nerve damage from the preexisting glaucoma may also be a factor in poor visual outcome. Less than half of the eyes achieve 20/400 or better vision. The treatment is similar to that for acute-onset postoperative endophthalmitis.

Endophthalmitis after penetrating trauma should be suspected whenever a greater than expected inflammatory response is observed. Because the organisms (eg, *Bacillus* species and *Streptococcus* species) causing posttraumatic endophthalmitis are, in general, more virulent than organisms causing postoperative endophthalmitis, the final visual outcome is often poor. The associated trauma to the eye and the frequent delay in diagnosis also contribute to a poor visual prognosis. A high index of suspicion and early diagnosis are important, because even traumatized eyes infected with virulent organisms can sometimes be salvaged when treatment is promptly initiated. Prophylactic antibiotic treatment from high-risk injuries (rural setting, injuries involving vegetable matter or soil, contaminated eating utensils, retained foreign bodies) should be administered. The management of posttraumatic endophthalmitis is similar to other endophthalmitis categories and often includes vitrectomy and intravitreal, subconjunctival, and topical antibiotics and steroids.

Endogenous endophthalmitis results from hematogenous spread of organisms to the eye. Fungi are a more common cause than bacteria and *Candida albicans* is the most common fungus isolated. The classic ocular finding is white vitreous opacities attached to each other by inflammatory vitreous bands in a configuration termed "string of pearls" (Figure 15.6). The second most frequently encountered fungus is *Aspergillus* species. *Streptococcus* species, *Staphylococcus aureus*, and *Bacillus* species are the most common cause of endogenous bacterial endophthalmitis. These patients are frequently debilitated or immunocompromised with indwelling catheters, although endogenous endophthalmitis can occur in drug abusers and rarely in otherwise healthy patients after dental procedures or childbirth. The infection may be caused by a transient bacteremia or fungemia in which case blood cultures may be negative. Sepsis with deep organ involvement may also be present. When the source of infection is not apparent, a systemic workup is indicated.

Endophthalmitis can occur from direct spread of organisms into the eye from an infected corneal ulcer (Figure 15.7). Factors predisposing to the development of endophthalmitis associated with microbial keratitis

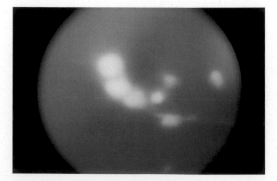

Figure 15.6 White inflammatory vitreous opacities in a "string of pearls" configuration in a patient with endogenous *Candida* endophthalmitis.

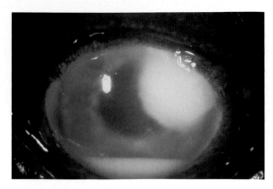

Figure 15.7 Infectious corneal ulcer associated with endophthalmitis.

include corticosteroid use, systemic immune dysfunction, as well as local ocular factors such as prolonged wear of contact lenses or contaminated lens solutions. Visual outcomes are poor due to the unusual and virulent nature of the infecting organisms.

Endophthalmitis may also occur following intravitreal injection of medications. The greater utilization of this route of therapy to treat various retinal diseases has increased the prevalence of this subgroup of endophthalmitis. Despite the growing number of intravitreal injections administered, endophthalmitis remains an uncommon complication. It has been reported most often after intravitreal injection of triamcinolone acetonide (IVTA) with the incidence ranging from 0.2% to 0.9% of injections. The clinical findings are similar to other forms of infectious endophthalmitis and include iritis, vitritis, hypopyon, pain, red eye, and decreased vision. The median time to presentation is 7.5 days. A sterile inflammatory uveitis may also occur after IVTA and must be distinguished from true infection. The noninfectious cases usually present earlier following the injection (median 1.5 days) and the external inflammatory signs such as redness and purulent discharge are usually less apparent. In addition, pain is much less common in noninfectious cases. Characteristics that may increase the risk of infection include immunosuppression, decreased ocular barrier function (presence of filtering bleb), multiuse triamcinolone acetonide bottles, and poor sterile techniques.

DIAGNOSIS

Two important factors in the diagnosis of endophthalmitis include the clinical recognition and microbiological confirmation. Endophthalmitis should be suspected in any eye that has a marked inflammatory response out of proportion to that usually seen in the typical clinical course. Because of the potential for significant visual loss, diagnostic tests are usually performed concurrently with treatment.

The clinical diagnosis is confirmed by obtaining aqueous fluid and vitreous specimens. Although vitreous specimens are more likely to yield a positive culture than simultaneously acquired aqueous specimens, both are important because either one can be positive without the other. Aqueous cultures are obtained by needle aspiration. Vitreous cultures can be obtained using needle aspiration or using an automated vitrectomy instrument, which simultaneously cuts and aspirates the vitreous. Vitreous obtained by needle aspiration can be directly inoculated onto appropriate culture media including chocolate agar, 5% blood sheep agar, thioglycollate broth, or Sabouraud agar. A specimen obtained during vitrectomy can be concentrated by filtration though a 0.45-μ filter, which is then placed on culture media. An alternative method for processing the vitrectomy specimen involves inoculating approximately 10 mL of the diluted vitrectomy specimen into standard blood culture bottles. The culture technique has been shown to yield a similar rate of culture positivity when compared with the traditional membrane filter technique. Gram stains are usually performed on aqueous and vitreous samples. In suspected fungal cases, additional information may be obtained using the Giemsa, Gomori's methenamine silver, and periodic acid-Schiff stains.

TREATMENT

Endophthalmitis can lead to rapid intraocular tissue destruction and irreparable damage. The mainstay of treatment for bacterial endophthalmitis is intraocular antibiotic therapy. The unique properties of the eye, including the fact that it is an enclosed cavity, as well as the presence of a blood ocular barrier, make intraocular injection of antibiotic an ideal way of achieving rapid and high antibiotic concentrations within the eye (Table 15.2).

Systemic antibiotics have traditionally been used to supplement intravitreous antibiotic injections in the management of endophthalmitis. The EVS randomized patients received ceftazidime and amikacin versus no systemic antibiotic therapy, but all patients received intravitreal antibiotics. The results of that study demonstrated there was no beneficial effect

Table 15.2 Treatment for Acute-Onset Postoperative Endophthalmitis

Route	Drug	Dose
Intravitreal	1. Vancomycin 2. Ceftazidime or Amikacin 3. Dexamethasone	1.0 mg/.1mL 2.25mg/.1mL 0.4mg/.1mL 0.4mg/.1m
Subconjunctival (optional)	1. Vancomycin 2. Ceftazidime 3. Dexamethasone	25 mg/.5mL 100 mg/.5mL 10 to 24 mg/1.0mL
Topical (optional)	1. Vancomycin and 2. Ceftazidime 3. Steroids and cycloplegics	50 mg/mL 100 mg/mL
Systemic (for more severe cases) (optional)	1. Vancomycin 2. Ceftazidime (or fourth generation quinolone for appropriate organism)	1.0 g IV q12h 1.0 g IV q12h

on final visual outcome or media clarity when these systemic antibiotics were used.

In addition to intravitreal antibiotics as the recommended treatment for suspected endophthalmitis, intravitreal dexamethasone (0.4 mg/0.1 mL) may also be used. Although both animal studies and small retrospective clinical trials have shown improved endophthalmitis treatment results when intravitreal steroids were combined with intravitreous antibiotic injection, definitive proof of the value of intravitreal steroids is not available. The EVS protocol did not utilize intravitreal steroids, but EVS patients were placed on oral prednisone (60 mg daily) for 5 to 10 days. In addition to intravitreal dexamethasone, we also recommend a 10 to 24 mg subconjunctival injection of dexamethasone at the time of initial treatment.

Vitrectomy surgery (Figures 15.1, 15.3 and 15.8) has traditionally been recommended for more severe cases of endophthalmitis (eg, initial visual acuity of light perception only and rapid-onset within 2 days of surgery, more severe intraocular inflammation). Theoretical advantages of vitrectomy include the rapid removal of infecting organisms, intraocular toxins, removal of vitreous opacities and membranes that may lead to traction retinal detachment, and more rapid clearing of the vitreous cavity. Vitrectomy also allows for collection of a greater volume of material for culture and the potential for enhanced distribution of intravitreal antibiotics. In both animal models of infectious endophthalmitis and in some retrospective studies, eyes treated with vitrectomy combined with intravitreal antibiotics had better results than eyes treated with intravitreal antibiotics alone.

The management of endogenous fungal endophthalmitis depends on the specific fungus isolated and the severity of infection (Figure 15.8). When a diagnosis of endogenous fungal endophthalmitis is suspected, a work-up to look for other organ involvement is recommended. This should usually be done in cooperation with an internist or infectious disease subspecialist. The use and type of systemic antifungal therapy depends on the presence or absence of systemic fungal infection. In suspected endogenous *Candida* endophthalmitis cases, the management approach is tailored to the clinical situation. When the infection is limited to the choroid and retina, systemic therapy alone may be adequate. Fluconazole or voriconazole may be used instead of amphotericin B as the systemic drug of choice for treating *Candida* endophthalmitis not associated with significant systemic involvement. Both fluconazole and voriconazole are systemically less toxic than amphotericin B and have better intraocular penetration. When moderate to severe vitreous involvement is present, a pars plana vitrectomy and intravitreal injection of amphotericin B (5–10 μg) is usually recommended. Intravitreal steroids may be injected simultaneously with intravitreal amphotericin.

Endogenous *Aspergillus* endophthalmitis more often occurs in immunocompromised patients, patients with *Aspergillus* endocarditis or pulmonary disease, or patients with a history of intravenous drug abuse. This organism has a propensity to involve the macular area resulting in macular abscess and a layering of white blood cells under the retina or internal limiting membrane (Figure 15.9). A combination of local ocular

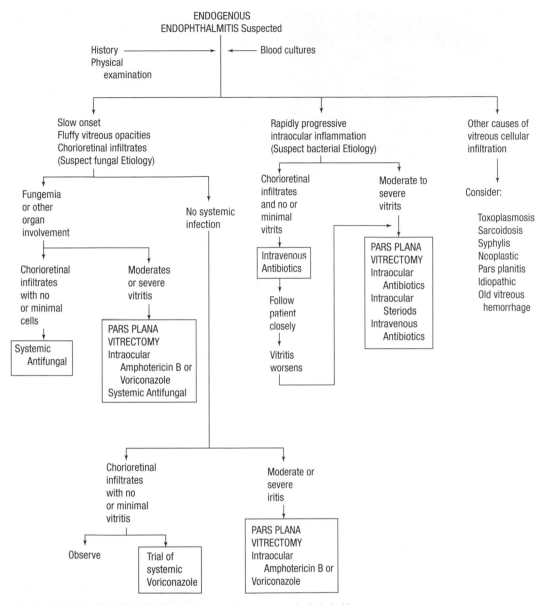

ENDOGENOUS
ENDOPHTHALMITIS Suspected

History → ← Blood cultures
Physical
examination

Slow onset
Fluffy vitreous opacities
Chorioretinal infiltrates
(Suspect fungal Etiology)

Rapidly progressive
intraocular inflammation
(Suspect bacterial Etiology)

Other causes of
vitreous cellular
infiltration

Fungemia
or other
organ
involvement

No systemic
infection

Chorioretinal
infiltrates
and no or
minimal
vitrits

Moderate to
severe
vitrits

Consider:

Toxoplasmosis
Sarcoidosis
Syphylis
Ncoplastic
Pars planitis
Idiopathic
Old vitreous
hemorrhage

Chorioretinal
infiltrates
with no
or minimal
cells

Moderates
or severe
vitritis

Intravenous
Antibiotics

PARS PLANA
VITRECTOMY
Intraocular
Antibiotics
Intraocular
Steriods
Intravenous
Antibiotics

Systemic
Antifungal

PARS PLANA
VITRECTOMY
Intraocular
Amphotericin B or
Voriconazole
Systemic Antifungal

Follow
patient
closely

Vitritis
worsens

Chorioretinal
infiltrates
with no
or minimal
vitritis

Moderate or
severe
iritis

Observe

Trial of
systemic
Voriconazole

PARS PLANA
VITRECTOMY
Intraocular
Amphotericin B or
Voriconazole

Figure 15.8 Algorithm for management of endogenous endophthalmitis.

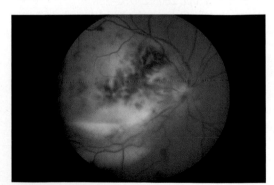

Figure 15.9 Macular abscess with a pseudohypopyon caused by endogenous *Aspergillus* infection.

therapy and systemic antifungal therapy (amphotericin B or voriconazole) is often recommended for treatment of this virulent organism.

PREVENTION

Because the ocular surface and adnexa are the primary sources of bacteria in exogenous endophthalmitis cases, the rate of postoperative endophthalmitis could theoretically be reduced by minimizing the ocular surface flora. The administration of topical 5% povidone-iodine solution to the conjunctival surface significantly reduces the conjunctival bacterial colony count. Reduction of conjunctival organisms may also

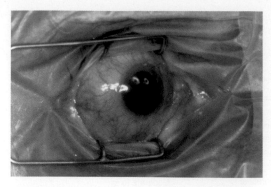

Figure 15.10 Eye undergoing surgery demonstrating plastic drape covering eyelid margin.

be enhanced with the addition of 3 days of topically applied, broad-spectrum antibiotics. Additional preventive measures include covering the eyelashes completely with a sterile plastic drape (Figure 15.10), meticulous surgical technique, including careful wound closure, and aseptic technique. Minimizing excessive pooling of fluid around the wound may also be helpful.

The role of prophylactic antibiotics added to the irrigating solution during the surgery is controversial. A multicentered European study demonstrated a significant reduction in the risk of developing endophthalmitis after cataract surgery when intracameral cefuroxime was administered at the time of surgery. In the EVS, 10 enrolled patients with endophthalmitis had a history of receiving intraocular antibiotics in the irrigating fluid during the cataract surgery. In addition, the potential for intraocular toxicity and development of resistant organisms limit the potential value of this method of prophylaxis. Postoperative periocular antibiotic injections are commonly used, but again are unproven in reducing the incidence of postoperative endophthalmitis.

SUGGESTED READING

Brod RD, Flynn HW Jr, Miller D. Endophthalmitis management. In: Spaeth G. ed. *Ophthalmic Surgery: Principles and Practice.* Philadelphia, PA: Lippincott; 2002.

Durand ML, Kim IK, D'Amico DJ, et al. Successful treatment of Fusarium endophthalmitis with voriconazole Aspergillus endophthalmitis with voriconazole and caspofungin. *Am J Ophthalmol.* 205;140: 552–554.

Endophthalmitis Vitrectomy Study Group. Results of the Endophthalmitis Vitrectomy Study: a randomized trial of immediate vitrectomy and of intravenous antibiotics for the treatment of postoperative bacterial endophthalmitis. *Arch Ophthalmol.* 1995; 113: 1479–1496.

Josephberg RG. Endophthalmitis: The latest in current management. *Retina.* 2006;26(suppl):47–50.

Miller JT, Scott IU, Flynn HW Jr, et al. Acute-onset endophthalmitis after cataract surgery (2000-2004): incidence, clinical settings, and visual outcomes after treatment. *Am J Ophthalmol.* 2005; 139:983–987.

Rosenberg KD, Flynn HW Jr, Alfonso EC, et al. Fusarium endophthalmitis following keratitis associated with contact lenses. *Ophthalmic Surg Lasers.* Imaging. 2006;37:310–313.

Schiedler V, Scott IU, Flynn HW Jr., et al. Culture-proven endogenous endophthalmitis: clinical features and visual outcomes. *Am J Ophthalmol.* 2004;137:725–731.

Seal BP, Gettinby G, Lees F, et al. ESCRS Endophthalmitis Study Group. ESCRS study of prophylaxis of postoperative endophthalmitis after cataract surgery: preliminary report of principal results from a European multicenter study. *J Cataract Refract Surg.* 2006;32:407–410.

Smiddy WE, Smiddy RJ, BA'Arath B, et al. Subconjunctival antibiotics in the treatment of endophthalmitis managed without vitrectomy. *Retina.* 2005;25:751–758.

Westfall AC, Osborn A, Kuhl D, et al. Acute endophthalmitis incidence: intravitreal triamcinolone. *Arch Ophthalmol.* 2005;123: 1075–1077.

16. Periocular Infections

Marlene L. Durand

Periocular infections are infections of the soft tissue surrounding the globe of the eye. These include infections of the eyelids, lacrimal system, and orbit. These are often managed by ophthalmologists with oculoplastics expertise; orbital infections are usually managed in conjunction with otolaryngologists and infectious disease physicians.

EYELID INFECTIONS

Each eyelid contains a fibrous tarsal plate that gives structure to the lid. Within each tarsal plate are 20 to 25 vertical meibomian glands that secrete sebum at the lid margins. Glands of Zeis, smaller sebaceous glands adjacent to the lid margin hair follicles, also secrete sebum. Sebum prevents ocular surface drying by keeping the tear film from evaporating too quickly.

Hordeolum

An internal hordeolum is an acute infection of a meibomian gland. Patients present with a tender area of swelling and erythema within the lid, pointing either to the skin or conjunctival surface. An external hordeolum (or stye) is an acute infection of a gland of Zeis and points to the lid margin. Both are usually caused by *Staphylococcus aureus* and respond to frequent warm compresses and topical bacitracin or erythromycin ointment.

Chalazion

A chalazion is a nontender nodule within the lid that points to the conjunctival surface and is due to a sterile granulomatous reaction to inspissated sebum within a meibomian gland. Most chalazia resolve spontaneously within 1 month, but persistent or recurrent chalazia should be biopsied to exclude squamous cell carcinoma.

Marginal Blepharitis

Marginal blepharitis is a diffuse inflammation of the lid margins and is usually due to hypersecretion of meibomian glands, although superinfection with *S. aureus* may play a role. The blepharitis is often recurrent and associated with seborrheic dermatitis or rosacea. It may be treated with gentle lid scrubs and topical bacitracin; oral tetracycline may be helpful if there is associated rosacea.

INFECTIONS OF THE LACRIMAL SYSTEM

Tears are mainly produced by the lacrimal gland, which is located beneath the upper outer rim of orbit. Tears flow medially across the eye, collect via the puncta, canaliculi, lacrimal sac, and lacrimal duct and drain into the nose beneath the inferior nasal turbinate. The only visible portions of the lacrimal system are the puncta and occasionally the lower portion of the lacrimal gland.

Dacryocystitis, or infection of the lacrimal sac, is the most common infection of the lacrimal system. It results from obstruction of the lacrimal duct and secondary infection of the pooled tears in the lacrimal sac. Patients often give a history of chronic tearing (epiphora) in the involved eye prior to presentation with acute dacryocystitis. Acute dacryocystitis presents as a painful, red swelling near the nasal corner of the eye. The most common bacteria involved are *S. aureus* and streptococci, although gram-negatives such as *Escherichia coli* may occasionally be present. Treatment often requires intravenous antibiotics (such as ampicillin-sulbactam) and incision and drainage. A dacryocystorhinostomy may be needed to treat the underlying chronic duct obstruction when the acute infection has subsided.

Dacryoadenitis, or infection of the lacrimal gland, is uncommon. Acute infection is most often due to *S. aureus* or streptococci and is treated with systemic antibiotics such as nafcillin.

Canaliculitis is usually a chronic infection of the canaliculi due to *Actinomyces israelii*, which forms concretions ("sulfur granules"). Treatment is usually office curettage of the concretions. See also Chapter 9, Infection of the Salivary and Lacrimal Glands.

PERIORBITAL INFECTIONS

The term *periorbital cellulitis* is commonly used but is imprecise, as it does not distinguish between preseptal cellulitis and orbital cellulitis. The term *orbital cellulitis* is often used to include subperiosteal and orbital abscesses as well as orbital cellulitis. The barrier between the preseptal and orbital soft tissues is the orbital septum, a fibrous membrane that arises from the periosteum of the orbital rim and extends to the tarsal plates of the lids. The distinction between preseptal and orbital infections is important, as preseptal infections are not vision threatening and almost never extend deeper, whereas orbital infections may rapidly cause vision loss. The distinction may be made clinically, as orbital infections have at least one of the following: proptosis, limitation of extraocular movement, or vision loss. Preseptal infections have none of these signs (See Table 16.1). Both preseptal and orbital cellulitis occur more often in children than in adults. Sinusitis is the etiology of 80% to 90% of these infections in any age group. The ethmoid sinus is the source of most infections, as it is separated from the orbit by the "paper-thin" bone, the lamina papyracea.

Preseptal cellulitis is similar to facial cellulitis, and is an infection of the superficial lid skin and preseptal soft tissues. It presents as unilateral redness and swelling of the eyelids, but with normal vision and extraocular movements. There is no proptosis. The etiology is ethmoid sinusitis in most cases. The bacterial etiology of the cellulitis is unknown but presumed to reflect the common causes of acute sinusitis, *Streptococcus pneumoniae* and *Haemophilus influenzae*, in addition to *S. aureus*. Some cases of preseptal cellulitis are due to superinfection of a break in the lid skin (eg, insect bite, rash, and abrasion), and these cases are usually caused by *S. aureus* or group A streptococci. Methicillin-resistant *S. aureus* (MRSA) should also be considered in areas where this organism is prevelant. A third etiology of preseptal cellulitis is bacteremic seeding. This is now very rare, although it was more common in the pre-Hib vaccine era when most cases were due to *H. influenzae* bacteremia. The entity is seen only in young children, usually younger than age 3, and is now caused by *S. pneumoniae*, group A streptococci, other streptococci, or occasionally by nontypable *H. influenzae*. These children should be hospitalized for treatment with intravenous antibiotics directed against the cause of the bacteremia.

Orbital cellulitis is an infection of the soft tissues of the orbit. Patients present with unilateral eyelid swelling and erythema, eye pain, and some degree of ophthalmoplegia or proptosis or both. There is often pain with eye movement. The proptosis may not be obvious and should be measured with a Hertel's exophthalmometer. A difference of 2 mm or more between the eyes signifies proptosis. Vision may be decreased, and there may be an afferent pupillary defect. Fever and leukocytosis are usually present in pediatric cases but may be absent in adults. Nearly all cases of orbital cellulitis in children and most in adults are caused by sinusitis, and many patients give a history of recent sinusitis symptoms. Occasional cases in adults are caused by extension of infection from acute dacryoadenitis, dacryocystitis, endophthalmitis, or penetrating orbital trauma. Diagnosis of orbital cellulitis is by physical examination and computed tomography (CT) scan of the orbit. The CT scan shows inflammation in the orbital soft tissues (eg, fat "stranding") but no abscess. Treatment is with intravenous broad-spectrum antibiotics directed against *S. aureus*, streptococci, anaerobes, and *H. influenzae*. Sinus drainage surgery is occasionally necessary as well.

Orbital subperiosteal abscess presents like orbital cellulitis, although symptoms are usually more severe. Because the ethmoid sinus is the source of infection in nearly all cases, the purulent collection is usually beneath the medial orbital periosteum. The periosteum bulges into the orbit, limiting medial rectus movement and causing the eye to look "down and out." Orbital CT scan demonstrates the collection. Nearly all cases in older children and adults require immediate surgical drainage of the abscess in addition to intravenous antibiotics. The need for immediate drainage surgery in children younger than 9 with normal vision is controversial, and some authors argue that they may be observed initially on intravenous antibiotics alone. Broad-spectrum antibiotics (eg, vancomycin, metronidazole, and ceftriaxone) are needed initially in all cases until culture results are available. Most cases are caused by a mixture of anaerobes and aerobes, with aerobes including one or more of the following: *S. aureus*, *Streptococcus anginosis (milleri)* group, group A streptococci, *H. influenzae*, *Moraxella catarrhalis*.

Orbital abscess has clinical and microbiologic features identical to those of orbital subperiosteal abscess. The abscess is usually medial or superomedial in the orbit, so the eye typically looks in the "down and out" direction, as in subperiosteal abscess. An orbital CT scan

Table 16.1 Preseptal Cellulitis and Bacterial Orbital Infections: Typical Signs and Etiologies (see text for exceptions).

	Lid Erythema and Edema	Limitation of EOM	Proptosis[a]	Decreased Vision	Usual Etiology
Preseptal cellulitis	+ to +++	0	0	0	Sinusitis[b], break in lid skin, bacteremia (only in young children, rare)
Orbital cellulitis	+++	+ to ++	+ to ++	0 to ++	Sinusitis[b]
Orbital abscess	+++	+++	+++	0 to +++	Sinusitis[b]
Subperiosteal abscess	+++	+++	+++	0 to +++	Sinusitis[b]
CST[c]	Bilateral	Bilateral	Bilateral	Often bilateral	Infection in "danger triangle"

Abbreviations: CST = cavernous sinus thrombophlebitis. EOM = extraocular movement.
[a] Proptosis = at least 2 mm difference as measured by Hertel's exophthalmometer.
[b] Usually ethmoid sinusitis.

reveals the collection, and treatment is immediate surgical drainage and broad-spectrum intravenous antibiotics. Delay in drainage of the abscess may lead to permanent loss of vision.

Cavernous sinus thrombophlebitis is a very rare complication of orbital infections or of other infections in the midface "danger triangle." The two cavernous sinuses are venous plexuses that are connected by intercavernous sinuses; involvement of one sinus can rapidly spread to the opposite side. Cranial nerves III through VI run through the cavernous sinus (Figure 16.1), and symptoms of cavernous sinus thrombosis are related to involvement of these nerves and are typically bilateral, as infection spreads to the opposite cavernous sinus. Patients with orbital cellulitis who then develop hypesthesia of forehead and cheek (cranial nerve V branches V1 and V2) and findings of orbital cellulitis in the opposite eye should be suspected of having cavernous sinus thrombophlebitis. Patients are usually febrile, complain of headache, and appear very ill (Figure 16.2). Diagnosis is by magnetic resonance imaging (MRI) and MRV. The most common bacterial etiology is *S. aureus*, but streptococci, anaerobes, and gram-negative bacilli may be present depending on the origin of infection. Treatment is with broad-spectrum intravenous antibiotics. The value of anticoagulation is unknown (see also Chapter 76, Intracranial Suppuration).

Invasive fungal infections, due to mucormycosis or aspergillosis, may mimic bacterial

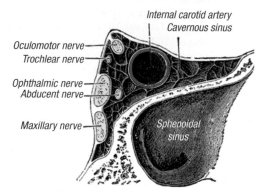

Figure 16.1 Oblique section through the cavernous sinus. (Figure from www.bartelby.com)

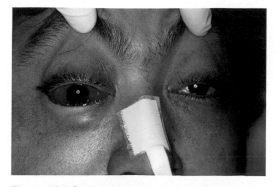

Figure 16.2 Septic cavernous sinus thrombosis; note palpebral edema, exophthalmos, and chemosis. (With permission of Arq. Neuro-Psiquiatr. vol.57 n.3A, São Paulo Sept. 1999, Trombose Séptica do Seio Cavernoso)

orbital cellulitis and/or bacterial cavernous sinus thrombophlebitis. Mucormycosis should be suspected in any patient with appropriate risk factors who presents with symptoms and signs of orbital cellulitis. Risk factors include diabetes (70% of cases), hematologic malignancies, immunosuppression (eg, organ transplant and chronic corticosteroid use), or deferoxamine therapy. Patients with orbital cellulitis due to mucormycosis present with ophthalmoplegia, proptosis, and lid edema. In contrast with bacterial orbital cellulitis, lid erythema and eye pain may be less prominent, whereas pain located outside the orbit (eg, temple and forehead) may be present. Hypesthesia of the cheek and forehead may be seen in mucormycosis and signifies involvement of the first and second divisions of cranial nerve V. Aspergillus infections of the orbit and cavernous sinus usually arise from invasive sphenoid sinus aspergillosis. Patients may present subacutely, with gradual onset of proptosis, ophthalmoplegia, and visual loss and with minimal lid swelling and erythema. The orbital apex may be involved first, leading to an orbital apex syndrome. The optic nerve and cranial nerves III, IV, VI, and V1 run through the orbital apex, so patients with this syndrome present with unilateral blindness, ptosis, proptosis, a fixed dilated pupil, and ophthalmoplegia.

SUGGESTED READING

Ambati BK, Ambati J, Azar N, et al. Periorbital and orbital cellulitis before and after the advent of *Haemophilus influenzae* type B vaccination. *Ophthalmology*. 2000;107:1450–1453.

Bhattia K, Jones NS. Septic cavernous sinus thrombosis secondary to sinusitis: are anticoagulants indicated? A review of the literature. *J Laryngol Otol*. 2002;116:667–676.

Boruchoff SA, Boruchoff SE. Infections of the lacrimal system. *Infect Dis Clin North Am*. 1992;6:925–932.

Colson AE, Daily JP. Orbital apex syndrome and cavernous sinus thrombosis due to infection with *Staphylococcus aureus* and *Pseudomonas aeruginosa*. *Clin Infect Dis*. 1999;29:701–702.

Donahue SP, Schwartz G. Preseptal and orbital cellulitis in childhood: a changing microbiologic spectrum. *Ophthalmology*. 1998;105:1902–1905.

Ferguson MP, McNab AA. Current treatment and outcome in orbital cellulitis. *Austr N Z J Ophthalmol*. 1999;27:375–379.

Harris GJ. Subperiosteal abscess of the orbit: age as a factor in the bacteriology and response to treatment. *Ophthalmology*. 1994;101:585–595.

Hartikainen J, Lehtonene OP, Saari KM. Bacteriology of lacrimal duct obstruction in adults. *Br J Ophthalmol*. 1997;81:37–40.

Patt BS, Manning SC. Blindness resulting from orbital complications of sinusitis. *Otolaryngol Head Neck Surg*. 1991;104:789–795.

Younis RT, Anand VK, Davidson B. The role of computed tomography and magnetic resonance imaging in patients with sinusitis with complications. *Larnygoscope*. 2002;112:224–229.

PART IV

Clinical Syndromes –
Skin and Lymph Nodes

17. Fever and Rash

John W. Sensakovic and Leon G. Smith

Patients presenting with fever and rash are one of the common symptom complexes presenting in medical practice. Because of the wide range of diseases that can present with this complex, the patient presenting with fever and rash is also one of the most challenging clinical syndromes.

Although both infectious and noninfectious disease processes can present with fever and rash, infectious causes are considered here. Nevertheless, noninfectious causes such as drug reactions, systemic vasculitis, serum sickness, erythema multiforme, toxic epidermal necrolysis, and Sweet's syndrome are often in the differential diagnosis.

The approach to the patient with infectious fever and rash should begin with the appreciation that causes include common infections that are often benign, serious emergent infections that can be rapidly fatal, and unusual infections that can pose a diagnostic challenge. Key features in the history and physical can be particularly important. These include childhood diseases and immunization history, seasonal diseases, travel history and geography, exposure, sexual history, and medication usage, as well as prodromal and accompanying symptoms. Physical examination, with particular attention to the characteristics of the rash, can be key, along with vital signs to assess severity of the illness, and particular attention to meningeal signs, lymph nodes, mucus membranes, conjunctiva, and joint examination.

When faced with the patient with fever and rash, the physician must be acutely aware of those several very serious infections that are commonly fulminant and that can be rapidly fatal. Thus, the physician must quickly address a series of important issues simultaneously (Table 17.1). These include the question of contagious potential to the medical staff, the need for rapid resuscitation in those patients who can present in shock, the rapid recognition of and therapeutic intervention for those infections that tend to be fulminant, and the need for a thorough evaluation and work-up for the extensive list of diagnostic possibilities that can present with fever and rash.

EMERGENT CONDITIONS PRESENTING WITH FEVER AND RASH

Rapid recognition and therapeutic intervention are essential in certain diseases presenting with fever and rash to minimize as much as possible the associated morbidity and mortality. The major conditions involved include meningococcemia, Rocky Mountain spotted fever, staphylococcal toxic shock syndrome, streptococcal toxic shocklike syndrome, bacteremia or endocarditis with septic emboli, and the rapidly spreading cellulitis (Tables 17.2 and 17.3). All of these conditions can present with fever and rash in a fulminant, rapidly progressive form, requiring expedient therapeutic intervention, often on an empiric basis, before confirmation of the diagnosis, if the associated mortality rates are to be minimized.

Generally, the most serious and rapidly progressive of these are associated with a petechial rash. These 1- to 2-mm purple lesions do not blanch with pressure, often coalesce to form larger ecchymotic areas, and usually are in the presence of leukocytosis and thrombocytopenia. Meningococcemia, Rocky Mountain spotted fever, and bacteremia/endocarditis with septic emboli are perhaps the most notable. However, other causes include gonococcemia, typhus, and rat-bite fever; viral infection, including dengue, hepatitis B, rubella, and Epstein-Barr virus (EBV); and noninfectious causes, including thrombotic thrombocytopenia purpura, Henoch-Schönlein purpura, vasculitis, and scurvy.

Rapidly progressive diseases with erythematous rash include staphylococcal toxic shock syndrome and streptococcal toxic shocklike syndrome, as well as the rapidly progressive cellulitis, which often have a vesicobullous component.

MENINGOCOCCEMIA

Of all the diseases presenting with fever and rash, meningococcemia is the one most likely to be rapidly fatal without early recognition and treatment. The ominous palpable purpura

Table 17.1 Major Issues in Patients with Fever and Rash

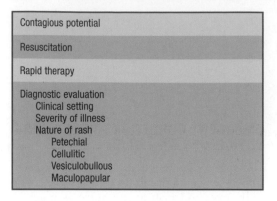

Contagious potential
Resuscitation
Rapid therapy
Diagnostic evaluation
Clinical setting
Severity of illness
Nature of rash
Petechial
Cellulitic
Vesiculobullous
Maculopapular

in an acutely ill, febrile patient characteristically suggests this disease. Other features that may be helpful in earlier diagnosis include sore throat, fever, muscle tenderness, and headache in the presence of significant leukocytosis and thrombocytopenia. The illness tends to occur in late winter and early spring and is well known to occur under crowded living conditions. The initial rash may be maculopapular, with the earliest petechial lesions occurring over pressure points such as the small of the back, and can easily be overlooked. The rash can progress rapidly over a few hours to the more classic, petechial form with peripheral acrocyanosis. Management requires immediate recognition, vigorous fluid replacement, and rapid therapy with aqueous penicillin, 12 to 24 million units daily intravenously (IV). Patients presenting with signs of adrenal insufficiency also require steroid replacement. The use of γ-globulin is controversial for patients with meningitis. Dexamethasone for 2 days started just before or with the first dose of antibiotics is indicated.

ROCKY MOUNTAIN SPOTTED FEVER

Rocky Mountain spotted fever can also present with fever and petechial rash in an acutely ill patient, yet is different from meningococcemia in several respects. The illness begins with fever and severe headache, occurs between May and September in temperate-zone states, and there is a history of tick exposure in 75% of the cases. The rash appears several days into the illness, begins as a maculopapular rash on wrists and ankles, and progresses to a petechial form and spreads to palms, soles, and trunk. A leukocytosis with thrombocytopenia is commonly present. Therapy is doxycycline, 100 mg every 12 hours, and must be instituted early on

a presumptive basis, before serologic confirmation, if mortality is to be significantly reduced. Alternative therapy is with chloramphenicol, 50 mg/kg/d IV. In institutions where available, immunofluorescence staining of a skin biopsy specimen of the rash can yield a rapid diagnosis. A review from Duke University Medical Center cited 10 cases of illness without rash or with fleeting atypical skin eruptions, emphasizing the need for a high index of suspicion in acutely ill patients.

TOXIC SHOCK SYNDROME

Toxic shock syndrome caused by the pyrogenic exotoxin of phage group 1 *Staphylococcus aureus* classically presented in a young menstruating female using a tampon. However, cases have also occurred as a result of nonvaginal foci of staphylococcal infection, including surgical wound infections and infectious endocarditis. The rash tends to be diffuse and scarlatiniform in character, with associated conjunctival hyperemia and a "strawberry tongue." The rash is associated with fever, hypotension, and evidence of multisystem derangement. Therapy requires vigorous fluid replacement, removal of the infected tampon or drainage of an identified infected focus, and nafcillin or oxacillin at 8 to 12 g/d. Some experts also recommend vaginal lavage with a betadine solution as a local antibacterial agent as well as for removal of any nonabsorbed exotoxin.

Staphlococcal scalded skin syndrome can be seen in young children infected with a staphylococcal strain producing epidermolysin A or B. The result is a superficial sloughing of the skin with a painful erythema. Nikolsky's sign, "onion skin" peeling of the skin with gentle pressure is seen.

A somewhat similar noninfectious entity, toxic epidermal necrolysis, is seen in adults. This typically is drug induced, and the sloughing of the skin occurs deeper, at the dermal-epidermal junction.

GROUP A STREPTOCOCCAL TOXIC SHOCKLIKE SYNDROME

The changing epidemiology of group A streptococcal infections has been recognized as a resurgence in rheumatic fever and an increase in the frequency of invasive infections and bacteremia. In addition, the group A streptococcal toxic shocklike syndrome has been recently defined by its characteristic early onset of shock and multiorgan failure in the presence of group

Table 17.2 Approach to Seriously Ill Patients with Fever and Rash

Clues	Disease	Diagnosis
Multiple purpuric lesions Earliest lesions small of back Rapid progression over hours	Meningococcemia	Gram stain of pustules Blood cultures
Tick exposure headache, fever, rash 2nd–6th days Wrists, ankles, progressing to palms, soles, trunk	Rocky Mountain spotted fever	DFA of skin biopsy Serology (CF)
Fever, rash, hypotension, menstruating female using tampons Surgical wound or skin infection	Toxic shock syndrome	Isolation of phage group I staphylococci
Fever, rash, hypotension, rapid onset of organ dysfunction	Group A streptococcal toxic shocklike syndrome	Evidence of group A streptococcal infection
Elderly or immunocompromised patient Several lesions, macular to necrotic pustules	Bacteremia with septic emboli	Gram stain of pustules Blood cultures Gram stain of buffy coat
Painful spreading lesions Local trauma	Rapidly spreading cellulitis	Clinical

Table 17.3 Characteristics of Serious Rashes

Onset with or after fever
Petechial lesions
Rapid spread
Purpuric lesions
Palmar/plantar involvement

A streptococcal infection, often with a generalized erythematous rash that may desquamate. Most of the isolates produce pyrogenic exotoxin A, and some cases have been associated with necrotic soft-tissue infections.

Septic Emboli

The diagnosis of septic emboli associated with bacterial bloodstream infection must be considered in any seriously ill patient with fever and rash. Such infections most commonly present in elderly or immunocompromised patients. Solitary or widely scattered purplish lesions, nonblanching and often with necrotic centers, suggest the diagnosis. The lesions often involve the digits. Ecthyma gangrenosum is one such lesion seen with *Pseudomonas aeruginosa* bacteremia. Such lesions are also seen most often in *Staphylococcus aureus* bacteremia, *Candida albicans* fungemia, and infectious endocarditis. Gram stain of aspirates from the skin lesions and of the buffy coat of the blood can be rapidly diagnostic; blood cultures are confirmatory. Presumptive therapy should be with nafcillin and gentamicin pending cultural confirmation. In institutions where methicillin-resistant *S. aureus* is a problem, a regimen of vancomycin, 1 g IV every 12 hours, and ceftazidime, 1 g IV every 8 hours, is recommended.

Rapidly Spreading Cellulitis

The various types of rapidly spreading cellulitis associated with fever and rash are not difficult to recognize in most instances because of the painful spreading inflammatory lesion on the skin. The diagnostic difficulty involves differentiating the various types of rapidly spreading cellulitis based on probable causative organism or organisms and whether infection is confined to the surface or extends to deeper structures, including fascia and muscle. With deep extension, case adequate surgical debidement is essential, along with appropriate antibiotic therapy. "Flesh-eating" necrotizing fasciitis from group A streptococcus can be difficult to diagnose, and it is increasing in frequency.

COMMON INFECTIONS PRESENTING WITH FEVER AND RASH

The most common infections presenting with fever and rash also fortunately include conditions that are generally benign.

Table 17.4 Rare Causes of Fever and Rash

Infectious		
Viral		
Parvovirus	Hand-foot-mouth	West Nile
EBV	Herpes Simplex	R.S.V.
CMV	Herpes Zoster	HHV6
Coxsackie	HIV	Smallpox
Enterovirus (echo)	Hepatitis B and C	Vaccina
Dengue	Monkey Pox	
Ebola	Rubella	
Bacteria		
Rat-bite fever	Leptospirosis	Neisseria
Mycoplasma pneumoniae	Lyme	Gonorrhea
BCG	Bartonella	Salmonella
Mycobacteria	Borrelia	
Fungal		
Candida	Coccidiomycosis	Histoplasmosis
Sportrichosis		
Non-Infectious		
Erythema multiforme	Vasculitis	Porphyria
Kawasaki	Sweets syndrome	Drug reaction
Graft vs host	Pyoderma gangrenosa	

Many of these febrile exanthems are due to viral illnesses of children or inadequately immunized adults. Such illnesses as measles, varicella, rubella, erythema infectiosum due to parvovirus B 19, and roseola infantum due to HSV 6 are typical. Kawasaki syndrome and streptococcal scarlet fever should also be considered in this age group.

In older children presenting with fever, rash, sore throat, and adenopathy, Epstein-Barr virus infection is common. In young adults presenting in such fashion where EBV and group A *Streptococcus* have been ruled out, pharyngitis with fever and rash due to a recently described organism, *Arcanobacterium*, should be considered. This gram-positive bacillus is usually very sensitive to erythromycin.

Enteroviral infections due to coxsackie viruses and echoviruses frequently present with febrile exanthem and should especially be considered during summer months and when accompanied with gastrointestinal symptoms.

UNUSUAL INFECTIONS THAT CAN POSE A DIAGNOSTIC CHALLENGE

A wide variety of less common infections that can present with fever and rash should also be considered, especially if associated with geographic or seasonal exposure (Table 17.4).

Lyme borreliosis can present with fever and a characteristic erythema migrans rash, resulting from geographic tick exposure. Diagnosis can be difficult early in the infection when serology can be negative and the rash can be atypical or missed. Follow-up serology may be diagnostic.

The recently recognized syndromes of West Nile virus infection, including West Nile fever, encephalitis, and facial paralysis, can present with fever and rash. The disease has a summer-fall prevalence and is associated most often with exposure to infected household mosquitoes. Other uncommon infections to be considered, also with geographic and seasonal occurrence, include Ehrlichiosis, dengue fever, tularemia, plague, leptospirosis, and typhoid fever.

Although a wide variety of diagnostic tests and procedures can be helpful in the workup of the patient presenting with fever and rash, none of these is as important as a careful history and physical examination.

SUGGESTED READING

Drage L. Life-threatening rashes: dermatologic signs of four infectious diseases. *Mayo Clin Proc*. 1999;74:68.

Kingston M, Mackey D. Skin clues in the diagnosis of life-threatening infections. *Rev Infect Dis*. 1986;8:1.

Clinical Syndromes – Skin and Lymph Nodes

Mackenzie A, et al. Incidence and pathogenicity of Arcanobacterium hemolyticum during a two year study in Ottawa. *Clin Infect Dis.* 1995;21:1–77.

Oblinger M, Sands M. Fever and rash. In Stein JH, ed. *Integral Medicine.* Boston, MA: Little, Brown; 1983.

Schlossberg D. Fever and rash. *Infect Dis Clin North Am.* 1996;10:101.

Valdez L, Septinus E. Clinical approach to rash and fever. *Infect Dis Pract.* 1996;20:1.

The Working Group on Severe Streptococcal Infections. Defining the group A streptococcal toxic shock syndrome. *JAMA.* 1993;269:390.

18. Staphylococcal and Streptococcal Toxic Shock and Kawasaki Syndromes

Aristides P. Assimacopoulos and Patrick M. Schlievert

TOXIC SHOCK SYNDROME

Staphylococcal and streptococcal toxic shock syndromes (TSS) are acute-onset multiorgan illnesses defined by the criteria listed in Tables 18.1 and 18.2. Staphylococcal TSS is caused by *Staphylococcus aureus* strains that make pyrogenic toxin superantigens (PTSAgs); coagulase-negative strains do not make the causative toxins. Streptococcal TSS is caused mainly by toxin-producing group A strains but occasionally by groups B, C, F, and G strains. Several subsets of staphylococcal TSS exist, with two major categories being menstrual and nonmenstrual.

Menstrual TSS (Figure 18.1), which occurs within a day or two of and during menstruation, primarily has been associated with use of certain tampons, notably those of high absorbency, and is associated with production of TSS toxin-1 (TSST-1) by the causative bacterium. Three theories have been proposed to explain the role of tampons in menstrual TSS: (1) Tampons introduce oxygen, which is required for production of TSST-1, into the vagina; (2) tampons bind magnesium, which alters growth kinetics of *S. aureus* and thus alters the time when TSST-1 is made; and (3) pluronic L-92, a surfactant present in the Rely tampon, which was highly associated with TSS, amplifies production of TSST-1. Certain other surfactants may have similar effects.

Nonmenstrual TSS occurs in both males and females, adults and children, and it is associated with *S. aureus* strains that make TSST-1 or staphylococcal enterotoxins, notably enterotoxin serotypes B and C. The illness occurs in association with nearly any kind of staphylococcal infection, but major forms have been identified: postsurgical, influenza associated, RED syndrome (see below), and occasionally with use of contraceptive diaphragms. Postsurgical TSS is often associated with *S. aureus* infections that do not result in pyogenic responses, and thus the source of infection may be difficult to find. Influenza TSS may

Table 18.1 Diagnostic Criteria for Staphylococcal Toxic Shock Syndrome

1. Temperature greater than 38.8° C

2. Systolic blood pressure ≤90 mm Hg for adults, less than the 5th percentile for childern, or greater than a 15 mm Hg orthostatic drop in diastolic blood pressure or orthostatic dizziness/syncope

3. Diffuse macular rash with subsequent desquamation

4. Three of the following organ systems involved:
   Liver: bilirubin, AST, ALT more than twice the upper normal limit
   Blood: platelets <100,000/mm^3
   Renal: BUN or cretinine more twice the upper normal limit or pyuria without urinary tract infection
   Mucous membranes: hyperemia of the vagina, oropharynx, or conjunctivae
   Gastrointestinal: diarrhea or vomiting
   Muscular: myalgias or CPK more than twice the normal upper limit
   Central nervous system: disorientation or lowered level of consciousness in the abesence of hypotension, fever, or focal neurologic defiicits

5. Negative serologies for measles, leptospiroisis, and Rocky Mountain spotted fever, Blood or CSF cultures negative for organisms other than *Staphylococcus aureus*

Abbreviations; AST = Aspartate transaminase; ALT = alanine aminotransferase; BUN = blood urea nitrogen; CPK = creatine phosphokinase; CSF = cerebrospinal fluid.

occur as a consequence of influenza or parainfluenza damage to the respiratory tract epithelium and superinfection with toxin-producing *S. aureus* (Figures 18.2 and 18.3). This illness is highly fatal in children. RED syndrome is a recalcitrant erythematous desquamating disorder in patients with acquired immunodeficiency syndrome (AIDS) that may last 70 days or more or until the patient succumbs. Finally, nonmenstrual TSS associated with use of diaphragms may be similar to menstrual TSS, although the reason for the association is unclear.

Streptococcal TSS primarily is associated with group A streptococcal infections, particularly M types 1 and 3. The illness may or

Table 18.2 Diagnostic Criteria for Streptococcal Toxic Shock Syndrome

1. Isolation of group A streptococci:
   From a sterile site for a *definite* case
   From a nonsterile site for a *probable* case

2. Clinical criteria:
   Hypotension *and* two of the following:

Renal dysfunction	Coagulopathy
Liver involvement	ARDS
Erythematous macular rash	Soft-tissue necrosis

Abbreviation; ARDS = Adult respiratory distress syndrome.

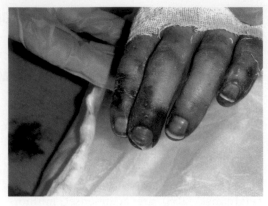

Figure 18.2 Gangrenous fingers and skin peeling with nonmenstrual staphylococcal toxic shock syndrome (pulmonary infection). (Courtesy of Gary R. Kravitz, MD St. Paul Infectious Disease Associates, St. Paul, MN.)

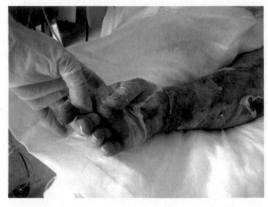

Figure 18.3 Same patient as in Figure 18.2, demonstrating extensive peeling and tissue damage. (Courtesy of Gary R. Kravitz, MD, St. Paul Infectious Disease Associates, St. Paul, MN.)

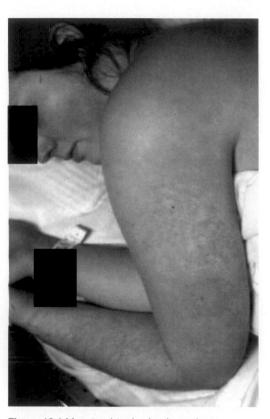

Figure 18.1 Menstrual toxic shock syndrome (vaginal colonization): diffuse blanching erythema. (Courtesy of David Schlossberg, MD.)

may not be associated with necrotizing fasciitis and myositis (Figures 18.4A-C). Occasionally, streptococcal TSS is caused by other groups of streptococci, primarily groups B, C, and G.

Group A streptococcal strains that cause TSS produce streptococcal pyrogenic exotoxins. The major association has been with SPE serotype A, but other members of the family may also contribute significantly. Non-group A streptococci associated with TSS also make PTSAgs,

only one of which has been characterized—that made by some group B strains.

Major risk factors for development of streptococcal TSS include chickenpox in children, penetrating and nonpenetrating wounds, use of nonsteroidal anti-inflammatory agents, and pregnancy.

KAWASAKI SYNDROME

Kawasaki syndrome (KS) is an acute multisystem vasculitis that occurs primarily in children younger than 4 years of age (Table 18.3). KS shares many features with scarlet fever and TSS, except that hypotension is absent; KS is a leading cause of acquired heart disease in this age group. Coronary artery abnormalities, including aneurysms, develop in 15% to 25% of patients.

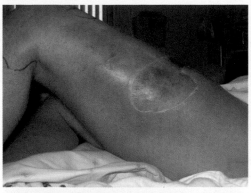
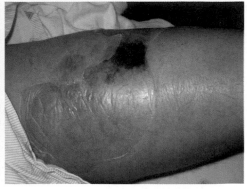
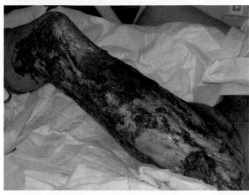

Figure 18.4 Necrotizing Fasciitis: Note the extensive edema, erythema, bullae formation, and necrosis in this patient's thigh (A and B). At the time of presentation, this patient was hypotensive with multisystem organ failure, with severe pain at the site of infection. (C) Leg after extensive debridement down to and below the level of the fascia. (With permission from the Regents of the University of California. Taken from http://medicine.ucsd.edu/Clinicalimg/Necrosis4)

The causative agent of KS remains unclear, but studies suggest that *S. aureus* and streptococcal PTSAgs may have important causal roles in many cases.

EVALUATION AND TREATMENT OF TOXIC SHOCK SYNDROMES

Differential Diagnosis of Toxic Shock Syndrome

- Viral disease, including measles, rubella, parvovirus B19
- Spotted fever group rickettsiae
- Leptospirosis
- Drug reactions, including Stevens-Johnson syndrome
- Collagen-vascular diseases, including systemic lupus erythematosus and Still's disease
- Scarlet and rheumatic fever
- Syphilis
- Typhoid fever

The physician should consider myositis or necrotizing fasciitis in any patient who presents with severe local pain, especially in an extremity, and other nonspecific influenza-like or gastrointestinal symptoms. Fever, erythema, and edema are usually absent. Early intervention is life-saving for patients with necrotizing soft tissue infections, so it is important to maintain a very high index of suspicion. An elevated creatinine, elevated creatine kinase (CK), or significant bandemia may suggest the diagnosis.

Initial Evaluation

Possible sources of infection or foreign bodies must be identified. The physician should perform a vaginal examination, remove any tampon, and culture for *S. aureus*. Any wounds should be unpacked and inspected. A thorough examination of the skin and soft tissues should be undertaken, paying special attention to any painful areas, even if typical signs of inflammation are absent. Cultures of blood and other sites, as appropriate, should be obtained. Early surgical intervention is extremely important. MRI may be used to identify deep soft-tissue necrosis and guide surgical intervention.

Table 18.3 Clinical Criteria for Kawasaki Syndrome*

1. Fever, usually of at least 5 days' duration

2. Four of five of the following:
   Extremity changes, induration, edema, erythema
   Oropharyngeal and lip changes, strawberry tongue, cracked lips
   Cervical lymphadenopathy: at least one node >1.5 cm
   Injected conjunctivae
   Rash, erythematous and polymorphous

3. Other diseases excluded

* Strict fulfillment is not always necessary; see Suggested Reading.

Supportive Care

Supportive care is of primary importance. Patients often require large amounts of intravenous fluids, vasopressors, and management of associated co-morbidities, such as acute renal failure, adult respiratory distress syndrome, disseminated intravascular coagulation, or myocardial suppression.

Antibiotics

Antistaphylococcal therapy decreases the risk of recurrence of staphylococcal TSS and will treat any active infection with *S. aureus* or β-hemolytic streptococci. One of the antistaphylococcal penicillins such as nafcillin (adults: 2 gm IV every 4 hours; children: 150 mg/kg/d IV divided every 6 hours) is an appropriate empirical choice. Alternative therapy, especially for patients with a non-anaphylactic penicillin allergy, is cefazolin (adults: 1–2 g IV every 8 hours; children: 50–100 mg/kg/d IV divided every 8 hours). For the patient with an anaphylactic penicillin allergy or cephalosporin allergy, or in areas with a high prevalence of community-associated methicillin-resistant *S. aureus*, vancomycin (adults: 1 g IV every 12 hours; children 40 mg/kg/d IV divided every 6 hours) can be used, and newer agents such as daptomycin or linezolid may be considered. Clindamycin, a protein synthesis inhibitor (adults: 900 mg IV every 8 hours; children: 40 mg/kg/d IV divided every 6–8 hours), may be given in addition as experimental data suggest that it inhibits exotoxin and M protein production. Dosage adjustments for renal failure may be required.

Once a microbiologic diagnosis has been established, the spectrum of therapy can be narrowed using penicillin (adults: 4 million units V every 4 hours; children: 250 000 U/kg/d IV divided every 4 hours) ampicillin (adults: 2 g every 6 hours; children: 50 mg/kg/d divided every 6 hours), ceftriaxone (adults: 2 gm IV every 24 hours; children: 50–75 mg/kg/d IV divided every 12–24 hours), or clindamycin alone, as appropriate. Therapy should be given for approximately 10 to 14 days unless a diagnosis, such as osteomyelitis, is made that requires extended therapy.

Intravenous Immunoglobulin

Lack of neutralizing antibodies seems to be a risk factor for staphylococcal and streptococcal TSS. Human and animal studies appear to support the use of intravenous immunoglobulin (IVIG) in these diseases. Preparations of IVIG may vary not only by manufacturer but also by batch in their ability to neutralize superantigenic toxins. Therefore, retreatment with a different preparation may be warranted in a patient who has not responded to initial therapy. Various IV doses have been used as follows: 1 g/kg on day one followed by 0.5 g/kg each day on days 2 and 3, 0.4 g/kg IV once daily for 5 days, or a single dose of 2 g/kg with a repeat dose at 48 hours if the patient remains unstable.

Steroids

The clinician should not miss the patient with absolute or relative adrenal insufficiency who requires both glucocorticoid and mineralocorticoid replacement therapy.

Surgical Intervention

Any obvious source of infection should be drained. There should be a low threshold to explore other sites as expected signs of inflammation may be absent, especially in streptococcal myositis. Radionuclide WBC scanning has been used to identify undrained foci of necrotizing fasciitis in a nonresponding patient.

Prevention

Up to 30% recurrence has been suggested. A course of rifampin is sometimes given in hopes of eliminating staphylococcal colonization. Avoidance of further tampon use is prudent after menstrual TSS. Close contacts of an index case of streptococcal TSS may be colonized with toxin-producing streptococci. Individuals with HIV, diabetes, recent chicken pox, cancer, heart disease, injection drug use, and those on steroids are at increased risk for sporadic invasive group A streptococcal disease and might be considered for prophylaxis.

TREATMENT OF KAWASAKI SYNDROME

Differential Diagnosis of Kawasaki Syndrome

- Acute adenoviral infection
- Other viral exanthemata, especially measles
- Scarlet fever
- Drug reactions, Stevens-Johnson syndrome, erythema multiforme
- Spotted fever group rickettsiosis
- TSS
- Staphyloccocal scalded skin syndrome
- Juvenile rheumatoid arthritis
- Leptospirosis
- Mercury poisoning

Differential Diagnosis

Irritability and gastrointestinal symptoms are common. Adenoviral infection may present the most common diagnostic dilemma. Incomplete Kawasaki Syndrome, more common in children less than 12 months of age, may be diagnosed when the patient has 5 or more days of fever and two or more criteria for diagnosis. The risk of coronary artery aneurysms increases significantly in patients not treated within 10 days.

Supportive Care

Cardiorespiratory monitoring, close clinical observation, and attention to fluid balance are required.

Aspirin

The physician should give high doses of aspirin (80-100 mg/kg/d in four divided doses) until fever is gone and then maintain low doses (3–5 mg/kg/d in single dose) for 6 to 8 weeks or until the platelet count and sedimentation rate are normal. Consider monitoring of serum salicylate levels in nonresponders. Some prefer high doses until day 14. Aspirin therapy should be continued indefinitely in any patient with coronary artery abnormalities. Influenza or varicella exposure may prompt discontinuation of aspirin therapy for up to 14 days because of the risk of Reye's syndrome.

Dipyridamole (4–9 mg/kg/d divided BID or TID) may substitute during this time in high-risk patients. Give influenza vaccination yearly while on aspirin.

Intravenous Immunoglobulin

The recommended dose is 2 g/kg IV given over 12 hours. Retreatment may be necessary in those whose fever persists or recurs. Measles, mumps, and rubella vaccines should be delayed for 11 months after IVIG unless there is high risk. If so, give the vaccination on schedule and repeat 11 months later.

Steroids

Intravenous methylprednisolone will hasten the resolution of fever and improve laboratory markers of inflammation when given in 1–3 pulse doses of 30 mg/kg. This should be considered especially for patients who fail treatment with IVIG.

Monitoring for Cardiac Complications

Inpatient and outpatient serial exams are important. Obtain electrocardiogram and cardiac echo early and repeat at 6 and 8 weeks. Pediatric cardiology consultation should be obtained. Stress testing and coronary angiography have value in specific clinical situations. The patient with coronary artery lesion (CAL) requires more intensive monitoring.

Evaluation of Therapy

Ten percent of patients may not respond. If fever or signs of inflammation persist or recur, consider retreatments with IVIG (1–2 g/kg over 10–12 hours). Pulsed doses of corticosteroids have been used in nonresponders with success despite initial reports that corticosteroids may increase the risk for CALs.

Long-Term Management

Restrict physical activity for 6 to 8 weeks. Determine frequency of follow-up on an individual basis. It is possible to identify a group of low-risk patients that may not require intensive follow-up. Complicated management issues, such as use of warfarin, calcium channel blockers, and angiography, are beyond the scope of this text. The reader is referred to the excellent reviews of Kawasaki Syndrome found in the Suggested Reading section.

Other Issues

Antibiotics are not routinely used. Pentoxifylline has been tried experimentally but is of no proven benefit.

SUGGESTED READING

Darenberg J, Soderquist B, Henriques Normark B, et al. Differences in potency of intravenous polyspecific immunoglobulin G against streptococcal and staphylococcal superantigens: Implications for therapy of toxic shock syndrome. *Clin Infect Dis.* 2004;38:836–842.

Mason WH, Takahashi M. Kawasaki syndrome. *Clin Infect Dis.* 1999;28:169–1878.

Pickering LK, et al., eds. 2006 *Report of the Committee on Infectious Diseases of the American Academy of Pediatrics (The Red Book).* 27th ed. Elk Grove, IL: American Academy of Pediatrics; 2006:412–415.

Newburger JW, Takahashi M, Gerber MA, et al. Diagnosis, treatment and long-term management of Kawasaki disease: A statement for health professionals from the Committee on Rheumatic Fever, Endocarditis, and Kawasaki Disease, Council on Cardiovascular Disease in the Young, American Heart Association, *Circulation.* 2004;110:2747–2771.

The Prevention of Invasive Group A Streptococcal Infections Workshop Participants. Prevention of invasive group A streptococcal disease among household contacts of case patients and among postpartum and postsurgical patients: recommendations from the Centers for Disease Control and Prevention. *Clin Infect Dis.* 2002;35:950–959.

19. Classic Viral Exanthems

Henry M. Feder, Jr., and Jane M. Grant-Kels

During the early 1900s, six common childhood exanthematous infections were defined by the numbers 1 through 6. The etiologic agents of these infections were unknown. Over the next century, the etiologies of these exanthems were defined, and 4 of the 6 were demonstrated to be caused by viruses (Table 19.1). The first exanthem was caused by the measles virus, the third by the rubella virus, the second and fourth by bacterial toxins, the fifth by parvovirus, and the sixth by human herpesvirus-6 (HHV-6).

In developed countries where most children have received measles and rubella vaccinations, other viral exanthems are often confused with breakthrough measles or rubella. For example, in a study of 2299 Finnish children with exanthems thought to be measles or rubella, only 6% actually had measles or rubella. When acute and convalescent serologies were performed, other diagnoses, including parvovirus (20%), enterovirus (9%), adenovirus (4%), and human herpesvirus (4%), were defined.

This chapter discusses the classic childhood viral exanthems: measles (rubeola), German measles (rubella), and exanthem subitum (roseola). Parvovirus infection is discussed in Chapter 189, Parvovirus Infection (Acute and Chronic).

RUBEOLA

Rubeola (measles) is caused by an RNA virus with one antigenic type and is classified in the genus *Morbillivirus* in the Paramyxoviridae family. The licensure of both a live attenuated and killed measles vaccine in 1963 resulted in a 98% diminution in incidence rates. The killed vaccine proved problematic, and only the live vaccine has remained available since 1967. Most cases of measles occur in the fall, winter, or spring, with the highest number of cases occurring in early spring. The measles virus is highly contagious and, like chickenpox, can be spread as tiny infectious droplets through the air without direct contact. If a patient is hospitalized with measles, airborne precautions are indicated for 4 days after the onset of rash. However, if the patient with measles is immunosuppressed, airborne precautions are required until the illness completely resolves. Measles and chickenpox are perhaps the two most contagious infectious diseases. The measles virus is labile and survives only a short time on fomites. The highest rates of transmission occur in the home, day-care centers, nursery schools, primary and secondary schools, and colleges and universities. School outbreaks can occur despite greater than 95% immunity among students. Most cases of measles occur after face-to-face contact. Thus, when a physician suspects measles, a defined or potential exposure should be identified.

Clinical and Laboratory Diagnosis

Measles demonstrates a characteristic clinical presentation, which makes the diagnosis straightforward. The incubation period is 10 to 12 days. There is a prodrome of low-grade fever, malaise, and headache. This is followed or accompanied by cough, coryza, and conjunctivitis. During the prodrome, Koplik spots, the enanthem of measles, appear on the buccal mucosa. Koplik spots are punctate white spots (like grains of sand) on erythematous bases. As the infection evolves, the number of Koplik spots increases and they appear as salt on a red background. They begin to resolve at the onset of the rash. After about 4 days of increasing prodromal symptoms, the patient develops high fever (103° to 105°F) and rash. The rash (Figure 19.1) begins as erythematous macules and papules at the hairline, on the forehead, behind the ears, and on the upper neck. This characteristic morbilliform rash occurs in almost 100% of normal individuals. The rash spreads to the trunk and extremities over the next 3 days. This erythematous rash blanches on pressure and may coalesce, and when it resolves, it may leave brownish staining that results from capillary hemorrhage. The characteristic morbilliform rash may not occur in up to 30% of patients who are immunosuppressed. When present, the high fever and rash persist for 2 to 4 days. When the rash fades, the coryza and conjunctivitis clear, but the cough may persist for another 5 days. A patient is contagious

Table 19.1 Classic Exanthems of Childhood

Order	Exanthems	Agent
First	Rubeola or measles	Measles virus
Second	Scarlet fever	Streptococcal toxin
Third	Rubella or German measles	Rubella virus
Fourth	Filatow-Dukes' disease	Streptococcal or Staphylococcal toxin
Fifth	Erythema infectiosum	Parvovirus
Sixth	Exanthem subitum or roseola	Human herpesvirus-6

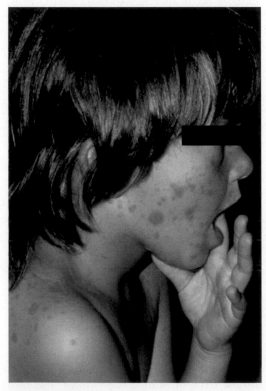

Figure 19.1 Measles in a 9-year-old child presenting as morbilliform lesions on the face, trunk, and palms.

from the onset of the prodrome until approximately 4 days after the onset of the rash.

The most common complications of measles are secondary bacterial infections, including pneumonia and otitis media. Diarrhea may also occur as a complication. The risk of complications is highest for infants younger than 1 year of age. A rare complication is postinfectious encephalomyelitis. This is a demyelinating disease that occurs in 1 per 1000 measles cases and has a mortality rate of 10% to 20%. Clinically, it begins with vomiting, and then obtundation and seizures develop. Measles has a mortality rate of less than 0.1% in normal patients; however, this increases to up to 50% with immunosuppression.

Measles can be confirmed by viral cultures of the nasopharynx, conjunctiva, blood, or urine. However, culture is technically difficult and not readily available. Sera may be obtained for measles antibody determinations both at the onset of the rash and 2 to 4 weeks later. A 4-fold or greater increase of measles antibody is diagnostic. Finally, a measles-specific IgM antibody test is also available. This IgM antibody is detectable from about 7 to 30 days after the onset of the rash. However, some measles antibody assays are not as sensitive as others. Immunity after measles infection is life long, and a second attack is very rare.

Treatment and Prevention

Treatment of measles is usually symptomatic—acetaminophen or a nonsteroidal anti-inflammatory drug (NSAID) is used for pain and fever. There are data to suggest that oral vitamin A supplementation lessens morbidity and mortality in malnourished patients. The dose is 100000 IU in a single oral dose for infants 6 months to 1 year of age and 200000 IU for patients older than 1 year. The use of vitamin A in infants less than 6 months old has not been adequately studied. For reasons that are not defined, malnourished patients may suffer acute vitamin A deficiency when infected with measles. Vitamin A is necessary for the maintenance of epithelial cell integrity and for normal immune function. Vitamin A supplementation for measles infection is recommended in patients who are malnourished and in immigrants from countries where malnourishment (and a high measles mortality rate, 1% or higher) is common. Because measles may be complicated by secondary bacterial infection, prophylactic antibiotics are sometimes prescribed, although not generally recommended. The most common bacterial complication is pneumonia cased by *Streptococcus pneumoniae, Hemophilus influenzae*, or *Staphylococcus aureus*.

Measles virus is susceptible in vitro to the antiviral agent ribavirin. However, ribravirin has not been studied in patients for the treatment of measles. There are anecdotal reports of successful use of intravenous and/or aerosolized ribavirin to treat severely ill, immunosuppressed patients with measles.

Measles vaccine is routinely recommended at ages 12 to 15 months. This vaccine is a live attenuated strain grown in chick embryo cells. In infants, the efficacy of this vaccine is hindered by passive maternal antibody, which is no longer present by 12 months. If the mother is immune via natural infection, not immunization, then maternal antibody can persist in the infant until 15 months. A second measles vaccine dose is recommended at 5 to 12 years of age. Unimmunized children and adults should be given two measles doses at least 1 month apart. Following one measles vaccine dose approximately 95% of patients will show a positive measles antibody response. This response rate increases to >99% following two measles vaccine doses. Because of the high immunization rates in the United States, reported cases of measles have usually been less than 100 cases per year over the last decade. After exposure to measles, in an unimmunized person, measles vaccine may be efficacious if given within 72 hours of exposure. Measles vaccine should be administered to patients with human immunodeficiency virus (HIV) because of the potentially devastating outcome of measles in this group. Because measles inoculation is a live vaccine, it is not recommended for immunosuppressed patients (see Table 19.2 for contraindications for measles vaccine).

Patients traveling to foreign countries should be immune to measles. For infants traveling to developing countries where measles is endemic, the measles vaccine can be given as early as 6 months of age.

Immunoglobulin (IG) may prevent or reduce the severity of measles if given within 6 days of an unimmunized patient's exposure. The recommended dose is 0.25 mL/kg given intramuscularly (0.50 mL/kg for immunocompromised patients) with a maximum dose of 15 mL. IG is also recommended for HIV-positive patients who are exposed to measles even if they have been previously immunized.

RUBELLA

Rubella is a togavirus with a single strand of RNA at its core. Rubella vaccine is a live attenuated virus that was licensed in 1969. Before the rubella vaccine, the major danger posed by rubella virus was the specter of infection during pregnancy, which could cause congenital rubella syndrome in the newborn. Before the vaccine

Table 19.2 Contraindications for Measles Vaccine

Pregnancy
Immunodeficiency or immunocompromised except for human immunodeficiency virus infection
History of anaphylaxis to eggs
History of anaphylaxis to neomycin

was available, thousands of cases of congenital rubella were reported each year in the United States. The vaccine was very successful. From 1985 through 1996, 122 cases of congenital rubella were reported to the National Congenital Rubella Syndrome Registry in this country. Since 2001, there have been ≤25 cases per year of rubella (and almost no cases of congenital rubella syndrome) reported in the United States. Rubella is no longer endemic in the United States. Congenital rubella in the United States is limited to unimmunized pregnant women who emigrate to the United States and were rubella infected in their country of origin.

Clinical and Laboratory Diagnosis

Rubella infection in infants and children is usually mild, and up to 50% of infections in children are asymptomatic. A prodrome characterized by tender posterior auricular, posterior cervical, and suboccipital adenopathy with malaise is common among adolescents and adults with rubella. The adenopathy may persist for weeks. The rubella exanthem begins on the face, neck, and scalp and spreads downward. The rash may be associated with fever, headache, myalgias, and arthralgias. The rash consists of pink macules and papules that range in diameter from 1 to 4 mm. The exanthem fades as it spreads; thus it may be absent on the face when it is prominent on the trunk. The exanthem, Forchheimer's sign, occurs in 20% of patients and is characterized as petechiae or red spots on the soft palate. It occurs during the prodrome or at the onset of the exanthem. Rubella is most commonly seen during late winter and early spring.

Rubella is spread by small droplets from the respiratory mucosa. Patients are most contagious from a few days before until up to 7 days after the onset of rash. Viral shedding can occur for up to 14 days after the onset of rash. Prolonged exposure usually is necessary for transmission of rubella. The incubation period is 14 to 23 days.

Complications of rubella are unusual. The most common complication is arthritis, which occurs almost exclusively in females and has an increasing incidence with older age groups. Rare complications include thrombocytopenia and encephalitis. The most devastating complication is congenital rubella syndrome. The frequency of congenital rubella is 50% if rubella infection occurs during the first 12 weeks of pregnancy. This incidence diminishes to 25% for infections occurring from 13 to 24 weeks. Congenital rubella syndrome is rare if maternal infection occurs after 24 weeks' gestation. Congenital rubella syndrome is commonly characterized by deafness, congenital cataracts, and patent ductus arteriosus. Severe involvement is often fatal, and infection involves many organs, including the skin (described as a blueberry muffin because of bluish areas of extramedullary hematopoesis).

Rubella can be diagnosed by the typical exanthem and the associated adenopathy. Posterior auricular adenopathy is suggestive of rubella. Rubella virus can be isolated from nasal secretions, but most laboratories do not have the proper reagents needed for isolation. Acute and convalescent (2 to 4 weeks after rash) serology should show a 4-fold or greater rise in rubella antibodies. A rubella-specific IgM antibody test is also available. The IgM antibody persists for several months after acute infection.

Treatment and Prevention

Typical rubella infection is mild and requires no therapy. The occasional patient with severe arthralgias or arthritis should respond to therapy with NSAIDs. Arthralgias and arthritis are much more common in females. The routine administration of IG after exposure is not recommended. However, if a pregnant patient is exposed to rubella in early pregnancy and termination of the pregnancy is not an option; the administration of IG may be considered. Limited data suggest that IG may decrease the manifestations of clinical rubella, but this does not guarantee a diminution in the incidence or severity of congenital rubella.

Rubella vaccine should be given with measles and mumps vaccine (MMR) in the same two-dose schedule: the first dose at 12 to 15 months and the second at 5 to 12 years of age. Contraindications for rubella vaccine are listed in Table 19.3. Because rubella is a live vaccine and can potentially infect the fetus, it should not be given during pregnancy, although the risk of fetal infection is low. In a study of 226 susceptible women who were inadvertently immunized with rubella vaccine during the first

Table 19.3 Contraindications for Rubella Vaccine

| Pregnancy |
| Immunodeficiency or immunocompromised except human immunodeficiency virus infection |
| Immunoglobulin in the last 3 months |

trimester, there were no congenital abnormalities in the offspring and two offspring showed asymptomatic infection. This benign outcome may reflect the fact that this is an attenuated viral vaccine.

ROSEOLA

Roseola, or exanthem subitum, is the sixth of the classic exanthems and is caused by HHV-6. This is a double-stranded DNA herpesvirus, and after the initial infection, the virus becomes latent. At birth, passively acquired HHV-6 antibody usually is present in the newborn. This protects the infant until about 6 months of age. From 6 to 24 months of age, about 80% of infants become infected with HHV-6. Cases of roseola occur throughout the year. The mode of transmission is unknown. It is unusual to demonstrate roseola spreading from one infant to another. After acute infection, HHV-6 can often be isolated from saliva. Saliva transmission from an asymptomatic contact to a susceptible infant may be the common route of transmission. HHV-6 can also be isolated from both peripheral blood lymphocytes and cerebrospinal fluid.

HHV-6 is a herpesvirus distinct from herpes simplex 1 and 2, varicella-zoster virus, cytomegalovirus, and Epstein-Barr virus. HHV-6 was first isolated in 1986. This was followed by the isolation of human herpesvirus-7 (which may also cause roseola) in 1990 and the subsequent isolation of human herpesvirus-8 (the cause of Kaposi's sarcoma) in 1994. HHV-6 may be divided into two major groups: variants A and B. Primary infection may be associated with roseola and is caused by variant B strains. In addition to causing roseola, HHV-6 causes a febrile illness without rash, a febrile illness with lymphadenopathy, gastroenteritis, upper respiratory infection, and inflamed ear drums; see Chapter 186, Human Herpesvirus 6, 7, 8.

Clinical and Laboratory Diagnosis

The incubation period of roseola is 9 to 10 days, and the disease has no prodrome. Clinical illness begins with a high fever (102°

to 105°F). Febrile seizures can occur. Roseola or other HHV-6 illnesses account for at least 10% of visits to the emergency room for infants younger than 2 years old. In addition, roseola accounts for 33% of febrile and recurrent febrile seizures seen in emergency rooms. The fever typically lasts 3 days. Clinically, when the fever resolves, the exanthem appears. The exanthem may also begin before the fever resolves. The exanthem is characterized by discrete, pale pink macules, varying in size from 1 to 5 mm in diameter. Around each lesion, there is a pale areola. The rash commonly begins on the trunk, on the neck, and behind the ears and spreads to the proximal extremities. The rash may become confluent. It rarely involves the face or distal extremities. The rash usually lasts for 2 to 48 hours. Before the rash appears, an exanthem of erythematous macules may be present on the soft palate. Vertical transmission of HHV-6 occurs in 1% to 2% of births. The significance of vertical transmission of HHV-6 is unknown.

Acute HHV-6 infection may be diagnosed by seroconversion from HHV-6 antibody negative to HHV-6 positive. A specific IgM antibody peaks 7 to 14 days after the onset of illness and usually becomes undetectable in several weeks. However, HHV-6 IgM antibody may persist in some patients and, thus, may be present without acute infection. Specific IgG antibody develops 2 to 4 weeks after the onset of illness and remains detectable indefinitely. Also, the IgG antibody may intermittently rise and fall, especially in association with cytomegalovirus or Epstein-Barr virus infections. Almost all children are seropositive for HHV-6 by age 4. In research laboratories, HHV-6 can be cultured from saliva and from mononuclear cells and can be detected by polymerase chain reaction (PCR).

Treatment and Prevention

At present, no treatment or prevention strategies are available for HHV-6 infection occurring in normal children and adults. In immunosuppressed patients possible therapies include ganciclovir, foscarnet, and cidofovir (please see also Chapter 87, Infection in Transplant Patients and Chapter 186, Human Herpesviruses 6, 7, 8). However, because HHV-6 is a common cause for febrile seizures in infants between 6 months and 2 years of age, an immunization would be valuable. Finally, it is not known how HHV-6 is spread. Thus there are no recommendations for isolation of infected hosts either in or out of the hospital.

SUGGESTED READING

Pickering LK, ed. *Red Book: Report of the Committee on Infectious Diseases*. 27th ed. Elk Grove Village, IL: American Academy of Pediatrics; 2006.

Bialecki C, Feder HM Jr, Grant-Kels JM. The six classic childhood exanthems: a review and update. *J Am Acad Dermatol*. 1989;21:891.

Davidkin I, et al. Etiology of measles and rubella-like illnesses in measles, mumps and rubella-vaccinated children. *J Infect Dis*. 1998;178:1567.

DeBolle L, et al. Update on human herpesvirus 6 biology, clinical features. *Clin Microbiol Rev*. 2005;18:217.

Hall CB, et al. Human herpesvirus-6 infection in children. *N Engl J Med*. 1994;331:432.

Hussey G. Managing measles. *Br Med J*. 1997;314:316.

Kaplan LJ, et al: Severe measles in immunocompromised patients. *JAMA*. 1992;267:1237.

Mulholland EK. Measles in the United States, 2006. *N Engl J Med*. 2006;355:440.

Parker AA et al. Implications of a 2005 measles outbreak in Indiana for sustained elimination of measles in the United States. *N Engl J Med*. 2006;355:447.

Pickering LK, ed. *Red Book: Report of the Committee on Infectious Diseases*. 27th ed. Elk Grove Village, IL: American Academy of Pediatrics; 2006.

Reef SE, Cochi SL. The evidence for the elimination of rubella and congenital rubella syndrome in the United States: a public health achievement. *Clin Infect Dis*. 2006;43:S123.

20. Skin Ulcer and Pyoderma

Joanne T. Maffei

Skin lesions are important clues to systemic diseases and, conversely, host factors make patients susceptible to skin infections caused by certain organisms. The skin has a limited response to insults from the microbial world, forming vesicles and pustules that eventually rupture and leave exposed dermis. Accurate diagnosis and appropriate treatment depend on a detailed history that includes systemic complaints, history of exposure and travel, and the initial appearance of the skin lesions. Sound diagnosis of difficult cases also depends on appropriate cultures and histopathology. When possible, cultures should be obtained by aspirating pus or blister fluid from under intact skin; cultures from ulcerated skin are less reliable because of colonization by nonpathogenic skin flora. A Gram stain and routine culture should be done first; if the ulcer persists despite a course of antibiotics, a skin biopsy with histopathology and cultures for routine agents, acid-fast organisms, and fungal pathogens is appropriate. If the lesion has multiple thin-walled vesicles with interspersed shallow ulcers and crusts or is on a mucus membrane, a direct fluorescent antibody (DFA) test or Tzank smear for herpes and viral culture should be considered.

Most superficial skin infections and ulcers can be treated empirically according to the typical clinical presentation of the lesions. A workup is required for lesions that do not respond to routine therapy, that are rapidly progressive, or that occur in an immunocompromised host.

SKIN ULCERS

Skin ulcers are superficial defects in the tissues of the epidermis and dermis, with surrounding inflammation. Infection, collagen vascular diseases, and malignancy can cause cutaneous ulcerations. Information on host factors, exposure history, and the clinical course of the lesions is critical to narrowing the differential diagnosis. The lesion's anatomic location also may offer clues to the cause. Facial ulcers may be caused by syphilis, herpes, or blastomycosis, whereas ulcers of the arms or hands may be caused by sporotrichosis, nocardia, atypical mycobacteria,

herpetic whitlow, or cutaneous anthrax. Ulcers on the chest wall from underlying pulmonary involvement, or associated with intravenous catheters may be caused by aspergillosis. Ulcers in the groin or perineum may result from sexually transmitted diseases such as syphilis, chancroid, and herpes, as well as from Behçet's disease or fixed drug eruption.

Ulcers on the lower extremities result from venous insufficiency in 70% to 90% of cases and occur below the knee but never on the bottom of the foot. The patient with venous stasis ulcers has good peripheral pulses and no peripheral neuropathy. Ulcers in patients with poor peripheral pulses, an ankle/brachial pressure index less than 0.9, or sensory loss must be investigated further because venous stasis is not the cause. Any ulcer on the leg that does not respond to treatment for venous stasis ulcers should be further investigated by biopsy and culture, as should any ulcer that is rapidly progressive or appears on an immunocompromised host. Figure 20.1 outlines the steps in evaluating and treating leg ulcers.

A history of unusual occupation, hobby, or exposure can suggest causes of skin ulcers such as tularemia in rabbit hunters, *Mycobacterium marinum* in aquarium enthusiasts, and leishmaniasis in travelers to endemic areas of the Middle East, North Africa, and Central and South America. Host factors also may predispose individuals to any of several types of ulcers. Patients with malignancies can be at risk for ecthyma gangrenosum caused by *Pseudomonas aeruginosa* or dense neutrophilic infiltration of the dermis that is noninfectious but responds to steroids (Sweet's syndrome, discussed later). Ecthyma gangrenosum caused by *P. aeruginosa* is a rapidly progressive (12 to 24 hours), necrotic ulceration with hemorrhagic bullae and skin sloughing in the setting of gram-negative sepsis and neutropenia. Empiric agents for ecthyma gangrenosum should include tobramycin plus piperacillin, ceftazidime, or imipenem.

Treatment of skin ulcers depends on the cause of the lesion. For venous stasis ulcers, local care with occlusive dressings on the wounds and compression bandages to aid venous return

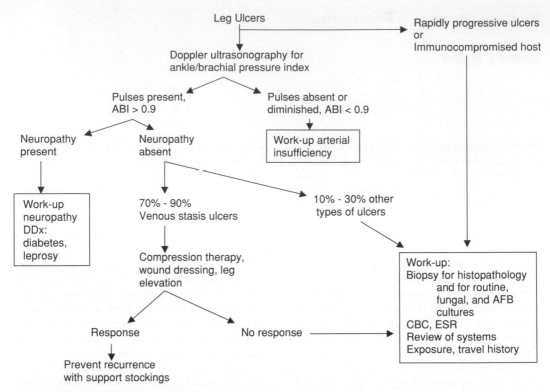

Figure 20.1 Algorithm for the evaluation of leg ulcers. ABI, ankle/brachial index; DDX, differential diagnosis; CBC, complete blood count; ESR, erythrocyte sedimentation rate; AFB, acid-fast bacilli.

is necessary. If cellulitis or folliculitis is present, antibiotics to cover *Staphylococcus aureus* (including methicillan-resistant *Staphylococcus aureus* [MRSA], streptococci, and gram-negatives should be administered empirically pending cultures. After the ulcer has healed, compression stockings should be worn to prevent new ulcers. Therapy for other types of ulcers should address their cause; Table 20.1 outlines the clinical presentation and epidemiology of infectious ulcers.

Noninfectious Ulcers

Noninfectious causes of cutaneous ulcers include drug reactions, collagen-vascular diseases, and malignancy. Drugs reported to cause ulcerations include methotrexate, etretinate, and warfarin. Wegener's granulomatosis, a systemic disease with involvement of the respiratory tract and kidneys, can form necrotizing ulcerations of the skin. Biopsy of these lesions may be positive for leukocytoclastic vasculitis, granuloma, and inflammatory infiltrates. Serology for immunoglobulin G (IgG) antibodies against neutrophilic cytoplasmic components (c-ANCA) are highly specific for Wegener's granulomatosis. Treatment includes corticosteroids and cyclophosphamide. Behçet's disease is another systemic condition

that involves recurrent oral and genital aphthous ulcerations, arthritis, and uveitis; in some cases it attacks the central nervous system. Treatment includes corticosteroids alone or in combination with colchicine, interferon-α, or azathioprine. Malignancy should always be considered as a possible cause of ulcers that have not responded to antimicrobial therapy because basal cell carcinoma, hematologic malignancies, and metastatic cancers may form skin ulcers.

PYODERMA

Pyoderma is a general term used to describe superficial disruption of the skin with pus formation in response to a bacterial infection. Generally caused by a single organism, pyoderma can be primary or secondary. Similar lesions can be produced by neutrophilic dermatoses such as pyoderma gangrenosum and Sweet's syndrome. Table 20.2 outlines the clinical presentation of pyoderma and suggested treatment.

Primary Pyoderma

Primary pyoderma is an infection of previously healthy skin, usually caused by *S. aureus* or *Streptococcus pyogenes*.

Clinical Syndromes – Skin and Lymph Nodes

Table 20.1 Clinical Presentation of Skin Ulcers Caused by Infectious Agents

Cause	Laboratory Work-up	Epidemiology	Clinical Clues to Diagnosis
Bacterial	Routine culture and Gram stain		
Bacillus anthracis (anthrax)	Gram (+) rod	Wool handler; Western Asia, West Africa	Lesions on face and arms; painless papule develops into vesicle that dries, forming black eschar that then separates from the base to form an ulcer with marked surrounding gelatinous edema; LN common
Corynebacterium diphtheriae (diphtheria)	Gram (+) rod	Tropical climates; rare in the United States	Ulcer with sharp margins and clean base; preexisting skin lesions may become infected
Francisella tularensis (tularemia)	Gram (–) coccobacillus, serology	Rabbit hunter	Systemic febrile illness; tender ulcer with painful LN
Nocardia sp.	Branching, beaded Gram (+) rod, modified AFB (+)	Immunocompromised patients, soil exposure	Ulcer with purulent drainage, nodular lymphangitis
Pseudomonas aeruginosa (ecthyma gangrenosum)	Gram (–) rod, may have associated bacteremia	Neutropenic or immunocompromised patients	Rapidly progressive eruption from papules to hemorrhagic vesicles or bullae that undergo central necrosis and ulceration
Polymicrobial	Mixed Gram (+), Gram (–), and anaerobes	Debilitated, immunocompromised, diabetic patients	Pressure sores, decubitus ulcers, foot ulcers
Yersinia pestis (plague)	Gram (–) coccobacillus, serology	Rodent zoonosis transmitted to humans via fleas; Far East, India, Africa, Central and South America	Bubonic plague with classic inguinal painful LN; may have skin lesions on lower extremities; pustule, papule, vesicle, or eschar may occur at inoculation site
Spirochetes			
Treponema pallidum (syphilis)	Serology	Sexually transmitted disease	Tertiary syphilis; nodular, ulceronodular, gummas; punched-out ulcer with gummy discharge
Fungal	Fungal smear, culture		
Aspergillus sp.	Septate hyphae	Immunocompromised, HIV positive	Ulcers, plaques, nodules, pustules; may be associated with trauma, intravenous catheter sites, secondary colonization of existing wounds, or direct extension from lung to chest wall
Blastomyces dermatitidis	Broad-based budding yeast, dimorphic fungus	Sugar cane worker, HIV positive, immunocompromised; North America, Africa	Subcutaneous nodule that enlarges and ulcerates, forming a crusted, verrucous plaque; may resemble squamous cell carcinoma

(continued)

Table 20.1 *(continued)*

Cause	Laboratory Work-up	Epidemiology	Clinical Clues to Diagnosis
Coccidioides immitis	Dimorphic fungus, serology	Soil exposure, HIV positive; Southwestern United States, Northern Mexico, Central and South America	Usually single nodule or plaque; may form pustules, subcutaneous nodules, or abscesses
Cryptococcus neoformans	India ink, encapsulated yeast, mucicarmine (+) capsule, cryptococcal antigen (serum and CSF)	Exposure to pigeons, soil exposure, HIV positive, immunocompromised	Papule with crust resembling molluscum contagiosum; also forms ulcers on skin, mouth, and genitalia; may have lung or CNS involvement
Histoplasma capsulatum	Dimorphic fungus, histoplasma antigen (urine and serum)	Bats, birds, and soil exposure; HIV positive, immunocompromised; Eastern and Central United States in Ohio/Mississippi river valleys, Central and South America, West Indies, Africa, Madagascar	Papule with crust resembling molluscum contagiosum; ulcerative plaques and oral ulcerations
Sporothrix schenckii	Dimorphic fungus	Rose gardening, soil exposure	Papule or pustule at inoculation site develops into subcutaneous nodules or ragged-edged ulcer with proximal nodular lymphangitis; usually on upper extremities
Mycobacterial	AFB smear, cx		
Mycobacterium marinum	AFB (+)	Aquarium enthusiasts	Ulcer with thin seropurulent drainage, nodular lymphangitis
Mycobacterium ulcerans (Buruli ulcer)	AFB (+), PCR for the insertion sequence IS *2404* in swabs or tissue samples	Africa, Australia, South East Asia, South America, North America (Mexico)	Subcutaneous nodule that ulcerates with extensive scarring and contracture formation; edematous lesion rapidly progresses to extensive ulceration, may have osteomyelitis contiguous to ulcer
Mycobacterium avium complex	AFB (+)	HIV positive, immunocompromised; soil, water	Multiple subcutaneous nodules or ulcers; may be associated with cervical lymphadenitis drainage to skin, or direct inoculation
Mycobacterium haemophilum	AFB (+), requires iron-supplemented culture medium and incubation at 30–32°C	Australia, United States, Canada, France; HIV positive, transplantation	Papules develop into pustules which form deep ulcers, usually on extremities overlying joints; may have septic arthritis +/– osteomyelitis, may have LN
Mycobacterium tuberculosis	AFB (+), PPD helpful if positive	Worldwide	Nodules or ulcers especially in HIV-positive patients
Viral			
Herpes simplex	DFA, viral cx, Tzank prep	Sexually transmitted disease	Oral, perineal, genital ulcers; whitlow on hands; lesions with thin-walled vesicles; shallow painful ulcers

Cause	Laboratory Work-up	Epidemiology	Clinical Clues to Diagnosis
Parasitic			
Leishmaniasis	Punch biopsy, aspirates, or scrapings of skin for culture, histopathology and touch prep using Wright's and Giemsa stains looking for amastigotes at base of lesion; serology; PCR of tissue aspirates or peripheral blood	Sandfly bites	Papule at the site of insect bite enlarges to form a nodule, which then develops into a punched-out ulcer; may have associated LN; rarely nodules form without ulceration; may involve nasal or oral mucosa
Old World *L. major* *L. tropica* *L. (L) aethiopica*		Mediterranean, Middle East, Africa, Southern Asia, India	
New World *L. mexicana* complex *Viannia subgenus: L* *(V) braziliensis, L (V)* *panamensis, L (V) guanensis,* *L (V) peruviana*		Latin America, Central and South America	

LN = lymphadenopathy; G (+)= gram-positive; G (–); = gram-negative; AFB = acid-fast bacilli; cx = culture; CNS = central nervous system; DFA = direct fluorescent antibodies; PCR = polymerase chain reaction; PPD = purified protein. derivative CSF = cerebrospinal fluid.

Impetigo

Impetigo is a superficial infection of the skin involving only the epidermis (see Figure 20.2.). Impetigo is highly contagious and usually occurs in young children following minor skin trauma. Nonbullous impetigo, the classic honey-colored crusts on the face or extremities, is caused by *S. pyogenes* or *S. aureus*; toxin-producing strains of *S. aureus* cause bullous impetigo (varnish-like crust). Treatment of bullous and nonbullous impetigo requires coverage of methicillin-sensitive *S. aureus* (MSSA): dicloxacillin 500 mg orally every 6 hours, or first-generation cephalosporins such as cephalexin 500 mg orally every 6 hours for 7 days; the oral cephalosporins cefixime, ceftibuten, and cefetamet pivoxil have no activity against MSSA. For penicillin-allergic patients, clindamycin 300 to 450 mg orally every 6 hours or clarithromycin 500 mg orally every 12 hours is appropriate. Because most areas have seen the emergence of community-acquired methicillin-resistant *S. aureus* (MRSA), empiric therapy targeting MRSA with trimethoprim-sulfamethoxazole 2 double strength tablets orally every 12 hours, or minocycline 100 mg orally every 12 hours is warranted. Topical mupirocin ointment 2% applied to the lesion 3 times daily is an equally effective alternative to systemic therapy.

Ecthyma

Ecthyma (Figure 20.3) is impetigo that extends through the epidermis, forming shallow ulcers with crusts. It occurs in immunocompromised patients and is caused by *S. pyogenes* or *S. aureus*. Gram stain and culture of the lesion must be performed to rule out MRSA or ecthyma gangrenosum, which is caused by *P. areuginosa* sepsis. Treatment of ecthyma due to streptococci or staphylococci is the same as that for impetigo, but duration of therapy may be longer. Unlike impetigo, ecthyma may heal with scarring.

Folliculitis

Folliculitis is an inflammation of the hair follicles, usually caused by *S. aureus*. Topical therapy with mupirocin 3 times daily for 7 days is usually adequate. If the infection does not respond, oral therapy with agents used for impetigo should be adequate. Lesions that do not respond to antistaphylococcal antibiotics should be cultured because they may be caused by MRSA or other pathogens. Therapy should be tailored to antimicrobial sensitivities. On rare occasions, gram-negative organisms cause folliculitis, typically in association with either superinfection in patients taking long-term antibiotics for acne vulgaris or hot-tub bathing. Gram-negative folliculitis in acne patients is caused by *Klebsiella*, *Enterobacter*,

Table 20.2 Clinical Presentation and Therapy of Pyoderma

Type Of Disease	Distinguishing Features	Causative Organism	Treatment
Primary Pyoderma			
Impetigo			For MSSA: Ampicillin-clavulanic acid 875 mg PO q12h or Dicloxacillin 500 mg PO q6 h or Cephalexin 500 mg PO q6h *(Not cefixime)* or Clindamycin 300 – 450 mg PO q6h or Clarithromycin 500 mg PO BID or Mupirocin ointment 2% topically TID For MRSA: Mupirocin ointment 2% topically TID or Minocycline 100 mg PO bid or Trimethoprim-sulfamethoxazole (TMP/SMX) 2 double strength tablets (TMP 160 mg) PO BID
Nonbullous Impetigo	Superficial honey-colored crusts	*Streptococcus pyogenes*, *Staphylococcus aureus*	
Bullous Impetigo	Thin vesicles and bullae, when ruptured produce varnish-like crust	Toxin-producing strains of *S. aureus*	
Ecthyma	Ulcer with crust	*Streptococcus pyogenes*, *S. aureus*	Treat as impetigo with oral agents, may need longer duration of therapy
Folliculitis	Hair follicle with pustules, erythema	*S. aureus*	*Topical:* Clindamycin or Erythromycin or Mupirocin or Benzoyl peroxide lotion *Unresponsive:* Treat as impetigo
Gram-negative folliculitis	Usually on face in patients with acne vulgaris on chronic suppressive antibiotic therapy	*Klebsiella, Enterobacter, Proteus* species	Ampicillin-clavulanic acid 875 mg PO q12h or TMP/SMX one double strength tablet (TMP 160 mg) PO BID
Hot-tub folliculitis	Pustules and vesicles on an erythematous base in bathing-suit distribution	*Pseudomonas aeruginosa*	Self-limited in normal hosts; decontaminate and chlorinate hot tub
Furuncle/Carbuncle	Abscess formation in dermis, subcutaneous tissue that may coalesce and drain; if cellulitis or sepsis associated, needs intravenous antibiotics; patients may have recurrences; suggest culture to rule out MRSA or gram-negative organisms	*S. aureus* both MSSA and MRSA, now many community-acquired strains are MRSA	Careful incision and drainage, and warm compresses; Antistaphylococcal antibiotics targeting MRSA including: TMP/SMX

Clinical Syndromes – Skin and Lymph Nodes

Type Of Disease	Distinguishing Features	Causative Organism	Treatment
			2 double strength (TMP 160 mg) PO bid +/– Rifampin 300 mg PO BID or Minocycline 100 mg PO BID If associated with cellulitis or sepsis: Vancomycin 1 g IV q12h or Daptomycin 4 mg/kg IV q 24h (dosed for skin/soft tissue only, not bacteremia) If recurrent, eradicate nasal carriage of *S. aureus* by: Mupirocin (topical 2%) intranasally BID X 5 d or Rifampin 600 mg PO q day plus either dicloxacillin 500 mg PO QID X 10 days (for MSSA) *or* TMP/SMX 2 double strength tablets PO BID × 10 days (for MRSA)
Neutrophilic			
Pyoderma gangrenosum	Rapidly progressive painful ulcers, ragged violaceous edges with necrotic centers, usually on lower legs; Underlying IBD, malignancy, arthritis, monoclonal gammopathy *Biopsy*: PMN, lymphocytic infiltration, +/– vasculitis	No organisms seen, culture negative	Methylprednisolone 0.5–1 mg/kg/d (+/– cyclosporine) or Cyclosporine 5 mg/kg/day (+/– methylprednisolone) For PG associated with Chrohn's disease: infliximab Other agents used include: mycophenolate mofetil, clofazimine, azathioprine, methotrexate, tacrolimus, thalidomide, dapsone (contraindicated in G6PD-deficient patients) Localized PG: topical or intralesional corticosteroids, or tacrolimus ointment
Sweet's syndrome	Fever, neutrophilia, prompt response to steriods, painful erythematous plaques, may form bullae and ulcerate; located on head, neck, arms; 20% have associated malignancy, usually AML, elevated sedimentation rate *Biposy*: dense PMN infiltration of the dermis, no vasculitis	No organisms seen, culture negative	Prednisone 1 mg/kg/d, slow taper over 4–6 wks; dramatic response. or Potassium iodide or Colchicine If steroids contraindicated, may use indomethacin, clofazimine, cyclosporine, dapsone
Secondary Pyoderma	Pre-existing lesions of dermatitis such as eczema, psoriasis, or surgical/traumatic wounds		Based on culture data. Note increasing rates of community-acquired MRSA

Abbrevialtions: AML = Acute myelogenous leukemia; G6PD = glucose-6-phosphate dehydrogenase; IBD = inflammatory bowel disease; MSSA = methicillin-sensitive *S. aureus*; MRSA = methicillin-resistant *S. aureus*; PG = pyoderma gangrenosum; PMN = polymorphonuclear leukocytes.

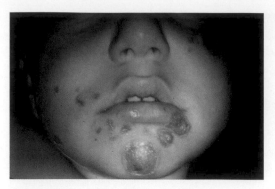

Figure 20.2 Impetigo. This is a superficial streptococcal or staphylococcal infection that occurs just beneath the stratum corneum. It generally occurs in the paranasal or perioral area in young people. Note typical honey-colored crusts, which heal without scarring. (Reproduced with permission from Sanders CV, Nesbitt L.T, eds. *The Skin and Infection: A Color Atlas and Text*. Baltimore: Williams & Wilkins; 1995: page 35.)

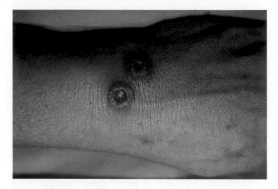

Figure 20.3 Ecthyma. This is a more serious form of impetigo in which the infection penetrates to the dermis. Scarring is common. (Reproduced with permission from Dr. Charles V. Sanders in Sanders CV, Nesbitt LT, eds. *The Skin and Infection: A Color Atlas and Text*. Baltimore: Williams & Wilkins; 1995: page 35.)

and *Proteus* species and usually occurs on the face. Treatment depends on susceptibilities, but ampicillin-clavulanic acid or trimethoprim-sulfamethoxazole may be used empirically. Hot-tub folliculitis caused by *P. aeruginosa* is usually self-limiting in a normal host, and no action is necessary beyond decontaminating the water and ensuring proper chlorination.

Furuncles and Carbuncles

Furuncles are skin abscesses caused by *S. aureus*; they may be begin as folliculitis that extends into the surrounding dermis and subcutaneous tissue. Carbuncles comprise several furuncles that coalesce to form loculated abscesses with draining pus. Treatment of

furuncles and carbuncles includes antistaphylococcal antibiotics targeting MRSA, along with careful incision and drainage of the abscess. Some patients with recurrent furuncles and carbuncles and may require elimination of nasal *S. aureus* carriage with nasal applications of mupirocin, or rifampin plus either dicloxacillin (for MSSA) or trimethoprim-sulfamethoxazole (for MRSA). Bathing with antibacterial soap also helps decrease *S. aureus* carriage.

Secondary Pyoderma

Secondary pyoderma is a bacterial superinfection of skin previously disrupted by trauma, surgery, or chronic skin conditions such as eczema or psoriasis. The usual organism is *S. aureus,* which can be methicillin-resistant whether community acquired or healthcare associated. Empiric treatment for serious wound infections is intravenous vancomycin pending culture results. Mild to moderate infections can be treated with oral trimethoprim/sulfamethoxazole (+/- rifampin) or minocycline. Secondary pyoderma caused by pressure sores and diabetic foot ulcers is usually polymicrobial and requires broad-spectrum therapy with piperacillin-tazobactam, imipenem, or a combination of ciprofloxacin and clindamycin. Table 20.2 summarizes suggested therapy for pyoderma.

Neutrophilic Dermatoses

Pyoderma caused by neutrophilic infiltrates usually is associated with underlying disease such as cancer or inflammatory bowel disease (IBD). The main entities are pyoderma gangrenosum and Sweet's syndrome.

Pyoderma Gangrenosum

The diagnosis of pyoderma gangrenosum is clinical. The lesion begins as a small erythematous papule, rapidly progressing to tender pustules that undergo central necrosis and ulceration. The border of the ulcers is ragged, violaceous, and surrounded by erythema. Distinguishing characteristics include severe pain at the ulcer site, lesions at the site of minor trauma, parchment scarring, and an associated systemic disease such as IBD, rheumatologic disease, or malignancy. Biopsy of the lesions is done to exclude infection, vasculitis, malignancy, and vascular occlusive disease because histopathologic findings are nonspecific. Central necrosis and lymphocytic and neutrophilic infiltrates with or without vasculitic changes are seen on histopathology of pyoderma gangrenosum lesions; lymphocytes and plasma cells around vessels are common findings. Pyoderma gangrenosum usually occurs on the lower extremities over bony prominences, where repeated trauma aggravates the condition (pathergy); its cause is unknown. Treatment for disseminated pyoderma gangrenosum includes methylprednisolone 0.5-1 mg/kg by mouth daily or cyclosporine 5 mg/kg/d given separately or together. For pyoderma gangrenosum associated with Chrohn's disease, the tumor necrosis factor-α inhibitor infliximab is recommended as first-line therapy. Mycophenolate mofetil, clofazimine, azathioprine, methotrexate, tacrolimus, thalidomide, dapsone, and many other drugs and modalities have been used to treat pyoderma gangrenosum; response to therapy varies.

Sweet's Syndrome

Sweet's syndrome is an acute febrile neutrophilic dermatosis that may be idiopathic or associated with a malignancy. Lesions are painful erythematous plaques usually on the upper extremities, head, and neck. These lesions are classically associated with fever and neutrophilia, but some patients have myalgia, arthralgia, proteinuria, and conjunctivitis. Nearly all patients with Sweet's syndrome have an elevated erythrocyte sedimentation rate. Dense neutrophilic infiltration of the dermis without vasculitis is the classic finding on biopsy, and it is important to exclude bacteria, mycobacteria, and fungi, because steroids are the appropriate therapy for Sweet's syndrome. The response to prednisone 1 mg/kg/d is dramatic; constitutional symptoms improve within hours, and skin lesions improve over 1 to 2 days. Steroids should be tapered slowly over 4 to 6 weeks. Other first-line agents used to treat Sweet's syndrome include potassium iodide or colchicine. If steroids are contraindicated, alternative treatments include clofazimine, indomethacin, cyclosporine, and dapsone.

Herpetic Whitlow

Herpetic whitlow, a herpes simplex infection of the pulp of the finger, may occur in anyone who has mucocutaneous herpes or who comes in contact with herpetic lesions (ie, health care workers). The initial lesion is a tender vesicle filled with turbid fluid. Lesions may be multiple and may ulcerate and become secondarily infected, developing purulent drainage. Axillary and epitrochlear lymphadenopathy with erythema of the proximal forearm also may occur. Diagnosis can be made by aspirating a vesicle and sending the fluid for viral culture, doing a Tzank test, or performing a DFA test on the blister fluid. Treatment includes acyclovir, and surgery should be avoided. Some lesions may be superinfected, so clinicians should consider coverage for *S. aureus* (targeting MRSA) with trimethoprim-sulfamethoxazole (TMP/SMX) 2 double strength (TMP 160 mg) tablets orally every 12 hours or minocycline 100 mg orally every 12 hours, if the lesion does not respond to acyclovir therapy alone.

SUGGESTED READING

Burton CS III. Treatment of leg ulcers. *Dermatol Clin.* 1993;11:315–323.

Cohen PR, Kurzrock R. Sweet's syndrome revisited: a review of disease concepts. *Int J Dermatol.* 2003;42:761–778.

Cohen PR, Talpaz M, Kuzrock R. Malignancy-associated Sweet's syndrome: review of the world literature. *J Clin Oncol.* 1988;6: 1887–1897.

De Araujo T, Valencia I, Federman DG, et al. Managing the patient with venous ulcers. *Ann Intern Med.* 2003;138:326–334.

Feingold DS. Staphylococcal and streptococcal pyodermas. *Semin Dermatol.* 1993;12: 331–335.

Fitzgerald RL, McBurney EI, Nesbitt LT Jr. Sweet's syndrome. *Int J Dermatol.* 1996; 35(1):9–15.

Fitzpatrick TB, Johnson RA, Wolff K, et al. Suurmond D. *Color Atlas and Synopsis of Clinical Dermatology Common and Serious Diseases.* 3rd ed. New York: McGraw-Hill; 1997.

Kostman JR, DiNubile MJ. Nodular lymphangitis: a distinctive but often unrecognized syndrome. *Ann Intern Med.* 1993;118:883–888.

Murakawa GJ, Harvell JD, Lubitz P, et al. Aspergillosis and acquired immunodeficiency syndrome. *Arch Dermatol.* 2000;136: 365–369.

Murray HW, Berman JD, Davies CR, et al. Advances in leishmaniasis. *Lancet.* 2005;366: 1561–1577.

Myskowski PL, White MH, Ahkami R. Fungal disease in the immunocompromised host. *Dermatol Clin.* 1997;15(2):295–305.

Powell FC, Su WPD, Perry HO. Pyoderma gangrenosum: classification and management. *J Am Acad Dermatol.* 1996;34(3): 395–409.

Reichrath J, Bens G, Bonowitz A, et al. Treatment recommendations for pyoderma gangrenosum: an evidence-based review of the literature based on more than 350 patients. *J Am Acad Dermatol*. 2005;53: 273–283.

Sadick NS. Current aspects of bacterial infections of the skin. *Dermatol Clin*. 1997;15(2): 341–349.

Sanders CV, Nesbitt LT, eds. *The Skin and Infection: A Color Atlas and Text*. Baltimore, MD: Williams & Wilkins; 1995.

Shelley WB, Shelley ED. *Advanced Dermatologic Diagnosis*. Philadelphia, PA: WB Saunders; 1992.

Wansbrough-Jones M, Phillips R. Buruli ulcer: emerging from obscurity. *Lancet*. 2006:367:1849–1858.

21. Cellulitis and Erysipelas

Mandi P. Sachdeva and Kenneth J. Tomecki

Skin and soft-tissue infections (SSTIs) are routinely encountered by physicians in the office setting and can vary in both clinical presentation and severity. Erysipelas is a more superficial SSTI involving the dermal lymphatics; cellulitis is a deeper infection extending into the deep dermis and subcutaneous tissues.

ERYSIPELAS

Clinical Manifestations

Erysipelas is a superficial SSTI with dermal lymphatic involvement and a distinct clinical presentation. The legs are the most common affected sites, but erysipelas can occur anywhere on the body. Young, elderly, and immunocompromised patients are particularly susceptible to erysipelas, especially if predisposing factors such as venous insufficiency, lymphedema, obesity, or any epidermal defect that impairs barrier function (eg, ulcers, operative or traumatic wounds, fissures) exist. Erysipelas is more common in older women and young men.

Erysipelas classically presents as a tender, sharply demarcated, bright-red edematous plaque with a raised, indurated advancing border (Figure 21.1). Abrupt onset of fever, chills, and malaise may precede skin disease by a few hours to a day. Some patients have associated regional lymphadenopathy with or without lymphatic streaking, in addition to edema with possible bullae formation.

Because erysipelas can produce lymphatic obstruction, it tends to recur in areas of earlier infection. Such recurrences are the most common complication occurring in approximately 30% of cases. Other complications including sepsis and progression to deep cellulitis are uncommon and are usually restricted to debilitated patients with underlying diseases.

Microbiology

Most cases of erysipelas are caused by β-hemolytic group A streptococci (GAS), including *Streptococcus pyogenes*. Less often groups C, D, and G streptococci are the causative organisms in adults. Group B streptococcus is often the cause of erysipelas in newborns and postpartum women. Other less common causative agents include *Staphylococcus aureus*, *Pneumococcus* species, *Klebsiella pneumoniae*, *Yersinia*, *enterocolitica*, and *Haemophilus influenzae*, which is now less common due to type B vaccination in infants. More recently, community- and hospital-acquired pathogens such as methicillin-resistant *S. aureus* (CA-MRSA, HA-MRSA) have emerged as potential causes of erysipelas.

Diagnosis and Differential Diagnosis

Characteristic skin disease usually suggests the diagnosis. Swabs for Gram stain and culture from a suspected portal of entry may be helpful but are usually not necessary. Skin biopsy for tissue culture and the injection-reaspiration method of tissue fluid collection both yield poor results and have little diagnostic value. Blood cultures are positive in only 5% of patients. Routine lab tests are usually unrevealing, but some patients will have leukocytosis.

Differential diagnosis includes allergic or photosensitive contact dermatitis, especially for patients with facial erysipelas, but fever, pain, and leukocytosis do not occur. Autoimmune diseases, including systemic lupus erythematosus and dermatomyositis, often exhibit facial rash and fever, but they evolve slowly and both are typically bilateral, less sharply demarcated, and lack intense erythema. Other diagnostic considerations include erythema infectiosum, Sweet's syndrome, angioedema, and erysipeloid.

CELLULITIS

Clinical Manifestations

Cellulitis is an infectious inflammation of the soft tissues. In contrast to erysipelas, cellulitis is a deeper infection of the dermis with variable depth of extension into subcutaneous tissue.

Clinically, cellulitis differs from erysipelas. Cellulitis typically presents as an ill-defined, erythematous firm plaque occurring in conjunction

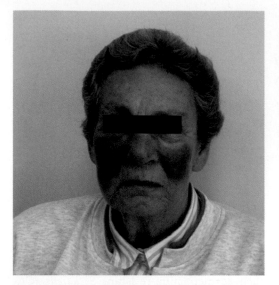

Figure 21.1 Bilateral facial erysipelas. Note discrete, raised edge of erythema.

with the four cardinal signs of inflammation: rubor, calor, dolor, and tumor (Figure 21.2). Affected patients often have associated fever, chills, and malaise.

In healthy patients, antecedent trauma often produces a defect in the skin barrier leading to cellulitis, in contrast to a bloodborne route in immunocompromised patients. If the leg is affected, interdigital tinea pedis is often the portal of entry. Other predisposing factors include peripheral vascular disease, alcoholism, intravenous drug abuse, malignancy, diabetes, or a concomitant skin disease such as stasis dermatitis or ulceration of any type.

Fever, lymphangitis, regional lymphadenopathy, focal abscess formation, and bullae may accompany cellulitis. In addition, necrosis of the skin and subcutaneous tissues may be a complication. Sepsis is a more common complication in children or immunocompromised adults. Many patients have leukocytosis. If the causative organism is GAS, cellulitis may lead to acute glomerulonephritis and a streptococcal toxic shock-like syndrome.

Microbiology

Streptococcus pyogenes and *Staphylococcus aureus* are the most frequent causes of cellulitis. Both CA-MRSA and HA-MRSA have become increasingly prominent causative pathogens in cellulitis as well. Other specific causes of cellulitis should be considered in particular clinical situations or because of certain patient exposures; these are listed in Table 21.1.

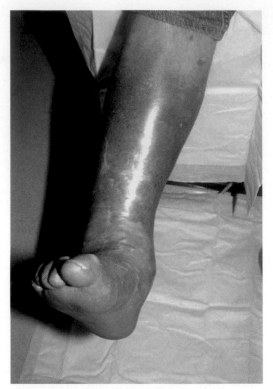

Figure 21.2 Right leg cellulitis. Note irregular margin.

Diagnosis and Differential Diagnosis

Clinical presentation should suggest the diagnosis, but a positive culture is confirmatory. Swabs from exudate, erosions, ulcerations, abscesses, and surgical wounds, as well as tissue biopsy for culture, have a high yield, more so than aspirate or blood cultures. Additional laboratory studies, including complete blood count, anti-DNase antibody, antistreptolysin titer, and blood cultures, can be performed but are not usually helpful or specific.

Imaging studies may be helpful. Conventional radiography can delineate pockets of gas in anaerobic cellulitis, especially clostridial cellulitis. Magnetic resonance imaging (MRI) can also aid in the diagnosis of SSTI. T2-weighted images highlight disease process best. Cellulitis of the periocular soft tissue warrants ophthalmologic evaluation to differentiate preseptal SSTI from orbital cellulitis, a medical emergency. Computed tomographic (CT) scanning can quickly differentiate these two entities.

The differential diagnosis of cellulitis, especially if localized to the lower extremity, includes other inflammatory diseases such as stasis dermatitis, superficial thrombophlebitis,

Table 21.1 Likely Causes of Cellulitis in Specific Clinical Situations or Related to Specific Exposures

Type/Scenario	Likely Organism
Postsurgical cellulitis	*Staphylococcus aureus*
Perianal cellulitis	Group B streptococcus
Preseptal cellulitis	*S. aureus, S. pyogenes*
Orbital cellulitis	*S. aureus, S. pyogenes*
Facial cellulitis	*Haemophilus influenzae*[a]
Neonatal cellulitis	Group B streptococcus
Crepitant cellulitis	*Clostridium* species
Salt water exposure	*Vibrio vulnificus*
Fresh water exposure	*Aeromonas hydrophilia*
Hot tub exposure	*Pseudomonas aeruginosa*
Soil exposure	*Clostridium* species
Dog/cat bite	*Pasteurella multocida*
Human bite	*Eikenella corrodens*
Immunocompromised	Often mixed infection, consider gram-negative organisms, fungi
Nosocomial	*Pseudomonas*
Handling of raw poultry, meat	*Erysipelothrix rhusiopathiae*
Handling of raw fish	*Streptococcus iniae Erysipelothrix rhusiopathiae*
Intravenous drug use	*S. aureus*

[a] Less common since advent of vaccine.

lipodermatosclerosis, vasculitis, and deep venous thrombosis.

THERAPY

Systemic antimicrobial therapy is the treatment of SSTIs, and many appropriate choices exist for uncomplicated cases (Table 21.2). Due to the emergence of resistant organisms, treatment considerations have changed somewhat in recent years. Being familiar with particular patient populations and regional variations in bacterial susceptibility patterns are critical in selecting appropriate antimicrobial therapy. If standard therapy fails, a resistant or less common organism (Table 21.3) may be the causative agent, and cultures with drug sensitivity are necessary to guide therapy.

For both uncomplicated erysipelas and cellulitis, empiric therapy should target *S. pyogenes* and *S. aureus*. Penicillins or other beta-lactam antibiotics, including first and second generation or the newer extended spectrum cephalosporins, are typically considered the treatment of choice for uncomplicated SSTIs. For penicillin-allergic patients, alternate therapies include either a cephalosporin if the penicillin allergy is not type I (immunoglobulin G [IgE]-mediated immediate hypersensitivity) or a macrolide, such as erythromycin, clarithromycin, or azithromycin. All of these have good but varied activity against gram-positive organisms. Clarithromycin is the most effective, followed by azithromycin and erythromycin. Compared to erythromycin, azithromycin and clarithromycin have fewer gastrointestinal side effects and better Gram-positive activity; therefore they may be better therapeutic options.

Clindamycin, a lincosamide, has good activity against *S. pyogenes* in addition to methicillin-susceptible *S. aureus* (MSSA) and CA-MRSA, although inducible resistance to clindamycin has become a concern. Resistance to erythromycin indicates the possibility of inducible resistance to clindamycin, which can be screened for in the laboratory by the D test.

The family of tetracycline antibiotics, including tetracycline, minocycline, and doxycycline, is effective in treating uncomplicated SSTIs with satisfactory coverage of common causative organisms as well as CA-MRSA. Specific issues including variable susceptibility based on both individual tetracycline drug and region, reduced absorption due to binding with food and cations, gastrointestinal upset, dizziness or vertigo, and photosensitivity may limit their use.

Fluoroquinolones have demonstrated efficacy similar to β-lactam antibiotics, but increasing resistance has limited their use as an alternative therapy.

Sulfamethoxazole-trimethoprim is a reasonable choice for SSTIs, especially if infection with MRSA is suspected. Risk of severe hypersensitivity reactions such as erythema multiforme, Stevens-Johnson syndrome, or even toxic epidermal necrolysis limits its use as a first-line agent.

In addition to systemic antimicrobial therapy, local measures including immobilization and elevation of the affected area can be important adjuvant therapies in uncomplicated SSTIs. If fluctuance is present, moist heat may help localize infection. All abscesses require incision and drainage with culture.

Table 21.2 Oral Antimicrobial Therapeutic Options for the Treatment of Uncomplicated SSTIs

Class	Medication	Adult Dosage
Penicillins[a]	Penicillin V	500 mg BID-QID
	Amoxicillin	500 mg TID
	Amoxicillin/clavulanate	875/125 mg BID
	Dicloxacillin	500 mg BID-QID
Cephalosporins	Cephalexin[b]	500 mg BID-QID
	Cefaclor[c]	250–500 mg TID
	Cefuroxime[c]	250–500 mg BID
	Cefprozil[c]	250 mg BID
	Cefdinir[d]	300 mg BID
	Cefpodoxime[d]	400 mg BID
Macrolides	Erythromycin	500 mg BID-QID
	Azithromycin	500 mg on day one, then 250 mg QD days 2–5
	Clarithromycin	500 mg QD-BID
Tetracyclines	Tetracycline	500 mg BID-QID
	Doxycycline	100 mg BID
	Minocycline	100 mg BID
Lincosamide	Clindamycin	300 mg BID-QID
Fluoroquinolones	Ciprofloxacin	500 mg BID
	Levofloxacin	500 mg QD
Other	Sulfamethoxazole-trimethoprim	800/160 mg (DS) BID

All treatment for 7 to 14 days unless otherwise specified.
[a] Adjustment in dosages required for renal impairment.
[b] First generation.
[c] Second generation.
[d] Extended spectrum.
Abbreviation: SSTIs = skin and soft-tissue infections

Hospitalization for intravenous antimicrobial therapy and supportive care is warranted for immunocompromised patients, patients with extensive skin disease with or without signs of sepsis, patients with systemic symptoms including fever, rigors, hypotension, or tachycardia, patients who have failed appropriate initial therapy or are rapidly progressing, and when necrosis is present. Vancomycin is typically considered the treatment of choice in this setting, especially with MRSA infection.

Polymicrobial infection should be suspected in immunocompromised patients, and broader coverage for gram-negative organisms is warranted. In such cases, combined treatment with vancomycin plus either an extended spectrum antipseudomonal penicillin, such as piperacillin-tazobactam or an extended-spectrum cephalosporin or clindamycin and a fluoroquinolone, is appropriate. If tissue necrosis is present, immediate surgical evaluation is required. Early and complete surgical debridement extending

Table 21.3 Recommended Antimicrobial Therapies for Specific Organisms

Organism	First Line Therapy	Alternative Therapies
Aeromonas hydrophila	Fluoroquinolone	TMP-SMX
Clostridium perfringens	Penicillin G +/− clindamycin	Doxycycline
Eikenella corrodens	Penicillin G, ampicillin	Amoxicillin/clavulanate, TMP-SMX, fluoroquinolone
Erysipelothrix rhusiopathiae	Penicillin G, ampicillin	Fluoroquinolone
Haemophilus influenzae	Cefotaxime, ceftriaxone	Cefuroxime, TMP-SMX, fluoroquinolone
Pasteurella multocida	Penicillin, ampicillin, amoxicillin	Doxycycline, TMP-SMX
Staphylococcus aureus	Dicloxacillin, oxacillin, nafcillin	Clindamycin, macrolide
HA-MRSA	Vancomycin	Linezolid, daptomycin, tigecycline
CA-MRSA	TMP-SMX	Minocycline, tetracycline, clindamycin, rifampin[a]
Streptococcus pyogenes	Penicillin	Other beta-lactams, macrolide
Vibrio vulnificus	Doxycycline + ceftazidime	Cefotaxime, fluoroquinolone

[a] Not recommended as monotherapy.

beyond the areas of necrosis to reach healthy tissue is necessary. Indicators of deep infection requiring debridement include gangrenous changes, severe pain or anesthetic skin, crepitus, poor response to antibiotic therapy, or abscess formation with multiple tracts.

Although not recommended for first- line therapy, other appropriate medications that can be used in the hospital setting if vancomycin allergy is present or vancomycin- resistant organisms are confirmed include linezolid, daptomycin, or tigecycline (Table 21.4).

Linezolid is currently approved for the treatment of complicated SSTIs due to MRSA and other drug-resistant gram-positive organisms. The ability to convert from intravenous to oral therapy makes this an attractive option. Daptomycin, a cyclic lipopeptide with an unclear mechanism of action, is known to be bactericidal against gram-positive bacteria, including MRSA. Tigecycline is a glycylcycline derived from tetracyclines; it offers broader coverage, including gram-positive, gram-negative, anaerobic, and multidrug-resistant organisms, and has also recently been approved for the treatment of complicated SSTIs.

Table 21.4 Intravenous Dosing Regimens for Complicated SSTIs

Medication	Adult Dosage
Vancomycin[a]	1 g q12h
Piperacillin/tazobactam[a]	3.375 g q6h
Clindamycin	600–900 mg q8h
Linezolid[b]	600 mg q12h
Daptomycin[b]	4–6 mg q24h
Tigecycline[c]	50 mg q12h after 100-mg loading dose

[a] Adjustment in dosage interval required for renal impairment.
[b] Same dose for oral conversion.
[c] Adjustment in dosage required for severe hepatic impairment.
Abbreviation: skin and soft-tissue infections = SSTIs

Recurrence is especially common in patients with SSTIs of the legs who have impaired circulation. In such instances, continuous antimicrobial prophylaxis may be necessary, coupled with weight reduction, support stockings to reduce edema, and good skin hygiene with emollients and possibly topical antifungal therapy.

SUGGESTED READING

Bisno AL, Stevens DL. Streptococcal infections of skin and soft tissues. *N Engl J Med.* 1996;334(4):240–245.

Elston DM. Community-acquired methicillin-resistant Staphylococcus aureus. *J Am Acad Dermatol.* 2007;56(1):1–16.

Rogers RL, Perkins J. Skin and soft tissues infections. *Prim Care.* 2006;33(3):697–710.

Rosen T. Update on treating uncomplicated skin and skin structure infections. *J Drugs Dermatol.* 2005;4(suppl 6):9–14.

22. Deep Soft-Tissue Infections: Necrotizing Fasciitis and Gas Gangrene

Stephen Ash

Necrotizing fasciitis (NF) and gas gangrene (GG) are serious infections of the deep soft tissue. They both carry a high morbidity and mortality. Early diagnosis and treatment is important and is the key to improving outcome. Broadly speaking, NF is an infection primarily of the fascia and deep soft tissue of the skin, whereas GG is usually an infection of the skeletal muscle.

Previously, NF has been subdivided into different categories based on anatomical site, but such classification is not helpful regarding the diagnosis and management of these dangerous conditions. Both GG and, particularly, NF are strongly associated with numerous underlying, premorbid risk factors (Table 22.1), each of which requires medical management to improve the prognosis of an individual patient.

Again, both conditions may be caused by one bacterial organism or, more commonly with NF, they may be polymicrobial and require treatment with broad spectrum or multiple antibiotics.

NECROTIZING FASCIITIS

Diagnosis

Necrotizing fasciitis is an uncommon, but severe, infection with a fulminant course and high mortality often following a history of trauma or surgery. The patient may go into rapid decline with necrosis of soft tissue and multisystem organ failure. The latter would appear to result from superantigenic overstimulation of the immune system and excessive production of cytokines.

Necrotizing fasciitis can affect any part of the body but has a predilection for the limbs, abdominal wall, perineum, and occasionally the neck and periorbital area. Although to begin with, there may be only slight redness, or other discoloration, and swelling, the clue to the patient having NF is often the disproportionate severity of pain as well as systemic upset. The condition is rapidly progressive, with systemic inflammatory responses, shock, and multiorgan failure. Early diagnosis is crucial in optimizing outcome. The diagnosis is predominantly clinical, but both ultrasonography and magnetic resonance imaging (MRI) scans may be of use in supporting such a diagnosis. These tests as well as plain x-ray may sometimes show gas in the soft tissue. Differentiating early NF from the more common cellulitis may be difficult; one clue may be the severe pain that often accompanies NF (Figure 22.1). Occasionally, one may find an area of anesthetic skin overlying the inflamed and indurated area. One report suggests tissue oxygen saturation of the affected limb may help distinguish between cellulitis and NF.

If left untreated, there is progressive discoloration and darkening of the tissue with subcutaneous hemorrhage accompanied by tachycardia, hypotension, acidosis, and fever or occasionally a fall in body temperature.

Some authorities have used a laboratory scoring system: the *Laboratory Risk Indicator for NECrotizing fasciitis* (LRINEC) to determine and assist in the diagnosis of NF. This uses a panel of hematological and biochemical test results (C-reactive protein [CRP], serum creatinine, total white cell count, hemoglobin, blood glucose, and serum sodium) to provide a scoring system for the risk of having NF.

Treatment

The principles of management of NF are outlined in Figure 22.2. Rapid resuscitation takes precedence, followed by the empiric administration of broad-spectrum antibiotics. The choice of antibiotic is further discussed below and summarized in Table 22.2. Surgery with exploration and excision of necrotic tissue should not be delayed. Surgery should involve thorough debridement of all nonviable and affected tissue; there is no role for an "incision and drainage" approach to surgery. Repeat surgical explorations on subsequent days should be considered.

Samples for microbiology such as blood cultures should be taken at presentation and also at the time of surgery. Administration of

Table 22.1 Factors Predisposing to Deep Soft-Tissue Infection (Necrotizing Fasciitis and Gas Gangrene)

Trauma, sometimes trivial and including insect bites
Recent surgery
Malignancy, particularly intra-abdominal and carcinoma of colon
Diabetes mellitus
Intra-abdominal sepsis
Alcoholism
Injecting drug use
Obesity
Malnutrition
Recent chickenpox
Immunocompromised states
Chronic renal failure
Systemic steroid use
Peripheral vascular disease
Old age

Table 22.2 Empiric Antibiotic Choices for Necrotizing Fasciitis

Benzyl penicillin + nafcillin + metronidazole + quinolone
Clindamycin + quinolone
Carbapenem, eg, Meropenem (+/–fluconazole)
Piperacillin with tazobactam
Consider vancomycin or linezolid or daptomycin or tigecycline for possible methicillan-resistant *Staphylococcus aureus* (MRSA)

antibiotics should not be delayed while waiting for results. Treatment of comorbidities such as diabetes and malnutrition is important.

Some clinicians suggest considering the following three adjuvant measures to try to improve outcome, although their usefulness remains controversial:

1. The use of hyperbaric oxygen has been tried in many cases of NF. It is not clear from reports whether the outcome is influenced by this therapy.
2. Topical negative pressure or vacuum-assisted wound healing has been tried in patients after surgical excision to promote efficient wound healing of what is often a large surface area of tissue.
3. Because it is thought that some of the systemic proinflammatory effects of NF, mediated by cytokines, are a result of superantigenic effects of bacteria, such as group A streptococci, there is a hypothesis that the administration of pooled, polyvalent intravenous immunoglobulin (IVIG) may be beneficial in modifying this response. There is no good evidence that this is of value so far, however.

Choice of Antibiotic

Possible choices of antibiotic are given in Table 22.2 and may be modified according to local policies and the circumstances around individual patients. The initial choice of antibiotic is likely to be empiric and should cover gram-positive and -negative organisms as well as anaerobic bacteria and should be administered intravenously, as absorption from the gut is likely to be unreliable in patients with severe systemic upset.

Over the past few years there have been reports of MRSA as the causative agent in some cases of NF, both in patients with infections

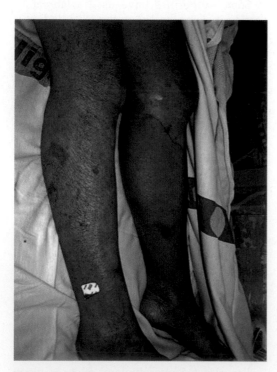

Figure 22.1 A 32-year-old man with early necrotizing fasciitis of the leg following minor trauma 3 days earlier.

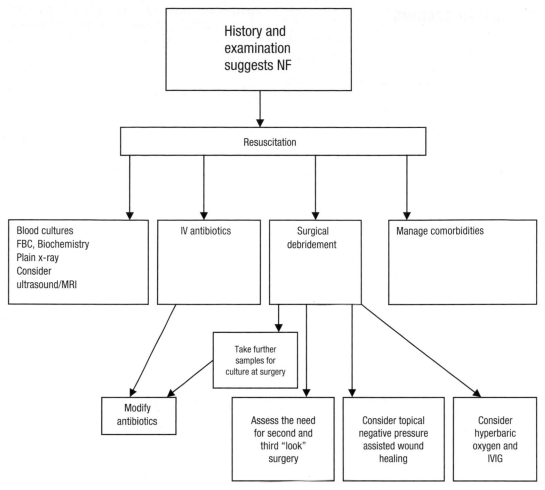

Figure 22.2 Management of necrotizing fasciitis.

acquired nosocomially and from the community. Some of the newer antibiotic agents with activity against MRSA may have use in this scenario, such as linezolid, tigecycline, and daptomycin.

GAS GANGRENE (CLOSTRIDIAL MYONECROSIS)

Gas gangrene is most often caused by the anaerobic spore-forming bacillus *Clostridium perfringens*, an organism that causes infection of skeletal muscle following surgery or trauma. Necrosis and gas formation are characteristic features of the infection. There is rapid advancement of infection and muscle necrosis over just a few hours, if untreated. Myonecrosis can also occur spontaneously, caused in this case by *Clostridium septicum*. This occurrence may be associated with underlying colonic abnormalities or leukemia.

The first symptom of posttraumatic or postsurgical GG is the sudden onset of pain at the infected site. The area becomes tender and discolored, although it may be pale to begin with. Gas may be detected in the muscle on plain X rays and also both computed tomography (CT) and MRI scans. However, with all but deep-seated infections, crepitus is palpable demonstrating the presence of gas in the muscle tissue. The patient will become systemically unwell, with a bacteremia in many instances. Hemolysis may ensue, and renal failure may follow as a consequence.

Urgent surgical debridement and antibiotic therapy are the essential mainstays of treatment and the prognosis may well be improved with the additional use of hyperbaric oxygen. Antibiotic therapy may be chosen from penicillins, clindamycin, and metronidazole. Tetracyclines and chloramphenicol can also be used. Antitoxin is no longer available.

SUGGESTED READING

Edlich RF, Winters KL, Woodard CR, Britt LD, Long WB. Massive soft tissue infections: necrotising fasciitis and purpura fulminans, *J Long Term Eff Med Implants.* 2005;15: 57–65.

Hasham S, Matteucci P, Stanley PRW, Hart NB. Necrotising fasciitis. *Br Med J.* 2005;330:830–833.

Wang TL, Hung CR. Role of tissue oxygen saturation monitoring in diagnosing necrotising fasciitis of the lower limbs. *Ann Emerg Med.* 2004;44:222–228.

Wong CH, Khin LW, Heng KS, Low CO. The LRINEC (Laboratory Risk Indicator for Necrotising Fasciitis) score: a tool for distinguishing necrotising fasciitis from other soft tissue infections. *Crit Care Med.* 2004;32:1535–1541.

Wong CH, Wang YS. The diagnosis of Necrotising fasciitis. *Curr Opin Infect Dis.* 2005;18:101–106.

Wong CH, Wang YS. What is subacute necrotising fasciitis? A proposed clinical diagnostic criteria. *J Infect.* 2006;52:415–419.

23. Human and Animal Bites

Ellie J. C. Goldstein

Annually, in the United States, more than 5 million animal and untold numbers of human bite wounds occur and account for 10 000 persons hospitalized and 1% (300 000) of all emergency department visits. Patients with bite wounds are also commonly seen as outpatients in primary care physician and specialist (orthopedics, plastic/hand surgery, infectious diseases physicians) offices. Some patients will attempt to conceal the nature of the injury with human bite wounds. The bacteriology of these wounds is diverse and comprises oral flora organisms, both aerobic and anaerobic, of the biting animal/human, the victim's skin flora, and occasionally environmental isolates.

ANIMAL BITES

Microbiology

An extensive number of bacterial species are isolated from infected dog and cat bite wounds. *Pasteurella* species, especially *Pasteurella multocida* and *Pasteurella septica,* will be present in 75% and 65% of cat bite and dog bite wounds, respectively. Anaerobes will be present in 50% of dog bite wounds and 67% of cat bite wounds. Streptococci, excluding group A β-hemolytic streptococci *(Streptococcus pyogenes)* are present in 46% of dog and cat bite wounds, whereas *Staphylococcus aureus* is present in 20% of dog bites but only 4% of cat bites. *Streptococcus pyogenes* (group A), if present, usually comes from the victim's skin because it is rarely isolated from dog oral flora. *Streptococcus aureus* is also a secondary invader originating as skin flora. *Capnocytophaga canimorsus* is an uncommon wound isolate but has been associated with bacteremia, some fatal, in asplenic and cirrhotic patients. Other veterinary species are often isolated but are difficult for the routine laboratory to identify.

WOUND CARE EVALUATION AND CARE

The elements of wound care are outlined in Table 23.1. The most important principle of

Table 23.1 Components of Care for Human and Animal Bites

History—situation, pet ownership/identity   Geographic location

Examination—nerve function
    Tendon function
    Blood supply (pulses)
    Presence of edema, crush injury
    Proximity to joint
    Bone penetration

Diagram of wound(s)
    Wound care—irrigation
    Debridement
    Elevation
    Immobilization/exercise

Antimicrobials
    Prophylaxis, 3 to 5 days (PO)
    Therapy for established infection (PO versus IM initial dose)
    Empirical versus specific (animal specific)

Culture (if infected)
Baseline radiograph
Tetanus toxoid (0.5 mL IM) if required
Rabies prophylaxis (RIG/human diploid cell vaccine) if needed
Health department report (if required)
Decision regarding need for hospitalization

immediate wound care is for the patient to wash the wound with soap and water as soon as possible after the injury. This will reduce any bacterial or viral (rabies prevention) inoculum. The addition of topical antiseptics or other remedies does not appear to affect the outcome or the incidence of infection. Washing the wound and keeping the wound clean and dry are sufficient for minor wounds. Minor injuries to compromised hosts (Table 23.2) can cause serious infection. Wounds that are on the hands, have associated crush injury or edema, are near a joint or may have penetrated a bone or a joint, and are moderately extensive should be treated aggressively. Bites, especially those around the head and neck, may penetrate a

Table 23.2 Compromised Hosts Requiring Prophylactic Antimicrobial and Aggressive Care for Animal Bite Wounds

Local defense defects
  Preexisting edema
  Prior lymph node dissection
  Prior radiation therapy

Medications
  Steroids
  Immunosuppressives

Diseases/conditions
  Alcoholism
  Asplenia
  Cirrhosis
  Leukemia
  Lymphoma
  Mastectomy (radical or modified radical)
  Myeloma
  Neutropenia
  System lupus, erythematosus

blood vessel and cause exsanguination. In addition, nerves and tendons may be injured or severed, and their function must always be evaluated, especially when wounds involve the hand. If edema is present, develops, or is preexisting, 24-hour-a-day elevation to reduce the edema is an important component of primary therapy. The use of slings is mandatory, and they should be worn to heart level when hand injury results in edema.

Cat scratches are more prone to infection than dog scratches, which are generally minor and rarely cause infection. Any eschar of a wound should be removed if there is more than 1 to 2 mm of erythema surrounding it or it is obviously infected. Puncture wounds are prone to infection, especially when associated with edema. They should be irrigated with sterile normal saline (no added iodine or antimicrobials) using an 18-gauge needle or catheter tip with a 20-mL syringe. The puncture is entered in the direction of injury and care taken to neither extend injury nor create a new one. This system functions as a high-pressure jet and reduces bacterial inoculum, whereas surface cleansing does not. Tears or avulsion should be copiously irrigated, any debris removed, and necrotic tissue cautiously debrided. Overly aggressive debridement can cause a defect that requires subsequent surgery.

Closure of infected wounds is contraindicated. Wounds to the head and neck seen less than 8 hours after injury may be closed if there is copious irrigation, debridement, no undue tension on the suture lines, and antimicrobials are given. The risks of closure with early presenting wounds to other parts of the body have not been studied. Approximating the edges with a tape bandage or delayed primary closure are often used.

Elevation is vital to decrease edema and prevent spread of infection and cannot be overemphasized. The failure of the patient to properly elevate the area is a common cause of therapeutic failure. In the hospital, elevation of a hand should be carried out using a 4-inch tubular stockinette, numerous safety pins, and an intravenous (IV) pole. A knot is placed at the elbow and the forearm placed between two layers of uncut stockinette held together by strategically placed safety pins.

If a tetanus booster has not been given within 10 years, 0.5 mL of tetanus toxoid should be given intramuscularly. Rabies prophylaxis will depend on local patterns of infection, and the local department of health should be consulted (refer to Chapter 190, Rabies, for details of rabies prophylaxis).

Antimicrobial Selection

The empirical selection of antimicrobials should take into account the microbiology of these wounds. Fortunately, most dog and cat bite isolates are susceptible to penicillin and ampicillin. Antimicrobial selections are outlined in Table 23.3. Of note is the relatively poor activity of cephalexin, cefaclor, cephadroxil, and erythromycin against *P. multocida*. Patients who present more than 24 hours after injury without clinical signs of infection rarely require antibiotics. Patients who present for care less than 8 hours after injury and without signs of established infection should be given prophylactic antibiotics for 3 to 5 days if they have moderate to severe wounds; have had a prior splenectomy or have splenic dysfunction; are immunocompromised; have cirrhosis or severe liver dysfunction; have multiple puncture wounds, especially to the hands; have wounds over a bone or joint; or have developed edema or have preexisting edema or crush injury. Unreliable patients should also be managed more aggressively and may require intramuscular (IM) antimicrobials and/or inpatient observation. Follow-up should be within 24 to 48 hours, and the patient should be instructed to call before that if the condition worsens. The most common complications are septic arthritis, osteomyelitis, and residual joint stiffness. Immediate pain out of proportion to the injury when in proximity to a bone or joint should raise the issue of periostium penetration.

Table 23.3 Activity of Selected Antimicrobials against Animal Bite Isolates

	Pasteurella multocida	*Staphylococcus aureus*[a]	Streptococci	Capnocytophaga	Anaerobes
Penicillin	+	−	+	+	V
Ampicillin	+	−	+	+	V
Amoxicillin-clavulanate	+	+	+	+	+
Ampicillin-Sulbactam	+	+	+	+	+
Dicloxacillin	−	+	+	−	−
Ertapenem/Carbapenems	+	+	+	+	+
Cephalexin	−	+	+	−	−
Cefuroxime	+	+	+	+	−
Cefoxitin	+	+	+	+	+
Tetracyclines	+	V	−	V	V
Moxifloxacin	+	+	+	+	+
Erythromycin	−	+	+	+	−
Azithromycin	+	+	+	+	−
Clarithromycin	V	+	+	+	−
Sulfa-trimethoprim	+	+	V	+	−
Clindamycin	−	+	+	−	+

Legend: +, Active;−, poor or no activity; *V*, variable activity against listed pathogen.
[a] Beta-lactams and moxifloxacin not active against MRSA; macrolides, clindamycin, and tetracyclines have variable activity.

Table 23.4 Criteria for Hospitalization of an Animal Bite Patient

Fever (>38°C [100.5°F])
Sepsis
Compromised host (see Table 23.1)
Advance of cellulitis
Patient noncompliance
Acute septic arthritis
Acute osteomyelitis
Severe crush injury
Tendon/nerve injury or severance
Tenosynovitis

Table 23.5 Causes of Therapeutic Failure for Animal Bite Wound Infections

Incorrect antimicrobial selection
Short antimicrobial duration
Insufficient antimicrobial dosage
Resistant isolates
Failure to elevate
Failure to recognize joint/bone involvement
Unrecognized abscess

Patients who present with established infection should receive proper wound care with irrigation, cautious debridement, tetanus and rabies evaluation, and courses of antibiotics. The decision to hospitalize a patient should follow the items in Table 23.4.

Table 23.6 Activity of Selected Antimicrobials against Human Bite Wound Isolates

	Eikenella corrodens	*Staphylococcus aureus*[a]	Streptococci	*Haemophilus* species	Anaerobes
Penicillin	+	–	+	–	–
Ampicillin	+	–	+	V	–
Amoxicillin-clavulanate	+	+	+	+	+
Ampicillin-sulbactam	+	+	+	+	+
Dicloxacillin	–	+	+	–	–
Cephalexin	–	+	+	–	–
Cefuroxime	+	+	+	+	–
Cefoxitin	+	+	+	+	+
Carbapenems	+	+	+	+	+
Tetracyclines	+	V	–	V	V
Moxifloxacin	+	+	+	+	+
Erythromycin	–	+	+	–	–
Azithromycin	+	+	+	+	–
Clarithromycin	V	+	+	-	–
Sulfa-trimethoprim	+	+	V	+	–
Clindamycin	–	+	+	–	+

Abbreviations: +, Activity = –, poor or no activity; *V* = variable activity against listed pathogen.
[a] β-lactams and moxifloxacin not active against methicillan-resistant staphylococcus aureus (MRSA); macrolides, clindamycin, and tetracyclines have variable activity.

The course for antimicrobial therapy for cellulitis is 7 to 14 days, for septic arthritis 3 to 4 weeks, and for osteomyelitis 4 to 6 weeks. Abscesses should be drained, and wounds should be cultured. Therapeutic failure of outpatient therapy, including those listed in Table 23.5, should lead to consideration of hospitalization.

HUMAN BITES

Human bites are either occlusional, where the teeth bite directly into flesh, or clenched-fist (closed-fist) injuries. Most occur during fights, and the patient often has a delayed presentation. They tend to be more severe than other animal bites but are managed similarly.

Occlusional bites may be to any part of the body and include "love nips." Bites to children or the elderly may be the result of abuse and should be paid particular attention. Occlusional injuries to the hand are often particularly severe and result in abscess or osteomyelitis. The bacteria associated with infection include viridans streptococci, especially *Streptococcus anginosus*, and *Streptococcus pyogenes* (group A), *S. aureus*, *Haemophilus* species, *Eikenella corrodens*, and, in more than 55% of cases, oral anaerobes. Antimicrobial therapy is outlined in Table 23.6. Of note is the poor activity of cephalexin and erythromycin against *E. corrodens* and anaerobes.

Clenched-fist injuries (CFIs) are the most severe of human bite wounds, and the

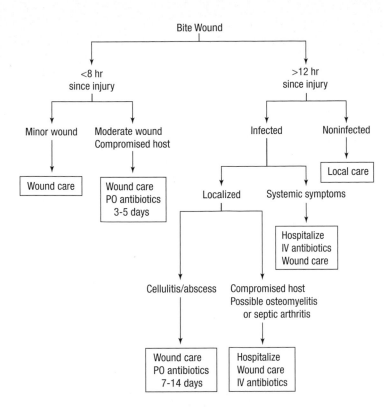

Figure 23.1 Bite wound therapy.

patients often require hospitalization. CFIs are often complicated by septic arthritis and osteomyelitis. Their management should include an evaluation by a surgeon familiar with hands to determine whether the joint capsule was penetrated. Elevation and splinting are usually required, as are intravenous antimicrobials.

An algorithmic summary of the approach to bite wounds is presented in Figure 23.1.

SUGGESTED READING

Center for Disease Control. Nonfatal dog-bite injuries treated in emergency departments-United States-2001. *Morb Mort Weekly Rep.* 2003;52:605–610.

Chuinard RG, D'Ambrosia RD. Human bite infections of the hand. *J Bone Joint Surg.* 1977;59:416–418.

Goldstein EJC. Bite wounds and infection. *Clin Infect Dis.* 1992;14:633–638.

Goldstein EJ. New horizons in the bacteriology, antimicrobial susceptibility, and therapy of animal bite wounds. *J Med Microbiol.* 1998;47:1.

Langley RL. Animal-related fatalities in the United States-an update. *Wilderness Environ Med.* 2005;16:67–74.

Talan DA, Citron DM, Abrahamian FM et al., Bacteriologic analysis of infected dog and cat bites: The bacteriology and management of dog and cat bite wound infections presenting to Emergency Departments. *N Engl J Med.* 1999;340:85.

Talan DA, Abrahamian FM, Moran GJ, et al. Clinical presentation and bacteriologic analysis of infected human bites in patients presenting to emergency departments. *Clin Infect Dis.* 2003;37:1481.

Wallace CG, Robertson CE. Prospective audit of 106 consecutive human bite injuries: the importance of history taking. *Emerg Med J.* 2005;22:883.

24. Lice, Scabies, and Myiasis

William L. Krinsky

Arthropod infestations of humans are most commonly caused by head or body lice (pediculosis), pubic lice (pthiriasis), fly larvae (myiasis), or mites. Although many mite species may feed on human tissue, sarcoptid mites (scabies) are the most common mites living on human hosts. All of these arthropods can cause irritation and inflammation of the skin, but fly larvae may penetrate more deeply into the body. Diagnosis of each of these parasitic problems is dependent on accurate identification of the infesting arthropod. Lice and scabies mites are readily transmitted between close contacts, whereas myiasis is not a contagious condition.

PEDICULOSIS CAPITIS

The most common form of louse infestation in North America is caused by the head louse, *Pediculus humanus* (designated *Pediculus humanus capitis* in the past to differentiate it from the body louse, formerly designated *Pediculus humanus humanus,* which has now been found to be genetically identical to the head louse). The presence of louse eggs (nits) cemented to the hairs of the scalp, or of lice themselves, is diagnostic. Many other bite lesions are caused by arthropods, such as spiders, rodent or bird mites, bed bugs, or biting flies, such as mosquitoes, but none of these are found infesting the affected person. The stage of the louse most commonly seen is the nit. Each nit is oval, opaque, and white (about 0.8×0.3 mm) and attached individually to a single hair by the female louse (Figure 24.1). Each nit is laid about 1 mm from the scalp surface. Screening of large numbers of individuals is expedited by use of a Wood's light, because nits fluoresce under ultraviolet (UV) light. Infested individuals usually first notice itching of the scalp, most often in the postauricular and occipital regions. Adult and immature lice are wingless and, as in all insects, have six legs. Each leg ends in a claw used for gripping hair. The adult lice are about 2 to 3.5 mm long and are white or cream in color (Figure 24.2).

Three immature stages (nymphs) precede the formation of the adult louse. All immatures and adults require blood and, as a result of feeding, produce erythematous, papular lesions that are the cause of the pruritus. Some patients react to louse saliva with urticaria or lymphadenopathy. Erythematous lesions on the trunk, and postauricular and posterior cervical lymph node enlargement in the absence of other lymphadenopathy, should lead to suspicion of head louse infestation. Nits are firmly attached to the hair shafts and will not readily slide off, as will most other contaminants, such as dandruff, hair casts, dried serous secretions, or dried hair spray, with which they may be confused (pseudopediculosis).

Head lice are not known to transmit any human pathogens, so treatment is solely aimed at ridding the infested individual of the insect parasites.

Therapy

Treatment of pediculosis capitis includes the use of various insecticidal shampoos and rinses, most of which contain insecticides. Permethrin, a synthetic pyrethrin, is still one of the safest treatments. Permethrin (1%) cream rinse (Nix® and others) is applied to clean, towel-dried hair and scalp for 10 minutes and then rinsed off. Both permethrin and malathion are pediculicidal and ovicidal, but the latter has an unpleasant odor, may sting the skin and eyes, and is very flammable. However, recent occurrences of louse resistance to pyrethroid preparations have led to recommendations for greater use of malathion (Ovide®). Unlike past recommendations of lengthy treatment regimens, just 1 or 2 20-minute applications of malathion lotion (0.5%) have been shown to be effective. Malathion should not be used with a hair dryer or curling iron, and it should not be used on infants (see Table 24.1). Recently, a nonchemical treatment involving a 30-minute application of hot air (58-59°C) was effective in killing 98% of eggs and 80% of lice in a controlled study of 18 patients.

All family members and close contacts should be examined and those with signs of infestation should be treated. Dead nits,

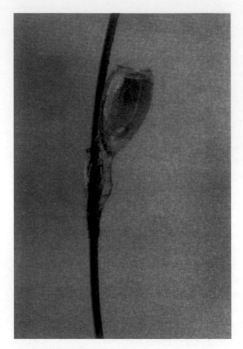

Figure 24.1 Nit (egg) of human louse Pediculus humanus. [Reprinted, from *Skin Disease Diagnosis and Treatment* by Habif, T.P., Campbell, J.L., Quitadamo, M.J. and Zug, K.A. (2001), p.243 (with permission from Elsevier.)]

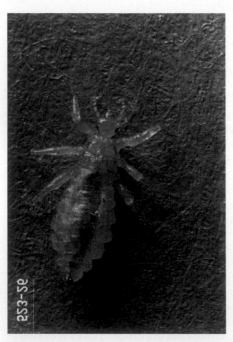

Figure 24.2 Adult human louse Pediculus humanus. [Reprinted, from *Skin Disease Diagnosis and Treatment* by Habif, T.P., Campbell, J.L., Quitadamo, M.J. and Zug, K.A. (2001), p.242 (with permission from Elsevier.)]

which will eventually drop off when the hair to which they are attached falls out or is cut, may be removed (with difficulty) for cosmetic purposes with a fine-toothed comb or forceps. All materials that touched the heads of infested persons, such as hats, scarves, bedding, and cushions, should be thoroughly washed in hot water or dry cleaned. Lice eggs require 6 to 10 days to hatch, and lice will not survive without blood for more than 10 days, so any infested materials kept in plastic bags for 4 weeks may be safely used. Hair grooming aids, such as brushes, combs, and curlers, should be discarded or soaked in a pediculicide for about 20 minutes or left in Lysol (2% in water) or isopropyl alcohol for about 1 hour and then thoroughly washed in hot, sudsy water.

PEDICULOSIS PUBIS (PTHIRIASIS)

Pubic louse infestation is caused by the crab louse (*Pthirus pubis*), named for its crablike appearance caused by the enlargement of the second two pairs of legs (Figure 24.3). Adult crab lice are 1 to 2 mm long and equally wide and are gray, yellow, or brown. Extreme pruritus in the inguinal region is usually the first sign of infestation. Dried serous fluid, blood, or louse feces in the pubic hair are indicative of an infestation. Heavily infested individuals may have blue or gray macules that do not blanch under pressure. Nits are usually laid on the pubic and perianal hair, but infestations of facial hair, including eyebrows, eyelashes, mustache, and beard, may occur, as do less frequent infestations of the axilla. Transmission occurs most often during sexual contact. Definitive diagnosis requires identification of the nits or lice. As with head lice, pubic lice are not known to

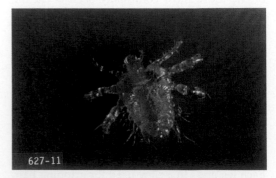

Figure 24.3 Human pubic (crab) louse Pthirus pubis. [Reprinted, from *Skin Disease Diagnosis and Treatment* by Habif, T.P., Campbell, J.L., Quitadamo, M.J. and Zug, K.A. (2001), p.243 (with permission from Elsevier.)]

transmit any pathogens to humans, so the sole aim of therapy is removal of the insect parasite infestation.

Therapy

Pubic lice are treated with insecticidal creams or shampoos applied to the inguinal region. Infestations of the eyelashes should be treated by an ophthalmologist. Conservative treatment with petrolatum (applied twice a day for 8 days), followed by mechanical removal of the nits, is most often recommended.

As in other louse infestations, all intimate contacts should be examined and treated when necessary. Undergarments and other clothing that touched infested persons should be thoroughly washed in hot water or dry cleaned. Infested materials placed in sealed plastic bags may be safely used after 1 month. Prepubertal children presenting with pubic louse infestations of facial hair or eyelashes should be evaluated with regard to possible child abuse or sexual molestation.

PEDULOSIS CORPORIS

Body louse infestation is caused by *Pediculus humanus* (sometimes incorrectly called *Pediculus corporis*), a louse species virtually identical in morphology to the head louse, except that it is usually slightly larger, about 2 to 4 mm long. Body lice feed on blood, but retreat to hide in clothing on which the nits are laid. Infestations are recognized by extreme pruritus in conjunction with observation of nits firmly attached to clothing fibers. Lice are rarely seen. The erythematous, maculopapular feeding lesions are often scratched beyond recognition, leaving only serous or bloody crusts, or secondary infection.

Unlike head and pubic lice, body lice may act as vectors of human bacterial pathogens in those areas of the world where these organisms are endemic. Louse-borne (epidemic) typhus, caused by *Rickettsia prowazekii*, still occurs in parts of Africa, Central and South America, and northern China. It is a serious, and sometimes fatal, disease that may become epidemic in crowded, unsanitary living conditions. Louse-borne relapsing fever, caused by *Borrelia recurrentis*, is also sometimes fatal but has been rarely seen in recent years, except in Ethiopia. Trench fever, caused by *Bartonella quintana,* is rarely fatal, and, as the name implies, was most common during World War I and reemerged in epidemic form in Europe during World War II. Since that war,

trench fever has been seen in Europe, Africa, Japan, Taiwan, Mexico, Bolivia, and Canada. It is becoming more prevalent in populations of homeless and displaced persons.

Therapy

Unlike the other forms of louse infestations, the lesions caused by body lice are the main focus of treatment. Antipruritics and antibiotics (for secondary infections) are used to treat the skin lesions. Ivermectin, a synthetic derivative of a macrocyclic lactone, has been used for various parasitic infestations. Recently, the drug (3 doses of 12 mg each, given at 7-day intervals) greatly reduced the number of body lice infesting a population of homeless men. Such treatment may be effective in limiting the viability of body lice in patients living in an institution or routinely returning to a treatment center or shelter (see Table 24.1). Depending on the geographic location of the infested individual and his or her contact with other similarly infested individuals, the physician should consider the possibility of louse-borne disease and notify the appropriate public health authorities if such disease occurs. Louse eggs that are laid on clothing (especially in seams) may be destroyed by pressing with a hot iron. Washing clothes in hot water and dry cleaning will kill lice and nits as in other forms of louse infestation. Lice have been killed in infested clothing with various pesticide treatments (10% DDT, 1% malathion, and 1% permethrin powders). Infested furniture, mattresses, and box springs should be discarded or fumigated to destroy lice and nits. Infested materials sealed in plastic bags may be used safely after 4 weeks.

SCABIES

Scabies dermatitis is caused by the mite *Sarcoptes scabiei* and its secretions and excretions. Direct skin-to-skin contact with an infested person is the most common form of transmission. The mites are microscopic; the adult female is the largest stage, 300 to 400 μm long (Figure 24.4). The female mites burrow into the skin and lay eggs. Skin lesions and intense pruritus are first noted 2 to 6 weeks after initial infestation and in as little as 1 to 3 days in cases of reinfestation. The most common lesions in order of frequency are papules, vesicles, crusted lesions, pustules, mite burrows, and wheals. Scratching in response to the extreme pruritus often results in excoriations and lesions appearing as eczema;

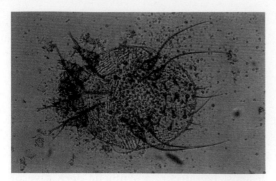

Figure 24.4 Scabies mite Sarcoptes scabiei female. [Reprinted from Skin Disease Diagnosis and Treatment by Habif, T.P., Campbell, J.L., Quitadamo, M.J. and Zug, K.A. (2001), p.238, with permission from Elsevier.]

therefore, definitive diagnosis requires identification of the mite. Mite burrows, which have been observed in less than 25% of patients, are linear (5 to 15 mm long) or serpentine and gray, erythematous, slightly swollen, or scaly. Burrows, when observed, are seen most often in interdigital areas, wrists, elbows, and lateral aspects of the hands, feet, and ankles. The burrows may be highlighted by applying mineral oil, ink, or tetracycline (which fluoresces under a UV lamp) and wiping off the excess that is not retained in the skin. A mite can be removed by gently lifting the top off of its burrow with a scalpel or needle and placing the debris from the burrow on a microscope slide. Observations of the material at 50–100× magnification can reveal living mites, ova, and mite feces. Mineral oil or immersion oil placed on the burrow material on the slide may enhance identification of the mite.

Therapy

As in pediculosis, treatment involves use of any of various lotions or creams, or in cases where the skin is extensively damaged and stinging or burning or percutaneous absorption may be a risk, oral ivermectin has been administered. Permethrin (5%) is currently the most often recommended treatment. It is rinsed off after 8 to 14 hours and administered again 1 week after the first treatment. Permethrin, which lacks the potential toxicity associated with lindane use, most often seen in infants, children, and pregnant or nursing women, is the treatment of choice for infants 2 months of age and older and these other patients. Special care should be made to coat the subungual areas and intertriginous spaces, such as the

intergluteal cleft, with scabieticide. When oral ivermectin is used, 200 μg/kg is recommended, with a repeat treatment 2 weeks later. Many patients, especially those with heavy mite burdens, as in crusted scabies, may continue to experience pruritus for up to 4 weeks after the repeat treatments suggested above. If pruritus persists for longer than this, another treatment should be given only if examination reveals the persistence of mites (see Table 24.1).

As in pediculosis, all close contacts should be treated. Although transmission via infested clothing or bedding is rare except in cases of crusted scabies, laundering clothing and bedding in hot water or dry cleaning will destroy the mites. Suspect materials may be safely used after storage for 10 days in sealed plastic bags.

MYIASIS

Myiasis is the invasion of living vertebrate (including human) tissue by fly larvae. Various species of flies that normally deposit eggs or larvae on garbage, carrion, or corpses may occasionally deposit these stages on wounds or skin adjacent to draining infections. Other fly species deposit eggs that hatch into larvae that penetrate intact skin. Flies in the former group include various house flies, blow flies (greenbottles and bluebottles), and flesh flies. The true myiasis producers in the second group are bot flies and warble flies. Although bot fly and warble fly larvae usually infest nonhuman hosts, such as sheep, cattle, horses, rodents, deer, and other wild mammals, these larvae occasionally invade human tissues. Myiasis is most often cutaneous, but fly larvae may also invade the nose and throat, eye, ear, and intestinal and genitourinary tract.

Dermal (furuncular) myiasis, arising in intact skin, as caused by the human bot fly (*Dermatobia hominis*) in Central and South America and the tumbu fly (*Cordylobia anthropophaga*) in Africa, appears as a painful or itching swelling with an opening at the skin surface. Observation of the opening under low magnification will reveal the posterior end of a moving larva, on which will be two dark circular areas, the respiratory openings (spiracular plates), which allow the larva to breathe while it is feeding with its anterior end embedded in the skin. If the larva is left in the skin, it will continue to feed just below the skin surface for several days to weeks and eventually back out and drop to the ground to complete development.

Table 24.1 Therapeutic Regimens for Lice and Scabies

Infestation	Treatment	Repeat Treatment (Precautions)
Head lice	Topical: Permethrin (1%) cream rinse or lotion—applied to clean, towel-dried hair and scalp for 10 minutes and then rinsed off.	Second application 7–10 days later, if lice persist.
	Malathion (0.5%) lotion—one or two applications of 20 minutes each.	(Contraindicated in infants; flammable; skin and eye irritation possible.)
Scabies	Topical: Permethrin (5%) cream rinsed off after 8–14 hours.	Second application 7 days later, if mites are still present.
	Oral: Ivermectin (200µg/kg).	Second dose 14 days later. (Not approved for children ≤15 kg or for pregnant or nursing mothers.)
Body Lice	Improved hygiene (changing clothes and bedding regularly). Oral: Ivermectin used in indigent population to reduce re-infestation.	

Therapy

Myiasis of the nose and throat, eye, ear, or internal organs may require surgical intervention or at least the use of anesthetics for manual removal of the larvae with forceps. Invasive rhino-orbital myiasis has been treated successfully with oral ivermectin prior to surgery.

In dermal myiasis, early diagnosis and removal of the larva will relieve the irritation and discomfort caused by its movements and feeding under the skin. Direct removal involves application of a local anesthetic, followed by grasping the larva with a forceps and pulling with constant pressure to dislodge its hold, which may be strong because of the retrorse teeth or spines surrounding the anterior part of its body (Figure 24.5). Indirect methods of removal involve application of an occlusive dressing containing petrolatum or even a piece of meat or animal fat if medical supplies are not readily available. Within a few hours, the suffocating larva will back out of the opening into the dressing or embed itself in the occlusive tissue. Secondary infections are rare, and little further treatment beyond disinfection is usually needed. Wound myiasis, which may even occur in modern medical facilities, can be prevented by frequent changes of dressings and isolation of patients, especially immobile ones, within screened rooms. Myiasis of wounds is treated by removal of the feeding maggots, irrigation, and disinfection. Because fly larvae feed on dead tissue, secrete antibiotic chemicals, and may even expedite healing, sterile maggot therapy (with greenbottle fly larvae)

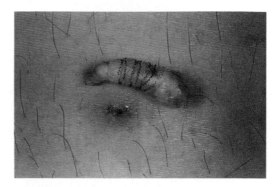

Figure 24.5 Human bot fly larva Dermatobia hominis lying on skin above the opening from which it was excised. The narrow posterior end of the larva is on the left and the widened anterior end with retrorse spines is on the right. [Reprinted, from *Skin Disease Diagnosis and Treatment* by Habif, T.P., Campbell, J.L., Quitadamo, M.J. and Zug, K.A. (2001), p.245 (with permission from Elsevier.)]

has been used successfully in the treatment of persistent surgical wounds, diabetic ulcers, and other surface lesions.

SUGGESTED READING

Brewer TF, Wilson ME, Gonzalez E, Felsenstein D. Bacon therapy and furuncular myiasis. *JAMA*. 1993;270(17):2087–2088.

Chosidow O. Scabies. *N Engl J Med*. 2006;354 (16):1718–1727.

Dourmishev AL, Dourmishev LA, Schwartz RA. Ivermectin: pharmacology and application in dermatology. *Int J Dermatol*. 2005;44(12): 981–988.

Drugs for head lice. *Med Lett*. 2005;47(1215/1216), August 15/29:68–70.

Foucault C, Ranque S, Badiaga S, Rovery C, Raoult D, Brouqui P. Oral ivermectin in the treatment of body lice. *J Infect Dis*. 2006;193:474–476.

Goates BM, Atkin JS, Wilding KG, et al. An effective nonchemical treatment for head lice: a lot of hot air. *Pediatrics*.2006;118(5): 1962–1970.

Leung AKC, Fong JHS, Pinto-Rojas A. Pediculosis capitis. *J Pediatr Health Care*. 2005;19(6):369–373.

Sherman RA. Wound myiasis in urban and suburban United States. *Arch Intern Med*. 2000;160:2004–2014.

25. Superficial Fungal Diseases of the Hair, Skin, and Nails

Evelyn K. Koestenblatt and Jeffrey M. Weinberg

The vast majority of fungal infections of the skin, hair, and nails are caused by the dermatophytes, and yeasts including *Candida* species and *Malassezia furfur*. Because these entities can mimic nonfungal diseases, proper diagnosis is essential. Some fungi causing systemic infections may begin as cutaneous lesions. In most cases, potassium hydroxide (KOH) preparation, culture, and/or biopsy can give a definitive diagnosis. Treatment may involve topical and/or systemic antifungal therapy.

THE DERMATOPHYTES

The dermatophytes are keratinophilic organisms that are found in specific ecological niches. Those found in the soil are referred to as geophilic organisms. Some primarily infect hair, skin, and nails of humans and are transmitted human to human (anthropophilic), and others are mainly found in fur, feathers, skin, and nails of animals (zoophilic). When transmitted to humans, zoophilic and geophilic organisms tend to be much more inflammatory than anthropophilic organisms. Factors precluding dermatophycosis include inoculum size, host immune status, the particular organism, a suitable environment, fungal growth rate exceeding epidermal turnover, and in certain instances the host genetics.

The term *tinea* refers to dermatophycosis or a dermatophyte infection due to one of the following genera: *Epidermophyton*, *Trichophyton*, or *Microsporum*. Dermatophyte infections are described by their location on the body: tinea capitis (scalp), tinea corporis (glabrous skin), tinea faciei (face), tinea cruris (groin), tinea manuum (hand), tinea pedis (feet), tinea barbae (beard), and tinea unguium (nails). Onychomycosis refers to any fungal infection (dermatophytes and nondermatophyte organisms) of the nails. Most infections in the United States are due to five species: *Trichophyton rubrum*, *Trichophyton tonsurans*, *Trichophyton mentagrophytes*, *Microsporum canis*, and *Epidermophyton floccosum*.

Tinea Capitis

In the United States, tinea capitis (scalp ringworm) is most commonly due to *Trichophyton tonsurans*. Clinically, this form of tinea capitis may appear as an area of alopecia with small black dots (Figure 25.1) and have some seborrheic scaling. The black dots are due to spore-filled hairs (endotrix invasion) breaking at the surface of the scalp. This type of infection is seen more frequently in African American and Hispanic children than in whites. An inflammatory boggy, tender, purulent mass called a kerion may be present especially in African American children. A short course of systemic steroids along with antifungal treatment will reduce the inflammation and chance of scarring alopecia. Other organisms causing black dot tinea, including *Trichophyton soudanense* and *T. violaceum*, are being recovered with greater frequency in the United States.

Microsporum canis and *M. audouinii* are among the organisms causing "gray patch ringworm." In this case the fungus is on the outside of the hair shaft (ectothrix invasion), causing it to have a grayish appearance. Some of these organisms produce a yellow-green fluorescence visible with a Wood's lamp. Favus is generally associated with malnutrition and poor hygiene, is rarely seen in the United States, and is most frequently due to *T. schoenleinii*. Clinically, favus appears as diffuse alopecia with yellow crusts or scutula, which are made up of hyphae and skin debris. Microscopically, hyphae and air spaces are seen within the hair shaft.

The most common methods for diagnosing tinea capitis are KOH preparation and fungal culture. Collection of infected hair is necessary for diagnosis of tinea capitis. The hairs may be obtained for both KOH prep and culture in two ways: a scalpel blade or glass slide (Figure 25.2) may be used scrape the area or a soft toothbrush or moist gauze can be firmly rubbed over the involved scalp. The hairs are placed onto a glass slide and mixed with 10% to 20% KOH, a coverslip is applied,

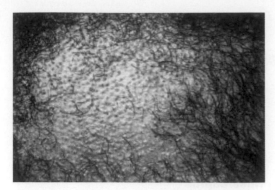

Figure 25.1 "Black dot tinea capitis" due to *T. tonsurans*. (Courtesy of Evelyn Koestenblatt.)

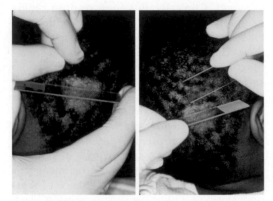

Figure 25.2 Tinea capitis techniques for collecting hair for KOH and culture. (Courtesy of Evelyn Koestenblatt.)

and the sample is then examined with a microscope. The hairs are inspected for evidence of fungal infection with spores either inside (endothrix) or outside (ectothrix) of the hair shaft. For culture the hairs are gently placed on the surface of the fungal media. Nothing but the specimen should be placed inside of the media tube.

The gold standard of therapy for tinea capitis is oral griseofulvin. Topical therapy is most often unsuccessful because the medication cannot penetrate the hair follicle. The dosage of microsized griseofulvin oral suspension is 20 to 25 mg/kg/d for 6 to 8 weeks. Griseofulvin is usually given to young children as a 125 mg/5 mL suspension, in conjunction with a fatty meal. Ultramicronized griseofulvin is given at a dose of 10 to 15 mg/kg/d.

Because many children and caretakers are asymptomatic carriers of infection, it is important for all family members to use 2.5% selenium sulfide or 2% ketoconazole shampoo 3 times per week to reduce the spread of infectious spores.

For patients who fail therapy with griseofulvin or cannot tolerate the medication, treatment with itraconazole (Sporanox) or terbinafine (Lamisil) is an option (Table 25.1). The dosing for itraconazole depends on the weight of the patient: 100 mg every other day for ≤20 kg, 100 mg/d for 20 to 40 kg, and 200 mg/kg for >40 kg. Similarly, terbinafine is dosed as follows: 62.5 mg/d for ≤20 kg, 125 mg/d for 20 to 40 kg, and 250 mg/d for >40 kg. The duration of treatment for the newer antifungals varies from 2 to 8 weeks in different studies. Microsporum infections require higher and longer dosing with terbinafine. Brushes, combs, hats, hair ribbons, barrettes, and bed linens should be thoroughly washed. All members of the patient's family should be evaluated for infection to prevent recurrences.

Tinea Corporis

Tinea corporis (Figures 25.3 and 25.4) refers to dermatophycosis of the glabrous skin. Types of clinical presentations include the following: sharply demarcated annular lesions with a scaly border, bullous lesions, granulomatous eruptions, pustular lesions, psoriasiform plaques, and verrucous lesions. The disease occurs worldwide and is generally more prevalent in tropical areas. *T. rubrum* is the most common cause of tinea corporis in the United States. *T. mentagrophytes* and *M. canis* are also common. Zoophilic organisms such as *M. canis* and some strains of *T. mentagrophytes* frequently present as multiple lesions that tend to be more inflammatory and symptomatic than infections caused by anthropophilic dermatophytes such as *T. rubrum*.

Tinea Cruris

Tinea cruris refers to dermatophyte infection of the groin, including the suprapubic areas, proximal medial thighs, perineum, gluteal cleft, and buttocks. Infection is most often seen in men and commonly caused by *T. rubrum*, *T. mentagrophytes*, and *E. floccosum*. Women less commonly develop tinea cruris, with candidiasis occurring more frequently.

Tinea Pedis

Athlete's foot or tinea pedis (Figure 25.5) is the most common fungal infection. This environment of moisture, friction, maceration, heat, darkness, and occlusion are perfect for fungal growth. *T. rubrum* is most frequently recovered

Table 25.1 Treatment for Tinea Capitis

Griseofulvin	Terbinafine	Itraconazole	Fluconazole
20–25 mg/kg/d for 6–8 weeks (liquid microsize)	62.5 mg/d ≤20 kg 125 mg/d 20–40 kg 250 mg/d >40 kg For 2–4 weeks	5 mg/kg/d For 4–8 weeks	6 mg/kg/d for 3–6 weeks

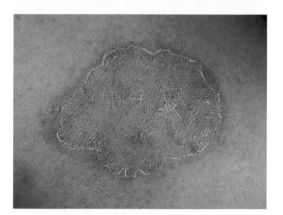

Figure 25.3 Tinea corporis. (Courtesy of Evelyn Koestenblatt.)

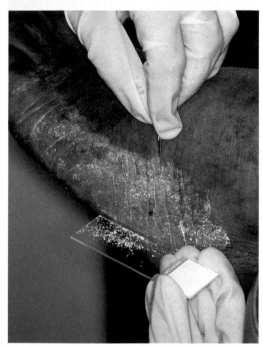

Figure 25.5 Moccasin type tinea pedis. Scrape the active border with a #15 blade for KOH preparation and culture. (Courtesy of Evelyn Koestenblatt.)

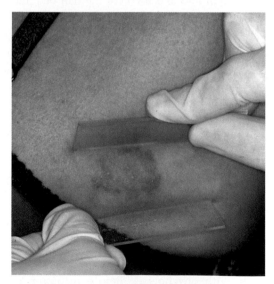

Figure 25.4 Erythematous tinea corporis with small pustules. (Courtesy of Evelyn Koestenblatt.)

and causes a "moccasin" distribution of scale and erythryma. *T. rubrum* is associated with an autosomal-dominant predisposition to this type of infection. Dermatophytosis may occur in between the toes and is referred to as interdigital tinea pedis. *T. mentagrophytes, T. rubrum,* or *E. floccosum* may be recovered with or without bacterial organisms and/or yeast. *T. mentagrophytes* may also cause an inflamma-

tory vesicular response especially on the plantar surface.

Tinea Manuum

The patients commonly have dermatophycosis of both feet and one hand. Clinically tinea manuum appears as fine scale with some erythema covering the surface of the palm, like the feet; *T. rubrum* is usually recovered.

Tinea Faciei and Tinea Barbae

Tinea faciei (Figure 25.6) occurs in women and children generally on the upper lip and chin and may be due to animal exposure. *T. rubrum, T. mentagrophytes,* and *M. canis* usually recovered. Topical therapy may be adequate in most cases. In the event of deep or widespread infection oral antifungal may be warranted. Tinea barbae or ringworm of the beard is seen

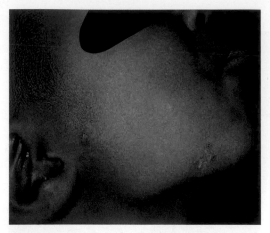

Figure 25.6 Tinea faciei. (Courtesy of Evelyn Koestenblatt.)

in men and associated with exposure to animals. The inflammatory type causes a deep nodular, pyogenic reaction. *T. mentagrophytes* and *T. verrucosum* tend to cause this kerion-like response, whereas *T. violaceum* and *T. rubrum* are likely to cause a more superficial infection with scaling and loss of hair. Like tinea capitis, extracted hairs are necessary for diagnosis by KOH and culture. In some instances biopsy may be necessary. Because the organisms affect the hair, oral antifungal therapy is necessary.

TREATMENT

First-line therapy for tinea corporis, cruris, manuum, faciei, and pedis consists of topical antifungals. Topical antifungal agents (Table 25.2) utilized in the treatment of dermatophytosis include several classes of medications: imidazoles, allylamines, benzylamines, and hydroxypyridones.

Commonly used imidazoles include clotrimazole (Lotrimin, Mycelex), miconazole (Micatin, Monistat), econazole (Spectazole), ketoconazole (Nizoral), oxiconazole (Oxistat), sertaconazole (Ertaczo), and sulconazole (Exelderm). The allylamines are fungicidal and include terbinafine (Lamisil AT), naftifine (Naftin), and butenafine (Mentax). Ciclopirox (Loprox) is fungicidal and has antibacterial, anti-inflammatory, and antifungal properties. Treatment regimens for topical medication are generally for 2 to 4 weeks twice a day. Treatment with oral antifungals may be necessary, especially when infection is widespread or involves hair-bearing areas. Effective adult dosing for terbinafine is 250 mg/day for 1 to 2 weeks, itraconazole 200 mg/day 1 week, and fluconazole 150 mg a week for 4 weeks.

ONYCHOMYCOSIS

Onychomycosis is more than just a cosmetic problem. It can be painful and embarrassing, and can cause more serious infections especially in the diabetic and immunocompromised populations. The dermatophytes account for approximately 90% of toenail infections, whereas yeasts account for the majority of fingernail onychomycosis. Up to 50% of nail dystrophy is due to fungal infections. There are four types of onychomycosis: (1) distal subungual onychomycosis, (2) white superficial onychomycosis, (3) proximal subungual onychomycosis, and (4) candida onychomycosis.

The most common form is distal subungual onychomycosis, most frequently caused by *T. rubrum*. The nail appears thickened, with subungual debris, discoloration, and onycholysis (separation of the nail plate from the nail bed). The infection begins at the distal and/or lateral nail fold and involves the nail bed and hyponychium. Both fingernails and toenails may present with this picture.

White superficial onychomycosis involves the surface of the toenail, giving it a chalky white appearance. It may be due to *T. mentagrophytes* or nondermatophytes such as *Acremonium, Aspergillus, Cephalosporium, Fusarium, or Scopulariopsis*. In the HIV population *T. rubrum* is generally recovered.

Proximal subungual onychomycosis is the least common form; it begins at the proximal nail fold, causing an opaque white area near the lunula. The opaque areas grow distally along with the nail. *T. rubrum* and occasionally *T. megninii* are the etiologic agents. This presentation may be a sign of HIV infection.

Candida onychomycosis is mainly due to *Candida albicans* and causes yellowing of the nails with onycholysis. Before initiation of therapy, it is important to document the presence of fungi utilizing one or more diagnostic techniques, including KOH preparation, fungal culture, and nail plate biopsy with PAS (periodic acid-Schiff) stain. The lab results are only as good as the way the specimen was taken. When dealing with distal and lateral onychomycosis (Figures 25.7 and 25.8), it is important to cut the nail back as far as possible to the juncture of the nail plate and nail bed. A curette is used to collect thin small pieces of nail and debris for KOH and culture.

Table 25.2 Anti Fungal Topical Agents

Name	Concentration/ Vehicle	Formulation/ Class	Antibacterial Activity	Anti-inflammatory Activity	Pregnancy Category	Indications	Dosage	Activity
Ertaczo	2% cream	Sertaconazole Imidiazole	Gram (+) Gram (−)	Yes	C	T. pedis	BID 4 wks	Efloc, Tment, Trub
Exelderm	1% cream 1% solution	Sulconazole Imidiazole	No	No	C	T. pedis/cruris/ corporis TV	QD-BID 3–4 wks QD-BID 3 wks	Efloc, Mcanis, Tment, Trub Calb Mfur
Lamisil AT	1% cream, spray solution	Terbinafine topical Allylamine	Gram (+)	No	B	T. pedis/cruris/ corporis TV (solution only)	QD-BID 1–4 wks BID 2 wks	Efloc, Tment, Trub Mfur
Loprox	0.77% cream, gel, suspension, 1% shampoo	Ciclopirox Hydroxypyridone	Gram (+) Gram (−)	Yes	B	T. pedis/cruris/ corporis TV (cream or suspension)	BID 1–4 wks BID 2–4 wks	Efloc, Mcanis, Tment, Trub, Calb Mfur
Lotrimin	1% cream, lotion, solution	Clotrimazole Imidiazole	Gram (+)	No	B	T. pedis/cruris/ corporis TV	BID 2–4 wks BID 2–4 wks	Efloc, Tment, Trub, Calb Mfur
Lotrisone	0.05%, 1%, cream, lotion	Betamethasone/ clotrimazole Imidiazole	Gram (+)	Yes	C	T. pedis T. cruris/ corporis	BID 4 wks BID 2 wks	Efloc, Mcanis, Trub, Calb
Mentax	1% cream	Butenafine HCl Benzylamine	No	Yes	B	T. pedis T. cruris/ corporis TV	BID 7 days QD 14 days QD 14 days	Efloc, Tment, Trub, Tton Efloc, Tment, Trub, Tton Mfur
Mycelex	1% cream, solution	Clotrimazole Imidiazole	No	No	B	T. pedis/cruris/ corporis TV	BID 2–4 wks	Efloc, Tment, Trub, Calb Mfur
Naftin	1% cream, gel	Naftifine Allylamine	Gram (+) Gram (−)	Yes	B	T. pedis/cruris corporis	BID 1–4 wks (gel) QD 1–4 wks (cream)	Efloc, Tment, Trub,
Nizoral	2% cream 2% shampoo	Ketoconazole Imidiazole	Gram (+)	No	C	T. pedis T. cruris/ corporis Cutaneous Candidiasis TV	QD 6 wks QD 2 wks QD 2 wks QD 2 wks	Efloc, Tment, Trub Efloc, Tment, Trub Calb Mfur
Oxistat	1% cream, lotion	Oxiconazole Imidiazole	Gram (+)	Yes, weak activity	B	T. pedis T. cruris/ corporis TV	QD/BID 4 wks QD/BID 2 wks QD 2 wks	Efloc, Tment, Trub Mfur
Penlac Nail Lacquer	8% solution	Ciclopirox Hydroxypyridone	No	No	B	T. unguium finger/toe nails	QD 48 wks	Trub
Spectazole	1% cream	Econazole Imidiazole	Gram (+) Some gram (−) No Pseudomonas	No	C	T. pedis T. cruris/ corporis Cutaneous Candidiasis TV	QD 4 wks QD 2 wks BID 2 wks QD 2 wks	Maud, Mcanis, Mgyp, Tment, Trub, Tton Maud, Mcanis, Mgyp, Tment, Trub, Tton

Abbreviations: TV = Tinea versicolor; Maud = *Microsporum audounii;* Mcanis = *Microsporum canis;* Mgyp = *Microsporum gypseum;* Tment = *Trichophyton mentagrophytes;* Trub = *Trichophyton rubrum;* Tton = *Trichophyton tonsurans;* Calb = *Candida albicans;* Mfur = *Malassezia furfur;* QD = once a day; BID = twice a day.

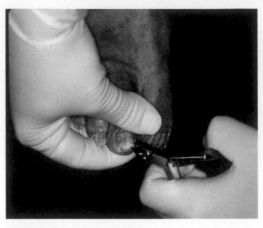

Figure 25.7 Clip back the nail as far as possible to the juncture of the nail plate and nail bed. (Courtesy of Evelyn Koestenblatt.)

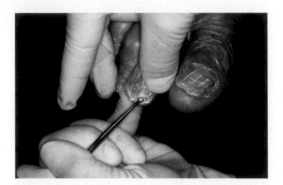

Figure 25.8 Curette small thin pieces of nail and debris for KOH preparation and culture. (Courtesy of Evelyn Koestenblatt.)

In white superficial (Figure 25.9), a curette can be uses to scrape the white chalky material off the surface of the nail. Material from proximal white can be obtained by a punch biopsy into the affected area, or use a curette to scrape the surface of the nail and discard the initial material and use the deeper scraping for KOH and culture.

KOH (Figures 25.10 and 25.11) is a simple, inexpensive, and reliable way to diagnose fungal infections. The scraping is collected on a clean glass slide; a couple of drops of 10% to 20% KOH are added and mixed with the specimen. A coverslip is applied, and the slide is gently heated to permit breakdown of the keratin. The slide is microscopically examined for hyphael elements and yeast cells.

Material for culture (Figure 25.12) should be gently placed on the surface of the agar using a wooden applicator stick premoistened with condensation from the tubed media. Sticks

and blades should not find their way into the culture media tubes.

Proper diagnosis is necessary because other disorders can mimic onychomycosis, including psoriasis, irritant dermatitis, and trauma. Topical treatment of onychomycosis will not generally cure the infection. Naftin gel and 8% solution of ciclopirox have been used with moderate success. In the past, patients with onychomycosis were treated with griseofulvin, with a cure rate of about 25% after 1 year of therapy for toenail disease. Over the past several years, the emergence of itraconazole and terbinafine has allowed much shorter and more effective courses of therapy.

Itraconazole has a broad spectrum of activity and shows activity against dermatophytes and nondermatophyte molds as well as yeasts and can be administered in a continuous or pulse fashion. In the continuous regimen, the dosage of itraconazole is 200 mg daily for 3 months for toenail disease and 2 months for fingernail disease. Pulse dosing of the medication involves a dosage of 200 mg twice daily for 1 week per month, with no therapy for the remaining 3 weeks. Toenails are treated with three pulses, whereas fingernails are treated with two pulses (Table 25.3). Unlike itraconazole, terbinafine is fungicidal, blocking cell membrane synthesis. This may account for terbinafine's higher efficacy for both mycological and clinical cure rates as compared to other systemic antifungals. Terbinafine dosage is 250 mg daily for 6 weeks for fingernails and 12 weeks for toenails.

Combination of systemic antifungal treatment and mechanical means such as clipping and debridement of the nail seem to clear infection more quickly. Other important measures

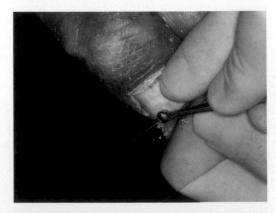

Figure 25.9 White superficial onychomycosis on the surface of the nail is scraped and small pieces are used for KOH preparations and culture. (Courtesy of Evelyn Koestenblatt.)

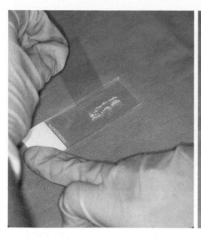

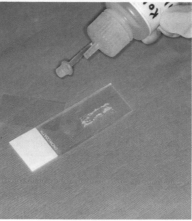

Figure 25.10 Method for KOH: Gather material on a clean glass slide and add a couple of drops of 10–20% KOH and mix with specimen add a coverslip. (Courtesy of Evelyn Koestenblatt.)

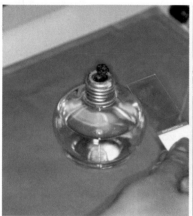

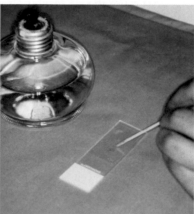

Figure 25.11 Heat slide gently and press coverslip to flatten scale. (Courtesy of Evelyn Koestenblatt.)

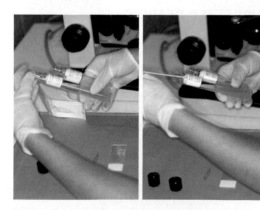

Figure 25.12 Specimen should be placed on the surface of the culture media with a wood applicator stick. (Courtesy of Evelyn Koestenblatt.)

are to wear white cotton socks, use antifungal powder, wear properly fitting shoes, throw away old fungus-laden shoes, and do not walk around barefoot in public areas.

With both itraconazole and terbinafine it is recommended that liver function tests be performed prior to and during treatment. Serious liver failure has been reported with the use of both drugs. Patients taking medication metabolized by the cytochrome P450 pathway should not take itraconazole due to serious drug interactions. There is a slight risk of developing congestive heart failure with itraconazole use. Interactions have been reported in patients taking terbinafine and tricyclic antidepressants.

Although not approved by the U.S. Food and Drug Administration fluconazole is used to treat onychomycosis at a dose of 150 mg/week for 6 months for fingernails and 9 to 12 months for toenails.

PITYRIASIS VERSICOLOR

Pityriasis versicolor is also known as tinea versicolor (TV) but this is a misnomer because it is due to yeast, not to one of the dermatophytes. The etiologic agent is *Malassezia furfur*. The skin lesions appear as sharply demarcated superficial macules that may be hyper- or hypopigmented with fine scaling and are found on the trunk, shoulders, neck, upper

Table 25.3 Treatment for Onychomycosis

	Fingernails	Toenails
Itraconazole	200 mg/day for 12 consecutive weeks OR 200 mg twice a day for 1 week per month for 2–3 months	200 /day for 6 consecutive weeks OR 200 mg twice a day for 1 week per month for 3–4 months
Terbinafine	250 mg/day 6 weeks	250mg/day 12 weeks
Fluconazole	150–200 mg/week for 6 months	150–200 mg/week 9–12 months

arms, back, abdomen, and occasionally on the face. Malassezia furfur appears as round to oval yeast forms on normal skin in sebum-rich areas. Predisposing factors that cause the yeast form to convert to phialides and spores include Cushing's disease, malnutrition, systemic steroid therapy, genetic predisposition, use of oral contraception, application of oils to the skin, immunosuppression, heat, and humidity.

Diagnosis can be easily made by KOH preparation. Phialides (short hyphae with a fertile end) and round short chains or clusters of budding thick-walled spores, commonly referred to as "spaghetti and meatballs," are seen microscopically. These organisms require an exogenous source of lipids for growth, so that culturing is generally not performed. Examination of the lesions with a Wood's lamp produces a pale yellow fluorescence.

A biopsy will show a thick basket-weave stratum corneum with phialides and spores. Treatment may be topical or systemic. For 1 week apply 2.5% selenium sulfide lotion daily for 10 minutes and then wash off. To prevent recurrence use the lotion monthly for 3 months and shampoo with selenium sulfide to prevent colonization of the scalp.

Ketoconazole shampoo, imidiazoles, triazoles, terbinafine spray, and propylene glycol are useful topical treatments. Itraconazole 200 mg/day for 5 to 7 days is effective, followed by 200 mg twice a day on a monthly base for prophylaxis. Ketoconazole 200 mg/day for 10 days or single dose 400 mg repeated monthly can be effective. Fluconazole has been shown to be effective taken as a single dose of 300 to 400 mg.

Patients must be advised that normal pigmentation may take awhile to return and that prophylaxis is necessary to avoid recurrence of infection.

CANDIDIASIS

Candida infections of the skin appear as erythematous, sometimes erosive, areas with satellite pustules. It is most commonly seen in intertriginous zones (submammary, inguinal creases, finger spaces), nails, scrotum, and diaper area. Topical therapy including the azoles, nystatin, and ciclopirox are generally effective. Fluconazole and itraconazole are useful if systemic therapy is required.

SUGGESTED READING

Elewski, BE, Hazen, PG. The superficial mycoses and the dermatophytes. *J Am Acad Dermatol*. 1989;21:655–73.

Finch JJ, Warshaw EM. Toenail onychomycosis: current and future treatment options. *Dermatol Ther*. 2007 Jan-Feb;20(1):31–46.

Kwong-Chung, KJ, Bennett, JE. *Medical Mycology*. Philadephia: Lea and Febiger, 1992.

Rinaldi, MG. Dermatophytosis: epidemiological and microbiological update. *J Am Acad Dermatol*. 2000;43:S120–4.

Rippon, JW. *Medical Mycology: the Pathogenic Fungi and the Pathogenic Actinomycetes*. 3rd ed. Philadelphia: WB Saunders Co., 1988.

26. Mycetoma (Madura Foot)

David M. Brett-Major and Kenneth F. Wagner[1]

Madura foot, or mycetoma, is a chronic localized infection of the skin, subcutaneous tissue, fascia, and muscle. Tumefaction, draining sinuses, and grains that are made up of aggregates of organisms characterize it. Although it is a well-defined clinical entity, it may be caused by a wide array of bacteria and fungi.

EPIDEMIOLOGY

Mycetomas are seen most commonly in countries with tropical and hot temperate climates that lie between the tropics of Cancer and Capricorn. Mycetoma is relatively common in Mexico, where it is the most common manifestation of deep mycotic infection. Other locations in the Western Hemisphere where the incidence is high include Central and South America. It is an uncommon disease in the United States, where it is seen mostly in the Southeast. Other locations worldwide where mycetomas are reported with some frequency include Senegal, Sudan, Somalia, India, and Southern Asia.

Men are affected about 4 to 5 times as often as women, with the peak incidence between ages 20 and 40 years. Farmers and other rural workers who work outdoors or go barefoot are most commonly affected.

CAUSES

Mycetomas fall into two broad categories based on the causative organism: *actinomycetomas*, which account for 60% of all mycetomas worldwide, are caused by aerobic bacteria, including *Nocardia*, *Streptomyces*, and *Actinomadura* species (Table 26.1); *eumycetomas* are caused by true fungi, and many organisms have been implicated (Table 26.2). The distribution of agents varies with geographic location. *Nocardia brasiliensis* is the most common cause in Mexico and Central and South America, where 98% of mycetomas are actinomycotic. *Madurella*

[1] This chapter reflects the work and views of the authors and does not necessarily represent that of the National Naval Medical Center, U.S. Navy, or the Department of Defense.

mycetomatis and *Streptomyces somaliensis* predominate in Africa and India. The most common cause of mycetoma in the United States is *Pseudallescheria boydii*.

PATHOGENESIS

The inciting event in a mycetoma is the traumatic inoculation of the causative agent into the skin or subcutaneous tissues of an otherwise healthy individual. This most often occurs to people who walk barefoot and receive penetrating injuries from thorn pricks, splinters, and animal and insect bites. Truncal infections develop after carrying sacks containing contaminated branches, leaves, and plants without wearing protective clothing. Head and neck mycetomas may result from carrying contaminated wood bundles on the head and shoulders. The sex, occupational, and geographic predilections likely reflect greater opportunity for soil contact and predisposition to injury in these groups.

CLINICAL MANIFESTATIONS

Some 60% to 70% of mycetomas involve the lower limbs (Figures 26.1 and 26.2), but any region of the body can be affected. The most common site is the foot, followed by the hands. Other fairly common sites include the torso (Figure 26.3), thighs, head, neck, and buttocks.

The disease starts as a hard, usually painless, papule or subcutaneous nodule. The initial lesion progressively increases in size and forms sinuses that communicate with the surface of the skin. Granules composed of aggregates of organisms are discharged through these sinuses. As old sinuses close up and scar, new ones develop. Over time, new nodules form adjacent to the original lesion. Direct extension along fascial planes leads to deep abscesses and bony involvement. This eventuates in bone destruction and remodeling, though pathologic fractures represent less than 1% of cases. Untreated, this process is chronic and progressive with continued cycles of swelling, suppuration, and scarring.

Table 26.1 Causative Agents and Treatment of Actinomycetomas

Organism	Grain Color	Treatment
Nocardia asteroides Nocardia brasiliensis Nocardia otitidis-caviarum or Nocardia caviae	White or yellow	Initial: 16 mg/kg/day TMP and 80 mg/kg/day SMX PO in divided doses and/or dapsone, 3 mg/kg/day in divided doses Severe disease: Add amikacin, 15 mg/kg/day × 3 wk IM or IV for 2–3 cycles with 15 days between cycles
Actinomadura madurae Actinomadura pelletieri Streptomyces somaliensis	White or yellow Red Yellow	Streptomycin, 14 mg/kg/day, and TMP-SMX or dapsone at above dosages

Abbreviations: TMP = Trimethoprim; SMX = sulfamethoxazole.

Table 26.2 Causative Agents of Eumycetomas

Black Grain	White Grain
Exophiala jeanselmei	Acremonium falciforme
Leptosphaeria senegalensis	Acremonium kiliense
Leptosphaeria tompkinsii	Acremonium recifei
Madurella mycetomatis	Aspergillus flavus
Madurella grisea	Aspergillus nidulans
Pseudochaetospharanema larense	Arthrographis kalrae
Pyrenochaeta romeroi	Curvularia lunata
Pyrenochaeta mackinnonii	Cylindrocarpon destructans
	Fusarium sp.
	Neotestudina rosati
	Pseudallescheria boydii (Scedosporium apiospermum)
	Trichophyton sp.
	Microsporum sp.

An emerging concern has been the presence of disseminated infection by classic mycetoma causing organisms in immunocompromised hosts, particularly those with prolonged periods

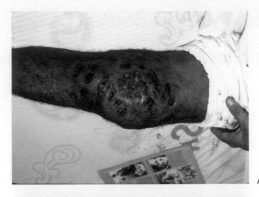

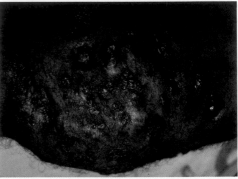

Figure 26.1 (A and B) Multiple active and scarred sinus tracts of knee and lower leg in a Panamanian native with mycetoma caused by *Nocardia brasiliensis.*

of neutropenia, such as transplant and liquid tumor patients. Although many approaches described here remain relevant, it is not the focus of this chapter.

DIAGNOSIS

The combination of tumefaction and multiple sinuses that drain grain-filled serosanguinous fluid in a typical anatomic location such as the foot is highly characteristic of mycetoma. After a thorough history, the initial diagnostic step should be the gross and microscopic examination of the grains. A crush preparation of the fluid in 20% potassium hydroxide and a Gram stain should be performed, with organisms initially being separated by the color and size of the grains. A biopsy should be obtained for histology and culture. The grain for culture should be rinsed quickly in 70% alcohol and washed in sterile saline to eliminate fungal and bacterial contamination. Hematoxylin-eosin (H&E) stain will detect grains in tissue specimens. Typically, they are surrounded by a ring of inflammatory cells tending to neutrophils with age, all of which

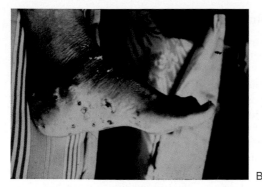

Figure 26.2 (A) Mycetoma (Madura foot) caused by *Nocardia brasiliensis* in a classic location on a Panamanian patient.

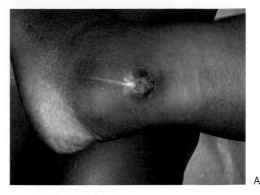

Figure 26.3 (A) Recurrence of *S. apiospermum* mycetoma of the left ankle in a young woman during pregnancy, 10 years following initial treatment and excision.

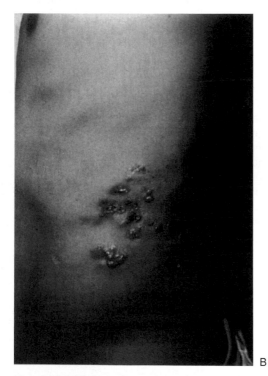

Figure 26.2 (B) Truncal mycetoma demonstrating multiple tumors and sinus tracts.

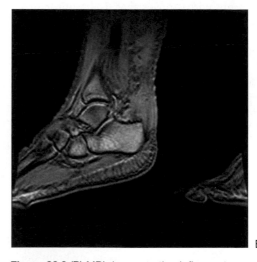

Figure 26.3 (B) MRI demonstrating inflammatory encasement of the Achilles tendon in the same woman. This patient presented with plantar contracture.

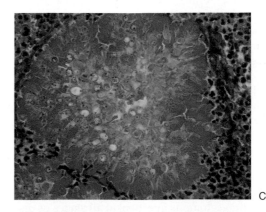

Figure 26.3 (C) Histopathology slide of a biopsy specimen from this patient demonstrating the characteristic white grain of her infecting organism. Note the neutrophilic infiltration of the grain suggesting chronicity.

are encased by dense fibrous tissue. Gram stain, Gomori methenamine silver, and periodic acid-Schiff (PAS) stains may be helpful in identifying hyphae. Tissue cultures for primary isolation on Lowenstein-Jensen medium, 7H12B medium, and brain-heart infusion with blood agar with and without antibiotics and subculture on Sabouraud's medium usually will lead to specific identification of the causative organism. Newer molecular diagnostic and typing methods such as restriction length fragment polymorphism (RFLP) typing and 16S ribosomal RNA sequencing may provide improved diagnostic identification of members of clinically significant species, although their principal use remains in molecular epidemiology. Although one small study supports a local test for *Nocardia*-associated mycetomatous infection, broad use of serodiagnostics has not been validated. Radiographs of the affected area should also be obtained to evaluate for bony involvement, and both magnetic resonance imaging (MRI) and ultrasound have been used for perioperative planning when biopsy or excision is desired.

DIFFERENTIAL DIAGNOSIS

Actinomycosis is similar to mycetoma. It presents with sinuses that drain sulfur granules. Unlike mycetomas, which are externally induced, actinomycosis is caused by organisms that are normal flora of the oral cavity, such as *Actinomyces israelii*. The differentiation between these two processes is important because the management and prognosis for actinomycosis is significantly different from that for a mycetoma.

Other processes that can clinically mimic mycetoma are botryomycosis, cutaneous tuberculosis, squamous cell carcinoma, and, less commonly, Kaposi's sarcoma, atypical melanoma, and cutaneous leishmaniasis. Botryomycosis is a chronic bacterial infection in which the sinuses drain granules composed of clusters of bacteria. Although the most common agent is *Staphylococcus aureus*, many gram-positive and gram-negative organisms may cause this disorder. If mycetoma has invaded bone, it can be confused with chronic bacterial osteomyelitis, syphilis, or osteosarcoma. Again, an accurate diagnosis using Gram and acid-fast bacilli stains, cultures, and histopathology is important so that the appropriate treatment regimens can be instituted.

Leprosy and mycetoma share areas of endemicity, and co-infecting mycetoma in nonhealing lepromatous lesions has been reported in India.

THERAPY

Despite continued use of aggressive surgical resection in resource-poor areas in the setting of eumycetomous infection, at all stages of disease, mycetoma can be cured or contained by medical treatment alone or in combination with limited surgery. However, prolonged antimicrobial therapy may be required.

Actinomycetoma

Several agents are effective in the treatment of actinomycetomas (see Table 26.1). The selection of medication depends on the causative agent, antimicrobial susceptibility, severity of disease, possible side effects, and cost. In the Western Hemisphere, where *Nocardia* is the major cause of mycetomas, sulfonamides are a good initial therapeutic choice. Trimethoprim with sulfamethoxazole (TMP-SMX), given orally at a dosage of 16 mg/kg/day trimethoprim and 80 mg/kg/day sulfamethoxazole, has proved to be successful in 60% to 70% of cases. Dapsone at an oral dosage of 3 mg/kg/day has also been useful either alone or in combination with TMP-SMX. These have been used for an average of 4 months to 2 years and should be continued until at least 6 months after all detectable signs of active disease have disappeared. The main side effects of sulfonamides in general include hematologic, gastrointestinal, and allergic skin reactions. The use of dapsone specifically may be limited by the development of methemoglobinemia, hemolytic anemia, and leukopenia. Therefore, when dapsone is used, close monitoring with serial complete blood counts is necessary. Resistance to TMP-SMX has been noted recently.

Several newer antibiotics, including fluoroquinolones, carbapenems, broad-spectrum cephalosporins, and minocycline, have shown in vitro activity and some clinical efficacy when used alone or in combination against *Nocardia*. Linezolid and several late-generation fluoroquinolones each have demonstrated good in vitro activity against both *Actinomadura madurae* and *Nocardia braziliensis*. The cost of these drugs has limited their clinical experience, as the greatest burden of mycetomatous disease is in poor areas.

Amikacin, either alone or in combination with TMP-SMX, has also been shown to be effective in the treatment of mycetoma caused by *Nocardia*. Amikacin is administered intramuscularly at a dosage of 15 mg/kg/day for 3 weeks. Two to three cycles with 15 days between each cycle are usually necessary. However, because of the associated risks of nephrotoxicity and ototoxicity, the need to follow peak and trough levels, and its cost, amikacin is best viewed as a second-line agent. It is most useful when there is resistance to prior therapy and when the extent or activity of the disease is severe and there is risk of dissemination to an adjacent organ.

In the Eastern Hemisphere, where *S. somaliensis* and *Actinomadura* are considerations, streptomycin sulfate given intramuscularly at a dosage of 14 mg/kg/day has been used. This generally is used in combination with TMP-SMX or dapsone. When streptomycin is used, the patient must be monitored for ototoxicity.

Eumycetoma

The medical management of eumycetomas is less successful and predictable than that of actinomycetomas. Small eumycetomas can be surgically excised, although recurrence may result if the lesion is incompletely excised. In more extensive lesions, surgical debulking followed by a prolonged course of an antifungal medication is likely to yield the best results. For eumycetomas, miconazole has demonstrated some effect in the past, but side effects and poor outcome limit its use. The most experience is with ketoconazole, 200 to 400 mg orally twice a day. Although many of these cases were caused by *M. mycetomatis*, successes have been seen with other fungi, including *Madurella grisea*, *Acremonium falciforme*, *Acremonium kiliense*, and *Pyrenochaeta romeroi*. However, therapeutic failures have also been noted. In vitro studies and accumulating clinical experience suggest that the newer triazole antifungal agents, especially itraconazole, may be more potent than ketoconazole against the fungi that cause eumycetomas. Itraconazole, 100 to 400 mg/day, has been successful in treating the same fungi previously treated with ketoconazole and in some instances effective in cases where ketoconazole had failed. There are also recent reports of successful treatment of eumycetomas with itraconazole for *Aspergillus nidulans*, *Aspergillus flavus*, *Aspergillus recife*, *Arthrographis kalrae*, *Fusarium*, and *Pseudallescheria boydii*. The new itraconazole cyclodextrin solution achieves higher serum itraconazole and hydroxyitraconazole concentrations than the capsule formulation, which may translate into better clinical outcomes. It appears that itraconazole may be more effective than fluconazole for mycetomas. Amphotericin B and griseofulvin have been used with limited success. A recent, small open label trial of terbinafine (500 mg by mouth twice daily) showed efficacy in 16 of 20 patients. The use of these agents is constrained by the high minimal inhibitory concentrations for these fungi and the adverse reactions that they cause. Because of the cost and limited clinical improvement by liposomal amphotericin B preparations at dosages up to 3 mg/kg/day, these agents have minimal use for eumycetomas.

Voriconazole, posaconazole, and caspofungin have good in vitro activity against many of the agents that cause mycetoma. Both voriconazole and posaconazole have been used successfully in reported cases, although more data are available with voriconazole. Its fungicidal activity is greater than itraconazole though it carries both a higher cost and risk of toxicity. Nonetheless, extended courses of therapy usually are well tolerated with the most common side effect being chromatic visual disturbance and less commonly hepatic enzyme elevation. Weight-based dosing may be necessary even with the oral formulation. One option in difficult cases may be to induce regression with a several-month-long course of voriconazole (3 mg/kg by mouth twice daily) or posaconazole and then transition to itraconazole for chronic suppression if relapse is noted, but such techniques have not been validated.

As response rates of different agents of mycetoma to the same antifungal may be different, it is at present unclear whether the newer drugs will be equally potent and have a similar range of applications as current therapy either used alone or in combination. In all cases of mycetoma, prolonged medical therapy will be necessary to accomplish a cure.

SUGGESTED READING

Abd Bagi ME, Fahal, AH, Sheik HE, et al. Pathological fractures in mycetoma. *Trans R Soc Trop Med Hyg*. 2003;97(5):582–584.

Ahmed AO, Mukhtar MM, Kools-Sijmons M, et al. Development of a species-specific PCR-restriction fragment length polymorphism analysis procedure for identification of Madurella mycetomatis. *J Clin Microbiol*. 1999;37(10):3175–3178.

Boiron P, Locci R, Goodfellow M, et al. Nocardia, nocardiosis and mycetoma. *Med Mycol*. 1998;36(suppl)1:26.

Elamin EM, Guerbouj S, Musa AM, et al. Uncommon clinical presentations of cutaneous leishmaniasis in Sudan. *Trans R Soc Trop Med Hyg*. 2005; 99(11):803–808.

Fahal AH. Mycetoma: a thorn in the flesh. *Trans R Soc Trop Med Hyg*. 2004;98(1):3–11.

Gomez-Flores A, Welsh O, Said-Fernández S, et al. In vitro and in vivo activities of antimicrobials against Nocardia brasiliensis. *Antimicrob Agents Chemother*. 2004;48 (3):832–837.

Husain S, Muñoz P, Forrest G, et al. Infections due to Scedosporium apiospermum and Scedosporium prolificans in transplant recipients: clinical characteristics and impact of antifungal agent therapy on outcome. *Clin Infect Dis*. 2005;40(1): 89–99.

Lewis RE, Wiederhold NP, Klepser ME. In vitro pharmacodynamics of amphotericin B, itraconazole, and voriconazole against Aspergillus, Fusarium, and Scedosporium spp. *Antimicrob Agents Chemother*. 2005;49(3): 945–951.

Lupi O, Tyring SK, McGinnis MR. Tropical dermatology: fungal tropical diseases. *J Am Acad Dermatol*. 2005;53(6):931–951.

Mancini N, Ossi CM, Perotti M, et al. Molecular mycological diagnosis and correct antimycotic treatments. *J Clin Microbiol*. 2005;43(7):3584; author reply 3584–3585.

McGinnis MR: Mycetoma, *Dermatol Clin*. 1996; 14(1):97.

N'diaye B, Dieng MT, Perez A, Stockmeyer M, Bakshi R. Clinical efficacy and safety of oral terbinafine in fungal mycetoma. *Int J Dermatol*. 2006;45(2):154–157.

Negroni R, Tobón A, Bustamante B, et al. Posaconazole treatment of refractory eumycetoma and chromoblastomycosis. *Rev Inst Med Trop Sao Paulo*. 2005;47(6): 339–346.

Pfaller MA, Marco F, Messer SA, et al. In vitro activity of two echinocandin derivatives, LY303366 and MK-0991 (L-743, 792), against clinical isolates of *Aspergillus, Fusarium, Rhizopus,* and other filamentous fungi, *Diagn Microbiol Infect Dis*. 1998;30(4):251.

Schaenman JM, Digiulio DB, Mirels LF, et al. Scedosporium apiospermum soft tissue infection successfully treated with voriconazole: potential pitfalls in the transition from intravenous to oral therapy. *J Clin Microbiol*. 2005;43(2):973–977.

Welch O: Treatment of eumycetoma and actinomycetoma. *Curr Top Med Mycol*. 1995;6:47.

Wildfeuer A, Seidl HP, Paule I, et al. In vitro evaluation of voriconazole against clinical isolates of yeasts, moulds and dermatophytes in comparison with itraconazole, ketoconazole, amphotericin B and griseofulvin. *Mycoses*. 1998;41(7–8):309.

27. Fever and Lymphadenopathy

Gustine Liu-Young and Gerald Friedland

FEVER AND LYMPHADENOPATHY

The occurrence of fever and lymphadenopathy is fairly common in clinical practice, thus it is important to have a logical and systematic approach for the accurate diagnosis and treatment of patients with this syndrome (Figure 27.1).

Careful history-taking and physical examination are essential in the initial evaluation of the patient and the following basic questions need to be answered:

1. Is the adenopathy local or generalized?
2. Is the process acute or chronic?
3. Is the cause infectious or noninfectious?
4. Is there a primary peripheral lesion?

Important elements of the history should also include occupational and animal exposures, geographic residence, travel history, high-risk sexual and/or drug use behavior, and presence or absence of systemic symptoms. A thorough examination must include the location and duration of lymphadenopathy, size, consistency, tenderness, and whether it is matted.

As a general rule, a node larger than 1 cm should be considered abnormal. Pain is usually the result of an inflammatory process or suppuration but may also represent hemorrhage into the necrotic center of a malignant node. The presence or absence of tenderness does not reliably differentiate benign from malignant nodes. Stony-hard nodes are usually a sign of malignancy. Very firm, rubbery nodes suggest lymphoma. Softer nodes are the result of infectious or inflammatory conditions and when suppuration is present, these nodes may tend to be fluctuant. The term *shotty* refers to small nodes that feel like "buckshot" under the skin, as found in the cervical nodes of children with viral illnesses.

A group of nodes that feel connected and seem to move as a unit is said to be *matted* and can be either benign (eg, tuberculosis [TB], sarcoidosis, lymphogranuloma venereum, and human immunodeficiency virus [HIV]) or malignant (eg, metastatic carcinoma and lymphoma).

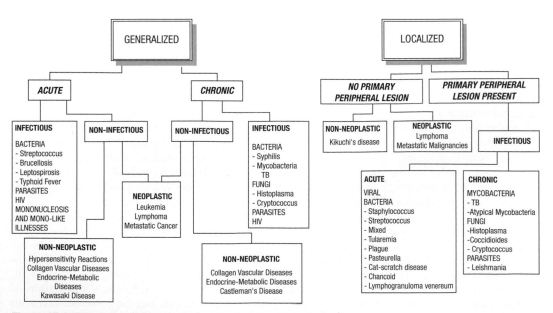

Figure 27.1 Differential diagnostic scheme for fever and lymphadenopathy.

Table 27.1 Localized Lymphadenopathy: Areas Drained and Associated Conditions

Lymph Node Area	Anatomic Area	Areas Drained	Associated Conditions/Comments
Head and neck	Occipital and posterior auricular	Scalp, face	Local infections with skin pathogens: *Staphylococcus, Streptococcus,* acute viral illnesses Children: secondarily infected insect, tick, or spider bites, dermatophyte infections (ringworm), viral infections
	Anterior auricular	Eyelids, palpebral conjunctivae, external auditory meatus, pinna	Conjunctivitis, oculoglandular syndrome (Francisella tularensis, N. gonorrhea, B. henselae), keratoconjunctivitis
	Tonsillar, submaxillary, submental	Pharynx, mouth, teeth, lips, tongue, and cheeks	Infections of the head, neck, sinuses, ears, scalp, pharynx, teeth, and oral mucosa
	Posterior cervical	Scalp & neck, skin of arms and pectorals, thorax, cervical, and axillary nodes	Mononucleosis, Kikuchi disease, tuberculosis, lymphoma, head and neck malignancies
Axillary		Upper extremity Thoracic wall, breasts, and back	Acute pyogenic infection, cat scratch disease, brucellosis, melanoma, breast malignancy
Inguinal		Lower extremities Abdominal wall Genitalia: penis, scrotum, vulva, vagina, perineum and perianal region	Pyogenic infections of the lower extremities Sexually transmitted diseases: herpes simplex, syphilis, Chancroid, lymphogranuloma venereum Pelvic and perianal malignancy
Mediastinal-hilar		Lungs, trachea, esophagus	Granulomatous disease (infectious and noninfectious), Malignancies
Abdominal Retroperitoneal Para-aortic		Abdominal viscera Reptroperitoneal organs: kidneys Pelvic organs	Usually granulomatous disease: *M. tuberculosis, M. avium* complex Malignancies: lymphoma

LOCALIZED LYMPHADENOPATHY

Lymphadenopathy is considered localized if no more than two contiguous lymph node groups are involved. Anatomically and clinically, the node-bearing areas are divided into five major groups, namely (1) the head and neck area, (2) the axilla, (3) the inguinal area, (4) the mediastinal-hilar areas, and (5) the retroperitoneal and para-aortic areas.

Basic knowledge of the anatomy and areas drained by these lymph nodes can help in narrowing the differential diagnosis (see Table 27.1). Infectious local adenopathy may be acute or chronic. It is usually associated with a primary lesion. At times, the peripheral lesion may be subtle or inapparent. In patients with unexplained localized lymphadenopathy and a reassuring clinical picture, a 3- to 4-week period of observation may be appropriate before considering biopsy.

The lymph nodes of the head and neck are collectively called cervical nodes and are more accurately subdivided into several anatomic and clinical areas (see Figure 27.2.). The occipital and posterior auricular nodes drain large areas of the scalp and face. Adenopathy of these groups may be associated with primary infectious lesions in these areas (usually from staphylococcal and streptococcal infections) but can be a common feature of acute viral illnesses as well. In children, secondarily infected wounds from insect bites and ringworm (dermatophyte infection) are common causes.

The anterior auricular nodes drain the eyelids, palpebral conjunctivae, external auditory meatus, and pinna of the ear. Conjunctivitis and anterior auricular adenopathy (the oculoglandular syndrome) is classically associated with *Francisella tularensis* via direct inoculation of the conjunctival sac but may also be seen with conjunctival infection from *Neisseria gonorrhoea*,

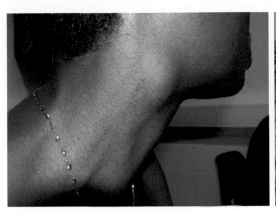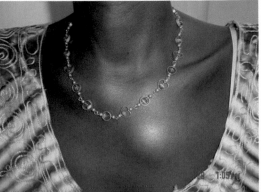

Figure 27.2 These pictures demonstrate palpable lymph nodes in the anterior cervical area (left image) and left parasternal areas (right image).

Bartonella henselae (cat scratch disease), and epidemic keratoconjunctivitis.

The tonsillar, submaxillary, and submental nodes drain the tonsils and other structures in the pharyngeal area. Enlargement of these nodes should prompt careful inspection of the mouth, dentition, and pharynx. In addition, this group also drains the external structures of the medial face including the lips, chin, cheeks, and medial aspects of the conjunctivae.

The posterior cervical nodes are in the occipital triangle of the neck above the inferior belly of the omohyoid muscle and posterior to the sternocleidomastoid muscle. These are commonly involved in infectious mononucleosis and mononucleosis-like syndromes, including HIV infection.

Kikuchi disease or histiocytic necrotizing lymphadenitis, is a fairly common self-limited disorder involving the cervical lymph nodes. This condition was first recognized in Japan and has now been reported in the United States. It has been predominantly described in females of Asian and Middle Eastern origin, commonly younger than 40 years of age. Clinical manifestations of this entity include fever or flulike symptoms, rash, localized and sometimes tender cervical lymphadenopathy, elevated erythrocyte sedimentation rate, and leukopenia. The involved nodes are usually rubbery or firm, discrete, and rarely greater than 2 cm in diameter. Its etiology is still obscure, but it has been associated with Kaposi's sarcoma-associated herpesvirus (KHSV-HHV-8). This condition does not respond to antibiotics but usually resolves spontaneously in 1 to 2 months. Because of its association with systemic lupus erythematosus (SLE) and Still's disease, it is also thought to be autoimmune in origin. Recognition of this disease is important because

this is commonly mistaken for other conditions that require treatment such as malignant lymphoma and Kawasaki's disease by pathologists who are unfamiliar with this condition.

The inferior deep cervical nodes lie below the level of the inferior belly of the omohyoid muscle and anteroposterior to the sternocleidomastoid muscle. These nodes receive drainage from the scalp, the superior deep cervical nodes, the axillary nodes and the nodes of the hilum of the lung, the mediastinum, and abdominal viscera. Adenopathy in this area is usually subtle but may be detected with the Valsalva maneuver.

Supraclavicular lymphadenopathy has been associated with malignancy in the majority of patients older than 40 years of age. The left supraclavicular (Virchow) node receives lymphatic flow from the thorax and abdomen and may indicate pathology involving the testes, ovaries, kidneys, pancreas, prostate, stomach, or gallbladder.

Mediastinal and hilar adenopathies are usually detected only on radiography. These nodes are rarely involved in acute suppurative disease. A useful diagnostic criterion is whether the lymphadenopathy is unilateral or bilateral. Unilateral enlargement most frequently suggests granulomatous disease of both infectious (eg, *Mycobacterium tuberculosis* and histoplasmosis) and noninfectious (eg, sarcoidosis) origin (see Figure 27.3). Bilateral hilar adenopathy is seen in approximately three-fourths of patients with sarcoidosis.

Acute suppurative mediastinal lymphadenitis can be a fulminant process, typically a complication of progressive infections of the upper respiratory tract, or perforation of the esophagus or bronchial tree as a result of trauma or surgery. When dealing with mediastinal and hilar adenopathy, the diagnostic approach includes

M. tuberculosis skin test (purified protein derivative [PPD]), sputum cultures (routine, fungal, acid-fast bacillus [AFB]), lymph node culture (routine, AFB, anaerobic) as well as cytology. Computed tomography (CT) is useful in assessing the size and location of these lymph nodes. Biopsy should be considered in any node >1 cm in the absence of a primary diagnostic lesion. Tissue for histologic examination may be obtained through inferior cervical node biopsy, transbronchial lung biopsy, mediastinoscopy, or percutaneous or surgical biopsy of hilar nodes (see Figure 27.4).

The axillary nodes drain the entire upper extremity as well as the lateral parts of the chest

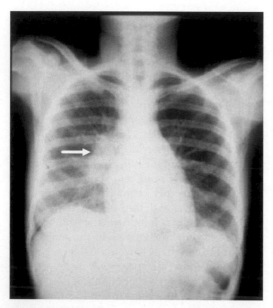

Figure 27.3 This chest X ray depicts unilateral (right) hilar lymphadenopathy (as indicated by the arrow) in a patient with pulmonary tuberculosis.

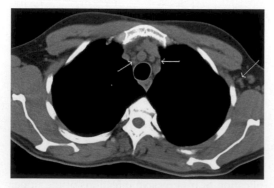

Figure 27.4 An example of chest CT in a patient with HIV and atypical mycobacterial pulmonary infection who presented with multiple hilar and left axillary lymphadenopathy (as indicated by the arrows).

wall, back, and breasts. This cluster of nodes is most frequently involved in acute pyogenic infections of these drainage areas. By far, the most common etiologic organisms include staphylococci and streptococci, associated with furunculosis, cellulitis, or lymphangitis. The extremities are also often the site of zoonotic infections from other organisms acquired from the environment, including *Francisella tularensis* (Tularemia), *Yersinis pestis* (Plague), *Pasteurella multocida*, *Erysipelothrix rhusiopathiae* (Erysipelothrix), and *Bartonella henselae* (cat scratch disease).

Some degree of inguinal lymphadenopathy is relatively common, partly due to frequency of trauma or prior infections in the lower extremities. These nodes not only drain the lower extremities but also the lower abdominal wall, the genitalia, perineum, and perianal areas. Acute pyogenic bacterial infection caused by the same organisms encountered in axillary adenopathy are the usual culprits. The drainage of the perineum and the perianal area suggests that enteric aerobic and anaerobic gram-negative organisms as well as gram-positive organisms are present. Because of the drainage of the genitalia, sexually transmitted infections often involve the inguinal nodes as well. Those most likely to present with prominent inguinal adenopathy are syphilis, lymphogranuloma venereum, chancroid, and genital herpes simplex.

The abdominal and retroperitoneal nodes drain the abdominal viscera, retroperitoneal and pelvic organs. They receive drainage from the inguinal nodes as well. Neither the nodes nor the primary site of infection, except the testes, are directly accessible thus making assessment difficult. Radiologic procedures must be employed for evaluation, most often CT or magnetic resonance imaging (MRI) (see Figure 27.5.).

GENERALIZED LYMPHADENOPATHY

Generalized lymphadenopathy is present if nodes in two or more noncontiguous major lymph-node–bearing areas are enlarged. It is frequently a manifestation of disseminated infection. Clues may be provided by the age of the patient, presence or absence of rash, geographic factors (eg, dengue fever, filariasis, localized leishmania lymphadenitis, histoplasmosis), occupation and dietary history (brucellosis, toxoplasmosis), and exposure to animals and their excreta or standing water (leptospirosis).

Acute generalized infectious lymphadenopathy, which is most often viral, is a common

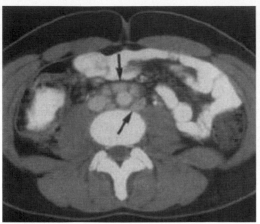
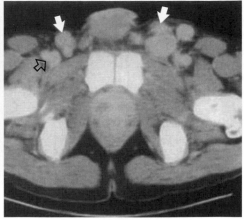

Figure 27.5 An example of high-attenuation lymph nodes (solid arrows) in the (A) retroperitoneum and (B) inguinal areas of patients with Acquired Immunodeficiency Syndrome (AIDS) and Kaposi's sarcoma. Contrast-enhanced femoral vessels are seen on the right (open arrow).

feature of many childhood viral infections, including rubella, measles, and varicella. Generalized lymph node enlargement may also be seen in the prodromal period of hepatitis A and B, Epstein-Barr virus (EBV), cytomegalovirus (CMV), HIV, and toxoplasmosis. These conditions initially present with the mononucleosis-like syndrome and generalized lymphadenopathy. Bacterial pathogens are much less often the cause of generalized lymphadenopathy, except in brucellosis and leptospirosis. In all these infections, the nodes are typically tender, discrete, firm to touch, and without fluctuance.

Acute generalized noninfectious lymphadenopathy is frequently due to hypersensitivity reactions, most commonly drug induced. Sulfonamides, hydralazine, carbamazepine, and phenytoin are among the agents that have been implicated in such reactions. This condition rapidly disappears on withdrawal of the offending drug. Other offending medications include allopurinol, atenolol, captopril, quinine, primidone, and sulindac. Collagen vascular diseases, including rheumatoid arthritis (RA) and SLE, may also cause acute generalized lymphadenopathy and fever. Kawasaki's syndrome (acute febrile mucocutaneous lymph node syndrome) is a disease of uncertain origin that is seen almost exclusively in infants and young children, also present with nonsuppurative cervical lymphadenopathy that may be unilateral.

Chronic generalized infectious lymphadenopathy is less likely to be viral, except for HIV. Its presence suggests more serious diagnostic possibilities. Disseminated bacterial and fungal diseases, including TB, syphilis, histoplasmosis, and cryptococcosis, should be considered. In children, persistent lymphadenopathy and fever may suggest an immunodeficiency state, including chronic granulomatous disease. Castleman's disease, associated with HHV-8, the same etiologic agent as for Kaposi's sarcoma, also presents with fever and chronic lymphadenopathy and is discussed later in this chapter.

Chronic generalized noninfectious lymphadenopathy is most often neoplastic. Lymphoreticular neoplasms (eg, Hodgkin's disease, non-Hodgkin's lymphoma, chronic lymphocytic leukemia) predominate. Fever, when present, may be due to the underlying malignant disease or to secondary infection. Nonneoplastic diseases (with variable frequency) cause chronic generalized lymphadenopathy and fever and these include sarcoidosis, Still's disease, and hyperthyroidism. In patients receiving immunosuppressive therapy following a solid organ or bone marrow transplant, one should consider the diagnosis of posttransplant lymphoproliferative disorder (PTLD), which is a heterogeneous group of lymphoid proliferations, most of which are of B-cell lineage and associated with EBV. These disorders can occur months to years after transplantation and would require reduction in immunosuppressive therapy with or without antiviral therapy.

ADENOPATHY AND HIV INFECTION

Acute retroviral infection is a mononucleosis-like syndrome that occurs 2 to 10 weeks after exposure to HIV. Acute bilateral generalized lymphadenopathy, which may be accompanied by fever, maculopapular rash, headache, mucosal ulcerations, myalgias, and malaise, are common features of this syndrome. Sometimes, there are signs and symptoms of meningitis, because HIV involves the neural tissues soon after infection. Because tests for HIV antibody are negative during the early stage of primary infection, the diagnosis is best made by testing for HIV RNA in plasma (viral load). Titers are extremely high during the initial infection and may be assayed by the reverse transcription–polymerase chain reaction (RT–PCR) method, branched-DNA testing, or amplification based on nucleic acid sequence. PCR tests for HIV DNA and cultures of circulating mononuclear cells or other tissues should also be positive during primary infection. The mean interval between the onset and resolution of symptoms during primary HIV infection is approximately 25 days.

The long period of asymptomatic infection that follows may last for years. During this time, many infected individuals exhibit persistent generalized lymphadenopathy (PGL). The nodes are typically nontender and firm to rubbery in consistency. PGL may persist for several years, into the period of early symptomatic HIV infection. Symptoms at this stage may include fevers, night sweats, weight loss, and diarrhea.

As HIV disease progresses, more severe complications including opportunistic infections and malignancies, may develop. This period defines acquired immunodeficiency syndrome, commonly known as AIDS. In contrast to earlier stages, lymphadenopathy is not a common finding in those with advanced HIV disease, and its presence suggests an infectious or neoplastic process involving the reticuloendothelial system. Of infectious causes, disseminated *Mycobacterium avium* intracellulare infection, *M. tuberculosis*, histoplasmosis, cytomegalovirus infection, toxoplasmosis, syphilis, and cryptococcosis are most common. Although high-grade B-cell lymphomas are common in AIDS, they are typically extranodal. Kaposi's sarcoma may involve lymph nodes, occasionally without apparent skin lesions.

Multicentric Castleman's disease, associated with HHV-8, presents with persistent fever, marked splenomegaly, generalized lymphadenopathy in over 90% of patients, weight loss in 70%, and pancytopenia in 35%. These symptoms usually last more than 6 months and may represent acute infection with HHV-8 or reactivation of HHV-8 in the setting of immune suppression in AIDS. For more details on HIV and AIDS, please refer to Chapter 99, Differential Diagnosis and Management of Opportunistic Infections Complicating HIV Infection.

General Diagnostic Approaches

In most cases of infectious lymphadenopathy, clinical and laboratory findings short of biopsy often suggest the causative agent in the enlarged nodes. Some of these findings are as follows:

1. Primary site of infection, eg, streptococcal cellulitis, staphylococcal furuncle, syphilitic chancre
2. Associated symptoms: "B" symptoms with lymphomas, rash, serositis with systemic lupus; arthritis with Still's disease, or rheumatoid arthritis
3. Characteristic rash, eg, rubella, rubeola, drug eruption, acute HIV infection
4. Characteristic physical findings, eg, splenomegaly in mononucleosis, lymphoma
5. Typical hematologic findings, eg, eosinophilia (drug reactions), atypical lymphocytosis (mononucleosis syndrome), high ESR (rheumatologic diseases)
6. Skin tests, eg, tuberculosis
7. Serologic tests, eg, EBV, hepatitis, syphilis, HIV, tularemia
8. Stains and cultures of material from peripheral primary lesions and pulmonary lesions (atypical mycobacteria, tuberculosis, plague)

LYMPH NODE BIOPSY VS FINE-NEEDLE ASPIRATION BIOPSY

The simplicity, safety, and cost-effectiveness of fine-needle aspiration (FNA) make it a useful test for the evaluation of persistent lymphadenopathy. The advent of radiologically guided FNA makes biopsy of the nodes of the hilum and retroperitoneum accessible, thus avoiding extensive surgical procedures. The presence of a cytopathologist on site to determine the adequacy of the specimen has been shown to increase the yield of FNA considerably. However, there are limitations to the procedure.

FNA is useful in the diagnosis of benign reactive processes, certain infections, or metastatic disease, yet its accuracy in the diagnosis of lymphoma and primary malignancies remain controversial. Technical difficulties pose an obstacle for the effective differentiation of certain malignancies. Because the chemotherapeutic agents used for treatment of patients with lymphoma are selected on the basis of the specific type of lymphoma, excisional biopsy remains necessary for definitive subclassification of lymphoma in the majority of patients.

Another limitation of FNA is insufficient material for histology, special stains, and culture, particularly when mycobacterial disease or other granulomatous infections are under consideration. These additional tests are often necessary to establish the diagnosis and select appropriate therapy. This is especially important for *M. tuberculosis* when establishing the species and resistance pattern is critical.

The following general guidelines are intended to suggest to the clinician circumstances in which excisional biopsy is appropriate:

1. Undiagnosed chronic lymphadenopathy of 1 month in adults, 3 months in children
2. Localized nonsuppurative lymphadenopathy without an accessible or apparent peripheral lesion
3. Enlarging undiagnosed lymphadenopathy after 2 weeks of observation
4. Nontender, matted to hard lymphadenopathy or a high clinical suspicion of neoplastic disease
5. Radiologic findings or systemic signs and symptoms suggesting granulomatous or lymphoproliferative disease when noninvasive tests are unrevealing
6. Positive tuberculin test in the absence of diagnostic pulmonary tuberculosis
7. New adenopathy in immunocompromised patients; although otherwise, asymptomatic patients with HIV and PGL do not need biopsies
8. Lymphadenopathy in the setting of fever of undetermined origin
9. Persistently nondiagnostic or inconclusive FNA results

Technique

Approximately half of all lymph node biopsies lead to a specific diagnosis. Careful attention to several rules maximizes the usefulness of the invasive diagnostic procedure.

1. Discuss the differential diagnosis with the surgeon, pathologist, and the microbiology laboratory ahead of time so that any special considerations (eg, fixation, staining, and special culture media) can be identified.
2. Select the best site. Lymph nodes frequently involved in minor inflammatory processes, such as the inguinal and submandibu-

lar nodes, should be avoided. In the presence of generalized lymphadenopathy, the inferior or posterior cervical nodes are preferred. The second choice is the axillary node.

3. The largest node in a cluster of enlarged nodes should be removed.
4. Remove nodes in their entirety with capsules intact. Dissect them, sending half of the specimen to the pathology laboratory and the other half to the microbiology laboratory for stains and culture of common pathogens, mycobacteria, fungi, and other suspected organisms (see Figure 27.6).
5. Request that the pathologist make additional sections of the excised tissue if the node is abnormal but not diagnostic.
6. Consider a repeat biopsy and the excision of more tissue if the node is abnormal but not diagnostic and the clinical picture is unclear.

Interpretation

Entities discussed in this chapter that have a characteristic histologic pattern and for which a specific or strongly suggestive diagnosis can be made histologically are lymphoma, other neoplasms, tuberculosis, fungal disease, sarcoidosis, toxoplasmosis, and cat scratch disease. Most noninfectious nonneoplastic disorders and most acute viral infections show nonspecific lymphadenitis or hyperplasia only. However, a significant number of patients with initially nondiagnostic lymph node biopsies and persistent lymphadenopathy will ultimately prove to have a serious underlying disease. If the biopsy is not initially diagnostic,

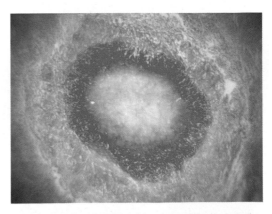

Figure 27.6 An example of a supraclavicular lymph node biopsy stained by H&E. This is a granuloma, with extensive necrosis in the center, caused by Mycobacterium tuberculosis. (Courtesy of Theresa Liu-Dumlao, MD.)

it is essential to follow the patient carefully and to consider repeat biopsy if adenopathy persists.

SUGGESTED READING

Ferrer R. Lymphadenopathy: Differential Diagnosis and Evaluation. *Am Fam Physician*. 1998;58(6):1313–1320.

Feigin RD, Schleien CI. Kawasaki disease. In: *Current Clinical Topics in Infectious Disease*. Vol. 4. 1983;30, New York: McGraw-Hill.

Fijten GH, Blijham GH. Unexplained lymphadenopathy in family practice: an evaluation of the probability of malignant causes and the effectiveness of physicians' workup. *J Fam Pract*. 1988;27:373–376.

Libman H. Generalized Lymphadenopathy. *J Gen Intern Med*. 1987;2:48–58.

Mason WH, Takahashi M. Kawasaki syndrome. *Clin Infect Dis*. 1999;28:169–185.

Morgenstern L. The Virchow-Troisier node: a historical note. *Am J Surg*. 1979;138:703.

Oksenhandler E, Cazals-Hatem D, Sculz TF, et al. Transient angiolymphoid hyperplasia and Kaposi's sarcoma after primary infection with human herpesvirus 8 in a patient with human immunodeficiency virus infection. *N Engl J Med*. 1998;338:1585–1590.

Oksenhandler E, Duarte M, Soulier J, et al. Multicentric Castleman's disease in HIV infection: a clinical and pathological study of 20 patients. *AIDS*. 1996;10:61–67.

Pasternack M, Swartz M. Lymphadenitis and lymphangitis. In: *Mandell's Principles and Practice of Infectious Diseases*. 6th ed. 2005; 1205–1211.

Scadden D, Muse V, Hasserjian R et al. A 41-yr old man with dyspnea, fever and lymphadenopathy. *N Engl J Med*. 2006;355: 1358–1368.

Spies J, Foucar K, Thompson CT, LeBoit PE. The histopathology of cutaneous lesions of Kikuchi's disease (necrotizing lymphadenitis): a report of five cases. *Am J Surg Pathol*. 1999;23:1040–1047.

Tsang WYW, Chan JKC, Ng CS. Kikuchi's lymphadenitis: a morphologic analysis of 75 cases with special reference to unusual features. *Am J Surg Pathol*. 1999;18:218–231.

Unger PD, Rappaport KM, Strauchen JA. Necrotizing lymphadenitis (Kikuchi's disease). *Arch Pathol Lab Med*. 1987;111: 1031–1034.

PART V

Clinical Syndromes – Respiratory Tract

Clinical Syndromes – Respiratory Tract

28. Acute and Chronic Bronchitis

Sanford Chodosh

Bronchial infections with viral and bacterial microorganisms are responsible for a significant percentage of ambulatory care visits and are among the principle causes of time lost from work. These infections occur in individuals with and without underlying chronic bronchial disease, each with important differences in etiology, clinical presentation, laboratory findings, and requirements for therapy.

ACUTE BRONCHITIS

Acute infectious bronchitis in individuals without underlying chronic lung disease is most commonly caused by viral pathogens, with a lesser contribution by *Mycoplasma, Chlamydophila,* and *Legionella.* The relative frequencies of these etiologies vary with time and place and have epidemic-like characteristics in the population. The clinical presentation is usually abrupt and is characterized by the onset of cough, which may be productive of scanty sputum. There are variable associated symptoms, including coryza, sore throat, burning sensation in tracheal area, malaise, feverishness, chilliness, and other symptoms of viremia. Wheezing and dyspnea are unusual symptoms in adults but may be present in young children, in which case it can be confused with asthma. All of these symptoms are most troublesome in the first few days of the infection and should significantly improve or resolve within 1 week. Medical intervention is rarely sought or required, and symptomatic therapy usually suffices. Routine laboratory studies are rarely indicated and are not likely to be useful. If the patient produces sputum, the cytologic findings are of neutrophils with swollen bronchial epithelial cells, which may demonstrate vacuolization. A Gram stain is characteristically free of bacteria. Treatment with antiviral agents is rarely indicated. However, if symptoms worsen or persist beyond a week, a nonviral etiology should be suspected. If the Gram stain now reveals significant bacterial types morphologically consistent with *Haemophilus, Streptococcus pneumoniae,* or *Moraxella,* antimicrobial therapy would be appropriate. The choice of antimicrobial would be similar to what will be covered under acute exacerbations of chronic bronchitis, but the duration of therapy can be reduced. If *Mycoplasma, Chlamydophila,* or *Legionella* infection were suspected, a 7-day course of a macrolide, tetracycline, or a selected quinolone would be appropriate. If *Bordetella pertussis* infection is suspected, macrolide therapy would be appropriate. Experience has shown that patients who seek medical care for acute bronchitis should be suspected of having unrecognized chronic bronchial disease, which usually delays the course of resolution observed in normal individuals.

ACUTE BRONCHITIS ASSOCIATED WITH CHRONIC BRONCHIAL DISEASE

Exacerbations caused by bacterial bronchitis are more common and more severe in patients with chronic bronchitis and chronic bronchial asthma. Because the incidence of both diseases is common, bacterial exacerbations represent one of the most common indications for prescribing an antimicrobial agent. Chronic bronchitis affects an estimated 15% to 25% of adults, many of whom have both acute exacerbations of chronic bronchitis (AECB) and acute bacterial exacerbations of chronic bronchitis (ABECB) over the course of their illness with the associated increased morbidity associated with such events. In addition to the deleterious individual effects, the costs to society are measured in billions of dollars. Despite this, the diagnosis and therapy of such episodes are often haphazard. The pathologic and physiologic abnormalities of the bronchial system that may predispose patients with chronic bronchial disease to bacterial infection include impaired mucociliary clearance, bronchi obstructed by abnormal secretions, and bronchoconstriction, and in patients with chronic bronchitis, an indolent presence of pathogenic bacteria in the bronchial epithelium as well as impaired host defenses. For example, bacterial phagocytosis and intracellular bactericidal activity by polymorphonuclear neutrophils is impaired, macrophage recruitment is decreased, and sputum immunoglobulin levels are subnormal.

Most acute bacterial exacerbations (ABE) present without an identifiable precipitating event. However, many occur following acute viral respiratory infections, excessive cigarette smoking, thickened secretions secondary to reduced humidity associated with winter heating, alcohol consumption, and anesthesia. The latter factor likely accounts for the increased frequency of postoperative bronchopulmonary infections noted in patients with underlying, but often undiagnosed, chronic bronchitis. All acute exacerbations of chronic bronchitis present with similar bronchopulmonary symptoms, which may include increased frequency and severity of cough, greater sputum production that is usually purulent, chest congestion, chest discomfort, increased dyspnea and wheezing, and scant hemoptysis. Systemic symptoms of malaise, anorexia, chilliness, or feverishness may also be present. However, shaking chills, fever, or pleuritic pain usually indicates the presence of pneumonia. Physical examination may reveal rhonchi, coarse rales, wheezes, decreased breath sounds, tachypnea, and tachycardia. Patients with chronic bronchitis who are admitted to hospital or treated in emergency rooms with compromised pulmonary function usually have had a preceding acute exacerbation.

Bacterial infection is the etiology of approximately 50% of the acute exacerbations suffered by patients with chronic bronchitis. Other common etiologies are acute viral tracheobronchitis, inhalation of toxic gases or particles (eg, cigarette smoke), thickened secretions, inhalation of allergens, or discontinuation of background therapy. The differentiation of ABE from other types of exacerbations is only occasionally possible from history, physical examination, blood tests, urine tests, chest roentgenograph, pulmonary function tests, or the gross appearance of the sputum. Although purulence of the sputum is often equated with infection, the characteristic yellow to green color of purulence is caused by myeloperoxidase released from polymorphonuclear neutrophils and eosinophils and reflects the stasis of secretions in the bronchial tree, which is a common factor in most types of exacerbations. Microscopic assessment of the sputum by means of a Gram stain and simple wet preparation reveal the two essential characteristics of bacterial infection: increased numbers of bacteria and increased bronchial neutrophilic inflammation. The Gram stain must have bacteria in numbers over 10 to 20 per oil immersion field, significantly above the average of two when the patient is stable. In addition, the wet preparation of the sputum should reveal that the majority of the inflammatory cells are neutrophils. This with an associated increase of the volume of sputum expectorated reflects the outpouring of neutrophils into the bronchial lumen in response to the bacterial infection. Microscopic screening of the sputum is essential to the selection of aliquots for evaluation that are free of oropharyngeal admixture. Much of the distrust of sputum findings commented on in the literature can be related to the failure to adhere to this simple procedure. If sputum is not selected for examination, the results will not reflect the bronchial pathology.

Table 28.1 details the distinguishing characteristics of the cellular population and Gram stain findings in the most common etiologically different types of acute exacerbations seen in chronic bronchitis or asthma. The identification of the specific etiology allows for selection of appropriate therapy and avoids the costs and adverse effects associated with the use of unnecessary medications.

Bacteriologic cultures and sensitivity testing are rarely indicated to determine treatment for ambulatory ABE. Exceptions to this rule are when gram-negative bacilli (other than *Haemophilus*-like organisms) or staphylococcal-like bacteria are noted on Gram stain. However, staphylococcal ABE are rare in ambulatory chronic bronchitis outpatients. Gram stains can provide immediate information with which to initiate therapy; waiting for cultures is not justified. In patients with chronic bronchitis, culture results from poorly selected aliquots are often falsely positive or negative and can lead to inappropriate choice of therapy.

Table 28.2 details the critical primary treatment modalities for the various types of acute exacerbations as well as those that are important supportive measures. Antimicrobials are not indicated for any of the acute exacerbations (AE), which are not bacterial in etiology. Their use can only add adverse side effects and contribute to the development of resistance to antimicrobials. A recent trend to treat all types of exacerbations empirically with both antimicrobials and corticosteroids should be discouraged. The decrease of host defenses associated with corticosteroids can be detrimental if the bacteria responsible for the ABE are not covered by the arbitrarily chosen antimicrobial.

Numerous comments in the literature claim that the need for antimicrobial therapy for ABECB is not proven. This is based on the reliance on the numerous published investigations with inadequate study design and the inappropriate inclusion of subjects with AECB without

Table 28.1 Key Sputum Characteristics in the Differential Diagnosis of Acute Exacerbations of Chronic Bronchitis or Asthma

	Neutrophils[a,b]	Eosinophils[a,b]	Type of Bronchial Epithelial Cells[b]	Bacteria on Gram Stain[c]
Acute bacterial bronchitis	Increased	No change	Pyknotic	Increased
Acute viral bronchitis	Increased	No change	Swollen	No change
Inhalation of toxic gases or particles	Increased	No change	Pyknotic	No change
Thickened secretions	No change	No change	Pyknotic	No change
Inhalation of allergens	Variable	Increased	Swollen	No change
Discontinuation of background therapy	No change	No change	Pyknotic	No change

[a] Percentage of all cell types and numbers excreted per day.
[b] As observed in wet sputum preparations.
[c] Numbers per oil immersion field with 0 to 2 as the average numbers seen in nonacute patients.

Table 28.2 Therapy for Acute Exacerbations of Chronic Bronchitis with or without Asthma

	Antimicrobial	Corticosteroids	Hydration and Humidification	Avoidance of Inhaled Irritants	Expectorant	Bronchodilation
Acute bacterial bronchitis	1	NA	2	2	2	2
Acute viral bronchitis	NA	NA	2	2	2	2
Inhalation of toxic gases particles	NA	NA[a]	2	1	2	2
Thickened secretions	NA	NA	1	2	1	2
Inhalation of allergens	NA	1	2	2	2	1
Discontinuation of background therapy	NA	NA	Renew appropriate background therapy			

Key: 1 = Primary or very important therapy; 2 = secondary or supportive therapy; NA = not applicable.
[a] Exception for acute inhalation of toxic materials known to cause serious acute inflammatory response.

demonstrated bacterial infection that would not be affected by the antimicrobial therapy. Data from well-designed investigations limited to subjects with ABECB provide more than sufficient evidence that antimicrobials are indicated for ABECB. The characteristics desirable in the chosen antimicrobial should include coverage of the major pathogens etiologic in ABE, a dosage regimen that favors compliance, and a low incidence of undesirable side effects. Educating patients at risk of developing ABE to recognize early symptoms can lead to early initiation of adequate antimicrobial therapy that decreases morbidity, unnecessary visits to emergency rooms, and expensive hospitalizations. The signs and symptoms of ABE should be significantly improved within 5 to 7 days after starting antimicrobial therapy. Patients should be reevaluated if this does not occur, and therapy may need to be modified.

Published investigations should help clinicians decide on an appropriate antimicrobial for

ABECB. Unfortunately, such publications can be misleading because of poorly conceived study designs. Deficiencies that should be looked for include the use of nonbacterial AECB cases mixed in with true ABECB cases obscuring any true differences among agents, investigations specifically designed to only demonstrate equivalence between antibiotics, and the exclusion of cases with in vitro–resistant bacteria from the analysis of efficacy. These types of investigations can lead clinicians to believe that all antibiotics are equally effective. Conversely, because little or no advantage of any antibiotic can be demonstrated in such studies—despite marked differences noted in in vitro activities—it is easy to incorrectly conclude that antibiotic therapy is unimportant in the treatment of ABECB. In addition, when all AECB are treated as if they were ABECB, the true cause of an AECB may not be identified and the specific therapy that could benefit the patient is not used.

Carefully controlled investigations in which a bacterial etiology is an absolute prerequisite demonstrate that there may be profound differences of outcome of ABECB between antibiotics. Selection of the proper antimicrobial once bacterial infection is identified as the cause of the AECB should assume that any of the four major pathogens might be present. *Haemophilus influenzae, Moraxella catarrhalis, S. pneumoniae,* and *Haemophilus parainfluenzae* make up more than 90% of the organisms etiologic in ABECB, with a predominance of *Haemophilus* species. During the 1990s, the older antimicrobials lost a significant degree of their original efficacy because of the increasing incidence of β-lactamase active *M. catarrhalis* (80%) and *H. influenzae* (40%) and of penicillin-resistant *S. pneumoniae.*

The goals of therapy for ABE are the expeditious resolution of the acute infection without significant early relapses and with a long infection-free posttreatment period. Success and compliance will be facilitated by selection of an antimicrobial drug with the best antibacterial sensitivity pattern, having few adverse effects and a simple dosage regimen. A first-choice antibiotic should provide prompt resolution of the acute infection in more than 94% of patients with ABECB, have less than a 10% relapse rate in the first 2 weeks after therapy, and keep most patients infection free for at least 5 to 6 months (Table 28.3). Recommendations to treat ABECB in which the severity of the underlying chronic bronchitis is mild with less effective antimicrobials is not based on adequate comparison studies. Use of low dosages and short periods of treatment are also of questionable validity.

Table 28.3 Ranking Criteria for Assessing Antimicrobial Therapy in ABECB

Ranking	1	2	3	4
Positive response during therapy (% of cases)	94–100	88–93	75–87	≤74
Continued positive response 2 weeks after therapy (% of cases)	83–88	72–82	61–71	≤60
Duration of infection-free period in days (based on mean values)[a]	>200	156–200	100–150	≤100
Probable sensitivity of infecting pathogens to the antimicrobial (%)	>95	85–95	75–85	≤75

[a] These data are from double-blind and crossover studies in which the same subjects were treated with different antimicrobials for separate ABECB.
Abbreviation: ABECB = acute bacterial exacerbations of chronic bronchitis.

The few data that exist strongly suggest that these practices lead to higher early relapses and shorter infection-free intervals. The tenacity of bacterial infection in chronic bronchitis is usually underestimated.

Prompt and adequate antimicrobial therapy will decrease the period of morbidity and the chances of progression to pneumonia and/or respiratory failure. All episodes of ABECB should be treated to achieve these positive outcomes. The vast majority of ABECB are treatable in the ambulatory setting with orally administered antimicrobials. If the patient is not already receiving adequate background therapy for his or her underlying disease, these measures should be instituted concomitant with the antimicrobial therapy. Resolution of the acute bacterial exacerbation should be defined as a return to the preexacerbation level of symptoms and bronchial inflammation. Acceptance of partial improvement can lead to a protracted period of morbidity and a higher level of bronchial mucosal damage and inflammation than was present before the infection. Insufficient improvement after 7 days of therapy, or worsening prior to this, is an indication for reevaluation. Persistence of the original bacteria or the emergence of new bacterial types in association with continued elevation of sputum neutrophilic inflammation indicates that the antimicrobial agent needs to be changed.

Oral agents used for ABECB come from most of the major antimicrobial classes (eg, penicillins, tetracyclines, quinolones, macrolides, cephalosporins, and sulfonamides). Efficacy of representative antimicrobials can be ranked from 1 (best results) to 4 (poorest results) using the criteria noted in Table 28.3 for the three major clinical and bacteriologic outcomes. Treatment failures are defined as failure to respond during treatment, early relapses as recurrences within 2 weeks of stopping therapy, and the infection-free period defined from the mean values from double-blind studies as the average number of days from stopping therapy to the next ABECB. A fourth criterion relates to the current sensitivity of the common ABECB pathogens to the antimicrobial. The best choice should be an antimicrobial with documentation of best results for all four criteria.

Table 28.4 details the efficacy and sensitivity patterns of antimicrobials that have been or are being commonly used to treat ABECB. Only data in which the cases evaluated had bacterial pathogens identified in double-blind–designed studies are listed. Efficacy data from parallel assignment studies are noted in parentheses, whereas data from crossover assignment studies are not. Crossover study comparisons benefit from having the same host for the two separate ABECB, diminishing some of the variability related to host factors. Antimicrobials are not listed in Table 28.4 if they are not commonly used for ABECB, if published data do not meet the criteria of having identified pretherapy pathogens for all analyzed cases, or if the study excluded cases with bacteria resistant to the antimicrobials being tested. Many of the studies were done before 1990, so it is important to consider the current sensitivity pattern when selecting an antimicrobial. These values will likely continue to change with time and vary because of locality differences.

The once highly efficacious penicillins have lost their preeminence as the drugs of choice for treatment of ABECB because of the significant increase of β-lactamase–active *H. influenzae* (40%) and *M. catarrhalis* (80%) and the rising incidence of penicillin-resistant *S. pneumoniae*. The rankings for ampicillin and amoxicillin (see Table 28.4) were established before the emergence of these factors and are included for their historical perspective. Even without current studies of these agents, the assumption should be that neither agent alone would now

be as efficacious for ABECB. The addition of a β-lactamase inhibitor (eg, clavulanic acid) to amoxicillin or ampicillin should theoretically restore their previous efficacy for *M. catarrhalis* and *H. influenzae*, but critical studies comparing these with and without inhibitors are not available. Not all β-lactamase subtypes are covered by the available inhibitors, suggesting that full theoretical advantage may not be realized. These inhibitors will not eliminate the problem of penicillin-resistant *S. pneumoniae*. The available data suggest that amoxicillin/clavulanic acid is comparable in efficacy to the synthetic tetracyclines for ABECB.

The fluoroquinolone class of antimicrobials has demonstrated the positive attributes that ampicillin once possessed. These are very effective against *H. influenzae* and *M. catarrhalis* and not affected by β-lactamase activity. The relative activity against *S. pneumoniae* by the various quinolones has defined those most efficacious for ABECB. Fluoroquinolones with poor activity against *S. pneumoniae* are not indicated for treatment of ABECB. Ciprofloxacin at the higher recommended dosage (750 mg twice daily) is quite effective in eradicating *S. pneumoniae* in clinical outcome studies, whereas at a lower dosage (500 mg twice daily), activity against pneumococci becomes marginal. Ofloxacin and levofloxacin appear to be slightly less efficacious at the dosage schedules generally recommended. Published reports of these agents do not usually address relapse rates and infection-free intervals for pathogen-proven cases. A number of newer quinolones have in vitro profiles suggesting a greater potential against *S. pneumoniae*. However, as activity against *S. pneumoniae* improves, efficacy against organisms such as *Pseudomonas aeruginosa* generally declines. Of these new quinolones, moxifloxacin appears to have the best efficacy and safety profile. Outcome studies in ABECB with this quinolone have not evaluated all of the important efficacy criteria or whether the recommended dosage schedules provide optimal results. A number of other studied and/or approved fluoroquinolones have been withdrawn due to safety issues or inadequate sales performance. Based on the available published experience, ciprofloxacin, 750 mg twice daily for 10 to 14 days, appears to be the quinolone of choice for treatment of ABECB pending definitive studies of the other quinolones.

When quinolones are contraindicated, one of the synthetic tetracyclines can be used. Doxycycline and minocycline are comparable in efficacy but doxycycline has fewer annoying

Table 28.4 Oral Antimicrobials for Acute Bacterial Exacerbation in Chronic Bronchitis[a,b]

	Dose/day (mg)	Schedule Duration (Days)	Response During Therapy	Early Relapse After Therapy	Infection-free Interval	Bacterial Susceptibility
Penicillins						
Ampicillin	500 qid	14	1	1	1	4
Amoxicillin	500 tid	14	2	1	2	4
Amoxicillin-clavulanic acid	500/125 tid	14	1	2	2	2
Amoxicillin-clavulanic acid	500/125 bid	7	(2)	ND	ND	2
Quinolones						
Ciprofloxacin	750 bid	14	1	1	1	1
Ciprofloxacin	500 bid	14	1	2	2	2
Ofloxacin	400 bid	10	(1)	ND	ND	2
Tetracyclines						
Doxycycline	100 bid	14	1	1	2	2
Doxycycline	200 qd	1				
	100 qd	9–13	(2)	(4)	ND	2
Tetracycline	1000 qid	14	2	4	3	3
Macrolides						
Clarithromycin	500 bid	14	2	3	2	2
Azithromycin	500 qd	1				
	250 qd	4	(2)	ND	ND	2
Azithromycin	500 qd	3	(3)	ND	ND	2
Erythromycin	250 qid	7	(3)	(4)	ND	4
Cephalosporins						
Cefuroxime	500 bid	14	(2)	ND	(2)	2
Cefaclor	500 tid	14	4	4	4	4
Cephalexin	500 tid	14	3	4	4	4
Cefprozil	500 bid	10	(4)	ND	ND	3
Sulfonamides						
Trimethoprim-sulfamethoxazole	800/160 bid	14	1	2	3	3

Abbreviations: ND = no data available.
[a] Ranking 1 to 4; see Table 28.3.
[b] Parallel assignment studies noted by numbers in parenthesis. All others from crossover assignment studies.

side effects. They have convenient dosage schedules not dependent on food restriction, have few adverse effects to restrict compliance, and are not limited by β-lactamase–active microorganisms. The side effects of regular tetracycline at adequate therapeutic dosages make compliance difficult and contribute to their poor efficacy. Although tetracycline-resistant *S. pneumoniae* have been reported, the clinical impact of this has not been evident in ABECB.

The newer macrolides, clarithromycin and azithromycin, are superior to erythromycin for ABECB. Telithromycin, a ketolide, is closely related to the macrolides. However, critical published data on efficacy of these agents for ABECB are scant. Clinical and bacteriologic outcome data suggest a role as second-choice therapy for ABECB. This is primarily related to a relatively lesser ability to eradicate *H. influenzae.* Although the macrolides have low degrees of toxicity, interactions with other therapeutic agents may cause some confusion regarding indications in individual patients. Recent reports of serious adverse events with telithromycin make its routine use for ABECB questionable. Macrolides have significant activity against *Chlamydia pneumoniae, Mycoplasma pneumoniae,* and *Legionella,* but although these pathogens are important in community-acquired pneumonia, they play a lesser role in ABECB. Erythromycin is not indicated for ABECB.

Trimethoprim-sulfamethoxazole is efficient during active treatment for ABECB, but it has a significant incidence of early relapse rate, and the infection-free interval is considerably shorter than with first-choice antibiotics. Although the low initial cost is favorable, the need to treat a new infection within an average of 3 months is not cost-effective. There are also concerns relating to increased toxicity in older patients.

Cephalosporins have variable success in treating ABECB. The efficacy of individual cephalosporins is difficult to assess from most of the published data. Resistant bacteria were commonly excluded from analysis in earlier studies. The appearance of equivalence with virtually any effective or ineffective comparative antibiotic is an inevitable outcome. Of the few properly studied cephalosporins, cefuroxime compared favorably with low-dose ciprofloxacin. Well-controlled studies with older cephalosporins, such as cephalexin and cefaclor, indicate a level of ineffectiveness in all outcome criteria approaching what would be expected from placebo therapy. Results from studies with ineffective agents like these strongly support the need for effective antibiotic therapy for ABECB. If antibiotic therapy was not important, the results of even carefully designed investigations should never demonstrate any differences.

Acute exacerbations, particularly ABECB, have been demonstrated to adversely affect the progression of chronic bronchitis. Prompt and effective treatment of ABECB will shorten the immediate morbidity and likely decrease the long-term detrimental decline in function. Recommendations to treat mild to moderate ABECB, particularly in chronic bronchitics mild disease, with less effective antimicrobials does not appear to be justified. Because chronic bronchitis is a progressive disease, it makes sense to treat ABECB in mild bronchitics with the most

effective antimicrobial therapy one would use in the more severe cases.

The effectiveness of even the best antimicrobial may be significantly affected by the use of an insufficient daily dose, too short a period of therapy, or both. Lower dosages often decrease the incidence of troublesome side effects, and shorter duration of therapy promotes better compliance. However, this must be balanced against a higher rate of early relapses and a more frequent occurrence of ABE in these chronically ill patients. Unfortunately, very few investigations have addressed this issue directly. Inference from a variety of studies strongly suggests that the higher recommended dosages given for at least 10 to 14 days are advantageous in treating ABECB. Examples from Table 28.4 support this. Ciprofloxacin, 750 mg twice daily, provides fewer relapses and a longer infection-free interval than does a dosage of 500 mg twice daily when both are given for 14 days. Azithromycin, 500 mg/day for 3 days, is not as effective during therapy as a 5-day course at a lower daily dose. Doxycycline, 100 mg twice daily, is more effective during and immediately after therapy than a lower (standard) regimen for the same duration of therapy.

When parenteral therapy is necessary in hospitalized patients, it is more important to identify the causative pathogen(s). Depending on the pathogen, ampicillin, ciprofloxacin (particularly for gram-negative infections), or doxycycline would be common choices. Multiple-drug therapy, including cephalosporins and aminoglycosides, may be necessary. Switching to oral therapy should be considered as early as possible in these circumstances as being cost-effective and permitting earlier discharge from hospital.

Antimicrobial therapy should always be accompanied by good supportive therapy. This should include the avoidance of smoking or other inhalation irritants, hydration, humidification, expectorants, bronchodilators, and adequate treatment of any associated asthma. When secretion clearance is particularly difficult, chest physiotherapy and mucolytic therapy are appropriate. Patients who have both chronic bronchitis and asthma will often note an exacerbation of asthmatic symptoms as the infection is controlled. Prompt recognition of this possibility should lead to vigorous treatment of the asthma and not be misdiagnosed as a failure of the antimicrobial. This can be easily detected by examination of the sputum, which would show a shift to a predominance of eosinophils and an absence of significant bacterial flora on Gram stain.

In summary, the first choice antimicrobials for ABECB are ciprofloxacin, 750 mg twice daily, or one of the other new quinolones when *Pseudomonas* infection is not a concern. Second-choice agents are ciprofloxacin, 500 mg twice daily; amoxicillin with clavulanic acid; and doxycycline. Other agents should be considered only when contraindications for the main antimicrobials exist.

SUGGESTED READING

Chodosh S. Treatment of acute exacerbations of chronic bronchitis: state of the art. *Am J Med.* 1991;91:87S–92S.

Chodosh S. Sputum production and chronic bronchitis. In Takishima T, Shimura S, eds. *Airway Secretion: Physiological Bases for the Control of Mucus Hypersecretion.* New York, NY: Marcel Dekker; 1994.

Chodosh S. Clinical significance of the infection-free interval in the management of acute bacterial exacerbations of chronic bronchitis. *Chest.* 2005;127:2231–2236.

Chodosh S, McCarty J, Farkas S, et al. Randomized double-blind study of ciprofloxacin and cefuroxime axetil for the treatment of acute bacterial exacerbations of chronic bronchitis. *Clin Inf Dis.* 1998; 27:722–729.

Wenzel RP, Fowler AA III. Clinical Practice. Acute bronchitis. *N Engl J Med.* 2006;355: 2125–2130.

29. Croup, Supraglottitis, and Laryngitis

Irmgard Behlau

CROUP

Croup is a clinical syndrome characterized by a seal-like barking cough, hoarseness, inspiratory stridor, and often some degree of respiratory distress. The term *croup* is usually used to refer to acute laryngotracheobronchitis. Other crouplike syndromes can include spasmodic croup and bacterial tracheitis (Table 29.1). Other potential infectious causes of stridor include supraglottitis (epiglottitis), peritonsillar abscess, retropharyngeal abscess, and rarely diphtheria, whereas noninfectious etiologies include angioneurotic edema, foreign body obstruction, hemangioma, trauma, neoplasm, subglottic stenosis, or extrinsic compression. Croup is primarily a disease of children between the ages of 1 to 6 with peak incidence between 6 months and 3 years. The parainfluenza viruses (1, 2, and 3) are the most frequent cause with outbreaks occurring predominantly in the winter months. Other occasional causes include respiratory syncytial virus (RSV), influenza, and adenovirus with rare cases secondary to *Mycoplasma, Corynebacterium diphtheriae,* and herpes simplex virus (HSV). In adults, the causes are also predominantly viral, including reported cases of influenza, parainfluenza, RSV, HSV, and cytomegalovirus (CMV). In either children or adults, most likely secondary bacterial infections with *Haemophilus influenzae* type b (Hib), staphylococci, *Moraxella catarrhalis,* and *Streptococcus pneumoniae* can be seen.

Croup usually follows a relatively mild upper respiratory infection. Its onset is commonly abrupt and occurs in the late evening and night. Viral infection with associated inflammation of the nasopharynx spreads inferiorly to the respiratory epithelium of the larynx and trachea. The subglottic region in children is normally narrow and surrounded by a firm ring of cartilage. Small swelling of this narrow subglottic area will significantly restrict air flow and produce audible inspiratory stridor, while the impairment of the mobility of the vocal cords will produce hoarseness.

Rapid, objective, and calm assessment of severity must be done to determine management and without respiratory compromise. The presence of chest wall retractions and stridor at rest are most critical (Table 29.2). Anteroposterior radiologic examination of the soft tissues of the neck (with medical monitoring) may be useful when the diagnosis is in question. The classic steeple sign is produced by the cone-shaped narrowing of the proximal 1-cm subglottic area of the trachea, at the conus elasticus to the level of the true vocal cords. It is produced by edema with elevation of the tracheal mucosa and the loss of the normal lateral convexities (shoulders) of the air column (Figure 29.1). Direct visualization of the airway can be attempted if the symptoms are not typical and the child is stable. If intubation appears imminent or there is a strong suspicion of epiglottitis, this should be performed under anesthesia. In croup, the supraglottic region appears normal.

Therapy

Management includes corticosteroids, nebulized budesonide, and nebulized epinephrine. Humidified oxygen and heliox are often used as supportive treatment and are equally effective. No clear data exist on the benefits of mist or humidified air; therefore, the use of mist tents, which separate children from their parents and impair the observation of the child's respiratory status, are discouraged. Analgesics improve sore throat and overall comfort. Antitussives, decongestants, and "prophylactic" antibiotics are not beneficial.

Due to the sustained anti-inflammatory effects of corticosteroids, they have been shown to improve the status of not only severe croup but also mild to moderate croup. Dexamethasone in doses of 0.15 to 0.6 mg/kg has been shown to be beneficial and decreases the need for hospitalizations and unscheduled medical visits even in mild croup. Oral, intramuscular, and intravenous routes of administration are all effective, with nebulized dexamethasone possibly less effective. Nebulized budesonide, 2 mg, has been shown to be as effective as dexamethasone but is often reserved for patients with intractable vomiting or due to the simultaneous need to

Table 29.1 Comparison of Crouplike Syndromes

Characteristic	Spasmodic Croup	Laryngeotracheobronchitits	Bacterial Tracheitis	Supraglottitis
Age range	6 mo–3 y	0–6 y (peak, 6 mo–3 yr)	1 mo–6 yr	Infants ≤2 mo, older children and adults
Etiology	? Viral ? Airway reactivity	Parainfluenza virus (1,2, 3) Influenza Respiratory syncytial virus Adenovirus	*Staphylococcus aureus* *H. influenzae* *C. diphtheriae*	*H. influenzae*(Hib/non-b) *S. pneumoniae* Group A streptococcus *H.parainfluenzae*
Onset	Sudden	Insidious	Rapid deterioration	Sudden
Clinical manifestations	Afebrile Nontoxic Barking cough Stridor Hoarse	Low-grade fever Nontoxic Barking cough Stridor Hoarse	High fever Toxic Barking cough Stridor Hoarse	High fever Toxic Nonbarking cough Muffled voice Drooling Dysphagia Sitting, leaning forward
Endoscopic findings	Pale mucosa Subglottic swelling	Deep-red mucosa Subglottic swelling	Deep-red mucosa Copious tracheal secretions	Cherry-red epiglottis Arytenoepiglottic swelling
Complete blood count, differential	Normal	Mild leukocytosis Lymphocytosis	Normal to mild leukocytosis; marked bandemia	Marked leukocytosis Bandemia
Radiographic findings	Subglottic narrowing	Subglottic narrowing	Subglottic narrowing Irregular tracheal border	Large epiglottis Thick arytenoepiglottic folds
Therapy	Mist Calm ?Racemic epinephrine ?Steroids	Corticosteroids Racemic epinephrine Nebulized budesonide Intubation (if necessary)	Intubation Antibiotics	Intubation Antibiotics
Response	Rapid	Transient	Slow (1–2 wk)	Variable (hrs-days)
Intubation	Rare	Occasional	Usual	Usual

administer with epinephrine in severe respiratory distress because it is substantially more expensive and more difficult to administer. The combination of oral dexamethasone and nebulized budesonide is no better than either alone. For the management of outpatient croup, oral prednisolone, 2 mg/kg/day as 2 divided doses per day, may be considered as an alternative, but comparison studies have been limited to oral dexamethasone.

Due to the rapid onset of action, the use of nebulized racemic epinephrine has markedly reduced the need for intubation, even in hospitalized patients, to less than 2%. L-epinephrine (1:1000) is as effective as racemic epinephrine. Improvement occurs within minutes, but symptoms can recur within 2 hours; therefore, patients must be observed in the emergency room for 3 hours.

The administration of oxygen should be reserved for children with significant respiratory distress and hypoxia (oxygen saturation on room air ≤92%). Heliox, a lower density gas that is a mixture of oxygen (20%–30%) and helium (70%–80%), has been proposed to help reduce the need for intubation in the severely ill child by improving laminar gas flow through a narrowed airway. There remains insufficient evidence to advocate its general use.

If intubation is deemed necessary, an endotracheal tube one to two sizes smaller than would be used for the same-size healthy child will be needed to prevent pressure necrosis and resulting subglottic stenosis. For those children who appear to have a secondary bacterial infection, antibiotic therapy similar to that recommended for epiglottitis should be considered to treat the possibility of a

Clinical Syndromes – Respiratory Tract

Table 29.2 Recommended Table Algorithm for the Management of Croup (Laryngotracheobronchitis)

Condition	Treatment
Mild	
No stridor *No* chest wall retractions *No* respiratory distress at rest	Analgesics, hydration as needed Single dose of oral dexamethasone (0.6mg/kg body weight) Educate parents (illness, when to seek medical assessment)
Moderate	
Stridor at rest Mild chest wall retractions No agitation or significant respiratory distress	Above including oral dexamethasone, 0.6 mg/kg Observe in emergency room If improved with no stridor or retractions, educate, home If no or minimal improvement by 4h, hospitalization
Severe	

Stridor may decrease with worsening airway obstruction
Significant respiratory distress
Severe chest wall retractions
Agitation or lethargy
Decreased air movement
Possibly cyanosis
	Nebulized racemic epinephrine 2.25% (0.5 mL/2.5mL saline)
	  or L-epinephrine 1:1000 (5 mL), may repeat
	Oral or parenteral dexamethasone 0.6 mg/kg, may repeat
	If contraindications to oral medication, consider nebulized
	  budesonide 2 mg with epinephrine
	Humidifed oxygen (≤92% room air O$_2$ sat, consider heliox)
	ICU care, intubation as necessary

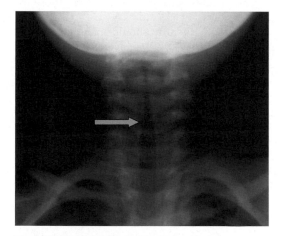

Figure 29.1 The "steeple sign" of croup. Anteroposterior radiograph of the upper airway (arrow) of a patient with croup. (Courtesy of Drs. A. Weber and H.D. Curtin, Dept. of Radiology, Massachusetts Eye and Ear Infirmary, Boston, MA)

secondary bacterial process. Table 29.2 outlines therapy recommendations depending on the clinical state of the patient.

ACUTE SUPRAGLOTTITIS (EPIGLOTTITIS)

Supraglottitis is characterized by inflammation and edema of the supraglottic structures, including the epiglottis, arytenoepiglottic folds, arytenoids, and false vocal cords; paradoxically, the epiglottis may be spared.

In children, acute supraglottitis is typically characterized by a fulminating course of severe sore throat, high fever, dysphagia, drooling, low-pitched inspiratory stridor, and airway obstruction, which, if left untreated, can lead to death. The child appears toxic and prefers an airway-preserving posture—sitting upright, jaw protruding forward, while drooling. In adults, the presentation is more variable; most adults have mild illness with a prolonged prodrome. In immunocompromised patients, there may be a paucity of physical findings.

Definitive diagnosis is made by examination of the epiglottis and supraglottic structures. No attempt should be made to visualize the epiglottis in an awake child; therefore a severely ill child must be examined in the operating room at the time of control of the airway. In children, the epiglottis is typically fiery red and extremely swollen, but occasionally the major inflammation involves the ventricular bands and arytenoepiglottic folds, and the epiglottis appears relatively normal. In adults, awake indirect laryngoscopy may be performed, but only when it is possible to establish an artificial airway. In adults, the supraglottic structures may appear pale with watery edema. If indirect laryngoscopy is unavailable, lateral neck radiographs are also useful for evaluating supraglottitis (Figure 29.2), but they are not as sensitive and should never delay protecting the airway. The classic appearance is of an enlarged epiglottis bulging from the anterior wall of the hypopharynx with straightening of the cervical spine from the usual mild lordosis.

The epidemiology of acute supraglottitis has changed dramatically since the introduction of the Hib vaccines in the mid- to late 1980s. Supraglottitis, which most commonly had affected children 2 to 7 years of age, is now rarer in young children than adults, is primarily a disease of older children adults, and is increasingly being caused by other microbial pathogens. The incidence of invasive Hib has decreased more than 99% compared to the pre-vaccine era. The organisms typically involved, in addition to Hib, are *Streptococcus pneumoniae, Staphylococcus aureus,* β-hemolytic streptococci, *H. influenzae* type non-b, *H. parainfluenzae,* rarely in adults *Pasteurella multocida,* and possibly increasing reports of *Neisseria meningitidis* since 1995. There are very rare reports of children developing Hib epiglottitis despite vaccination. The role respiratory tract viruses play as primary pathogens remains unclear. There have been reports of herpes simplex virus (HSV) type 1 and varicella as primary pathogens in immunocompromised hosts. Noninfectious causes include thermal and corrosive injury, lymphoproliferative disorders, and graft-versus-host disease.

Therapy

Treatment of acute supraglottitis is directed at establishing an airway and administering appropriate antibiotics. Children with epiglottitis should routinely have an artificial airway established; observation cannot be routinely rec-

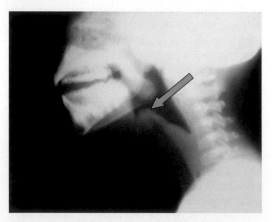

Figure 29.2 The "thumb sign" of supraglottitis. Lateral radiograph of the neck in a patient with supraglottitis; arrow indicates thickened epiglottitis. (Courtesy of Drs. A. Weber and H. Curtin, Department of Radiology, Massachusetts Eye and Ear Infirmary, Boston, MA)

ommended because the mortality rate is 6% to 25% and increases to 30% to 80% for those who develop obstruction. Most deaths occur within the first hours after arrival. The use of a "prophylactic airway" has reduced the mortality rate to less than 1%. The management of the airway in adult supraglottitis reflects the greater variability of clinical presentation and course. It has a range of mortality rates from 10% to 32%. Vigilant airway monitoring and continuous staging are needed for adults whose disease may progress to respiratory compromise. A formal written "acute airway obstruction protocol" should be followed. Factors associated with airway obstruction include symptomatic respiratory difficulty, stridor, drooling, shorter duration of symptoms, enlarged epiglottis on radiograph, and *H. influenzae* bacteremia.

An endotracheal tube is preferred over a tracheotomy for the following reasons: (1) ease of removal of the tube 2 to 3 days after the edema has subsided, thereby shortening the hospital stay; (2) no surgery; and (3) mortality and complication rates equal to or lower than those for tracheotomy.

Antibiotic therapy should include coverage for *H. influenzae, S. pneumoniae,* group A β-hemolytic streptococci, other streptococci, *H. parainfluenzae,* and *S. aureus.* Second- and third-generation cephalosporins are first-line agents. Pediatric dosages are intravenous cefuroxime, 150 mg/kg, 3 doses per day; cefotaxime, 150 mg/kg, 3 doses per day; or ceftriaxone, 50 mg/kg/day, or ampicillin-sulbactam, 200 to 400 mg/kg, ampicillin at 4 doses per day. The recommended adult dosages are intravenous cefuroxime, 0.75 to 1.5 g given 3 times per day; ceftriaxone, 2 g/day; cefotaxime, 2 g every 4 to 8 hours, or ampicillin/sulbactam 1.5 to 3 g every 6 hours. Antibiotic therapy should be continued for 10 to 14 days. In patient populations with a significant prevalence of infection with community-acquired methicillin-resistant *S. aureus* (MRSA) or highly penicillin-resistant *S. pneumoniae,* clindamycin, 30 to 40 mg/kg divided in 3 doses (max 2400 mg/day) or vancomycin, 40 to 60 mg/kg per day in 3 to 4 doses in children or 2 g/day in adults dependent on renal function should be considered. Duration of therapy is usually 7 to 14 days, depending on patient response.

Steroids are commonly used for supraglottitis to theoretically decrease inflammation. There has been no evidence for any significant benefit, and in adults, there is no indication that steroids prevent the need for airway intervention. With epiglottitis being so uncommon and therefore all studies being small, it will be difficult to evaluate any beneficial role. The use of steroids remains controversial.

Prevention

Prophylaxis is indicated for supraglottitis secondary to Hib. Rifampin, 20 mg/kg, not to exceed 600 mg/day, for 4 doses is recommended for: (1) all household contacts (except pregnant women) when there is a child younger than 12 months irrespective of vaccine status or there is a child younger than 4 years of age with incomplete vaccination; (2) day-care and nursery school classroom contacts (including adults) if (a) two or more cases of invasive disease have occurred within 60 days and unvaccinated or incompletely vaccinated children attend or (b) with one case and susceptible children 2 years or younger who attend for 25 hours or more per week and susceptible children should be vaccinated; if children are older than 2 years, rifampin prophylaxis need not be given irrespective of vaccination status. (3) The patient should receive prophylaxis before discharge if treated with ampicillin or chloramphenicol to prevent reintroduction of the organism into the household. Prophylaxis is not needed for those treated with the aforementioned recommended cephalosporins because they eradicate Hib from the nasopharynx.

Since the introduction of conjugated vaccines for infants beginning at 2 months of age, the incidence of supraglottitis resulting from Hib in this age group has declined by 99%, along with other invasive forms of Hib. There have been isolated rare reports of supraglottitis in children who have been vaccinated, but in general, we are seeing a near-eradication of Hib supraglottitis in young children. Supraglottitis caused by Hib occurs now in this country primarily in undervaccinated children, infants too young to have completed the primary series of vaccinations, and older children and adults who have never been immunized.

LARYNGITIS

The larynx rests in the hypopharynx and consists of: (1) the supraglottic larynx, which includes the laryngeal inlet formed by the epiglottis anteriorly and the arytenoepiglottic folds bilaterally merging inferiorly into false cords, and (2) the glottic larynx, which consists of the true vocal cords.

Acute laryngitis often presents with hoarseness, odynophagia, and localized pain, which may also be referred and manifests as otalgia. Obstruction of the airway is uncommon in adults but more common in young children, especially if associated with tracheal inflammation as in croup, and must be distinguished from acute supraglottitis. Examination of the larynx reveals erythema, edema, secretions, and occasionally superficial mucosal ulcerations. The presence of exudate or membrane on the pharyngeal or laryngeal mucosa should raise the suspicion of streptococcal infection, mononucleosis, or diphtheria; granulomatous infiltration may be compatible with tuberculosis, sarcoidosis, fungal infection, or syphilis.

The respiratory viruses such as influenza virus, parainfluenza virus, rhinovirus, and adenovirus are most often isolated in cases of laryngitis (90%). *Moraxella catarrhalis* has been isolated from the nasopharynx of 50% to 55% and *H. influenzae* from 8% to 15% of adults with laryngitis. It remains unclear whether these may represent a secondary bacterial invasion. Group A and G streptococci, *Chlamydia pneumoniae,* and *Mycoplasma pneumoniae* have also been associated with acute laryngitis. Laryngeal diphtheria is very rare and usually results from extension of pharyngeal involvement. It may occur in previously immunized persons.

Fungal infections such as histoplasmosis, coccidioidomycosis, blastomycosis, and cryptococcosis may cause laryngitis. Candidiasis is most often seen in immunosuppressed patients. *T. pallidum,* herpes simplex virus, and herpes zoster virus may also be causes of acute laryngitis. Laryngeal tuberculosis is very rarely seen in the United States since the advent of effective antimycobacterial therapy. It is associated with a large tuberculous load, and patients often have very active pulmonary involvement. Sarcoidosis, Wegener's granulomatosis, and rhinoscleroma may be considered causes of laryngitis.

Therapy

Because most cases of acute laryngitis are viral in etiology and self-limited, treatment usually consists of resting the voice and inhaling moistened air. The role of empiric antibiotic therapy of laryngitis has been examined by prospective double-blinded studies. Penicillin V had no effect on the clinical course. Patients treated with erythromycin (0.5 g twice a day for 5 days) had a marked reduction of *M. catarrhalis* carriage in the nasopharynx and reported a significant improvement of subjective voice disturbances after 1 week and cough after 2 weeks; however, there was no difference in laryngoscopic examination and voice evaluation. Because acute laryngitis in adults is self-limiting and subjective symptoms are spontaneously reduced after 1 week in most cases, empiric antibiotic treatment does not seem warranted as a general policy.

Antimicrobial therapy is indicated only in those patients with a bacterial infection or superinfection; therapy is directed toward the believed causative agent. Usual duration is for 10 to 14 days. The use of corticosteroids should be avoided due their ability to mask vocal cord pathology.

Immunosuppressed patients who present with hoarseness or patients whose hoarseness has persisted longer than 10 to 14 days should have a laryngoscopic examination to exclude other more atypical causes such as herpes simplex virus, bacterial, fungal, mycobacterial, and malignant etiologies of laryngitis.

SUGGESTED READINGS

Cherry JD. State of the evidence for standard-of-care treatments for croup: are we where we need to be? *Pediatr Infect Dis J.* 2005;24: S198–S202, discussion S201.

Frantz TD, Rasgon BM, Quesenberry CP: Acute epiglottis in adults. Analysis of 129 cases. *JAMA.* 1994;272(17):1358–1360.

Klassen TP. Recent advances in the treatment of bronchiolitis and laryngitis in new frontiers in pediatric drug therapy. *Pediatr Clin North Am.* 1997;44:(1)249–261.

Klassen TP, Craig WR, Moher D, et al. Nebulized budesonide and oral dexamethasone for treatment of croup: a randomized controlled trial. *JAMA.* 1998;279(20):1629–1632.

Kortepeter MG, Adams BL, Zollinger WD, Gasser RA, Jr. Fulminant supraglottitis from *Neisseria meningitidis, Emerg Infect Dis.* 2007; 13(3):502–504.

Mayo-Smith MF, Hirsch PJ, Wodzinski SF, et al. Acute epiglottitis: an 18 year experience in Rhode Island, *Chest.* 1995;108:1640.

Russell K, Wiebe N, Saenz A, et al. Glucocorticoids for croup. *Cochrane Database Syst Rev.* 2004;1:CD001955.

Schalen L, Eliasson I, Kamme C, et al. Erythromycin in acute laryngitis in adults, *Ann Otol Rhinol Laryngol.* 1993;102(3 Pt 1):209–214.

Schwam E, Cox J. Fulminant meningococcal supraglottitis: an emerging infectious syndrome? *Emerg Infect Dis.* 1999;5(3):464–467.

Shah RK, Roberson DW, Jones DT. Epiglottitis in the *Hemophilus influenzae* type B vaccine era: changing trends. *Laryngoscope.* 2004; 114(3):557–560.

Vernacchio L, Mitchell AA. Oral dexamethasone for mild croup. *N Engl J Med.* 2004;351:2768–2769.

The Croup Working Group. Guideline for the diagnosis and management of croup. Alberta Medical Association Clinical Practice Guidelines (Canada). Available at http://www.albertadoctors.org/bcm/ama/ama-website.nsf Accessed June 2007.

30. Atypical Pneumonia

Thomas M. File, Jr.

INTRODUCTION

The term *atypical pneumonia* was first coined in the early 1950s to describe cases of pneumonia caused by an unknown agent(s) and which appeared clinically different from pneumococcal pneumonia. It was initially characterized by constitutional symptoms, often with upper and lower respiratory tract symptoms and signs, a protracted course with gradual resolution, the lack of typical findings of consolidation on chest radiograph, failure to isolate a pathogen on routine bacteriologic methods, and a lack of response to penicillin therapy. In the 1940s an agent that was believed to be the principal cause was identified as *Mycoplasma pneumoniae*. Subsequently, other pathogens have been linked with atypical pneumonia because of similar clinical presentation, including a variety of respiratory viruses, *Chlamydophila psittaci, Coxiella burnetti,* and, more recently, *Chlamydophila pneumoniae*. Less common etiologic agents associated with atypical pneumonia include *Francisella tularensis, Yersinia pestis* (plague), and the sin nombre virus (hantavirus pulmonary syndrome), although these agents are often associated with a more acute clinical syndrome. In addition, although presently exceedingly rare, inhalation anthrax is included in part because of the concern for this pathogen as an agent of bioterrorism. Finally, pneumonia caused by *Legionella* species, albeit often more characteristic of pyogenic pneumonia, is also included because it is not isolated using routine microbiologic methods.

Although the original classification of atypical and typical pneumonia arose from the perception that the clinical presentation of patients was different, recent studies have shown that there is considerable overlap of clinical manifestations of specific causes that does not permit empiric therapeutic decisions to be made solely on this basis. Thus, the designation of atypical pneumonia is controversial in relation to scientific and clinical merit, and many authorities have suggested that the term *atypical* be discontinued. However, the term remains popular among clinicians and investigators and remains prevalent in recent literature regardless of its clinical value. Moreover, options for appropriate antimicrobial therapy for the most common causes are similar, which is considered justification by some to lump these together.

Mycoplasma pneumoniae, Chlamydophila pneumoniae, and *Legionella pneumophila* are the most common causes of atypical pneumonia. The results of recent studies indicate that they cause from 15% to as much as 50% (in selected outpatient populations) of cases of community-acquired pneumonia (CAP). However, these pathogens (with the exception of *L. pneumophila*) are not identified often in clinical practice, because there is not a specific, rapid, or standardized test for their detection. The "other" causes of atypical pneumonia occur with much less frequency.

Recently published North American guidelines for management of CAP acknowledge the significance of these pathogens by suggesting the need for empiric therapy that is active against these organisms. The North American approach is to use initial antimicrobial therapy that provides coverage for *S. pneumoniae* plus atypical pathogens (particularly *M. pneumoniae* or *C. pneumoniae,* which are common causes of outpatient CAP). Although the clinical course of *M. pneumoniae* or *C. pneumoniae* infection is often self-limited, these pathogens can cause severe CAP, and appropriate treatment for even mild CAP due to *Mycoplasma* reduces the morbidity of pneumonia and shortens the duration of symptoms. In several observational studies of patients who require hospitalization, antimicrobial regimens that have activity against atypical pathogens have been associated with better outcomes. Although these findings are not definitive, they support an important role for atypical pathogens. In contrast, the British Thoracic Society approach places less significance than the North American approach on the need to treat the atypical pathogens empirically in ambulatory patients, most of whom have mild disease. A policy for initial empirical therapy that covers *M. pneumoniae* is considered unnecessary, because the pathogen exhibits epidemic periodicity every 4 to 5 years and largely affects younger persons.

The possible value of regimens that cover atypical pathogens was addressed in two recent meta-analyses that addressed patients with mild to moderate CAP and those requiring hospitalization. Both analyses found no statistically significant advantage of antibiotics active against atypical pathogens over β-lactam antibiotics. However, most of the studies in these analyses were designed to show noninferiority and used end points of mortality or standard test of cure criteria (usually 7 to 10 days after discontinuation of therapy) that would not detect a faster resolution of disease between the various arms. Many infections due to *M. pneumoniae* or *C. pneumoniae* are self-limited or part of mixed infections (which might respond to a β-lactam). Furthermore, subgroup analysis in patients with *Legionella* species found a significantly lower failure rate in those who were treated with antibiotics active against atypical pathogens. A well-designed, prospective study will be required to more definitively determine the optimal approach to empiric therapy in relation to the need to treat initially for the atypical pathogens.

The association of the atypical pathogens and acute exacerbations of chronic bronchitis (AECB) is less clear than for CAP. Numerous reproducible studies have found *Haemophilus influenzae* to be the most common organism associated with AECB. *Streptococcus pneumoniae* and *Moraxella catarrhalis* are found in lesser frequency. In approximately one half of all cases no bacterial pathogens are isolated, suggesting other causes of AECB, such as environmental factors. Enterobacteriaceae and *Pseudomonas* spp. are predominant pathogens in patients with more severe lung disease. Viral infections may trigger AECB in as many cases. Although *M. pneumoniae* with AECB has not been associated, various reports link *C. pneumoniae* with AECB.

There is increasing information concerning the association of *Chlamydophila* and *Mycoplasma* and asthma pathogenesis, although most studies investigating this have been uncontrolled.

CLINICAL MANIFESTATIONS

Although the diagnosis of these specific pathogens is difficult to establish on clinical manifestations alone, there are several generalizations which may be helpful to the clinician in considering these infections.

Mycoplasma pneumoniae

Mycoplasma pneumoniae is a common cause of respiratory infections that include inapparent infection, upper respiratory infection, tracheobronchitis, and pneumonia. Infection is transmitted from person to person by respiratory droplets with a usual incubation period of several weeks. It is estimated that only 3% to 10% of infected persons develop pneumonia.

M. pneumoniae infections are ubiquitous and can affect all age groups. Although commonly perceived as a cause of CAP predominantly in young healthy patients, the incidence of *M. pneumoniae* pneumonia increases with age, highlighting the importance of this pathogen in the elderly as well.

M. pneumoniae pneumonia is considered to be the classic atypical pneumonia. Many of the pathogenic features of infection with *M. pneumoniae* are believed to be immune mediated rather than induced directly by the bacteria (antibodies produced against the glycolipid antigens of *M. pneumoniae* may cross-react with human red cells and brain cells). The onset is usually insidious, over several days to a week. Constitutional symptoms including headache (usually worse with cough), malaise, myalgias, and sore throat are frequently present. Cough is typically initially dry, may be paroxysmal and frequently worse at night, and may become productive of mucopurulent sputum. Sinus and ear pain are occasionally reported. The physical findings often are minimal, seemingly disproportional to the patient's complaints. Auscultation of the lungs usually reveals variable scattered rales or wheezes. Bullous myringitis, first described in volunteer subjects infected with *M. pneumoniae*, has been infrequent in naturally occurring infection and is not a diagnostic sign. Chest radiograph findings are variable. Most common is peribronchial pneumonia. Other patterns include atelectasis, nodular infiltration, and hilar adenopathy.

The course of *M. pneumoniae* pneumonia is usually mild and self-limiting. However, significant pulmonary complications may occur and include pleural effusion, pneumatocele, lung abscess, pneumothorax, bronchiectasis, chronic interstitial fibrosis, respiratory distress syndrome, and bronchiolitis obliterans.

M. pneumoniae pneumonia is often associated with extrapulmonary manifestations including rash, neurological involvement (ie, aseptic meningitis, meningoencephalitis, cerebral ataxia,

Guillain-Barre syndrome, and transverse myelitis), hemolytic anemia (associated with cold agglutinins), myopericarditis, polyarthritis, and pancreatitis.

Chlamydophila pneumoniae

Pneumonia caused by *C. pneumoniae* may be sporadic or epidemic. *C. pneumoniae* infections are often acquired early in life. Transmission is by person to person via respiratory secretions with an incubation period of several weeks. Reinfections or recrudescent processes, both referred to as recurrent infection, may occur throughout one's lifetime. Most adults who are hospitalized with *C. pneumoniae* pneumonia have recurrent infection.

The clinical manifestations of *C. pneumoniae* pneumonia remain somewhat unclear because of the lack of a gold standard of diagnosis and the contributing effect of copathogens. The onset is usually insidious. Infections often present initially with sore throat, hoarseness, and headache as important nonclassic pneumonic findings. A subacute course is common and fever is low grade. Cough is prominent but unproductive and may last, if not treated early and effectively, for weeks or even months. Clinical characteristics, however, are generally not predictive of *C. pneumoniae* as etiology. Chest radiographs of patients with *C. pneumoniae* pneumonia tend to show less extensive opacifications in relation to clinical findings than other processes. However, extensive infiltrates have been reported.

The clinical characteristics associated with primary infection may be difficult to distinguish from those of reinfection because of the confounding effect of comorbid conditions on age. However, patients with primary infection are usually younger and tend to have higher fever. For older patients with reinfection, the presence of comorbid illness and the requirement for supplemental oxygen therapy are often the reason for hospital admission.

Legionella pneumophila

Legionellosis is primarily associated with two clinically distinct syndromes: legionnaire's disease (LD), a potentially fatal form of pneumonia, and Pontiac fever, a self-limited, nonpneumonic illness. Many of the clinical features of LD are more typical of pyogenic (bacterial) pneumonias than the previously described atypical pneumonia. However, as LD has become increasingly recognized, less severely ill patients are seen earlier in the course of disease, and thus clinical manifestations of unusual severity once considered distinctive LD are now known to be less specific. *Legionella* is not spread person to person but usually by exposure to water. Outbreaks may be associated with infected water sources. The incubation period is 2 to 10 days.

The onset is often acute, accompanied by high fever, myalgias, anorexia, and headache. Temperature often exceeds 40°C. Gastrointestinal symptoms are prominent, especially diarrhea, which occurs in 20% to 40% of cases. Relative bradycardia, which had been purported to be a common finding in earlier studies, has been overemphasized as a diagnostic finding. Hyponatremia and elevated lactate dehydrogenase levels (LDH) were commonly observed in our Ohio Study.

Other Causes of Atypical Pneumonia

Several of the less common causes of the atypical pneumonia syndrome are infections transmitted from animals to humans. In such cases epidemiological clues may be very important; and although specific manifestations cannot be considered diagnostic of a specific etiology, there are general findings that are characteristic of these diseases (Table 30.1).

Coxiella burnetii may be associated with exposure via any mammal but most commonly cattle, goats, sheep, and pets, including cats and dogs. The mode of transmission is either aerosol or by tick bite; high concentrations of the organism can be found in birth products of infected animals. The incubation period is approximately 3 weeks. The acute disease is a self-limiting "flulike" illness characterized by high fever, rigor, headache, myalgia, cough, and arthralgia. Pneumonia may be accompanied by granulomatous hepatitis. Radiological findings include lobar or segmental alveolar opacities that may be multiple. Other manifestations may include maculopapular or purpuric rash, aseptic meningitis or encephalitis, hemolytc anemia, endocarditis, pericarditis, pancreatitis, or epididymoorchitis.

Pneumonia due to *Chlamydophila psittaci* usually occurs after exposure to infected birds. The onset is often insidious with nonproductive cough, fever, and headache but may be abrupt. The incubation period is usually 5 to 15 days. Clinical clues include pharyngeal erythema, splenomegaly (which tends to occur toward the end of the first week), and a specific rash (Horder spots; pink blanching

Table 30.1 Common Characteristics and Therapy for the Other Atypical Pneumonias

Pathogen	Epidemiological or Underlying Condition	Clinical Features	Recommended Therapy
Chlamydophila psittaci	Exposure to birds	HA, myalgia prominent, liver involvement, horder spots (see text)	Tetracycline, doxycycline, macrolides
Coxiella burnetii[a] (Q Fever)	Exposure to farm animals (especially parturient)	HA prominent, liver involvement	Tetracycline, doxycycline, macrolides
Francisella tularensis[a] (Tularemia)	Exposure to rabbits	HA, chest pain prominent, hilar adenopathy	Streptomycin or gentamicin considered as drug of choice; Doxycycline effect for most cases (especially if nonsevere)
Yersinia pestis[a] (Pneumonic plague)	Exposure to infected animals (rodents, cats, squirrels, chipmunks, prairie dogs)	For inhalation, acute onset with rapidly severe pneumonia; blood-tinged sputum	Streptomycin, gentamicin, tetracycline, doxycycline
Bacillus anthracis[a]	Wood mill worker	Biphasic (see text); hallmark radiographic finding- mediastinal widening	Ciprofloxacin plus one of the following for initial therapy: Rifampin, vancomycin, β-lactam, or clindamycin; switch to monotherapy with ciprofloxacin or doxycycline when clinically appropriate
Viruses			
Influenzae	Influenza in community	Influenza pneumonia usually follows tracheo-bronchitis	Oseltamivir (orally), zanamivir (via inhalation)[b]
Adenovirus		Pharyngitis prominent Bronchospasm	
Respiratory syncytial virus	Adults: Cardiopulmonary disease, COPD		No recommended antiviral agent currently available for adults
Hantavirus pulmonary syndrome	Exposure to rodent excreta	Febrile prodrome; followed by noncardiogenic pulmonary edema with shock; thrombocytopenia	Supportive care

[a] Potential infectious agent for biological warfare.
[b] Benefit for primary influenza pneumonia is unknown.
Abbreviations: HA = headache; COPD = chronic obstructive pulmonary disease.

maculopapular eruption resembling rose spots of typhoid fever) that are seen in a minority of cases.

Primary tularemic pneumonia occurs after direct inhalation of infected aerosols and is most common in persons in a high-risk occupation or avocation. In a recent outbreak of tularemic pneumonia, a significant risk factor was mowing grass (presumably in close contact to rabbit habitats). Pneumonia may also occur from hematogenous spread after vector-borne (eg, tick) infection. The most important reservoirs and vectors are ticks, hares, and rabbits. The onset is usually abrupt with high fever, chills, cough (usually nonproductive, occasionally with hemoptysis), pleuritic chest pain, and diaphoresis. Signs and symptoms may be mild and persist for several weeks especially when occurring as a complication of ulceroglandular disease.

The clinical illness of hantavirus pulmonary syndrome (HPS) typically begins with a prodromal phase, which is followed by a cardiopulmonary phase in patients with prior exposure to rodent excreta. Typically the incubation period is 3 weeks after exposure. The earliest clinical manifestation occurs during the prodrome phase and is characterized by nonspecific manifestations such as fever myalgia, headache, nausea, vomiting, abdominal pain (often severe and may be mistaken as acute abdomen), and cough. This phase typically lasts 3 to 8 days and is followed by the cardiopulmonary phase, which starts suddenly with tachypnea and shortness of breath and is followed by respiratory failure and shock. Chest radiograph shows noncardiogenic bilateral interstitial edema during this phase. Characteristically, the patient is hemoconcentrated and manifests significant thrombocytopenia.

Pneumonic plague and inhalation anthrax syndrome are of increasing recent interest because of concern as possible agents of bioterrorism. Plague pneumonia may occur after hematogenous spread during bacteremia of bubonic or septicemic plague or after inhalation of bacteria after coming in contact with a person or animal (most often a cat) with plague pneumonia. The incubation is usually 2 to 3 days. The disease may have an abrupt onset and usually begins with a painless cough with shortness of breath. Sputum is thin, watery, and blood tinged, and the Gram stain reveals typical *Yersinia pestis* (bipolar gram-negative bacilli). Untreated pneumonic plague has a 40% to 90% mortality.

In the natural setting, inhalation anthrax is exceedingly uncommon and is classically referred to as woolsorters disease, because of the association with workers in wool mills who may inhale *B. anthracis* spores. However, the potential use as a biological weapon has brought increased interest to this pathogen, particularly because of the environmental stability of spores, small inoculum necessary to produce fulminant infection, and high mortality rate. In the recent outbreak of probable bioterrorism-associated anthrax conducted through the U.S. postal system, 9 cases of inhalation anthrax were identified, resulting in 4 deaths. The incubation is variable, often less than 1 week, but it can be 6 weeks or longer. Initial symptoms are nonspecific with fever, malaise, chest pain, and nonproductive cough. This may be followed by brief improvement and then severe respiratory distress, shock, and death. Widened mediastinum (associated with hemorrhagic mediastinitis) without parenchymal infiltrates found on radiographic imaging (computed tomography scan is most sensitive) is characteristic of inhalation anthrax. The diagnosis is often established with positive blood cultures that may initially be dismissed as contaminants.

Viruses account for an important number of pneumonias in adults, especially during the winter months and among the elderly. One recent study found that 18% of hospitalized CAP patients had a viral etiology. Influenza and respiratory syncytial virus (RSV) are the most commonly identified viral pathogens; others include parainflunza virus, rhinovirus, coronavirus, and possibly human metapneumovirus (although pneumonia is uncommon). Influenza should be considered during periods of peak activity within a community and is often associated with sudden fever, myalgias, and cough. RSV is a more common cause of pneumonia in immunocompetent adults than previously appreciated. Characteristics include seasonal occurrence (winter) and association of bronchospasm.

DIAGNOSIS

Laboratory tests used for the diagnosis of the etiologic agents associated with atypical pneumonia are listed in Table 30.2. In general, there is a lack of rapid, accessible, and accurate diagnostic tests for the most common causes, *C. pneumoniae* and *M. pneumoniae*. Rapid diagnostic tests and accessible culture methods are available for *Legionella* and influenza virus but must be specifically requested from the clinical microbiology lab because they are not routinely performed. Hopefully newer tests such as DNA amplification tests (ie, polymerase chain reaction), which are not yet available for rapid diagnosis in most settings, might become increasingly available in the future to provide a cost-effective and rapid means of diagnosis. Serologic tests are less valuable, given the requirement for measurement during acute and convalescent specimens (Table 30.2); however, this remains the most common means of laboratory diagnosis for most pathogens associated with atypical pneumonia.

ANTIMICROBIAL THERAPY

Antimicrobial agents generally considered effective for these atypical pathogens are included in Tables 30.1, 30.3, and 30.4. Because most cases of atypical pneumonia are treated empirically, clinicians also need to consider the possibility of other so-called standard pathogens (ie, *S. pneumoniae*, *H. influenzae*) when deciding on antimicrobial therapy.

Mycoplasma and *Chlamydophila*

Therapy of *Mycoplasma* and *Chlamydophila* has been the subject of some conjecture. A common view is that it really does not matter whether antibiotics are given for most of these

Table 30.2 Diagnostic Studies for Pathogens Associated with Atypical Pneumonia

Pathogen	Rapid Test	Standard Culture or Microbiologic Test(s)	Serology, Other Tests
M. pneumoniae	PCR [95][a,b]	Throat or NP swab [90] (requires 7–10 days for preliminary growth)	ELISA, CF[c] [75-80] (IgM may be present after 1 week but can persist 2–12 months) Diagnostic criteria: Definite: 4-fold titer rise Possible: IgG ≥ 1:64 (CF) IgM ≥ 1:16 (ELISA) Cold agglutinin [50] [less than 50% specificity; takes several weeks to develop]
C. pneumoniae	PCR[b] [80–90]	Throat or NP swab[d] [50–90]	MIF[c] (IgM may take up to 4–6 weeks to appear in primary infection) Diagnostic criteria: Definite: 4-fold titer rise Possible: IgG ≥ 1:512 IgM ≥ 1:32
Legionella pneumophila	Urine antigen[e] [60–70] PCR[b], DFA[f] [25–75]	Sputum, bronchoscopy [75–99] (selective media required, 2–6 days)	IFA[c] [40–75] Diagnostic criteria: Definite: 4-fold titer rise Possible: IgG or IgM ≥ 1:512 (titer of 1:256 has positive predictive value of only 15%)
C. psittaci	PCR[b]	Usually not done (considered laboratory hazard)	CF (presumptive IgG ≥ 1:32) MIF for IgM
Coxiella burnetii	PCR[b]	Usually not done (considered laboratory hazard)	ELISA, IFA, CF
Viruses Influenza	Antigen detection (EIA), DFA stain PCR	Virus isolation	CF or HAI
RSV	Antigen detection (EIA), DFA stain PCR	Virus isolation	ELISA
Adenovirus	DFA stain, PCR	Virus isolation	ELISA or RIA
Francisella tularensis		Culture (selective media)	ELISA preferred Passive hemagglutination
Yersinia pestis	Gram stain, morphology, gram-negative coccobacillus exhibiting bipolar staining ("safety pin"); PCR	Culture	Serology available
Bacillus anthracis (Inhalation Anthrax)	PCR	Culture (may be dismissed as *Bacillus* contaminant)	

[a] [] = % sensitivity of test. [b] Available in selected laboratories, reagents are not FDA cleared.
[c] Paired sera generally required. ELISA = enzyme-linked immunosorbent assay; CF = complement fixation; MIF = microimmunofluorescence; IFA = indirect fluorescence Ab.
[d] Rarely done, requires specialized culture techniques.
[e] Only for *L. pneumophila* serogroup 1 (≈ 60–70% of cases); can be positive for months.
[f] Direct fluorescence Ab; primarily for *L. pneumophila* serogroup one; some false positives with other species, technically demanding.

Table 30.3 Authors Recommendation for Antimicrobial Therapy of *M. pneumoniae* and *C. pneumoniae* (Adult Doses[a])

Antimicrobial	Dose	Duration (days)
Erythromycin[b]	500 mg QID	10–14
Clarithromycin (Biaxin)	500 mg BID	7–10
Azithromycin (Zithromax)[b]	500 mg initially then 250 mg QD (alternative 500 mg QD)	5 (3)
Dirithromycin (Dynabac)	500 mg QD	10–14
Telithromycin (Ketek)	800 mg QD	7
Tetracycline	500 mg QID	10–14
Doxycycline[b]	100 mg BID	7–10
Levofloxacin (Levaquin)[b]	500 mg QD / 750 mg QD	5–14[c] / 5
Moxifloxacin (Avelox)[b]	400 mg QD	5–14[c]
Gemifloxacin (Factive)	320 mg QD	5[c]

[a] Oral except where noted.
[b] Also can be administered intravenously in equivalent dose.
[c] See text.

Table 30.4 Parenteral Therapy for Serious *Legionella* Infections[a]

Preferred Antimicrobial	Alternative Antimicrobial
Fluoroquinolone	
Levofloxacin (Levaquin) 500 mg IV q24h (750 mg QD for 5 days possible for immunocompetent patients)	Erythromycin 1 g IV q6h +/– rifampin[b,c]
Moxifloxacin (Avelox) 400 mg IV q24h	Doxycycline (Vibramycin) 100 mg IV q12h +/– rifampin
Azithromycin (Zithromax) 500 mg IV q24h	

[a] Requiring hospitalization or in immunocompromised patients; can change to orally when clinically stable and can take orally.
[b] 300–600 mg IV q12h.
[c] Not FDA approved for this indication.

infections because the mortality is low, these infections are often self-limiting, there may be ambiguity of diagnosis (especially for *C. pneumoniae*), the confounding effects of copathogens, and a question of antimicrobial efficacy. However, there are data that indicate treatment (especially for *M. pneumoniae*) reduces the morbidity of pneumonia and shortens duration of symptoms.

Erythromycin and tetracyclines have been the old standbys in the treatment of *M. pneumoniae* infections and have been considered effective therapy according to the early reports of *C. pneumoniae* infections. From studies that have assessed the microbiologic efficacy against *M. pneumoniae* or *C. pneumoniae*, it is apparent that these pathogens may persist in respiratory secretions despite good clinical response to these agents. The new macrolides clarithromycin and azithromycin and the azalide telithromycin have good in vitro activity against these organisms and have shown good results in clinical studies. Although the clinical significance is uncertain, emergence of macrolide-resistant *M. pneumoniae* with a 23S rRNA gene mutation has been recently reported from Japan.

The newer fluoroquinolones (ie, levofloxacin, moxifloxacin, gemifloxacin) are bactericidal, are more active in vitro than ciprofloxacin, and have been shown to be effective in clinical trials.

Legionella

There is little debate concerning the need for therapy of *Legionella* pneumonia. Delay in instituting appropriate antimicrobial therapy for *Legionella* pneumonia significantly increases mortality. Therefore, empirical anti-*Legionella* therapy should be included in treatment of severe CAP. Erythromycin initially had been considered accepted as the treatment of choice for legionnaire's disease. However, intracellular models as well as animal models of *Legionella* infection indicate that the systemic fluoroquinolones and the newer macrolides (especially azithromycin) show superior activity compared with erythromycin. These newer agents have better pharmacokinetic properties: better bioavailability, longer half-life requiring fewer doses per day, better intracellular penetration into macrophages, and better tolerability. On the basis of greater activity in intracellular models and several observational studies, the quinolones may produce a superior clinical response compared with macrolides. The addition of rifampin to erythromycin has been suggested for patients who are severely ill; however, there are no convincing laboratory data to show that adding rifampin to fluoroquinolones or the more active macrolide therapy improves bacterial killing. Although uncontrolled clinical reports show that ciprofloxacin has effectively treated patients with LD, I prefer the newer fluoroquinolones because of greater activity in vitro against *S. pneumoniae* (including drug-resistant strains) and other common causes of CAP that need to be considered for empirical therapy. Doxycycline has also been shown to be effective in limited, well-documented cases. Recommendations for initial parenteral therapy are listed in Table 30.4. Oral therapy for less serious cases or for step-down from intravenous therapy includes the oral macrolides and fluoroquinolones as well as doxycycline.

The duration of therapy for optimal response of *C. pneumoniae* and *M. pneumoniae* has not been well established. In initial descriptions of *C. pneumoniae* pneumonia, observers found that respiratory symptoms frequently recurred or persisted after short courses (5 to 10 days) of erythromycin or tetracycline. In recent recommendations, the usual duration of therapy for *C. pneumoniae* or *M. pneumoniae* using more recently approved agents has been 7 to 10 days (shorter for azithromycin because of the longer half-life); however, recent studies (mostly with the fluoroquinolones) have suggested that a minimum of 5 days may be adequate for immunocompetent patients if the patient has had a good clinical response within 48 to 72 hours. Similarly, the usual duration of therapy for legionnaire's disease of immunocompetent adults has been 7 to 14 days; one recent study showed good efficacy of 750 mg every day of levofloxacin for 5 days. For therapy of immunocompromised patients or more severe disease, longer duration is recommended.

Therapy for Other Pathogens Associated with Atypical Pneumonia (See Table 30.1)

CHLAMYDOPHILA PSITTACI

The tetracyclines are generally considered the drugs of choice with the macrolides as appropriate alternatives (similar duration as for *C. pneumoniae*). The newer fluoroquinolones are active in vitro and in animal models but their efficacy for human infection is unknown.

COXIELLA BURNETII

The tetracyclines and macrolides are both considered effective (usually for 10 days). In one small prospective study, doxycycline was slightly more effective than erythromycin, but most cases were benign and self-limiting. Combination therapy (eg, doxycycline plus ciprofloxacin or rifampin) has been used for Q fever endocarditis.

FRANCISELLA TULARENSIS

No prospective controlled clinical trials have defined optimal antimicrobial therapy. The traditional choice of therapy for pneumonic tularemia is streptomycin (1 g every 12 hours if severely ill or 500 mg every 12 hours in milder disease) or gentamicin (3 to 5 mg/kg/day) for 7 to 14 days. Doxycycline (100 mg IV or orally BID) has often been used with good success, particularly in nonsevere pneumonia, and is easier to administer.

HANTAVIRUS PULMONARY SYNDROME

Treatment options are limited. The use of ribaviran has not been shown to be effective in one small study. Optimal cardiopulmonary and fluid management is critical for appropriate management.

YERSINIA PESTIS

Streptomycin (similar dose/day as for tularemia) is considered the drug of choice, with 10 days being the minimum recommended course of therapy. Alternatives include gentamicin, tetracycline, and chloramphenicol. Close contacts of patients with pneumonic plague should receive tetracycline (500 mg for times daily) or doxycycline (100 mg twice daily) for 5–7 days for prophylaxis.

INHALATION ANTHRAX

The mortality rate remains high if treatment is not initiated prior to the development of clinical symptoms. Penicillin intravenously in high doses has historically been the preferred therapy, but reports of resistance have been published so that many authorities now recommend ciprofloxacin (500 mg twice daily) as preferred empiric treatment prior to susceptibility tests. Because of possible resistance, recent recommendations for initial therapy of inhalation anthrax are to use a multidrug regimen that can be switched to monotherapy once the patient has stabilized and possible susceptibility test results are known (Table 30.1). Treatment should be continued for 60 days due to the potential problem of prolonged incubation with delayed, but lethal, disease. There is no known person to person transmission; however, if anthrax is a concern as an agent of bioterrorism, it is important to provide prophylaxis to the population at risk. The preferred regimens are ciprofloxacin (500 mg orally twice daily) or doxycycline (100 mg orally twice daily), depending on the the susceptibility of the epidemic strain. Prophylaxis should be continued for 60 days. Other fluoroquinolones are probably equally effective.

INFLUENZA

The impact of specific antiviral treatment on patients with influenza pneumonia is unclear. However, because such patients often have recoverable virus (median duration of 4 days) after hospitalization, antiviral treatment seems reasonable from an infection control standpoint alone. Because of its broad influenza spectrum, low risk of resistance emergence, and lack of bronchospasm risk, oseltamivir, a neuramidase inhibitor that is effective for both influenza A and B, is an appropriate choice. The M2 inhibitors amantadine and rimantadine are active only for influenza A. In addition, viruses recently circulating in the United States and Canada are often resistant to the M2 inhibitors based on antiviral testing. Therefore, neither amantadine nor rimantadine should be used for the treatment or chemoprophylaxis of influenza A in the United States until susceptibility to these antiviral medications has been reestablished among circulating influenza A viruses.

RSV

The routine use of ribavirin is not recommended for infants and children with RSV LRTI. Several authorities recommend therapy in selected infants and young children who are at high risk for serious RSV disease (ie, infants with congenital heart disease, lung disease, immunodeficiency or immunosuppressive therapy; infants who are severely ill with decreased PaO$_2$). The benefit of ribavirin therapy for healthy or immunocompromised adults has not been established.

SUGGESTED READING

Cunha BA. The atypical pneumonias: clinical diagnosis and importance. *Clin Microbiol Infect*. 2006;12 (suppl 3):12–24.

Dunbar LM, Khashab MM, Kahn JB et al. Efficacy of 750 mg, 5-day levofloxacin therapy in the treatment of community-acquired pneumonia caused by atypical pathogens. *Curr Med Res Opin*. 2004;20:555–563.

File TM Jr, Garau J, Blasi F, et al. Guidelines for empiric antimicrobial prescribing in community-acquired pneumonia. *Chest*. 2004; 125:1888.

File TM Jr, Tan JS, Plouffe JF Jr. The role of atypical pathogens: Mycoplasma pneumoniae, Chlamydia pneumoniae, and Legionella pneumophila in respiratory infection. *Infectious Dis Clin North Am*. 1998; 12:569–592.

Infectious Diseases Society of America and the American Thoracic Society. Consensus guidelines on the management of community-acquired pneumonia. *Clin Infect Dis*. 2007;44(Suppl 2):527–572.

Johnston SL, Martin RJ. Chlamydophila pneumoniae and Mycoplasma pneumoniae: a role in asthma pathogenesis? *Am J Resp Crit Care Med*. 2005;172:1078–1089.

Marrie TJ, Poulin-Costello M, Beecroft MD, Herman-Gnjidic Z. Etiology of community-acquired pneumonia treated in an ambulatory setting. *Resp Med*. 2005;99:60–65.

Mills GD, Oehley, MR, Arrol, B. Effectiveness of beta lactam antibiotics compared with antibiotics active against atypical pathogens in non-severe community acquired pneumonia: meta-analysis. *Br Med J*. 2005;330:456.

Morozumi M, Hasegawa K, Kobayashi R, et al. Emergence of macrolide-resistant Mycoplasma pneumoniae with a 23S rRNA gene mutation. *Antimicrob Agents Chemother*. 2005;49:3100.

Pedro-Botet L, Yu VL. Legionella: macrolides or quinolones? *Clin Microbiol Infect*. 2006;12(suppl 3):25–30.

Shefet D, Robenshtok E, Paul M, et al. Empirical atypical coverage for inpatients with community-acquired pneumonia: a systematic review of randomized controlled trials. *Arch Intern Med*. 2005;165:1992–2000.

Tan JS. The other causes of 'atypical' pneumonia. *Curr Opin Infect Dis*. 1999;12:121–126.

Templeton KE, Schelting SA, van den Eeden WC, et al. Improved diagnosis of the etiology of community-acquired pneumonia with real-time polymerase chain reaction. *Clin Infect Dis*. 2005;41:345–351.

31. Community-Acquired Pneumonia

Rebecca Edge Martin

Community-acquired pneumonia (CAP) is a significant cause of morbidity and mortality in the United States. Most episodes occur after the sixth decade of life in patients with one or more chronic underlying diseases. Mortality from CAP averages 14% and has not decreased significantly since the early 1950s, despite advances in antibiotic and intensive care therapy.

Making the diagnosis of pneumonia is usually not difficult; deciding which patients should be admitted to the hospital and selecting appropriate therapy, however, can be challenging. The purpose of this chapter is to assist the clinician in deciding which patients should be admitted to the hospital and in selecting antibiotic therapy for CAP in immunocompetent patients who are not residents of chronic care facilities.

DIAGNOSIS AND TREATMENT

The diagnosis of pneumonia is suspected when one or more of the following clinical findings are present: cough, purulent sputum, dyspnea, pleuritic pain, fever, leukocytosis, chest auscultation findings consistent with pneumonia, or a new pulmonary infiltrate. Once the diagnosis is made, the physician must decide whether hospitalization is necessary and, if hospitalized, whether intensive care unit (ICU) monitoring is advised.

A number of risk factors predict a complicated course (Table 31.1). Two published sets of criteria may assist the physician in deciding if hospitalization is necessary: the CURB-65 score from the British Thoracic Society and the Pneumonia Severity Index (PSI) from the Pneumonia Patient Outcomes Research Team (PORT). The PSI calculates risk by giving points to 19 variables based on age and comorbidities similar to those listed in Table 31.1. Patients are then assigned to one of five risk categories. Patients falling in risk groups I and II can be managed as outpatients, whereas risk groups III–V should be hospitalized. The modified CURB-65 criteria includes confusion, blood urea nitrogen (BUN) ($\geq$ 20 mg/dL), respiratory

Table 31.1 Predictors of a Complicated Course in Patients with Community-Acquired Pneumonia

Suspicion of high-risk cause (*Staphylococcus aureus*, gram-negative bacilli, aspiration, or postobstructive process)
Age > 50 years
Prior episode of pneumonia
Consolidation, multilobe involvement, or pleural effusion on chest radiograph
Abnormalities on physical examination: 　Temperature ≤ 95°F (35°C) or >104°F (40°C) 　Systolic or diastolic blood pressures ≤90 mm Hg or ≤60 mm Hg, respectively 　Respiratory rate ≥30 breaths/minute 　Heart rate >125 beats/minute 　Extrapulmonary areas of infection
Laboratory factors 　Abnormal renal function (BUN >20 mg/dl or serum creatinine >1.2 mg/dL) 　Sodium ≤130 mg/dL 　Glucose ≥250 mg/dL 　Hematocrit ≤30% 　WBC count ≤4000/mm³ or >30,000/mm³ 　Metabolic acidosis (pH ≤7.35) 　PaO₂ ≤60 mm Hg breathing room air
Comorbid conditions 　Renal insufficiency 　Congestive heart failure 　Liver disease 　Diabetes mellitus 　Altered mental state 　Neurologic disease 　Alcoholism 　Immunosuppression 　Malignancy 　Splenectomy
No responsible person in the home to assist the patient
Abbreviations: BUN = Blood urea nitrogen; WBC = white blood cell.

rate ($\geq$ 30 breaths/ minute), blood pressure (systolic ≤90 mm Hg or diastolic ≤60), and age ≥65 years. Patients with 0–1 of these findings can be managed as outpatients. Those with a score of 2 should be admitted to a hospital ward, whereas those with 3 or more should be cared

Table 31.2 Relevant Clinical History Related to Specific Pathogens

Anaerobes (oral)	Alcoholism, aspiration, lung abscess, recent dental work, endobronchial obstruction
Bordetella pertussis	Cough ≥2 weeks with whoop or vomiting after cough
Burkholderia cepacia	Bronchiectasis
Chlamydia pneumoniae	COPD, smokers, biphasic illness
Chlamydia psittaci	Bird exposure
Coccidioides immitis	Travel to Southwest United States
Coxiella burnetti	Farm animal or pregnant cat exposure, hepatosplenomegaly
Francisella tularensis	Exposure to wild mammals, esp. rabbits and ticks in endemic areas
Haemophilus influenzae	COPD, smokers, HIV, postinfluenza
Hantavirus pulmonary syndrome	Pulmonary edema, hemoconcentration, thrombocytopenia esp. after travel to Southwest United States
Histoplasmosis capsulatum	Bat or bird droppings, cave exploration
Influenza	Seasonal outbreak. Travel to or residence in Asia: avian influenza
Klebsiella pneumoniae	Alcoholics
Legionella species	Hotel or cruise ship
Moraxella catarrhalis	COPD, smokers
Mycobacterium tuberculosis	Alcoholics, HIV, elderly, injection drug use
Mycoplasma pneumoniae	Prominent cough, hyperreactive airways, hemolytic anemia
Pneumocystis jiroveci	HIV
Pseudomonas aeruginosa	COPD, bronchiectasis
SARS	Travel to or residence in Asia or with outbreak in other countries
Staphylococcus aureus	Postinfluenza, endobronchial obstruction, injection drug use
Streptococcus pneumoniae	Most common through all age groups, alcoholics, postinfluenza

[a] *Bacillus antracis*, (anthrax), *Yersinia pestis* (plague), and *Francisella tularensis* (tularemia) would be the most likely bacterial bioterrorism agents to cause pneumonia.
Adapted from Infectious Diseases Society of America and American Ihoracic Society Consensus Guidelines 2007.

for in an ICU. The CURB-65 is less cumbersome and easier to use in the outpatient setting. The PSI, which has been studied more extensively, perhaps gives a more accurate prediction of which patients can be safely managed outside the hospital. These risk stratification guides are helpful, but in the final analysis, the clinician's assessment and instinct must be the ultimate decision-making tool.

The exact microbial cause of an episode of CAP is rarely known when antibiotics are started. Accurate historical information, including occupation; travel; exposure to animals, birds, and insects; recent dental work; and history of alcohol or drug abuse may suggest a cause (Table 31.2). Anaerobic infection is often accompanied by foul-smelling sputum and a history of seizure disorder or alcoholism. Hantavirus pulmonary syndrome (HPS), which has been reported in most areas of the United States, is usually associated with fever, myalgia, and subsequent pulmonary edema, hemoconcentration, thrombocytopenia, and leukocytosis. There are, however, no unique clinical features of any pathogen that allow a specific identification by history alone. Human immunodeficiency virus (HIV) disease should be a diagnostic consideration in most patients hospitalized with CAP and HIV serology should be obtained.

The laboratory studies found in Tables 31.3 and 31.4 may be useful in the diagnosis

Table 31.3 Routine Studies Useful in the Diagnosis and Management of Patients Hospitalized with Community-Acquired Pneumonia

Chest radiograph (posterior and lateral)
Arterial blood gas values (for hospitalized patients. Pulse oximetry should be obtained for patients judged suitable for outpatient therapy.)
Complete blood count with differential
Chemistry panel, including electrolytes, glucose, blood urea nitrogen, and creatinine
Aminotransferases
Blood culture (2 sets drawn 10 minutes or more apart) Not necessary for all patients. See Table 31.4.
Pleural fluid stain, culture, leukocyte count with differential, pH

Sputum studies (for pneumonia unresponsive to usual antibiotics, see Table 31.4):
    Acid-fast stain and culture
    Fungal stains and culture
    Legionella spp. culture
    Immunofluorescent antibody, Gomori's methanamine silver, or Giemsa stain for *Pneumocystis jirovecii* (formerly *Pneumocystis carinii*)
    A Gram stain (from an appropriately obtained specimen, examined by an expert within 2 h of collection before the patient has received antibiotics)

Urinary antigen
    Streptococcus pneumoniae
    Legionella spp.

Serology (for patients with appropriate epidemiological history)
    HIV serology
    Legionella spp.
    Francisella tularensis
    Mycoplasma pneumoniae
    Chlamydia (pneumoniae and psittacosis) spp.
    Coxiella burnetii

Abbreviation: HIV = human immunodeficiency virus.

and management of CAP. The extent of the evaluation should depend on the severity of illness and the likelihood that test results will influence therapy. Diagnostic studies are usually unnecessary for the patient who is to be treated on an outpatient basis because empiric antimicrobial choices are adequate. Hospitalized patients should have, at a minimum, routine laboratory studies that include a complete blood count with differential, a chest radiograph, and arterial blood gases. Many other common diagnostic methods are expensive and technically difficult to perform. Blood cultures are diagnostic in up to 14% of patients hospitalized for CAP. They are most useful in patients with severe CAP and need not be obtained in all patients hospitalized (see Table 31.4). The value of the Gram stain and culture of expectorated sputum is controversial. They are most useful in patients with severe CAP (Table 31.4) and are not necessary in all hospitalized patients. The sputum specimen should be grossly purulent, obtained by deep cough (or tracheal aspirate), and processed in less than 2 hours. Minimum criteria for a specimen suitable for culture are fewer than 10 squamous epithelial cells or more than 25 polymorphonuclear neutrophils (PMNs) per low-power field. Timely and correct processing of sputum is a challenge in most clinical settings.

Sputum studies can be diagnostic for disease caused by *Legionella* species, mycobacteria, fungi, influenza, respiratory syncytial virus, and *Pneumocystis jiroveci,* formerly *Pneumocystis carinii* (see Table 31.3). A parapneumonic pleural effusion is a common complication of pneumonia, and cultures of the fluid will often give a positive result. The incidence of pleural effusion accompanying pneumonia depends on the etiologic agent. Effusions accompany *Streptococcus pyogenes* infections around 95% of the time but accompany only 10% of *Streptococcus pneumoniae* infections. Bronchial alveolar lavage may be useful but should not be relied on to determine a bacterial agent. Protected brush specimens obtained by bronchoscopy are more accurate than expectorated sputum. The gold standards of transthoracic needle aspiration and open lung biopsy are definitive when an organism is found, but they place the patient at added risk.

Urinary antigens (UAT) may be useful in the diagnosis of severe *Legionella* spp. and *S. pneumoniae* infections. Both tests have a greater than 90% specificity. The *S. pneumoniae* UAT may yield a diagnosis even after antibiotics have been started. The *Legionella* UAT detects only serogroup I, which is responsible for most cases of community-acquired legionnaire's disease in the United States. Further studies are needed to demonstrate whether a positive *Legionella* UAT in a patient with CAP will allow the antibiotic regimen to be narrowed to a macrolide alone without increase in morbidity or mortality. Serologic studies may aid in diagnosis but rarely in antibiotic choice. A 4-fold rise in serologic titer is necessary for confirmation, and an appropriate serologic response will often take several weeks. Cross-reactivity among some organisms lessens the specificity of serology. A definitive microbial cause can be identified in patients only 50% of the time, even after extensive testing.

Table 31.4 Clinical Indications for More Extensive Diagnostic Testing[a]

Indication	Blood Culture	Sputum Culture[b]	*Legionella* UAT	Pneumococcal UAT
ICU admission	X	X	X	X
Failure of outpatient antibiotic therapy		X	X	X
Cavitary infiltrates	X	X[c]		
Leukopenia	X			X
Active alcohol use	X	X	X	X
Chronic severe liver disease	X			X
Severe obstructive/structural lung disease		X		
Asplenia (anatomic or functional)	X			X
Recent travel (within 2 weeks)			X	
Positive *Legionella* UAT result		X[d]	NA	
Positive pneumococcal UAT result	X	X		NA
Pleural effusion	X	X	X	X

Abbreviations: NA = not applicable; UAT = urinary antigen test.
[a] Adapted from Table 5, IDSA/ATS Consensus Guidelines.
[b] A Gram stain should be obtained as well.
[c] Fungal, tuberculosis and bacterial cultures.
[d] Special media for *Legionella*.

RECOMMENDATION FOR EMPIRIC SELECTION OF ANTIMICROBIAL AGENTS

Because a definitive pathogen usually will not have been identified when therapy for pneumonia must be started, empiric selection of antimicrobials is necessary. Selection of appropriate antibiotics may be facilitated by categorizing patients according to age and severity of illness, taking into consideration any comorbidities and epidemiologic factors present. Some microbes cause disease in all ages and types of patients; others are common only in patients with certain comorbidities. Tables 31.5 to 31.8 list these categories of patients along with common pathogens and appropriate antibiotic therapy.

Among patients with mild pneumonia not requiring hospitalization (see Table 31.5), *S. pneumoniae* is the most common bacterial pathogen. The atypical pneumonias (*Mycoplasma pneumoniae* and *Chlamydia pneumoniae*) are common in this group as well. Atypical pneumonia generally is benign, with systemic complaints often more prominent than respiratory ones. Fever, headache, and myalgia are common. Leukocytosis is rare, and chest

Table 31.5 Guidelines for Empiric Antibiotic Therapy for Community-Acquired Pneumonia in Outpatients Younger than 50 Years with No Comorbid Illness

Common Pathogens
Streptococcus pneumoniae
Mycoplasma pneumoniae
Chlamydia pneumoniae
Respiratory viruses
Antibiotics

Erythromycin, 500 mg PO QID, or
     Azithromycin, 500 mg PO day 1, then 250 mg daily
     Clarithromycin, 250 mg PO BID

If macrolide intolerant: Doxycycline 100 mg PO BID

[a] If > 25% *S. pneumoniae* macrolide resistant [MIC ≥16 µg/mL] in a community: levofloxacin 750 mg PO daily, or moxifloxacin 400 mg PO daily.

infiltrates consist primarily of segmental lower lobe or hilar infiltrates. Although *M. pneumoniae* is more common among patients younger than 30 years of age, it is recognized with increasing

Table 31.6 Guidelines for Empiric Antibiotic Therapy for Community-Acquired Pneumonia in Patients Older than 50 Years or with Comorbid Illness Not Requiring Hospitalization

Common Pathogens
Streptococcus pneumoniae
Legionella spp.
Haemophilus influenzae
Moraxella catarrhalis
Other gram-negative bacilli
Respiratory viruses

Antibiotics

Fluoroquinolone as a single agent
  Levofloxacin 750 mg PO daily
  Moxifloxacin 400 mg PO daily

or

Macrolide[a]
  Azithromycin, 500 mg PO day 1, then 250 daily
  Clarithromycin, 250 mg BID

and

β-lactam
  Amoxycillin 1 gram 3 times daily
  Amoxycillin-clavulanate 2 grams BID
  Ceftriaxone, cefpodoxime, cefuroxime

[a] Doxycycline 100 mg BID may be substituted in macrolide-intolerant patients.

Table 31.7 Guidelines for Empiric Antibiotic Therapy for Community-Acquired Pneumonia in Patients Requiring Hospitalization (Not Intensive Care)

Common Pathogens
Streptococcus pneumoniae
Mycoplasma pneumoniae
Chlamydia pneumoniae
Haemophilus influenzae
Legionella spp.
Aspiration
Respiratory viruses

Antibiotics

Fluoroquinolone[a]
  Levofloxacin 750 mg IV/PO daily
  Moxifloxacin 400 mg IV/PO daily

or

Macrolide[b]
  Azithromycin, 500 mg PO day 1, then 250 daily
  Clarithromycin, 250 mg BID

and
β-lactam   Cefotaxime, ceftriaxone, ampicillin, ertapenem

[a] Second regimen should be substituted if fluoroquinolones have been used in the previous 3 months.
[b] Doxycycline 100 mg BID may be substituted in macrolide-intolerant patients.

frequency in older persons. *M. pneumoniae* is characterized by a prominent cough, often occurs in slowly evolving epidemics, and can precipitate reactive airway disease, especially in children. *C. pneumoniae* is a common cause of mild, often biphasic illness. Upper respiratory symptoms and pharyngitis predominate initially. After recovery, pneumonia may develop 2 or 3 weeks later. Reinfection is common. Macrolides (eg, erythromycin, azithromycin, and clarithromycin) are the drugs of choice for treating outpatient pneumonia in low-risk patients. Doxycycline should be used for those who are macrolide intolerant.

Patients who are older than 50 years of age or have comorbid illnesses (see Table 31.6) are more likely to require hospitalization. Some can be managed as outpatients but will require frequent follow-up visits. Gram-negative organisms, such as *Haemophilus influenzae* and *Moraxella catarrhalis,* are more common in this group, particularly in persons who smoke or have chronic obstructive pulmonary disease. A

respiratory fluoroquinolone, such as levofloxacin or moxifloxacin, is the drug of choice for this group of patients. If the patient has been treated with a fluoroquinolone in the previous 3 months or has an allergy to them, then azithromycin or clarithromycin plus a β-lactam should be given.

Patients admitted to the hospital with pneumonia of moderate severity require empiric therapy to cover the organisms listed in Table 31.7. Recent guidelines from the Infectious Diseases Society of America (IDSA) and American Thoracic Society (ATS) recommend that the first antibiotic dose be given in the emergency department.

Empiric antimicrobial therapy should include either a respiratory fluoroquinolone alone or a macrolide (azithromycin or clarithromycin) combined with a β-lactam. If fluoroquinolones have been used in the previous 3 months, the second regimen, which omits a fluoroquinolone, is preferred. Ertapenem is as efficacious

Table 31.8 Guidelines for Empiric Antibiotic Therapy for Community-Acquired Pneumonia in Patients Requiring Intensive Care Hospitalization

Common Pathogens
Streptococcus pneumoniae
Legionella spp.
Staphylococcus aureus[a]
Haemophilus influenzae
Pseudomonas aeruginosa
Enterobacteriacae spp.
Gram-negative bacilli
Aspiration
Respiratory viruses
Antibiotics[a]
β-lactam[b]   Ceftriaxone, cefotaxime, or ampicillin-sulbactam
and
Azithromycin or respiratory fluoroquinolone

[a] If *S. aureus* infection is suspected, either vancomycin or linezolid should be added to above regimen.
[b] If *P. aeruginosa* is a likely organism, an antipseudomonal β-lactam (piperacillin-tazobactam, cefepime, imipenem, or meropenem) should be substituted for the β-lactams listed above. Either ciprofloxacin or levofloxacin should accompany the antipseudomonal β-lactam or the combination of an aminoglycoside with azithromycin.

as ceftriaxone but has not been as extensively studied. It is useful when a more broad spectrum agent is necessary to cover anaerobes and gram-negative organisms; it is not, however, active against *Pseudomonas aeruginosa*. When the etiologic agent and its sensitivity are known, the antibiotic regimen should be as narrow and as cost-effective as possible.

The importance of subdividing hospital admissions for pneumonia into moderate and severe illness lies in the recognition of increased mortality in patients with severe pneumonia, especially during the first 7 days. Mortality ranges from 50% to 70% in some studies. Severe pneumonia manifests as hypoxia, tachypnea, multilobe involvement or consolidation, and signs of septic shock. These patients should be managed in an ICU. Organisms listed in Table 31.8 may cause more severe disease, although the severity of the pneumonia and ultimate outcome is more a function of the immune response of the host. Initial antimicrobial

therapy should include either a macrolide or fluoroquinolone plus a β-lactam. Persons requiring ICU monitoring should have blood cultures drawn and sputum studies for Gram stain and culture. Although the organisms seen on a sputum Gram stain may not be the actual bacterial cause of the pneumonia, empiric antibiotic choices should take into account what is found on the Gram stain. Gram-positive cocci in clusters should alert the physician to possible *Staphylococcus aureus* pneumonia. *S. aureus* pneumonia is most often seen as a complication of influenza. Methicillin-resistant *S. aureus* is now commonly found in the community and, if associated with the Panton-Valentine leukocidin toxin, can produce severe necrotizing pneumonia. For persons admitted to the ICU with severe pneumonia and clusters of gram-positive cocci in the sputum or cavitary lesions in the lung, initial therapy should include either vancomycin or linezolid. Linezolid has the advantage of decreasing toxin production. When a patient admitted to the ICU has severe structural defects of the lung (COPD or bronchiectasis) and gram-negative organisms are seen in the sputum, initial antibiotics should have activity against *P. aeruginosa* (see Table 31.8).

A few other organisms deserve special mention. Although rare in most of the United States, tularemic pneumonia should be considered in endemic areas among patients with exposure to wild mammals, especially rabbits, and exposure to ticks. Intravenous gentamicin should be given to a hospitalized patient when tularemic pneumonia is in the differential. *Coxiella burnetii* causes an atypical pneumonia often accompanied by hepatosplenomegaly. It is endemic in many hot, dry areas such as southern Texas. The most common reservoirs are sheep, goats, cattle, and ticks. Tetracycline or doxycycline is the recommended therapy. *Chlamydia psittaci* is another atypical pneumonia that should be considered in patients with exposure to infected birds, especially parrots. Splenomegaly in conjunction with an atypical pneumonia suggests psittacosis. Again, the drug of choice is tetracycline or doxycycline. *Mycobacterium tuberculosis* should be considered early in the differential diagnosis of pneumonia not responding to usual antibiotics. Endemic fungal infections, such as blastomycosis, histoplasmosis, cryptococcocosis, and coccidioidomycosis, may also present as a CAP.

Viruses are responsible for up to one-third of the cases of CAP. The viruses most commonly associated are influenza, rhinoviruses, coronaviruses, and parainfluenza. Human metapneumovirus (hMPV) is a recently discovered virus from the family Paramyxoviridae. It most commonly occurs in late winter or early spring in young children and in adults over the age of 65 years. Symptoms range from mild disease to severe pneumonia, and hMPV may be responsible for an exacerbation of asthma. Respiratory syncytial virus (RSV) can also cause pneumonia in adults, particularly those who are immunocompromised. Severe acute respiratory syndrome (SARS), which was first identified in the spring of 2003, is caused by a coronavirus. It manifests as a biphasic illness with fever, myalgia, chills, and headache. Up to 20% of the patients diagnosed with SARS have a diarrheal illness as well. Leukopenia, thrombocytopenia, elevated LDH, creatine kinase, and aminotransferases are commonly seen. SARS should be considered in a patient with a respiratory illness who has traveled to a country with recently documented SARS cases or in a patient with known exposure to a patient with SARS, and strict respiratory isolation should be instituted. Treatment for all these viruses, except for RSV and influenza, is supportive. Early use of inhaled ribavirin in bone marrow transplant patients with RSV may reduce morbidity and mortality. If given within the first 48 hours, neuraminidase inhibitors may be effective in lowering the complications seen with influenza and the spread of influenza to other patients. Oseltamivir is the recommended drug for hospitalized patients because it is less likely to acquire resistance and to cause bronchospasm. Amantidine and rimantidine are not recommended because of widespread resistance.

THERAPEUTIC RESPONSE

As a rule, antibiotic choices should not be altered during the first few days of therapy unless there is marked deterioration or cultures indicate the need for a change. Usually 48 to 72 hours are required for significant clinical improvement. Fever usually lasts 2 to 4 days but may last longer, especially if bacteremia accompanies the pneumonia. The white blood cell count generally returns toward normal after 4 days, and blood cultures become negative 24 to 48 hours after treatment is begun. Dur-ation of therapy should be individualized according to the infecting organism and overall health of the patient. Generally, treatment of bacterial pneumonia requires 7 to 10 days of antibiotics, whereas atypical pneumonia requires a longer period, ranging up to 21 days. Patients should receive a minimum of 5 days of antibiotic therapy for CAP. Because of its long tissue half-life, azithromycin may be given for a shorter duration. Patients with pneumonia caused by *S. pneumonia* should usually receive antibiotic therapy for 72 hours after the resolution of fever. Bacteremic patients will require a 10- to 14-day course of treatment. Immunocompromised patients usually require 21 days of treatment. When the patient is hemodynamically stable and improving clinically, oral antimicrobials should be considered, assuming the patient has adequate absorption. It is not necessary that the patient be afebrile, but the fever curve should be trending down.

Resolution of abnormal radiographic findings usually lags behind clinical improvement. It is slower in elderly patients, smokers, and those with comorbidities or multilobe involvement. Multiple chest radiographs in the hospital are unnecessary except for intubated patents and those with clinical deterioration. Patients who are older than 40 years of age or are smokers should be followed until complete radiographic resolution of the infiltrate is demonstrated. Follow-up chest radiographs should be obtained between 7 and 12 weeks after completion of therapy. If abnormalities have not resolved or greatly improved, the possibility of an occult neoplasm should be considered.

There are a number of reasons for failure in the treatment of CAP. The serum level of the chosen antibiotics may not be high enough. Correct dosage and route of administration should be reevaluated when the patient does not respond appropriately. Some antibiotics, such as the aminoglycosides, may not achieve high enough concentrations in the lung tissue. The etiologic agent may be resistant to the antibiotics, or less likely, the organism may develop resistance during therapy. An initial response followed by recurrent fever may be due to thrombophlebitis at the intravenous infusion site, an emerging empyema, or drug fever. In addition, lack of clinical improvement should raise the suspicion of a cause other than routine bacteria, such as viruses, mycobacteria, fungi, or parasites. Clinicians must always keep in mind the possibility of a noninfectious illness that mimics pneumonia, such as pulmonary infarction carcinoma, pulmonary edema, atelectasis, sarcoidosis, hypersensitivity pneumonitis, and drug-induced pulmonary disease.

SUGGESTED READING

Bates JH, Campbell GD, Barron AL, et al. Microbial etiology of acute pneumonia in hospitalized patients. *Chest.* 1992;101: 1005–1012.

Bartlett JG. Diagnostic test for etiologic agents of community-acquired pneumonia. *Infect Dis Clin North Am.* 2004;18:809–827.

Bartlett JG, Mundy L. Community-acquired pneumonia. *N Engl J Med.* 1995;333: 1618–1624.

British Thoracic Society Research Committee. Community-acquired pneumonia in adults in British hospitals in 1982–1983: a survey of aetiology, mortality, prognostic factors and outcome. *Q J Med.* 1987;62: 195–220.

Fine MJ, Auble TE, Yealy DM et al. A prediction rule to identify low-risk patients with community-acquired pneumonia. *N Engl J Med.* 1997;336:243–250.

Fine MJ, Smith MA, Carson CA et al. Prognosis and outcomes of patients with community-acquired pneumonia. A meta-analysis. *JAMA.* 1996;275(2):134–141.

Lim WS, van der Eerden MM, Laing R, et al. Defining community-acquired pneumonia severity on presentation to hospital: an international derivation and validation study. *Thorax* 2003;58:377–382.

Mandell LA, Wunderink RG, Anzueto A. et al: Infectious Diseases Society of America/ American Thoracic Society consensus guidelines on the management of community-acquired pneumonia in adults. *Clin Infect Dis* 2007;44(suppl 2):S27–S72.

Micek ST, Dunne ST, Kollef MH, et al. Pleuropulmonary complications of Panton-Valentine leukocidin-positive community-acquired methicillin-resistant *Staphylococcus aureus*: importance of treatment with antimicrobials inhibiting exotoxin production. *Chest.* 2005;128:2732.

32. Nosocomial Pneumonia

Burke A. Cunha

INTRODUCTION

Nosocomial pneumonia (NP) may be defined as a pneumonia that occurs in the hospital. Nosocomial pneumonia is synonymous with hospital-acquired pneumonia (HAP). There is a subset of NP and HAP of patients who are on ventilators, and this subset of patients are referred to as ventilator-associated pneumonias (VAP). NP/HAP may be considered as early NP/HAP, ie, occurring ≤5 days after hospital admission, or as late NP/HAP occurring ≥5 days after hospital admission. There is little clinical rationale for this distinction except that it can skew the data in studies and affect mortality outcomes and initial empiric therapy that differ between the "early" and "late" NP/HAP. "Early" NP/HAP really represents incubating community-acquired pneumonia (CAP) that has become clinically manifest within 5 days of admission to the hospital. Therefore, the organisms in the early NP/HAP group are really CAP pathogens, predominantly *Streptococcus pneumoniae*. In the traditional group of NP/HAP, ie, the late-onset NP/HAP, the organisms are reflective of the aerobic gram-negative bacillary flora of the hospital. Because early NP/HAP is really CAP manifesting in the hospital, henceforth it will be termed *late onset* NP/HAP. The most important, albeit not the most frequent, pathogen in the NP/HAP group is *Pseudomonas aeruginosa*. Other gram-negative bacilli are also major pathogens in NP/HAP, eg, *Klebsiella pneumoniae* and *Serratia marcescens*.

RESPIRATORY SECRETION COLONIZATION VERSUS NOSOCOMIAL PNEUMONIAS

Particularly in VAP, the secretions of intubated patients rapidly become colonized due to several factors. Being in the intensive care setting over time predisposes to colonization by the aerobic gram-negative bacilli (GNB) of the intensive care unit (ICU). Empiric antimicrobial therapy with some agents selected GNBs to colonize the patient's body fluids. Antimicrobial therapy, if not carefully chosen, can increase colonization of respiratory secretions not only with GNB but also with *Staphylococcus aureus*, either methicillin-sensitive *S. aureus* (MSSA) or methicillin-resistant *S. aureus* (MRSA). Relatively avirulent organisms that are predominantly colonizers of respiratory secretions, rarely ever cause NP/HAP, ie, *Enterobacter* species, *Citrobacter freundii*, *Burkholderia cepacia*, *Stenotrophomonas maltophilia*. These organisms recovered from respiratory secretions in ventilated patients should be considered as "colonizers" and ordinarily should not be treated with antibiotics (Table 32.1). More difficult to evaluate is the presence in respiratory secretions in ventilator patients of organisms that are predominantly colonizers but are virulent and have the pathogenic potential to cause invasive disease. Organisms that are predominantly colonizers but occasionally are pathogens in NP/HAP include *P. aeruginosa*, *Acinetobacter baumannii*, and *K. pneumoniae*. *Acinetobacter baumannii* NP/HAP, like *Legionella* NP/HAP, typically occurs in clusters originating as part of a common source outbreak and does not present as isolated cases. Similarly, gram-positive organisms that are relatively virulent and rarely, if ever, associated with pneumonia are enterococci. *Staphylococcus aureus*, either MSSA/MRSA, commonly colonizes respiratory secretions, but is a rare cause of NP/HAP/VAP. The majority of *S. aureus* pneumonias found in the ICU are postviral influenza CAPs. Literature based on National Nosocomial Infections Surveillance system (NNIS) data is misleading and greatly exaggerates the true incidence of MSSA/MRSA NP/HAP/VAP (Table 32.2).

DIAGNOSIS OF *S. AUREUS* AND *P. AERUGINOSA* PNEUMONIA

The definitive diagnosis of NP/HAP/VAP is difficult without invasive diagnostic tests. Patients are often regarded as having NP/HAP/VAP if the patient has fever, leukocytosis, and pulmonary infiltrates compatible with bacterial pneumonia. Obviously, there are many non-infectious disease disorders that present with the same clinical syndrome complex that

Table 32.1 Nosocomial Respiratory Colonizers and Pathogens

Common Colonizers of Respiratory Secretions	Respiratory Pathogens in Nosocomial Pneumonias
Common	**Common**
Pseudomonas aeruginosa	*Pseudomonas aeruginosa*
Enterobacter species	*Klebsiella pneumoniae*
Stenotrophomonas	*Serratia marcescens*
(*Xanthomonas*) *maltophilia*	*Escherichia coli*
Burkholderia (*Pseudomonas*) *cepacia*	
Citrobacter freundii	
Acinetobacter baumannii [a]	
Staphylococcus aureus	**Uncommon**
(MSSA/MRSA)	*Acinetobacter* [a]
	Legionella
	Staphylococcus aureus
	(MSSA/MRSA)

[a] Cause of nosocomial pneumonia usually as part of an outbreak.
Abbreviations: MRSA = methicillin-resistant Staphylococcus aureus
MSSA = methicillin-susceptible Staphylococcus aureus

Table 32.2 Epidemiologic Diagnosis of Nosocomial Pneumonia

Appearance of New Pulmonary Infiltrates >5 Days In Hospital with:
Fever > 101°F
Leukocytosis ± left shift
Pulmonary infiltrates *consistent* with bacterial pneumonia

mimic NP/HAP/VAP but are clearly not diagnostic of pneumonia. *P. aeruginosa* and *S. aureus* in particular have readily recognizable clinical presentations. When either of these two organisms is responsible for pneumonia (ie, CAP, NP/HAP or VAP), such patients rapidly become critically ill with high spiking fevers accompanied by cyanosis and rapid cavitation on the chest x-ray within 72 hours after the initial appearance of the infiltrate. Both *P. aeruginosa* and *S. aureus,* when causing lung infection, present as a fulminant necrotizing pneumonia, which is nearly often fatal. Such patients may or may not have *P. aeruginosa* or MSSA/MRSA in their respiratory secretions. Aside from lung biopsy or autopsy proven diagnosis of *P. aeruginosa* or *S. aureus* pneumonia, the clinical presentation reflects the underlying pathology rather than epidemiological data. NNIS data indicates the prevalence of MSSA/MRSA is as high as 25% in respiratory secretions which is inconsistent

with the clinical presentation and mortality data. Because *S. aureus* CAP or NP/HAP/VAP remains rare. If the clinical presentation is discordant with the clinical manifestations of the organism recovered from respiratory secretions, the pulmonary infiltrates should not be ascribed to either *P. aeruginosa* or *S. aureus*. NP/HAP/VAP. *Pseudomonas aeruginosa* and *S. aureus,* common colonizers of respiratory secretions, may cause tracheobronchitis that should be treated.

SELECTION OF OPTIMAL EMPIRIC MONOTHERAPY FOR NOSOCOMIAL PNEUMONIA

Because of the difficulty in clinically diagnosing NP/HAP/VAP, necessarily a certain level of over treatment must be accepted until there are better methods available to accurately diagnose NP/HAP/VAP. Because we must accept a certain degree of overtreatment due to misdiagnosis, the clinician should try to use antibiotics as selectively as possible and for the shortest duration of time. Most importantly, the antibiotics selected for empiric treatment of NP/HAP/VAP should, in addition to the appropriate spectrum, have a "low resistance" potential to prevent the emergence of multidrug-resistant (MDR) GNBs or the selecting out of *S. aureus* in the patient's respiratory flora. Antibiotics that are most likely to result in the emergence of MDR GNBs are ceftazidime, imipenem, and ciprofloxacin. In addition, ceftazidime and ciprofloxacin are likely to select out MSSA/MRSA as colonizers in the patient's respiratory secretions, particularly in ventilated patients. Agents with the appropriate spectrum for NP/HAP/VAP (ie, with a high degree of anti-*P. aeruginosa*) activity include meropenem, piperacillin, tazobactam, or cefepime. Meropenem is optimal monotherapy for NP/HAP/VAP because of its high degree of antipseudomonal and its minimal or no resistance potential, even if used for extended periods of time. None of meropenem, levofloxacin, or piperacillin/tazobactam predispose to *Clostridium difficile* diarrhea/colitis. Meropenem may be safely used in the penicillin-allergic patient. Meropenem is a carbapenem and not a β-lactam and there is no cross reactivity with penicillin-allergic patients and may be safely used in patients who have had penicillin anaphylactic reactions (Table 32.3).

It has been shown that well-selected monotherapy is optimal treatment for NP/HAP/VAP. There is no advantage in double drug therapy.

Table 32.3 Factors in Antibiotic Selection of Empiric Therapy for Nosocomial Pneumonia

Important Factors
High degree of activity against *Pseudomonas aeruginosa*
Penetrates lung parenchyma in therapeutic concentrations
"Low resistance" potential
Good safety profile 　　No ↑ resistance activity aerobic gram-negative bacilli 　　No ↑ prevalence of MSSA/MRSA 　　No ↑ prevalence of VRE 　　No ↑ *C. difficile* diarrhea/colitis
Relatively modest cost
Nonimportant Factors
Anti-MSSA/MRSA activity
Penetration into epithelial lung/fluid, alveolar macrophages (unless due to *Legionella*)
Abbreviations: MSSA = methicillin-susceptible *Staphylococcus aureus* MRSA = methicillin-resistant *Staphylococcus aureus*

Table 32.4 Empiric Therapy of Nosocomial Pneumonia

Non-Multidrug-Resistant Gram-Negative Nosocomial Pneumonia
Preferred Therapy
Meropenem 1 g (IV) q8h × 2 weeks Piperacillin/tazobactam 4.5 g (IV) q6h + amikacin 1 g (IV) q24h × 2 weeks Levofloxacin 750 mg (IV) q24h × 2 weeks Cefepime 2 g (IV) q8h ± amikacin 1 g (IV) q24h × 2 weeks
MDR Gram-Negative Nosocomial Pneumonia **MDR *Klebsiella Pneumoniae***
Tigecycline 100 mg (IV) x 1 dose, then 50 mg (IV) q12h × 2 weeks Colistin 1.7 mg/kg (IV) q8h x 2 weeks ± rifampin 600 mg (IV) q24h × 2 weeks Polymyxin B 1.25 mg/kg (IV) q12h × 2 weeks
MDR *Acinetobacter Baumannii*
Tigecycline 100 mg (IV) x 1 dose, then 50 mg (IV) q12h × 2 weeks Ampicillin/sulbactam 3 g (IV) q6h × 2 weeks Colistin 1.7 mg/kg (IV) q8h ± rifampin 600 mg (IV) q24h × 2 weeks Polymyxin B 1.25 mg/kg (IV) q12h × 2 weeks
MDR *Pseudomonas Aeruginosa*
Colistin 1.7 mg/kg (IV) q8h ± rifampin 600 mg (IV) q24h × 2 weeks Polymyxin B 1.25 mg/kg (IV) q12h × 2 weeks
Abbreviation: MDR = multidrug resistant. Adapted from: Cunha BA. *Pneumonia Essentials*. 6th ed. Royal Oak, MI: Physicians' Press; 2007.

Double drug therapy was used when the only antibiotics available were those that had relatively little activity against difficult to treat pathogens (ie, *K. pneumoniae, P. aeruginosa*) had to be used in combination to achieve acceptable therapeutic effect. At the present time, there is no need for double drug therapy of *K. pneumoniae, Enterobacter* species, or *P. aeruginosa* because antibiotics currently available have such a high degree of activity against these organisms.

ANTIBIOTIC THERAPY OF MDR NOSOCOMIAL PNEUMONIA GNB

If MDR *K. pneumoniae, A. baumannii,* or *P. aeruginosa* therapy are encountered, then effective antimicrobial drug therapy is relatively limited. Meropenem remains the most reliable agent against most of MDR GNBs. For the strains that are meropenem resistant, other organisms are available and effective. For MDR *K. pneumoniae* and *A. baumannii,* tigecycline has been effective. For MDR *Pseudomonas, Acinetobacter,* and *K. pneumoniae,* colistin or polymyxin B are highly effective. Again, clinicians are advised to avoid attempting to treat these organisms in respiratory secretions just because they are there. Therapy for MDR *K. pneumoniae, A. baumannii,* or *P. aeruginosa* should be reserved for those with purulent tracheobronchitis or highly likely/proven pathogens in NP/HAP/VAP (Table 32.4).

The treatment of NP/HAP/VAP is ordinarily 2 weeks. Some patients may be treated for fewer than 2 weeks, but longer than 2 weeks of therapy suggests an incorrect diagnosis/alternate diagnosis rather than inappropriate antimicrobial therapy.

HSV-1 NOSOCOMIAL PNEUMONIA

A common complication in ventilated patients with persistent fever, leukocytosis, and minimal pulmonary infiltrates is herpes simplex virus 1 (HSV-1) NP. HSV-1 NP presents as "failure to wean" on patients who have received ≥2 weeks of appropriate antimicrobial therapy and have failed to improve. Otherwise unexplained "failure to wean" off a ventilator in a patient without severe preexisting cardiopulmonary disease, after 2 weeks of appropriate antimicrobial therapy, should suggest the diagnostic possibility of HSV-1 NP. HSV-1 NP is a common but underrecognized clinical entity. Most clinicians change antibiotic therapy after 2 weeks and continue for 1 or more additional

Table 32.5 Characteristics of Nosocomial HSV-1 Pneumonia in Immunocompetent Hosts

Symptoms
Failure to wean off respirator (in patients without advanced preexisting lung disease)

Signs
Low-grade fever
Unexplained hypoxemia with normal/near normal chest x-ray
No HSV vesicles in respiratory passages

Laboratory Tests
Leukocytosis (± left shift)
$\downarrow pO_2 / \uparrow$ A-a gradient (>30)
Serology: negative HSV-1 IgM/±↑ titers or HSV-1 ↑ IgM/± ↑ IgG titers
Chest x-ray: normal or diffuse "ground glass" opacities
Gallium/indium scan: bilateral symmetrical diffuse uptake
Spiral chest CT: diffuse "ground glass" opacities
Bronchoscopy: ± HSV-1 virus cultured from respiratory secretions
Cytology: HVS-1 intranuclear inclusion bodies (Cowdry type A)

Therapy
Acyclovir 10 mg/kg (IV) q8h × 7–10 days
Results in rapid improvement as manifested by
$\downarrow F_{I\,02}$
$\uparrow P_{02}$
$\downarrow$ A-a gradient

Adapted from: Cunha BA: *Pneumonia Essentials*. Royal Oak, MI: Physicians' Press; 2007.

weeks, hoping that the patient will eventually improve and be able to be weaned off the ventilator. If HSV-1 NP is suspected, diagnostic bronchoscopy should be performed. Bronchial lavage (BAL)–obtained cytological specimens of respiratory cells are necessary for diagnosis. Respiratory secretions serology, the presence of herpetic vesicles in the bronchials, and culture of HSV from respiratory secretions are not diagnostic. Cytopathic changes in distal respiratory epithelial cells indicate tissue invasion and not viral colonization/reactivation. Cytology diagnostic of HSV NP is the finding of Cowdry type A intranuclear intrusion bodies in respiratory epithelial cells from BAL specimens. If cytopathic changes of HSV-1 are found in BAL specimens, empiric therapy with acyclovir should be initiated (Table 32.5). Initiation of acyclovir therapy usually results in a rapid improvement in oxygenation as manifested by a decrease in the FiO_2, and increase in the PO_2, and a decrease in the A-a gradient 3 to 5 days after initiation of therapy. Patients then can be weaned off the ventilators over the next several days.

SUGGESTED READING

Alvarez Lerma F and Serious Infection Study Group. Efficacy of meropenem as monotherapy in the treatment of ventilator-associated pneumonia. *J Chemother*. 2001;13:70–81.

American Thoracic Society/Infectious Diseases Society of America. Guidelines for the management of adults with hospital-acquired, ventilator-associated and healthcare-associated pneumonia. *Am J Respir Crit Care Med*. 2005;171:388–416.

Berman SJ, Fogarty CM, Fabian T, et al. Meropenem monotherapy for the treatment of hospital-acquired pneumonia: results of a multicenter trial. *J Chemother*. 2004;16:362–371.

Chastre J, Fagon JY. Ventilator-associated pneumonia. *Am J Respir Crit Care Med*. 2002;165:867–903.

Cunha BA. Monotherapy for nosocomial pneumonias. *Antibiot Clin*. 1998;2:34–37.

Cunha BA. Strategies to control antibiotic resistance. *Semin Respir Crit Care Med*. 2000;21:3–8.

Cunha BA. Effective antibiotic resistance and control strategies. *Lancet*. 2001;357:1307–1308.

Cunha BA. Nosocomial pneumonia: diagnostic and therapeutic considerations. *Med Clin N Am*. 2001;85:79–114.

Cunha BA. *Pseudomonas aeruginosa*: antibiotic resistance and antimicrobial therapy. *Semin Respir Ther*. 2002;17:231–239.

Cunha BA. Herpes simplex-1 (HSV-1) pneumonia. *Infect Dis Pract*. 2005;29:375–378.

Eisenstein L, Cunha BA. Herpes simplex virus type 1 (HSV-1) pneumonia presenting as failure to wean. *Heart Lung*. 2003;32:65–66.

Laforce FM. Systemic antimicrobial therapy of nosocomial pneumonia: monotherapy versus combination therapy. *Eur J Clin Microbiol Infect Dis*. 1989;8:61.

Levin AS, Barone AA, Penco J, et al. Intravenous colistin as therapy for nosocomial infections caused by multidrug-resistant Pseudomonas aeruginosa and Acinetobacter baumannii. *Clin Infect Dis*. 1999;28:1008–11.

Linden PK, Paterson DL. Parenteral and inhaled colistin for treatment of ventilator-associated pneumonia. *Clin Infect Dis*. 2006;43:S89–S94.

Lode HM, Raffenberg M, Erbes R, et al. Nosocomial pneumonia: epidemiology, pathogenesis, diagnosis, treatment and prevention. *Curr Opin Infect Dis*. 2000;13:377–384.

Simoons-Smit AM, Kraan EM, Beishuizen A, et al. Herpes simplex virus type 1 and respiratory disease in critically-ill patients: real pathogen or innocent bystander? *Clin Microbiol Infect*. 2006;12:1050–1059.

33. Aspiration Pneumonia

Arash Heidari and Matthew Bidwell Goetz

INTRODUCTION

Aspiration is the introduction of oropharyngeal or gastric contents into the respiratory tract. Three major syndromes may develop as a consequence of aspiration: chemical pneumonitis, bronchial obstruction secondary to aspiration of particulate matter, and bacterial aspiration pneumonia. Less commonly, interstitial lung disease occurs in persons with chronic aspiration. Which of these consequences emerges is determined by the amount and nature of the aspirated material as well as by the integrity of host defense mechanisms. Aspiration is the main means of bacterial contamination of the lower airways.

The term *aspiration pneumonia* is used to refer to the infectious consequences of introduction of relatively large volumes of material (macroaspiration). Although healthy persons frequently aspirate small volumes of pharyngeal secretions during sleep, the development of pneumonia after such microaspiration is normally prevented by mechanical (eg, cough and mucociliary transport) and immunological responses. Pneumonia arises when these host defenses are not able to limit bacterial proliferation either because of microaspiration of highly virulent pathogens to which the host lacks specific immunity (eg, *Streptococcus pneumoniae* or enteric gram-negative bacteria) or because of macroaspiration of lower or higher virulence organisms.

Aspiration may be clinically obvious, as when acute pulmonary complications follow inhalation of vomited gastric contents. Such acute chemical pneumonitis is often referred to as Mendelson syndrome. On the other extreme, so-called silent aspiration, as occurs in persons with neurological impairment who lack cough responses, is often followed by the indolent onset of infectious pneumonia consequent to the inhalation of the low virulence mixtures of aerobic and anaerobic microorganisms normally resident in the oropharynx.

In evaluating patients who have aspirated, it is important to bear in mind that there is considerable overlap between chemical pneumonitis and aspiration pneumonia. Aspiration of gastric contents is inevitably accompanied by aspiration of the oropharyngeal flora that may result in the emergence of infection within several days if high virulence organisms have colonized the oropharynx or in the delayed emergence of mixed aerobic/anaerobic pneumonia caused by normal oral flora.

RISK FACTORS

Several groups of factors increase the risk of aspiration pneumonia. First is disturbance of the normal oropharyngeal or gastric flora. The presence of gingivitis, dental plaque, and decayed teeth combined with poor oral hygiene or decreased salivary flow (eg, due to tube feedings or anticholinergic medications) increases the predisposition to developing pneumonia following an aspiration event by increasing colonization of the oropharynx by relatively low virulence bacteria. Similarly, decreased gastric acidity, enteral feeding, gastroparesis, or small-bowel obstruction increase colonization of gastric contents by pathogenic microorganisms. Moreover, replacement of normal oral flora by more virulent microorganisms such as *Staphylococcus aureus*, *Pseudomonas aeruginosa*, and *Klebsiella pneumoniae* as a consequence of alcoholism, malnutrition, diabetes, and other severe comorbidities or prior antimicrobial therapy also increases the risk of pneumonia following an aspiration event.

For self-evident reasons, conditions that impair cough and other normal mechanical oropharyngeal reflexes that prevent aspiration increase the risk of aspiration pneumonia. These include cerebrovascular and other neurological diseases, alcoholism, drug abuse, general anesthesia, seizures, disorders of the gastrointestinal tract, and uncontrolled postoperative pain (see Table 33.1). In addition, pulmonary clearance defects at the mucociliary level (eg, secondary to tobacco smoking or influenza), and impairment of normal humoral and cellular host defenses, particularly those conditions that decrease immunoglobulin production (eg, hematological malignancies) or result in severe neutropenia, also increase the risk of developing pneumonia after aspiration.

CLINICAL EPIDEMIOLOGY

In 2004 there were approximately 180 000 inpatient admissions in the United States for which the principal diagnosis was food/vomit (or aspiration) pneumonitis (ICD-9 507.0). These hospitalizations accounted for more than 28 000 inpatient deaths with a total medical care cost of 6 billion dollars. Another 228 000 persons received a secondary diagnosis of aspiration pneumonitis. Swallowing disorders due to neurologic diseases affect 300 000 to 600 000 people each year in the United States. Nearly 40% of stroke patients with dysphagia aspirate and develop pneumonia. Overall, aspiration pneumonitis accounts for approximately 0.5% of all hospitalizations, 3% to 4% of inpatient mortality, and 5% to 23% of all cases of community-acquired pneumonia.

More than 70% of cases of aspiration pneumonia are in persons older than 65 years of age. As a corollary, aspiration pneumonia is the second most frequent principal cause of hospitalizations among United States Medicare patients. Among nursing home patients, aspiration pneumonia accounts for up to 30% of cases of pneumonia, occurs at a rate three times that of age-matched patients in the community and markedly increases the risk of death. Among such patients, difficulty swallowing food, use of tube feedings, requiring assistance with feeding, delirium, and use of sedative medications are the most frequent risk factors for aspiration pneumonia. While the debilitated elderly are at particularly high risk, prior silent aspiration is also common in apparently healthy elderly patients with community-acquired pneumonia.

Aspiration complicates the course of approximately 10% of persons admitted to hospitals for overdosage with sedative or hypnotic agents and 0.05% to 0.8% of persons receiving general anesthesia for surgical procedures. Patient characteristics independently associated with an increased risk of aspiration following general anesthesia include male sex, nonwhite race, age of >60 years, dementia, chronic obstructive pulmonary disease, renal disease, malignancy, moderate to severe liver disease, and emergency surgery.

CLINICAL COURSE AND DIAGNOSIS

Aspiration of gastric contents results in acute inflammation of the major airways and lung

Table 33.1 Risk Factors for Aspiration

Altered Level of Consciousness

General anesthesia
Narcotic and sedative drugs
Drug overdose and ethanol toxicity
Metabolic encephalopathies (electrolyte imbalances, liver failure, uremia, sepsis)
Hypoxia and hypercapnia
Central nervous system (CNS) infections
Dementia

Abnormal Glottic Closure

Anesthetic induction or postanesthetic recovery
Postextubation
Structural lesions of the CNS (tumors, cerebrovascular accident, head trauma)
Seizures
Infection (eg, diphtheria, pharyngeal abscess)

Gastroesophageal Dysfunction

Alkaline gastric pH
Gastrointestinal tract dysmotility
Esophagitis (infectious, postradiation)
Hiatal hernia
Scleroderma
Esophageal motility disorders (achalasia, megaesophagus)
Tracheoesophageal fistula
Ascites (increased intra-abdominal pressure)
Intestinal obstruction or ileus
Diabetes (functional gastric outlet obstruction)

Neuromuscular Diseases

Guillain-Barré syndrome
Botulism
Muscular dystrophy
Parkinson's disease
Polymyositis
Amyotrophic lateral sclerosis
Multiple sclerosis
Myesthenia gravis
Poliomyelitis
Tardive dyskinesia

Mechanical Factors

Nasogastric or enteral feeding tubes
Upper endoscopy
Emergency and routine airway manipulation
Surgery or trauma to the neck and pharynx
Tumors of the upper airway
Tracheostomy
Endotracheal tube
Zenker's diverticulum

Other Factors

Obesity
Pregnancy

parenchyma. Animal models demonstrate maximal hypoxemia within 10 minutes of aspiration. In these models, the severity of lung injury is greatest when the pH is less than 2.5, but gastric materials can cause severe pulmonary injury even at higher pH. Local injury results in complement activation as well as release of TNF-α, IL-8, and other proinflammatory cytokines that in turn are primarily responsible for the acute nonobstructive complications of chemical aspiration.

Acute symptoms and signs of chemical pneumonitis include respiratory distress, fever, cough, reflex bronchospasm, leukocytosis, and pulmonary infiltrates. Life-threatening hypoxemia may develop as a consequence of atelectasis, pulmonary capillary leak, and direct alveolar damage. These early findings are easily attributable to chemical pneumonitis rather than bacterial infection if they follow witnessed vomiting and aspiration of gastric acidic contents. If the event is not witnessed, detection of gastric enzyme pepsin in tracheal aspirate may be used as a marker for gastric aspiration pneumonitis.

Many patients with chemical pneumonitis improve without any specific antimicrobial therapy. Other patients develop progressive clinical symptoms and worsening radiographic findings for several days after an aspiration event. Such progression indicates the emergence of the acute respiratory distress syndrome and/or bacterial pneumonia. Alternatively, patients may initially improve for several days but then worsen with the onset of recurrent symptoms and signs indicative of secondary bacterial pneumonia.

The differentiation of aspiration pneumonia from progressive chemical pneumonitis is often challenging as there is frequent overlap between these two syndromes. This distinction is important given the desirability of avoiding unnecessary antibiotic use, especially as pneumonia fails to develop in approximately half of all aspiration events. Furthermore, given the differences in microbial etiology of aspiration pneumonia versus community-acquired pneumonia, it is important to consider aspiration in persons with pneumonia who have the risk factors listed in Table 33.1 even if an aspiration event has not been witnessed.

The clinical presentation of aspiration pneumonia is much less dramatic than that of chemical pneumonitis. Clinical characteristics include fever, alteration of general well-being, and respiratory symptoms such as productive cough, dyspnea, and pleuritic pain. However, in elderly patients who are at greatest risk for aspiration, the early signs and symptoms of pulmonary infection may be muted and overshadowed by nonspecific complaints such as general weakness, decreased appetite, altered mental status, or decompensation of underlying diseases. Many episodes of aspiration pneumonia, especially those involving normal oral flora (ie, mixed aerobic/anaerobic infections), result from silent aspiration. These patients may have an indolent disease and not develop fever, malaise, weight loss, and cough for 1 to 2 weeks or more after aspiration. This is an especially common presentation for patients who present with mixed aerobic/anaerobic lung abscesses or empyemas after an aspiration event.

Radiographic evaluation is necessary to establish the diagnosis of pneumonia as there is no combination of historical data, physical findings, or laboratory results that reliably confirms the diagnosis. Limitations of chest radiography for the diagnosis of pneumonia include poor specificity in patients with the acute respiratory distress syndrome and decreased sensitivity in persons with previous structural lung disease, very early infection, severe dehydration, or profound granulocytopenia. Otherwise, the failure to detect an infiltrate essentially rules out the diagnosis of pneumonia. Although spiral computed tomography (CT) of the chest provides a more sensitive means of detecting infiltrates than chest radiography, such infiltrates may not actually represent pneumonia. Esophagography and CT are especially useful in the evaluation of aspiration disease related to tracheoesophageal or tracheopulmonary fistula.

Radiologic findings do not distinguish between chemical pneumonitis and aspiration pneumonia save for the fact that radiological abnormalities have more rapid onset with chemical pneumonitis. Pneumonia complicating aspiration most often involves the posterior segment of the right upper lobe, the superior segment of the right lower lobe, or both, as well as the corresponding segments on the left. Manifestations of mixed aerobic/anaerobic infection include necrotizing pneumonia, lung abscess, and empyema (Figures 33.1–33.4). Foreign body aspiration typically occurs in children and manifests as obstructive lobar or segmental overinflation or atelectasis. An extensive, patchy bronchopneumonic pattern may be observed in patients following massive aspiration of gastric contents.

Although the utility of sputum examination is much debated, pleural fluid (if present) and two sets of blood cultures should always be obtained and efforts to obtain sputum should be pursued before initiation of antimicrobial therapy in hospitalized patients with aspiration pneumonia. Sputum samples must be carefully collected, transported, and processed

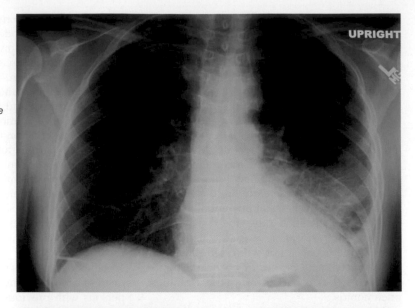

Figure 33.1 *K. pneumoniae* infection causing left lower lobe pneumonia in a 47-year-old woman who aspirated during a period of depressed consciousness due to alcohol intoxication.

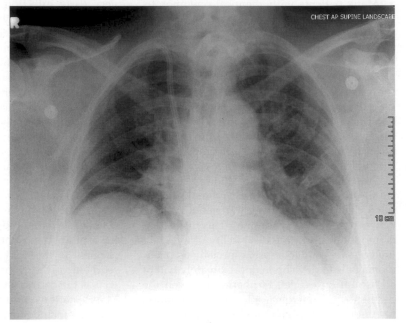

Figure 33.2 Bilateral lower lobe pneumonia due to *P. aeruginosa* in a dialysis-dependent nursing home patient following episode of vomiting.

to optimize the recovery of common aerobic bacterial pathogens such as *S. pneumoniae*. Because anaerobic cultures are not performed for sputum specimens, the presence of mixed bacterial flora on the sputum Gram stain should be used to diagnose polymicrobial infection typical of the mixed aerobic-anaerobic infections. Inspection of the sputum Gram stain is also necessary to ensure that the materials being cultured are not unduly contaminated by saliva. Bronchoscopic sampling of the lower respiratory tract (with a protected specimen brush or by bronchoalveolar lavage) and

quantitative culture are particularly useful in critically ill patients with hospital-acquired aspiration pneumonia. Such interventions are especially warranted in persons who do not respond to initial antimicrobial therapy.

Unfortunately, despite extensive evaluation, the microbial cause of pneumonia can be identified in only 40% to 60% of hospitalized patients. Nevertheless, identification of the infecting microorganism serves to verify the clinical diagnosis of infection and facilitates the use of specific therapy instead of unnecessarily broad-spectrum antimicrobial agents.

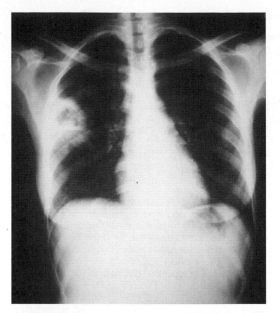

Figure 33.3 Mixed aerobic/anaerobic lung abscess following aspiration.

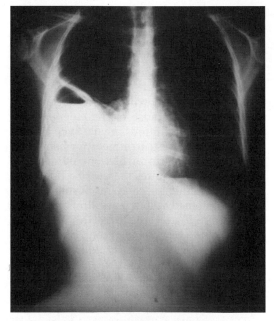

Figure 33.4 Mixed aerobic/anaerobic empyema following aspiration.

MICROBIOLOGY

The microbial etiology of aspiration pneumonia is complex and variable. The distribution of responsible pathogens differs in persons with community- versus hospital-acquired illness and varies with the presence or absence of previous antimicrobial exposure, comorbidities, or odontogenic disease.

In many studies performed during the 1970s, bacteriologic specimens were obtained by percutaneous transtracheal sampling or thoracentesis, and rigorous laboratory methods were used to optimize the recovery of anaerobic bacteria. Although typical causes of bacterial pneumonia such as *S. pneumoniae* were often recovered, these studies demonstrated that viridans streptococci and anaerobic organisms, including *Peptostreptococcus, Bacteroides, Prevotella,* and *Fusobacteria,* were the predominant pathogens in aspiration pneumonia. In most of these studies the specimens were obtained in the later stages of the disease when complications such as abscesses or empyema were present.

Although some recent studies show a decreased prevalence of anaerobic bacteria as causes of aspiration pneumonia, the adequacy of attention to anaerobic culture techniques is often uncertain, leaving in doubt whether the true frequency of anaerobic infection has been underestimated. Well-performed studies continue to demonstrate anaerobes in up to 20% of nursing home patients with aspiration pneumonia; increased rates are found in patients with greater levels of debility. Conversely, the frequency of anaerobic infection is somewhat less in edentulous patients. In recent studies, the most frequently recovered aerobic organisms from persons with community-acquired aspiration pneumonia have been *S. pneumoniae, Hemophilus influenzae, Staphylococcus aureus,* and *Enterobacteriaceae* (eg, *Escherichia coli, Klebsiella* species and *Enterobacter* species).

Aerobic bacteria, particularly *S. aureus,* enteric gram-negative bacilli (ie, *Enterobacteriaceae*), and occasionally *P. aeruginosa,* are more common causes of aspiration pneumonia in persons who develop disease while hospitalized or in a nursing home setting. At least 40% of hospital-associated pneumonias, many of which are due to aspiration, are caused by *S. aureus* and *Enterobacteriaceae.* Patients admitted to a respiratory or intensive care unit have the highest risk of nosocomial gram-negative bacillary pneumonia. *P. aeruginosa* is most common in persons who have received prior intensive antimicrobial therapy or who have underlying bronchiectasis or severe immunological compromise. Polymicrobial infection is common in patients with aspiration pneumonia.

CLINICAL MANAGEMENT

Although corticosteroids have long been used in the treatment of acute chemical pneumonitis due to aspiration, this treatment cannot be

Table 33.2 Suggested Empiric Therapy for Inpatients with Aspiration Pneumonia

Suspected Pathogens	Preferred Agents	Alternative Agents
Mixed aerobic/anaerobic flora	β-lactam plus metronidazole, β-lactam/β-lactamase inhibitor[a]	Clindamycin, moxifloxacin, ertapenem
Enterobacteriaceae	β-lactam/β-lactamase inhibitor[a], cefepime, carbapenem[b]	Third-generation cephalosporin[c] or fluoroquinolone[d], both +/− aminoglycoside[f]
P. aeruginosa	Antipseudomonal β-lactam[e] +/− aminoglycoside[f], carbapenem +/− aminoglycoside[f]	Ciprofloxacin + aminoglycoside, ciprofloxacin + antipseudomonal β-lactam[f]
S. aureus	Vancomycin	Linezolid, quinupristin/dalfopristin

Note: Therapy should be modified when the identity and susceptibility of the responsible pathogen(s) is determined.
[a] Ticarcillin/clavulanate and piperacillin/tazobactam are the preferred β-lactam/β-lactamase inhibitors for the treatment of nosocomial pneumonia due to *Enterobacteriaceae*. Ampicillin/sulbactam lacks adequate activity against many nosocomial enteric gram-negative bacilli.
[b] Ertapenem, imipenem, and meropenem have equivalent activity against *Enterobacter* spp. mixed aerobic/anaerobic flora. Only imipenem and meropenem have activity against *P. aeruginosa*.
[c] Third-generation cephalosporins: cefotaxime, ceftriaxone, and ceftazidime.
[d] Levofloxacin and ciprofloxacin generally have equivalent activity against *Enterobacter* spp. and *P. aeruginosa*. High resistance rates, particularly for nosocomial isolates of limit the empiric usefulness of these agents in many settings.
[e] Antipseudomonal β-lactams: ceftazidime, cefepime, imipenem, meropenem, mezlocillin, piperacillin or piperacillin-tazobactam.
[f] Addition of an aminoglycoside should be strongly considered in serious ill patients to ensure adequate breadth of antimicrobial therapy.

recommended. Prospective studies have failed to show a benefit in animal models of acid lung injury or in patients with either aspiration pneumonitis or the acute respiratory distress syndrome.

Antibiotic use is not warranted in most patients who acutely develop fever, leukocytosis, and pulmonary infiltrates following aspiration as these consequences are caused by chemical irritation and inflammation rather than to established infection. Antibiotic use in such patients is essentially prophylactic and may facilitate colonization and infection by more resistant pathogens. However, there may be some benefit in selected populations such as persons with acute life-threatening complications of aspiration or those who have aspirated heavily colonized gastric contents (eg, in the setting of small bowel obstruction). Antibiotics should generally be administered to patients whose symptoms do not resolve within 48-72 hours or in whom new or progressive signs of pulmonary infection later emerge.

The need to select antibiotics with robust anaerobic activity in the treatment of patients with aspiration pneumonia is controversial. Vigorous antianaerobic therapy may not offer meaningful benefit to patients with simple pneumonia, especially if therapy is not unduly delayed. However, antimicrobial therapy with antianaerobic therapy should be given to persons with aspiration events with necrotizing pneumonias, lung abscesses, or empyemas or who present following the indolent onset of pneumonia. Because of the emergence of β-lactamase-mediated resistance among anaerobes, empirical treatment for aspiration pneumonia likely to involve mixed aerobic/anaerobic flora requires the use of a β-lactam/β-lactamase inhibitor, clindamycin, or metronidazole combined with a penicillin, ampicillin, or an appropriate cephalosporin (Table 33.2). Because of the very frequent concomitant presence of aerobes, metronidazole monotherapy should not be given.

Considering the range of pathogens and antimicrobial resistance, initial therapy of aspiration pneumonia that develops in nursing home or hospitalized patients must be carefully selected. Although monotherapy may be reasonable for immunocompetent patients with mild to moderate diseases who are known or likely to be infected by susceptible strains of *Proteus, Morganella, K. pneumoniae*, or *E. coli*, broad-spectrum multidrug therapy is often necessary to ensure coverage of the likely pathogens. The choice of a particular combination must depend on the severity of infection, presence or absence of immunocompromise, and hospital-specific patterns of antimicrobial resistance and rates of isolation by specific microorganisms. Therapy can be made more specific when the pathogen(s) has been identified and susceptibilities are known.

With appropriate antimicrobial therapy, 50% of patients treated for aspiration pneumonia defervesce within 2 days of initiation of antibiotic therapy and 80% do so within 5 days. Prolonged fever is more common in patients with lung abscess or with infections by aggressive pathogens such as *P. aeruginosa*.

PREVENTION

Precautions should be taken to minimize the possibility of aspiration in hospitalized patients. Avoidance of the recumbent position and hypopharyngeal suctioning prevent aspiration by intubated patients. Guidelines from the American College of Chest Physicians and the American Gastroenterology Association provide specific recommendations regarding the evaluation of patients who are at risk for aspiration due to dysphagia. These guidelines recommend a multidisciplinary approach to patient evaluation and note the need to design and test therapy on an individual-patient basis. Patients with documented aspiration during swallowing studies have a 4- to 10-fold increased risk of pneumonia depending on the magnitude of aspiration.

Placement of gastrostomy tubes in persons with dysphagia is not superior to the use of a nasogastric tube for preventing aspiration. The failure of this intervention is likely related to ongoing aspiration of oral secretions and the observation that aspiration of gastric contents still occurs in persons fed by gastrostomy tubes. Nonetheless, decreased local irritation, fewer mechanical problems, and improved nutrition justify the use of gastrostomy tubes in many patients. When used, the residual volume of tube feedings in the stomach should be monitored, and tube feedings should be held if the residual volume exceeds 50 mL.

Good periodontal care decreases the burden of pathogenic bacteria in oral secretions and thereby may prevent aspiration pneumonia.

In contrast, prophylactic antibiotic use is not recommended for patients in whom aspiration is suspected or witnessed.

SUGGESTED READING

Guidelines for the management of adults with hospital-acquired, ventilator-associated, and healthcare-associated pneumonia. *Am J Respir Crit Care Med.* 2005;171;388–416.

Centers for Disease Control and Prevention. Guidelines for prevention of nosocomial pneumonia. MMWR *Morb Mortal Wkly Rep.* 1997; 46(RR-1):1–79.

Cook IJ, Kahrilas PJ. AGA technical review on management of oropharyngeal dysphagia. *Gastroenterology.* 1999;116:455–478.

El Solh AA, Pietrantoni C, Bhat A, et al. Microbiology of severe aspiration pneumonia in institutionalized elderly. *Am J Respir Crit Care Med.* 2003;167:1650–1654.

Gudiol F, Manressa F, Pallares R, et al. Clindamycin vs. penicillin for anaerobic lung infections. High rate of penicillin failures associated with penicillin-resistant *Bacteroides melaninogenicus. Arch Intern Med.* 1990;150:2525–2529.

Mandell LA, Bartlett JG, Dowell SF, et al. Update of practice guidelines for the management of community-acquired pneumonia in immunocompetent adults. *Clin Infect Dis.* 2003;37:1405–1433.

Marik PE. Aspiration pneumonitis and aspiration pneumonia. *N Engl J Med.* 2001;344: 665–671.

Marik PE, Kaplan D. Aspiration pneumonia and dysphagia in the elderly. *Chest.* 2003;124:328–336.

Smith Hammond CA, Goldstein LB. Cough and aspiration of food and liquids due to oral-pharyngeal dysphagia: ACCP evidence-based clinical practice guidelines. *Chest.* 2006;129:154S–168S.

Terpenning MS, Taylor GW, Lopatin DE, Kerr CK, Dominguez BL, Loesche WJ. Aspiration pneumonia: dental and oral risk factors in an older veteran population. *J Am Geriatr Soc.* 2001;49:557–563.

34. Lung Abscess

Lisa L. Dever

Lung abscess is a chronic or subacute lung infection initiated by the aspiration of contaminated oropharyngeal secretions. The result is an indolent, necrotizing infection in a segmental distribution limited by the pleura. Except for infections with unusual organisms such as *Actinomyces,* the process does not cross interlobar fissures, and pleural effusion is uncommon. The resultant cavity is usually solitary, with a thick, fibrous reaction at its periphery. So defined, lung abscess is almost always associated with anaerobic bacteria, although microaerophilic and aerobic bacteria are frequently present as well.

In contrast, necrotizing pneumonia is an acute, often fulminant, infection characterized by irregular destruction of alveolar walls and therefore multiple cavities. This infection spreads rapidly through lung tissue, frequently crossing interlobar fissures, and is often associated with pleural effusion and empyema. The duration of illness before recognition is usually only a few days. Causative organisms include *Staphylococcus aureus, Streptococcus pyogenes, Klebsiella pneumoniae, Pseudomonas aeruginosa,* and, less commonly, other gram-negative bacilli, *Legionella* species, *Nocardia* species, and fungi.

The focus of this discussion will be the diagnosis and therapy of anaerobic lung abscess. Diagnosis can usually be made from the clinical presentation and chest radiograph findings. Many patients have conditions such as seizure disorders, neuromuscular diseases, alcoholism, or other causes for impaired consciousness that predispose them to aspiration of oropharyngeal secretions. Additionally, patients with impaired local and systemic host defenses are at greater risk. Gingival disease and poor dental hygiene, which promote higher concentrations of anaerobic organisms in the mouth, are common. Patients usually give a several-week history of fever and cough; putrid sputum occurs in less than 50% of patients. With chronic infection, patients will often experience weight loss and anemia, mimicking malignancy. Chest radiographs show consolidation in a segmental or lobar distribution with central cavitation, and air-fluid levels are often present (Figure 34.1).

Chest tomography can further define the extent and location of the abscess (Figure 34.2). The lung segments most commonly involved are those that are dependent when the person is supine (ie, posterior segments of the upper lobes and superior segments of the lower lobes). Aspiration and resulting lung abscess are uncommonly found in anterior lung segments because of the uphill angulation of the trachea when the subject lies prone.

The etiologic diagnosis of lung abscess is hampered by contamination of specimens by the normal anaerobic flora of the mouth. Although the Gram stain of sputum may be helpful in suggesting an etiologic diagnosis, routine sputum cultures are of no value because all contain anaerobic organisms. Techniques that have been used to obtain uncontaminated lower-airway specimens for anaerobic cultures include transtracheal needle aspiration, transthoracic needle aspiration, and open lung biopsy. Using these techniques, early investigators demonstrated anaerobic bacteria in virtually all untreated patients. These invasive techniques are seldom warranted in the clinical management of patients today. More recently, investigators have used quantitative cultures of bronchoalveolar lavage or other bronchoscopically obtained lower-airway specimens, such as those obtained with a protected specimen brush. Although these methods may prove useful in the occasional patient suspected of having lung abscess, they are not needed in most. Transthoracic fine-needle aspiration guided by either ultrasound or computed tomography (CT) has been used increasingly for diagnostic purposes. Although generally safe in experienced hands, serious complications such as pneumothorax and bacterial contamination can result and greatly prolong the recovery period.

Anaerobic organisms most commonly recovered from lung abscesses are listed in Table 34.1. Multiple anaerobic organisms are commonly present along with aerobic or microaerophilic organisms. The viridans streptococci, particularly the *S. milleri* group, appear to be significant pathogens. *Klebsiella pneumoniae* was the most common pathogen in a retrospective

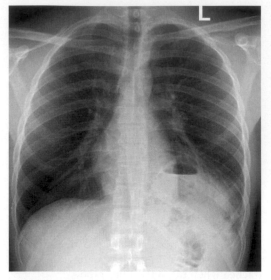

Figure 34.1 Chest radiograph showing a large cavitating lung abscess with air-fluid level in the left lower lobe.

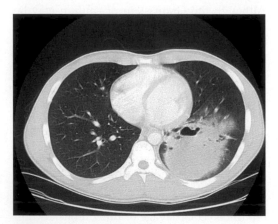

Figure 34.2 Computed tomography scan of the chest further defines the location and extent of the abscess cavity measuring 12 × 9 cm.

review of 90 cases of community-acquired lung abscess from Taiwan. *K. pneumoniae* was recovered from 30 patients (33%), compared to 28 patients with anaerobic organisms. Although there are likely several explanations for these findings, including prior antibiotic therapy and the geographic location, the results are intriguing and bear further investigation. Other than determination of β-lactamase production, susceptibility testing of anaerobic organisms is usually not required.

THERAPY

Most lung abscesses are treated empirically. Table 34.2 provides therapeutic options for

Table 34.1 Anaerobes Most Commonly Isolated in Lung Abscess

Organism
Gram-Negative Bacilli
Pigmented *Prevotella* spp.
Pigmented *Porphyromonas* spp.
Nonpigmented *Prevotella* spp.
Bacteroides fragilis group
Fusobacterium nucleatum
Fusobacterium spp.
Gram-Positive Cocci
Peptostreptoccus spp.
Peptococcus spp.
Gram-Positive Bacilli
Clostridium perfringens
Clostridium spp.
Propionibacterium acnes
Actinomyces spp.

intravenous treatment of lung abscess. Selection of agents should be guided by the spectrum of pathogens suspected or isolated from appropriate collected specimens. Historically, penicillin has been the antibiotic of choice because of its good in vitro activity against most anaerobic and microaerophilic bacteria present in the oral cavity. Early studies showed excellent responses when either parenteral or oral penicillin was used as a single agent in the treatment of anaerobic lung infections. Two randomized clinical trials found that clindamycin is superior to penicillin. In both of these studies, the time to resolution of symptoms and the failure rate were significantly lower in clindamycin-treated patients. Failure of penicillin therapy was associated with the isolation of penicillin-resistant *Bacteroides* species in one of these studies. Although increasing resistance of anaerobes and gram-positive bacteria to clindamcyin has also been reported, it is still preferred over penicillin for treatment of lung abscess when anaerobes or microaerophilic streptococci are likely to be predominant pathogens.

The combination of metronidazole and penicillin has been used with success for the treatment of anaerobic pulmonary infections. It should not be used if aerobic gram-negative bacilli may be part of the infectious process. Metronidazole has excellent bactericidal activity against virtually all anaerobes but lacks activity against microaerophilic and aerobic streptococci, as well as *Actinomyces* species, and should not be used as a single agent in the treatment of lung abscess.

Table 34.2 Intravenous Antibiotic Therapy of Anaerobic Lung Abscess[a]

Antibiotic	Intravenous Dosage	Frequency
Clindamycin	900 mg	q8h
Penicillin G plus metronidazole	2–3 million U 500 mg	q4h q6h
Alternative Regimens with Broader-Spectrum Activity[b]		
Ampicillin-sulbactam	3 g	q6h
Ticarcillin-clavulanate	3.1 g	q6h
Piperacillin-tazobactam	3.375 g	q6h
Cefoxitin	2 g	q6h
Ertapenem	1 g	q24h
Imipenem	500 mg	q6h
Meropenem	1 g	q8h
Moxifloxacin	400 mg	q24h
Tigecycline	100 mg first dose then 50 mg	q12h

[a] All dosages are for adults with normal renal function.
[b] Includes activity against gram-negative aerobic bacilli.

A number of other agents have good in vitro activity against anaerobic organisms, including β-lactamase producers, and may pose less risk for the development of *Clostridium difficile*-associated disease than clindamycin. These agents include second-generation cephalosporins, carbapenems, β-+/β-lactamase inhibitor combination drugs, the newer fluoroquinolones, and tigecycline, a new glycycline antibiotic. In addition, these drugs are attractive for the treatment of lung abscess because of their activity against many of the aerobes that may be present in mixed infections. Drugs that have little or no anaerobic activity should not be used in the treatment of lung abscess; such agents include aminoglycosides, aztreonam, and the older fluoroquinolones, levofloxacin and ciprofloxacin. A recent study found that ampicillin-sulbactam was as effective as clindamycin with or without an added cephalosporin in the treatment of aspiration and lung abscess. Although a number of newer antimicrobials have a suitable spectrum of activity in vitro, it is unlikely that any of them will ever prove to be more efficacious than current therapy in prospective clinical trials. This is because of the difficulties inherent in conducting trials in this condition – no single institution sees large numbers of patients with lung abscess, it is difficult to isolate anaerobic organisms from uncontaminated respiratory specimens for accurate diagnosis and susceptibility testing, and the patients' response to treatment varies widely but is often slow, which can lead to the erroneous conclusion of treatment failure if that decision is made too early.

Duration of Therapy

The duration of therapy for lung abscesses must be individualized, but extended therapy is usually required. Parenteral therapy is recommended initially in seriously ill patients and should be continued until the patient is afebrile and clinically improving. A prolonged course of oral antibiotics follows initial parenteral therapy. Less severely ill patients can be treated effectively with oral antibiotics alone. Options for oral therapy are provided in Table 34.3. Therapy should be continued until there is complete resolution or at least stabilization of chest radiograph lesions—this may require 8 weeks or more of therapy. Relapses have been reported when therapy has been discontinued before resolution of chest radiograph findings, even when patients are clinically asymptomatic.

Table 34.3 Oral Antibiotic Therapy of Anaerobic Lung Abscess

Antibiotic	Dosage (mg)	Frequency
Clindamycin	300	QID
Penicillin G plus	750	QID
Metronidazole	500	QID
Amoxicillin/ clavulanate	875	BID
Moxifloxacin	400	Daily
Note: All dosages are for adults with normal renal function.		

Other Therapy

As with all abscesses, the patient with lung abscess will not improve until drainage has been accomplished. Ideally, drainage is effected via the tracheobronchial tree. Postural drainage may be a useful adjunct. Bronchoscopy should be performed in patients who have unchanged air-fluid levels (or increasing levels) and who remain septic after 3 to 4 days of antibiotic therapy. Bronchoscopy rarely results in direct drainage of the abscess cavity; rather, drainage occurs over hours to days after suctioning of secretions and manipulation of the involved bronchopulmonary segments. The presence of a large abscess cavity (>6 to 8 cm diameter) requires special consideration. Some authorities prefer to drain such abscesses surgically because of the fear of an unplanned and uncontrolled sudden evacuation of the abscess contents into the bronchial tree with resultant asphyxiation. Another approach is to use a rigid bronchoscope to examine and open the involved airways because of the greater capacity for suctioning. A third approach is to perform fiberoptic bronchoscopy through an endotracheal tube with large-bore suction catheters at the ready. Successful drainage through pigtail catheters placed directly in abscess cavities using a flexible bronchoscope has been reported. It must be remembered that the gross appearance of the bronchial orifice and the results of cytologic examinations may falsely suggest the presence of an underlying malignancy because of intense and long-lived inflammation. However, nearly 50% of lung abscesses in adults older than 50 years of age are associated with carcinoma of the lung, either because of cavitation of the neoplasm or cavitation behind a proximal bronchial obstruction. Such patients should be followed to resolution with great care.

The drainage approach that has gained the most popularity in recent years is percutaneous catheter drainage, usually guided by CT or ultrasound. Although there are no controlled trials evaluating the role of this procedure in the treatment of lung abscess, a review of the literature would suggest that, in appropriately selected patients, those in whom medical therapy has failed and/or are not suitable for surgery, this approach is safe and effective. The safety of this approach, however, depends critically on the degree of synthesis of the two pleural surfaces. If the visceral pleura has not been firmly adhered to the chest wall, a pyopneumothorax results, often with bronchopleural fistula—a true disaster that is to be avoided. In that regard, transthoracic drainage should be reserved for patients who have failed attempts at endobronchial drainage.

SUGGESTED READING

Allewelt M, et al. Ampicillin + sulbactam vs. clindamycin±cephalolsporin for the treatment of aspiration pneumonia and primary lung abscess. *Clin Microbiol Infect.* 2004;10:163–170.

Bartlett JG. Anaerobic bacterial infections of the lung and pleural space. *Clin Infect Dis.* 1993;16(Suppl 4):S248–S255.

Bartlett JG. The role of anaerobic bacteria in lung abscess. *Clin Infect Dis.* 2005;40:923–925.

Gudiol F, et al. Clindamycin vs. penicillin for anaerobic lung infections: High rate of penicillin failures associated with penicillin-resistant *Bacteroides melaninogenicus. Arch Intern Med.* 1990;150:2525–2529.

Herth F, et al. Endoscopic drainage of lung abscesses: Technique and outcome. *Chest.* 2005; 127:1378–1381.

Wali SO, et al. Percutaneous drainage of pyogenic lung abscess. *Scand J Infect Dis.* 2002;34:673–679.

Wang JL, et al. Changing bacteriology of adult community-acquired lung abscess in Taiwan: *Klebsiella pneumoniae* versus anaerobes. *Clin Infect Dis.* 2005;40:915–922.

35. Empyema and Bronchopleural Fistula

Charlotte E. Bolton and Dennis J. Shale

Infection of the pleural space leading to empyema formation, and the importance of clearing infection and pus from this space, has been recognized since ancient times. Historically, empyema was associated with pneumococcal pneumonia, with *Streptococcus pneumoniae* causing up to 70% of pleural space infections. With effective antibiotic treatment for pneumonia, the incidence of empyema has decreased markedly, and the spectrum of causative organisms has widened, with *S. pneumoniae* now accounting for as few as 10% to 20%. However, parapneumonic effusions occur in 30% to 60% of pneumonia cases, and, when empyema occurs, it is associated with an overall mortality of 20%.

Parapneumonic effusions are classified as simple or uncomplicated, complicated, and empyema, based on the appearance and biochemical characteristics of aspirated fluid, which supports the clinical impression of a continuum of disease (Table 35.1).

This classification also has clinical utility in that, during the early acute phase, with free flowing fluid, treatment is simpler than in the more chronic fibropurulent stage associated with multiple loculations and the need for greater interventional therapy. Empyema may be defined as the presence of organisms and numerous host defense cells, neutrophils, in the pleural fluid, or, more narrowly, as pus apparent to the naked eye. Bronchopleural fistula (BPF) may be caused by an empyema or may be associated with empyema following surgery, penetrating lung injuries, or a lung abscess.

ETIOLOGY

Empyema occurs most commonly in association with bacterial pneumonia, either in a community- or hospital-acquired setting. In a recent study in 434 pleural infections in the United Kingdom using standard culture and nucleic amplifications techniques a causative organism was identified in 74%. Of the 336 isolates in the community-acquired setting 52% were of the genus *Streptococcus*,

approximately 20% were anaerobes, 10% were staphylococcal, and 10% were gram-negative organisms. In the hospital acquired infections (60 isolates) *Staphylococcus* was the major genus isolated (35%) of which 71% were methicillin-resistant forms, 23% were gram-negative organisms, 18% were *Streptococcus*, and 8% were anaerobes. Other organisms isolated included *Actinomyces* spp., *Enterococcus* spp., and *Mycobacterium tuberculosis*. This large study supports smaller studies suggesting the spectrum of organisms in pleural infections differs from that in pneumonia. Local events such as thoracic surgery, rupture of the esophagus, hepatic or subphrenic abscesses and all penetrating injuries may introduce organisms, especially gram-negative or anaerobic organisms, into the pleural space. Ameba may enter the pleural space from an amebic abscess in the liver. Tuberculous empyema is a minor problem in the developed world, but is still seen in reactivation of tuberculosis in the elderly. However, in the third world, with rapid urbanization, continued population increase, and greater levels of human immunodeficiency virus infection, there is an increasing incidence of tuberculous empyema. Pleural space infections may cause a BPF or may occur secondary to a BPF. Lung resection surgery remains the major cause of BPF, occurring in 3% to 5% of these operations.

CLINICAL FEATURES

There are no specific features to differentiate simple from uncomplicated parapneumonic effusions. The main features are fever, chest pain, sputum production, appropriate physical signs of an effusion, and peripheral blood leukocytosis. Progression to an empyema is usually indicated clinically by the persistence or recurrence of fever and features of systemic upset with a lack of resolution of physical signs, because differentiation of consolidation from a small- to medium-volume effusion may not be possible. Other physical features include dyspnea with large effusions, rapid-onset finger clubbing, lethargy, and marked weight loss.

Table 35.1 Classification of Parapneumonic Effusions and Empyema

	Appearance	Biochemistry and Bacteriology	Risk Category for Poor Outcome
Simple parapneumonic	Clear fluid	pH >7.2 LDH ≤1000 IU/L Glucose >3.3 mmol/L Negative Gram smear or culture	1 and 2 Very low or low
Complicated parapneumonic	Clear fluid or turbid	pH ≤7.2 LDH >1000 IU/L Glucose ≤3.3 mmol/L Positive Gram smear or culture likely	3 Moderate
Empyema	Frank pus	Positive Gram smear or culture likely Biochemistry unnecessary	4 High

Purulent sputum may indicate the development of a BPF. However, more insidious onset may occur with the presentation occurring over weeks to months after the original pneumonia or injury.

INVESTIGATIONS

A chest radiograph usually shows collection of fluid, although a localized, loculated collection may resemble an intrapulmonary mass. Differentiation between these possibilities may be resolved by the addition of a lateral chest radiograph to the standard posteroanterior film or by ultrasound or computed tomographic (CT) scanning. Ultrasonography can also be used to guide a percutaneous diagnostic aspiration if there is pleural thickening or loculation. It is occasionally difficult to distinguish between empyema with a BPF and a lung abscess. In this setting, the use of CT scanning may guide both investigation and management approaches.

Aspirated material should be collected under anaerobic conditions and a portion submitted for anaerobic culture and a sample in a blood culture bottle can increase the anaerobic yield. Routine bacterial and mycobacterial culture should be undertaken with cytological examination. If appropriate, fungi and parasites should be sought. Other investigations including pH, glucose concentration, and lactate dehydrogenase activity of the fluid may be of use if there is little evidence of purulence to the naked eye. A meta-analysis of pleural fluid biochemistry, based on user characteristics, demonstrated that pH, especially ≤7.2, was a guide

to the need for tube drainage and that glucose or lactate dehydrogenase (LDH) determination conferred no extra benefit; however, if pH assessment is unavailable, a glucose ≤60 mg/dL (3.3 mmol/L) is an alternative guide. Pleural pH is measured in nonpurulent samples taken into a heparinized syringe and determined in a blood gas analyzer. There is no need to determine the pH of purulent samples. Litmus paper assessment is not an alternative. It should be remembered that lidocaine can lower the pH of samples and hence the sampling syringe should not be contaminated by this.

Generally, percutaneous pleural biopsy is not helpful and potentially harmful, although the diagnosis of tuberculosis is often made only from such material.

The literature on the value of individual investigations in guiding management is very limited. The American College of Chest Physicians (ACCP) analysis of risk of a poor outcome is based on pooled data, a small number of randomized controlled trials, and expert consensus but provides a framework to guide management of treatment (Table 35.1).

THERAPY

There has been a paucity of evidence on which to base therapeutic decisions. However, the recent ACCP and the British Thoracic Society (BTS) UK guidelines have both reviewed evidence and graded it to develop management recommendations. These documents represent current good practice, but both emphasize the need for more robust studies in the area of the management of pleural space infections.

Management options are summarized in Table 35.2 with summary notes. All patients with a pleural effusion in the presence of sepsis or pneumonia require diagnostic aspiration. Patients with parapneumonic effusion or empyema require antibiotics, usually, commenced empirically and subsequently guided by culture results. Many will have received antibiotics already, and negative cultures do not indicate cessation of antimicrobial therapy.

Small or insignificant effusions, the maximal thickness of which is ≤10 mm on ultrasound scanning or decubitus radiograph (category 1) may not need thoracocentesis and are unlikely to need tube drainage. However, if the volume increases up to 50% hemithorax (category 2), or a positive Gram stain or culture is reported, further thoracocentesis is recommended, though in a very small effusion such results are often false positives. In these categories the risk of a poor outcome is low, and they equate to the former simple or uncomplicated parapneumonic effusions.

Larger effusions occupying more than 50% hemithorax with evidence of loculation or parietal pleural thickening or with a pH ≤ 7.2 or evidence of infection in the pleural space (category 3) require closed tube drainage and carry a moderately high risk of a poor outcome. Generally, such drainage is effective, though negative low-pressure suction may be needed if flow is slow and will hasten the obliteration of the pleural space. This approach is contraindicated in patients with a neoplasm causing airway obstruction, which is the only indication for bronchoscopy in such patients. Full characterization of this category, which corresponds to the complicated parapneumonic effusions in other classifications, requires more extensive investigation to develop an appropriate management plan (Table 35.2). Effective antibiotic choice and closed tube drainage should lead to radiologic and clinical improvement within 24 to 36 hours. Failure to respond requires further investigation, including imaging to assess tube position, any residual collection, or the formation of loculation, and should include contrast-enhanced CT scanning as loculation and parietal pleural thickening are indicators of a poor outcome. A slow response to lack of improvement will allow an empyema to form and may require surgical intervention, while increasing the risk of prolonged morbidity and a higher mortality.

The presence of pus defines an empyema (category 4), which carries a high risk of a poor outcome and requires closed tube drainage and antibiotic treatment. Frequently in empyema, the chest tube can become blocked, requiring saline flushes to maintain patency. As many infections will be of mixed organisms, antibiotic coverage for both anaerobic and nonanaerobic organisms is required. Surgical options are likely to be needed in this group. It requires a cautious and balanced decision so that surgery is not contemplated too late, a widely reported problem, when the patient's condition may reduce the chance of a satisfactory outcome. Medical or surgical thoracoscopy have been reported to reduce the time to recovery and to be as effective as formal surgical intervention, but the design of comparisons is inadequate to make firm recommendations other than that surgical options should be pursued if there is evidence of continuing sepsis and a collection after 7 days of antibiotic treatment and drainage.

Decortication aims to remove pus and fibrous tissue lining the pleural cavity but is a major surgical procedure and is unsuitable for debilitated patients, who should be considered for fibrinolytic therapy or open drainage. Decortication has the benefit of a quicker resolution of the empyema over methods of open drainage, which have a median healing period of 6 to 12 months. In general, decortication is not needed for residual pleural thickening from the successful management of categories 3 or 4, unless it persists for longer than 6 months or where there is extensive pleural thickening or respiratory symptoms secondary to restrictive effects.

The evidence for using fibrinolytic agents has been inconclusive due to small, often open, studies. A recent double-blind study in 454 patients with complicated pleural infection and at category 3 or 4 risk compared streptokinase with placebo, with all other treatment options as per routine. The primary end point of death or surgical drainage at 3 months was no different between treatment groups, $p = .43$. Similarly, secondary endpoints of death rate, requirement for surgery, radiographic outcome, and length of hospital stay were also no different between the streptokinase or placebo groups, whereas serious adverse events were increased in the streptokinase group, relative risk 2.49 (95% CI 0.98-6.36). Important contraindications include BPF, coagulation disorders, and allergy.

Currently fibrinolytic therapy is not recommended for routine care of infected pleural effusions but remains an option for the patient unfit for surgery. Treatment with streptokinase

Table 35.2 Management Options for Pleural Space Infection

Therapeutic Option	Comment
Observation and antibiotics	Acceptable option for small volume category 1 or 2 low-risk collections.
Therapeutic thoracentesis	Repeated treatment used in complicated effusions and empyema. Small studies suggest benefits, but no comparison with tube drainage.
Tube thoracostomy	Most commonly used drainage method. Combined with antibiotics can improve clinical and radiological status in 24–36 hours.
Fibrinolysis	Probably not of value in most complicated effusions. Can be used in patients unfit for required surgical intervention.
Medical or surgical thoracoscopy	Allows complete drainage and inspection of the pleural space. Small studies suggest leads to more rapid resolution of effusion.
Decortication	Allows removal of all pus, tissue debris, and connective tissue. Is major surgery and requires the patient to be fit for surgery. Appropriately used, will reduce management period. Not for routine management of residual pleural thickening.
Open drainage	An alternative option to decortication for patients unfit for surgery, but leads to a prolonged recovery period.

250 000 international units twice daily for 3 days or urokinase 100 000 international units daily for 3 days has been recommended. The latter is less likely to produce allergic side effects. Studies are underway to compare the use of streptodornase (DNase) with tissue plasminogen activator and saline in complicated parapneumonic effusions.

This classification of empyema has the value of matching a spectrum of clinical status to a plan of escalating therapeutic options but remains only a guide based on limited evidence. Patients may move in either direction along this spectrum, so careful and repeated assessment of the patient's status is required, particularly soon after a therapeutic intervention is made, to ensure a continuing appropriate management response.

The aim with BPF is to deal with the air leak and any subsequent empyema. Air in the pleural cavity indicates the presence of a BPF and need for tube drainage. The air leak may be dealt with either by surgical or nonsurgical intervention, largely depending on the size and duration of the BPF (Table 35.3).

Table 35.3 Management of Bronchopleural Fistula (BPF)

Small BPF

Some may close spontaneously:
Without empyema
    Transbronchoscopic fibrin glue
    Transbronchoscopic tissue glue
    Transbronchoscopic vascular occlusion coils
    Transbronchoscopic laser/tetracycline/gel foam
    Thoracoscopic sealing
With empyema
    Antibiotic/tube drainage and attempted closure of BPF

Large BPF

Typically associated with empyema:
    Surgical options include decortication or open drainage of empyema and occlusion of the BPF by direct closure or well-vascularized muscle or omental flaps

Pleural space infections demand major management decisions of physicians. There are various approaches to the patient with empyema and bronchopleural fistula, and the heterogeneity of the response means that the management of this problem should be individualized to the patient. There is considerable literature relating to such problems, but most studies until recently have been too small to demonstrate clear beneficial options.

SUGGESTED READING

Colice GL, Curtis A, Deslauriers J, et al. Medical and surgical treatment of parapneumonic effusions: an evidence-based guideline. *Chest.* 2000;118:1158–1171.

Davies CWH, Gleeson FV, Davies RJO. British Thoracic Society guidelines for the management of pleural infection. *Thorax.* 2003;58 (suppl ii):18–28.

Light RW. Parapneumonic effusions and empyema. *Proc Am Thorac Soc.* 2006;3: 75–80.

Maskell NA, Batt S, Hedley EL, et al. The bacteriology of pleural infection by genetic and standard methods and its mortality significance. *Am J Respir Crit Care Med.* 2006;174:817–823.

Maskell NA, Davies CW, Nunn AJ, et al. First Multicenter Intrapleural Sepsis Trial (MIST1) Group. U.K. Controlled trial of intrapleural streptokinase for pleural infection. *N Engl J Med.* 2005;352(9): 865–874.

PART VI

Clinical Syndromes –
Heart and Blood Vessels

36. Endocarditis of Natural and Prosthetic Valves: Treatment and Prophylaxis

Mashiul H. Chowdhury and Paola R. Solari

DEFINITION AND PATHOGENESIS

The term *infective endocarditis* (IE) denotes an infection of the endothelial surface of the heart. This is usually a valvular surface, but nonvalvular extracardiac endothelium can also be infected.

In the past, IE was classified as acute or subacute, depending on the severity of clinical presentation. Since the advent of antibiotics, classification and therefore therapeutic decisions are based on the bacteriology and the valvular tissue involved, that is, native valve versus prosthetic valve.

The animal model of endocarditis has improved the understanding of the in vivo aspect of the pathogenesis of this disease. Any structural abnormalities that cause turbulent blood flow across a high to low pressure gradient denude epithelium from surfaces impacted on by the turbulence. Such damaged areas (most commonly valvular surfaces) are predisposed to platelet and fibrin deposition and eventually to the formation of sterile vegetation, also known as *nonbacterial thrombotic endocarditis* (NBTE).

When transient bacteremia occurs after injury to mucosal surfaces in the oropharynx, genitourinary tract, or gastrointestinal tract, organisms are deposited onto the NBTE, where they adhere firmly, multiply, and stimulate further deposition of platelets and fibrin. The infected site is sustained by inaccessibility of the organisms to host defenses. Enlargement of the lesion into a mature vegetation may result in destruction of valves and may cause complications through local bacterial spread or through embolization of fragments of the vegetation. The endovascular location of the lesions causes multiorgan bacterial seeding as well as organ damage through immune complex deposition.

NATIVE VALVE ENDOCARDITIS

In most cases of native valve endocarditis, there is an identifiable predisposing cardiac lesion. Mitral valve prolapse is now the most commonly identified underlying cardiac abnormality in patients with IE in the United States. The risk of IE is estimated to be 5 to 8 times greater than that of individuals with a normal mitral valve. Men with mitral valve prolapse are at considerably greater risk than women, although the frequency of mitral valve is 3 times greater in women than in men. Rheumatic heart disease is still the most common underlying heart condition for bacterial endocarditis in developing countries. Other recognized predisposing cardiac lesions are ventricular septal defects, subaortic and valvular aortic stenosis, tetralogy of Fallot, coarctation of the aorta, Marfan syndrome, and pulmonary stenosis, but not uncomplicated atrial septal defects.

Although the overall incidence of infective endocarditis, 1.7 to 6.2 cases per 100 000 person-years, has remained relatively stable over time, since the late 1960s the epidemiologic features of infective endocarditis have changed in the developed world as a result of increasing longevity and the introduction of more invasive procedure within the health care system. The steady increase in the median age (47 to 69 years compared to 30 to 40 years in preantibiotic era) has given rise to degenerative valvular diseases (calcified aortic stenosis, calcified mitral valve annulus, and mitral valve prolapse) and increased exposure to health care–associated infections. *Staphylococcus aureus* has surpassed viridans group streptococci as the leading cause of infective endocarditis. In recently published data from the International Collaboration of Endocarditis-Prospective Cohort study (ICE-PCS) *S. aureus* was the most commonly identifiable pathogen among the 1779 cases of definitive infective endocarditis (31.4%). *Staphylococcus aureus* IE remains the most aggressive form of native valve infection; patients have a higher mortality rate and are more likely to experience an embolic and/or a central nervous system (CNS) event (Figures 36.1A–C). Enterococci (10% of cases of native valve IE) present an enhanced risk to elderly men and young women with genitourinary disease. In recent years, both enterococci and staphylococci have become

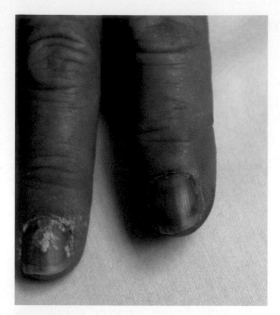

Figure 36.1(A) Splinter hemorrhage of nails in patient with Staphylococcus aureus infective endocarditis.

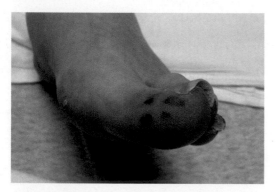

Figure 36.1(B) Embolic lesions in a patient with Staphylococcus aureus infective endocarditis.

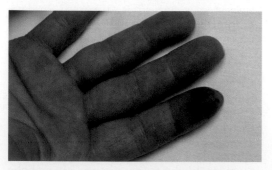

Figure 36.1(C) Embolic lesions in a patient with Staphylococcus aureus infective endocarditis.

major pathogens in infections originating from intravascular catheters. Occasionally, almost all species of bacteria can cause infective endocarditis. Fastidious oropharyngeal organisms such as the HACEK group (*Haemophilus parainfluenzae, Haemophilus influenzae, Haemophilus aphrophilus, Haemophilus paraphrophilus, Actinobacillus actinomycetemcomitans, Cardiobacterium hominis, Eikenella corrodens,* and *Kingella kingae,* and *Kingella denitrificans*) cause 10% of community-acquired IE. Fungi rarely cause IE on a native valve (2%) except in intravenous drug abusers (13%).

PROSTHETIC VALVE ENDOCARDITIS

The overall incidence of prosthetic valve endocarditis (PVE) is 1% to 4% during the first 12 months following valve surgery. The causative organisms differ in early and late PVE. Infection within 60 days of valve insertion is considered to be early PVE and is usually caused by *Staphylococcus epidermidis* (25% to 30%) or *S. aureus* (15% to 20%). In a recent prospective study of patients with prosthetic valves and *S. aureus* bacteremia conducted at Duke University Medical Center, 26 of 51 patients (51%) developed PVE. The risk of endocarditis in this study was independent of the type of valve (mechanical vs. bioprosthetic), location (mitral vs. aortic), or onset of bacteremia after prosthetic valve implantation. The remaining cases of PVE are caused by gram-negative aerobic organisms, enterococci, diphtheroids, and streptococci. Fungal endocarditis may develop in patients with prolonged hospitalization with indwelling central venous catheters and long-term antibiotic use. Organisms that cause late PVE closely resemble those of native valve endocarditis, although staphylococci remain predominant.

NOSOCOMIAL ENDOCARDITIS

Infective endocarditis can occur as a complication of nosocomial bacteremia. Since the mid-1980s, the increased use of intravascular devices and invasive diagnostic procedures, with their consequent complications, has increased the risk of health care-associated endocarditis. *Staphylococcus aureus*, including methicillin-resistant *S. aureus* (MRSA), *S. epidermidis*, and enterococcus are the predominant pathogens. A retrospective study in Europe showed a 10-fold increase in the incidence of nosocomial endocarditis from 1978 to 1992, compared with cases from 1960 to 1975. According to recent analysis of 262 patients with hospital-acquired *S. aureus* bacteremia at Duke University Medical Center 13% developed *S. aureus* endocarditis. In most studies, an intravascular device has been implicated as the source of bacteremia.

INFECTIVE ENDOCARDITIS IN THE INTRAVENOUS DRUG ABUSER

Endocarditis in intravenous drug abusers (IVDAs) involves mainly normal valves. Only 20% of the patients have an underlying valvular abnormality when IE is diagnosed. Infection is believed to result from the deposition of bacteria on valves that have sustained microscopic injury through bombardment with drug-associated contaminants injected intravenously. The tricuspid valve is predominantly involved in IVDAs, but aortic and mitral valves may also be damaged. Although *S. aureus* is known to be the most common causative organism in patients with IE associated with IVDAs, a variety of microorganisms and fungi, including unusual and fastidious organisms (eg, the HACEK group), are not uncommon in IVDAs, particularly in the patients who are not meticulous in their injection practices. Because of the higher incidence of right-sided lesions and the generally younger age of the affected group, prognosis for recovery in treated IVDAs' IE is better than in the general population. However, valvular damage sustained in the course of the infection confers an extremely high risk of recurrent IE in those patients who continue to indulge in intravenous drugs.

DIAGNOSIS OF INFECTIVE ENDOCARDITIS

Definitive diagnosis of IE requires documentation of sustained bacteremia with microorganism typical for endocarditis in a patient with an underlying valvular cardiac lesion or by direct demonstration of the pathogen by culture or histopathology of the vegetation or an embolus. The Duke criteria, in use since 1994 to diagnose IE clinically, were primarily developed to facilitate epidemiological and clinical research. The Duke criteria incorporate echocardiographic findings and IVDA as an important epidemiologic risk factor into the previously formulated Von Reyn criteria for IE and expanded their sensitivity and specificity. Patients with suspected endocarditis were stratified in 3 categories: definite, possible, and rejected cases. Although its high sensitivity was confirmed by several subsequent studies, some problems emerged with the original criteria with the broad classification of cases as "possible," the increased relative risk of endocarditis with *S. aureus* bacteremia, the widespread use of transesophageal echocardiography (TEE) for diagnosis (Figure 36.1D), and the classification of culture negative endocarditis. Modifications of the Duke criteria were proposed in 2000 (Table 36.1) because they have been used as a clinical guide for the diagnosis of infective endocarditis.

THERAPY

A vegetation consists of microorganisms in high density ($>10^8$ organisms/g of tissue) and in a reduced metabolic state inside an acellular lesion with impaired host defenses. Eradication of IE is thus almost totally dependent on the efficacy of the antimicrobial therapy. To achieve this end, certain principles of therapy are critical:

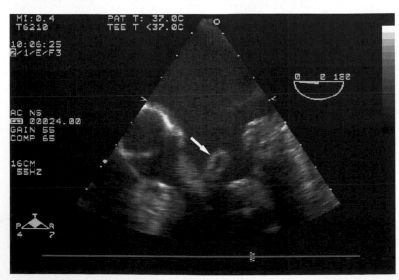

Figure 36.1(D) Transesophageal echocardiogram of a patient with Haemophilus parainfluenzae infective endocarditis showing large vegetation in mitral valve chordae apparatus (*arrow*).

Table 36.1 Modified Duke Criteria for Diagnosis of Infective Endocarditis

Definitive Infective Endocarditis	
Pathological Criteria	
Microorganism demonstrated by culture or histology of vegetation or emboli or intracardiac abscess, Histopathologically proven at autopsy or surgery	
Clinical Criteria	
2 major; 1 major and 3 minor criteria; or 5 minor criteria	
Possible Infective Endocarditis	
1 major and 1 minor or 3 minor criteria[a]	
Rejected	
Alternative diagnosis, resolution of syndrome with ≤4 days of antibiotic; no histopathological evidence with ≤4 days of antibiotic therapy; does not meet criteria for "Possible" IE.	

Major Criteria	Minor Criteria
Positive blood cultures	Predisposing heart condition or intravenous drug use
Typical microorganism for IE from 2 separate blood cultures, as follow: Viridans streptococci, *Streptococci bovis*, HACEK group, *Staphylococcus aureus*[a], or community-acquired enterococci with no primary focus	Fever (>38°C)
	Vascular phenomena
	Immunologic phenomena
Persistently positive blood cultures with microorganism consistent with IE: At least 2 positive blood cultures drawn >12 h apart	Positive blood cultures but short of major criteria or serologic evidence of infection; excludes single positive blood cultures with coagulase-negative staphylococci and organism consistent with IE
All of 3 or a majority of 4 or more separate blood cultures: First and last sample at least 1 h apart	
Single blood culture positive for *Coxiella burnetii* or positive serology: Antiphase 1 IgG ab titer >1:800[a]	Echocardiogram consistent with IE but short of major criteria was eliminated[a]
Endocardial involvement by showing vegetation; or abscess; or new prosthetic valve dehiscence; or *de novo* valvular regurgitation in echocardiogram. TEE recommended for prosthetic valve, "Possible IE" cases, or complicated IE with intracardiac abscess[a]	

Abbreviations. TEE = transesophageal echocardiogram; IE = infective endocarditis; IgG = immunoglobulin G; ab = antibody.
[a] Modifications from the original Duke Criteria.

1. Parenteral antibiotics are usually required to provide a predictably high serum antibiotic level and thus to optimize penetration of the antibiotic into tissue.
2. Bactericidal rather than bacteriostatic antibiotics should be used to compensate for impaired host defenses in the vegetation.
3. Prolonged therapy is required for complete eradication of microorganisms.

In a patient with suspected IE but in whom culture results are not available, empiric antimicrobial therapy should be directed against staphylococci, streptococci, and enterococci unless epidemiologic data point at alternative etiologies. Nafcillin or oxacillin, 2 g IV every 4 hours, and gentamicin, 1 mg/kg IV every 8 hours, may be used as initial therapy. Vancomycin, 15 mg/kg every 12 hours, should be used if the patient is allergic to penicillin. Vancomycin should also be the drug of choice in suspected nosocomial endocarditis because of the high incidence of MRSA and coagulase-negative *S. epidermidis* (CoNS) in such setting.

Viridans Streptococci and *Streptococcus bovis*

Antibiotic selection of the therapy of streptococcal endocarditis is based on the minimal inhibitory concentration (MIC) of the isolated organism to penicillin (Table 36.2). Viridans streptococci or *S. bovis* are generally highly

Table 36.2 Antibiotic Therapy for Streptococcal Endocarditis

Viridans Streptococci or *S. bovis* MIC ≤0.12 µg/mL	Viridans Streptococci or *S. bovis* MIC >0.12 µg/ml to ≤0.5 µg/mL	Viridans Streptococci or *S. bovis* MIC >0.5 µg/mL
Native Valve		
PCN G, 12–18 mU/24 h IV -4 wk or Ceftriaxone, 2 g/24 h IV/IM -4 wk	PCN G, 24 mU/24 h IV 4 wk or Ceftriaxone, 2 g/24 h IV/IM 4 wk plus	PNC G, 18–30 mU/24 h IV 4–6 wk or Ampicillin, 12 g/24 h IV 4–6 wk plus
PCN G, 12–18 mU/24 h IV 2 wk or Ceftriaxone, 2 g/24 h IV/IM 2 wk plus Gentamicin, 1 mg/kg q8h IV/IM for the first 2 wk	Gentamicin 1mg/kg IV/IM q8h for the first 2 wk	Gentamicin, 1 mg/kg q8h IV/IM 4–6 wk
Prosthetic Valve		
PCN G, 24 mU/24 h IV 6 wk or Ceftriaxone, 2 g/24 h IV/IM 4wk with or without Gentamicin 1 mg/kg IV/IM q8h for the first 2 wk*	PCN G, 24 mU/24 h IV 6 wk or Ceftriaxone, 2 g/24 h IV/IM 6 wk plus Gentamicin 1 mg/kg IV/IM q8h for 6 wk	PCN G, 24 mU/24 h IV 6 wk or Ceftriaxone, 2 g/24 h IV/IM 6wk plus Gentamicin 1mg/kg IV/IM q8h for 6 wk
If Patient is Allergic to PCN		
Vancomycin, 30 mg/kg q24h IV divided in 2 doses, no more than 2 g /24 h unless concentration inappropriately low 4 wk	Vancomycin, 30 mg/kg q24h IV divided in 2 doses, no more than 2 g /24 h unless concentration inappropriately low 6 wk	Vancomycin, 30 mg/kg q24h IV divided in 2 doses, no more than 2 g /24 h unless concentration inappropriately low 6 wk plus Gentamicin, 1 mg/kg q8h IV/IM 4–6 wk

Abbreviations: MIC = minimal inhibitory concentration; PCN = penicillin.
[a] Combination therapy has not demonstrated superior cure rates compared to monotherapy

susceptible to penicillin (MIC ≤0.12 µg/mL) and can be treated with aqueous penicillin G or ceftriaxone for 4 weeks. The addition of gentamicin can shorten therapy to 2 weeks, but such therapy should be reserved for patients with normal renal function and uncomplicated (ie, short duration, minimal distal disease) endocarditis. The same regimen applies to the therapy of streptococcal PVE, but the duration of treatment is prolonged to 6 weeks. For streptococci with moderate resistance to penicillin (MIC >0.12–≤ 0.5 µg/ mL), the addition of gentamicin for the first 2 weeks is always recommended to prevent relapse. Infective endocarditis caused by highly penicillin-resistant viridans streptococci (MIC >0.5 µg/ mL) and newly named *Abiotrophia defectiva* and *Granulicatella* species (formally known as nutritionally variant streptococci) are difficult to treat and should be treated with the same regimen as recommended for enterococcal endocarditis. Vancomycin is an option only for penicillin-allergic patient.

Staphylococci

Most strains of *S. aureus* are resistant to penicillin by virtue of β-lactamase production. Therapy is based on antistaphylococcal penicillins (ie, nafacillin, oxacillin) or first-generation cephalosporins (ie, cefazolin) administered for 6 weeks (Table 36.3). The addition of gentamicin to nafcillin enhances the rate of killing of bacteria and the sterilization of blood, but no clinical advantage results from longer than 3- to 5-day use, whereas toxicity increases significantly. Currently its use continues to be optional. Vancomycin should be used only in cases of serious β-lactam allergy (immunoglobulin E [IgE]-mediated hypersensitivity) or if a methicillin-resistant isolate is suspected or documented; otherwise cefazolin can be substituted for nafcillin for a less frequent dosing regimen. Increasing rates in methicillin-resistant strains in both hospital and community obligates the use of vancomycin as empiric antibiotic therapy. In a

Table 36.3 Antibiotic Therapy for Staphylococcal Endocarditis

S. aureus or Coagulase-Negative Staphylococcus Native Valves	*S. aureus* or Coagulase-Negative Staphylococcus Prosthetic Valves
Methicillin Sensitive	
Nafcillin, 12 g q24h IV 6 wk plus (optional) gentamicin, 1 mg/kg q8h IV 3–5 days or Cefazolin, 6 g q24h IV 6 wk plus (optional) Gentamicin, 1 mg/kg q8h IV 3–5 days	Nafcillin, 12 g q24h IV ≥6 wk plus Rifampin, 300 mg PO q8h ≥6 wk plus Gentamicin, 1 mg/kg q8h IV first 2 wk
Methicillin-Resistant or PCN Allergic	
Vancomycin, 30 mg/kg q24h IV divided in 2 doses, no more than 2 g/24 h unless concentration inappropriately low 6 wk	Vancomycin, 30 mg/kg q24h IV divided in 2 doses ≥6 wk plus Rifampin, 300 mg PO q8h ≥6 wk plus Gentamicin, 1 mg/kg q8h IV first 2 wk
Daptomycin, 6 mg/kg q24 IV 4–6 wk (for right-sided endocarditis only).	

recent noninferiority clinical trial, daptomycin (a cyclic lipopeptide; 6 mg/kg intravenously daily) has been approved by the U.S. Food and Drug Administration (FDA) for treatment of *S. aureus* bacteremia and right-sided endocarditis caused by methicillin susceptible *S. aureus* (MSSA) or MRSA. Although another new agent, linezolid, (a bacteriostatic oxazolidinone) has been suggested to be equivalent or superior to vancomycin in certain MRSA infections, data are limited in treatment for infective endocarditis in humans at the present time. In a patient with uncomplicated right-sided *S. aureus* endocarditis (only tricuspid valve involved) resulting from IVDA, 2 weeks of intravenous nafcillin with gentamicin for 2 weeks may be adequate therapy. These findings do not extrapolate to treatment with vancomycin.

In prosthetic valve endocarditis, the most common causative agents are *S. aureus* and coagulase-negative *S. epidermidis* (see Table 36.3). Both species are commonly resistant to β-lactam antibiotics; thus, until sensitivity to methicillin can be confirmed, vancomycin should be used as the primary therapy of native valve endocarditis. Bacteriologic failures are common, and surgical valve replacement may be necessary.

Enterococci and Vancomycin-Resistant Enterococcus

The enterococcus is becoming a serious gram-positive nosocomial pathogen. Enterococci are streptococci intrinsically resistant to the bactericidal effect of penicillin or vancomycin. Therefore, for the treatment of endocarditis, the addition of aminoglycoside is needed to promote bactericidal effect. Cephalosporins are always inactive against enterococci and cannot be used interchangeably with penicillin in this setting. Emergence in nosocomial settings of strains of enterococci highly resistant to penicillin, aminoglycosides, and vancomycin has seriously compromised the efficacy of available treatment. To guide the choice of the most effective regimen, all enterococcal isolates in cases of suspected IE should be subjected to in vitro sensitivity testing.

The established course of treatment for patients with native valve endocarditis caused by a community-acquired enterococcus (ie, one relatively sensitive to penicillin and susceptible to synergistic killing with aminoglycosides) is 4 to 6 weeks of penicillin (18 to 30 mU $\times 10^6$ U/day) or vancomycin, 1 g every 12 hours, plus gentamicin, 3 mg/kg/day in divided doses (Table 36.4). Patients with prosthetic valve infection should have therapy prolonged for minimal of 6 weeks. When enterococcal strains are gentamicin-resistant, streptomycin should be used as alternative combination therapy whenever susceptible. For enterococci highly resistant to ampicillin and highly resistant to aminoglycosides, treatment is based on vancomycin alone. The relapse rate may increase substantially.

Vancomycin-resistant enterococcus (VRE) now accounts for 15% of infections in critical care units. *Enterococcus faecium* is much more

Table 36.4 Antibiotic Therapy for Enterococcal and PCN-Resistant Strain Streptococcal Endocarditis

Enterococci and PCN-Resistant Strain Streptococci, Native Valves or Prosthetic Valves[a]
Penicillin Sensitive
PNC G, 18–30 mU/24 h IV plus gentamicin, 1 mg/kg q8h IV 4–6 wk or Ampicillin, 12 g q24h IV, plus gentamicin, 1 mg/kg IV q8h 4–6 wk
Penicillin Resistant or PCN Allergic (β-lactamase-producing strain)
Ampicillin-sulbactam, 12 g q24h IV 6 wk, plus gentamicin, 1 mg/kg IV q8h 6 wk or Vancomycin, 30 mg/kg q24h IV divided in 2 doses 6 wk, plus gentamicin[b], 1 mg/kg q8h IV 6 wk
Enterococci PCN and Vancomycin-Resistant Native Valves or Prosthetic Valves

E. faecium	*E. faecalis*
Linezolid, 600 mg IV/PO q12h ≥ 8 wk or Quinapristin-dalfopristin 22.5 mg/kg 24 h divided in 3 doses ≥8 wk	Imipenem/cilastatin, 2 g q24h IV ≥8 wk, plus ampicillin 12 g q24h IV ≥8 wk or Ceftriaxone, 2 g q24h IV/IM ≥8 wk, plus ampicillin 12 g q24 h IV ≥8 wk

Abbreviation: PCN = penicillin.
[a] Prosthetic valve or intracardiac material; recommended therapy for 6 weeks.
[b] Substitute gentamicin for streptomycin, 15 mg/kg q24 h IV/IM divided in 2 doses 4–6 wk, whenever enterococci are gentamicin resistant but streptomycin sensitive.

commonly vancomycin resistant than *E. faecalis*. Occasional cases of VRE endocarditis have been reported. Few therapeutic options are available for the treatment of multiply resistant enterococci, thus there is no standard regimen for VRE endocarditis. From compassionate use data, linezolid resulted in a cure rate of 77% in VRE infective endocarditis. Clinical success rates for treatment of vancomycin-resistant *E. faecium* (VREF) infections with quinapristine-dalfopristin (synercid) are as high as 73%, although data are extremely limited with regard to VREF endocarditis. Double β-lactam combination therapies have a synergistic bactericidal activity in vitro and in vivo for *E. faecalis*; these combinations have been used to treat high-level aminoglycoside-resistant strains and some cases of multidrug-resistant *E. faecalis* endocarditis (Table 36.4). The clinical efficacy of daptomycin for VRE infective endocarditis is as yet undetermined. Studies evaluating such agents are warranted. Figure 36.2 presents an algorithm that may be helpful in managing enterococcal endocarditis.

Other Treatment Considerations

Gram-negative organisms of the HACEK group grow slowly on standard culture medium and may require >2 weeks of incubation; susceptibility testing is therefore difficult. β-lactamase–

Table 36.5 Antibiotic Therapy for Endocarditis Caused by HACEK[a] Microorganisms

Native and Prosthetic Valve
Ceftriaxone 2 g/24 h IV/IM 4 wk or Ampicillin-sulbactam 12 g/24 h IV 4 wk or Ciprofloxacin 1 g/24 h PO or 400 mg q12h IV 4 wk (need close monitoring)

[a] *Haemophilus parainfluenzae, H. influenzae, H. aphrophilus, H. paraphrophilus, A. actinomycetemcomitans, C. hominis, E. corrodens, K. kingae, and K. denitrificans*

producing HACEK organisms have emerged; therefore ampicillin can no longer be recommended. At this time, third- or fourth-generation cephalosporines or ampicillin-sulbactam should be the regimen of choice. Fluoroquinolones (ciprofloxacin, levofloxacin, gatifloxacin, or moxifloxacin) could be used as an alternative regimen in patients who cannot tolerate β-lactam therapy, although there are limited clinical data (Table 36.5).

Most streptococci other than viridans or enterococci (ie, pneumococcus, group A to G streptococci) remain susceptible to penicillin, but therapy before the availability of their susceptibility profile must take into

ENTEROCOCCAL ENDOCARDITIS

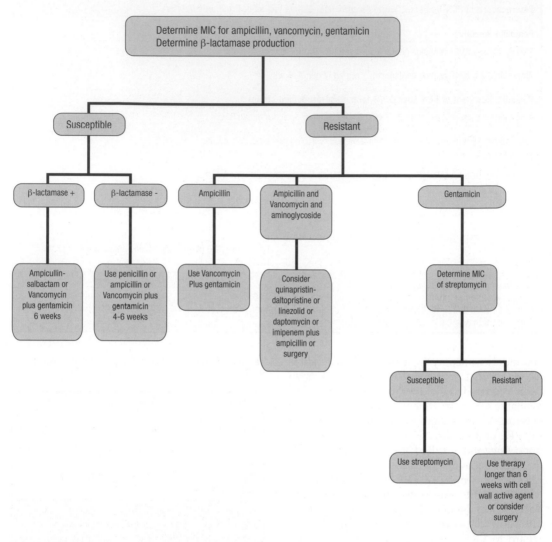

Figure 36.2. Algorithm for the treatment of enterococcal endocarditis.

account the possibility of a resistance isolate. Although pneumococcal endocarditis is rare (≤1%), its fulminant course and the increasing incidence of penicillin and cephalosporin resistance have mandated vancomycin with or without ceftriaxone as the empiric regimen. Nongroup A strains of streptococci may need gentamicin in addition to penicillin to ensure synergistic killing. *Enterobacteriaceae* and *P. aeruginosa* are uncommon causes of endocarditis. Therapy should be determined by in vitro susceptibility testing. Adequacy of the regimen may require monitoring via serum bactericidal activity.

Treatment of PVE is generally longer than native valve IE. If infection occurs within a

year after surgery, empiric therapy should particularly target *S. epidermidis* and *S. aureus*. Combination triple therapy is recommended (Table 36.3) based on limited clinical data, but many experimental animal models of endocarditis have shown benefit of rapid sterilization of vegetation with the additional use of rifampin. Thus, when PVE is clinically suspected, the combination of vancomycin, gentamicin, and rifampin should be initiated empirically. For staphylococcal infection, nafcillin or oxacillin should be substituted for vancomycin if susceptibility results allow. If the pathogen is resistant to all available aminoglycosides, a fluoroquinolone may be used as an alternative. Duration of aminoglycoside use

Table 36.6 Antibiotic Therapy for Culture-Negative Endocarditis

Native Valve	Prosthetic Valve
Ampicillin-sulbactam 12g/24h IV 4–6 wk plus Gentamicin 1 mg/kg IV/IM q8h for 4–6 wk or Vancomycin 30 mg/kg q24h IV divided in 2 doses 4–6 wk plus Gentamicin 1mg/kg IV/IM q8h for 4–6 wk plus Ciprofloxacin 1g/24h PO or 400 mg q12h IV 4–6 wk	**Early infection (≤1 y)** Vancomycin 30mg/kg q24h IV divided in 2 doses 6 wk plus Gentamicin 1mg/kg IV/IM q8h 2 wk plus Cefepime 2 g q8h IV 6 wk plus Rifampin 300 mg q8h PO/IV 6 wk
If _Bartonella_ suspected, Ceftriaxone, 2 g/24 h IV/IM 6 wk plus Gentamicin 1mg/kg IV/IM q8h 2 wk with or without Doxycycline 100 mg PO/IV q12h 6 wk	

is similar to recommendations for infection of native valves.

Due to higher mortality and valvular complications of PVE, especially when due to _S. aureus_, surgery is more frequently considered than in native valve infection; consultation with both infectious diseases and cardiothoracic surgery is advisable.

Fungal endocarditis is poorly responsive even to the gold standard treatment, that is, amphotericin B for ≥6 weeks. Surgical valve replacement is usually necessary. In patients with hemodynamically stable valves and candida or aspergillus infections susceptible to imidazoles, long-term suppression with fluconazole (_Candida albicans_) or itraconazole (_Aspergillus_ species) may be the preferred therapeutic choice. In prosthetic valve endocarditis, valve replacement is usually mandatory regardless of the fungal organism.

Culture-negative endocarditis (CNE) remains an important category of infective endocarditis and therapeutic choice often is challenging. Administration of antibiotics before collection of blood cultures and fastidious bacterial pathogens are commonly encountered etiology in CNE. Epidemiological features should always guide the choice of therapy (Table 36.6).

Traditionally, oral regimens have not had a role in the treatment of endocarditis because adequate antibiotic serum levels could not be achieved. With newer agents such as the quinolones, the serum concentration after oral administration is equivalent to that seen with parenteral dosing. These agents have been used for the oral treatment of highly susceptible gram-negative pathogens. Also, a 4-week oral regimen of ciprofloxacin plus rifampin has

Table 36.7 Cardiac Conditions Warranting Endocarditis Prophylaxis

Prophylaxis Recommended
Prosthetic heart valves Previous history of endocarditis Certain congenital heart conditions, including • unrepaired or incompletely repaired cyanotic congenital heart disease, including those with palliative shunts and conduits • a completely repaired congenital heart defect with prosthetic material or device, whether placed by surgery or by catheter intervention, during the first six months after the procedure • any repaired congenital heart defect with residual defect at the site or adjacent to the site of a prosthetic patch or a prosthetic device Valvular disease in cardiac transplant recipients.
Prophylaxis no Longer Recommended
Mitral valve prolapse Rheumatic heart disease Bicuspid valve disease Calcified aortic stenosis Congenital heart conditions such as ventricular septal defect, atrial septal defect and hypertrophic cardiomyopathy.

been used to treat uncomplicated right-sided endocarditis in IVDAs. Close monitoring of patients with adequate gastrointestinal function and compliance is mandatory. Clinical outcome data are limited.

PROPHYLAXIS

The American Heart Association's (AHA) most recent guideline in April 2007 made substantial changes in recommending preventive antibiotics. Most individuals will no longer need prophylactic antibiotics before dental procedures

Table 36.8 Procedures Warranting Endocarditis Prophylaxis

Prophylaxis Recommended
All dental procedures that involve manipulation of gingival tissue or the periapical region of teeth or perforation of the oral mucosa
Tonsillectomy and/or adenoidectomy
Invasive respiratory procedures to treat infection
Surgical procedures involving infected skin and soft tissues

Prophylaxis not Recommended
Injection of local intraoral anesthetic through non-infected tissue
Taking dental radiograph
Placement of removable prosthodontic or orthodontic appliances
Adjustment orthodontic appliances
Placement of orthodontic brackets
Shedding of deciduous teeth
Bleeding from trauma to the lips or oral mucosa
Endotracheal intubation
Bronchoscopy without biopsy
Tympanectomy tube insertion
Transesophageal echocardiogram
Gastrointestinal or genitourinary procedures
Vaginal delivery or vaginal hysterectomy
Cesarean section
Dilatation and curettage
Ear and body piercing
Tattooing

Table 36.9 AHA-Recommended Prophylactic Regimens

Single Dose 30–60 Minutes Before Procedure
Oral   Amoxicillin 2g
Unable to take oral medications   Ampicillin 2g IV/IM or cefazolin/ceftriaxone* 1g IV/IM
Allergic to penicillin   Clindamycin 600mg or Azithromycin/clarithromycin 500 mg or cephalexine 2g
Allergic to penicillin and unable to take oral medications   Clindamycin 600 mg IV or cefazolin/ceftriaxone* 1g IV/IM
* Use only if non-IgE mediated allergic reaction

to prevent infective endocarditis. This recommendation is based on recent evidence that suggests that the risks of prophylactic antibiotics outweigh the benefits for most patients. Data also suggest that endocarditis is much more likely to result from random bacteremias associated with daily activities than from dental, gastrointestinal, or genitourinary instrumentation; currently, there is no compelling evidence to link endocarditis risk with bacteremia from invasive and dental procedures. The new guidelines consider only cardiac conditions with the highest risk of adverse outcome from endocarditis for which prophylaxis should be recommended (Table 36.7). The procedures are limited to dental and invasive respiratory procedures and surgery of infected soft tissues (Table 36.8).

The antibiotic regimens are listed in Table 36.9. Prophylaxis for gastrointestinal and genitourinary procedures are no longer recommended because of insufficient data to support current practice.

SURGICAL INDICATIONS IN THE MANAGEMENT OF INFECTIVE ENDOCARDITIS

In certain cases of infective endocarditis, surgery is associated with improved patient outcomes. Some of these indications are strongly supported by evidence. Other indications are more relative and have conflicting evidence, but expert opinion often favors surgical intervention (Table 36.10). Congestive heart failure resulting from acute aortic insufficiency remains the major indication for immediate valve replacement because of the unacceptable high mortality rate in medically treated patients. Nonresponse to antimicrobial therapy may mandate valve removal if no alternative source for the continued bacteremia or fungemia is found. Fungal endocarditis on a prosthetic valve almost always requires valve replacement. With aggressive preoperative and postoperative antibiotic therapy, valve replacement with a mechanical prosthesis during active IE is a safe procedure. The risk of relapse of endocarditis in a newly implanted prosthetic valve is minimal.

Local cardiac complications of IE may require surgical intervention. Transesophageal echocardiography is a powerful tool for detection of valvular dehiscence, rupture, fistula, perforation, perivalvular extension of abscess, a large abscess, or a large vegetation (>10 mm) on an anterior mitral valve leaflet. Because large vegetations tend to embolize, valve replacement or vegetectomy may be indicated in a patient with suspected or documented recurrent CNS or large vessel emboli.

Anticoagulation during IE is a considerable risk for intracerebral hemorrhage. Anticoagulation is not recommended as a therapeutic option; however, maintenance anticoagulation in a patient with a prosthetic

Table 36.10 Indications for Surgical Intervention in Native and Prosthetic Valve Infective Endocarditis

Surgery Usually Recommended	Surgery to Be Considered
Congestive heart failure from acute aortic insufficiency	Large (>10 mm) anterior mitral leaflet vegetation
Infective endocarditis caused by organism that may respond poorly to antimicrobial therapy (eg, fungal or *Brucella* sp.)	Increase in vegetation size despite adequate treatment (after 4 weeks of antibiotic)
Persistent bacteremia after 1 week of adequate antibiotic therapy	Periannular extension on infection or myocardial abscesses
More than one embolic event occurring within the first 2 weeks of antibiotic therapy	IE caused by resistant enterococci species when effective bactericidal therapy is not available
Presence of echocardiography finding consistent with local cardiac complications such as valve dehiscence, large perivalvular abscess, rupture, or perforation of a valve	Uncontrolled infection caused by highly antibiotic-resistant pathogens despite optimal therapy (enterococci or gram-negative bacilli)
Staphylococcus aureus prosthetic valve endocarditis complicated by perivalvular abscess or dehiscence (reduces mortality rates)	
PVE or left-sided IE caused by gram-negative bacteria like *Serratia marcescens, Pseudomonas* sp.	

valve should be continued regardless of the diagnosis of endocarditis because of the risk of mechanical thrombosis.

SUGGESTED READING

Baddour LM, et al. Infective endocarditis: diagnosis, antimicrobial therapy, and management of complications: a statement for healthcare professionals from the Committee on Rheumatic Fever, Endocarditis, and Kawasaki disease, Council on Cardiovascular Disease in the Young, and the Councils on Clinical Cardiology, Stroke, and Cardiovascular Surgery and Anesthesia. *Circulation.* 2005;111:e394–e434.

Chu VH, et al. Native valve endocarditis due to coagulase-negative staphylococci: Report of 99 episodes from the International Collaboration on Endocarditis Merged Database. *Clin Infect Dis.* 2004; 39:1527.

Dajani AS, et al. Prevention of bacterial endocarditis: recommendations by the American Heart Association. *JAMA.* 1997; 96:358.

Ellis, ME, et al. Fungal endocarditis: evidence in the world literature, 1965-1995. *Clin Infect Dis.* 2001;32:50–62.

Fowler VG Jr, et al. Daptomycin versus standard therapy for bacteremia and endocarditis caused by *Staphylococcus aureus. N Engl J Med.* 2006;355:653–665.

Fowler VG Jr, et al. Infective endocarditis due to *S. aureus* bacteremia: 59 prospectively identified cases with follow-up. *Clin Infect Dis.* 1999;28:106–114.

Miro JM, et al: *Staphylococcus aureus* native valve infective endocarditis: report of 566 episodes from the International Collaboration on Endocarditis Merged Database, *Clin Infect Dis.* 2005;41:507–514.

Mylonakis E, Calderwoal SB. Infective endocarditis in adults. *N Engl J Med.* 2001;345:1318–1330.

Rybak MJ, Coyle EA. Vancomycin-resistant enterococcus: infectious endocarditis treatment, *Curr infect Dis Rep.* 1999;1:(2): 148–152.

Stevens MP, Edmond MB. Endocarditis due to vancomycin-resistant enterococci: case report and review of literature. *Clin Infect Dis.* 2005;41:1134–1142.

Strom BL, et al. Dental and cardiac risk factors for infective endocarditis: A population-based, case-control study. *Ann Intern Med.* 1998;129:761–769.

Wilson W, et al. Prevention of infective endocarditis: guidelines from the American Heart Association. *J Am Dent Assoc.* 2007; 138(6) 739–45, 747–60.

37. Acute Pericarditis

Richard A. Martinello and Michael Cappello

INTRODUCTION

The pericardium serves to protect the heart from physiologic changes in intracardiac pressure related to respiration and postural change, and it may also serve to augment the mechanical function of the cardiac chambers. The pericardium is composed of a visceral layer that directly adheres to the epicardium and a parietal layer separated by 10 to 35 mL of serous fluid.

EPIDEMIOLOGY AND ETIOLOGIC AGENTS

Both infectious and noninfectious processes have been identified as causes of pericarditis (inflammation of the pericardium). Most cases are due to viral pathogens and are self-limited, and the specific pathogen remains unidentified. In one series, pericarditis was diagnosed in 5% of adults presenting for emergency care due to chest pain that was not associated with myocardial infarction. Because the majority of cases of acute pericarditis are caused by viruses, most patients present in the spring and summer months, overlapping with the peak prevalence of enteroviruses. During the winter months, influenza virus is a frequent cause of pericarditis, whereas pericarditis due to bacterial or atypical pathogens occurs throughout the year.

In areas of the world where the incidence of infection with *M. tuberculosis* remains high, tuberculosis is responsible for more than 50% of cases of acute pericarditis. Tuberculosis should be considered in persons who have spent significant time in endemic countries, including international adoptees, immigrants, and refugees. Patients with human immuno-deficiency virus (HIV) are more likely to experience nonpulmonary manifestations of tuberculosis, such as pericarditis, and have been shown to experience higher rates of mortality due to tuberculous pericarditis than their non-HIV counterparts.

Pericarditis may also develop following cardiothoracic surgery. This may be due to a bacterial surgical site infection or postpericardiotomy syndrome, a noninfectious inflammatory condition that generally develops 2 to 6 months following cardiac surgery. In immunocompromised hosts, the range of potential pathogens that can cause pericarditis is quite broad and includes viruses, bacteria, fungi/yeasts, and parasites (Table 37.1) Acute pericarditis can also be due to noninfectious causes (Table 37.2).

PATHOGENESIS

Microbial pathogens may gain entry into the pericardial space by direct extension from the chest (eg, in the context of pneumonia or mediastinitis), through direct extension from the heart itself (eg, endocarditis), through hematogenous spread (bacteremia or viremia), or via direct inoculation (eg, surgery, trauma). The presence of an adjacent or concurrent infection, as well as a history of recent surgery or trauma, may provide significant clues to specific pathogens. For example, purulent pericarditis due to *N. meningitidis* has been diagnosed in patients with concurrent bacterial meningitis. In a review of 162 children with purulent pericarditis, all but 10 patients had at least one additional site of infection, suggesting that isolated cardiac disease occurs infrequently in those with purulent pericarditis. In cases where either *S. aureus* or *H. influenzae* type B was the responsible pathogen, pneumonia, osteomyelitis, and cellulitis were the most frequently identified additional sites of infection. Tuberculous pericarditis usually occurs in the absence of identifiable pulmonary disease, which suggests that the pathogenesis involves the spread of mycobacteria from adjacent mediastinal lymph nodes into the pericardium.

The inflammatory response in the pericardial space leads to extravasation of additional pericardial fluid, polymorphonuclear white blood cells, and monocytes. During bacterial or fungal pericarditis, the inflammatory process may be sufficient to lead to loculation and fibrosis. Significant fibrosis may lead to constrictive pericarditis, which is manifest

Table 37.1 Infectious Causes of Acute Pericarditis

Viruses
Coxsackievirus A
Coxsackievirus B[a]
Echoviruses
Mumps virus
Influenza viruses
Cytomegalovirus
Herpes simplex virus
Hepatitis B virus
Measles virus
Adenovirus
Human immune deficiency virus
Varicella virus

Bacteria
Staphylococcus aureus[a]
Streptococcus pneumoniae[a]
Haemophilus influenzae[a]
Neisseria meningitidis[a]
Streptococcus pyogenes
α-Hemolytic streptococci
Klebsiella spp.
Pseudomonas aeruginosa
Escherichia coli
Salmonella spp.

Anaerobes
Listeria monocytogenes
Neisseria gonorrhoeae
Coxiella burnettii
Actinomyces spp.
Nocardia spp.
Mycoplasma pneumoniae

Mycobacteria
Mycobacterium tuberculosis
Mycobacterium avium complex

Fungi
Histoplasma capsulatum
Blastomyces dermatitidis
Candida spp.
Aspergillus spp.
Cryptococcus neoformans
Coccidioidomycosis

Parasites
Toxoplasma gondii
Entamoeba histolytica
Toxocara canis
Schistosomes

[a] Most common causes of acute bacterial or viral pericarditis in North America.

Table 37.2 Major Noninfectious Causes of Acute Pericarditis

Collagen Vascular Diseases
Systemic lupus erythematosus
Rheumatoid arthritis
Scleroderma
Rheumatic fever

Drugs
Procainamide
Hydralazine

Myocardial Injury
Acute myocardial infarction
Chest trauma (penetrating or blunt)
Postpericardiotomy syndrome

Sarcoidosis

Familial Mediterranean Fever

Uremia

Neoplasia
Primary
Metastic

Irradiation

pericardial space prevents adequate right atrial filling and leads to reduced stroke volume, low output cardiac failure, and shock. If the accumulation of pericardial fluid occurs more slowly, as is common with viral pericarditis, large amounts may be present without hemodynamic effect.

SYMPTOMS AND CLINICAL MANIFESTATIONS

Chest pain is the most common presenting symptom of acute pericarditis. Due to the relationship between the phrenic nerve and pericardium, pain resulting from inflammation of the pericardium may be retrosternal with radiation to the shoulder and neck or may localize between the scapulae. Often, the pain is worsened by swallowing or deep inspiration or when the patient is supine. Dyspnea is also a common presenting symptom. If pericarditis has resulted from contiguous spread of bacteria or fungi from an adjoining structure, the signs and symptoms of the primary infectious process may predominate. Purulent pericarditis due to a bacterial pathogen tends to be more acute and severe in nature, whereas viral pericarditis is typically of lesser severity. Symptoms of tuberculous pericarditis tend to be insidious in presentation.

by signs and symptoms associated with compromised ventricular filing. The rapid accumulation of exudative fluid, as is often seen in purulent pericarditis, frequently leads to hemodynamic changes. Cardiac tamponade occurs when increased fluid within the

Clinical Syndromes – Heart and Blood Vessels

In infants, the presenting signs and symptoms of pericarditis may be nonspecific and include fever, tachycardia, and irritability. Older children may complain of chest and/or abdominal discomfort. A study by Carmichael et al. in 1951 showed that more than half of patients diagnosed with "nonspecific" pericarditis of presumed viral origin described a respiratory illness preceding the diagnosis of pericarditis by 2 to 3 weeks.

On physical exam, nearly all patients with pericarditis, regardless of cause, will have tachycardia. Those with bacterial pericarditis are also likely to have fever and tachypnea, as well as possible evidence of at least one additional site of infection (eg, pneumonia, surgical site infection, and osteomyelitis). Perhaps the most characteristic physical finding in acute pericarditis is the presence of a friction rub on cardiac auscultation. The rub may be confused with a high-pitched murmur, particularly when it is only present in systole. Pericardial friction rubs may have as many as three components, which correspond with atrial systole, ventricular systole, and rapid ventricular filling during early diastole. A rub may be best appreciated with the patient leaning forward or even in the knee-chest position. Although more than one component of a pericardial rub may be present, all three components were noted in less than 50% of patients in one case series.

The presence of a pulsus paradoxus or jugular venous distention suggests the possibility of cardiac tamponade, which may require emergent intervention. This is most frequently seen in the presence of a large or rapidly accumulating pericardial effusion but can also result from constrictive disease due to long-standing pericarditis with fibrosis.

DIAGNOSIS

An acutely enlarged cardiac silhouette on chest radiograph, particularly in the absence of increased pulmonary vascularity, suggests the presence of pericardial effusion. However, there may be no radiographic abnormalities detected in patients with small, but rapidly accumulating, effusions, as well as in those with constrictive disease.

Although the pericardium is not involved in the electrical activity of the heart, pericarditis is associated with classic electrocardiographic changes, which are likely due to concomitant inflammatory changes in the epicardium and outer myocardium. Electrocardiographic changes may be present in 50% of patients with acute pericarditis, and the specific changes evolve over time. Elevation or depression of the ST and/or depression of the PR segments may occur early in the disease process (Figure 37.1). Over subsequent days, the ST segment returns to baseline. Late ECG changes in pericarditis include flat or inverted T waves. These EKG changes can be differentiated from those due to myocardial infarction as it is uncommon for T-wave inversions to be detected until the ST segment changes resolve. Large pericardial effusions may result in reduced voltage or electrical alternans due to beat-to-beat variation in the position of the heart within the pericardial fluid.

Echocardiography is the diagnostic study of choice for detecting excess pericardial fluid and is recommended for all patients in whom pericarditis is suspected. In patients with poststernotomy pericarditis, computed tomography (CT) scan and magnetic resonance imaging (MRI) are both extremely useful for identifying mediastinal fluid collections and potential abscesses.

Pericardiocentesis is the most reliable means of determining the etiology of pericarditis. Drainage of pericardial fluid should be performed when there is evidence for cardiac tamponade or a suspicion of tuberculous, neoplastic, or purulent pericarditis. The fluid should be transported quickly to the microbiology laboratory for Gram, acid fast, and silver stains, as well as culture for bacteria (aerobic and anaerobic), fungi, mycobacteria, and viruses. It should also be analyzed for cell count and differential, glucose, total protein, red blood cell count, and cytology. When tuberculous pericarditis is suspected, biopsy of the pericardium for histology is useful, and an adenosine deaminase level should be measured in the pericardial fluid.

For patients in whom a viral etiology is suspected, swabs from the nasopharynx, throat, and rectum should also be sent for culture or polymerase chain reaction (PCR) as these sites are more likely to yield a positive culture for enterovirus than pericardial fluid. In the setting of pneumonia, sputum or tracheal aspirates can be cultured for bacteria, and diagnostic studies for influenza A or B virus should be obtained. Acute and convalescent antibody titers may be measured for the common enterovirus serotypes.

In patients with purulent pericarditis, blood cultures are frequently positive. These patients should be carefully evaluated for other infectious processes, including pneumonia, osteomyelitis, and meningitis. A positive

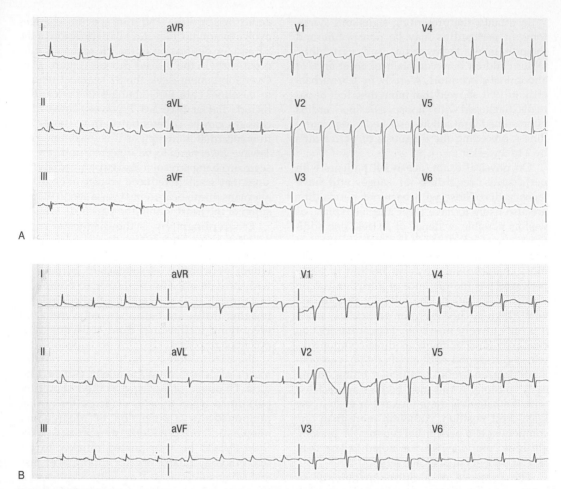

Figure 37.1 (A) Electrocardiogram (EKG) in acute pericarditis. ST segment elevation is noted with an upward concave appearance in all leads except I, aVR, and aVL. PR segment depression is noted in I, II, III, aVF, and the precordial leads (Courtesy Dr. Thuy Le). (B) EKG from the same patient as in A, but 3 days later. Note that PR segment depression persists in II, III, and aVF. Some ST elevation persists but has markedly diminished compared with the initial EKG (Courtesy Dr. Thuy Le).

bacterial culture from one of these alternative sites is strongly suggestive of the identity of the pericardial pathogen.

The diagnosis of tuberculous pericarditis can be particularly challenging. Although a study by Strang et al. found cultures of pericardial fluid to be positive in 75% of suspected cases, results may not be available for weeks. In this setting, pericardial biopsy may yield a more rapid diagnosis of *M. tuberculosis* infection, particularly if the characteristic granulomatous changes are present. Cigielski et al. have recently shown that a PCR-based assay was nearly as sensitive as culture (81% vs 93%) for detecting *M. tuberculosis* in pericardial biopsy specimens. The obvious advantage to PCR is the speed with which results can be obtained, although false-positive results may occur more frequently than with culture.

TREATMENT

Urgent drainage of pericardial fluid should be considered in any patient with a possible diagnosis of purulent pericarditis or if hemodynamic compromise is identified. The outcome in these patients is generally poor without surgical drainage, even when appropriate antibiotics are administered. Likewise, purulent infections contiguous with the mediastinum should be drained. If the Gram stain of pericardial fluid does not suggest an etiologic agent in the setting of purulent pericarditis, then empiric antibiotic coverage should be initiated while awaiting the results of cultures. The antibiotic(s) for empiric coverage should be chosen according to whether the patient has evidence for a contiguous site of infection, history of recent cardiothoracic surgery, trauma, or other relevant risk factors. In patients with community-acquired purulent pericarditis and no history of antecedent surgery or trauma, empiric treatment directed at *S. aureus* (oxacillin) and common respiratory pathogens (ceftriaxone) would be appropriate. Depending on the prevalence of methicillin-resistant *S. aureus* within the community, vancomycin may be appropriate for initial empiric therapy.

If a viral etiology is suspected, nonsteroidal anti-inflammatory drugs (NSAIDs) are used as first-line therapy and have been found to relieve chest discomfort in 85% to 90% of patients. Typically, ibuprofen (1600 mg to 3200 mg divided per day) is the drug of choice due to its low incidence of adverse events compared with other NSAIDs. Some experts favor the use of aspirin (650 mg to 975 mg every 6 to 8 hours) in patients who have experienced a recent myocardial infarction, as evidence from animal studies have led to concern that other NSAIDs may impair scar formation. Indomethacin has been shown to decrease coronary artery blood flow and therefore should be avoided in persons with coronary artery disease.

Colchicine (600 mg to 1000 mg twice daily, initially then 500 mg twice daily) has been shown to effectively decrease the incidence of recurrent pericarditis. Some experts recommend its use during first episodes of pericarditis if NSAIDs are unable to completely abate symptoms. A recent study comparing treatment with aspirin plus colchicine versus aspirin alone in patients with acute pericarditis demonstrated that those receiving both drugs experienced a significantly greater rate of symptom control at 72 hours and a significantly lower rate of recurrence at 18 months. Treatment with systemic corticosteroids has been found to decrease inflammation and control symptoms effectively but appears to be associated with greater rates of relapse and therefore should be reserved for the most recalcitrant cases.

It is recommended that patients avoid strenuous activity during the initial weeks after diagnosis of acute pericarditis, but patients may then reintroduce activities after complete resolution of symptoms. Treatment with NSAIDs, with or without cholchicine, is generally continued for 4 weeks and 3 months, respectively.

Tuberculous pericarditis should be treated with four active antimicrobial agents until susceptibilities are known. The recommended duration of therapy for pericarditis caused by *M. tuberculosis* is 6 to 12 months, with the longer durations reserved for patients who appear to improve more slowly. Though many experts recommend concurrent use of corticosteroids to decrease the risk of cardiac tamponade and death, currently available data fail to conclusively support corticosteroid use. Likewise, it is not clear that there is a role for routine pericardial drainage or pericardiectomy in the treatment of tuberculous pericarditis.

COMPLICATIONS

Increased intrapericardial pressure due to an accumulating effusion may result in cardiac tamponade. Tamponade should be suspected if the patient's hemodynamic status is unstable, heart sounds are diminished, jugular venous pressure is raised, or if pulsus paradoxus is present. Echocardiography may note significant variation in blood flow across the mitral and tricuspid valves with respiration and collapse of the right-sided chambers during diastole. Drainage of the pericardial effusion is essential in the setting of purulent pericarditis or in the presence of tamponade. Patients with purulent pericarditis should be treated with a combination of both antimicrobial therapy and drainage. High mortality rates have been observed for patients with purulent pericarditis who have received only medical or surgical management.

A minority of patients may experience recurrent pericarditis involving reaccumulation of the pericardial effusion, fever, and chest pain. These episodes may relapse and remit for several years and are most commonly diagnosed in patients with prior viral pericarditis. Recurrent episodes are rarely complicated by either tamponade or constriction and are effectively treated with NSAIDs with or without cholchicine. Corticosteroids have been used in patients with more severe manifestations, in which case pericardiectomy should be considered.

Constrictive pericarditis occurs due to the development of a thickened fibrous exudate within the pericardium, and the pericardium itself may calcify. The reduced compliance of the pericardial sac may impair diastolic filling and result in hemodynamic compromise. Constrictive pericarditis has most commonly been associated with antecedent tuberculous pericarditis, cardiac surgery, and radiation-induced pericarditis, though patients with a history of prior pericarditis of any etiology are at risk for developing constrictive disease. Constrictive pericarditis typically presents within 3 to 12 months of the initial episode, though the time interval may be days to years. Less severe cases may be managed medically by careful monitoring of the patient's fluid status, but pericardiectomy remains the definitive therapy.

SUGGESTED READING

Adler Y, Finkelstein Y, Guindo J, et al. Colchicine treatment for recurrent pericarditis: a decade of experience. *Circulation*. 1998;97:2183–2185.

Imazio M, Demichelis B, Parrini I, et al. Management, risk factors, and outcomes in recurrent pericarditis. *Am J Cardiol*. 2005;96:736–739.

Lange RA, Hillis LD. Clinical practice: acute pericarditis. *N Engl J Med*. 2004;351:2195–2202.

Levy PY, Corey R, Berger P, et al. Etiologic diagnosis of 204 pericardial effusions. *Medicine (Baltimore)*. 2003;82:385–391.

Little WC, Freeman GL. Pericardial disease. *Circulation*. 2006;113:1622–1632.

Mayosi BM, Wiysonge CS, Ntsekhe M, et al. Clinical characteristics and initial management of patients with tuberculous pericarditis in the HIV era: the Investigation of the Management of Pericarditis in Africa (IMPI Africa) registry. *BMC Infect Dis*. 2006;6:2.

Ntsekhe M, Wiysonge C, Volmink JA, Commerford PJ, Mayosi BM. Adjuvant corticosteroids for tuberculous pericarditis: promising, but not proven. *QJM*. 2003;96:593–599.

Oakley CM. Myocarditis, pericarditis and other pericardial diseases. *Heart*. 2000;84:449–454.

Permanyer-Miralda G. Acute pericardial disease: approach to the aetiologic diagnosis. *Heart*. 2004;90:252–254.

Soler-Soler J, Sagrista-Sauleda J, Permanyer-Miralda G. Relapsing pericarditis. *Heart*. 2004;90:1364–1368.

Spodick DH. Acute pericarditis: current concepts and practice. *JAMA*. 2003;289:1150–1153.

38. Myocarditis

Catherine Diamond and Jeremiah G. Tilles

ETIOLOGY

The majority of cases of idiopathic lymphocytic myocarditis (ILM) in the United States and Western Europe are thought to be viral in origin (Table 38.1) but there is considerable etiologic variation depending on the geographic location, season, and age of the host. The most commonly associated viruses are enteroviruses, particularly coxsackie B viruses. In research studies, enteroviral genomic sequences have been detected in approximately 25% of endomyocardial biopsies (EMB) from patients with either active myocarditis or dilated cardiomyopathy. Adenovirus and parvovirus are also common, particularly in children. Hepatitis C virus (HCV), echovirus, influenza virus, human immunodeficiency virus (HIV), and herpesviruses such as cytomegalovirus (CMV), Epstein–Barr virus (EBV), herpes simplex virus (HSV), and varicella zoster virus (VZV) also are among the more frequent viral etiologies. The myocardium sometimes demonstrates more than one virus by polymerase chain reaction (PCR) exam, but concurrent or past viral infection unrelated to the current myocarditis may be the cause of such findings. In the 2003 U.S. government program in which smallpox (vaccinia) vaccine was administered to approximately 38000 potential first responders during a bioterrorism event, the incidence of myo/pericarditis was 5.5 per 10000 vaccinees. Nonviral infectious causes such as *Corynebacterium diphtheriae* (diphtheria), *Borrelia burgdorferi* (Lyme disease), and American trypanosomiasis (Chagas disease) are found in the appropriate epidemiologic setting. Noninfectious causes (Table 38.2), such as sarcoidosis, peripartum, and drug-induced myocarditis and celiac disease, can manifest myocarditis. In one study of 187 consecutive patients with myocarditis, 9 (4.8%) had celiac disease by duodenal endoscopy and biopsy, compared to 1 of 306 controls without myocarditis (0.3%). All nine had cardiac autoantibodies in the serum and refractory iron deficiency, but none had typical gastrointestinal symptoms of celiac disease. Unfortunately, clinicians usually are unable to determine the cause of most cases of myocarditis.

PATHOGENESIS

The pathogenesis of ILM is complex and can differ depending on the infective agent. The latter typically causes an inflammatory infiltrate and injury to adjacent myocardial cells. Some viruses such as coxsackie B infect the myocytes themselves; others, for instance, CMV and VZV, may injure vascular endothelial cells. Susceptibility to coxsackie B in mice is genetically dependent. In an animal model of viral myocarditis, when 2- to 3-week-old mice receive intraperitoneal injections with coxsackie B virus, the virus can be isolated from the heart and blood during the acute phase of viral replication. Induced proinflammatory cytokines such as tumor necrosis factor-α (TNFα), interlevkin I-β (IL-1-β), and nitric oxide also play an essential role in the pathogenesis of myocarditis. In humans, coronary artery microvascular spasm may cause myocardial hypoperfusion. Cardiac histology during this phase may show inflammatory infiltrates and myocyte necrosis. Further tissue damage occurs later in a percentage of patients with infiltration of T lymphocytes and antibodies to cardiac proteins. Finally, dilated cardiomyopathy (DCM) may develop with fibrosis and ventricular remodeling.

The role of enterovirus in the pathogenesis of myocarditis is an evolving research area. In the late 1990s, investigators reported that adenovirus and coxsackie B virus bind to a common receptor, the coxsackie-adenovirus receptor (CAR), expressed on the surface of cardiac myocytes. This receptor has been considered a potential target for interventional therapy of myocarditis. Investigators also discovered a new mechanism for enteroviral myocyte injury. Enterovirus protease 2A cleaves dystrophin resulting in disruption of the dystrophin–glycoprotein complex, a component of the cytoskeleton of cardiac myocytes. It is also known that genetic defects in dystrophin cause Duchenne's muscular dystrophy, a condition that has been associated with DCM.

Table 38.1 Major Infectious Causes of Myocarditis

Viral

Adenovirus
Dengue
Enterovirus
    Echovirus
    Coxsackie A and B
    Polio
Herpesvirus
    Cytomegalovirus
    Epstein–Barr virus
    Herpes simplex
    Varicella-zoster virus
Hepatitis B or C virus
Human immunodeficiency virus
Influenza A and B
Lymphocytic choriomeningitis virus
Measles
Mumps
Parvovirus
Rabies
Respiratory syncytial virus
Rubeola
Rubella
Vaccinia (smallpox vaccine)
Variola (smallpox)
Yellow fever

Bacterial

Actinomyces
Brucella
Chylamydia psittaci, Chlamydia pneumoniae
Clostridium perfringens
Corynebacterium diphtheriae (diptheria)
Legionella
Listeria monocytogenes
Mycobacterium tuberculosis
Mycoplasma pneumoniae
Staphylococcus aureus
Streptococcus pneumoniae
Vibrio cholerae

Spirochetes

Borrelia burgdorferi (Lyme disease)
Treponema pallidum (Syphilis)

Rickettsial

Coxsiella burnetti (Q fever)
Rickettsia rickettsii (Rocky Mountain spotted fever)
Rickettsia tsutsugamushi (scrub typhus)

Fungal

Endemic fungi (blastomyces, cryptococcus, coccidioides, histoplasma)
Aspergillus
Candida

Protozoal or Parasitic

Entamoeba histolytica
Trypanosoma cruzi (Chagas' disease), *Trypanosoma gambiense, Trypanosoma rhodesiense* (African sleeping sickness)
Toxoplasma gondii
Trichinella spiralis

Table 38.2: Selected Noninfectious Causes of Myocarditis

Immune

Celiac disease
Sarcoidosis
Giant cell myocarditis
Systemic lupus erythematosus
Systemic sclerosis (scleroderma)
Rheumatoid arthritis
Dermatomyositis/polymyositis
Still's disease
Rheumatic fever

Hypereosinophilia

Endocrine

Thyrotoxicosis/hypothyroidism
Pheochromocytoma

Toxic

Alcohol
Cocaine
Emetine
Catecholamines
Arsenic
Carbon monoxide
Heavy metals (copper, lead, iron)
Anthracyclines
Cyclophosphamide

Drug-induced Hypersensitivity

Clozapine
Lithium
Tetracycline
Sulfonamides
Methyldopa
Hydrochlorothiazide

Radiation

Insect Bite (bee, wasp, spider, scorpion)

Peripartum

Kawasaki Disease

EPIDEMIOLOGY, NATURAL HISTORY, AND PROGNOSIS

Because myocarditis is often undiagnosed and the clinical and histologic definitions of the disease are poorly correlated, the actual incidence of histologic myocarditis is unknown. In a study of 1230 cases of initially unexplained cardiomyopathy in the United States, the investigators ultimately attributed 9% to myocarditis. Because of the variation in presentation, it is unclear how often myocarditis progresses to dilated cardiomyopathy. Most patients with mild disease recover completely over time. However, it is known that ventricular arrhythmia may be the sole sign of myocarditis. It has been estimated that myocarditis accounts for 20% of cases of sudden death among active young individuals without known heart disease. In a small fraction of patients who recover from myocarditis, the disease recurs. This occasionally has been related to withdrawal of immunosuppressive therapy.

In the Myocarditis Treatment Trial (MTT) a better left ventricle ejection fraction (LVEF) and shorter duration of disease at baseline and less intensive conventional therapy were predictors of improvement in LVEF. Although there was an initial improvement in mean LVEF from 25% at baseline to 34% at 28 weeks, the mortality rate was found to be 20% at 1 year and 56% at 4 years. The placebo-controlled Intervention in Myocarditis and Acute Cardiomyopathy (IMAC) trial of the effect of intravenous immune globulin (IVIG) on LVEF in adults with recent onset of idiopathic DCM or myocarditis demonstrated 14% improvement of left LVEF with conventional heart failure therapy at 6 months regardless of treatment assignment. The transplant-free survival rate was 88% at 2 years of follow-up. The IMAC and MTT study populations differed in that all MTT but only a minority of IMAC subjects had cellular inflammation by histologic exam. In addition, MTT subjects could have a history of heart failure for up to 2 years at randomization, whereas IMAC subjects had no more than 6 months of symptoms.

Patients with fulminant myocarditis (including severe hemodynamic compromise) have a significantly better transplant-free survival than those with acute myocarditis of ordinary severity (93% vs 45%). Thus, it appears that patients with fulminant myocarditis should be allowed sufficient time for a nonsurgical recovery prior to consideration of heart transplantation. In another study using molecular diagnostics, patients with persistent viral genomes had a reduction in LVEF from 54% to 51%, whereas patients with clearance of the viral genome improved from 50% to 58%, suggesting that viral persistence is a poor prognostic factor. Clinically, elevated baseline mean pulmonary artery pressure may indicate an increased risk of death.

CLINICAL PRESENTATION

Most individuals with myocarditis are asymptomatic or suffer a mild viral prodrome. Some have a subacute presentation with mild ventricular dysfunction and heart failure. A minority of patients present with cardiogenic shock or even sudden death. Others present late with chronic dilated cardiomyopathy. Patients with viral myocarditis may give a history of a preceding flulike illness with symptoms such as muscle aches, fever, or sore throat. Pleuritic chest pain and pericardial effusion with a pericardial friction rub may occur with concomitant pericarditis. The physical examination may be normal or there may be sinus tachycardia (or an S3, S4, or summation gallop) or a mitral regurgitant murmur with ventricular dilation. In contrast with adults, most children with myocarditis present with acute or fulminant disease. Individuals with vaccinia myocarditis will have a history of smallpox vaccination in the prior month. Myocarditis can mimic myocardial ischemia and/or infarction, for instance, in young patients with chest pain and creatinine phosphokinase (CPK) elevation without coronary artery disease. Ventricular tachycardia may be the sole clinical manifestation of myocarditis.

DIAGNOSIS

Table 38.3 includes diagnostic options for infectious myocarditis. There are no laboratory, electrocardiographic (ECG), or echocardiographic features that distinguish between patients with or without histologic evidence of myocarditis. Patients may have an elevated erythrocyte sedimentation rate (ESR) and, less commonly, either leukocytosis or leukopenia. The ECG may show tachycardia, partial or complete heartblock, diffuse ST elevation, T-wave inversion, or nonspecific ST-segment and T-wave abnormalities and can simulate the ECG pattern of either acute myocardial infarction or pericarditis. Holter monitoring may detect atrial or ventricular arrhythmias or ectopy. The MB fraction of creatinine kinase (CK-MB) or troponin may be elevated with myocardial damage.

The clinician may attempt to identify the etiologic virus through serologic testing either by demonstrating a four-fold increase in antibody titer during convalescence or by initial detection of specific immunoglobulin M (IgM). However, because the viral infections that cause myocarditis are common, serologic evidence of infection does not provide hard evidence of causation. It is good practice to use serologies to exclude certain infectious etiologies because some conditions, such as Chagas or HIV-related myocarditis, have specific treatments. Alternatively, it may be possible to isolate an enterovirus by cell culture from a remote site such as from throat or rectal swabs, stool, blood, or cerebrospinal fluid despite a several week lapse in time since the onset of the infection. Virus isolation from

Table 38.3 Diagnostic Clues and Options for Infectious Myocarditis

History
Chest pain
Palpitations
Shortness of breath/cough
Fever
Arthralgias
Antecedent upper respiratory tract infection
Physical Examination
Tachycardia
S3, S4, or summation gallop
Mitral regurgitant murmur
Pericardial friction rub
Congestive heart failure (jugular venous distension, hepatomegaly, edema)
Cardiac Testing
Electrocardiogram
Chest x-ray study
Echocardiogram
Cardiac catheterization
Magnetic resonance imaging
Endomyocardial biopsy
Light microscopy
Polymerase chain reaction
Immunohistochemistry (viral stains, T-cell markers)
Viral cultures
Laboratory Testing
Creatinine phosphokinase
Troponin
Erythrocyte sedimentation rate
White blood cell count
Isolation of virus from throat or rectal swabs, stool, blood, cerebrospinal fluid, or tissue
Serologic testing (four-fold rise in antibody titer or positive IgM)

myocardial tissue is rare unless the patient is a neonate or immunocompromised. Studies have shown that a significant minority of patients with myocarditis or dilated cardiomyopathy have evidence of viral infections such as enterovirus or adenovirus by PCR of cardiac tissue. However, false-positive PCR may be due to concurrent or previous unrelated viral infection or specimen contamination, and treatments for enteroviral and adenoviral infections are not currently available. Thus, it is difficult to assess the clinical utility of PCR testing at this time. Laboratory tests to exclude noninfectious causes such as autoimmune disease, amyloidosis, or hemochromatosis may be clinically appropriate (Table 38.2).

Routine chest radiographs may show an enlarged heart or signs of heart failure. Echocardiography evaluates wall motion, estimates LVEF, and detects the presence of pericardial effusion. It generally shows diffuse ventricular dilation with globally reduced contractility. In cases of rapid onset, the left ventricle may be hypokinetic with minimal dilation. Serial echocardiograms can provide evidence of deterioration or improvement. Currently available nuclear imaging tests are not clinically useful but MRI can be helpful in both the diagnosis and follow-up of myocarditis and as a guide for biopsy procedures. Cardiac catheterization may rule out causes of cardiac disease other than myocarditis.

The histologic diagnosis of myocarditis during life must be based on the interpretation of endomyocardial biopsy. The Dallas criteria are a histopathological categorization for the diagnosis of myocarditis proposed in 1986 and the historical gold standard. Active myocarditis comprises an inflammatory infiltrate of the myocardium with necrosis and/or degeneration of adjacent myocytes inconsistent with the typical appearance of ischemic heart disease. Borderline myocarditis occurs when the inflammatory infiltrate is spare or there is no myocyte injury. The inflammatory infiltrates in myocarditis are typically focal and transient, and thus endomyocardial biopsy is relatively insensitive. Also, pathologists may disagree on the interpretation of biopsy results. In certain diseases such as toxoplasmosis, Chagas, Lyme, and trichinosis, the histopathology may be diagnostic. Table 38.4 lists indications for EMB in adults. EMB may be necessary to diagnose some collagen vascular diseases; infiltrative and storage disease such as amyloid, sarcoid, or hemochromatosis; giant cell myocarditis; or malignancy. Transvenous EMB of the right ventricular septum (the preferred

Table 38.4 Potential Indications for Endomyocardial Biopsy in Patients with Myocarditis and Heart Failure

Rapidly progressive symptoms of heart failure or deteriorating left ventricular ejection fraction despite optimal medical management
Acutely worsening, hemodynamically significant rhythm disturbances, eg progressive heart block and ventricular tachycardia
Peripheral eosinophilia, rash, and fever
Clinical suspicion of secondary causes that might be revealed by biopsy and alter therapy, eg, sarcoidosis or giant cell arteritis

approach) has a 1 in 250 risk of perforation and a 1 in 1000 risk of death in experienced operators. There is also a risk of embolic stroke with biopsy of the left ventricle. Pediatricians may have a lower threshold for performing EMB because of the differing clinical features between adults and children. Given that no specific effective treatments are known for the most common causes of myocarditis and that the clinical manifestations of myocarditis usually resolve with conservative therapy, EMB generally is not necessary in adults.

THERAPY
Conventional Therapy

Patients should rest in bed with oxygen supplementation and avoid strenuous exercise (Figure 38.1). Exercise has been shown to be deleterious in mouse models. Cardiac monitoring is necessary to detect rhythm disturbances. Because most antiarrhythmics are negative ionotropes, they should be employed cautiously, eg, in the setting of high-grade ventricular ectopy. Although complete heart block requires transvenous pacing, often the conduction abnormality is transient and will not require a permanent pacemaker. Patients with congestive heart failure respond to standard measures such as diuretics and salt and fluid restriction. Dobutamine, dopamine, and other inotropic agents may also be useful. Ideally, all heart failure patients should receive an angiotensin-converting enzyme (ACE) inhibitor. Captopril may be more effective than other ACE inhibitors due to its oxygen radical–scavenging properties. In cardiogenic shock, aggressive supportive therapies, including intensive care, intra-aortic balloon pumps, extracorporeal membrane oxygenation, or left ventricular assist devices, may be necessary. Anticoagulation

is contraindicated in acute viral myopericarditis because of the danger of inducing cardiac tamponade but may be considered in the setting of atrial fibrillation or intracardiac thrombi. Although stable patients with heart failure and reduced LVEF generally should receive β-blockers, the role of β-blockers in the therapy of acute myocarditis is less clear, recognizing their negative inotropic effects. Although calcium channel blockers might prevent the coronary microvascular spasm of myocarditis and have been ameliorative in animal models of myocarditis, they are not recommended in the routine treatment of human myocarditis. Digoxin and spironolactone are not therapy for acute heart failure but could play a useful role in chronic heart failure. Salicylates and nonsteroidal anti-inflammatory drugs (NSAIDs) increase viral replication and mortality in mouse models of myocarditis and should be avoided. After hospital discharge, the patient should receive clinical and echocardiographic follow-up and avoid alcohol and strenuous exercise.

Specific Antiviral Therapy

If diagnostic studies or epidemiologic data point to a virus for which specific therapy is available, use of such therapy would be reasonable although efficacy in human myocarditis is unproven. Thus, in the initial viral phase, antiviral agents such as ganciclovir for CMV, neuraminidase inhibitors for influenza, or antiretrovirals for HIV could be beneficial. Although pleconaril inhibits replication of enterovirus in vitro, the drug currently is not available in the United States.

Immunosuppressants

In the murine model immunosuppression during the viral replication phase increases myocardial damage and worsens survival. In the best-designed study in humans thus far (the MTT, described above), immunosuppressive therapy did not improve LVEF or survival. However, the study was limited by the small number of biopsies that showed histologic myocarditis by the Dallas criteria and by the lack of agreement in biopsy interpretation between local pathologists and study panel cardiac pathologists. In another study, 84 patients with dilated cardiomyopathy with human leukocyte antigen (HLA) upregulation on biopsy were randomized to receive either immunosuppression with corticosteroids and azathioprine or placebo for 3 months. After 2 years,

Clinical Syndromes – Heart and Blood Vessels   **275**

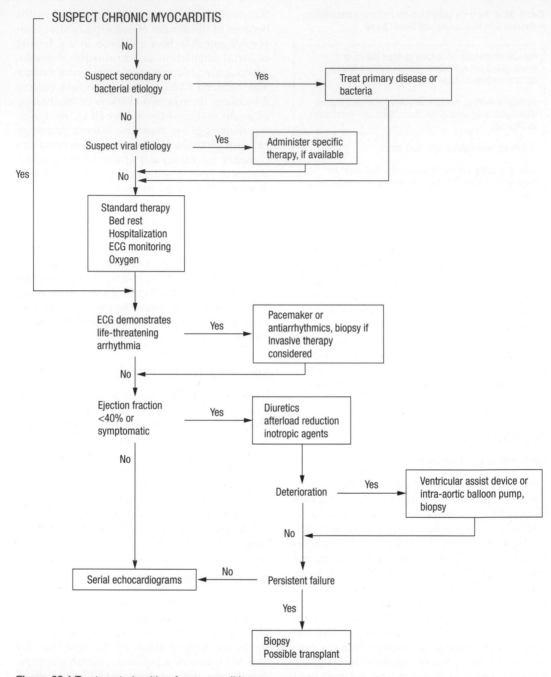

Figure 38.1 Treatment algorithm for myocarditis.

there were no significant differences in the primary end point (a composite of death, heart transplantation, and hospital readmission) between the 2 study groups, but LVEF and New York Heart Association class were significantly better in the immunosuppression group compared with the placebo group. Although these data are consistent with a long-term benefit of immunosuppressive therapy in patients with dilated cardiomyopathy and HLA upregulation, the utility of these finding is uncertain because the etiologic agents were not identified and the laboratory tests performed in the study may not be widely available clinically. A matched-cohort study in children demonstrated clinical, hemodynamic, and histologic improvement with prednisone combined with azathioprine or cyclosporine in children with active myocarditis and severe hemodynamic dysfunction. However, the study had methodologic flaws, including lack of blinding, questionable histologic criteria, and a small number of patients. Because of the conflicting results noted, we advise that the use of immunosuppressive therapy in myocarditis be limited to clinical trials.

Immunomodulators

In mice, IVIG suppresses cardiac damage, reduces inflammation, and improves survival. In a small, retrospective study of IVIG treatment of presumed acute myocarditis in children, treatment with high-dose (2 g/kg) IVIG was associated with superior recovery of left ventricular function compared with historical controls; there was a trend toward improved survival 1 year after presentation. In the adult IMAC trial mentioned previously, 62 patients with recent onset dilated cardiomyopathy (LVEF ≤40%) randomly received 2 g/kg IVIG or placebo. Notably, only 16% of IMAC subjects had cellular inflammation on EMB. Regardless of treatment assignment, slightly more than half of patients had an increase in LVEF ≥10% by 1 year from study entry, and 36% normalized their LVEF to ≥50%. These results suggest that IVIG does not augment improvement in LVEF in adults with recent-onset dilated cardiomyopathy. Pediatricians continue to use high-dose IVIG (2 g/kg over 24 hours) in children with acute myocarditis on EMB. Animal studies suggest IVIG is most effective in the early viremic stage of disease and children tend to have more acute, febrile disease with positive EMB results than adults, consistent with an earlier presentation.

Interferon-α, given close to the time of viral innoculation, reduces mortality and myocardial lesions in mouse models of coxsackie B myocarditis. Because patients with viral myocarditis typically do not present as early in their course, it is difficult to know how applicable these data are to human myocarditis. In a series of 22 patients with left ventricular dysfunction, symptomatic heart failure, and enteroviral or adenoviral persistence in the myocardium by PCR, 18×10^6 IU per week of β-interferon for 24 weeks was associated with viral clearance and a significant decrease in left ventricular size and improvement in left ventricular function. A randomized placebo-controlled study with Beta Interferon for Chronic Cardiomyopathy (BICC) is underway to determine the validity of the smaller, earlier study.

THE FUTURE OF MYOCARDITIS THERAPY

The application of immunohistochemical methods such as monoclonal antibodies to identify white blood cell subsets allows more sensitive characterization and localization of infiltrating cells. Polymerase chain reaction (PCR) allows amplification of distinct viral gene regions from endomyocardial biopsies with high sensitivity and specificity but does not allow localization. However, in situ hybridization using enterovirus probes can localize viral genomes to infected myocardial cells. The European Study of Epidemiology and Treatment of Cardiac Inflammatory Disease (ESETCID) is a multicenter, prospective, placebo-controlled, double-blind study that will enroll 250 subjects with biopsy-proven myocarditis and separate them into three subgroups (autoimmune myocarditis, enteroviral myocarditis, and CMV-induced myocarditis). In contrast to prior intervention studies, ESETCID will use new laboratory techniques such as PCR and in situ hybridization as well as conventional histologic methods. Specific therapy will include immunoglobulin with ganciclovir for CMV myocarditis, interferon-α for enterovirus, and prednisolone with azathioprine for autoimmune myocarditis. Vaccination development and usage against viruses such as coxsackie B, adenovirus, and parvovirus B19 might reduce the incidence of myocarditis in the future.

SUGGESTED READING

Cappola TP, et al. Pulmonary hypertension and risk of death in cardiomyopathy: patients with myocarditis are at higher risk. *Circulation.* 2002;105:1663–1668.

Felker GM, et al. Underlying causes and long-term survival in patients with initially unexplained cardiomyopathy. *N Engl J Med.* 2000;342:1077–1084.

Kuhl U, et al. Interferon-beta treatment eliminates cardiotropic viruses and improves left ventricular function in patients with myocardial persistence of viral genomes and left ventricular dysfunction. *Circulation.* 2003; 107:2793–2798.

Kuhl U, et al. Viral persistence in the myocardium is associated with progressive cardiac dysfunction. *Circulation.* 2005;112:1965–1970.

Magnani JW, Dec GW. Myocarditis: current trends in diagnosis and treatment. *Circulation* 2006; 113:876–890.

Mason JW, et al. A clinical trial of immunosuppressive therapy for myocarditis, *N Engl J Med*. 1995;333:269–275.

McCarthy RE III, et al. Long-term outcome of fulminant myocarditis as compared with acute (nonfulminant) myocarditis. *N Engl J Med*. 2000;342:690–695.

McNamara DM, et al. Controlled trial of intravenous immune globulin in recent-onset dilated cardiomyopathy. *Circulation*. 2001; 103:2254–2259.

Wojnicz R, et al. Randomized, placebo-controlled study for the treatment of inflammatory dilated cardiomyopathy. *Circulation*. 2001; 104:39–45.

Wu, LA, Lapeyre AC III, Cooper LT. Current role of endomyocardial biopsy in the management of dilated cardiomyopathy and myocarditis. *Mayo Clin Proc*. 2001;76:1030–1038.

39. Mediastinitis

Keith S. Kaye and Ravi Karra

The mediastinum is defined as the space in the thorax between the lungs; it houses the heart, great vessels, esophagus, trachea, thymus, and lymph nodes. The connective tissues of the mediastinum are continuous with the long fascial planes of the head and neck, one reason why until the advent of thoracic surgery, mediastinitis was primarily a complication of odontogenic infections. By virtue of its deep position within the thorax, the mediastinum is a relatively protected organ space. There are four major portals of entry into the mediastinum: (1) direct inoculation of the mediastinum following sternotomy (ie, postoperative mediastinitis (POM)); (2) spread along the long fascial planes of the neck (ie, descending mediastinitis); (3) rupture of mediastinal structures, such as the esophagus; and (4) contiguous spread of infection from adjacent thoracic structures.

POSTOPERATIVE MEDIASTINITIS

Postoperative mediastinitis (POM) is classified as an organ space infection by Centers for Disease Control and Prevention (CDC) criteria and is a dreaded complication of median sternotomy. POM classically presents as a febrile illness with sternal wound dehiscence and purulent drainage, usually 2 to 4 weeks after sternotomy. Occasionally POM presents as a more chronic, indolent infection months to years after sternotomy. Sometimes, only superficial signs of infection are present, making POM difficult to diagnose. Frequently, a high index of clinical suspicion is required to differentiate POM from a more superficial sternal wound infection.

Pathogenesis

Infection most often occurs as the result of direct inoculation of host bacteria into the mediastinum during surgery. Bacteria that colonize the skin and oral mucosa, such as coagulase-negative *Staphylococcus* (CoNS) and *Staphylococcus aureus* are the most common causes of POM. Gram-negative bacilli, a less common cause of POM, are believed to spread to the mediastinum from the abdomen. Infrequently, pathogens such as *S. aureus* might be introduced into the mediastinum by a member of the surgical team after a break in sterile technique or by contaminated operative instruments. Whether bacterial contamination develops into full-blown infection is a combination of three major factors: (1) inoculum of bacterial contamination, (2) the degree of local tissue and vascular damage, and (3) host immunity. Larger inoculum and greater perioperative tissue damage both increase the risk for infection. Decreased host immunity increases susceptibility to the development of POM.

Epidemiology and Outcomes

POM has been estimated to occur following 0.7% to 3.4% of all sternotomies. Despite advances in surgical techniques and the use of preoperative prophylactic antibiotics, rates of POM in the modern era remain around 1.0%. The high number of median sternotomies performed annually makes POM a frequently encountered problem.

Risk factors for the development of POM have been well chronicled and can be grouped into three categories: (1) host-related factors, (2) hospital-related factors, and (3) technical or operative factors. Host-related factors that increase the risk for POM include obesity, increased age, history of diabetes, history of prior sternotomy, concurrent perioperative infection (such as cellulitis), and New York Heart Association (NYHA) class III or IV heart failure. Hospital factors that increase the risk for POM include prolonged postoperative mechanical ventilation and prolonged postoperative stay in an intensive care unit (ICU). Operative factors that increase risk for POM include an increased duration of surgery and surgical complexity of a given case. Complex surgeries with increased risk of POM include simultaneous coronary artery bypass grafting (CABG) and valve repair, "repeat" or "redo" median sternotomy, and surgical reexploration following initial sternotomy.

POM is a serious infection and is associated with significant attributable morbidity and mortality. Estimates of postoperative mortality range from 11.8% to 14% in patients with POM compared to 2.7% to 5.5% in uninfected operative controls. Risk factors for mortality in the immediate postoperative period include host factors (advanced age and postoperative bacteremia), hospitalization-related factors (such as need for postoperative intra-aortic balloon pump and prolonged postoperative mechanical ventilation), technical factors (prolonged operative duration and need for surgical reexploration), and pathogen-related factors. *Staphylococcus aureus* is a particularly virulent pathogen, and POM due to methicillin-resistant *S. aureus* (MRSA) is associated with particularly adverse clinical outcomes. Patients with POM are not only at increased risk for mortality during the immediate postoperative period but also carry a two- to four-fold increased risk for death for up to 10 years following cardiothoracic surgery. Risk factors for long-term mortality in patients with POM have recently been described and include >65 years, serum creatinine >2.0 mg/dL prior to surgery, infection with methicillin-resistant *S. aureus* (MRSA), delay of sternal closure more than 3 days following therapeutic debridement for POM, and failure to treat POM with effective antimicrobial agents within 7 days of therapeutic sternal debridement.

DESCENDING NECROTIZING MEDIASTINITIS

Mediastinitis arising from the migration of pathogens from head or neck infection, as opposed to direct inoculation of the mediastinum, is classified as descending necrotizing mediastinitis. Odontogenic infections cause nearly 60% of all descending necrotizing mediastinitis. However, virtually any infection of the head and neck can spread into the mediastinum. If infections of the head and neck are treated with appropriate antimicrobial agents, descending necrotizing mediastinitis can be prevented. In the modern age of antibiotics, descending mediastinitis has becoming increasingly rare.

Pathogenesis

Spread to the mediastinum can occur via each of the three spaces of the head and neck: the pretracheal space (suppurative thyroid and tracheal infections), the perivascular space (oropharyngeal infections), and the retrovisceral space (oropharyngeal infections). Negative intrathoracic pressure during inspiration acts to draw infection into the mediastinum from these spaces. The retropharyngeal space houses the "danger" space, so named because it extends from the base of the skull all the way to the diaphragm. Spread within the retropharyngeal space is involved in the pathogenesis of approximately 70% of cases of descending mediastinitis. Infections of the perivascular space can also be complicated by thrombophlebitis of the jugular vein (Lemierre disease) and direct extension of infection into the carotid artery. (See also Chapter 10, Deep Neck Infections.)

Epidemiology and Outcomes

The microbiology of descending necrotizing mediastinitis reflects the types of bacteria that usually colonize or infect the head and neck. Often, descending necrotizing mediastinitis is a polymicrobial infection involving anaerobes. Common anaerobes include *Fusobacterium*, *Prevotella*, *Vellionella*, *Peptostreptococcus*, and other oral anaerobes. *Streptococci* spp. are common pathogens. *Actinomyces* can also cause descending mediastinitis.

Patients with descending necrotizing mediastinitis often present with fevers, signs of an underlying head and neck infection, and sometimes sepsis. However, in immunocompromised patients, obvious clinical signs and symptoms may not be readily apparent. Signs of associated neck infection can provide clues to the presence of descending mediastinitis and include trismus, pain of the oropharynx, pain on movement of the neck, dysphagia, hoarseness, stridor, and occasionally erythema of the overlying skin. Overall, the diagnosis of descending necrotizing mediastinitis requires a high degree of clinical suspicion. Early recognition and treatment is important, as this syndrome can be rapidly fatal.

MEDIASTINITIS ORIGINATING FROM MEDIASTINAL STRUCTURES

Mediastinitis can also occur as a result of direct spillage of bacteria from mediastinal structures. Perforation of any of the organs or vessels housed in the mediastinum, most commonly the esophagus, can lead to mediastinitis. Perforation of the esophagus can occur after heavy emesis (as in Boerhaave's syndrome); following ingestion of sharp objects such as glass; or following procedures involving the esophagus such as endoscopy, myotomy, or esophageal stenting. Mediastinitis can develop following tracheal perforation, which sometimes occurs as a complication of endotracheal intubation

Clinical Syndromes – Heart and Blood Vessels

and bronchoscopy. Rare cases of mediastinitis have been reported as a consequence of spread of infection from the aorta following surgical repair.

In cases of mediastinitis originating from mediastinal structures, particularly in Boerhaave's syndrome, patients often present with acute chest pain and fever. If mediastinitis is suspected, special attention in the history should be focused on any recent procedures involving the trachea or esophagus or episodes of heavy retching.

MEDIASTINITIS FROM CONTIGUOUS THORACIC INFECTIONS

Another mechanism of mediastinal infection involves contiguous spread of infection from thoracic structures into the mediastinum. If untreated, pulmonary infections due to bacteria, fungi, and *Mycobacteria* can cause secondary mediastinitis. Mediastinitis caused by bacterial pathogens usually presents as an acute, severe infection. Mediastinitis due to tuberculosis or histoplasmosis tends to have a subacute or chronic course compared to bacterial infection. These infections can lead to granulomatous mediastinitis or immune-related deposition of collagen within the mediastinum and resultant fibrosing mediastinitis.

EVALUATION OF SUSPECTED MEDIASTINITIS

It is important to obtain historical information from the patient regarding antecedent events that might have predisposed to mediastinitis such as median sternotomy, head and neck illness, or a recent prior endoscopic or bronchoscopic intervention.

Patients with mediastinitis classically present with chest pain and fever. The chest pain is sometimes pleuritic in nature. On exam, patients with mediastinitis usually display signs of severe systemic illness such as hypotension and sepsis. In some instances, patients may not present with overwhelming systemic signs and symptoms of infection. Often, a high degree of clinical suspicion is needed to differentiate POM from superficial infection.

There are many other diverse signs and symptoms of mediastinitis that present with varying frequencies depending on the type of mediastinitis present in a given case. For example, patients with POM classically present within 3 weeks of surgery with erythema or frank purulent drainage at the sternal incision site. If the sternum is firmly depressed on either side of the incision, a sternal "click" is sometimes elicited, representing the instability of the sternum secondary to damage of underlying tissue planes. Unfortunately, acute signs and symptoms of POM might not be present and sometimes patients present with only mild signs of infection, such as small amounts of drainage or erythema from a median sternotomy site. In contrast, patients with descending necrotizing mediastinitis often have signs of head and neck infection, making evaluation of the head and neck a critical component of the physical exam. Sometimes, in cases of dental abscess, fluctuant masses are present at the base of the teeth. Other signs to evaluate on examination include the presence of tonsillar exudates, pharyngeal irritation, or cervical lymphadenopathy. Pain on palpation of the neck may also be helpful in recognizing the tracking of infection from the head and/or neck to the mediastinum. "Hamman crunch" is a physical exam finding that is present in some cases of mediastinitis. This finding is characterized by crunching sounds heard on cardiac auscultation with each heartbeat and is indicative of air in the mediastinum. Patients with mediastinitis secondary to spread of infection from adjacent organs often have signs or symptoms associated with infection of the adjacent organ space (eg, findings of pulmonary consolidation in cases of pneumonia).

When considering mediastinitis, diagnostic evaluation initially should include a complete blood count, white blood cell differential, blood cultures, and radiographic imaging. Chest x-ray should be obtained and may show a widened mediastinum (most commonly seen in cases of descending necrotizing mediastinitis). Rarely, chest x-ray might demonstrate pneumomediastinum. Chest computed tomography (CT) and magnetic resonance imaging (MRI) are the most useful radiographic tests for evaluating potential cases of mediastinitis, particularly descending mediastinitis, mediastinitis caused by rupture of mediastinal structures, and mediastinitis due to contiguous spread of infection from adjacent thoracic structures. Computed tomography and MRI sometimes demonstrate the presence of fluid in the mediastinum indicative of inflammation or the presence of abscess. Computed tomography and MRI are also more sensitive than chest x-ray for identifying pneumomediastinum. However, in cases of POM, MRI and CT are less useful in the diagnosis of mediastinitis during the immediate postoperative period. Postoperative inflammation in the mediastinum is usually present following median sternotomy and can be difficult to differentiate from infection or abscess. Currently, indium-labeled leukocyte scans and thermography are being studied in efforts to enhance the specificity of thoracic imaging in cases of POM, but the utility of these tests in POM diagnosis remains unknown.

PREVENTION AND TREATMENT OF SUSPECTED MEDIASTINITIS

Postoperative Mediastinitis

In patients undergoing sternotomy, preoperative antibiotic prophylaxis is recommended. First- or second-generation cephalosporins can be administered within 60 minutes of surgery. In patients or institutions with high rates of MRSA or in patients with a penicillin allergy, vancomycin can be considered as prophylactic agent.

Optimal treatment of POM involves a combination of definitive surgical debridement and appropriate antimicrobial therapy. In POM, the most common pathogens are gram-positive cocci (*Staphylococcus* spp. and *Streptococcus* spp.) and gram-negative bacilli. Therefore, initial antimicrobial therapy typically includes two agents: one with activity against aerobic gram-positive cocci and one with activity against aerobic gram-negative bacilli. Gram-positive coverage usually includes a β-lactam (such as nafcillin or cefazolin) or glycopeptides (such as vancomycin). At institutions where MRSA is a notable POM pathogen, vancomycin should be used for empiric gram-positive therapy. Empiric coverage for gram-negative pathogens usually involves treatment with a fluoroquinolone, aminoglycoside, or extended-spectrum cephalosporin. Pseudomonas is a rare pathogen in mediastinitis and, therefore, antipseudomonal drugs are not required for empiric therapy. Antimicrobial therapy should be tailored to culture results. Culture specimens, ideally obtained in the operating room, are usually available within 3 to 5 days after they are submitted.

Immediate surgical debridement is needed to confirm the diagnosis of mediastinitis (by demonstrating the presence of pus in the mediastinum), to obtain tissue for microbiologic culture, and to remove purulent material and devitalized or grossly infected tissue. Sternectomy usually is necessary due to concurrent sternal osteomyelitis. After initial debridement and sternectomy, various therapeutic operative approaches can be

implemented. Historically, the sternum was left open and packed until granulation tissue visibly developed. However, this approach was felt to lead to considerable morbidity and mortality, often due to superinfection of the open mediastinum. More recently, preferred approaches have included closure with a muscle flap, usually derived from the pectoralis or omentum, and placement of fenestrated drains in the mediastinum. Closure of the sternum with a muscle flap typically occurs either immediately after sternectomy and debridement or soon afterward. Occasionally, the sternum is closed primarily without use of a muscle flap, although this approach occurs infrequently.

More recently, other approaches to therapy after initial debridement have included utilization of Wound Vacs, which seal the thoracic cavity and provide continuous suction of necrotic tissue and fluid. Other surgeons have implanted antibiotic-laden beads into the mediastinum after debridement. However, there are few data supporting the efficacy of the Wound Vacs or mediastinal beads in treatment of POM.

Descending Necrotizing Mediastinitis, Mediastinitis Originating from Mediastinal Structures, and Mediastinitis from Contiguous Thoracic Infections

In descending necrotizing mediastinitis, empiric antimicrobial therapy should provide activity against gram-positive cocci, anaerobes, and gram-negative rods. When the infection is restricted to the upper mediastinum, transcervical drainage is recommended. However, when infection includes the lower mediastinum, open drainage after sternotomy is often necessary.

Mediastinitis following rupture of a mediastinal viscous requires open surgical drainage and repair of the perforated viscous. In the case of Boerhaave's syndrome, antibiotics with activity against aerobic gram-negative bacilli and anaerobes should be used. For example, an extended generation cephalosporin in combination with metronidazole or clinidamycin would be a reasonable empiric regimen. Other single-drug regimens might include a β-lactam/β-lactamase inhibitor combination such as piperacillin–tazobactam or a carbapenem. Surgical intervention is guided by the degree of infection and the perforation. Large collections of infection require drainage, and large esophageal tears require local esophagectomy and repair.

Mediastinitis secondary to spread of a contiguous thoracic infection should be empirically treated with broad-spectrum antibiotics with activity against pulmonary pathogens such as *Streptococcus pneumoniae*, *S. aureus*, and gram-negative bacilli. In cases of suspected aspiration pneumonia, anaerobes should also be covered. An appropriate empiric regimen might include a third-generation cephalosporin or aztreonam in combination with vancomycin and either clindamycin or metronidazole. Definitive therapy requires debridement of the mediastinum and drainage of infected thoracic collections, usually via chest tube. Antibiotic regimens should be tailored based on intraoperative culture results.

Fibrosing mediastinitis due to either mycobacterial infection or fungal infection is a therapeutic challenge. Empiric therapy for *M. tuberculosis* typically includes standard three or four drug regimens (eg, isoniazide, rifampin, pyrazinamide, and ethambutol). For the treatment of fungal infections, itraconazole, sometimes in combination with amphotericin for histoplasmosis is used. However, the utility and effectiveness of antimicrobial therapy in the treatment of fibrosing mediastinitis due to these pathogens remains unclear. Surgical debridement is primarily used to relieve vascular and airway obstruction.

SUGGESTED READING

Eklund AM, Lyytikainen O, Klemets P, et al. Mediastinitis after more than 10,000 cardiac surgical procedures. *Ann Thorac Surg.* 2006;82:1784–1789.

Karra R, McDermott L, Connelly S, et al. Risk factors for 1-year mortality after postoperative mediastinitis. *J Thorac Cardiovasc Surg.* 2006;132:537–543.

Port JL, Kent MS, Korst RJ, et al. Thoracic esophageal perforations: a decade of experience. *Ann Thorac Surg.* 2003;75:1071–1074.

Robicsek F. Postoperative sterno-mediastinitis. *Am Surg.* 2000;66(2):184.

40. Vascular Infection

Susan E. Beekmann and David K. Henderson

Diagnosis and treatment of vascular infections is complex and depends on a variety of factors, including the location of the infected tissue, the microbiology of the infection, and patient-specific factors, such as anatomy and immune status. Purulent or suppurative thrombophlebitis is inflammation of a peripheral or central venous wall because of the presence of microorganisms. Endarteritis (or infective arteritis) and mycotic aneurysms are infections of the arterial walls; arterial aneurysms or pseudoaneurysms are usually present because endarteritis may be difficult to diagnose unless an aneurysm is present. The term *mycotic aneurysm* is a misnomer that refers to any arterial aneurysm of infectious cause, fungal or bacterial, and may also include secondary infections of preexisting aneurysms or pseudoaneurysms. Vascular graft infections present an even wider spectrum of disease that depends on the type and location of the graft. Management of infections located on vascular prostheses is further complicated by the fact that prosthesis excision can jeopardize a patient's life and organ function, and alternative grafting techniques, including ex situ bypass, autologous reconstruction, and a variety of other graft materials must be considered. Finally, endovascular repair of aneurysms has resulted in a variety of infectious complications of endovascular stents, stent-grafts, and other intra-arterial devices.

PURULENT PHLEBITIS OF PERIPHERAL AND CENTRAL VEINS

Pathogenesis and Diagnosis

Septic thrombophlebitis is characterized by inflammation with suppuration of the vein wall. The various anatomic sites of this serious condition determine the clinical significance and manifestations. Superficial suppurative thrombophlebitis is most often a complication of indwelling intravenous catheters or intravenous substance use. Suppurative thrombophlebitis due to intravenous catheters occurs more commonly with plastic than with steel cannulas. Irritation of the vein wall and

subsequent development of purulent thrombophlebitis occurs more often with polyethylene catheters than with Teflon or Silastic catheters and is higher in lower extremity cannulation. Central vein thrombosis is a relatively common complication of central venous catheterization, occurring in as many as one-third of patients in some autopsy and clinical series. Suppurative thrombophlebitis of the thoracic central veins results from the bacterial or fungal contamination (sepsis) of these often asymptomatic thrombi. The second major type of septic thrombophlebitis occurs by invasion from adjacent primary nonvascular infections and includes Lemierre's syndrome (internal jugular vein septic thrombophlebitis) as well as other entities discussed elsewhere. Lemierre's syndrome, although rare, usually follows an oropharyngeal infection and occurs most often in previously healthy patients aged 16 to 25 years.

Diagnosis of peripheral suppurative thrombophlebitis may be difficult if local findings of inflammation are absent, as often occurs in lower extremity cannulization. Local findings are much more common in suppurative thrombophlebitis of the upper extremities. Bacteremia is present in as many as 90% of patients with peripheral suppurative thrombophlebitis, and gross pus within the vein may be apparent in half of the patients. Suppurative thrombophlebitis of the thoracic central veins should be considered in any septic patient with a central venous catheter when bacteremia (or fungemia) fails to resolve after removal of the catheter and institution of appropriate antimicrobial therapy. Diagnosis can be established by venography with the demonstration of thrombi in a patient with bacteremia or fungemia. Computed tomography (CT) with contrast is also likely to be diagnostic; presence of gas in the venular lumen is typical of this condition. Magnetic resonance imaging (MRI) may be even more sensitive for diagnosis. In Lemierre's syndrome, the course is described by the triad of pharyngitis, a tender/swollen neck, and noncavitating pulmonary infiltrates. Septic pulmonary emboli occurred in 97% of cases in two series. Oropharyngeal findings alone, however, are not diagnostic, and a tender and/or swollen neck occurs in only about 50% of patients. Computed tomography, ultrasound or MRI can document this syndrome.

Therapy

Treatment of superficial suppurative thrombophlebitis traditionally has consisted of surgical excision plus parenteral antimicrobials. Most of the literature, which is derived primarily from burn center studies, strongly recommends vein excision, indicating that patients treated with antibiotics alone had a much higher death rate than patients who underwent surgical exploration. Other studies suggest that local incision and drainage of the involved site plus appropriate antimicrobial therapy may be sufficient in many nonburn cases. Patients who fail less radical surgery should then be referred for extensive surgical excision with total removal of all involved veins and drainage of contiguous abscesses.

Enterobacteriaceae caused more than half of all cases of suppurative thrombophlebitis in recent reviews, followed by *Pseudomonas aeruginosa*, *Staphylococcus aureus*, and *Candida* species. Initial empiric treatment might include vancomycin and either an aminoglycoside or a third- or fourth-generation cephalosporin with antipseudomonal activity to cover the *Enterobacteriaceae*, *Pseudomonas*, and *S. aureus* (both methicillin resistant and methicillin sensitive) until a culture of the infected material can be performed. Blood cultures should always be drawn before antibiotics are initiated. Empiric antibiotic choices should be tailored for known resistance patterns within hospitals and in geographic areas and may be adjusted based on Gram stain results. For example, a Gram stain of venular material showing gram-negative rods should result in discontinuation of vancomycin. Therapy with an appropriate antibiotic(s) should be continued once culture results are available. Treatment of suppurative thrombophlebitis caused by *C. albicans* is controversial because most of these infections can be cured by vein excision alone. Nonetheless, fluconazole, 400 to 800 mg/day, may be used, and amphotericin B or fluconazole is mandatory in the immunosuppressed patient or if metastatic complications occur.

Treatment of central suppurative thrombophlebitis consists of catheter removal and parenteral antibiotics. The addition of full-dose anticoagulation is more controversial, although a recent review concluded that the administration of heparin in these settings may be beneficial. Empiric antibiotic treatment is the same as for peripheral suppurative thrombophlebitis with the potential addition of an antipseudomonal penicillin. The antibiotics appropriate for the organisms identified from cultured material should be continued for at least 2 weeks after catheter removal. A minimum of 4 weeks of antimicrobial treatment is recommended after catheter removal when *S. aureus* is involved. Amphotericin B to a total dosage of at least 22 mg/kg ± 5 FC is recommended for suppurative thrombophlebitis of the great central veins caused by *Candida* species; for the intrinsically resistant species, including *C. glabrata* and *C. krusei*, fluconazole may be an acceptable alternative. Lemierre's syndrome should be treated with a prolonged course of either clindamycin or metronidazole. Surgical treatment is usually not necessary.

ARTERIAL INFECTIONS (MYCOTIC ANEURYSMS AND ARTERITIS)
Pathogenesis and Diagnosis

Mechanisms of arterial infection include (1) embolomycotic aneurysm secondary to septic microemboli (underlying infective endocarditis), (2) extension from a contiguous infected focus, (3) hematogenous seeding during bacteremia originating from a distant site, and (4) trauma to the vessel wall with direct contamination, with the latter mechanism occasionally associated with iatrogenic manipulation of the artery (eg, cannulation). Normal arterial intima is quite resistant to infection, but congenital or acquired malformation or disease (eg, atherosclerosis) lowers resistance to infection, and hematogenous seeding of a previously damaged arteriosclerotic vessel currently constitutes the most common mechanism of infection (Figure 40.1). Mycotic aneurysms complicate infective endocarditis in approximately 5% to 10% of cases, with about half of these aneurysms involving the brain. Gram-positive organisms are the most common pathogens, with *S. aureus* accounting for approximately 30% to 40% of cases when bacteria seed an atherosclerotic vessel. Gram-negative bacteria are the causative organisms in approximately one-third of cases, with *Salmonella* species found in about 20% of all cases. When aneurysms are associated with

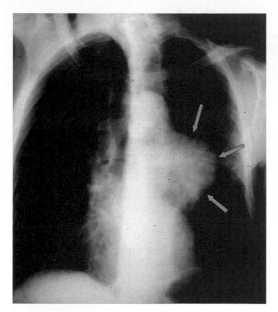

Figure 40.1 Infected atherosclerotic aneurysm of descending thoracic aorta (*arrows*): blood cultures grew Salmonella. (Courtesy of David Schlossberg, MD.)

endocarditis, gram-positive organisms account for at least 80% of pathogens.

Clinical manifestations depend to a large extent on the site of the aneurysm (Table 40.1). Although most infected aortic aneurysms occur in elderly atherosclerotic men (4:1 ratio, men > women), symptoms are nonspecific and may overlap with those of uninfected aneurysms. Fever and continuing bacteremia despite seemingly appropriate antimicrobial therapy are suggestive of an infected intravascular site.

A variety of intra-arterial prosthetic devices are now being used in cardiovascular medicine, including arterial closure devices, prosthetic carotid patches, coronary artery stents and endovascular stents, and stent-grafts. Infections of these devices remain either uncommon or extremely rare, but infectious complications associated with the placement of these devices are often devastating. *Staphylococcus aureus* has been implicated in as many as three-quarters of these cases, and has been the primary pathogen, even in late-onset infections. Blood cultures should be obtained from all patients who have a history of endovascular stent placement and local or systemic signs of infection.

Therapy

Despite improved prognosis for infected aneurysms of the thoracoabdominal vessels associated with earlier diagnosis and treatment, the case fatality rate for aortic aneurysms infected with gram-negative organisms is extraordinary and may be as high as 75%. Currently accepted management is intravenous antibiotic therapy, excision and debridement of the artery or aneurysm, and extraanatomic vascular reconstruction along an uncontaminated path, where possible. As a general principle, antibiotic therapy alone usually is insufficient without surgical resection of the infected tissue. Despite this axiom, surgical management of asymptomatic intracranial mycotic aneurysms does depend on their size and location, because small lesions may resolve with antibiotic therapy alone. A reasonable approach would be to monitor by MRI every 2 to 3 weeks for 2 months. Surgery is indicated if the infected vessel is accessible or the lesions increase in size and should be considered if the lesions fail to decrease in size.

Basic principles of grafting in this situation include the use of autogenous rather than synthetic grafts and insertion only in clean, noninfected tissue planes. Use of cryopreserved allografts allows in situ reconstruction and may be acceptable for cases involving the thoracic or suprarenal aorta. Direct reconstruction with synthetic or autologous grafts has become increasingly common, and short- and midterm outcomes of this approach appear to be acceptable. At surgery the aneurysm must be sectioned, Gram stained, and cultured; appropriate antibiotic therapy must be individualized and based on culture and sensitivity results. Bactericidal antibiotics should be continued for 6 to 8 weeks postoperatively. Endoluminal stenting for mycotic aneurysms is an additional alternative that reduces hospital stay and frequency of surgical complications but that raises significant concern because of persistent infection. In many cases, these endovascular stents are short-term solutions, and chronic oral antimicrobial therapy is required. Nonetheless, endovascular grafts may now be used preferentially in patients for whom conventional surgical methods carry extremely high risk.

VASCULAR GRAFT INFECTIONS
Pathogenesis and Diagnosis

Reported incidence of vascular graft infections ranges from 0.8% to 6% and varies with the site of graft placement and the prosthetic graft material selected for insertion. For example, procedures

Table 40.1 Diagnosis and Management of Mycotic Aneurysms

Site	Frequency of Diagnosis (Range)	Clinical Presentation
General		
All infected aneurysms	100%	Fever common (70%–94%) Malaise, weight loss Pain (100%) Rapidly expanding mass Leukocytosis (65%–85%) Positive blood cultures (50%–75%)
Specifics		
Aorta Infrarenal abdominal aorta[a] Ascending aorta and arch (secondary to endocarditis)	27% (11%–75%)	Abdominal or back pain Palpable abdominal lesions (about 50%–65%) Vertebral osteomyelitis (lumbar/thoracic)
Visceral artery Superior mesenteric,[a] splenic, hepatic, celiac, renal	24% (0%–29%)	Colicky abdominal pain Jaundice (hepatic artery) Hemoptysis or hemothorax (celiac artery)
Iliac	4% (0%–25%)	Thigh pain, quadriceps wasting, depressed knee jerk Arterial insufficiency of extremity
Arm Radial artery[a] Brachial artery Subclavian artery	10% (0%–9%)	Pain over site of lesion About 90% palpable May appear as cellulitis, abscess; distal embolic lesions; skin changes common
Leg Femoral artery[a]	12% (4%–44%)	Pain over site of lesion About 90% palpable Pulsatile mass, decreased peripheral pulses Possible local suppuration, distal embolic lesions; petechiae, purpura
Intracranial Peripheral middle cerebral artery[a]	4%	Usually clinically silent May appear as severe unremitting headache Usually secondary to endocarditis

Abbreviations: CT = computed tomography; MRI = magnetic resonance imaging; WBC = white blood cell; IV = intravenous; IVDU = intravenous drug user.
[a] Most common site or manifestation.

requiring an inguinal incision have an incidence of infection that is 2 to 3 times higher than procedures not requiring an inguinal incision; use of a vascular prosthesis results in significantly higher infection rates than autologous reconstruction. Most contamination likely occurs at the time of implantation, although both hematogenous seeding as well as bacteria harbored in atherosclerotic plaques may account for some late graft infections. Prophylactic systemic antibiotics at time of graft placement have been associated with a decrease in vascular graft infections in recent years. Prophylactic antibiotics should be considered mandatory with placement of vascular grafts.

Staphylococci remain the most prevalent pathogens, with *S. epidermidis* infections often presenting months to years after the operation

Imaging	Microbiology	Management
Findings: Aneurysm with lack of intimal calcification Perianeurysmal fluid/gas collection *Studies:* CT with contrast, MRI Ultrasonography (if accessible) Radionuclide-tagged WBC scans	*Staphylococcus* 40% (at least 66% *S. aureus*) *Salmonella* 20% *Streptococcus* 20% *Escherichia coli* 6% IVDU: *S. aureus*, *Pseudomonas* sp. *Enterococcus* sp., *S. viridans*	*Surgical:* Wide debridement, irrigation with antibiotic solution of involved tissues, complete resection of aneurysm if possible *Antibiotic:* Empiric treatment with IV antibiotics for 6-8 wk after surgery based on culture results of resected tissue Follow-up blood cultures Consider chronic suppressive oral antibiotic therapy when extra-anatomic bypass is not performed (ie, for in situ repairs)
Frontal, lateral abdominal x-ray studies Abdominal ultrasound	*Salmonella* sp. have predilection for suprarenal aorta *Staphylococcus* predominates in infrarenal aorta	Extra-anatomic arterial reconstruction (axillofemoral or aortofemoral)
Ultrasound may exclude other causes (eg, pancreatic masses)	*Bacteroides fragilis* reported from supraceliac aorta and celiac artery	Complete excision may be hazardous; careful drainage and longer-term antibiotic therapy may be necessary
		Excision and arterial ligation; reconstruction usually can wait until infection has resolved
		Proximal ligation of the vessel, resection of the aneurysm, and appropriate drainage should be followed by antibiotic therapy.
	S. aureus incidence as high as 65%	Excision and arterial ligation; reconstruction usually can wait until infection has resolved Autogenous grafting may allow reconstruction through the bed of the resected aneurysm if anastomoses performed in clean tissue planes
Four-vessel cerebral arteriography invaluable MRI	*Enterococcus* sp. *S. viridans* *Pseudomonas* sp. *Candida albicans*	

and *S. aureus* most commonly causing early infections (Table 40.2). More than 70% of infections involving vascular grafts of the groin and lower extremities develop within 1 to 2 months of surgery, whereas 70% of intra-abdominal graft infections do not manifest until months or years after surgery.

Appropriate imaging of the infected area is vital to diagnosis because the extent of local infections may not be recognized if imaging techniques are inadequate. Angiography often is unhelpful in the diagnosis of vascular graft infections, but it is useful for identifying aortoenteric fistulas as well as for guiding the surgical procedure. An anatomic imaging study should be performed. Ultrasound can be used for superficial grafts, including dialysis shunts; a CT with contrast or an MRI

Table 40.2 Diagnosis and Management of Vascular Graft Infections

Site	Clinical Presentation	Microbiology	Imaging	Management
General				
Any infected vascular graft	*Early (≤4 mo):* Immediate postoperative infections rare; usually associated with wound sepsis Fever, leukocytosis, bacteremia Anastomotic bleeding (most common with gram-negative organisms) Wound healing complication *Late:* Systemic signs few or absent; WBC count often normal Tenderness, erythema of skin over prosthesis Anastomotic false aneurysm Graft-enteric erosion, fistula	*Staphylococcus aureus* Coagulase-neg'ative staphylococci *Streptococcus* *Escherichia coli* *Klebsiella* *Pseudomonas*	*Findings:* Perigraft fluid, gas collection; abnormal appearance of perigraft soft tissues; abscess; pseudoaneurysm formation *Studies: Anatomic imaging study:* 1. CT with contrast, or 2. MRI with contrast and fat saturation; or, for superficial grafts: 3. Ultrasonography *Radioisotope studies that may be useful:* 1. WBC-labeled indium scan, or 2. Tc99-HMPAO-labeled WBC, if available	*Surgical:* Wide debridement, irrigation with antibiotic solution of involved tissues (commonly used but efficacy data not available), graft excision when possible with ex situ bypass reconstruction Consider thorough debridement with myocutaneous flap for patients with a patent graft, intact anastomoses, absence of hemorrhage, and sterile blood cultures *Antibiotic:* Empiric treatment with IV antibiotics for 4-6 wk after surgery based on culture results of resected tissue Follow-up blood cultures Consider chronic suppressive oral antibiotic therapy if infected graft not removed
Specific				
Aortoiliac	Higher incidence in months 8–15 First symptoms, fever, slightly increased WBC count Later, abdominal, back pain, false aneurysm formation Finally, hemorrhage	*E. coli* *S. aureus* *Streptococcus* *S. epidermidis* (or coagulase-negative staphylococci)	MRI more sensitive than CT for aortal graft infection	Place axillofemoral or bifemoral graft, then remove entire aortic graft Close arteriotomy sites with monofilament sutures, irrigate with antibiotic solution (no efficacy data)
Aortofemoral	False aneurysm in groin site Wound infection or abscess in inguinal incision Pulsatile mass at groin site	*S. aureus* *S. epidermidis* *Proteus* sp. *E. coli* *Streptococcus* Other gram-negative bacilli	Ultrasonography can be useful in femoral area	May be possible to remove only infected part of graft (one limb), although continued infection likely without removal of entire graft Extra-anatomic bypass when possible
Axillofemoral	Same as for aortofemoral	Same as for aortofemoral	Same as for aortofemoral	Remove entire graft Intra-abdominal graft may suffice for revascularization; high amputation and death rates

Site	Clinical Presentation	Microbiology	Imaging	Management
Axillofemoral	Same as for aortofemoral	Same as for aortofemoral	Same as for aortofemoral	Remove entire graft Intraabdominal graft may suffice for revascularization; high amputation and death rates
Femoropopliteal	Higher incidence in first 3 mo Small sinus tract, abscess, cellulitis in inguinal incision	*S. aureus* *Streptococcus* *S. epidermidis* Other gram-negative bacilli		Remove entire graft Nonviable limbs must be revascularized or amputated; delay amputation as long as possible to allow maximum development of collaterals

Abbreviations: WBC = white blood cell; MRI = magnetic resonance imaging; CT = computed tomography; IV = intravenous.

with contrast and fat saturation should be performed for deeper grafts. If doubt about infection still exists, radioisotope imaging can be performed using either indium-111-labeled leukocytes or, if available, technetium-99 hexamethylpropyleneamine oxime (HMPAO)-labeled leukocytes. These studies, although sensitive, are limited by low specificity, particularly in the early postoperative setting (ie, in the period up to 12 weeks following surgery). Imaging findings that suggest the presence of graft infection include the presence of fluid around the graft, air, the defionition of abnormal tissue planes, extensive soft tissue swelling, and the identification of pseudoaneurysms, especially when more than one are apparent.

Therapy

Conventional treatment after vascular graft infection remains the gold standard and is defined as intensive antibiotic therapy and graft excision with extra-anatomic bypass revascularization if distal ischemia is present. Revascularization should be delayed, if possible, to establish potential collateral circulation and to decrease bacterial levels. Although antibiotic treatment and local wound care usually are unsuccessful when used alone, very specific criteria are now defining a subset of patients who may be managed without removal of the entire graft or with in situ grafting. These criteria include the following (at a minimum): a patent graft, intact and uninvolved anastomoses, absence of hemorrhage, and sterile blood cultures. Diabetic patients

and those receiving long-term systemic steroid therapy should be considered at highest risk for continued infection without graft removal and extra-anatomic bypass. Likelihood of successful graft preservation appears to be highest with early, low-grade infections (eg, early coagulase-negative staphylococcal infection) and lowest with gram-negative infections and *S. aureus*. Muscle flap coverage after aggressive perigraft debridement should be considered a vital component during attempts to salvage grafts. The optimal therapy of infected vascular grafts remains removal of the entire graft and revascularization where necessary through uninfected tissue planes.

If a new graft must be placed in the infected field (in situ grafting), use of autogenous artery or vein grafts may decrease susceptibility to infection. In the absence of available autologous vessels, prosthetic conduits (including rifampin-bonded prostheses), or cryopreserved arterial allografts may be used. Parenteral antibiotics should be administered for 4 to 6 weeks after the infected graft is removed, and some authorities have recommended administering oral antibiotics for an additional 1 to 3 months. Because of the risk of reinfection regardless of the treatment chosen, surveillance ultrasound examination should be performed every 3 to 6 months for life.

SUGGESTED READING

Antonios VS, Baddour LM. Intra-arterial device infections. *Curr Infect Dis Rep.* 2004;6:263–269.

Chirinos JA, et al. Septic thrombophlebitis: diagnosis and management. *Am J Cardiovasc Drugs.* 2006;6:9–14.

Perera GB, Fujitani RM, Kubaska SM. Aortic graft infection: update on management and treatment options. *Vasc Endovasc Surg.* 2006;40:1–10.

Pounds LL, et al. A changing pattern of infection after major vascular reconstructions. *Vasc Endovascular Surg.* 2005;39:511–517.

Zetrenne E, et al. Managing extracavitary prosthetic vascular graft infections: a pathway to success. *Ann Plastic Surg.* 2006;57: 677–682.

41. Pacemaker, Defibrillator, and VAD Infections

Stacey A. Rizza and James M. Steckelberg

Implantable cardiac pacemakers and defibrillators have greatly decreased the morbidity and mortality rates associated with cardiac arrhythmias. Increasing numbers of people are receiving these devices as the procedures for implantation and device technology improve; as a result, increasing numbers of devices are at risk for infection. The cumulative risk of pacemaker- and defibrillator-related infections after implantation has been estimated to be between 1% and 19% over the lifetime of the device. Infection of these implantable devices is associated with excess morbidity, including prolonged hospital stays and mortality rates as high as 30% in one series.

The first single-chamber permanent pacemakers were introduced for clinical use in the late 1950s. Today, it is estimated that more than 1 million people in the United States have permanent pacemakers. The pacemaker itself consists of a generator, placed below the pectoral muscle, that serves as the power source. An electrical stimulus from the generator travels through an insulated electrical conductor to the electrodes, which deliver the impulse to the endocardium or epicardial surface.

Early implantable cardioverter defibrillator devices (ICDs) required surgical placement of epicardial defibrillation patches, which was facilitated by sternotomy, lateral thoracotomy, or subxiphoid approach. Since 1988, transvenous placement of endocardial coils, similar to pacemakers, has become routine practice. In addition, generator packs have become smaller, allowing for pectoral placement as opposed to the traditional abdominal placement of larger, older generators. These technologic advances have reduced the morbidity rates associated with implantation and lowered the incidence of infection. In some cases, however, subcutaneous mesh patch electrodes are necessary for adequate defibrillation thresholds. These patches have been associated with a three-fold higher infection rate.

PACEMAKER AND DEFIBRILLATOR INFECTION

Several risk factors that predispose patients to developing infections of their pacemakers or defibrillators have been identified (Table 41.1). Infection of pacemakers occurs more often among patients with diabetes than among nondiabetic patients. However, studies have not adequately determined whether the greater number of device infections in diabetic patients is secondary only to a greater prevalence of implantable antiarrhythmic devices in this population or to an increased incidence of infection among diabetic patients with pacemakers. Other common risk factors include surgical procedure–related issues, skin disorders such as a rash or acne, systemic steroid use, and postinsertion hematomas at the generator site.

The microbiology of pacemaker and defibrillator infections is similar to that of other implantable prosthetic devices (Table 41.2). Early infections, within 4 weeks of implantation of the device, generally are related to device or wound contamination at the time of surgery. *Staphylococcus aureus* is the most common microbial cause. Infections occurring more than 4 weeks after device implantation typically are caused by less virulent organisms, such as coagulase-negative staphylococci. Other gram-positive organisms such as *Enterococcus* species, *Peptostreptococcus* species, or less commonly, gram-negative bacilli such as *Klebsiella* species, *Escherichia coli*, and *Pseudomonas* species, have also been reported. *Aspergillus* species, *Candida* species, and *Mycobacterium avium-intracellulare* infections have also been described but are rare.

CLINICAL PRESENTATION AND DIAGNOSIS

Implantable antiarrhythmic device infections are associated with several different clinical syndromes. Infection can involve the generator

Table 41.1 Patient Risk Factors for Infection of Implantable Pacemakers or Defibrillators

Diabetes mellitus
Number of operations
Total number of device-related procedures
Temporary pacing wires prior to implantation
Postinsertion hematoma
Implanted central catheter
Systemic steroids
Renal insufficiency at time of implantation
Skin disorders

pocket, the lead wires, native valve endocarditis, or a combination of these. Infections at the generator pocket are most common and may present with localized pain, erythema, and erosion of the skin over the generator or drainage from the pocket. A thick, yellowish, purulent drainage from the pocket with surrounding erythema is more often caused by *S. aureus*, whereas clear drainage without erythema is generally caused by less virulent organisms such as *Staphylococcus epidermidis*. The fibrous scar tissue surrounding the generator pocket is relatively avascular. This avascular tissue combined with a foreign body has been postulated to predispose the patient to persistent local infection. Patients with electrode or cardiac valve infection may have nonspecific symptoms such as fevers, chills, arthralgias, or wasting.

In patients with local symptoms of infection at the generator pocket, diagnosis is relatively straightforward. Sterilely obtained samples of fluid or drainage from the pocket should be cultured when possible. Blood cultures should also be obtained before beginning antimicrobial treatment to exclude an associated bacteremia. Positive blood cultures strongly suggest lead infection or endocarditis. Endocarditis related to pacemaker or defibrillator lead infections is rare and usually involves the tricuspid valve.

Several series have investigated the ability of echocardiography to identify lead vegetations. Transthoracic echocardiography has a sensitivity of about 30%, and transesophageal echocardiography has a sensitivity of about 95%. Other diagnostic tests that can be used to identify infections on implantable antiarrhythmic devices include computed tomography (CT) and gallium scans. Computed tomography

scans are most helpful in identifying inflammation at the site of epicardial defibrillator patches, and gallium scans have been used to delineate the extent of pacemaker or defibrillator infection; however, gallium scans are more useful when negative.

After appropriate cultures have been obtained, antimicrobial treatment should begin (Table 41.3). Empiric coverage should include antimicrobials with activity against *S. aureus* and coagulase-negative staphylococci. For methicillin-susceptible staphylococci, a β-lactamase–resistant penicillin such as oxacillin is appropriate. However, if sensitivities are unknown or the staphylococcus is methicillin resistant, vancomycin should be used. Enterococci are intrinsically resistant to cephalosporins and require penicillin or vancomycin, depending on sensitivities. If vancomycin cannot be clinically tolerated, daptomycin and linezolid are reasonable second-line agents for methicillin-resistant staphylococcus or vancomycin-resistant enterococcus. Daptomycin is U.S. Food and Drug Administration (FDA) approved for staphylococcal bacteremia and right-sided infective endocarditis at 6 mg/kg. Linezolid is active against these bacterium in vitro and although it has not been studied in vivo in this setting, would be a reasonable second-line agent to vancomycin. Treatment for infections caused by gram-negative organisms should be directed by the susceptibilities. Cephalosporins, quinolones, or expanded-spectrum penicillins are often appropriate choices.

MANAGEMENT

Most series report high relapse rates without complete explantation of the pacing or defibrillating system; therefore, guidelines, including those of the American Heart Association, recommend complete removal of the cardiac device for cardiac device infections. However, there are a few case reports of salvage of an infected generator, using intravenous antibiotics and 5 days of continuous irrigation to the pocket.

The least invasive surgical procedure possible should be used to explant the device. Removing the leads transvenously with traction through the original site has been shown to be adequate in several series. However, this procedure can be very difficult and result in avulsion of the tricuspid valve, arteriovenous fistulas, or retention of the lead tip. Recent advances with laser treatment has improved transvenous lead extraction greatly. A laser sheath is slid over the length of the electrode and used to excise

Table 41.2 Most Common Site of Infection and Associated Organism According to Time after Device Implantation

	Time of Onset After Placement	Site of Infection	Symptoms	Most Common Organism
Early	2–4 wk	Pocket	Local	*Staphylococcus aureus*
Late	>4 wk	Pocket and/or electrodes	Local and/or systemic	Coagulase-negative *Staphylococcus*

Table 41.3 Recommended Initial Antimicrobial Choice According to the Organism and Its Susceptibilities

Organism	Susceptibility	Primary	Alternative
Staphylococcus aureus	Penicillin sensitive	Penicillin G, 2–5 mU q4–6h[a]	Cefazolin, 1–2 g q8h Ceftriaxone, 1 g q24h
Staphylococcus epidermidis	Penicillin resistant Methicillin sensitive Methicillin resistant	Oxacillin, 1–2 g q4–6h Nafcillin, 1–2 g q4–6h Vancomycin, 15 mg/kg q12h[b]	Cefazolin, 1–2 g q8h
Enterococcus spp.	Penicillin sensitive Penicillin resistant	Penicillin G, 2–5 mU q4–6h[a] Ampicillin, 1–2 g q4–6h[a] Vancomycin, 15 mg/kg q12h[b]	Vancomycin, 15 mg/kg q12h[b]
Enterobacteriaceae[c]	Empiric treatment Directed treatment (based on cultures)	Cefepime, 1–2 g q12h[a] Ceftazidime, 1–2 g q8h[a] Least expensive, least toxic active agent	Quinolone[d] Imipenim, 500 mg q6h[a]
Pseudomonas aeruginosa[d,e]		Cefepime, 1–2 g q12h[a] Ceftazidime, 1–2 g q8h[a]	Quinolone[d] Imipenem, 500 mg q6h[a] Aztreonam, 0.5–2 g q8h[a]

[a] Dosages adjusted for renal function.
[b] Monitor and adjust dosage.
[c] For some organisms, combination therapy is appropriate.
[d] For example, ciprofloxacin, 200–400 mg q12h IV/250–750 mg bid PO,[a] or levofloxacin, 500–750 mg qd IV or PO.[a]
[e] Based on susceptibilities.

the implanted lead, allowing the entire lead to be withdrawn with little trauma. If complete lead removal is not possible transvenously, if large vegetations are present on the lead, or if epicardial patches need to be removed, an open surgical procedure is required. The risk of untreated infection compared with the risks of thoracotomy must be weighed for each clinical scenario. In one small nonrandomized study, 8 patients remained infection free after 4 weeks total of antimicrobial therapy despite retained lead tips after attempted transvenous lead removal.

The new pacing or defibrillating system (when required) should be implanted at a distant site. It is common practice to delay reimplantation and treat with intravenous antibiotics; however, a one-stage procedure was effective in one series of 31 patients. In another small nonrandomized study, 2 weeks of antimicrobial therapy before reimplantation, followed by 10 days of additional antimicrobial treatment, was successful. After the new device is implanted, antimicrobial therapy should be continued for 10 days to 2 weeks for less virulent organisms associated with rapid fever resolution and clinical improvement. A longer course of therapy should be used for more virulent organisms or in patients with prolonged fevers, persistent bacteremia, or endocarditis. Up to 6 weeks of antimicrobial therapy may be appropriate in these latter settings.

VAD INFECTION

Ventricular assist devices (VAD) are sometimes necessary for people who require myocardial support and, with new advances in technology, can be worn on the body outside the hospital for prolonged periods of time. Similar to other implantable cardiac devices, infection is relatively common with VAD and associated with significant morbidity. The incidence of infection ranges from 13% to 80%. The highest risk of infection is during the first 30 days and initial episodes of infection are rare after 90 days.

Several risk factors are associated with VAD infections, including length of surgery, hemorrhage, malnutrition, diabetes, and obesity. Because a VAD requires that a drive line exit the skin to be attached to an external device, this may prevent healing around the exit site and allow entry of skin flora into the implantable device. One study suggests that placing the device in the abdominal cavity instead of the peritoneal area decreases the chance of infection.

VAD infections can present as local drive line or pocket infections that result in pain, erythema, or purulence at the exit site. More severe infections can involve blood contact with intracorporeal VAD components or endocarditis. The average time between device placement and bacteremia was 23 days in one study.

The most common pathogens described with VAD infections have been *S. aureus*, *S. epidermidis*, *Enterococcus* sp., *Pseudomonas aeruginosa*, and *Candida* sp. One study reported that bacteremias that caused VAD infections resulted from vascular catheters (16%), lower respiratory tract infections (6%), abdominal infections (6%), and urinary tract infections (1%). In the remainder, no source was identified.

The most common VAD infections are localized to the cutaneous exit site. These infections can be treated with local wound care and antibiotics alone. Infections that involve the abdominal wall or the drive line should be treated with local debridement and rerouting the drive line through a clean site before antibiotic therapy. Although no randomized controlled studies clearly define how long antimicrobial should be used, 2 to 4 weeks was adequate for most reported cases. If a deeper infection involving the pumping system develops, systemic antimicrobials should be used for 4 to 6 weeks,

followed by oral suppressive antibiotics until the pump is removed.

PREVENTION

Preventing infections of implantable antiarrhythmic devices is fundamental. Because most early infections result from wound contamination at the time of surgery, a good skin preparation before surgery is essential. It remains standard practice to give antistaphylococcal antimicrobial prophylaxis before implantation. Although the evidence for this recommendation remains inconclusive, preoperative antimicrobial prophylaxis has proven successful for other intravascular implantable devices. Regarding endocarditis prophylaxis, the American Heart Association does not recommend antimicrobial prophylaxis for patients with implantable antiarrhythmic devices undergoing dental or other procedures associated with transient bacteremias.

SUGGESTED READING

Baddour LM, et al. Nonvalvular cardiovascular device-related infections. *Clin Infect Dis.* 2004;38:1128–1130.

Gandelman G, et al. Intravascular device infections: epidemiology, diagnosis, and management. *Cardiol Rev.* 2007;15:13–23.

Klug D, et al. Systemic infection related to endocarditis on pacemaker leads: clinical presentation and management. *Circulation.* 1997;95:2098–2107.

Molina JE. Undertreatment and overtreatment of patients with infected antiarrhythmic implantable devices. *Ann Thorac Surg.* 1997;63:504–509.

Smith PN, et al. Infections with nonthoracotomy implantable cardioverter defibrillators: can these be prevented? Endotak Lead Clinical Investigator: *Pacing Clin Electrophysiol.* 1998;21:42–55.

Uslan D, et.al. Cardiac devise infections: getting to the heart of the matter. *Curr Opin Infect Dis.* 2006;19:345–348.

Victor F, et al. Pacemaker lead infection: echocardiographic features, management, and outcome. *Heart.* 1999;81:82–87.

42. Acute Viral Hepatitis

Harmit Kalia and Paul Martin

Acute viral hepatitis is a systemic infection that affects predominantly the liver and remains a significant cause of morbidity and mortality in the United States despite the availability of effective vaccination against hepatitis A and B, the two major causes of viral hepatitis. There are five major hepatotropic viruses (A, B, C, D, and E) that cause acute hepatitis, resulting in acute hepatic necrosis and inflammation. Acute viral hepatitis typically runs its course in 6 months or less, in contrast to chronic hepatitis, which persists for longer. However, with modern serological and molecular diagnostic testing, the time course is less important in distinguishing acute from chronic viral hepatitis. The clinical illness produced by these viruses can range from asymptomatic and clinically inapparent to a fulminant and fatal acute infection. A major distinction between hepatitis A and E compared to hepatitis B, C, and D is that the former cause acute hepatitis only in contrast to the latter three, which are also important causes of chronic hepatitis and cirrhosis. Other viral infections, such as Epstein–Barr virus (EBV) and cytomegalovirus (CMV), can present with prominent hepatic dysfunction, although they are usually multisystem disorders. Hepatitis G virus and TT virus (TTV) have also been implicated in causing hepatic dysfunction, but their clinical significance remains dubious.

HEPATITIS A VIRUS

The hepatitis A virus (HAV) is an RNA virus, identified in 1973, transmitted via the fecal–oral route and is a common cause of acute hepatitis in North America. Community outbreaks due to contaminated water or food (eg, shellfish and green onions) are well recognized. It is more prevalent in low-socioeconomic areas, where a lack of adequate sanitation and poor hygienic practices facilitate its spread. In the United States, the incidence has decreased remarkably since the availability (1995) of an HAV vaccine and implementation of vaccination in children in regions with rates above the national average. In underdeveloped countries, HAV infection typically occurs in childhood and is subclinical

(age ≤6 years, 70% are asymptomatic), with most of the population infected before adulthood and acquiring immunity. HAV infection, occurring in older children and adults, is more likely to be symptomatic and associated with morbidity and even mortality. The average incubation period is 28 days (range 15 to 50 days), with peak fecal viral shedding and infectivity before the onset of clinical symptoms, which can include anorexia, fever, malaise, fatigue, nausea, vomiting, diarrhea, and right upper quadrant discomfort. In acute HAV infection, these symptoms tend to occur 1 to 2 weeks before the onset of jaundice and can last ≤2 months, although a significant number of these patients will have prolonged or relapsing disease.

The typical serologic course of acute HAV is shown in Figure 42.1. Injury to the hepatocytes is due to the host's immune response. Replication of HAV occurs exclusively within the cytoplasm of the hepatocyte, where the virus causes a noncytopathic infection. Recovery is usually uneventful. However, the illness occasionally is bimodal, with apparent recovery followed by return of symptoms before eventual recovery. A prolonged cholestatic phase may also occur, with clinical symptoms illustrated by persistent jaundice with prominent pruritis. It is important to recognize the rare fulminant case of HAV infection that more frequently occurs in adulthood. Features that suggest its onset include a prolonged prothrombin time, hypoglycemia, deepening jaundice, or hepatic encephalopathy. Prompt evaluation for liver transplant should be initiated if these ominous signs appear in a patient with acute HAV infection. The overall case fatality rate is 0.3% to 0.6% but reaches 1.8% among adults >50 years. Patients with chronic liver disease who contract hepatitis A are at increased risk for acute liver failure that has led to the recommendation that patients with chronic liver disease who are HAV naïve should undergo vaccination against HAV.

Routine diagnosis of acute HAV infection is made by detection of immunoglobulin M (IgM) anti-HAV antibody in serum (Table 42.1). IgM anti-HAV, which becomes detectable 5 to 10

Figure 42.1 Course of acute hepatitis A. HAV = hepatitis A virus; ALT = alanine aminotransferase; anti-HAV = antibody to hepatitis A virus. (Adapted from Martin P, Friedman LS, Dienstag JL. Diagnostic approach to viral hepatitis. In: Thomas HC, Zuckerman AJ, eds. *Viral Hepatitis.* Edinburgh: Churchill Livingstone; 1993.)

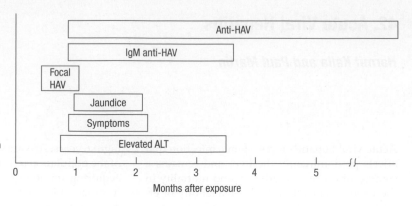

Table 42.1 Diagnostic Testing for Viral Hepatitis

Type	Diagnostic Tests	Comments
Hepatitis A virus (HAV)	IgM anti-HAV	Acute infection
	IgG anti-HAV	Resolved infection, immunity
Hepatitis B virus (HBV)	HBsAg	Indicates infection
	IgM anti-HBc	Acute infection
	HBeAg, HBV DNA	Indicates replication
	Anti-HBs	Indicates immunity
	IgG anti-HBc	Current or prior infection
Hepatitis C virus (HCV)	Anti-HCV	Indicates infection
	HCV RNA	Indicates infection/viremia
Hepatits D virus (HDV)	IgM anti-HDV	IgM anti-HBc positive indicates co-infection
		IgG anti-HBc positive indicates superinfection
	Anti-HDV	Indicates infection
	HDV RNA and HDV Antigen	Research tools at present
Hepatitis E virus (HEV)	IgM anti-HEV	Acute infection
	IgG anti-HEV	Resolved infection
EBV	EBV IgM and PCR	Indicates infection
CMV	CMV IgM and PCR	Indicates infection

Abbreviations: EBV = Epstein–Barr virus; CMV = cytomegalovirus

days before the onset of symptoms, persists for 3 to 12 months after infection. IgG anti-HAV antibody presents early in infection and persists indefinitely. The presence of IgG anti-HAV alone indicates previous infection with development of immunity to HAV either as a result of prior infection or vaccination.

Hepatocellular damage is due to the host's immune response that is mediated by CD8+T lymphocytes and natural killer cells. Infected hepatocytes are cleared under the influence of interferon-γ. Severe acute hepatitis is sequelae of an excessive host response that is clinically observed by marked reduction of HAV RNA during the infection.

Therapy

Acute HAV infection is self-limited without chronic sequelae. About 85% of patients who

Table 42.2 Therapy of Acute Viral Hepatitis

Type	Major Focus	Comments
Hepatitis A	Symptomatic therapy only	Recognition of FHF and referral for orthotopic liver transplantation important
Hepatitis B	Symptomatic therapy for acute disease; consider oral therapy for severe acute HBV	Observe for FHF
Hepatitis C	Interferon-α for acute infection	Treatment efficacious in acute hepatitis C virus
Hepatitis D	Vaccination against HBV	Liver disease clinically more severe than hepatitis B virus alone
Hepatitis E	Symptomatic therapy only	FHF can be seen in pregnant women
EBV	Symptomatic therapy only	Important factor in development of lymphoproliferated disease in post liver transplantation
CMV	Immunocompetent patients: none Immunocompromised: ganciclovir, forscarnet, and cidofovir	

Abbreviations: EBV = Epstein–Barr virus; CMV = cytomegalovirus; FHF = fulminant hepatic failure

are infected with HAV have unremarkable clinical and biochemical recovery within 3 months of onset of infection, and nearly all have complete recovery by 6 months. Therapy, as in all forms of acute viral hepatitis, is mainly supportive and includes bed rest if the patient is symptomatic, a high-calorie diet, avoidance of hepatotoxic medications, and abstinence from alcohol (Table 42.2). Fatalities due to HAV are more common with advancing age and in those with chronic liver disease. Because acute HAV is more likely to lead to hepatocellular failure in adults, these patients need close follow-up until symptoms resolve.

Because HAV is transmitted predominantly by the fecal–oral route, prevention includes good personal hygiene and immunization. General measures include careful handwashing practices, especially with food preparation and handling; proper disposal of waste and sewage; and access to clean water. Passive prophylaxis with intramuscular (IM) polyclonal serum immune globulin before and after exposure has been shown to be safe and efficacious. Preexposure prophylaxis should be reserved for nonimmune patients who are at risk for HAV or those who are allergic to HAV vaccine. Postexposure prophylaxis with immune globulin is recommended for the following high-risk groups: (1) close household and sexual contacts of an index patient with documented acute HAV, (2) staff and patients of institutions for the developmentally disabled with outbreaks of HAV, (3) children and staff of day-care centers with an index case of HAV, (4) those exposed

to protracted community outbreaks, and (5) travelers and military personnel who plan to visit countries endemic for HAV. A vaccine made with inactivated HAV has been available in the United States since 1995. It is recommended for travelers to endemic areas, nonimmune residents of such areas, others with potential occupational exposures such as caretakers in institutions for the developmentally challenged, and any person with underlying chronic liver disease. Persons with clotting-factor disorders should also be immunized. A dose of 1 mL as an IM injection into the deltoid muscle should be followed by a booster dose 6 to 12 months later. The initial dose should be given at least 1 month before possible exposure.

Treatment decisions regarding postexposure prophylaxis with immune globulin along with vaccination should be individualized. Concurrent administration of HAV immunoglobulin and vaccine is recommended for preexposure and postexposure prophylaxis in high-risk individuals. Antiviral therapy has no established role in the treatment of hepatitis A given the high rate of uneventful sponataneous recovery.

HEPATITIS B VIRUS

Hepatitis B virus (HBV) is the most common cause of chronic viral hepatitis worldwide and is also a major cause of acute viral hepatitis. There are an estimated 400 million people chronically infected with HBV. In the Far East and sub-Saharan Africa, up to 20% of the population has serologic evidence of current or prior HBV infection. In the United States, although HBV infection is less frequent, 0.5% of the population is chronically infected. Importantly, the prevalence of chronic HBV is much higher in certain immigrant communities, including Asian Americans. After acute HBV infection, the risk of chronic infection varies inversely with age. Thus, children younger than the age of 5 have a high risk of chronicity after acute HBV infection, whereas an immunocompetent adult has ≤5% likelihood of developing chronic infection after acute infection.

HBV is a DNA virus transmitted predominantly by intimate contact or percutaneous exposure. In Asia and other hyperendemic areas, vertical transmission is an important transmission route, whereas other important modes of transmission such as sexual and percutaneous are predominant in the Western world. The incubation period is 45 to 160 days. The usual course of a patient with acute HBV infection is shown in Figure 42.2. Typically, elevated alanine aminotransferase (ALT) levels and clinical symptoms appear earlier than jaundice. However, not all patients with acute HBV infection develop jaundice. About 70% of patients with acute HBV infection have subclinical or anicteric hepatitis, whereas 30% develop icteric hepatitis. Paradoxically, the patient with anicteric and less clinically severe acute HBV infection is more likely to become chronically infected than the individual with more symptomatic acute infection because a brisk immune response causes more hepatic dysfunction but also a greater likelihood of ultimate clearance of HBV infection.

The symptomatic patient should be reassured that full recovery is likely but should be warned to report back if symptoms such as deepening jaundice, severe nausea, or somnolence develop because these symptoms may herald fulminant hepatic failure. Fulminant hepatic failure occurs in approximately 0.1% to 0.5% of acute HBV cases. Like acute HAV, acute infection may be more severe in patients with underlying chronic liver disease.

The diagnosis of acute HBV hepatitis is made by the detection of hepatitis B surface antigen (HBsAg) and IgM antihepatitis B core antibody (anti-HBc IgM) in the serum (Table 42.3). Resolution of HBV infection is characterized by the loss of HBsAg. Development of the corresponding neutralizing antibody anti-HBs IgG ("total") antihepatitis B core antibody (anti-HBc IgG) with IgM anti-HBc and persists even after resolution of infection. Detection of IgG anti-HBc distinguishes immunity-acquired prior infection rather than vaccination in a patient with detectable anti-HBc.

As noted above, more than 95% of adults with acute HBV infection have successful clearance of HBV; the remainder develop chronic infection. Individuals who are immunocompromised or have another chronic condition such as renal failure are more likely to develop chronic infection. Children younger than 5 years and the elderly also have a greater likelihood of becoming chronically infected. The absence of a brisk immune response during acute HBV infection, implied by a relative absence of symptoms, with modest aminotransferase elevation in an anicteric patient, indicates that infection is more likely to become chronic. Chronic HBV infection

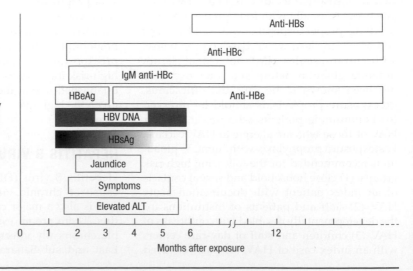

Figure 42.2 Typical course of acute hepatitis B. HBsAg = hepatitis B surface antigen; ALT = alanine aminotransferase; HBV DNA = hepatitis B virus DNA; HBeAg = hepatitis B e antigen; Anti-HBc = antibody to hepatitis B core antigen; Anti-HBe = antibody to hepatitis B e antigen; Anti-HBs = antibody to hepatitis B surface antigen. (Adapted from Martin P, Friedman LS, Dienstag JL. Diagnostic approach to viral hepatitis. In: Thomas HC, Zuckerman AJ, eds. *Viral Hepatitis*. Edinburgh: Churchill Livingstone; 1993.)

Table 42.3 Initial Serologic Workup of Suspected Acute Hepatitis

IgM anti-HAV
HBsAg
(If positive, then IgM anti-HBc)
Anti-HCV HCV RNA
Consider testing for CMV and EBV if A, B, and C tests are negative

is suggested by HBsAg positivity for longer than 6 months with absence of IgM anti-HBc. However, in severe reactivation of chronic HBV infection (spontaneous or iatrogenic due to administration of corticosteroids or chemotherapy) to an infected patient, IgM anti-HBc may reappear in serum although usually in low titer. The presence of HBeAg and HBV DNA in the serum suggests ongoing active viral replication or "high replicative state" in a patient with chronic infection. The absence of these markers of active replication in a chronically infected patient with no clinical evidence of liver disease is sometimes referred to as the *low* or *nonreplicative state.*

Therapy

Interferon-α, pegylated interferon-α 2a, lamivudine, adefovir, dipivoxil, entecavir, and telbivudine are currently approved therapies in the United States for the treatment of chronic HBV infection. Given the high rate of spontaneous resolution of acute HBV in otherwise healthy adults, no randomized controlled trials have been undertaken to assess efficacy of antiviral therapy for this indication. Anecdotal benefits from therapy of severe acute HBV have been reported. Therapy is indicated for chronically infected patients with active viral replication. Therapy for chronic HBV infection is discussed in Chapter 43, Chronic Hepatitis.

The highly effective recombinant HBV vaccine is recommended for all newborns, infants, adolescents, health care workers, hemodialysis patients, household contacts, and sexual partners of HBV-infected individuals, international travelers to endemic areas, injection drug users, men having sex with men or heterosexuals with multiple sexual partners, patients with chronic liver disease, and those who are potential organ transplant recipients. Postexposure prophylaxis

should consist of a combination of HBV vaccination and passive protection with hepatitis B immunoglobulin (HBIG).

Prompt referral to a transplant center is indicated for symptoms of fulminant acute HBV infection such as hepatic encephalopathy, worsening coagulopathy, or ascites. Outcomes of posttransplant for HBV have been favorable. There has been a very low rate of recurrence of viral infection with current immunoprophylaxysis regimens by using an oral antiviral agent with high-dose HBIG. However, indefinite HBIG therapy is both cumbersome and expensive. Accordingly, transplant programs are evaluating the use of alternative schedules of HBIG administration and combinations of antiviral agents to prevent allograft reinfection.

HEPATITIS C VIRUS

The hepatitis C virus (HCV) is a single-stranded RNA virus and is the major cause of what was formerly known as posttransfusional non-A, non-B hepatitis. It is estimated that about 170 million people in the world are chronically infected with HCV. Acute HCV is typically subclinical, with fewer than 25% of patients developing jaundice, and thus acute illness usually escapes medical attention. If symptomatic, acute HCV is less likely to lead to chronicity. HCV infection is usually transmitted parenterally. In the past, this was often by contaminated blood products. Now, most HCV infection is contracted by sharing contaminated needles among intravenous drug abusers or by other percutaneous or high-risk practices such as tattooing or possibly intranasal cocaine use, although the latter is contoversial. Sexual and maternal–neonatal transmission can occur but are generally less efficient routes of transmission although maternal human immunodeficiency virus (HIV) co-infection appears to increase the risk of perinatal transmission. Acute HCV infection results in a high rate of chronicity, up to 85% in some series.

Figure 42.3 shows the course of a patient with acute HCV infection progressing to chronicity. The incubation period is 14 to 180 days, after which elevation of ALT levels occurs and symptoms may appear, although, as noted, the acute illness is frequently subclinical. Fulminant hepatic failure due to acute HCV infection is very rare but may be more common in patients with underlying chronic HBV infection.

Figure 42.3 Typical course of acute hepatitis C progressing to chronic hepatitis C. HCV = hepatitis C virus; anti-HCV = antibody to the hepatitis C virus. (Adapted from Martin P, Friedman LS, Dienstag JL. Diagnostic approach to viral hepatitis. In: Thomas HC, Zuckerman AJ, eds. *Viral Hepatitis*. Edinburgh: Churchill Livingstone, 1993.)

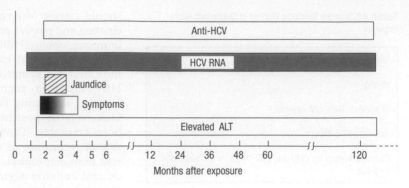

Routine diagnosis is made by detection of antibodies in serum to HCV (anti-HCV) by enzyme-linked immunosorbent assay (ELISA) testing in the serum. The recombinant immunoblot assay (RIBA) test was formerly used to enhance specificity as a supplemental test in ELISA-positive individuals. However, it has been supplanted by polymerase chain reaction (PCR) testing to confirm by viremia. Fluctuating ALT levels are characterisitic of chronic HCV infection. Perhaps a fifth of chronically infected patients have ALT levels regarded as within the normal range, although this reflects a lack of sensitivity of aminotransferases in detecting lesser degrees of necroinflammatory activity in the liver rather than an absence of liver injury. PCR techniques vary in their sensitivity in detecting HCV RNA. The even more sensitive transcription-mediated amplification (TMA) technique can detect even more minute quantities of HCV RNA (0.9-5.2 copies/mL).

Therapy

At present, indications for therapy in chronic HCV infection include persistent viremia and evidence of liver injury. Therapy of chronic HCV infection is discussed in more detail in Chapter 43 Chronic Hepatitis. Importantly, treatment of HCV during the acute phase is highly effective and results in a sustained virological response in up to 95% of treated patients. Absence of resolution of documented acute HCV within 12 weeks of onset is an indication to start interferon therapy. Acute HCV infection is most typically recognized in a health care worker after a needlestick injury. Although ribavirin is not required in treatment of acute HCV, it should be used in patients who do not respond to 3 months of interferon monotherapy. It has been reported that delaying antiviral therapy for 2 to 4 months after acute HCV infection does not compromise efficacy. This time frame allows spontaneous resolution of HCV without embarking on unnecessary treatment with interferon.

An HCV vaccine is not yet available because of the virus' heterogeneity, and until recently, lack of a cell culture system made its development difficult. There is no benefit from γ globulin administration following a needlestick exposure to HCV. In the health care setting, universal precautions are mandatory because the risk of HCV transmission by needlestick to health care workers is substantial, averaging about 3% particularly with hollow-bore needles. Routine screening by blood banks for HCV has reduced the risk of transmission by transfusion to a negligible level. Following liver transplant, HCV reinfection of the transplanted liver occurs in almost all the patients, with a subset of patients developing early severe recurrence of viral infection.

HEPATITIS D VIRUS

The hepatitis delta virus (HDV) is an incomplete RNA virus, requires HBsAg to complete its replicative cycle, and thus can occur only in the presence of HBV infection. The incubation period is 2 to 8 weeks. HDV may be transmitted simultaneously with HBV (co-infection) or acquired in chronic HBV carriers (superinfection). It is estimated that 5% of the HBV carriers in the world are infected with HDV. In the United States, HDV is spread mainly through intravenous drug abuse, whereas in other areas of high endemicity, such as the Mediterranean, intimate contact is implicated in transmission. Most cases of co-infection of HDV and HBV are self-limited, as in HBV infection, but patients are more likely to develop fulminant hepatitis than with HBV infection alone. If HDV is acquired by superinfection, progression to cirrhosis is more likely than with HBV alone. Superinfection often results in a flare in disease activity and clinical deterioration.

The diagnosis of HDV co-infection is made if serum IgM anti-HDV, HBsAg, and IgM anti-HBcAb are all present in serum. HDV superinfection is denoted by IgM anti-HDV, HBsAg, and IgG anti-HBcAb with absent IgM anti-HBc. During the acute phase of infection with HDV, serologic detection of antibodies to HDV is often insensitive. The only commercial assay available is a blocking radioimmunoassay for total anti-HDV; however, anti-HDV appears late in the course of acute delta virus infection. If HDV is clinically suspected, repeat testing may be required (see Table 42.1). HDAg can be detected by direct immunofluorescence or immunohistochemical staining. Direct serologic tests for delta virus include molecular hybridization techniques and reverse transcriptase–PCR-based assays, but these techniques are not widely available for clinical use.

Therapy

There is no specific treatment for acute HDV infection. Vaccination against HBV prevents HDV infection. The risk of HDV exposure by illicit intravenous drug use must be stressed to HBsAg-positive patients.

Patients with chronic HDV infection tend to present with progressive and often advanced liver disease, and HDV infection should be considered in a patient with clinically severe disease and HBV infection. The only medications with efficacy in the treatment of chronic HDV are the interferons, and generally treatment needs to be long-term. The oral agents used for HBV infection are ineffective in HDV as HBV replication is already suppressed by HDV. Liver transplantation is an option for patients with a fulminant presentation of acute HDV infection as well as decompensated cirrhosis. Liver transplant outcomes are better in patients with HDV than in those transplanted for HBV. HDV infection appears to have a protective effect against HBV reinfection, possibly via suppression of HBV replication.

HEPATITIS E VIRUS

The hepatitis E virus (HEV) is an RNA virus spread by fecal–oral transmission, similarly to HAV. The incubation period is 15 to 60 days and there is a high infection rate found in adults between the ages of 15 and 40. HEV disease occurs in developing countries, primarily through fecal contamination of water supplies. Several geographic regions, including China, India, Pakistan, and Mexico, have been identified as endemic. HEV infection is self-limited, without chronic sequelae. The highest attack rate appears to be among individuals between 15 and 40 years of age. A unique feature of this disease is that fulminant hepatic failure occurs more frequently in pregnancy. The illness carries a high mortality rate (15%–25%) among pregnant women in the third trimester. The United States is not an endemic region for the disease, but HEV should be considered in patients with hepatic dysfunction who have traveled to areas endemic for the disease within the last 1 to 2 months. Rare cases have been described in the United States in the absence of foreign travel. Selected reference laboratories can detect HEV RNA by PCR and acute infection by IgM anti-HEV antibodies.

Therapy

As with acute HAV, the disease is self-limited, and therapy is supportive only. Pregnant patients should be discouraged from traveling to endemic areas. During travel to an endemic area, common sense precautions include careful handwashing, drinking bottled water only, and abstaining from fresh raw vegetables or fruits and uncooked shellfish.

EPSTEIN–BARR VIRUS

EBV, the causative agent for infectious mononucleosis (fever, pharyngitis, and lymphadenopathy), is common and produces a wide spectrum of clinical manifestations. In 80% to 90% of cases, it causes asymptomatic liver enzyme elevation. Serum aminotransferases, alkaline phosphatase, and lactate dehydrogenase increase to 2 to 3 times the upper limits of normal. Clinical manifestations can include abdominal pain, hepatomegaly, splenomegaly, and, rarely, jaundice. The serum aminotransferases typically rise over 1 to 2 weeks, and in most patients the disease is self-limited with resolution of symptoms and normalization of enzymes over the subsequent 4 to 6 weeks. Severe hepatitis and fulminant hepatic failure, although rare, have been reported. This tends to occur more commonly in patients older than 30 years of age. The diagnosis of EBV hepatitis is suggested by clinical features of mononucleosis and laboratory data suggestive of acute EBV infection. Leukocytosis with a predominance of lymphocytes and monocytes is commonly seen. Up to half of these patients may have mild thrombocytopenia. EBV IgM antibodies peak early and can persist for months, after which EBV IgG develops. Although the Monospot is sensitive in detecting heterophile antibodies, it is not specific for EBV infection. EBV DNA quantification can be accomplished through PCR assays on blood or plasma. Liver biopsy is not usually indicated, but if the case is a diagnostic challenge, in situ hybridization or PCR of the biopsy sample may be used to confirm the diagnosis. Treatment is supportive as no specific treatment exists. Acyclovir has been used without effect on symptoms or outcome. EBV may rarely cause chronic infection in immunocompetent patients. EBV infection is an important factor in the development of posttransplantation lymphoproliferative disease in organ transplant recipients.

CYTOMEGALOVIRUS

CMV infection frequently involves the liver, manifesting commonly as asymptomatic elevation of serum aminotransaminases. It can be a result of a primary infection or reactivation of a latent infection in an immunocompromised host. In immunocompetent children and adults, primary CMV infection usually is subclinical but may cause an illness that can mimic mononucleosis. The clinical course is typically mild and self-limited, but CMV has been implicated in hepatic granulomata, cholestatic hepatitis, and even rare cases of fatal hepatic necrosis. CMV can be severe and even life-threatening in patients with impaired cellular immunity. The infection is typically disseminated, and liver involvement can be in the form of hepatitis or cholangiopathy (mimicking primary sclerosing cholangitis). Routine diagnosis of acute infection can be made by detecting IgM antibodies to CMV. Liver biopsy may be indicated in an immunocompromised patient, for instance, following liver transplant where the characteristic owl eye inclusions help establish the diagnosis. Another reliable and fast method to detect CMV viremia is by PCR. Therapy for immunocompetent patients with mild CMV infection is not needed. For immunocompromised patients, effective therapies include ganciclovir.

HEPATITIS G VIRUS

The hepatitis G virus (HGV) is a single-stranded RNA virus with some genomic similarity to HCV. HGV is a blood-borne virus transmitted by transfusion of contaminated blood products or parenteral exposure to blood among intravenous drug abusers or hemodialysis patients. Accordingly, HGV often occurs as a co-infection with other hepatitis viruses (especially 10%–20% of HCV patients) because of similar modes of transmission. Vertical transmission from mother to infant and sexual transmission are rare. HGV can be diagnosed by testing the serum using PCR, but the sensitivity and specificity of this test is unknown. The role of HGV as a cause of acute or chronic hepatic dysfunction has not been established. Indeed, persistent viremia for many years has been documented in the absence of aminotransferase elevations. There is no indicated test for it at this time in suspected viral hepatitis.

TT VIRUS

TT virus is a single-stranded, nonenveloped circular DNA virus first isolated in Japan in 1997 from the serum of a patient (initials, T.T.) with posttransfusion, non-A-to-G hepatitis. It is highly prevalent in the general population. Since its initial discovery, TTV has been increasingly reported to be highly prevalent worldwide. TTV DNA titers are high in the liver compared to the serum, but the correlation with viremia and serum elevations in aminotransferases have not been consistently demonstrated. Co-infection with other chronic viral hepatitis viruses commonly occurs and most likely reflects similar modes of transmission. However, TTV does not alter the natural history of the co-infected patient. Although TTV was implicated as the causative virus in the patient in whom it was first identified, other studies have not been able to support this. Therefore, despite early interest in TTV as a possible etiologic agent in viral hepatitis and cirrhosis, current data suggest that TTV does not play a significant role in the genesis of acute or chronic liver disease.

SUGGESTED READING

Keeffe EB, Dieterich DT, Hans SH, et al. A treatment algorithm for the management of chronic hepatitis B virus infection in the United States: an update. *Clin Gastroenterol Hepatol.* 2006;4(8):936–962.

Keeffe EB, Iwarson S, McMahon BJ, et al. Safety and immunogenicity of hepatitis A vaccine in patients with chronic liver disease. *Hepatology.*1998; 27(3):887–888.

Saab S, Martin P. Tests for acute and chronic viral hepatitis: finding your way through the alphabet soup of infection and superinfection. *Postgrad Med*. 2000;107(2):123–126, 129–130.

Sjogren MH. Serologic diagnosis of viral hepatitis. *Med Clin North Am*. 1996;80(5): 929–956.

Sjogren MH. Prevention of hepatitis B in nonresponders to initial hepatitis B virus vaccination. *Am J Med*. 2005;118(suppl 10A):34S–39S.

Taylor RM, Davern T, Munoz S, Han SH, et al. Fulminant hepatitis A virus infection in the United States: incidence, prognosis and outcomes. *Hepatology*. 2006;44(6):1397–1399.

Tran TT, Martin P. Hepatitis B: epidemiology and natural history. *Clin Liver Dis*. 2004;8(2):255–266.

Weston SR, Martin P. Serologic and molecular testing in viral hepatitis: an update, *Can J Gastroenterol*. 2001;15(3):177–184.

43. Chronic Hepatitis

Michelle E. Freshman and Lawrence S. Friedman

Chronic hepatitis is defined as chronic necroinflammation of the liver of more than 3 to 6 months' duration, demonstrated by persistently abnormal serum aminotransferase levels and characteristic histologic findings. The causes of chronic hepatitis include hepatitis B, C, and D viruses (HBV, HCV, and HDV) as well as alcoholic and nonalcoholic steatohepatitis (NASH), autoimmune hepatitis, chronic hepatitis associated with certain medications (such as isoniazid and nitrofurantoin), Wilson disease, α_1-antitrypsin deficiency, and, rarely, celiac sprue. In addition to etiology, chronic hepatitis is characterized by the grade of portal, periportal, and lobular inflammation (minimal, mild, moderate, or severe) and the stage of fibrosis (none,

mild, moderate, severe, cirrhosis). This chapter focuses on the infectious causes of chronic hepatitis—HBV, HCV, and HDV.

CHRONIC HEPATITIS B

Chronic hepatitis B afflicts nearly 400 million people worldwide (Figure 43.1) and 1.5 million, with a predominance of men, in the United States. It may be identified initially as acute hepatitis B that does not resolve or diagnosed in a patient who is evaluated because of persistently elevated serum aminotransferase levels. Early in the course of chronic hepatitis B, hepatitis B e antigen (HBeAg) and high levels of HBV DNA are present in serum, indicative

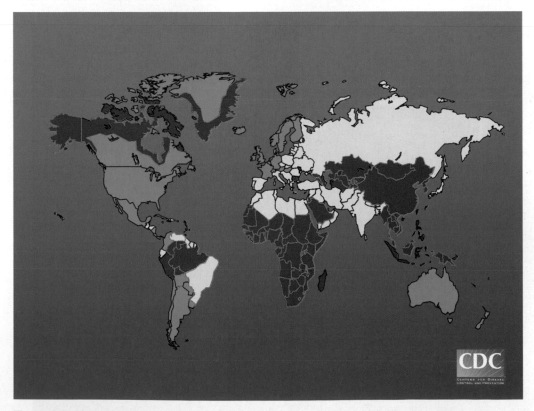

Figure 43.1 Map of the world showing the prevalence of the chronic hepatitis B carrier state in low- (green, ≤2%), medium- (yellow, 2%–7%), and high- (red, ≥ 8%) prevalence areas. Adapted from the Centers For Disease Control Web site, Viral Hepatitis B, Educational Materials, CDC Viral Hepatitis Brochures/Posters, Hepatitis B 101, slide 3/20 2005. [http://www.cdc.gov/mmwr/Pdf/rr/rr5416.pdf].

of active viral replication and necroinflammatory activity in the liver. The risk of progression to cirrhosis (at a rate of 2%–5.5% per year) and hepatocellular carcinoma (at a rate of >2% per year in those with cirrhosis) correlates with the patient's baseline serum HBV DNA level. Antibody to hepatitis B core antigen of the immunoglobulin G (IgG) class (IgG anti-HBc) is typically present in patients with chronic hepatitis B, but some patients may have low levels of IgM anti-HBc, a marker more typical of acute hepatitis B (Table 43.1). In some patients, clinical and biochemical improvement coincides with disappearance of HBeAg (occurring in 9%–20% of patients per year), reduced HBV DNA levels (≤10^5 copies/mL), and appearance of anti-HBe in serum (Figure 43.2). If cirrhosis has not yet developed, such persons with the *inactive HBsAg carrier state* are at a low risk for the subsequent development of cirrhosis and hepatocellular carcinoma.

Mutations of the HBV genome may develop during the course of chronic hepatitis B. Certain mutations of the precore or core promoter region of the HBV genome typically lead to reduced or absent production of HBeAg but high serum levels of HBV DNA (*HBeAg-negative chronic hepatitis B*). Co-infection with HCV or human immunodeficiency virus (HIV) with a low CD4

Table 43.1 Clinical Significance of Serologic Markers Used in the Diagnosis of Hepatitis B Virus (HBV) Infection

Serologic Marker	Clinical Significance
HBsAg	Acute or chronic infection
IgM anti-HBc	Acute infection
HBeAg	High infectivity
Anti-HBe	Low infectivity (with exceptions)
Anti-HBs	Immunity
IgG anti-HBc (and HBsAg)	Chronic infection
IgG anti-HBc (and anti-HBs)	Resolved infection

Abbreviations: Anti-HBe = antibody to hepatitis B e antigen; anti-HBs = antibody to hepatitis B surface antigen; HBeAg = hepatitis B e antigen; HBsAg = hepatitis B surface antigen; IgG anti-HBc = IgG antibody to hepatitis B core antigen; IgM anti-HBc = IgM antibody to hepatitis B core antigen.

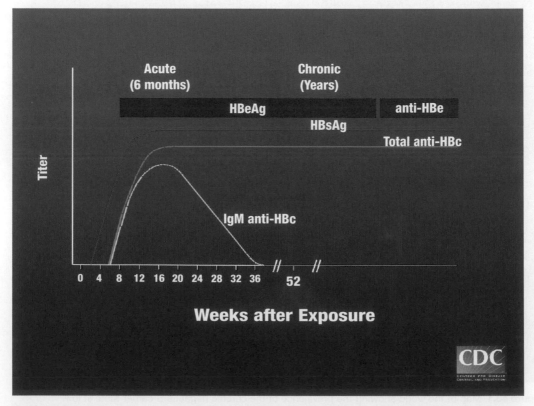

Figure 43.2 Typical serologic course of chronic hepatitis B virus infection. Adapted from the Centers for Disease Control Web site, Viral Hepatitis B, Educational Materials, CDC Viral Hepatitis Brochures/Posters, Hepatitis B 101, slide 10/20.

count is also associated with an increased frequency of cirrhosis.

Treatment

Treatment of chronic hepatitis B is generally indicated in patients with active viral replication characterized by a serum HBV DNA level of $>10^5$ copies/mL and elevated serum aminotransferase levels. Treatment options include interferon-based therapy as well as nucleoside or nucleotide analogs (Table 43.2).

The interferon formulations approved for the treatment of chronic hepatitis B are pegylated interferon (peginterferon) α-2a, 180 μ subcutaneously once weekly for 48 weeks, and recombinant human interferon α-2b, 5 million or 10 million units by subcutaneous injection, once daily or 3 times weekly for 4 to 6 months. Because of once-weekly administration and higher response rates, peginterferon is preferred. The definition of a treatment response is shown in Table 43.3, and specific goals of therapy are listed in Table 43.4. Up to 40% of treated patients will respond with sustained normalization of aminotransferase levels, disappearance of HBeAg and HBV DNA from serum, appearance of anti-HBe, and improved survival (see Table 43.3). A response is most likely in patients with a low baseline HBV DNA level and high aminotransferase levels and is more likely in those infected with HBV genotype A (prevalent in the United States) than with D (prevalent in the Middle East and South Asia). Moreover, some responders may eventually clear HBsAg from serum and liver tissue, develop anti-HBs in serum, and thus be cured (see Table 43.4). Relapses are uncommon in such complete responders. However, the need for self-injection and high frequency of side effects (Table 43.5) limit the attractiveness of interferon therapy for HBV infection (see also Chronic Hepatitis C, Treatment). Moreover, interferon cannot be used to treat patients with cirrhosis because of the risk of precipitating decompensation.

Nucleoside and nucleotide analogs may be used instead of interferon for the treatment of chronic hepatitis B and are much better tolerated (Table 43.6). The first available nucleoside analog was lamivudine, which, in a dose of 100 mg orally daily, reliably suppresses HBV DNA in serum, improves liver histology in 60% of patients, and leads to normal serum alanine aminotransferase (ALT) levels in over 40% as well as HBeAg-to-anti-HBe seroconversion in 20% of patients after 1 year of therapy (Table 43.7). The drug is continued for at least 6 months

Table 43.2 Therapeutic Agents Used to Treat Chronic Hepatitis B Virus (HBV) Infection

Immune Modulators	Nucleoside and Nucleotide Analogs
Interferon α	Lamivudine
Peginterferon α	Adefovir dipivoxil
Thymosin[a]	Entecavir
Therapeutic vaccines[a]	Telbivudine
α-glucosidase inhibitor derivatives[a]	Tenofovir[a]
Monoclonal antibodies[a]	Clevudine[a]
	Emtricitabine[a]
	Famciclovir[a]
	Pradefovir[a]

[a] Under investigation.

Table 43.3 Definition and Criteria of Treatment Responses in Chronic Hepatitis B Virus (HBV) Infection

Biochemical	Decrease in serum ALT level to normal
Virologic	Decrease in serum HBV DNA level to ≤10^5 copies/mL
Histologic	Decrease in necroinflammatory score by 2 points or more
Sustained virologic response: Biochemical, virologic, and histologic responses ≥ 6 months posttreatment	
Abbreviations: ALT = alanine aminotransferase.	

after HBeAg-to-anti-HBe seroconversion has occurred, and rates of response increase with longer treatment duration. In patients with advanced fibrosis or cirrhosis, treatment with lamivudine reduces the risk of hepatic decompensation and hepatocellular carcinoma. By the end of the first year of treatment, however, 15% to 30% of responders become resistant to lamivudine, as a result of a mutation in the polymerase gene (YMDD motif) of HBV DNA. These patients may experience a relapse of hepatitis, as demonstrated by a rise in serum aminotransferase and HBV DNA levels. The rate of resistance to lamivudine rises to 70% when the drug is continued for 5 years. Interferon used in combination with lamivudine may reduce the rate of resistance but does not appear to be more

Table 43.4 Goals of Therapy for Chronic Hepatitis B Virus (HBV) Infection

Sustained Suppression of HBV Replication
HBV DNA undetectable in serum HBeAg to anti-HBe seroconversion HBsAg to anti-HBs seroconversion
Remission of Liver Disease
Normalization of serum ALT levels Improvement in liver histology
Improvement in Clinical Outcome
Prevention of liver failure and hepatocellular carcinoma Improved survival
Abbreviations: ALT = alanine aminotransferase; anti-HBe = antibody to hepatitis B e antigen; anti-HBs = antibody to hepatitis B surface antigen hepatitis B virus; HBeAg = hepatitis B e antigen; HBsAg = hepatitis B surface antigen.

Table 43.5 Adverse Effects of Standard and Pegylated Interferon

Flu-like symptoms
Neuropsychiatric side effects
Exacerbation of underlying autoimmune diseases
Myalgia and arthralgia
Immunosuppression
Nausea, anorexia, weight loss
Bone marrow suppression
Thyroid dysfunction
Pulmonary disorders
Retinal changes (reversible)
Injection-site reactions

effective in achieving long-term suppression of viral replication than either drug alone.

A nucleotide analog, adefovir dipivoxil, has activity against both wild-type and lamivudine-resistant HBV. The standard dose is 10 mg orally once a day. As with lamivudine, only a small number of patients achieve sustained suppression of HBV replication with adefovir, and long-term therapy is often required. Resistance to adefovir is less frequent than with lamivudine and is seen in up to 20% of patients treated for 5 years. Patients with underlying renal dysfunction are at risk of nephrotoxicity from adefovir.

Entecavir is another nucleoside analog approved for the treatment of chronic hepatitis B and is more potent than lamivudine and adefovir. The dose is 0.5 mg orally once a day or, for patients who have become resistant to lamivudine, 1 mg daily. Histologic improvement is observed in 70% of treated patients, and HBV DNA is suppressed in serum in up to 80%. Resistance to entecavir does not occur when entecavir is used as a first-line therapy but occurs in 9% of lamivudine-resistant patients after 1 year and up to 40% after 4 years.

The most recently approved nucleoside analog is telbivudine given in a dose of 600 mg orally once a day. It is more potent than lamivudine, but resistance to the drug may develop, and there is some cross-resistance in patients who have become resistant to lamivudine.

Tenofovir, a drug used for the treatment of HIV infection, also has substantial activity against HBV but has not been approved for use in HBV infection. Other nucleoside analogs, including emtricitabine and clevudine, are under study, and strategies using multiple drugs are being investigated.

Nucleoside and nucleotide analogs are well tolerated even in patients with decompensated cirrhosis (for whom the treatment threshold is an HBV DNA level of 10^4 copies/mL) and may be effective in patients with rapidly progressive hepatitis B (*fibrosing cholestatic hepatitis*) following organ transplantation. Although therapy with these agents leads to biochemical, virologic, and histologic improvement in patients with HBeAg-negative chronic hepatitis B and baseline HBV DNA levels $\geq 10^4$ copies/mL, relapse is frequent when therapy is stopped, and long-term treatment is often required. The relative efficacy rates of the agents used to treat chronic hepatitis B are shown in Table 43.8. Sequential addition of a second antiviral agent (eg, adefovir added to lamivudine) or substitution of an alternative agent (eg, entecavir for adefovir) is usually effective after resistance to the first agent has developed. The development of resistance occasionally results in hepatic decompensation. Combined use of peginterferon and a nucleoside or nucleotide analog has not been shown convincingly to have substantial advantage over the use of either type of drug alone.

Treatment with a nucleoside analog is also recommended for inactive HBV carriers prior to the initiation of immunosuppressive therapy or cancer chemotherapy to prevent reactivation. In patients infected with both HBV and HIV, antiretroviral therapy, including two drugs

Table 43.6 Pros and Cons of Drugs Used to Treat Chronic Hepatitis B virus (HBV) infection

	Peginterferon	Lamivudine	Adefovir	Entecavir	Telbivudine
Pros	Finite duration	Oral	Oral	Oral	Oral
	Durable response	Negligible side effects	Negligible side effects	Negligible side effects	Negligible side effects
	No resistant mutants	Has been used in pregnancy and prior to chemotherapy	Effective against lamivudine-resistant mutants	More potent than other oral agents; little resistance	
	Shown to lead to HBsAg → anti-HBs seroconversion in responders				
Cons	Injection	Indefinite duration of therapy in incomplete responders	Indefinite duration of therapy in incomplete responders	Indefinite duration of therapy in incomplete responders	Indefinite duration of therapy in incomplete responders
	Side effects (see Table 5)		Renal toxicity in higher doses		Elevated CK
			Resistant mutants (20% at 4 years)		
		High rate of resistant mutants (>70% after 4 years)		10% cross-resistance with lamivudine	Some cross-resistance with lamivudine

Abbreviations: CK = creatine kinase; HBsAg = hepatitis B surface antigen.

Table 43.7 Features of Therapy with Nucleoside/Nucleotide Analogs for Chronic Hepatitis B Virus (HBV) Infection

HBeAg-to-anti-HBe seroconversion in 12%–21% at 1 year
HBeAg-to-anti-HBe seroconversion increases over time
Serum ALT level predicts HBeAg loss
HBeAg-negative patients are more likely than HBeAg-positive patients to become HBV DNA-negative, but response is much less durable
Liver histology improves
Degree of viral suppression varies among drugs
Rate of serum HBsAg loss is low (≤1%) after 1 year
Resistance profiles vary

Abbreviations: ALT = alanine aminotransferase; anti-HBe = antibody to hepatitis B e antigen; anti-HBs = antibody to hepatitis B surface antigen; HBeAg = hepatitis B e antigen; HBsAg = hepatitis B surface antigen.

Table 43.8 Rates of Suppression of Serum Hepatitis B Virus (HBV) DNA to Undetectable Levels after 1 Year of Treatment in Patients with Chronic Hepatitis B

	HBeAg-Positive Patients (%)	HBeAg-Negative Patients (%)
Placebo	0	0
Peginterferon	25	63
Lamivudine	36	72
Adefovir dipivoxil	21	51
Entecavir	67	90
Telbivudine	58	79

Abbreviation: HBeAg = hepatitis B e antigen.

active against both agents (eg, lamivudine and tenofovir), has been recommended when the CD4 count is less than 500/mm^3. Guidelines for the treatment of chronic hepatitis B are summarized in Figures 43.3A, 43.3B , and 43.3C.

CHRONIC HEPATITIS C

Chronic hepatitis C develops in up to 85% of patients with acute hepatitis C. It is clinically indistinguishable from chronic hepatitis of other causes and may be the most common cause of chronic hepatitis. Worldwide, 200 million

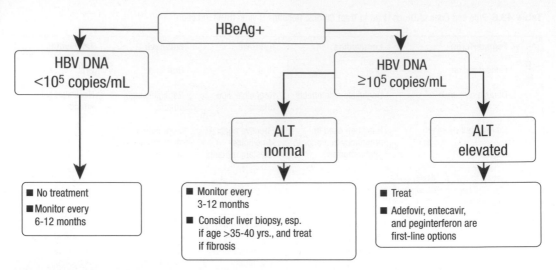

Figure 43.3A Suggested treatment algorithm for HBeAg-positive patients with compensated chronic hepatitis B virus (HBV). Adapted from Keeffe EB, Dieterich DT, Han SH, et al. A treatment algorithm for the management of chronic hepatitis B virus infection in the United States: an update. *Clin Gastroenterol Hepatol.* 2006;4:936–962, with permission. ALT = alanine aminotransferase; HBeAg = hepatitis B e antigen.

people are infected with HCV, with 1.8% of the U.S. population infected. In approximately 40% of cases, serum aminotransferase levels are persistently normal. The diagnosis is confirmed by detection of antibody to HCV (anti-HCV) by enzyme immunoassay (EIA). In rare cases of chronic hepatitis C, the anti-HCV is negative by EIA, but HCV RNA is detected by polymerase chain reaction (PCR) testing.

Patients with chronic hepatitis C should undergo baseline measurement of the HCV RNA level and genotype testing; HCV genotypes 1a and 1b, by far the most prevalent in the United States, are less responsive to antiviral treatment than genotypes 2 and 3 (see later). Liver biopsy is often recommended to assess the stage of fibrosis, particularly in patients infected with HCV genotype 1. Because of high response rates to treatment in patients infected with HCV genotype 2 or 3, liver biopsy is often deferred in these patients. Progression to cirrhosis occurs in 20% of affected patients after 20 years, with an increased risk in men, those who drink more than 50 g of alcohol daily, and possibly those who acquire HCV infection after age 40. Blacks have a higher rate of chronic hepatitis C but lower rates of fibrosis progression and response to therapy than whites. Immunosuppressed persons, including patients with hypogammaglobulinemia, HIV infection with a low CD4 count, and organ transplants, appear to progress more rapidly to cirrhosis than immunocompetent persons with chronic hepatitis C. Cannabis and tobacco

smoking and hepatic steatosis also appear to promote progression of fibrosis. Persons with chronic HCV infection and persistently normal serum aminotransferase levels usually have mild chronic hepatitis with little fibrosis, but up to 10% of these patients have cirrhosis.

Treatment

Treatment of chronic hepatitis C is generally considered in patients under age 70 with more than minimal fibrosis on a liver biopsy specimen. Peginterferon taken once a week is more effective than standard interferon, presumably because of sustained high blood levels, and is used in combination with oral ribavirin, a nucleoside analog. Two formulations of peginterferon are available: peginterferon α-2b, with a 12-kDa polyethylene glycol (PEG), and peginterferon α-2a, with a 40-kDa PEG. Whether there are clinically important differences between the two formulations is unclear. The addition of ribavirin results in higher sustained response rates than interferon or peginterferon alone. Overall, sustained response rates (SVRs) with a combination of peginterferon and ribavirin are as high as 55% (46% for HCV genotype 1 and up to 82% for genotypes 2 or 3). Response rates are lower in patients with advanced fibrosis, high levels of viremia, alcohol consumption, large body habitus, male sex, HIV coinfection, and severe steatohepatitis. SVRs are also lower in blacks than whites, in part because of higher rate of genotype 1 among infected black

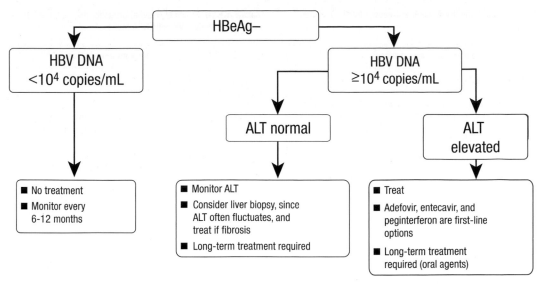

Figure 43.3B Suggested treatment algorithm for HBeAg-negative patients with compensated chronic hepatitis B virus (HBV). Adapted from Keeffe EB, Dieterich DT, Han SH, et al. A treatment algorithm for the management of chronic hepatitis B virus infection in the United States: an update. *Clin Gastroenterol Hepatol*. 2006;4:936–962, with permission. ALT = alanine aminotransferase; HBeAg = hepatitis B e antigen.

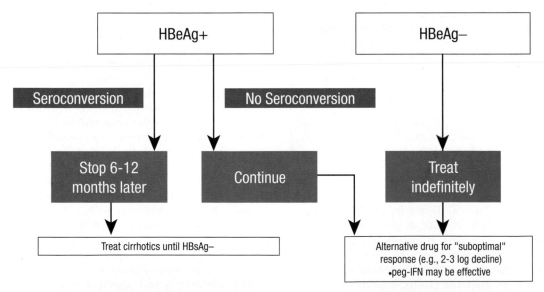

Figure 43.3C Treatment end points for patients with hepatitis B e antigen-positive (HBeAg+) and hepatitis B e antigen-negative (HBeAg-) chronic hepatitis B. Adapted from Keeffe EB, Dieterich DT, Han SH, et al. A treatment algorithm for the management of chronic hepatitis B virus infection in the United States. *Clin Gastroenterol Hepatol*. 2004;2:87–106, and Marcellin P, Boyer N, Piratvisuth T, et al. Efficacy and safety of peginterferon alpha-2a (40KD) (Pegasys) in patients with chronic hepatitis B who had received prior treatment with nucleos(t)ide analogues—the Pegalam cohort. *J Hepatol*. 2006;44(suppl 2):S187. IFN = interferon.

patients. For prior nonresponders to standard interferon and ribavirin, sustained response rates to retreatment with peginterferon and ribavirin are only 10% to 15%. Contraindications to treatment with interferon and ribavirin are shown in Table 43.9.

When used with peginterferon α-2b, ribavirin is given in a dose based on the patient's weight, with a range of 800 to 1400 mg daily divided into two doses (Table 43.10). When used with peginterferon α-2a, the daily ribavirin dose is 1000 or 1200 mg, depending on whether the patient's weight is less than or greater than 75 kg. Patients infected with HCV genotype 1a or 1b are treated for 48 weeks. In patients who achieve a rapid virologic response

Table 43.9 Contraindications to Treatment with Interferon and Ribavirin[a]

Clinically decompensated liver disease[b]
History of solid organ transplant
Severe extrahepatic disease (malignancy, blood disorders, unstable angina, severe chronic lung disease)
Uncontrolled autoimmune disorders
Pregnancy or planned pregnancy by the patient or patient's sexual partner
Unwillingness or inability to use adequate birth control
Documented nonadherence to prior medical treatment, procedures, and follow-up
Inability to self-administer or to arrange appropriate medication injection
Severe uncontrollable psychiatric disease, particularly depression with current suicidal risk
Ongoing injection drug use[c]
Ongoing alcohol abuse[c]

[a] Adapted From National Institutes of Health Consensus Development Conference Statement. Management of hepatitis C: 2002—June 10–12, 2002. *Hepatology.* 2002; 36:S3–S20.
[b] Bilirubin > 1.5 mg/dL; prothrombin time > 15 seconds; international normalized ratio > 1.7; albumin ≤ 3.4 g/dL; ascites; bleeding esophageal varices; hepatic encephalopathy. As defined by Hoofnagle JH, Seeff LB. Peginterferon and ribavirin for chronic hepatitis C. *N Engl J Med.* 2006;355:2444–2451.
[c] If high risk for relapse exists.

Table 43.10 Principal Antiviral Drugs for the Treatment of Chronic Hepatitis C Virus (HCV) Infection

Drug	Recommended Dose[a]
Peginterfon α-2a (Pegasys)	180 μg subcutaneously once weekly
Peginterferon α-2b (PEG-Intron)	1.5 μg/kg subcutaneously (up to 150 μg/week) once weekly
Ribavirin (Copegus, Rebetrol)	Genotype 1: 1,000 mg if ≤ 75 kg OR 1200 mg if > 75 kg orally daily (in two divided doses) Genotype 2 and 3: 800 mg orally daily (in two divided doses)
Hemodialysis	Peginterfon α-2a 135 μg subcutaneously once weekly
Renal dysfunction	Reduce dose of peginterferon α-2b by 25% if creatinine clearance is 30–50 mL/min; Reduce dose by 50% if creatinine clearance is 10–29 mL/min
Severe anemia	Reduce dose of ribavirin in decrements of 200 mg or hold temporarily

[a] Adjusted regimens (necessary in up to 30%–40% of cases).

(RVR), defined as a decrease in the serum HCV RNA level to ≤50 IU/mL by week 4, treatment for 24 weeks results in an SVR of 90%; in practice, treatment is usually given for a total of 48 weeks. For those who do not achieve an RVR, but who meet the threshold for an early virologic response (EVR), a reduction in viral load of at least 2 logs by 12 weeks, treatment is continued for the full 48 weeks. If an EVR is not achieved, but viral levels decline substantially by 12 weeks and become undetectable by 24 weeks, treatment may be extended to 72 weeks. In the absence of an EVR, treatment is typically discontinued, because an SVR is unlikely. Patients with cirrhosis or a high viral level in serum (>400000 IU/mL), including those infected with genotype 3, require at least 48 weeks of treatment.

Patients infected with genotype 2 or 3 (without cirrhosis and with low levels of viremia) are treated for 24 weeks and require a ribavirin dose of only 400 mg twice daily. Preliminary findings suggest that for patients infected with these genotypes who clear the virus within 4 weeks, treatment for 12 to 16 weeks may be sufficient, especially in patients who have pre-treatment RNA levels ≤400 000 IU/mL. In patients with HCV RNA levels >400000 IU/mL or steatosis, treatment extending beyond 24 weeks may improve the likelihood of an SVR.

For patients infected with HCV genotype 1 and without any fibrosis on liver biopsy, expectant management and a repeat liver biopsy in 3 to 5 years are often recommended.

Peginterferon α and ribavirin may be beneficial in the treatment of cryoglobulinemia associated with chronic hepatitis C. *Chronic HCV carriers* with normal serum aminotransferase levels respond just as well to treatment as do patients with elevated aminotransferase levels. Patients with both HCV and HIV infections may benefit from treatment of HCV if the CD4 count is not low, because in HCV/HIV–co-infected persons, long-term liver-related mortality increases as mortality from HIV infection is reduced by highly active antiretroviral therapy.

Treatment with peginterferon α plus ribavirin is costly (between $30,000 and $40,000 for a

48-week course), and side effects, which include flulike symptoms, are almost universal; more serious toxicity includes psychiatric symptoms (irritability, depression), thyroid dysfunction, and bone marrow suppression. Discontinuation rates are around 10% and higher in persons over age 60 than in younger patients. A blood count is obtained at weeks 1, 2, and 4 after therapy is started and monthly thereafter (Table 43.11). Interferon is contraindicated in patients with decompensated cirrhosis, profound cytopenias, severe psychiatric disorders, and autoimmune diseases.

Patients taking ribavirin must be monitored for hemolysis, and, because of teratogenic effects in animals, men and women taking the drug must practice strict contraception during and for 6 months after conclusion of therapy. Ribavirin should be avoided in persons over age 65 and in others in whom hemolysis could pose a risk of angina or stroke. Rash, itching, headache, cough, and shortness of breath also occur with the drug (Table 43.12). Lactic acidosis is a concern in patients also taking highly active antiretroviral therapy for HIV infection.

Erythropoetin (eg, epoetin alfa) and granulocyte colony-stimulating factor may be used to treat therapy-induced anemia and leukopenia. Interferon is generally contraindicated for heart, lung, and renal transplant recipients because of an increased risk of organ rejection. Selected liver transplant recipients with recurrent hepatitis C may be treated with peginterferon and ribavirin, but response rates are low.

In nonresponders to interferon-based therapy, long-term *maintenance* peginterferon therapy as a strategy to prevent liver fibrosis and reduce the risk of cirrhosis and hepatocellular carcinoma is under study. Consensus interferon, a synthetic recombinant interferon known as alfacon, 15 mcg/day subcutaneously for 12 weeks and then 15 mcg three times a week for 36 weeks, plus ribavirin has been reported to lead to a sustained virologic response in 37% of nonresponders to peginterferon and ribavirin, but these findings require confirmation. Ribavirin analogs that cause little hemolysis and new antiviral drugs such as protease inhibitors are under study.

CHRONIC HEPATITIS D

HDV (also called the delta agent) is a defective RNA agent that infects (either concurrently or sequentially) only persons also infected with HBV. An estimated 15 million HBsAg carriers are infected with HDV, although the rate

Table 43.11 Monitoring Parameters for Interferon-Based Therapy with or without Ribavirin

Parameter	Interval
WBC with differential, Hb, Hct, platelets, serum creatinine	Before treatment, wk 1 or 2, wk 4, then monthly or bimonthly during therapy or more frequently as indicated
Serum ALT	Before treatment, month 1, then every 1–2 months
Pregnancy test	Before treatment, monthly during therapy, and for 6 months after completing therapy
Thyroid-stimulating hormone	Before treatment and at least every 12 wk during therapy
Blood glucose	Before treatment and at least every 12 wk during therapy
HCV RNA by quantitative and/or qualitative assay	Before treatment, 4, 12, and 24 wk during therapy, at end of therapy, and 6 months following the completion of therapy
Assess for adverse effects and adherence	At each routine visit
Depression screen	At baseline and each routine visit
Substance use assessment (alcohol, cocaine, opiate, heroin, or amphetamine use)	At baseline and each routine visit, if appropriate

Abbreviations: ALT = alanine aminotransferase; ANC = absolute neutrophil counts; EVR early virologic response; Hb = hemoglobin; Hct = hematocrit; WBC = white blood cell count; wk = week.

Table 43.12 Adverse Effects of Ribavirin

Teratogenicity
Hemolytic anemia
Headache
Gastrointestinal distress
Skin rash, itching
Conjunctivitis
Cough
Insomnia
Pancreatitis (rare)

of infection appears to be declining in the Mediterranean basin, especially in Italy. In the Pacific Islands, the rate of HDV infection among HBV carriers is as high as 90%, whereas the rate is as low as 5% in Japan. Acute HDV infection superimposed on chronic HBV infection may result in severe chronic hepatitis, which may progress rapidly to cirrhosis and may be fatal. The diagnosis is confirmed by detection of antibody to HDV (anti-HDV) or hepatitis D antigen in serum.

Treatment

High-dose recombinant interferon α-2a (9 million units subcutaneously 3 times weekly for 48 weeks) has been the standard of treatment of HDV infection, leading to normalization of serum aminotransferase levels, histologic improvement, and elimination of HDV RNA from serum in about 20 to 50% of patients with chronic hepatitis D. However, relapse rates approach 80% to 90% once therapy is stopped. Recently, peginterferon α-2b, 1.5 µg/kg/week subcutaneously for 48 weeks, has been shown to produce an SVR in 43% of patients. For slow responders, the duration of peginterferon monotherapy may need to be extended. Nucleoside and nucleotide analogs are not effective in treating chronic hepatitis D. Newer pharmaceutical and vaccine strategies are under investigation.

PROGNOSIS OF CHRONIC VIRAL HEPATITIS

The course of chronic viral hepatitis is variable and unpredictable. The sequelae of chronic viral hepatitis include cirrhosis, liver failure, and hepatocellular carcinoma. In patients with chronic hepatitis B, the 5-year mortality rate is 0% to 2% in those without cirrhosis, 14% to 20% in those with compensated cirrhosis, and 70% to 86% following decompensation. Antiviral treatment appears to improve the prognosis in responders. Chronic hepatitis C is an indolent, often subclinical, disease that may lead to cirrhosis in 20% to 30% of cases and hepatocellular carcinoma after decades, at a rate of 1%–4% per year. The mortality rate from transfusion-associated hepatitis C may be no different from that of an age-matched control population. Nevertheless, mortality rates clearly rise once cirrhosis develops, and mortality from cirrhosis and hepatocellular carcinoma due to hepatitis C is expected to triple in the next 10–20 years. Peginterferon plus ribavirin appears to have a beneficial effect on survival and quality of life, is cost-effective, and appears to retard and even reverse fibrosis and in responders may reduce the risk of hepatocellular carcinoma.

PRIMARY AND SECONDARY PREVENTION

Newborns of HBV-infected mothers should receive hepatitis B immunoglobulin within 12 hours of birth as well as the hepatitis B vaccine series to significantly reduce the likelihood of viral transmission. Pregnant patients with chronic hepatitis B and extremely high serum HBV DNA levels are potential candidates for antiviral treatment with a nucleoside analog during the third trimester to reduce the serum HBV DNA level prior to delivery, but this strategy requires further study. In healthy patients, efforts to prevent HBV and HDV infection are focused on reducing the opportunity for sexual transmission or exposure from intravenous drug use. Intravenous drug use is by far the most significant source of HCV infection worldwide, particularly in countries where blood transfusion products are screened for HCV.

Patients with chronic hepatitis B or C should be vaccinated against hepatitis A. Those with chronic hepatitis C should receive the HBV vaccine. In HDV-endemic areas, HBsAg-negative patients should receive the HBV vaccine. Furthermore, patients with chronic hepatitis should receive the pneumococcal and influenza vaccines. Finally, in patients with chronic hepatitis B and active viral replication as well as in those with chronic hepatitis C and advanced liver fibrosis, serum alpha-fetoprotein testing and abdominal ultrasonography are recommended every 6 months to screen for hepatocellular carcinoma. (For management of occupational exposure to HBV and HCV, see Chapter 102, Percutaneous Injury: Risks and Management.)

SUGGESTED READING

Castelnau C, Le Gal F, Ripault MP, et al. Efficacy of peginterferon alpha-2b in chronic hepatitis delta: relevance of quantitative RT-PCR for follow-up. *Hepatology*. 2006;44:728–735.

Chang T-T, Gish RG, de Man R, et al. A comparison of entecavir versus lamivudine for HBe-Ag positive chronic hepatitis B. *N Engl J Med*. 2006;354:1001–1010.

Dienstag JL, McHutchinson JG. American Gastroenterological Association technical review on the management, and treatment of hepatitis C. *Gastroenterology*. 2006;130: 231–264.

Hoofnagle JH, Doo E, Liang TJ, et al. Management of hepatitis B: Summary of a clinical research workshop. *Hepatology*.2007; 45:1056–1075.

Hoofnagle JH, Seeff LB. Peginterferon and ribavirin for chronic hepatitis C. *N Engl J Med*. 2006;355:2444–2451.

Keeffe EB, Dieterich DT, Han S-HB, et al. A treatment algorithm for the management of chronic hepatitis B virus infection in the United States. *Clin Gastroenterol Hepatol*. 2004;2:87–106.

Keeffe EB, Dieterich DT, Han SH, et al. A treatment algorithm for the management of chronic hepatitis B virus infection in the United States: an update. *Clin Gastroenterol Hepatol*. 2006;4:936–962.

Keeffe EB, Zeuzem S, Koff RS, et al. Report of an international workshop: roadmap for management of patients receiving oral therapy for chronic hepatitis B. *Clin Gastroenterol Hepatol*. 2007;5:890–897.

Lai C-L, Shouval D, Lok AS, et al. Entecavir versus lamivudine for patients with HBeAg—negative chronic hepatitis B. *N Engl J Med*. 2006;354:1011–1020.

Liaw YF, Leung N, Guan R, et al. Asian-Pacific consensus statement on the management of chronic hepatitis B: a 2005 update. *Liver Int*. 2005;25:472–489.

Locarnini S, McMillan J, Bartholomeusz A. The hepatitis B virus and common mutants. *Semin Liver Dis*. 2003;23:5–20.

Lok AS, McMahon BJ. Practice Guidelines Committee, American Association for the Study of Liver Diseases (AASLD): chronic hepatitis B: update of recommendations. *Hepatology*. 2004;39:857–861.

Lok AS, McMahon BJ. Chronic hepatitis B. *Hepatology*. 2007;45:507–509.

National Institutes of Health Consensus Development Conference statement: management of hepatitis C: 2002—June 10–12, 2002. *Hepatology*. 2002;36:S3–S20.

Niro GA, Ciancio A, Gaeta GB. Pegylated interferon alpha-2b as monotherapy or in combination with ribavirin in chronic hepatitis delta. *Hepatology*. 2006;44:713–720.

Strader DB, Wright TL, Thomas DL, et al. Diagnosis, management, and treatment of hepatitis C: AASLD practice guideline. *Hepatology*. 2004;39:1147–1171.

Yee HS, Currie SL, Darling JM, et al. Management and treatment of hepatitis C viral infection: recommendations from the Department of Veterans Affairs Hepatitis C Resource Center Program and the National Hepatitis C Program Office. *Am J Gastroenterol*. 2006;101: 2360–2378.

44. Biliary Infection: Cholecystitis and Cholangitis

Robert V. Rege

Infectious and inflammatory disorders of the gallbladder and bile ducts are referred to, respectively, as cholecystitis and cholangitis. Most of these disorders involve acute bacterial infections and can be quite serious or even life-threatening problems that require prompt diagnosis and treatment. This chapter discusses the pathogenesis, diagnosis, and current treatment of both acute cholecystitis and acute cholangitis.

ACUTE CHOLECYSTITIS

Acute cholecystitis refers to acute inflammation of the gallbladder. Ninety-eight percent of episodes of acute cholecystitis exhibit cystic duct obstruction on radionucleotide (hydroxy iminodiacetic acid; HIDA) scan, indicating that the process most often begins with obstruction of the cystic duct by a gallstone. In about 2% to 5% of cases termed acute acalculous cholecystitis, no gallstones are present, although some cases still exhibit obstruction of the cystic duct from fibrosis or edema. Acute acalculous cholecystitis is most often found in debilitated or critically ill patients who have not been fed by mouth for extended periods of time leading to nonemptying of the gallbladder and stasis of bile in its lumen. A cascade of events triggered by gallstones, stasis, or cystic duct obstruction result in inflammation in the wall of the gallbladder, superinfection with bacteria, and eventually compromise of the gallbladder wall (Figure 44.1).

If unchecked, gangrene of the gallbladder develops and perforation of the gallbladder with abscess formation or generalized perforation ensues. It should be understood that complicated acute cholecystitis is much more morbid than uncomplicated acute cholecystitis and can be a potentially life-threatening emergency. It is therefore imperative that acute cholecystitis be diagnosed and effectively treated before it reaches this stage.

Diagnosis

Patients with acute cholecystitis experience right upper quadrant abdominal pain and demonstrate systemic signs of inflammation such as fever and elevated white blood cell count. The duration of pain, usually more than 12 hours, and the presence of abdominal tenderness distinguish acute cholecystitis from biliary colic. On physical examination, tenderness is well localized in the right upper quadrant of the abdomen directly over the gallbladder. More diffuse right upper quadrant tenderness is more suggestive of a liver problem, complicated cholecystitis such as gallbladder perforation, or another upper abdominal cause of pain. Tenderness that increases with inspiration, as the gallbladder descends to touch the examiner's hand (Murphy's sign), is characteristic of acute cholecystitis. The presence of dark urine, acholic stool, and jaundice raises the question of a gallstone in the common bile duct, also called choledocholithiasis, or, less frequently, a malignant obstruction of the duct, which is more often characterized by painless jaundice. Back pain and epigastric tenderness heightens one's suspicion of biliary pancreatitis or choledocholithiasis.

Some patients show fewer signs and symptoms of acute cholecystitis, resulting in later presentation or delayed diagnosis. The severity of the disease may be much greater than appreciated, leading to conversion from laparoscopic to open operation or, more significantly, to complicated acute cholecystitis. Patients presenting with advanced disease but minimal findings are more likely to be elderly and male. They also more often relate a history of cardiac disease and exhibit a higher than expected white blood cell count (Figure 44.1).

Laboratory testing should include complete blood count (CBC) with differential, liver function tests, serum amylase, and serum lipase. The latter tests help differentiate acute cholecystitis from choledocholithiasis or biliary pancreatitis. CBC usually demonstrates moderately elevated white blood count, reflecting the inflammatory nature of the problem. White blood cell counts exceeding 13 000/mm^3, and certainly greater than 15 000/mm^3, suggest complicated acute cholecystitis. Gangrene of the gallbladder and perforated gallbladder should be considered, and treatment should be expedited.

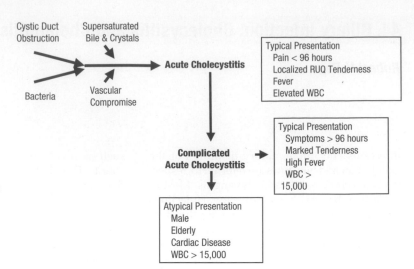

Figure 44.1 The pathogenesis of acute cholangitis is outlined on the left side of the figure, whereas differences in clinical presentation between acute cholecystitis and complicated acute cholecystitis are shown on the right.

Ultrasound of the right upper quadrant of the abdomen reliably demonstrates gallstones in the majority of patients. A typical clinical presentation coupled with a "positive" ultrasound suffices for the diagnosis of acute cholecystitis. In addition, ultrasound may demonstrate more specific signs of acute cholecystitis in some patients, including thickening of the gallbladder wall and pericholecystic fluid. A technetium radionucleotide cholecintography (HIDA scan) may be helpful if the patient does not have gallstones on ultrasound or if the presentation is otherwise atypical. Nonvisualization of the gallbladder on HIDA scan indicates cystic duct obstruction and is specific for acute cholecystitis. Only about 2% of patients with acute cholecystitis demonstrate visualization of the gallbladder on this study, and demonstration of the gallbladder argues strongly against acute cholecystitis (Figure 44.1).

Bacteriology

Interestingly, bacteria are not cultured from bile in the great majority of patients undergoing operation early in the course of the disease. Isolation of bacteria from bile increases as the duration from the onset of symptoms increases; the majority of patients demonstrate bacterobilia by 3 days. The most common organisms isolated are gram positives, especially *Enterococcus* (Table 44.1), but gram-negative bacteria, *Klebsiella*, *Proteus*, and *Pseudomonas*, are also frequently cultured. Isolation of multiple species of bacteria is common. Anaerobic bacteria are isolated in only about 10% of cases but may be more common because of difficulties culturing these organisms using standard techniques. Some estimate that *Bacteroides* and *Clostridium*

species may be evident in as many as 50% of cases of biliary disease. *Candida* species are very uncommon in normal patients but are frequently found in immunosuppressed patients and patients with malignancy. Considering the possible bacteria involved, patients with acute cholecystitis require broad-spectrum antibiotic coverage, and immunosuppressed patients and those with malignancy require even broader coverage (Table 44.1).

Treatment

Initial therapy for the patient with acute cholecystitis includes fluid resuscitation, intravenous fluid replacement, bowel rest, and antibiotics. The patient should be prepared for operation because this may be required at any time if the disease progresses. Cephalosporin antibiotics cover the spectrum of bacteria found in most patients, but complicated cholecystitis and immunosuppressed patients require wider spectrum coverage (Table 44.2).

Surgical removal of the gallbladder is necessary, but the timing of cholecystectomy is debatable. Laparoscopic cholecystectomy is the standard of care, but open operation or conversion to open operation should be used liberally in patients with marked inflammation or fibrosis. Failure to do so could result in bile duct injuries. Laparoscopic cholecystectomy is usually successful in the early course of the disease and may even be facilitated by edema, but complications of acute cholecystitis and the rate of conversion from laparoscopic to open operation increase markedly 96 hours after the onset of symptoms.

Because of this, it is my preference to perform early cholecystectomy. Most patients are

Table 44.1 Broad Spectrum Penicillin as Adequate Therapy for Acute Cholangitis

	Total (N = 96% of Patients)	Benign Causes (N = 42% of Patients)	Malignant Causes (N = 54% of Patients)
Gram Negative			
Klebsiella species	54	31	72
Escherichia coli	39	43	35
Enterobacter species	34	17	48
Pseudomonas species	24	12	33
Citrobacter species	21	17	24
Proteus species	13	12	13
Aeromonas species	5	2	7
Serratia species	3	0	6
Gram Positive			
Enterococcus	34	36	33
Streptococcal species	38	24	48
Anaerobes			
Bacteroides species	15	17	13
Clostridium species	5	2	7
Fungi			
Candida species	18	5	28
Others	14	19	9

Adapted from Thompson JE Jr, Pitt HA, Doty JE, et al. Broad spectrum penicillin as adequate therapy for acute cholangitis. *Surg Gynecol Obstet.* 1990;171(4):279.

admitted to the hospital and placed on medical therapy. Operation is performed within 24 to 72 hours from the onset of symptoms. Patients with more severe disease and those who present late in their course require early, or even emergent, intervention. Early operation is safe in the hands of experienced biliary surgeons and avoids progression of the disease and recurrence of cholecystitis sometimes observed in those treated medically. As many as 30% of patients treated medically exhibit persistent symptoms or progressive disease and require emergent operation. Laparoscopic cholecystectomy may still be performed in the majority of these patients but is more difficult and requires conversion in 10% to 30% of patients.

Some surgeons recommend a delay of 6 weeks from the time of presentation to surgical resection, if medical treatment is successful. Their rationale is that elective operation is safer than an emergent procedure, but data have not shown this to be the case, except in seriously ill patients who have contraindications to surgery. Medical treatment with delayed cholecystectomy is certainly a consideration for critically ill patients or those with severe comorbidities who are expected to improve with time. Percutaneous drainage of the gallbladder is an option for patients who fail medical therapy and are high risk for surgical therapy.

ACUTE CHOLANGITIS

Acute cholangitis refers to infection and inflammation of the intra- and extrahepatic biliary tree. Bacteria are the most frequent cause, but

Table 44.2 Summary of Antibiotic Regimens for Acute Cholecystitis and Acute Cholangitis

Acute Cholecystitis
Cefoxitin 1–2 g IV q6–8h
Ampicillin-sulbactam (Unasyn) 3 g IV q6h
Acute Cholangitis
Single Agents
Ciprofloxacin 400–800 mg IV q12h or Piperacillin-Tazobactam (Zosyn) 3.375 g IV q6h or Imipenem 500 mg IV q6h
Multidrug Therapy
Ampicillin 2 g IV q6h + gentamicin 5–7 mg/kg IV q24h or Cefazadime 1–2 g IV q8-12h + Ampicillin 2 g IV q6h + Metronidazole 500 mg IV q6h

cholangitis can result from parasitic infections, autoimmune disease, and chemical irritants. Past terms, including *suppurative cholangitis* and *ascending cholangitis*, used for the most critically ill patients with acute cholangitis, have been replaced by the term *toxic cholangitis*. Toxic cholangitis occurs when the bacteria in bile gain access to the sinusoids in the liver and are rapidly disseminated, causing sepsis.

The pathogenesis of acute cholangitis involves several abnormalities: obstruction of the biliary tree, injury to the biliary epithelium, and bacteria in bile. Most patients harboring bacteria in their bile do not have an infection. In fact, colonization of bile with bacteria increases with advancing age and is asymptomatic. Asymptomatic bactobilia places patients at high risk for acute cholangitis should they develop biliary obstruction or injury to the epithelium, as might occur during an invasive biliary tract procedure.

Most cases of cholangitis are secondary to either partial or complete biliary obstruction, but the incidence of iatrogenic cholangitis is rising with the increased use of endoscopic and radiological procedures on the bile duct. Obstruction of the bile duct by gallstones is the most common cause of cholangitis in the United States. Malignant obstruction of the bile duct is also common, but most patients with malignant obstruction present with painless jaundice and sterile bile. Care must be taken to avoid converting patients with malignant obstruction from sterile to colonized bile by using prophylactic antibiotics with invasive diagnostic tests or therapeutic interventions. When obstruction occurs, bile duct pressure increases and eventually disrupts the intracellular junctions between epithelial cells in the proximal biliary ducts. Bacteria gain access to the sinusoids of the liver and to the blood stream, causing bacteremia, high fevers, and sepsis. Acute cholangitis is a life-threatening disorder that requires prompt diagnosis and treatment.

Diagnosis

The classic description of patients with acute cholangitis—termed Charcot's triad—consists of abdominal pain, fever, and jaundice. Unfortunately, only about 50% of patients present with all three symptoms and signs. The most consistent signs of acute cholangitis are fever and chills, which are present in 90% of patients. Fevers are most often high and spiking. Reynolds' pentad, which consists of Charcot's triad plus hypotension and altered sensorium, is indicative of toxic cholangitis. Unfortunately, all five features are present in the minority of patients with toxic cholangitis.

Physical examination most often reveals tenderness in the right upper quadrant of the abdomen and jaundice. However, as many as 20% of patients with acute cholangitis have a serum bilirubin level of less than 2.0 mg/dL, so the lack of jaundice does not exclude a diagnosis of acute cholangitis. Physical findings are usually accompanied by leukocytosis and abnormal liver function tests, but septic patients may have a low white blood count. Ultrasound should be performed urgently to distinguish "medical" from "surgical" jaundice: Dilated bile ducts are indicative of obstruction and surgical jaundice. Endoscopic retrograde cholangiography (ERC; see treatment) is usually diagnostic but can also be therapeutic. Percutaneous transhepatic cholangiography is helpful when ERC is unsuccessful.

Bacteriology

Similar organisms are isolated from the bile of patients with acute cholangitis and acute cholelithiasis. However, the infections are more severe. Blood cultures are often positive with isolates typical of those found in bile. Differences exist between malignant versus benign causes of acute cholangitis. Table 44.1 outlines the main organisms that are found in bile with acute cholangitis as discussed for acute cholecystitis, Bacteriology.

Treatment

The treatment of acute cholangitis requires aggressively addressing both the infection and the biliary obstruction. Acute cholangitis is a life-threatening problem and patients with this disorder require placement in the intensive care unit and aggressive monitoring. Intravenous hydration should be started, and urine output should be followed closely. Patients with biliary obstruction are often hypovolemic and require restoration of normal intravascular volumes before undergoing invasive diagnostic and therapeutic procedures. If this is not done, they are at high risk to develop renal failure. Patients also often exhibit coagulation defects that must be corrected with vitamin K, fresh frozen plasma (FFP), and platelets. Antibiotic therapy is essential and, like fluids, should be instituted immediately before diagnostic and therapeutic interventions.

Broad-spectrum coverage should be started initially and later tailored to match the sensitivities of isolated organisms. The longstanding regimen of ampicillin and an aminoglycoside continue to provide excellent coverage for the major culprits, including *Enterococcus* species, but nephrotoxicity of the aminoglycoside may be a problem. Although first- and second-generation cephalosporins provide good prophylaxis for elective biliary surgery, they lack the breadth of gram-negative coverage required for treatment of patients with severe infections, such as acute cholangitis. Third-generation cephalosporins provide excellent gram-negative coverage but do not treat *Staphylococcus* and *Enterococcus* species and anaerobic bacteria well, and these species have been isolated in 34% of patients with acute cholangitis. Triple therapy with ceftazadime, ampicillin, and metronidazole has been used for many years, but more recently single drug therapy with ciprofloxacin has been shown to be as efficacious as triple drug therapy. This regimen is particularly helpful in patients with recurrent cholangitis, because it can be administered long term as an outpatient. Pipericillin may also be considered as a single agent because it has been shown to be as effective as ampicillin and tobramycin, while some newer combinations, such as piperacillin-tazobactam (Zosyn), also appear to be quite effective (Table 44.2). In patients with biliary obstruction secondary to *Ascaris* or *Clonorchis*, specific antiparasitic therapy is indicated (see specific chapters).

After adequate resuscitation and antibiotic administration, the primary goal is to relieve obstruction of the biliary tree if it is present.

Although this commonly required, emergent operative intervention in the past with drainage of the common bile duct with a t-tube, currently, this is accomplished quite effectively using either endoscopic retrograde cholangiopancreatography (ERCP)-mediated drainage or percutaneous transhepatic cholangiography (PTC). The risk of ERCP is less than PTC in these sick patients and is usually the method of first choice. Effective drainage of the biliary tree has been accomplished by removal of obstructing gallstones or by stenting the duct. Cancers of the biliary tree can be visualized and biopsied. Stents can usually be placed across the obstructing lesion. If ERCP fails to provide adequate drainage, PTC should be undertaken. This may be the procedure of choice for patients with cholangiocarcinoma in the proximal bile duct because, in this case, PTC may actually be safer than ERCP. Once the acute obstruction has been managed by drainage, the patient should improve.

If appropriate, the patient should then undergo an elective, definitive procedure to treat the cause of biliary obstruction, because recurrent cholangitis is common. Cholecystectomy should be performed if choledocholithiasis was the inciting event. Curable malignancies should be resected. Benign strictures require balloon dilatation or choledochointestinal bypass, whereas unresectable tumors are either bypassed or palliated with internal or external stents.

Timing of operation for patients who present with a transient episode of biliary pancreatitis or with low or moderate risk of choledocholithiasis (transient elevation of liver function tests) is somewhat controversial. Interestingly, most stones pass from the common duct spontaneously. The incidence of retained common bile duct stones is highest early after an attack and decreases with time. However, there is a risk of recurrent pancreatitis, obstructive jaundice, and acute cholangitis in patients who do not pass their stones. The timing of treatment then depends on a balance between intervention for those stones that do not pass and recurrence of the disease. Patients with mild pancreatitis and a low risk of common bile duct stones may be taken to the operating room for laparoscopic cholecystectomy with intraoperative cholangiography, if the surgeon is prepared to perform laparoscopic common bile duct exploration. The standard of care in this country is to intervene in these patients during or shortly after the index admission.

However, patients who present with severe, complicated pancreatitis may be poor candidates for surgery. Most surgeons would allow them to recover from their episode of pancreatitis before definitive intervention. Patients with unrelenting pancreatitis, persistently elevated liver enzymes, or jaundice are at high risk for common bile duct stones and should be considered for ERCP. This modality should be considered both diagnostic and therapeutic, as stones can be extracted. Cholecystectomy is performed later to avoid recurrent complications of stones.

SUGGESTED READING

Jeyarajah DR, Rege RV. Operative management of cholangitis, choledocholithiasis, and bile duct strictures in the septic patient. In: *Shackelford's Surgery of the Alimentary Tract*. 5th ed, Vol III. Philadelphia, PA, Saunders; 2001.

Jeyarajah DR, Rege RV. Antibiotic selection in biliary surgery. In: Cameron JL, ed. *Current Surgical Therapy*. 8th ed. New York, NY: Elsevier Mosby; 2004:444–447.

Lipsett PA, Pitt HH. Acute cholangitis. *Front Biosci*. 2003;8:s1229–s1239.

Rege RV. Biliary colic and acute cholecystitis. In: Afdhal NH, ed. *Gallbladder and Biliary Tract Diseases*. Madison, NY: Marcel Dekker;2000:471–490.

Rege RV, Jeyarajah DR. Biliary infection: cholecystitis and cholangitis. In: Schlossberg D, ed. *Current Therapy of Infectious Disease*. 2nd ed. St. Louis, MO: Mosby; 2000: 157–159.

Rege RV. Cholecystitis and cholelithiasis. In: Rakel and Bope, ed. *Conn's Current Therapy*. New York, NY:Elsevier Science; 2004:510–513.

Rutledge D, Jones DJ, Rege RV. Consequences of delay in surgical treatment of biliary disease. *Am J of Surg*. 2000;180:466–469.

Sinanan MN. Acute cholangitis. *Infect Dis Clin North Am*. 1992;6:571.

Thompson JE Jr, Pitt HA, Doty JE, et al. Broad spectrum penicillin as an adequate therapy for acute cholangitis. *Surg Gynecol Obstet*. 1990;171:275.

Yusoff IF, Barkun JS, Barkun AN. Diagnosis and management of cholecystitis and cholangitis. *Gastroenterol Clin North Am*. 2003;32:1145–1168.

45. Pyogenic Liver Abscess

H. Franklin Herlong

First described by Hippocrates, pyogenic liver abscess is an uncommon but important hepatic infection. The relative infrequency of abscess formation, despite the extensive exposure of the liver to bacteria from its dual blood supply, is related to the efficiency of the Kupffer cells in filtering bacteria. Over the past several decades with easily accessible imaging techniques enabling prompt diagnosis, potent antibiotics and effective drainage procedures, the mortality from pyogenic liver abscess has declined dramatically.

EPIDEMIOLOGY

In the first large published series of cases of pyogenic liver abscess in the United States, based on patients at Charity Hospital in New Orleans, there was an incidence of 8 cases per 100 000 admissions. There was a 2:1 male predominance with a mortality rate of 72%. Several studies published around 40 years later show significant demographic changes. In the initial report most patients were in their 3rd decade of life compared to the 5th to 6th decades in later series. Although the incidence of abscesses appears to be increasing by a factor of 2, the male predominance has disappeared and the mortality rate has fallen to approximately 12%. These differences probably reflect changes in the underlying factors causing the abscesses. Most of the earlier cases likely resulted from intra-abdominal infections such as diverticulitis or appendicitis. With better diagnostic imaging techniques, along with the availability of potent antibiotics, complications from abscess formation after intra-abdominal infections has diminished significantly. In more recent series, biliary tract disorders and their treatments account for most of the predisposing factors. This shift probably accounts for the age and gender differences.

ETIOLOGY

Pyogenic liver abscesses result from seeding of the liver from direct extension (peritonitis, subphrenic abscess), pyelophlebitis of the portal vein (appendicitis, diverticulitis, colon cancer, inflammatory bowel disease (IBD)), biliary tract disorders (cholecystitis, cholangitis complicating malignancy or stones), penetrating trauma, or bacteremia (pneumonia, endocarditis). Rarely abscesses develop after arterial embolization or radiofrequency ablation of hepatic tumors. In most series, no identifiable source can be documented in around 25% of cases. Most abscesses are solitary with the majority in the right lobe of the liver. Of all of the predisposing conditions, biliary tract disorders are currently the most common, accounting for 30% to 50% of cases. Cholangitis from obstructing cholangiocarcinomas is more common than infections resulting from calculus obstruction.

CLINICAL PRESENTATION

Most patients with pyogenic liver abscesses appear acutely ill with fever, chills, and right upper quadrant pain. However, in elderly, debilitated patients, clinical signs may be minimal, potentially delaying diagnosis. The majority of patients have tender hepatomegaly, occasionally with focal tenderness over the intercostal spaces of the right upper quadrant. However, in patients with liver transplants, denervation may prevent the pain of hepatic enlargement. Fatigue, malaise, and weight loss are common; however, jaundice is unusual unless the abscess compresses the biliary tact. An associated pleural effusion may obliterate breath sounds at the right bases. Laboratory abnormalities include the typical findings seen in systemic infection or many other liver diseases. Modest elevations of the alkaline phosphatase, aminotransferases, and bilirubin concentrations are common. A leukocytosis with a left shift is present in most patients, and half will have positive blood cultures. No single tests or combinations of tests can accurately predict the outcome, size, or number of abscesses or complications.

Cultures from liver abscesses usually yield polymicrobial flora with microbiologic profiles reflecting the source of the liver abscess. Enteric aerobic gram-negative bacilli and enterococcus suggest the biliary tract. *Staphylococcus aureus* is a common cause of liver abscess in children and trauma patients. A single organism indicates hematogenous spread. Mixed enteric flora containing anaerobes like *Bacteroides fragilis* originate from portal bacteremias. An unusual pathogen, *Yersinia enterocolitica*, causes abscesses in patients with diabetes or underlying liver disease, particularly hemochromatosis. Initially described in Taiwan, a distinct clinical entity caused by monomicrobial *Klebsiella pneumoniae* infection is emerging as an important cause of pyogenic liver abscess in this country. These patients present with classic symptoms of hepatic abscess; most have underlying diabetes mellitus and no coexisting intra-abdominal pathology. Species of *Candida* cause abscesses in immunosuppressed patients, particularly those receiving chemotherapy. The abscess may not be apparent until the neutrophil count rebounds (Table 45.1).

DIAGNOSIS

The availability of accurate imaging techniques is one of the most important factors accounting for the reduction in mortality rates from pyogenic liver abscess. Ultrasonographic examination of the abdomen shows a focal defect with variable appearance of echogenicity. Typically the abscesses are cystic, round lesions with irregular walls. They may be septated and multiloculated and contain internal echoes cause by debris. Although the sensitivity is usually about 75%, small abscesses may go undetected. Computed tomography (CT) is the most widely used modality to confirm the presence of pyogenic liver abscesses. When performed with contrast, sensitivities approach 95%. Computed tomography can detect smaller lesions than ultrasonography and may also help identify other sites of intra-abdominal infections. Technetium-99m sulfa colloid and gallium citrate scans are rarely used because they can not reliably detect small lesions or distinguish abscesses from neoplasm. There is no evidence that magnetic resonance imaging is superior to CT.

TREATMENT

Antibiotic therapy should be initiated promptly when pyogenic liver abscess is suspected. Because no randomized controlled trials are available to govern empiric therapy, antibiotic regimens are based on the most probable source of infections (Table 45.2). Initial antibiotic therapy can obviously be adjusted based on information obtained

Table 45.1 Clinical Findings in Pyogenic Liver Abscess

Signs and Symptoms	Incidence (%)
Fever	75
Chills	60
Abdominal pain	60
Weight loss	30
Hepatomegaly	50
Right upper quadrant tenderness	40
Jaundice	25
Laboratory Values	
Leukocytosis	70
Elevated bilirubin	40
Elevated alkaline phosphatase	50
Elevated aminotransferases	60

from the Gram stain and cultures of aspirated abscess contents and blood cultures.

Although there are anecdotal reports of successful treatment of pyogenic liver abscesses with antibiotics alone, some form of drainage procedure is advocated in most patients unless the abscess is less than 3 cm in diameter. Multiple small abscesses are not amenable to surgical or catheter drainage and must be treated with intravenous antibiotics alone. Not surprisingly, this group has a very high mortality.

Several studies have compared percutaneous, closed aspiration, and surgical drainage techniques. However, differences in location, etiologic disorders, and comorbidities make comparisons difficult. Closed aspiration is the simplest and least costly approach. However, reaccumulation often requires repeat procedures or surgical intervention. Placement of a catheter into the abscess cavity under ultrasound guidance is a popular method of drainage at many centers. This technique is often used if closed aspiration is unsuccessful.

Surgical therapy is rarely required but may be necessary when concomitant causative conditions require surgical correction or the abscess ruptures. Through a transperitoneal approach, a suction catheter is inserted into the abscess cavity, making sure all loculated pockets are effectively drained. If necessary, biopsies of the wall can be taken to exclude a tumor. The

Table 45.2 Empiric Antibiotic Therapy for Pyogenic Liver Abscess

Potential Source	Suggested Regimen
Biliary	Pip/Tz 4.5 g q8h IV or
	AM/SB 3.0 g q6h IV or
	ERTA 1.0 g IV qd or
	MER 1.0 g q8h IV or
	CIP 400 mg IV BID + metro 1.0 g IV then 0.5 g q6h
Intra-abdominal	IMP 500 mg IV q6h or
	MER 1 g IV q8h or
	AMP 2 g IVq6h + Metro 500 mg IVq 6h + CIP 400 mg IVq12h

Abbreviations: AMP = ampicillin; AAM/SB = ampicillin/sulbactam (Unasyn); CIP = ciprofloxacin; ERTA = ertapenem; IMP = imipenem cilastatin (Primaxin); MER = meropenem; Pip/Tz = piperacillin/tazobactam.

catheter is brought out through a stab incision for additional drainage or irrigation. After several weeks the catheter is removed.

PROGNOSIS

Since the mid-1960s there has been a dramatic decline in the number of deaths from pyogenic hepatic abscesses. Current mortality rates range from 5% to 20%. The differences are largely related to variations in the percentage of patients who have multiple abscesses, associated septicemia, or underlying malignancy. At present, with prompt diagnosis and drainage, few patients die from complications of the abscess itself. Instead mortality results from comorbidities like biliary tract or intra-abdominal malignancies.

SUGGESTED READING

Derosier LC, Canon CM, Vickers SM. Liver abscess. In: Yeo CJ, ed. *Shackelford's Surgery of the Alimentary Tract*. Philadelphia, PA: Saunders Elsevier; 2007:1640.

Huang C-J, Pitt HA, Lipsett PA, et al. Pyogenic hepatic abscess: changing trends over 42 years. *Ann Surg*. 1996;223:600–607; discussion 607–609.

Lederman ER, Crum HF. Pyogenic liver abscess with a focus on Klebsiella pneumoniae as a primary pathogen: an emerging disease with unique clinical characteristics. *Am J Gastroenterol*. 2005;100:322–331.

46. Infectious Complications of Acute Pancreatitis

Daniel Wolfson and Jamie S. Barkin

Acute pancreatitis (AP) is an acute inflammatory process of the pancreas in which pancreatic enzymes are released and autodigest the gland with effects ranging from edema to necrosis. Acute pancreatitis has a wide spectrum of disease from a mild, transitory illness to a severe, rapidly fatal disease. Approximately 80% of patients with the disease have a mild acute interstitial edematous pancreatitis with a low morbidity and mortality rate (≤1%). Mild pancreatitis is usually self-limiting, subsiding in most cases uneventfully within 3 to 4 days and rarely needing intensive care treatment or pancreatic surgery. Severe or necrotizing pancreatitis develops in about 20% of patients, early death within 1 week of admission is related to systemic inflammatory response syndrome (SIRS), with infection of pancreatic and peripancreatic necrosis representing the single most important risk factor for a fatal outcome. Overall, AP is complicated by infection in approximately 10% of patients and is associated with 70% to 80% mortality. The greater the amount of necrotic reaction, the greater the risk of subsequent infection of the gland.

The prognosis and severity of a pancreatitis attack may be assessed by monitoring clinical signs and symptoms. The clinical findings in severe disease may include the presence of hypotension, hypoxemia, renal failure, and hemoconcentration reflective of intravascular volume loss. Other findings may include abdominal pain and nausea, fever (>38.6°C [101.5°F]), ascites, and ecchymosis. Several classification systems have been developed in an attempt to provide reliable prognostic classification for patients with acute pancreatitis. The APACHE II scale (*a*cute *p*hysiological *a*ssessment and *c*hronic *h*ealth *e*valuation), multiple organ system failure (MOSF) scale (Table 46.1), and the Ranson's criteria (Table 46.2) have all been used. The MOSF and APACHE II scales can usually be performed within a few hours after admission. The APACHE II scores are generated from multiple parameters and are considered highly accurate. Furthermore, APACHE II scores allow prediction of severity from the day of admission and may be recalculated on a daily basis.

Unfortunately, because of the time-consuming and cumbersome nature of the APACHE II evaluation, it is rarely used in clinical practice. The MOSF system has better clinical utility for evaluating patients at admission and at 48 hours than the APACHE II score. The Ranson's criteria are the scale assessment both at admission and at 48 hours and require 2 days to assess patient prognosis.

COMPUTED TOMOGRAPHY

Rapid bolus computed tomography (CT) scanning using intravenous (IV) contrast effectively and accurately (>95%) detects pancreatic necrosis. Computed tomography scanning should be restricted to patients who have severe acute pancreatitis, who do not show signs of clinical improvement despite supportive care over several days, and in whom infection is suspected, by either fever or positive blood cultures. Computed tomography scan with IV contrast should be utilized only after volume repletion to prevent renal damage. The severity of AP can be estimated by the findings on the CT scan such as the presence of pancreatic enlargement, peripancreatic inflammatory changes, and the presence of fluid collections within the pancreas parenchyma.

NATURAL HISTORY OF ACUTE PANCREATITIS

Since the mid-1990s it has become evident that there are two phases in the natural course of severe or necrotizing acute pancreatitis. It includes an early vasoactive and toxic phase and a late phase dominated by septic complications. The first 14 days after onset of the disease are characterized by SIRS. Inflammatory mediators released into the systemic circulation are associated with the development of cardiorespiratory and renal failure, fever, and tachycardia. In the late phase, infection of pancreatic necrosis develops usually after the first week, peaks in the second and third week after onset of the disease, and is reported in 40% to 70% of patients with necrotizing pancreatitis.

Table 46.1 Criteria for Organ System Failure[a]

Organ System	Criteria
Cardiovascular	Mean arterial pressure $\leq = 50$ mm Hg. Need for volume loading and/or vasoactive drugs to maintain systolic blood pressure above 100 mm Hg. Heart rate $\leq = 50$ beats per minute. Ventricular tachycardia/fibrillation. Cardiac arrest. Acute myocardial infarction.
Pulmonary	Respiratory rate $\leq = 5$ per minute or $> = 50$ per minute. Mechanical ventilation for 3 or more days or $Fio_2 > 0.4$ and/or positive end-expiratory pressure >5 mm Hg.
Renal	Serum creatinine $> = 3.5$ mg/dL (280 mmol/L). Dialysis/ultrafiltration needed.
Neurologic	Glasgow Coma Scale ¾ 6 (in the absence of sedation).
Hematologic	Hematocrit $\leq = 20\%$. Leukocyte count $\leq = 300$ per mm³ (0.3 3 10⁹ per L). Platelet count $\leq = 50$ 3 10³ per mL (50 3 10⁹ per L). Disseminated intravascular coagulation
Hepatic	Total bilirubin level $> = 3.5$ mg/dL (51 mmol/L) in the absence of hemolysis. ALT >100 U/L
Gastrointestinal	Stress ulcer necessitating transfusion of more than 2 units of blood per 24 hours. Acalculus cholecystitis. Necrotizing enterocolitis. Bowel perforation.

[a] From Larvin M, McMahon M. *Lancet.* 1989;22:201–204.

Table 46.2 Predictors of Severity in Acute Pancreatitis

Ranson's Criteria on Admission

Age >55 years
A white blood cell count of >16,000/µL
Blood glucose >11 mmol/L (>200 mg/dL)
Serum LDH >350 IU/L
Serum AST >250 IU/L

Ranson's Criteria After 48 h of Admission

Fall in hematocrit by >10%
Fluid sequestration of >6 L
Hypocalcemia (serum calcium ≤ 2.0 mmol/L [≤ 8.0 mg/dL])
Hypoxemia ($PO_2 \leq 60$ mm Hg)
Increase in BUN to >1.98 mmol/L (>5 mg/dL) after IV fluid hydration
Base deficit of >4 mmol/L

The Prognostic Implications of Ranson's Criteria are as Follows

Score 0 to 2: 2% mortality
Score 3 to 4: 15% mortality
Score 5 to 6: 40% mortality
Score 7 to 8: 100% mortality

[a] From Banks PA. Predictors of severity in acute pancreatitis. *Pancreas.* 1991;6(suppl 1):S7–12.

Sepsis-related multiple organ failure induced by infected pancreatic necrosis is the main life-threatening complication, with mortality rate of up to 70%. Infected necrosis has been recognized as the single most important risk factor in death from necrotizing pancreatitis.

TYPES OF INFECTIONS

There are two distinctive forms of infection in acute pancreatitis: infected pancreatic necrosis and pancreatic abscess. At the Atlanta consensus conference 1992, these terms were defined as follows: pancreatic necrosis is a diffuse or focal area of nonviable pancreatic parenchyma that is typically associated with pancreatic fat necrosis. Contrast-enhanced

CT scans, currently the gold standard for clinical documentation of pancreatic necrosis, will demonstrate the nonperfused areas of pancreatic parenchyma, indicating necrosis (Figure 46.1 and 46.2).

A pancreatic abscess is a circumscribed intra-abdominal collection of pus, usually in the proximity of the pancreas and containing little or no pancreatic necrosis. A pancreatic abscess is a consequence of severe acute pancreatitis. It is likely that pancreatic abscesses are a consequence of limited necrosis, with subsequent liquification and secondary infection during the course of severe acute pancreatitis. This definition includes infected pseudocysts. A pseudocyst is a collection of pancreatic juice, enclosed by a wall of fibrous or granulated tissue, which may develop in severe acute pancreatitis and may become infected. By CT, abscesses are well-circumscribed fluid collections that may or may not contain foci of air (Figure 46.3).

It is important to distinguish between infected pancreatic necrosis and pancreatic abscesses, because significantly lower mortality rates are described for patients with pancreatic abscesses. Furthermore, pancreatic abscesses, in general, develop later in the course of the disease (usually after 5 weeks), whereas infected pancreatic necrosis may already be found within the first week after the onset of

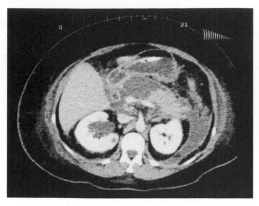
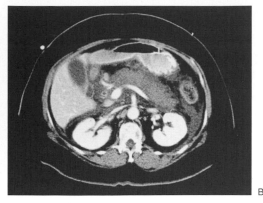

A

B

Figure 46.1 Contrast-enhanced computed tomography of pancreatic necrosis. (A) Focal pancreatic necrosis. There is lack of enhancement of the pancreatic head, neck, and body. Note the lower attenuation of the necrotic pancreas relative to the normally enhanced pancreatic tail. (B) Diffuse pancreatic necrosis. There is complete loss of the normal enhancement pattern of the pancreas.

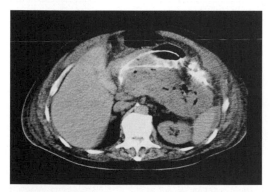

Figure 46.2 On this unenhanced computed tomography, there are foci of air seen in the pancreatic bed suggestive of infected pancreatic necrosis.

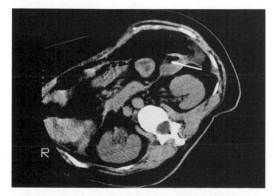

R

Figure 46.3 Pancreatic abscess. There is a focal fluid collection just inferior to the pancreatic tail and posterior to the descending colon. Computed tomography-guided aspiration revealed bacterial contamination thus making it an abscess.

symptoms. Infected necrosis could be thought of as a sponge of tissue with purulent material, thus it has a solid and liquid component, whereas an abscess is mostly infected fluid.

PATHOGENESIS

The pathophysiology of infection of peripancreatic necrosis is essentially unknown. Upper gastrointestinal dysmotility has been observed in AP as well as in cholestasis and sepsis. There are several hypothetical mechanisms by which bacteria can enter pancreatic and peripancreatic necrosis leading to the infection (Figure 46.4) and include (1) the hematogenous route via the circulation, (2) transmural migration through the colonic bowel wall either to the pancreas (translocation), (3) via ascites to the pancreas, (4) via the lymphatics to the circulation, (5) via the biliary duct system, and/or (6) from the duodenum via the main pancreatic duct. Most pathogens in pancreatic infection are the gastrointestinal gram-negative bacteria; therefore, the colon seems to be the main source of pancreatitis-related infections. It is, therefore, possible that bacterial translocation is the most important mechanism for contamination of pancreatic necrosis.

Several studies have examined the frequency of bacterial infection of necrotic areas in the natural course of severe AP, without antibiotic intervention. Beger et al. showed an overall contamination rate of 24% within the first week of the onset of acute pancreatitis in patients undergoing surgery for severe acute pancreatitis, increasing to 46% and 71%, respectively, in the second and third weeks. Thus, patients with severe AP have the highest risk of pancreatic infection in the third week after onset of the disease. The overall infection rate in this series was 39%.

Thus pancreatic necrosis may become infected after the 5th day of disease and is dependent on the extent of intra- and extrapancreatic

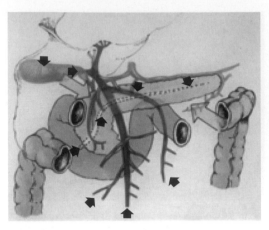

Figure 46.4 Possible infection routes in severe acute pancreatitis.

Table 46.3 Microorganisms Cultured from Pancreatic Necrosis in the Preantibiotic era: Results from 45 Patients with Necrotizing Pancreatitis

Bacteria Isolated	Number of Patients
Gram-negative	
Escherichia coli	24
Enterobacter aerogenes	16
Pseudomonas aerogenes	5
Proteus spp	5
Bacteroides spp	5
Klebsiella pneumonia	3
Citrobacter freundii	1
Gram-positive	
Streptococcus faecalis	6
Staphylococcus aureus	4
Streptococcus viridans	1
Staphylococcus epidermidis	1
Others	
Candida species	3
Mycobacterium tuberculosis	1

necrosis. Through morphological analysis by contrast-enhanced CT scanning, Beger et al. found a higher rate of infection in patients with extensive pancreatic necrosis. Two-thirds of the patients with infected pancreatic necrosis had a total amount of necrosis of more than 30%, whereas 60% of patients with sterile necrosis had necrotic areas of less than 30%. Therefore, it seems that the presence of a significant extent of necrosis (>50% on CT scanning) is predictive of severe disease and helps to identify patients who might develop septic complications.

MICROBIOLOGY

Prior to the era of prophylactic use of antibiotics in acute pancreatitis, the predominant pathogens found in pancreatic infection were gastrointestinal gram-negative bacteria. The culture of infected pancreatic necroses yielded monomicrobial flora in 60% to 87% of cases. A preponderance of gram-negative aerobic bacteria was usually present (*Escherichia coli*, *Pseudomonas* spp., *Proteus*, *Klebsiella* spp.), which suggested an enteric origin, but gram-positive bacteria (*Staphylococcus aureus*, *Streptococcus faecalis*, *Enterococcus*), anaerobes, and, occasionally, fungi had also been found. The incidence of fungi in long-term disease may increase, especially after prolonged antibiotic treatment (Table 46.3).

PREDICTIVE FACTORS

Several factors have been associated with the infection rate of pancreatic necrosis. It has been demonstrated that the frequency of infected necrosis correlates with the duration of the disease. In patients with necrotizing pancreatitis, the proportion of patients who had proven infected necrosis at the time of surgery rose from 24% in the first week to 36% and 72% in the second and third weeks, respectively. Gerzof et al., using CT-guided fine-needle aspiration (FNA), reported infection in 22% of their patients within the first week after the onset of pancreatitis and in 55% within 2 weeks.

Infection also correlates with the extent of pancreatic necrosis. The highest infection rate has been reported in patients who had more than 50% necrosis of the pancreas. Therefore, it appears that the presence of a significant extent of necrosis (>50% on CT scanning) is predictive of severe disease and helps to identify patients who might develop septic complications. Thus severity correlates with infection that may be a primary or secondary indicator of organ system failure.

Overall there seem to be no differences with regard to clinical course and infection rate depending on the etiological factor in acute pancreatitis. This was shown in another prospective study with 190 patients that analyzed the severity of the disease, serum enzyme elevation, indicators for necrosis, systemic complications, and mortality with regard to etiology of the pancreatitis. They found that there were no differences based on the etiology of the pancreatitis.

DIAGNOSIS

Infection of necrotic pancreatic tissue is usually suspected in patients who develop clinical signs of sepsis or ongoing organ system failure. These patients should undergo CT or endoscopic ultrasound-guided FNA of pancreatic necrosis or adjacent fluid. This is an accurate, safe, and reliable approach to differentiate between sterile and infected necrosis. Complication rates of this procedure are low, with only very few serious complications such as bleeding, aggravation of acute pancreatitis, or death reported in the literature. Bacterial testing of the aspirate, including Gram staining and culture of the aspirated material, yields diagnostic sensitivity and specificity of 88% and 90%. It is important to emphasize that only those patients who present with clinical signs of sepsis or ongoing organ system failure should undergo FNA, as FNA bears a potential risk of secondary infection.

TREATMENT

Local infection of necrotic areas of the pancreas influences the course of the disease, its prognosis, and the clinical management. Bacterial infection of pancreatic necrosis is usually suspected in patients who develop signs of sepsis and is confirmed by a bacteriologically positive FNA. Conservative treatment has previously been said to lead to almost 100% mortality in patients with signs of local and systemic septic complications. Even after surgery, patients with infected necrosis have a mortality rate ranging from 15% to 82%, which is 3 times higher than the mortality of those patients with sterile necrosis. Infected pancreatic necrosis is a definitive indication for surgery or drainage. Conversely, the management of sterile pancreatic necrosis is usually nonoperative. Surgical intervention in patients with sterile pancreatic necrosis is limited to patients with a deteriorating clinical course that does not respond to intensive care.

Nevertheless, there is general agreement that surgical treatment of severe acute pancreatitis, whether infected or not, should be postponed for as long as possible, and the second or third week seems to guarantee optimal operative conditions for necrosectomy. Surgical methods for the treatment of necrosis are varied, and the best method has yet to be determined. The recommended, and currently accepted, surgical management technique should be an organ-preserving approach that involves debridement or necrosectomy, combined with a postoperative management concept that maximizes evacuation of retroperitoneal debris and exudate. Three comparable techniques are available: (1) closed continuous lavage of the retroperitoneum, (2) management by planned, staged relaparotomy, and (3) the open packing technique. In experienced hands these approaches have reduced mortality from severe acute pancreatitis to ≤15%. Other strategies include percutaneous CT-guided catheter drainage, endoscopic transoral intrapancreatic drainage and irrigation lavage, and laparoscopic necrosectomy. Those undergoing a minimally invasive retroperitoneal approach have a reduced need for postoperative intensive care and less systemic inflammatory response (Figure 46.5).

PREVENTION

The role of prophylactic antibiotics to prevent secondary infection of pancreatic tissue remains controversial. A multicenter trial of 102 patients with severe AP randomized patients to either selective gut decontamination (oral and rectal norfloxacin, colistin, and amphotericin; and IV cefotaxime 500 mg every 8 hours) or standard treatment found that selective decontamination decreased the need for laparoscopy and reduced late (>2 weeks) mortality owing to a significant reduction of gram-negative pancreatic infection ($P = .003$). Overall mortality fell from 35% in controls to 22% ($P \le .05$) in the selective decontamination group.

Previous investigations indicated that systemic antibiotics alone were ineffective in preventing secondary infection, but these studies included patients without necrosis and used antimicrobial agents with poor penetration into pancreatic tissue. A recent trial found fewer infectious complications and lower mortality among patients with alcohol-induced necrotizing pancreatitis randomized to prophylactic IV cefuroxime (4.5 g/day) versus no antibiotics. Agents such as imipenem and fluoroquinolones have an even more favorable pharmacologic profile, demonstrating both outstanding penetration into pancreatic tissues and excellent activity against the most prevalent

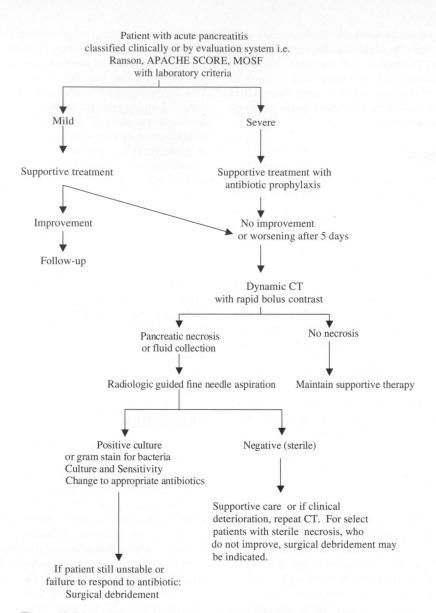

Figure 46.5 Approach to the patiente with necrotizing pancreatitis. Acute pancreatitis classified clinically or by evaluation system (Ranson, APACHE score, MOSF) with laboratory criteria.

organisms. A retrospective study found that 75 patients with necrotizing pancreatitis who received 4 weeks of imipenem had a significant decrease in the incidence of pancreatic infection (27% versus 76%) and a trend toward improved mortality compared with historical controls. A controlled trial of 74 patients with necrotizing pancreatitis by CT scan found that patients randomized to imipenem (500 mg administered IV every 8 hours) had a 2.5-fold reduction in pancreatic infectious complications and a trend toward reduced mortality (7% versus 12%).

The clinical course of patients with necrotizing pancreatitis who received antibiotics within 36 hours versus those in whom antibiotic therapy was delayed up to 4.8 days found that early antibiotic treatment is associated with a significant improvement in the prognosis of necrotizing acute pancreatitis. The early group had a significant decrease in both pancreatic and extrapancreatic infections. Therefore current evidence would seem to justify early prophylactic administration of an antibiotic concentrated by the pancreas (for example, imipenem) in patients with clinically severe AP.

NUTRITIONAL SUPPORT OF PATIENTS WITH NECROTIZING PANCREATITIS

Classically, patients with severe AP were treated with total parenteral nutrition (TPN) because enteral feeding was thought to stimulate the pancreas and worsen pancreatic injury. In contrast, recent data suggest that TPN does not hasten pancreatic recovery and that enteral feeding is actually well tolerated. Potential benefits of enteral feeding include decreased gut permeability, prevention of bacterial translocation, and therefore a reduction in secondary pancreatic infection. Enteral feeding is also significantly less expensive than TPN and is associated with fewer cases of catheter-related sepsis.

Several prospective randomized studies have examined the role of enteral feeding, initiated within 48 hours of the onset of severe acute pancreatitis, administered via a tube advanced into the jejunum under radiographic guidance. These studies, which included approximately 100 patients in total, suggest that enteral nutrition results in fewer total and septic complications, significantly improves acute phase responses and disease severity scores, and can be delivered at one-third to one-fifth the cost of TPN. Therefore in patients who are unable to take in oral nutrition by day 5 evaluation for enteral feedings should be initiated.

INFECTED PANCREATIC COLLECTIONS AND PSEUDOCYSTS

Up to 40% of patients with AP have acute fluid collections that consist of enzyme-rich pancreatic secretions that occur during the first 2 weeks of the episode. These acute collections are usually peripancreatic, without a capsule, and confined to the anatomic space within which it arises. Extrapancreatic fluid collections can also occur in the lesser sac, perirenal and spleen and liver. These collections, which can be single or multiple, result from pancreatic and gastrointestinal fistulas that usually close spontaneously. If these collections do not resolve spontaneously, they may become a pseudocyst that can become infected. Most acute fluid collections resolve spontaneously so they do not need to be drained unless they become infected. If infected, percutaneous or endoscopic drainage of the infected pseudocyst or collection can be performed. Once drainage ceases, the infection is controlled, and the collection is resolved via CT scan, we perform a fistulogram to document that its ductular communication has closed and then the catheter is removed.

SUMMARY

In conclusion, our goal in patients with severe acute pancreatitis is to prevent infection with prophylactic antibiotics and early initiation of nutrition via the enteral route. If the patient is clinically suspected of having infected necrosis, CT-guided FNA with culture and sensitivity of the aspirate directs our antibiotic therapy. Support for organ system failure is ongoing, and our goal is to prolong the time to surgery, if needed, until the second week or thereafter.

SUGGESTED READING

Banks PA. Predictors of severity in acute pancreatitis. *Pancreas*. 1991;6:S7–S12.

Beger HG, Rau B, Mayer J, Pralle U. Natural course of acute pancreatitis. *World J Surg*. 1997;21:130–135.

Schmid SW, Uhl W, Friess H, et al. The role of infection in acute pancreatitis. *Gut*. 1999;45:311–316.

Buchler P, Reber HA. Surgical approach in patients with acute pancreatitis. Is infected or sterile necrosis an indication–in whom should this be done, when and why? *Gastroenterol Clin North Am*. 1999;28(3): 661–671.

Choe KA. Imaging in pancreatic infection. *J Hepatobiliary Pancreat Surg*. 2003;10: 401–405.

Connor S, Raraty MG, Howes N, et al. Surgery in the treatment of acute pancreatitis–minimal access pancreatic necrosectomy. *Scand J Surg*. 2005;94:135–142.

Gerzof SG, Banks PA, Robbins AH, et al. Early diagnosis of pancreatic infection by computed tomography guided aspiration. *Gastroenterology*. 1987;93:1315–1320.

Hartwig W, Werner J, Uhl W, et al. Management of infection in acute pancreatitis. *J Hepatobiliary Pancreat Surg*. 2002;9: 423–428.

Larvin M, McMahon MJ. APACHE-II score for assessment and monitoring of acute pancreatitis. *Lancet*. 1989;2:201–205.

Manes G, Uomo I, Menchise A, et al. Timing of antibiotic prophylaxis in acute pancreatitis: a controlled randomized study with meropenem. *Am J Gastroenterol.* 2006;101:1348–1353.

Uhl W, Isenmann R, Büchler MW. Infections complicating pancreatitis: diagnosing,

treating, preventing. *New Horiz.* 1998;6 S72–S79.

Uhl W, Schrag HJ, Wheatley AM, et al. The role of infection in acute pancreatitis. *Dig Surg.* 1994;11: 214–219.

47. Esophageal Infections

Joshua Forman and Jean-Pierre Raufman

Esophageal infections are encountered frequently in clinical practice, particularly in patients with impaired host defenses, and are an important contributor to morbidity and mortality. The acquired immunodeficiency syndrome (AIDS) epidemic and the increasing use of organ transplantation with its attendant immunosuppresive therapy have precipitated an increased incidence of esophageal infections. Although *Candida albicans* is typically the etiologic agent in mildy immunosuppressed patients with infectious esophagitis, a variety of fungal, viral, and bacterial pathogens are capable of causing infection (see Table 47.1). Regardless of the organism, infection causes mucosal inflammation resulting in the hallmark clinical complaint of odynophagia and potentially resulting in erosions, ulcers, or fistulae. Rapid identification and treatment of the infecting organism is of paramount importance because, in contrast to underlying clinical states that predispose to their occurrence, esophageal infections generally respond rapidly and completely to appropriate treatment.

FUNGAL INFECTIONS OF THE ESOPHAGUS

Candida Species

Candida albicans is the fungal organism most frequently implicated in infectious esophagitis. Other *Candida* species (*Candida tropicalis, Candida parapsilosis, Candida krusei,* and *Candida glabrata*) are less commonly involved. *Candida* organisms are normal components of the oral flora, and colonization of the esophagus is not unusual. A population-based study revealed esophageal colonization in approximately 20% of healthy, ambulatory adults. Colonization involves adherence and proliferation of *Candida* organisms within the superficial mucosa. Progression to infectious esophagitis requires invasion of the epithelium. Invasion usually occurs in the setting of defective cellular immunity. The spectrum of esophageal infection with *Candida* species is broad, ranging from scattered white plaques accompanied by mild or no symptoms

to dense pseudomembranes consisting of fungi, sloughed mucosal cells, and fibrin overlying severely damaged mucosa. The latter are usually accompanied by severe symptoms.

Infection with human immunodeficiency virus (HIV) is the most significant risk factor for the development of candidal esophagitis, although the prevalence of esophageal *Candida* infection is decreasing with the widespread use of highly active antiretroviral therapy. Infection is primarily seen with CD4 counts below 200/μL and represents an AIDS-defining illness. The risk of infection increases with the degree of immune compromise. Infection occurs most frequently in patients with persistently low CD4 counts. Additional risk factors include hematologic malignancies, diabetes mellitus, adrenal insufficiency, alcoholism, advanced age, radiation therapy, systemic chemotherapy, and the use of oral and inhaled steroid therapy. Esophageal motility disorders (eg, achalasia) may also predispose to infection. Immunosuppression in organ transplant recipients imparts significant risk although the prevalence of infection is reduced by the frequent use of systemic fungal prophylactic therapy. Immunomodulatory and biologic therapy, increasingly utilized in the management of immunologic conditions such as inflammatory bowel disease and rheumatoid arthritis, does not appear to increase the risk for esophageal candidiasis.

CLINICAL PRESENTATION AND COMPLICATIONS

Candida esophagitis may not cause symptoms, particularly in those who are immunocompetent with few adherent esophageal plaques. When symptomatic, the most common complaint is odynophagia, and the pain is usually localized to a discrete retrosternal area. Odynophagia may impair swallowing minimally, or the pain may be so intense that the patient avoids eating and is unable to tolerate secretions. In severe cases, retrosternal chest pain or burning may be present without swallowing. In granulocytopenic patients, fungal infection may be disseminated, thereby resulting in fever, sepsis, and signs and symptoms related to hepatic, splenic, or renal fungal abscesses.

Table 47.1 Organisms Associated with Infectious Esophagitis

Fungi
Candida species (especially *C. albicans*)
Aspergillus species
Histoplasma capsulatum
Blastomyces dermatitides
Viruses
Herpes simplex virus type 1
Cytomegalovirus
Varicella-zoster virus
Human immunodeficiency virus
Bacteria
Mycobacterium tuberculosis and *M. avium*
Actinomyces israelii
Staphylococcus aureus
Streptococcus viridans
Lactobacillus acidophilus
Treponema pallidum
Idiopathic ulcerative esophagitis in AIDS

In AIDS, esophageal candidiasis is commonly associated with oropharyngeal thrush. In this setting, the presence of esophageal symptoms (odynophagia or dysphagia) plus oral candidiasis predicts the presence of *Candida* esophagitis in 71% to 100% of cases. Nevertheless, *Candida* esophagitis occurs independent of thrush at least 25% of the time.

It is important to recognize that mucosal *Candida* infections frequently coexist with other esophageal infections. For example, in published case series, oral thrush was present in 7 of 14 patients with herpes simplex virus (HSV) esophagitis and in 2 of 10 with HIV-associated idiopathic ulcers. In a study of 110 HIV-infected patients with esophageal symptoms, 72 were diagnosed with esophagitis. Among the 52 diagnosed with *Candida* esophagitis, concomitant infection with cytomegalovirus (CMV) and HSV was noted in 22 and 2 patients, respectively.

Severe complications of esophageal candidiasis include esophageal bleeding from ulceration; luminal obstruction from a fungus ball; mucosal scarring and stricture; fistulization into the trachea, bronchi, or mediastinum; and esophageal mucosal sloughing with replacement by pseudomembranes. Although life-threatening hemorrhage has been reported, bleeding from esophageal candidiasis is usually mild, not requiring transfusion.

DIAGNOSIS

Candida esophagitis should be suspected when at-risk patients complain of odynophagia or dysphagia, particularly in the setting of AIDS. In this setting, many authorities recommend empiric therapy. Because of the high frequency of co-infection, further evaluation is reserved for those who do not respond within 7 days.

The most accurate method for diagnosing fungal esophagitis is endoscopy with directed brushing and biopsy of lesions (Figure 47.1). Endoscopic appearance alone may be suggestive but is insufficient to diagnose *Candida* esophagitis. Typical candidal plaques are creamy white or pale yellow (Figure 47.2A). At endoscopy, the gross appearance is graded: grade 1, a few raised white plaques up to 2 mm wide without ulceration; grade 2, multiple raised white plaques more than 2 mm wide without ulceration; grade 3, confluent, linear, and nodular elevated plaques with superficial ulceration; and grade 4, finding of grade 3 plus narrowing of the esophageal lumen.

Brushings from involved surfaces and ulcers can be obtained with a sheathed cytology brush spread onto slides and stained by the periodic acid–Schiff (PAS), silver, or Gram methods. Mycelial forms and masses of budding yeast are consistent with *Candida* infection (Figure 47.2B). Fungal cultures are generally not helpful unless an unusual pathogen (eg, a resistant *Candida* species, such as *C. glabrata*) is suspected.

Because findings are often nonspecific and concurrent infections (eg, *C. albicans* plus a virus) will be missed, radiographic studies of the esophagus are not helpful in establishing an accurate diagnosis of esophageal infection. Nonetheless, barium esophagrams may reveal a "shaggy" esophagus, plaques, pseudomembranes, cobblestoning, nodules, strictures, fistulae, or mucosal bridges. Radiographic examination may be useful when endoscopy is not available, when endoscopic biopsies are precluded because of coagulopathy, or when dysphagia or coughing associated with eating are prominent symptoms, thereby suggesting the presence of perforation, stricture, or fistula.

TREATMENT

Patients at risk for *Candida* esophagitis who present with odynophagia or dysphagia can be

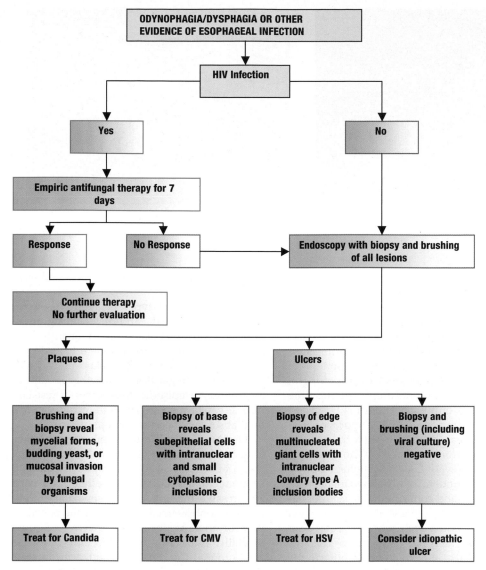

Figure 47.1 Suggested diagnostic approaches to common esophageal infections. HIV – Human immunodeficiency virus; CMV = cytomegalovirus; HSV = herpes simplex virus type 1.

treated with an empiric course of antifungal therapy without endoscopic confirmation of disease. Empiric therapy is particularly indicated in the presence of oral thrush. If symptoms do not improve after 7 days, further evaluation is necessary.

Antifungal treatment options for esophageal candidiasis include the imidazoles, echinocandins, and amphotericin B. Imidazoles alter fungal cell membrane permeability by inhibiting the synthesis of ergosterols. Potential agents in the imidazole class include fluconazole, itraconazole, and voriconazole. Fluconazole (100 to 200 mg daily for 14 to 21 days orally or intravenously) is favored due to its excellent efficacy, ease of administration, low toxicity, and low cost. Itraconazole oral solution (200 mg daily) appears as effective as fluconazole in randomized trials but is associated with more adverse events. Itraconazole inhibits the cytochrome P450 enzymes and thus has the potential for drug interactions. Itraconazole capsules are also available, but absorption is less predictable compared to the liquid formulation. In a large, randomized, double-blind, muticenter trial, voriconazole (200 mg twice daily orally or 4 mg/kg every 12 hours intravenously) was as effective as fluconazole and may be effective in cases that are refractory to fluconazole. Transient visual disturbance was the most

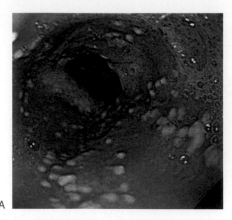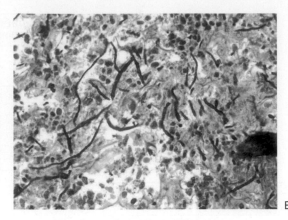

Figure 47.2 (A) Endoscopic appearance of *Candida* esophagitis with multiple raised white plaques. **(B)** Biopsy revealing budding yeast cells, hyphae, pseudohyphae, and mucosal invasion by the organisms (periodic acid–Schiff 60×; courtesy of Harris Yfantis, MD, Baltimore VA Medical Center, Md.).

frequently reported side effect, occurring in 23% of patients. Guidelines published by the Infectious Disease Society of America (IDSA) indicate that topical therapies are ineffective for the treatment of esophageal candidiasis.

Echinocandins inhibit the synthesis of β(1,3)-D-glucan, an essential component of *Candida* cell walls. Options include caspofungin, micafungin, and anidulafungin. At the time of this writing, only caspofungin is U.S. Food and Drug Administration (FDA) approved. The echinocandins are administered intravenously and are therefore utilized in hospitalized patients with severe *Candida* esophagitis. In a double-blind, randomized trial of patients with advanced HIV and confirmed *Candida* esophagitis, caspofungin (50 mg daily intravenously) was efficacious and well tolerated compared to fluconazole (200 mg daily intravenously). Caspofungin also appears to be effective in the treatment of esophageal candidiasis resistant to fluconazole and is a much less toxic alternative to amphotericin B. Studies with micafungin (150 mg daily intravenously) and anidulafungin (100 mg on day 1 followed by 50 mg daily intraveneously) also suggest similar efficacy and tolerability compared to fluconazole.

Amphotericin B binds irreversibly to fungal membrane sterols, thereby altering membrane permeability. Amphotericin B (0.3 to 0.7 mg/kg daily intraveously) has similar efficacy compared to fluconazole but, due to increased toxicity relative to other agents, its use should be limited in patients with *Candida* esophagitis. Current indications for amphotericin B include drug-resistant candidal infections and candidiasis during pregnancy. Imidazoles are teratogenic and should not be used during the first trimester of pregnancy. No data are currently

available regarding the use of echinocandins in pregnancy.

Of the different types of agents used for treating esophageal candidiasis, drug resistance has been associated predominantly with imidazoles. Risk factors include advanced immunosupression and chronic exposure to imidazole therapy, regardless of whether therapy is continuous or episodic. Most cases of resistant disease can be managed with the echinocandins or, if absolutely necessary, amphotericin B.

For chronically immunosuppressed patients, long-term therapy with fluconazole (100 mg daily) effectively prevents oropharyngeal and esophageal candidiasis. Whether long-term suppressive therapy with fluconazole is indicated is controversial. Because of the effectiveness of therapy for acute infection, limited mortality associated with infection, cost, and the potential for resistance and drug interactions, most specialists do not favor primary or secondary prophylaxis. Nonetheless, secondary prophylaxis may be appropriate for patients with frequent or severe infections.

Other Fungal Infections of the Esophagus

Esophageal aspergillosis, histoplasmosis, and blastomycosis, acquired from the environment rather than from endogenous flora, are much less common than infection with *Candida* species. Blastomycosis and histoplasmosis commonly invade the esophagus from paraesophageal lymph nodes. *Aspergillus* infection results in large, deep ulcers, whereas esophageal histoplasmosis and blastomycosis are characterized by focal lesions and abscesses. With involvement of muscle layers, severe odynophagia results. Complications of these noncandidal fungal infections include esophageal stricture and tracheoesophageal fistula. *Aspergillus* species have a distinctive microscopic appearance. *Histoplasma* organisms usually do not invade the esophageal mucosa. Hence, endoscopic brushing and biopsy specimens may be nondiagnostic, and bronchoscopy, mediastinoscopy, or surgery may be needed to diagnose this infection. Intravenous amphotericin B is the preferred treatment for *Aspergillus* infection and is also used for complicated histoplasmosis and blastomycosis. Itraconazole, voriconazole, and caspofungin may also play a role in treating noncandidal fungal esophageal infections. However, the role of these agents has yet to be defined.

VIRAL INFECTIONS OF THE ESOPHAGUS

Herpes Simplex Virus Type 1

HSV type 1 (HSV-1) is the most common of the three herpes viruses that infect the esophagus; the others are CMV and varicella-zoster virus (VZV). HSV-1 esophagitis usually occurs in the setting of immunocompromise although infection may also occur in immunocompetent individuals without predisposing risk factors. Most infections occur in those receiving immunosuppressive medications, such as solid organ and bone marrow transplant recipients. In two series, HSV was the sole cause of esophageal infection in only 5% of patients with HIV.

HSV is a large, enveloped, double-stranded DNA virus that infects squamous epithelium, inducing the characteristic painful herpetic vesicles with erythematous bases. Latency in the root ganglia of nerves supplying the affected regions may follow resolution of acute HSV infection. Although primary HSV esophagitis occurs, most cases result from virus reactivation as acute infection is followed by latency in the root ganglia of nerves that supply the affected regions, such as the laryngeal, superficial cervical, or vagus nerves.

The abrupt onset of severe odynophagia is a common presenting symptom of HSV esophagitis. Other symptoms include persistent retrosternal pain, nausea, and vomiting. Bone marrow transplant recipients may have continuous nausea and vomiting as the sole manifestation of HSV esophagitis. Herpes labialis (ie, cold sores) or skin involvement may precede or occur concurrent with esophageal infection. About 25% of HSV esophagitis cases are accompanied by either HSV or *Candida*

infection in the oropharyngeal or genital area. In untreated immunocompetent persons, HSV esophagitis generally resolves 1 to 2 weeks after the onset of symptoms, although early initiation of antiviral therapy may hasten recovery. In immunodeficient patients, esophageal infection with HSV can cause hemorrhage and perforation with tracheoesophageal fistulae or can disseminate to involve the liver, lungs, and central nervous system.

A diagnosis of HSV esophagitis is usually established by endoscopy (see Figure 47.1). Early, vesicular herpetic lesions (round 1- to 3-mm vesicles in the mid- to distal esophagus) are characteristic but rarely seen. More commonly, by the time endoscopy is performed, the vesicles have sloughed to reveal discrete, circumscribed ulcers with raised edges (Figure 47.3A). These "volcano" lesions result in the classic appearance of HSV esophagitis on double-contrast barium studies of the esophagus, although similar radiographic findings may rarely be seen in *Candida* esophagitis. Discrete HSV ulcers seen at early stages can coalesce into large lesions or, in severe cases, progress to near-total denudation of the esophageal epithelium. Hence, diffuse herpetic esophagitis results in cobblestoning or a "shaggy" mucosa that is similar in appearance to *Candida* esophagitis.

HSV infection is confirmed with viral culture and histologic or cytologic examination of brushings and biopsies from ulcer edges. Tissue from the ulcer edge is utilized because HSV preferentially infects squamous epithelial cells. Material from the ulcer base, where epithelial cells are absent, is not adequate to establish a diagnosis. Viral culture is more sensitive than routine histologic examination of brushings and biopsy specimens. Findings observed with histologic staining of HSV-infected epithelial cells include multinucleated giant cells, ballooning degeneration, "ground-glass" intranuclear Cowdry type A inclusions, and margination of chromatin (Figure 47.3B). Immunohistologic stains using monoclonal antibodies to HSV antigens and in situ hybridization are also available for select cases.

For immunocompromised patients able to tolerate oral medications, HSV esophagitis should be treated with acyclovir (400 mg 5 times daily) or valacyclovir (1000 mg three times daily). Therapy should be given for a total of 14 to 21 days. Those unable to swallow should be treated with intravenous acyclovir (5 mg/kg every 8 hours). Oral therapy should be instituted when feasible based on the patient's symptoms. Immunocompetent patients with

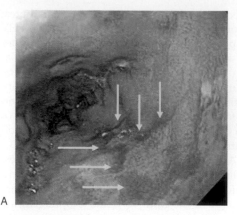 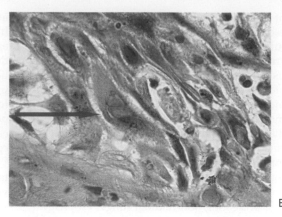

Figure 47.3 (A) Endoscopic photograph revealing a large sharply demarcated ulcer with raised edges in the middle third of the esophagus. Ulcer borders are defined by arrows. **(B)** Biopsy from the ulcer margin demonstrating a multinucleated giant cell (hemotoxylin and eosin stain, 100×; courtesy of Harris Yfantis, MD, Baltimore VA Medical Center, Md.).

HSV esophagitis may experience spontaneous resolution after 1 to 2 weeks although a more rapid response may be attained with a short course of oral acyclovir. Unfortunately, strains of HSV resistant to acyclovir have emerged. In the setting of acyclovir resistance, intravenous foscarnet at a dose of 40 mg/kg 3 times daily is required.

Acyclovir is also used for prophylaxis. Prophylaxis with oral acyclovir may be indicated for immunocompromised persons at high risk for reactivation of HSV such as HSV-seropositive transplant recipients and AIDS patients with recurrent herpetic infections. Famciclovir is an acyclovir analog with a similar spectrum of activity and better bioavailability that may also be employed for oral prophylaxis and treatment.

Cytomegalovirus

CMV, a ubiquitous herpesvirus, infects most of the world's adults. In healthy people with latent infection, CMV viral DNA can be detected in many tissues, including circulating leukocytes. Latent infection is responsible for the high transmission rate of the virus from CMV-seropositive donors to CMV-seronegative recipients after blood transfusion or organ transplantation. In contrast to HSV, esophageal infection with CMV, either primary or reactivation of latent virus, occurs only in immunodeficiency states (AIDS and others). In published series, CMV was an esophageal pathogen or copathogen in 33 of 110 patients with HIV infection and esophageal symptoms and in 7 of 21 symptomatic bone marrow transplant recipients. Other differences between these

herpesviruses is that, in CMV esophagitis, the virus infects subepithelial fibroblasts and endothelial cells of the esophagus, not squamous epithelial cells, and the onset of symptoms with CMV is typically more gradual than with HSV or *Candida* esophagitis. Because CMV disease is systemic and involves multiple organs, nausea, vomiting, fever, epigastric pain, diarrhea, and weight loss are prominent symptoms, whereas dysphagia and odynophagia are less commonly observed than in HSV infection.

To diagnose CMV esophagitis, it is necessary to obtain tissue for biopsy (see Figure 47.1). Neither clinical assessment, radiographic findings, nor endoscopic findings alone are sufficient or accurate to distinguish CMV esophagitis from other causes of viral esophagitis. For example, barium studies in CMV esophagitis may reveal focal ulcerations in the distal third of the esophagus that are indistinguishable from those seen with HSV. In some cases, radiographs may show flat elongated, tear-drop, or stellate giant ulcers that can be confused with those observed with HIV-associated idiopathic esophageal ulcers. Endoscopically, superficial erosions or deep ulcers with geographic, serpiginous, flat borders in the mid- to distal esophagus are suggestive of CMV esophagitis, but findings may be indistinguishable from HSV esophagitis. Deep ulcers may extend longitudinally for several centimeters and may reach the muscularis, occasionally resulting in stricture formation. Numerous biopsy samples should be taken from ulcer bases, where CMV-infected subepithelial fibroblasts and endothelial cells are most likely to be present. Specimens containing only squamous epithelium are not helpful, and superficial brushings for cytologic examination do not increase the diagnostic yield. Because CMV may infect gastric and intestinal epithelial and lamina propria cells, biopsy of abnormal mucosa in these areas should also be obtained for histology and viral culture. Biopsy specimens are important for confirmation of CMV infection and to exclude concurrent fungal, viral (HSV), or bacterial pathogens.

Histologic features indicative of CMV infection include the presence of large cells in the subepithelial layer with amphophilic intranuclear inclusions, a "halo" surrounding the nucleus, and, in contrast to HSV and VZV, multiple, small cytoplasmic inclusions (Figure 47.4A). Although immunohistochemical staining and in situ hybridization can confirm CMV infection (Figure 47.4B), viral cultures from tissue obtained from the ulcer base are more sensitive and less costly. CMV DNA polymerase chain reaction (PCR) is more sensitive than viral culture, but interpretation of a positive test may be difficult as latent CMV infection can yield a positive PCR result.

CMV esophagitis is effectively treated with ganciclovir and foscarnet, alone or in combination (see Table 47.2). Ganciclovir (5 mg/kg intravenously every 12 hours for 2 weeks) is highly effective in eliminating CMV from esophageal ulcers, but symptoms are slow to respond and large ulcers are slow to heal. Furthermore, without restoration of the normal immune system, recurrence after short courses of therapy is common. Therefore, it is recommended that full-dose antiviral therapy for 2 to 3 weeks be followed by maintenance therapy until immunosuppression resolves (see Table 47.2). Persons with AIDS and recurrent CMV infection often require indefinite maintenance therapy with ganciclovir. Bone marrow suppression is the major adverse effect of ganciclovir and may be particularly severe when ganciclovir is combined with other marrow-toxic agents. An additional concern with long-term therapy is emergence of ganciclovir-resistant CMV with long-term therapy. Ganciclovir-resistant CMV is usually responsive to foscarnet (90 mg/kg intravenously every 12 hours for 2 to 3 weeks) followed by maintenance therapy (90 to 120 mg/kg/d). Cidofovir, a highly nephrotoxic agent, may be used in the setting of CMV resistant to ganciclovir and foscarnet.

As CMV is an important cause of morbidity in transplant recipients, prophylaxis against the development of CMV-related disease is extremely important. Both morbidity and mortality related to primary CMV infection in CMV-naïve transplant recipients can be reduced by screening donor blood products for CMV antibodies. For patients who are CMV seropositive or who are recipients of organs from CMV-seropositive donors, CMV infection can be prevented by administering prophylactic ganciclovir.

Varicella-Zoster Virus

The frequency of VZV esophagitis during the course of chickenpox or herpes zoster infections is unknown. Symptomatic VZV esophagitis is extremely rare. Although VZV esophagitis may be severe in profoundly immunocompromised individuals, it is relatively minor compared with other manifestations of disseminated infection such as varicella encephalitis, pneumonitis, and fulminant hepatitis. The clinical presentation and esophageal findings with VZV mimic HSV esophagitis. Finding concurrent dermatologic VZV lesions (shingles) is often crucial for diagnosing VZV esophagitis.

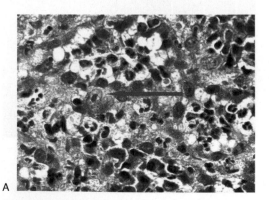

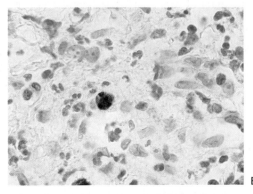

Figure 47.4 (A) Biopsy specimen from the base of an esophageal ulcer revealing a perinuclear "halo" suggestive of herpes simplex virus infection (hematoxylin and eosin stain, 100×, courtesy of Harris Yfantis, MD, Baltimore VA Medical Center, MD.). **(B)** Biopsy specimen revealing subepithelial cytomegalovirus by immunohistochemical staining (100×; courtesy of Harris Yfantis, MD, Baltimore VA Medical Center, Md.).

Table 47.2 Recommended Treatment of Common Esophageal Infections

Cause	Primary Treatment	Alternative Treatment
Candida	Fluconazole, 100–200 mg PO/IV daily for 14–21 days Itraconazole oral solution, 200 mg PO twice daily for 14–21 days	Voriconazole, 200 mg PO twice daily for 14–21 days or 4 mg/kg IV twice daily (change to PO when feasible) Caspofungin 50 mg IV once daily for 14–21 days Amphotericin B 0.3–0.7 mg/kg IV once daily for 14–21 days
Herpes simplex virus	Acyclovir, 400 mg PO 5 times daily for 14–21 days or 250 mg/m² IV q8h (change to PO when feasible) Valacyclovir, 1 g PO 3 times daily for 14–21 days	Foscarnet, 90 mg/kg IV q12h for 14–21 days (for acyclovir-resistant infection) Famciclovir, 500 mg PO twice daily for 14–21 days
Cytomegalovirus	Ganciclovir, 5 mg/kg IV q12h for 14–21 days, followed by maintenance therapy until immunosuppression resolves	Foscarnet, 90 mg/kg IV q12h for 14–21 days, followed by maintenance therapy with 90–120 mg/kg/d
Varicella-zoster virus	Acyclovir, 250 mg/m² IV q8h for 7–10 days Famciclovir, 500 mg PO twice daily for 14 days	Foscarnet, 90 mg/kg IV q12h for 14–21 days
HIV-idiopathic ulcers	Prednisone, 40 mg PO daily for 4 weeks, then taper	Thalidomide, 200 mg PO daily for 4 weeks

VZV esophagitis may be treated with acyclovir or famciclovir. Foscarnet is an alternative for acyclovir-resistant VZV (see Table 47.2).

Idiopathic Ulcerative Esophagitis in AIDS

HIV infection is often associated with esophageal ulcers that lack identifiable pathogens. These lesions, called *HIV-associated* or *idiopathic esophageal ulcers*, appear as multiple, small aphthoid ulcers during seroconversion in early HIV infection and, later, as giant, deep ulcers extending up to several centimeters (Figure 47.5). The latter are associated with severe, incapacitating odynophagia. Radiologic and endoscopic studies reveal ulcers that mimic those caused by CMV. Clinical and endoscopic improvement have been reported following systemic prednisone (40 mg/ day for 4 weeks followed by a 1-month taper) or intralesional corticosteroid therapy. A thorough search for infectious pathogens, including endoscopic brushing and biopsy, must be undertaken before corticosteroid therapy is initiated. Thalidomide (200 mg daily for 4 weeks), a

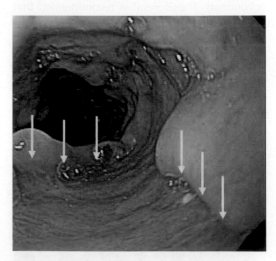

Figure 47.5 Endoscopic photograph of a large idiopathic esophageal ulcer crater in a patient with acquired immunodeficiency syndrome and odynophagia. Ulcer borders are defined by arrows.

sedative with immunomodulatory properties related to inhibition of tumor necrosis factor-α, has also been used successfully to treat these ulcers.

Bacterial, Mycobacterial, and Treponemal Infections

Esophageal infection with normal oropharyngeal flora rarely occurs, although invasive bacteria may account for 11% to 16% of infectious esophagitis in immunodeficient patients, especially those with granulocytopenia. Use of gastric acid–suppressing medications, such as proton pump inhibitors, may also increase the risk of bacterial esophagitis. As with other organisms, symptoms of bacterial esophagitis include dysphagia and odynophagia. Fever is an uncommon finding, probably because of agranulocytosis. Endoscopic findings are nonspecific, including mucosal friability, plaques, pseudomembranes, and ulcerations. Diagnostic biopsies reveal sheets of confluent bacteria invading subepithelial tissues. Bacterial culture of biopsy material is often contaminated by multiple organisms and consequently of little utility. Bacterial esophagitis is treated with a broad-spectrum, β-lactam antibiotic combined with an aminoglycoside.

Formerly, esophageal infection with *Mycobacterium tuberculosis* or *Mycobacterium avium* was considered a rare finding that occurred in fewer than 0.15% of autopsies. However, with the advent of the AIDS epidemic, the prevalence of tuberculosis has increased. Esophageal involvement with tuberculosis almost always results from direct extension of infection from adjacent mediastinal structures, with few cases of primary esophageal tuberculosis. Symptoms of esophageal mycobacterial infection include odynophagia, dysphagia, weight loss, cough, chest pain, and fever, depending on the extent of involvement. Fistulae within the wall of the esophagus (so-called double-barrelled esophagus) and connecting to the mediastinum, trachea, or bronchi are not infrequent. Contrast radiology findings, including ulcers, fistulae, and strictures, are not specific. Gross endoscopic findings include shallow ulcers, heaped-up lesions mimicking cancer, and extrinsic compression of esophagus from adenopathy (the latter can also be evaluated by computed tomography of the chest). Lesions should be biopsied and brushed. Specimens should be sent for histology, routine culture, mycobacterial culture, acid-fast stain, and PCR. Mycobacterial infection of the esophagus can be confirmed when endoscopic biopsies reveal granulomas or acid-fast bacilli. A positive PCR is also diagnostic. Esophageal infection with mycobacteria is treated with standard multidrug therapy, guided in part by the sensitivity profile in the community. In addition to pharmacologic therapy, endoscopic stenting or surgery is sometimes required to treat fistulas and perforations.

In the current era, esophageal syphilis is rare. Tertiary syphilis may be associated with gummas, diffuse ulceration, fistulas, and stricture of the upper third of the esophagus. Syphilitic esophagitis may be considered in a patient with tertiary syphilis and an inflammatory esophageal stricture. The diagnosis may be suspected if syphilitic periarteritis is present on endoscopic biopsy specimens; however, specific immunostaining for *Treponema pallidum* should be performed for definitive diagnosis.

SUGGESTED READING

Anderson LI, Frederiksen HJ, Appleyard M. Prevalence of esophageal Candida colonization in a Danish population: special reference to esophageal symptoms, benign esophageal disorders, and pulmonary disease. *J Infect Dis.* 1992;165:389–392.

Baehr PH, McDonald GB. Esophageal infections: risk factors, presentation, diagnosis, and treatment. *Gastroenterology.* 1994;106:509–532.

Bonacini M, Young T, Laine L. The causes of esophageal symptoms in human immunodeficiency virus infection: a prospective study of 110 patients. *Arch Intern Med.* 1991;151:1567–1572.

Graman PS. Esophagitis. In: Mandell GL, Bennett JE, Dollin R, eds. *Mandell, Bennet, and Dolin's Principles and Practice of Infectious Diseases.* 6th ed. New York, NY: Churchill Livingstone; 2005.

Kearney DJ, McDonald GB. Esophageal disorders caused by infection, systemic illness, medications, radiation, and trauma. In: Feldman M, Tschumy W, Friedman L, Sleisenger M, eds. *Sleisenger & Fordtran's Gastrointestinal and Liver Disease.* 7th ed. Philadelphia, PA: WB Saunders; 2002.

Mocroft A, Oancea C, Lunzen JV, et al. Decline in esophageal candidiasis and use of antimycotics in European patients with HIV. *Am J Gastroenterol.* 2005;100:1446–1454.

Raufman JP. Declining gastrointestinal opportunistic infections in HIV-infected persons: a triumph of science and a challenge of our HAARTS and minds. *Am J Gastroenterol.* 2005;100:1455–1458.

Rex JH, Walsh TJ, Sobel JD, et al. Practice guidelines for the treatment of candidiasis.

Infectious Disease Society of America (IDSA). *Clin Infect Dis.* 2000;30:662–678.

Wilcox CM. Esophageal infections. In: Yamada T, ed. *Textbook of Gastroenterology.* 3rd ed. Philadelphia, PA: Lippincott; 1999.

Wilcox CM, Schwartz DA, Clark WS. Esophageal ulceration in HIV infection: causes, response to therapy, and long-term outcome. *Ann Intern Med.* 1995; 123:143–149.

48. Gastroenteritis

Douglas R. Morgan and Robert L. Owen

GASTROENTERITIS

Gastroenteritis, broadly defined, refers to any inflammatory process of the stomach or intestinal mucosal surface. However, the term usually refers to acute infectious diarrhea, a diarrheal syndrome of less than 2 weeks' duration that may be accompanied by fever, nausea, vomiting, abdominal pain, dehydration, and weight loss. This chapter provides an overview of the infectious enteritides. Other chapters consider food poisoning, traveler's diarrhea, antibiotic-associated diarrhea, sexually transmitted enteric infections, and *Helicobacter pylori* disease.

In developed countries, gastroenteritis, similar to upper respiratory infections, is common and annoying, but it usually does not require a physician visit, laboratory evaluation, or antibiotic treatment. Globally, it is the second-leading cause of mortality, after cardiovascular disease. Gastroenteritis is the leading worldwide cause of childhood death and of years of productive life lost, with approximately 12 600 deaths per day. Annual per-person attack rates range from 1 to 5 in the United States and Europe and up to 5 to 20 in the developing world. There are approximately 100 million cases per year among adults in the United States, nearly 50% of which require subjects to limit their activities for more than 24 hours, whereas 8% require consultation with a physician and fewer than 0.3% result in hospitalization.

PATHOPHYSIOLOGY

The gastrointestinal (GI) tract is remarkably efficient at fluid reabsorption. Normally, of the 1 to 2 L of fluid ingested orally and the 7 L that enter the upper tract from saliva, gastric, pancreatic, and biliary sources, less than 200 mL of fluid are excreted daily in the feces. Thus, small increases in secretory rate or decreases in the absorptive rate can easily overwhelm the colonic absorptive capacity of about 4 L/day—leading to diarrhea, defined as increased frequency (more than three bowel movements) or increased volume (>200 mL/day).

Intestinal infection with bacteria, viruses, and parasites that produce gastroenteritis usually follows fecal–oral transmission. Host defenses, which protect the human intestine, are reviewed in Table 48.1. The principal defenses include gastric acidity and the physical barrier of the mucosa. A gastric pH below 4 will kill more than 99% of ingested organisms, although rotavirus and protozoal cysts can survive. Patients with achlorhydria from gastric surgery, human immunodeficiency virus (HIV) infection, chronic atrophic gastritis, or use of proton pump inhibitors (PPIs) are at increased risk of developing infectious diarrhea. Disruption of the mucosal barrier, as with mucositis associated with chemotherapy or irradiation, predisposes patients to gram-negative sepsis. Increased peristalsis in gastroenteritis propels organisms along the GI tract, analogous to the cough reflex with clearing of the lungs. The intestinal flora forms an important element of the host defense, both in terms of quantity and composition. The small intestine and colon contain approximately 10^4 and 10^{11} organisms/g, respectively. More than 99% of the colonic bacteria are anaerobes. Their production of fatty acids with an acidic pH and their competition for mucosal attachment sites prevent colonization by invading organisms. At the extremes of age, in children and the elderly, and after recent antibiotic use, the flora are altered and the risk for gastroenteritis increased. Impairment of intestinal immunity is also a risk factor for intestinal infections.

Virulence factors play a complementary role in acute infectious diarrhea. Whether an individual ingests an inoculum sufficient to establish clinical gastroenteritis is directly related to community sanitation and personal hygiene. Most organisms require an inoculum of 10^5 to 10^8 to establish infection. Exceptions include *Shigella* and protozoa such as *Giardia, Cryptosporidium*, and *Entamoeba*, which may cause diarrhea when only 10 to 100 organisms are ingested. Bacteria produce several types of toxins, which lead to different clinical syndromes, including enterotoxin (watery diarrhea), cytotoxin (dysentery), and neurotoxin. Botulinum toxin is the classic example of a

Table 48.1 Host Defenses

Host Defense Factor	Example Disease State
Barrier	
Gastric acid	Achlorhydria (PPI, HIV, gastric surgery)
Mucosal integrity	Mucositis (chemotherapy)
Intestinal motility	
Peristalsis	Blind loop, antimotility drugs, hypomotility states (diabetes, scleroderma)
Commensal microflora	Antibiotics, age extremes
Sanitation	Contaminated water
Intestinal immunity	
Phagocytic	Neutropenia
Cellular	HIV
Humoral	IgA deficiency

Abbreviations: PPI = Proton pump inhibitor; HIV = human immunodeficiency virus; IgA = immunoglobulin A.

Table 48.2 Virulence Factors

Virulence Factors	Examples
Inoculum size	*Shigella, Entamoeba, Giardia*
Adherence	Cholera, EPEC
Invasion	*Shigella, Salmonella typhi, Yersinia,* EIEC
Toxins	
Enterotoxin	Cholera, *Salmonella,* ETEC
Cytotoxin	*Shigella, Clostridium difficile,* EHEC
Neurotoxin	*Clostridium botulinum, Staphylococcus aureus, Bacillus cereus*

Abbreviations: EPEC = enteropathogenic *Escherichia coli*; EIEC = enteroinvasive *E. coli*; ETEC = enterotoxigenic *E. coli*; EHEC = enterohemorrhagic *E. coli*.

preformed neurotoxin, but interestingly, both *Staphylococcus aureus* and *Bacillus cereus* also produce neurotoxins that act on the central nervous system to produce emesis. Adherence and invasion factors facilitate colonization and contribute to virulence. Various forms of *Escherichia coli* express the gamut of virulence factors (Table 48.2).

CLINICAL SYNDROMES

The acute infectious diarrheas can be divided into noninflammatory, inflammatory, and invasive (Table 48.3). Although most attacks are noninflammatory and caused by viruses, more severe attacks are often bacterial. The bacteria causing a noninflammatory diarrhea, such as *Vibrio cholerae* and enterotoxigenic *E. coli* (ETEC), typically secrete an enterotoxin that affects the small intestine, producing a large volume of watery diarrhea without fecal leukocytes. Most forms of viral gastroenteritis (eg, *Rotavirus* and *Norovirus* [Norwalk agent]) also fall into this group. The inflammatory diarrheas typically infect the colon, causing frequent small-volume stools, often with fecal white cells and either gross or occult blood. Fever, tenesmus, and bloody diarrhea are characteristic of dysentery. Some bacteria that cause inflammatory diarrhea produce cytotoxins. The invasive diarrheas may be considered a subset of the inflammatory

diarrheas because there is invasion of the intestinal mucosa, and with a propensity to cause bacteremia and distant disease. *Salmonella typhi* is the prototype. Typhoid bacteria invade the Peyer's patches of the distal ileum then disseminate and multiply in the reticuloendothelial system to produce systemic disease.

Patients with an absolute neutrophil count ≤500/μL secondary to immunodeficiency or cytotoxic drugs, particularly during treatment of malignancies or stem cell transplantation, may develop neutropenic enterocolitis or typhlitis (from *typhlon*, the Greek term for cecum). In these patients, cytotoxic mucosal injury and neutropenia decrease host defenses allowing various microorganisms to invade, producing fever, abdominal pain (often in the right lower quadrant), watery or bloody diarrhea, and thickening of the bowel wall on computed tomography (CT) imaging.

Certain subpopulations of patients with gastroenteritis merit surveillance because of the organisms involved, the potential for severe disease, and the possible need for intervention. These are listed in Table 48.4. Foodborne disease should be considered in outbreaks of acute GI symptoms affecting two or more persons. The most common causes include *Salmonella* species, *S. aureus, Shigella* species, *B. cereus,* and *Clostridium perfringens.* Patients with the acquired immunodeficiency syndrome (AIDS) are predisposed to a number of unique infections (microsporidia, cytomegalovirus) or more severe manifestations of otherwise common infections (*Salmonella, Campylobacter,*

Table 48.3 Clinical Syndromes

	Noninflammatory	Inflammatory	Invasive
Syndrome	Watery diarrhea, emesis	Dysentery	Enteric fever
Site	Small intestine	Colon	Ileum, colon
Stool			
Volume	Large	Small	Small
Fecal WBCs	Absent	Present	Present
Common Organisms			
Bacteria	*Vibrio cholerae* ETEC	*Shigella* spp. *Salmonella* spp. *Campylobacter jejuni*	*Salmonella typhi* *Yersinia* spp. *Brucella*
Viruses	Rotavirus Norovirus[a] Adenovirus Astrovirus	—	—
Parasites	*Giardia* *Cryptosporidium*	*Entamoeba*	*Entamoeba*

Abbreviations: WBC = white blood cell; ETEC = enterotoxigenic *E. coli;*
EIEC = enteroinvasive *E. coli.*
[a] Formerly known as the Norwalk agent or calicivirus.

Cryptosporidium). The microbial pathogens responsible for traveler's diarrhea are dependent on the region visited. Enterotoxigenic *E. coli* is the most commonly isolated organism, ranging between 20% and 60% of isolates in areas of Asia and Latin America, respectively. Acute infectious proctitis, which is often sexually transmitted, leads to tenesmus, hematochezia, and rectal pain. Syphilis, gonorrhea, and chlamydia are additional organisms to consider. The incidence of sexually transmitted proctitis is decreasing in the AIDS era with safer sex practices. Other important subpopulations include patients with antibiotic-associated diarrhea, especially those from hospitals or chronic care facilities.

Gastroenteritis is a major cause of global mortality and morbidity among infants and children. In developed countries, acute diarrheal illnesses account for 7% of pediatric ambulatory visits as well as hospitalizations. Peak attack rates involve young schoolchildren and their younger siblings. Most cases are caused by viral agents: rotaviruses (10% to 50%), *Norovirus* (Norwalk agent, 10% to 30%), and the enteric adenoviruses (2% to 5%). Bacterial agents cause less than 15% of disease

but may cause severe disease in patients with *Campylobacter* species, *E. coli* species, *Salmonella* species, or *Yersinia* species. EHEC O157:H7 is an important cause of hemolytic–uremic syndrome in children. *Yersinia* causes a watery diarrhea in children ages 1 to 5, but it may mimic appendicitis in older children and adolescents. Important pathogens in day-care and institutional settings are the above-mentioned bacterial species, as well as *Giardia lamblia*, *Cryptosporidium* species, and *Clostridium difficile*.

Helicobacter pylori infection is a form of GI infection localized to the stomach. This gram-negative spiral bacterium is the principal cause of chronic gastritis, atrophic gastritis, and peptic ulcer disease. Based on epidemiologic data, it is also a major etiologic factor in the development of gastric adenocarcinoma and low-grade, mucosa-associated lymphoid tissue (MALT) lymphoma. It is likely acquired in childhood via gastro-oral transmission, and the prevalence within a population is directly related to the socioeconomic status of the cohort in childhood. Nearly 60% of the world's population is chronically infected; in the United States, 30% to 40% of adults and 5% to 10% of adolescents are infected. More

Table 48.4 Etiologic Agents by Clinical Presentation

Population	Bacteria	Viruses	Parasites	Other
Food poisoning	Salmonella	Norwalk	Trichinella	Ciguatera
	Staphylococcus aureus	Hepatitis A	Giardia	Histamine fish
	Shigella		Cryptosporidium	
	Clostridium perfringens			
	Bacillus cereus			
	Listeria			
AIDS	Salmonella	CMV	Cryptosporidium	AIDS
	Campylobacter		Isospora belli	enteropathy
	Shigella		Microsporidia	
	MAC			
Traveler's diarrhea	Escherichia coli ETEC	Rotavirus	Giardia	No pathogen (40%)
	Shigella		Cyclospora	
	Aeromonas			
	E. coli, other			
Acute proctitis	Gonorrhea	HSV	Entamoeba	
	Chlamydia	Condyloma, HPV	Cryptosporidium	
	Treponema pallidum	CMV		
	Shigella			
	Salmonella			
Day-care centers	Shigella	Rotavirus	Giardia	
	Campylobacter jejuni		Cryptosporidium	
Antibiotic associated	Clostridium difficile			Candida albicans
Seafood ingestion	Vibrio spp.		Anisakidae	

Abbreviations: AIDS = acquired immunodeficiency virus; CMV = cytomegalovirus; MAC = *Mycobacterium avium* complex; ETEC = enterotoxigenic *E. coli;* HSV = herpes simplex virus; HPV = human papilloma virus.

than 50% of peptic ulcers are caused by *H. pylori,* and there is substantial prospective evidence that eradication of the organism significantly decreases the recurrence risk. Studies to date fail to demonstrate a strong association between *H. pylori* and functional dyspepsia or that its eradication in this setting relieves symptoms. Diagnostic tests include serology enzyme-linked immunosorbent assay (ELISA), urea breath test, stool antigen exam, and gastric biopsy (rapid urease tests, histology).

PATIENT EVALUATION

Most cases of acute gastroenteritis are self-limited and do not require medical attention. Physician consultation generally is advised for patients with a fever (>38.5°C [101.3°F]), dysentery (bloody stools), significant abdominal pain, dehydration, and risk factors for disease requiring intervention. Initial evaluation consists of the history, physical examination, and screening stool examination. Laboratory testing and antimicrobial therapy are recommended in a limited subset of patients based on this initial evaluation.

The history should focus on the severity of disease and the risk factors for specific types of infectious diarrhea. The patient should be questioned regarding symptom duration, fever, abdominal pain, tenesmus, and dehydration. The description of the diarrhea is important: frequency, volume, and any blood, pus, or mucus. Diarrhea persisting longer than 2 to

4 weeks qualifies as chronic, has an alternate differential, and should be fully investigated. Inquiry should also be made into factors that may place the patient in a specific subpopulation at increased risk for significant infection. Examples include age over 70, recent international travel or camping, recent antibiotic use, HIV disease or risk factors, other immunosuppression (including prednisone therapy), anal eroticism, seafood consumption, household contacts of day-care workers or children, and the potential for a common source outbreak (eg, friends or relatives with similar symptoms). Short incubation periods of fewer than 6 hours, or 6 to 16 hours, suggest ingestion of an enterotoxin produced by *S. aureus* and *B. cereus* or *C. perfringens,* respectively. A viral infection or food poisoning is suggested when vomiting is the dominant complaint.

A broad differential diagnosis is considered initially because acute diarrhea may be the initial presentation of noninfectious and potentially life-threatening diseases. Important diagnoses to consider include inflammatory bowel disease, mesenteric vascular disease, bowel obstruction, and GI hemorrhage. Patients should be questioned regarding medications that may cause diarrhea, such as metformin, colchicine, diuretics, angiotensin-converting enzyme (ACE) inhibitors, PPIs, and magnesium-containing antacids.

The physical examination is important to gauge the severity of the disease. Orthostasis, tachycardia, decreased skin turgor, and dry mucous membranes are signs of significant dehydration. The presence of fever, abdominal tenderness, and skin rash should be documented. All patients should undergo a rectal examination when rectal bleeding is suggested.

The majority of patients who present for medical evaluation warrant a screening stool examination. A fresh-cup specimen is preferred because there is evidence that swab and diaper specimens have decreased sensitivity. The stool should be evaluated for fecal leukocytes and fecal occult blood. Fecal leukocytes are detected in the clinical laboratory either with staining techniques or lactoferrin testing. In the office or at the bedside, microscopic examination of the stool is facilitated by the methylene blue stain. A wet mount is prepared with two drops of methylene blue mixed with fecal mucus; 2 minutes should be allowed for adequate staining of the leukocyte nuclei before high-power microscopy of the cover-slipped slide. The presence of three or more fecal leukocytes per high-powered field in at least 4 fields is

Table 48.5 Fecal Leukocytes

Present	Variable	Absent
Campylobacter	*Salmonella*	Toxigenic bacteria
Shigella	*Yersinia*	ETEC, EPEC
EIEC, EHEC	*Clostridium difficile*	Viruses
	Vibrio parahemolyticus	Parasites
	Noninfectious causes Ischemic colitis IBD	

Abbreviations: EIEC = Enteroinvasive *E. coli*; EHEC = enterohemorrhagic *E. coli*; IBD = inflammatory bowel disease; ETEC = enterotoxigenic *E. coli*; EPEC = enteropathogenic *E. coli*.

considered a positive examination. The fecal lactoferrin latex agglutination assay may be a more precise marker of fecal leukocytes. Table 48.5 lists the degree of association of the usual enteric pathogens with fecal leukocytes. With fecal leukocytes, there is some overlap between the inflammatory and noninflammatory diarrheas. The finding on screening stool examination of fecal leukocytes, lactoferrin, or occult blood have equal predictive values for diffuse colonic disease, positive stool cultures, and disease requiring antimicrobial therapy. The organisms most commonly associated with a positive screening test include *Salmonella, Shigella, Campylobacter, Yersinia, Aeromonas, Vibrio,* and *C. difficile.*

The history, physical examination, and office stool evaluation serve as screening steps before further laboratory evaluation and possible need for treatment. As noted, most patients have self-limited noninflammatory infectious diarrhea and require only symptomatic therapy. Laboratory evaluation is indicated as follows: patients with severe or persistent disease (fever greater than 38.5°C [101.3°F], dehydration, grossly bloody stools, duration of more than 1 week), patients from the aforementioned subpopulations, and patients with positive stool screening examinations (fecal leukocytes or occult blood). The initial laboratory evaluation should include a complete blood count, serum electrolytes, and stool processed for bacterial culture. Stool cultures will identify *Salmonella, Shigella,* and *Campylobacter* and, in some labs, *Yersinia and Aeromonas.* Many stool cultures are ordered inappropriately. The probability of a positive culture is less than 2% to 5% for patients without fever, occult blood, or fecal leukocytes. The yield increases to approximately 20% and 50%, respectively, when 1 or 2 of the 3 findings are present. Formed stools should not be sent for testing. Patients hospitalized for more than 3 days who subsequently develop diarrhea are unlikely to have a bacterial or parasitic pathogen, and stool cultures are inappropriate.

Additional laboratory or diagnostic evaluation depends on the clinical situation. Routine stool examination for ova and parasites are not recommended. Studies for parasites are indicated in the setting of persistent diarrhea, international or wilderness travel, AIDS, and infants attending a day-care center (or persons exposed to such infants). In addition, fecal leukocyte-negative, bloody diarrhea is associated with *Entamoeba histolytica*, *Schistosoma*, *Dientamoeba fragilis*, and *Balantidium coli*. The sensitivity of 3 ova and parasite examinations on 3 separate days is 95% to 98%. Stool testing for *C. difficile* cytotoxin, previously reserved for those with a history of antibiotic use or hospitalization, is now broadened with advent of community-acquired infection. Differentiation of pathogenic and nonpathogenic strains of *E. coli* requires serotyping in specialized laboratories and is not generally indicated, except in an outbreak situation in which *E. coli* O157: H7 may be involved. Commercial Enzyme Immuroassay kits are available for detection of rotavirus and enteric adenovirus and may be useful in the pediatric population and in elderly patients who have lost their acquired immunity. Sigmoidoscopy with biopsy should be considered for cases of acute proctitis, dysentery, and persistent infectious diarrhea. Endoscopy (colonoscopy/ileoscopy, capsule endoscopy) or abdominal imaging (CT scan, small-bowel-follow-through) may be helpful in complex presentations to help differentiate infectious and noninfectious causes of acute diarrhea.

The initial evaluation of AIDS-associated diarrhea should include stool examination for culture, ova and parasites, and acid-fast stain. Specialized stool studies are required for the detection of *Cryptosporidium, Cyclospora*, microsporidiosis, and *Isospora belli*. Mucosal biopsies are required for the diagnosis of cytomegalovirus and *Mycobacterium avium-intracellulare* complex (MAC). Sigmoidoscopy may be considered for persistent or severe cases in patients with CD4 counts of less than 100 or those who have experienced weight loss. Colonoscopy/ileoscopy and upper endoscopy generally are reserved for refractory cases.

MANAGEMENT

Rehydration is the focus of initial management. This can be accomplished with oral fluids. Oral rehydration solutions (ORS) have decreased worldwide cholera mortality rates from 50% to 1%. The World Health Organization (WHO) ORS is made up of 3.5 g of sodium chloride, 2.5 g of sodium bicarbonate, 1.5 g of potassium chloride, and 20 g of glucose/L water. Rice-based ORS also may be used. Prepared forms are available in solution (eg, Pedialyte, Rehydrolyte) and packets (eg, Orlyte). Various homemade recipes exist. One example includes alternating a glass of fruit juice (8 oz) with honey (½ tsp) and salt (¼ tsp), with a second glass of water (8 oz) with baking soda (¼ tsp). Sport drinks such as Gatorade are reasonable for nondehydrated adults. The goal is the passage of relatively dilute urine every 2 to 4 hours. Patients are advised to eat judiciously until stools are again formed. Cereals (rice, pasta), boiled foods (potatoes, vegetables), bananas, and crackers are recommended initial foods. Alcohol (cathartic effect), caffeine (increases intestinal motility), and carbonated drinks (gastric distension with reflex colonic contraction) should be avoided. Recommendations vary regarding dairy products, as transient lactose intolerance may occur.

In addition to rehydration, symptomatic therapy includes administering agents to control the diarrhea. These agents include bulking agents, antimotility drugs, and antisecretory medications. They are outlined in Tables 48.6 and 48.7. Antimotility agents should not be used if there is a possibility of a severe inflammatory bacterial diarrhea, particularly a febrile dysentery syndrome. Loperamide (Imodium) is the drug of choice in most situations because of its efficacy and safety. Bismuth subsalicylate (BSS) has antisecretory and antibacterial properties and is the drug of choice when vomiting is a significant part of the patient's presentation. It should not be used in the immunosuppressed patient, particularly the HIV population, because bismuth encephalopathy may occur. Diphenoxylate-atropine (Lomotil), which has both antimotility and antisecretory activity, may cause central nervous system depression, especially in children. Despite their popularity, kaopectate, cholestyramine, lactobacilli, and the anticholinergics have not been shown to be consistently effective. Severe AIDS diarrhea should be treated in stepwise fashion with Imodium (2 to 4 mg orally 4 times daily), lomotil (1 to 2 tablets orally 4 times daily), morphine (MS Contin 30 mg twice daily) or tincture of

Table 48.6 Symptomatic Therapy for Diarrhea

General	Intraluminal	Antimotility	Antisecretory
Rehydration	Bulking agents	Opiates	BSS
ORS	Psyllium	Loperamide	Octreotide
IV	Adsorbents	Diphenoxylate	
Diet therapy	Kaolin-pectin	Codeine	
	Attapulgite	Tincture of opium	
	Cholestyramine	Anticholinergics	
	Bacterial agents	Atropine	
	Lactobacilli	Scopolamine	
	Saccaromyces		

Abbreviations: ORS = oral rehydration solution; IV = intravenous; BSS = bismuth subsalicylate.

Table 48.7 Antidiarrheal Therapy

Agent	Dosing	Comments
Loperamide[a] (Imodium)	2 mg PO q3h	Initial dose, 4 mg Maximum, 16 mg/day
Diphenoxylate (Lomotil)	2 tablets or 10 mL PO QID	Maximum, 8 tablets/day
BSS[b] (Pepto-Bismol)	2 tablets or 30 mL PO QID	Maximum, 8 tablets/day
Tincture of opium	0.5–1.0 mL PO q4–6h	
Octreotide	100–500 µg SC TID	

Abbreviations: BSS = bismuth subsalicylate; SC = subcutaneously.
[a] Loperamide is the drug of choice. BSS may be used in presentations with significant vomiting.
[b] BSS should not be used in patients with human immunodeficiency virus because of the risk of bismuth encephalopathy.

opium (DTO 0.5 to 1 mL orally 4 times daily), and octreotide (100 to 500 µg subcutaneously (SC) 3 times daily, increasing the dosage 200 µg every 3 days until response is seen).

Antibiotic therapy is indicated in a limited subset of patients with acute infectious diarrhea, as outlined in Table 48.8. Empiric therapy with a quinolone (norfloxacin, ciprofloxacin, levofloxacin) pending stool studies is recommended for severe traveler's diarrhea, for patients with fever, and for patients with a positive stool-screening study (leukocytes or blood). Macrolides (eg, azithromycin) may be used when drug allergies or quinolone resistance are factors. Patients with a positive stool culture or parasite examination should be treated in specified situations. Standard indications include symptomatic infections with certain bacteria (*Shigella*, enteroinvasive *E. coli*, *C. difficile*, *V. cholerae*), sexually transmitted pathogens, and parasites. Therapy is reserved for specific situations for *Salmonella, Campylobacter, Yersinia, Aeromonas,* noncholera *Vibrio,* and other strains of *E. coli* (enteropathogenic *E. coli* (EPAC) enteroaggregative *E. coli* (EAEC)). Treatment of *Salmonella* and *Campylobacter* is indicated for patients with dysentery, systemic illness, bacteremia, or significant comorbidity (immunosuppression, malignancy, sickle cell anemia, prosthetic device, age extremes). Although controversial because of the possible association with the hemolytic-uremic syndrome, antimicrobial therapy is not recommended for enterohemorrhagic *E. coli,* including *E. coli* O157:

Table 48.8 Antibiotic Therapy by Etiologic Agent

Etiologic Agent	Therapy	Duration	Comments
Bacteria			
Empiric therapy[a]	Quinolone[b]	5–7 days	Indications: Fever and positive stool screen[c] Dysentery syndrome Traveler's diarrhea, severe
Campylobacter	Erythromycin, 500 mg PO QID Quinolone[b] Azithromycin, 500 mg PO qd	5 days	See text for treatment indication.
Clostridium difficile[a]	Metronidazole, 250 mg PO QID Vancomycin, 125 mg PO QID	7–10 days	Metronidazole is the drug of choice given VRE risk.
EIEC, ETEC[a]	Quinolone[b] TMP-SMX-DS PO BID	5 days	Treatment is not indicated for EHEC, including O157:H7.
EPEC	Quinolone[b]	5 days	
Salmonella	Quinolone[b] TMP-SMX-DS PO BID Chloramphenicol, 500 mg PO QID	3–7 days	See text for treatment indication.
Shigella[a]	Quinolone[b] TMP-SMX-DS PO BID Azithromycin, 250–500 mg PO qd	3–5 days	
Vibrio cholerae[a]	Doxycycline, 300 mg PO Ciprofloxacin, 1 g PO	1 dose	
Yersinia	Ceftriaxone, 2 g IV qd Quinolone[b]	5 days	For severe infection
Parasites			
Cyclospora	TMP-SMX-DS PO BID	7 days	
Entamoeba[a]	Metronidazole, 750 mg PO TID	10 days	Follow with cyst-eradication regimen.
Giardia[a]	Metronidazole, 250 mg PO TID	5 days	
Isospora	TMP-SMX-DS PO BID	7 days	

Abbreviations: VRE = vancomycin-resistant enterococcus; EIEC = enteroinvasive *E. coli;* ETEC = enterotoxigenic *E. coli;* TMP-SMX-DS = trimethoprim-sulfamethoxazole, 160–800 mg double-strength tablet; EHEC = enterohemorrhagic *E. coli;* EPEC = enteropathogenic *coli.*
[a] Treatment clearly indicated. Treatment for the other listed microbes will depend on the clinical situation.
[b] Quinolone oral therapy options include: ciprofloxacin 500 mg BID, ofloxacin 300 mg BID, levofloxacin 250 mg qd.
[c] Positive stool screen: fecal leukocytes or hemoccult positive.

H7. Metronidazole is the drug of choice for *C. difficile* colitis, given the risk of vancomycin-resistant enterococcus. Three standard regimens have evolved for *H. pylori* eradication: PAC (PPI, amoxicillin, clarithromycin), PMC (PPI, metronidazole, clarithromycin), and PBMT (PPI, bismuth, metronidazole, tetracycline). PAC is the usual first line therapy, with PBMT used for retreatment.

In summary, acute gastroenteritis, although common, is usually a self-limited disease. Oral rehydration and symptomatic therapy are appropriate for most patients. Medical evaluation is advised for patients with significant fever, dysentery, abdominal pain, dehydration, or risk factors for disease requiring intervention. Laboratory evaluation and antibiotic treatment should be limited to specific situations.

SUGGESTED READING

Centers for Disease Control and Prevention (CDC). Severe Clostridium difficile-associated disease in populations previously at low risk: four states, 2005. *Morb Mortal Wkly Rep.* 2005; 54:1201–1205.

DuPont HL. Practice guidelines on acute infectious diarrhea. *Am J Gastroenterol.* 1997;92: 1962–1975.

Guerrant RL, Van Gilder T, Steiner TS, et.al. Practice guidelines for the management of infectious diarrhea. *Clin Infect Dis.* 2001; 32:331–351.

Hines J, Nachamkin I. Effective use of the clinical microbiology laboratory for diagnosing diarrheal diseases. *Clin Infect Dis.* 1996;23:1292.

Musher DM, Musher BL. Contagious acute gastrointestinal infections. *N Engl J Med.* 2004;351:2417–2427.

Shaheen NS, Hansen R, Morgan DR, et al. The burden of gastrointestinal and liver diseases, 2006. *Am J Gastroenterol.* 2006;101:2128–2138.

Thielman NM, Guerrant RL. Acute infectious diarrhea. *N Engl J Med.* 2004;350:38–47.

49. Food Poisoning

Andrew T. Pavia

Foodborne illnesses are caused by ingestion of foods containing microbial and chemical toxins or pathogenic microorganisms. This chapter concentrates on toxin-mediated syndromes, usually called *food poisoning,* rather than on syndromes reflecting enteric infection, such as salmonellosis, shigellosis, vibriosis, and *Escherichia coli* O157:H7 infection. Treatment of these infections is covered in Chapter 48, Gastroenteritis, and in chapters on the specific organisms.

CLINICAL PRESENTATION AND DIAGNOSIS

Initially, the diagnosis of specific food poisoning syndromes is suggested by the clinical presentation, the incubation period from exposure to onset of symptoms, and the food consumed. The incubation periods, symptoms, and commonly associated foods for specific syndromes are shown in Table 49.1. Incubation periods range from a few hours or less in the case of preformed chemical and bacterial toxins, such as histamine poisoning (scombroid), staphylococcal food poisoning, and *Bacillus cereus,* to several days for bacterial infections (eg, *Campylobacter jejuni, Salmonella, Yersinia enterocolitica,* and *E. coli* O157:H7 or other enterohemorrhagic *E. coli*) and some types of mushroom poisoning. Therefore it is essential to obtain a diet history covering 3 to 4 days before the onset of symptoms. A careful history of illness in meal companions may help point to the responsible food. It is clinically useful to consider syndromes grouped by incubation period and symptoms.

Nausea and Vomiting within 1 Hour

Symptoms developing within 5 to 15 minutes of exposure that resolve over 1 to 2 hours are typical of contamination of food or drink with heavy metals or other nonspecific chemical irritants.

Nausea, Vomiting, or Diarrhea within 1 to 16 Hours

When gastrointestinal symptoms develop 1 to 16 hours after exposure, the likely agents include *Staphylococcus aureus, B. cereus,* and *Clostridium perfringens.* Vomiting is the dominant feature

of *S. aureus* and short-incubation, or emetic, *B. cereus* food poisoning. These syndromes result from preformed centrally acting toxins elaborated by the organisms in food when the food is mishandled. In contrast, abdominal cramps and diarrhea are most prominent in long-incubation, or diarrheal, *B. cereus* poisoning and *C. perfringens* food poisoning. In these syndromes, toxins are also elaborated in the small intestine. The duration of illness is usually less than 24 hours. Diagnosis of these syndromes is usually made on epidemiologic and clinical grounds. Laboratory confirmation of *S. aureus* food poisoning is based on isolation of *S. aureus* from food handlers and demonstration of more than 10^5 colonies per gram of the same strain in food or enterotoxin production. Laboratory confirmation of *B. cereus* and *C. perfringens* can be performed in epidemiologic investigations; it requires collection of food and stool for quantitative cultures.

Watery Diarrhea and Cramps within 16 to 48 Hours

Diarrhea following a slightly longer incubation period is typical of viral foodborne illness, particularly Norovirus (Norwalk virus), and enterotoxin-producing bacteria, including enterotoxigenic *E. coli* (ETEC), *Vibrio cholerae* O1 and non-O1, and other *Vibrio* species. Most microbiology laboratories can diagnose *Vibrio* infections from stool culture provided the laboratory is aware that *Vibrio* is being considered. Diagnosis of ETEC infection requires detection of enterotoxin production by *E. coli* isolates and is limited to reference laboratories. Antigen detection–based enzyme immunoassays using recombinant antigens have been developed for the diagnosis of Norwalk and other gastroenteritis-causing viruses; these are limited to research laboratories but may soon become commercially available.

Fever, Diarrhea, and Abdominal Cramps within 16 to 96 Hours

Bacterial infections of the gastrointestinal tract and gut-associated lymphatics with *Salmonella,*

Table 49.1 Incubation Period, Symptoms, and Common Vehicles for Microbial Causes of Food Poisoning

Organism	Incubation Period (Hours) Median (Range)	Vomiting	Diarrhea	Fever	Common Vehicles
Staphylococcus aureus	3 (1–6)	+++	++	0	Ham, poultry, cream-filled pastries, potato and egg salad
Bacillus cereus (emetic syndrome)	2 (1–6)	+++	++	0	Fried rice
Bacillus cereus (diarrheal syndrome)	9 (6–16)	+	+++	0	Beef, pork, chicken, vanilla sauce
Clostridium perfringens	12 (6–24)	+	+++	0	Beef, poultry, gravy
Vibrio parahemolyticus	15 (4–96)	++	+++	++	Fish, shellfish
Vibrio cholerae O1 and non-O1	24 (12–120)	++	+++	+	Shellfish
Norovirus	24 (12–48)	+++	++	++	Shellfish, salads, ice
Shigella	24 (7–168)	+	+++	+++	Egg salads, lettuce, sandwiches
Clostridium botulinum	24 (12–168)	++	+	0	Canned vegetables, fruits, sauces and fish; salted fish; bottled garlic, baked potatoes
Salmonella	36 (12–72)	+	+++	++	Beef, poultry, pork, eggs, dairy products, fruit and vegetables, sprouts
Campylobacter jejuni	48 (24–168)	+	+++	+++	Poultry, raw milk
Entereohemorrhagic Escherichia coli (eg, O157:H7)	96 (48–120)	++	+++	+	Beef (especially hamburger), raw milk, salad dressings, lettuce, sprouts, apple cider
Yersinia enterocolitica	96 (48–240)	+	+++	+++	Pork, chitterlings, tofu, milk
Cyclospora cayatensis	168 (24–336)	+	+++	++	Raspberries, basil, lettuce

Key: 0 = Rare (≤10%); + = infrequent (11%–33%); ++ = frequent (33%–66%); +++ = classic (>67%).

Shigella, C. jejuni, Y. enterocolitica, and enterohemorrhagic *E. coli* (EHEC) typically follow a longer incubation period and are marked by more prominent signs of colonic inflammation or systemic illness. Diarrhea that becomes bloody after 12 to 36 hours is typical of *E. coli* O157:H7 and other EHEC. These organisms are now among the most common causes of bacterial gastroenteritis in North America (see Chapter 48, Gastroenteritis).

Diarrhea, Fatigue, and Weight Loss within 1 to 14 Days

Cyclospora infection should be suspected in a patient with diarrhea of several days' duration associated with loss of appetite and weight and prominent fatigue. The incubation period is highly variable, ranging from 1 to 14 days, with a median of 7 days. Recent outbreaks have definitively shown that *Cyclospora* infections in developed countries can result from consumption of contaminated foods, notably fresh raspberries, mesclun lettuce, and basil.

Paresthesias within 6 Hours

Chemical food poisoning caused by niacin, Chinese restaurant syndrome (monosodium glutamate), histamine fish poisoning, ciguatera poisoning, and neurotoxic and paralytic shellfish poisoning present with paresthesias and other symptoms after a brief incubation period. Chinese restaurant syndrome is characterized by a burning sensation in the neck, chest, and abdomen with chest tightness and occasionally facial flushing, headache, nausea, and abdominal cramps.

The features of fish and shellfish poisoning are summarized in Table 49.2. Histamine fish poisoning (scombroid) is caused by bacterial decarboxylation of histidine in fish that are inadequately refrigerated, resulting in production of large amounts of histamine. Signs and symptoms are facial flushing, headache, nausea, and, less commonly, urticaria or diarrhea. The fish is often reported to have a peppery or bitter taste. Demonstration of high levels of histamine in the implicated fish confirms the diagnosis.

Ciguatera fish poisoning results from ingestion of fish containing toxins produced by the dinoflagellate *Gambierdiscus toxicus*. Predatory fish such as grouper, amberjack, snapper, and barracuda are usually implicated. The symptoms, which are quite distinctive, usually involve the combination of gastrointestinal and neurologic symptoms, most commonly perioral and distal extremity paresthesias, and reversal of hot and cold sensation. Other symptoms include sensation of loose teeth, arthralgias, headaches, muscle weakness, pruritus, lancinating pains, and hallucinations. Bradycardia, hypotension, and respiratory paralysis may occur. The symptoms may last from a few days to 6 months. The diagnosis is based on the clinical picture; detection of ciguatoxin in the fish by high-performance lipid chromatography (HPLC), radioimmunoassay (RIA) or enzyme linked immunoassay (EIA), or bioassay is confirmatory.

Paralytic shellfish poisoning (PSP) and neurotoxic shellfish poisoning (NSP) are closely related syndromes caused by heat-stable neurotoxins produced by dinoflagellates (*Gonyaulax catonella* and *Gonyaulax tamarensis* cause PSP; *Gymnodinium breve* causes NSP). During periodic blooms of the dinoflagellates, which may cause red tides, shellfish concentrate the heat-stable toxins. PSP is more severe and occurs in colder waters. Patients develop symptoms a median of 30 minutes after exposure. Symptoms consist of paresthesias and dysesthesias, beginning with the lips, mouth, and face and progressing to the extremities, and then dysphonia, dysphagia, ataxia, muscle weakness, and, in severe cases, respiratory paralysis occur. NSP occurs primarily near warmer waters and is characterized by similar paresthesias, reversal of hot and cold sensation, nausea, vomiting, and ataxia. Toxin

can be detected in samples of the shellfish by bioassay. Anamnestic shellfish poisoning is a recently described syndrome associated with mussels contaminated with domoic acid elaborated by *Nitzchia pungens*. In some patients, gastrointestinal symptoms are followed by memory loss, coma, cardiac arrhythmias, and death. Haff disease is a syndrome of acute rhabdomyolysis that is caused by an unidentified toxin in certain bottom-feeding fish, notably buffalo fish and burbot. Patients present 6 to 21 hours after ingestion with vomiting, severe myalgia, and stiffness. Elevated creatine phosphokinase (CPK) and other muscle enzyme levels confirm the diagnosis.

Nausea, Vomiting, Diarrhea, and Paralysis within 18 to 36 Hours

Foodborne botulism results from exposure to one of three distinct botulinum toxins, A, B, and E, produced when *Clostridium botulinum* spores germinate in food in an anaerobic environment. Gastrointestinal symptoms occur before the onset of neurologic symptoms in about 50% of patients with acute foodborne botulism. Descending paralysis begins with cranial nerve weakness manifested as dysphonia, dysphagia, diplopia, and blurred vision, followed by muscle weakness and respiratory insufficiency. Larger doses of toxin result in shorter incubation periods and more severe symptoms. Botulism can be differentiated from acute myasthenia gravis and Guillain–Barré syndrome (which may follow *C. jejuni* infection) by botulism's normal cerebrospinal fluid protein, the descending nature of the paralysis, absence of sensory symptoms, normal nerve conduction studies, and typical electromyographic findings of increase in the action potential with rapid repetitive stimulation. Confirmation is based on detection of toxin in food or in serum or stool of patients by mouse toxicity assay or of *C. botulinum* spores in the stool by selective culture.

Mushroom Poisoning Syndromes

Syndromes of food poisoning from mushrooms fall into eight major categories, outlined in Table 49.3. Parasympathetic syndromes, delirium, disulfiram (Antabuse)-like symptoms, hallucinations, or gastroenteritis may occur after a short incubation period. The more serious syndromes of monomethylhydrazine poisoning, hepatorenal failure from amatoxin-containing mushrooms, and

Table 49.2 Clinical Features of Fish and Shellfish Poisoning

Syndrome	Incubation Period	Symptoms	Vehicles	Duration
Histamine (scombroid)	5 min–1 h	Facial flushing, headache, nausea, cramps, diarrhea, urticaria	Tuna, mackerel, bonito, mahi-mahi, bluefish	Hours
Ciguatera	1–6 h	Diarrhea, nausea, vomiting, myalgia, arthralgia, shooting pains, perioral and extremity paresthesias, hot-cold reversal, fatigue	Barracuda, snapper, grouper, amberjack	Days to months
Neurotoxic shellfish poisoning	5 min–4 h	Paresthesias, nausea, vomiting, ataxia	Shellfish	Hours to days
Paralytic shellfish poisoning	5 min–4 h	Paresthesias, cranial nerve weakness, ataxia, muscle weakness, respiratory paralysis	Shellfish	Hours to days
Domoic acid	15 min–38 h	Vomiting, cramps, diarrhea, confusion, amnesia, cardiac irritability	Mussels	Indefinite
Haff disease		Muscle pain, stiffness, brown urine	Buffalo fish	2–3 days

tubulointerstitial nephritis develop after longer incubation periods and may not be suspected initially. If available, specimens of the mushrooms should be examined promptly by a mycologist or poison control expert to confirm the diagnosis. Toxins can be detected in gastric contents, blood, or urine by thin-layer chromatography.

THERAPY

Nonspecific Therapy

Most food poisoning syndromes are self-limited, and for the majority of episodes, non-specific supportive therapy is all that is required. Exceptions include botulism, listeriosis, some enteric infections in infants and compromised hosts, and some types of mushroom poisoning.

The mainstay of treatment is fluid and electrolyte replacement to prevent and treat dehydration. The first step is to assess the degree of volume depletion by examining the skin turgor, mucous membranes, vital signs, and mental status. Measuring postural changes in pulse and blood pressure is also helpful in quantifying the volume loss. Slightly dry mucous membranes and thirst indicate mild dehydration (5% to 6% deficit, or 50 to 60 mL/kg); loss of skin turgor, very dry mucous membranes, postural pulse increases, and sunken eyes indicate moderate dehydration (7% to 9%); and the additional presence of weak pulse, postural hypotension, cold extremities, or depressed consciousness indicates severe volume depletion, above 10%.

Most children and adults with diarrhea can be treated successfully with oral rehydration. This therapy is possible because of the coupled transport of glucose with water and sodium even in severely damaged small bowel. Diarrheal stool contains significant concentrations of sodium, potassium, and bicarbonate, and fluid therapy should replace these losses.

One liter of the World Health Organization's recommended replacement solution contains 90 mmol of sodium, 20 g of glucose, 20 mmol of potassium, 80 mmol of chloride, and 30 mmol of citrate (as a bicarbonate source); this is close to an ideal solution. Commercial solutions such as Rehydralyte, Ricelyte, and Pedialyte have a slightly lower sodium concentration, but they are convenient and readily available, if expensive. A homemade approximation of the oral solution can be made by adding a pinch of salt, a pinch of baking soda, and a spoonful of sugar or honey to an 8-oz glass of fruit juice. For patients with altered consciousness or uncontrolled vomiting, intravenous rehydration with Ringer lactate should be used initially. The estimated volume deficit should be replaced over 4 hours; after that, ongoing losses should be replaced. Gatorade and commercial soft drinks are poor choices because the low sodium content can lead to hyponatremia and the high osmolarity can exacerbate diarrhea.

Table 49.3 Clinical Syndromes of Mushroom Poisoning

Syndromes (Toxins)	Incubation Period	Symptoms	Mushrooms
Parasympathetic (muscarine)	30 min–2 h	Sweating, salivation, lacrimation, blurred vision, diarrhea, bradycardia, hypotension	*Inocybe* spp *Clitocybe* spp.
Delirium (ibotenic acid, muscimol)	30 min–2 h	Dizziness, incoordination, ataxia, hyperactivity, visual disturbance, stupor	*Amanita muscaria, Amanita pantherina*
Disulfuram-like (coprine)	30 min after alcohol	Flushing, metallic taste, nausea, vomiting, sweating, hypotension	*Coprinus atramentarius, Clitocybe clavipes*
Hallucinations (psilocybin)	30–60 min	Mood elevation, anxiety, muscle weakness, hallucination	*Psilocybe cubensis, Panaleolus* spp.
Gastroenteritis	30 min–2 h	Nausea, vomiting, abdominal cramps, diarrhea	Various
Methemoglobin poisoning (monomethylhydrazine gyromitrin)	6–12 h	Nausea, vomiting, bloody diarrhea, abdominal pain, convulsion, coma, liver failure, hemolysis	*Gyromitra* spp.
Hepatorenal failure (amatoxins, phallotoxins)	6–24 h	Nausea, vomiting, abdominal pain, diarrhea; then jaundice, liver and kidney failure, coma, death	*Amanita phalloides, Amanita verna, Amanita virosa, Galerina autumnalis, Galerina marginata*
Tubulointerstitial nephritis (orellanine)	36 h–14 days	Thirst, nausea, vomiting, flank pain, chills, oliguria	*Cortinarius orellanus, Cortinarius speciosissimus*

Water intake should be allowed ad lib, and solid food can be introduced as soon as it is tolerated. Some patients will develop lactose intolerance after severe or protracted diarrhea, and dairy products should be avoided if they appear to exacerbate symptoms.

Phenothiazine antiemetics may be useful for severe or prolonged vomiting. Promethazine (Pheneragan), 12.5 to 25 mg, and prochlorperazine (Compazine), 5 to 10 mg orally or intramuscularly (IM), 25 mg rectally, can be given orally, as suppositories, or intramuscularly. Alternatively, droperidol (Inapsine), 1 to 2 mL, can be used intravenously (IV). Antidiarrheals should be used cautiously, especially in children. Pepto-Bismol 30 mL orally every 4 to 6 hours may be reasonable if an antidiarrheal is used because it has been shown to bind some enterotoxins. Care must be taken because of the salicylate content.

Specific Therapy

Specific therapies for food poisoning are outlined in Table 49.4. Gastric emptying and administration of active charcoal and cathartics are important for virtually all cases of mushroom poisoning. If vomiting has not occurred spontaneously in patients with botulism or ciguatera, the remaining food should be removed from the gut. In botulism, paralytic shellfish poisoning, and ciguatera, death from respiratory failure is the major risk, and monitoring the vital capacity can be lifesaving.

Polyvalent equine antitoxin, which binds botulinum toxins A, B, and E, is available in the United States through state health departments and the Centers for Disease Control and Prevention (770-488-7100, 24 hours a day). It may prevent further paralysis but does not reverse established symptoms. To be effective, it should be administered early. Dosage and a protocol for desensitization in the case of a positive skin test are listed in the package insert.

In ciguatera poisoning, analgesia and avoidance of unpleasant stimuli such as warm baths are usually adequate. Anecdotal reports in the literature suggest that amitriptyline, 25 to 50 mg/day orally, and tocainide may be useful for dysesthesias. Intravenous mannitol has also been reported to be effective for severe neurologic manifestations. For histamine fish poisoning, conventional antihistamines, such as diphenhydramine, 25 to 50 mg IM or IV, are

Table 49.4 Specific Treatment for Food Poisoning Syndromes

Syndrome	First-Line Treatment	Comment
Staphylococcus aureus, Bacillus cereus, Clostridium perfringens, Norwalk virus	Fluid replacement, antiemetics (eg, promethazine [Phenergan], prochlorperazine [Compazine], droperidol [Inapsine])	Oral rehydration is usually adequate if vomiting can be controlled.
Bacterial gastroenteritis	Fluid replacement; antimicrobials helpful for some syndromes	See chapters on specific organisms and Chapter 48, Gastroenteritis, for specific antimicrobial therapy.
Clostridium botulinum	Gastric empying, cathartics if food still in gastrointestinal tract; respiratory support, polyvalent antitoxin[a]	Antitoxin should be given as soon as possible.
Cyclospora	Trimethoprim-sulfamethoxazole (160 mg trimethoprim component bid for 7 days)	If not treated, symptoms may be protracted and relapsing.
Histamine (scombroid)	Antihistamine (eg, diphenhydramine 25–50 mg IM or IV)	H2 receptor antagonists (cimetidine) have been helpful for refractory symptoms.
Ciguatera	Empty stomach if vomiting has not occurred; analgesia, antiemetics, supportive measures; atropine for symptomatic bradycardia	Amitryptiline (25–50 mg/d) or tocainide may help paresthesias; mannitol infusion, calcium gluconate infusion have been used
Neurotoxic shellfish poisoning	Supportive therapy	
Paralytic shellfish poisoning	Supportive therapy, monitor vital capacity	
Haff disease	IV hydration	Mannitol and bicarbonate have also been used to protect renal tubules.
Muscarine-containing mushrooms	Gastric emptying, activated charcoal, cathartics; atropine 0.01 mg/kg IV up to 1 mg	Titrate atropine to drying of secretions
Muscimol- and ibotenic acid-containing mushrooms	Gastric emptying, activated charcoal, cathartics; supportive measures	Physostigmine may be used if anticholinergic symptoms are severe.
Hallucinogen-containing mushrooms	Reassurance, quiet room; diazepam for severe agitation	
Monomethylhydrazine-containing mushrooms (*Gyromitra* spp.)	Gastric emptying, activated charcoal, cathartics; for delirium, pyridoxine, 25 mg/kg IV	For methemoglobinemia, methylene blue 1% solution 0.1–0.2 mL/kg over 5 min
Amatoxin-containing mushrooms	Gastric emptying, activated charcoal, cathartics; correction of fluid and electrolytes; monitoring glucose, liver, and renal function	Thioctic acid[b], silibinin, high dosages of steroids, and IV penicillin have been advocated, but controlled data are lacking; hemodialysis, charcoal hemoperfusion, and liver transplantation may be necessary.
Orellanine-containing mushrooms	Gastric emptying, activated charcoal, cathartics; cautious correction of fluid and electrolyte problems	Hemodialysis is often necessary.

[a] Available through State Health Department, or Foodborne and Diarrheal Diseases Branch, Centers for Disease Control and Prevention 404-639-2206 8:00 to 4:30 EST workdays; 404-639-2888 nights, weekends, and holidays.
[b] Assistance in obtaining thioctic acid can be sought through regional poison control centers.

helpful. Epinephrine or albuterol should be given for bronchospasm. Intravenous cimetidine can be tried for refractory symptoms.

Atropine is a specific antidote for poisoning from muscarine-containing mushrooms, but the dosage (0.01 mg/kg up to a maximum of 1 mg) should be titrated to control excess respiratory secretions and bradycardia rather than other symptoms.

Specific treatment is usually not necessary for poisoning caused by acid-containing ibotenic or muscimol-containing mushrooms. If severe anticholinergic symptoms such as hyperpyrexia, hypertension, or severe agitation are present, physostigmine, 0.01 mg/kg IV, should be used. Cardiac and blood pressure monitoring are necessary because hypotension and bradycardia can result.

For poisoning caused by monomethylhydrazine-containing mushrooms, pyridoxine, 25 mg/kg IV, should be given; the dose can be repeated every 5 to 10 minutes. The methemoglobin level should be measured if possible. If there is symptomatic methemoglobinemia with central cyanosis, methylene blue, 0.1 to 0.2 mL/kg of a 1% solution, should be given over 5 minutes.

The high fatality rate associated with poisoning by *Amanita phalloides* and related amatoxin-containing mushrooms makes it a special concern. Toxin removal should be attempted with activated charcoal and cathartics even after several days because of the extensive enterohepatic cycling. During the initial phase, gastrointestinal symptoms may cause hypotension. This first stage often is followed by a stage of apparent improvement, but hepatic transaminases usually are elevated by 24 to 48 hours. Fulminant hepatic necrosis and acute renal failure begin after 48 to 96 hours. Supportive treatment consists of careful fluid replacement and monitoring of serum glucose and liver function tests. Thioctic acid may be partially effective at 300 mg/kg/day IV with glucose infusion in divided doses every 6 hours; contact the regional poison control center for help in obtaining it. The roles of IV penicillin, silibinin, and high-dose steroids are unclear. Charcoal hemoperfusion is theoretically attractive if it can be begun within the first 10 to 16 hours. Liver transplant has been successful in some cases. Assistance from the regional poison control center should always be sought for help with mushroom identification and for the latest treatment information.

REPORTING

Reporting of suspected foodborne outbreaks to local or state health departments is an important part of management because epidemiologic investigation can clearly establish the responsible food and may prevent many additional cases.

SUGGESTED READING

Diaz JH. Syndromic diagnosis and management of confirmed mushroom poisonings. *Crit Care Med.* 2005;33:427–436.

King CK, Glass R, Bresee JS, Duggan C; Centers for Disease Control and Prevention. Managing acute gastroenteritis among children: oral rehydration, maintenance, and nutritional therapy. *MMWR Recomm Rep.* 2003;52(RR-16):1–16.

Pavia AT. Foodborne and waterborne disease. In: Long S, Pickering L, Prober C, eds. *Principles and Practices of Pediatric Infectious Disease.* 2nd ed. New York, NY: Churchill Livingstone; 2002.

Scallan E. Activities, achievements, and lessons learned during the first 10 years of the Foodborne Diseases Active Surveillance Network: 1996–2005. *Clin Infect Dis.* 2007;44:718–725.

Sobel J. Botulism. *Clin Infect Dis.* 2005;41:1163.

Tauxe RV. Emerging foodborne pathogens. *Int J Food Microbiol.* 2002;78:31–41.

50. Antibiotic-Associated Diarrhea

John G. Bartlett

Diarrhea is a relatively common complication of antibiotic use. Nearly all agents with an antibiotic spectrum of activity have been implicated. The great majority of cases are either enigmatic or caused by *Clostridium difficile*.

DIAGNOSTIC STUDIES

Clostridium difficile–associated disease should be suspected in any patient who has diarrhea in association with antibiotic exposure. The most common inducing agents are clindamycin, fluoroquinolones, and cephalosporins. Nevertheless, nearly any antimicrobial agent with an antibacterial spectrum of activity can cause this complication.

The usual method for identifying cases of diarrhea caused by *C. difficile* is the toxin assay. The original technique was with a tissue culture assay for detection of cytotoxin or toxin B; more recently 95% of laboratories in the United States have used the enzyme immunoassay (EIA) for detection of toxin A or toxin A plus B. Occasional labs screen for *C. difficile* by culture (which takes 3 days) or by detecting the common antigen (which takes hours) to be followed by testing for the toxin by the more sensitive tissue culture method. Studies of the EIA compared with the tissue culture assay indicate that it is relatively specific and has the advantage of providing results within 2 to 3 hours, but it is only about 75% sensitive, so there are many false negatives.

Anatomic studies, usually sigmoidoscopy or colonoscopy, were far more common before the general availability of *C. difficile* toxin assays in the late 1970s. This also was when pseudomembranous colitis (PMC) was a relatively common complication because of the lack of treatment to interrupt the natural history of the disease. Endoscopy is still indicated in some patients who have negative toxin assays and/or pose other problems in diagnosis. Computed tomography (CT) and x-ray studies with contrast are sometimes done for other conditions and will occasionally show changes that are highly suggestive of antibiotic-associated colitis caused by *C. dif-*

ficile; nevertheless, these are substantially less sensitive and toxin testing is clearly preferred for the vast majority of cases.

CLOSTRIDIUM DIFFICILE: TREATMENT

The first principle of treatment is discontinuation of the implicated antimicrobial agent. Supportive measures include fluid and electrolyte restoration and avoidance of antiperistaltic agents such as loperamide. Some patients respond to simple withdrawal of the implicated antimicrobial agent and appropriate supportive care.

If the condition being treated requires continued antibiotic treatment, the recommendation is to change to an agent that is infrequently associated with this complication, such as sulfonamide, tetracycline, aminoglycoside, vancomycin, a macrolide, a narrow-spectrum β-lactam, or a urinary antiseptic.

Antibiotic treatment directed against *C. difficile* is readily available and highly effective using vancomycin or metronidazole (Table 50.1). Response is impressive; generally, fever resolves within 24 hours and diarrhea over an average of 4 to 5 days. Overall response rates are usually reported at 95% to 100%. Vancomycin has ideal pharmacokinetic properties because it is poorly absorbed with oral administration, so levels in the colon lumen are several hundred-fold higher than the minimum inhibitory concentration. All strains are sensitive. This is a disease the putative agent of which is entirely restricted to the colon lumen, so tissue levels are irrelevant to therapy. The disadvantages of vancomycin treatment are relatively high rates of relapse, relatively high costs, occasional poor response to the drug due to ileus, and possible role in promoting vancomycin-resistant *Enterococcus faecium*.

Metronidazole is active against virtually all strains of *C. difficile* and has a track record of efficacy comparable with that of vancomycin in comparative trials. Theoretic disadvantages are the low levels of the drug in the colon lumen because of almost complete absorption. This drug is substantially less expensive than

Table 50.1 Treatment of *C. difficile* Diarrhea and Colitis

Nonspecific Measures
Discontinue the implicated antibiotic; if continued antibiotic treatment is necessary, change to an alternative agent that is unlikely to cause or promote *C. difficile*–associated enteric disease.
Change to another agent infrequently associated with this complication.
Provide supportive measures.
Avoid antiperistaltic agents.
Use enteric precautions for hospitalized patients.
Specific Treatments
Antimicrobial Agents if Symptoms are Severe or Persist
Oral Agent (Required)
Vancomycin, 125 mg PO QID, 10 days[a] Metronidazole, 250 mg PO QID or 500 mg PO TID, 10 days[a]
Parenteral Agents: (efficacy not established)
Metronidazole, 500 mg IV q12h (efficacy not established)
Alternative Treatments
Anion Exchange Resins
Cholestyramine, 4 g packet PO TID, 7–14 days[a] Cholestipol, 5 g packet PO TID, 7–14 days
Alter fecal flora with fecal transplant
Lactinex or alternative lactobacillus preparation, 1 g packet Gr *Saccharomyces boulardii*

[a] Established efficacy.

Table 50.2 Methods to Manage Multiple Relapses of *C. difficile* Diarrhea or Colitis

Metronidazole or vancomycin PO × 10 days followed by:
Vancomycin, 125 mg PO QID × 10 days, followed by vancomycin, 125 mg PO QID × ≥4 wk
Vancomycin, 125 mg PO QID × 10 days, then taper over 4 wk
Vancomycin, 125 mg PO QID, plus *Saccharomyces boulardii* (not FDA-approved) × 14 days, then *Saccharomyces boulardii* for 4 wk
Intravenous γ globulin, 400 mg/kg q3wk (supporting data are anecdotal).

vancomycin. Most guidelines recommend it as initial therapy for most patients with *C. difficile*–associated disease. Vancomycin is reserved for patients who fail to respond to metronidazole or for initial treatment of patients who are seriously ill due to this complication. The rate of relapse for metronidazole is comparable with that for vancomycin.

Relapses of *C. difficile* diarrhea are seen only with antibiotic therapy. The typical clinical presentation is recurrence of the initial symptoms 3 to 10 days after discontinuation of metronidazole or vancomycin. Patients generally respond to readministration of either agent, but occasional patients have multiple relapses that can be a major therapeutic problem; several therapeutic options are summarized in Table 50.2.

Clostridium difficile–associated enteric disease is now largely a nosocomial problem. Recommendations to control spread include (1) isolating patients, especially those with in-continence; (2) enforcing handwashing with soap or detergent; and (3) replacing electronic thermometers. With outbreaks, it may be necessary to restrict use of selected antimicrobials.

NAP1 STRAIN

This strain was rare until the early 2000s, when it was first recognized in Quebec and then the United States and Europe. Distinguishing features are that it (1) produces more toxin A and B in vitro than the strains seen previously and (2) in contrast to earlier strains, it is resistant to fluoroquinolones. The consequences of these two properties is that it appears to (1) cause more disease including outbreaks, possibly due to the enormous use of fluoroquinolones, and (2) more serious disease that is more likely to be refractory to standard therapy. As a consequence, early diagnosis and prompt treatment is emphasized.

OTHER CAUSES

Most patients with antibiotic-associated diarrhea or colitis have negative diagnostic studies for *C. difficile* toxin and have no established agent or mechanism. Some believe the best explanation is dysbiosis of the colonic flora, resulting in failure of this flora to metabolize carbohydrate in the gut resulting in an osmotic diarrhea. The antimicrobial agents implicated are the same that cause *C. difficile* disease. However, some of the clinical differences include the facts that this osmotic form of diarrhea is usually dose related, symptoms usually resolve when the implicated agent is discontinued or reduced in dose, systemic symptoms are unusual, it is rarely serious or life threatening, and colitis (fecal leukocytes, fever, or evidence of colitis by endoscopy or CT scan) is unusual. This form of diarrhea also tends to be spora.dic, whereas *C. difficile* may be endemic or epidemic within hospitals or nursing homes.

The usual treatment for antibiotic-associated diarrhea with a negative toxin assay is to discontinue the implicated agent; most patients respond. Patients with serious disease, evidence of colitis, or persistent symptoms after discontinuation of antibiotics should have repeat toxin assays for *C. difficile* due to the high rate of false-negative results. Patients with persistent or serious symptoms in the face of negative assays should undergo anatomic studies using endoscopy and exploration of alternative causes such as, for example, idiopathic inflammatory bowel disease, other enteric pathogens, and diarrhea caused by other medications.

SUGGESTED READING

Bartlett JG. *Clostridium difficile*: clinical considerations. *Rev Infect Dis.* 1990;12:S243–S251.

Bartlett JG. Narrative review: the new epidemic of Clostridium difficile-associated enteric disease. *Ann Intern Med.* 2006;145:758–764.

Fekety R, Shah AB. Diagnosis and treatment of *Clostridium difficile* colitis. *JAMA.* 1993; 269:71–75.

Gerding DN, Johnson S, Peterson LR, et al. *Clostridium difficile*—associated diarrhea and colitis. *Infect Control Hosp Epidemiol.* 1995;16:495–477.

Johnson S, Sasmore MH, Farrow KA, et al. Epidemics of diarrhea caused by a clindamycin-resistant strain of *Clostridium difficile* in four hospitals. *N Engl J Med.* 1999;341:1645–1651.

McDonald LC, Killgore GE, Thompson A, et al. an epidemic, toxin gene-variant strain of *Clostridium difficile*. *N Engl J Med.* 2005;353:2433–2441.

Merz CS, Kramer C, Forman M, et al. Comparison of four commercially available rapid enzyme immunoassays with cytotoxin assay for detection of *Clostridium difficile* toxin(s) from stool specimens. *J Clin Microbiol.* 1994;32:1142–1147.

Tsutaoka B, Hansen J, Johnson D, et al. Antibiotic-associated pseudomembranous enteritis due to *Clostridium difficile*. *Clin Infect Dis.* 1994;18:982–984.

51. Sexually Transmitted Enteric Infections

Thomas C. Quinn

INTRODUCTION

A wide variety of microbial pathogens may be transmitted sexually by the oral–anal or genital–anal routes. Sexually transmitted enteric infections may involve multiple sites of the gastrointestinal tract, resulting in proctitis, proctocolitis, and enteritis. These infections occur primarily in men who have sex with men (MSM) and heterosexual women who engage in anal–rectal intercourse or in sexual practices that allow for fecal–oral transmission. Anorectal infections with syphilis, gonorrhea, condyloma acuminata (human papillomavirus, HPV), lymphogranuloma venereum (LGV), and granuloma inguinale (donovanosis) have been recognized for many years. Over the past 2 decades, other sexually transmitted pathogens such as herpes simplex virus (HSV) and *Chlamydia trachomatis* have also been recognized as causing anorectal infection. Enteric pathogens traditionally associated with food or waterborne acquisition but that also may be transmitted sexually include *Giardia lamblia, Entamoeba histolytica, Campylobacter, Shigella,* and *Salmonella*. In patients with acquired immunodeficiency syndrome (AIDS), other opportunistic infections, including *Candida, Microsporida, Cryptosporidia, Isospora, Cyclospora, Mycobacterium avium* complex, and cytomegalovirus (CMV), may also cause intestinal disorders.

Depending on the pathogen and the location of the infection, symptoms and clinical manifestations vary widely. Perianal lesions are usually caused by syphilis, HSV, granuloma inguinale, chancroid, and condyloma acuminata. Rectal infections cause inflammation of the rectal mucosa, commonly referred to as *proctitis*. Symptoms include constipation, tenesmus, rectal discomfort or pain, hematochezia, and a mucopurulent rectal discharge. Proctitis can be caused by gonorrhea, chlamydia, syphilis, and HSV. Proctocolitis involves inflammation extending from the rectum to the colon, and in addition to the organisms causing proctitis, other enteric pathogens such as *Shigella, Salmonella, Campylobacter, E. histolytica,* and CMV may be involved. Enteritis is an inflammatory illness of the duodenum, jejunum, and/or ileum. Sigmoidoscopy results are often normal, and symptoms consist of diarrhea, abdominal pain, bloating, cramps, and nausea. Additional symptoms may include fever, weight loss, myalgias, flatulence, urgency, and, in severe cases, melena. Sexually transmitted pathogens usually associated with enteritis include *Shigella, Salmonella, Campylobacter, Giardia,* CMV, and, potentially, *Cryptosporidia, Isospora,* and *Microsporida.*

The large number of infectious agents that cause enteric and anorectal infections necessitate a systematic approach to the management of these conditions. While obtaining the medical history, the clinician should attempt to differentiate between proctitis, proctocolitis, and enteritis and should assess the constellation of symptoms that suggest one or another likely infectious cause. The history should be used to investigate types of sexual practices and possible exposure to the pathogens known to cause intestinal infections. Examination should include inspection of the anus, digital rectal examination, and anoscopy to identify general mucosal abnormalities. Initial laboratory tests should include a Gram stain of any rectal exudate obtained with the use of an anoscope. The demonstration of leukocytes provides objective evidence of the presence of an infectious or inflammatory disorder. Cultures for gonorrhea should be obtained from the rectum, urethra, and pharynx, and, if possible, rectal culture for chlamydia should be performed. Serologic tests for syphilis should be performed in all cases. Dark-field examination of any ulcerations and a rapid plasma reagin test should be performed. Cultures for HSV should be performed if ulcerative lesions are present. If proctocolitis is present, additional stool cultures for *Campylobacter, Salmonella,* and *Shigella* should be obtained, and stool examination for *E. histolytica* is indicated. For human immunodeficiency virus (HIV)-positive patients, other pathogens, including *Microsporida,* CMV, atypical *Mycobacteria, Cryptosporidia,* and *Isospora,* should be screened for by stool examination and cultured. Specific information on clinical presentation, diagnosis, and therapy is provided in other chapters on gastroenteritis, intestinal protozoa, and individual enteric pathogens.

GONOCOCCAL PROCTITIS

Rectal infection with *Neisseria gonorrhoeae* occurs predominantly among homosexual men and women engaging in anal–rectal intercourse. In many cases of women, the patient has no history of rectal intercourse and the infection is thought to have resulted from contiguous spread of infected secretions from the vagina. Symptoms, when present, develop approximately 5 to 7 days after exposure. Symptoms are usually mild and include constipation, anorectal discomfort, tenesmus, and a mucopurulent rectal discharge that may cause secondary skin irritation, resulting in rectal itching and perirectal erythema. Although asymptomatic or mild local disease is common, complications such as fistulas, abscesses, strictures, and disseminated gonococcal infection may occur.

Findings of rectal gonorrhea during anoscopy are nonspecific and limited to the distal rectum. The most common finding is the presence of mucopus in the rectum. The rectal mucosa may appear completely normal or demonstrate generalized erythema with local areas of easily induced bleeding, primarily near the anal–rectal junction. Diagnosis is usually made by Gram stain and culture of material obtained by swabbing the mucosa of the rectal area. The sensitivity of Gram stain of rectal exudate for identification of gram-negative intracellular diplococci is approximately 80% when obtained through an anoscope versus 53% for blindly inserted swabs. Cultures inoculated on selective media provide the definitive diagnosis; however, the precise sensitivity of a single rectal culture for gonorrhea may be no greater than 80%. DNA detection assays are now widely available for detection of gonorrhea in urogenital specimens and appear to be equally sensitive as culture.

Therapy for *N. gonorrhoeae* has focused on a single-dose therapy effective against β-lactamase–inducing strains. A single dose of ceftriaxone, 125 mg intramuscularly (IM), or cefixime, 400 mg orally, are recommended regimens for uncomplicated anal infection. These regimens are effective in treating more than 95% of rectal infections. Quinolones are not recommended due to increasing resistance, especially among MSM. Cotreatment for chlamydia with doxycycline, 100 mg orally twice a day for 7 days (or azithromycin 1.0 g orally) is recommended. Because of the established efficacy of these regimens, routine repeat testing for cures generally is not recommended unless therapeutic compliance is questionable or symptoms persist after treatment. If there is continued evidence of proctitis, further evaluation for other agents such as chlamydia, syphilis, enteric bacterial pathogens, and HSV should be considered.

CHLAMYDIA PROCTITIS

Rectal infection with LGV and non-LGV immunotypes of *C. trachomatis* have been well documented. LGV infections are endemic in tropical countries, but they have also been seen in the United States and Europe and more often in homosexual men than in heterosexual men and women. LGV infections usually cause a severe proctocolitis characterized by severe anorectal pain, bloody mucopurulent discharge, and tenesmus. Inguinal adenopathy, which is characteristic of genital LGV, is often present. Sigmoidoscopy typically reveals diffuse friability with discrete ulcerations in the rectum that occasionally extend to the descending colon. Strictures and fistulas may become prominent and can be easily misdiagnosed clinically as Crohn's disease or carcinoma. Histologically, rectal LGV may be confused with Crohn's disease because giant cells, crypt abscesses, and granulomas may be present.

The non-LGV immunotypes of *C. trachomatis* are less invasive than LGV and cause a mild proctitis characterized by rectal discharge, tenesmus, and anorectal pain. Many infected individuals may be asymptomatic and can be diagnosed only by routine cultures. However, even in asymptomatic cases, abnormal numbers of fecal leukocytes are usually present. Sigmoidoscopy results may be normal or may reveal mild inflammatory changes with small erosions or follicles in the lower 10 cm of the rectum.

Diagnosis of chlamydia proctitis is best made by isolation of *C. trachomatis* from the rectum, together with an appropriate response to therapy. Serology is useful for the diagnosis of LGV with a complement fixation titer of >1:64. Direct fluorescent antibody staining with monoclonal antibody of rectal secretions can also be used to establish the diagnosis. Nucleic acid amplification tests (NAATs) have been used with good reported sensitivity and specificity but are not currently U.S. Food and Drug Administration (FDA) approved for rectal specimens. Azithromycin, tetracycline, and doxycycline are the drugs of choice for infection with *C. trachomatis*. Azithromycin,

1.0 g as a single dose, is effective for urethritis and cervicitis and has been recommended for uncomplicated rectal infections. Doxycyline, 100 mg twice a day for 7 to 10 days, is effective, except for treating LGV infection, which should be treated for 3 weeks with doxycycline. Patients should be followed carefully with repeat sigmoidoscopy, particularly when there is any question about the differential diagnosis of LGV versus inflammatory bowel disease.

ANORECTAL SYPHILIS

Treponema pallidum can be seen in its early infectious stages, with a primary anorectal lesion appearing 2 to 6 weeks after exposure to rectal intercourse. However, clinicians often fail to recognize anorectal chancres, and consequently, syphilis in MSM is diagnosed in a secondary or early latent stage much more often than in the primary stage. Careful perianal examination can reveal unsuspected perianal chancres, but digital rectal examination and anoscopy may be required to detect asymptomatic chancres higher in the anal canal or rectum. When anorectal syphilis causes symptoms, it is often misdiagnosed as a traumatic lesion, fissure, or hemorrhoiditis. When symptoms are present, they include mild anal pain or discomfort, constipation, rectal bleeding, and occasionally a rectal discharge. Primary anorectal syphilis may appear as a single or multiple, mirror-image perianal ulcers ("kissing chancres"). It can also present as an ulcerated mass typically located on the anterior wall of the rectum. Inguinal adenopathy with rubbery, nonsuppurative, painless nodes may be associated with anorectal syphilis; it helps distinguish it from fissures. Secondary syphilis may cause discrete polyps, smooth lobulated masses, mucosal alterations, and nonspecific mucosal erythema or bleeding. In secondary syphilis, condyloma lata may be found near or within the anal canal. These are smooth, warty masses and should be differentiated from the more highly keratinized condyloma acuminata.

Diagnosis of anorectal syphilis is based on serology, perirectal and digital rectal examination, and anoscopy. Detection of motile treponemes by dark-field examination is useful for evaluation of perianal and anal lesions but may be less specific for rectal lesions because pathogenic treponemes can be found in the intestine. Biopsies of rectal lesions or masses should be processed for silver staining if syphilis is suspected. Serologic diagnosis of syphilis is based on the presence of antibodies to nontreponemal

and treponemal antigens. A positive Venereal Disease Research Laboratory (VDRL) test or rapid plasma reagin (RPR) test must be confirmed by a positive specific test such as the fluorescent treponemal antibody absorption test (FTA-ABS) or the microhemagglutination assay (MHA). Concomitant HIV infection may alter serologic manifestations of syphilis. There has been delayed or absent RPR reactivity in some patients infected with HIV and proven secondary syphilis.

Treatment for anorectal syphilis is standard treatment for early syphilis and consists of benzathine penicillin, 2.4 million U IM. Penicillin-allergic patients may be treated with a 15-day course of doxycycline, 100 mg twice daily, or tetracycline, 500 mg 4 times a day.

SHIGELLA, SALMONELLA, AND CAMPYLOBACTER INFECTIONS

Shigellosis presents with an abrupt onset of diarrhea, fever, nausea, and cramps. Diarrhea is usually watery but may contain mucus or blood. Sigmoidoscopy usually reveals an inflamed mucosa with friability not limited to the distal rectum, and histologic examination shows diffuse inflammation with bacteria scattered throughout the submucosa. *Shigella sonnei* and *S. flexneri* account for most of the *Shigella* infections in the United States. Diagnosis is made by culturing the organism from the stool on selective media. Treatment is usually supportive with fluid replacement, and antimotility agents should be avoided. Antibiotics are useful in the management of shigellosis because use of appropriate therapy has reportedly shortened the period of fecal excretion and limited the clinical course. However, some authorities believe that antibiotic therapy should be reserved for the severely ill only or the immunocompromised patient because the infection is typically self-limited and resistance has been common. HIV-infected patients who develop *Shigella* infections may require prolonged treatment or suppressive therapy similar to those infected with salmonella. Antibiotic therapy should be chosen according to the sensitivity pattern of the *Shigella* species isolated. Ciprofloxacin, 500 mg twice a day for 7 days, is usually effective unless resistance is evident.

Campylobacter jejuni and *Campylobacter*-like organisms such as *Helicobacter cinaedi* and *Helicobacter fennelliae* have also been associated with proctocolitis in homosexual men. Clinical manifestations of infections resulting from all *Campylobacter* species appear nearly identical. There is often a prodrome with fever, headache, myalgia, and malaise 12 to 24 hours before the onset of intestinal symptoms. The most common symptoms are diarrhea, malaise, fever, and abdominal pain. Abdominal pain is usually cramping and may be associated with 10 or more bowel movements per day. *Campylobacter enteritis* is often self-limiting with gradual improvement in symptoms over several days. Illnesses lasting longer than 1 week occur in approximately 10% to 20% of patients seeking medical attention, and relapses are often seen in HIV-infected patients. Fecal leukocytes are uniformly present, and diagnosis is confirmed by isolation of the organisms on selective media in a microaerophilic atmosphere. Therapy consists of fluid and electrolyte replacement and antibiotic treatment. Erythromycin at a dosage of 500 mg 4 times daily for 1 week, azithromycin 500 mg once daily for 3 days, or ciprofloxacin 500 mg twice a day for 7 days has also been used for treatment successfully, but resistance to these antibiotics has also been increasing within recent years.

Salmonella infections of the intestinal tract are primarily caused by *S. typhimurium* and *S. enteritidis.* Salmonella has been reported among homosexual male partners, suggesting sexual transmission and salmonella bacteremia in an HIV-infected individual are now diagnostic of AIDS. Clinical presentation often depends on the host-immune status. In an immunocompetent person, salmonellosis is usually self-limited and causes gastroenteritis. No antibiotic therapy is recommended because symptoms fade within days, and antibiotics have been associated with prolonged salmonella intestinal carriage. In HIV-infected individuals, salmonella infections may cause severe invasive disease and often result in bacteremia with widespread infection. The fluoroquinolones are effective drugs of choice for *Salmonella* infections in immunocompromised individuals. Despite adequate therapy for bacteremia, virtually all HIV-infected patients may suffer recurrent salmonella septicemia. Ciprofloxacin, 500 to 750 mg twice daily, has been effective in suppressing recurrences in such patients.

PARASITIC INFECTIONS

Homosexual men engaging in sexual activities involving fecal contamination such as oral–anal sex are at increased risk for a number of parasitic infections, including *Giardia lamblia, Iodamoeba butschlii, Dientamoeba fragilis, Enterobius vermicularis, Cryptosporidia, Isospora,* and *Microsporidia.* Of these infections, *Giardia* and *E. histolytica* appear to be the most common sexually transmitted parasitic infections. *Giardia lamblia* is associated with symptoms of enteritis, and *E. histolytica* may cause proctocolitis. Most *E. histolytica* infections are asymptomatic and less than 10% of those infected develop invasive disease with amoebic dysentery or liver abscess. Most *E. histolytica* strains isolated from homosexual men are the nonpathogenic strains that are not usually associated with gastrointestinal symptoms. However, when symptoms are present, they may vary from mild diarrhea to fulminant bloody dysentery. These symptoms may wax and wane for weeks to months.

Diagnosis is based on demonstration of *E. histolytica* in the stool in a wet mount of a swab or in biopsy of rectal mucosal lesions. Occasionally, multiple fresh stool examinations are necessary to demonstrate the cysts or trophozoites or *E. histolytica.* For noninvasive disease limited to the lumen only, paromomycin 25 to 30 mg/kg/day in 3 doses for 7 days is the regimen of choice. Invasive intestinal disease should be treated with metronidazole, 750 mg 3 times daily for 10 days.

Giardia lamblia also appears to be sexually transmitted through oral–anal contact. Giardiasis is typically an infection of the small intestine, and symptoms vary from mild abdominal discomfort to diarrhea, abdominal cramps, bloating, and nausea. Multiple stool examinations may be necessary to document infection with *G. lamblia.* When stool examination is negative, sampling of the jejunal mucus by the Enterotest or small-bowel biopsy may be necessary to confirm the diagnosis. Metronidazole 250 to 500 mg 3 times a day for 7 days is recommended. Alternative regimens include tinidazole, 2 g only single dose, or paromomycin, 500 mg 3 times daily for 7 to 10 days.

Although sexual transmission of *Cryptosporidia, Isospora belli,* and *Microsporida* are commonly seen in HIV-infected homosexual men, evidence for sexual transmission is limited. These protozoa primarily infect the small bowel and cause nonspecific watery diarrhea, abdominal cramping, and bloating. Diagnosis is established by a modified acid-fast stain or fluoramine stain of the stool or by concentration and identification of the organism by the sugar-flotation method. A commercially available fluorescein monoclonal antibody assay increases the sensitivity for detection of *Cryptosporidia.* Treatment of *Cryptosporidia* or *Isospora* infections in immunocompetent patients with self-limited diarrhea is rarely required. Among HIV-infected individuals, treatment should be directed toward symptomatic treatment of the diarrhea with dehydration and repletion of electrolyte losses by either oral or intravenous route. Although several antibiotics have been used, including paromomycin and azithromycin, chronic infection and relapses are common. The most effective therapy currently is a reversal of immunosuppression with the use of highly active antiretroviral therapy. It is common for patients with severe diarrhea from *Cryptosporidia* and *Microsporida* to clear their infections by taking combination antiretroviral agents with reduction in the viral load below detectable limits. Successful treatment of the infection presumably results from a subsequent rise in CD4 count and restoration of immune competence sufficient to clear the intestinal infection.

SUGGESTED READING

Benson CA, Kaplan JE, Masur H, Pau A, Holmes KK. Treating opportunistic infections among HIV-infected adults and adolescents: recommendations from CDC, the National Institutes of Health, and the HIV Medicine Association/Infectious Diseases Society of America. *Clin Infect Dis*. 2005;40: S131–S235.

Centers for Disease Control and Prevention. 2006 guidelines for treatment of sexually transmitted diseases, MMWR 55, August 4, 2006. www. cdc.gov/std/treatment/2006/ rr5511.pdf, accessed September 4, 2007.

Fenton KA, Imrie J. Increasing rates of sexually transmitted disease in homosexual men in Western Europe and the United States: why? *Infect Dis Clin North Am*. 2005; 19:311–331.

Kent CK, Chaw JK, Wong W, et al. Prevalence of rectal, urethral, and pharyngeal Chlamydia and gonorrhea detected in 2 clinical settings among men who have sex with men: San Francisco, California, 2003. *Clin Infect Dis*. 2005;41:67–74.

Klausner JD, Kohn R, Kent C. Etiology of clinical proctitis among men who have sex with men. *Clin Infect Dis*. 2004;38:300–302.

Thom K, Forrest G. Gastrointestinal infections in immunocompromised hosts. *Curr Opin Gastroenterol*. 2006;22:18–23.

Van der Bij AK, Spaargaren J, Moree SA, et al. Diagnostic and clinical implications of anorectal lymphogranuloma venereum in men who have sex with men: a retrospective case-control study. *Clin Infect Dis*. 2006;42:186–194.

52. Acute Appendicitis

S. Frank Redo[†]

Acute appendicitis may occur in all age groups but is most common in older children and young adults. It is rare in infants, probably because of the conical nature of the appendix, which permits easier entry and exit of stool. In children up to 4 to 6 years of age and in the elderly, diagnosis is difficult and often not made until perforation has occurred. The incidence is equal in males and females but increases in males during early adulthood, after which the sex ratio again becomes equal.

PATHOGENESIS

Acute appendicitis is initiated by obstruction of the lumen by stool (fecalith), fibrous band, lymphoid hyperplasia, or a foreign body. The normal mucosal secretion of the appendix collects distal to the site of the obstruction, which leads to an increase in intraluminal pressure. This causes first interference with venous outflow and subsequently, as pressure increases, with arterial blood inflow. Ulceration of the mucosa occurs with infiltration of the wall of the appendix by bacteria. The resultant infection may lead to gangrene, necrosis, and perforation.

DIAGNOSIS

Symptoms and Signs

In a classical case of acute appendicitis, the patient gives a history of periumbilical pain associated with nausea and vomiting that migrates and localizes in the right lower quadrant. This may occur within 1 to 2 or 12 to 18 hours. Vomiting usually consists of only 1 or 2 episodes and begins after the onset of pain. If vomiting precedes the pain, the patient probably does not have appendicitis. Anorexia is common.

Unfortunately, this classical history does not exist in all cases. If the appendix is retrocecal, the pain may be described as being in the right flank or right back. When the appendix lies in the pelvis, the pain may be in the testicle or suprapubic (bladder) region. Diarrhea, in such instances, may be a presenting associated problem.

On physical examination, the abdomen usually is tense with spasm and guarding in the right lower quadrant. If the pain has had moderately long duration, the entire abdomen may be rigid, suggesting peritonitis and probable perforated appendix. Discrete tenderness at McBurney's Point diagnostic for acute appendicitis. Rebound, shake, and toe–heel tenderness are indicative of peritoneal irritation. When the appendix is retrocecal, rebound tenderness may not be evident. In such instances, however, there usually is a positive psoas sign.

The abdomen should be palpated for a mass in the right lower quadrant and auscultated for bowel sounds. Bowel sounds may be normal in the early phase of infection but become less active or quiet as the process progresses.

Percussion over the flank and back may cause pain when the appendix is retrocecal. Temperature rarely exceeds 38.5°C (101.3°F) unless there has been perforation and peritonitis has developed.

On rectal examination, a mass may be palpable in the right lower quadrant. Pain may be elicited in this region by pressure of the examining finger on the anterior aspect of the right rectal wall.

Laboratory

Laboratory work-up should begin with a complete blood count, urinalysis, serum electrolyte determinations, and supine and upright radiographs of the abdomen. The hemoglobin and hematocrit levels are helpful in assessing dehydration and hemoconcentration. The white blood cell (WBC) count is usually elevated to 15 000 or more with a differential high in polymorphonuclear cells and bands.

The urinalysis provides another clue with respect to degree of hydration. In addition, results of microscopic examination reveal WBC count, red blood cell (RBC) count, and bacteria content. A small number of WBCs or RBCs may be seen in the urine, especially when the appendix lies on or near the ureter. Large numbers of bacteria or pus in urine, not found in appendicitis, indicate probable urinary tract infection.

Abdominal radiographs confirm or rule out small-bowel obstruction, right lower quadrant mass, or fecalith. If the presentation and clinical and laboratory findings are not diagnostic, sonography, computed tomography (CT), or barium enema may be required for the diagnosis.

Differential Diagnosis

Many conditions may present with symptoms and signs that mimic acute appendicitis. These conditions include mesenteric adenitis ("pseudoappendicitis"), usually in younger patients and most frequently associated with enterocolitis from *Yersinia enterocolitica, Salmonella enteriditis,* and *Campylobacter jejuni; Yersinia pseudotuberculosis;* and occasionally urinary tract infections, constipation, intussusception, primary peritonitis, duodenal ulcer, measles, Epstein–Barr Virus (EBV) mononucleosis, Crohn disease, sickle cell disease, hemophilia, leukemia, Meckel's diverticulum, pneumonia, pelvic inflammatory disease, ovarian pathology, or mittelschmerz in females. In most instances, history and physical and laboratory findings may differentiate these problems from acute appendicitis, although the gastroenteritis and mesenteric adenitis syndromes just referred to may be particularly misleading, and their mimicry is often termed *pseudoappendicitis.* In patients with acquired immunodeficiency syndrome (AIDS), pseudoappendicitis also may be caused by bacterial typhlitis, cecal cytomegalovirus (CMV) infection, or tuberculosis.

Types of Appendicitis

Appendicitis is seen in five forms: simple acute, suppurative, gangrenous, perforated, and abscess (Table 52.1).

THERAPY

Although the literature describes treatment with antibiotics alone in selected patients with nonperforated appendicitis, in the author's opinion the optimal treatment of appendicitis is surgical removal of the affected organ. Surgery should be performed as soon as possible after diagnosis. Patients with signs of peritonitis with dehydration and electrolyte abnormalities should have fluid and electrolyte resuscitation for a few hours before surgery. This should be started promptly, but complete restoration of normality before the operation is not necessary. Ringer lactate solution and normal saline may

Table 52.1 Types of Appendicitis

Type	Characteristics
Simple acute	Mild hyperemia, edema, no serosal exudate
Suppurative	Edematous, congested vessels, fibrinopurulent exudate; peritoneal fluid increased, clear or turbid; may be early walling off by omentum and adjacent bowel or mesentery
Gangrenous	As above plus areas of gangrene, microperforations, increased and purulent peritoneal fluid
Perforated	Obvious defect in wall of appendix; peritoneal fluid thick and purulent; ileal obstruction possible
Abscess	Appendix may be sloughed; abscess at site of perforation: right iliac fossa, retrocecal, subcecal, or pelvic; may present rectally; thick, malodorous pus

be infused to correct fluid and electrolyte abnormalities. If there is evidence to suggest a ruptured appendix with peritonitis, a nasogastric tube should be inserted and placed on suction.

The operation is performed using a McBurney or Rocky-Davis incision, except in those instances in which the diagnosis is in doubt, especially in females. In those cases, a lower midline or right paramedian approach is preferred.

If there is an associated abscess, the appendix should be removed, unless extensive dissection is required to locate the appendix. The peritoneal cavity is irrigated copiously with saline. There is some question about the efficacy of antibiotics in the irrigant.

The abscess cavity should be drained and the drains brought out through a separate stab wound, not the incision. Usually three soft rubber (Penrose) drains are placed, one up to the subhepatic region on the right, a second into the pelvis, and a third down to the right gutter near the base of the cecum. The drains are left in place for 7 days, after which they are gradually removed over the next 2 to 3 days, by which time a definite tract should have developed. The tract should be allowed to close from the deeper to the superficial portion. The skin edges must not be allowed to seal until the tract has closed.

If the patient is not seen early in the course of the disease and when seen is improving and there is a palpable, nonobstructing right lower quadrant mass, nonoperative treatment is used by some. In such cases, an interval appendectomy is usually done 2 to 3 months after the patient has recovered and is free of abdominal complaints. Similarly, in patients in whom surgery reveals a well walled-off peri-appendiceal abscess, many surgeons simply drain the abscess to avoid general peritoneal contamination and perform an elective appendectomy 2 to 3 months later. This can be done laparoscopically.

Given the minimal morbidity of the procedure, some investigators believe that interval appendectomy done laparoscopically should be considered for most patients. Laparoscopic appendectomy may replace conventional appendectomy. In the pediatric surgery literature, it is suggested that laparoscopic appendectomy be avoided in children who have complicated appendicitis because of the increased risk for postoperative intra-abdominal abscesses. Laparoscopic appendectomy is currently widely used and has been reported as a safe alternative to open appendectomy in uncomplicated cases of acute appendicitis, but because of an increased rate of postlaparoscopic complications, it may be contraindicated in patients with gangrenous appendicitis, peritonitis, or abscess. The advocates of laparoscopic appendectomy stress that it can be done safely with minimal morbidity. The procedure takes more time and costs more. However, postdischarge recovery is shortened, and there is a better cosmetic result. There is no significant difference in length of hospital stay, oral feedings, or wound complications between open and laparoscopic appendectomy.

Antibiotic Regimens

The use of antibiotic prophylaxis for appendicitis is controversial. Many surgeons think antibiotics are not needed for a patient suspected of having acute appendicitis without evidence of peritonitis to suggest perforation or abscess. However, the efficacy of preoperative antibiotics in decreasing the infectious complications of appendicitis has been demonstrated. Also, the possibility of perforation at the time of initial evaluation of a patient has led to widespread use of preoperative antibiotics.

Antibiotic therapy should be given within 4 hours of surgery (usually 1 hour before). For acute, nonperforated appendicitis, antibiotics may not be necessary for more than 24 hours. In most instances, the single preoperative dose is all that is given. If an acute perforated appendix is found, antibiotics are given for 10 days. If a definite abscess is encountered, in addition to adequate drainage, antibiotic

Table 52.2 Duration of Antibiotic Regimens in Appendicitis

Type of Appendicitis	Duration of Therapy
Simple acute	Preoperatively and for 12–24 h postoperatively
Acute with perforation	Preoperatively and for 10 days postoperatively
Acute with abscess	Preoperatively and for as long as 21 days postoperatively

therapy should be continued for as long as 21 days (Table 52.2). This is a conservative regimen. The patient may be discharged when there are no longer signs of active disease and continue the remainder of the course of antibiotics on a home intravenous program or on an appropriate oral regimen.

There is no universal regimen for antibiotic use, though coverage should include activity against anaerobes, gram-negative enteric bacilli, and streptococci, in view of the polymicrobial nature of the infection. Thus, a single drug such as cefoxitan, cefotetan, ertapenem, ampicillin–sulbactam, ticarcillin–clavulanate or moxifloxacin may be employed, as well as combination regimens such as metronidazole combined with cefazolin or ceftriaxone or metronidazole combined with levofloxacin or ciprofloxacin. (For more detailed considerations of antimicrobial therapy of perforation or abscess, please see Chapter 56, Peritonitis.)

SUGGESTED READING

Fuchizaki U, Machi T, Kaneko S. Clinical challenges and images in GI. Yersinia enterocolitica mesenteric adenitis and terminal ileitis. *Gastroenterology*. 2006;131(5):1379, 1659.

Morrow SE, Newman KD. Current management of appendicitis. *Semin Pediatr Surg*. 2007;16(1):34–40.

Sauerland S, Lefering R, Neugebauer EA. Laparoscopic versus open surgery for suspected appendicitis. *Cochrane Database Syst Rev*. 2004;18(4):CD001546.

Styrud J, Erikssin S, Nilsson I, et al. Appendectomy versus antibiotic treatment in acute appendicitis: a prospective multicenter randomized controlled trial. *World J Surg*. 2006;30(6):1033–1037.

Thoeni RF, Cello JP. CT imaging of colitis. *Radiology*. 2006;240(3):623–638.

53. Diverticulitis

Ronald Lee Nichols and James R. Korndorffer, Jr.

Diverticulosis coli is an anatomic abnormality of the large bowel wall that manifests itself in various ways. Its occurrence varies greatly with such factors as geographic location, dietary habits, race, and age. In the United States, a third of the population over age 50 is affected.

The diagnosis of diverticulosis coli is often made incidentally in otherwise asymptomatic patients at the time of routine surveillance endoscopy or barium enema x-ray examination. However, unless a stricture is present, most of these patients require only counseling about possible infectious or hemorrhagic complications of the disease and the need for prophylactic measures such as a fiber-rich diet, adequate fluid consumption, and the prevention of constipation.

When clinical manifestations of diverticulosis occur, surgical intervention is necessary in only a minority of patients. These patients may have massive, or recurrent, gastrointestinal bleeding but more commonly have localized intra-abdominal abscess or generalized peritonitis that has developed after diverticular perforation.

Clinically significant diverticular disease and its complications continue to tax the diagnostic and therapeutic skills of physicians. Physical findings range from diffuse slight abdominal tenderness to shock secondary to either massive hemorrhage or overwhelming sepsis. During such life-threatening emergencies, the physician must be prepared to resuscitate the patient quickly and proceed to surgical intervention without benefit of a definite diagnosis.

DIAGNOSIS OF INFECTION

The most common clinically significant manifestations of diverticulosis are hemorrhage and infection (diverticulitis). In patients with signs of abdominal infection, including fever and abdominal pain and tenderness, usually in the left lower quadrant, it is often possible to make a presumptive diagnosis of acute diverticulitis on the basis of history, physical examination, and initial laboratory tests. This allows for the initiation of resuscitative measures, including empiric antibiotic therapy. Although further diagnostic radiographic procedures can be delayed for up to 2 days, if the patient continues to show signs of improvement, it is best to perform them as soon as possible to confirm the presumptive diagnosis.

Although ultrasonography is an effective and relatively inexpensive method of evaluating the abdomen and pelvis, particularly for imaging abscesses and their relationship to adnexal structures, most consider computed tomography (CT) to be superior, notably in the evaluation of right colon lesions, and safer than contrast enema studies. Others prefer the contrast enema as the most effective method of colonic imaging. Water-soluble contrast materials are preferred to barium to avoid barium peritonitis in case of perforation or leakage.

Once diverticulitis has been documented radiographically, further clinical decisions depend on the resolution of signs and symptoms of infection. If they resolve completely and the patient is stable, examine the entire large bowel endoscopically for neoplastic disease. Colonoscopy is best performed approximately 6 weeks after symptoms of diverticulitis have subsided so that enough time passes for resolution of any partial obstruction secondary to inflammatory changes in the bowel wall.

MANAGEMENT OF COMPLICATIONS

The greatest number of complications in colonic diverticular disease result from infection. They range from localized short segments of diverticulitis to abscesses and/or fistulas to free perforation with generalized peritonitis and overwhelming intra-abdominal sepsis (Figure 53.1). The cause of the diverticular perforation is not clear. Some authorities postulate that a surge in intraluminal pressure is often the cause, and others suggest ulceration, ischemia, and foreign-body perforation.

Peridiverticulitis

When ulceration or ischemia is not accompanied by free communication with the peritoneal

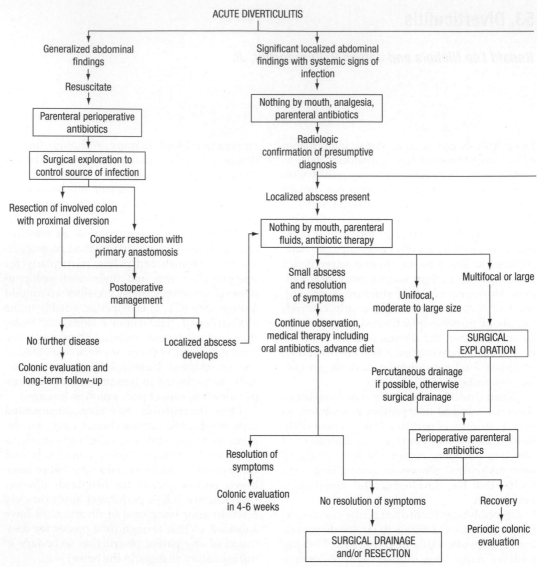

Figure 53.1 Algorithm for the work-up and treatment of acute diverticulitis.

cavity, penetration of mixed bacterial flora into the wall initiates peridiverticular infection.

Patients with localized peridiverticular disease usually complain of abdominal pain localized to the left lower quadrant. In some cases, however, a redundant sigmoid colon may have sufficient mobility to produce local symptoms in the right lower or right upper abdominal quadrant as well as in the midepigastrium. These patients are often febrile and have mild leukocytosis. However, they respond well to bowel rest, parenteral fluids, and antibiotic therapy. Nasogastric tube insertion is usually unnecessary unless obstructive signs and symptoms are present.

It is important that patients take nothing by mouth to abolish the gastrocolic reflex.

Most patients require a 3- to 5-day course of appropriate parenteral antimicrobials (Table 53.1). If they continue to improve, with normalization of the white blood cell (WBC) count, temperature, and abdominal examination, we discontinue their parenteral antibiotics and advance them to a regular diet that is devoid of poorly digestible foods (eg, whole corn).

Patients must be followed carefully after resolution of abdominal symptoms. If no disease other than diverticulosis is found on follow-up endoscopy, each patient should follow a fiber-supplemented diet with a generous consumption of fluids.

We do not recommend surgery after a single, uncomplicated episode of diverticulitis

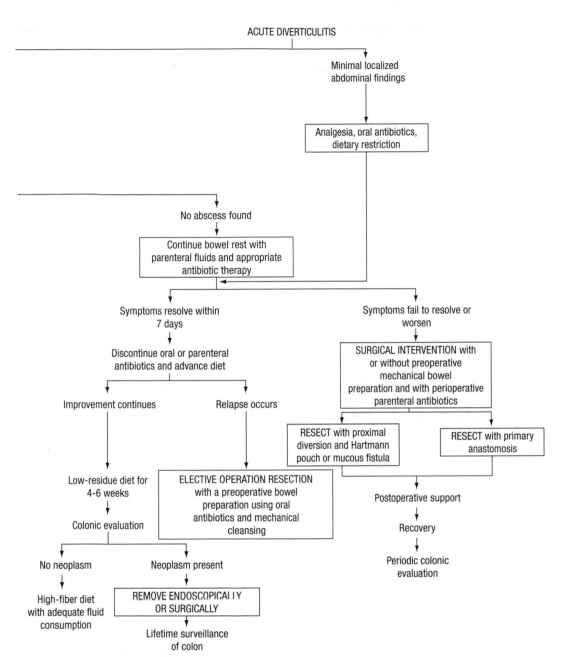

ACUTE DIVERTICULITIS

Minimal localized abdominal findings

Analgesia, oral antibiotics, dietary restriction

No abscess found

Continue bowel rest with parenteral fluids and appropriate antibiotic therapy

Symptoms resolve within 7 days

Symptoms fail to resolve or worsen

Discontinue oral or parenteral antibiotics and advance diet

SURGICAL INTERVENTION with or without preoperative mechanical bowel preparation and with perioperative parenteral antibiotics

Improvement continues

Relapse occurs

RESECT with proximal diversion and Hartmann pouch or mucous fistula

RESECT with primary anastomosis

Low-residue diet for 4-6 weeks

ELECTIVE OPERATION RESECTION with a preoperative bowel preparation using oral antibiotics and mechanical cleansing

Postoperative support

Colonic evaluation

Recovery

No neoplasm

Neoplasm present

Periodic colonic evaluation

High-fiber diet with adequate fluid consumption

REMOVE ENDOSCOPICALLY OR SURGICALLY

Lifetime surveillance of colon

in otherwise healthy patients. Rather, we recommend medical therapy when the first episode is mild and uncomplicated and advise patients younger than 40 years of age that a more aggressive form of the disease may develop.

Although the medical approach rarely fails to control the signs and symptoms of peridiverticulitis, surgical resection may become necessary if the infection does not resolve with prolonged parenteral antibiotic therapy. Occasionally, a major complication such as liver abscess or bacteremia develops and requires

colonic resection. However, patients with very limited symptoms and no signs of systemic sepsis may respond to oral regimens of antibiotics aimed at covering these colonic aerobes and anaerobes (Table 53.2).

Pericolic Disease

If the peridiverticular process fails to respond to antibiotic therapy or the patient presents in a late stage of the infectious process, an abscess may be present. Such a pericolic abscess can often be demonstrated by ultrasound or CT.

Table 53.1 Intravenous Antibiotics for Aerobic and Anaerobic Human Colonic Microflora

Drug	Dosage	Frequency
Combination Therapy		
Aerobic Coverage[a]		
Amikacin	15 mg/kg/d	BID-TID
Aztreonam	1–2 g	q8–12h
Ceftriaxone	1–2 g	qd
Ciprofloxacin	200–400 mg	ql2h
Gentamicin	3 mg/kg/d	q8h
Tobramycin	3 mg/kg/d	q8h
Anaerobic Coverage[b]		
Clindamycin	600–900 mg	q8h
Metronidazole	7.5 mg/kg	q6h
Single-Drug Therapy		
Aerobic-Anaerobic Coverage		
Ampicillin–sulbactam	1.5–3 g	q6h
Cefotetan	1–2 g	q8–12h
Cefoxitin	1–2 g	q6–8h
Imipenem–cilastatin	500 mg	q6h
Meropenem	1 g	q8h
Piperacillin–tazobactam	3.375–4.5 g	q6h
Ticarcillin–clavulanic acid	3.1 g	q6h
Tigecyline	100 mg (initial dose) then 50 mg	q12h

[a] To be combined with a drug exhibiting anaerobic activity.
[b] To be combined with a drug exhibiting aerobic activity.
Abbreviations: BID = twice a day.
TID = three times a day.

Table 53.2 Oral Antibiotic Regimens for Treatment of a Mild Episode of Acute Diverticulitis

Antibiotic	Dosage (mg)	Frequency-Duration
Ciprofloxacin	500	BID
Ciprofloxacin and Metronidazole	500 500	BID BID
TMP-SMX DS and Metronidazole	800 500	BID BID
Amoxicillin-clavulanic acid	250–500	TID
Doxycycline	100	q24h

Abbreviations: BID = twice a day.
TID = three times a day.
TMS-SMX DS = trimethoprim-sulfamethoxazole (Bactrim) double strength.

If these studies reveal a small cavity and the patient is improving dramatically, continuation of medical therapy and antibiotics may be warranted. In selected patients, percutaneous drainage of the abscess may be a useful adjunct to surgery. Decompressing the purulent contents of an abscess via CT-guided percutaneous catheter placement gains time to improve the patient's status with volume replacement, parenteral hyperalimentation, and appropriate antibiotic therapy. Once the abscess cavity has been resolved by catheter drainage, it is possible to prepare the bowel for elective resection of the diseased colon, often with primary anastomosis (Table 53.3).

Collections not accessible to percutaneous techniques or those associated with peritonitis are best treated surgically. There are two essential operative goals. The first is to resect the inflamed colon and control the associated septic complications; we believe surgical resection of the infectious source is superior to simple diversion of colonic contents (colostomy) and drainage. The second goal is to restore intestinal continuity. Although this may require a second procedure in some cases, we believe it can be accomplished safely during the same operation (single-stage procedure) in most patients. This is particularly true in individuals who are not hemodynamically compromised, who have localized diverticulitis, or who have diverticulitis with an associated mesocolonic abscess amenable to en bloc resection and with no intra-abdominal spillage of purulent material.

Another somewhat controversial technique is resection of the involved colon, usually the sigmoid, intraoperative lavage, and primary anastomosis. This procedure requires a team effort to keep control of either the proximal or distal colon during lavage, preventing gross peritoneal fecal contamination with its accompanying disastrous effects.

In summary, if emergency surgery is necessary for localized diverticulitis, we try to remove the inflamed colon, most often performing a primary anastomosis. If this is inadvisable because of hemodynamic instability or gross evidence of peritoneal contamination, we do an end colostomy with a distal pouch, usually using the Hartmann procedure or distal mucous

Table 53.3 Suggested Approach to Preperative Preparation for Elective Colon Resection

Two Days Before Surgery (at Home)

1. Low-residue or liquid diet *plus*
   sodium phosphate (Phosphosoda), 1½ oz PO at 6 PM
   or
2. Nothing additional until next day

One Day Before Surgery (at Home or in Hospital if Necessary)

Admit in morning (if necessary and allowed)
1. Continue clear liquid diet, IV fluids as needed *plus*
   sodium phosphate (Phosphosoda), 1½ oz PO at 6 AM
   or
2. Start clear liquid diet *plus*
   whole-gut lavage with polyethylene glycol, 1 L/h PO starting at 8 AM until diarrhea is clear (no longer than 3–4 h)
No enemas
All patients receive 1 g of neomycin PO and 1 g of erythromycin base PO at 1 PM, 2 PM, and 11 PM

Day of Surgery
Operation at 8 AM A single dose of antibiotic with broad-spectrum aerobic/anaerobic activity given IV by anesthesia personnel in the operating room just before incision; repeat dosage if operation lasts more than 2 h

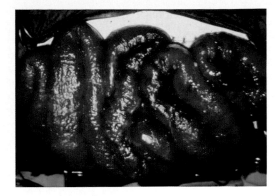

Figure 53.2 Generalized peritonitis occurring after free perforation of a sigmoid diverticula. Open midline incision reveals erythematous distended small intestine.

fistula. In modern surgery, diversion alone is rarely done as it has shown to result in a high mortality rate.

Generalized Intra-abdominal Sepsis

The cause of generalized abdominal findings suggesting intra-abdominal sepsis is often unknown before exploratory laporatomy. These patients require prompt fluid resuscitation and empiric antibiotic coverage with an agent or combination of agents that will control both aerobic and anaerobic enteric organisms (see Table 53.1). If there is evidence of perforation or if the patient is in shock, laparotomy as soon as the patient is stable is often necessary. Laparotomy often reveals fibrinous exudate, free pus, or abscesses throughout the abdominal cavity (Figure 53.2). If we find diverticulitis, we resect the involved segment and perform a proximal colostomy. Under these conditions, we do not consider performing a primary anastomosis. We prefer to leave a closed distal pouch, but only if there is no other obstructing or significant neoplastic lesion present. Such a lesion could produce a blind-loop syndrome and leakage of the distal pouch or could require another operation for its removal.

After resection, we copiously irrigate the abdominal cavity with normal saline. We strongly believe that if gross peritonitis is present, the skin wound should not be closed tightly if at all. Patients who have undergone such surgery usually require careful monitoring in an intensive care unit and appropriate antibiotic coverage.

Many of these patients develop secondary intra-abdominal or pelvic abscesses, which are detectable with CT or ultrasound. If percutaneous drainage is not succesful a feasible repeat laparotomy will likely be necessary. Many of these patients will also have prolonged ileus and therefore require parenteral hyperalimentation to meet the extraordinary metabolic demands of controlling intra-abdominal sepsis. Of course, enteral nutrition should be resumed as soon as possible. See also Chapter 54, Abdominal Abscess.

SUGGESTED READING

Krukowski ZH, Matheson NA. Emergency surgery for diverticular disease complicated by generalized and faecal peritonitis: a review. *Br J Surg.* 1984;17:921–927.

Nichols RL. Bowel preparation. In: Wilmore DW, et al. eds. *Care of the Surgical Patient.* New York, NY: Scientific American; 1995.

Nichols RL, Smith JW, Garcia RY, et al. Current practices of preoperative bowel preparation among North American colorectal surgeons. *Clin Infect Dis.* 1997;24:609–619.

Nichols RL. Current strategies for prevention of surgical site infections. *Curr Infect Dis Rep* 2004;6:426–434.

Nichols RL, Peritonitis. In: Gorbach SL, Bartlett JG, Blacklow NR, eds. *Infectious Diseases.*

3rd ed.Philadelphia, PA: Lippincott Williams & Wilkins; 2004:723–731.

Nichols RL, Choe RL, Weldon CB. Mechanical and antibacterial bowel preparation in colon and rectal surgery. *Chemotherapy*. 2005;51(Suppl 1):115–121.

The Standards Task Force of the American Society of Colon and Rectal Surgeons. Practice parameters for the treatment of sigmoid diverticulitis. *Dis Colon Rectum*. 2000;43: 289–297.

Clinical Syndromes – Gastrointestinal Tract, Liver, and Abdomen

54. Abdominal Abscess

Donald D. Trunkey

Abdominal abscess can follow primary intra-abdominal disease such as diverticulitis, appendicitis, biliary tract disease, pancreatitis, or perforated viscus; abdominal surgery; penetrating and blunt abdominal trauma; and bacteremic spread of infection from a distant source to an intra-abdominal site, particularly in the immunocompromised patient. The mortality rate is reported as high as 40%; however, recent studies suggest a mortality rate of 20%, with the reduction most likely the result of earlier diagnosis. The three distinct anatomic locations of abdominal abscesses are intraperitoneal, retroperitoneal, and visceral, the last developing in liver, gallbladder, spleen, pancreas, and kidney. Liver abscesses are covered in Chapter 45, Pyogenic Liver Abscess and pancreatic abscesses in Chapter 46, Infectious Complications of Acute Pancreatitis.

Bacteria in the peritoneal cavity are subject to the normal influences of gravity and pressure gradients. If the patient is upright, peritoneal fluid will collect within the dependent portion of the pelvis. Patients who are sick with an intra-peritoneal process such as peritonitis typically are supine, and their dependent positions are the subphrenic space and the pericolic gutters. Pressure gradients within the peritoneal cavity are due to motion of the diaphragm. With expiration, relative negative pressure beneath the diaphragm sets up a current of movement that favors fluid moving from the pericolic space to the subhepatic and subphrenic space. These currents allow the bacteria to come into contact with the diaphragmatic surface, which has lymphatic fenestrations and is an important means of clearing bacteria from the celomic cavity. Equally important is the clearance of bacteria by macrophages and neutrophils.

Initially, macrophages are the primary white cells in peritonitis; they are followed in a few hours by neutrophils. The exudate typically associated with peritonitis may approach 300 to 500 mL of fluid per hour. This contributes not only to hypovolemia and shock but perhaps also to impaired clearance of bacteria when fibrin blocks the fenestrations in the diaphragm.

Other factors contributing to abscess formation are adjuvants, which include hemoglobin, hematoma, dead tissue, and foreign bodies. Hypovolemia and hemorrhagic shock also enhance the frequency and severity of infection. Blood transfusion has been indicated as a potential contributor to intraperitoneal sepsis because it is immunosuppressive. The diabetic patient may be at increased risk because some host defense mechanisms are impaired. Protein–calorie malnutrition and antecedent steroid therapy also may contribute to formation of intra-abdominal abscess.

Finally, abdominal abscess should be viewed as a continuum in the systemic inflammatory response syndrome. On one hand, formation of an abdominal abscess may represent a success from the host defense viewpoint because the infection is now localized and walled off. On the other hand, many abdominal abscesses progress to severe sepsis and septic shock, particularly when left untreated. Furthermore, low pH, larger bacterial inocula, poor perfusion, the presence of hemoglobin, and large amounts of fibrin make the abscess an ideal environment that is penetrated poorly by many antimicrobial therapies.

CLINICAL FEATURES

The clinical presentation of an abdominal abscess is greatly influenced by the immunocompetence of the host. The nonimmunocompromised patient typically has a spiking fever, abdominal pain, and tenderness. There is a leukocytosis of 15 000 to 25 000/mm^3. Pleural fluid is present in about 80% of patients with subphrenic abscess. Occasionally, there is intrathoracic spread of an abdominal abscess, which presents as empyema, cough, and even formation of a bronchopleural fistula with resultant thick, foul-smelling sputum. Less often, the patient may develop a chronic intra-abdominal abscess that smolders for many weeks or even months. These patients have a fever of unknown origin and as time progresses often become cachectic. Similarly, patients with tuberculosis splenic abscesses often present as a chronic cachectic disease.

In contrast, the immunocompromised patient has blunting of the clinical symptoms. Fever may be absent, rebound tenderness and guarding are markedly diminished or absent, and leukocytosis is not a reliable indicator of sepsis. Unfortunately, intra-abdominal abscess is increasing in the immunocompromised patient, and mortality is significantly higher than in the nonimmunocompromised patient.

DIAGNOSIS

At present, computed tomography (CT) is the gold standard for diagnosis of abdominal abscess. CT has a sensitivity of 78% to 100%, and ultrasound has a sensitivity of 75% to 82%. Magnetic resonance imaging (MRI) is no better than CT; however, there are recent articles expressing some concern for repeated CT scans and increased risk later for cancer particularly in children. Computed tomography is superior to ultrasound for all anatomic sites with the possible exception of the pelvis. Computed tomography scan can be done in almost all patients, including those with wounds, dressings, ostomies, and drains. In an era of managed care, it is imprudent from a cost standpoint to do plain films, which help with fewer than 50% of patients. Similarly, scintigraphy, arteriograms, and radio contrast studies lack sensitivity and specificity. Sequential testing is more costly than CT scanning, and with spiral CT, time is no longer a major consideration. The interventional radiologist should be aware when the CT is done that abdominal abscess is being considered. If an abscess is found, the patient can often have percutaneous drainage immediately upon diagnosis.

THERAPY

There are three major considerations for optimal management of the patient with abdominal abscess. First and foremost is drainage of the abscess. Second is appropriate antibiotic therapy, and third is physiologic support for the patient.

Since 1980, there has been a shift from open abdominal to percutaneous drainage. The results of percutaneous drainage appear to be equal clinically and more cost-effective in the nonimmunocompromised patient. Although there have been no randomized trials, the only advantage of abdominal drainage is that the length of stay in the hospital is shorter than with percutaneous drainage. However, percutaneous drainage has been more problematic in the immunocompromised host. This may be because of a higher incidence of fungal infections which are associated with tissue invasion.

Percutaneous drainage is done with CT or ultrasound guidance. If the patient's symptoms have not improved within 48 to 72 hours, open abdominal drainage should be strongly considered. In certain high-risk immunocompromised patients, open abdominal drainage may be the procedure of choice. This depends on the infecting organism and the extent of the abscess. Percutaneous drainage can also be used for splenic and renal abscess. A contraindication to percutaneous drainage is lack of a safe access route. A safe drainage route is identified in 85% to 90% of patients. Pelvic abscess may be best drained by transrectal technique. Percutaneous drainage results are problematic for abscesses in the posterior subphrenic space or in the porta hepatica, for those abscesses among loops of small bowel, for suspected echinococcal cysts, and for abscesses containing necrotic or neoplastic tissue.

In complex abscesses and immunocompromised patients, open drainage allows debridement of the abscess wall. A modification of open abdominal drainage is planned relaparotomy (etappenlavage). One study suggests a diminishing point of return after three laparotomies or when the bacterial count falls below 10^5 organisms/mL. Another review recommends initial antimicrobial therapy only for abscesses less than 3 cm in size; those greater than 3 cm require drainage.

Antimicrobial Treatment

In the nonimmunocompromised patient, anaerobic bacteria are isolated in up to 60% to 70% of abdominal abscesses. Commonly isolated bacteria include *Bacteroides fragilis*, peptostreptococci and peptococci, *Clostridium* species, *Escherichia coli*, *Enterobacter* and *Klebsiella* organisms, and enterococci. *Staphylococcus aureus* is uncommon in intra-abdominal abscess and suggests bacteremic seeding, an immunocompromised patient, or vertebral osteomyelitis. *Candida* also suggests an immunocompromised host or previous antimicrobial therapy. *Pseudomonas* species, *Serratia* species, cytomegalovirus, *Coccidioides immitis*, *Cryptococcus neoformans*, and *Mycobacterium avium* are also found in the immunocompromised patient.

Antimicrobial therapy for abdominal abscesses should be based on specific cultures when possible. If the organism is not known, therapy should be directed by Gram stain.

Broad-spectrum coverage should be avoided when possible, and when it does become necessary, cyclic administration of antibiotics within the institution may avoid resistance problems and opportunistic infections. Until definitive cultures are available, broad-spectrum antibiotics, including anaerobic coverage, are indicated. An aminoglycoside plus metronidazole is a good choice for the patient who is only mildly to moderately ill. *Bacteroides fragilis* has an increasing prevalence of resistance to clindamycin, making clindamycin less dependable as a first-line agent. If the patient is at risk for aminoglycoside toxicity (antecedent renal failure, hypovolemic shock, severe trauma), an alternative therapeutic regimen is the substitution of a quinolone or a third-generation cephalosporin for the aminoglycoside. The monobactam aztreonam is also a good choice when *Pseudomonas* is strongly suspected; however, anaerobic coverage must be added to this drug. Additional agents useful as monotherapy are the combinations piperacillin–tazobactam, imipenem–cilastatin, or ampicillin–sulbactam. If the patient is immunocompromised or has recent isolation of *Candida* from the urine or tracheobronchial tree, amphotericin B or fluconazole should accompany the initial treatment. A Gram stain and fungal preparations should always be obtained from the abscess cavity. If the Gram stain shows a predominance of gram-positive cocci in chains, ampicillin may be added for activity against *Enterococcus* species.

COMPLICATIONS

Open drainage of the abdominal abscess has been associated with enteric fistula formation. Percutaneous drainage has a small but predictable failure rate; failure requires open drainage. All abdominal abscesses may progress to septicemia, septic shock, and sequential organ failure. Abdominal abscess can be a major cause of adult respiratory distress syndrome, renal failure, and liver failure. In addition to the appropriate individual organ support measures carried out in an intensive care setting, attention must be directed to adequate nutrition. Studies show that enteral nutrition is superior to parenteral nutrition.

SUGGESTED READING

Barie PS, Hydo LJ, Eachempati SR. Longitudinal outcomes of intra-abdominal infection complicated by critical illness. *Surg Infect.* 2004;5(4):365–373.

Bone RC. Sepsis, the sepsis syndrome, multiorgan failure: a plea for comparable definition. *Ann Intern Med.* 1991;114:332–333.

Kumar RR, Kim JT, Haukoos JS, et al. Factors affecting the successful management of intra-abdominal abscesses with antibiotics and the need for percutaneous drainage. *Dis Colon Rectum.* 2006;49(2):183–189.

Siewert B, Tye G, Kruskal J, Sosna J, Opelka F. Impact of CT-guided drainage in the treatment of diverticular abscesses: size matters. *Am J Radiol.* 2006;186(3):680–686.

Sirinek KR. Diagnosis and treatment of intra-abdominal abscesses. *Surg Infect.* 2000;1(1):31–38.

Swartz MN, Simon HB. Peritonitis and intraabdominal abscesses. *Sci Am.* 1995;23:1.

Thompson AE, Marshall JC, Opal SM. Intraabdominal infections in infants and children: descriptions and definitions. *Ped Crit Care Med.* 2005;6:S30–S35.

55. Splenic Abscess

Naveed Saqib and Thomas R. Howdieshell

The diagnosis of splenic abscess is often over-looked because of its rarity and misleading clinical features, as well as the presence of pre-disposing conditions that obscure its clinical presentation. Hence, it is not surprising that splenic abscess is often diagnosed during post-mortem examinations (0.2% to 0.7% incidence in various autopsy series), even in the era of antibiotics. Contributing factors to an apparent increase in the incidence of splenic abscess in-clude advances in radiologic imaging, comfort with nonoperative management of blunt splenic trauma, and a greater number of patients who have cancer or are immunocompromised.

INCIDENCE AND PREDISPOSING FACTORS

Splenic abscesses occur more commonly in males (55% to 60% in several series), with the average age ranging from 25 to 54 years. Nelken et al. describe a bimodal distribution: patients younger than 40 years of age; gener-ally immunosuppressed or drug addicts, who usually present with a multilocular abscess; and patients older than 70 years of age who are suf-fering from diabetes and/or a nonendocarditic septic focus and develop a unilocular abscess.

The primary predisposing causes of splenic abscess include metastatic hematogenous infec-tion, contiguous disease processes extending to the spleen, splenic trauma, hematologic disor-ders (collagen-vascular diseases, hemoglobin-opathies, malignancy), and immunodeficiency states (acquired, congenital). The incidence of these predisposing causes or risk factors is shown in Table 55.1.

METASTATIC HEMATOGENOUS INFECTIONS

Infective endocarditis is the most common con-dition predisposing a patient to splenic abscess (Figure 55.1). Although the exact incidence is difficult to determine, several studies demon-strated the occurrence of splenic embolization in 31% to 44% of the patients with endocarditis. Histologic examination disclosed splenitis in at

Table 55.1 Primary Predisposing Causes or Risk Factors for Splenic Abscess

Factors	Percentage
Infectious etiology	**68.8**
Endocarditis	15.3
Septic syndrome	11.9
Miscellaneous	11.9
Urinary infection	7.1
Otitis	3.3
Appendicitis	2.8
Pneumonia	2.8
Brucellosis	2.3
Lung abscess	2.3
Malaria	1.9
Diverticulitis	1.9
Amebiasis	0.95
Noninfectious etiology	**31.2**
Contiguous diseases	23.0
Trauma	16.7
Hemoglobinopathies	11.9

least 20% of patients. Splenic infarction occurred in 30% to 67% of patients with endocarditis dur-ing the preantibiotic era and in 33% to 44% of these patients during the antibiotic era. In 1977, Pelletier and Petersdorf reported the incidence of splenic abscess in patients with subacute bac-terial endocarditis to be approximately 2.4%. Mycotic aneurysms are seen angiographically within abscesses, but whether these predispose a patient to, or result from, splenic abscess re-mains uncertain.

In addition to endocarditis, a multitude of other infections have been reported as primary causes of splenic abscess (see Table 55.1). Miscellaneous infections include dental abscess,

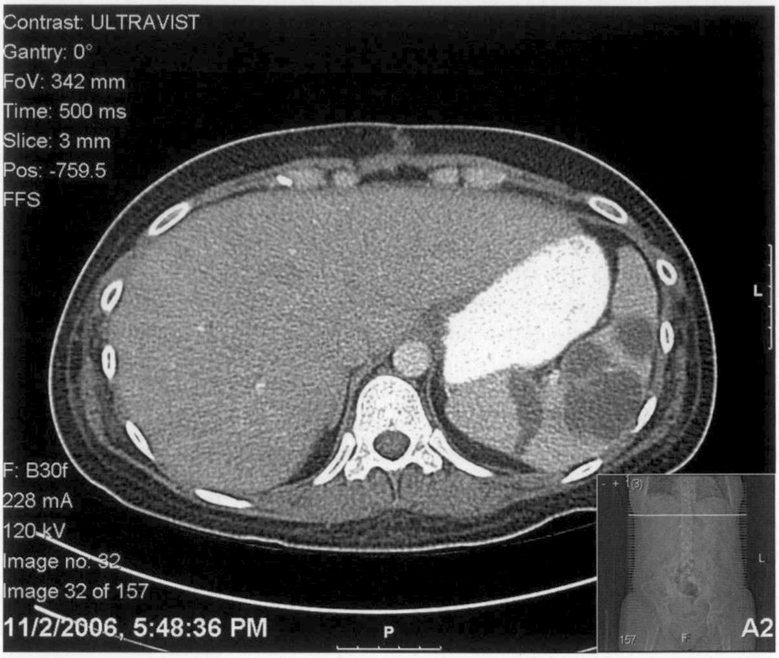

Figure 55.1 Multilocular splenic abscess in an intravenous drug abuse patient with bacterial endocarditis.

bacteremia after dental extraction, tonsillectomy, peritonsillar abscess, acute parotitis, bronchiectasis, perinephric abscess, decubitus ulcer, complicated infectious mononucleosis, tuberculosis, yellow fever, typhoid fever, diphtheria, and anthrax.

CONTIGUOUS INFECTION

On occasion, splenic abscess can result from the direct extension of disease having its primary focus in adjacent organs. Contiguous extension from diverticulitis, pancreatic pseudocyst or carcinoma, gastric ulcer, carcinoma of the stomach, perihepatic abscess, perinephric and subphrenic abscess, and carcinoma of the descending colon have been reported.

TRAUMATIC ABSCESS

Traumatic abscess results from secondary infection and suppuration of contused parenchyma or of a hematoma arising from injury to splenic tissue. In a report by Phillips et al., the initial traumatic injury was not easily recognized or reported, and most patients developed signs and symptoms of splenic infection after a latent period of 2 weeks to 4 months after sustaining injuries to the left upper quadrant. Splenic abscess has been reported after operative repair of splenic injury (splenorrhaphy) and nonoperative management of blunt splenic injuries diagnosed by computed tomography (CT) scan (Figure 55.2). On

occasion, radiologic procedures such as splenic artery embolization for hemorrhage control following traumatic injury or splenoportography for portocaval shunt evaluation have been implicated as causes of splenic abscess.

HEMATOLOGIC DISORDERS

Hemoglobinopathies accounted for approximately 12% of splenic abscesses reported by Alonso Cohen et al. Patients with sickle cell disease have an increased risk of acquiring invasive bacterial infections as a result of hyposplenism, including functional defects in opsonization, phagocytic function, and cell-mediated immunity. If a patient with sickle cell disease and prior splenic infarcts develops a transient bacteremia from a central line infection or cholecystitis, bacteria may seed the infarcted regions with resultant abscess formation.

The spleen may also be a site of infection in patients with collagen-vascular diseases. Splenic abscesses have been reported in patients with rheumatoid arthritis, systemic lupus erythematosus, and polyarteritis nodosa. Pathologic features of the spleen in these illnesses include capsulitis and small infarcts.

IMMUNODEFICIENCY STATES

Splenic abscess has been reported complicating acquired immunodeficiency syndrome (AIDS), chemotherapy, cancer (leukemia,

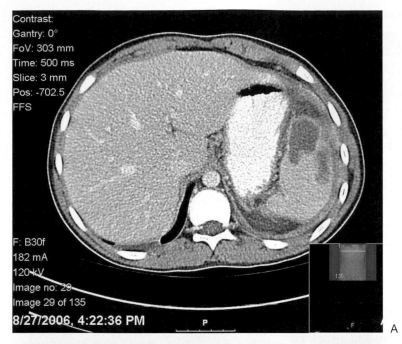

A

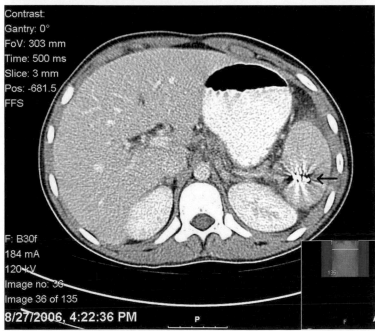

B

Figure 55.2 (A and B) Splenic abscess following nonoperative management of blunt splenic injury including splenic artery embolization. Note embolization coil (B, see arrow).

lymphoma), bone marrow and solid organ transplantation, long-term steroid use, and conditions such as diabetes mellitus and alcoholism.

DIAGNOSIS

History and Physical Examination

The signs and symptoms of a splenic abscess are often insidious, nonspecific, and related to the underlying disease. Table 55.2 characterizes the clinical findings in 227 patients. Fever is the most common symptom, but pain in the left hypochondrium appears in a minority of cases, with vague abdominal pain being more common. Pain is probably caused by splenitis with capsular involvement. Abscesses located in the upper pole of the spleen tend to irritate the diaphragm causing radiation of pain toward the left shoulder (Kehr sign) and an elevated, immobile

Table 55.2 Clinical Findings in Splenic Abscess

Clinical Feature	Percentage
Fever	92.5
Abdominal tenderness	60.1
Abdominal pain	57.5
Splenomegaly	56.0
Left upper quadrant pain	39.2
Pleuritic pain	15.8
Toxic syndrome	15.4
Vomiting	14.0

left hemidiaphragm. Splenic rupture also commonly manifests as left shoulder pain. An abscess located in the lower pole of the spleen more often irritates the peritoneal surface, resulting predominantly in signs and symptoms of peritonitis. A deep-seated abscess that does not involve the splenic capsule may be accompanied only by nonspecific symptoms of infection without pain or other localizing signs.

Laboratory Findings

Leukocytosis is present in 70% to 80% of patients, but is a variable finding. In several series, the white cell count varied between 2400 and 41000 cells/mm^3. In general, other serum laboratory studies were not helpful. Blood cultures were positive in 50% to 70% of patients. Of these positive blood cultures, 60% to 75% grew the same organisms as those subsequently isolated from the splenic abscess.

The infecting organisms and their incidence from a review of 189 patients of Nelken and others are reported in Table 55.3. The increasing number of splenic abscesses resulting from gram-negative organisms appears to be related to the widespread use of broad-spectrum antibiotics, the improved survival of critically ill patients colonized with these bacteria, and prolonged hospitalization, each increasing the risk of nosocomial infection. *Candida* abscesses of the spleen are seen almost exclusively in neutropenic patients with the exception of disseminated candidiasis as a complication of abdominal surgery. Fungal abscesses due to *Candida* are also more likely to complicate the use of broad-spectrum antibiotics, indwelling central venous lines, total parenteral nutrition, systemic steroids, cytotoxic chemotherapy, or immunosuppression

Table 55.3 Infecting Organisms and Their Incidence in Splenic Abscess

Organism	Percentage
Aerobic bacteria ($n = 90$)	**56**
All *Staphylococcus*	20
All *Salmonella*	15
Escherichia coli	15
Enterococcus	8
Salmonella typhi	7
Unspecified *Streptococcus*	6
Unspecified coliforms	6
Staphylococcus epidermidis	4
α-*Streptococcus*	4
Klebsiella	3
Enterobacter	2
Proteus	2
Pseudomonas aeruginosa	2
Shigella	2
Diphtheroids	2
β-Hemolytic *Streptococcus*	1
Nonhemolytic *Streptococcus*	1
Fungi ($n = 41$)	**26**
Candida albicans	42
Candida tropicalis	21
Aspergillus	10
Blastomycosis	5
Aureobassidium pullulans	2
Anaerobic bacteria ($n = 28$)	**18**
Mixed	30
Bacteroides	23
Propionobacterium species	20
Clostridium	13
Streptococcus	10
Fusobacterium	4
Actinomyces	0

after organ transplantation. Organisms responsible for AIDS-related splenic abscesses include *Salmonella, Mycobacterium avium-intracellulare, Candida, Aspergillus,* and *Pneumocystis carinii.* In several series, approximately one fourth of patients with a splenic abscess did not have an organism cultured from the abscess cavity, possibly related to the use of intravenous antibiotic therapy prior to abscess drainage.

Radiographic Findings

The most common findings on chest radiography are an elevated left hemidiaphragm (31%), pleural effusion (28%), and left basilar pulmonary consolidation (18%). Plain abdominal films reveal an abnormal soft tissue density or gas pattern in only 35% of patients. Computed tomography scanning, with a sensitivity of 96% and an associated specificity between 90% and 95%, is currently the best diagnostic test for splenic abscess. Computed tomography scan may show a homogeneous low-density area, with or without rim enhancement; lucent areas within the spleen containing fluid levels of different densities; and intrasplenic gas formation. This gas may be dispersed diffusely through the abscess as fine, low-attenuation bubbles or may coalesce into one or more larger collections. Computed tomography scan may also be a therapeutic choice, aiding or guiding percutaneous abscess drainage.

Ultrasonography has a sensitivity of 60% to 75% in the detection of splenic abscess. The ultrasound appearance of splenic abscess is characterized as a hypoechoic or nearly anechoic, ovoid- or round-shaped area in the spleen, with varying internal echogenicity, irregular wall, and mild to moderate distal acoustic enhancement. Ultrasonic examinations are not specific, and the findings are highly variable and may be difficult to interpret. However, ultrasonography is low cost, noninvasive, and readily repeatable to evaluate for interval change or resolution.

Differential Diagnosis

The differential diagnosis should include intraparenchymal hematoma, splenic infarction, parasitic and nonparasitic splenic cysts, subphrenic abscess, pulmonary empyema, perinephric abscess, neoplasm, and leukemic infiltration. In a review of 3372 subphrenic abscesses, Ochsner and Graves found a primary lesion in the spleen in approximately 4% of the cases. Therefore, the possibility of coexistent

splenic abscess should be considered in the presence of a subphrenic abscess. Pulmonary empyema as a complication of splenic abscess (4%) may also divert the clinician's attention from the primary lesion.

TREATMENT

There is no place for long-term medical management of a clinically overt splenic abscess. The mainstay of treatment consists of splenectomy and appropriate antibiotics, with a success rate of 86% to 94%. Recent evidence has shown that percutaneous drainage plus effective antibiotics is a safe and efficacious therapy. Percutaneous drainage may be used if the patient has a unilocular abscess, is in unstable condition from a recent operation, has had multiple previous operations, or has significant risks for general anesthesia or standard surgical drainage. The catheter can be removed when the drainage is minimal and the cavity has decreased in size as evidenced by sinogram, ultrasound, or CT scan. If the patient does not improve clinically, splenectomy is recommended. Percutaneous drainage is most likely to succeed when the abscess collection is unilocular, has a discrete wall, and has no internal septation. Abscesses containing thick, tenacious, necrotic debris are less likely to be successfully drained percutaneously, as are phlegmons, poorly defined cavities, microabscesses, multiple abscesses, and abscesses originating from a contiguous process. However, for a single loculation, percutaneous drainage has been reported to be effective in 68% to 75% of cases. Complications associated with percutaneous drainage include hemorrhage, pleural empyema, pneumothorax (transpleural catheterization), and fistula.

Broad-spectrum antibiotics should be initiated when a splenic abscess is diagnosed. This therapy should include agents effective against staphylococci (including methicillin-resistant *Staphylococcus aureus* [MRSA] if local resistance patterns make this a reasonable possibility), streptococci, and gram-negative bacteria. A semisynthetic penicillin or advanced generation cephalosporin plus an aminoglycoside are recommended. If a contiguous abdominal process is suspected, anaerobic agents such as clindamycin or metronidazole should be added. In immunosuppressed patients, antifungal coverage such as fluconazole should be initiated early in the disease process. Some authors recommend continuing antibiotics for 2 to 3 weeks after splenectomy or discontinuation of percutaneous drainage.

The optimal management of fungal splenic abscess remains to be defined. Some authors have suggested prolonged courses of amphotericin B with a total dose ranging from 500 mg to 2 g. Others have suggested splenectomy in conjunction with amphotericin B for the treatment of fungal splenic abscess. The argument in support of splenectomy for fungal abscess is based primarily on reports of bacterial splenic abscess in which nonoperative therapy was associated with high mortality. However, because most cases of splenic candidiasis represent disseminated infection, splenectomy does not address the problem of *Candida* present in other tissues, most notably the liver. There are many reports of confirmed splenic fungal abscesses resolving with antifungal drugs alone. Several case reports and a recent multicenter randomized trial in patients without neutropenia or major immune deficiency indicate that fluconazole may be as efficacious as amphotericin B. Patients suspected of having a fungal abscess should have a specific diagnosis made by percutaneous aspiration of the liver or spleen or laparoscopic or open biopsy of the lesions. This is important because the differential diagnosis includes leukemic infiltrates, metastatic tumor, and fungal and bacterial abscesses.

Splenic abscess may rupture into the peritoneal cavity, thus causing acute peritonitis. A mortality rate of 50% has been reported in cases of splenic abscess rupture. A splenic abscess may also drain into the stomach, colon, or pleura. However, splenic abscesses most commonly produce repeated bacteremia, which ends in septic shock if not treated. Two thirds of all splenic abscesses in adults are solitary, and one third are multiple. In children, however, the opposite is true. Solitary abscesses generally are easier to diagnose and treat, and usually are caused by streptococci, staphylococci, or *Salmonella*. Multiple abscesses tend to be caused by gram-negative bacilli or *Candida*. The prognosis is clearly related to patient age, associated diseases, and development of multisystem organ failure.

With early diagnosis and treatment of splenic abscess, the mortality rate can be as low as 7%. Medical therapy appears appropriate for patients with mycobacterial, *Pneumocystis carinii*, and fungal disease. Percutaneous drainage appears reasonable for patients with a singular, unilocular abscess without associated intra-abdominal disease. In patients in whom there is any question as to the accessibility, locularity, or singularity of the abscess, or if there is a question of intra-abdominal pathology, splenectomy remains the treatment of choice.

SUGGESTED READING

Alonso Cohen MA, Galera MJ, Ruiz M, et al. Splenic abscess. *World J Surg*. 1990;14:513–516; discussion 516–517.

Chang KC, Chuah SK, Changchien CS, et al. Clinical characteristics and prognostic factors of splenic abscess: a review of 67 cases in a single medical center of Taiwan. *World J Gastroenterol*. 2006;12:460–464.

Ekeh AP, McCarthy MC, Woods RJ, et al. Complications arising from splenic embolization after blunt splenic trauma. *Am J Surg*. 2005;189:335–339.

Johnson JD, Raff MJ, Barnwell PA, et al. Splenic abscess complicating infectious endocarditis. *Arch Intern Med*. 1983;143:906–912.

Nelken N, Ignatius J, Skinner M, et al. Changing clinical spectrum of splenic abscess. A multicenter study and review of the literature. *Am J Surg*. 1987;154:27–34.

Ochsner A, Graves AM. Subphrenic Abscess: An analysis of 3,372 collected and personal cases. *Ann Surg*. 1933 Dec; 98(6):961–90.

Pelletier LL Jr, Petersdorf RG. Infective endocarditis: a review of 125 cases from the University of Washington Hospitals, 1963–72. *Medicine (Baltimore)*, 1977 Jul; 56(4):287–313.

Phillips GS, Radosevich MD, Lipsett PA. Splenic abscess: another look at an old disease. *Arch Surg*. 1997;132:1331–1335, discussion 1335–1336.

Rex JH, Bennett JE, Sugar AM, et al. A randomized trial comparing fluconazole with amphotericin B for the treatment of candidemia in patients without neutropenia. *N Engl J Med*. 1994;331:1325–1330.

Thanos L, Dailiana T, Papaioahnou, et al. Percutaneous CT-guided drainage of splenic abscess. *AJR Am J Roentgenol*. 2002;179:629–632.

Tung CC, Chen FC, Lo CI. Splenic abscess: an easily overlooked disease? *Am Surg*. 2006;72:322–325.

56. Peritonitis

Linda A. Slavoski and Matthew E. Levison

Peritonitis is inflammation of the serous lining of the peritoneal cavity. This inflammation may result from a response to microorganisms and/or chemical irritants, such as blood, bile, and pancreatic secretions. The peritoneal cavity is lubricated with 20 to 50 mL of clear yellow transudative fluid, normally with fewer than 300 cells/mm^3 (consisting of mainly mononuclear cells), a specific gravity below 1.016, and protein (consisting of mainly albumin) below 3 g/dL.

In this chapter infectious causes of peritonitis are considered. Two major types of infective peritonitis exist: (1) primary (spontaneous or idiopathic) and (2) secondary. When signs of peritonitis and sepsis persist after treatment for secondary peritonitis and no pathogens or usually only low-grade pathogens are isolated, the clinical entity has been termed *tertiary peritonitis*. Intraperitoneal abscesses can result from (1) localization of the initially diffuse peritoneal inflammatory response to one or more dependent sites (ie, the pelvis, the right or left subphrenic spaces, which are separated by the falciform ligament, and Morrison's pouch, which is the most posterior superior portion of the subhepatic space and is the lowest part of the paravertebral groove when the patient is recumbent) or (2) at the site of the intra-abdominal source of the infection (eg, periappendiceal, pericholecystic, or peridiverticular abscess). Peritonitis may also result from the use of a peritoneal catheter for dialysis or central nervous system ventriculo-peritoneal shunting. For management of peritoneal catheter-related peritonitis, see Chapter 94, Dialysis-Related Infection.

PRIMARY PERITONITIS

Primary peritonitis is best defined as infection of the peritoneal cavity without an evident source in the abdominal cavity. Primary peritonitis occurs at all ages. In children it particularly occurs in association with postnecrotic cirrhosis and with nephrotic syndrome. Primary peritonitis, also called *spontaneous bacterial peritonitis*, in the adult is seen most commonly in association with ascites from any cause but most commonly alcoholic cirrhosis, especially in its end stage. It has been seen also with ascites caused by postnecrotic cirrhosis, chronic active hepatitis, acute viral hepatitis, congestive heart failure, malignancy, systemic lupus erythematosus, and nephrotic syndrome. Rarely, primary peritonitis occurs with no apparent underlying disease. Primary peritonitis has been reported in 10% of all hospitalized patients with alcoholic cirrhosis and ascites.

Primary peritonitis is a monomicrobial infection and only very rarely involves obligate anaerobes; if ascitic fluid cultures reveal a polymicrobial or anaerobic infection, secondary peritonitis should be suspected. The organisms reported to cause primary peritonitis in children are *Streptococcus pneumoniae* and group A streptococci. These organisms are much less important now and have been replaced by gram-negative bacilli and, to a lesser extent, staphylococci. In adults gram-negative bacilli also predominate, followed by streptococci and other gram-positive cocci. *Escherichia coli* is the most frequently isolated pathogen, followed by *Klebsiella* species, *S. pneumoniae*, and other streptococcal species, including enterococci. *Staphylococcus aureus* is rare in primary peritonitis. Cases with positive ascitic fluid culture but with low leukocyte counts and no clinical findings of peritonitis have been designated as bacterascites. This may represent early colonization of the peritoneal cavity. Conversely, some patients have clinical evidence of peritonitis, elevated leukocyte counts in the ascitic fluid, but negative cultures in the absence of recent antibiotic use. These have been called *culture-negative neutrocytic ascites*.

The route of infection in primary peritonitis may be hematogenous, lymphogenous, via transmural migration through the intact bowel wall, or, in women, from the vagina via the fallopian tubes. Seeding of ascitic fluid during bacteremia is probably the most common route. Pathogenetic mechanisms in cirrhosis are likely to be bacterial overgrowth in the upper intestinal tract, alterations in the intestinal mucosal barrier, translocation to the regional mesenteric lymph nodes, and from there into the blood stream. In addition, clearance of bacteria from blood is delayed in patients with cirrhosis due to decreased phagocytic activity within the reticuloendothelial system, impaired intracellular killing by neutrophils and monocytes, impaired opsinization, and low serum and ascitic complement levels.

The clinical features of primary peritonitis are variable. In children it is often confused with acute appendicitis. The most common sign is fever (often low grade) reported to occur in up to 80% of patients. Fever may be present without abdominal signs or symptoms, or the intraperitoneal infection may be clinically silent. Ascites that predates the infection is almost always present. Other signs and symptoms include abdominal pain, nausea, vomiting, diarrhea, diffuse abdominal tenderness, rebound tenderness, and hypoactive to absent bowel sounds. Atypical signs such as hypothermia, hypotension, and unexplained decline in renal function may be present, as well as unexplained encephalopathy, hepatorenal syndrome, and variceal bleeding in cirrhotic patients. Because peritonitis may be clinically inapparent in a patient with ascites and decompensated liver disease, routine paracentesis is necessary in every hospitalized cirrhotic patient with ascites, especially if febrile, to disclose its presence.

The diagnosis of primary peritonitis requires that the possibility of an intra-abdominal source of infection be excluded, usually by means of contrast-enhanced computed tomography (CT). Examination of the ascitic fluid is required. The ascitic fluid leukocyte count is generally greater than 250 polymorphonuclear leukocytes/mm^3. Gram stain of the fluid is commonly negative because of the low bacterial density in ascitic fluid. The diagnostic yield of ascitic fluid culture can be enhanced by culturing a relatively large volume (eg, 10 mL). Blood cultures should also be obtained because concurrent bacteremia is often present.

Because the Gram stain is often negative in primary peritonitis, the initial choice of antimicrobial agents is often empiric and is modified once results of cultures and susceptibility testing are available. Initial therapy should be directed against enteric gram-negative bacilli and gram-positive cocci. Acceptable regimens include the third-generation cephalosporins ceftriaxone and cefotaxime, the fourth-generation cephalosporin cefepime, or one of the newer generation of fluoroquinolones (eg, levofloxacin or moxifloxacin) that have improved activity against *S. pneumoniae*, including those strains that are relatively penicillin resistant, and β-lactam

antibiotic-β-lactamase inhibitor combinations (eg, ampicillin–sulbactam, ticarcillin–clavulanate, or piperacillin–tazobactam). If peritonitis develops during hospitalization, antimicrobial therapy should have activity against more antibiotic-resistant *Enterobacteriaceae* and *Pseudomonas aeruginosa*.

Streptococcus pneumoniae and group A streptococci are best treated with high-dose penicillin G, ceftriaxone, or cefotaxime. Methicillin-sensitive *S. aureus* is best treated with a penicillinase-resistant penicillin (nafcillin) or with a first-generation cephalosporin (cefazolin). If the strain is methicillin resistant or the patient is allergic to penicillin, vancomycin is used. If *Pseudomonas aeruginosa* is isolated, an aminoglycoside can be given in combination with an antipseudomonal penicillin or cephalosporin, aztreonam, or imipenem or meropenem, or, preferrably to avoid the nephrotoxic and ototoxic potential of an aminoglycoside-containing regimen, ciprofloxacin combined with another antipseudomonal agent should be used if results of susceptibility testing permit. Antimicrobial therapy should be continued for 10 to 14 days if improvement is noted; however, shorter-course (5 day) therapy has been shown to be efficacious if rapid clinical improvement occurs. Intraperitoneal antimicrobial administration has not been shown to be beneficial. A clinical response should be evident by 48 to 72 hours in patients receiving appropriate antimicrobial therapy. Failure to respond in this manner should prompt an examination for an alternative or additional diagnoses.

Cirrhotic patients who have had an upper gastrointestinal bleed are at high risk of primary peritonitis and may benefit from primary antibiotic prophylaxis with a fluoroquinolone or trimethoprim–sulfamethoxazole. Similarly, recurrence of primary peritonitis is relatively common in patients with advanced liver disease; 70% of patients will have a recurrence in the first year after their initial episode. Secondary prophylactic maintenance therapy with norfloxacin (400 mg daily), ciprofloxacin (750 mg once a week), or trimethoprim-sulfamethoxazole (one double-strength tablet once daily for 5 days each week) can reduce the frequency of recurrent episodes, perhaps by selective decontamination of the bowel, and may be an option in patients awaiting liver transplantation but may not otherwise prolong survival in this population with end-stage liver disease. Indeed long-term antibiotic use may increase risk of secondary infection with multiply antibiotic-resistant pathogens.

Occasionally, peritonitis may be caused by *Mycobacterium tuberculosis,* usually from hematogenous dissemination from remote foci of tuberculous infection or extension of infection in mesenteric lymph nodes intestine, or, in women, fallopian tubes or ovaries. The diagnosis of tuberculous peritonitis can usually be confirmed by histologic examination and culture of a peritoneal biopsy specimen and fluid. Diagnosis of *Coccidioides immitis* peritonitis can be made by wet mount of ascitic fluid, histology, and culture of the peritoneal biopsy specimen and fluid.

SECONDARY PERITONITIS

By definition, secondary peritonitis is associated with a predisposing intra-abdominal lesion, and it usually involves components of the gastrointestinal flora. Any of numerous intra-abdominal processes may give rise to secondary peritonitis; a partial list includes perforation of a peptic ulcer; traumatic perforation of the uterus, urinary bladder, stomach, or small or large bowel; appendicitis; pancreatitis; diverticulitis; bowel infarction; cholecystitis; biliary sepsis; rupture of an intra-abdominal abscess; operative contamination of the peritoneum; and female genital tract infection such as septic abortion, postoperative uterine infection, endometritis, or salpingitis.

Although any type of microorganism may be responsible, secondary peritonitis is usually an endogenously acquired polymicrobial infection. On average, about five bacterial species are isolated, and they include both obligate and facultative anaerobes. The species of organisms vary with the primary source of the infection. When community-acquired peritonitis is secondary to a breach in the integrity of the stomach and duodenum in the absence of obstruction usually involves mouth flora, ie, mainly β-lactam–susceptible gram-positive cocci and anaerobic gram-negative bacilli, such as *Prevotella melaninogenica* (formerly a member of the *Bacteroides melaninogenicus* group) and *Candida* species. When community-acquired peritonitis is secondary to a breach in the integrity of the lower small bowel or colon or is secondary to a breach of more proximal portions of the gastrointestinal tract when obstruction is present, components of the colonic flora with particular pathogenic potential predominate. In descending order of frequency they include *E. coli, Bacteroides fragilis,* enterococci, other *Bacteroides* species, *Fusobacterium, Clostridium perfringens*, other clostridia, *Peptostreptococcus,* and *Eubacterium.* Similar organisms (*E. coli,*

enterococci, *Clostridium,* and *B. fragilis*) are also responsible for peritonitis complicating cholecystitis and biliary sepsis. Concomitant bacteremia has been reported in 20% to 30% of patients. Organisms most frequently recovered from the blood are *E. coli* and *B. fragilis.* In patients who acquire their infection after admission to a hospital, more antibiotic-resistant organisms such as *Enterobacter, Serratia, Acinetobacter,* vancomycin-resistant enterococci, and *P. aeruginosa* are more frequently isolated.

The presenting symptoms are similar to those of primary peritonitis. The rapidity of onset and initial location and extent of peritoneal involvement vary with the inciting event; for example, sudden massive intraperitoneal spillage of gastric contents secondary to traumatic injury produces severe epigastric pain that, within minutes, spreads to involve the entire abdomen. In contrast, the spread of pain from a lesion such as a ruptured appendix or colonic diverticulum is much more gradual and limited as the inflammatory process usually has time to wall off.

Pain is the predominant symptom. Pain and abdominal tenderness to palpation are usually maximal over the organ in which the process originated (eg, epigastrium for a ruptured peptic ulcer, right upper quadrant for cholecystitis, right lower quadrant for appendicitis, and left lower quadrant for diverticulitis). Other findings include fever, nausea, vomiting, and abdominal distension. The patient often lies motionless with the legs drawn up to the chest; any motion is likely to exacerbate the abdominal pain. Blood pressure is usually normal early but may fall with onset of septic shock, and there may be an increase in respiratory rate and tachycardia. Direct and rebound abdominal tenderness and abdominal wall rigidity are often present. Bowel sounds are absent. Rectal and vaginal examinations, and in women in whom an ectopic pregnancy is suspected, a urinary beta–human chorionic gonadotropin (β-HCG) determination, are necessary.

Often, the diagnostic evaluation must be brief but thorough because of the patient's critical condition. Laboratory studies include a complete blood count, serum chemistry profile, liver profile, and amylase and lipase determinations. Appropriate cultures should be done promptly (eg, blood), although culture of peritoneal fluid is often delayed until the time of laparotomy. Chest radiographs should be obtained to exclude chest conditions that might simulate clinically an intra-abdominal process. Plain radiographs of the abdomen may also be helpful, sometimes revealing free air or fluid, bowel distention, ileus, or bowel wall edema. However, CT of the abdomen and pelvis with contrast is most helpful to localize the infection and indicate its probable source.

Antimicrobial therapy is initiated early to control bacteremia and to minimize the local spread of infection. Patients with hemodynamic, respiratory, renal, and other critical organ system dysfunction require immediate appropriate supportive therapy. Surgery is often necessary to drain purulent material that contains bacteria, excessive levels of proinflammatory cytokines and adjuvants (eg, fecal matter, food, blood, bile, barium) that would enhance the virulence of peritoneal infection; debride devitalized tissues that foster anaerobic conditions; and control continued peritoneal contamination with bacteria and adjuvants by removing the initiating process (eg, cholecystitis, appendicitis, and diverticulitis). Optimal management also includes bowel decompression (eg, by proximal colostomy for perforation, diverticulitis, or colonic carcinoma).

Antibiotic therapy should be begun as soon as blood cultures are obtained but often before peritoneal fluid can be obtained for culture. Peritoneal fluid cultures should be obtained at the time of paracentesis, percutaneous drainage of an intraperitoneal abscess, or laparotomy. Recent data suggest that survival of patients is diminished if initial therapy is inadequate, regardless of the adequacy of subsequent therapy. Initial therapy is consequently empirical and must have broad-spectrum activity against the suspected pathogens.

Inclusion of enterococcal coverage in empiric regimens for polymicrobial intraperitoneal infection is somewhat controversial. Both animal models of experimental polymicrobial intraabdominal infection and clinical data emphasize the importance of enterococci as a component of the polymicrobial infectious inoculum. For example, a multicenter study of intraabdominal infection found that the presence of enterococci in the initial culture, independent of the APACHE II (acute physiology and chronic health evaluation) score, predicted treatment failure with broad-spectrum antimicrobial regimens that lacked specific enterococcal activity. APACHE II score, age, length of preinfection hospital stay, and postoperative infections predicted the presence of enterococci. Therefore, it is prudent to include empiric antienterococcal therapy in an attempt to improve outcome in high-risk patients and in patients with cardiac valvular lesions that place them at high risk for

a bad outcome of endocarditis (eg, prior endocarditis, prosthetic cardiac valves, or complex cyanotic heart disease).

Similarly, treatment of *Candida* in polymicrobial infection is controversial. Isolation of *Candida* from blood cultures or as the sole organism within residual or recurrent intraabdominal infection, or as the predominant organism on Gram staining of peritoneal exudate, represents an indication for additional specific antifungal therapy.

Clindamycin–aminoglycoside combination or cefoxitin had been standard regimen for community-acquired secondary peritonitis. However, a significant proportion of *B. fragilis* are now resistant to clindamycin, cefoxitin, and cefotetan, and aminoglycosides have significant nephrotoxicity and ototoxicity; these drugs therefore can no longer be recommended for empiric coverage now that more reliable and less toxic agents are available. For example, although *Bacteroides fragilis*, as well as many *P. melaninogenica*, produce β-lactamase and are thereby resistant to ampicillin, ticarcillin, and piperacillin, these organisms are sensitive to the β-lactam–β-lactamase inhibitor combinations ampicillin–sulbactam, piperacillin–tazobactam, and ticarcillin–clavulanate, as well as the carbapenems imipenem, meropenem, and ertapenem, the fluoroquinolone moxifloxacin, and metronidazole. Narrower-spectrum antimicrobial regimens that are appropriate for community-acquired secondary intraperitoneal infections in less severely ill patients include (1) ampicillin–sulbactam alone and (2) cefazolin or ceftriaxone combined with metronidazole.

Because nosocomial intraperitoneal infections are caused by more resistant flora, which may include *P. aeruginosa*, *Enterobacter* species, *Proteus* species, and enterococci, and early institution of adequate empirical therapy appears to be important in reducing mortality, broaderspectrum empiric regimens are appropriate for nosocomial infections, as well as for more severely ill or immunocompromised patients. The local prevalence of certain nosocomial pathogens and their susceptibility patterns should also be taken into account when selecting appropriate empiric regimens for nosocomial infections. Broader-spectrum single and combination antimicrobial regimens that are appropriate for these nosocomial or severe intraperitoneal infections include the following:

1. A third- or fourth-generation cephalosporin (ceftazidime or cefepime) plus metronidazole

2. Levofloxacin or ciprofloxacin plus metronidazole
3. A newer fluoroquinolone moxifloxacin alone*
4. A β-lactam–β-lactamase inhibitor alone (ampicillin–sulbactam*, piperacillin–tazobactam* and ticarcillin–clavulanate)
5. A carbapenem alone (imipenem*, meropenem or ertapenem)
6. Aztreonam plus vancomycin plus metronidazole*
7. Tigecycline

Empiric regimens with activity against E. faecalis (indicated by asterisks above) are preferred for these severe or nosocomial infections.

The monobactam aztreonam lacks activity against anaerobes and gram-positive cocci. The carbapenems and fluoroquinolones, but not third-generation cephalosporins or β-lactamase–β-lactamase inhibitor combinations, are frequently active against ampC β-lactamase–producing and extended-spectrum β-lactamase (ESBL)-producing aerobic–facultative gram-negative bacilli. Ertapenem, however, does not cover P. aeruginosa, and ticarcillin–clavulanate, meropenem, ertapenem, and cephalosporin- or some fluoroquinolone-containing regimens do not adequately cover enterococci.

Tigecycline, a twice-daily intravenously administered antibiotic, in a new class called glycylcyclines that are related to the tetracycline minocycline, has been recently approved as monotherapy for complicated intra-abdominal infections in adults. It is active against a broad spectrum of Gram-positive and Gram-negative bacteria, including anaerobes, such as Bacteroides fragilis, and drug-resistant pathogens such as methicillin-resistant Staphylococcus aureus, vancomycin-resistant enterococci, and penicillin-resistant pneumococci. However, tigercycline is not active against P. aeruginosa.

Fluoroquinolone-or aztreonam-containing regimens can be used in penicillin-allergic patients. Empiric regimens should be subsequently modified once results of cultures and susceptibility testing of aerobic–facultative pathogens isolated in the individual patient become available. However, empiric antimicrobial therapy directed against anaerobes should be maintained, even if anaerobes are not recovered from clinical specimens, because of the unreliability of clinical anaerobic methodology.

If vancomycin-resistant (VRE) E. faecium are isolated, the oxazolidinone linezolid, the lipopeptide daptomycin, or the streptogramin combination quinupristin–dalfopristin is appropriate, and if the more penicillin-susceptible VRE E. faecalis is isolated, ampicillin, the oxazolidinone linezolid, or the lipopeptide daptomycin is appropriate (E. faecalis are inherently streptogramin resistant). Azoles and caspofungin are relatively nontoxic alternatives to amphotericin; however, non-albicans Candida species such as Candida glabrata and Candida krusei show decreased susceptibility to fluconozole but are sensitive to caspofungin. Use of fluconozole for non-albicans Candida should be based on in vitro susceptibility testing. If methicillin-sensitive S. aureus is isolated, an antistaphylococcal β-lactam such as nafcillin is preferred, unless the patient is penicillin allergic, when vancomycin is preferred. If methicillin-resistant S. aureus is isolated, vancomycin is preferred, unless the patient cannot tolerate vancomycin, when the following antibiotics are alternatives: daptomycin, linezolid, quinupristin–dalfopristin, trimethoprim–sulfamethoxazole, and minocycline.

The duration of antimicrobial therapy after adequate surgery is usually 5 to 10 days but depends on severity of infection, clinical response to therapy, and normalization of the white blood cell count. Only a short course of antimicrobial therapy (about 24 hours) is required for sterile peritonitis that occurs around an infected but resected intra-abdominal organ, such as an appendix or gallbladder. Once the patient can tolerate oral therapy, antimicrobial agents can be given orally rather than intravenously, if oral agents are available that have antimicrobial activity equivalent to that of the intravenous regimen.

The main therapy for any intraperitoneal abscess is early and adequate drainage. Effective management depends on accurate localization of the abscess and discrimination between single and multiple abscesses. In recent years, successful therapy has been accomplished using percutaneous catheter drainage as an alternative to surgery. This method has become possible with the use of refined imaging techniques, especially ultrasonography and CT. The general requirements for CT- or ultrasound-guided percutaneous catheter drainage include (1) an abscess that can be adequately approached via a safe percutaneous route; (2) an abscess that is unilocular; (3) an abscess that is not vascular and the patient has no coagulopathy; (4) joint radiologic and surgical evaluation, with surgical backup for any complication or failure; and (5) the possibility of dependent drainage via the percutaneously placed catheter. Computed tomography also allows detection of an unsuspected additional intra-abdominal problem that would otherwise require surgical intervention. Percutaneous catheter drainage can be used as an initial approach in a patient too unstable to withstand immediate surgery. Definitive surgery can then be postponed until the patient is in better condition.

Peritoneal catheter-related peritonitis usually results from contamination of the catheter by skin flora. The most common pathogens include *Staphylococcus epidermidis, S. aureus, Streptococcus* species, and diphtheroids. Other less frequently isolated pathogens include *E. coli, Klebsiella, Enterobacter, Proteus,* and fungi. Symptoms include abdominal pain and tenderness, nausea, and vomiting.

SUGGESTED READING

Burnett RJ, Haverstock DC, Dellinger EP, et al. Definition of the role of enterococcus in intraabdominal infection: analysis of a prospective randomized trial. *Surgery.* 1995;188:716–721; discussion 721–723.

Cavaillon JM, Annane D. Compartmentalization of the inflammatory response in sepsis and SIRS. *J Endotoxin Res.* 2006;12:151–170.

Chong AJ, Dellinger EP. Current treatment of intraabdominal infections. *Surg Technol Int.* 2005;14:29–33.

Gines P, Rimola A, Planas R, et al. Norfloxacin prevents spontaneous bacterial peritonitis recurrence in cirrhosis: results of a double-blind, placebo-controlled trial. *Hepatology.* 1990;12:716–724.

Holzheimer RG, Gathof B. Re-operation for complicated secondary peritonitis — how to identify patients at risk for peritoneal sepsis. *Eur J Med Res.* 2003;8:125–134.

Levison ME, Bush LM. Peritonitis and other intra-abdominal infections. In Mandell GL, Bennett JE, Dolin R, eds. *Principles and Practice of Infectious Diseases.* 6th ed. New York, NY: Churchill Livingstone; 2005.

Malangoni MA, Song J, Herrington J, Choudri S, Pertel P. Randomized control trial of moxifloxacin compared with piperacillin-tazobactam and amoxicillin-clavulanate for the treatment of complicated intra-abdominal infections. *Ann Surg.* 2006;244:204–211.

Marshall JC, Maier RV, Dellinger EP, Jiminez MF. Source control in the management of severe sepsis and septic shock: an evidence-based review. *Crit Care Med.* 2004;32(suppl 11):S513–S526.

Montravers P, Dupont H, Gauzit R, et al. Candida as a risk factor for mortality in peritonitis. *Crit Care Med.* 2006;34:646–652.

Nathens AB, Rotstein OD, Marshall JC. Tertiary peritonitis: clinical features of a complex nosocomial infection. *World J Surg.* 1998;22:158–163.

Pacelli F, Doglietto GB, Alfieri S, et al. Prognosis in intraabdominal infections: multivariate analysis on 604 patients. *Arch Surg.* 1996;131:641–645.

Sanna A, Adani GL, Anani G, Donini A. The role of laparoscopy in patients with suspected peritonitis: experience of a single institution. *J Laparoendosc Adv Surg Tech A.* 2003;13:17–19.

Solomkin JS, Mazuski JE, Baron EJ, et al. Guidelines for selection of anti-infectives for complicated intra-abdominal infections. *Clin Infect Dis.* 2003;37:997–1006.

Solomon JS, Yellin AE, Rotstein OD, et al. Protocol 017 Study Group. Ertapenem versus piperacillian/tazobactam in the treatment of complicated intraabdominal infections: results of a double-blind, randomized comparative phase III trial. *Ann Surg.* 2003;237:235–245.

Sotto A, Lefrant JY, Fabbro-Peray P, et al. Evaluation of antimicrobial therapy management of 120 consecutive patients with secondary peritonitis. *J Antimicrob Chemother.* 2002;50:569–576.

Strauss E, Caly WR. Spontaneous bacterial peritonitis: a therapeutic approach. *Expert Rev Anti-infect Ther.* 2006;4:249–260.

57. Whipple's Disease and Sprue

Phillip B. Amidon

WHIPPLE'S DISEASE

Whipple's disease is a rare multisystem disease with only 664 known cases before 1985 and less than 30 new cases being reported per year worldwide. Prior to antibiotic therapy the disease was uniformly fatal. Symptoms typically precede diagnosis by 5 to 10 years. Because of the many clinical findings shared by other common disorders, considering a diagnosis of Whipple's disease is one of the most important steps regarding therapy. Beginning insidiously with complaints of arthralgia, myalgia, fever, and weight loss and progressing to diarrhea, it is usually diagnosed during the work-up of the malabsorption, which is the hallmark of Whipple's disease. Joint pain and swelling are common, followed by steatorrhea with protein, carbohydrate, vitamin, and mineral malabsorption. Microcytic, iron-deficiency anemia is common, as is macrocytic anemia, from B-12 and folate deficiency. Cardiac involvement includes endocarditis of any valve, myocarditis, and pericarditis. The eye is sometimes involved, with uveitis, choreoretinitis, or keratosis. The most feared manifestation, central nervous system (CNS) Whipple's disease, is associated with headache, personality change, ataxia, ophthalmoplegia, seizures, and dementia.

The etiologic agent, *Tropherma whipplei*, is a gram-positive, periodic acid–Schifff (PAS)-positive, non-acid-fast, rod-shaped bacillus with typical electron microscopy morphology. The organism is grown only in cell culture, using peripheral blood monocytes. Host interaction is likely involved in the pathogenesis of Whipple's disease. In autopsy series, the frequency is less than 0.1%; 40- to 50-year old men predominate, and 97% are white. Human leukocyte antigen (HLA)-B27 is found in 28% to 44% of patients, compared with an HLA-B27 incidence of 8% in the general population. Polymerase chain reaction (PCR) technology has identified the unique gene segment that encodes the 16S ribosomal RNA of the bacillus. PCR testing has a very high sensitivity (96.6%) and specificity (100%) and has identified *T. whippeli* in tissues that demonstrate no evidence of disease.

Biopsy and tissue PCR are necessary to make the diagnosis. The intestine is nearly always involved, with endoscopic biopsy of the distal duodenum or proximal jejunum being sufficient. Upper GI endoscopy reveals shaggy yellow-white granulated mucosa between Kerckring folds. Wireless capsule endoscopy may show similar changes throughout the small intestine. Histologic findings, partial villous atrophy, is demonstrated by flattened villi, cuboid deformation of the epithelium, excess extracellular fat accumulation, and PAS-positive macrophages in the lamina propria, adjacent to the lumen. PAS-positive macrophages are detectable in the joint, bone marrow, spleen, adrenal, kidney, heart, and brain tissue. Infected mesenteric lymph nodes may be present. PCR testing is confirmatory. Because the CNS is considered the most serious site of involvement in Whipple's disease, treatment should always include PCR analysis of cerebrospinal fluid (CSF). This test is useful for diagnosis and for monitoring response to therapy, even in patients without neurological symptoms.

Before antibiotic therapy, the disease was invariably fatal. Because of the rarity of the disease, no large-scale controlled studies have been done to determine optimal therapy. Treatment is based on clinical experience and retrospective studies involving small numbers of patients. The first cure was reported with chloramphenicol in 1952. Later, tetracycline was commonly used. However, the problem of relapse and CNS involvement has led to re-evaluation of therapy. The now-recognized high prevalence of CNS disease requires drugs that cross the blood-brain barrier. A look-back study of 88 patients by Keinath found a 35% relapse occurring on average 4 years after stopping antibiotic treatment. Of those, 43% of the relapsers had been treated only with tetracycline and 68% of that group had a CNS relapse. No CNS relapses were noted in the group treated initially with parenteral penicillin and streptomycin followed by oral trimethoprim-sulfamethoxazole (TMP-SMX). In other reports, some patients had developed symptomatic Whipple's disease of the CNS while undergoing treatment with

TMP-SMX alone. Two such patients were found to be CSF PCR positive and were treated with ceftriaxone and chloramphenicol with conversion to PCR-negative status. There is a case report of a patient presenting with neurologic symptoms and a magnetic resonance imaging (MRI) scan suggesting Whipple's disease in whom a relapse occurred 7 years after the onset of symptoms. The CSF PCR was negative, but the symptoms and MRI findings improved with antibiotic therapy.

Based on clinical findings published to date, recommended treatment is parenteral streptomycin, 1 g, and penicillin G, 1.2 million U daily for 14 days, followed by TMP-SMX double-strength (DS), orally twice daily for 1 year (Table 57.1). Alternative therapies that have been used are ampicillin, 2 g orally 3 times daily, and ceftriaxone, 2 g daily intravenously (IV) for 14 days, followed by twice-daily TMP-SMX DS for 1 year. Also, parenteral ceftriaxone, 2 g daily, streptomycin, 1 g daily for 14 days, followed by TMP-SMX DS, twice daily orally for 1 year.

With treatment, the steatorrhea may persist for up to 7 months. The bacteria may be visible by electron microscopy for up to 4 months. The mucosal changes seen by light microscopy take an average of 14 months to normalize, and PAS-laden macrophages can still be found up to 2 years after therapy. Currently, the optimal length of treatment is unknown, and proof of cure does not exist. Follow-up should continue for at least 20 years. Relapses occur on average after 4 years (20 months to 20 years). Therapy for relapse is outlined in Table 57.2. CNS relapses typically occur late and are not associated with intestinal symptoms. It is not yet clear that CNS PCR is an accepted criterion, but recent experience suggests a potential value of monitoring the CSF PCR as a parameter of the therapeutic response; a positive result often turns negative with successful therapy.

SPRUE

Sprue is general term applied to disorders of intestinal malabsorption. Only two of these disorders, tropical sprue and small intestinal bacterial overgrowth syndrome, have infectious causes.

Tropical Sprue

Tropical sprue affects the entire length of the small intestine and causes diarrhea and malabsorption with multiple and severe nutritional deficiencies. The diagnosis requires demonstration of intestinal malabsorption of at least two nutrients, exclusion of other diseases that cause malabsorption, a compatible jejunal biopsy, and response to therapy. Tropical sprue occurs between the tropics of Capricorn

Table 57.1 Recommended Regimens of Antibiotic Therapy for Whipple's Disease; Initial Presentation

A. Penicillin G 1.2 million U/day IM × 14 days
plus
Streptomycin 1 g daily IM × 14 d
(followed by)
TMP-SMX 1 DS tab BID PO × 1 y
or
B. Ampicillin 2 g TID PO × 14 d
plus
Ceftriaxone 2 g daily IV × 14 d
(followed by)
TMP-SMX 1 DS tab BID PO × 1 y
or
C. Ceftriaxone 2 g daily IV × 14 d
plus
Streptomycin 1 g daily IM × 14 d
(followed by)
TMP-SMX I DS tab BID PO × 1 y
Abbreviations: IM = intramuscularly; TMP–SMX = trimethoprim–sulfamethoxazole; DS = double strength; BID = twice a day; PO = orally; IV = intravenously; TID = three times a day.

Table 57.2 Recommended Regimens of Antibiotic Therapy for Whipple's Disease; Relapse

A. Chloramphenicol 1 g QID IV × 2–4 wk
B. Penicillin G 1.2 million U/day IM × 2–4 wk
C. Streptomycin 1 g daily IM × 2–4 wk
D. Ceftriaxone 2 g daily IV × 2–4 wk (followed by)
TMP-SMX 1 DS tab BID PO × 1–2 y
Abbreviations: QID = four times a day; IV = intravenously; IM = intramuscularly; TMP–SMX = trimethoprim–sulfamethoxazole; DS = double strength; BID = twice a day; PO = orally.

Table 57.3 Recommended Therapy for Tropical Sprue

Tetracycline 250 mg QID PO × 3–6 m
plus
Folic acid 5 mg daily PO × 3–6 m
plus
Vitamin B-12 1000 µg weekly IM × 3–6 m
Abbreviations: QID = four times a day; PO = orally; IM = intramuscularly.

Table 57.4 Recommended Therapy for Small Bowel Bacterial Overgrowth Syndrome

A. Amoxicillin–clavulinate 875 mg BID PO × 7–10 d
or
B. Cephalexin 250 mg QID PO × 7–10 d
or
C. Metronidazole 250 mg TID PO × 7–10 d
Abbreviations: BID = twice a day; PO = orally; QID = four times a day; TID = three times a day.

and Cancer. Visitors to these areas can develop disease within weeks, but it is more likely to occur in those who have lived there for more than a year. An illness resembling tropical sprue appears in the Indian medical literature between 1600 and 1300 BC. Tropical sprue occurred in British troops in Singapore during the 1700s and in American soldiers and service personnel in the Philippines, Puerto Rico, and Vietnam. Patients have malabsorption of fat with steatorrhea and abnormal D-xylose absorption, with deficiencies of folate, B-12, vitamins A and D, protein, magnesium, and calcium. Jejunal biopsies normally demonstrate finger-shaped villi with a paucity of intraepithelial lymphocytes, delicate subendothelial basement membrane, and sparse mononuclear cell population of the villous core. In tropical sprue the jejunal biopsy reveals thick, leaf-shaped villi, infiltration of the epithelium with lymphocytes, thickened and collagenous basement membrane, and infiltration of the villous core by chronic inflammatory cells. The mucosal lesion coincides with the onset of tissue folate deficiency. Persistent contamination of the small bowel by enterotoxigenic *Escherichia coli*, which are unusually adherent to the mucosa, may be the precipitating cause. Tropical sprue should be considered in anyone returning from the tropics with persistent diarrhea. Demonstrating malabsorption of fat, B-12, and D-xylose, along with a compatible jejunal biopsy, should result in a response to therapy. Treatment with tetracycline, 250 mg orally 4 times daily, and folic acid, 5 mg daily for 3 to 6 months, is usually effective (Table 57.3). Vitamin B-12, 1000 µg, is recommended weekly for several weeks to replenish tissue stores. Treatment typically results in subjective and objective improvement within weeks, although up to 2 years of therapy may be required for complete resolution of tropical sprue.

SMALL-BOWEL BACTERIAL OVERGROWTH SYNDROME

Small-bowel bacterial overgrowth syndrome condition occurs when the normal flora of the small intestine is repopulated in numbers and species by the flora of the colon. The colonic flora compete with the human host for ingested nutrients, and the toxic by-products of colonic fermentation in the small bowel cause a wide spectrum of symptoms. These symptoms include diarrhea, malabsorption, and malnutrition. Conditions associated with small-bowel bacterial overgrowth syndrome are as follows:

1. Profound gastric hypochlorhydria
2. Structural changes in the small bowel such as jejunal diverticulae, afferent loop, blind loop, gastrocolic and jejunocolic fistula
3. Disordered intestinal motility from idiopathic intestinal pseudoobstruction and scleroderma
4. Immunodeficiency syndromes and occasionally in cirrhosis and chronic pancreatitis with narcotic overuse.

Therapy of symptomatic disease requires reduction of the bacterial overgrowth in the small bowel. Surgical correction of an underlying structural abnormality responsible for the intestinal stasis is seldom possible. Patient management is therefore medical, with broad-spectrum antibiotic therapy, often for the patient's lifetime. Traditional therapy has been tetracycline, but the high incidence of bacterial resistance, especially with *Bacteroides* organisms, limits its effectiveness. Aerobic and anaerobic flora can be suppressed with amoxicillin–clavulanate, 875 mg twice daily; cephalexin, 250 mg 4 times daily; or metronidazole, 250 mg 3 times daily (Table 57.4). Antibiotics are given for 7 to 10 days. If

---

Clinical Syndromes – Gastrointestinal Tract, Liver, and Abdomen

symptoms are recurrent, cyclic therapy of 1 week of every 4 with rotating coverage to avoid bacterial resistance is often necessary. Currently available prokinetics have not been found useful. Attention to the nutritional status is important. Vitamin B-12, 1000 μg parenterally, (intramuscularly, IM), calcium, and vitamin K are very often necessary to correct secondary deficiency states.

SUGGESTED READING

Fritscher-Ravens A, Swain CP, von Herbay A. Refractory Whipple's disease with anemia: first lessons from capsule endoscopy. *Endoscopy.* 2004;36:659–662.

Muir-Padilla J, Myers JB. Whipple disease: a case report and review of the literature. *Arch Pathol Lab Med.* 2005;129: 933–936.

Muller SA, Vogt P, Altwegg M, Seebach JD. Deadly carousel or difficult interpretation of new diagnostic tools for Whipple's disease: case report and review of the literature. *Infection.* 2005;33:39–42.

Nath SK. Tropical sprue. *Curr Gastroenterol Rep.* 2005;7:343–349.

Olmos M, Smecuol E, Maurino E, Bai JC. Decision analysis: an aid to the diagnosis of Whipple's disease. *Aliment Pharmacol Ther.* 2006;23:833–840.

Pereira SP, Gainsborough H, Dowling RH. Drug induced hypochlorhydria causes high duodenal bacterial counts in the elderly. *Aliment Pharmacol Ther.* 1998;12: 99–104.

Clinical Syndromes – Genitourinary Tract

58. Urethritis and Dysuria

Georgios Pappas and Matthew E. Falagas

The term *urethritis* refers to inflammation of the urethra, which can be attributed both to infectious and noninfectious processes. The urethral canal essentially represents the first site of the body to be exposed to a variety of sexually transmitted pathogens, and the interaction of these pathogens with the epithelial cells of the urethra gives rise to the syndrome's symptoms.

Dysuria refers to the experience of pain, burning sensation or discomfort in urination and is a subjective symptom related to varying pathology of the urinary tract. Urethra being the terminal pathway of urine flow, its inflammation most often accounts the for experience of dysuria.

ETIOLOGY

Traditionally urethritis has been divided into gonococcal urethritis (GU) and nongonococcal urethritis (NGU). *Neisserria gonorrhoeae* as a cause of urethritis has been recognized since ancient years, and in fact its name represents a description, in Greek, of the syndrome's symptoms as defined by Galen: "gono" referring to semen, which was supposed to be the main constituent of the urethral discharge, and "rrhea" a term for flow. Descriptions of urethritis exist in the Old Testament, in the Book of Leviticus, in ancient Chinese documents, and in the Hippocratic Corpus.

Nongonococcal urethritis has been often considered synonymous to *Chlamydia trachomatis* infection, although a continuously increasing number of pathogens are also implicated (Table 58.1). *Chlamydia trachomatis* is generally thought of as the commonest cause of NGU, especially in younger patients, although some studies suggest that *Ureaplasma urealyticum*, biovar 2, may be a more prevalent cause of infection. Numerous other pathogens have been associated with NGU: *Mycoplasma genitalium* as a cause of urethritis was recognized in the early 1980s and has since gained significant scientific interest. Its etiological role as a sexually transmitted pathogen has been confirmed recently. *Trichomonas vaginalis* is

Table 58.1 Etiology and Relative Frequency of Infectious Urethritis

Pathogen	Reported Frequency in Cases of Urethritis
Neisseria gonorrhoeae	12%–34%
Chlamydia trachomatis	15%–55% of NGU
Mycoplasma genitalium	3%–38% of NGU
Ureaplasma urealyticum	6%–60% of NGU
Trichomonas vaginalis	≤5% of NGU
Gardnerella vaginalis	12% of NGU in a single study
Mycoplasma hominis	Rare, frequency vaguely defined
Herpes simplex virus	Rare
Gram-negative bacteria	Rare
Adenoviruses	Rare
Other: mycobacteria, syphilis, lymphogranuloma venereum, streptococci, *Neisseria meningitides*, anaerobes, fungi	Very rare/Isolated reports

Abbreviation: NGU = nongonococcal urethritis.

invariably isolated in clinical series of urethritis. *Gardnerella vaginalis* has been considered a frequent cause of urethritis in certain series. Herpes simplex virus (HSV) is also a potent cause, both as HSV1 and HSV2. More rare causes include adenoviruses, lymphogranuloma venereum, mycobacteria, and syphilis, as well as gram-negative pathogens (usually *Esherichia coli*, usually implicated in cases of strictures or accompanying cystitis). Even rarer causes include other viral infections, cytomegalovirus (CMV) implicated in immunocompromised patients, streptococcal species (especially *Streptococcus pyogenes*), *Neisseria meningitides*, fungi, and anaerobes such as *Bacteroides* species.

EPIDEMIOLOGY

The global annual incidence of urethritis is enormous: An estimated 62 million cases of GU and 89 million cases of NGU occur annually. In the United States, 5 million annual cases are estimatedly reported, the majority of which are NGU. Gonococcal urethritis accounts for 600 000 cases annually according to the Centers for Disease Control and Prevention, although underreporting may exist. The incidence of GU has been declining in the United States since 2000, whereas inverse trends have been observed for NGU. The latter are accompanied though by a declining incidence of chlamydial NGU and may actually reflect the increasing recognition of other etiologies of NGU. A steady increase of the total urethritis cases reported in males has been observed in France in recent years. The increasing availability of sophisticated diagnostic techniques in third-world countries has also augmented in underlining the magnitude of the problem.

There seems to be no racial predilection for the incidence of the syndrome, although certain socioeconomic factors may apply, urethritis being more common in low-income populations. Gender predilection seems also not to exist, although the difference in the syndrome's clinical presentation between males and females (subsequently discussed) may account for a larger percentage of female cases that are asymptomatic and thus not reported; however, although male urethritis is a distinct syndrome, female disease is often misdiagnosed in the context of, or coexists undiagnosed with, inflammation of other sites of the female urogenital tract, most importantly cervicitis. Due to urethritis being a sexually transmitted disease, the age group of 20–24 years predominates in reported cases. The use of condoms has been inversely related to the incidence of urethritis. Other risk factors include the use of spermicides (which though may predispose to chemical urethritis only), the number of sexual partners, homosexuality in males, unprotected anal sex for heterosexual males, and history of other sexually transmitted diseases.

COMPLICATIONS

The importance of urethritis as a medical entity lies not in the severity of the syndrome per se but in its potential complications: these complications may be rare in male patients but do include formation of strictures or abscesses, prostatitis, epididymitis, infertility, disseminated gonococcal infection, and proctitis. In female patients complications (or coexistence of inflammation for that matter) are more common and may lead to pelvic inflammatory disease (PID), which may be of considerable severity. Disseminated gonococcal infection can also follow urethritis in females. In pregnant women, chlamydial infection can lead to transmission of the pathogen to neonates leading to ophthalmia neonatum. Another important parameter of urethritis is that local inflammation results in disruption of the integrity of the epithelial barrier, thus urethritis confers an increased risk for human immunodeficiency virus (HIV) transmission. Reiter's syndrome, the coexistence of urethritis with ocular inflammation occurring as an autoimmune process after gastrointestinal or genitourinary infections, is another complication to be taken into account.

DIFFERENTIAL DIAGNOSIS

Differential diagnosis includes traumatic urethritis, occurring after catheterization manipulations, the already-mentioned chemical urethritis, and Reiter's syndrome.

The disease is often asymptomatic, particularly so in female patients and in cases of chlamydial etiology. Up to 75% of women with chlamydial urethritis experience no symptoms. Gonococcal urethritis exhibits a shorter incubation period than NGU and a more abrupt onset and is usually symptomatic. Incubation period lies between a few days, for gonococcal disease, and up to 2 weeks for the nongonococcal one. Urethral discharge, dysuria, and urethral pruritus are the cardinal symptoms: Discharge is a product of the polymorphonuclear cell influx in the region as part of the immune response and epithelial cell apoptosis, is usually mucopurulent, most often observed in the morning, may be blood-tinged, and is a result of the inflammatory interplay following entry of the pathogen. This inflammatory response is more pronounced in cases of gonococcal urethritis compared to chlamydial infection, thus discharge and overall symptoms are more pronounced in gonococcal disease in males (the syndrome remains asymptomatic in the majority of females). Other causes of nongonogoccal urethritis though, as *Mycoplasma genitalium*, tend also to cause symptomatic disease. *Trichomonas* infection in males tends to be asymptomatic, but when symptomatic, it may be more clinically severe than GU.

Dysuria should be differentiated from frequency or urgency, which point to other diagnoses. It is reported that dysuria may be aggravated by alcohol consumption or during

Table 58.2 Diagnostic Tools for Pathogens Involved in Urethritis

Pathogen	Diagnostic Tools	Comments
Neisseria gonorrhoeae	Gram stain Culture NAHT NAAT	Culture and NAHT require urethral swab specimens, whereas NAAT can be performed on urine specimens
Chlamydia trachomatis	Culture Direct immunofluorescence Enzyme immunoassays NAHT NAAT	NAHT require urethral swab specimens, whereas NAAT can be performed on urine samples/ in females addition of cervical samples increases sensitivity NAAT more sensitive and 100% specific
Mycoplasma genitalium	NAAT	NAAT can be performed on urine samples/ in females addition of cervical samples increases sensitivity
Ureaplasma urealyticum, *Mycoplasma hominis*	Culture	Cultures need specialized media, not performed in everyday practice Urethral swabs preferred to urine samples
Trichomonas vaginalis	Wet preparation Culture NAAT	Wet preparation is 60% sensitive, often negative in males Anaerobic culture of urethral swab or first-void urine, 95% sensitive NAAT is considered superior to cultures (97% sensitivity and 98% specificity), but needs multiple samples in males

Abbreviations: NAAT = nucleic acid amplification tests; NAHT = nucleic acid hybridization tests.

menstruation in females. There are no systemic symptoms as fever, and presence of such symptoms should orientate the diagnosis elsewhere. Because dysuria may be attributed not only to infectious processes of the whole genitourinary tract, including pyelonephritis or even prostatitis, but also to noninfectious causes of flow obstruction (including anatomical malformations, neoplasms, or even hormonal causes such as endometriosis and neurogenic, and psychogenic conditions), the significance of this subjective symptom is mainly in localizing the clinician's interest in the genitourinary tract.

DIAGNOSIS

The diagnosis of urethritis is based on the presence of relevant clinical symptoms (discharge and dysuria) accompanied by laboratory findings: Gram stain microscopy of urethral secretions that exhibits five or more white blood cells (WBC) per oil-immersion field, a positive WBC esterase test of first-void urine, or a first-void urine sample exhibiting 10 or more WBC per high-power field (HPF). The latter though has been considered inadequate by various studies reporting that 12% of chlamydial infections and 5% of gonococcal ones may be undiagnosed by this criterion.

Gram stain microscopy allows for initial etiologic work-up, because the observation of gram-negative intracellular diplococci may allow for a rapid diagnosis of gonococcal urethritis, with a sensitivity and specificity of >95% and >99%, respectively. Yet, absence of these findings on a Gram smear does not rule out gonococcal infection. Although, as will be subsequently discussed, isolation of the specific pathogen implicated may not alter therapeutic choices significantly, further diagnostic work-up is usually performed. Cultures may allow for isolation of the specific pathogen and evaluation of its antimicrobial susceptibility. Molecular diagnostic methods have been increasingly applied to urethritis diagnosis, nucleic acid amplification tests (NAAT) being the most popular choices, because they can be performed with urine specimens as well as urethral samples. These assays have shown exquisite sensitivity and sensibility both for *Gonococci* and *Chlamydia*. Other NAAT exist for less common pathogens, as *Mycoplasma genitalium*, but their standard application in clinical practice has been in dispute. Trichomonas diagnosis can be easily performed with a wet preparation, whereas fungal etiology can be outlined by a potassium hydroxide preparation. Table 58.2 summarizes current diagnostic facilities for each pathogen and specific data about each assay's sensitivity and specificity. Laboratory tests should also include testing for other sexually transmitted diseases, including

HIV and syphilis, and, in female patients, pregnancy should be ruled out before specific antibiotic recommendations.

TREATMENT

Table 58.3 summarizes the suggested antibiotic regimens used in the treatment of urethritis, according to the Centers for Disease Control and Prevention. It should be stated that many cases of urethritis may resolve spontaneously or evolve, in cases of NGU, in asymptomatic infection. Nevertheless, antibiotic treatment of urethritis should always follow the diagnosis, for reasons pertaining to the patient and the overall incidence of the disease: Treatment prevents the evolution of complications associated with the disease and, furthermore, prevents further sexual transmission of the pathogen from the patient to his/her partners.

Another important aspect that should be kept in mind regarding treatment decisions is that gonococcal and chlamydial infection frequently coexist; thus, a diagnosis of gonococcal infection through a Gram smear showing gram-negative intracellular diplococci will warrant treatment of both gonococcal and chlamydial disease. This observation has further raised questions regarding the utility of sophisticated diagnostic assays when Gram smear shows gonococcal disease: it simply is cheaper to treat both for gonococcal and chlamydial urethritis than confirm or exclude chlamydial disease through further testing.

Various antibiotics have been shown as effective in the treatment of different etiologic forms of urethritis: For chlamydial infection, azithromycin, and doxycycline have proven equally successful according to a recent meta-analysis, with microbial cure rates of 97% and 98%, respectively. Azithromycin is superior in terms of compliance because it can be directly administered on diagnosis, but doxycycline is of considerably lower cost. Azithromycin may be superior for treatment of *Mycoplasma genitalium* infections. There is no difference in the percentage or severity of adverse events between the two antibiotic classes. None of the various alternatives has proven superior, although not all of them have been evaluated in randomized trials. Erythromycin is marred by low compliance due to frequent gastrointestinal adverse events.

Regimens of choice for gonococcal disease include third-generation cephalosporins administered as a single dose. Ceftriaxone exhibits higher blood microbicidal levels and

Table 58.3 Optimal Treatment of Urethritis and Alternative Approaches[a].

Gonococcal Urethritis (always in Conjunction with Treatment for *Chlamydia*)
Ceftriaxone, 125 mg IM, single dose, or
Cefixime, 400 mg PO, single dose, or
In settings where *Neisseria gonorrhoeae* resistance to quinolones is low, ciprofloxacin or ofloxacin or levofloxacin, 500/400/250 mg, respectively, PO, single dose
Alternative regimens
Spectinomycin, 2 g IM, single dose, or
Ceftizoxime, 500 mg IM, single dose, or
Cefoxitin, 2 g IM, single dose, plus probenecid, or
Cefotaxime, 500 mg IM, single dose
Regimens of inferior or unproven efficacy
Gatifloxacin, or norfloxacin, or lomefloxacin, 400/800/400 mg, respectively, PO, single dose, or
Cefpodoxime, 200 mg PO, single dose, or
Cefuroxime axetil, 1 g PO, single dose
Chlamydial Infection
Azithromycin, 1g PO, single dose, or
Doxycycline, 100 mg PO, 2× daily for 7 d
Alternative regimens
Erythromycin base, 500 mg PO, 4× daily, for 7 d, or
Erythromycin ethylsuccinate, 800 mg PO, 4 times daily, for 7 d, or
Ofloxacin, 300 mg PO, 2× daily for 7 d, or
Levofloxacin, 500 mg PO, once daily, for 7 d
***Mycoplasma Genitalium* Infection**
Azithromycin, 1 g orally, single dose, or
Doxycycline, 100 mg PO, 2× daily for 7 d
***Ureaplasma Urealyticum* Infection**
Azithromycin, 1g PO, single dose, or
Doxycycline, 100 mg PO, 2× daily for 7 d (possibility of resistant strain), or
Quinolones, as used for *Chlamydia trachomatis* infection
***Mycoplasma hominis* Infection**
Doxycycline, 100 mg PO, 2× daily for 7 d (possibility of resistant strain), or
Quinolones, as used for *Chlamydia trachomatis* infection, or
Clindamycin, dose varying

Trichomonas Vaginalis Infection
Metronidazole, 2 g PO, single dose, or
Tinidazole, 2 g PO, single dose
Pregnancy
Azithromycin, 1 g PO, single dose, or
Amoxicillin, 500 mg PO 3× daily for 7 d
Alternatively: any erythromycin regimen, apart from erythromycin estolate
[a] Major recommendations from Workowsky and Berman, 2006. Abbreviations: IM = intramuscularly; PO = orally.

for a more sustained period than cefixime and should be considered as the optimal regimen. Tetracycline and older β-lactams have no place in the current therapeutic regimens of gonococcal infection (even with the adjuvant use of probenecid for β-lactams) due to the increased resistance patterns observed worldwide. Quinolones might be viewed as potential single-dose monotherapy candidates that could treat both gonococcal and chlamydial infection, but the increasing rates of gonococcal resistance to these agents observed in Europe, the Middle East, and Asian and Pacific countries as well as the Western United States (California and Hawaii, in particular, and especially in homosexual males) prohibits such a recommendation, at least in infections related to the above mentioned parameters. In populations based on areas with low levels of quinolone resistance, ciprofloxacin in a single oral dose of 500 mg has proven efficient in treatment of gonococcal infection, with a microbiological eradication rate above 99% and sustained blood levels. Similar efficacy, with microbiological cure rates above 98% for gonococcal urogenital infections has been proven for ofloxacin. However, ciprofloxacin's efficacy against *Chlamydia* is doubtful. Azithromycin may be efficacious against both gonococci and *Chlamydia*, although at different doses.

Other alternative drugs for the treatment of gonococcal infection exhibit certain drawbacks: Spectinomycin, although of exquisite microbiological efficacy (>98%), is expensive and needs parenteral administration; thus its only role lies in treatment of patients who cannot tolerate cephalosporins or quinolones. Other cephalosporins and other quinolones have not proven advantageous compared to the suggested regimens. Oral cephalosporins have proven microbicidally inferior to the suggested regimens. However, there is increasing concern regarding azithromycin's efficacy against *Mycoplasma genitalium*, because recent studies have underlined emergence of resistance and therapeutic failures in cases of urethritis treated with azithromycin. These studies have shown a potent role for moxifloxacin in such cases. *Ureaplasma urealyticum* follows the susceptibility patterns of *Chlamydia*, although the risk of tetracycline resistance is significant. *Mycoplasma hominis* is resistant to azithromycin and macrolides but sensitive to tetracyclines, quinolones, and clindamycin.

In pregnancy, gonococcal infection can be treated with the usual cephalosporin regimens, and azithromycin can be considered a safe regimen for chlamydial infection. Amoxicillin can be administered safely and efficaciously in these patients too.

Patients should be advised to abstain from sexual practices for the following week post treatment initiation, and previous sexual contacts should be traced and tested, extending to a period of 6 weeks prior to diagnosis. If the patient reports no contacts during this period, then the last sexual partner should be notified and tested. Alternatively, sexual partners can be treated on the responsibility of the patients, a practice that has been supported inconsistently as effective. Retesting is not advisable: yet, there is an increased prevalence of gonococcal infections in patients with a recent previous gonococcal infection, and a similar risk exists for a new chlamydial infection after an initial one in female patients, with reinfection possessing greater potential for complications such as PID. Therefore, female patients with previous gonococcal or chlamydial infections should be retested if opportunity arises during the following months, although this test is distinct from a test seeking evidence of microbiological eradication. Gonococcal infection in males is usually symptomatic and would orientate the patient toward seeking medical advice, if re-infection occurs. Follow-up testing for microbiological eradication is suggested for pregnant women at 3 weeks after treatment completion.

Recurrence may be attributed to noncompliance with the initial treatment or re-exposure to a nontreated partner, to *Trichomonas* infection in patients not treated with azithromycin, which should be treated with metronidazole or tinidazole or azithromycin, to infection by *Ureaplasma urealyticum* strain resistant to tetracycline (when this antibiotic category has been initially used), or to emergence of resistant strains of other pathogens (see above for resistance of *Mycoplasma genitalium* to azithromycin). Another possible diagnosis in male patients may be chronic nonbacterial prostatitis, which in a significant percentage is accompanied by sterile urethral inflammation.

PREVENTION

Prevention through screening has been often advocated: The Centers for Disease Control and Prevention advocate the annual screening for chlamydial infection in sexually active females aged 24 years or younger and in older females who belong to certain risk groups (eg, multiple partners and sex workers). Screening for gonococcal infection should also be advocated for sexually active females aged 24 years or younger, patients with a history of gonococcal infection or other sexually transmitted disease, sexually active females with new or multiple sexual partners, inconsistent users of condoms, sex workers, and intravenous drug users. The active research in the field of development of a *Chlamydia* vaccine may offer further prospects in the future for control of urethritis incidence. Until then, public health policies should be vigorously implemented.

SUGGESTED READING

Bradshaw CS, Jensen JS, Tabrizi SN, et al. Azithromycin failure in *Mycoplasma genitalium* urethritis. *Emerg Infect Dis.* 2006;12:1149–1152.

Bradshaw CS, Tabrizi SN, Read, TRH, et al. Etiologies of nongonococcal urethritis: bacteria, viruses, and the association with orogenital exposure. *J Infect Dis.* 2006;193:336–345.

Bremnor JD, Sadovsky R. Evaluation of dysuria in adults. *Am Fam Physician.* 2002;65:1589–1596.

Centers for Disease Control and Prevention. Sexually Transmitted Disease Surveillance, 2004. Atlanta, GA: Department of Health and Human Services, CDC, National Center for HIV, STD, and TB Prevention; 2005.

Falagas ME, Gorbach SL. Prostatitis, epididymitis, and urethritis: Practice guidelines. *Infect Dis Clin Practice.* 1995;4:325–333.

Iser P, Read TH, Tabrizi SN, et al. Symptoms of non-gonococcal urethritis in heterosexual men: a case control study. *Sex Transm Infect.* 2005;81:163–165.

Jacobson GF, Autry AM, Kirby RS, et al. A randomized controlled trial comparing amoxicillin and azithromycin for the treatment of *Chlamydia trachomatis* in pregnancy. *Am J Obstet Gynecol.* 2001;184:1352–1356.

Johnson RE, Newhall WJ, Papp JR, et al. Screening tests to detect *Chlamydia trachomatis* and *Neisseria gonorrhoeae* infections, 2002. *MMWR Recomm Rep.* 2002;51:1–38.

Kissinger P, Mohammed H, Richardson-Alston G, et al. Patient-delivered partner treatment for male urethritis: a randomized, controlled trial. *Clin Infect Dis.* 2005; 41:623–629.

Lau CY, Qureshi AK. Azithromycin versus doxycycline for genital chlamydial infections: a meta-analysis of randomized clinical trials. *Sex Transmit Dis.* 2002;29:497–502.

Lyss SB, Kamb ML, Peterman TA, et al. Project RESPECT study group *Chlamydia trachomatis* among patients infected with and treated for *Neisseria gonorrhoeae* in sexually transmitted disease clinics in the United States. *Ann Intern Med.* 2003;139:178–185.

Taylor SN Mycoplasma genitalium. *Curr Infect Dis Rep.* 2005;7:453–457.

U.S. Preventive Services Task Force. Screening for chlamydial infection: recommendations and rationale. *Am Fam Physician.* 2002;65:673–676.

U.S. Preventive Services Task Force. Screening for gonorrhea: recommendation Statement. *Ann Fam Med.* 2005;3:263–267.

Workowski KA, Berman SM. Sexually transmitted diseases treatment guidelines, 2006. *MMWR Recomm Rep.* 2006;55:1–94.

59. Vaginitis and Cervicitis

Sebastian Faro

INTRODUCTION

To understand vaginitis and cervicitis one must understand what has been defined as a healthy vaginal microflora. The assumption is that *Lactobacillus* is a key factor in maintaining a healthy vaginal ecosystem; however, there are likely other important factors that are at play that maintain the vaginal ecosystem in a healthy state. Although there is still a significant void in our knowledge of all components of the vaginal ecosystem needed to maintain it in a healthy state, we do know that *Lactobacillus* does apparently have a significant role in maintaining dominance and suppresses the pathogenic bacteria. A healthy vaginal ecosystem is defined as an ecosystem that exhibits no symptoms (odorless; no itching, burning, or discomfort), discharge is white to slate gray, and microscopically the squamous epithelial cells are well estrogenized and there are ≤5 white blood cells seen microscopically at 40× magnification per field. The bacteria observed at 40× magnification are mostly large bacilli, and other bacterial morphotypes are rarely observed.

An understanding of the dynamics of endogenous vaginal microflora and its interaction with the vaginal ecosystem is emerging. The available data enable us to begin to understand the role of *Lactobacillus* in maintaining a healthy vaginal flora and possibly preventing infection of the lower as well as the upper genital tract. Lower genital infection or alterations of the endogenous vaginal microflora result in vaginitis. Vaginitis is not only the most common benign condition that affects women but results in extremely high costs for treatment, significant morbidity as a cause of postoperative pelvic infection, and possible impact on pregnancy.

A great deal has been written about abnormalities of the vaginal ecosystem, especially bacterial vaginosis, and it possible role in premature labor and premature delivery. However, the data have not been forthcoming in explaining how or if bacterial vaginosis is one of the etiologies of premature labor and delivery. Treating pregnant patients with bacterial vaginosis has not been demonstrated to reduce or prevent premature labor or delivery in this group of patients. These observations reflect that there is a lack of understanding of bacterial vaginosis and its possible effect on pregnancy. There is a lack of understanding other causes of vaginitis that is exemplified by the poor treatment outcomes for candidiasis, bacterial vaginosis, bacterial vaginitis, inflammatory vaginitis, and so on.

HEALTHY VAGINAL ECOSYSTEM

The vaginal ecosystem is complex and consists of various constituents that are produced by the patient and by members of the endogenous microflora. The ecosystem contains carbohydrates, amino acids, sugars, organic acids, fatty acids, hormones, immunoglobulins, cytokines, and fragments of nuclei acids, cellular metabolites, and constituents as well as a variety of microorganisms. The endogenous bacteriology consists of gram-positive and gram-negative bacteria. The ratio of gram-positive to gram-negative bacteria, especially nonpathogenic bacteria to pathogenic bacteria, is important. This ratio determines the status of the endogenous vaginal microflora, that is, whether *Lactobacillus* maintains dominance or other specific bacteria gain dominance.

Lactobacillus crispatus appears to be the dominant bacterium in the healthy vaginal ecosystem and is present in a concentration of 10^6 bacteria/mL of vaginal fluid. The other bacteria that make up the endogenous vaginal microflora are present in a concentration of 10^3 bacteria/mL of vaginal fluid. The endogenous microflora is made up of a variety of gram-negative and positive facultative and obligate anaerobic bacteria (Table 59.1). Maintaining a low number of pathogenic bacteria allows the host defensive system to ward off infection, especially at the time of surgery. This low number of pathogenic bacteria, although not causing infection, does stimulate the patient's immune system at a low level and can be considered to be primed. Therefore, when infection becomes a threat and there are no other factors to burden the immune system, infection can be successfully prevented. The pathogenic bacteria

Table 59.1 Characteristics of Vaginal Discharge

Characteristic	Healthy	Bacterial Vaginosis	Candida	Bacterial Vaginitis	Trichomoniasis
Discharge Color	White	Dirty gray	White	Gray to green	Dirty-gray, green
Odor	None	Fishy	None to	None	Fishy
WBC	≤5/HPF	≤45	≤5	≤5	>5
Squamous cells	Estrogenized				Estrogenized
Bacterial morphotypes	Bacilli	Mixed	Bacilli	Mixed to unimicro	Mixed

Abbreviations: WBC = white blood cells; HPF = high power field

provide stimulation to the patient's immune system by releasing endotoxins and exotoxins into the vaginal ecosystem.

Although there are gaps in the knowledge of the vaginal ecosystem, it is known that *Lactobacillus* maintains the ecosystem in a healthy state by the production of organic acids, mainly lactic acid, hydrogen peroxide, and a protein, lactocin. This bacteriocin, lactocin, is a low-molecular-weight protein that inhibits the growth of bacteria. It appears that the critical factor in maintaining *Lactobacillus* as the dominant bacterium is the acidity of the vagina. Maintaining the pH >3.8 and ≤4.5 will allow *Lactobacillus* to be dominant. The facultative and obligate bacteria do not grow well at acidic pH below 4.5. *Lactobacillus* by the production of organic acids, especially lactic acid, maintains the vaginal ecosystem in a very acidic state. Maintenance of an acidic environment results in a significant decrease in the growth rate of the facultative and obligate anaerobic bacteria. Once the pH rises >4.5, the growth rate of *Lactobacillus* decreases significantly, the pathogenic bacteria begin to grow at an increased rate, and one or more bacteria gains dominance.

EVALUATING THE VAGINAL MICROFLORA

The evaluation of the patient with complaints of suspected vaginitis begins with taking a detailed history. This should include the patient's sexual behavioral practices. Attempt to determine all the medications that have been used to treat her vaginitis. Questions should also be directed at the use of herbal and home remedies. The use of medications could have driven the endogenous vaginal microflora away from a *Lactobacillus*-dominant microflora to any number of bacterial conditions (eg, bacterial vaginosis, group B *Streptococcus*, and *Escherichia coli*).

Question the patient with regard to the precise anatomic site where her symptoms originate. It is helpful to have a diagram of the vulva, vestibule, and the vagina so the patient can point to the anatomic area where her symptoms are. At the beginning of the pelvic examination have her point where she is experiencing her symptoms. Having a mirror available for the patient view her own genitalia can be of significant assistance in identifying the exact location of her symptoms in most instances.

The pelvic examination begins with inspection of the skin of the vulva looking for color and texture changes and thickening or thinning of the skin. In addition, inspect the vulva and vestibule for lesions (eg, fissures, blisters, ulceration, pustules, and masses). If a lesion is identified, a specimen should be obtained for culture of bacteria and herpes virus. If indicated, a skin punch biopsy should be obtained.

The vaginal examination begins with noting if there is discharge exiting the vagina. Note should be made of the color, consistency, and quantity. When inserting a speculum to open the vagina care should be taken to avoid traumatizing the cervix and cause bleeding, which will cause an increase in pH and can obscure microscopic examination. The vaginal epithelium should be examined for rugae, color, the presence of erythema, or petechiae. The vaginal discharge should be characterized as to color, consistency, and whether there is an odor. The pH of the vagina can be determined by applying a pH strip to the lateral vaginal wall and comparing the color change of the strip to the color chart that comes with the box of pH strips. A cotton- or Dacron-tipped applicator should be used to obtain a specimen of the vaginal discharge from the lateral vaginal wall. The specimen of the discharge is placed on a glass slide, and 1 or 2 drops of 10% potassium hydroxide is mixed with the discharge to determine if a fishlike odor is given off. This indicates that there are large numbers of obligate anaerobes present in the vagina, indicating the presence of bacterial vaginitis or large numbers of obligate anaerobes in association with *Trichomonas vaginalis*. The swab is placed in a test tube and 2 mL of normal saline is added. The swab is vigorously agitated to remove some of the discharge; the swab is removed and pressed on the surface of a glass slide. A cover slip is placed over the diluted discharge and examined under 40× magnification.

Patients most frequently complain of vaginal itching and or burning. These patients associate these symptoms with candidiasis and often call their physician requesting a prescription be telephoned into their pharmacy. However, not all itching is vaginal and is due to infection with *Candida*. Once again, the physician must determine the precise anatomical site where her symptoms are located. Repeated exposure to vaginal antifungal agents can cause a shift in the endogenous microflora away from *Lactobacillus*. Therefore, you should avoid prescribing vaginal or oral medication over the telephone but should have the patient come into the office for an examination.

BACTERIAL VAGINOSIS

Bacterial vaginosis (BV) is considered not an infection but an alteration in the endogenous bacterial make-up of the vagina. Thus, BV is, if the above concept is accepted, the result of a disruption in the vaginal ecosystem. The alteration in the endogenous microflora results in *Lactobacillus* being replaced by a variety of obligate anaerobic bacteria that have assumed dominance. Lactobacilli are significantly depressed, and the numbers (concentration) of facultative anaerobes occupy a position between the lactobacilli and obligate anaerobes. Obligate anaerobes number $\geq10^8$ bacteria/mL of vaginal fluid, and facultative anaerobes number $\geq10^5$ but $\leq10^6$ bacteria/ mL of vaginal fluid. Microscopic examination of the vaginal discharge will reveal the presence of an extremely dense amount of bacteria of various morphotypes, an absence of white blood cells (WBC), and clue cells. Clue cells are well-estrogenized squamous epithelial cells with numerous bacteria adhering to the cytoplasmic membrane

obscuring the cytoplasmic membranes and intracellular organs.

The etiology responsible for the shift in dominance away from *Lactobacillus* to a predominantly obligate anaerobic bacterial microflora is not known. However, one important and probably the earliest change is a decrease in hydrogen ion concentration. This rise in pH results in a decrease in growth of lactobacilli and increase in the growth in *Gardnerella vaginalis*.

The growth in *G. vaginalis* results in a further increase in pH and a decrease in oxygen concentration in the vaginal ecosystem. Along with a decrease in growth of lactobacilli, the facultative anaerobic bacteria switch from an aerobic metabolism to an anaerobic metabolism, further reducing the oxygen concentration and hydrogen ion concentration in the vaginal ecosystem. When pH 5 is reached the obligate anaerobic bacteria begin to grow more rapidly. Once the obligate anaerobes become dominant the condition known as bacterial vaginosis (BV) is established.

The diagnosis of BV is established when the following criteria are met:

1. The discharge is a dirty gray color
2. The discharge is typically liquid but can vary in consistency
3. pH ≥5
4. Mixing potassium hydroxide (KOH) with the vaginal discharge causes the release of amines that emits a fishy odor
5. Microscopic examination of the discharge reveals the following:
   a. Noticeable paucity of WBC (≤5/40× magnification)
   b. Well-estrogenized squamous epithelial cells
   c. Presence of clue cells (squamous epithelial with bacteria densely; adherent to the cytoplasmic membranes, the bacteria are so numerous that the cytoskeleton of the squamous cell is obliterated
   d. There are numerous individual bacteria floating in the vaginal fluid
   e. There is a noticeable absence of large bacilli

There is no one good treatment for BV that has a long-lasting effect. However, the available treatments (Table 59.2) have an efficacy rate slightly over the short term that is approximately 75%. Many patients state that their BV resolves when treated but returns within 2 to 4 weeks following treatment or quickly following sexual intercourse. This indicates or suggests

Table 59.2 Treatments for Bacterial Vaginosis

Metronidazole 2 g PO taken as a single dose
Metronidazole 500 mg taken twice a day for 7 d
Metronidazole gel 0.75% introduced into the vaginal daily for 5 d
Clindamycin 2% cream introduced into the vagina daily for 7 d
Clindamycin 2% emulsion introduced into the vagina once
Clindamycin ovules introduce once a day for 3 d
Tinidazole 2 g PO taken as a single dose (not currently FDA approved)

that sexual intercourse may be a mechanism of transmission altering a weakly stabilized vaginal ecosystem.

FAILURE TO RESOLVE BV

The patients treated for BV should be evaluated within 2 weeks of completing a course of treatment. The vaginal pH should be determined and if the pH has not returned to ≤4.5 and microscopic examination of the vaginal discharge does not reveal the presence of large bacilli (*Lactobacillus*), a healthy vaginal ecosystem has not been restored. The patient should be treated again. Although retreatment data are not available, the approach should be directed at lowering the vaginal pH. It is important to understand that administering repeated course of antibiotics will have an adverse effect on the endogenous vaginal microflora. Antibiotics such as clindamycin and metronidazole can (1) suppress the obligate anaerobic bacteria allowing facultative bacteria to gain dominance and (2) select for resistant bacteria among the population of obligate anaerobic bacteria.

Therefore, administration of agents to retreat patients with recurrent BV should not rely solely on antimicrobial agents. It seems logical to administer an agent that would acidify the vagina (eg, boric acid, 600 mg twice daily for 14 days). Introducing acidifying agents into the vagina will lower the pH and allow *Lactobacillus* to grow and suppress the growth of all other bacteria. It has been shown, in the laboratory, that subjecting facultative and obligate anaerobic bacteria to media at a pH ≤4.5 inhibits their growth, but not the growth of *Lactobacillus*. Administration of boric acid gelatin capsules, 600 mg, twice a day for 14 days, can result in a reduction of the vaginal pH. It may be necessary to administer a second course of boric acid to restore *Lactobacillus* to dominance.

The significance of BV is the number of genera present and the large numbers of bacteria in each genus. Although the obligate anaerobic bacteria dominate there are also a large number of facultative anaerobes. There are a large number of virulent pathogenic bacteria within each of these groups of bacteria. These pathogenic bacteria pose a threat to both the obstetric and gynecologic patient, especially if the patient is to undergo pelvic surgery. Bacterial vaginosis has been associated with postoperative pelvic infection, postpartum endometritis, chorioamnionitis, premature labor, premature rupture of amniotic membranes, and premature delivery.

BACTERIAL VAGINITIS

This is an area of some degree of controversy. Patients often present with "vaginitis," but the symptoms are not consistent from patient to patient, as they are in patients with BV, candidiasis, and trichomoniasis. There are no significant data regarding bacterial vaginitis, its etiology, microbial pathophysiology, diagnosis, and treatment. However, bacterial vaginitis is most likely to appear in patients who have been treated repeatedly with antibiotics either orally, intravenously, or intravaginally. The endogenous vaginal microflora is easily disrupted and shifted away from *Lactobacillus* dominance to another bacterium or bacteria becoming dominant.

Bacterial vaginitis apparently evolves when the pH of the vaginal ecosystem rises above 4.5. This results in a shift in bacterial dominance away from *Lactobacillus* and there is selection for one or more bacteria to gain dominance. The dominant bacterium can be any one or more of the bacteria that are already present, that is, a resident bacterium or a member of the endogenous vaginal microflora (eg, *Escherichia coli*, *Klebsiella*, and *Streptococcus agalactiae*).

Symptoms associated with bacterial vaginitis include a copious discharge, varying in color, and the patient states that her vagina feels irritated or is uncomfortable or feels like "sandpaper." The clinical findings are as follows: (1) pH ≥4.5, usually >5; (2) a copious vaginal discharge; (3) color of the discharge green, yellow, cream colored, or dirty gray; (4) WBC ≥10 cells/40× magnification; (5) squamous epithelial cells are well estrogenized; (6) the absence of large bacilli morphotypes (*Lactobacillus*); (6) the presence of numerous bacteria (eg, small bacilli and cocci); and (7) the absence of a pathogen (eg, *Trichomonas vaginalis*).

The diagnosis of bacterial vaginitis is based on an elevated pH, the absence of clue cells, and the absence of large bacillary morphotypes. Culture of the vagina can be of assistance in determining which bacterium or bacteria gained dominance. There is a tendency to treat bacterial vaginitis with antibiotics; however, the use of antibiotics can result in selection of another bacterium. Therefore, it appears that treatment should be initiated with boric acid vaginal capsules or suppositories twice a day for 14 days. The patient should be re-evaluated within 2 to 4 days after completing the therapy to determine if the pH decreased to ≤4.5, did large bacillary morphotypes resume dominance. The patient may require a second course of intravaginal boric acid capsules, 600 mg, twice a day for 14 days.

The significance of bacterial vaginitis is that one or more virulent bacteria may become dominant. If the patient with bacterial vaginitis undergoes a procedure that invades the upper genital tract via the lower genital tract there is significant potential for serious infection. This situation becomes significant if the dominant bacterium or bacteria is a gram-negative facultative bacterium.

VULVOVAGINAL CANDIDIASIS

Vulvovaginal candidiasis (VVC) is probably the most common type of vaginitis, and approximately 75% of women will experience at least one episode in their lifetime. Approximately 25% will experience a recurrence and 5% will develop chronic recurrent or persistent VVC. The difficulty in treating VVC is 2-fold: (1) although the "infecting" yeast may test sensitive to the antifungal administered, VVC does not respond to this agent when administered; and (2) approximately 20% to 40% of healthy and asymptomatic women are colonized with *Candida*. Therefore the goal of successful treatment of VVC should not be eradication of yeast but complete resolution of the signs and symptoms of disease.

Typically, the patient with VVC presents with complaints of vulva and or vaginal burning and itching. There is usually erythema, edema, and excoriations of the vulva. There can be a thick white or pasty discharge on the vulva. The vagina can also appear erythematous. The discharge may be liquid to pasty and is usually white. The pH is usually ≤ 4.5 but can be higher. Microscopic examination of a diluted portion of the vaginal discharge can reveal the presence of hyphal forms or budding yeast.

Candida albicans is the most common species causing VVC but other species can cause vulvovaginitis. *Candida albicans* is a unique yeast in that it can grow as a hyphal form or as a budding yeast. It is not known which form, if at all, is resistant to antifungal treatment. Many other species can cause vulvovaginitis and these species tend to be resistant to the commonly employed antifungal treatments, both over the counter and prescription antifungal agents. Therefore, patient suspected of or documented with VVC should have a specimen of the vaginal discharge submitted for isolation and identification of the yeast causing VVC. If the isolated specimen is identified as a species other than *C. albicans*, it is unlikely to respond to the usual antifungal agents (Table 59.3) administered in the standard dosing regimens.

However, if one of these agents is selected, it should be administered for an extended period of time. The agent selected, preferably terconazole, butaconazole, or tioconazole, should be administered as follows: Terconazole for 14 to 21 days, and butaconazole or tioconazole repeated weekly for 3 weeks.

Following completion of therapy, the patient should be re-examined at 1, 4, and 8 weeks following treatment to determine if there is short-term and long-term efficacy of the treatment. Successful treatment is defined as resolution of the signs and symptoms of a yeast infection. In addition, microscopic examination of the vaginal discharge should be devoid of hyphal elements or yeast cells. A specimen for culture should not be obtained. In the absence of the signs and symptoms of a yeast infection as well as the absence of yeast on microscopic examination of the vaginal discharge, a positive culture should not be interpreted as a treatment failure. These findings should be regarded as the patient being colonized by yeast, and the yeast is part of the patient's endogenous vaginal microflora.

Examination of the patient suspected of VVC begins with inspection of the vulva for erythema, swelling, edema, excoriations, and the presence of discharge. The vaginal examination begins with insertion of the speculum into the vagina without traumatizing the vagina or the cervix. The vaginal pH is determined, and a portion of the discharge should be examined microscopically. If there is difficulty in determining if yeasts are present, a drop of concentrated KOH can be mixed with a drop of the vaginal discharge. KOH will dissolve all constituents in the vaginal discharge

Table 59.3 Antifungal Agents for the Treatment of WC

Agent	Dosage
Intravaginal	
Butaconazole 2% cream	
Gynazole-1	1 applicator full × 1
Mycelex-3	1 applicator full daily × 3 d
Clotrimazole	
Gyne-Lotrimin 3	1 applicator full daily × 3 days or 200 mg suppository daily × 3 d
Gyne-Lotrimin combination	100 mg suppository daily × 7 d and application of 1% cream to vulva as needed
Clotrimazole cream 1`%	1 applicator full daily × 7 d
Miconazole cream	
Monistat-7 2% cream	one applicator full daily × 7 d
Monistat-3 4% cream	one applicatorful daily × 3 d
Suppository	100 mg suppository daily × 7 d
Suppository	200 mg suppository daily × 3 d
Terconazole	
Terazole 0.4% cream	1 applicator full daily × 7 d
Terazole 0.8% cream	1 applicator full daily × 3 d
Suppository	80 mg suppository daily × 3 d
Tioconazole	
Vagistate-1	1 applicator full × 1
Monistat-1	1 applicator full × 1
Gentian violet dye 2%	Paint vagina and vulva weekly until resolution of signs and symptoms of yeast infection
Fluconazole	
100 mg	2 tablets PO on day 1 followed by one tablet daily for 4 d
150 mg	1 tablet PO weekly × 1 dose
150 mg	Suppression therapy, one tablet PO monthly at the onset of menses × 6 months; patients not menstruating take 150 mg every 30 d × 6 mo
Ketoconazole	
200 mg	1 tablet PO × 7 d

except the chitinous cell walls of the fungus. Therefore, the hyphae and spore of *Candida* will be intact and easily identified. A specimen should be obtained from the vaginas of all patients being evaluated for symptomatic vaginitis. This will prove especially helpful in those cases where yeast as well as other possible causes of vaginitis are not identified by microscopic examination. It is not uncommon to examine a patient with symptoms of vaginal burning and itching and not find yeast present on microscopic examination. A negative pelvic and microscopic examination and a negative culture will essentially rule out yeast as a cause of vaginitis.

Only one species can be identified on microscopic examination of the vaginal discharge from a patient with VVC and that is nonhyphal spore-forming species, *C. glabrata*. This species is resistant to the usual antifungal agents and therefore requires the use of other agents that must be compounded and are not obtained from a commercial pharmacy (Table 59.4).

Another treatment option is to paint the vagina and vulva with gentian violet dye weekly until the condition has resolved.

Patients who have been successfully treated but experience recurrent episodes of VVC should be considered for suppressive therapy. Chronic recurrent VVC is defined as the occurrence of 4 episodes in a 12-month period. The presence of recurrent, chronic, or persistent VVC can be an indicator of diabetes or an immunosuppressive disorder. The patient's chronic use of medication may also play a role in the evolution of VVC. The patient's sexual partner should also be considered as serving as a vector for reinfection. The male partner should be suspected of having a yeast infection if he has penile burning or itching, especially if these symptoms occur shortly after having sexual intercourse. The male may report the presence of erythema of his genitalia. The patient being treated for recurrent, chronic, or persistent VVC should be treated simultaneously with a vaginal preparation and oral nystatin, 200 000 or 400 000 units 4 times a day for 10 days. This is intended to diminish the rectal carriage of *Candida*. The sexual partner should be treated with nystatin plus triamcinelone cream 3 times a day for 10 days to reduce penile colonization and decrease the chance for transferring the yeast to his sexual partner.

Once the patient with recurrent, chronic, or persistent VVC has been cured of his or her acute episode, he or she should be placed on suppressive therapy (Table 59.3). Suppressive therapy can be as follows: fluconazole, 150 mg monthly for 6 months to be taken orally at the time of the menses; if menstruation has ceased, then the patient should take the medication on the same day of each month for 6 months. An alternative regimen is to take fluconazole, 150 mg orally weekly for 6 weeks.

Pregnant patients with recurrent VVC can be treated with either terconazole vaginal suppositories, 80 mg weekly for 6 weeks. An alternative suppressive antifungal regimen is butaconazole 2% intravaginal cream weekly for 6 weeks. Fluconazole is contraindicated in pregnancy.

Patients who fail to respond to therapy and have persistent VVC can be treated with boric acid capsules or suppositories, amphotericin B cream, or flucytosine cream administered intravaginally. Once the patient responds

Table 59.4 Antifungal Agents Used for the Treatment of *C. glabrata* Vaginitis

Agent	Dose
Boric acid vaginal capsules	600 mg twice daily for 14 days
Amphotericin B cream 30 %	1 applicator full q hs × 10 days
Flucytosine	

to treatment, suppressive therapy should be instituted.

TRICHOMONIASIS

Trichomonas vaginalis is a flagellated protozoan that is found in genital tracts of females and males. Humans are the only known host for *T. vaginalis*. Studies have demonstrated that *T. vaginalis* can survive outside the human host, albeit for extremely short periods time, on inanimate objects (eg, towels, washcloths, and toilet seats). However, there are no data to support transmission from an inanimate object to a human that causes urogenital infection. Transmission from an inanimate object to a human remains a possibility but is highly unlikely.

The most common route of transmission other than sexual intercourse is via passage through an infected birth canal to the delivering fetus. Neonatal infection has been reported in 1% to 17% of female infants born to mothers with vaginal trichomoniasis.

Trichomonas vaginalis infection typically presents with a green to gray vaginal discharge (Table 59.5). The discharge can be minimal or copious and seen exiting from the vagina covering the vestibule. The discharge can be frothy. The presence of the discharge on the labia and the vestibule may be indicative of infection involving Skene glands and Bartholin glands. Infection with *T. vaginalis* can be asymptomatic, mildly symptomatic, or very symptomatic (Table 59.6).

The diagnosis of *T. vaginalis* is based on either microscopic identification of the protozoan in the vaginal discharge or any one of several commercially available tests. However, if a patient presents with the clinical symptoms and signs listed in Tables 59.5 and 59.6, but *T. vaginalis* cannot be identified on microscopic examination of the vaginal discharge, an aliquot of the vaginal discharge can be used to inoculate Diamond medium. This medium can be purchase from a

Table 59.5 Characteristics of Vaginal Discharge due to *T. vaginalis* Infection

1. The color of the vaginal discharge can range from green, yellow, gray, or dirty gray.

2. The discharge is usually odorless unless bacterial vaginosis is present, then there is typically a fishlike odor.

3. The whiff test is negative, unless bacterial vaginosis is present.

4. Consistency of the discharge is usually liquid.

5. pH ≥ 5

6. Microscopic analysis

   a. Well-estrogenized squamous cells

   b. WBC > 5/40× magnification field

   c. Clue cells are not present unless bacterial vaginosis is present.

   d. There are typically a variety of bacterial morphotypes present.

   e. Flagellated protozoans (*T. vaginalis*) are present.

Table 59.6 Clinical Findings Associated with *T. vaginalis* Vaginitis

Symptoms	(%)
None	9–60
Odorless discharge	90
Irritation, pruritis	20–80
Dyspareunia	10–50
Dysuria	30–50
Lower abdominal pain	5–12
Signs	**(%)**
None	15
Vulvar erythema	10–20
Excessive discharge	50–75
Frothy discharge	10–20
Vaginal erythema	40–75
Strawberry cervix	45

Adapted from Rein MF: Trichomonas vaginalis. In: Mandell GI, Douglas PG, Bennett JE, eds. *Principles and Practice of Infectious Diseases*. 4th ed. New York, NY: Churchill Livingstone; 1995: 2493.

number of different supply sources. The cost of this medium is approximately 50 cents to 1 dollar per tube. The inoculated medium can sit at room temperature and be examined daily for the presence of *T. vaginalis*.

Patients who present with a dirty-gray to green to yellow discharge, and in whom *T. vaginalis* is not identified on microscopic examination of the vaginal discharge, should be evaluated and treated as follows:

1. Obtain a specimen from the endocervix for the detection of *Chlamydia trachomatis* and *Neisseria gonorrhoeae*.
2. Perform a whiff test on the vaginal discharge if the pH ≥5.
3. Perform a bimanual pelvic examination to determine if there is tenderness on palpation of the cervix, uterus, and adnexa.
4. Institute therapy with either metronidazole 500 mg, 3× daily or tinidazole 500 mg daily plus levofloxacin 500 mg daily for 7 to 10 days.

The tentative diagnosis is cervicitis, especially if no vaginal pathogen is established. Treatment should be instituted if there is evidence of tenderness in the uterus or one or both adnexa. *Trichomonas vaginalis* is a sexually transmitted organism, and it is not unusual to find more than one sexually transmitted infection present simultaneously.

Cervicitis typically presents with hypertrophy of the endocervical columnar epithelium. In addition, endocervical mucopus may be present. When the cervix is gently touched with a cotton- or Dacron-tipped swab, it may bleed briskly. Patients found to have a positive test for *T. vaginalis*, *C. trachomatis*, and/or *N. gonorrhoeae* should be further evaluated for human papillomavirus, herpes simplex, hepatitis B, hepatitis C, HIV, and syphilis. Further sexually transmitted infection (STI) testing is indicated because the finding of one or more STIs is indicative of sexual risky behavior and places the individual at risk for contracting other STIs.

Treatment of *T. vaginalis* vaginitis is with metronidazole or tinidazole. Metronidazole continues to be the first-line agent because it is less costly than tinidazole. However, other than the one-time dose of metronidazole, compliance with tinidazole is likely to be higher because of once-a-day dosing and fewer side effects versus 3-times-a-day dosing. Standard treatment with metronidazole is either a one-time oral dosage of 2 g, 250 mg 3 times a day, or 500 mg 2 times a day for 7 days. The newer drug in the United

States, tinidazole, can be administered in an oral single dosage of 2 g or 500 mg daily for 7 days. Tinidazole is touted as being more effective in those cases where metronidazole-resistant *T. vaginalis* is suspected.

Individuals not responding to a metronidazole regimen should be instructed to complete the course of medication prescribed. They should also be encouraged to discontinue sexual intercourse until therapy is completed and re-examination can established that a cure has been achieved. If this can be accomplished, then she must insist that her partner wear a condom when they have sexual intercourse. In addition, her sexual partner or partners must be treated during the same period. If her sexual partner or partners are not treated, then the probability of reinfection is high.

If an individual treated for *T. vaginalis* vaginitis continues to be infected and has been compliant with the treatment and management, then the possibility of resistance should be entertained. The treating physician should contact either an infectious disease specialist or Centers for Disease Control and Prevention (CDC) for assistance in treating this patient. The physician should not automatically increase the dose of metronidazole.

INFLAMMATORY VAGINITIS

Inflammatory vaginitis is a difficult diagnosis to establish because it may be the result of an infection of the cervix, endometrium, and fallopian tubes. Inflammatory vaginitis may be the result of an infection with *T. vaginalis*, although no protozoans are seen on microscopic examination of the vaginal discharge. Inflammatory vaginitis may overlap with desquamative vaginitis, bacterial vaginitis, or trichomonas vaginitis. Whenever a large number of WBCs (>10/high-powered field [HPF]) are seen in the vaginal discharge, a pathologic condition (eg, bacterial vaginitis, trichomonas vaginitis, cervicitis, endometritis, and/or salpingitis) should be sought. When all these conditions have been eliminated, then a diagnosis of inflammatory vaginitis can be made.

Patients with inflammatory vaginitis can present with a copious yellow, cream-colored, or green vaginal discharge. There is no odor associated with the discharge of inflammatory vaginitis (Table 59.7). The patient frequently complains of nonspecific vaginal discomfort that is usually associated with pressure or friction in inserting a tampon or during sexual intercourse.

Table 59.7 Characteristics of Inflammatory Vaginitis

1. Discharge yellow, cream colored, green.

2. Discharge is odorless.

3. pH ≥5

4. Whiff test is negative.

5. Cervix does not show any evidence of inflammation, and test negative for *C. trachomatis* and *N. gonorrhoeae*.

6. There is no evidence of endocervical mucopus.

7. The uterus is not tender to palpation.

8. No history of irregular uterine bleeding.

9. Adnexa are not tender to palpation.

10. The patient is afebrile.

The evaluation of the patient should include a complete blood count with a WBC differential and sedimentation rate. The results of these tests will indicate whether there is an infection or and inflammatory condition present in the patient with inflammatory vaginitis. It is possible that the vaginal presentation may indicate that there is a systemic process (eg, lupus) that is causing vaginitis.

Once the diagnosis of inflammatory vaginitis is established and no pathogen is present, therapy with hydrocortisone can be initiated. Antibiotic therapy should be avoided in the patient with inflammatory vaginitis. Therapy with hydrocortisone, 25 mg vaginal suppositories administered twice a day for 14 days, is usually effective. The patient who does not respond to this therapy requires a second evaluation for the possible existence of a pathogen; this may require an endometrial biopsy. The endometrial specimen is divided into two portions. One portion is processed for bacteria, and the other specimen is processed for histological analysis. Again, when no pathogen is identified, reinstitution of hydrocortisone, 25 mg vaginal suppositories twice a day for 21 days, should be initiated. At the completion of this regimen, the patient should be tapered off the hydrocortisone vaginal suppositories over the next several weeks. For example, the treatment is as follows: one vaginal suppository daily for 7 days followed by one vaginal suppository every other day, and then every second day, and so on, until the patient inserts one vaginal suppository per week and then stops. The patient should be examined 1 week after completing therapy to determine if a healthy vaginal ecosystem has been restored.

CYTOLYTIC VAGINITIS OR VAGINOSIS

Cytolytic vaginitis or vaginosis has also been referred to as Döderlein cytolysis vaginitis. The distinction between vaginitis and vaginosis is based on whether an inflammatory response is present. Cytolytic vaginitis is uncommon and therefore often goes unrecognized and is treated empirically with antifungal agents or as BV.

Cytolytic vaginitis or vaginosis can be asymptomatic, or the patient may describe vague symptoms (eg, vaginal burning and or pruritus). No pathogen is identified when the vaginal discharge is examined with the aide of the microscope. The patient may also complain of dyspareunia and dysuria. It is thought that the dyspareunia occurs because there is a degree of inflammation of the vaginal epithelium and this epithelium is easily traumatized during sexual intercourse. Dysuria occurs when urine comes into contact with the tissue of the vestibule. Characteristics of cytolytic vaginitis/vaginosis are listed in Table 59.8. The diagnosis of cytolytic vaginitis/vaginosis is difficult to establish but should be suspected when the vaginal pH ≤4.0 and there is a noticeable increase in bacteria (ie, large bacilli and an absence of other bacterial morphotypes). The cytoplasm of intact vaginal epithelial cells is not homogenous but is heterogeneous and appears granular. Many of the squamous epithelial cells are disrupted, resulting a significant amount of cellular debris floating in the vaginal fluid.

There is no adequate treatment for this condition. A logical approach to treatment is to reduce the hydrogen ion concentration, making the vaginal ecosystem less acidic. The pH should be raised above 4.5 because this would lead to an inhibition in the growth of lactobacilli and permit the growth of the other bacteria that constitute the endogenous vaginal microflora. Clindamycin cream or ovules administered intravaginally should decrease the numbers of lactobacilli, thereby decreasing the amount of organic acids, especially lactic acid, and the numbers of obligate anaerobic bacteria. This should allow the pH to rise and permit the ecosystem to achieve equilibrium.

An alternate treatment is to douche with baking soda, 30 to 60 g of sodium bicarbonate in 1 L of warm water 2 to 3 times a week. This should be repeated until symptoms abate; then the frequency of douching should be

Table 59.8 Characteristics of Cytolytic Vaginitis/Vaginosis

1. Pruritus
2. Burning
3. Increase in the amount of discharge
4. The color of the discharge is white to slate-gray.
5. Consistency of the discharge ranges from liquid to pasty.
6. The number of lactobacilli is increased compared to the number present when the vaginal ecosystem is balanced.
7. WBC ≤5/HPF
8. No pathogen is present (yeast, *Trichomonas*).
9. There is no evidence of BV or an altered vaginal microflora.
10. Cytoplasm within the squamous epithelial cells is not homogenous.
11. Many of the squamous epithelial cells appear disrupted.
12. pH ≥3.5 but ≤4.5
13. Lactobacilli can be seen adhering to the membrane of the squamous epithelial cells.
14. There is a noticeable absence of other bacterial morphotypes in the vaginal discharge.

decreased to once a week until it can be confirmed that a healthy vaginal ecosystem has been re-established.

DESQUAMATIVE VAGINITIS

Desquamative vaginitis is characterized by the presence of erythema of the vaginal epithelium that can be mild to severe. When severe, the epithelia walls of the vagina appear beefy red, and shallow ulcers may develop. Typically the number of WBCs does not exceed 5/HPF. Occasionally a thin gray membrane develops over the ulcerated epithelium, and the patient complains of vaginal burning. The presence of a large number of WBCs >10/HPF can indicate that there is an infection or inflammatory vaginitis.

The diagnosis of desquamative vaginitis is based on a pH ≥5, the presence of sheets of squamous cells floating in the vaginal fluid, and WBC ≤5/HPF. The vaginal discharge is usually abundant, odorless, white, and thick to pasty and contains sheets of squamous epithelium. The dominant bacterial morphotype is large bacilli.

There is no adequate treatment for this condition, but success has been achieved with clindamycin, 2 to 4 g intravaginally every night for 2 weeks. Clindamycin should be effective in lowering the concentration of lactobacilli and obligate anaerobic bacteria without significantly affecting the other bacteria present in the vaginal microflora.

An alternative treatment is to place an acidifying agent in the vagina to lower the pH. If the pH is lowered to below 4.5, this should result in slowing of the growth of lactobacilli. Slowing the growth of lactobacilli should result in a slowing of the metabolism of the bacterium and a decrease in the production of organic acids. The end result should be a restoration in the balance of the ecosystem and a decrease in sloughing of the vaginal epithelium.

ATROPHIC VAGINITIS

Atrophic vaginitis is a condition that arises when there is insufficient estrogen, resulting in a failure of the maturation of the vaginal epithelium. This is seen in any condition in which there is a significant decrease in estrogen production (eg, breast-feeding, natural menopause, women younger than 50 who have had a bilateral salpingo-oophorectomy, and women receiving progesterone therapy in the absence of estrogen). Atrophic vaginitis can also result from women receiving therapy that suppresses ovarian function thereby causing depletion in estrogen.

The patient with atrophic vaginitis typically presents with vulvovaginal burning, itching, dysuria, dyspareunia, and vaginal bleeding. The introitus and vagina become stenoic, and these areas easily become traumatized during sexual intercourse. These patients often experience bleeding during and after sexual intercourse. The bladder, urethra, and vagina share a common embryonic origin. These organs are all hormone dependent and suffer the same consequences when estrogen is no longer available. The estrogen-deprived patient can develop urinary frequency, urgency, bladder irritation, and dysuria.

The diagnosis can be established by noting that the vaginal epithelium is pale pink to almost white, rugae are absent, and the vaginal walls appears smooth. The pH >5, and discharge is dirty gray to green. Microscopic examination of the vaginal discharge reveals numerous WBCs and rare estrogenized squamous epithelial cells. There are numerous immature squamous cells (ie, the cells appear rounded not naviculated, the nuclei are large with a reduction in the amount of cytoplasm). Lactobacilli are typically absent, and there is no one dominant bacterial morphotype.

Treatment is with estrogen replacement either systemically or intravaginally. The quickest relief is achieved with intravaginal estrogen, either a cream or vaginal tablet.

SUGGESTED READING

Amsel R, Totten PA, Holmes KK, et al. Nonspecific vaginitis: epidemiologic, diagnostic, and therapeutic considerations. *Am J Med*. 1983;74:14–22.

Aroucheva A, Gariti D, Simon M, et al. Defensive factors of vaginal lactobacilli. *Am J Obstet Gynecol*. 2001;185:375–379.

Aroutcheva A, Simoes JA, Shott S, Faro S. The inhibitory effect of clindamycin on Lactobacillus in vitro. *Infect Dis Obstet Gynecol*. 2001;9:239–244.

Eschenbach DA, Davick PR, Holmes KK, et al. Prevalence of hydrogen peroxide producing Lactobacillus species in normal women and women with bacterial vaginosis. *J Clin Microbiol*. 1989;27:251–256.

Faro S. *Vaginitis: Differential Diagnosis and Management*. New York, NY: Parthenon; 2004.

Heine P, McGregor JA. Trichomonas vaginalis: a re-emerging pathogen. *Clin Obstet Gynecol*, 1993;38:137–144.

Kaufman RH, Faro S, Brown D. *Benign Diseases of the Vulva and Vagina*. St. Louis, MO: Mosby; 2004:260–282.

Sobel JD. Epidemiology and pathogenesis of recurrent vulvovaginal candidiasis. *Am J Obstet Gynecol*. 1985;152:924–935.

Sobel JD, Faro S, Force RW, et al. Vulvovaginal candidiasis: diagnostic criteria and microbial and epidemiologic associations. *Obstet Gynecol*. 1998;178:203–211.

Sobel JD, Nyirjesy P, Brown W. Tinidazole therapy for metroniodazole resistant vaginal trichomoniasis. *Clin Infect Dis*. 2001;33:1341–1346.

60. Epididymo-Orchitis

Brandon Palermo and Thomas Fekete

INTRODUCTION

Infectious and inflammatory processes involving the contents of the scrotum are uncommon. They are usually easy for patients to identify because they cause symptoms of pain and swelling. However, most clinicians other than urologists are unfamiliar with the range of problems that can affect the testis and epididymis and rarely see boys or men with orchitis or epididymitis.

ANATOMY/DEFINITION

The epididymis is a tightly coiled tubular structure on the posterior aspect of the testes that connects the efferent ducts of each testis to the vas deferens. The three regions of the epididymis – the head, body, and tail – serve as sequential sites for sperm transport, maturation, and storage.

Epididymitis involves inflammation or infection of the epididymis, usually accompanied by pain and swelling. It is the most common cause of intrascrotal inflammation. Acute epididymitis is characterized by symptoms lasting for less than 6 weeks, whereas chronic epididymitis involves symptoms persisting for 3 months or longer. Orchitis, or inflammation of the testes, is less common than epididymitis. However, the two structures can be involved together making it difficult to distinguish the clinical entities involving them, thus the term *epididymo-orchitis* is used to capture these combined inflammatory processes. In patients with acute epididymo-orchitis, inflammatory responses in adjacent structures, such as the seminal vesicles, can occur and can lead to abscess formation.

EPIDEMIOLOGY

Overall, studies suggest that acute epididymo-orchitis is relatively uncommon. However, the true incidence in the general population is difficult to ascertain because studies often aggregate acute and chronic presentations into a single diagnostic category. A national survey of physician visits in the United States military showed that epididymo-orchitis accounted for 0.29% of ambulatory visits in men less than 50 years old; these statistics may be unreliable because they were based on billing code data. A prospective Canadian study demonstrated that 0.9% of men who presented to outpatient urology clinics in 2004 had epididymitis, which was less common than prostatitis or interstitial cystitis. Only a small fraction had acute symptoms because approximately 80% of men with epididymitis in this study reported symptoms lasting for longer than 3 months.

Acute epididymo-orchitis tends to involve only one side at a time, with right and left being equally susceptible. Bilateral inflammation is exceedingly rare. The average age of patients in the prospective Canadian study was 41 years. Other studies report variable mean ages, but the incidence of epididymitis tends to peak in younger, sexually active men. The majority of cases occur between 20 and 39 years.

PREDISPOSING FACTORS

The exact pathogenesis of epididymitis has not been clearly elucidated. Epididymo-orchitis is clearly associated with a sexually transmitted infection, urinary tract infection, or systemic infection. It is presumed that infecting organisms usually reach the epididymis via retrograde extension from the prostate or seminal vesicles, but hematogenous and lymphatic spread may also occur. It has been proposed that voiding dysfunction in the form of higher voiding pressures may result in urethrovasal reflux. Acute epididymitis is rare in prepubescent boys and, when present, is usually associated with abnormalities of the urinary tract, including vesicoureteral reflux.

Urological factors – including lower urinary tract obstruction from benign prostatic hyperplasia (BPH), prostate cancer, or urethral stricture – have been associated with epididymitis in older patients, and the presumption is that they lead to infection via the ascending route or by not permitting normal drainage of the proximal internal genital structures.

Invasive prostate procedures, including biopsy, transurethral resection, brachytherapy, laser prostatectomy, and radical prostatectomy have been associated with epididymitis; reported rates are approximately 1% to 2%. No controlled studies have been conducted to evaluate the efficacy of prophylactic antibiotics for these procedures. Other mechanical insults such as direct trauma or pressure (eg, from bicycle riding) have been associated with epididymitis even after vasectomy. In fact, vasectomy itself has been associated with persistent tenderness and a nodular presence in the scrotum—presumably the result of sperm extravasation ("sperm granuloma").

ETIOLOGY

Infectious

Pathogens were rarely isolated from the urinary tract of patients with epididymitis until the 1970s, so a debate raged about the causes of epididymitis. Some believed that reflux of sterile urine during lifting or straining caused the inflammation, whereas others believed that virtually all cases of epididymitis were due to infection of an adjacent structure. Since then, improved diagnostic testing and multiple studies have supported infection as the predominant etiology. Harnisch et al. published the first study to show that pathogens that caused acute epididymitis were associated with age: epididymitis in younger men was usually associated with urethritis caused by *Neisseria gonorrhoeae* and *Chlamydia trachomatis*, whereas in older men it was associated with *Escherichia coli, Klebsiella* spp., or *Pseudomonas aeruginosa* bacteriuria. Berger et al. later demonstrated that the majority of "idiopathic" epididymitis was caused by *Chlamydia trachomatis*.

Subsequent studies have confirmed the general relationship between age and pathogen. In children below the age of sexual activity, the microbial flora of epididymitis is a mix of skin and urinary flora. Among sexually active adolescents and men aged less than 35 years, acute epididymitis is likely associated with a sexually transmitted infection caused by *C. trachomatis* or *N. gonorrhoeae*. Gram-negative enteric organisms tend to cause epididymitis in older men, although sexually transmitted infections are still very common. Gram-negative enteric organisms should also be considered in men who have insertive anal intercourse.

Many other less common infectious causes of acute epididymitis have been reported

Table 60.1 Causes of Acute Epididymo-Orchitis

Cause	Organism/Disease
Sexually Acquired	
Major	*Chlamydia trachomatis* *Neitsseria gonorrhoeae*
Other	*Ureaplasma urealyticum* *?Mycoplasma genitalium*
Assoicated with Bacteriuria	
Major	*E. coli* *Proteus* spp. *Klebsiella pneumoniae* *Pseudomonas aeruginosa*
Other	*Haemophilus influenzae* type b *Salmonella* spp. Staphylococci Streptococci
Other Infections	
Bacterial	*M. tuberculosis* *Brucella* spp. *Nocardia asteroides*
Fungal	*Blastomyces dermatitidis* *Histoplasma capsulatum* *Coccidioides immitis* *Candida albicans* *Candida glabrata*
Viral	Mumps Mumps vaccine Cytomegalovirus (in HIV)
Parasitic	*Schistosoma haematobium* [18] *Wucherenia bancroffi* filariasis [19]
Non-infective Causes	
	Amiodarone therapy Vasculitis Behçet's disease Polyarteritis nodosa Henoch–Schönlein purpura
Idiopathic	

(see Table 60.1). *Staphylococcus* and *Streptococcus* spp. may cause acute epididymitis. Endemic fungi, including *Histoplasma capsulatum, Coccidioides immitis,* and *Blastomyces dermatitidis,* have been described. *Candida* spp. have been

Clinical Syndromes – Genitourinary Tract

reported to cause epididymitis in patients with diabetes. Suppurative epididymo-orchitis and chronic prostatitis due to *Burkholderia pseudomallei* have been recently reported in a patient who traveled to Myanmar.

Mumps virus is a well-known cause of orchitis, but epididymitis may develop as a complication. Mumps orchitis tends to occur in prepubertal boys several days after they have parotitis from the mumps virus; it is rarely seen in men. Mumps is uncommon in developed countries with broad uptake of MMR vaccination, but it still occurs in pockets where there is incomplete vaccination or when a new case is introduced even into a highly vaccinated population Mumps vaccine can occasionally also cause orchitis that is rare and mild. Mumps orchitis rarely leads to infertility.

Brucella is a relatively common cause of epididymo-orchitis in endemic areas, particularly in Mediterranean and Middle Eastern countries. Most patients have acute brucellosis when epididymo-orchitis occurs and have impressive fevers punctuated by periods of apyrexia. Patients may have a history of occupational contact with animals or consuming unpasteurized milk or cheese. Urinalysis and culture are often normal, and blood cultures are positive in about 50% of cases.

Tuberculosis epididymitis is rare and difficult to diagnose. Patients may present with a painful or painless scrotal mass or swelling. Urinalysis usually reveals a sterile pyuria, but secondary bacterial infection may be present. Diagnosis is made via identification of *M. tuberculosis* from the urine. Because few organisms are present in the urine, direct smears are usually negative and sensitivity of cultures may be only 50%. The sensitivity of urinary polymerase chain reaction (PCR) has been reported as 84% to 97%, although this test is not widely available.

Distinct etiologies of epididymo-orchitis have been reported in patients with human immunodeficiency virus (HIV) infection and in transplant recipients receiving immunomodulating drugs. Epididymo-orchitis with bacteremia has been caused by *Haemophilus influenzae* and *Chryseobacterium* (formerly *Flavobacterium*) *meningosepticum*. *Plesiomonas shigelloides* infection has become recognized as an opportunistic pathogen; a case of bacteremia and epididymo-orchitis was reported in a patient with HIV and chronic hepatitis C. *Nocardia* infection is a rare cause of epididymo-orchitis and usually involves other organs at the same time. Cytomegalovirus was isolated from the urine and semen in a patient with HIV infection who had epididymitis that was refractory to antibiotics. HIV infection may also increase the risk of genitourinary tuberculosis (TB) with involvement of scrotal contents, although such infections are more often seen in settings where patients are already at higher risk for TB.

Noninfectious

Although most cases of epididymo-orchitis are of an infectious etiology, several noninfectious causes have been described. Amiodarone can rarely cause a reversible epididymitis. Epididymitis has been reported in patients with polyarteritis nodosa (PAN); one case report has described bilateral epididymitis that did not respond to antimicrobial therapy as the presenting symptom of PAN. Epididymitis is a rare manifestation of Behcet's disease and may be associated with more severe disease. Other systemic vasculitides, including Henoch–Schönlein purpura, have been associated as well. The etiology of some cases of acute epididymitis remains "idiopathic," but advances in microbiology and molecular diagnostic techniques may elucidate specific infectious causes in the future.

CLINICAL FEATURES AND DIFFERENTIAL DIAGNOSIS

Exquisite unilateral testicular tenderness, scrotal edema, and swelling occur early and are often the dominant features of epididymo-orchitis. Fever, rigors, and leukocytosis may be present. In a retrospective study of 121 patients with acute epididymitis, dysuria was present in 33% of patients, urethral discharge was present in only 5%, and positive urine cultures were found in less than 25% of patients. Urethritis or pyuria, in the absence of bacteriuria, is usually associated with sexually transmitted acute epididymitis. Bacteriuria and irritative voiding symptoms—such as dysuria, frequency, and urgency—tend to be associated with urinary obstruction and/or structural urogenital disease in older men.

The differential diagnosis of an acutely painful, swollen scrotum includes acute epididymo-orchitis, torsion of the spermatic cord, torsion of testicular appendages, testicular tumor, incarcerated hernia, acute hydrocele, or trauma. Although these entities have overlapping signs and symptoms, identifying testicular torsion is important because it necessitates immediate surgical intervention. Testicular torsion cannot be excluded based on physical examination alone, but the absence of a cremasteric reflex in a patient with acute, unilateral scrotal tenderness suggests the diagnosis. Elevation of the scrotum usually relieves the pain of acute epididymitis but not torsion.

DIAGNOSTIC WORK-UP

Evaluation of suspected epididymo-orchitis is initially based on clinical suspicion of disease from patient complaints of pain and/or swelling within the scrotum. Although referred scrotal pain from other pelvic processes can occur, the first challenge is ruling out testicular torsion. The distinction between torsion and inflammation or infection needs to made quickly, particularly in prepubescent boys, because untreated torsion can jeopardize the testis. Expert urologic consultation may be urgently required. There are two useful noninvasive tests for blood flow to the testes. Radionuclide scanning is sensitive but not routinely available; markedly increased perfusion of technetium is associated with infection, whereas perfusion is never increased with testicular torsion. Doppler ultrasound showing normal to increased testicular blood flow is 70% sensitive and 88% specific in patients with epididymitis.

If torsion is not considered likely, the best initial diagnostic study is urine collection for urinalysis and culture. If urethral secretions are present, Gram stain is highly sensitive and specific for diagnosing urethritis (>5 leukocytes/oil-immersion field) and can establish gonococcal infection by demonstrating leukocytes containing intracellular gram-negative diplococci. Nucleic acid amplification tests of urine specimens are highly sensitive for *N. gonorrhoeae* and *C. trachomatis* and have largely supplanted urethral cultures to diagnose these infections.

In patients who do not respond to empirical therapy, particularly in those who have unique risk factors based on host immune status, travel history, or geographic location, a more exhaustive work-up should be performed in conjunction with urological consultation. This may include further imaging, additional cultures (eg, acid-fast bacillus (AFB) and fungal cultures), and direct sampling of the epididymis in some cases.

TREATMENT

Treatment includes antimicrobial therapy in combination with analgesics, bed rest, and scrotal elevation. Empirical therapy should be initiated before laboratory results are available.

For acute epididymitis likely caused by *N. gonorrhoeae* or *C. trachomatis* infection, the Centers for Disease Control and Prevention (CDC) recommends ceftriaxone 250 mg IM in a single dose plus doxycycline 100 mg orally twice a day for 10 days. For patients with cephalosporin and/or tetracycline allergies, fluoroquinolone therapy can be used with the proviso that gonococcal resistance to fluoroquinolones is spreading and thus patients will need close follow-up (particularly in areas where resistance is known to be a problem). Sex partners of patients with epididymitis caused by *N. gonorrhoeae* or *C. trachomatis*, who had contact within 60 days of symptoms, should be referred for evaluation and treatment. Although it is prudent to counsel patients that sexual intercourse should be avoided until they and their sex partners have completed therapy and are without symptoms, the optimal duration of this period of abstinence has never been studied.

When non-sexually transmitted disease (STD) infection is suspected, treatment for epididymitis mirrors that for urinary tract infection (UTI) in men. Because there are no controlled trials of epididymitis treatment, it is not known which antibiotics are most effective. Fluoroquinolones have good oral bioavailability, spectrum of activity and penetration of genitourinary tissues and have been widely used for prostatitis and UTI in men; by extension, they have been proposed as drugs of first choice for epididymitis. The CDC recommends either ofloxacin, 300 mg orally twice a day, or levofloxacin, 500 mg orally once daily for 10 days, but antibiotic choice and duration should be tailored to the specific pathogen if one is cultured. Other agents active against uropathogens (eg, trimethoprim–sulfamethoxazole, amoxicillin) can be tried in the event of fluoroquinolone failure or intolerance.

Patients should respond clinically in the first few days of treatment, and failure to improve may indicate abscess, tumor, vasculitis, or fungal, mycobacterial, or more exotic etiology. Kashiwagi et al. described 3 cases of acute epididymitis-orchitis due to *Pseudomonas aeruginosa* infection. In each case, several weeks of empirical antibiotic therapy failed, and an abscess was discovered when orchiectomy was performed. Thus, persistence of symptoms should prompt a more exhaustive work-up.

CONCLUSION

Diseases of the epididymis and testis are uncommon as compared to other andrological and urinary problems of boys and men. However, their management can be challenging because tests to make a specific etiologic diagnosis are often invasive and hard to perform in the office or even the emergency room. Once the diagnosis of testicular torsion has been ruled out, the management of epididymal disease can begin with a limited set of diagnostic tests and an empirical trial of antibiotics. For patients with more complex or chronic disease, comanagement with a urologist can allow for access to better clinical and diagnostic tools. Uncommon problems such as noninfectious diseases related to connective tissue disease or vasculitis can be challenging in patients who do not already have such a diagnosis. Unusual or exotic infections such as brucellosis or regional fungal infection should be considered in patients with the appropriate travel history. The only drug that has been strongly associated with epididymitis is amiodarone. Pure orchitis is sometimes viral and should be considered in any male with mumps (particularly if mumps virus is known to be in circulation or if there is an outbreak of febrile disease with parotitis). If patients do not respond to initial therapy, further work-up should be pursued.

SUGGESTED READING

Berger RE, Alexander ER, Monda GD, Ansell J, McCormick G, Holmes KK. Chlamydia trachomatis as a cause of acute "idiopathic" epididymitis. *N Engl J Med.* 1978;298(6):301–304.

Centers for Disease Control and Prevention. Sexually transmitted diseases treatment guidelines, 2006. *MMWR Recomm Rep.* 2006; 55 (RR-11):1–94.

Cho YH, Jung J, Lee KH, Bang D, Lee ES, Lee S. Clinical feature of patients with Behcet's disease and epididymitis. *J Urol.* 2003;170:1231–1233.

Demar M, Ferroni A, Dupont B, Eliaszewicz M, Bouree P. Suppurative epididymo-orchitis and chronic prostatitis caused by *Burkholderia pseudomallei*: a case report and review. *J Travel Med.* 2005;12:108–112.

Harnisch JP, Berger RE, Alexander ER, Monda G, Holmes KK. Etiology of acute epididymitis. *Lancet.* 1977;819–821.

Hoffelt SC, Wallner K, Merrick G. Epididymitis after prostate brachytherapy. *J Urol.* 2003;63:293–296.

Kashiwagi B, Okugi H, Morita T, et al. Acute epididymo-orchitis with abscess formation due to Pseudomonas aeruginosa: report of 3 cases. *Hinyokika Kiyo.* 2000;46(12):915–918.

Liu HY, Fu YT, Wu CJ, Sun GH. Tuberculous epididymitis: a case report and literature review. *Asian J Androl.* 2005;7(3):329–332.

Luzzi GA, O-Brien TS. Acute epididymitis. *BJU Int.* 2001;87:747–755.

Nickel JC, Teichman JMH, Gregoire M, Clark J, Downey J. Prevalence, diagnosis, characterization, and treatment of prostatitis, interstitial cystitis, and epididymitis in outpatient urological practice: the Canadian PIE study. *Urology.* 2005;66:935–940.

Rosenstein D, McAninch JW. Urologic emergencies. *Med Clin North Am.* 2004;88:495–818.

61. Genital Ulcer Adenopathy Syndrome

Allan Ronald

Control of genital ulcer disease (GUD) has become an important public health priority. Ulcerative lesions may produce significant local genital pain, some pathogens may be transmitted from mothers to their infants, and genital lesions increase the risk of human immunodeficiency virus (HIV) acquisition and transmission during sexual intercourse. Table 61.1 lists the infectious and noninfectious etiologies that may produce genital ulcerations with or without adenopathy. The most common sexually transmitted etiologies of GUD include syphilis, which is caused by *Treponema pallidum*; genital herpes caused by herpes simplex viruses (HSV) 1 and 2; chancroid, caused by *Hemophilus ducreyi*; lymphogranuloma venereum (LGV), caused by the L1, L2, and L3 serovars of *Chlamydia trachomatis*; and granuloma inguinale (donovanosis), caused by *Calymmatobacterium granulomatis*. Trauma, erosive balanitis, and fixed-drug eruptions are the most common nontransmissible causes of GUD. Neoplasia, fungi, and mycobacteria should be excluded by biopsy if the ulcer persists. Because of the limitations of diagnostic tests, a specific diagnosis is obtained in about 80% of patients.

Considerable geographic variation exists in the etiology and prevalence of GUD (Table 61.2). In Europe and North America, fewer than 10% of patients present to sexually transmitted disease (STD) clinics with a genital ulcer compared with 20% to 40% of patients presenting to these clinics in Africa and Asia. HSV is the most common cause of genital ulcerations in Europe and North America, whereas chancroid has been the most common cause of genital ulcerations in regions of Africa and Asia. However, genital herpes is now much more common in patients co-infected with HIV, whereas chancroid has largely disappeared from most African and Asian countries where it was previously common. LGV is endemic in some areas of the tropics and since 2003 has reappeared as an epidemic among men in developed countries who have sex with men, many of whom are HIV positive. Donovanosis has been endemic in Papua, New Guinea, India, and Southern Africa but it appears to be increasingly rare.

Table 61.1 Etiologies of Genital Ulcer Disease

Infectious
Bacterial
Haemophilus ducreyi (chancroid)
Treponema pallidum (syphilis)
Chlamydia trachomatis (lymphogranuloma venereum)
Calymmatobacterium granulomatis (donovanosis)
Balanitis (often polymicrobial but *C. albicans* is often present)
Viral
Herpes simplex
Varicella zoster[a]
Epstein-Barr virus
Cytomegalovirus[a]
Parasitic
Sarcoptes scabiei[a]
Phthirus pubis[a]
Entamoeba histolytica[a]
Trichomonas vaginalis[a]
Noninfectious
Trauma
Fixed drug eruptions
Pyoderma gangrenosum[a]
Behçet's disease[a]
Reiter's syndrome[a]
Wegener's granulomatosis[a]
Neoplasms[a]
Unknown
[a] Unusual.

Syphilis persists as a global pandemic that has recently reappeared with substantial disease outbreaks among homosexual men with an increased incidence in HIV-positive populations.

CLINICAL PRESENTATIONS

Clinical features of GUD are listed in Table 61.3. The incubation period is usually less than 1 week for genital herpes and chancroid, 1 to 3 weeks for LGV, and 2 to 6 weeks for syphilis and donovanosis. Depending on the etiology, the initial lesion can be a papule, pustule, or vesicle, but this lesion usually erodes to form an ulcer. In men the ulcers are often located on the coronal sulcus but may also be found on the glans, prepuce, and shaft of the penis or less often on the scrotum or surrounding skin. Herpes and chancroid have a predilection for involving the frenulum. In women the ulcers may occur on the labia, in the vagina, on the cervix, on the fourchette, or on the perianal area. Perianal and intrarectal ulcers are common in homosexual men.

Genital Herpes

HSV-1 is transmitted primarily by oral contact and in most of the developing world, primary infections occur in infancy and genital HSV-1 infections are uncommon. However, in the developed world most adolescents have not acquired HSV-1, and this virus is frequently transmitted sexually particularly with oral–genital sexual contact. In all societies, HSV-2 is almost always transmitted by sexual contact. Genital herpes due to both viruses presents as multiple, small vesicles that rapidly become superficial ulcers with erythematous margins. Dysuria, urethritis, and gynecologic symptoms may predominate depending on the site of vesicles. Systemic symptoms of fever, myalgias, and headache can occur with a primary infection. A prodome of paresthesias 12 to 48 hours before the appearance of vesicles is often reported with recurrences. Painful lymphadenopathy can be present with the primary infection. Following primary infection, both viruses remain latent in the sensory ganglions but recur unpredictably and are usually less severe than the initial infection. Recurrences tend to be more severe and persistent in HIV-infected individuals. Large, painful, often single, ulcers are commonly seen in immunocompromized HIV-infected individuals, particularly in the perianal area.

Syphilis

The ulcer seen with primary syphilis is classically solitary, painless, and minimally tender and has elevated, well-demarcated margins with an indurated nonpurulent base. Multiple ulcers are common in women.

Table 61.2 Geographic Variation in the Prevalence of Genital Ulcer Diseases

	Southeast Asia/India	Africa	North America/ Europe
Chancroid	+/−	+/−	+/−
Syphilis	+++	+++	++
Genital herpes	++++	++++	++++
Lymphogranuloma venereum	+	+	+
Donovanosis	+/−	+/−	+/−

Lymphadenopathy, if present, is usually bilateral with firm, nontender nodes. Secondary syphilis can have many cutaneous features, including condyloma and superficial ulcers.

Chancroid

Chancroid typically produces painful, excavated ulcers with irregular, undetermined margins and a purulent base (Figure 61.1). The ulcers can be superficial and may resemble herpetic ulcers. Approximately 50% of the patients will develop painful inguinal lymphadenopathy, which is often unilateral. Lymph nodes may become fluctuant and rupture. Untreated ulcers may persist for months and heal with scarring.

Lymphogranuloma Venereum

The ulcer of LGV is a small, transient, usually superficial, painless lesion that precedes the development of inguinal lymphadenopathy by 7 to 30 days; fewer than a third of the patients remember having had an ulcer. The lymph nodes are tender and may become fluctuant with eventual rupture and formation of draining sinuses. A "groove" sign may be present if nodes above and below Poupart's ligament are involved. Women and homosexual men may have involvement of perianal and perirectal tissues with clinical features of proctitis. Complications of untreated infection include genital elephantiasis, rectal strictures, and perianal fistulas. Other manifestations include meningoencephalitis, hepatitis, erythema nodosum, and erythema multiforme.

Donovanosis

The patient presents with slowly progressive disease of the genital area characterized by heaped-up granulomatous tissue

Table 61.3 Clinical Characteristics of Genital Ulcer Adenopathy Syndromes

	Syphilis	Herpes Simplex Virus	Chancroid	Lymphogranuloma Venereum	Donovanosis
Incubation period	9–90 d	2–7 d	1–14 d	7–21 d	8–80 d
Primary lesion	Papule	Vesicle	Papule or pustule	Papule, pustule, or vesicle	Papule
Number of lesions	Usually solitary	Multiple	Multiple	Usually solitary	Variable
Classical Ulcer Characteristics					
Size (mm)	5–15	1–10	2–20	2–10	Variable
Margins	Well demarcated Elevated Round or oval	Erythematous	Ragged, irregular Undetermined	Elevated Round or oval	Variable Elevated, irregular
Depth	Superficial or deep	Superficial	Excavated	Superficial or deep	Elevated
Base	Red, smooth, nonpurulent	Red, smooth, serous discharge	Purulent exudate	Variable	"Beefy" red, rough
Induration	++	—	—	—	++
Pain	—	++	++	±	—
Lymphadenopathy	++[B]	++[B]	++[U]	++[U]	—[P]
Characteristics of Lymphadeopathy					
Consistency	Firm	Firm	Fluctuant	Fluctuant	—
Tenderness	—	++	++	++	—

[B] Bilateral; [U] unilateral; [P] pseudolymphadenopathy.

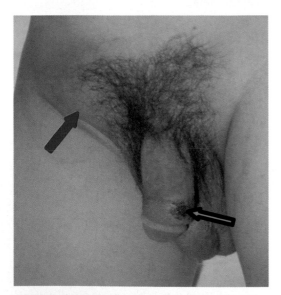

Figure 61.1 Chancroid; note penile lesion (*green arrow*) and inguinal adenopathy (*red arrow*). Public Health Image Library; content provider CDC/Susan Lindsley.

and painless genital ulceration. Local extension, healing, and fibrosis may occur simultaneously. Lymphadenopathy is unusual, but "pseudobuboes" caused by subcutaneous extension of the granulomatous process into the inguinal area are common. Systemic spread with involvement of liver, thorax, and bones has been reported but is rare.

LABORATORY DIAGNOSIS OF GUD

Clinical diagnosis of GUD is imprecise because of overlap between the clinical syndromes, the frequent presence of mixed infections, and atypical presentations. Because of these limitations, the diagnosis must be confirmed whenever possible using the relevant laboratory tests (Table 61.4). Specimens should be collected for *H. ducreyi*, *C. trachomatis*, and *H. simplex* cultures and, if available, DNA identification with polymerase chain reaction (PCR). If possible, a dark-field examination should be performed

Table 61.4 Recommended Tests for Diagnosing Genital Ulcer Diseases

	Recommended Tests	Other Tests
Chancroid	Culture	Gram stain/PCR
Syphilis	Dark-field examination	PCR
	Direct fluorescent antibody test	
	Serology (eg, RPR/VDRL, FTA–ABS, MHA–TP)	
Genital herpes	Viral culture	Antigen detection (ELISA), PCR
		Serology
Lymphogranuloma venereum	PCR	Chlamydia culture
		Serology (complement fixation, microimmunofluorescence)
Donovanosis	Giemsa or Wright stains of tissue smears	
	Histopathology	

Abbreviations: PCR = polymerase chain reaction; RPR = rapid plasma reagin; VDRL = Venereal Disease Research Laboratories; FTA–ABS = Fluorescent treponemal antibody absorption; MHA–TP = Microhemagglutination test for *Treponema palladum*; ELISA = enzyme-linked immunosorbent assay.

in all patients presenting with GUD unless classical vesical lesions in clusters provide definite evidence of herpes genitalis. The ulcer base is washed with saline, dried with a cotton gauze, and squeezed between the thumb and forefinger until an exudate appears. This can be collected directly onto a coverslip for dark-field microscopy. Vesicles and pustules should be aspirated with a fine-gauge needle or deroofed and swabbed for viral culture. Fluctuant lymph nodes should be aspirated for *H. ducreyi* and *C. trachomatis* culture. Both fluorescent treponemal antibody absorption [FTA–ABS] Treponema pallidum particle Agglutination [TPPA] and nontreponemal rapid plasma reagin [RPR], Venereal Disease Research Laboratories [VDRL] serologic tests should be obtained in all patients with GUD to exclude syphilis. LGV diagnosis is confirmed by PCR or by rising antibody titers or a single titer of 1:64 by complement fixation or 1:512 by microimmunofluorescence.

APPROACH TO THE PATIENT WITH GUD

An algorithm for investigating a patient with genital ulceration is given in Figure 61.2. The history is crucial. Information should be collected about the sexual risk factors, demographics, medication, and travel. Risk factors such as sex work or recent prostitute contact are associated with syphilis and chancroid. Travel may suggest the diagnosis of an otherwise uncommon cause such as donovanosis. Self-medication with topical or systemic antibiotics may lead to a false-negative dark-field examination.

TREATMENT

The drug regimens currently recommended for treating GUD are given in Table 61.5. Treatment traditionally has been initiated only once a laboratory diagnosis has been established; however, the delay inherent in obtaining laboratory results makes it necessary to initiate empiric syndromic therapy at the time of the initial visit. Syndromic therapy should usually be effective for syphilis. Fluctuant bubos should be incised or aspirated. All patients with GUD should be tested for HIV infection.

Patients should be reassessed at 7 days to assess response to therapy. Most patients will show improvement; failure of the lesions to respond should prompt a search for an alternative diagnosis. The RPR or VDRL as well as a treponemal test should be repeated in all patients who had a negative test on initial evaluation because the test may give a false-negative result

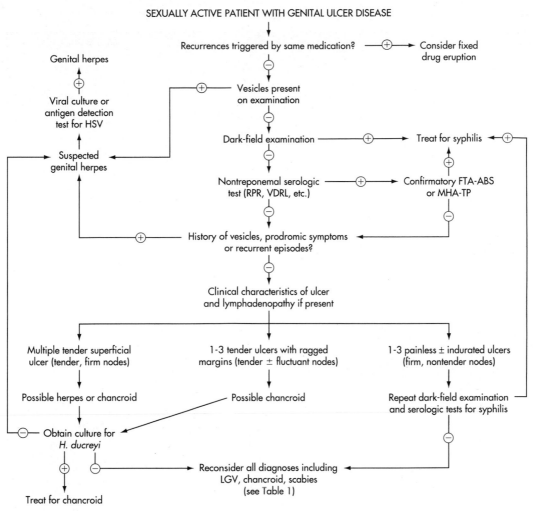

SEXUALLY ACTIVE PATIENT WITH GENITAL ULCER DISEASE

Figure 61.2 Diagnostic algorithm for patients with genital ulcer disease.

when the patient first presents with primary syphilis. Specific treatment recommendations for the common causes of GUD are given in the following sections.

Syphilis

A single intramuscular (IM) injection of benzathine penicillin G, 2.4 million U, is the treatment of choice for both HIV-infected and -uninfected patients with primary or secondary syphilis. Doxycycline or tetracycline can be used in patients with a documented penicillin allergy. All patients should be followed with a quantitative RPR or VDRL at 3, 6, 12, and 24 months after treatment. Treatment failure is diagnosed if clinical signs persist or recur, a sustained 4-fold rise in titer occurs, or an initially high titer (>1/8) fails to decline by at least 4-fold

at 6 months. Patients who fail treatment as determined by the criteria outlined should undergo a lumbar puncture and be treated with benzathine penicillin G, 2.4 million U IM weekly for 3 weeks, if the cerebrospinal fluid (CSF) is normal. Patients with CSF abnormalities should be treated for neurosyphilis. Because tetracyclines are contraindicated in pregnancy, pregnant patients with a true penicillin allergy must be desensitized and treated with penicillin. All persons who had sexual contact during the preceding 90 days should be treated as well as being followed with serology.

Chancroid

Trimethoprim-sulfamethoxazole (TMP–SMX) is no longer recommended for the treatment of chancroid because *H. ducreyi* is resistant

Table 61.5 Treatment Regimens for Infectious Causes of the Genital Ulcer Adenopathy Syndrome

Disease	Recommended Regimen	Alternative Regimens	Comments
Primary syphilis	Benzathine penicillin G (2.4 million U IM)	Doxycycline (100 mg PO BID × 14 days) or Tetracycline (500 mg PO QID × 14 days)	The Jarisch-Herxheimer (J-H) reaction (acute onset of fever accompanied by headache, myalgia, malaise, nausea, and tachycardia) may occur 2–24 h after initiating therapy for syphilis. Although the J-H reaction may produce fetal distress or premature labor in a pregnant woman; this is not an indication to delay therapy.
Chancroid	Erythromycin (250 mg PO QID × 7 days) Erythromycin (500 mg PO QID × 7 days)	Azithromycin (1 g PO × 1 dose) or Ciprofloxacin (500 mg PO × 1 dose) or Amoxicillin-clavulanic acid (500/125 mg PO TID × 7 days)	Single-dose regimens are contraindicated in HIV-seropositive patients because of unexpectedly high failure rates.
Lymphogranuloma venereum	Doxycycline (100 mg PO BID × 21 days)	Erythromycin (500 mg PO QID × 21 days) or Sulfisoxazole (500 mg PO QID × 21 days)	Contacts may require treatment.
Donovanosis	Doxycycline (100 mg PO BID)	Cotrimoxazole (TMP–SMX 160/800 PO BID) Ciprofloxacin (500 mg PO BID) Tetracycline (500 mg PO QID)	Treat until all lesions are healed (may take up to 4 wk).
Genital herpes (primary)	Acyclovir (200 mg PO 5 × daily × 10 days) Famciclovir (250 mg PO TID × 5–10 days) Valacyclovir (1 g PO BID × 5–10 days)		Recurrences require treatment only if severe.

Abbreviations: HIV = human immunodeficiency virus; IM = intramuscularly; PO = orally; BID = twice a day; QID = four times a day; TID = three times a day; TMP–SMX = trimethoprim–sulfamethoxazole.

to this regimen in most areas of the world. Erythromycin, 500 mg orally 4 times daily for 7 days, has been the treatment of choice. However, erythromycin, 250 mg 3 times daily for 7 days, is as effective in both HIV-infected and -uninfected patients. Both a single dose of azithromycin, 2 g, and ciprofloxacin, 500 mg, are also effective, with cure rates of over 90%. All chancroid patients with initially negative serologies for HIV and syphilis should have these tests repeated at 3 months. All persons who had sexual contact with the patient in the preceding 3 weeks should be treated regardless of evidence of infection. Erythromycin can be used in pregnant patients.

Lymphogranuloma Venereum

Doxycycline for 21 days is the treatment of choice for LGV, but treatment failures may occur, especially in the presence of proctitis and repeated even longer courses should be prescribed. Pregnant patients should be treated with erythromycin. All sexual contacts within

Clinical Syndromes – Genitourinary Tract

the last 30 days should be investigated for rectal, urethral, or cervical chlamydial infection and treated regardless of laboratory confirmation.

Donovanosis

Doxycycline remains the treatment of choice for donovanosis, although treatment failures occur. When therapy fails, patients should be treated with TMP–SMX or ciprofloxacin.

Genital Herpes

Acyclovir, valacyclovir, or famciclovir should be used to treat the initial clinical episode of genital herpes, and for severe cases, intravenous acyclovir therapy may be required. Prophylaxis is indicated for patients with concomitant HIV infection or frequent recurrences. Acyclovir, 400 mg twice daily, famciclovir, 250 3 times daily, or valacyclovir, 1 g once daily, each prevents 90% or more of recurrences. See Chapter 185, Herpes Simplex Viruses 1 and 2 for more details of treatment.

SUGGESTED READING

Chen CY, Chi KH, Alexander S, et al. The molecular diagnosis of lymphogranuloma venereum: evaluation of a real-time multiplex polymerase chain reaction test using rectal and urethral specimens. *Sex Transm Dis.* 2007; 34(7): 451–455.

Klint M, Lofdahl M, Ek C, et al. Lymphogranuloma venereum prevalence in Sweden among men who have sex with men and characterization of Chlamydia trachomatis ompA genotypes. *J Clin Microbiol.* 2006;44(11): 4066–4071.

Mackay IM, Jeoffreys N, Bastian I, et al. Detection and discrimination of herpes simplex viruses, Haemophilus ducreyi, Treponema pallidum, and Calymmatobacterium (Klebsiella) granulomatis from genital ulcers. *Clin Infect Dis.* 2006;42:1431143–148.

Orroth KK, White RG, Korenromp EL, et al. Empirical observations underestimate the proportion of human immunodeficiency virus infections attributable to sexually transmitted diseases in the Mwanza and Rakai sexually transmitted disease treatment trials: simulation results. *Sex Transm Dis.* 2006;33:536–544.

Paz-Bailey G, Rahman M, Chen C, et al. Changes in the etiology of sexually transmitted diseases in Botswana between 1993 and 2002: implications for the clinical management of genital ulcer disease. *Clin Infect Dis.* 2005;41:1304–1312.

Peterson TA, Furness BW The resurgence of syphilis among men who have sex with men. *Curr Opin Infect Dis.* 2007;20 :54–59.

Ray K, Bala M, Gupta SM, et al. Changing trends in sexually transmitted infections at a regional STD centre in North India. *Indian J Med Res.* 2006;124:559–568.

Ward H, Martin I, Macdonald N, et al. Lymphogranuloma venereum in the United kingdom. *Clin Infect Dis.* 2007;44:26–32.

62. Prostatitis

Jonathan M. Zenilman

Prostatitis is a common clinical problem and can be due to infectious or noninfectious etiologies. Data from the U.S. National Center for Health Statistics and other sources, including population-based studies, suggest that nearly 9% of the male population suffer from prostatitis and pelvic pain symptoms and that there are more than 2 million physician's visits annually for prostatitis, most of which are to internists and family practitioners.

Prostatitis is thought to represent the clinical syndrome correlating with inflammatory exudate within the ducts and prostate gland tissue. In acute prostatitis, the inflammatory cells are polymorphonuclear (PMN) leukocytes. In chronic prostatitis, a lymphocytic and mononuclear inflammatory process is present. Chronic prostatitis is often focal. Furthermore, noninfectious events may contribute to the chronic prostatitis syndrome. For example, prostatic concretions may serve as a nidus for the development of chronic bacterial prostatitis. Focal prostatic necrosis (as part of benign prostatic hyperplasia) may cause prostatic inflammation, even without infection.

The majority of bacterial prostatitis cases occur due to reflux of infected urine into the prostatic ducts and canaliculi. Although large-scale formal epidemiologic studies have not been done, prostatitis not surprisingly is seen most commonly in older men. Bacterial prostatitis is more common in patients with previous prostate disease, diabetes mellitus, and a history of urethral instrumentation (such as catheterization).

Because urethritis is the initial symptom of gonococcal and chlamydial infection, patients seek care early, and with the widespread availability of effective treatments, they are eradicated. Nevertheless, Sexually transmitted diseases (STDs), especially chlamydia, have been increasingly implicated in chronic prostatitis. Most of these are cases where the organism has been identified by nucleic acid amplification assays such as polymerase chain reaction (PCR).

Prostatitis due to hematogenously disseminated organisms is usually seen as part of those disease syndromes. Organisms implicated have been *Mycobacterium tuberculosis, Cryptococcus neoformans, Coccidioides immitis, Histoplasma capsulatum, Aspergillus* spp., and *Candida*. With the exception of *Candida,* these infections present as granulomatous disease and are often confused with malignancy.

PROSTATITIS: CLINICAL SYNDROMES

Except for acute prostatitis, the accurate clinical diagnosis of prostatitis is difficult. Clinical symptoms are typically nonspecific, and the differential diagnosis often includes a host of noninfectious urological problems. Many patients seek urological or infectious disease consultation for prostatitis evaluation after previous diagnoses of lower urinary tract infection or STD syndromes; therefore, they have been often treated with antibiotics previously. Because of the gland's location, definitive histopathological diagnosis by biopsy is rarely an option, unless malignancy is strongly suspected.

In 1995, a National Institutes of Health (NIH) Consensus Conference differentiated 4 types of prostatitis. The Mears-Stamey prostatitis localization protocol (see below) can be especially helpful in differentiating these types, especially types II-IV.

Type 1

Acute prostatitis is usually caused by an ascending urinary tract bacterial infection and is characterized by an abrupt, febrile illness with symptoms referable to the lower genitourinary tract. Chills, leukocytosis, urinary frequency, and occasional bladder outlet obstruction are present. A rectal examination typically shows an enlarged, boggy, exquisitely tender prostate.

Type 2

Chronic bacterial prostatitis is diagnosed on the basis of prostatic or pelvic pain symptoms, including lower genitourinary tract symptoms such as perineal, penile, scrotal, and lower back pain, urinary urgency, feeling of incomplete voiding, frequency, nocturia, and dysuria.

Diagnosis is based on culture of a pathogen in the expressed prostatic secretions (EPS) or postprostatic massage voided bladder specimen (see below).

In both acute and chronic prostatitis caused by ascending urinary tract infection, the organisms present are typically *E. coli*, with others, such as *Klebsiella* and *Proteus.*

Type 3

Chronic prostatitis/pelvic pain syndrome is defined as the presence of symptoms of chronic prostatitis, similar to those found in type 2 prostatitis, but where no bacterial etiology is found after careful investigation, including culture of expressed prostatic secretions and postprostatic massage urine. Systemic symptoms are unusual, and rectal examination of the prostate is typically unremarkable. In practice, most men come for evaluation after being treated initially with antibiotics for community-acquired urinary tract infection. In many studies, type 3 prostatitis is subdivided into two categories—those patients with symptoms who have evidence of inflammation (white cells found in expressed prostatic secretions) and those without physical evidence of prostatic inflammation (formerly termed *prostadynia*). The etiology of chronic prostatitis is not known in most cases. Inflammatory cytokines and prostaglandins have been implicated, but even if this is the case, the ultimate causal pathway and inciting event is not known.

Although prostatitis/pelvic pain syndrome is common, the important differential diagnosis includes ruling out prostatic hyperplasia due to either benign prostatic hypertrophy or tumor and urethral stricture due to previous undertreated urethritis. Carcinoma of the bladder should be considered, especially in patients with hematuria. Urine cytology is useful in ruling out this diagnosis. Neuromuscular urologic disorders may also be involved and should be considered in consultation with the urologist if laboratory investigations fail to reveal an etiology for the symptoms.

Type 4

Asymptomatic prostatitis is defined as physical evidence of prostatic inflammation in the prostatic secretions but absent symptoms. This is typically diagnosed as an incidental finding in persons being evaluated for other, noninflammatory prostate or lower genitourinary tract disorders, such as benign prostatic hypertrophy.

LABORATORY EVALUATION

The only way chronic bacterial prostatitis can be diagnosed and differentiated is by evaluating the expressed prostatic secretions for inflammatory cells and bacterial pathogens. Stamey and Meares's technique of segmental urinary tract culture is widely accepted.

Procedure

The patient should have a full bladder and should not have taken antibiotics for 48 hours. The penis is washed with sterile water (no antibacterial are used because they may reduce culture yield). In uncircumcised men, the foreskin is retracted. The patient is then asked to void. The first 10cc are collected (VB_1) and a midstream sample is collected (VB_2). After voiding 200cc, the patient is instructed to kneel. The physician vigorously massages the prostate, and the expressed prostatic secretions (EPS) are collected in a sterile container as they drip from the urethral meatus. The patient is then asked to empty his bladder, and the first 10cc of this final void (VB_3) are collected. Gram stain smear is prepared from the EPS specimens, and leucorrhea is defined as the presence of 12 white blood cells per high-powered field (WBC/HPF). The midstream urine and prostatic secretions are sent to the laboratory (chilled) for culture. The laboratory should be asked to perform low colony count cultures.

Because of the complexity of the test, some investigators have proposed modifying the test protocol to two steps—using initial midstream urine and the postmassage prostatic secretions. These results have been found to correlate well with the full 4-step procedure.

Evaluation of Results

Differential diagnosis and staging of prostatitis is achieved by using the data from the expressed prostatic secretions and the midstream urine (VB_2), and are summarized in Table 62.1. The number of white cells in prostatic secretions necessary to make the diagnosis varies in the literature. However, nearly all have >12 WBC/HPF. Type I acute bacterial prostatitis has a large number of organisms and PMN; the diagnosis is seldom subtle. Chronic prostatitis is diagnosed by presence of PMNs in the expressed prostatic secretions. Culture results from the EPS differentiate bacterial (type II) and noninfectious bacterial causes (type III).

Table 62.1 Differential Diagnosis of Prostatitis

	Midstream Urine WBC	Culture	EPS WBC	Culture
I. Acute Bacterial				
Prostatitis	++	+	++	+
II. Chronic Bacterial				
Prostatitis	+	+	+	+
III. Chronic Nonbacterial Prostatitis				
Inflammatory	−	−	+	−
Noninflammatory	−	−	−	−

Treatment of Bacterial Prostatitis (Types I and II)

For types I and II (acute and chronic bacterial prostatitis), determination of bacterial etiology is desirable because antimicrobial therapy for prostatitis is usually required for at least 4 weeks. If the patient has taken antibiotics prior to evaluation, false-negative cultures will occur. Except in cases of acute prostatitis, the clinician may want to consider discontinuing antibiotics, waiting for 48 to 72 hours, and then obtaining the prostatic fluid and urine cultures.

The organisms typically isolated are those associated with lower urinary tract infection (Table 62.2). Enteric gram-negative rods are most common, followed by *Enterococcus, S. saprophyticus,* and *Pseudomonas.* Streptococci and anaerobes are rarely involved. If the patient has been recently instrumented or catheterized in a hospital setting, especially if he or she has been treated with antibiotics, *Pseudomonas* and *Enterococcus* would be the major concerns. In some studies, *Mycoplasma hominis* and *Ureaplasma urealyticum* have been cultured in up to 25% of cases. Routine culture for these organisms is not recommended as special media, and bacteriological techniques are required. Furthermore, both of these organisms are found frequently as commensals in normal hosts and their role as pathogens is controversial.

In sexually active patients, especially those with multiple partners, *Chlamydia* and *Trichomonas* are rarely found. These organisms are difficult to culture. Fungal and mycobacterial causes can be usually diagnosed only by prostatic biopsy.

ISSUES IN TREATMENT

Evaluating treatment efficacy of prostatitis is complicated by the following:

Table 62.2 Organisms Implicated in Bacterial Prostatitis

Gram-Negative
Escherichia coli
Proteus mirabilis
Klebsiella
Pseudomonas aeruginosa
Gram-Positive
Enterococcus
Staphylococcus saprophyticus

1. The difficulties in making an accurate clinical diagnosis, especially in the substantial fraction of patients with prior antibiotic therapy for lower tract urinary tract infection.
2. The lack of a standardized definition of cure. Most studies of treatment, even those which evaluate prostatic secretions for bacteriology, do not repeat the procedure at posttherapy evaluation.
3. The optimal duration of therapy is not definitively known.
4. There are few longitudinal, randomized controlled trials which have evaluated prostatitis treatment efficacy.

Acknowledging these difficulties, most authorities believe that treatment regimens for bacterial prostatitis should include the following:

1. An antimicrobial effective against the most likely organisms.
2. An antimicrobial that is well absorbed into prostate tissue and has an acid dissociation coefficient (pK_a) that is favorable to trap the

drug in prostate tissue (compared to the acidic urinary tract environment).

3. The treatment duration should be 4–6 weeks. Therefore, drugs that require less frequent dosing would be preferred to facilitate compliance.

The quinolones and sulfa-trimethoprim (Table 62.3) meet these criteria. I prefer to use the quinolones because they are associated with fewer side effects, especially in older patients, and are more active against the gram-positive organisms. Adequate regimens include ciprofloxacin 500 mg twice daily and levofloxacin 500 mg once daily. Moxifloxacin *should not* be used because this drug is excreted primarily in the bile and does not achieve high urinary concentrations. If enterococcus is suspected, then my preference is to use amoxicillin/clavulanate (amoxicillin 875 mg/clavulanate 125 mg 3 times daily. The amoxicillin is active against enterococcus (which is resistant to quinolones), and the clavulanate inhibits the β-lactamase secreted by the enteric genitourinary pathogens.

Recurrent disease is common – reported in as many as 40% of patients. In patients with well-documented disease, antimicrobials should be resumed for a minimum of 3 months. If a second recurrence occurs, chronic prophylaxis should be considered. Recurrence after cessation of antibiotics in patients with poorly documented disease should be viewed as an opportunity to fully evaluate the syndrome.

Treatment of Type III (Nonbacterial) Prostatitis

Treatment of nonbacterial chronic prostatitis is notoriously difficult. Patients often present having had multiple evaluations and procedures; in one study, over half of patients had cystoscopic evaluation. Three approaches have been used, in each, the data either demonstrate no effect or are equivocal.

1. Antimicrobials. In carefully controlled studies, antimicrobial therapy for treatment of putative noncultivable organisms has not been shown to be effective, and is *not* recommended.

Table 62.3 Therapy Options for Prostatitis Types I and II

Trimethoprim-Sulfa DS (160/800mg) BID
Ciprofloxacin 500 mg twice daily
Levofloxacin 500 mg once daily
Amoxicillin/clavulanate (875 mg/125 mg)
Oral therapy duration is 4–6 wk

Abbreviations: DS = double strength; BID = twice a day.

2. α-Blockers. A number of smaller studies have suggested effects of α-blockers such as alfuzosin (10 mg twice daily for 12 weeks), doxazosin (1–4 mg daily for 12 weeks), tamsulosin (0.4 mg daily for 12 weeks) or terazosin (1–5 mg daily for 12 weeks). Careful studies, which have included double blind studies that used a validated prostate symptom scoring instrument and compared the drug(s) with placebo or with antimicrobials, have demonstrated minimal, if any effect. These drugs are also associated with a host of side effects, including dizziness, hypotension, headache, and decreased ejaculate volume.

3. Finasteride. Finasteride has also been evaluated in small studies, one of which has shown a modest effect in reducing symptoms but not pain, and cannot be evaluated as therapy at this time.

SUGGESTED READING

Alexander RB, Propert KJ, Schaeffer AJ, et al. Ciprofloxacin or tamsulosin in men with chronic prostatitis/chronic pelvic pain syndrome. *Ann Int Med.* 2004;141:581–589.

Domingue GJ, Hellstrom WJG. Prostatitis. *Clin Microbiol Rev.* 1998;11:604–613.

Hua VN, Schaeffer AJ. Acute and chronic prostatitis. *Med Clin N Am.* 2004;88:483–494.

Meares EM, Stamey EA. Bacteriologic localisation patterns in bacterial prostatitis and urethritis. *Invest Urol.* 1968;5:492–518.

Schaeffer AJ. Chronic prostatitis and the chronic pelvic pain syndrome. *N Engl J Med.* 2006; 356:1690–1698.

63. Pelvic Inflammatory Disease

William J. Ledger

INTRODUCTION

The current emphasis on evidence-based medicine has poorly served our approach to pelvic inflammatory disease. On paper, the goal of determining the best therapeutic strategy by prospective randomized double-blind studies is laudable, but it makes the assumption that patients with similar risk factors can be grouped into large study groups for such endeavors. It is increasingly apparent that this has not been the case.

Pelvic inflammatory disease (PID) is a classification that attempts to encompass too-wide a range of clinical syndromes. It includes seriously ill women with a tubo-ovarian abscess, who require hospitalization, intravenous antibiotics, and sometimes operative intervention for a cure. In contrast, most women with PID either are asymptomatic or have such mild symptoms that they do not seek medical care. To address these concerns, the International Infectious Disease Society for Obstetrics-Gynecology (I-IDSOG-USA) suggested the term *upper genital tract infection* (UGTI) be used with the designation of the etiologic agent. In addition, the UGTI can be placed in stages, depending on the clinical severity of the infection.

Epidemiologic studies have added to the confusion about risk factors for PID. Since the early 1980s, study after study has shown bacterial vaginosis (BV) and douching as risk factors for the development of PID, but in separate prospective studies on BV and douching, no increased risk was seen.

In addition, epidemiologic studies that suffer from inaccurate reporting of condom use and imperfect diagnosis of sexually transmitted disease (STD) infection have been used to bolster the faith-based emphasis on abstinence over condoms to prevent infection.

MICROBIOLOGY

The diversity of the clinical picture of PID is matched by the variety of microbiologic findings. There are infections in which a single pathogen dominates, such as *Neisseria gonorrhoeae*, *Chlamydia trachomatis*, and the group A *Streptococcus*. In contrast, most infections are polymicrobial with aerobes, *Mycoplasma hominis*, *Ureaplasma urealyticum*, or anaerobes involved. Gram-negative anaerobes are particularly important in those women who develop a tubo-ovarian abscess.

CLINICAL DIAGNOSIS

The clinical diagnosis of PID remains a work in progress. More sensitive and more specific invasive techniques to diagnose PID, including laparoscopy, endometrial biopsy, and needle culdocentesis have been confined to research studies and are not used routinely by clinicians. There is a dependence on clinical findings, which are variable. In some women, the diagnosis is obvious. This is particularly true in patients requiring care in urban emergency departments. When *N. gonorrhoeae* is one of the pathogens, the patient usually has severe lower abdominal discomfort, excruciating pain on pelvic examination, and an elevated temperature. This is what a clinician expects with a bacterial infection. Patients seen in the early stages of a gonococcal infection, however, may present with minimal symptoms, including a new discharge, abnormal bleeding, or urinary urgency and frequency. Another group with an obvious diagnosis are those women with a pelvic abscess. These patients are usually febrile and have tender pelvic masses detected on pelvic examination and confirmed by imaging study such as a pelvic ultrasound. In contrast, in women infected with *C. trachomatis* with PID have minimal or no symptoms, usually afebrile without an elevated white blood cell count. Many do not seek medical care. Because of this, I share the concerns of the Centers for Disease Control and Prevention (CDC) about the validity of the minimal criteria for physician diagnosis. These criteria—lower abdominal tenderness, adnexal tenderness, and cervical motion tenderness—exclude more women who do not have PID, but they also reduce the number of women with PID who are identified.

Table 63.1 Parenteral Treatment

Recommended Parenteral Regimen A
Cefotetan 2 g IV q12h
or
Cefoxitin 2 g IV q6h
plus
Doxycycline 100 mg PO or IV q12h
Parenteral treatment can be discontinued 24 h after a patient improves. Clinical oral therapy with doxycycline 100 mg twice a day to complete 14 d of therapy.
Recommended Parenteral Regimen B
Clindamycin 900 mg IV q8h
plus
Gentamicin loading dose IV or IM (2 mg/kg of body wt), followed by a maintenance dose (1.5 mg/kg) q 8h. Single daily dosing may be substituted.
Parenteral treatment can be discontinued 24 h after a patient improves. Oral therapy should then be given to complete 14 d of therapy, either clindamycin 450 mg 4× per d or doxycycline 100 mg 2× per d
Alternative Parenteral Regimen
Ampicillin/sulbactam 3 g IV q6h
plus
Doxycycline 100 mg PO or IV q12h
Abbreviations: IV = intravenous; PO = orally; IM = intramuscularly.

Table 63.2 Oral Treatment

Recommended Oral Regimen A
Ceftriaxone 250 mg IM in a single dose
plus
Doxycycline 100 mg PO 2× per d for 14 d
with or without
Metronidazole 500 mg PO 2× per d for 14 d
or
Cefoxitin 2 g IM in a single dose and Probenecid, 1 g orally administered concurrently in a single dose
Recommended Oral Regimen A
plus
Doxycycline 100 mg PO 2× per d for 14 d
with or without
Metronidazole 500 mg PO 2× per d for 14 d
or
Other parenteral third-generation cephalosporin (eg, ceftizoxime or cefotaxime)
plus
Doxycycline 100 mg PO 2× per d for 14 d
with or without
Metronidazole 500 mg PO 2× per d for 14 d
[a] Quinolones should not be used in persons with a history of recent foreign travel or partners' travel, infections acquired in California or Hawaii, or infections acquired in other areas with increased QRNG prevalence. Abbreviations: IM = intramuscularly; PO = orally; QRNG = Fluoroquinolone-resistant *Neisseria gonorrhoeae*.

There are other signs of early infection that should be called into play by clinicians. Suspect a pelvic infection in a young sexually active woman who has either a new sexual partner or a promiscuous male partner who does not use condoms. Consider this diagnosis whenever these women complain of urgency and frequency of urination, whose urination culture shows no significant growth of bacteria, irregular vaginal bleeding with no obvious cause found on pelvic examination, or, most commonly, a new vaginal discharge.

Another problem is that more relaxed physician standards that increase the likelihood of a diagnosis of PID are of no value if the patients do not present for care. The current reality in the United States is that many of these women with few or no symptoms do not consider themselves sick enough to seek medical care. We need a new direction in patient care. Women need to be educated and made aware of the risks of infection if exposed to a new male partner who does not use a condom. They also should be made aware of the subtle signs of pelvic infection and to seek medical care. One possible future strategy will be to have these women test themselves with a vaginal swab that will be polymerase chain reaction (PCR) tested for the presence of *C. trachomatis*. Studies indicate that this would be a feasible strategy.

TREATMENT

There are no prospective studies available with the statistical power to dictate absolute criteria to determine hospital admission or the best choice of antibiotics to prevent long-term morbidity. One study to compare inpatient versus outpatient therapy had 78.1% of the patients with well-established infections, with symptoms for more than 3 days, before treatment was begun. Well-established infections are not as responsive to antibiotic therapy. In addition, the current clinical reality of care is that treatment regimens have to be initiated before culture or PCR studies identify the pathogens present. Because of this, initial regimens should include antibiotics effective against *N. gonorrhoeae, C. trachomatis*, and gram-negative anaerobes. Changes in initial choices can be made if bacterial identification suggests that other agents should be used.

In Sexually Transmitted Diseases Treatment Guidelines, 2006, the CDC provide the following options (Tables 63.1 and 63.2). Patients who fail to respond to systemic antibiotic treatment should be evaluated to see whether pelvic abscess formation has occurred. In women in whom an abscess is discovered, aspiration can be done under direct laparoscopic vision or ultrasonography guided needle aspiration. The patients who fail to respond to this intervention are few in number, but they may need operative removal of infected tissue to achieve a cure.

SUGGESTED READING

Centers for Disease Control and Prevention. Sexually transmitted diseases treatment guidelines 2006. 2006;55(RR-11):1.

Hemsel DL, Ledger WJ, Martens M, Monif GRG, Osborne NG, Thomason JL. Concerns Regarding the Centers for Disease Control's published guidelines for pelvic inflammatory disease. *Clin Infect Dis*. 2001;32:103.

Montgomery RS, Wilson SE. Intra-abdominal abscesses: image-guided diagnosis and therapy. *Clin Infect Dis*. 1996;23:28.

Ness RB, Soper DE, Holley RL, et al. Effectiveness of inpatient and outpatient treatment strategies for women with pelvic inflammatory disease: results from the Pelvic Inflammatory Disease Evaluation and Clinical Health (PEAH) Randomized Trial. *Am J Obstet Gynecol*. 2002;186:929.

Ness RB, Hillier SL, Kip KE, et al. Bacterial vaginosis and risk of pelvic inflammatory disease. *Obstet Gynecol*. 2004;104:761–769.

Peipert JF, Boardman L, Hogan JW, Mayer KH. et al. Laboratory evaluation of acute upper genital tract infection. *Obstet Gynecol*. 1996;87:730.

Polaneczky M, Quigley C, Pollock L, et al. The use of self-collected vaginal introital specimens for the detection of Chlamydia trachomatis infections in women. *Obstet Gynecol*. 1998;91:375.

Reich H, McGlynn F. Laparoscopic treatment of tubo-ovarian and pelvic abscess. *J Reprod Med*. 1987;32:747.

Rothman KJ, Funch DP, Alfredson T, et al. Randomized field trial of vaginal douching, pelvic inflammatory disease and pregnancy. *Epidemiology* 2003;14(3):340.

Sweet RL. Role of bacterial vaginosis in pelvic inflammatory disease. *Clin Infect Dis*. 1995;20:S271.

Witkin SS, Jeremias J, Toth M and Ledger WJ. Cell-medicated immune response to the recombinant 57-kDa heat-shock protein of Chlamydia trachomatis in women with Salpingitis. *J Inf Dis*. 1993;167:1379.

Wølner-Hanssen P, Eschenbach DA, Paavonen J, et al. Association between vaginal douching and acute pelvic inflammatory disease. *JAMA*. 1990;263(14):1936

64. Urinary Tract Infection

Henry M. Wu, Judith A. O'Donnell, and Elias Abrutyn[†]

Urinary tract infections (UTIs) are exceedingly common in both the outpatient and inpatient settings. They occur in patients of all ages, affecting females throughout life and males at each end of the age spectrum. In 2000, there were an estimated 8.27 million outpatient physician visits with UTI as the primary diagnosis. In addition, UTIs are the most common nosocomial infection and the leading cause of gram-negative bacillary sepsis in hospitalized patients. The phrase *urinary tract infection* encompasses a broad array of diagnoses, including cystitis, pyelonephritis, asymptomatic bacteriuria, complicated infections associated with nephrolithiasis or bladder catheters, and recurrent infections. The appropriate management of a patient with a UTI entails the consideration of several factors, including the patient's age and sex, the presence of underlying diseases or pregnancy, the history and timing of prior UTIs, the differentiation between cystitis and pyelonephritis, and the expected microbial uropathogen involved.

The delineation of upper versus lower tract infection is essential to understanding the approach to therapy. *Lower urinary tract infection* is infection involving the bladder (cystitis) and describes the syndrome of dysuria, pyuria, increased urinary frequency, or urgency. *Upper urinary tract infection,* or *pyelonephritis,* is infection involving the bladder and kidney that classically presents with fever and flank pain, with or without the symptoms of lower tract infection. The pathogenesis of most upper and lower UTIs is related to the ability of microorganisms to establish colonization in the periurethral area and subsequently ascend into the urinary tract, thus causing infection. The hematogenous route is a less common mechanism for establishing UTIs.

Distinguishing uncomplicated from complicated UTI is critical to developing an appropriate treatment strategy. An uncomplicated infection of the urinary tract occurs in an otherwise healthy individual who has no functional or structural abnormalities of the kidneys, ureters, bladder, or urethra. Most adult women with cystitis fall into this category. Complicated infections of the urinary tract are those infections occurring in the setting of functional or anatomic abnormalities of the upper or lower tract (such as urinary retention from anatomic obstruction or neurogenic bladder) that are associated with nephrolithiasis, occur in the presence of an indwelling bladder catheter, or are seen in patients with underlying conditions such as pregnancy, diabetes mellitus, renal transplantation, or sickle cell anemia. Infections with unusual or multidrug-resistant bacteria are also often considered complicated. These conditions are recognized as factors that conceptually affect response to therapy adversely. UTIs in adult men are uncommon without complicating factors (such as urinary obstruction or prostatitis), and most cases should be treated as complicated infections.

Uncomplicated lower UTIs respond well to therapy of short duration (3–7 days) and are not associated with sequelae. Complicated infections are often associated with factors that may predispose the patient to bacteremia or recurrence, and they are thought to require longer courses of therapy (7–14 days or more). It is important to recognize that different authors often define complicated UTIs differently, and that few studies have been performed to determine the best treatment courses for specific types of complicated UTIs.

The vast majority of both upper and lower tract infections are monomicrobial. *Escherichia coli* by far is the single most common pathogen among all UTIs. Other members of the *Enterobacteriaceae* family such as *Proteus* species, *Enterobacter* species, and *Klebsiella* species are also common UTI pathogens. *Staphylococcus saprophyticus* is the second most common cause of uncomplicated lower tract UTI in women. Among the other gram-positive organisms, *Enterococcus* species are frequently encountered. Many other bacteria have been implicated as UTI pathogens, especially when an indwelling bladder catheter is present. A polymicrobial infection in the absence of a bladder catheter may suggest an enterovesical fistula, although urine cultures contaminated in the collection process are often polymicrobial. Fungi can also be pathogens, usually when a bladder catheter is chronic. *Candida albicans* and other *Candida* species are the most common isolates when funguria is identified. Several sexually transmitted infections (STIs), including *Chlamydia trachomatis, Neisseria gonorrhoeae, Trichomonas vaginalis,* and genital herpes simplex virus infection, can present similarly to UTI. Appropriate diagnostic evaluation for STIs should be a part of a UTI work-up in sexually active patients with symptoms that may also be consistent with an STI.

LOWER UTI: CYSTITIS

Women are much more likely to develop cystitis than men, in part because bacteria are able to ascend into the bladder of women with greater efficiency, and uncomplicated cystitis in women represents the most common UTI encountered in the outpatient setting. Typical symptoms include dysuria, urinary frequency, urgency, and, occasionally, hematuria or lower abdominal pain. The presence of fever or flank pain should raise the concern for pyelonephritis or complicated UTI. In addition to history and physical exam findings, laboratory tests, including rapid dipstick testing, microscopic analysis of urine sediment, and urine culture, are often used in the diagnosis of cystitis and other UTIs.

Diagnosis

Studies suggest that the pretest probability of UTI in women who present with UTI symptoms is very high, with estimates ranging from 35% to over 50%. Specific symptoms (dysuria, frequency, and hematuria) have been found to raise the likelihood of UTI in women who present for evaluation. However, other findings such as the absence of dysuria or back pain, and the presence of vaginal irritation or discharge (by history or physical examination) decrease the likelihood of UTI. The presence of more than one symptom of UTI such as dysuria and frequency combined with the absence of vaginal discharge or irritation can raise the likelihood of UTI sufficiently to make empiric treatment without further testing reasonable in a woman with no complicating factors in her history. However, testing with dipstick tests, microscopic urinalysis, or culture is often necessary to confirm the diagnosis. A urine culture should be obtained from patients with suspected pyelonephritis or evidence of complicated UTI, recurrent UTIs, or treatment failures. Urine cultures should also be obtained for patients with risk factors

for antibiotic resistant uropathogens (including recent antibiotic use, recent hospitalization, or residence in a long-term care facility).

Laboratory diagnosis of all UTIs involves the screening for significant pyuria and bacteriuria. Pyuria is present in virtually all cases of symptomatic UTIs in nonneutropenic patients. Bacteriuria can be difficult to assess given the ease of specimen contamination with periurethral flora during collection, as well as, the overgrowth of bacteria that may result from the improper handling of specimens. Although suprapubic aspiration or straight catheterization has the best chance of minimizing contamination, midstream, "clean-catch" urine collection remains the most practical method of obtaining urine samples in the ambulatory adult.

Dipstick tests are commonly used because of their rapid results and ease of use. The performance characteristics of the dipstick leukocyte esterase (LE, an indirect indicator of pyuria) and nitrite tests (an indicator for the presence of bacteria in the family Enterobacteriaceae, including *E. coli*) have been extensively studied, although their accuracy varies significantly depending on the patient population and the standard used to define UTI. A positive result for either LE or nitrite testing has shown to have limited sensitivity for the detection of UTI. A negative test for both is also limited in its specificity for the absence of UTI. The ideal role of dipstick testing in the work-up of UTIs remains unclear, though the predictive value of positive or negative results clearly varies widely depending on the pretest likelihood of UTI. For example, in a woman with a typical UTI presentation without vaginal symptoms, the pretest probability of UTI is very high; therefore, a positive urine LE or nitrite test would add little to the already high level of suspicion for UTI, whereas negative tests for both cannot rule out infection confidently enough to withhold further work-up or treatment. The dipstick may be most useful for rapid rule-out of UTI among women with a moderate to low pretest likelihood of infection, such as minimally symptomatic patients or those with both bladder and vaginal symptoms.

Pyuria can be assessed with more direct methods. Hemocytometer (counting chamber) measurement of urine leukocytes can give an accurate assessment of pyuria. A urine leukocyte count ≥ 10 leukocytes/mm^3 is considered significant. Another method involves the microscopic examination of urine sediment from centrifuged samples, counting the number of leukocytes observed per high-powered field. The accuracy of this method depends significantly on the skill of the operator and the level of laboratory procedural standardization. Readers are encouraged to determine the method used by their laboratory.

Bacteria can be readily seen by examining a wet mount preparation or by Gram stain of unspun urine. The gram-stained preparations are particularly useful in severe UTIs, where early identification of the uropathogen morphology (ie, gram-negative vs gram-positive) may be helpful. Although not always necessary in the work-up of uncomplicated cystitis in women, quantitative urine cultures provide the gold standard for microbiologic diagnosis of UTIs. Growth, identification, and susceptibility testing of the uropathogen can offer the most effective means for establishing infection and determining appropriate therapy.

Traditionally, bacteriuria with $\geq10^5$ colony-forming units (CFU) of bacteria per milliliter of urine has been considered indicative of UTI. This threshold was extrapolated from studies of pyelonephritis or asymptomatic bacteriuria in women. However, based on more recent studies, lower colony counts (10^2 to 10^4 CFU/mL) in association with signs and symptoms of cystitis in young women have also been accepted as significant and diagnostic of infection. It remains unclear what quantitative threshold is ideal for complicated infections or UTIs in men, although some authorities recommend a threshold of 10^3 CFU/mL of urine for the latter.

Therapy

Therapy of uncomplicated cystitis is directed at eradicating pathogenic bacteria from the bladder as well as the periurethral area, and this can be accomplished with a short course of an effective antimicrobial agent. Therapy is usually started without available culture results, and empiric antibiotic treatment is directed against the most common uropathogens. For healthy women with uncomplicated cystitis, empiric treatment targeting *E. coli* and *S. saprophyticus* is recommended. Trimethoprim-sulfamethoxazole (TMP–SMX) and fluoroquinolones (eg, ciprofloxacin, ofloxacin, and levofloxacin) have been most extensively studied, and 3-day treatment courses have been shown to be as effective as longer courses for uncomplicated UTI in women. TMP–SMX is generally well tolerated and inexpensive, justifying its historic role as a first-line agent. TMP as a single agent appears to be as effective as TMP–SMX, and it

may be considered in patients with a history of sulfa allergy. Fluoroquinolones have gained much popularity due to their wide spectrum of activity and excellent tolerability. It should be noted that oral fluoroquinolones cannot be taken concomitantly with preparations containing divalent or trivalent cations (eg, iron salts or antacids containing magnesium or aluminum) or sucralfate. Among the newer fluoroquinolones, moxifloxacin and gemifloxacin achieve poor levels in the urine and are not approved for treatment of UTI.

Ampicillin and amoxicillin, which were once mainstays of UTI therapy, should no longer be considered first-line agents. Thirty to forty percent of community-acquired *E. coli* strains are resistant to these β-lactam drugs. Moreover, TMP–SMX and the fluoroquinolones appear to be more effective cystitis treatments even when resistance is not present. TMP–SMX and fluoroquinolones appear to be more effective than β-lactam drugs at eliminating *E. coli* and other pathogens from the vaginal reservoir while causing less disruption of normal vaginal and fecal flora. Other drugs approved for the treatment of uncomplicated cystitis are nitrofurantoin (given for 7 days) and single-dose fosfomycin. Their efficacy appears to be somewhat inferior compared to TMP–SMX and fluoroquinolones, but evaluation of these treatments are less complete. Nitrofurantoin and fosfomycin have only been studied for treatment of lower UTIs, and they should not be used to treat upper UTIs. It should also be noted that these antibiotics each have relatively narrow spectrums of coverage.

The rapidly increasing rate of resistance of *E. coli* to TMP-SMX since the early 1980s has raised significant concern about its empiric use for UTI. This has led to the general recommendation from experts that TMP-SMX should not be used as a first-line agent when local resistance rates are greater than 10%–20%. Fluoroquinolones are usually recommended as the alternative first-line agent, though the increasing rates of resistance to these drugs are also concerning.

Studies have suggested that the highest risk of UTI caused by TMP–SMX–resistant *E. coli* is associated with recent TMP–SMX or other systemic antibiotic use. Other studies have found similar associations between recent fluoroquinolone use and the development of fluoroquinolone-resistant infections. Recent infection with drug-resistant bacteria, hospitalization, or residence in a long-term care facility can also increase the risk of UTI caused by drug-resistant bacteria. When local outpatient uropathogen resistance rates are not available, it is reasonable to limit first-line use of TMP–SMX to patients without recent antibiotic treatment in the past 3 months and no recent hospitalization. For mild infections, nitrofurantoin or fosfomycin may be reasonable alternatives to TMP–SMX in patients who have not received these antibiotics recently. Table 64.1 outlines general treatment recommendations and drug dosages for uncomplicated cystitis.

Complicated UTI

A detailed discussion of the diagnosis and management of individual types of complicated UTIs is beyond the scope of this chapter. The management of funguria and UTIs occurring in catheterized patients are discussed in detail in Chapter 106, Infections Associated with Urinary Catheters. Generally, urine culture and sensitivity should be performed for all patients with complicated UTIs. Treatment duration for complicated UTIs, including UTIs in men, is usually 7 to 14 days, due to the potential for higher rates of treatment failure and relapse in complicated infections treated for short courses.

The issues regarding antibiotic choice in light of increasing rates of resistance are similar to those discussed previously for uncomplicated UTIs; however, one must remember the potentially higher risk of resistant pathogens in many populations with complicated UTIs, particularly those who have had recent antibiotic use, recurrent infections, or recent hospitalization. Therefore, TMP–SMX, nitrofurantoin, and fosfomycin are generally not recommended for the empiric treatment of complicated infections, and it is recommended to initiate treatment with a broad-spectrum antibiotic such as a fluoroquinolone. Coverage should be modified as needed, or narrowed where possible, once the culture and susceptibility results are available. Consultation with an infectious diseases expert should be considered in severe cases or those with highly resistant pathogens.

UPPER UTI: PYELONEPHRITIS

Causative organisms for pyelonephritis are similar to those causing uncomplicated cystitis. Typical symptoms and signs include fever (>38°C), nausea, vomiting, flank pain, or costovertebral angle tenderness. Symptoms of cystitis are often present. The diagnosis of pyelonephritis can often be made clinically; however, it is important to remember that pyelonephritis may present similarly to other intra-abdominal and gynecologic conditions, including appendicitis, cholecystitis, and pelvic inflammatory disease. Therefore, a careful history and physical exam are essential, and a pelvic examination should be considered in women who present with vaginal symptoms or atypical presentations.

As is true with other types of UTI, pyuria is almost always present. Urine dipstick tests for LE and nitrites can be used to screen for the presence or absence of infection but they cannot differentiate upper from lower tract diseases. Furthermore, they are generally not sensitive enough to rule out pyelonephritis; therefore, urinalysis with a quantitative measurement for pyuria should be performed (ie, with a hemocytometer or microscopic examination of urine sediment). A urine Gram stain may be helpful to direct initial empiric treatment; however, urine culture and sensitivity are essential in all cases. The accepted diagnostic threshold for significant bacteriuria in pyelonephritis is $\geq 10^5$ CFU/mL of urine, although colony counts as low as 10^3 CFU/mL of urine may be seen. Blood cultures should be performed in patients with high fever or severe disease. Pregnancy should be ruled out in all women of childbearing age. Pregnancy is a predisposing condition for pyelonephritis, and many antibiotics, including fluoroquinolones, are contraindicated during pregnancy.

Many patients with uncomplicated pyelonephritis may be treated as outpatients with oral antibiotics. Indications for hospitalization include severe nausea or vomiting requiring intravenous antibiotics or hydration, signs of sepsis or severe disease (high fevers, hypotension, etc.), diagnostic uncertainty, or concerns regarding ability to adhere to treatment plans or follow-up. If the patient is deemed an appropriate candidate for outpatient oral therapy, fluoroquinolones are generally recommended as the first-line agent given the rising rates of resistance to TMP–SMX in *E. coli* (Table 64.2). If a urine Gram stain reveals gram-positive cocci (suggesting a possible enterococcal infection), amoxicillin should be added at 500 mg orally 3 times daily. Antibiotics should be narrowed or adjusted according to culture and susceptibility results, and TMP–SMX can be used if the causative pathogen is shown to be susceptible. Fourteen-day treatment courses have traditionally been recommended for pyelonephritis, but courses as short as 7 days may be appropriate in mild to moderate cases when fluoroquinolones are used. Patients usually improve quickly over the first 48 to 72 hours of therapy, and it is important for follow-up to occur within this period to review clinical

Table 64.1 Antibiotics for Uncomplicated Lower Urinary Tract Infections

Drug	Dose	Comments
TMP–SMX	1 DS (160/800) tablet 2× for 3 d	First-line agents unless:≥ 10%-20% rate of *E. coli* resistance to TMP-SMX locally, or History of recent[a] antibiotic use, or History of recent hospitalization TMP may be considered as an alternative to TMP-SMX in patients with sulfa allergy. FDA pregnancy category C
TMP	100 mg 2× for 3 d	
Ciprofloxacin	250 mg 2× for 3 d	Consider fluoroquinolones as first line agents if: ≥10%–20% rate of *E. coli* resistance to TMP-SFX locally, or History of sulfa allergy, or Recent[a] history of antibiotic use other than fluoroquinolones FDA pregnancy category C
Extended-release ciprofloxacin	500 mg daily for 3 d	
Levofloxacin	250 mg daily for 3 d	
Ofloxacin	200 mg × for 3 d	
Nitrofurantoin (macrocrystals)	50–100 mg 4× daily for 7 d	May be less effective but consider for patients with mild to moderate symptoms, and: ≥10–20% rate of *E. coli* resistance to TMP–SMX locally, or History of sulfa allergy, or Recent[a] history of antibiotic use other than nitrofurantoin FDA pregnancy category B
Nitrofurantoin (monohydrate macrocrystals)	100 mg 2× daily for 7 d	
Fosfomycin	3 gm single dose	May be less effective but consider for patients with mild to moderate symptoms, and: ≥10%–20% rate of *E. coli* resistance to TMP–SMX locally, or History of sulfa allergy, or Recent[a] history of antibiotic use other than fosfomycin FDA pregnancy category B

[a] Within the previous 3 months.
Note. Antibiotic dose recommendations assume normal renal function.
Abbreviations: TMP–SMX = trimethoprim–sulfamethoxazole; DS = double strength; FDA = Food and Drug Administration.

response and culture results. In the absence of improvement, further diagnostic evaluation is required to determine if there is an abscess or urinary tract obstruction.

Patients requiring hospitalization for management and initial treatment of pyelonephritis can be given parenteral therapy with any of several anti-infective agents (Table 64.2). Therapy with a parenteral fluoroquinolone, extended-spectrum cephalosporin, or aminoglycoside with or without ampicillin should be considered. If gram-positive cocci are found on Gram stain, therapy with ampicillin (or ampicillin–sulbactam) with an aminoglycoside is recommended. Local resistance patterns, if available, should direct empiric antibiotic choices. Increasingly, multidrug-resistant *Enterobacteriaceae* and enterococci are

encountered, particularly in inpatient settings. Coverage with broader spectrum agents (eg, cefepime, ceftazidime, piperacillin–tazobactam, ticarcillin-clavulanate, amikacin, imipenem, or meropenem) should be considered in severe cases or in patients with risk factors for drug-resistant uropathogens. Consultation with an infectious diseases expert should be considered in such cases.

Antibiotic coverage should be narrowed, if possible, when culture and sensitivity results are available. After clinical improvement, oral therapy with a fluoroquinolone, TMP–SMX, amoxicillin, or amoxicillin–clavulanate can be considered for susceptible infections. A 14-day course of therapy is generally recommended for hospitalized patients. In the event that no response to therapy is seen within the first

Table 64.2 Antibiotics for Uncomplicated Pyelonephritis

Description	Therapy	Comments
Outpatient	Ciprofloxacin, 500 mg 2× daily Levofloxacin, 250–500 mg daily	Fluoroquinolones are first-line agents in most situations. Must follow-up in 48–72 h to assess response.
	TMP-SMX, 1 DS (160/800) tablet twice daily	Use TMP-SMX only if causative organism is shown to be susceptible.
Hospitalized	Ciprofloxacin, 400 mg IV q12h Levofloxacin, 250–500 mg IV daily Ceftriaxone, 1 g q24h Cefotaxime, 1 g q8h Aztreonam, 1 g q8h Ampicillin[a] 1–2 g q6h + aminoglycoside (Gentamicin or tobramycin, 5 mg/kg q24h) Gentamicin or tobramycin, 5 mg/kg q24h	Streamline therapy based on culture and sensitivity data; can switch to orals once patient responds. Empiric use of broader spectrum agents may be necessary in severe disease or if the risk of antibiotic-resistant bacteria is present.

[a] If enterococcus suspected use an ampicillin-based regimen.
Abbreviation: C/S = culture and sensitivity.
Note. Antibiotic dose recommendations assume normal renal function.

72 hours, renal ultrasound or computed tomography (CT) scan is suggested to evaluate for obstruction, abscess, or other complication.

ASYMPTOMATIC BACTERIURIA

Asymptomatic bacteriuria is defined as the presence of significant bacteriuria ($\geq 10^5$ CFU/mL) in the absence of signs or symptoms of UTI. The diagnosis of asymptomatic bacteriuria is made in women after *two* separate clean-voided urine specimens demonstrate the same organism. Only *one* sample is required to make the diagnosis in males. When urine is obtained via straight catheterization in men or women, one sample with bacteriuria $\geq 10^2$ CFU/mL is considered diagnostic. Asymptomatic bacteriuria can be common in certain populations. Reported prevalence rates range from 1.0% to 5.0% among healthy premenopausal women to 1.9% to 9.5% among pregnant women and up to 16% of elderly ambulatory women. The prevalence of asymptomatic bacteriuria is even greater among elderly persons in long-term care facilities and patients with spinal cord injuries. The rate of asymptomatic bacteriuria reaches 100% in patients with chronic urinary catheterization.

Various studies have shown no clinical benefit in the treatment of asymptomatic bacteriuria in most patient populations, including diabetics, patients with spinal cord injury, and patients with an indwelling catheter. Notable exceptions are pregnant women and patients undergoing urologic procedures with expected mucosal bleeding. Pregnant women with asymptomatic bacteriuria have an increased risk of pyelonephritis and are more likely to experience premature delivery. Patients with asymptomatic bacteriuria undergoing urologic procedures with mucosal bleeding such as transurethral prostate resection have a high rate of bacteremia and sepsis. Therefore, the Infectious Diseases Society of America (IDSA) *Guidelines for the Diagnosis and Treatment of Asymptomatic Bacteriuria* recommend screening and treatment for asymptomatic bacteriuria in pregnant women and prior to urologic procedures where mucosal bleeding is expected. Pregnant women should be screened early in pregnancy and treated with 3 to 7 days of an antibiotic that may be safely administered during pregnancy. Empiric choices include amoxicillin, 500 mg orally 3 times daily, or cephalexin, 500 mg orally four times daily. TMP–SMX (one double-strength tablet twice daily) may also be used if the pregnancy is not in the third trimester. Pregnant women should be periodically screened for recurrent bacteriuria after treatment, but the proper screening interval is not known. Patients undergoing urologic procedures should be screened and, if culture positive, treated prior to the procedure. IDSA guidelines indicate that antibiotics should be discontinued at the completion of the procedure, unless an indwelling catheter is left in place.

There is no evidence to support the routine screening for asymptomatic bacteriuria in most other patient populations. However, studies on

Table 64.3 Summary of Treatment Recommendations for Recurrent Urinary Tract Infections

Prophylaxis	Antimicrobial Agent	Dose	Comments
Postcoital (Single Dose)	TMP–SMX	40/200 mg (1/2 single-strength tablet)	Eliminates vaginal reservoir without disturbing other flora FDA pregnancy category C
	Nitrofurantoin (macrocrystals)	50–100 mg	FDA pregnancy category B
	Cephalexin	250 mg	Disrupts vaginal flora FDA pregnancy category B
	Ciprofloxacin	125 mg	FDA pregnancy category C
Continuous[a]	TMP–SMX	40 mg/200 mg (1/2 single-strength tablet)	May be give daily or 3× a wk Eliminates vaginal reservoir without disturbing other flora Safe with years of use FDA pregnancy category C
	TMP	100 mg	See above
	Nitrofurantoin (macrocrystals)	50–100 mg	FDA pregnancy category B
	Cephalexin	125–250 mg	Disrupts vaginal flora FDA pregnancy category B
	Cefaclor	250 mg	Disrupts vaginal flora FDA pregnancy category B
	Ciprofloxacin	125 mg	FDA pregnancy category C

[a] All doses are given daily unless otherwise specified.
Note. Antibiotic dose recommendations assume normal renal function.
Abbreviations: TMP–SMX = trimethoprim–sulfamethoxazole; FDA = Food and Drug Administration.

the management of asymptomatic bacteriuria in patients who have received solid organ transplantation are sparse, and no specific recommendation on screening can be made at this time.

RECURRENT CYSTITIS

Recurrent cystitis is defined as 2 episodes over 6 months, or ≥3 more infections per year. Recurrent cystitis can be categorized into two types, relapse and reinfection, although the distinction between the two can be difficult. A recurrent infection is considered a relapse if it occurs within 2 weeks of finishing treatment for the previous infection and the pathogen is the same strain. Reinfection is defined as recurrent infection with a different strain of bacteria, or if the infection is with the same strain greater than 2 weeks after finishing a course of treatment for a UTI. Reinfection accounts for the majority of recurrent infections. Relapsing

UTIs usually result from inadequate length of therapy, structural abnormalities, abscess formation, or chronic bacterial prostatitis. When relapse occurs despite appropriate treatment, further investigation of the genitourinary tract is warranted.

For women with frequent recurrent uncomplicated cystitis secondary to reinfection, various management strategies may be considered. Patient-initiated self-treatment may be used with short-course regimens in the educated patient with 2 or fewer episodes per year. Only patients who will reliably contact their physicians if their symptoms do not improve in 48 hours should be considered for this strategy. Alternatively, postcoital prophylaxis can be offered to patients who can temporally associate their UTI recurrences with sexual activity. Recommended regimens for postcoital prophylaxis are listed in Table 64.3.

In the remainder of women with 3 or more UTIs per year, continuous low-dose antimicrobial prophylaxis can be considered. Continuous prophylaxis has been shown to be highly effective, although the benefits must be weighed against the expense and the risks of adverse drug reactions. Continuous prophylaxis may be given for 6 to 12 months, prescribed either nightly or 3 times weekly, and a variety of agents may be used (Table 64.3). As noted earlier, only TMP-SMX and the fluoroquinolones have the advantage of being less disruptive on normal vaginal flora. In general, when prophylaxis is discontinued, women with recurrent UTI usually revert back to their baseline pattern of recurrent infection. If this occurs, prophylaxis can be reinitiated if the uropathogens remain susceptible.

Other strategies to prevent recurrent cystitis have been proposed. Although postcoital voiding in women has not been studied in controlled trials, it is often recommended based on biologic plausibility and anecdotal evidence. Given the minimal costs and side effects, it is reasonable to suggest postcoital voiding to women with postcoital UTIs. Cranberry juice has long been suggested as a preventative measure for UTIs, and a natural compound present in cranberry juice has been shown to inhibit the binding of uropathogens to uroepithelial cells. Although clinical studies have shown some evidence that cranberry juice and cranberry products can prevent recurrent cystitis, the ideal amounts and duration of treatment remains undetermined. It should also be noted that cranberry products may increase the effect of warfarin.

Finally, in postmenopausal women with recurrent UTIs, estrogen replacement therapy has been studied. Loss of estrogen with menopause leads to an elevated vaginal pH, a loss of lactobacilli in the vagina, and a more uropathogen-dominant vaginal flora. Limited clinical data suggest that topical estrogens can help prevent recurrent UTI. However, pending further study, the role of hormonal therapy in UTI prevention remains undetermined.

SUGGESTED READING

Bent S, Nallamothu BK, Simel DL, et al. Does this woman have an acute uncomplicated urinary tract infection? *JAMA*. 2002;287(20): 2701–2710.

Cardozo L, Lose G, McClish D, et al. A systematic review of estrogens for recurrent urinary tract infections: third report of the hormones and urogenital therapy (HUT) committee. *Int Urogynecol J*. 2001;12(1):15–20.

Fihn SD. Clinical practice: acute uncomplicated urinary tract infection in women. *N Engl J Med*. 2003;349(3):259–266.

Hooton TM, Besser R, Foxman B, et al. Acute uncomplicated cystitis in an era of increasing antibiotic resistance: a proposed approach to empirical therapy. *Clin Infect Dis*. 2004;39(1):75–80.

Nicolle LE, Bradley S, Colgan R, et al. Infectious Diseases Society of America guidelines for the diagnosis and treatment of asymptomatic bacteriuria in adults. *Clin Infect Dis*. 2005;40(5): 643–654.

Sobel JD, Kaye D. Urinary tract infection. In: Mandell GL, Bennett JE, Dolin R, eds. *Principles and Practice of Infectious Diseases*. 6th ed. Philadelphia, PA: Elsevier; 2005.

Talan DA, Stamm WE, Hooton TM, et al. Comparison of ciprofloxacin (7 days) and trimethoprim-sulfamethoxazole (14 days) for acute uncomplicated pyelonephritis in women: a randomized trial. *JAMA*. 2000;283 (12):1583–1590.

Warren JW, Abrutyn E, Hebel JR, et al. Guidelines for antimicrobial treatment of uncomplicated acute bacterial cystitis and acute pyelonephritis in women. Infectious Diseases Society of America (IDSA). *Clin Infect Dis*. 1999;29(4):745–758.

Wilson ML, Gaido L. Laboratory diagnosis of urinary tract infections in adult patients. *Clin Infect Dis*. 2004;38(8):1150–1158.

Wright OR, Safranek S. Urine dipstick for diagnosing urinary tract infection. *Am Fam Physician*. 2006;73(1):129–130.

65. Candiduria

Jack D. Sobel

Since the early 1980s, the prevalence of candiduria in hospitals has increased by 200% to 300% such that in a community hospital, 5% of urine cultures may yield *Candida,* and in tertiary care centers, *Candida* accounts for almost 10% of urinary isolates, including a quarter of Foley catheter–associated infections. Most positive *Candida* urine cultures are isolated or transient findings of little significance and represent colonization of catheters rather than true infection. Although less than 10% of candidemias are the consequence of candiduria, *Candida* urinary tract infections (UTIs) have emerged as important nosocomial infections.

Candida albicans is the most common species isolated from the urine, whereas non-*albicans Candida* species account for almost half the *Candida* urine isolates. *Candida glabrata* is responsible for 25% to 35% of infections.

PREDISPOSING FACTORS

Candiduria is rare in the absence of predisposing factors. Most infections are associated with use of Foley catheters, internal stents, and percutaneous nephrostomy tubes. Diabetic patients, especially when their diabetes is poorly controlled, are particularly at risk primarily because of increased instrumentation, urinary stasis, and obstruction secondary to autonomic neuropathy. Concomitant bacteriuria is common and bacterial adherence to bladder epithelium may play a key role in pathogenesis of *Candida* infection. Antimicrobials similarly play a critical role in that candiduria almost always emerges during or immediately after antibiotic therapy. Antibiotics, especially broad-spectrum agents, act by suppressing protective indigenous bacterial flora in the gastrointestinal (GI) tract and lower genital tract, facilitating *Candida* colonization of these sites with ready access to the urinary tract. Nosocomial candiduria is more common in intensive care unit (ICU)-based catheterized women with concomitant contributory vaginal *Candida* colonization. The pool of critically ill, immunosuppressed medical, and surgical patients has increased, and this increase, together with improved technology,

provides an expanded population at risk of developing *Candida* infection.

Most lower UTIs are caused by retrograde infection from an indwelling catheter or genital or perineal colonization. The upper urinary tract is uncommonly involved during ascending retrograde infection and then only in the presence of urinary obstruction, reflux, or diabetes. Renal candidiasis is usually the consequence of secondary hematogenous seeding of the renal parenchyma; *Candida* species have a unique tropism for the kidney and results in anterograde candiduria.

CLINICAL ASPECTS

Most patients with candiduria are asymptomatic, especially those with indwelling bladder catheters. Clinical manifestations depend on the site of infection. *Candida* cystitis may present with frequency, dysuria, urgency, hematuria, and pyuria. Ascending infection resulting in *Candida* pyelonephritis is characterized by fever, leukocytosis, and rigors and is indistinguishable from bacterial pyelonephritis. Excretory urography may reveal ureteropelvic fungus balls or papillary narcosis. Renal candidiasis is difficult to diagnose when secondary to hematogenous spread and presents with fever and other signs of sepsis. By the time renal candidiasis is considered, blood cultures are usually no longer positive; however, unexplained deteriorating renal function is often evident.

Because isolation of *Candida* from a urine specimen may represent contamination, colonization, or superficial or deep infection of the lower or upper urinary tract, diagnosis is difficult and management depends on the site of infection. Contamination of the sample is particularly common in women with vulvovaginal colonization and may be excluded by repeating urine culture with special attention to proper collection techniques. Differentiating infection from colonization may be extremely difficult if not impossible in some patients, especially if they are catheterized. Accordingly, I often rely on accompanying clinical features to determine the significance of candiduria; unfortunately these are often nonspecific in critically ill patients, and fever and leukocytosis may have several other sources.

Quantitative urine colony counts have some value in separating infection from colonization but only in the absence of a Foley catheter. The latter negates any diagnostic value of quantitative cultures. In noncatheterized patients, counts greater than 10^4 colony-forming units (CFU)/mL are usually associated with infection. It is rare for patients with invasive disease of the kidney, pelvis, or bladder to have 10^3 CFU/mL or less. Most patients with urinary tract *Candida* infection have pyuria, but the value of this finding is similarly diminished in the presence of a catheter or concomitant bacteriuria and in neutropenic subjects. Serologic tests of *Candida* tissue invasion are not available. Treatment is preceded by attempts to localize the source or anatomic level of infection. Unfortunately, no reliable tests to differentiate renal candidiasis from the more frequent lower tract infections exist. The extremely rare finding of *Candida* microorganisms and pseudohyphae enmeshed in renal tubular casts is useful when present. Ultrasonography and computed tomography (CT) scans have a useful but limited role in localization. A 5-day bladder irrigation with amphotericin B may be of value in localizing the source of candiduria in catheterized subjects in that postirrigation persistent candiduria originates from above the bladder, thus identifying patients with need for further studies. Unfortunately, the lengthy nature of this diagnostic test excludes its utility in most febrile, critically ill subjects.

PROGNOSIS

Prognosis depends on the anatomic site of *Candida* infection and the presence of urinary drainage tubes, obstruction, and concomitant renal failure. A high mortality rate of 20% is found in candiduria patients, which is more a reflection of the multiple serious illnesses found in these patients than the consequence of candiduria per se.

MANAGEMENT

More important than the knowledge of antifungal agents for treating candiduria is understanding the indications and rational basis for initiating treatment. Regrettably, despite the availability of a variety of potent antifungal agents, data from controlled studies are scant.

ASYMPTOMATIC CANDIDURIA

No antifungal therapy is required for asymptomatic candiduria in catheterized adult patients, a common condition, because candiduria often is transient only, and even if persistent rarely results in serious morbidity. Moreover, relapse of candiduria following therapy is common if the patient remains catheterized: In catheterized patients, removal of the catheter and discontinuation of antibiotics often results in cessation of candiduria (40%). Change of catheter results in elimination of candiduria in only approximately 20% of patients.

In contrast, persistent candiduria in non-catheterized patients should be investigated because the likelihood of obstruction and stasis is high. Persistent asymptomatic candiduria in catheterized, low-birth-weight infants, as well as in afebrile neutropenic patients, requires antifungal therapy and investigation to exclude the possibility of renal or systemic involvement. Patients with asymptomatic candiduria in whom urologic instrumentation or surgery is planned should have candiduria eliminated or suppressed before and during the procedure to prevent precipitating invasive candidiasis and candidemia. Successful elimination can be achieved by amphotericin B irrigation using a concentration of 50 μg/dL of sterile water for 7 days or with systemic therapy using amphotericin B, flucytosine, or fluconazole. Fluconazole, 200 to 400 mg/day, oral therapy should continue for at least 14 days to maximize cure rates. The management of asymptomatic candiduria in the renal transplant patient is perplexing. Many recipients are diabetic, are receiving perioperative antibiotics and immunosuppressive agents, and have Foley catheters and temporary ureterocystic stents. The risk of ascending infection is high given the above and frequent reflux. Fortunately, occurrence of symptomatic renal infection and candidemia is rare. A recent large study by Safdar et al. found that treatment and eradication of candiduria did not enhance graft on patient survival.

CANDIDA CYSTITIS

Symptomatic cystitis requires treatment with either amphotericin B bladder irrigation (50μg/dL) or systemic therapy, once more using intravenous (IV) amphotericin B, flucytosine, or oral fluconazole. Oral azole agents ketoconazole, itraconazole, and voriconazole are poorly excreted in the urine, and there is limited and suboptimal clinical experience only. In contrast, fluconazole is water soluble, well absorbed orally with more than 80% excreted unchanged in the urine, achieving high urine concentrations, and is highly effective. The optimal dose and duration of fluconazole therapy has yet to be determined, but usually 200 to 400 mg/day is prescribed for 7 to 10 days. Similarly, the duration of therapeutic bladder irrigation with amphotericin B is arbitrary, lasting 5 to 7 days. Amphotericin B bladder irrigation is extremely labor intensive and has largely fallen out of favor, even in symptomatic patients, being replaced by oral fluconazole except in the presence of azole-resistant *Candida* strains. Flucytosine is also excreted unchanged in high concentrations in the urine and is highly active against most *Candida* species, including *C. glabrata*; nevertheless, because resistance develops rapidly to flucytosine when used alone, this agent is rarely used especially because its use is precluded in renal insufficiency.

Single-dose IV amphotericin B, 0.3 mg/kg, has also been shown to be highly efficacious in the treatment of lower urinary tract candidiasis, achieving therapeutic urine concentrations for considerable time after the single administration. More prolonged systemic IV amphotericin B (7 to 10 days) and at conventional dosage of 0.5 to 0.7 mg/kg/day is preferable for resistant fungal species.

ASCENDING PYELONEPHRITIS AND CANDIDA UROSEPSIS

Invasive upper UTI requires systemic antifungal therapy as well as immediate investigation and visualization of the urinary drainage system to exclude obstruction, papillary necrosis, and fungus ball formation. Previously favored therapy consisted of IV amphotericin B, 0.5 to 0.7 mg/kg/day, for a variable duration depending on severity of infection, presence of candidemia, and response to therapy, in general 1 to 2 g total dose. However, systemic therapy with fluconazole, 5 to 10 mg/kg/day (IV or oral) for at least 2 weeks offers an effective and less toxic alternative regimen. Moreover, although the echinocandin class of antifungals (caspofungin, micafungin, and anidulafungin) achieve low urinary concentrations, they are effective for kidney parenchymal infections and particularly useful for *Candida* species resistant to azoles. Infection refractory to medical management should be treated surgically with drainage, or in cases of a nonviable kidney, nephrectomy may be indicated. An obstructed kidney with hydronephrosis requires a percutaneous nephrostomy.

In some cases, nephrostomy drainage must be combined with local amphotericin B irrigation (50 µg/dL) or fluconazole, particularly with end-stage renal disease and low urinary levels of antifungal agents.

RENAL AND DISSEMINATED CANDIDIASIS

Management of renal candidiasis secondary to hematogenous spread is that of systemic candidiasis, including IV amphotericin B, 0.6 to 1.0 mg/kg/day, or IV fluconazole, 5 to 10 mg/kg/day. More recently IV voriconazole, 4 mg/kg twice a day, or any of the echinocandins could be used in preference to amphotericin B. Dosage modifications of fluconazole are necessary in the presence of moderate to severe azotemia. Prognosis depends on correction of underlying factors, that is, resolution of neutropenia, removal of responsible intravascular catheters, and susceptibility of the *Candida* species, but most importantly the nature and prognosis of the underlying disease per se. Systemic candidiasis involving metastatic sites of infection requires prolonged therapy for approximately 4 to 6 weeks.

SUGGESTED READING

Ang BSP, Telenti A, King B, et al. Candidemia from a urinary tract source: microbiological aspects and clinical significance. *Clin Infect Dis.* 1993;17:662–666.

Como JA, Dismukes WE. Oral azole drugs as systemic antifungal therapy. *N Engl J Med.* 1994;330:263–272.

Drew RH, Arthur RR, Perfect JR. et al. Is it time to abandon the use of amphotericin B bladder irrigation? *Clin Infect Dis.* 2005;40:1465–1470.

Fisher JF, Chew WH, Shadomy S, et al. Urinary tract infections due to *Candida albicans. Rev Infect Dis.* 1982;4:1107.

Kauffman CA Vazquez JA, Sobel JD, Candiduria. *Clin Infect Dis.* 2005;41 suppl; 6:S371.

Kauffman CA, et al. A prospective multicenter surveillance study of funguria in hospitalized patients. *Clin Infect Dis.* 2000;30:14–18.

Pappas PG. Infectious Diseases Society of America: Guidelines for treatment of candidiasis. *Clin Infect Dis.* 2004;38:161–189.

Rivett AG, Perry JA, Cohen J. Urinary candidiasis: a prospective study in hospitalized patients. *Urol Res.* 1986;14:183–186.

Safdar N, Slattery WR, Knasinski V, et al. Predictors and outcomes of candiduria in renal transplant recipients. *Clin Infect Dis.* 2005;40:1413–1421.

Shay AC, Miller LG. et al. An estimate of the incidence of Candiduria among hospitalized patients in the United States. *Infect Control Hosp Epidemiol.* 2004;25:894–895.

Sobel JD, Kauffman CA, McKinsey D, et al. Candiduria—a randomized double-blind study of treatment with fluconazole and placebo. *Clin Infect Dis.* 2000;30:19–24.

Wise GJ, Silver DA. Fungal infections of the genitourinary system. *J Urol.* 1993; 149:1377–1388.

66. Focal Renal Infections and Papillary Necrosis

Louise M. Dembry and Vincent T. Andriole

Focal infections of the kidney can be divided into intrarenal and perirenal pathology (Table 66.1). The classification of intrarenal abscess encompasses renal cortical abscess and renal corticomedullary abscess; the latter includes acute focal bacterial nephritis, acute multifocal bacterial nephritis, and xanthogranulomatous pyelonephritis. Perirenal abscesses are found in the perinephric fascia external to the capsule of the kidney, generally occurring as a result of extension of an intrarenal abscess. Papillary necrosis is a clinicopathological syndrome that develops during the course of a variety of syndromes, including pyelonephritis, affecting the renal medullary vasculature that in turn leads to ischemic necrosis of the renal medulla.

RENAL CORTICAL ABSCESS

A renal cortical abscess results from hematogenous spread of bacteria from a primary focus of infection outside the kidney, often the skin. The most common causative agent is *Staphylococcus aureus* (90%). Predisposing conditions include entities associated with an increased risk for staphylococcal bacteremia, such as hemodialysis, diabetes mellitus, and injection drug use. The primary focus of infection may not be apparent in up to one-third of cases. Ascending infection is an infrequent cause of renal cortical abscess formation. Ten percent of renal cortical abscesses rupture through the renal capsule forming a perinephric abscess.

Patients present with chills, fever, and back or abdominal pain, with few or no localizing signs (Table 66.2). Most patients do not have urinary symptoms as the process is circumscribed in the cortex and does not generally communicate with the excretory passages. Costovertebral angle tenderness and involuntary guarding in the upper lumbar and abdominal musculature are often present on physical examination. A flank mass or bulge in the lumbar region with loss of lumbar lordosis may be present.

Radiological techniques are useful in characterizing the renal mass and making the

Table 66.1 Focal Renal Infections

Intrarenal Abscesses
Renal cortical abscesses
Renal corticomedullary abscesses
Acute focal bacterial nephritis
Acute multifocal bacterial nephritis
Xanthogranulomatous pyelonephritis
Perinephric Abscesses

diagnosis. Ultrasonography is useful in the diagnosis of this entity and may be used to drain the abscess percutaneously and follow its response to therapy. Computed tomography (CT) is the most precise noninvasive technique for diagnosis as it yields the most accurate anatomic information. It may also be used as a guide to percutaneous aspiration.

Renal cortical abscesses often respond to antistaphylococcal antibiotics alone and surgical intervention is usually not required. If the diagnosis of renal cortical abscess is suspected and bacteriologic evaluation of the urine reveals large, gram-positive cocci or no bacteria, antistaphylococcal therapy should be started promptly (Table 66.3). A semisynthetic penicillin (oxacillin or nafcillin), 1 to 2 g every 4 to 6 hours, is appropriate empiric therapy. For penicillin-allergic patients, a first-generation cephalosporin, such as cefazolin 2 g every 8 hours, may be used. Vancomycin (15 mg/kg every 12 hours) should be used for patients with a severe immediate β-lactam allergy. Parenteral antibiotics are administered for 10 days to 2 weeks, followed by oral antistaphylococcal therapy for at least 2 to 4 more weeks. Fever generally resolves after 5 to 6 days of antimicrobial therapy. If there is no response to therapy in 48 hours, percutaneous aspiration should be considered, and, if unsuccessful, open drainage should be undertaken. The prognosis is good if the diagnosis is made promptly and effective therapy is instituted immediately.

Table 66.2 Clinical and Laboratory Findings of Renal and Perirenal Abscesses

	Renal Cortical Abscess	Renal Corticomedullary Abscess	Perinephric Abscess
Epidemiology	Males 3× > Females, 2nd–4th decades, hematogenous seeding of the kidneys	Males = Females (females > males in xanthogranulomatous pyelonephritis), incidence increases with age, associated with an underlying abnormality of the urinary tract	Males = Females, 25% of patients are diabetic, rupture of an intrarenal suppurative focus into the perinephric space
Clinical presentation	Chills, fever, localized back or abdominal pain	Chills, fever, flank or abdominal pain, nausea and vomiting (65%)	Insidious onset over 2–3 wk: fever (early), flank pain (late)
Urinary symptoms	None[a]	Dysuria/other urinary tract symptoms variably present	Dysuria 40%
Physical exam	Flank mass	Flank mass in 60%, hepatomegaly in 30%	Flank or abdominal mass in ≤50%, 60% have abdominal tenderness
Organisms	*S. aureus*	Enteric aerobic gram-negative rods (*E. coli, Klebsiella* species, *Proteus mirabilis*	Enteric aerobic gram-negative rods and *S. aureus*; occasionally *Pseudomonas* species, gram-positive bacteria, obligate anaerobic bacteria, fungi, mycobacteria; 25% polymicrobial
Urinalysis	Normal[a]	Abnormal in 70% of patients	Abnormal in 70% of patients
Urine cultures	Negative[a]	Generally positive	Positive in 60%
Blood cultures	Often negative	Often positive	Positive in 40%

[a] If there is no communication between the abscess and the collecting system

RENAL CORTICOMEDULLARY ABSCESS

Renal corticomedullary abscesses occur most commonly as a complication of bacteriuria and ascending infection accompanied by an underlying urinary tract abnormality. The most common abnormalities include obstructive processes, genitourinary abnormalities associated with diabetes mellitus or primary hyperparathyroidism, and vesicoureteral reflux. Enteric aerobic gram-negative bacilli, including *Escherichia coli, Klebsiella* species, and *Proteus* species, are commonly responsible for this infection. Acute focal bacterial nephritis, a severe form of acute bacterial interstitial nephritis involving a single renal lobe, represents focal inflammation of the kidney without frank abscess formation and may be an early phase of acute multifocal bacterial nephritis. Xanthogranulomatous pyelonephritis is an uncommon but severe chronic infection of the renal parenchyma. It may be related to a combination of renal obstruction and chronic urinary tract infection. Predisposing factors include renal calculi, urinary obstruction,

lymphatic obstruction, partially treated chronic urosepsis, renal ischemia, and secondary metabolic alterations in lipid metabolism, abnormal host immune response, diabetes mellitus, and primary hyperparathyroidism.

Patients typically present with fever, chills, and flank or abdominal pain. Two-thirds of patients have nausea and vomiting, and dysuria may not be present. Patients may have a history of recurrent urinary tract infections, renal calculi, or prior genitourinary instrumentation. On exam, 60% of patients will have a flank mass and 30% will have hepatomegaly. Patients with acute focal or multifocal bacterial nephritis are frequently bacteremic. Many patients (75%) are anemic, and up to 50% of patients with xanthogranulomatous pyelonephritis have hyperuricemia.

The nonspecific clinical presentation is associated with a variety of renal processes, including renal cortical abscess, perinephric abscess, renal cysts, and tumors. Radiographic techniques are necessary to differentiate these various processes. Ultrasonography and CT scanning are both used for diagnosing renal

Table 66.3 Therapy of Renal and Perirenal Abscesses

	Empiric Therapy	Duration	Drainage	Surgery
Renal Cortical Abscess	Semisynthetic penicillin: oxacillin or nafcillin (1–2 g IV every 4–6 h) Penicillin allergy: First generation cephalosporin (cefazolin 2 g IV every 8 h, cephalothin 2 g IV every 4 h) or vancomycin (15 mg/kg IV every 12 h) if severe immediate β-lactam allergy.	Intravenous antibiotics for 10 days to 2 wks followed by 2–4 wks of an oral antistaphylococcal antibiotic (dicloxacillin 500 mg every 6 hours, cephalexin 500 mg every 6 hours).	If no response to treatment after 48 h → percutaneous drainage followed by open drainage if no response.	
Renal Corticomedullary Abscess				
Acute focal bacterial nephritis	Extended spectrum penicillin (piperacillin 3–4 g IV every 4–6 h), extended spectrum cephalosporin (ceftriaxone 1 g IV every 24 h, cefotaxime 1 g every 8 h), fluoroquinolone (ciprofloxacin 200–400 mg IV every 12 h), ampicillin (1 gram IV every 4–6 hours) with gentamicin or cefazolin (1 g every 8 h) with gentamicin.	Intravenous for 24–48 h after resolution of symptoms and fever followed by 2 wks of oral antibiotics based on results of susceptibility testing (cefpodoxime 200 mg every 12 h or ciprofloxacin 500 mg every 12 h).	Generally not necessary.	
Acute multifocal bacterial nephritis	Same as acute focal bacterial nephritis	Intravenous for 24–48 h after resolution of symptoms and fever followed by 2 wks of oral antibiotics.	If slow response to antibiotics or large abscess, presence of obstructive uropathy, urosepsis or advanced age.	
Xanthogranulomatous pyelonephritis	Same as acute focal bacterial nephritis	Intravenous for 24–48 h after resolution of symptoms and fever followed by 2 wks of oral antibiotics		Surgical excision usually necessary for cure (partial nephrectomy or total nephrectomy)
Perinephric Abscess	Antistaphylococcal agent with an aminoglycoside or an extended spectrum β-lactam agent. If *P. aeruginosa* is isolated, an anti-pseudomonal beta-lactam (piperacillin, cefoperazone 2 g IV every 12 h, ceftazidime 2 g IV every 8 hours) should be added to the aminoglycoside. Alternatively, ciprofloxacin 200–400 mg IV every 12 hours can be added and the aminoglycoside discontinued. For enterococcus the treatment of choice is ampicillin 2 g IV every 4–6 h (or vancomycin 15 mg/kg IV every 12 h for penicillin allergic patients) plus gentamicin.	Initial parenteral therapy until clinical improvement, change to appropriate oral therapy until radiographic studies indicate resolution of process.	Requires percutaneous drainage followed by open surgical drainage if no resolution.	Nephrectomy in cases that do not resolve with antibiotics and drainage.

corticomedullary abscesses except for xanthogranulomatous pyelonephritis for which ultrasound findings are less specific than CT findings. Magnetic resonace imaging (MRI) may be considered for patients with renal insufficiency or allergy to iodinated contrast material but otherwise it is not better than CT for imaging of renal corticomedullary abscesses.

Most patients with acute focal and multifocal bacterial nephritis manifest a clinical response to antibiotic treatment alone within 1 week of starting therapy. Patients generally have no sequelae following treatment. Radiological techniques should be used to ensure resolution of the parenchymal abnormalities after clinical resolution. A large, well-established abscess may be more difficult to treat successfully with antimicrobial agents alone than an abscess identified early. An intensive trial of appropriate antibiotic therapy can be attempted before considering surgical drainage for lesions localized to the renal parenchyma. Parenteral antimicrobial agents and intravenous hydration should be administered promptly when the diagnosis is considered. Empiric antimicrobial therapy is directed against the common bacterial organisms in this setting, including *E. coli*, *Klebsiella*, and *Proteus* species (Table 66.3). An extended spectrum penicillin (such as piperacillin), an extended spectrum cephalosporin (ceftriaxone or cefotaxime), or ciprofloxacin are all appropriate choices. Alternatively, an intravenous β-lactam antibiotic, such as ampicillin or cefazolin, along with an aminoglycoside can be administered until culture and sensitivity results are known. Antimicrobial therapy should be modified based on the results of culture and sensitivity testing. Duration of therapy should be determined on a case-by-case basis. Current recommendations are to continue parenteral antimicrobial therapy for at least 24 to 48 hours after clinical improvement of symptoms and resolution of fever. Oral antibiotic therapy, based on antimicrobial susceptibility results, can then be administered for an additional 2 weeks.

Acute focal bacterial nephritis typically responds to antimicrobial therapy alone, with follow-up radiographic studies showing complete resolution of the intrarenal lesion. Most patients with acute multifocal bacterial nephritis improve with antibiotics alone, albeit slowly, and only occasionally is a drainage procedure necessary. Factors associated with failure to respond to antimicrobial therapy alone include large abscesses, obstructive uropathy, advanced age, and urosepsis. Percutaneous aspiration of the abscess combined with parenteral antibiotics has been successful in those requiring drainage. If obstructive uropathy is present, prompt drainage by percutaneous nephrostomy until the patient is stable and afebrile is appropriate at which time the lesion should then be corrected. If open drainage is required, incision and drainage are done when possible. Nephrectomy is reserved for patients with diffusely damaged renal parenchyma or patients requiring urgent intervention for survival.

Patients with xanthogranulomatous pyelonephritis generally require surgical excision of the xanthogranulomatous process for cure of the disease, although there have been several case reports of successful treatment without surgical intervention. Once the tissue is removed, the xanthogranulomatous process ceases and does not recur; however, bacteriuria may recur and require treatment. After excision, the prognosis in those without other urinary pathologic conditions is excellent.

PERINEPHRIC ABSCESS

The common etiologic agents of intrarenal abscesses, *E. coli*, *Proteus* species, and *S. aureus*, are also the common organisms associated with perinephric abscesses. Other gram-negative bacilli associated with this entity are *Klebsiella* species, *Enterobacter* species, *Pseudomonas* species, *Serratia* species, and *Citrobacter* species. Occasionally enterococci are implicated and anaerobic bacteria may account for culture-negative abscesses. Fungi, particularly *Candida* species, are also important, as is *Mycobacterium tuberculosis*. Perinephric abscesses may be polymicrobial in up to 25% of cases.

A perinephric abscess is a collection of suppurative material in the perinephric space between the renal capsule and Gerota's fascia. Most perirenal abscesses result from the rupture of an intrarenal abscess into the perinephric space, chronic or recurrent pyelonephritis, particularly in the presence of obstruction, and xanthogranulomatous pyelonephritis. Predisposing conditions for perinephric abscesses are similar to those for intrarenal abscesses. Most patients have underlying urinary tract abnormalities, usually obstruction. Patients with chronic or recurrent urinary tract infections, with or without calculi, may also be at increased risk. Up to 25% of patients are diabetic.

The symptoms develop insidiously over a period of 2 to 3 weeks (Table 66.2). Fever is the most common presenting symptom and is present in virtually all patients. Unilateral flank pain is common (70%–80%), whereas chills and dysuria are less common (40%). Flank and costovertebral angle tenderness is often present on exam, and 60% of patients may have abdominal tenderness. Half the patients have a flank or abdominal mass, and referred pain is not uncommon.

The key to making this diagnosis is considering this entity in the differential and doing the appropriate radiographic studies. Computed tomography scanning is the study of choice as it identifies the abscess and defines its extent beyond the renal capsule and the surrounding anatomy, including extension into the psoas muscle. The diagnosis should be strongly considered in any patient with a febrile illness and unilateral flank pain that does not respond to therapy for acute pyelonephritis.

Early recognition, prompt drainage, and antimicrobial therapy have all contributed to decrease the mortality associated with this entity. However, antimicrobial therapy alone is not adequate and should be used in conjunction with percutaneous drainage performed under CT or ultrasound guidance. Surgical drainage is considered when percutaneous drainage fails or is contraindicated. Acute nephrectomy is occasionally indicated. Empiric antimicrobial therapy should be directed against the most common gram-negative pathogens and S. aureus (Table 66.3). An aminoglycoside (gentamicin or tobramycin) and an antistaphylococcal β-lactam (oxacillin, nafcillin, or cefazolin) are appropriate initial antibiotics. An extended spectrum β-lactam may be used in place of an aminoglycoside for gram-negative coverage in patients with abnormal renal function. Once culture results are obtained, therapy should be modified accordingly. When P. aeruginosa is cultured, an antipseudomonal β-lactam (piperacillin, cefoperazone, or ceftazidime) should be added to the aminoglycoside; alternatively, the aminoglycoside may be discontinued and ciprofloxacin given. If enterococcus is isolated, ampicillin plus gentamicin is the treatment of choice. Isoniazid plus rifampin is indicated for M. tuberculosis infections; ethambutol and streptomycin may also be used in combination with these. Amphotericin B is necessary for treatment of fungal abscesses. Perirenal abscesses may cause ureteral compression giving rise to hydronephrosis. Even after drainage, ureteral stenosis from periureteritis may evolve during the healing process, which is a late complication of this disease.

RENAL PAPILLARY NECROSIS

Renal papillary necrosis is an uncommon severe complication of pyelonephritis (2%–5% of patients) that occurs most often in patients with underlying structural renal abnormalities or host immunocompromise (over half of

Table 66.4 Conditions Associated with Development of Papillary Necrosis

Diabetes mellitus
Pyelonephritis
Obstruction
Analgesic abuse
Sickle cell disease
Renal transplantation

patients are diabetic) (Table 66.4). When papillary necrosis is caused by infection, both kidneys are frequently affected with one or more pyramids involved. As the lesion progresses, a portion of the necrotic papilla may break off, producing a calyceal deformity that results in a recognizable radiological filling defect. The sloughed portion may be voided and in some instances can be recovered from the urine.

Patients present with worsening symptoms of pre-existing pyelonephritis. They may have lumbar pain, hematuria, and fever. The diagnosis should be considered in diabetic patients with active pyelonephritis who experience a rapid clinical deterioration and/or worsening renal function. Multiphasic helical CT is helpful in identifying early papillary necrosis.

Therapy is directed toward control of infection generally caused by the common uropathogens including E. coli, Proteus species, and Klebsiella species (see recommendations for treatment of renal corticomedullary abscesses, Table 66.3). If the patient does not respond promptly to appropriate antimicrobial therapy and infection is not controlled, nephrectomy may need to be considered.

SUGGESTED READING

Brown BS, Dodson M, Weintraub PS. Xanthogranulomatous pyelonephritis: report of nonsurgical management of a case and review of the literature. *Clin Infect Dis*. 1996; 22:308–314.

Dalla Palma L, Pozzi-Mucelli F, Ene V. Medical treatment of renal and perirenal abscesses: CT evaluation. Clin Radiol. 1999;54:792–797.

Dembry LM, Andriole VT. Renal and perirenal abscesses. *Infect Dis Clin North Am*. 1997; 11:663–680.

Eknoyan G, Qunibi WY, Grissom RT, Tuma SN, Ayus JC. Renal papillary necrosis: an update. *Medicine*. 1982;61:55–73.

Kaplan DM, Rosenfield AT, Smith RC. Advances in the imaging of renal infection. *Infect Dis Clin North Am*. 1997;11:681–705.

Lang EK, Maccia RJ, Thomas R, et al. Multiphasic helical CT diagnosis of early medullary and papillary necrosis. *J Endourol*. 2004;18:49–56.

PART IX

Clinical Syndromes – Musculoskeletal System

67. Infection of Native and Prosthetic Joints

Shahbaz Hasan and James W. Smith

NATIVE JOINT INFECTIONS

Infections of native joints generally occur in patients with predisposing factors such as trauma, underlying arthritis, immunosuppressive therapy, diabetes mellitus, malignancies, intravenous drug abuse, and other infections (eg, endocarditis, skin infections, and urinary tract infections). Hematogenous spread of the organism through the highly vascular synovial space leads to an influx of polymorphonuclear leukocytes (PMLs) into the synovium and then to a release of enzymes that destroy the articular surface.

Diagnosis

Patients present with pain and limited motion of the joint. Fever may be mild, with only a few patients having a temperature higher than 39°C (102.2°F). Joint tenderness can be minimal to severe, but most patients have swelling as a result of joint effusions in response to the infection. Involvement of multiple joints is seen in 10% to 20% of cases, especially in viral arthritis and rheumatoid arthritis. Laboratory findings suggestive of septic arthritis include an elevated erythrocyte sedimentation rate and synovial fluid cell counts exceeding 50 000/mL, with more than 75% PMLs. In no individual case do any of these findings distinguish infected from inflammatory arthritis, such as rheumatoid or crystalline arthropathy, so the diagnosis is based on cultures of synovial fluid. On occasion, blood cultures may be positive. In patients with a chronic monarticular process caused by mycobacterial or fungal organisms, synovial tissue cultures provide a better yield than synovial fluid cultures. Serum antibody tests provide the diagnosis of Lyme or viral arthritis. Polymerase chain reaction (PCR) assay of the joint fluid may yield the diagnosis in partially treated patients or in patients' infections caused by fastidious organisms such as *Mycoplasma, Chlamydia,* or *Borrelia burgdorferi* (Lyme disease). Plain radiographs are seldom of use diagnostically. Computed tomography (CT) and magnetic resonance imaging (MRI) provide more detail of the surrounding soft tissue and may reveal adjacent osteomyelitis. Radionuclear scans may be needed to visualize the sacroiliac joint; however, they are unable to distinguish septic arthritis from other inflammatory arthritis.

Staphylococcus aureus is the most common organism isolated in native bacterial arthritis. However, a variety of other gram-positive and gram-negative organisms have been reported as agents in monarticular bacterial arthritis. *Neisseria gonorrhoeae* is the main cause of bacterial arthritis in sexually active individuals with no underlying joint disease. It presents with a syndrome of fever, skin lesions, and polyarticular involvement, often with associated tenosynovitis. Any of a number of mycobacterial and fungal organisms can cause a chronic, slowly progressive infection of a single joint with tenosynovitis. Viral agents commonly associated with arthritis include rubella and parvovirus B19 (erythema infectiosum or fifth disease) in women and mumps in men. Hepatitis B infection may manifest as a prodromal syndrome consisting of arthritis and urticaria that disappear with the onset of jaundice.

Therapy

Empiric antimicrobial therapy for suspected bacterial arthritis is started after obtaining appropriate fluid specimens for analysis and culture. The choice of antibiotics depends on the patient's age, risk factors, and results of the synovial fluid Gram stain (Figure 67.1). The antibiotics are modified after obtaining the culture results. The usual course of antibiotics is 2 weeks. Infections from staphylococci and gram-negative bacilli require 3 weeks of treatment. Mycobacterial and fungal infections are treated for up to a year. Initial therapy by causative organism is given in Table 67.1.

Infected joint effusions require repeated needle aspirations of recurrent joint effusions during the first 5 to 7 days of antimicrobial therapy. Most patients respond to needle aspiration. If the volume of fluid and number and percentage of PMLs decrease with each aspiration, no drainage is required. However, if the effusion persists for more than 7 days or the cell count does not decrease, surgical drainage

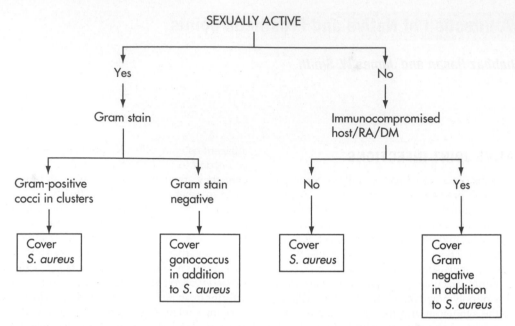

Figure 67.1 Empiric antibiotic coverage for nontraumatic, acute monoarticular arthritis.

is indicated. Surgical drainage is also indicated when effective decompression with needle aspiration is unlikely (hip joint) or when the joint is not accessible for aspiration (sternoclavicular and sacroiliac joints); if the joint space has become loculated as a result of formation of adhesions; or if thick, purulent material resisting aspiration is encountered. Arthroscopic drainage is an alternative to open drainage for the knee, shoulder, and ankle joints.

Prognosis

Bacterial arthritis is associated with a mortality of 10% to 15%. Up to 25% to 50% of surviving patients are left with residual loss of joint function. Poor outcomes are commonly seen in the elderly and those with severe underlying joint disease, hip infections, or infections caused by mycobacterial or fungal agents.

PROSTHETIC JOINT INFECTIONS

Prosthetic joint surgery has been used with increasing frequency over the past 3 decades. About 400 000 arthroplasties are performed in the United States each year. Although most procedures involve the hip and knee joints, arthroplasties of the elbow, shoulder, and wrist are also being performed. Primary indications for surgery generally include rheumatoid arthritis, degenerative joint disease, fractures, and septic arthritis.

Ten-year implant survival rates of 70% to 90% are being achieved at most centers as a result of recent technical advances. Most failures result from aseptic loosening of the prosthesis, with infectious complications accounting for fewer than 1% of implant failures. These prosthesis infections necessitate extensive surgical procedures and prolonged use of antibiotics, all of which result in increased cost, morbidity, and rarely, mortality. Risk factors for the development of prosthesis infection include rheumatoid arthritis, previous surgeries at the joint, postoperative wound infection, hematoma, and unhealed or draining wounds at hospital discharge. Other risk factors reported by some authors include skin ulcers, obesity, age, use of steroids, diabetes mellitus, and distant site infections, especially urinary tract and skin infections. Varying frequency of infection is noted with different joints: Incidence of infections for hip arthroplasties is less than 1%; for knees 1% to 2%; and for elbows 4% to 9%.

Direct inoculation of the joint at the time of surgery and intraoperative airborne contamination probably account for most infections. Evidence of the importance of this is demonstrated by the preponderance of infections caused by skin commensals (Table 67.2) and by reduction in frequency of infection that accompanies the use of prophylactic antibiotics. Hematogenous seeding of the implants is implicated in infections occurring more than 2 years postoperatively.

Table 67.1 Therapy for Bacterial Arthritis of Native Joints

Microorganism/Infection	Treatment	Duration
Staphylococcus aureus	Penicillinase-resistant penicillins,[a] first-generation cephalosporin,[b] or cefuroxime, 1.5 g q8h	3 wk
Methicillin-resistant *S. aureus* or patient allergic to penicillin	Vancomycin, 1 g q12h daptomycin 4–6 mg/kg/d, or linezolid 600 mg q12h	3 wk
Streptococci	Penicillin G, 4 million units q6h, or first-generation cephalosporin[b] or clindamycin, 300 mg q8h	2 wk
Gram-negative bacilli	Antipseudomonal cephalosporins,[c] carbapenem,[d] quinolone[e]	3 wk
Disseminated gonococcal infection	Ceftriaxone, 1 g q24h until response, then cefixime, 400 mg PO BID	7–10 d
Septic gonococcal arthritis	Ceftriaxone, 1 g q24h, or quinolone	3 wk
Lyme arthritis	Doxycycline, 100 mg PO BID, or ceftriaxone, 2 g q24h IV	4 wk, 2 wk
Mycobacterium tuberculosis	Isoniazid, 300 mg/day, plus rifampin, 600 mg/day, with ethambutol, 15 mg/kg/day, and pyrazinamide, 1500 mg/day for the first 2 mo	1 y
Fungal arthritis	Amphotericin B, 0.5–0.7 mg/kg/day for a total of 2 g, then itraconazole, 200–400 mg/day PO, or fluconazole, 200–400 mg/day PO	1 y

[a] Nafcillin, 2 g q6h IV.
[b] Cefazolin, 1 g q8h IV, or cephalothin, 1–2 g q6h IV.
[c] Ceftazidime, 2 g q8h IV, or cefepime, 1 g q12h IV.
[d] Imipenem-cilastatin, 500 mg q6h IV, or meropenem, 500 mg q8h IV.
[e] Ciprofloxacin, 400 mg q12h IV, or levofloxacin, 500 mg q24h IV.
Abbreviations: PO = orally; BID = twice a day; IV = intravenously.

Diagnosis

The diagnosis of acute prosthetic joint infection is suspected in those who develop pain and fever within 6 months of the procedure. These findings are similar to those of acute septic arthritis in a native joint. However, most infections tend to be indolent and manifest with local pain and mechanical loosening of the prosthesis. Clinical features, laboratory tests, and imaging techniques may be insufficient to differentiate between aseptic and septic complications (Table 67.3). Infection must be suspected because aseptic loosening would be managed with a one-stage revision, whereas infections require extensive debridement, prolonged antibiotics, and often delayed reimplantation. Hence, the diagnosis of an infection often has to be confirmed on the basis of the intraoperative appearance of the tissues and the presence or absence of acute inflammatory reaction on the intraoperative histopathology specimens. Given the heterogeneity of organisms (see Table 67.2), the joint fluid and tissues must be submitted for aerobic and anaerobic bacterial, fungal, and mycobacterial cultures.

Table 67.2 Microbiology of Prosthetic Joint Infections

Organism	Percentage
Staphylococcus aureus	25
Coagulase-negative staphylococci	25
Streptococci	5–10
Enterococci	3–5
Gram-negative bacilli	8–10
Anaerobes	5–10
Mixed	10–15
Others (fungi, mycobacteria, actinomyces, brucella)	1–2

Therapy

The object of successful management of prosthetic joint infections is 2-fold: eradication of infection and maintenance of functional integrity of the joint. Two-stage reimplantations offer the best possible outcome. However, not

Table 67.3 Diagnostic Features of Prosthetic Joint Infections

	Suggestive Findings	Comments
History	Rest pain; lack of postoperative pain-free interval; difficult wound healing; fever	These findings are not specific; they may also be found in aseptic loosening of the prosthesis. Infected prosthesis may be asymptomatic.
Physical findings	Swelling; tenderness; limitation of motion; fever	As above.
Laboratory tests	Leukocytosis; ESR >30 mm; raised CRP	Elevations in these parameters noted in most acute infections but may be normal in chronic, indolent infections.
Radiology	Periostitis; endosteal scalloping; focal or diffuse osteolysis	Radiologic findings may be normal. Cannot distinguish mechanical loosening from septic arthritis.
Nuclear imaging	Enhanced uptake in the region of the prosthesis	Subjective and reader dependent. Sequential bone and tagged white cell scans provide greater sensitivity and specificity than if done alone. Provides no information about organisms.
Joint aspiration	Positive cultures	Sensitivity 60%–80%; specificity 85%–95%; dry taps 10%–15%. More useful in symptomatic cases; provides specific information about organisms and sensitivities; detection of previously undetected infections.

Abbreviations: ESR = erythrocyte sedimentation rate; CRP = C-reactive protein.

all patients may be suitable candidates for this extreme surgical undertaking because of poor bone stock, inability to withstand prolonged immobilization, or inability to eradicate the infectious agent. Such cases may call for other salvage techniques that usually sacrifice joint function for microbiologic cure (Table 67.4). Antibiotic selection is based on the susceptibility pattern of the organisms isolated through joint aspiration or intraoperative joint tissue and fluid cultures. The antibiotics of choice for the isolated organisms are similar to those used in native joint infections (see Table 67.1). Unlike native joint infections, the most common organisms isolated in prosthetic joint infections are coagulase-negative staphylococci (see Table 67.2). Therefore this organism should not be considered a contaminant but should be treated with vancomycin, 1 g intravenously (IV) twice daily, to which some would add rifampin. If the prosthesis is removed, parenteral antibiotics are administered for 6 weeks; however, if management includes retention of the prosthesis, a prolonged course of oral antibiotics (6 months to 1 year) should be given after the completion of the course of parenteral antibiotics. With regard to staphylococci, oral agents may include quinolones, if susceptible, such as ciprofloxacin, 750 mg twice daily, or levofloxacin, 500 mg once daily, combined with rifampin, 600 mg once daily. Other alternatives include minocycline or doxycycline, 100 mg twice daily.

Prevention

Prophylactic antibiotic coverage generally includes agents directed against the most common causative agents, that is, gram-positive cocci. A penicillinase-resistant penicillin or a

Table 67.4 Treatment Options for Prosthetic Joint Infections

Technique	Method	Comments
Reimplantation (exchange arthroplasty)	Removal of prosthesis and cement, immediate reimplantation (one stage) or delayed reimplantation (two stages)	Technique of choice. Excellent functional results and good microbiologic cure. Patient must be physically able to undergo major surgery and prolonged immobilization. Adequate bone stock necessary for reimplantation.
Resection arthroplasty	Removal of prosthesis and cement, extensive debridement of adjacent bone	Used if reimplantation not possible because of major bone loss, recurrent infections, poorly responsive organisms (e.g., fungi) and patient mobility not essential. Provides good microbiologic cure at the expense of joint function.
Arthrodesis	Removal of prosthesis and cement and fusion of joint	If mobility is needed but patient cannot undergo reimplantation. May require prolonged immobilization.
Amputation		Radical treatment may be necessary following multiple revision attempts, intractable pain, or life-threatening infection.
Implant salvage	Chronic antibiotic suppression, alone or with local debridement and retention of prosthesis	Indicated if patient is unable or refuses to undergo major surgery. May be successful in ≤20% provided duration of symptoms ≤2 wk, no sinus drainage, no radiologic evidence of loosening, and the microorganism is highly susceptible to antibiotics.

first-generation cephalosporin may achieve this. The antimicrobial agents are administered within 30 to 60 minutes of surgery and are continued for up to 24 postoperatively. Antibiotic-impregnated beads and cement have also been used extensively because they have the advantage of delivering high local levels of antibiotics with minimal systemic toxicity. Laminar air-flow devices and body exhaust suits have been recommended to prevent intraoperative contamination; however, it is unclear whether these considerably expensive techniques are cost-effective.

There is no convincing evidence of benefit of routine prophylaxis with antibiotics for patients with prosthetic joints undergoing uncomplicated dental, urinary, or gastrointestinal procedures. The risk of infection is similar to that of endocarditis developing in the general population. In a joint advisory statement, however, the American Dental Association and the American Academy of Orthopedic Surgeons have suggested prophylaxis regimens similar to those set out by the American Heart Association for endocarditis in certain high-risk patients undergoing high-risk dental procedures. See Chapter 111, Nonsurgical Antimicrobial Prophylaxis.

SUGGESTED READING

Berbari EF, Osman, DR, Duffy MC, et al. Outcome of prosthetic joint infection in patients with rheumatoid arthritis: impact of medical and surgical therapy in 200 episodes. *Clin Infect Dis.* 2006;42:216–223.

Donatto KC. Orthopedic management of septic arthritis. *Rheum Dis. Clin North Am.* 1998;24:275–286.

Garvin KL, Hanssen AD. Infection after total hip arthroplasty: past, present and future. *J Bone Joint Surg.* 1995;77-A:1576–1588.

Kaandorp CJE, Van Schaardenburg D, Krijnen P, et al. Risk factors for septic arthritis in patients with joint disease: a prospective study. *Arthritis Rheum.* 1995;38:1819.

Lentino JR. Prosthetic joint infections: bane of orthopedists, challenge for infectious disease specialists. *Clin Infect Dis.* 2003;36:1157.

Marculescu CE, Berbari EF, Hanssen AD, et al. Outcome of prosthetic joint infections treated with debridement and retention of components. *Clin Infect Dis.* 2006;42:471–478.

Smith JW, Piercy E. Infectious arthritis. *Clin Infect Dis.* 1995;20:225–230.

68. Bursitis

Richard H. Parker

Inflammation of bursal sacs, or bursitis, is a common condition. Bursae are fluid-filled sacs that act as cushions between tendons and either bone or skin. There are more than 150 bursae in the human body. Most cases of bursitis involve either the olecranon or the prepatellar bursa, and the majority are related to trauma. About one-third are infected and a few are secondary to inflammation associated with rheumatologic disorders. Trauma can result in both septic and nonseptic bursitis. Septic bursitis can occur as a complication of bacteremia without a history of trauma to the involved area. A common cause of septic bursitis is the injection of medication, often corticosteroids, into a bursa as treatment for nonseptic bursitis. Septic bursitis is less common in the pediatrics patient but does occur and is usually associated with acute trauma such as sports-related injuries.

Septic and nonseptic bursitis of superficial bursae such as at the olecranon and prepatellar sites may present as both red and tender (Figure 68.1). Clinical features, including fever or infection at another site, may help differentiate infected from noninfected. Bursitis of deeper bursae is usually nonseptic, but tuberculous bursitis of the greater trochanter and other sites has occurred. Microorganisms from the skin cause most infectious bursitis. Although *Staphylococcus aureus* is the most common single microorganism isolated from infected bursa, if introduced any microorganism (hemolytic streptococci or gram-negative bacilli) can infect these spaces. As with other infectious diseases, the immunocompromised host may be infected with unusual opportunistic microorganisms.

Diagnosis of septic bursitis requires aspiration of fluid for microscopy, culture, cell counts, and glucose (Table 68.1).

THERAPY

Therapy is started following a decision as to whether the inflammation is infectious or noninfectious (Figure 68.2). Noninfectious bursitis is treated with immobilization, heat, and anti-inflammatory agents and referred to orthopedics depending on the severity or response to therapy. Septic bursitis might require hospitalization for surgical drainage and intravenous antimicrobial therapy. However, if the patient is not septic, toxic, or immunocompromised and is considered compliant, therapy can be initiated with oral antimicrobial agents and the patient is followed closely as an outpatient. Home intravenous infusion therapy is an option but should be restricted to therapy of methicillin-resistant *S. aureus* (MRSA) or other pathogens that require use of drugs that can be given only intravenously or when patients cannot tolerate oral medications.

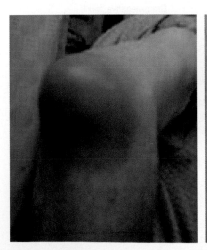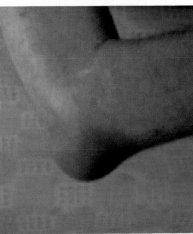

Figure 68.1 Red, swollen olecranon bursa.
(From *Resident and Staff Physician*, March 2006)

Table 68.1 Findings in Bursal Fluid Related to Causes of Bursitis

Finding	Normal	Trauma	Sepsis	Rheumatoid Inflammation	Microcrystalline Inflammation
Color	Clear yellow	Bloody xanthochromic	Yellow, cloudy	Yellow, cloudy	Yellow, cloudy
WBC	0–200	≤5000	1000–200 000	1000–20 000	1000–20 000
RBC	0	Many	Few	Few	Few
Glucose	Normal[a]	Normal[a]	Decreased	Decreased (slight)	Variable
Gram stain, culture	Negative	Negative	Positive	Negative	Negative

Abbreviations: WBC = white blood cell; RBC = red blood cell.
[a] Fluid glucose/blood glucose = 0.6–1.

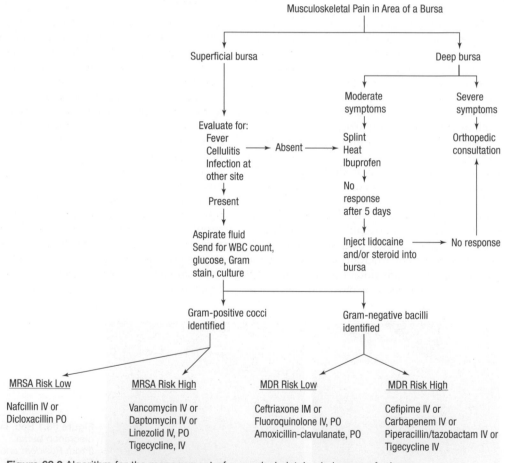

Figure 68.2 Algorithm for the management of musculoskeletal pain in area of a bursa.

Initial therapy must use a good antistaphylococcal agent. In areas where MRSA are common, intravenous vancomycin, daptomycin, or linezolid should be initiated. Linezolid has excellent biovailability with equal efficacy for MRSA either IV or orally. Clindamycin may be useful in community-acquired MRSA provided inducible clindamycin resistance has been ruled out by appropriate studies. Therapy to cover an infection caused by gram-negative bacilli and/or anaerobes should be started if the septic bursitis occurs in the lower extremity or in an immunocompromised patient. Oral antimicrobial agents, if not started initially, can be used within 48 to 72 hours. Depending on Gram stain and culture results, an oral drug could be selected (Figure 68.2). Well-tolerated, once-a-day therapy is considered preferable for compliance. Total duration of therapy is usually 3 to 4 weeks. The recurrence of fluid after initial aspiration requires reaspiration and consideration for surgical drainage or bursectomy.

SUGGESTED READING

Barham GS, Hargreaves DG. Mycobacterium kansasii olecranon bursitis. *J Med Microbiol.* 2006;55:1745–1746.

Garcia-Porrua C, González-Gay MA, Ibañez D, et al. The clinical spectrum of severe septic bursitis in northwestern Spain: a 10 year study. *J Rheumatol.* 1999; 26:663–667.

Harwell JI, Fischer D. Pediatric septic bursitis: Case report of retrocalcaneal infection and review of the literature. *Clin Infect Dis.* 2001;32:E102–E104.

Ho G, Tice AD. Comparison of nonseptic and septic bursitis. *Arch Intern Med.* 1979;139:1269–1273.

Jaovisidha S, Chen C, Ryu KN, et al. Tuberculous tenosynovitis and bursitis: imaging findings in 21 cases. *Radiology.* 1996;201:507–513.

Khazzam M, Bansal M, Fealy S. Candida infection of the subacromial bursa. *J Bone Joint Surg.* 2005;87:168–171.

Small LN, Ross JJ. Suppurative tenosynovitis and septic bursitis. *Infect Dis Clin North Am.* 2005;19:991–1005.

Stell IM. Septic and non-septic olecranon bursitis in the accident and emergency department—an approach to management. *J Accid Emerg Med.* 1996;13:351–353.

69. Acute and Chronic Osteomyelitis

Daniel P. Lew and Francis A. Waldvogel

Osteomyelitis is a progressive infectious process involving the various components of bone, namely periosteum, cortical bone, and the medullary cavity. The disease is characterized by progressive, inflammatory destruction of bone; by necrosis; and by new bone apposition.

Acute osteomyelitis evolves over several days to weeks: the term *acute* is used in opposition to *chronic* osteomyelitis, a disease characterized by clinical symptoms that persist for several weeks followed by long-standing infection evolving over months or even years, by the persistence of microorganisms, by low-grade inflammation, by the presence of necrotic bone (sequestra) and foreign material, and by fistulous tracts. The terms *acute* and *chronic* do not have a sharp demarcation and are often used somewhat loosely. Nevertheless, they are useful clinical concepts in infectious diseases because they describe two different patterns of the same disease, caused by the same microorganisms, but with different evolutions.

CLINICAL MANIFESTATIONS AND CHARACTERISTICS OF THE PATHOGEN

From a practical point of view, it is useful to distinguish three types of osteomyelitis, which are described separately. Hematogenous osteomyelitis follows bacteremic spread, is seen mostly in prepubertal children and in elderly patients, and is characterized by local proliferation of bacteria within bone during septicemia. In most cases, infection is located in the metaphyseal area of long bones or in the spine. Osteomyelitis secondary to a contiguous focus of infection without vascular insufficiency follows trauma, organ perforation, or an orthopedic procedure. It implies an initial infection, which by continuity gains access to bone. By definition, it can occur at any age and can involve any bone. It is useful to distinguish in this group those patients with a foreign body implant: Foreign material has a high susceptibility to infection and often requires removal to achieve cure.

Diabetic foot osteomyelitis has several important contributing factors leading to bone destruction: diabetes and its metabolic consequences, neuropathy, tissue ischemia resulting from poor vascularization, and infection.

TREATMENT
Basic Principles

The many pathogenic factors, modes of contamination, clinical presentations, and types of orthopedic procedures related to osteomyelitis have precluded a very scientific approach to therapy, with well-controlled, statistically valid studies; however, experimental models have helped clinicians to understand some basic principles of antibiotic therapy. Thus, except for the fluoroquinolones, which penetrate particularly well into bone, bone antibiotic levels 3 to 4 hours after administration are usually low compared with serum levels; consequently, antibiotic treatment given parenterally has to be given for several weeks to achieve an acceptable cure rate; and early antibiotic treatment, given before extensive bone destruction has occurred, produces the best results. Finally, a combined antimicrobial and surgical approach should at least be discussed in all cases: Whereas at one end of the spectrum (eg, hematogenous osteomyelitis) surgery is usually unnecessary, at the other end (a consolidated infected fracture) cure may be achieved with minimal antibiotic treatment provided that the foreign material is removed.

Microbiologic and Pathologic Criteria

If there is one area where adequate sampling for bacteriology is important, this is the case of osteomyelitis, because treatment will be given for many weeks, most often by a parenteral route based on the results of the initial culture. Adequate sampling of deep infected tissue is thus extremely useful (in contrast to specimens obtained superficially from ulcers or from fistulae, which are often misleading).

Results of Gram stain and culture, obtained ideally before therapy, should be analyzed carefully. The importance of histology (and intraoperative frozen section histology searching for neutrophil infiltrates) has also been shown in the setting of prosthetic joint infection.

Antimicrobial Therapy

Single-agent chemotherapy is usually adequate for the treatment of osteomyelitis of any type. A conventional choice of antimicrobial agents for the most commonly encountered microorganisms is given in Table 69.1. As a general principle, these antibiotics should be given parenterally for 4 to 6 weeks, as substantiated by experimental models.

In recent years, new approaches to antimicrobial therapy have been developed experimentally and validated clinically. Thus, in hematogenous osteomyelitis of childhood, initial parenteral administration of antibiotics may be followed with an equal success rate by completion of treatment with oral therapy for several weeks, provided that the organism is known, clinical signs abate rapidly, patient compliance is good, and serum antibiotic levels can be monitored. This approach has now also been validated in small series of adult patients. Another approach that is gaining acceptance because of its reduced cost is parenteral administration of antibiotics, first in the hospital and then on an outpatient basis (outpatient parenteral therapy, OPAT). Since the early 1990s, the oral combination of rifampin–quinolone (mainly ciprofloxacin or levofloxacin combined with rifampin) has been used with success for the therapy of staphylococcal osteomyelitis and particularly staphylococcal prosthetic joint infections. The fluoroquinolones have indeed been one of the most interesting developments in this domain and have been shown to be quite efficient in experimental infections and in several randomized and nonrandomized studies in adults. However, several caveats remain: Whereas their efficacy in the treatment of osteomyelitis caused by most Enterobacteriaceae seems undisputed, their advantage over conventional therapy in osteomyelitis caused by *Pseudomonas* or *Serratia* species remains to be demonstrated.

In general, long-term oral therapy extending over months and more rarely years is aimed at palliation of acute flare-ups of chronic, refractory osteomyelitis.

Local administration of antibiotics, either by instillation or by gentamicin-laden beads, has its advocates both in the United States and in Europe but has not been submitted to critical, controlled studies; antibiotic diffusion is limited in time and space; and it could be of some additional benefit in osteomyelitis secondary to a contiguous focus of infection.

Finally, considerable progress has been achieved in the development of novel surgical approaches (bone graft, revascularization procedure, muscle flaps) that allow more rapid formation of new bone.

CLINICAL RESPONSE

Because of the protracted clinical characteristics of osteomyelitis, *cure* is defined as the resolution of all signs and symptoms of active disease at the end of therapy and after a minimal posttreatment observation period of 1 year. By contrast, *failure* is defined as a lack of apparent response to therapy, as evidenced by one or more of the following: (1) persistence of drainage, (2) recurrence of a sinus tract or failure of a sinus tract to close, (3) persistence of systemic signs of infection (chills, fever, weight loss, bone pain), and (4) progression of bone infection shown by imaging methods (eg, radiography, computed tomography [CT], or magnetic resonance imaging [MRI]).

HEMATOGENOUS OSTEOMYELITIS

Historically, hematogenous osteomyelitis has been described in children. It involves mostly the metaphysis of long bones (particularly tibia and femur), usually as a single focus. In adults, it most commonly involves the vertebral plateaux.

The clinical features of hematogenous osteomyelitis in long bones are quite typical: chills, fever, and malaise reflect the bacteremic spread of microorganisms; pain and local swelling are the hallmarks of the local infectious process.

Bacteria responsible for hematogenous osteomyelitis reflect essentially their bacteremic incidence as a function of age, so the organisms most commonly encountered in neonates include *Staphylococcus aureus*, group B streptococci, and *E. coli*. Later in life, *S. aureus* predominates, whereas in elderly persons, who are often subject to gram-negative bacteremias, an increased incidence of vertebral osteomyelitis caused by gram-negative rods is found.

Fungal osteomyelitis is a complication of intravenous device infections, neutropenia, or profound immune deficiency; *Pseudomonas aeruginosa* hematogenous osteomyelitis is often

Table 69.1 Antibiotic Treatment of Osteomyelitis in Adults

Microorganisms Isolated	Treatment of Choice	Alternatives
Staphylococcus aureus		
Penicillin sensitive	Penicillin G (4–6 million units q6h)	A cephalosporin II[a], clindamycin (600 mg q6h), or vancomycin[b]
Penicillin resistant	Nafcillin or Flucloxacillin (2 g q6h)	A cephalosporin II, clindamycin (600 mg q6h), or vancomycin
		Ciprofloxacin (750 mg q12h oral) and[b] Rifampin (600 to 900 mg q24h oral)
Methicillin resistant	Vancomycin (1 g q12h)	Teicoplanin[c] (400 mg q24h, first day q12h)
Various streptococci (group A or B β-hemolytic; *Streptococcus pneumoniae*)	Penicillin G (3 million units q4–6h)	Clindamycin (600 mg q6h), erythromycin (500 mg q6h), or vancomycin
Enteric gram-negative rods	Quinolone (ciprofloxacine, 500–750 mg q12h oral)	A wide spectrum cephalosporin[d]
Serratia sp. *Pseudomonas aeruginosa*	Piperacillin[e] (2–4 g q4h) and initial gentamycin[f] (1.5 mg/kg/day)	A wide spectrum cephalosporin or a quinolone (with initial aminoglycosides)
Anaerobes	Clindamycin (600 mg q6h)	Amoxicillin-clavulanic acid 1.2 q6h to 2.2 q8h) or metronidazole for gram-negative anaerobes (500 mg q8h)
Mixed infection (aerobic and anaerobic microorganisms)	Amoxicillin-clavulanic acid (2.2 g q8h)	Imipenem[g] (500 mg q6h)

[a] II, Second generation (eg, cefuroxime).
[b] For sensitive *S.aureus* strains an IV switch to oral therapy combining ciprofloxacin 500–750 mg q12h and rifampin 600 mg q24h is common practice.
[c] Teicoplanin is presently available only in Europe. The role of novel glycopeptides remains to be assessed.
[d] Third or fourth generation (ceftazidime or cefepime).
[e] Depends on sensitivities: piperacillin/tazobactam and imipenem are useful alternatives.
[f] Due to potential nephrotoxicity or otoxicity an association containing aminoglycosides is less often used, and only during the initial phase of treatment.
[g] In cases of aerobic gram-negative microorganisms resistant to amoxicillin-clavulanic acid.

seen in drug addicts and has a predilection for the cervical vertebrae.

Treatment of Acute Hematogenous Osteomyelitis

Hematogenous osteomyelitis of the long bones rarely occurs in adults. When it develops, debridement and/or incision and drainage of soft-tissue abscesses are usually required. Appropriate deep-tissue samples should be obtained, and parenteral administration of an antimicrobial regimen may be begun as empirical therapy aimed at the clinically suspected pathogen(s). Once the organism is isolated, in vitro susceptibility testing can be done as a guide to treatment. The current standard of care is parenteral antimicrobial treatment for 4 to 6 weeks (for oral therapy see above), with the start of this interval dating from the first day of treatment judged to be appropriate in light of in vitro susceptibility results.

VERTEBRAL OSTEOMYELITIS

The management of vertebral osteomyelitis requires effective antimicrobial therapy and may necessitate early surgery and stabilization of the spine. The choice of an antimicrobial drug is guided by the culture results of specimens obtained by biopsy or during debridement. Needle biopsy obtained through CT guidance is currently the process of choice to obtain samples, which are submitted in parallel to bacteriologic and pathologic evaluation. Pathology is particularly useful in patients with previous antibiotic therapy or suspected mycobacterial or fungal disease. If the first biopsy is culture negative, a second biopsy guided by CT scan should be obtained. In case of a second failure to establish diagnosis the physician faces the choice to propose empirical therapy or to request a surgical biopsy for diagnosis.

Depending on the pharmacologic characteristics of a specific antibiotic, it may be administered by the oral or the parenteral route. The antimicrobial agent should be given for 6 weeks. The duration of treatment is usually dated either from the initial use of an effective antimicrobial agent or from the last major debridement. The indications for surgery in vertebral osteomyelitis are similar to those in hematogenous infections of long bones: failure of medical treatment, formation of soft-tissue abscesses, impending instability, or neurologic signs indicating spinal cord compression. In this last case, surgery is an emergency procedure. The neurologic status of the patient must therefore be monitored frequently. Eventual fusion of adjacent infected vertebral bodies is a major goal of therapy.

OSTEOMYELITIS SECONDARY TO A CONTIGUOUS INFECTION WITHOUT VASCULAR DISEASE

The situation and the clinical picture are more complex in cases of osteomyelitis associated with a contiguous focus of infection, for example, as a complication of the insertion of a total hip prosthesis. After a few days' pain following surgery, the situation improves and the patient is progressively mobilized. In infected patients, the pain reappears progressively, mostly on weight bearing. The patient is mildly febrile, and the wound is slightly erythematous with a slight discharge. At this stage, no other clinical sign points toward the diagnosis of osteomyelitis, and no radiographic examination or other imaging procedure is fully diagnostic. A similar clinical reasoning has to be used to diagnose osteomyelitis secondary to a contiguous infection subsequent to a comminuted fracture, which can become contaminated by wound infection. Any prosthetic material can become contaminated during surgery and produce similar signs of infection during the ensuing weeks.

Other episodes of osteomyelitis may arise secondary to a tooth, or sinus infections, pressure sores or punctive wounds, as exemplified by the following: (1) acute purulent frontal sinusitis can lead to bone involvement, with a characteristic edema of the forehead (Pott's puffy tumor); (2) dental root infection can lead to local bone destruction, (3) deep-seated pressure sores can lead to local bone destruction, usually of the sacrum.

Under all these conditions, the inflammatory reaction may be mild, and the bone destruction difficult to assess.

Staphylococcus aureus and coagulase-negative staphylococci are the most frequently reported microorganisms in prosthetic joint infections. Various types of mixed infections due to streptococci, *Propionibacterium acnei,* anaerobic microorganisms, Enterobacteriaceae, and *Pseudomonas aeruginosa* (the last mostly in the setting of chronic osteomyelitis, comminuted fractures, and puncture wounds to the heel) may be encountered. Finally, osteomyelitis of the mandible and secondary to pressure sores often also contains anaerobic flora. These organisms may also be encountered in bone infections due to human and animal bites.

Practical Approach and Therapy

Adequate drainage, thorough debridement, obliteration of dead space, wound protection, and specific antimicrobial therapy are the mainstays of management. After clinical evaluation, a bone biopsy should be performed, and the sample obtained should be submitted for aerobic and anaerobic cultures (fungal or mycobacterial when appropriate) and histopathologic evaluation. Often, the patient receives antimicrobial agents only after the results of cultures and susceptibility tests become available. However, if immediate debridement is required, the patient should receive empirical antimicrobial therapy before the bacteriologic data are reported. This antimicrobial regimen can be modified, if necessary, on the basis of culture and susceptibility results Most of the time surgical debridement is an important adjunctive therapy. Ideally, specific antimicrobial therapy is initiated before debridement is undertaken, particularly if microbiology specimens have been obtained. Debridement includes removal of orthopedic appliances (when possible or indicated), except those deemed absolutely necessary for stability. Often, debridement must be repeated for the removal of all nonviable tissue.

Posttraumatic infected fractures are especially difficult to treat. A variety of techniques have evolved for the management of the exposed bone and/or the dead space(s) created by the trauma and debridement (ie, use of local tissue flaps and of vascularized tissue transferred from a distant site). Other experimental modalities that are occasionally used include cancellous bone grafting and implantation of acrylic beads impregnated with one or more antibacterial agents. Finally, in patients with chronic extensive and difficult to treat osteomyelitis, the Ilizarov fixation device allows major segmental resections, in combination with new bone growth to fill in the defect. The bone growth process is very protracted, extending over months to years.

Antimicrobial agents are used to treat viable infected bone and to protect bone that is undergoing revascularization. Because revascularization of bone after debridement takes 3 to 4 weeks, as discussed above the patient should be treated with parenteral antimicrobial agents for 4 to 6 weeks, often followed by oral therapy for several additional weeks. The duration of this prolonged antimicrobial therapy is usually dated from the last major debridement.

DIABETIC FOOT OSTEOMYELITIS

Diabetic foot osteomyelitis is a special entity observed in patients with diabetes and is located almost exclusively on the lower extremities. Diabetic neuropathy is the most important causal factor. The infection starts insidiously in an area of previously traumatized skin and increased local pressure. In a patient who has complained of intermittent claudication, cellulitis may remain at a minimum, and infection progressively burrows its way to the underlying bone (eg, toe, metatarsal head, or tarsal bone). Physical examination elicits either no pain (in case of advanced neuropathy) or excruciating pain if bone destruction has been acute; an area of cellulitis may or may not be present; and crepitus can be felt occasionally, which points toward the presence of either anaerobes or Enterobacteriaceae. Physical examination includes a careful examination of the vascular supply to the affected limb and the evaluation of a concomitant neuropathy.

Here again, the whole gamut of human pathogenic bacteria can be isolated, often in multiple combinations. *Staphylococcus aureus* and β-hemolytic streptococci still predominate in acute soft-tissue infections leading to osteomyelitis, but any other gram-positive or gram-negative aerobic or anaerobic bacteria may be involved, particularly in chronic or nosocomial infection. To distinguish between superficial colonization/infection and bone infection, several experts propose bone biopsy for histopathology and culture. This procedure is aimed at firmly establishing diagnosis and at optimizing therapy.

The ability to reach bone by gently advancing a sterile surgical probe combined with plain radiography is the best initial approach to the diagnosis of diabetic foot osteomyelitis. If bone is detected on probing, treatment for osteomyelitis is recommended. If bone cannot be detected by probing and the plain radiography does not suggest osteomyelitis, the recommended treatment is a course of antibiotics directed at soft-tissue infection. Because occult osteomyelitis may be present, radiography should be repeated at 2 to 4 weeks. Further studies, such as nuclear magnetic resonance (MRI) are recommended in doubtful cases.

Practical Approach and Therapy

The prognosis for cure of diabetic foot osteomyelitis is poor because of the local impaired ability of the host to favor the eradication of the infectious agent.

The vascular insufficiency is due to the atherosclerotic peripheral vascular disease, a secondary manifestation of diabetes mellitus. It is important to determine the amount of vascular compromise. This assessment can be made by measurement of transcutaneous oximetry (once inflammation has been controlled) and of pulse pressures with Doppler ultrasonography. If serious ischemia is suspected, arteriography of the lower extremity, including the foot vessels, should be performed.

The patient may be managed by antimicrobial therapy with debridement surgery or ablative surgery. The type of treatment offered depends on the oxygen tensions of tissue at the infected site, the extent of osteomyelitis and time damage, the potential for revascularization, and the preference of the patient.

Revascularization often proves to be useful before bone resection or extensive amputation is considered. There is no convincing evidence that hyperbaric oxygen is useful for the treatment of diabetic osteomyelitis. Poor prognostic factors on admission include fever, increased serum creatinine levels, prior hospitalization for diabetic foot lesions, and gangrenous lesions.

SUGGESTED READING

Caputo GM, Cavanagh PR, Ulbrecht JS, et al. Assessment and management of foot disease in patients with diabetes. *N Engl J Med.* 1994;331:854–860.

Lew DP, Waldvogel FA. Osteomyelitis. *N Engl J Med.* 1997;336:999–1007.

Lew DP, Waldvogel FA. Use of quinolones in osteomyelitis and infected orthopeadic prosthesis. *Drugs.* 1999;58(suppl 2):85–91.

Lew DP, Waldvogel FA. Osteomyelitis. *Lancet* 2004;364:369–379.

Lipsky BA. Osteomyelitis of the foot in diabetic patients. *Clin Infect Dis.* 1997;25:1318–1326.

Lipsky BA, Berendt AR, Deery HG, et al. Diagnosis and treatment of diabetic foot infections. *Clin Infect Dis.* 2004;39: 885–910.

Pittet D, Wyssa B, Herter–Clavel C, et al. Outcome of diabetic foot infections treated conservatively. *Arch Intern Med.* 1999;159:851–856.

70. Polyarthritis and Fever

Robert S. Pinals

Polyarthritis and fever may be manifestations of a wide variety of infectious and noninfectious diseases (Table 70.1). Prompt identification of treatable infectious diseases is important; even the diagnosis of nontreatable infections may have important consequences for the individual or for public health. In all cases, treatment is based on specifics that apply to the known or presumptive pathogen.

BACTERIAL INFECTIONS

Suppurative bacterial arthritis caused by *Staphylococcus aureus*, group A streptococci, and gram-negative bacteria usually is monoarticular, but 10% of patients have polyarticular involvement, occurring simultaneously or within 1 to 2 days. Risk factors for bacterial polyarthritis are listed in Table 70.2. Septic joints in such persons are not always red, hot, or exquisitely painful. The mortality rate is higher with polyarticular infection (>30%) than with monoarticular infection (≤10%) and has not changed in recent years. Therefore, just as for a monoarticular arthritis, prompt arthrocentesis of a polyarthritis is essential because delay in the diagnosis and treatment is the best predictor of an unfavorable outcome. Broad-spectrum antibiotic treatment should be started immediately.

The bacteria listed in Table 70.2 are more likely than others to produce polyarthritis. Neisserial arthritis, which is most often polyarticular, presents as migratory arthritis with chills, fever, and tenosynovitis in the wrist and ankle extensor tendon sheaths. Characteristic pustular or vesicular skin lesions often aid in diagnosis. Disseminated gonococcal infections occur more often in women, especially during menses and the second and third trimesters of pregnancy. Therapy should be started immediately after cultures are obtained. Dramatic improvement in fever and joint symptoms within 24 hours supports a presumptive diagnosis of gonococcal arthritis even when cultures are negative. Chronic or episodic meningococcemia can present in a similar fashion.

In bacterial endocarditis, musculoskeletal symptoms may be the initial manifestation of

Table 70.1 Causes of Polyarthritis and Fever

Bacterial Infections	Rheumatoid arthritis
Septic arthritis	
Bacterial endocarditis	Still's disease
Brucella species	
Lyme disease	Systemic Rheumatic Illnesses
Syphilis	Systemic vasculitis
Whipple's disease	Systemic lupus
	erythematosus
Mycobacteria	
M. tuberculosis	Crystal-induced arthritis
Atypical organisms	Gout and pseudogout
Leprosy	
	Mucocutaneous disorders
Mycoplasma infections	Dermatomyositis
	Behçet's disease
Viral infections	Henoch–Schönlein purpura
	Kawasaki disease
Fungal infections	(mucocutaneous lymph
	node syndrome)
Parasitic infections	
	Erythema nodosum
Postinfectious or	
reactive arthritis	Erythema multiforme
Enteric infection	
Chlamydia	Pyoderma gangrenosum
Rheumatic fever	
	Pustular psoriasis
Inflammatory bowel	
disease	Other diseases
Serum sickness	Familial Mediterranean fever
Antibiotics and other	
drugs	Leukemia, lymphoma, and
	other malignancies
	Sarcoidosis

infection. Low back pain and arthralgias are most common, but polyarthritis with effusions may occur. The synovial fluid cell count generally is lower than with septic arthritis, and the fluid usually is sterile. In suspect cases, blood cultures should be held 2 weeks to increase the yield of fastidious organisms. Rheumatoid factor is present in about one-third of patients.

Brucellosis is an acute, chronic, or undulant febrile illness. Joint involvement is frequent; sacroiliitis and a peripheral monoarthritis are most common. A nondestructive polyarthritis similar to a reactive arthritis occurs in about 1% of arthritis cases.

Table 70.2 Risk Factors for Polyarticular Infection

Pathogens	Host Factors
Neisseria gonorrhoeae	Intravenous drug abuse
Neisseria meningitidis	Immunosuppression
Streptocobacillus moniliformis	Rheumatoid arthritis
Streptococcus pneumoniae	Gout
Haemophilus influenzae	Other polyarthropathies
Group G streptococcus	
Bacteroides fragilis	

In early Lyme disease, disseminated infection with *Borrelia burgdorferi* can cause fever and polyarthralgias. Frank arthritis is uncommon, but when it is present, pain and restriction of movement in the temporomandibular joints are highly suggestive. Immunoglobulin M (IgM) antibodies may be detected 4 to 6 weeks after the tick bite. If the patient lives in or has traveled to an endemic area, presumptive treatment should be given even when there is no diagnostic erythema chronicum migrans (ECM) lesion and the serology is negative. Late Lyme arthritis, occurring weeks to months after the tick bite, usually is monoarticular and most often involves a knee. Less often, it is episodic and polyarticular, involving both small and large joints. Serology usually is strongly positive.

Rarely, another spirochetal infection, secondary syphilis, presents with a febrile symmetric polyarthritis that can mimic rheumatoid arthritis. Most patients have a maculopapular rash on the palms and soles, and the serology is always positive.

Whipple's disease is caused by an intracellular bacillus that has never been grown in culture but was recently characterized by amplification of an RNA sequence obtained from involved tissue. The clinical picture resembles that of inflammatory bowel disease, but arthritis is a common early complication, with several patterns, including migratory and persistent oligoarticular synovitis. The diagnosis is made by biopsy of the intestinal mucosa or lymph nodes. Long-term antibiotic treatment is required for cure.

MYCOBACTERIA

Tuberculosis causes indolent monoarthritis (85%) or oligoarthritis (15%). Rarely, a patient with pulmonary or visceral tuberculosis will manifest an acute polyarthritis without evidence of joint infection (Poncet's disease). The symptoms resolve within weeks of starting conventional treatment.

Atypical mycobacteria can also infect joints, tendon sheaths, and bursae. Only occasionally is the infection polyarticular and then usually in patients who have underlying joint problems from trauma, surgery, steroid injections, acquired immunodeficiency syndrome (AIDS), or systemic arthritis. Diagnosis is by culture, and treatment includes multiple drugs. Synovectomy may be necessary.

Lepromatous leprosy can cause acute polyarthritis with fever, and all forms (lepromatous, tuberculoid, borderline) can be associated with an indolent polyarthritis. Therefore, this diagnosis must always be considered in evaluating polyarthritis in residents of endemic areas.

MYCOPLASMAS

Arthralgias are common with *Mycoplasma pneumoniae* infection, and rarely a true migratory polyarthritis occurs. Most reported cases with a prominent rheumatic syndrome have been in children with obvious respiratory infection, and the arthritis has lasted for weeks or even months.

A distinctly different syndrome of septic arthritis is caused by *Mycoplasma hominis*, *Ureaplasma urealyticum*, and other members of the family in variously immunocompromised persons. This septic arthritis usually is monoarticular, although a few patients with hypogammaglobulinemia have a polyarthritis resembling rheumatoid arthritis. If mycoplasmal joint infection is suspected, both blood and joint fluid should be cultured using commercial enriched media.

VIRAL ARTHRITIS

Arthritis can occur with infection caused by any of several viral agents (Table 70.3). Viral invasion per se, joint damage from normal immune responses, and alteration of the host immune system by the virus have all been identified or proposed as mechanisms of injury. Symmetric and asymmetric polyarthritis and polyarthralgia are the most common patterns of joint involvement. Diagnosis is usually made by serology, but polymerase chain reaction on joint fluid is occasionally available.

In hepatitis B infection, polyarthritis with or without a rash may precede any symptoms

Table 70.3 Viral Infections Associated with Arthritis

Often	Occasionally
Parvovirus B19	Hepatitis C virus
Hepatitis B virus	Adenoviruses
Rubella virus and vaccine	Herpesviruses
Alphaviruses	Enteroviruses
Mumps	Lymphocytic choriomeningitis virus

Table 70.4 Polyarthritis Associated with HIV Infection

Type	Characteristic Features
Nonspecific synovitis (HIV-associated arthritis)	Lower extremity oligoarthritis often with noninflammatory synovial fluid despite severe pain and signs of inflammation; persistent symmetric polyarthritis
Seronegative spondyloarthropathy Psoriatic arthritis Reactive arthritis	Frequent heel pain and other enthesopathy; strong association with HLA-B27; more severe than in patients without HIV
Septic arthritis	Infection may be opportunistic, related to intravenous drug abuse, or sexually transmitted; axial joints likely to be affected

Abbreviations: HIV = human immunodeficiency virus; HLA = human leukocyte antigen.

of hepatitis. At the time of arthritic symptoms, transaminases usually are elevated and hepatitis B surface antigen (HbsAg) is present in serum in very high titer. Hepatitis B infection should be considered in any sexually active person or suspected drug user with an acute polyarthritis. Occasionally, hepatitis C can cause polyarthritis without fever. Painful small-joint nondestructive synovitis and tenosynovitis are the typical presentation.

Rubella and parvovirus B19 can cause a similar clinical syndrome, especially in young women. Because rubella is now uncommon and rubella vaccine has been modified to reduce arthritogenic strains, parvovirus arthropathy, which can occur in epidemics, is probably more common. An acute-onset, symmetric polyarthritis involving the hands and feet is typical. Rash is more common in children, but the arthritis is more prominent in adults. The presence of serum IgM antibody to parvovirus B19 is diagnostic.

Several causes of polyarthritis are recognized with human immunodeficiency virus (HIV) infection (Table 70.4). Many are secondary processes, but an HIV-related arthritis has been described. Whatever the cause, arthritis can be a presenting feature of HIV disease, and patients with an obscure polyarthritis of new onset should be asked about risk factors for HIV exposure and testing with consent advised as necessary.

FUNGAL INFECTIONS

A polyarthralgia or polyarthritis sometimes accompanies acute histoplasmosis and coccidioidomycosis. When erythema nodosum is a presenting feature, acute synovitis and periarthritis of both ankles is the usual pattern. Both types resolve without sequelae. Chronic pathogenic fungal infections occasionally lead to arthritis, but they are almost always monoarticular or pauciarticular.

Among opportunistic fungi only *Candida* species are reported to cause arthritis with any frequency. Disseminated candidiasis of immunocompromised neonates, infants, and adults can produce polyarthritis as well as monoarthritis or oligoarthritis. Diagnosis is by culture of joint fluid, synovium, adjacent bone, or other extra-articular sites.

PARASITIC INFECTIONS

Joint inflammation is relatively rare in these diseases, but because hundreds of millions of people are afflicted by them, they occasionally must be considered in the differential diagnosis of polyarthritis occurring in migrants, travelers, and immunocompromised persons from endemic regions. The parasites most likely to be associated with polyarthritis are listed in Table 70.5. Identification of the parasite and improvement after antiparasitic treatment support the diagnosis.

POSTINFECTIOUS OR REACTIVE ARTHRITIS

Rheumatic fever is the prototype for postinfectious polyarthritis. Adults with arthritis and fever after group A streptococcal pharyngitis seldom have carditis and often do not

Table 70.5 Parasites and Arthritis

Organism
Giardia lamblia
Cryptosporidium
Toxoplasma gondii
Strongyloides
Taenia saginata
Toxocara canis
Schistosoma species
Filaria species

Table 70.6 Causes of Reactive Arthritis

Chlamydia trachomatis
Ureaplasma urealyticum
Yersinia enterocolitica, Yersinia pseudotuberculosis
Campylobacter species
Salmonella species
Shigella species
Clostridium difficile

demonstrate the classical migratory pattern, high fever, and dramatic response to salicylates. This poststreptococcal reactive arthritis may be additive and asymmetric, primarily affecting the lower extremities. A similar reactive arthritis pattern is also seen after various genitourinary and enteric infections (Table 70.6). Fever may accompany the primary infection but is mild or absent during the subsequent polyarthritis except in a few patients with intense joint inflammation. A genetic predisposition is an important determinant for the rheumatic syndrome. Except in rheumatic fever, human leukocyte antigen (HLA)-B27 is found with high frequency, especially in patients of northern European ancestry, with the triad of urethritis, conjunctivitis, and arthritis. In some infections, bacterial antigen may be identified in the synovial fluid or membrane, but there are no viable organisms. This suggests that dissemination has resulted in an immune reaction in synovial and other tissues. There is very little evidence that anitbiotics modify the course of reactive arthritis.

NONINFECTIOUS CAUSES

Polyarthritis and fever may be presenting features of many noninfectious systemic illnesses (see Table 70.1).

Still's disease is the systemic form of juvenile rheumatoid arthritis, which occasionally occurs in adults. High spiking fever, chills, and marked polymorphonuclear leukocytosis, often preceded by a nonstreptococcal sore throat, are highly suggestive of a bacterial infection. Arthralgia and myalgia are early

features; joint swelling appears days or weeks after the onset of fever. There are no diagnostic laboratory tests, but a typical evanescent pink macular rash that accompanies fever spikes is a useful finding. Its recognition may obviate unnecessary imaging and the invasive diagnostic procedures and multiple courses of antibiotics to which patients with persistent high fever are often subjected. The diagnosis of Still's disease is confirmed by the course, in which chronic polyarthritis is the dominant feature. Most patients have elevations of serum ferritin levels well in excess of those seen with infectious and inflammatory reactions. This finding is nonspecific but may be a useful diagnostic clue.

Adult rheumatoid arthritis rarely has a febrile presentation. When fever accompanies exacerbations of synovitis, a superimposed septic arthritis must be ruled out by joint aspiration. Some patients have episodes of severe monoarticular or oligoarticular sterile inflammation accompanied by fever and synovial fluid white blood cell counts greater than 50000/mm³. This "pseudosepsis" improves either spontaneously or with anti-inflammatory medication.

Systemic vasculitis may present with polyarthritis and fever, but there are usually other diagnostic clues such as skin lesions and neuropathy or indicators of multiorgan involvement.

Systemic lupus erythematosus may feature high fever and polyarthritis, but the latter usually includes more small than large joints, in contrast to the pattern in septic arthritis. In lupus induced by procainamide and other drugs, this presentation is particularly common.

In crystal-induced arthritis (gout and pseudogout), acute monoarticular or polyarticular synovitis resembling septic arthritis may occasionally be accompanied by high fever. A few of these patients may indeed have bacterial super-infection, but most have sterile synovial fluids in which polarizing microscopy will identify the causative crystals. Patients with polyarticular gout are often normouricemic at the time of the acute episode. Therefore, serum uric acid is not a useful diagnostic test.

Inflammatory bowel disease may present with fever and/or with an oligoarticular arthritis in large joints, but the two features are usually not simultaneous. The synovitis is low grade with prominent effusion and little pain.

Polymyalgia rheumatica may present with low-grade and occasionally high fever. Proximal myalgia and arthralgia are seldom accompanied by joint swelling, and morning stiffness is generally a prominent symptom. Joint effusions are most commonly observed in the knee; these are seldom confused with septic arthritis because pain is much less severe and cell counts fall in the low inflammatory range.

Familial Mediterranean fever presents in childhood with brief episodes that may include fever, arthritis, serositis, and an erysipelas-like rash. An infectious etiology may be suspected initially, but a history of prior episodes and familial occurrence point away from this.

Sarcoidosis may present acutely, particularly in young women with the triad of erythema nodosum, arthritis, and hilar adenopathy (Lofgren syndrome). Low-grade fever usually accompanies the skin lesions and inflammatory arthritis and tenosynovitis in both ankles. The syndrome is self-limited, but steroid therapy for several weeks is often indicated to control disabling symptoms. The involved joints do not show sarcoid granulomas on biopsy, and there is no residual inflammation or fibrosis in the joints or other tissues.

SUGGESTED READING

Dubost JJ, Fis I, Denis P, et al. Polyarticular septic arthritis. *Medicine (Baltimore)*. 1993;72: 296–310.

Goldenberg DL. Septic arthritis. *Lancet.* 1998;351:197–202.

Harris ED Jr, Sledge CB, Budd RC, et al., eds. *Kelley's Textbook of Rheumatology*. 7th ed. Philadelphia, PA: Elsevier Saunders;2005.

Pinals R. Polyarthritis and fever. *N Engl J Med.* 1994;330:769–774.

71. Infectious Polymyositis

Upinder Singh

Infectious polymyositis is an entity in which there is generalized muscle damage (rhabdomyolysis) caused by an infectious agent. The syndrome of rhabdomyolysis is characterized by elevated serum creatinine phosphokinase (CPK) concentrations and myoglobinuria leading to renal dysfunction. The muscle injury in rhabdomyolysis occurs in a generalized pattern and lacks a specific focus of abscess or infection as is seen in pyomyositis. The entity of pyomyositis is discussed in a separate chapter, Chapter 22, Deep Soft-Tissue Infections: Necrotizing Fasciitis and Gas Gangrene.

A variety of precipitating factors can lead to rhabdomyolysis. These include crush and compression injuries, drug and alcohol ingestion, metabolic and electrolyte disturbances, hypothermia and hyperthermia, and a variety of miscellaneous infections. This review focuses on infectious causes. It is important to distinguish rhabdomyolysis caused by a pathogen from that caused by sepsis, hypotension, or electrolyte imbalances that accompany a severe systemic infection.

VIRAL INFECTIONS

The wide spectrum of viral infections that have been reported to cause rhabdomyolysis are listed in Table 71.1. Influenza is the most common viral etiology reported to precipitate rhabdomyolysis, followed by human immunodeficiency virus (HIV) and enteroviral infection. The presenting symptoms in these patients include myalgias, weakness, muscle tenderness, and edema. Whether the association with influenza results primarily from a special predilection of the virus for the muscle tissue or frequent reporting of the association because of physician awareness and relative ease of diagnosis is unclear. Severe renal dysfunction in rhabdomyolysis secondary to influenza infection is common and apparently not related solely to the level of CPK elevation. The precise mechanism predisposing to renal damage from influenza-induced rhabdomyolysis is unclear; however, the association is intriguing and clinically significant, and aggressive measures

Table 71.1 Viral Causes of Rhabdomyolysis

Influenza virus A and B
Influenza A H5N1 (avian)
Human immunodeficiency virus
Coxsackie virus
Epstein-Barr virus
Echovirus
Cytomegalovirus
Adenovirus
Herpes simplex virus
Parainfluenza virus
Varicella-zoster virus
Picornavirus, including coxsackie and echovirus
Measles virus
Hepatitis C
Severe acute respiratory syndrome (SARS)-associated coronovirus
Flavivirus (Dengue virus; West Nile virus)
Rotavirus

should be taken to preserve renal function in these individuals.

Rhabdomyolysis caused by HIV infection adds to the spectrum of clinical presentations of HIV infection. Many musculoskeletal syndromes associated with HIV infection have been documented, ranging from myopathy to rhabdomyolysis. Muscle damage can occur in a variety of clinical scenarios in association with HIV infection, including acute seroconversion and antigenemia, end-stage disease with myopathy, and myositis resulting from medication side effects. Muscle biopsies of patients with HIV-induced rhabdomyolysis reveal a nonspecific inflammatory myopathy with focal necrotic areas and regenerating fibers.

The precise pathophysiology underlying virus-induced myoglobinuria is unknown; however, two mechanisms have been postulated: direct viral invasion and toxin generation. Some authors have suggested that direct viral invasion of muscle fibers causes muscle necrosis. Data to support this hypothesis include the identification of viral inclusions, viral DNA, and the isolation of viruses in tissue culture from the muscles of infected patients. In addition, electron microscopy has identified viral particles, and biopsies reveal a lymphocytic infiltrate in the infected muscles. This evidence strongly suggests that direct viral invasion may have a causative role in precipitating rhabdomyolysis. However, various reports documenting normal muscle biopsies or hyaline degeneration and myonecrosis but no viral particles by immunofluorescence and electron microscopy are used to refute this theory. Biopsies of clinically affected musculature that are essentially normal raise the possibility of a circulating "toxin" or cytokine causing rhabdomyolysis. However, to date no putative toxins have been isolated from cases of virus-induced rhabdomyolysis.

BACTERIAL INFECTIONS

Many bacterial agents have been reported to cause rhabdomyolysis (Table 71.2). The most common associations are with *Legionella* species, followed by *Streptococcus* species, *Francisella tularensis,* and *Salmonella* infections. An ever-increasing number of bacterial agents are being associated with this entity, probably because of many factors, including better diagnostic techniques, an increasing population of immunocompromised individuals susceptible to infection, and increasing physician awareness. Individuals with bacterial infections resulting in rhabdomyolysis have significant morbidity (57% with renal failure in one study) and mortality (38% in one series).

Many other infections have been reported to result in muscle damage and include fungal, rickettsial, spirochetal, and protozoal infections (Tables 71.3 to 71.6). In these cases, the clinician will most likely identify the infectious agent through obtaining epidemiologic, environmental, and exposure histories. However, once the infectious agent is identified, a high index of suspicion must be maintained for concomitant muscle injury, and therapies (eg, antibiotics, antifungals, contrast agents) that may exacerbate renal dysfunction must be carefully considered.

Two proposed mechanisms of muscle injury by bacteria include toxin generation and direct

Table 71.2 Bacterial Causes of Rhabdomyolysis

Gram-Positive Bacteria	Gram-Negative Bacteria
Streptococcus pneumoniae	*Legionella* spp.
Staphylococcus aureus	*Francesella tularensis*
Group B streptococcus	*Salmonella* spp.
Streptococcus pyogenes	*Vibrio* spp.
Listeria spp.	*Brucella* spp.
Staphylococcus epidermidis	*Escherichia coli*
Bacillus spp.	*Herbicola lathyri*
Clostridium spp.	*Klebsiella* spp.
Viridans streptococci	*Aeromonas*
Streptococcus suis	*Haemophilus influenzae*
β-hemolytic streptococci	*Neisseria* spp.
Streptococcus pyogenes	

Table 71.3 Fungal Causes of Rhabdomyolysis

Candida spp.
Aspergillus spp.
Mucor spp.

Table 71.4 Protozoal and Helminthic Causes of Rhabdomyolysis

Plasmodium spp.
Toxoplasma gondii
Trichinosis

Table 71.5 Miscellaneous Infectious Causes of Rhabdomyolysis

Spirochetes	Rickettsial	Mycoplasma
Leptospira spp.	*Rickettsia conorii*	*Mycoplasma pneumoniae*
Borrelia burgdorferi	*Rickettsia tsutsugamushi* *Ehrlichia equi* *Ehrlichia chaffeensis* *Coxiella burnetti* *Anaplasma phagocytophilum*	

Table 71.6 Other Infections and Related Causes of Rhabdomyolysis

Intravesical instillation of bacille Calmette-Guérin
Tuberculosis

Table 71.7 Envenomations Reported to Cause Rhabdomyolysis

Snakes	Other
South American rattlesnake	Hornets
Tiger snake	Wasps
Mojave rattlesnake	Bees
Russel viper	Desert centipede
	Redback spider
	Taipan

bacterial invasion. *Legionella* is believed to release an endotoxin or exotoxin that causes rhabdomyolysis. Biopsies that are negative for the organism by immunofluorescence (IF) support this hypothesis. Organisms such as *Streptococcus* and *Salmonella* cause muscle damage by direct bacterial invasion as well as by decreasing the oxidative and glycolytic enzyme activity of skeletal muscle and activating lysosomal enzymes. A number of bacterial pathogens, including *Staphylococcus aureus, Streptococcus pyogenes, Vibrio* species, and *Bacillus* species, have been demonstrated in muscle biopsy specimens, lending credence to the hypothesis of direct bacterial invasion. Rickettsial illnesses such as Q fever and Rocky Mountain spotted fever can cause muscle injury through vasculitis, as well as direct muscle invasion. A variety of cytokines, such as tumor necrosis factor-α and interleukin-1, released during systemic infections from a broad range of infections, can result in skeletal muscle proteolysis.

ENVENOMATIONS

Envenomations reported to cause rhabdomyolysis are listed in Table 71.7. Snake bites are commonly reported to cause muscle injury and include bites inflicted by the Mojave rattlesnake, Russel viper, *Croatus durissus terrificus* (South American rattlesnake), Australian snake, tiger snake, and seasnake. These patients present with obviously swollen, tender muscles and high CPK levels. In contrast to viral and bacterial causes of rhabdomyolysis, envenomations generally cause a larger myotoxic insult. A large proportion of these patients also subsequently develop acute renal failure, presumably directly related to the increased renal toxicity from myoglobin. The mechanism of muscle damage in these cases appears to be a direct myotoxic activity of the various venoms. Muscle biopsies from patients reveal myonecrosis, loss of cross-striations, contraction band formation, and mitochondrial swelling.

RENAL FAILURE IN RHABDOMYOLYSIS

The renal dysfunction associated with rhabdomyolysis arises from a variety of interrelated factors. In muscle injury, both myoglobin and heme proteins are released, although neither is directly toxic to the glomerulus. Heme protein can result in renal tubular injury through a variety of mechanisms: (1) renal vasoconstriction, (2) direct renal tubular cell cytotoxicity, or (3) intraluminal cast formation and tubular obstruction. Therapeutic measures that increase renal blood flow and decrease tubular obstruction are useful in preventing renal injury in these patients.

In a variety of case series, an interesting association of rhabdomyolysis from influenza infection resulting in renal failure has been noted. This association is not the result of higher levels of muscle injury as measured by CPK levels and may point to another mechanism of renal injury in influenza infection. In *Legionella* infection, a variety of renal pathologies have been observed, including acute tubulointerstitial nephritis, acute pyelonephritis, mesangioglomerulonephritis, and rapidly progressive glomerulonephritis. The organism has also been demonstrated in renal tissue by electron microscopy and indirect immunofluorescence. Thus renal injury in rhabdomyolysis may be caused by a combination of heme-induced injury and direct effect of the infectious agent.

THERAPY AND MANAGEMENT

General issues in the management of rhabdomyolysis include supportive care and treatment of the underlying predisposing condition or infection. These measures would apply to the infectious etiologies just discussed. For detailed information on the management of renal failure from rhabdomyolysis, see reviews by Visweswaran and Guntupalli and Huerta-Alardin et al. The general approach is as follows: (1) maintenance of a high degree of suspicion for rhabdomyolysis in the appropriate clinical setting; (2) appropriate diagnostic work-up, including CPK levels, urinalysis, and urine myoglobin levels; (3) rapid institution of organism-specific drug therapy; and (4) supportive renal care. The renal function can be protected by maneuvers such as volume expansion and urine alkalinization. Other metabolic disturbances resulting from muscle injury, such as hyperkalemia and metabolic acidosis, also may need specific therapy.

SUGGESTED READING

Falasca GF, Reginato AJ. The spectrum of myositis and rhabdomyolysis associated with bacterial infection. *J Rheumatol.* 1994;10:1932–1937.

Gabow PA, Kaehny WD, Kelleher SP. The spectrum of rhabdomyolysis. *Medicine.* 1982;61:141–152.

Huerta-Alardin AL, Varon J, Marik PE. Bench-to-bedside review: rhabdomyolysis—an overview for clinicians. *Crit Care.* 2005;9:158–169.

Joshi MK, Liu HH. Acute rhabdomyolysis and renal failure in HIV-infected patients: risk factors, presentation, and pathophysiology. *AIDS Patient Care STDS.* 2000;14:541–548.

Knochel JP. Mechanisms of rhabdomyolysis. *Curr Opin Rheumatol.* 1993;5:725–731.

Mannix R, Tan ML, Wright R, Baskin M. Acute pediatric rhabdomyolysis: causes and rates of renal failure. *Pediatrics.* 2006;118:2119–2125.

Melli G, Chaudhry V, Cornblath DR. Rhabdomyolysis: an evaluation of 475 hospitalized patients. *Medicine.* 2005;84:377–385.

Singh U, Scheld WM. Infectious etiologies of rhabdomyolysis: three case reports and review. *Clin Infect Dis.* 1996;22:642–649.

Visweswaran P, Guntupalli J. Rhabdomyolysis. *Crit Care Clin.* 1999;15:415–428, ix–x.

72. Psoas Abscess

Pamela A. Lipsett

INTRODUCTION

Iliopsoas abscess is an uncommon but important and potentially life-threatening infection that is typically difficult to recognize. Even today, most of the literature on psoas abscess includes case reports and small case series with few institutions seeing more than one case of iliopsoas abscess in a year. Large review series have been published by Ricci et al. and more recently by De and Pal. Originally described by Abeille in 1854 as an abscess of the psoas muscle, the etiology of the disease has changed substantially in the Western world since *Mycobacterium tuberculosis* has decreased in frequency. The incidence of iliopsoas abscess has increased from 3.9 cases per year to more than 12 per year in 1995. At our institution, 1 to 4 cases of iliopsoas abscess are currently seen each year.

ANATOMY

An iliopsoas abscess occurs in the retroperitoneal space that contains both the iliopsoas and iliacus muscle. The psoas major muscle is a long broad muscle that originates in the retroperitoneum from the lateral borders of T12 to L5 vertebrae. The muscle courses along the vertebral and lumbar regions to the pelvic brim, passing beneath the inguinal ligament and in front of the capsule of the hip joint, ending in a tendon that inserts into the lesser trochanter of the femur. The iliacus contributes fully to the tendinous insertion at the femur, which is often why the muscles are referred to as a single muscle, the iliopsoas. The fascia that envelops the iliopsoas compartment covers the iliacus, psoas major, and psoas minor and courses through the retroperitoneum from the lower part of the thorax to the lower lumbar vertebrae and defines the iliopsoas compartment. The psoas muscle is susceptible to both hematogenous spread and local direct extension of infectious processes. Local structures that may cause direct spread of infection include the spine, colon, small bowel, pancreas, iliac lymph nodes, and genitourinary tract structures. An endofascia

envelops the psoas muscle, and an infectious process that involves the psoas muscles via direct extension lies outside this fascial envelope, whereas a hematogenously spread infection lies within this fascia. The psoas muscle is extremely rich in vascular supply with venous supply from the lumbar spine and lymphatic channels from overlying muscle. Thus, venous drainage from an infected spine, such as Potts's disease, or from lymphatic spread, such as can occur with *Salmonella* sp., are seen with an iliopsoas abscess.

ETIOLOGY

The general cause of an iliopsoas abscess is considered to be either primary or secondary (Table 72.1). An iliopsoas abscess arising from another local source has been termed a secondary iliopsoas abscess, whereas those without an identified or suspected local direct extension are termed primary in origin. Tuberculosis infections of the spine and intra-abdominal pathology such as Crohn's disease, appendicitis, diverticulitis, postsurgical, trauma, and genitourinary are all possible causes of an iliopsoas abscess. Crohn's disease is the most common cause of a secondary iliopsoas abscess.

The anatomy of the psoas muscle described above appears to predispose the area to infection via both the local direct extension route and via hematogenous dissemination. Although the etiology and predisposing factors associated with this disease have changed since the early 1950s, today "primary" or hematogenous dissemination and infection of the psoas compartment accounts for about 40% of all cases. In such primary cases, patients may use intravenous drugs as a means of contaminating the blood and retroperitoneum, or they may have chronic debilitating diseases, such as severe malnutrition and immunosuppression. Secondary iliopsoas abscesses occur as related to the gastrointestinal or genitourinary tract or from contamination of the musculoskeletal tree via injury or operation. Gastrointestinal diseases known to be associated with psoas

Table 72.1 Conditions Associated with an Iliopsoas Abscess

Condition
Primary Abscess
Intravenous drug use Human immunodeficiency virus Immunosuppression Renal failure Diabetes
Secondary Abscess
Gastrointestinal disease: Crohn's disease, appendicitis, diverticulitis, colon cancer, rectal cancer Genitourinary disease: Urinary tract infection, urinary tract cancer, renal stones Musculoskeletal disease: Vertebral osteomyelitis, septic arthritis, infectious sacroiliitis Vascular disease: Endocarditis, infected aortic aneurysm (usually following a repair), mycotic femoral pseudoaneurysm or aneurysm, infected hardware (catheter or stent) Gynecologic disease: Tubo-ovarian abscess, perforated uterus from septic abortion, intrauterine contraceptive device Lymphatic: Suppurative lymphadenitis

abscess include Crohn's disease, enteric fistula from any cause, perforating cancer, and *Salmonella* enteritis. Local extension from a genitourinary source such as from a prostatic or renal abscess is the origin of a few cases. Direct spread from spinal or hip surgery or osteomyelitis from this area can explain additional case series of iliopsoas abscess.

Because of its rich vascular supply and endovascular fascia, a primary iliopsoas abscess is presumed to arise from the hematogenous spread of pathogens from an occult source of infection in the body. The pathogens causing a secondary and primary iliopsoas abscess differ substantially with a primary iliopsoas due to a *Staphylococcus* species in more than 85% of all patients. A primary iliopsoas abscess can be quite similar to tropical myositis in clinical appearance. Today in some centers, especially those with a large population of patients with intravenous drug abuse, primary iliopsoas abscesses are the single most common type of iliopsoas abscesses seen. In areas where human immunodeficiency virus (HIV) disease is prevalent, one should be concerned about *Staphylococcus, Mycobacterium tuberculosis*, and *Mycobacterium avium* as possible causes. As noted above, following the control of *M. tuberculosis* in some countries, iliopsoas abscess is most commonly associated with gastrointestinal and genitourinary tract abnormalities.

CLINICAL PRESENTATION

The clinical presentation of a patient with an iliopsoas abscess is protean. The age of presentation in reported series ranges from neonates to >80 years, depending on associated risk factors. However, the median age at presentation is 45 years, and the disease is more common in younger patients than in the elderly. In children the disease is most commonly confused and must be distinguished from a septic hip. Clinical presenting signs and symptoms are shown in Table 72.2. The vast majority of patients present with a somewhat vague history of fever; flank, hip, back, or abdominal pain; and a limp. They may present with a mass in the back, flank, or groin. Symptoms of associated gastrointestinal, genitourinary, recent injury, or surgery should be specifically sought. In addition to fever, night sweats and weight loss may also be seen. Pain may be radiating down the leg from nerve compression and can confuse the health care provider that a neurological disease is present. Complaints of leg swelling can be related to compression of the venous outflow of the leg, or a deep venous thrombosis may even develop.

On physical examination the patient classically will present with a unilateral flexion deformity of the lower extremity on the side of the psoas abscess. As many as 24% of patients will have swelling in the flank with local erythema. As noted, a mass may be seen in the back, flank, hip, groin, or abdomen. Pain is almost uniformly present on attempted hip extension (psoas sign). Because the symptoms are nonspecific and nonlocalizing, patients often present for examination 2 weeks after the onset of symptoms and the diagnosis may not be obvious for 5 to 7 days after presentation until alternative, more common diagnoses are excluded. Thus the differential diagnosis is extremely broad with causes of musculoskeletal pain from the back, flank, and hip being the most common. In a secondary iliopsoas abscess the patient may complain of urinary or gastrointestinal symptoms primarily with flank or back pain as an associated or secondary complaint. The classic triad of fever, flank pain, and a limp (or flexion deformity) is seen in fewer than one-third of all patients.

Laboratory abnormalities are typically present but are highly variable. Signs of infection such as an elevated erythrocyte sedimentation rate are typical, and usually an elevated white blood cell count is seen, often in the range of 12 000 to 16 000/mm^3. Because the patient may

Table 72.2 Clinical Signs and Symptoms of Patients with an Iliopsoas Abscess

Clinical Sign or Symptom	Percentage of Patients with Sign or Symptom
Fever	82–90

Pain
  Abdominal
  Flank/back
  Hip
	64–100
	35–100
	30–35
	29

Psoas sign	100
Unilateral flexion deformity	29
Mass	18–80
Swelling or erythema	24
Nausea and vomiting	30
Chills and night sweats	6
Elevated white blood cell count	90–100
Positive blood cultures	70

be ill and dehydrated for some time before the diagnosis is suspected, an elevated blood urea nitrogen and creatinine may be seen. Blood cultures when obtained are positive in almost 70% of all patients. Blood cultures should be obtained in a patient with the symptom complex of fever and back, flank, or abdominal pain. The type of microorganism isolated from the blood may well provide additional insight as to the underlying etiology of the iliopsoas abscess because etiologies are linked to specific microbial pathogens.

DIAGNOSIS AND CLINICAL MANAGEMENT

The diagnosis of an iliopsoas abscess is relatively easy to confirm once it is considered. As mentioned above, however, the diagnosis is often delayed in prehospital presentation and in considering an iliopsoas abscess as the underlying condition responsible for fever and flank, back, abdominal, or hip pain. Diagnosis and localization of disorders of the psoas muscle are most efficiently and accurately made using computed tomography (CT) scans. The CT scan ensures a reliable differentiation of iliopsoas disorders but is less reliable in differentiating neoplasms, abscesses, and hematomas. Some characteristics are helpful in distinguishing among these possibilities; although the

sensitivity for any single CT finding is reported to be between 67% and 100%, depending on the characteristic (Table 72.3), with specificity ranging between 57% and 80%. An iliopsoas neoplasm is more likely (67%) if irregular borders of the lesion were seen on CT scan. If the entire iliopsoas compartment is diffusely involved and the muscle is hyperdense, a hematoma is most likely. All three lesions, a neoplasm, a hematoma, and an abscess, can cause destruction of tissue planes. The most reliable way to distinguish among the three possibilities is that an abscess is most likely to be a low-attenuation lesion. Although classically when gas is seen on a CT scan it is associated with an abscess, this finding is actually more common in neoplasms (20%) than in abscesses (10%). Without aspiration and/or biopsy the exact etiology of an iliopsoas abnormality is difficult to determine. Thus the CT scan can point to the iliopsoas compartment as an etiology for symptoms and signs, but subsequent diagnostic aspiration, biopsy, or drainage should be considered. One of the additional benefits to CT as a diagnostic modality is that the CT scan may identify additional intra-abdominal or retroperitoneal structures that are involved and contributing to the formation of the abscess (Figures 72.1 and 72.2). Both intravenous and oral contrast administration are indicated to help distinguish additional concurrent pathology from the CT scan. Magnetic resonance imaging (MRI) is generally better for defining soft-tissue involvement, and this test may offer better anatomic definition of the retroperitoneum. However, MRI cannot delineate air bubbles in an abscess, and concurrent gastrointestinal pathology when present may be difficult to determine using MRI. In patients in whom a spinal process, such as an epidural abscess, is contributing to the development of an abscess, the MRI may be preferable over the CT scan. A flat abdominal roentgenogram may show the absence of the iliopsoas shadow or distortion and or medial displacement of the cecum. Of course, this is a nonspecific finding.

Some authors recommend an abdominal ultrasound in establishing this diagnosis because it is easy to obtain and is noninvasive and less costly than a CT scan. Ultrasound may be used in an emergency department as a screening tool. Depending on the patient's body habitus, an ultrasound maybe helpful and even diagnostic. Overlying bowel gas may also obscure pathology in the iliopsoas compartment. The ultrasound has been used effectively in some institutions as a screening examination in patients with fever, flank, hip, back, or abdominal pain

Table 72.3 Comparison of Different CT Features in Distinguishing Abscesses from Neoplasms and Hematomas of the Iliopsoas Compartment

CT Feature	Sensitivity (%)	Specificity (%)	Accuracy (%)
Enlargement of both psoas and iliacus muscle	29	52	41
Low attenuation of the lesion	100	43	70
Diffuse involvement of the entire muscle by lesion	19	52	36
Irregular lesion margins	52	43	48
Fat infiltration	62	48	55
Fascial disruption	57	57	57

Modified from Lenchik L, Dogvan DJ, Kier R. CT of the iliopsoas compartment: value in differentiating tumor, abscess, and hematoma. *AJR Am J Roentgenol*. 1994;162:83–86.
Abbreviation: CT = computed tomography

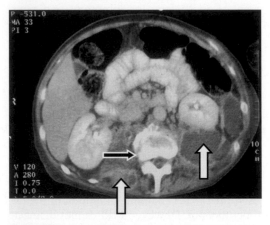

Figure 72.1 Computed tomography (CT) scan with oral and intravenous contrast of a 35-year-old human immunodeficiency virus (HIV) positive patient with evidence of bilateral iliopsoas abscesses. The vertebral body also has signs of beginning destruction. *Mycobacterium tuberculosis* was isolated from the abscess.

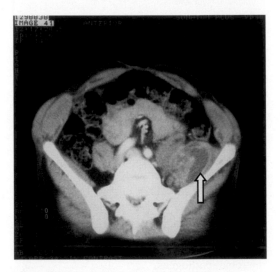

Figure 72.2 Computed tomography (CT) scan with oral and intravenous contrast that shows involvement of the left iliopsoas compartment, in this case the iliacus. The complex collection was drained via an operative approach and grew *Staphylococcus aureus*.

and may lead to a more expedient consideration of this diagnosis. The gallium-67 uptake scan is occasionally used in patients with fever of unknown origin and may indicate a gallium-67 avid lesion oriented in the direction of the psoas muscle. However, this study contributed to the diagnosis or management of patients with an iliopsoas abscess only 54% of the time and therefore cannot be routinely recommended. Gastrointestinal studies with barium or contrast studies through sinus tracks may provide some additional information if it is a suspected source of the abscess, especially when there is a history of inflammatory bowel disease or recent surgery.

THERAPY

Immediately on diagnosis of an iliopsoas abscess, prompt treatment is necessary. Blood cultures should have been obtained and, because they are often positive, should assist in directing antimicrobial therapy. Determining the ultimate appropriate antimicrobial therapy of course depends on the results of systemic and direct cultures obtained from the abscess. The organisms likely to be causative are determined principally by the etiology of the infection. Thus identifying risk factors for primary infections (intravenous drug abuse, chronic disease, immunosuppression, HIV disease) and for secondary disease (gastrointestinal or pancreatic illness, urinary symptoms, recent trauma, hip or back surgery) will help determine likely pathogens (Table 72.4). In our study population, 75% of patients with a primary iliopsoas abscess had a *Staphylococcus aureus* infection, thus empiric therapy for this disease must include adequate staphylococcal coverage. Community-acquired methicillin-resistant *Staphylococcus aureus* was recently described as the bacterial cause of a primary iliopsoas abscess in a military recruit. In patients with a secondary abscess, enteric organisms were present in 78%, therefore empiric antimicrobial therapy should include enteric organisms when a secondary abscess is suspected or until a secondary abscess (especially when related to the gastrointestinal tree) is identified or likely. In one series, *Staphylococcus aureus* was also seen even in secondary abscess. Cultures should generally be sent for common bacterial pathogens, but *Mycobacterium* species and enteric pathogens such as *Salmonella* should be specifically considered.

Once the etiology of the abscess is known and pathogens are identified by blood culture and direct aspiration, antibiotics can be tailored. Because most of these patients are ill and bacteremic at the time of initial presentation, most commonly initial antimicrobial therapy should be given intravenously. Later, appropriate oral therapy can be utilized when indicated by the patient's clinical course. For a primary abscess, staphylococcal coverage can be instituted by a variety of appropriate agents, including the penicillins oxacillin and nafcillin, the cephalosporins, clindamycin, or the fluroquinolones. In institutions where methicillin-resistant staphyloccoci are prominent, irrespective of the organism ultimately being identified as *S. aureus* or coagulase-negative staphylococci, vancomycin therapy may be required. Vancomycin therapy should be considered empirically when the patient is thought to have a primary abscess, a large proportion of staphylococcal organisms (either community- or nosocomially acquired depending on the patient history) are methicillin resistant, *and* the patient is critically ill. Patients with an iliopsoas abscess following hip or back surgery or those with lumbar osteomyelitis are also likely to have infection with a gram-positive organism, although certainly infection with *Mycobacterium tuberculosis* or *Brucella* sp. must be suspected when spinal pathology is present. Specific stains and cultures should be obtained to rule out this possibility. The

Table 72.4 Pathogens Found in Iliopsoas Abscesses

Iliopsoas Etiology	Pathogen
Primary	
Intravenous drug abuse	*Staphylococcus aureus*, coagulase-negative Staphylococcus, especially methicillin resistant
Immunocompromised	*S. aureus, Mycobacterium tuberculosis, Mycobacterium avium* Occasional gram negatives
Secondary	
Gastrointestinal, ie, Crohn, fistula, cancer, pancreatic, recent operation	*Escherichia coli, Klebsiella, Enterococcus* sp, *Proteus* sp.,*Bacteriodes* sp., *Peptostreptococcus, Clostridium, Salmonella enteriditis*
Genitourinary	*E. coli, M. tuberculosis, Enterococccus* sp.
Lumbar/Back	*M. tuberculosis, S. aureus*, coagulase negative staphylococcus
Trauma	Enteric and *Staph* organisms

presence of concurrent hepatosplenomegaly may indicate that spinal brucellosis is present, and the agglutination test should be obtained. In children, an iliopsoas abscess is more often related to the hip, and gram-positive organisms predominate.

For patients with a secondary abscess, enteric organisms, most commonly *E. coli, Klebsiella*, and *Enterococcus* sp., are present (Table 72.4). Occasionally *Pseudomonas* species have been isolated. However, much like intra-abdominal abscesses, the microbiology of a secondary iliopsoas abscess when an enteric or pancreatic source is likely usually is polymicrobial in nature. Anaerobes certainly can be present under these circumstances when cultures are carefully obtained and processed. When a gastrointestinal source is suspected or identified, broad-spectrum coverage, including the facultative gram-negative aerobes and anaerobes, should be utilized. Thus either monomicrobial therapy or combination therapy can be utilized as long as the agent covers both aerobes and anaerobes (Table 72.5). Total duration of antimicrobial therapy should be determined by clinical course, but usually signs and symptoms of infection take 5 to 10 days to completely resolve. Antibiotics probably should be continued for 48 to 72 hours beyond the resolution of fever, white blood cell, and any local signs of erythema. Antibiotics are not necessary

Table 72.5 Treatment Options for Iliopsoas Abscesses

Iliopsoas Etiology	Treatment Option
Primary	
Intravenous drug abuse Immunocompromised	Initial coverage should include specific coverage for *S. aureus* but should also include gram-negative coverage until the final organism(s) are known. *Options:* Oxacillin (or nafcillin) and aminoglycoside, cephalosporins, especially cefipime, fluoroquinolones, clindamycin, and aminoglycoside. Vancomycin should be considered for critically ill patients and those with high risk of methicillin resistance.
Secondary	
Gastrointestinal, ie, Crohn's, fistula, cancer, pancreatic, recent operation Genitourinary Lumbar/Back Trauma	Initial empriric coverage for all secondary abscesses should be broad spectrum and should include gram-negative aerobes and anaerobes. *Options: Monotherapy: Moderate Illness:* Cefotetan (cefoxitin), ertapenem, pipercillin–tazobactam; *Severe illness:* Pipercillin–tazobactam, imipenem, meripenem, *Combination Therapy:* Clindamycin + aminoglycoside, clindamycin and third-generation cephalosporin (cefotaxime, ceftriaxone), clindamycin and aztreonam, clindamycin and fluoroquinolone

for the entire duration of the drainage catheter, only while clinical signs are present; usually this is at least 7 days and most typically 10 days to 18 days total. Oral antibiotics may be used if the patient has a susceptible organism(s) and the gastrointestinal tract is functional.

Patients with an iliopsoas abscess typically must undergo some sort of drainage procedure, either operative or percutaneous, usually with radiological guidance. The decision regarding which of the two approaches should be utilized is individualized and is based in part on the presence of concurrent disease that would require treatment such as with an enteric source. Other factors that might favor operative drainage include multiple loculations within the abscess and the need for debridement of local tissue. Percutaneous drainage certainly can temporize and stabilize a critically ill patient and has been part of the routine management of this problem for more than 20 years. In the absence of intra-abdominal pathology that requires open operative treatment, percutaneous drainage with a 10 or 12 French catheter is typically employed. In some cases, percutaneous aspiration of a small abscess cavity may be curative without drain insertion. If the patient is treated with percutaneous drainage, the cavity must be completely obliterated before the catheter is removed. Failure to obliterate the abscess cavity prior to removing the catheter most often leads to a recurrent abscess. A sinogram, or dye study through the catheter, along with a CT confirming complete resolution of the collection should be obtained prior to removal of the catheter.

OUTCOME

The outcome from an iliopsoas abscess depends on the underlying etiology, associated diseases, a prompt diagnosis and timely treatment. Survival is certainly complicated by the presence of underlying cancer and also by the presence of immunosuppression. In our study between 1987 and 1994, of 18 patients with iliopsoas abscess, 17 patients survived to hospital discharge. The one patient death was related to metastatic renal carcinoma. A recent series from Bengal described 70 patients with an iliopsoas abscess; 60 were from nontubercular causes, and 33 were due to *Staphylococcus aureus*. All patients were treated with open extraperitoneal drainage, with an average of 275 cc of purulence evacuated initially (100 to 500 range). The series morbidity included 3 patients with a recurrent abscess and incisional hernia development in 3 patients, but there was no mortality seen. However, in a recent series of 40 patients with an iliopsoas abscess, the overall mortality was 15% and was associated with a higher severity of illness at presentation as well as a postoperative etiology. In this and several other series, especially in those with Crohn's disease, recurrence of the abscess is not uncommon (>15%), thus patients should be specifically followed for this possibility.

If an iliopsoas abscess is identified early in its course before the onset of septic shock, intravenous antibiotics and either open or percutaneous drainage will be likely to offer long-term survival. In 169 cases in children summarized by Song et al., 142 (84%) were treated by open drainage, 17 (10%) were treated percutaneously, and 10 (6%) cases were treated with antibiotics alone.

SUMMARY

An iliopsoas abscess should be suspected in patients with fever and flank, back, hip, or abdominal pain with or without a limp or hip flexion deformity. Patients with chronic illness; immunosuppression; intravenous drug abuse; gastrointestinal, genitourinary, or surgical treatment; or injury to the back, flank, or hip should be suspected of having an iliopsoas abscess. The physical appearance of the patient is usually with fever, and localizing findings of the abdomen, flank, and back depend on underlying etiology of the abscess. A unilateral flexion deformity may be seen. A groin swelling may be noted. Microbiology of the abscess depends on the etiology, with a primary abscess today in the United States the single most important etiology, with *S. aureus* the causative organism. Secondary abscesses are often enteric or genitourinary in etiology and thus broad-spectrum coverage, including anaerobes, is warranted. Once considered, the diagnosis of an iliopsoas abscess is easily established with a CT scan, although an ultrasound may be an excellent screening tool. Treatment includes a prolonged course of antibiotics and adequate operative or nonoperative drainage.

SUGGESTED READING

Baier PK, Arampatizis, Imdahl A, Hopt UT. The iliopsoas abscess: aetiology, therapy and outcome. *Lagenbecks Arch Surg.* 2006;391:411–417.

Cantasdemir M, Kara B, Cebi D, Selcuk ND, Numan F. Computed tomography-guided percutaneous catheter drainage of primary and secondary iliopsoas abscesses. *Clin Radiol.* 2003;58(10):811–815.

Chern CH, Hu SC, Kao WF, Tsai Y, Yen D, Lee CH. Psoas abscess: making an early diagnosis in the ED. *Am J Emerg Med.* 1997;15:83–88.

De U, Pal DK. Seventy cases of non-tubercular psoas abscess at a rural referral centre in South Bengal. *Trop Doct.* 2006;36(1):53–54.

Lenchik L, Dogvan DJ, Kier R. CT of the iliopsoas compartment: value in differentiating tumor, abscess, and hematoma. *AJR Am J Roentgenol.* 1994;162:83–86.

Macgillvray DC, Valentine RJ, Johnson JA. Strategies in the management of pyogenic psoas abscesses. *Am Surg.* 1991;57:701–705.

Mallick IH, Thoufeeq MH, Rajendran TP. Iliopsoas abscess. *Post Grad Med J.* 2004;80:459–462.

Mückley T, Schutz T, Kirschner M, et al. Psoas abscess: the spine as a primary source of infection. *Spine.* 2003;28(6):E106–E113.

Navarro Lopez V, Lopez Garcia F, Gonzalez Escoda E, Gregori Colome J, Munoz Perez A. Psoas abscess in patients infected with the human immunodeficiency virus. *Eur J Clin Microbiol Infect Dis.* 2004;23(8):661–663.

Neufeld D, Keidar A, Gutman M, Zissin R. Abdominal wall abscesses in patients with Crohn's disease: clinical outcome. *J Gastrointest Surg.* 2006;10:445–449.

Santaella RO, Fishman EK, Lipsett PA. Primary vs secondary iliopsoas abscess presentation. *Microbiol Treat Arch Surg.* 1995;130:1309–1313.

Song J, Letts M, Monson R. Differentiation of psoas muscle abscess from septic arthritis of the hip in children. *Clin Orthopaed Rel Res.* 2001;391:258–265.

Ricci MA, Rose FB, Meyer KK. Pyogenic psoas abscess: worldwide variations in etiology. *World J Surg.* 1986;10:834–843.

Walsh TR, Reilly JR, Hanley E, Webster M, Peitzman A, Steed DL. Changing etiology of iliopsoas abscess. *Am J Surg.* 1992;163:413–416.

Wells RD, Bebarta VS. Primary iliopsoas abscess caused by community-acquired methicillin-resistant *Staphylococcus aureus. Am J Emerg Med.* 2006;24(7):897–898.

Clinical Syndromes – Neurologic System

73. Bacterial Meningitis

Allan R. Tunkel

CLINICAL PRESENTATION

The classic clinical presentation in patients with bacterial meningitis is that of fever, headache, meningismus, and signs of cerebral dysfunction (confusion, delirium, or a declining level of consciousness). In a review of 493 cases of acute bacterial meningitis in adults, the classic triad (ie, fever, nuchal rigidity, and change in mental status) was found in only two-thirds of patients, but all had at least one of these findings. The meningismus may be subtle, marked, or accompanied by Kernig's and/or Brudzinski's signs. However, in a recent prospective study that examined the diagnostic accuracy of meningeal signs in adults with suspected meningitis, the sensitivity of these findings was only 5% for Kernig's sign, 5% for Brudzinski's sign, and 30% for nuchal rigidity, indicating that they did not accurately distinguish patients with meningitis from those without meningitis, and the absence of these findings did not rule out the diagnosis of bacterial meningitis. Cranial nerve palsies and focal cerebral signs are seen in 10% to 20% of cases. Seizures occur in about 30% of patients. Papilledema is observed in less than 5% of cases early in infection, and its presence should suggest an alternative diagnosis. As meningitis progresses, patients may develop signs of increased intracranial pressure (eg, coma, hypertension, bradycardia, and palsy of cranial nerve III).

To further characterize the accuracy and precision of the clinical examination in adult patients with acute meningitis, patient data on 845 episodes of acute meningitis (confirmed by lumbar puncture or autopsy) in patients aged 16 to 95 years was reviewed. The results demonstrated that individual items of the clinical history (ie, headache, nausea, and vomiting) had a low accuracy for the diagnosis of meningitis in adults. However, on review of the accuracy of physical examination findings, the absence of fever, neck stiffness, and altered mental status effectively eliminated the likelihood of acute meningitis; the sensitivity was 99% to 100% for the presence of one of these findings in the diagnosis of acute meningitis. Despite these findings, physicians should have a low threshold for performance of lumbar puncture in patients at high risk for bacterial meningitis.

Certain symptoms or signs may suggest an etiologic diagnosis in patients with bacterial meningitis. About half of the patients with meningococcemia, with or without meningitis, present with a prominent rash that is localized principally to the extremities. The rash typically is macular and erythematous early in the course of illness, but it quickly evolves into a petechial phase with further coalescence into a purpuric form; the rash may evolve rapidly, with new petechiae appearing during the physical examination. Patients with *Listeria monocytogenes* meningitis have an increased tendency toward focal deficits and seizures early in the course of infection; some patients may present with ataxia, cranial nerve palsies, or nystagmus as a result of rhombencephalitis. In a large review of 367 episodes of central nervous system (CNS) infection caused by *L. monocytogenes*, the most frequent findings were fever (92%) and altered sensorium (65%), with headache reported in only about 50% of patients.

Furthermore, some patients may not present with many of the classic symptoms or signs of bacterial meningitis. Elderly patients, particularly those with underlying medical conditions (eg, diabetes mellitus, cardiopulmonary disease) may present insidiously with lethargy or obtundation, no fever, and variable signs of meningeal inflammation. Neutropenic patients may also present in a subtle manner because of the impaired ability of the patient to mount a subarachnoid space inflammatory response.

DIAGNOSIS

Bacterial meningitis is diagnosed by examination of cerebrospinal fluid (CSF) obtained via lumbar puncture. In virtually all patients with bacterial meningitis, the opening pressure is elevated (>180 mm H_2O), with values greater than 600 mm H_2O suggesting the presence of cerebral edema, intracranial suppurative foci, or communicating hydrocephalus. The CSF white blood cell count is elevated (usually 1000 to 5000 cells/mm^3, with a range of ≤100 to >10 000/mm^3); patients with low CSF white blood cell counts (from 0 to 20/mm^3), despite high CSF bacterial concentrations, tend to have a poor prognosis. There is usually a neutrophilic predominance (≥80%), although approximately 10% of patients with acute bacterial meningitis will present with a lymphocytic predominance in CSF (more common in neonates with gram-negative bacillary meningitis and patients with *L. monocytogenes* meningitis). A decreased CSF glucose concentration (≤40 mg/dL) is found in about 60% of patients; a CSF-to-serum glucose ratio of less than 0.31 is observed in about 70% of patients. The CSF protein is elevated in virtually all cases (usually 100 to 500 mg/dL). Gram stain examination of CSF permits a rapid, accurate identification of the causative microorganism in about 60% to 90% of patients with bacterial meningitis; the specificity is nearly 100%, and the likelihood of detecting the organism is greater with higher CSF bacterial densities. CSF cultures are positive in 70% to 85% of patients with bacterial meningitis. The yield of culture is decreased in patients who have received prior antimicrobial therapy.

In patients with bacterial meningitis and a negative CSF Gram stain, several rapid diagnostic tests for detection of specific bacterial antigens in CSF have been developed to aid in the etiologic diagnosis. Currently available latex agglutination techniques have a sensitivity ranging from 50% to 100% (although these tests are highly specific) and detect the antigens of *Haemophilus influenzae* type b, *Streptococcus pneumoniae*, *Neisseria meningitidis*, *Escherichia coli* K1, and *Streptococcus agalactiae*. However, the routine use of latex agglutination for the etiologic diagnosis of bacterial meningitis has recently been questioned and is no longer routinely recommended, because bacterial antigen testing does not appear to modify the decision to administer antimicrobial therapy and false-positive tests have been reported; this test may be useful, however, in the patient pretreated with antimicrobial therapy and whose Gram stain and CSF cultures are negative. Polymerase chain reaction (PCR) has been used to amplify DNA from patients with meningitis caused by several meningeal pathogens. The clinical utility of PCR for the diagnosis of bacterial meningitis was assessed in one study with a broad range of bacterial primers, yielding a sensitivity of 100%, specificity of 98.2%, positive predictive value of 98.2%, and negative predictive value of 100%. Further refinements are needed before this technique can be used in patients with presumed bacterial meningitis when CSF Gram stain, bacterial antigen tests, and cultures are negative.

THERAPY
Initial Approach to Management

In patients with the clinical presentation of acute bacterial meningitis, the initial management includes performance of a lumbar puncture. If the CSF formula is consistent with the diagnosis of bacterial meningitis, targeted antimicrobial therapy and adjunctive dexamethasone (see below) should be initiated based on results of Gram stain (Table 73.1). However, if no etiologic agent can be identified on initial CSF analysis, empiric antimicrobial therapy and adjunctive therapy should be initiated rapidly based on the patient's age (Table 73.2). In patients with a clinical presentation of bacterial meningitis in whom there is a delay in performance of lumbar puncture or if there is suspicion of an intracranial mass lesion that is causing their neurologic presentation (ie, those with focal neurologic deficits, abnormal level of consciousness, new onset seizure, or papilledema on funduscopic examination or those who are immunocompromised or have a history of CNS disease), a computed tomography (CT) scan of the head should be performed before lumbar puncture. In these patients, blood cultures must be obtained and appropriate antimicrobial and adjunctive therapy given prior to lumbar puncture, or before the patient is sent to the CT scanner, to potentially reduce the increased morbidity and mortality associated with bacterial meningitis when initiation of appropriate antimicrobial and adjunctive therapy is delayed. Although there are no prospective data on the timing of administration of antimicrobial therapy in patients with bacterial meningitis, a retrospective cohort study in patients with community-acquired bacterial meningitis demonstrated that a delay in initiation of antimicrobial therapy after patient arrival in the emergency room was associated with an adverse clinical outcome when the patient's condition advanced to a high stage of prognostic severity, supporting the assumption that treatment of bacterial meningitis before it advances to a high level of clinical severity improves clinical outcome. Although the yield of positive CSF cultures may decrease with initiation of antimicrobial therapy prior to obtaining CSF for analysis, the pretreatment blood cultures, CSF formula, and/or Gram stain will

Table 73.1 Recommended Antimicrobial Therapy for Acute Bacterial Meningitis Based on Presumptive Identification by Positive Gram Stain

Microorganism	Therapy
Streptococcus pneumoniae	Vancomycin plus a third-generation cephalosporin[a,b]
Neisseria meningitidis	Third-generation cephalosporin[a]
Listeria monocytogenes	Ampicillin or penicillin G[c]
Haemophilus influenzae type b	Third-generation cephalosporin[a]
Streptococcus agalactiae	Ampicillin or penicillin G[c]
Escherichia coli	Third-generation cephalosporin[a]

[a] Cefotaxime or ceftriaxone.
[b] Addition of rifampin may be considered.
[c] Addition of an aminoglycoside should be considered.

Table 73.2 Common Bacterial Pathogens and Empiric Therapeutic Recommendations Based on Age in Patients with Meningitis

Age	Common Bacterial Pathogens	Empiric Antimicrobial Therapy
<1 mo	*Streptococcus agalactiae, Escherichia coli, Listeria monocytogenes, Klebsiella pneumoniae*	Ampicillin plus cefotaxime, or ampicillin plus an aminoglycoside
1–23 mo	*S. agalactiae, E. coli, Haemophilus influenzae, Streptococcus pneumoniae, Neisseria meningitidis*	Vancomycin plus a third-generation cephalosporin[a]
2–50 y	*S. pneumoniae, N. meningitidis*	Vancomycin plus a third-generation cephalosporin[a,b]
>50 y	*S. pneumoniae, N. meningitidis, L. monocytogenes,* aerobic gram-negative bacilli	Vancomycin plus ampicillin plus a third-generation cephalosporin[a,b]

[a] Cefotaxime or ceftriaxone.
[b] Some experts would add rifampin if dexamethasone is also given.

likely provide evidence for or against a diagnosis of bacterial meningitis.

Adjunctive Therapy

Because of the unacceptable morbidity and mortality rates in patients with bacterial meningitis, even in the antibiotic era, investigators have been studying the pathogenic and pathophysiologic mechanisms operable in bacterial meningitis in the hopes of improving outcome from this disorder. Initial experimental studies focused on the subarachnoid space inflammatory response that occurs during bacterial meningitis to determine whether attenuation of this response would improve outcome. Through the use of experimental animal models of infection,

it was determined that one corticosteroid agent, dexamethasone, was effective in reducing the CSF white blood cell response and CSF tumor necrosis factor concentrations, with a trend toward earlier improvement in CSF concentrations of glucose, protein, and lactate; these parameters improved without any apparent decrease in the rate of CSF bacterial killing.

Based on these and other studies in experimental animal models, numerous clinical trials were undertaken to determine the effects of adjunctive dexamethasone on the outcome in patients with bacterial meningitis. A meta-analysis of these clinical studies confirmed the benefit of adjunctive dexamethasone (0.15 mg/kg every 6 hours for 2 to 4 days) for *H. influenzae* type b meningitis and, if commenced with or before parenteral antimicrobial therapy, suggested benefit for pneumococcal meningitis in childhood. Evidence of clinical benefit was strongest for hearing outcomes. In adults with acute bacterial meningitis, a recent prospective, randomized, placebo-controlled, double-blind multicenter trial in 301 patients demonstrated that patients randomized to receive adjunctive dexamethasone were less likely to have unfavorable outcome and death; benefit was most evident among the subgroup of patients with pneumococcal meningitis. Based on the available evidence, adjunctive dexamethasone (0.15 mg/ kg every 6 hours for 2 to 4 days with the first dose administered 10 to 20 minutes before, or at least concomitant with, the first dose of an antimicrobial agent) should be utilized in adults with suspected or proven pneumococcal meningitis. Adjunctive dexamethasone should not be given to adults who have already received antimicrobial therapy, because administration in this setting is unlikely to improve patient outcome. The data are inadequate to recommend adjunctive dexamethasone in adults with meningitis caused by other meningeal pathogens, although some authorities would initiate dexamethasone in all adults because the etiology of meningitis is not always ascertained at initial evaluation.

Despite the studies that have demonstrated the benefits of adjunctive dexamethasone in patients with bacterial meningitis, the use of adjunctive dexamethasone is of concern in those with pneumococcal meningitis caused by highly penicillin- and cephalosporin-resistant strains, in which patients may require antimicrobial therapy with vancomycin. In this instance, a diminished CSF inflammatory response after dexamethasone administration might significantly reduce vancomycin penetration into CSF and delay CSF sterilization. The published trials have not examined outcome in patients with these resistant isolates who have received adjunctive dexamethasone, and it is unlikely that this question will be definitively answered in the near future, given the difficulty in enrolling adequate numbers of patients with these resistant strains into clinical trials. Therefore, for any patient receiving adjunctive dexamethasone who is not improving as expected, a repeat lumbar puncture 36 to 48 hours after initiation of antimicrobial therapy is recommended to document sterility of CSF.

Antimicrobial Therapy

Once the infecting meningeal pathogen is isolated and susceptibility testing known,

antimicrobial therapy can be modified for optimal treatment (Table 73.3). Recommended antimicrobial dosages for meningitis in adults with normal renal and hepatic function are shown in Table 73.4. The following sections review recommendations for use of antimicrobial therapy in patients with bacterial meningitis based on the isolated meningeal pathogen.

STREPTOCOCCUS PNEUMONIAE

The recommended therapy of pneumococcal meningitis has been changed based on pneumococcal susceptibility patterns. Pneumococcal strains with minimal inhibitory concentrations (MICs) less than 0.1 µg/mL are considered susceptible to penicillin, those with MICs ranging from 0.1 to 1.0 µg/mL are of intermediate susceptibility, and those with MICs 2.0 µg/mL or greater are highly resistant. Resistant strains have been reported from many countries throughout the world, including the United States, where the prevalence of penicillin-nonsusceptible S. pneumoniae ranges from 25% to more than 50%. Because initial CSF concentrations of penicillin are only approximately 1 µg/mL after parenteral administration of standard high dosages, penicillin cannot be recommended as empiric antimicrobial therapy when S. pneumoniae is considered a likely infecting pathogen in patients with purulent meningitis. Of additional concern is that pneumococcal strains resistant to the third-generation cephalosporins have also been described in patients with meningitis. Several alternative agents have been examined for the treatment of meningitis caused by penicillin-resistant pneumococci. Chloramphenicol is one agent that has been studied, although clinical failures with chloramphenicol have been reported in patients with penicillin-resistant isolates. Vancomycin has also been evaluated, but as a single agent is likely to be suboptimal for therapy of pneumococcal meningitis. Furthermore, S. pneumoniae strains tolerant to vancomycin have been described.

Based on these data, it is recommended that, for empiric therapy of suspected pneumococcal meningitis, the combination of vancomycin and a third-generation cephalosporin (either cefotaxime or ceftriaxone) should be used pending in vitro susceptibility results. This combination was synergistic in a rabbit model of penicillin-resistant pneumococcal meningitis and was synergistic, or at least additive, in the CSF of children with meningitis. If the organism is sensitive to penicillin (MIC <0.1 µg/mL), penicillin is the drug of choice.

Table 73.3 Specific Antimicrobial Therapy for Acute Bacterial Meningitis

Microorganism	Standard Therapy	Duration of Therapy
Streptococcus pneumoniae		10–14 d
Penicillin MIC <0.1 µg/mL	Penicillin G or ampicillin	
Penicillin MIC 0.1–1.0 µg/mL	Third-generation cephalosporin[a]	

Penicillin MIC ≥2.0 µg/mL, or cefotaxime
    or ceftriaxone MIC ≥1.0 µg/mL
	Vancomycin plus a third-generation
	    cephalosporin[a,b]	

Neisseria meningitidis		7 d
Penicillin MIC <0.1 µg/mL	Penicillin G or ampicillin	
Penicillin MIC 0.1–1.0 µg/mL	Third-generation cephalosporin[a]	
Listeria monocytogenes	Ampicillin or penicillin G[c]	≥21 d
Streptococcus agalactiae	Ampicillin or penicillin G[c]	14–21 d
Haemophilus influenzae		7 d
β-lactamase – negative	Ampicillin	
β-lactamase – positive	Third-generation cephalosporin[a]	
Escherichia coli and other Enterobacteriaceae[e]	Third-generation cephalosporin[a]	21 d
Pseudomonas aeruginosa	Cefepime[c] or ceftazidime[c]	21 d
Staphylococcus aureus		10–14 d
Methicillin-sensitive	Nafcillin or oxacillin	
Methicillin-resistant	Vancomycin	
Staphylococcus epidermidis	Vancomycin[d]	10–14 d

[a] Cefotaxime or ceftriaxone.
[b] Consider addition of rifampin if the ceftriaxone MIC is >2 µg/mL.
[c] Addition of an aminoglycoside should be considered.
[d] Addition of rifampin should be considered.
[e] Choice of a specific antimicrobial agent must be guided by in vitro susceptibility test results.
Abbreviation: MIC = minimal inhibitory concentration.

For intermediate susceptible strains (MIC 0.1 to 1.0 µg/mL), a third-generation cephalosporin is used. However, if highly resistant strains are documented by susceptibility testing, vancomycin plus the third-generation cephalosporin are continued for the entire treatment period. Some investigators have also recommended the addition of rifampin, although no clinical data support this recommendation; rifampin should be added only if the organism is susceptible and there is a delay in the expected clinical or bacteriologic response. In patients not responding, intrathecal or intraventricular vancomycin remains a reasonable option.

Several other antimicrobial agents appear promising for the therapy of penicillin-resistant pneumococcal meningitis. Meropenem, a new carbapenem with less proconvulsant activity than imipenem, has been utilized in children and adults with bacterial meningitis, including cases caused by *S. pneumoniae*, with microbiologic and clinical outcomes similar to those following treatment with cefotaxime or ceftriaxone. However, in one study of 20 cefotaxime-resistant pneumococcal isolates, 4 were intermediate and 13 were resistant to meropenem, suggesting that meropenem may not be a useful alternative agent for treatment of pneumococcal isolates that are highly resistant to penicillin and cephalosporins. Newer fluoroquinolones (eg, moxifloxacin) that have excellent in vitro activity against *S. pneumoniae* have also been shown to have efficacy in experimental animal models of penicillin-resistant pneumococcal meningitis, although only trovafloxacin has been shown in a clinical trial to be as efficacious as ceftriaxone, with or without vancomycin, in children with bacterial meningitis. Although trovafloxacin is no longer used because of concerns of liver toxicity, these data suggest the potential usefulness of the newer fluoroquinolones in the treatment of bacterial meningitis. However, further clinical

Table 73.4 Recommended Dosages of Antimicrobial Agents for Meningitis in Adults with Normal Renal and Hepatic Function

Antimicrobial Agent	Total Daily Dose (IV)	Dosing Interval (h)
Amikacin[a]	15 mg/kg	8
Ampicillin	12 g	4
Aztreonam	6–8 g	6–8
Cefepime	6 g	8
Cefotaxime	8–12 g	4–6
Ceftazidime	6 g	8
Ceftriaxone	4 g	12–24
Chloramphenicol[b]	4–6 g	6
Ciprofloxacin	800–1200 mg	8–12
Gentamicin[a,c]	5 mg/kg	8
Meropenem	6 g	8
Moxifloxacin[d]	400 mg	24
Nafcillin	9–12 g	4
Oxacillin	9–12 g	4
Penicillin G	24 million U	4
Rifampin	600 mg	24
Tobramycin[a]	5 mg/kg	8
Trimethoprim–sulfamethoxazole[e]	10–20 mg/kg	6–12
Vancomycin[f,g]	30–45 mg/kg	8–12

[a] Need to monitor peak and trough serum concentrations.
[b] Higher dosage recommended for pneumococcal meningitis.
[c] Intrathecal dosage is 1–8 mg; usual daily dose is 1–2 mg for infants and children, and 4–8 mg for adults. Intrathecal dosing should always be used in combination with a parenteral agent.
[d] No data on optimal dose needed in patients with bacterial meningitis.
[e] Dosage based on trimethoprim component.
[f] Maintain serum trough concentrations of 15–20 μg/mL.
[g] Intrathecal dosage is 5–20 mg; most studies have used a 10-mg or 20-mg dose.

trials are needed before these agents can be recommended as first-line therapy for patients with bacterial meningitis.

NEISSERIA MENINGITIDIS

The antimicrobial agent of choice for therapy of *N. meningitidis* meningitis is penicillin G or ampicillin. These recommendations may change in the future as a result of the emergence of meningococcal strains that are resistant to penicillin G, with an MIC range of 0.1 to 1.0 μg/mL. In a population-based surveillance study for invasive meningococcal disease in selected areas of the United States, 3 of 100 isolates had penicillin MICs of 0.125 μg/mL. However, the clinical significance of these isolates is unclear because patients with meningitis caused by these organisms have recovered with standard penicillin therapy. Some authorities would treat patients with meningococcal meningitis with a third-generation cephalosporin (either cefotaxime or ceftriaxone) pending susceptibility testing of the isolate. Single-dose ceftriaxone was also found to be noninferior compared with chloramphenicol when used against epidemic meningococcal meningitis in one study, suggesting that this agent should be utilized during meningococcal epidemics in the developing world.

LISTERIA MONOCYTOGENES

Despite their broad range of in vitro activity, the third-generation cephalosporins are inactive against *L. monocytogenes.* Therapy for *Listeria* meningitis should consist of ampicillin or penicillin G, with addition of an aminoglycoside considered in proven infection because of documented in vitro synergy. In the penicillin-allergic patient, trimethoprim–sulfamethoxazole, which is bactericidal against *Listeria* in vitro, should be used. Despite favorable in vitro susceptibility results, chloramphenicol and vancomycin are associated with unacceptably high failure rates, although intraventricular vancomycin was efficacious in one case of recurrent *L. monocytogenes* meningitis.

HAEMOPHILUS INFLUENZAE

The therapy of bacterial meningitis caused by *H. influenzae* type b depends on whether the strain produces β-lactamase. For β-lactamase–negative strains, ampicillin is recommended, and for strains that produce β-lactamase, a third-generation cephalosporin (either cefotaxime or ceftriaxone) should be used. In addition, a third-generation cephalosporin should be used as empiric therapy in all patients in whom *H. influenzae* type b is a possible pathogen. Chloramphenicol is not recommended because chloramphenicol-resistant isolates have been reported throughout the world, and even in patients with chloramphenicol-sensitive isolates, a prospective study found chloramphenicol to be bacteriologically and clinically inferior to ampicillin, ceftriaxone, or cefotaxime in the therapy of childhood bacterial meningitis caused predominantly by *H. influenzae* type b. Although cefuroxime, a second-generation cephalosporin, initially appeared to be efficacious in the therapy of *H. influenzae* type b meningitis, a recent study comparing cefuroxime with ceftriaxone for childhood bacterial meningitis documented delayed CSF sterilization and a higher incidence of hearing impairment in the patients receiving cefuroxime; other studies have reported the development of *H. influenzae* meningitis in patients receiving cefuroxime for nonmeningeal *H. influenzae* disease. Cefepime has been compared with cefotaxime in a prospective randomized trial for treatment of meningitis in infants and children; cefepime was found to be safe and therapeutically equivalent to cefotaxime and can be considered a suitable therapeutic alternative for treatment of patients with this disease.

AEROBIC GRAM-NEGATIVE BACILLI

Outcome from meningitis caused by enteric gram-negative bacilli has been greatly improved with the availability of the third-generation cephalosporins (cure rates of 78% to 94%). Ceftazidime, a third-generation cephalosporin with enhanced in vitro activity against *Pseudomonas aeruginosa,* led to a cure in 19 of 24 patients with *P. aeruginosa* meningitis in one study when used alone or in combination with an aminoglycoside. Similar results were observed in a study of pediatric patients in which 7 patients were cured clinically and 9 were cured bacteriologically when receiving ceftazidime-containing regimens. In patients with enteric gram-negative bacillary meningitis not responding to conventional parenteral antimicrobial therapy, concomitant intraventricular or intrathecal aminoglycoside therapy should be considered, although this mode of therapy was associated with a higher mortality rate than systemic therapy alone in infants with gram-negative meningitis and ventriculitis.

Several other antimicrobial agents (eg, imipenem, meropenem, cefepime, aztreonam, colistin) have been successfully used in isolated case reports and in small series of patients with meningitis caused by aerobic gram-negative bacilli. Imipenem has been efficacious, although a high rate of seizure activity (33% in one study) limits its usefulness in patients with bacterial meningitis. The fluoroquinolones (eg, ciprofloxacin, pefloxacin) have also been used in some patients with bacterial meningitis, although their primary usefulness is for therapy of meningitis caused by multidrug-resistant gram-negative organisms or when the response to conventional therapy is inadequate; these agents should not be used as first-line empiric therapy in patients with meningitis of unknown etiology because of their poor in vitro activity against *S. pneumoniae* and *L. monocytogenes.*

STAPHYLOCOCCI AND STREPTOCOCCI

Meningitis caused by *Staphylococcus aureus* should be treated with nafcillin or oxacillin; vancomycin is used for patients who are allergic to penicillin or when the organism is methicillin resistant. For meningitis caused by coagulase-negative staphylococci (eg, *S. epidermidis*), vancomycin is recommended; rifampin should be added if the patient fails to improve. In patients with meningitis caused by

S. agalactiae, ampicillin plus an aminoglycoside is recommended based on documented in vitro synergy and because of the emergence of penicillin-tolerant strains; alternatives include the third-generation cephalosporins and vancomycin.

PREVENTION

It has become clear in recent years that the spread of several types of bacterial meningitis can be prevented by chemoprophylaxis of contacts of patients with meningitis. The rationale is for eradication of nasopharyngeal colonization, thereby preventing transmission to susceptible contacts and the development of invasive disease in those already colonized. Chemoprophylaxis is recommended for contacts of a case of meningococcal meningitis. Therapy is recommended for close contacts of the index case, defined as household contacts, day-care center members, and anyone directly exposed to the patient's oral secretions (eg, through kissing, mouth-to-mouth resuscitation, endotracheal intubation, or endotracheal tube management); the index case may also need to receive prophylaxis if he or she is treated with an antimicrobial agent (eg, penicillin or chloramphenicol) that does not reliably eradicate meningococci from the nasopharynx of colonized patients. The optimal regimen to prevent invasive meningococcal disease is controversial. At present, the Centers for Disease Control and Prevention recommend rifampin (600 mg in adults, 10 mg/kg in children beyond the neonatal period, and 5 mg/kg in infants younger than 1 month of age) given at 12-hour intervals for 2 days. However, eradication rates are only 80% with rifampin, and adverse events, need for multiple dosing, and emergence of resistant organisms have made it less than an ideal agent. Alternatively, ceftriaxone (250 mg intramuscularly in adults and 125 mg intramuscularly in children) or a single dose of oral ciprofloxacin (500 mg) has been found to be efficacious. Ceftriaxone is probably the safest alternative in the pregnant patient. Azithromycin (500 mg orally once) was also shown to be as efficacious as the four-dose regimen of rifampin in the eradication of meningococci from the nasopharynx. Widespread chemoprophylaxis to low-risk contacts should be discouraged because of the concern over emergence of resistant organisms and possible future limitations on this approach.

SUGGESTED READING

Appelbaum PC. Resistance among *Streptococcus pneumoniae*: implications for drug selection. *Clin Infect Dis.* 2002;34:1613–1620.

de Gans J, van de Beek D; European Dexamethasone in Adulthood Bacterial Meningitis Study Investigators. Dexamethasone in adults with bacterial meningitis. *N Engl J Med.* 2002;347:1549–1556.

Hasbun R, Abrahams J, Jekel J, et al. Computed tomography of the head before lumbar puncture in adults with suspected meningitis. *N Engl J Med.* 2001;345:1727–1733.

McIntyre PB, Berkey CS, King SM, et al. Dexamethasone as adjunctive therapy in bacterial meningitis. A meta-analysis of randomized clinical trials since 1988. *JAMA.* 1997;278:925–931.

Thomas KE, Hasbun R, Jekel J, et al. The diagnostic accuracy of Kernig's sign, Brudzinski's sign, and nuchal rigidity in adults with suspected meningitis. *Clin Infect Dis.* 2002;35:46–52.

Tunkel AR. *Bacterial Meningitis.* Philadelphia, PA: Lippincott Williams & Wilkins; 2001.

Tunkel AR, Hartman BJ, Kaplan SL, et al. Practice guidelines for the management of bacterial meningitis. *Clin Infect Dis.* 2004;39:1267–1284.

Tunkel AR, Scheld WM. Corticosteroids for everyone with meningitis? *N Engl J Med.* 2002;347:1613–1615.

van de Beek D, de Gans J, Tunkel AR, et al. Community-acquired bacterial meningitis in adults. *N Engl J Med.* 2006;354:44–53.

Weisfelt M, van de Beek D, Spanjaard L, et al. Clinical features, complications, and outcome in adults with pneumococcal meningitis: a prospective case series. *Lancet Neurol.* 2006;5:123–129.

74. Aseptic Meningitis Syndrome

Burt R. Meyers and Mirella Salvatore

Aseptic meningitis syndrome is associated with symptoms, signs, and laboratory evidence of meningeal inflammation with spinal fluid findings that suggest a viral or noninfectious origin. Clinically, patients present with headache, nausea, meningismus, and photophobia, symptoms that are also common in patients with bacterial meningitis. A stiff neck, with or without a Brudzinski or Kernig sign, may be observed. Patients usually appear nontoxic but may have changes in mental status, including irritability. Other signs of possible viral infection may include pharyngitis, adenopathy, morbilliform rash, and evidence of systemic viral infection, including myalgia, fatigue, and anorexia. There are usually no signs of vascular instability, and the course is often self-limiting.

Aseptic meningitis is a syndrome of multiple etiologies, both infectious and noninfectious (Table 74.1). Infections are usually of viral origin but also may be due to mycobacteria, fungi, rickettsiae, and parasites. Group B coxsackieviruses (mostly serotypes 2 through 5) and echoviruses (mostly serotypes 4, 6, 9, 11, 16, and 30) are responsible for more than 90% of cases of viral meningitis. Herpes virus, arboviruses, lymphocytic choriomeningitis virus (LCM), Lyme disease, leptospirosis, and acute human immunodeficiency virus (HIV) are the etiologic agents that make up most of the remaining infectious cases. Noninfectious causes include drug reactions, collagen-vascular diseases (ie, lupus erythematosus granulomatous arteritis), sarcoidosis, cerebral vascular lesions, epidermal cysts, meningeal carcinomatosis, serum sickness, and nonfocal lesions of the central nervous system (CNS). Specific syndromes (ie, Mollaret's meningitis, Still's disease) may produce a similar clinical picture. The etiologic diagnosis of aseptic meningitis is often complicated by the numerous possible causes and the lack of specific diagnostic tests.

ETIOLOGY
Infectious Agents

The most common causes of viral meningitis are the enteroviruses, herpes viruses, and HIV.

Some viruses passively enter through the skin or respiratory, gastrointestinal, or urogenital tract and may cause initial infection at the entrance site. Some viruses spread through nerve endings by retrograde transmission via neuronal axons (ie, poliovirus, rabies virus, herpes virus). Enteroviruses, LCM, mumps, and arthropodborne viruses replicate initially in muscle cells or mesodermal cells. Other viruses enter via the nose, cause infection of the submucosa, and then enter the subarachnoid space. Most viruses probably enter the CNS following viremia with primary replication at the site of entry and dissemination into the systemic circulation to either anchor and grow in the choroid plexus or pass directly through it into the CNS. Enteroviruses and HIV are carried by this route.

Enteroviruses are the most common cause of viral meningitis occurring mostly during summer and fall but may continue to cause CNS infection also during the winter. The presentation is not distinctive, and the disease presents with abrupt onset and fever, nausea, vomiting, and photophobia. Rash and upper respiratory symptoms may be present. Another increasingly common cause of viral meningitis is represented by HSV. Although HSV encephalitis is mostly caused by HSV-1, meningitis is generally caused by HSV-2. In patients presenting with HSV meningitis genital lesions may be present, and one-quarter of the cases presenting with primary genital herpes have meningeal involvement. However, in the case of recurrent Mollaret meningitis, which is due to HSV-2 in 80% of cases, genital lesions are usually absent. Primary HIV can present as aseptic meningitis with headache, nausea, vomiting, fever, and stiff neck. This disease is self-limiting and can be the only manifestation of HIV for many years. Unfortunately, if patients are not diagnosed at the time of their acute illness, they may infect a number of sexual partners before the diagnosis is established. Interestingly, early onset of aseptic meningitis has not been associated with late neurologic manifestations in HIV-1 infection, and treatment is symptomatic. Other than during the acute phase, aseptic meningitis may also be present during different stages of the disease. The diagnosis may be later complicated by the fact that cerebrospinal fluid (CSF) pleocytosis is less common with advanced immunosuppression. Exposure to excretions of rodents can cause the exposure to the LCM, a human zoonosis caused by a rodentborne arenavirus. The infection, more common during the winter, presents often as an influenza-like syndrome.

Nonviral causes of meningitis have often a more complicated course than viral meningitis and must be recognized because they may have specific therapy. Agents such as bacteria, mycobacteria, and fungi enter the body through the respiratory tract, including the pharynx, sinuses, skin, or lung, and travel to the CNS via the bloodstream. Pneumonitis may be followed by fungemia or bacteremia. Coccidioides meningitis has to be considered in patients with indolent symptoms such as persistent fever and headache who live or traveled from the Southwestern United States and Central or South America. Meningitis is frequently not recognized in this population and may be lethal. *Treponema pallidum* and *Borrelia burgdorferi* enter the CNS after bloodstream invasion.

Noninfectious Etiologies

Entities that should be considered include neurosarcoidosis, connective-tissue disorders, meningeal carcinomatosis or lymphomatosis, CNS vasculitis, migraine-associated pleocytosis, and postviral or postvaccination syndromes. Mechanisms whereby meningeal carcinomatosis, collagen-vascular disease, brain tumors, and epidural or subdural abscess cause changes in the CSF have not been described. Antineoplastic agents, immunoglobulins, and immunosuppressants, including orthoclone (OKT-3), trimethoprim–sulfamethoxazole, and nonsteroidal anti-inflammatory drugs (NSAIDs), may produce aseptic meningitis syndrome; the pathophysiology is unknown.

DIAGNOSTIC WORK-UP

In establishing a diagnosis, clues in the history, physical examination, and CSF examination (Table 74.2) are important.

History

Time of the year may be an important clue because many viral infections are seasonal, occurring during late summer and early fall. Examples are the enteroviruses, whereas

Table 74.1 Causes of Aseptic Meningitis

Infectious	
Enterovirus	Echovirus Coxsackie virus A & B Poliovirus Enterovirus 68–71
Herpesvirus	Herpesvirus (HSV) 1 and 2 Varicella-zoster virus Epstein–Barr virus Cytomegalovirus HSV-6
Paramyxovirus	Mumps virus Measles virus
Togavirus	Rubella virus
Arbovirus	Eastern equine encephalitis virus Western equine encephalitis virus Venezuelan encephalitis virus
Flavivirus	Japanese encephalitis virus Murray Valley encephalitis virus St. Louis encephalitis virus West Nile virus Powassan
Bunyavirus	California encephalitis virus LaCrosse encephalitis virus
Reovirus	Colorado tick fever virus
Arenavirus	Lymphocytic choriomeningitis virus
Rhabdovirus	Rabies virus
Retrovirus	Human immunodeficiency virus human T-cell lymphotrophic virus (HTLV)-I
Adenovirus	
Mycoplasma	*Mycoplasma pneumoniae*
Fungi	*Cryptococcus neoformans* *Coccidiodes immitis* *Histoplasma capsulatum* *Candida* spp. *Aspergillus* *Blastocystis* *Sporothrix Schenckii*
Mycobacteria	*Mycobacterium tuberculosis*
Rickettsia	*Rickettsia rickettsii* Anaplasma
Mycoplasma	*Mycoplasma pneumoniae*
Spirochetes	*Treponema pallidum* (syphilis) *Borrelia burgdorferi* (Lyme) *Borrelia recurrentis* (Relapsing Fever) *Leptospira* spp. (leptospirosis)

Infectious	
Parasites	*Angiostrongylus cantonensis* (eosinophilic meningitis) *Toxoplasma gondii* Gnathostoma spinigerium
	Taenia solium (cysticercosis) *Trichinella spiralis* *Taenia canis* (visceral larva migrants) Negiceria fowleri Acanthamoeba spp
Bacteria	Partially treated bacterial meningitis *Listeria monocytogenes* *Brucella* *Nocardia* Acute or subacute bacterial endocarditis Parameningeal focus (brain or epidural abscess) *Chlamydia* spp. *Actinomyces* spp.
Noninfectious	
Drug reactions	Nonsteroidal anti-inflammatory agents Antineoplastic agents Antibiotics (trimethoprim–sulfamethoxazole) Immunosuppressants (orthoclone, azathioprime) Isoniazid Immunoglobulin
Malignancy	Primary medulloblastoma Metastatic leukemia Hodgkin's disease
Collagen vascular disease	Lupus erythematous Behçet's/Adult-onset Still's disease
Trauma	Subarachnoid bleed Traumatic lumbar puncture neurosurgery
Chemicals	Lead mercury Contrast agents Disinfectants, glove powder
Neurologic disorders	Cerebral vascular lesions Epidermal cysts Brain tumors
Systemic disorders	Sarcoidosis Vasculitis
Miscellaneous	Serum sickness Mollaret's meningitis Meningeal carcinomatosis Vaccination Postinfectious viral syndromes Post-transplantation lymphoproliferative disorder

Table 74.2 Diagnostic Work-up for Aseptic Meningitis Syndrome

Clinical Evaluation

History

Season (summer, enteroviruses, Rocky Mountain spotted fever)
Geographic area (Colorado tick fever, babesia, Lyme disease)
Exposure to other patients (mumps, varicella)
Tick, mosquito bites (malaria, Lyme disease), tsetse fly (trypanosomiasis)
Exposure to animals (rabies, hantavirus, LCM)
Sexual history (HIV, HSV, syphilis)
IVDU (endocarditis)
Drug reactions (immunoglobulin, OKT-3, NSAIDs, antibiotics)

Physical Examination

Spinal Fluid

Opening pressure
Leukocyte count predominance
    a. Neutrophils (initial echo, polio, HSV, Mollaret's, TB)
    b. Lymphocytes (Coxsackie, enterovirus)
    c. Eosinophils (angiostrongylus Gnathostoma)
    d. Abnormal cells (Mollaret's, lymphoma, WNV)
Protein ≤40 mg/dL
Glucose ≤40 mg/dL or ≤50% serum
Gram stain, AFB smear, Papanicolau stain (Mollaret's meningitis)
Cryptococcal antigen, India ink
Immunoelectrophoresis
Wet mount (toxoplasmosis, amebae)
Bacterial, mycobacterial, fungal cultures
PCR for enterovirus HSV, VZV (in immunocompromised patients), CMV, EBV
Antibodies to *Borrelia burgdorferi*, *Brucella*, *Histoplasma capsulatum* antigen and anti-histoplasma antibody testing by complement fixation, beginning with undiluted CSF, complement-fixing IgG antibodies, or immunodiffusion tests for IgM and IgG for *Coccidioides immitis* (chronic or recurrent presentation)

Serologic Testing

Cryptococcal antigen
Histoplasma urinary and serum antigen (MiraVista Diagnostics)
Lyme disease ELISA, Western blot
Rocky Mountain spotted fever indirect fluorescent antibody test (state health departments)
ANA
HIV-I/HIV-2 antibody
HTLV-1
Serum and CSF VDRL

Other

PPD
Chest x-ray film
Computed tomography, magnetic resonance imaging
Echocardiogram

Abbreviations: HIV = human immunodeficiency virus; HSV = herpes simplex virus; IVDU = intravenous drug use; OKT-3 = orthoclone; NSAIDs = nonsteroidal anti-inflammatory drugs; AFB = acid-fast bacilli; VDR =, Venereal Drug Research Laboratory; ELISA = enzyme-linked immunosorbent assay; ANA = antinuclear antibody.

mumps and LCM peak during winter and spring. Other viruses such as HSV-2 and HIV have to be considered in any season. West Nite virus (WNV) and equine-associated meningo-encephalitis outbreaks occur from late summer to early fall. Avian (for WNV) or equine sources (for equine encephalopathy) with spread via mosquitoes is the presumed route of infection to humans. Furthermore, a history of exposure to patients with known viral illness often suggests enteroviral infection. Similar presentation in association with genital lesions should suggest HSV-2 meningitis, although genital lesions are absent in about 15% of the cases.

Exposure to mice and rodents suggests infection with LCM, less commonly *Leptospira* species, or hantavirus, which may cause a severe pulmonary syndrome. History of sexual contacts should be elicited because HSV and, in appropriate risk groups, syphilis and HIV may present initially with aseptic meningitis. All patients, including the elderly, should be questioned about risk factors for HIV infection, including sexual promiscuity, intravenous drug use, sexual preference, and history of transfusions with blood or blood products. human T-cell lymphotrophic virus (HTLV)-I infection may also present with the diagnosis of spastic paraparesis.

Syphilitic meningitis has become a more common diagnostic consideration for the aseptic meningitis syndrome in the acquired immune deficiency syndrome (AIDS) era. Syphilitic meningitis may coexist with the primary or secondary infection or may follow it by as much as 2 years.

Geographic location, in terms of domicile and travel history, should be evaluated. Exposure to insects such as the tsetse fly in Africa could suggest trypanosomiasis, and mosquito bites in a traveler to India or Mauritius associated with fever and rash may suggest chikungunya (CHK). *Histoplasma capsulatum*, *Coccidioides immitis*, and *B. burgdorferi* occur mainly in certain sections of the United States. Those who have recently been in contact with a pet or have been camping may risk infection with Rickettsia, *Anaplasma*, or *Borrelia* related to a tick bite. Exposure to mosquito bites may result in WNV infection or equine meningoencephalitis virus infection. Rabies, although rare, should be considered if the patient was bitten or in contact with the secretions of an infected skunk, raccoon, dog, fox, or bat. Drinking untreated water on backpacking trips may result in *Leptospira* infection, ingestion of unpasteurized milk and cheeses may cause brucellosis, and contaminated processed meats (ie, frankfurters) may cause *Listeria monocytogenes* infection in pregnant women, elderly, and immunocompromised hosts.

Meningitis due to fungi is a consideration primarily in patients affected by HIV and in those who have organ transplantation, immunosuppressive chemotherapy, or chronic corticosteroid therapy. However, the most common pathogen, *Cryptococcus neoformans*, can occur in immunocompetent hosts.

Vasculitides found in patients of Mediterranean origin include Behçet's disease and familial Mediterranean fever. Certain drugs, including intravenous immunoglobulin, trimetropim–sulfamethoxazole, NSAIDs, and immunosuppressants, have been associated with aseptic meningitis syndrome. Intracranial infections often present with headache and fever. Brain, epidural, or subdural abscesses may be present in patients with a history of upper respiratory tract infection (ie, otitis media, sinusitis) or infection of the teeth or gums. Computed tomography (CT) scan or magnetic resonance imaging (MRI) may aid in this diagnosis. Aseptic meningitis syndrome has been associated with subacute bacterial endocarditis; physical stigmata, including conjunctival petechiae, cardiac murmurs, retinal lesions, and evidence of embolic phenomenon, may be found. Infection with either mycobacteria or fungi or a history of malignancy must be considered.

It is important to investigate recent antibiotic use. Partially treated bacterial meningitis should be suspected if the patient has received prior oral antimicrobial therapy and has persistently low CSF glucose or pleocytosis, with a negative Gram stain. Recurrent bouts of meningitis with a benign clinical picture and unknown etiology suggest Mollaret's meningitis.

Physical Examination

A physical examination may elicit findings that may suggest a specific agent. Generally the patient is febrile and nontoxic, pulse and respiration normal, with or without evidence of meningismus. Examination of the skin may reveal a morbilliform or vesicular rash consistent with enteroviral infection, primary HIV or syphilis, or evidence of a tick bite. However, a rash can be observed also in some cases of meningococcemia. The scalp should be examined carefully, especially the area behind the ears. Petechiae on the hands and feet usually suggest rickettsial infection. Examination of the eyes for conjunctival petechiae and funduscopic examination may reveal lesions typical of infectious endocarditis. Other lesions usually found by funduscopic examination are associated with cytomegalovirus (CMV) or *Toxoplasma*, especially if there is suspicion of HIV. The oral cavity may show thrush with or without cervical adenopathy. Presence of parotid or testicular swelling enlargement is consistent with mumps meningitis. The chest examination is usually normal, but a murmur in this setting suggests endocarditis; a pericardial rub suggests coxsackievirus infection or a collagen-vascular syndrome. Hepatomegaly, splenomegaly, or adenopathy may suggest a systemic disease, including disseminated viral or fungal infection. Genital ulcerative lesions may be present in vascular syndromes such as lupus erythematosus and may also be consistent with HSV-2 infection. Examination of the neck may reveal evidence of stiffness on flexion and a positive Brudzinski and/or Kernig sign. Focal or multiple cranial nerve involvement suggests lesions such as a brain, subdural, or epidural abscess; embolic phenomena may also produce these lesions. Asymmetric flaccid paralysis suggests WNV infection. Physical examination may also reveal a typical malar rash or other signs of collagen-vascular disease.

Laboratory Data

The CSF should be examined and opening pressure recorded; in aseptic meningitis the CSF is clear with a normal or mildly increased opening pressure. The white blood cell (WBC) count is usually less than 500/mL but it can reach 1000/mL with a predominance of lymphocytes. However, CSF differential cell counts may reveal a predominance of polymorphonuclear leukocytes mostly with Echovirus, poliovirus, mumps, HSV, *Mycobacterium. tuberculosis*, and Mollaret's meningitis. A shift toward a lymphocyte predominance during the first week of the disease occurs. Pleocytosis has been reported in 25% of patients with enteroviral infection. Eosinophils in the CSF suggest parasitic disease secondary to angiostrongylus, *Taenia* sp., or *Schistosoma*. Japonicum or paragonimus westemani meningeal carcinomatosis is suggested when abnormal cells are seen, and large granular cells with indistinct cytoplasm suggest Mollaret's meningitis. Fat droplets have been seen following epidermoid cyst rupture. Spinal fluid glucose should be compared with simultaneously drawn blood glucose. Normal levels of CSF glucose (40 mg/dL or >50% to 66% of the blood levels) suggest viral meningitis. However,

the glucose content may be lower than normal in 18% to 33% of cases, and viruses like herpes, mumps, LCM, and polio can cause hypoglycorrhachia (Table 74.3). A study of CSF from 334 cases of WNV infection showed that it usually presents with CSF pleocytosis, increased protein, and normal glucose. The protein levels in aseptic meningitis are usually normal or slightly elevated; levels greater than 800 mg suggest CSF block with infection or tumor, although this has also been associated with chemical meningitis. A wet prep of CSF should be examined to look for *Toxoplasma gondii* or amebae (eg, Histolytica). Gram stain and bacterial culture should be performed because a partially treated bacterial infection or infection with *Listeria monocytogenes* may occasionally present with a predominance of lymphocytes. Acid-fast smears, culture, and polymerase chain reaction (PCR) (non-U.S. Food and Drug Administration (FDA)-approved) should be done to rule out mycobacterial infections, and India ink stain or determination of cryptococcal antigen in the CSF should be performed.

The CSF should be also sent for routine fungal and mycobacterial cultures. With the increasing use of the nucleic acid detection tests, viral cultures from CSF are not useful and should not be performed routinely. Viral cultures are laborious and time consuming, and they need to be performed in four different cell lines that are then evaluated daily for cytopathic effect. The findings are then confirmed by a neutralizing or an immunofluorescence antibody test. The overall sensitivity of virus isolation from the CSF of patients with aseptic meningitis is between 3% and 40%. In a recent review of more than 20 000 CSF viral cultures, ≤0.1% recovered species were nonenteroviruses and non-Herpes, suggesting that when nucleic acid amplification testing is performed, viral cultures have no additional benefit. If indicated, simultaneous viral cultures are obtained from throat washings and stool specimens.

CSF should be sent for PCR, which is available for the detection of a range of pathogens, particularly viruses. This technique is highly sensitive and specific, with results available within 24 hours, requiring only small volumes of CSF. PCR is the best assay for the detection of HSV-1, HSV-2, varicella-zoster virus (VZV), human herpesvirus 6 and 7, CMV, Epstein–Barr virus (EBV), enteroviruses, respiratory viruses and HIV in CSF samples. PCR for *Chlamydia. pneumoniae* can also be performed from a CSF sample. Respiratory viruses, *Chlamydia pneumoniae*, and *Mycoplasma pneumoniae* can

Table 74.3 Differential Diagnosis of Cerebrospinal Fluid (CSF) Glucose Concentrations

Normal CSF Glucose Concentration	Decreased CSF Glucose Concentration
Enteroviruses	Partially treated bacterial meningitis
Mumps virus	*Listeria monocytogenes*
Arthropodborne viruses	
Herpes simplex virus-1 and -2	*Mycobacterium tuberculosis*
Human immunodeficiency virus	*Candida*
Influenza virus types A and B	*Cryptococcus neoformans*
Measles, subacute sclerosing panencephalitis	*Coccidioides immitis*
Varicella-zoster virus	*Histoplasma capsulatum*
Cytomegalovirus	*Blastomyces dermatitidis*
Treponema pallidum	Herpes simplex virus-1
Borrelia burgdorferi	Mumps virus
Leptospirosis	Lymphocytic choriomeningitis virus
Rickettsia rickettsii	Poliovirus
Human monocytic ehrlichiosis	
Anaplasma phagocytophilum	Sarcoidosis
Behçet's disease	Leptomeningeal carcinomatosis
Migraine	
Vasculitis	
Postinfectious encephalomyelitis	
Nonsteroidal anti-inflammatory agents	
Orthoclone	
Azathioprine	
Trimethoprim–sulfamethoxazole	
Isoniazid	
Intravenous immunoglobulin	

also be detected from throat samples and enterovirus nucleic acid from stool samples; however, these cannot confirm the etiology of the meningitis. The use of PCR for the diagnosis of infectious origins of aseptic meningitis has resulted in increased identification of the enterovirus, which allows the discontinuation of antimicrobial therapy, decreases hospital length of stay and costs, and enables patients to return to their usual environments.

The use of multiplex PCR is increasingly used for facilitating the assay of multiple viruses on the same sample. The sensitivity and specificities of this technique are similar to those of the single PCR. New development of specific microarrays is still experimental and quite expensive, but it allows the study and identification of several pathogens at the same time.

Examination of the peripheral blood reveals a WBC count that is usually normal or may be less than $5000/mm^3$. The differential is also normal, although occasionally a left shift of polymorphonuclear leukocytes has been observed. Eosinophilia has been described in parasitic infections and in drug and serum sickness reactions. Leukopenia associated with thrombocytopenia may suggest *Anaplasma* and Rickettsia Infection, and nonspecific changes in hepatic enzymes may be found in viral infections. Sedimentation rate may be normal or elevated. Blood cultures should always be performed, because *L. monocytogenes*, *Brucella*, and rarely some typical pathogens, such as *Streptococcus pneumoniae*, *Neisseria meningitidis*, and *H. influenzae*, may present with a predominance of lymphocytes in the CSF. Infectious endocarditis from either bacteria or fungi can be considered in the appropriate clinical setting when a patient has positive blood cultures.

If fungal disease is suspected, serologic studies should be performed for cryptococcal antigen and *C. immitis*. *Histoplasma capsulatum* urinary antigen should be tested. PCR for *Mycoplasma pneumoniae* is also warranted. Venereal Disease Research Laboratory (VDRL) test should be performed on CSF. PCR tests have been developed using a variety of syphilitic antigens. They are quite specific but do not distinguish live from dead organisms. When rickettsial diseases are suspected (ie, Rocky Mountain spotted fever or Lyme disease), appropriate serologic tests should be performed, but therapy should not be delayed while tests are pending. If rabies is suspected, an immunofluorescence test on conjunctival scrapings or subcutaneous neck fascial biopsy is the best method for establishing the diagnosis. Other serologic tests include antinuclear antibody (ANA) to rule out systemic lupus erythematosus. Given the appropriate clinical setting, HIV testing may be warranted. The virus in CSF may be detected through PCR.

If vesicular lesions are present, immunofluorescent staining for HSV-1, HSV-2, and VZV and viral culture from the lesion should be performed. If lesions other than vesicular lesions are found, careful examination by dark-field may reveal evidence of *T. pallidum*. Petechial lesions should be stained and cultured for bacteria and stained with immunofluorescence antibody for *R. rickettsii*. Throat and stool cultures should be obtained for confirmation of enteroviral infection.

A chest roentgenogram specifically looking for diffuse infiltrates, cavitation, and pleural or pericardial involvement may suggest mycoplasma, mycobacterial, or fungal infection in that order. Evidence of a mass lesion in this setting suggests carcinoma and possibly meningeal carcinomatosis. With physical findings of focal involvement, an MRI scan should be performed to look for evidence of an intracranial infection or malignancy.

THERAPY

The diagnosis and treatment of the aseptic meningitis syndrome is a challenge, because differentiating between infectious and noninfectious etiologies can be difficult. For patients with a suspected bacterial etiology or partially treated meningitis, antibiotic therapy should be promptly initiated. In case of aseptic meningitis in an elderly or immunocompromised patient or in case of an unclear picture, antibiotic therapy should be empirically initiated and discontinued if patient improves symptomatically and cultures are negative. If the patient deteriorates without a clear diagnosis, a repeat lumber puncture may be indicated. Although the management of patients with aseptic meningitis of viral origin includes supportive care in most cases, specific therapy exists for some viral pathogens. Acyclovir may be used to treat meningitis caused by HSV and VZV, and ganciclovir is used for CMV infection. Acyclovir, 10 mg/kg every 8 hours, is used for HSV and VZV; ganciclovir, 5 mg/kg twice a day, is the regimen for CMV. The newer oral antiviral compounds valacyclovir and famciclovir have a 5-fold higher bioavailability than acyclovir, allowing less frequent dosing.

No antiviral therapeutic agent for enteroviruses has demonstrated improved outcome in controlled clinical trials, and antiviral therapy of enteroviral meningitis is limited. The administration of γ globulin has led to improvement in patients with agammaglobulinemia who have chronic enteroviral meningitis as well as in neonates with enteroviral sepsis and meningitis. Pleconaril is an orally administered antiviral agent that inhibits enteroviral replication by binding the viral capsid. This drug may reach much higher concentrations within the CNS, suggesting its potential use to treat CNS infection. However, pleconaril induces CYP3A enzyme activity and has not been FDA approved because of its potential for drug interactions. Two large studies of aseptic meningitis due to enterovirus revealed that pleconaril shortened the course of illness compared to placebo, especially when administered early during the course of the disease. However, subgroup analysis showed only a modest benefit in patients with more severe disease.

Most viral meningitides are benign and require no therapy. For bacterial, fungal, and spirochetal disease, antimicrobial therapy directed against the offending agent is required (see specific chapters) and should not be delayed while awaiting the results of CSF assay. Treatment with doxycycline in association with two other agents may be indicated for patients suspected of having *Brucella* and with doxycycline or chloramphenicol is used for Rocky Mountain spotted fever. Specific therapy with ampicillin plus gentamicin is suggested when *L. monocytogenes* is the suspected agent, especially in elderly and immunocompromised hosts.

Because the differential diagnosis of aseptic meningitis syndrome is so broad, the initial evaluation of the patient in conjunction with the results of CSF studies will determine whether the patient requires antimicrobial therapy pending culture results from blood and CSF PCR. Patients who are toxic appearing, in the extremes of life, or with serious underlying disease should be admitted to the hospital and treated empirically until a clear diagnosis is made. Isolation precautions for contagious diseases should be instituted.

SUGGESTED READING

Chavanet P, Schaller C, Levy C, et al. Performance of a predictive rule to distinguish bacterial and viral meningitis. *J Infect*. 2007;54:328-336.

Desmond RA, Accortt NA, Talley L, et al. Enteroviral meningitis: natural history and outcome of pleconaril therapy. *Antimicrob Agents Chemother*. 2006;50:2409–2414.

Diaz-Hurtado M, Vidal-Tolosa A. Drug-induced aseptic meningitis: a physician's challenge. *J Natl Med Assoc*. 2006;98:457.

Hamrock DJ. Adverse events associated with intravenous immunoglobulin therapy. *Int Immunopharmacol*. 2006;6:535–542.

Khetsuriani N, Lamonte-Fowlkes A, Oberst S, et al. Enterovirus surveillance-United States, 1970–2005. *MMWR Surveill Summ*. 2006;55:1–20.

Kupila L, Vuorinen T, Vainionpaa R, et al. Etiology of aseptic meningitis and encephalitis in an adult population. *Neurology*. 2006;66:75–80.

Lee BE, Davies HD. Asephic meningitis curr. op. *Infect Dis*. 2007;20:272–277.

Marra CM, Maxwell CL, Smith SL, et al. Cerebrospinal fluid abnormalities in patients with syphilis: association with clinical and laboratory features. *J Infect Dis*. 2004;189:369–376.

Polage CR, Petti CA. Assessment of the utility of viral culture of cerebrospinal fluid. *Clin Infect Dis*. 2006;43:1578–1579.

Sendi P, Graber P. Mollaret's meningitis. *Can Med Assoc J*. 2006;174:1710.

Shalabi M, Whitley RJ. Recurrent benign lymphocytic meningitis. *Clin Infect Dis*. 2006;43:1194–1197.

Whitley RJ, Roizman B. Herpes simplex virus infections. *Lancet*. 2001;357:1513–1518.

75. Acute Viral Encephalitis

David N. Irani

INTRODUCTION

Viral infections of the central nervous system (CNS) are uncommon but potentially devastating clinical events. As a group, these infections range from benign, self-limited forms of meningitis to full-blown and often fatal cases of acute encephalitis to chronic, persistent diseases. Encephalitis literally refers to inflammation of the brain parenchyma, and such a host response is common with many viral infections that spread to this site (Figure 75.1). In contrast, meningitis results when infection and the associated inflammatory response are limited to the leptomeninges and the subarachnoid space. In reality, the two syndromes often occur together—hence the term *meningoencephalitis.* Acute viral encephalitis or acute viral meningoencephalitis is suggested by various signs and symptoms indicative of brain parenchymal invasion (mental status and behavioral changes, seizures, and focal neurological deficits) accompanied by fever. Such patients require emergent evaluation for what can be a life-threatening infectious illness that sometimes has a treatable cause.

ETIOLOGY

More than 100 different viruses can infect the human CNS, but a much smaller number cause the vast majority of viral encephalitis cases. The most relevant pathogens come from the Herpesviridae, Picornaviridae, Retroviridae, Paramyxoviridae, and a group of RNA viruses formerly called the *arboviruses,* now designated as the Togaviridae, Flaviviridae, Bunyaviridae, and Reoviridae families (Table 75.1). The acquired immunodeficiency syndrome (AIDS) epidemic and the therapeutic use of immunosuppression in transplant recipients and oncology patients have resulted in the identification of new infectious disease processes that can cause signs and symptoms consistent with acute encephalitis. A greater proportion of immunocompromised hosts now requires discrimination between an ever-expanding list of potential infectious and noninfectious causes

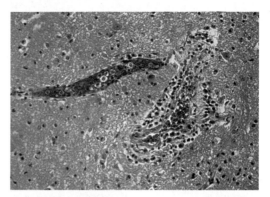

Figure 75.1 Mononuclear inflammatory cells accumulate around blood vessel in a fatal case of Japanese encephalitis. These perivascular "cuffs" are a characteristic histopathological finding in the central nervous system (CNS) during acute viral encephalitis. Hematoxylin & eosin, 100×. (Courtesy of Richard T. Johnson, MD, Department of Neurology, The Johns Hopkins University School of Medicine.)

of an acute encephalitis-like clinical picture (Table 75.2).

EPIDEMIOLOGY

The viruses that cause acute encephalitis vary widely in their epidemiology. In many cases, the identification of a particular causative agent can be aided by clues derived from the surrounding environment (geography, season) as well as from a careful review of the patient's background (sexual behavior, intravenous drug use, travel, occupation, arthropod or animal contacts, vaccine history, and exposure to ill persons). One important point is that many viruses causing acute encephalitis are transmitted to humans via infected mosquitos and thus produce disease in the summer or early fall months when the vectors are prevalent. A summary of the epidemiologic findings associated with the more common viral encephalitides is presented (Table 75.3).

PATHOGENESIS

Most viruses gain entry into the CNS either through hematogenous or intraneural spread.

Table 75.1 Significant Causes of Acute Viral Encephalitis in Humans

Herpesviridae	Reoviridae
Herpes simplex virus	Colorado tick fever virus
Varicella-zoster virus	**Picornaviridae**
Cytomegalovirus	Echovirus
Epstein-Barr virus	Coxsackievirus
Human herpes virus 6	Poliovirus
B virus	Enterovirus 71
Bunyaviridae	**Retroviridae**
	Human immunodeficiency
California serogroup	virus, type 1
viruses	**Papovaviridae**
La Crosse virus	JC virus
Jamestown Canyon virus	
Snowshoe hare virus	**Orthomyxoviridae**
Togaviridae (alphaviruses)	Influenza virus
Eastern equine encephalitis	**Paramyxoviridae**
virus	Measles virus
Western equine	Mumps virus
encephalitis virus	Nipah virus
Venezuelan equine	**Miscllaneous viruses**
encephalitis virus	Adenovirus
Flaviviridae	Lymphocytic
Japanese encephalitis virus	choriomeningitis virus
St. Louis encephalitis virus	Rabies virus
West Nile virus	
Tickborne encephalitis	
viruses	

Table 75.2 Nonviral Causes of an Acute Encephalitis-Like Clinical Presentation

Infectious	Noninfectious
Bacterial	**Parainfectious/**
Acute bacterial meningitis	**Autoimmune**
Brain abscess	Reye's syndrome
Parameningeal infection	Postinfectious
Subdural empyema	encephalomyelitis
Venous sinus	Postvaccination
thrombophlebitis	encephalomyelitis
CNS Lyme disease	
Neurosyphilis	**Neoplastic**
Whipple disease	Primary or metastatic brain
Bacterial toxin-mediated	tumor
process	Paraneoplastic disorder
	Neoplastic meningitis
Fungal	
Fungal meningitis	**Cerebrovascular**
Fungal brain abscess	Acute ischemic stroke
	Subdural hematoma
Parasitic	CNS vasculitis
Toxoplasma gondii	
abscess	**Systemic**
Cerebral malaria	Metabolic encephalopathy
Human African	Connective tissue disease
trypanosomiasis	Drug intoxication
Amebic	**Epileptic**
Naegleria fowleri	Seizures/postictal state
meningoencephalitis	
Acanthamoeba	**Traumatic**
meningoencephalitis	Acute head injury

Bunyaviridae, Flaviviridae, and Togaviridae seed the CNS from the bloodstream after subcutaneous inoculation by the insect vector and replication in local tissues. Other neurotropic viruses enter the host via the respiratory tract (eg, adenovirus, measles, influenza) or the gastrointestinal tract (eg, enteroviruses). Rabies virus reaches the CNS via intra-axonal transport in sensory nerves that innervate the skin. The pathogenesis of herpes simplex virus (HSV) encephalitis remains incompletely understood, but virus passage along the olfactory and trigeminal nerve tracts from ganglia where it can reactivate from latency likely explains the classic temporal lobe localization. Host factors play a role in both the susceptibility to and the severity of viral encephalitis. Chronic enteroviral meningoencephalitis occurs most commonly in patients with agammaglobulinemia, whereas acute measles, cytomegalovirus (CMV), and varicella-zoster virus (VZV) encephalitis usually occurs in patients with impaired cellular immunity.

Once inside the CNS, encephalitic viruses cause pathology either due to direct cytopathic effect or as a result of immune-mediated injury. The tropism of these pathogens for various parenchymal cell populations varies during acute encephalitis, but those infecting neurons often cause particularly severe disease (Figure 75.2). The ensuing histopathological changes reflecting the host response include the perivascular infiltration of mononuclear inflammatory cells (Figure 75.1), a reactive astrocytosis, the formation of glial nodules, and neuronophagia. Cytotoxic T cells and phagocytic macrophages may actually be the effectors of much of the resulting neural injury. It is also likely that soluble immune factors (cytokines, chemokines, nitric oxide, etc.) contribute to disease pathogenesis in complex ways, both to the benefit and the detriment of the infected host. While some of these factors such as the interferons (α, β, and γ) and their regulatory transacting proteins may act to limit local CNS virus replication, others such as interleukin (IL)-1, IL-6, and tumor necrosis factor (TNF)-α may have injurious properties in humans and clearly make viral encephalitis worse in animal models of these diseases.

In postinfectious encephalitis, disease occurs via immune-mediated mechanisms rather than through direct cytopathic effects and manifests as multifocal perivascular demyelination. Although poorly understood, it is assumed that the elicited antiviral immune response

Table 75.3 Clinical and Epidemiologic Characteristics of Major Causes of Viral Encephalitis in the United States

Family/Virus[a]	Affected Hosts	Peak Season/ Pattern	Geography/ Incidence	Clinical Presentation	Epidemiologic Clues
Herpesviridae					
HSV	All ages	Year-round; endemic	Ubiquitous (~2500 cases/y)	Focal neurological deficits; seizures; bizarre behavior	
VZV	Healthy and immunocompromised adults; infants	Year-round; endemic	Ubiquitous	Ataxia; stroke-like episodes; can have an accompanying myelitis	Recent primary varicella rash or herpes zoster dermatomal rash
CMV	Immunocompromised adults; infants	Year-round; endemic	Ubiquitous	Periventricular lesions on brain MRI; accompanying lumbosacral polyradiculitis	Known HIV+ individuals; posttransplant recipients (especially bone marrow recipients)
Retroviridae					
HIV	All ages	Year-round; endemic	Ubiquitous (3000–4000 cases/y)	Subacute cognitive deficits; psychomotor slowing	High-risk sexual practices; intravenous drug use
Papoviridae					
JC virus	Immunocompromised adults	Year-round; endemic	Ubiquitous (400–800 cases/y)	Focal neurological deficits; multifocal MRI lesions	HIV+ individuals; post-transplantion or chemotherapy
Togaviridae					
Eastern equine encephalitis virus	Young and elderly	Summer and fall; endemic/ sporadic	East and Gulf Coasts (5–10 cases/y)	Fulminant deficits; seizures; coma	Outdoor occupation or activities; proximity to marshes or standing water
Western equine encephalitis virus	Young and elderly	Summer and fall; endemic/ sporadic	Midwest and Western States (10–15 cases/y)	Nonfocal deficits; headache	Outdoor occupation or activities; travel or habitation in rural areas
Flaviviridae					
West Nile virus	All ages (but most cases in the young and the elderly)	Summer and fall; epidemic	Nationwide (2,000–4,000 cases/y over the last few years)	Nonfocal deficits; headache; ~20% with a poliomyelitis-like illness	Outdoor exposure (urban or rural); most cases are concentrated in a few states each season

(continued)

Table 75.3 *(continued)*

Family/Virus[a]	Affected Hosts	Peak Season/Pattern	Geography/Incidence	Clinical Presentation	Epidemiologic Clues
St. Louis encephalitis virus	Young and elderly	Summer and fall; epidemic	Nationwide (~100 cases/y; range 2–1967 cases/y)	Nonfocal deficits; headache	Outdoor exposure; endemic in rural areas in the West; sporadic urban outbreaks in the Eastern States
Bunyaviridae					
La Crosse virus	Young	Summer and fall; endemic and small case clusters	Midwest and Eastern States (75–100 cases/y)	Often asymptomatic; can cause seizures	Outdoor activities; suburban cases occur near wooded areas
Picornaviridae					
Echoviruses Coxsackieviruses Polioviruses Unclassified viruses (EV68–EV71)	Young, especially agammaglobulinemic children	Summer and fall; epidemic	Nationwide (~1000 cases/y)	Accompanying viral exanthem, conjunctivitis, myopericarditis, herpangina, hand-foot-and-mouth disease	Known community epidemic of picornavirus
Rhabdoviridae					
Rabies	All ages	Year-round; endemic	Nationwide (10–15 cases/y)	Prior animal bite or scratch; autonomic symptoms in ~80%; paralysis in ~20%	Animal contact

Abbreviations: AIDS = acquired immunodeficiency syndrome; HIV = human immunodeficiency virus; CMV = cytomegalovirus; MRI = magnetic resonance imaging; HSV = herpes simplex virus; VZV = Varicella-zoster virus.

somehow triggers pathogenic antimyelin autoimmunity through a process such as molecular mimicry. Viruses implicated in this type of encephalitis include measles, mumps, rubella, VZV, and Epstein–Barr virus (EBV). This form of encephalitis usually manifests itself within weeks of the triggering infection.

CLINICAL MANIFESTATIONS

Although the severity of deficits can range from very mild to extreme, most patients with acute viral encephalitis develop a progressive constellation of complaints that evolves over a period of several days and prompts them to seek medical attention. Manifestations typically include fever, symptoms of meningeal inflammation (headache, neck stiffness, nausea, and vomiting), and signs indicative of brain parenchymal involvement (seizures, behavioral changes, weakness, and an altered sensorium often progressing to coma over time). None of these signs or symptoms are pathognomonic of a particular virus, although an occasional extraneural manifestation may point to a specific pathogen when present. These might include parotitis with mumps infection, pharyngitis and lymphadenopathy with EBV, and a dermatomal rash with VZV. Nonspecific neuroendocrine complications of viral encephalitis may include inappropriate antidiuretic hormone secretion and diabetes insipidus.

More importantly, certain viral pathogens exhibit strong predilections to infect particular

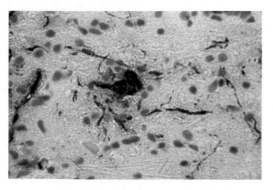

Figure 75.2 Immunohistochemical identification of viral antigens within neurons in a fatal case of Japanese encephalitis. Viruses tropic for neurons often cause severe forms of acute encephalitis. Immunoperoxidase with hematoxylin counterstain, 125×. (Courtesy of Richard T. Johnson, MD, Department of Neurology, The Johns Hopkins University School of Medicine.)

regions of the CNS, resulting in characteristic focal neurological deficits. Although CMV typically involves periventricular areas, rabies the limbic system, VZV the cerebellum, and Japanese encephalitis virus (JEV) the basal ganglia, the prototypic example of such a focal infection is HSV infection of the temporal and inferofrontal lobes of the brain. Accordingly, patients with herpes simplex encephalitis (HSE) commonly present with a hemiparesis, visual field cut, aphasia (if the dominant temporal lobe is involved), and complex-partial or generalized seizures. Because the mortality of untreated HSE exceeds 70%, and because morbidity and mortality can be significantly reduced with the prompt initiation of antiviral therapy, it is imperative that all patients with a fever and such focal neurological deficits be promptly evaluated for this infection and started on empiric therapy until the results of specific diagnostic tests are available.

DIAGNOSIS

Routine laboratory studies (serum chemistries, peripheral cell counts, etc.) have limited value in the diagnosis of acute viral encephalitis. Acute and convalescent serum samples can be sent for the measurement of specific antibodies against a number of viral pathogens to identify an etiologic agent (discussed below). In the acute stages of the illness, however, the main diagnostic tools are neuroimaging studies to confirm structural involvement of the CNS and a lumbar puncture (LP) to identify suspicious inflammatory changes in the cerebrospinal fluid (CSF) and to seek molecular evidence of

a particular viral pathogen within the intrathecal space.

Electroencephalography and Brain Imaging Studies

The electroencephalogram (EEG) may sometimes aid in the diagnosis of an acute focal encephalitis such as HSE. Periodic lateralized epileptiform discharges in the temporal lobe can be identified within the first days after symptom onset. Although of low specificity, encephalitis-induced EEG abnormalities can precede cranial computed tomography (CT) changes that may not be seen until several days later. Electroencephalographic evidence of seizures during the course of infection mandates the use of antiepileptic therapies. Furthermore, although diffuse slowing of background EEG activity or epileptiform features are common in the acute stages of viral encephalitis, the emergence of slow background activity at follow-up is often associated with a less favorable clinical outcome.

Brain imaging is essential in the evaluation of suspected viral encephalitis, and a contrast-enhanced cranial magnetic resonance imaging (MRI) scan is now the diagnostic procedure of choice. Conventional fluid-attenuated inversion-recovery (FLAIR) MRI sequences allow for the early radiographic detection of disease in the inferomedial temporal lobes indicative of HSE (Figure 75.3). Likewise, thalamic lesions that are hyperintense on T_2-weighted images are characteristic of Japanese encephalitis, and focal abnormalities in the basal ganglia have been associated with eastern equine encephalitis virus (EEEV)-induced disease. Recent comparative studies now demonstrate that diffusion-weighted MRI may be superior to more conventional sequences for the early detection of brain abnormalities in both HSE and West Nile virus (WNV) encephalitis. Thus, it seems likely that newer, more sensitive imaging modalities will continue to augment our ability to diagnose encephalitis patients, even though the main tools will always be the specific identification of viral pathogens using other molecular techniques.

In cases where MRI findings are equivocal, alternative brain imaging modalities such as single-photon emission computed tomography (SPECT) examination may sometimes be useful to identify areas of hyperperfusion. In one small study of patients with acute viral encephalitis, unilateral hyperperfusion as measured by SPECT was an independent predictor

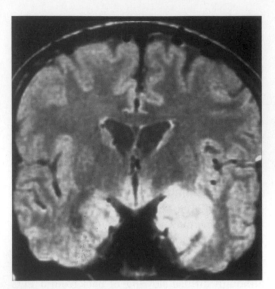

Figure 75.3 Coronal fluid-attenuated inversion-recovery magnetic resonance imaging (MRI) imaging from a patient with polymerase chain reaction (PCR)-proven herpes simplex encephalitis (HSE). Hyperintense signal is seen in the medial portion of both temporal lobes as well as in the inferior frontal lobes in a distribution that is highly characteristic of this disease.

of poor outcome. Still, the optimal application of this technique requires further investigation.

Cerebrospinal Fluid Analysis

Examination of the CSF is mandatory in all suspected cases of acute viral encephalitis. Routine CSF studies in these diseases will generally show a mononuclear cell pleocytosis of not more than 1000 cells/mm³, with cell counts usually ranging from 30 to 200 cells/mm³. Up to a third of patients with HSE and WNV encephalitis will have more than 50% neutrophils at the time of their initial LP. Although the total protein content may be normal in the first week of disease, levels are usually elevated thereafter, and 15% to 20% of encephalitis patients have CSF protein concentrations of greater than 100 mg/dL. Hypoglycorrhachia is relatively uncommon in viral encephalitis, but CSF glucose levels can sometimes be low with infections caused by lymphocytic choriomeningitis virus. Viral cultures of CSF are invariably negative in cases of encephalitis, but new molecular diagnostic modalities have been successfully used to identify specific pathogens. It cannot be overemphasized, however, that even in advance of a positive molecular assay for HSV, all patients with a fever, focal neurological deficits,

and a CSF pleocytosis should be treated for presumptive HSE until an alternative diagnosis is confirmed.

Pathogen-Specific Assays

Serologic assays are available for most neurotropic viruses, including the Herpesviridae, Bunyaviridae, Togaviridae, Flaviviridae, Picornaviridae, and Rhabdoviridae, and many of these tests can be applied to both serum and CSF samples. Unfortunately, viral-specific antibodies can be difficult to detect early in disease, and the process of comparing acute to convalescent serum titers is of limited utility when the initial therapeutic decisions are made.

Polymerase chain reaction (PCR)-based amplification techniques have recently been used to detect the nucleic acids of a number of neurotropic viruses in the CSF of patients with viral encephalitis. In particular, PCR assays can now routinely detect most Herpesviridae and Picornaviridae, as well as JC virus and certain Togaviridae and Flaviviridae. In HSE, the sensitivity and specificity of PCR for the detection HSV-specific DNA sequences is 95% and 98%, respectively, compared to the gold standard of direct brain biopsy. Positive results have been reported as early as a day after onset of symptoms and may persist for as long as 1 week after the initiation of antiviral therapy. Occasionally, HSV PCR can be negative early in disease, and serial testing of CSF samples is advised if the clinical suspicion remains high despite an initial negative assay. Beyond just the detection of viral nucleic acids in clinical samples, PCR is now being used to measure viral loads, to monitor the duration and adequacy of antiviral therapy, to identify determinants of drug resistance, and even to explore the etiology of brain diseases of uncertain causes. Future applications of nucleic acid detection methods for clinical samples such as CSF are likely to incorporate rapid methods that can screen a sample for many pathogen-specific sequences in a single reaction.

Brain Biopsy

The utility of diagnostic brain biopsy in the management of suspected encephalitis remains controversial. Proponents advocate that direct tissue analysis may sometimes confirm an alternative diagnosis of a treatable disorder in a proportion of PCR-negative cases, whereas those not in favor of its use argue that the yield of the procedure is unacceptably low. However, when a diagnosis remains elusive in a patient with a

Table 75.4 Treatment Regimens for Acute Viral Encephalitis Caused by *Herpesviridae*

Virus[a]	Drug of Choice	Major Toxicities	Alternate Regimen[b]	Major Toxicities
HSV	Acyclovir, 10 mg/kg IV q8h for 14–21 d	Nephrotoxicity, vomiting, diarrhea, mental status changes	Foscarnet, 60 mg/kg IV q8h or 90 mg/kg IV q12h for 14–21 d	Nephrotoxicity, electrolyte disturbances, nausea, fever
CMV	Induction: ganciclovir, 5 mg/kg IV q12h for 21 d, plus Foscarnet, 60 mg/kg IV q8h or 90 mg/kg IV q12h for 21 d	Bone marrow suppression, rash, fever Nephrotoxicity, electrolyte disturbances, nausea, fever	Cidofovir, 5 mg/kg IV qwk, plus probenecid, 2 g PO 3 h before cidofovir dose, 1 g 2 h immediately after dose, and 1 g 8 h after dose	Nephrotoxicity, rash, cardiomyopathy
CMV[c]	Maintenance: ganciclovir, 5 mg/kg IV qd, plus Foscarnet, 90 mg/kg IV qd	As above As above	Valganciclovir, 900 mg PO qd	Nephrotoxicity, bone marrow suppression, rash, fever
VZV	Acyclovir, 10 mg/kg IV q8h for 10–14 d	As above	Foscarnet, 60 mg/kg IV q8h for 14–21 d	As above
EBV	Acyclovir, 10 mg/kg IV q8h for 14 d	As above	Ganciclovir, 5 mg/kg IV q12h for 21 d	As above

[a] HSV = herpes simplex virus; CMV = cytomegalovirus; VZV = varicella-zoster virus; EBV = Epstein–Barr virus; IV = intravenously; PO = orally.
[b] Alternate regimens are indicated in the setting of known drug resistance (rare in immunocompetent hosts, but not uncommon in immunocompromised patients who have received extended prior antiviral therapy).
[c] Continue maintenance therapy in HIV-infected patients until CD4 count >100 cells/mm³ for >6 months.

deteriorating clinical course, brain biopsy continues to play an important role.

THERAPY

General Supportive Care

Because effective antiviral treatments are not yet available for many neurotropic viruses, attention must be focused on preventing and treating the many complications that can arise in a critically ill patient. Neurologically, seizures and elevated intracranial pressure may necessitate the use of anticonvulsants as well as interventions such as hyperventilation and osmotic agents. Systemically, the possibility of pneumonia, deep vein thrombosis, pulmonary embolism, gastrointestinal stress ulcers, decubitus ulcers, musculoskeletal contractures, and malnutrition all must be sought with rigor to limit disease morbidity and mortality.

Antiviral Therapy

There are few effective antiviral regimens for the treatment of patients with acute viral encephalitis. Nevertheless, several drugs have demonstrated activity against members of the herpesvirus family (Table 75.4).

HERPESVIRIDAE

Acyclovir remains the mainstay of treatment for the acute encephalitis caused by HSV. A previously used agent, vidarabine, has much more limited clinical benefit. In adults with HSE, treatment with 10 mg/kg of acyclovir intravenously every 8 hours for 21 days reduces overall mortality from over 70% to below 20%, and importantly, nearly 40% of treated patients recover to the point of returning to normal function. In contrast, clinical trials comparing acyclovir with vidarabine in neonatal HSV encephalitis have failed to show significant differences in outcome, and morbidity and mortality remain high. Relapses have occurred after the administration of acyclovir in a few cases outside of large clinical trials, and most are associated with persistent fever, suggesting an inadequate duration of therapy. Still, such treatment failures have also been attributed to viral drug resistance and postinfectious encephalomyelitis. Drug-resistant HSV occurs with thymidine kinase alternation or deficiency. Resistant strains have been described in cases of refractory HSE among HIV-infected individuals and should be considered in the setting of a worsening clinical picture and/or CSF persistence of HSV DNA despite appropriate therapy with acyclovir. Intravenous foscarnet is recommended in these cases.

In the era of the AIDS epidemic, CMV encephalitis has become a more common disease. It is invariably preceded by viremia and retinitis, and many patients have already received some antiviral therapy and may harbor drug-resistant virus by the time the encephalitis develops. Unfortunately, aggressive antiretroviral therapy is the optimal way to prolong survival in AIDS-related CMV encephalitis. Ganciclovir, one of the mainstays in the treatment of CMV retinitis, has yielded inconsistent results for brain involvement, and its use is limited by significant myelosuppression. Foscarnet crosses the blood–brain barrier more readily, attaining virustatic concentrations in CSF. It, therefore, is an alternative to ganciclovir despite significant renal and electrolyte effects. Unfortunately, although the combination of ganciclovir and foscarnet may transiently stabilize or improve the condition of most HIV-positive patients with acute CMV encephalitis, the regimen does not have an appreciable effect on survival that averages only 3 months in this setting.

High-dose parenteral acyclovir has been used in the treatment of VZV encephalitis, although the efficacy of antiviral drugs has yet to be proven in this disease. Immunocompetent patients with VZV encephalitis often have an associated granulomatous arteritis of the brain, and a brief course of corticosteroids is often empirically added for its anti-inflammatory effects. Encephalitis is a rare complication of EBV infection. The therapeutic benefit of acyclovir in EBV encephalitis remain unproven as well, but it should be strongly considered given the lack of alternative regimens and the relatively low toxicity of acyclovir.

PARAMYXOVIRIDAE

Infection with measles virus is associated with several distinct CNS syndromes, including two forms of acute encephalitis. One is a classic postinfectious encephalomyelitis that causes acute demyelination via immunologically mediated mechanisms. Corticosteroids are widely used in this situation, but are of unproven benefit in randomized studies. An inclusion-body encephalitis occurs in 5% to 10% of immunocompromised hosts within 1 to 6 months after exposure to measles, and anecdotal reports suggest that intravenous ribavirin has some effectiveness when administered early in the course of this disease. Subacute sclerosing panencephalitis is a chronic disease that occurs in about 1 per million normal hosts, usually years after measles exposure, and typically progresses to death. Intraventricular interferon-α,

intravenous or intraventricular ribavirin, and oral isoprinosine, either alone or in various combinations with each other, have been reported to increase disease remission rates in small case series. The rare nature of this disease, however, has precluded controlled trials and the development of a clearly established treatment regimen.

PAPOVAVIRIDAE

Several compounds have been employed for the treatment of JC virus, the etiologic agent of progressive multifocal leukoencephalopathy (PML), without success. Still, the recent identification of the 5HT2A subtype of serotonin receptors as a receptor for JC virus infection of glial cells has raised hope that the atypical antipsychotic agents—ziprasidone, risperidone, and olanzapine—that serve as selective blockers of this receptor subtype might have some efficacy against this otherwise uniformly fatal disease.

PICORNAVIRIDAE

Enteroviruses as a group are the most common cause of acute viral encephalitis, and although most patients with these infections recover uneventfully, they can be life threatening in infants and immunocompromised hosts. Pleconaril is a novel compound that integrates into the capsid of both enteroviruses and rhinoviruses and inhibits their replication. It shortens the duration of symptoms in enteroviral meningitis, and analysis of its compassionate use in more life-threatening situations suggests that 60% to 70% of patients have a favorable clinical and virological response to therapy. Older studies report that the intraventricular administration of gammaglobulin may be beneficial in the treatment of picornaviral encephalitis in agammaglobulinemic children.

BUNYAVIRIDAE, FLAVIVIRIDAE, TOGAVIRIDAE, AND REOVIRIDAE

Because effective antiviral therapies for the arthropod-transmitted encephalitides are lacking, treatment for these diseases is also generally supportive. Still, because both polyclonal antisera and monoclonal antibodies against the viral envelope glycoprotein can protect mice from otherwise fatal WNV encephalitis, a randomized, double-blind, placebo-controlled trial of intravenous immunoglobulin containing high titers of anti-WNV immunoglobulin G has been initiated for the treatment of patients with this disease. Enrollment for this trial finished in late 2006, but data are unpublished as of yet.

OUTCOME

Because cases of acute viral encephalitis range from benign, self-limited illnesses to full-blown and highly cytolytic infections, the clinical outcome for patients with these diseases varies widely. The prognosis in HSE is variable despite the availability of antiviral therapy; younger age (≤30 years), a higher level of consciousness at presentation (Glasgow Coma Scale score >10), and a shorter duration of disease before the initiation of acyclovir (≤4 days) all predict an improved chance of survival. Even among survivors in whom treatment is initiated soon after disease onset, nearly two-thirds have long-term neurological deficits. For patients with WNV encephalitis, recent epidemiological studies have shown that nearly 20% die in the acute stages of infection and another 50% to 60% have residual damage that requires chronic institutionalization or extended care in the home. Fortunately, most cases of enteroviral meningoencephalitis have a better prognosis, and these patients usually recover without major sequelae. Worldwide, annual outbreaks of Japanese encephalitis cause extensive morbidity and mortality, and several new viral encephalitides have appeared in tropical or subtropical regions. Some of these new viruses are quite neurovirulent, and the possibility that these infections might spread to more temperate regions means that ongoing efforts to monitor, prevent, and treat these diseases must continue for the foreseeable future.

SUGGESTED READING

Cinque P, Bossolasco S, Lundkvist A. Molecular analysis of cerebrospinal fluid in viral diseases of the central nervous system. *J Clin Virol.* 2003;26:1–28.

Davis LE, De Biasi R, Goade DE, et al. West Nile virus neuroinvasive disease. *Ann Neurol.* 2006;60:286–300.

Debiasi RL, Tyler KL. Molecular methods for diagnosis of viral encephalitis. *Clin Microbiol Rev.* 2004;17:903–925.

Griffiths P. Cytomegalovirus infection of the central nervous system. *Herpes.* 2004;11(suppl 2):95A–104A.

Johnson RT. *Viral Infections of the Nervous System.* 2nd ed. Philadelphia, PA: Lippencott-Raven; 1998.

Maschke M, Kastrup O, Forsting M, et al. Update on neuroimaging in infectious central nervous system disease. *Curr Opin Neurol.* 2004;17:475–480.

Solomon T. Flavivirus encephalitis. *N Engl J Med.* 2004;351:370–378.

Steiner I, Budka H, Chaudhuri A, et al. Viral encephalitis: a review of diagnostic methods and guidelines for management. *Eur J Neurol.* 2005;12:331–343.

Whitley RJ. Herpes simplex encephalitis: adolescents and adults. *Antiviral Res.* 2006;71:141–148.

Whitley RJ, Gnann JW. Viral encephalitis: familiar infections and emerging pathogens. *Lancet.* 2002;359:507–513.

76. Intracranial Suppuration

Brian Wispelwey and Kristine M. Peterson

BRAIN ABSCESS

A brain abscess begins as a localized area of cerebritis that develops into a collection of pus surrounded by a well-vascularized capsule. Brain abscesses are uncommon, with reported occurrence rates of 0.18% to 1.3% in large autopsy series. They most commonly result from contiguous septic foci, but hematogenous spread from a distant source and neurosurgical procedures or trauma are other risk factors. No predisposing factor can be found in approximately 20% of cases (Table 76.1).

The age distribution of patients with brain abscess varies with its cause. A brain abscess from an otogenic focus typically occurs in patients younger than 30 and shows a male predominance. Brain abscess secondary to sinusitis typically occurs in men in their second to third decade of life.

Pathogenesis

The location of a brain abscess is dependent on its predisposing cause. Abscess from a contiguous focus usually occurs in the cortical area of the brain near its causal site. The most common focus of contiguous infections are otitis or sinusitis. Infection from a contiguous site can either spread directly through intervening tissues, bone, and meninges or indirectly through retrograde thrombophlebitis of the diploic or emissary veins. An abscess may also result from an otogenic infection by spread through pre-existing channels such as the internal auditory canal, cochlear, and vestibular aqueducts. The majority of otogenic brain abscesses are located in the temporal lobe, followed by the cerebellum. Approximately 90% of cerebellar abscesses are secondary to an otogenic infection. Brain abscesses due to sinusitis are almost always found in the frontal lobe.

Brain abscesses secondary to hematogenous dissemination are often multiple and are located in the territory of the middle cerebral artery at the gray-white junction. They have a distant focus of infection, which is most often within the chest. These abscesses are poorly encapsulated and have a high mortality.

Table 76.1 Clinical Settings Associated with Brain Abscess

Spread from a Contiguous Focus
Otitis media, mastoiditis; 40% of all brain abscesses
Sinusitis, frontal
Dental infections (≤10%), typically with molar infections; abscesses usually frontal but may be temporal
Meningitis; rarely complicated by brain abscess (must be considered in neonates with *Citrobacter diversus* meningitis, of whom 70% develop brain abscess)

Hematogenous Spread from a Distant Focus of Infections
Empyema, lung abscess, bronchiectasis, cystic fibrosis, wound infections, pelvic infections, intra-abdominal sepsis

Trauma
After penetrating head trauma, brain abscess develops in about 3%, more commonly after gunshot wounds
Neurosurgical procedures; complicated by brain abscess in only 6 to 17 per 10,000 clean neurosurgical procedures

Cryptogenic
Asymptomatic pulmonary arteriovenous malformation (AVM), a consideration in cases of cryptogenic brain abscess
Cyanotic congenital heart disease is present in 5% to 10% of brain abscesses and is the most common predisposing factor in some pediatric series.

Brain abscesses rarely accompany bacteremia if the blood–brain barrier is intact. For example, despite the presence of persistent bacteremia in bacterial endocarditis, brain abscess is rare (9 brain abscesses reported in 218 cases of infective endocarditis).

Causes

Organisms isolated from brain abscesses are outlined in Table 76.2. Although a single organism is detected in the majority of bacterial brain abscesses, nearly 30% have mixed cultures. *Streptococci*, Enterobacteriaceae, and anaerobes are most commonly found. *Staphylococcus aureus* is commonly isolated in pure culture.

Fungal brain abscess has increased in incidence due to the prevalent use of immunosuppressive agents, corticosteroids, and

Table 76.2 Pathogens in Brain Abscess

Agent	Frequency (%)
Streptococci (*S. intermedius*, including *S. anginosis*)	60–70
Bacteroides and *Prevotella* spp.	20–40
Enterobacteriaceae	23–33
Staphylococcus aureus	10–15
Fungi[a]	10–15
Streptococcus pneumoniae	<1
Haemophilus influenzae	<1
Protozoa, helminths[b] (vary geographically)	<1

[a] Yeasts, fungi, *Aspergillus*, agents of mucor, *Candida*, cryptococci, coccidiodoides, *Cladosporium trichoides*, *Pseudallescheria boydii*
[b] Protozoa, helminths, *Entameba histolytica*, schistosomes, paragonimus, cysticerci

Table 76.3 Causes of Parenchymal CNS Lesions in Patients with AIDS

Toxoplasma gondii

Most common focal lesion
Occurs in about 10% of all AIDS patients
>1 lesion seen on MRI with surrounding edema, mass effect, and ring enhancement
Most common location is the basal ganglia; most Toxo IgG positive

Primary Lymphoma

Occurs in about 2% of AIDS patients
Lymphoma is B cell in origin
Lesions and hyperdense or isodense on CT with edema, mass effect, and variable enhancement CNS caused by Epstein–Barr virus

Progressive Multifocal Leukoencephalopathy

Occurs in 2% to 5% of AIDS patients
Lesions occur at gray-white junction and adjacent white matter—caused by JC virus (Papovavirus)
On imaging, lesions are hypodense without mass effect

Less Common

Cryptococcus neoformans[a]
Histoplasma capsulatum[a]
Coccidioides immitis[a]
Other fungi—*Aspergillus*, *Candida*, agents of mucor
Mycobacterium tuberculosis[a]
Mycobacterium avium complex
Cytomegalovirus[b]
Metastatic malignancy, notably KS
Acanthamoeba
Bacterial brain abscess of *Listeria*, *Nocardia*, *Salmonella*
Syphilis[a]

Abbreviations: CNS = central nervous system; AIDS = acquired immunodeficiency syndrome; MRI = magnetic resonance imaging; CT = computed tomography; KS = Kaposi's sarcoma; IgG = immunoglobulin G
[a] More commonly meningitis
[b] More commonly encephalitis

broad-spectrum antibiotics. *Candida* species are the most prevalent fungi in autopsy series. Risk factors for invasive *Candida* infection include the use of corticosteroids, broad-spectrum antimicrobials, and hyperalimentation. Cerebral aspergillosis occurs in 10% to 20% of all cases of invasive aspergillosis, although the brain is rarely the only site of infection. Most cases occur in neutropenic patients with underlying hematologic malignancy. Fungi of the *Zygomycetes* most often cause rhinocerebral mucormycosis, particularly in patients with diabetes mellitus and ketoacidosis, hematologic malignancies, or patients on immunosuppressive therapy. Isolated cerebral mucormycosis is most commonly seen in injection drug users. *Scedosporium apiospermum* is a common mold found in soil. Brain abscess with this organism is often associated with near drowning, trauma, or immunosuppression. Numerous other etiologic agents of fungal brain abscess exist.

There are several protozoa and helminths that produce brain abscess. The most common is *Toxoplasma gondii*, which typically causes an intracerebral mass or encephalitis in immunosuppressed hosts.

Infections more often found in patients with defects in cell-mediated immunity include *T. gondii*, *Nocardia asteroides*, *Crypto-coccus neoformans*, mycobacteria, and *Listeria monocytogenes*. Neutrophil defects are associated with an increased incidence of infections caused by Enterobacteriaceae, *Pseudomonas*, and fungi. Patients with acquired immunodeficiency syndrome (AIDS) may develop focal central nervous system (CNS) lesions as a result of a variety of pathogens (Table 76.3).

Clinical Manifestations

The clinical course of patients with brain abscess varies dramatically. In approximately 75% of patients, symptoms are present for fewer than 2 weeks. The prominent symptoms are secondary to mass effect, not infection (Table 76.4). Headache, the most common symptom, may be hemicranial or generalized. Varying degrees of altered mental status are present in most patients.

Table 76.4 Clinical Manifestations of Brain Abscess[a]

Headache	70%	Nuchal rigidity	≈25%
Fever	50%	Papilledema	≈25%
Altered mental status	>50%	Focal neurologic findings	≈50%
Seizures	25–35%		

[a] Fewer than half have classic triad of fever, headache, and neurologic deficits.

Table 76.5 Laboratory Tests and Imaging Studies

Laboratory Tests[a]

WBC: moderate leukocytosis present in about 50% (only 10% WBC >20,000) and normal WBC in 40%
Moderate increase in ESR
Chest x-ray film is useful in detecting the origin of hematogenous brain abscess
EEG abnormal in most patients, lateralizes to side of lesion

Imaging Studies

CT scan: useful in evaluating the brain, sinuses, mastoids, and middle ear
MRI: appears more sensitive early in illness and in detecting cerebral edema
^{99m}Tc very sensitive; useful where CT or MRI not available

Abbreviations: WBC = white blood cell count; ESR = erythrocyte sedimentation rate;
EEG = electroencephalograph; CT = computed tomography;
MRI = magnetic resonance imaging.
[a] Lumbar puncture is contraindicated in patients with known or suspected brain abscess.

Brain abscesses in certain locations may cause additional symptoms. For example, cerebellar abscesses are often associated with nystagmus, ataxia, vomiting, and dysmetria. Frontal lobe abscesses induce headaches, drowsiness, inattention, and decline in mental function. Temporal lobe abscesses are associated with early ipsilateral headaches and, if in the dominant hemisphere, aphasia. Intrasellar abscesses simulate pituitary tumors. Brainstem abscesses often cause facial weakness, headache, fever, hemiparesis, dysphagia, and vomiting.

Laboratory Findings

Most laboratory tests are not diagnostic for brain abscess (Table 76.5). Lumbar puncture is contraindicated in patients with known or suspected brain abscess. Not only are cerebrospinal fluid (CSF) findings nonspecific, but patients may herniate after the procedure. In one series, 41 of 140 patients deteriorated within 48 hours after lumbar puncture, and 25 died. Similar results have been reported in other studies.

Imaging studies are most useful in making a diagnosis of brain abscess. Computed tomography (CT) can be used to evaluate all cranial structures, including the paranasal sinuses, mastoids, and middle ear. It can detect edema, hydrocephalus, shift, or imminent ventricular rupture. Contrast enhancement is essential. A brain abscess appears as a hypodense center with an outlying uniform ring of enhancement following the injection of contrast. This is surrounded by a variable hypodense region of brain edema.

Magnetic resonance imaging (MRI) is the diagnostic procedure of choice to diagnose a brain abscess. It appears more sensitive than CT for detecting cerebral edema and early changes associated with brain abscess and is more accurate in differentiating the central necrosis of brain abscess from other fluid accumulations.

Gadolinium enhancement provides additional information about brain abscess structure. On T1-weighted images, enhancement of the abscess capsule occurs. On T2-weighted images, the zone of edema that surrounds the abscess has high signal intensity, and the capsule appears as a well-defined hypointense rim at the abscess margin.

Magnetic resonance spectroscopy and positron emission tomography (PET) may have better sensitivity and specificity for the diagnosis of brain abscess but are not currently available in most clinical settings. However, diffusion-weighted (DW) MRI is commonly available and useful to differentiate brain abscess from neoplasm. It typically shows a high signal and low apparent diffusion coefficient (ADC) values in the abscess cavity because the inflammatory dense cellular composition of the pus leads to restricted molecular motion. False-positive results may occasionally be seen in cases of cystic or necrotic cerebral metastases.

Therapy

Most patients with bacterial brain abscess require surgical management. The two available procedures are aspiration and excision. No prospective randomized trial has been performed to compare these procedures. Aspiration causes less tissue damage than excision, and stereotactic aspiration is particularly valuable for deep-seated abscesses and for those at critical locations. Medical therapy alone can be considered in the cerebritis stage prior to development of the abscess capsule, or when the abscess is small or inaccessible. However, it has been recommended that all abscesses larger than 2.5 cm in diameter or with significant mass effect should be aspirated or excised. In one series, no abscess larger than 2.5 cm resolved without surgical therapy. If the abscesses are smaller than 2.5 cm in diameter, the largest and/ or most accessible lesion should be aspirated for diagnostic purposes.

Approach to the Patient with Suspected Brain Abscess

Patients who present with altered consciousness, focal CNS signs, or seizures usually are candidates for contrast-enhanced CT or MRI. Lumbar puncture usually is postponed until a space-occupying CNS lesion is excluded. If rapid clinical progression is occurring, blood cultures for bacteria and fungi may be done and empiric antimicrobial therapy begun before neuroimaging. In every case, management should be done in conjunction with a neurosurgeon. A probable focus in the paranasal sinus or middle ear should prompt consultation also with an otolaryngologist. Empiric treatment depends on the presence or absence of immunosuppression, particularly AIDS, as follows.

Antibiotics for the treatment of brain abscess should be administered intravenously, be active against the most likely pathogens, reach adequate concentrations in the abscess fluid, and have bactericidal activity. A third-generation cephalosporin, such as cefotaxime 3 to 4 grams every 8 hours, or ceftriaxone, 2 grams every 12 hours, is recommended as first-line empirical therapy of community-acquired brain abscess due to its coverage of streptococci as well as its broad gram-negative spectrum of activity. This antibiotic should be used in conjunction with metronidazole, 7.5 mg/kg (often rounded out to 500 mg) every 6 hours, which attains high concentrations in brain abscess pus and has bactericidal activity against strict anaerobes. A high proportion of deep wound infections after neurosurgical procedures are due to methicillin-resistant *Staphylococcus aureus* (MRSA), *Staphylococcus epidermidis*, and multiresistant Enterobacteriaceae. Therefore, recommended emperic antibiotics for brain abscess after a neurosurgical procedure include meropenem or cefepime plus vancomycin. Emperic antibiotic therapy should be modified or extended based on culture results, clinical status, and radiological findings (Table 76.6).

Table 76.6 Antimicrobial Therapy for Brain Abscess

Antimicrobial Agent	Total Daily Dose
Cefotaxime	8–12 g
Ceftazidime	6–12 g
Ceftriaxone	4 g
Chloramphenicol	4–6 g
Metronidazole	30 mg/kg
Nafcillin	9–12 g
Penicillin G	24 million U
Vancomycin	2 g

Most patients require surgery. If the patient remains stable and the abscess is accessible, aspiration (CT guided, if possible) is desirable to make a specific bacteriologic diagnosis and narrow the antimicrobial regimen. Although delay may render cultures negative, aspiration during the cerebritis stage may be dangerous, causing hemorrhage. Certain poor prognostic parameters, clinical or radiographic, may necessitate earlier aspiration. If the lesion appears encapsulated by CT scan criteria, antibiotic treatment can be started and aspiration for diagnosis and drainage performed without delay. Subsequent management depends on clinical and radiographic (CT) parameters. Later neurologic deterioration, enlargement of an abscess after a 2-week interval, or failure of the abscess to decrease in size after 3 to 4 weeks of antibiotics are indications for further surgery. The duration of microbial therapy remains unsettled. Many authorities treat parenterally for approximately 6 to 8 weeks. Duration cannot be determined by resolution of all CT or MRI abnormalities. A cured brain abscess may continue to appear as nodular contrast enhancement on CT scans for 4 weeks to 6 months after completion of successful therapy.

AIDS Patients and Other Immunocompromised Patients

Patients with advanced HIV infection or AIDS and who have CNS lesions on MRI or contrast-enhanced CT consistent with toxoplasmosis are usually begun on empiric therapy with pyrimethamine and sulfadiazine. Pyrimethamine is given to adults as a single loading dose of 75 to

100 mg followed by 25 to 50 mg daily. Folinic acid is given, 10 mg daily, to decrease bone marrow suppression from pyrimethamine. Sulfadiazine is given, 1 g orally every 6 hours. If sulfadiazine is not available, clindamycin is an acceptable substitute at 600 mg intravenously (IV) every 6 hours. Low-grade fever and a gradual onset also prompt this approach. The limitation of empiric therapy is that radiologic distinction between toxoplasmosis and other lesions is not accurate. Progressive deterioration, an atypical CT or MRI, or failure to show clinical and imaging improvement during 2 weeks of therapy generally prompts biopsy or aspiration. Some physicians also use a negative *Toxoplasma* serology to prompt early neurosurgical intervention. Patients taking trimethoprim–sulfamethoxazole (TMP–SMX) prophylaxis for pneumocystosis may be at a lower risk of toxoplasmosis and are therefore more likely to have another diagnosis. Newer diagnostic modalities, such as single-photon emission computed tomography (SPECT), may allow immediate differentiation between *Toxoplasma* and other pathologic processes. (See Chapter 99, Differential Diagnosis and Management of Opportunistic Infections Complicating HIV Infection.)

The range of pathogens for brain abscess is so broad in other immunocompromised patients that empiric therapy has limited value. Early neurosurgical intervention is usually indicated.

Corticosteroids

The role of corticosteroids in the treatment of brain abscess remains controversial. They should be restricted to patients who have progressive neurologic deterioration or impending cerebral herniation and radiologic evidence that the abscess is causing significant cerebral edema and mass effect. The use of corticosteroids may delay the entry of antibiotics into the CNS, impair the clearance of bacteria, inhibit capsule formation, and alter the appearance of follow-up radiologic imaging.

Prognosis

Several factors are associated with a poor prognosis (Table 76.7). In addition, characteristics such as patient's age, large abscess, and metastatic lesions also influence outcome. Neurologic sequelae develop in 30% to 55% of patients, and in 17% they are incapacitating. Seizures develop in a variable percentage of patients (12% to >50%).

Table 76.7 Adverse Prognostic Factors in Brain Abscess

Delayed or missed diagnosis
Poor localization, especially in the posterior fossa (before CT)
Multiple, deep, or multiloculated abscesses
Ventricular rupture (80%–100% mortality)
Fungal cause
Inappropriate antibiotics
Abbreviation: CT = computed tomography.

SUBDURAL EMPYEMA

Subdural empyema is the most common sinusitis-associated intracranial infection. The frontal sinus is most frequently implicated, and the most common location of a subdural empyema is the frontal lobe. Other causes of subdural empyema include meningitis, otitis media, prior head trauma, infection of an existing subdural hematoma, or neurosurgical procedure. Subdural empyemas have a male predominance and most often occur in the second decade of life in otherwise healthy individuals. An intracerebral abscess occurs concomitantly in 6% to 22% of cases, and an epidural abscess in 9% to 17%.

Causes

Subdural empyemas are most often monomicrobial; however, polymicrobial infections are common. Organisms found in paranasal sinus cultures often do not correlate with subdural cultures. Aerobic and anaerobic streptococci are the most frequently isolated pathogens. *Staphylococci* are cultured less often, followed in frequency by aerobic gram-negative bacilli and nonstreptococcal anaerobes (Table 76.8). Sterile cultures occur in a substantial number of cases, possibly due to the prior administration of antibiotics or difficulties in culturing anaerobic organisms.

Clinical Presentation

Due to a lack of anatomical constraints to limit the spread of infection in the subdural space, the clinical manifestations can progress rapidly (Table 76.9). Headache and fever are common early symptoms. Altered mental status, focal neurological deficits, meningismus, papilledema, and vomiting may also result.

Table 76.8 Pathogens in Subdural Empyema

Aerobic streptococci	32%
Anaerobic streptococci	16%
Staphylococcus aureus	11%
coagulase-negative staphylococci	5%
Aerobic gram-negative bacilli	8%
Anaerobes	5%
No organism isolated	34%

Table 76.9 Clinical Presentation of Subdural Empyema

Headache	
Altered mental staus	≈50%
Fever (>39°C [102.2°F])	Majority
Focal neurologic findings Hemiparesis, ocular palsies, dysphagia, cerebellar signs	In all, eventually
Seizures	25%–80%
Meningismus	≈80%

Seizures are common and occur in 25% to 80% of cases.

Diagnosis

Diagnosis is made by imaging with contrast-enhanced CT or MRI. A subdural empyema appears as a crescent-shaped area of hypodensity adjacent to the falx cerebri or below the cranial vault. With contrast enhancement, an intense line can be seen between the subdural collection and the cerebral cortex. Edema can cause effacement of the basilar cisterns and flattening of the cortical sulci. MRI is more sensitive in detecting subdural empyemas, particularly at the base of the brain, in the posterior fossa, or along the falx cerebri. On MRI, T1-weighted images may reveal mass effect and a hypointense subdural lesion, which is hyperintense on T2-weighted imaging. On DWI, subdural empyemas have a high signal intensity, in contrast to sterile subdural effusions, which have a low signal intensity.

Therapy

Surgical intervention using either a burr hole versus craniotomy to drain the subdural empyema is an important part of therapy. Drainage is useful to both relieve mass effect and obtain cultures to guide antimicrobial therapy. Exploration of a sinus or otologic focus of infection should also be done.

A reasonable empiric antibiotic regimen for a community-acquired subdural empyema would be a third-generation cephalosporin plus metronidazole. Depending on the prevalence of MRSA or the likelihood of coagulase-negative staphylococci, the addition of vancomycin could be considered as well. Further antimicrobial therapy should be directed against pathogens revealed by Gram stain, culture of aspirated material, and knowledge of the primary site of infection. Parenteral antibiotics are continued for 3 to 6 weeks depending on the clinical response and associated conditions.

Prognosis

Prognosis is related to the degree of neurologic impairment at presentation. Mortality is about 7% in patients who are alert and well oriented, 21% in patients who are lethargic or comatose but respond purposefully, and 56% in patients who are unresponsive. Neurologic sequelae in the form of hemiparesis and aphasia are common, and up to 40% of patients may have seizures.

CRANIAL EPIDURAL ABSCESS

Cranial epidural abscesses (Figure 76.1) were traditionally the sequelae of sinusitis, mastoiditis, and otitis media. Currently, one of the most common causes of an intracranial epidural abscess is a neurosurgical procedure. The organisms responsible for epidural abscesses are similar to those that cause subdural empyemas.

The dura is essentially adherent to the inner lining of the skull, which constrains the epidural space and limits spread of purulence. Because of this, epidural abscesses are typically slow growing and have an indolent course. Headache may be the only presenting symptom. Over time, complications such as subdural empyema, brain abscess, or meningitis may result. It is the manifestations of these complications that may be the first indication of an intracranial process.

Contrast-enhanced CT or MRI may be used to diagnose an intracranial epidural abscess. Lentiform or crescentic collections overlying a cerebral convexity and/or in the interhemispheric fissure are seen. Treatment is the same as for subdural empyema.

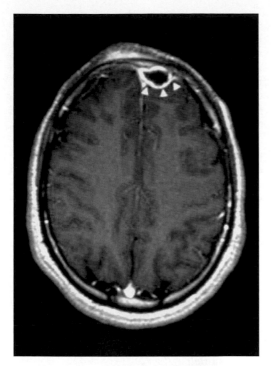

Figure 76. 1 Epidural abscess associated with frontal sinus disease. Postgadolinium axial T1W-MRI showing thick-walled enhancing epidural collection close to the inner table of the frontal bone (*arrowheads*) with adjacent soft tissue swelling. (From Bradley: *Neurology in Clinical Practice, 4th ed.*, Copyright © 2004 Butterworth-Heinemann, an imprint of Elsevier.)

SUPPURATIVE INTRACRANIAL THROMBOPHLEBITIS

Cavernous sinus thrombosis most commonly results from spread of infection from the sinuses, especially the sphenoid sinus. Infections of the middle third of the face, dental abscesses, otogenic infections, and orbital cellulitis are other sources of cavernous sinus thrombosis (see Chapter 16, Periocular Infections). Lateral sinus thrombosis is a serious complication of both acute and chronic otitis media. Infection of the superior and inferior petrosal sinuses may also result from otitis media or mastoiditis. Suppurative thrombophlebitis of the superior sagittal sinus may develop after infection of the face, scalp, or subdural or epidural space or after meningitis.

Pathogenesis

Suppurative thrombophlebitis occurs intracranially because of the close proximity of the dural venous sinuses to other structures in the skull. The transverse sinus receives several important supratentorial veins from the temporal and occipital lobes, as well as many infratentorial veins. The superior petrosal sinus, which receives venous channels from the tympanic structures, drains into the transverse sinus as well. The sigmoid sinus, which lies close to mastoid cells, is the inferior continuation of the transverse sinus.

The dural venous sinuses and cranial veins are valveless, and blood flow is determined by pressure gradients. Bacteria that enter the facial veins are carried through the cavernous sinuses to the petrosal sinuses and finally the internal jugular vein. Conditions that increase blood viscosity, such as trauma, dehydration, malignancy, and pregnancy, increase the likelihood of developing thrombosis. Predisposing conditions are not identified in every case.

Causes

The causative pathogen in suppurative intracranial thrombophlebitis depends on the site of the original infection (Table 76.10). *Staphylococcus aureus* is the most common pathogen in cavernous sinus thrombosis, but other gram-positive cocci such as *Streptococcus* species, gram-negative bacilli, and anaerobes can be seen. The most common bacteria in lateral sinus thrombosis include gram-negative bacilli and anaerobes. Mixed infections are frequent.

Clinical Presentation

The clinical presentation depends on the location of disease (Table 76.11). Cavernous sinus thrombosis can present with periorbital edema, chemosis, visual loss, restricted eye movement, and proptosis. Orbital cellulitis and orbital apex syndrome can present similarly. In contrast, preseptal cellulitis is confined to structures anterior to the orbit. Suppurative cavernous sinus thrombosis can spread via intercavernous sinuses to the contralateral cavernous sinus within 24 to 48 hours. The thrombus may also extend to other dural venous sinuses, adjacent vascular structures, or the brain parenchyma. Metastatic spread of septic emboli may occur and most commonly involves the lung.

Classic symptoms and signs of LST include severe headache, otalgia, spiking fevers, mastoid swelling, and tenderness. However, patient presentations may be highly variable and are influenced by the common occurrence

Table 76.10 Suppurative Intracranial Thrombophlebitis: Organism by Site of Infection

Sinusitis	Streptococci Staphylococci Anaerobes
Soft-tissue infections of the face	*Staphylococcus aureus*
Otitis, mastoiditis	Streptococci *Haemophilus influenzae* Gram-negative bacilli Staphylococci

Table 76.11 Symptoms of Suppurative Thrombophlebitis

Cavernous sinus thrombosis	Photophobia, ptosis, diplopia, proptosis, chemosis, weak extraocular muscles, papilledema, altered mental status, meningismus, decreased visual acuity, involvement bilaterally; same findings in opposite eye
Septic lateral sinus thrombosis	Headache >80%, earache, vomiting, vertigo associated with otitis, fever and abnormal ear findings, increased facial sensation, 6th nerve palsy, facial pain
Superior sagittal sinus	Altered mental status, motor deficits, papilledema, nuchal rigidity, seizures >50%
Inferior petrosal sinus	Gradenigo's syndrome (ipsilateral facial pain and lateral rectus weakness)

of concurrent intracranial complications and preadmission antibiotics. Symptoms and signs of raised intracranial pressure may result if the thrombosis significantly impairs CSF resorption or cerebral venous outflow. These include headache, nausea, vomiting, 6th nerve palsy, and papilledema. Nuchal rigidity has been reported to occur in 8% to 61% of patients. Unlike meningitis, the nuchal rigidity associated with lateral sinus thrombosis is often unilateral with negative Kernig and Brudzinski signs.

Diagnosis

On contrast-enhanced CT scan, the most accurate diagnostic finding of sinus thrombosis is the empty delta sign. This consists of a darkened area of thrombus in the vessel lumen, surrounded by the contrast-enhanced sinus wall. The thrombus formed within the lumen of the sinus may present different attenuations according to its developmental stage, and artifacts from adjacent bone structures are factors that may decrease the sensitivity of CT. Contrast-enhanced CT has a sensitivity of ~80% for the diagnosis of dural sinus thrombosis. On MRI, an acute thrombus (days 0 to 3) appears isointense on T1-weighted images and hypointense on T2-weighted images. In the subacute phase (days 3 to 15), there is increased intensity of the thrombus in both T1- and T2-weighted images. MR venography (MRV) is more sensitive then contrast-enhanced CT or MRI and demonstrates the loss of signal and then absence of flow in the sinus. Computed tomography venography may be as accurate as MRV. It is less impaired by motion artifact because of a rapid acquisition time. It more frequently depicts sinuses of smaller cerebral veins with low flow than MRV does. However its disadvantages include significant exposure to ionizing radiation and the need for IV contrast material.

Therapy

Initial IV treatment with antibiotics that have a broad spectrum of activity and good CSF penetration should be used. Surgical removal of the source of infection should also be undertaken. Mortality rates from LST have improved but are still approximately 10%.

Anticoagulation is controversial, and its major risk is intracranial hemorrhage. One study found anticoagulation with antimicrobial therapy may reduce mortality of cavernous sinus thrombosis, but only if used early in disease. It has not been proven to be beneficial in lateral sinus thrombosis.

SUGGESTED READING

Brock DG, Bleck TP. Extra-axial suppurations of the central nervous system. *Semin Neurol.* 1992;12:263–272.

Kastenbauer S, Hans-Walter P, Wispelwey B, Scheld WM. Brain abscess. In: Scheld WM, Whitley R, Marra CM, eds. *Infections of the Central Nervous System.* 3rd ed. Philadelphia, PA: Lippincott, Williams & Wilkins; 2004.

Manolidis S, Kutz JW Jr. Diagnosis and management of lateral sinus thrombosis. *Otol Neurotol* 2005;26:1045–1051.

Osborn MK, Steinberg JP. Subdural empyema and other suppurative complications of paranasal sinusitis. *Lancet Infect Dis.* 2007;7:62–67.

Prasad KN, Mishra AM, Gupta D, Husain N, Husain M, Gupta RK. Analysis of microbial etiology and mortality in patients with brain abscess. *J Infect.* 2006;53: 221–227.

Reddy JS, Mishra AM, Behari S, et al. The role of diffusion-weighted imaging in the differential diagnosis of intracranial cystic mass lesions: a report of 147 lesions. *Surg Neurol.* 2006;66:246–250.

Tunkel, AR. Brain abscess. In: Mandell GL, Dolin R, Bennett JE, eds. *Principles and Practices of Infectious Diseases.* 6th ed. New York, NY: Churchill-Livingstone; 2005.

Weon Y-C, Marsot-Dupuch K, Ducreux D, Lasjaunias P. Septic thrombosis of the transverse and sigmoid sinuses: imaging findings. *Neuroradiology.* 2005;47:197–203.

77. Spinal Epidural Abscess: Diagnosis and Management

Mark J. DiNubile

Epidural abscess is an unusual but important cause of back pain. Because this infection is a potentially crippling but treatable condition, early diagnosis and aggressive therapy are essential for good outcomes. Even with an indolent presentation, infected patients can still suffer devastating neurological complications related to delays in recognition and appropriate intervention.

CLASSIFICATION

Epidural abscesses can be separated anatomically into infections involving the spinal or cranial epidural space. Cranial epidural abscesses are recognized complications of cranial surgery or trauma; they may also complicate otorhinological infections or procedures. Because of the distinct differences between cranial and spinal infections, cranial epidural abscess and the related subdural empyema will not be discussed in the following review.

Spinal epidural infections can often be segregated into acute and chronic presentations. This simple categorization correlates, albeit imperfectly, with certain clinical and laboratory manifestations, bacteriology, cerebrospinal fluid (CSF) formulae, anatomic details, pathology, and pathogenesis (Table 77.1). The nontuberculous bacterial spinal epidural abscess constitutes the major focus of this review. Tuberculous, fungal, and parasitic abscesses of the spinal epidural space typically evolve more insidiously than pyogenic bacterial epidural abscesses. Other than candidial infections, these etiologies are more frequently encountered in tropical and subtropical resource-constrained regions of the world. Metastatic carcinoma and lymphoma represent common alternative diagnoses that can exactly mimic epidural infections but mandate very different treatments.

Another critical distinction with therapeutic implications concerns the route of epidural infection. Microbes most commonly access the epidural space by hematogenous dissemination from a distant, sometimes trivial, infectious focus. A substantial minority of cases arise from contiguous spread, usually but not invariably from adjacent vertebral osteomyelitis. Epidural abscesses of hematogenous origin are most often located in the dorsolateral thoracic or lumbar area, where the epidural space is widest. Abscesses that form secondary to adjacent osteomyelitis usually involve the epidural space anteriorly or circumferentially. Many times it is unclear whether the epidural space represents the primary or a secondary site of infection.

CLINICAL PRESENTATION AND COURSE

The manifestations of spinal epidural abscess were conceptualized by Heusner (1948) as progessing through four distinguishable but overlapping stages: (1) spinal ache (or back pain); (2) root (or radicular) pain; (3) weakness; and, finally, (4) paralysis. The actual time between the onset of back pain and development of neurologic deficits can be highly variable. The often rapid evolution from backache to neurologic catastrophe (or even death) forces physicians to consider this entity in the differential diagnosis of all patients with new or changing back pain, particularly when fever and localized spinal tenderness coexist. Other presenting complaints include paresthesias (sometimes described as "electric" in character), paresis, incontinence, constipation, and urinary retention. Atypical presentations include meningismus (with cervical involvement), acute abdominal pain (with thoracic infection), and hip pain (with lumbar disease).

In patients with epidural abscesses, an occult primary source of infection, such as endocarditis, adjacent osteomyelitis, or a distant visceral abscess, may be present. Initially inapparent infectious foci may ultimately dictate the length of antimicrobial treatment or mandate additional procedures. Not unexpectedly, bacteremia is more often documented in acute hematogenous than chronic locally advancing infections. Especially when *Staphylococcus aureus* is the pathogen, the infection may be multifocal due to seeding of distant sites during the primary or secondary bacteremia.

Table 77.1 Characteristic Findings in Acute versus Chronic Spinal Epidural Abscess

	Acute	Chronic
Duration of symptoms	Less than 2 wks	More than 2 wks
Fever	Often present	Low grade or absent
Systemic toxicity	Sometimes	Infrequently
Source	Hematogenous (often from minor skin infection)	Direct extension from vertebral osteomyelitis
Back pain	Always	Always
Localized spinal tenderness	Very common	Nearly universal
Root weakness	Common	Common
Peripheral leukocytosis	Usually present	Usually absent
Erythrocyte sedimentation rate	Greatly elevated	Greatly elevated
CSF leukocytes[a] (per mm^3)	Usually 50–1000	Often <50
CSF protein >100 mg/dL	Almost always	Almost always
Anatomic location	Usually posterior to spinal cord	Commonly anterior to spinal cord
Gross pathology	Purulent exudate	Granulation tissue

Abbreviation: CSF = cerebrospinal fluid.
[a] Frank pus may be encountered if a lumbosacral epidural abscess is entered during attempted lumbar puncture. If this occurs, the spinal needle must not be further advanced because introducing the needle into the subarachnoid space may precipitate meningitis. The aspirated purulent material should be sent immediately in the airless capped syringe for appropriate studies, including Gram stain and aerobic/anaerobic cultures.

The feared neurological complications of epidural abscess can arise from either pressure causing compression of the spinal cord or septic thrombophlebitis causing ischemic necrosis. The former mechanism is probably more common, but vascular compromise is likely responsible for sudden deterioration in heretofore stable patients.

RISK FACTORS

Patients with a history of back trauma are predisposed to seed the injured area during transient bacteremia and therefore constitute a special risk group for vertebral osteomyelitis and/or epidural abscess. Suspicion of epidural infection should also be raised when a patient with osteomyelitis or after recent back surgery, epidural anesthesia, or lumbar puncture reports increasingly severe back pain.

All patients with bacteremia or candidemia incur some risk of metastatic seeding. Patients with cutaneous infections, infected catheters, dental abscesses, decubitus ulcers, urinary tract infections, or endocarditis can develop a secondary epidural focus through hematogenous spread, even in the absence of recognized back injury. The risk appears highest in the aftermath of *Staphylococcus aureus* bacteremia and is not totally eliminated by the 2 to 4 weeks of antibiotic therapy usually given to such patients. Injection drug users with or without endocarditis may present with infections of the epidural space. Diabetic patients, patients receiving long-term parenteral nutrition, and patients undergoing hemodialysis also appear to be at increased risk for epidural infection.

MICROBIOLOGY

Staphylococcus aureus is the predominant bacterial species recovered from all types of epidural abscesses, often originating from an inapparent and otherwise inconsequential primary skin focus. Less common isolates include streptococci, anaerobes, *Candida* species, *Salmonella*, *Brucella*, and various gram-negative rods. The epidemiological context may provide essential clues to otherwise unsuspected pathogens. Gram-negative osteomyelitis, septic arthritis, and epidural infection in young adults are often complications of injection drug use, where both Enterobacteriaceae and *Pseudomonas aeruginosa* need to be considered among the possible pathogens. Enterobacteriaceae and occasionally enterococci can spread from urinary tract or pelvic infection to the lumbar spine and/or epidural space through vascular anastomoses in Batson's plexus.

Tuberculous spondylitis (Pott's disease) is frequently associated with epidural abscess and may be the presenting or sole manifestation of reactivation tuberculosis. Chronic osteomyelitis due to mycobacteria is often clinically and radiologically indistinguishable from that caused by pyogenic bacteria, although the course is generally more protracted. Histopathology typically reveals fibrous connective tissue studded with caseating granulomata containing multinucleated giant cells. Acid-fast bacilli (AFB) can often be demonstrated by appropriate stains. Operative intervention is not routinely required for Pott's disease in the absence of significant or progressive neurologic involvement. Candida osteomyelitis with or without epidural infection may present as a delayed complication of catheter-related candidemia despite short-course antifungal therapy. Other etiologies of epidural abscess have rarely included *Actinomyces*, *Nocardia*, *Cryptococcus*, *Blastomyces*, *Aspergillus*, *Rhizopus*, and *Echinococcus*.

DIAGNOSIS

Every patient who experiences acute or progressive back pain, fever, and local spine tenderness must be evaluated for the possibility of spinal epidural abscess. Despite its sometimes subtle and variable presentation, the diagnosis needs to be considered promptly after presentation. Not all of the symptoms and signs classically attributed to an epidural abscess are present in every patient; children especially may exhibit only atypical features. In patients with a chronic course, fever and systemic complaints may be minimal. In several series, roughly half of patients with spinal epidural abscesses were initially given unrelated diagnoses. Once diagnosed with an epidural abscess, patients should be treated with the same degree of urgency accorded patients with cancer and new back pain.

Conventional radiology of the spine may not be helpful because osseous destruction can be absent or inapparent. Although fever is often low grade or nonexistent in patients with chronic epidural abscess, they will have abnormal spine radiographs more commonly than those with acute disease. Bone and gallium scans and even computed tomography (CT) are rarely unequivocal and can delay definitive diagnostic testing.

Whether acute or chronic, all patients with suspected epidural space infection require magnetic resonance imaging (MRI) of the spine, a CT, or a conventional myelogram on an urgent basis. MRI is currently the preferred dianostic procedure. If myelographic contrast material is injected into the subarachnoid space, CSF should first be obtained for stains and cultures, glucose and protein levels, total and differential cell counts, and cytology. Spinal puncture should be performed at a site as far as safely possible from the area of suspected abscess. The needle should be advanced slowly, with frequent aspirations; if pus is encountered, the needle should be withdrawn and the aspirated material sent for appropriate tests. If nonsurgical management is planned, CT-guided aspiration of the epidural collection may be attempted to obtain specimens for culture.

TREATMENT

Traditional management of spinal epidural abscess usually requires a combined medical and surgical approach involving immediate surgical decompression and prolonged antibiotic therapy. Exposure of the entire length of the abscess with drainage, debridement, and irrigation has been standard practice.

In acute or rapidly progressing cases, antibiotic therapy ought to be initiated promptly and often empirically after blood and other readily accessible sites of infection are obtained for stains and cultures. An antistaphylococcal agent should be routinely included in an empirical antibiotic regimen. With the spread of nosocomial methicillin-resistant *S. aureus* (MRSA) and the advent of community-acquired MRSA, coverage with antistaphylococcal β-lactam agents is increasingly inadequate (as discussed below). Antibiotic agents active against gram-negative and strictly anaerobic bacteria should be added to the regimen if these organisms are suspected based on clinical grounds or epidemiological context. For example, a patient with a lumbar epidural abscess of suspected urinary tract origin would need broader coverage for gram-negative pathogens. For infections associated with injection drug use, coverage for *P. aeruginosa* and mouth anaerobes needs to be considered. The initial regimen should be modified once results of stains, cultures, and susceptibility tests from aspirates or operative specimens are available. Gram-stained specimens may provide rapid information that can lead to modifications of the planned antibiotic regimen before culture results return. Blood cultures, ideally obtained before antibiotic administration, may yield the causative organism. Aerobic and anaerobic cultures from appropriately processed specimens usually identify the pathogen(s) unless substantial antibiotic treatment has preceeded sampling.

Ultimately, culture and antimicrobial susceptibility dictate the final choice of antibiotic(s). Community-acquired *S. aureus* infections have traditionally been treated with nafcillin, 2 g intravenously (IV) every 4 hours, or cefazolin, 1 g IV every 8 hours, in patients not allergic to β-lactam agents. Clindamycin, 600 mg IV every 8 hours, and vancomycin, 1 g IV every 12 hours, remain the standard alternatives for seriously penicillin-allergic patients. Vancomycin, daptomycin, or linezolid are appropriate when methicillin-resistant staphylococci are recovered or strongly suspected unless susceptibilities to other agents (such as clindamycin, quinolones, or trimethoprim–sulfamethoxazole) are reasonably assured on epdemiological grounds or by testing the isolate in the clinical microbiology laboratory. There is emerging clinical experience at this time with the use of extended-spectrum quinolones (eg, levofloxacin) for the treatment of staphylococcal epidural abscesses. In susceptible staphylococcal infections associated with osteomyelitis, an oral regimen of rifampin 600 daily combined with either ciprofloxacin 750 mg twice daily or levofloxacin 750 mg once daily would be a reasonable choice for completion of a prolonged antibiotic course after successful acute management. For susceptible gram-negative infections, trimethoprim–sulfamethoxazole, an advanced-generation cephalosporin, or a quinolone may be used. Metronidazole is the drug of choice for most anaerobic infections. Quinolones, trimethoprim–sulfamethoxazole, and metronidazole should be given orally to patients who can tolerate medication by mouth. The incidence of iatrogenic complications (as well as the cost) would likely be dramatically reduced by removing IV catheters and administering antibiotic therapy by mouth when appropriate.

The optimal duration of antibiotic therapy has not been determined in controlled studies. Recommendations range from 2 to 8 weeks. Therapy for at least 6 weeks is usually recommended when vertebral osteomyelitis coexists.

Wheeler et al. first reported 38 cases of epidural abscess managed conservatively without surgery in 1992. Nearly half of these patients had an underlying condition predisposing to epidural abscess, and the majority of infections involved multiple vertebral levels. Overall, 23 patients (61%) recovered completely. Nonsurgical management was more consistently successful in stable patients who presented with localized back or radicular pain without objective neurological signs such as weakness, urinary retention, or urinary or bowel incontinence. Whether some patients with neurological deficits would have benefited from prompt surgical intervention remains unknown. Subsequent studies have both supported and refuted these observations. Controversy still rages over whether any patient with spinal epidural abscess should be managed without surgery.

Operative intervention still is the standard of care under most circumstances. Medical management alone may be an appropriate option for highly selected patients who have no significant neurologic deficits or have a contraindication to surgery (Table 77.2). Unfortunately, some patients will suffer neurologic progression despite appropriate antibiotics, which can ensue abruptly and unpredictably without warning. The resultant paresis or paralysis may not be reversible, even if surgery is then performed urgently. In addition to mass effect, vascular compromise from septic arterial or venous thrombosis with cord infarction may play a key pathophysiologic role in these tragic cases.

The role of medical, surgical, and other modalities of care for patients with spinal epidural abscess continues to evolve. Advances in radiologic and microbiologic techniques over the past decade make conclusions from earlier studies hard to apply today. Use of serial MRI examinations to follow a patient's course may obviate the need for invasive procedures in some patients, but the natural evolution of MRI findings has not been clearly delineated. Percutaneous drainage of epidural abscesses may be a compromise approach in some patients for both diagnosis and treatment, but the literature provides only anecdotal experiences supporting this procedure so far. Some experts have voiced a theoretical objection about the risk of seeding the subarachnoid space and inducing meningitis during the aspiration procedure.

All patients with epidural abscess, whether managed conservatively or not, must be

Table 77.2 Potential Candidates for Medical Management of Spinal Epidural Abscess Without Immediate Operative Intervention

No significant or progressive neurological dysfunction
or
Poor surgical candidate
or
Complete paralysis for >72–96 h
AND
Diagnosis is secure, and causative organism has been identified.

evaluated by careful and repeated physical examinations at least daily for signs of progression. A role for periodic imaging during the course (or at the conclusion) of therapy is not firmly established. Acute neurologic decompensation can lead to irreversible changes with frightening rapidity, even in patients clinically stable up to that point.

PROGNOSIS

Spinal epidural abscess was often a lethal infection prior to the antibiotic era. Consequent to advances in diagnostic and therapeutic modalities, poor outcomes are much less common today. Nevertheless, mortality rates of 10% to 30% continue to be reported. Up to a third of survivors have persistent weakness or paralysis. Khanna et al. performed a retrospective analysis of factors associated with poor neurologic prognosis and/or mortality in 41 cases. They found presenting symptoms of back pain or radiculopathy to be associated with the best functional outcome, regardless of symptom duration. For patients presenting with neurologic deficits, duration of symptoms ("acute" versus "chronic" presentations) has been awarded variable prognostic value in the published literature to date. Khanna et al. found that more severe presenting symptoms and signs heralded a poorer prognosis, with a trend to better outcome if treatment is initiated within 72 hours. Other poor prognostic indicators were patient age, "severe" thecal sac compression on imaging studies, operative findings of granulation tissue rather than pus, and lumbosacral involvement compared with thoracic or cervical sites. There was no attributable prognostic significance to anterior versus posterior location or craniocaudal extent.

SUMMARY AND CONCLUSIONS

Although uncommon, epidural abscess is a potentially devastating infection the neurologic consequences of which can often be prevented or reversed by prompt diagnosis and appropriate medicosurgical treatment. Spinal epidural abscess may present as an acute or chronic process. Typical symptoms of acute spinal epidural abscess include fever, backache, and root pain for less than 2 weeks. Pathogenesis often involves hematogenous spread, usually of *S. aureus,* from a distant, often trivial infection. Patients with a more chronic course usually have developed epidural infection by local extension from adjacent vertebral osteomyelitis. Their major complaints are backache and weakness; fever is typically low grade. Early diagnosis and combined aggressive medical-surgical intervention are still essential for optimal results in most patients because neurologic function may deteriorate at an unpredictable rate, often without any warning, leaving irreversible and incapacitating deficits.

SUGGESTED READING

Baker AS, Ojemann RG, Swartz MN, et al. Spinal epidural abscess. *N Engl J Med.* 1975;293:463–468.

Darouiche RO. Spinal epidural abscess. *N Engl J Med.* 2006;355:2012–2020.

Davis D, Wold RM, Patel Rj, et al. The clinical presentation and impact of diagnostic delays on emergency department patients with spinal epidural abscess. *J Emerg Med.* 2004;26:285–291.

Heusner AP. Nontuberculous spinal epidural infections. *N Engl J Med.* 1948;239:845.

Khanna RK, Malik GM, Rock JP, et al. Spinal epidural abscess: evaluation of factors influencing outcome. *Neurosurgery.* 1996;39: 958–964.

Pereira CE, Lynch JC. Spinal epidural abscess: an analysis of 24 cases. *Surg Neurol.* 2005;63 Suppl:S26–S29.

Reihsaus E, Waldbaur H, Seeling W, et al. Spinal epidural abscess: a meta-analysis of 915 patients. *Neurosurg Rev.* 2000;23:175–204; discussion 205.

Siddiq F, Chowfin A, Tight R, et al. Medical vs surgical management of spinal epidural abscess. *Arch Intern Med.* 2004;164: 2409–2412.

Wheeler D, Keiser P, Rigamonti D, et al. Medical management of spinal epidural abscesses: case report and review. *Clin Infect Dis.* 1992;15:22–27.

78. Myelitis and Peripheral Neuropathy

Rodrigo Hasbun and Newton E. Hyslop, Jr.

Myelitis and peripheral neuropathy complicate many infections. The following discussion covers the major infectious etiologies of myelitis (Table 78.1), peripheral neuropathy (Table 78.2), polymorphic syndromes (Table 78.3), which typically involve the central and peripheral nervous system as well as the spinal cord, and neuropathic syndromes seen in human immunodeficiency virus (HIV) infection (Table 78.4). In addition, an algorithm (Figure 78.1) suggests an approach to the clinical and laboratory diagnosis of myelitis and peripheral neuropathy.

MYELITIS

Myelitis is an infectious or noninfectious inflammation of the spinal cord. It may be divided into processes that directly attack cord structures, *primary* myelitis, and those which begin in adjacent structures but progress to alter cord function, *secondary* myelitis. Primary myelitis can present as one of three discrete clinical patterns: (1) anterior poliomyelitis, (2) leukomyelitis, or (3) transverse myelitis. Poliomyelitis is inflammation involving the gray matter; leukomyelitis is confined to the white matter. Transverse myelitis, inflammation of an entire cross section of the spinal cord, can affect more than one spinal segment. A number of infectious agents are known to cause or to be associated with myelitis. Myelitis can also occur after an infection or a vaccination as in the acute disseminated encephalomyelitis syndrome seen in children.

There are five cardinal manifestations of spinal cord disease: pain; motor deficits; sensory deficits; abnormalities of reflexes and muscle tone; and bladder dysfunction. The distribution of neurological deficits depends on the spinal segment(s) affected. Local pain occurs at the site of the lesion and can assume a radicular quality if the nerve roots are involved. Paresthesias have greater localizing value than radicular pain. Weakness is present in virtually all disorders of the spinal cord, and in myelitis may progress over hours, days, or weeks. Paraplegia and spinal shock are characterized by areflexia and atonia below the level of the lesion, and by absent plantar reflexes. More slowly progressive lesions are associated with hyperreflexia and hypertonia. Bladder dysfunction is usually not an early sign of spinal cord disease, although if spinal shock develops, flaccid bladder paralysis ensues with urinary retention and overflow incontinence. Chronic myelopathies cause a small spastic bladder and result in urgency, frequency, and incontinence.

Acute transverse myelitis of infectious origin must be distinguished from compressive myelopathies (eg, epidural abscess, tumor) and any other noninfectious cause of myelitis such as multiple sclerosis or systemic lupus erythematosus. Magnetic resonance imaging of the spinal cord with gadolinium contrast must be performed early to exclude a compressive lesion.

HIV

Vacuolar myelopathy is a diagnosis of exclusion. Although of distinctive neuropathology, it often coexists with the acquired immunodeficiency syndrome (AIDS)- associated dementia complex, also known as HIV encephalopathy or encephalitis. In some series vacuolar myelopathy has been found in up to 50% of AIDS patients undergoing autopsy before the era of highly active antiretroviral therapy (HAART). In severe cases patients develop spastic paraparesis of the lower extremities with or without involvement of the arms, mimicking human T-cell lymphotrophic virus, type 1 (HTLV-I) myelopathy. The weakness, which may be asymmetric, evolves over weeks. Coexisting neuropathy is often present. A discrete sensory level is unusual, and sphincter dysfunction occurs late in the course of the disease.

Tropical Spastic Paraparesis/HTLV-I–Associated Myelopathy

HTLV-I is a retrovirus associated with adult T-cell leukemia and tropical spastic paraparesis/HTLV-I–associated myelopathy (TSP/HAM). Approximately 10 to 20 million people

Table 78.1 Myelitis

Syndrome/ Disease	Organism	Symptoms, Signs & Neurologic Findings	CN	PN	Cord	Other Findings	Risk Factors
Anterior polio myelitis syndrome	Poliovirus 1,2,3	*Onset:* Acute *Clinical patterns:* Spinal & bulbar paralysis *Common features:* Asymmetric flaccid paralysis (AFP)	✓		✓	"Minor illness" (3–4d) influenza-like syndrome "Major illness" (5–7d) aseptic meningitis myeloencephalitis	Absence of protective immunity and travel in endemic areas
	Nonpolio Coxsackie A,B Echovirus Enterovirus West Nile virus (WNV)	*Onset:* Acute *Clinical patterns:* Similar to polio but milder disease *Asymptomatic infection:* Common except at extremes of age & in immunosuppressed	✓		✓	CNS phase aseptic meningitis, encephalitis, encephalomyelitis	Seasonal incidence in temperate climates (summer), year-round in tropical climates WNV: Vector borne (*mosquito*) & transmitted by breast milk, blood transfusions, and organ transplants
Ascending myelitis syndrome (leukomyelitis)	HIV-1	*Onset:* Acute/subacute *Clinical patterns:*	✓	✓	✓		See below
	HTLV-1	*Onset:* Subacute/chronic *Clinical patterns:* tropical spastic paraparesis (TSP) or HAM			✓	'Rosette cells" in CSF lymphocytes Coinfection with HIV in IVDUs	Injecting drug use Prior residence in endemic areas
	Herpesviruses: CMV, EBV HSV, VZV	*Onset:* Acute *Clinical patterns:* Ascending pattern w/initial plexitis Asymmetric commonly		✓	✓	Primarily seen in immunosuppressed	Related to epidemiology of primary infection
	Herpes B virus (Monkey B)	*Onset:* Subacute (5–30 d) *Clinical pattern:* Aseptic meningitis Ascending encephalomyelitis	✓		✓	Prodromal illness: Early *(vesicles);* Intermediate *(numbness, weakness, hiccups)*	Macaque monkey bite or exposure to tissues Laboratory workers exposed to contaminated cell cultures
Transverse myelitis syndrome	*Primary* myelitis VZV Spirochetes[1] Schistosomiasis Post-meningococcal	*Onset:* Acute (after prodrome) *Clinical patterns:* Sensory motor level Initial spinal shock Hyperreflexia below level of lesion			✓		Related to epidemiology of primary infection
	Secondary myelitis: Bacteria, fungi, mycobacteria	*Onset:* Acute/subacute *Clinical patterns:* Radicular-spinal cord syndrome Cauda equina syndrome			✓	Related to primary infection and organisms	Injecting drug use Hematogenous osteomyelitis Back surgery: Intra-operative contamination

Spirochetes include: Borrelia species (*B. burgdorferi* – Lyme, *B recurrentis* – relapsing fecer), *Leptospira sp., T. pallidum*;
Abbreviations: CMV = Cytomegalovirus; HSV = Herps simplex virus; EBV = Epstein-Barr virus; HIV = Human immunoodeficiency Virus; VZV = Varicella zoster virus; IDUs = injecting drug users; IVDU = intravenous drug use; inflammatory demyelinating polyneuropathy; CSF = cerebrospinal fluid; CNS = central nervous system; WNV = West Nile virus.

are infected worldwide with endemic areas in the Caribbean basin, southern Japan, Africa, and Italy. In New Orleans, 6% of HIV-positive patients are co-infected with HTLV-I, the majority of them having a history of intravenous drug use. HTLV-I causes a chronic meningo-myelitis with focal destruction of gray matter and demyelination, the latter occurring primarily within the posterior columns and corticospinal tracts. The mean age of onset

Table 78.2 Peripheral Neuropathy

Syndrome/ Disease	Organism/ Antibiotic	Symptoms, Signs & Neurologic Findings	CN	PN	Cord	Other Findings	Risk Factors
Polyneuritis: Acute (AIDP) Guillain-Barre Landry Miller-Fisher Chronic (CIDP)	1. Idiopathic 2. Infection-associated	*Onset:* Acute/ subacute & chronic *Common features:* Progressive, symmetric weakness Distal→proximal limbs Truncal→cranial muscles Paresthesias, hypotonia, areflexia *Clinical patterns:* Ascending, descending, bulbar	✓	✓		Variable autonomic dysfunction (ileus, cardiac)	Preceding viral illness or vaccination, prior episode Infection-associated: Viral (EBV, HIV, hepatitis) Bacterial *(Campylobacter)* Chlamydia (*C. psittaci*) Mycoplasma *(M. pneumoniae)* Spirochetes (Lyme borreliosis)
Neuropathy due to bacterial toxins	C. diphtheriae	*Onset:* Acute/ subacute *Clinical patterns:* Bulbar symptoms Ascending peripheral neuropathy	✓	✓		Pharyngitis with pseudomembrane Myocarditis Endocarditis	Absence of protective immunity, epidemic respiratory diphtheria, contaminated wound
	C. botulinum	*Onset:* Acute/ subacute (dose-related) *Clinical patterns:* Bulbar symptoms Myasthenia-like weakness	✓	✓		Autonomic dysfunction (dry tongue, ileus, urinary retention) Decreased vital capacity	Food sources Contaminated wounds (IDUs) Sinusitis in cocaine snorters
	C. tetani	*Onset:* Acute/ subacute (dose-related) *Clinical patterns:* Localized, cephalic, generalized	✓	✓	✓	Autonomic dysfunction Hypertensive crises Decreased vital capacity	Absence or loss of protective immunity Puncture/ contaminated wounds Infected neonatal cord stumps
Medication *Acute* Antibacterials	Aminoglycosides Polymyxins	*Onset:* Acute (concentration-related) *Clinical patterns:* Neuromuscular blockade	✓	✓		Decreased vital capacity Generalized paralysis	Excessive or unadjusted dosage for lean body mass
Subacute Anti-TB Antiretrovirals Antibacterials	Isoniazid ddl, ddC, d4T Chloramphenicol Metronidazole Nitrofurantoin	*Onset:* Subacute (dose & duration) *Clinical patterns:* Symmetric Distal paresthesias & weakness Progressive loss of distal DTRs		✓			Isoniazid: Lack of pyridoxine Nucleoside Anti-retrovirals: Pre-existing neuropathy Excessive or unadjusted dosage Antibiotics: Cumulative dosage

(continued)

Table 78.2 *(continued)*

Syndrome/ Disease	Organism/ Antibiotic	Symptoms, Signs Neurologic Findings	CN	PN	Cord	Other Findings	Risk Factors
Vasculitis	Polyarteritis nodosa (PAN) Wegener's	*Onset:* Subacute *Clinical patterns:* Mononeuritis multiplex *Common features:* Asymmetric weakness, paresthesias, loss of DTRs in affected areas		✓		PAN: Asymptomatic micro-aneurysms Wegener's: sinusitis, pulmonary & renal lesions, +/– eosinophilia	PAN: Chronic active hepatitis B Wegener's: Unknown etiology
Leprosy	*Mycobacterium leprae*	*Onset:* Insidious/ acute *Clinical patterns:* Mononeuritis multiplex Polyneuropathy *Common features:* Anesthetic lesions, enlarged nerves	✓	✓		Deformity Nerves most commonly affected: Median, ulnar, peroneal	General Genetic susceptibility Prior residence in endemic areas Neuropathy Tuberculoid Reversal reaction

Abbreviations: EBV = Epstein-Barr virus; HIV = human immunodeficiency virus; IDUs = injecting drug users.

of neurological disease is 40 to 50 years, with women more commonly affected than men (2.5:1 to 3:1). Patients typically complain of bilateral weakness and stiffness of the lower extremities but may also have difficulty walking and back pain. Later in the disease neurogenic bladder may develop. Physical examination shows spastic paraparesis, hyperreflexia, and extensor plantar reflexes. Vibratory sensation and proprioception are reduced. Typically the disease is slowly progressive, although the upper extremities are usually not affected. The cerebrospinal fluid (CSF) may demonstrate a lymphocytic pleocytosis, elevated CSF immunoglobulin (Ig) G, and oligoclonal banding. Anti-HTLV-I antibodies are also demonstrable in the CSF. Diagnosis is established clinically in the presence of HTLV-I seropositivity and characteristic with CSF findings. The differential diagnosis includes multiple sclerosis, syphilitic meningomyelitis, and adhesive arachnoiditis. Because the virus is also associated with polymyositis, weakness secondary to myopathy must also be excluded. No effective antiretroviral or adjunctive therapies have been established to date. Because the risk factors for HTLV-I infection overlap with those for HIV, patients should also be tested for HIV infection.

Herpesviruses

All herpesviruses have been implicated in acute transverse myelitis, especially in the setting of immunosuppression (AIDS or posttransplant). Herpes simplex virus (HSV) types I and II, varicella-zoster virus (VZV), cytomegalovirus (CMV), and Epstein–Barr virus (EBV) have all been associated with a nonspecific myelitis, although severe ascending necrosis of the cord appears to be most typical. Associated clinical findings of concurrent CMV retinitis, peripheral outer retinal necrosis, or active skin lesions characteristic of herpes simplex or zoster are helpful in suggesting CMV, HSV, or VZV, but the absence of these findings does not exclude them.

Patients may have fever and characteristically have rapidly progressive neurological deficits. The CSF usually shows a lymphocytic pleocytosis, elevated protein, and normal glucose. Early empiric therapy with intravenous acyclovir, ganciclovir or foscarnet may preserve cord function pending definitive diagnosis in immunocompromised patients presenting with acute transverse myelitis of unknown origin. Valacyclovir and valgancyclovir are attractive agents in suppressing herpes simplex and CMV myelitis, respectively,

Table 78.3 Polymorphic Neurologic Syndromes Associated With Infections

Syndrome/ Disease	Organism	Symptoms, Signs & Neurologic Findings	CN	PN	Cord	Other Findings	Risk Factors
HIV-associated	HIV-1	*Onset:* Acute, subacute, and chronic *Clinical Patterns:* Acute: GBS, Bell's palsy, mononeuritis multiplex Subacute/chronic: Vacuolar myelopathy: progressive spasticity; Ascending myelitis (leukomyelitis); Sensory peripheral neuropathy (CIDP)	✓	✓	✓	*Acute* infection: aseptic meningitis, infectious mononucleosis syndrome *Late disease:* concurrent HIV encephalopathy	IVDU, sexual transmission, exposure to contaminated blood or body fluids
Mycoplasma-associated	*Mycoplasma pneumoniae*	*Onset:* acute *Clinical Patterns :* Ascending myelitis (leukomyelitis), polyradiculitis	✓	✓	✓	Commonly associated with encephalitis	Recent upper respiratory infection in child or young adult
Neuro-brucellosis	*Brucella sp.*	*Onset:* Subacute/chronic *Clinical patterns:* Radiculitis, myelitis, CN palsies	✓	✓	✓	Encephalitis, meningitis, mycotic aneurysm; Leukoclastic vasculitis, thrombocytopenia and splenomegaly in children	Unpasteurized milk products, occupational exposure to livestock & cattle parturition
Neuro-borreliosis	*Borrelia burgdorferi*	*Onset:* Acute & chronic *Clinical patterns:* Acute: Bell's palsy, aseptic meningitis, encephalitis, transverse myelitis Chronic: weakness, paresthesias	✓	✓	✓	*Acute:* Erythema chronicum migrans	Tick-bite Travel or residence in endemic areas
Neuro-syphilis	*Treponema pallidum*	*Onset:* Acute & chronic *Clinical patterns:* Acute syphilitic meningitis Chronic asymptomatic Chronic symptomatic (meningovascular, behavioral, tabes dorsalis, myelopathy)	✓	✓	✓	Dementia Gumma (cord/meninges) Uveitis, optic atrophy Deafness	Asymptomatic (abnormal CSF) and symptomatic neurosyphilis occurs after early syphilis. Higher risk with HIV infection with or without standard treatment of primary syph
VZV-associated	VZV	*Onset:* Acute *Clinical patterns:* Bell's palsy, Ramsey Hunt syndrome Sensory radiculitis (CN & PN) Ascending & transverse myelitis	✓	✓	✓	Dermatonal vesicles Encephalitis Uveitis, corneal ulcer	Immunosuppression (with recrudescent VZV)
Herpes simplex-asocciated	HSV	*Onset:* Acute and recurrent *Clinical patterns:HSV-1:* Bell's palsy; *HSV-2:* sacral radiculitis (Elsberg syndrome)	✓	✓	✓	Ascending necrotizing myelitis Mollaret's meningitis	AIDS Primary genital HSV

Abbreviations: CMV = Cytomegalovirus; HSV = Herpes simplex virus; EBV = Epstein-Barr virus; HIV = Human immunodeficiency virus; VZV = Varicella zoster virus; IDUs = injecting drug users; IVDU = intravenous drug use; GBS = Guillain-Barre syndrome; CIDP = chronic inflammatory demyelinating polyneuropathy.

in immunosuppressed individuals. Oral gancyclovir is ineffective because of its limited bioavailability.

Cercopithecine herpesvirus 1 (B virus), *Herpesvirus simiae*, a naturally occurring virus among primates of the genus *Macaca*, can cause a fatal encephalitis in humans with associated ascending myelitis following a bite. Patients may develop vesicular lesions at the site of the bite before the development of neurological manifestations. Human B-virus infections are diagnosed by viral culture and serology, which must be performed in certified laboratories. The Centers for Disease Control and Prevention (CDC) should be consulted in cases of suspected or known human B-virus infection. Acyclovir has been used as prophylaxis and treatment.

Enteroviruses

The enteroviruses are well-known causes of infectious myelitis, of which poliovirus is most common worldwide. In developed nations, polio is now unusual, but sporadic cases of myelitis due to other enteroviruses still occur (eg, coxsackie A and B, echo, and enteroviruses 70 and 71). Myelitis due to the nonpolio enteroviruses, generally less severe than that due to polio, causes weakness rather than paralysis. In some cases of viral myelitis, it may be difficult to distinguish between postinfectious, immune-mediated cord injury and direct viral invasion. Detection of virus in the CSF is supportive of direct viral invasion. Enteroviruses can be recovered from CSF as well as from blood, pharynx, and stool. The most reliable diagnostic test is the CSF enteroviral polymerase chain reaction (PCR).

West Nile Virus

Since the initial appearance of West Nile virus (WNV) in 1999 in the United States, more than 20 000 WNV disease cases have been reported to the CDC. Although most WNV infection is either asymptomatic or self-limited, low morbidity illnesses, neuroinvasive disease (NID) occurs at the extremes of life and in immunosuppressed individuals. Acute flaccid paralysis (AFP) syndrome is one of the most serious neurological manifestations of NID and mimics poliomyelitis by injury to the anterior horn cells of the spinal cord. Commonly accompanying WNV encephalitis, AFP appears abruptly and often results in asymmetric lower extremity weakness. Areflexia, loss of bladder and bowel function, and signs of denervation (fasciculations, atrophy) may develop. There are currently no licensed agents to treat WNV disease.

Syphilis

Four types of spinal cord disease are associated with *Treponema pallidum* infection: tabes dorsalis, syphilitic meningomyelitis, anterior spinal artery syndrome, and gummas of the meninges and cord. Because of its varied pathogenesis, syphilis should be considered in the differential diagnosis of nearly all diseases of the spinal cord. The serum rapid plasma reagin (RPR) titer is usually above 1:32 in neurosyphilis, and the CSF usually shows a lymphocytic pleocytosis, elevated protein, and normal glucose. The CSF Venereal Disease Research Laboratory test (VDRL) is specific but generally insensitive. Other options for diagnosis include the CSF fluorescent treponemal antibody test and the *Treponema pallidum* PCR.

Mycoplasma pneumoniae

Central nervous system (CNS) complications of *Mycoplasma pneumoniae* infection are probably the most frequent extrapulmonary manifestation of this disease. Although encephalitis is the most common neurological complication, meningitis, polyradiculitis, and myelitis have also been reported. The exact pathogenesis of CNS disease is unknown, but it may be secondary to direct invasion, elaboration of neurotoxins, autoimmune complexes, or vasculitis. A history of recent or concurrent respiratory tract infection, especially in a child or young adult, should suggest the diagnosis. Diagnosis may be achieved by a positive CSF *Mycoplasma pneumoniae* PCR or retrospectively by observing a 4-fold rise in antibody titers. If active infection is present, antibiotic therapy may be effective. Tetracycline penetrates the CNS more effectively than erythromycin or other macrolides but is contraindicated in young children. Steroids and plasmapheresis have also been advocated but remain controversial.

Brucellosis

Approximately 2% to 5% of patients with brucellosis have neurological complications, often with considerable clinical overlap. Although meningitis with cranial nerve palsies and vasculitis are the most common neurological manifestations, direct involvement of the brain or cord can result in encephalitis or myelitis, respectively. Myelopathy typically involves the corticospinal tracts and produces a pure upper

Table 78.4 Etiology of Neuropathic Syndromes in HIV infection

---

Autoimmune/Idiopathic

Acute inflammatory demyelinating polyneuropathy (*AIDP - Guillain–Barre Syndrome*)
Chronic inflammatory demyelinating polyneuropathy (*CIDP*)

Vasculitis

Bell's palsy
Ataxic dorsal radiculopathy
Mononeuritis multiplex from hepatitis B virus (HBV)-associated cryoglobulinemia

Opportunistic Infections

Cryptococcal meningitis: bulbar palsies
Herpesviruses polyradiculopathy, sacral radiculitis, Bell's palsy
    Epstein-Barr virus
    Cytomegalovirus (CMV)
    Varicella zoster virus (VZV)
    Herpes simplex type 1 (HSV-2) type 2 (HSV-2)
Neurosyphilis: polyradiculopathy
Tuberculous meningitis: bulbar palsies

Drug Toxicity or Nutritional

Antiretroviral nucleoside analogues
    Dideoxycytosine (ddC)
    Dideoxyinosine (ddI)
    Stavudine (d4T)
Niacin analogue: isoniazid (INH) without B[6]
Neurotoxic antibiotics: aminoglycosides, chloramphenicol, metronidazole, nitrofurantoin, polymyxins
Vitamin deficiencies: folate, pyridoxine, B[12]

---

motor neuron syndrome without sensory findings. Brucella cause granulomatous spondylitis that can progress to epidural abscess with secondary myelitis. Similarly, radiculopathy due to chronic inflammatory entrapment of intrathecal nerve roots, particularly in the lumbosacral region, may complicate brucellosis. CSF usually reveals a lymphocytic pleocytosis, elevated protein, and hypoglycorrhachia. CSF cultures are positive in fewer than 50% of cases. Cultures of blood and tissue fluids may become positive in 2 to 4 days with modern automated liquid culture systems, particularly when specimens are first processed to release intracellular organisms. PCR methods are reportedly more sensitive than culture.

Treatment of neurobrucellosis currently consists of multidrug therapy for 2 to 4 months. If there is a symptomatic epidural abscess, surgical exploration and decompression may be advisable. Adjunctive use of steroids early in meningitis may reduce complications resulting from vasculitis.

NEUROPATHY

Although the manifestations of neuropathy include a number of disease patterns, the causes, both infectious and noninfectious, are often specific to one particular pattern. Consequently, the approach to the patient with peripheral neuropathy begins with identification of the pattern of illness. Initially, the history should focus on the duration of onset of symptoms and their relation to antecedent or comorbid illnesses. An acute onset is highly suggestive of an inflammatory, immunologic, vascular, or toxic cause. Because infectious diseases are known to mediate disease via all of these mechanisms, most neuropathies due to infectious diseases will present acutely or subacutely. Chronic neuropathies of infectious origin, although less common, do occur, particularly leprosy and Lyme borreliosis. In general, an acute onset suggests a more favorable prognosis and should prompt a timely search for the underlying cause to prevent permanent neurological sequelae. Diagnostic clues of infection may be suggested by a recent or current systemic illness, such as pharyngitis in diphtheritic neuropathy, *Campylobacter* gastroenteritis in Guillain–Barré syndrome (GBS), or epidemiologic exposures such as tick bites and sexual contact with persons at risk for sexually transmitted diseases. Travel and residence history is also of diagnostic importance in suggesting an entity such as Lyme borreliosis.

The four major anatomic patterns of neuropathy are *mononeuropathy, mononeuropathy multiplex, polyneuropathy,* and *plexopathy.* Neuropathies are further classified according to the type of functional nerve involvement: *purely motor, sensory, autonomic,* or *mixed,* with one functioning type predominating. Although motor dysfunction is the most obvious sign of peripheral nerve disease, sensory disturbances often herald it. In classifying the neuropathy, the physical exam should address the following questions. Does the involvement include more than one functional nerve type? Is involvement symmetric or asymmetric, distal or generalized, ascending or descending? Is there a sensory level on the trunk? Do motor and sensory deficits overlap, and do they match subjective complaints? What are the activity levels of the deep tendon reflexes and other reflexes (eg, Babinski, genitoanal, and abdominal responses)? Is sphincter function normal? Is there evidence of denervation (eg, fasciculation, atrophy, fatigability)? Are skin lesions associated with the nerve deficits? Establishing the anatomic pattern of illness and its rate of onset lets the neuropathic syndrome be identified and points to specific causes. Discussed next are some of the major infectious causes of peripheral neuropathy.

Leprosy

Leprosy (or Hansen's disease) is a chronic mycobacterial infection in which *Mycobacterium leprae* primarily affects the peripheral nervous system (PNS) and secondarily involves skin and other tissues. *M. leprae* is shed from skin and mucous membranes and transmitted from person to person by prolonged physical contact.

Worldwide, Hansen's disease is one of the most common causes of peripheral neuropathy. Although a rare endemic disease in the United States, new cases are still diagnosed in immigrants from Southeast Asia. Ranging from tuberculoid to lepromatous disease, leprosy is a spectrum of illness resulting from a complex interaction between the organism and the host's immune response. The three cardinal manifestations of leprosy are anesthetic skin lesions, palpably enlarged peripheral nerves, and, in lepromatous patients only, visible acid-fast bacilli on skin biopsy or slit skin smear that do not grow in conventional mycobacteriological cultures.

Although skin lesions have a variable appearance, anesthesia of the involved skin is the one characteristic feature in typical leprosy. Lepromatous leprosy usually results in symmetric anesthesia of the colder areas of the body (eg, pinnae, dorsa of hands and feet), whereas nerve involvement in indeterminate and tuberculoid leprosy is typically asymmetric.

The peripheral nerves most commonly involved are the facial, ulnar, median, common peroneal, and posterior tibial nerves. Superficial nerves, such as the ulnar and posterior auricular nerves, are readily accessible to palpation and are often enlarged and tender. Because neuropathic mutilation of the hands and feet is a significant cause of disability, a complete motor and sensory exam of the hands and feet should be performed before beginning therapy. Slit skin smears are usually positive in lepromatous and borderline lepromatous leprosy but are typically negative in tuberculoid and borderline tuberculoid disease. Where the disease is rare, such as in the United States, skin biopsy should be performed. Skin testing with lepromin is not useful in diagnosis. The most important recent advance in the diagnosis of leprosy is the development of an *M. leprae* DNA PCR, but it is not yet clinically available.

Treatment regimens for leprosy are based on the burden of infecting organisms and the host's immune status. Lepromatous patients are anergic, and tuberculoid patients are intensely immune. Borderline states fall in between. Specific details about therapy and prevention of neuropathy can be found in Chapter 140, Leprosy.

HIV-Associated Neuropathies

Neuropathy is the most common neurological disorder associated with HIV disease. Occasionally neuropathy is the initial manifestation of HIV infection itself, such as Bell's palsy or GBS.

Isolated cranial neuropathies may also occur at any stage of HIV infection. Acute facial weakness characteristic of Bell's palsy usually occurs early in HIV infection and is often associated with a lymphocytic meningitis. In advanced HIV infection the differential diagnosis of cranial neuropathies includes CNS opportunistic infections such as cryptococcosis, acute herpes zoster, and meningeal lymphomatosis.

Late-onset neuropathy is frequently overshadowed by the more striking CNS complications of HIV infection, such as vacuolar myelopathy and AIDS dementia complex, or by opportunistic infections, such as toxoplasmic encephalitis. However, subclinical neuropathy may be nearly universal at the time of death. Many causes of neuropathy have been described in HIV-infected persons (Table 78.4).

Predominantly sensory neuropathy is the most common neuropathy seen in AIDS and is one of the most debilitating aspects of advanced HIV infection. Its exact cause is unclear, although immune complex vasculitis has been suggested by pathology studies. Patients usually complain of painful paresthesias and burning of the distal extremities, primarily of the soles of the feet. On exam, only patients with progressive HIV neuropathy will exhibit a generalized decrease in sensation in the affected areas and atrophy of the intrinsic muscles of the feet. Deep tendon reflexes of the ankles are eventually lost, but patellar reflexes may be exaggerated by coexisting myelopathy. When reflexes are affected, nerve conduction studies are consistent with distal axonal degeneration. Reversible causes of neuropathy should be excluded. Treatment of HIV predominantly sensory neuropathy is generally unsatisfactory. Also, since subclinical disease is probably universal in advanced HIV infection, patients receiving chronic therapy with antiretroviral agents having dose-dependent neurotoxicity, such as the early nucleoside analogues dideoxyinosine (ddI), dideoxycytosine (ddC), and stavudine (d4T), should be regularly evaluated for clinical neuropathy.

Herpesvirus-Associated Causes of Peripheral Neuropathies: CMV, HSV, VZV, EBV, and B-Virus

CMV infection of the peripheral nerves, essentially unknown prior to AIDS, is the consequence of systemic CMV infection and is often associated with evidence of active CMV infection in other systems, particularly retinitis. The capacity of CMV to invade both endothelial and Schwann cells accounts for its varied clinical manifestations. Polyradiculopathy, the most dramatic of these syndromes, is caused by CMV more often than by other herpes viruses. It is characterized by a subacute onset of ascending motor weakness, areflexia, incontinence or urinary retention, paresthesias, and variable sensory dysfunction. Patients often complain of pain in the back and legs. Intense inflammation of the lumbar nerve roots, dorsal root ganglia, and spinal cord result in characteristic CSF findings mimicking bacterial meningitis: polymorphonuclear predominance (up to 90%), hypoglycorrhachia, and elevated protein. CSF white blood cell counts can vary from fewer than 50 to more than 3000. Diffuse enhancement of the cauda equina on post contrast magnetic resonance imaging (MRI) has been reported. PCR to detect the viral DNA of CMV in the CSF is the diagnostic method of choice. In some case reports CMV polyradiculopathy partially responded to ganciclovir (GCV) if therapy began early at dosages of 5 mg/kg intravenously twice a day for 2 weeks, followed by a maintenance dose of 5 mg/kg daily. Oral valgancyclovir is an attractive alternative for treatment and suppression of CMV polyradiculopathy. Intravenous foscarnet and cidofovir are reserved for patients with gancyclovir-resistant CMV infections.

Herpes simplex type 2 can cause a sacral radiculitis (Elsberg syndrome) manifested by urinary retention, constipation, erectile dysfunction, sensory loss in a lower sacral dermatome, and buttock pain. MRI of the lumbar spine may show sacral root edema and enhancement, and the CSF HSV-2 PCR is positive. In AIDS patients, the infection can progress to an ascending necrotizing myelitis. *Herpes simplex type 1* causes approximately 15% of Bell's palsy episodes. Antiviral therapy with either acyclovir or valacyclovir with concomitant steroids should be considered.

VZV is another herpes virus that can cause polyradiculopathy in AIDS patients. VZV classically involves the dorsal root ganglia, but spread of inflammation into the cord can reach anterior horn cells resulting in a combination of pain with motor paralysis. VZV has also been associated with transverse myelitis and myositis. Zoster-associated disease may occur in the absence of a vesicular rash (*Zoster sine herpete*). The diagnosis is established by obtaining a positive VZV DNA PCR on CSF. Treatment is intravenous acyclovir. As with HSV, VZV also causes approximately another 15% of Bell's palsy episode. Antiviral therapy with adjunctive steroids should be considered.

Additional herpesviruses that may cause peripheral neuropathy include EBV and B-Virus.

Treponema pallidum–Associated Neuropathy

CNS syphilis may also present as a subacute polyradiculopathy in HIV infection. In contrast to CMV and HSV, the CSF contains lymphocytes, and the CSF VDRL is usually but not always positive. Therefore, if other evidence points to prior syphilis but the CSF VDRL is negative, the patient should be treated empirically with high-dose penicillin G. Since HIV infection, irrespective of CD4 count, may contribute to an unacceptably high number of treatment failures, close follow-up of syphilis serologies and CSF VDRL is warranted.

Mononeuropathy Multiplex

Mononeuropathy multiplex is a syndrome of simultaneous or sequential neuropathy of noncontiguous nerve trunks evolving over days to years. Characterized by patchy and asymmetric motor and sensory nerve dysfunction, Mononeuropathy multiplex is possibly the result of ischemic injury from viral or other infection of the endothelium of the vasa nervorum and immune complex disease. Mononeuritis multiplex may be seen early in HIV infection even before immunosuppression has occurred. Some cases are associated with cryoglobulinemia in persons dually infected with hepatitis B, in which the course is often benign and generally does not require specific therapy. In patients with advanced HIV infection and CD4 counts ≤50, CMV is the most likely cause, and CMV replication in peripheral nerve is demonstrable. Neuroborreliosis is a common cause of Bell's palsy in areas endemic for *Borrelia burgdorferi*.

Inflammatory Demyelinating Neuropathies

Acute inflammatory demyelinating polyneuropathy (AIDP), or GBS, has a well known association with a variety of infectious diseases such as EBV, CMV, HIV, *Mycoplasma pneumoniae,* psittacosis, Lyme disease, and particularly *Campylobacter jejuni*. In over half of patients a mild respiratory or gastrointestinal tract illness precedes the onset of the disorder by 1 to 3 weeks. Patients usually have an ascending symmetric weakness that can progress to respiratory failure. Areflexia and a variable degree of sensory loss are also evident. Transient paresthesias and pain in the back and legs are frequent complaints. Constitutional symptoms are unusual. The CSF is typically acellular with elevated protein, but variations occur.

GBS must be distinguished from other neurological illnesses (such as myasthenia gravis) and two infectious diseases, botulism and acute flaccid paralysis of enteroviral or other etiology. In botulism the pupillary reflexes are lost early, and significant autonomic dysfunction (e.g. bradycardia, dry mouth, abdominal cramps, urinary difficulty) and progressive diaphragmatic weakness occurs before muscle strength is reduced symmetrically. Acute flaccid paralysis worldwide is caused by poliovirus and other enteroviruses, but cases due to WNV have increased as its territory has expanded. AFP clusters usually occur in outbreaks during the temperate seasons. Patients present with asymmetric paralysis and symptoms of fever and meningoencephalitis.

The treatment of GBS is multidisciplinary with respiratory monitoring and support. Both plasma exchange and high-dose intravenous immunoglobulin (IVIg) are effective in reducing both the severity of the disease and the residual deficits. Steroids are not effective in GBS.

Early plasma exchange (PE) shows significant benefit in 70% of patients in controlled, collaborative trials, which also showed the optimal number of PEs to be related to functional stage of the patient at the time of presentation. PE remains the current recommended treatment of choice for most patients. IVIg is equally effective as plasma exchange. IVIg is generally reserved for those who cannot tolerate plasmapheresis because of bleeding diathesis, hypotension, hypovolemia, or sepsis.

Chronic inflammatory demyelinating polyneuropathy (CIDP), associated with multiple predisposing factors, is also seen in patients infected with HIV. Like GBS, it presents primarily as weakness with varying degrees of sensory loss. Physical exam reveals proximal muscle weakness of the upper and lower extremities. Weakness of the neck flexors is particularly suggestive. As in GBS, CSF analysis is remarkable for elevated protein and the absence of cells. The presence of cells should raise suspicion of HIV infection. Plasmapheresis is the treatment of choice but its efficacy is less predictable than with GBS. Glucocorticosteroids do have a well-established role in CIDP as part of stabilization therapy following initial clinical response to PE or IVIg.

Lyme Neuroborreliosis

Borrelia burgdorferi infection can result in acute and chronic peripheral neuropathies. Acute disseminated disease is usually characterized by peripheral and/or cranial neuropathies and meningoencephalitis, usually 4 to 12 weeks after tick bite. Acute infection may also manifest as plexitis, mononeuropathy multiplex, or myelitis. Unilateral or bilateral facial palsies, the most frequent neurological manifestations, may be seen in 50% of patients. The pathogenesis of the neuropathies is currently unknown, but an autoimmune reaction between anti-Borrelia antibodies and peripheral nerves is proposed as a cause. In endemic areas, facial palsy with a history of tick bite is sufficient to warrant empiric therapy, even in the absence of meningitis. Peripheral nerve involvement, typically asymmetric, usually presents as a motor, sensory, or mixed radiculoneuropathy. Months to years after infection, chronic Lyme borreliosis can cause intermittent distal paresthesias and radicular pain. Physical exam may be normal, but nerve conduction studies demonstrate axonal neuropathy. Diagnosis and specific antibiotic therapy are discussed in Chapter 162, Lyme Disease.

Neuropathies Due to Bacterial Toxins

DIPHTHERIA

Diphtheria is rare in the United States but may still be seen in unimmunized children and in adults with waning immunity. However, travelers to areas with diphtheria outbreaks, or endemic diphtheria, continue to be advised to either have completed a primary immunization series or received a booster dose within the last 10 years. Travelers at substantial risk for exposure to toxigenic strains of *Corynebacterium diphtheriae* are those with prolonged travel, extensive contact with children, or exposure to poor hygiene.

Neurological, cardiac, and renal complications of diphtheria are due to the elaboration by the microorganism of the extremely potent protein toxin which acts on the elongation factor, a critical protein needed for mammalian protein synthesis. The two major fragments (A and B) of the toxin secreted by *C. diphtheria* are excluded by the blood–brain barrier, which explains the preferential involvement of peripheral and cranial nerves. The organism remains localized, either in the nose ("anterior nasal diphtheria"), throat ("faucial diphtheria"), larynx ("laryngeal diphtheria"), or cutaneous wounds ("skin diphtheria"), releasing its toxin for local and systemic effects. The toxin causes a noninflammatory demyelination of the cranial and peripheral nerves through its toxic effect on Schwann cells. Other toxigenic species include *Corynebacterium ulcerans*, which causes respiratory diphtheria and mastitis in cattle, *C. pseudotuberculosis,* and *C. ulcerans.*

In upper respiratory tract diphtheria, locally produced toxin causes the earliest neurological symptoms, which result from paralysis of the pharyngeal and laryngeal muscles. The patient may speak with a nasal voice and complain of dysphagia and nasal regurgitation. As the disease progresses, within days the trigeminal, facial, vagal, and hypoglossal nerves are affected ("*bulbar phase*"), and loss of ocular accommodation is followed in 1 to 2 months by a generalized ascending or descending sensorimotor polyneuropathy ("*systemic phase*"), frequently complicated by myocarditis and injury to other organs.

The initial diagnosis is primarily clinical. The diagnosis is established by recovering the organism from the source (from throat culture in pharyngitis or from wound in the case of cutaneous diphtheria) or by detection of circulating *C. diphtheriae* exotoxin in the blood, which is now the definitive test. Isolation of *C. diphtheriae* from blood cultures indicates possible endocarditis. If exotoxin testing is not available, assays for circulating antitoxin antibody support the diagnosis when the level is nonprotective (≤0.01 IU/mL). CSF is normal except for an elevated protein, comparable to GBS.

Early recognition, treatment of local infection with antibiotics, and administration of diphtheria antitoxin may avoid neurological and cardiac complications. Antibiotics are useful in eradicating the organism and thereby limiting both toxin production and transmissibility. Penicillin and erythromycin are of similar efficacy and render the patient noncontagious after 48 hours. Eradication should be documented. Close contacts also need antibiotic treatment.

As prompt administration of diphtheria antitoxin (equine) is the most important factor in reducing morbidity and mortality, the CDC will dispense antitoxin based on clinical presentation and presumptive diagnosis. Patients with diphtheria also must receive the complete series of diphtheria toxoid as appropriate for their age.

BOTULISM AND TETANUS

Botulism and tetanus are the other two neurological disorders caused by elaborated bacterial toxins. Both toxins exert their effects by interrupting normal nerve conduction rather than by directly damaging the nerve.

Botulism *Clostridium botulinum* is a ubiquitous, spore-forming, anaerobic gram-positive rod that lives in soil and aquatic habitats. It produces a potent neurotoxin, termed BoNT, capable of binding irreversibly and blocking acetylcholine release at the neuromuscular junction.

BoNT is readily destroyed by boiling, but *C. botulinum* spores require superheating to 121°C (250°F). Toxin-production has also been identified in other Clostridium species (*C. baratii* and *C. butyricum*) associated with toxico-infectious botulism. *C. argentinese* produce type G BoNT but have not yet been associated with outbreaks.

Eight subtypes of toxin are known: A, B, C_1, C_2, D, E, F, and G. Human disease usually results from ingestion of toxin containing contaminated food and rarely from contamination of a wound. Types A, B, E, and F are the toxins most frequently implicated in human disease, and a trivalent antitoxin (type ABE) is available in the United States for treatment. Purified botulinum neurotoxin has been mass-produced for aerosol use in biological warfare and for medical treatment of dystonias and cosmetic surgery through selective injection of toxin.

Epidemiological characteristics of clinical botulism include (1) *infant botulism* in babies between 1 and 6 months of age; (2) *hidden botulism* in adults following contamination of the gut by spores of *C. botulinum*; (3) *foodborne botulism*, usually involving several persons who share the same food and then develop disease; (4) *wound botulism,* arising from the proliferation of *C. botulinum* in a contaminated, anaerobic wound or paranasal sinus in cocaine snorters; (5) *inadvertent botulism*, or systemic complications from the therapeutic use of purified botulinus toxin; and (6) *bioterrorism*, where botulinus toxin is dispersed by aerosol or used to contaminate food and water supplies.

Neuromuscular symptoms of botulism vary with the age of the patient; by whether the exposure is the result of ingestion of preformed prototoxin or from active toxin production following colonization of gut or wound; and by toxin type. Infants first develop constipation, then hypotonia ("floppy baby syndrome") and ophthalmoplegia. In the adult form, most patients present as a "descending" symmetric form of paralysis, because the eye and facial muscles are relatively more sensitive than skeletal muscles to any form of neuromuscular blockade. Clinical features include symmetrical cranial neuropathies (i.e., drooping eyelids, diplopia, weakened jaw clench, difficulty speaking and swallowing), autonomic dysfunction (blurred vision and dry mouth), symmetrical descending weakness in a proximal to distal pattern, and respiratory dysfunction from respiratory paralysis or airway obstruction. Sensory exam is always normal. Wound botulism has the same clinical pattern as food botulism.

If the source is food, there is a predictable interval from exposure to onset of disease. In severe disease, paralysis involves the diaphragm and other muscles of respiration. Since neurological effects are dose-dependent, members of groups with a common source exposure will exhibit differing degrees of neurological findings depending on the amount of prototoxin ingested. Toxin type also affects rate and extent of progression of symptoms. Type E has the shortest incubation period, but type A produces more severe illness and requires intubation more frequently (67%).

Diagnosis can be confirmed by measuring toxin in serum, feces, gastric contents, or vomitus, and, if available, in the food source. Stool cultures may contain the organism in infant botulism and sporadic adult cases but rarely in foodborne disease. Any suspicious wounds should be gram-stained and cultured aerobically and anaerobically, and tissues and exudates collected for toxin analysis. CSF is normal. The edrophonium bromide (Tensilon®) test for myasthenia gravis is negative. Electrophysiological testing is helpful in distinguishing this disorder from other causes of motor weakness with preserved sensation. Public health authorities should always be notified immediately of any suspected case.

Specific treatment of adult botulism includes administration of polyvalent antitoxin, released upon request by the CDC. Antibiotics are commonly used with general wound management in wound botulism. Although immediate administration of antibiotic theoretically releases more prototoxin by bacterial lysis, it should not be withheld if anti-toxin is not readily available.

Tetanus Tetanus is caused solely by the toxic action on the nervous system of the potent neurotoxin, tetanospasmin, or tetanus neurotoxin (TeNT), produced by the anaerobic spore-forming rod *Clostridium tetani* which is widely distributed in nature. *C. tetani* is usually introduced into tissues as a spore. Disease only develops if anaerobic conditions obtain, which permits growth of the toxin-producing vegetative form. Tetanus toxin is the next most potent toxin after botulinum toxin. Like botulinus neurotoxin (BoNT), TeNT is a protein with three domains endowed with different functions: neurospecific binding, membrane translocation, and proteolysis for specific components of the neuroexocytosis apparatus. While tetanus neurotoxin acts mainly at CNS synapses, the seven (BoNT) subtypes act peripherally.

The tetanic syndrome originates from the toxin's disinhibitory action on spinal reflex arcs. TeNT acts within the CNS, in contrast to the specific action of BoNT on the peripheral nervous system. The spastic paralysis induced by the toxin is due to the blockade of neurotransmitter release from spinal inhibitory interneurons. When inhibitory impulses to the motor neurons are blocked, the uninhibited firing of motor nerve transmissions continues, resulting in prolonged muscle spasms of both flexor and extensor muscles that can persist for weeks. Disturbances of the sympathetic nervous system also occur, including labile hypertension, cardiac tachyarrythmias, peripheral vasoconstriction, and profuse sweating. Neuronal cell death may occur from unopposed excitation.

Despite availability of effective and inexpensive tetanus toxoid vaccines, cases of tetanus continue to occur in the United States with fatality rates up to 25%. Risk factors include failure of health care providers to use prophylactic tetanus toxoid as part of management of an acute wound injury in unimmunized or partially immunized immigrants, or in elderly persons with age-related waning specific immunity. Although penetrating necrotizing wounds, such as missile injuries and compound fractures, are especially supportive of growth of *C. tetani*, minor wounds are common portals of entry in cases of childhood and adult tetanus. Tetanus may occur in nonimmune or partially immune persons with chronic otitis media, decubitus ulcers, postpartum, postabortion uterine infections, and after nonsterile intramuscular injections, acupuncture, ear piercing, and tongue piercing. Tetanus, like botulism, also occurs when drug users produce an anaerobic local environment at a contaminated injection site.

Primary prevention of tetanus is accomplished by active immunization with vaccines. The recent shortage of tetanus and diphtheria vaccines provoked a cost-analysis evaluation, which led to a recommendation to abandon the decennial Td booster in favor of a single midlife booster between 50 and 65 years of age. *Secondary prevention* refers to post-wound tetanus prophylaxis, and varies with vaccine history and type of wound. To avoid unnecessary vaccinations, health care providers should inquire from patients presenting for wound management about the timing of their last tetanus-containing vaccine. All wound patients should receive Td if they have received ≤3 tetanus-containing vaccines, or if vaccination history is uncertain. These patients also should receive tetanus immunoglobulin passive immunity if wounds are contaminated with dirt, feces, soil, or saliva or have puncture wounds, avulsions, or wounds resulting from missiles, crushing, burns, or frostbite.

There are three alternate presentations of clinical tetanus: (1) local tetanus with muscular contraction at the site of injury, which may persist or progress to the generalized form; (2) cephalic tetanus affecting cranial nerves, mostly the VIIth pair; and (3) generalized tetanus with lockjaw, reflex spasms easily provoked by external stimuli, opisthotonos, and risus sardonicus. The patient is completely conscious during spasms and experiences intense pain. Glottal or laryngeal spasm and urinary retention may occur. Autonomic involvement results in generalized sympathetic overactivity with hypertension, tachycardia, and arrhythmias.

The "incubation period" is the time from inoculation to the first symptom, and reflects the quantity of toxin released and distance traveled to the CNS. The "period of onset," also referred to as the "invasion period" in older literature, is the time between the first symptom and start of spasms, and reflects rate of progression of neurological disease.

The most important prognostic factor for generalized tetanus is not the incubation period, but the rate of progression from onset of symptoms to full development of disease.

Diagnosis is based on clinical criteria and is confirmed by the characteristic neurophysiological findings and absence of serum anti-tetanus antibody. The CSF is normal. Gram stain and anaerobic cultures of the wound may or may not reveal the organism.

Acute treatment has four components: (1) appropriate care of the local wound with debridement and systemic antibiotics; (2) systemic (intramuscular.) administration of human antitoxin; (3) control of spasms, with associated intensive care support until the effects of bound toxin are no longer detectable, using sedation with benzodiazepines and adding neuromuscular blockade to the level of paralysis when necessary; and (4) alpha and beta-adrenergic blockade to prevent secondary autonomic hyperactivity. Details are provided elsewhere.

For tetanus survivors, prevention of future risk also requires a primary vaccination series for active immunization. Location and timing of initiation of the vaccine series should avoid interference with immune response when simultaneously administering therapeutic doses of antitoxin.

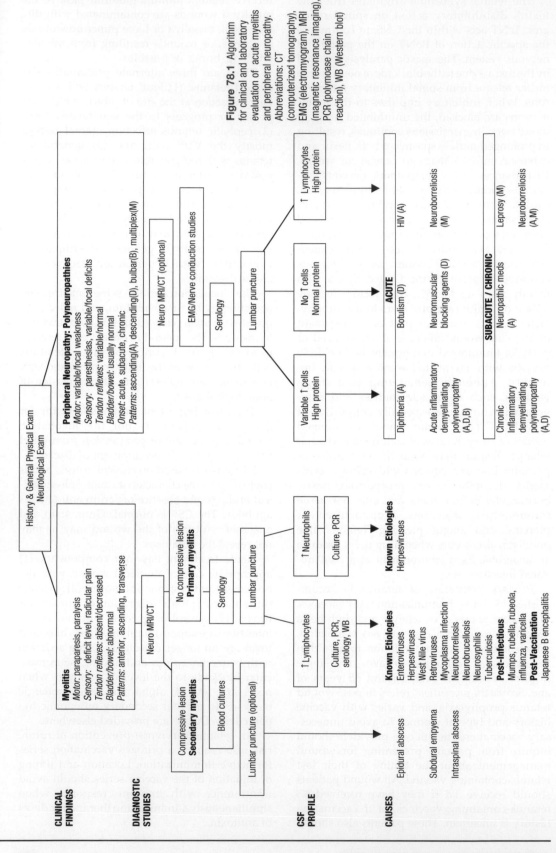

Figure 78.1 Algorithm for clinical and laboratory evaluation of acute myelitis and peripheral neuropathy. Abbreviations: CT (computerized tomography), EMG (electromyogram), MRI (magnetic resonance imaging), PCR (polymoase chain reaction), WB (Western blot)

CLINICAL FINDINGS

History & General Physical Exam
Neurological Exam

Myelitis
Motor: paraparesis, paralysis
Sensory: deficit level, radicular pain
Tendon reflexes: absent/decreased
Bladder/bowel: abnormal
Patterns: anterior, ascending, transverse

Peripheral Neuropathy: Polyneuropathies
Motor: variable/focal weakness
Sensory: paresthesias, variable/focal deficits
Tendon reflexes: variable/normal
Bladder/bowel: usually normal
Onset: acute, subacute, chronic
Patterns: ascending(A), descending(D), bulbar(B), multiplex(M)

DIAGNOSTIC STUDIES

Neuro MRI/CT

Compressive lesion
Secondary myelitis

No compressive lesion
Primary myelitis

Serology

Lumbar puncture

Blood cultures

Lumbar puncture (optional)

Neuro MRI/CT (optional)

EMG/Nerve conduction studies

Serology

Lumbar puncture

CSF PROFILE

↑ Lymphocytes

Culture, PCR, serology, WB

↑ Neutrophils

Culture, PCR

Variable ↑ cells
High protein

No ↑ cells
Normal protein

↑ Lymphocytes
High protein

CAUSES

Epidural abscess

Subdural empyema

Intraspinal abscess

Known Etiologies
Enteroviruses
Herpesviruses
West Nile virus
Retroviruses
Mycoplasma infection
Neuroborreliosis
Neurobrucellosis
Neurosyphilis
Tuberculosis
Post-Infectious
Mumps, rubella, rubeola, influenza, varicella
Post-Vaccination
Japanese B encephalitis

Known Etiologies
Herpesviruses

ACUTE

Diphtheria (A)

Acute inflammatory demyelinating polyneuropathy (A,D,B)

Botulism (D)

Neuromuscular blocking agents (D)

HIV (A)

Neuroborreliosis (M)

SUBACUTE / CHRONIC

Chronic Inflammatory demyelinating polyneuropathy (A,D)

Neuropathic meds (A)

Leprosy (M)

Neuroborreliosis (A,M)

SUGGESTED READING

Beilke M, Theall KP, O'Brien M, et al. Clinical outcomes and disease progression among patients coinfected with HIV and HTLV I and II. *Clin Infect Dis.* 2004;39:256–263.

Davis L, DeBiasi R, Goade D, et al. West Nile virus neuroinvasive disease. *Ann Neurol.* 2006;60:286–300.

Hyslop NE, Hasbun R. Infectious diseases of the spinal cord and peripheral nervous system. In: Gorbach SL, Bartlett JG, Blacklow NR, eds. *Infectious Diseases.* Philadelphia: Saunders;2004:1332–1373.

Kawaguchi K, Inamura H, Abe Y, et al. Reactivation of herpes simplex virus type 1 and varicella-zoster virus and therapeutic effects of combination therapy with prednisolone and valacyclovir in patients with Bell's palsy. *Laryngoscope.* 2007;117(1):147–156.

Scollard DM, Adams LB, Gillis TP, et al. The continuing challenges of leprosy. *Clin Microbiol Rev.* 2006;19(2):338–381.

Wormser GP, Dattwyler RJ, Shapiro ED, et al. The clinical assessment, treatment, and prevention of lyme disease, human granulocytic anaplasmosis, and babesiosis: clinical practice guidelines by the Infectious Diseases Society of America. *Clin Infect Dis.* 2006;43(9):1089–1134.

79. Reye's Syndrome

Omar Massoud and Rajiv R. Varma

Reye's syndrome (RS) is an acute, serious, postinfectious, metabolic encephalopathy and fatty infiltration of the liver. Despite prodromes related to viral illnesses, there is no encephalitis or viral invasion, and brain and liver tissue cultures show no viral growth. It typically affects children, but young and rarely older adults may be involved. Classic RS follows influenza B or chickenpox, but many respiratory and other viruses have been implicated. In the 1970s and early 1980s, it was recognized as a prominent cause of mental changes in children, and many infections, drugs, and toxins were suspected in the etiology. An association with the use of salicylates in children with febrile illnesses was recognized. Avoidance of salicylates has been followed by a dramatic decline in cases since the mid-1980s. Because aspirin is still used in combination in over-the-counter cold and other medicines, inadvertent use can occur. Aspirin is widely used in adults, including those with febrile illnesses; it raises at least a theoretical possibility of RS cases in adults. Salicylates most likely exacerbate an underlying disease in susceptible individuals rather than cause it. It is now suspected that at least some of the patients with RS may have had metabolic diseases or toxic exposures that were not recognized in the 1970s and 1980s. These heterogeneous groups of disorders are often labeled as Reye-like syndromes (RLS). RLS are now diagnosed more often and have largely replaced RS. It is, therefore, crucial to differentiate RS from RLS. Such a differentiation is also helpful in understanding the etiology and pathophysiology of these disorders.

CLASSICAL REYE'S SYNDROME

Reye's syndrome usually has a biphasic course. The first one is a prodromal phase during which a viral prodrome, typically an upper respiratory infection associated with fever, occurs. Fever may not be detectable if antipyretic agents are used. This may last between 3 and 5 days and may be related to influenza B, varicella-zoster or other viruses. The patient may temporarily improve for up to 1 to 2 days or progress directly to the second phase. Vomiting starts and becomes persistent and is followed by mental changes.

Viral prodrome followed by vomiting and then mental changes indicates a more serious illness and needs special attention promptly. Despite mental changes, there are no localizing signs. Mental status may deteriorate rapidly within hours. Both sexes are equally affected; it is more common in rural and suburban areas. Reye's syndrome is more likely in winter months but has been reported in all seasons. Patients have been generally in good health in prior years and are usually overweight. Cutaneous stigmata of liver disease are absent as is jaundice that may occur later in more severe cases. In patients with hepatic encephalopathy due to acute hepatocellular injury or cirrhosis, jaundice and cutaneous stigmata are usually seen. In Reye's syndrome, edema and ascites are undetectable. Patients are well built and well nourished. The liver is enlarged, smooth, and may be massive; spleen tip is not palpable and there are no other signs of portal hypertension. The National Institutes of Health–recommended staging system has been adopted to grade severity of mental changes (Table 79.1) and has been widely used since 1981.

Liver tests show an acute hepatocellular injury pattern and should be measured in children and young adults with unexplained mental changes. Elevation of blood ammonia is universal during the 24 to 48 hours of the onset of encephalopathy. Initial blood ammonia levels correlate with the severity, outcome, and development of sequelae later. The most reliable values are those obtained within 24 hours of onset of encephalopathy. Blood ammonia levels of 5 times or greater above normal and tested in early phases have a poor prognosis; those above 3 times normal are more likely to progress to coma. Initial blood ammonia levels less than twice normal and obtained within 24 hours of encephalopathy have an excellent prognosis. Blood ammonia levels decline later regardless of the outcome and should be measured regularly. Prothrombin time and serum albumin are near normal but vary and become

Table 79.1 Staging of Reye's Syndrome

	Stage I	Stage II	Stage III	Stage IV	Stage V
Level of consciousness	Lethargic; follows verbal commands	Combative or stuporous; verbalizes inappropriately	Coma	Coma	Coma
Posture	Normal	Normal	Decorticate	Decerebrate	Flaccid
Response to pain	Purposeful	Purposeful	Decorticate	Decerebrate	None
Pupillary reaction	Brisk	Sluggish	Sluggish	Sluggish	None
Oculocephalic reflex (doll's eyes)	Normal	Conjugate deviation	Conjugate deviation	Inconsistent or absent	None

Staging criteria adopted at the National Institutes of Health's NIH Reye's Syndrome Consensus Development Conference held in March 1981. Modified from the criteria proposed by Love-joy FH, et al.

more abnormal with the progression to coma. Hypoglycemia is seen in children younger than 2 years and occasionally in those with severe RS. Hypoglycemia raises the possibility for RLS.

Pathology

Liver is grossly yellow to white and enlarged but smooth. The fatty appearance of the liver is due to its high lipid content, especially triglycerides. Light microscopy shows microvesicular steatosis that is panlobular. Routine stains may miss these changes, which can be subtle as nuclei remain central within the hepatocytes; in macrovesicular steatosis, large fat droplets displace nuclei to the periphery. Special fat stains are helpful. Electron microscopy is pathognomonic in RS, especially the characteristic mitochondrial changes. Microvesicular steatosis is suggestive but not diagnostic and can be seen in other disorders of mitochondrial metabolism. Some cases reported as Reye's syndrome may have been due to inborn errors of metabolism mimicking RS; diagnosis remains in doubt without electron microscopy of the liver. Brain biopsy shows changes seen in cerebral edema; other findings are somewhat similar to those seen in the liver.

Pathophysiology

Reye's syndrome is an acquired form of mitochondrial disease. It is unclear as to why these patients develop RS, whereas others recover following a viral illness without changes in mentation. Mitochondrial structural abnormalities are associated with reduction of intramitochondrial enzymes such as carbamoyl phosphate synthetase (CPS), ornithine transcarbamylase (OTC), and pyruvate dehydrogenase. The cause

of mitochondrial injury remains an enigma. Aspirin certainly has a role, but it remains doubtful if salicylates alone cause RS. Mitochondrial inhibitors such as aspirin probably exacerbate the metabolic derangements. We speculate that very mild cases of RS probably still occur in children who almost always recover as use of aspirin or other inhibitors of mitochondrial function are now avoided in them.

Therapy

Early and accurate diagnosis is key to successful outcome. Early referral to a tertiary case facility is recommended. Reduction of cerebral edema is the primary goal along with correction of metabolic abnormalities. This requires a multidisciplinary team approach and should include neurologist, intensivist, hepatologist, and others as needed. Therapy is supportive. Monitoring for hypoglycemia, degree of encephalopathy, potential airway problems, other metabolic parameters such as ammonia, liver chemistries, including prothrombin time, electrolytes, osmolality, and renal function, is required. Intravenous 10% to 15% dextrose infusion should be started. Other hypertonic solutions such as mannitol may be needed to reduce cerebral edema but should be avoided or administered in low doses, if renal function is impaired. Elective intubation, hyperventilation, and monitoring of intracranial pressure may be necessary. Administration of L-carnitine intravenously in severe cases is often recommended. Hypothermia was not widely practiced in the 1970s and 1980s when RS was at its peak. Hypothermia has been found to be beneficial in cerebral edema associated with fulminant hepatic failure and other disorders;

it is relatively less invasive and safe and should be considered. Procedures and treatments such as inductions of pentobarbital coma, craniectomy corticosteroids, dialysis, and exchange transfusion have no established benefit. The authors have used exchange transfusion in the past. Vitamin K injection should be administered initially and repeat as needed. No food orally (NPO), placement of nasogastric tube, lactulose, neomycin, and elevation of head are also recommended.

REYE-LIKE SYNDROME

There is an increasing number of hereditary and acquired disorders that present with clinical and pathologic features that resemble Reye's syndrome. These disorders are collectively referred to as mitochondrial hepatopathies (Table 79.2).

With the decline in the incidence of Reye's syndrome, a patient presenting with the clinical picture suggestive of Reye's syndrome is more likely to have a Reye-like disorder. High index of suspicion and rigorous testing are indicated as many of Reye-like disorders are potentially treatable. Onset of symptoms before the age 3 years, family history of similar illness, and presence of precipitating factors as changes in diet or prolonged fasting are all suggestive of a Reye-like syndrome. Liver biopsy should be performed and reviewed by an experienced pathologist. The early diagnosis of potentially treatable inborn metabolic disorders may prevent subsequent serious life-threatening complications. Table 79.3 shows some of the distinctive features between Reye's syndrome and Reye-like syndrome.

REYE'S SYNDROME IN ADULTS

Diagnosis in adults has been reported but is more difficult due to the following reasons: physicians caring for adults are less familiar with the RS and RLS; as children become adults, the risk of drug abuse increases and the differential diagnosis somewhat changes; unrecognized inborn errors of metabolism become less likely in adults; liver biopsy and electron microscopy already recommended in children becomes even more crucial. Aspirin and other salicylates are still widely used in adults in a wide variety of diseases, including febrile illness.

PROGNOSIS

Grade 1 Reye's syndrome carries an excellent prognosis with complete recovery without

Table 79.2 Mitochondrial Hepatopathies

I. Primary (inherited) disorders
Disorders of oxidative phosphorylation
Complexes I, II, III, and IV deficiencies
Disorders of fatty acid oxidation:
Medium chain and short chain acyl CoA
dehydrogenase deficiency (MCAD and SCAD)
Long chain and short chain 3-OH acyl CoA
dehydrogenase deficiency (LCHAD and SCHAD)
Disorders of urea cycle
Carbamyl phosphate synthetase (CPS) deficiency
Ornithine transcarbamylase (OTC) deficiency

II. Secondary (acquired) disorders
Reye's syndrome
Copper overload syndromes (eg, Wilson's disease)
Iron overload syndromes (eg, Neonatal iron storage disease)
Drugs:
Aspirin
Amiodarone
Barbiturates
Chloramphenicol
Nonsteroidal anti-inflammatory drugs (Ibuprofen, piroxicam)
Nucleoside analogues (FIAU, DDI, AZT)
Riluzole
Tacrine
Tetracycline
Ticlopidine
Trimethoprim–sulfamethoxazole
Valproic acid
Toxins:
Antimycin A
Bacillus cereus toxin (cereulide)
Cyanide
Dimethylformamide
Ethanol
Hypoglycin
Iron
Perhexiline maleate
Rotenone
Selenium

sequelae. In grade 4 and 5 cases, complete recovery is unlikely and death is common. Prolongation of prothrombin time is common in severe cases. Initial blood ammonia levels predict severity and thus the prognosis. The prognosis of Reye-like syndrome depends on the etiology, stage, and severity of the primary disorder.

CONCLUSION

The CDC proposed the following criteria for case definition when epidemics of RS were common: the presence of acute, noninflammatory encephalopathy, clinical alterations of consciousness with either laboratory (low or normal leukocyte count in cerebrospinal fluid) or histologic (cerebral edema without inflammation) documentation; hepatopathy, diagnosed either

Table 79.3 Reye's Syndrome vs Reye-like Syndrome

	Reye's Syndrome	Reyes-like Syndrome
Age	Average age is 6 years	Varies with etiology, metabolic cause: <2 years, other cases: older
Sex	Both sexes equally affected	Varies with etiology
Family history	Negative	Positive in metabolic disorders
Failure to thrive	No	Maybe
Vomiting followed by mental changes	Prominent feature	Less common, vomiting may be absent
Hypoglycemia	Less common	More common
Recurrence	Highly unlikely	Likely in metabolic disorders
Lumbar puncture	Increased opening pressure	Increased or normal opening pressure
Cerebro spinal fluid	Normal	Abnormal in infections
Localizing signs	Absent	May be present
Jaundice	Rare	More common
Blood Ammonia		
Early	Elevated	Elevated or normal
Late	Improves regardless of outcome	Improves in many
Serum transaminases	Universally elevated; hepatocellular injury pattern	Elevated or normal; wide variations
Prothrombin time	Near normal or prolonged with severity	More prolonged in cirrhosis, normal in many
Serum albumin	Normal initially	Normal or low
Liver		
Histology	Microvesicular steatosis	Variable
Electron microscopy	Characteristic mitochondrial changes	Variable
Organic acids in urine	Detected	Characteristic or variable
Amino acids in serum	Dicarboxylic acids	Characteristic or variable

by biopsy or autopsy or a 3-fold or greater rise in aminotransferase or ammonia levels; no known other reasonable explanation. A great deal has been learned since the CDC proposed the criteria in the early 1970s. Reye's syndrome is no longer the prevalent disease it once was, thanks at least in part to the connection with aspirin use and its subsequent avoidance in children with febrile illnesses and progress made in the recognition of inborn errors of metabolism, mitochondrial diseases, hyperammonemia syndromes, drugs, toxins, and environmental factors that can present as illnesses mimicking RS. These are a heterogeneous group of disorders called RLS and have largely replaced RS in general. The CDC-proposed criteria can be a feature of both Reye's and Reye-like syndrome and thus serve a useful purpose. Reye's syndrome has facilitated the discovery of other mitochondrial disorders and exemplifies successful prevention of a devastating disease.

SUGGESTED READING

Ballistreri WF, Schubert WK. Liver diseases in infancy and childhood. In: Schiff ER, Schiff L, eds. *Diseases of the Liver*. Philadelphia, PA: Lippincott; 1993:1099.

Belay ED, Bresee JS, Holman, RC, et al. Reye's syndrome in the United States from 1981 through 1997. *N Engl J Med.* 1999;340:1377–1382.

Casteels-Van Dael M, Van Geet C, Wouters C, et al. Reye syndrome revisited: a descriptive term covering a group of heterogeneous disorders. *Eur J Paediatr.* 2000;159:641.

Garcia-Cazorla A, De Lonlay P, Rustin P, et al. Mitochondrial respiratory chain deficiencies expressing the enzymatic deficiency in the hepatic tissue: a study of 31 patients. *J Pediatr.* 2006;149 (3):401–405.

Jonas MM, Perez-Atayde AR. Liver disease in infancy and childhood. In: *Schiff's Disease of the Liver.* Philadelphia, PA: Lippincott Williams & Wilkins; 2003:1459–1496.

Meythaler JM, Varma RR. Reye's syndrome in adults: diagnostic considerations. *Arch Intern Med.* 1987;147:61–64.

Treem WR, Sokol RJ. Disorders of the mitochondria. *Semin Liver Dis.* 1998;18: 237–253.

Varma RR. Reye's syndrome: handbook of experimental pharmacology-m. In: Cameron RG, Feuerg, de la Igenia FA, eds. *Drug Induced Hepatotoxiaty.* Heidelberg: Springer-Verlag; 1995.

80. Progressive Multifocal Leukoencephalopathy

Joseph R. Berger

INTRODUCTION

In their seminal report in 1958, Astrom, Mancall, and Richardson described a progressive neurological syndrome with characteristic neuropathological findings of demyelination, giant astrocytes, and oligodendrocytes with abnormal nuclei. They named the disorder progressive multifocal leukoencephalopathy (PML). The viral etiology of this neurological disease was not determined until later. PML remained a vanishingly rare disorder seen almost exclusively in individuals with underlying immunosuppressive disorders until the advent of the acquired immunodeficiency syndrome (AIDS) pandemic. In developed countries, PML occurs in approximately 1 in 20 of all human immunodeficiency virus (HIV)-infected persons and AIDS is now the predisposing disorder for 90% of all PML cases. More recently, monoclonal antibodies that result in a highly specific alteration of immune function, such as natalizumab, an α-4 integrin inhibitor, and rituximab, a chimeric monoclonal antibody directed against CD20 receptors on B cells, and whose therapeutic applications have become increasingly prevalent, have been associated with PML.

JC VIRUS AND THE PATHOGENESIS OF PML

In 1965, Zu Rhein and Chou identified viral particles in glial nuclei resembling papovavirus. Subsequently, Padgett isolated polyoma virus from PML brain in glial cell cultures. This virus proved to be a double-stranded DNA virus of icosahedral symmetry. It has a simple DNA genome of 5.1 kilobases in a double-stranded, supercoiled form, encapsidated in an icosahedral protein structure measuring 40 nm in diameter. JC virus (JCV) DNA encodes for three capsid (VP1, VP2, and VP3) proteins and three regulatory proteins (agnoprotein, t, and T). Despite reports to the contrary, it appears that almost all, if not all, cases of PML are caused by the JC virus of the polyoma virus genus.

JC virus uses serotonin receptor 5 HT2a for binding to the cell surface. It is not unlikely that other receptors that remain yet to be identified can also permit JC virus binding. Following binding, the virus enters the cell through clathrin and eps15-dependent pathways, following which it is transported to the endoplasmic reticulum through caveosomes. From there, it enters the nucleus (Figure 80.1). Nuclear DNA binding proteins that selectively interact with the regulatory region of the genome are critical to the tropism of the virus. Cells that are not permissive to JCV infection probably do not have these same protein factors and/or have other proteins that bind the JCV regulatory sequences and block transcription.

Seroepidemiological studies demonstrate that the virus is ubiquitous. By the age of 20 years, 80% or more of the population has been exposed to JC virus and in some urban areas that number may exceed 90%. The mechanism of spread of JC virus remains uncertain. The detection of JC virus in tonsillar tissue suggests the possibility of a respiratory or oropharyngeal route, but studies of the expression of reactivated JC virus in saliva and oropharyngeal secretions by polymerase chain reaction (PCR) has not demonstrated its presence in immunologically normal individuals. No acute illness has been consistently identified with primary JC virus infection. Following infection, latent virus can be demonstrated in many extraneural sites, including kidneys, lymph nodes, tonsils, and lung. Urinary excretion of JC virus is frequently detected. Differences in the virus isolated from the kidney and that from the brain of patients with PML has led to the designation of the former as "archetypal" virus. The latter virus shares regulatory sequences with JCV virus that replicates in bone marrow–derived lymphocytes, and it has been suggested that these JCV-infected B lymphocytes migrate to the brain providing a route for central nervous system (CNS) penetration of the virus. As patients with PML have immunoglobulin (Ig)G antibodies to JC virus, not IgM, the disease is thought to be a consequence of reactivation of latent JCV rather than a new infection.

The virus is periodically reexpressed and can be detected in circulating peripheral blood mononuclear cells by PCR in 0% to 8% of normal individuals and in 30% to 50% of immunocompromised persons. The development of PML is likely a stochastic event in which several circumstances must apply including: (1) initial infection, (2) establishment of viral latency, (3) mutation to a strain that is neurotropic, (4) reexpression, (5) entry into the brain, and (6) failure of normal immune mechanisms to suppress and/or clear the virus from the brain.

The numbers of AIDS patients developing PML greatly exceeds those of patients developing other illnesses having similar degrees of impaired cell-mediated immunity suggesting that factors related to HIV infection may be amplifying the frequency of the disease. The upregulation of endothelial adhesion molecules for JC virus-infected B lymphocytes due to cytokines elaborated by HIV-infected macrophages and microglial cells in the brain may contribute to its increased frequency in this condition. Additionally, the HIV tat protein and HIV-induced chemokines may transactivate JC virus.

PATHOLOGY

As its name implies, the disease is characterized by multiple sites of demyelination with a distinctive microscopic triad of multifocal myelin and oligodendroglial cell loss with minimal inflammatory infiltrate; hyperchromatic enlarged oligodendroglial nuclei (Figure 80.2); and enlarged and bizarre appearing astrocytes with irregularly lobulated nuclei. The enlarged oligodendroglia are found mostly at the periphery of the lesion, whereas the atypical astrocytes are generally more centrally located. Ultrastructurally, the viral particles may be detected by electron microscopy. Alternatively, the virus can be detected by immunohistochemical staining or by PCR. The virus appears in three forms: a filamentous form in the nuclei of infected cells and in spherical or paracrystalline forms in either nucleus or cytoplasm. Virions are visualized mostly in oligodendrocytes and rarely in astrocytes. Infection of oligodendrocyte is productive, whereas the astrocyte is nonpermissive for viral replication.

EPIDEMIOLOGY

Prior to 1982, 200 cases of PML had been recorded by the National Center for Health Statistics. The overwhelming majority of these cases were the consequence of lymphoid

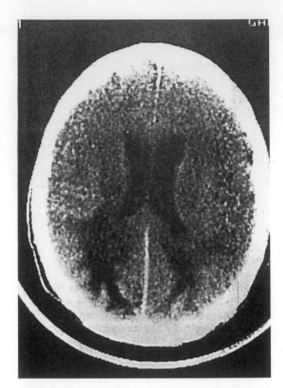

Figure 80.1 Computed tomography scan shows hypodense abnormalities in bilateral occipital lobes.

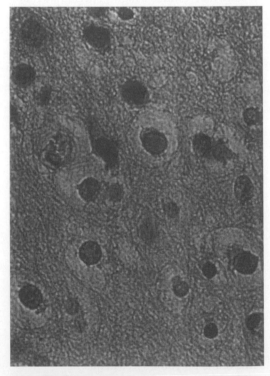

Figure 80.2 An abnormal infected oligodendrocyte with enlarged nuclei.

malignancies. Other neoplastic disorders, granulomatous disease, such as tuberculosis and sarcoidosis, and immunosuppressed conditions followed in frequency. About 5% of patients with PML in one large series from 1984 had no identifiable underlying disorder. From the beginning of the AIDS pandemic through the introduction of highly active antiretroviral therapy (HAART), the numbers of PML deaths has increased dramatically. From 1981 to 1990, 0.73% of AIDS deaths reported to the Centers for Disease Control and Prevention were associated with PML. However, most series suggest that approximately 5% of HIV-infected individuals ultimately develop PML. A striking 20-fold increase in the prevalence of PML was seen between the years 1980 to 1984 and 1990 to 1994 in south Florida with all but 2 of 156 cases of PML in this series occurring in association with HIV. Typically, AIDS patients with PML have significant lymphopenia and low CD4 lymphocyte counts; however, in one series, >10% had CD4 counts in excess of 200 cells/mm^3 at the time of presentation. The introduction of HAART may have led to a decline in the frequency with which PML complicates HIV infection, although this remains to be unequivocally established.

CLINICAL MANIFESTATIONS

The clinical manifestations of PML are varied and depend on the area of white matter involved. The most common signs and symptoms vary with the population studied. Common abnormalities include weakness, gait disturbance, speech and language disorders, cognitive dysfunction, and visual loss. Weakness, frequently hemiparesis, is the foremost manifestation of the disease at both onset and time of diagnosis. Ataxia, dysarthria, numbness, headaches, aphasia, seizures, and vertigo are occasionally noted. Rarely, focal cognitive deficits, such as prosopagnosia, apraxia, left-sided neglect, and Gerstmann's syndrome, are observed; however, global deficits such as memory disturbances and personality changes are more common. On rare occasion, magnetic resonance imaging (MRI) abnormalities due to PML may be detected in advance of any clinical features; however, they generally occur within weeks of this observation.

RADIOLOGY

The diagnosis of PML is strongly suggested by the typical appearance on imaging studies. On computed tomography (CT), multiple white matter hypodensities are revealed (Figure 80.2), but MRI is more sensitive. The lesions of PML appear hyperintense on T2 (Figure 80.3) and hypointense on T1. The scalloped appearance of these areas is due to subcortical "U" fiber involvement. Although any area can be affected, there is a predilection for the frontal and parieto-occipital regions, perhaps due to the large volume of white matter in these areas. About one-third of patients have posterior fossa involvement, and 5% have only cerebellar and brainstem lesions. Most patients have bilateral abnormal areas, and basal ganglia may be affected, chiefly due to involvement of myelinated fibers that course through this region. Enhancement is not typical, but up to 9% can have faint peripheral enhancement around the lesions.

PML must be differentiated from HIV leukoencephalopathy, although this can be difficult on a radiological basis. The MRI of HIV encephalopathy often shows atrophy and the white matter lesions do not enhance and are typically isointense on T1WI. Clinical distinguishing characteristics are its rapid course, focal features, and subcortical involvement. In contrast, HIV encephalopathy or dementia has a more protracted course, is of a cortical nature, and only rarely has focal features.

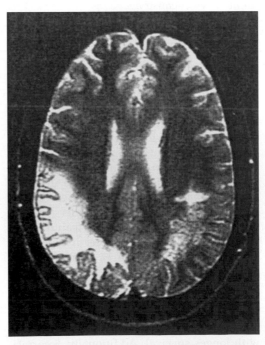

Figure 80.3 This T2-weighted magnetic resonance image shows extensive hyperintense signal abnormalities in the right hemisphere white matter and smaller subcortical lesions on the left.

CEREBROSPINAL FLUID

Routine studies on cerebrospinal fluid (CSF) are not particularly helpful diagnosing PML. A mild increase in protein as well as an increase myelin basic protein may be detected in the CSF. In HIV-infected individuals, the presence of oligoclonal bands and increased IgG synthesis (elevated CSF index) is not infrequently observed but is the consequence of HIV rather than JCV. PCR for JC virus is an indispensable test for diagnosing PML in persons with the appropriate clinical and radiographic features. CSF PCR has a specificity of 100% and has a sensitivity of 70% to 80%.

DIAGNOSING PML

A positive CSF PCR for JCV coupled with clinical and radiographic findings consistent with PML is considered to be sufficient to establish the diagnosis. However, in approximately 30% of patients with PML, the CSF PCR for JCV will be falsely negative. Therefore, brain biopsy may be required to establish the diagnosis. Tissue diagnosis is confirmed by the combination of the pathognomonic histopathological triad of PML and specific evidence of the presence of JCV. JC viral DNA can be detected by in situ hybridization and JC virus antigens by immunocytochemistry.

PROGNOSIS

In the absence of a reversible immunosuppressive disorder, the prognosis of PML is typically grim, with death occurring in most patients between 1 and 18 months (mean 4 months) after disease onset. Prior to the availability of effective antiretroviral therapy, there had been occasional reports of stabilization and improvement, clinically and radiologically, in AIDS patients with PML. Similarly, rare instances of "burnt out" PML have been observed with other immunosuppressive disorders in both HIV and non-HIV cases. Certain features seem to be associated with a greater likelihood of long survival (in excess of 12 months), including PML as the heralding illness of AIDS, lesser degree of immunosuppression (CD4 counts >300 cells/mm^3), enhancement on radiographic imaging, and any evidence of clinical recovery. Low CSF JC viral loads has also correlated with longer survival. Additionally, a correlation between low titers of JC viral DNA load in the CSF and prolonged survival has also been demonstrated. The longest reported survival

has been 92 months from onset of illness. The cellular immune response against JCV appears to tightly correlate with a favorable clinical outcome in PML. The presence of JCV-specific cytotoxic T lymphocytes (CTL) in these patients is likely related to the presence of inflammatory infiltrates in the PML lesions that are responsible for the alterations of the blood–brain barrier and marginal contrast enhancement seen on imaging studies. These JCV-specific CTLs are probably instrumental in destroying infected oligodendrocytes.

TREATMENT

To date there are no unequivocally successful therapeutic modalities for PML. Most of the extant literature consists of anecdotal reports. Anecdotal responses to antiretroviral therapy in the pre-HAART era led to the suggestion to administer zidovudine. However, in vitro assays failed to demonstrate an effect of zidovudine on JC virus replication. The survival of PML in the era of HAART has changed quite considerably, however, with as many as 50% of patients demonstrating long-term survival (>12 months). The benefit of HAART in AIDS-associated PML has not been universally observed, however, as the benefit seems to be chiefly confined to treatment-naïve patients. The remarkable success of HAART in the treatment of AIDS-related PML has had its downside as well. A syndrome referred to as the immune reconstitution inflammatory syndrome (IRIS) may result in new or worsening neurological deficits, an increased number or size of lesions observed by neuroimaging, contrast enhancement of these lesions, and brain edema. Fatal outcomes have been reported, and the development of this syndrome with infratentorial PML may be especially dangerous.

Nucleoside analogs have been employed because they impede the synthesis of DNA. In vitro studies have clearly demonstrated the ability of cytosine arabinoside (cytarabine, ARA-C), a cytosine analog, to inhibit JC virus replication, and anecdotal reports of intravenous and intrathecal administration suggested the value of this therapy in PML. However, a carefully conducted clinical trial of AIDS-related PML failed to show any value of either intravenous or intrathecal administration of ARA-C when compared to placebo. Theoretically, neither method of administration permitted adequate concentrations of the drug to reach the disease sites, and trials with novel intraparenchymal delivery systems have been suggested. Alternatively, higher doses of ARA-C than those employed in the randomized study may prove beneficial. Despite anecdotal reports of the value of other nucleoside analogs in PML, such as adenine arabinoside (vidarabine, ARA-A), none has been convincingly demonstrated to ameliorate the disease course.

Interferons have also had occasional positive results both subcutaneously and intrathecally when used in conjunction with ARA-C. The antiretroviral activity of the interferons may be the consequence of their ability to stimulate natural killer (NK) cells. In a pilot study of 17 patients with AIDS and PML treated with interferon-α2a and zidovudine, two had long-term clinical stabilization, although none improved. A retrospective study compared patients with AIDS-associated PML receiving a minimum treatment of 3 weeks of 3 million units of IFN-α daily to untreated historical controls and suggested that IFN-α treatment delayed the progression of the disease, palliated symptoms, and significantly prolonged survival. However, reexamination of that data indicated that the improved survival could be explained by the concomitant administration of HAART.

The antineoplastic drug camptothecin, a DNA topoisomerase I inhibitor, and its close relative, topotecan, have been demonstrated to block JC virus replication in vitro when administered in pulsed doses in amounts nontoxic to cells. The therapeutic effectiveness of topoisomerase I inhibitors for PML have been entirely anecdotal. They display significant systemic toxicity, and their value in the treatment of PML remains open to question.

Cidofovir [HPMPC; (S)-1-(3-hydroxy-2-phosphonylmethoxypropyl)cytosine] and its cyclic counterpart have demonstrated selective antipolyomavirus activity. The 50% inhibitory concentrations for HPMPC were in the range of 4 to 7 μg/mL, and its selectivity index varied from 11 to 20 for mouse polyomavirus and from 23 to 33 for SV40 strains in confluent cell monolayers. It has been proposed as an agent for the treatment of PML, and there is anecdotal evidence to support its use in AIDS and with other immunosuppressive conditions. However, several larger observational studies have failed to show any benefit. Better designed trials to address the value of cidofovir for PML are needed before it is widely adopted, particularly in light of the serious side effects that occur with the drug, including ocular hypotony, bone marrow depression, and renal disorders.

New technologies coupled with our increased understanding of the molecular biology of JC virus will likely result in novel strategies. The observation that the virus uses the 5HT2a serotonin receptor to bind to cells has led to the suggestion that inhibition of this binding by drugs such as zisprasidone, risperidone, and olanzapine may prove valuable. Similarly, inhibition of the clathirin-dependent endocytosis by drugs such as chlorpromazine may have a role treating the disorder. There is at least one anecdotal report alleging efficacy of risperidone in the treatment of PML arising following stem cell transplantation; however, these reports need to be viewed with a critical eye as long-term survival may be seen as part of the natural history of the disease.

Another possibility is the use of antisense oligonucleotides. An antisense oligonucleotide that is properly designed with a specific complementary base sequence that binds selectively to a targeted region of messenger RNA (mRNA) can prevent the translation of the mRNA into protein. Antisense oligonucleotide directed to JC virus T antigen may reduce viral expression by 80%. Antisense oligonucleotides that target other sites of the viral genome, such as transcription sites, may prove to be effective therapeutic strategies. As a strong JCV-specific cellular immunity has recently been associated with a favorable clinical outcome of PML, the enrichment of an autologous population of JCV-specific CTL populations using tetrameric MHC class-I/JCV peptide complexes may be demonstrated to be a therapeutic option. Koralnik and colleagues demonstrated the ability to boost immunity to JC virus with a vaccine based on a newly discovered JCV-specific CTL epitope. Conceivably, this approach, too, may have some therapeutic merit.

CONCLUSION

The occasional report of stabilization or remission and the growing understanding of the pathophysiology of the virus provide hope for the future development of curative strategies. The growing number of persons affected with PML has allowed the organization of carefully designed therapeutic trials to address this issue.

SUGGESTED READING

Astrom K, Mancall E, Richardson E. Progressive multifocal leukoencephalopathy. *Brain.* 1958;81:93–111.

Berger JR, Houff S. Progressive multifocal leukoencephalopathy: lessons from AIDS and natalizumab. *Neurol Res*. 2006;28(3): 299–305.

Berger JR, Pall L, Lanska D, Whiteman M. Progressive multifocal leukoencephalopathy in patients with HIV infection. *J Neurovirol*. 1998;4(1):59–68.

Clifford DB, Yiannoutsos C, Glicksman M, et al. HAART improves prognosis in HIV-associated progressive multifocal leukoencephalopathy. *Neurology*. 1999;52(3):623–625.

De Luca A, Giancola ML, Ammassari A, et al. The effect of potent antiretroviral therapy and JC virus load in cerebrospinal fluid on clinical outcome of patients with AIDS-associated progressive multifocal leukoencephalopathy. *J Infect Dis*. 2000;182(4): 1077–1083.

Elphick GF, Querbes W, Jordan JA, et al. The human polyomavirus, JCV, uses serotonin receptors to infect cells. *Science*. 2004;306(5700): 1380–1383.

Koralnik IJ. Progressive multifocal leukoencephalopathy revisited: has the disease outgrown its name? *Ann Neurol*. 2006;60(2):162–173.

Koralnik IJ, Du Pasquier RA, Letvin NL. JC virus-specific cytotoxic T lymphocytes in individuals with progressive multifocal leukoencephalopathy. *J Virol*. 2001;75(7): 3483–3487.

Major EO, Amemiya K, Tornatore CS, Houff SA, Berger JR. Pathogenesis and molecular biology of progressive multifocal leukoencephalopathy, the JC virus-induced demyelinating disease of the human brain. *Clin Microbiol Rev*. 1992;5(1):49–73.

Thurnher MM, Post MJ, Rieger A, Kleibl-Popov C, Loewe C, Schindler E. Initial and follow-up MR imaging findings in AIDS-related progressive multifocal leukoencephalopathy treated with highly active antiretroviral therapy. *AJNR Am J Neuroradiol*. 2001;22(5):977–984.

81. Cerebrospinal Fluid Shunt Infections

Elisabeth E. Adderson and Patricia M. Flynn

Cerebrospinal fluid (CSF) shunts are critical for many patients surviving congenital central nervous system anomalies, infection, or intracranial hemorrhage. Infection is a common complication of these devices and a leading cause of morbidity and hospitalization. Despite this, there is little consensus on the optimal means to prevent and treat these infections.

PATHOGENESIS

Most CSF shunts are silastic tubes inserted into the cerebral ventricles or subarachnoid space and connected to a pressure-regulating valve on the external skull. The proximal shunt is connected to tubing tunneled under the skin to the peritoneal cavity (ventriculoperitoneal shunt). In situations where intraperitoneal drainage is not feasible, the shunt may drain into the right atrium (ventriculoatrial shunt) or pleural cavity (ventriculopleural shunt).

The reported incidence of CSF shunt infections ranges from 1% to 30%, with an average of ≈10% in recent studies. Risk factors for infection include previous surgical revision, a short interval from the time of placement or revision, younger age (particularly premature neonates), a less-experienced surgeon, previous infection, endoscopic surgery, and the presence of a postoperative CSF leak. Shunt valve design does not appear to influence infection rates.

The majority (40% to 75%) of CSF shunt infections are caused by coagulase-negative *Staphylococcus* spp. *Staphylococcus aureus* and gram-negative bacilli are each responsible for between 6% and 35% of infections. *Escherichia coli*, *Klebsiella* spp., and *Pseudomonas aeruginosa* are the most commonly reported gram-negative pathogens. Anaerobic bacteria, especially *Propionibacterium* spp., and fungi are occasionally reported.

Most (50% to 70%) CSF shunt infections occur within 60 days of shunt insertion, and 90% occur in the first 6 months after placement. This timing, and the prominent role of bacteria that normally colonize the skin in causation, suggests that most infections result from the intraoperative contamination of shunt devices. Less commonly,

shunt infections may result from direct extension of surgical wound infections. Infections with delayed onset (after 2 to 3 months) and those caused by gram-negative bacilli may originate from an intra-abdominal focus (appendicitis, bowel perforation, or surgery/trauma) by retrograde spread or bacteremia. Organisms such as coagulase-negative *Staphylococcus* and *S. aureus* adhere specifically to medical devices or to host proteins that are rapidly deposited on these foreign bodies. Adherent bacteria are enveloped in biofilm, a complex mixture of carbohydrate and proteins that both augments adherence and protects the organism from host immune defenses. Bacteria in biofilm are less susceptible to antimicrobial killing than are planktonic organisms. In some cases, biofilm acts as a mechanical barrier to reduce the penetrance of drugs. Sessile organisms also have reduced growth rates and metabolic changes that may affect the expression and function of drug targets.

CLINICAL PRESENTATION

The clinical presentation of shunt infections may range from almost asymptomatic colonization of the shunt device to severe ventriculitis, depending on the infecting organism and patient's underlying medical condition. Illness is frequently nonspecific. It is imperative to exclude CSF shunt infections in patients with unexplained systemic illness or symptoms of shunt malfunction, because these infections cannot reliably be distinguished from systemic illnesses or noninfectious causes of shunt malfunction. The most common symptoms include fever, vomiting, lethargy or altered consciousness, and irritability. Fever may be absent initially in up to 40% of patients. Some patients have more obvious presentations, with evidence of wound infection, inflammation along the subcutaneous shunt tract, or signs of meningeal irritation or elevated intracranial pressure. Approximately 10% have symptoms and signs of distal infection, including abdominal pain, guarding, gastrointestinal obstruction, or a palpable peritoneal pseudocyst. Patients with infected ventriculoatrial shunts are generally bacteremic and have more prominent fever and other constitutional symptoms. Ventriculoatrial shunt infections are occasionally complicated by an immune-complex–mediated "shunt nephritis," characterized by hypocomplementemia, hematuria, proteinuria, and renal dysfunction.

DIAGNOSIS

CSF shunt infections are diagnosed by examination and culture of CSF obtained from the shunt reservoir or cerebral ventricles. The CSF white blood cell count is usually elevated (usually 100 to 2500 cells/mm^3, with a range of 0 to >18 000/mm^3); however, a mild pleocytosis is also commonly observed with mechanical shunt malfunction and hypersensitivity reactions to shunt material. There is typically a neutrophil predominance (range 0% to 93%) and CSF eosinophilia of >5% occurs in 15% to 25% of patients. The CSF protein is generally elevated (usually 150 to 400 mg/dL). CSF glucose concentrations are less frequently abnormal, typically ranging from 30 to 60 mg/dL.

Gram stain examination of CSF permits a rapid diagnosis in 70% to 90% of patients. CSF cultures are positive in approximately 85% of patients. Positive cultures are less common in patients who have received antimicrobial therapy prior to CSF sampling. The likelihood of a positive culture may also be reduced in patients with infections caused by unusual pathogens, including anaerobic bacteria and fungi. Polymerase chain reaction amplification of bacterial DNA may be more sensitive than culture, but the specificity of these tests has not been established and they are not widely available. Blood cultures are rarely positive in ventriculoperitoneal shunt infections. In one study, an elevated serum C-reactive protein was helpful in distinguishing shunt infections from mechanical obstruction.

THERAPY

Initial Approach to Management

In patients with suspected CSF shunt infections, initial management includes obtaining CSF from the shunt reservoir or ventricle for Gram stain, culture, and biochemical analysis. Patients with presentations suggestive of infection should begin antimicrobial therapy while awaiting results of CSF cultures. Patients who have mild illness, no evidence of shunt malfunction, a mild pleocytosis, and negative

CSF stains may be observed without empirical therapy. Contamination of diagnostic CSF samples is possible. It is prudent, therefore, to obtain a second CSF sample before instituting antibiotic therapy in cases where antimicrobials have not been administered and the patient's course is not consistent with infection.

Antimicrobial Therapy

Empirical antibiotic therapy should be based on the likely pathogen, clinical findings, and the severity of illness. Children with uncomplicated infections may be treated with vancomycin alone, in doses appropriate for intracranial infections (Table 81.1). Combination therapy with vancomycin and an agent effective against gram-negative bacilli (cefepime, ceftazidime, or meropenem) is recommended for initial treatment of adults, children with more severe clinical illness, patients with findings suggestive of intra-abdominal infection, and those with gram-negative bacilli seen on CSF stain. Definitive antimicrobial therapy should be based on the specific organism, *in vitro* susceptibility testing, and the ability of the antimicrobial agent to cross the blood–brain barrier.

Poor blood–brain barrier penetration is a significant problem with some antimicrobial agents used to treat shunt infections, most notably vancomycin. Serum vancomycin levels should be monitored, aiming for peak concentrations of 30 to 45 µg/mL and trough concentrations of 15 to 20 µg/mL. Effective CSF concentrations of vancomycin, aminoglycosides, and certain other antimicrobial agents can often be more easily achieved by antimicrobial administration into the cerebral ventricles. No prospective randomized trials have compared combined parenteral and intraventricular administration of antimicrobials to parenteral therapy alone. Intraventricular administration is commonly made use of, nonetheless, in patients with suboptimal responses to systemic antibiotics and patients for whom shunt removal is not feasible. Some authorities advocate the routine use of intraventricular antimicrobials in infection caused by susceptible organisms. No antimicrobial agents are currently licensed for intraventricular use. Intraventricular vancomycin and aminoglycosides, however, have few reported adverse affects when used at appropriate concentrations (Table 81.2). Preservative-free formulations of these drugs should be reconstituted in sterile normal saline for administration and the extraventricular drain (EVD) clamped for 15 minutes to permit diffusion throughout the ventricular

Table 81.1 Recommended Doses of Intravenous Antimicrobial Agents

Agent/Age[a]		Total Daily Dose	No. Daily Doses
Ampicillin	Neonate <7 days	150 mg/kg	3
	Neonate 8–28 days	200 mg/kg	4
	Children	300 mg/kg	4
	Adults	12 g	6
Cefepime	Neonate <7 days	–	
	Neonate 8–28 days	–	
	Children	150 mg/kg	3
	Adults	6 g	3
Cefotaxime	Neonate <7 days	100–150 mg/kg[a]	2–3
	Neonate 8–28 days	150–200 mg/kg	3–4
	Children	300 mg/kg	4–6
	Adults	8–12 g	4–6
Ceftazidime	Neonate <7 days	100–150 mg/kg[a]	2–3
	Neonate 8–28 days	150 mg/kg	3
	Children	150 mg/kg	3
	Adults	6 g	3
Ceftriaxone	Neonate <7 days	–	
	Neonate 8–28 days	–	
	Children	100 mg/kg	2
	Adults	4 g	2
Meropenem	Neonate <7 days	—	
	Neonate 8–28 days	—	
	Children	120 mg/mL	3
	Adults	6 g	3
Nafcillin	Neonate <7 days	75 mg/kg	2–3
	Neonate 8–28 days	100–150 mg/kg[a]	3–4
	Children	200 mg/kg	4–6
	Adults	9–12 g	6
Oxacillin	Neonate <7 days	75 mg/kg	2–3
	Neonate 8–28 days	150–200 mg/kg[a]	3–4
	Children	200 mg/kg	4
	Adults	9–12 g	6
Penicillin G	Neonate <7 days	150 000 U/kg	2–3
	Neonate 8–28 days	200 000 U/kg	3–4
	Children	300 000 U/kg	4–6
	Adults	24 000 000 U	6
Rifampin	Neonate <7 days	–	
	Neonate 8–28 days	10–20 mg/kg	2
	Children	10–20 mg/kg	1–2
	Adults	600 mg	1

(continued)

Table 81.1 *(continued)*

Agent/Age[a]		Total Daily Dose	No. Daily Doses
Vancomycin	Neonate <7 days	20–30 mg/kg	2–3
	Neonate 8–28 days	30–45 mg/kg	3–4
	Children	60 mg/kg	4
	Adults	30–45 mg/kg	2–3

[a] Lower doses and increased intervals are advisable for infants weighing <2000 g.

Table 81.2 Recommended Initial Doses and Cerebrospinal Fluid Concentrations of Intraventricularly Administered Antimicrobials

Agent/Age	Initial Dose (mg/day)	Peak Concentration[a] (mg/L)	Trough Concentration[b] (mg/L)
Vancomycin			
Infants and children	2–10	50–80	≤10
Adults	5–20		
Gentamicin			
Infants and children	1–4	5–20	≤2
Adults	4–8		
Tobramycin			
Infants and children	1–4	5–20	≤2
Adults	4–8		
Amikacin			
Infants and children	2–8	25–30	≤5
Adults	5–10		

[a] Peak concentrations measured 15 to 30 minutes after administration
[b] Initial trough concentration measured 24 hours after administration of the first dose

system. An alternative "flush" procedure has been described in which a more diluted antimicrobial solution is infused slowly through one EVD and allowed to drain through a second EVD placed in the contralateral ventricle. Antimicrobial CSF concentrations achieved by intraventricular administration are highly variable and should be monitored periodically to both ensure adequate levels and avoid toxicity. CSF antimicrobial trough concentrations that exceed pathogens' minimum inhibitory concentration by 10- to 20-fold are desirable.

Surgical Therapy

Three general approaches for surgical management of shunt infection are practiced. Most commonly, antimicrobial therapy is combined with shunt removal and, if required, an EVD placed for CSF drainage until the shunt can be replaced. A one-stage procedure combines antibiotic therapy with immediate replacement of the infected shunt.

Finally, some patients have been treated with antibiotics alone without shunt removal. The success rates for each of these management schemes are approximately 88%, 68%, and 33%, respectively. The poor cure rates observed with antibiotic therapy alone are likely to be attributable to the combination of persistent viable bacteria in biofilms and the limited achievable CSF concentrations of many antimicrobial agents. Clinical studies have also described a shorter duration of hospitalization and lower mortality rates with two-stage shunt management, although it is probable that patients with a poor overall prognosis are more likely to be treated with antibiotics alone. These data suggest that patients with CSF shunt infections are optimally treated by removal of infected hardware and antimicrobial therapy followed by delayed shunt replacement. Shunt removal is indicated for wound or shunt tract infections, which should also be treated with local debridement and in patients with evidence of intra-abdominal infection other than isolated infection of an abdominal pseudocyst without positive CSF cultures. The latter patients are treated by shunt externalization, drainage of fluid collections, and systemic antimicrobials appropriate for intra abdominal infection. Patients with a short life expectancy, an Ommaya reservoir, and with infections caused by coagulase-negative *Staphylococcus* spp. that respond promptly to aggressive medical therapy may be considered for conservative management without shunt removal. These patients should have EVD or ventricular reservoirs placed and be treated with systemic and intraventricular antimicrobial agents for a minimum of 14 days after CSF sterilization, with meticulous attention to ensuring CSF antimicrobial concentrations are optimal.

Continuing Management

After antimicrobial therapy is initiated, CSF should be sampled every 1 to 2 days for culture and Gram stain until its sterility is confirmed. If cultures remain positive after 48 hours of appropriate systemic therapy, CSF antimicrobial concentrations should be determined and the addition of intraventricular antimicrobial agents should be considered. In infections caused by susceptible gram-positive bacteria, combination therapy with rifampin, which has excellent CSF and biofilm penetration, may be helpful. The possibility that the EVD has become colonized, which occurs in 5% to 10% of cases, should also be taken into account. Routine changes of EVDs, however, have not been proven to reduce the risk of colonization or secondary infection.

The optimal duration of therapy for CSF shunt infections has not been systematically studied. Most infections caused by coagulase-negative *Staphylococcus* spp. and *S. aureus* can be treated for 7 to 10 days after CSF is sterile. Infections caused by gram-negative pathogens are generally treated for a minimum of 10 to 14 days after CSF sterilization. Published studies have described a variety of criteria for the timing of shunt replacement, but most practitioners consider this after the CSF is sterile for 7 to 10 days and CSF protein concentrations fall ≤200 mg/dL.

OUTCOMES

CSF shunt infections are an uncommon direct cause of death. These infections, however, may be a risk factor for mortality related to underlying medical conditions. Some studies in children have noted an increased incidence of intellectual impairment and learning disabilities in patients with CSF shunt infections compared to those with shunts and no history of infection.

PREVENTION

Strict attention to disinfection of skin and surgical technique at the time of shunt or EVD placement may prevent many shunt infections. EVDs should be removed at the earliest feasible time. The use of prophylactic antimicrobial agents at the time of shunt insertion is controversial. Although no randomized controlled trials have compared infection rates, many studies have suggested prophylaxis may reduce shunt infection rates without an increase in infections caused by resistant organisms. A recent analysis of these studies concluded that short term (≤24 hour) antimicrobial prophylaxis should be considered, an approach consistent with general recommendations for the prevention of surgical infections. Most studies have used cefazolin for prophylaxis, with the first dose of 1 g intravenously for adults and 20 mg/kg for children within 60 minutes before surgical incision, followed by 2 additional doses at 8-hour intervals. For patients with serious allergies to cephalosporins and in institutions with a high incidence of infections caused by methicillin-resistant *S. aureus,* vancomycin is an alternative (adults, 15 mg/kg within 120 minutes before surgical incision and 12 hours later; children, 10 to 15 mg/kg intravenously within 120 minutes before surgical incision and every 6 hours for a total of 4 doses).

Catheters impregnated with antimicrobial agents (clindamycin, minocycline, and/or rifampin) have been developed recently. Incorporation of these drugs has no apparent effect on shunt function and no significant toxicity in animal and limited human studies. Antibacterial activity gradually decays over a period of months, in some cases persisting for >90 days after shunt insertion. Preliminary trials of these devices have been promising, but their effects on antimicrobial resistance and long-term studies of efficacy are needed.

MENINGITIS IN PATIENTS WITH CSF SHUNT INFECTIONS

Rarely, patients with CSF shunts may develop hematogenous bacterial meningitis caused by common pathogens such as *Streptococcus pneumoniae*, *Neisseria meningitidis*, and *Haemo-philus influenzae* type b. These infections can generally be treated by systemic antimicrobial agents alone, without removal of the shunt.

SUGGESTED READING

Brown EM, Edwards RJ, Pople IK. Conservative management of patients with cerebrospinal fluid shunt infections. *Neurosurgery*. 2006;58:657–665.

Rarilal B, Costa J, Samaio C. Antibiotic prophylaxis for surgical introduction of intracranial ventricular shunts. *Cochrane Database Syst Rev.* 2006;3:CD005365.

Schreffler RT, Schreffler AJ, Wittler RR. Treatment of cerebrospinal fluid shunt infections: a decision analysis. *Pediatr Inf Dis J.* 2002;21:632–636.

Yogev R, Tan T. Infections related to prosthetic or artificial devices. In: Feigin RD, Cherry JD, Demmler GJ, Kaplan SL, eds. *Textbook of Pediatric Infectious Diseases*. 5th ed. Philadelphia, PA: Elsevier Science; 2004.

82. Prion Diseases

Richard T. Johnson

Transmissible spongiform encephalopathies or prion diseases are chronic neurological disorders characterized by long incubation periods; progressive noninflammatory disease of brain and spinal cord; transmissibility within species and, to a limited extent, across species barriers; a failure of any immune response; and a uniformly fatal course. The pathology is characterized by neuronal loss, gliosis, and vacuoles in cytoplasm of neural cells giving the spongiform appearance on microscopic exam. Infectivity copurifies with an isoform of a normal surface glycoprotein expressed primarily in the central nervous system. The function of the normal prion protein is unknown; but the misfolded protein—the prion—induces posttranslational conversion of normal prion protein with a helical structure into the infectious isoform rich in β-pleated sheets. This abnormal protease-resistant protein accumulates in brain leading to disease. To date no nucleic acid has been detected in the transmissible particle.

Prion diseases are recognized in animals (scrapie, bovine spongiform encephalopathy, and chronic wasting disease of deer and elk) and humans (kuru, Creutzfeldt-Jakob disease [CJD], and the variant of CJD related to bovine spongiform encephalopathy). The human forms of disease can be divided into three groups: (1) sporadic CJD represents 85% to 90% of cases, (2) familial CJD due to mutations in the gene coding for prion protein making up 10% of cases, and (3) transmitted CJD due to iatrogenic transmission, cannibalism in the case of kuru, and, recently, transmission of bovine spongiform encephalopathy to humans.

EPIDEMIOLOGY

Sporadic CJD occurs worldwide at a rate of about 1 per million population per year. Rates are equal in men and woman, and mean age of onset is about 65 with few cases younger than 55 or older than 80 years of age. No geographic or temporal clustering is evident; conjugal exposure does not increase risk; and no occupations such as meat preparer, medical worker, or farmer appear related to disease. The assumption is that the great majority of cases of CJD result either from random misfolds of the prion protein that then cause a cascade of misfolding or from an undetected environmental exposure.

Familial cases of CJD have been related to >25 point mutations, insertions, and deletions in the gene coding for the prion protein. They show a pattern of autosomal dominant inheritance. In addition, polymorphisms in the gene, particularly a methioine/valine polymorphism at codon 129, influence susceptibility to sporadic and transmitted CJD and determine the phenotype of some hereditary forms.

Transmitted diseases include kuru, which was transmitted through ritual endocannibalism among the Fore tribal group of central New Guinea, and variant CJD transmitted from bovine spongiform encephalopathy to young people predominantly in the United Kingdom. In addition, iatrogenic CJD has occurred with contaminated operating room tools, by injection of human growth hormone derived from cadaveric pituitaries, and from the use of dural grafts in neurosurgery. Although human growth hormone was replaced by safe recombinant growth hormone in 1985 and most neurosurgeons have abandoned the use of human dural grafts, exposure history must still be sought because incubation periods of up to 50 years may be anticipated. The outbreak of over 170 000 cows with bovine spongiform encephalopathy in the United Kingdom peaked in 1993 and has been declining since then; the ongoing point source epidemic was related to contaminated feed. Nearly 200 young adults have now developed variant CJD, which represents the spread of this bovine prion to humans; 80% of these cases have been in the United Kingdom. Rare cases of bovine and human disease are now being seen in many countries.

CLINICAL SYMPTOMS AND SIGNS

Sporadic CJD often begins insidiously with fatigue, loss of dexterity, distortion of vision, insomnia, and other nonspecific complaints. About 40% have early complaints of cognitive decline, and 40% have an early onset of movement disorders, particularly cerebellar ataxia. The progression is rapid. Dementia and severe motor abnormalities, particularly startle-sensitive myoclonus, develop within weeks or months. Aphasia, blindness, hemiparesis, and mutism may all develop. The mean survival is only 5½ months, and 90% of patients are dead within 12 months.

The familial cases may have distinctive phenotypes such as Gerstmann–Straussler–Scheinker disease with cerebellar ataxia and fatal familial insomnia with autonomic abnormalities, but most familial cases have presentations similar to sporadic cases. In general, familial cases have onsets at earlier ages and have more protracted courses.

Variant CJD occurs in older children and young adults and has a protracted course; mean age of onset is 29 years, and mean survival is 14 months. The clinical presentations are unique often with behavioral abnormalities, depression, and pain. Variant CJD and kuru, both of which are thought to be transmitted orally, present with early cerebellar ataxia and a delay in the development of cognitive changes.

Laboratory Tests

Blood counts and chemistries are generally normal. The cerebrospinal fluid is typically acellular, with normal or mildly elevated protein, normal sugar, and no abnormal antibody synthesis or oligoclonal bands. Elevations of spinal fluid 14–3–3 protein or neuron-specific enolase, both normal neuronal proteins, are common in sporadic disease but present in only half of familial or variant cases where progression of disease is slower.

The electroencephalogram (EEG) usually shows nonspecific slowing early in disease, but a pattern of periodic sharp wave complexes, characteristic but not diagnostic of CJD, is common late in disease, particularly after myoclonic jerking has begun. The typical EEG pattern usually does not develop in variant CJD.

Computerized tomography (CT) of the brain is usually normal except to show atrophy in the late stage of disease. In contrast, magnetic resonance imaging (MRI) may give very typical patterns early in disease using FLAIR and DWI imaging. A cortical ribbon pattern is common, and a characteristic increased signal in the caudate and putamen is frequent. In contrast, in variant CJD the pulvinar of the thalamus usually shows an increased signal.

Spinal fluid 14-3-3 protein, EEG, and MRI are all helpful, but none have perfect selectivity or sensitivity. Sensitivity is increased if tests are repeated during the course of disease.

Uncertainty of diagnosis may necessitate a brain biopsy. Adequate tissue should be obtained for standard histology as well as frozen tissue for immunocytochemistry, Western blots for prion protein, and genetic studies for mutations in the *PRNP* gene. This can be processed free of charge by the National Prion Disease Pathology Surveillance Center (see Suggested Reading). The same center can assist with autopsies and funeral arrangements when local concerns about infectiousness interfere with good medical practice.

DIFFERENTIAL DIAGNOSIS

Early in disease differentiation from Alzheimer disease and other degenerative diseases may be difficult, particularly in some cases of familial Alzheimer disease where myoclonus is seen. The rapid course of CJD and the development of focal neurological findings usually clarify this differential. It is early in disease that the finding of 14-3-3 protein in spinal fluid and MRI changes can be helpful.

Causes of subacute dementia such as neurosyphilis, fungal meningitis, and other inflammatory diseases are ruled out by spinal fluid examination. Localized vasculitis usually is accompanied by spinal fluid protein elevation but can pose the most difficult diagnosis to rule out in CJD. Cases of gliomatosis cerebri, intravascular lymphomatosis, and anti-GAD antibody cerebellar ataxia have been reported to clinically simulate CJD and show positive 14-3-3 protein in spinal fluid.

Toxic and metabolic diseases can mimic CJD. Cognitive impairment and myoclonus have been seen with bismuth and lithium intoxication and in Hashimoto encephalopathy. In these acute intoxications or metabolic disorders, seizures and myoclonic jerks often occur at the onset; in CJD, myoclonus usually develops after several months, and seizures are rare. A history of familial disease, travel, drug ingestion, blood transfusions, prior neurosurgical or ophthalmological procedures, thyroid disease, and toxin exposures should be pursued in all suspected cases.

TREATMENT

No long-term remission or survival has ever been documented with animal or human prion disease. Treatment, therefore, takes two forms:

palliative treatment and experimental treatment.

Patients in late stages of CJD are often mute and show limited voluntary motor activity. Agitation is not a common problem, so psychotropic drugs are seldom indicated. If myoclonic jerking is distressing to the patient, clonazepam (0.5 to 5 mg 3 times a day) can be given. Seizures are unusual, but, if they occur, treat with routine anticonvulsants. Swallowing may become impaired. Nutrition by feeding tube and hydration by the intravenous route may be considered after discussion with family.

Experimental treatment with amphotericin B, pentosan polysulfate, Congo red, quinacrine, and chlorpromazine has shown some beneficial effect in vitro and limited effects in mice with scrapie. Human experimental trials of several drugs are in planning or in progress.

No special isolation precautions are needed at home or in the hospital, except to mark spinal fluid and blood specimens for special handling because of hazard of prion disease. Masks, gowns, and gloves in hospital rooms are not only unnecessary but harmful. Family members suddenly seeing a parent treated as infectious who has been recently babysitting a grandchild are terrified, and subsequent nursing home or hospice placement may be jeopardized by isolation procedures.

SUGGESTED READING

Belay ED, Schonberger LB. The public health impact of prion diseases. *Ann Rev Publ Health*. 2005;26:191–212.

Johnson RT. Prion diseases. *Lancet Neurol*. 2005;4:635–642.

Seipelt M, Zerr I, Nau R, et al. Hashimoto's encephalitis as a differential diagnosis of Creutzfeldt-Jakob disease. *J Neurol Neurosurg Psychiat*. 1999;66:172–176.

Trevitt CR, Collinge J. A systematic review of prion therapeutics in experimental models. *Brain*. 2006;129:2241–2265.

National Prion Disease Pathology Surveillance Center, Case Western Reserve University, Cleveland OH; Telephone 216-368-0597 (studies of biopsy and autopsy tissue, 14-3-3 analysis on CSF, genetic studies; no charge) Patient support and information: www. cjdfoundation.com.

PART XI

The Susceptible Host

83. Evaluation of Suspected Immunodeficiency

Thomas A. Fleisher

The need to evaluate immunologic function has become a part of the standard practice of clinical medicine, resulting at least in part from the secondary immunodeficiency produced by human immunodeficiency virus (HIV) infection. In addition, since the early 1990s the molecular basis of primary immunodeficiency disorders has evolved, with now more than 120 genetic defects identified and an expanded range of clinical phenotypes associated with immune dysfunction. This chapter presents the general methods available to assess immune function linking these to the clinical infection scenaria that suggest specific types of immunodeficiency.

The primary clinical problem that sets the stage for initiating an immunologic evaluation is a history of increased susceptibility to infection. In general, the specific characteristics of the recurrent and/or chronic infections, including organism(s), sites, and response to therapy, provide critical insights into the most likely source of the immunodeficiency.

Defects in adaptive immunity involving antibody production (humoral immunity) lead to recurrent infections with high-grade encapsulated extracellular bacteria such as *Haemophilus influenzae* and *Streptococcus pneumoniae* usually affecting the sinopulmonary tract. The protective immune response depends on the production of antibodies against the capsular carbohydrate antigens present on these organisms. In contrast, the clinical picture of patients with defective T-cell (cellular) immunity typically consists of recurrent infections with opportunistic organisms, including *Pneumocystis jiroveci* (formerly *Pneumocystis carinii*), *Candida* species, and cytomegalovirus. This demonstrates that functional T cells are required to prevent or clear infection with these opportunistic intracellular microorganisms. A more recent focus of study has been the interface between the adaptive and innate immune systems directed at defects in the interferon-γ/interleukin (IL)-12 circuit found in certain patients with persistent nontuberculous mycobacterial (NTB) infection. The critical role of the lymphoid arm of the innate immune system (natural killer cells) in host defense has been clarified based on

defects affecting these cells producing clinical phenotypes that include increased susceptibility to herpes family (eg, Epstein–Barr virus [EBV] and herpes simplex virus [HSV]) viruses and in some cases uncontrolled inflammation. Abnormalities in the phagocytic arm of adaptive immunity (involving neutrophils), including cellular dysfunction and decreased cell numbers, result in cutaneous and deep-seated abscesses, pneumonia, periodontitis, and osteomyelitis. Typically these infections are caused by bacteria such as *Staphylococcus aureus* and fungi such as *Aspergillus* and *Nocardia* species. The clinical findings point to the critical role of mobile phagocytic cells in the normal host defense. Congenital defects in specific complement components of innate immunity can also be associated with recurrent infections although in many cases these are also linked to the development of autoimmune disease.

Clinical suspicion of a defect in immune function is primarily generated by the medical history, with careful attention to the frequency and sites of infections, the types of organisms involved, and the therapy required. Any patient with a history of increased susceptibility to infection must also be carefully questioned about risk factors for HIV infection. In addition, the family history may also prove important because many defined immune deficiencies are genetically linked. The physical examination can provide clues in the case of specific primary immunodeficiencies (eg, typical facies in the hyper-immunoglobulin E (IgE) [Job] syndrome, scars from abscess drainage sites) and may also provide clues to the evaluation of secondary immune disorders (eg, oral hairy leukoplakia or Kaposi's sarcoma in HIV infection).

EVALUATING B-CELL FUNCTION

Clinical findings that suggest an abnormality in antibody production are recurrent or chronic infections with encapsulated bacteria involving the sinopulmonary tract. Gastrointestinal, hematologic, and autoimmune disorders may also be associated with antibody deficiencies (Table 83.1).

Table 83.1 Evaluation of Suspected Antibody (B-Cell) Immunodeficiency

Screening Tests
Quantitative immunoglobulins
Specific antibody
Circulating specific antibodies
Postimmunization antibodies
Protein antigens
Carbohydrate antigens
IgG subclasses (+/−utility)
Human immunodeficiency virus testing

Secondary Tests
B-cell immunophenotyping
In vitro B-cell function tests (primarily research)

The clinical screening of antibody-mediated immune function can be accomplished by measuring the levels of the major immunoglobulin classes, IgG, IgA, and IgM. The results must be compared with age-matched reference intervals (normal ranges) that are typically expressed as 95% confidence intervals. The serum immunoglobulin levels are the net of protein production, utilization, catabolism, and loss.

There are no rigid standards regarding the diagnosis of immunoglobulin deficiency, although an IgG value below 3 g/L (300 mg/dL) generally suggests an increased risk for infection. Hypogammaglobulinemia associated with significant recurrent bacterial infection is a definitive indication for intravenous immunoglobulin replacement therapy after completing the evaluation.

Measurement of a functional antibody response is particularly useful when the total immunoglobulin levels are modestly depressed or normal in the face of a history of recurrent infection. The simplest method is evaluation for spontaneous antibodies (eg, antiblood group antibodies [isohemagglutinins] and antibodies to immunizations). The definitive method is immunizing and assessing preimmunization versus 3-week postimmunization antibody levels with both protein antigens (eg, tetanus toxoid) and polysaccharide antigens (eg, Pneumovac). Guidelines for normal responses, which are usually provided by the testing laboratory, typically consist of at least a 4-fold increase in antibody and/or protective levels of antibody following immunization.

An additional and readily available test is quantitation of IgG subclass levels; these are most useful in evaluating the IgA-deficient patient with significant recurrent infections. However, in many settings detection of an IgG subclass deficiency still requires the demonstration of an abnormality in functional antibody production before therapy such as intravenous immunoglobulin is indicated.

Despite the preponderance of recurrent opportunistic infections resulting from HIV infection, appropriate testing to rule this out should be considered even in the face of recurrent bacterial infection. This type of clinical presentation is particularly common among children infected with HIV. Testing focused on viral load may be needed to rule out HIV infection in the face of absent or diminished antibody production, because the screening tests depend on detecting anti-HIV antibodies (enzyme-linked immunosorbent assay [ELISA] and Western blot assays).

Additional tests focused on humoral immune function are generally performed in specialized centers and fall into two general categories: evaluation of the number and characteristics of B cells and testing the function of B cells in vitro. The former determines the number and specific surface characteristics of B cells generally performed by flow cytometry (immunophenotyping). The latter involves studies that test in vitro B-cell signaling and immunoglobulin biosynthesis.

EVALUATING T-CELL FUNCTION

A clinical history of recurrent opportunistic infections strongly suggests an abnormality in T-cell function. Immunodeficiency involving T cells has the highest prevalence as a secondary defect associated with HIV infection. Thus, initial screening assays should always include testing for HIV infection. In addition, the absolute lymphocyte count (generated from the white blood cell count and differential) and cutaneous delayed-type hypersensitivity (DTH) response to recall antigens are standard screening tests. The significance of the former relates to the fact that T cells constitute approximately three-fourths of the circulating lymphocytes. The DTH response provides an in vivo window of T-cell function in response to a previously encountered antigen. However, failure to respond may either reflect T-cell dysfunction (T-cell anergy) or indicate that the host has not been exposed (sensitized) to the antigen. Consequently, it is prudent to use more than one antigen for testing. Clinical correlates of a DTH response include the cutaneous response to poison ivy and other contact hypersensitivity reactions (Table 83.2).

The screening tests for T-cell function are often followed by additional testing to complete

Table 83.2 Evaluation of Suspected T-Cell Immunodeficiency

Screening Tests
Human immunodeficiency virus testing
Lymphocyte count
Delayed-type hypersensitivity skin tests
Secondary Tests
T-cell enumeration
T-cell proliferation (mitogen, alloantigen, antigen)
T-cell cytokine production

the assessment of cellular immunity. This parallels that of B cells with quantitation and characterization (immunophenotyping) of T cells by flow cytometry together with in vitro functional testing (eg, proliferation assays and cytokine production).

EVALUATING DEFECTS IN THE IL-12/23 AND INTERFERON-γ PATHWAYS

Recent data have identified abnormalities in specific components of a cytokine pathway of response involving T cells and monocytes/macrophages associated with recurrent infections to a limited range of opportunistic organisms, particularly NTB. The infections are typically invasive and fail to respond to long-term multiple-agent antimicrobial therapy. These findings led to a study demonstrating that interferon-γ is an effective adjunct to antimicrobials in treating some of these patients. This represents an area of active investigation that has identified specific defects in some patients and is now focused on clarifying the molecular basis of additional patients. This represents an expanding group of identified immune disorders associated with a clinical phenotype of recurrent infections involving a more limited range of microorganisms. The laboratory evaluation of the patients with persistent NTB is generally performed in specialized centers and is focused on defining defects in the cellular signaling pathways involving IL–12/23 and interferon-γ.

EVALUATING DEFECTS IN NATURAL KILLER CELL FUNCTION

The third arm of the lymphoid system consists of circulating cells distinct from B and T cells, the natural killer (NK) cells. Deficiency in NK cell function has been described in a limited number of patients with recurrent herpes infections. In addition, experimental models point to a role for the NK cell in allograft and tumor rejection.

Another category of NK cell (and cytotoxic T cell) defects is found in disorders with an uncontrolled inflammatory response initiated by specific infections that can lead to multiple organ damage (hemophagocytic lymphocytic histiocytosis [HLH] and the X-linked lymphoproliferative syndrome [XLP]). Testing of NK cell function includes immunophenotyping NK cells by flow cytometry and assaying killing activity using standard in vitro assays.

EVALUATING DEFECTS IN INNATE IMMUNE SIGNALING

An area of intense current investigation involves the identification of disorders associated with defective signaling by Toll-like receptors (TLR). This is a family of at least 10 receptors that represent a phylogenetically more primitive arm of the immune system-dependent signaling via pattern recognition of bacterial, fungal, and viral products. An example of such a process is the activation of monocytes and macrophages by bacterial lipopolysaccharide (LPS) binding TLR4. This pathway of activating the immune system appears to be one of the first lines in host defense as it does not require prior exposure to the pathogenic organism. Recently, two different clinical phenotypes have been identified with genetic defects involving TLR signaling. In one, there is a genetic susceptibility to serious bacterial infection that presents in childhood and generally improves during adolescence. The most recently described defect is associated with the development of herpes simplex encephalitis. Additional defects in TLR function are likely to be indentified, and this represents an evolving field in clinical immunology. Currently, the evaluation of TLR function is confined to a limited number of centers that usually screen by evaluating TLR-induced cytokine production using a series of ligands specific for one or more specific TLRs.

EVALUATING NEUTROPHIL FUNCTION

The clinical features of neutrophil dysfunction usually include recurrent bacterial and fungal infections of the skin, lymph node, lung, liver, bone, and, in some cases, the periodontal tissue. This clinical presentation is most commonly observed with neutropenia as a result of decreased production, altered localization, or increased destruction of the neutrophil. In addition, some primary and secondary abnormalities of neutrophil function also demonstrate patterns of increased susceptibility to infections (Table 83.3).

Table 83.3 Evaluation of Suspected Neutrophil Deficiency

Screening Tests
Multiple sequential neutrophil counts
Review of neutrophil morphology

Secondary Tests
CD11, CD18 assessment
Respiratory burst assessment
Nitroblue tetrazolium test
Flow cytometric test
Specific enzyme activity testing
Chemotaxis testing
In vivo (Rebuck skin window)
In vitro (Boyden chamber, soft agar assay)

The clinical pattern of infection often can help to discriminate the underlying problem. Patients with neutropenia and those with the leukocyte adhesion deficiency (LAD) tend to have recurrent cellulitis, periodontal disease, otitis media, pneumonia, and rectal or gastrointestinal abscesses. Although LAD is accompanied by a persistent granulocytosis, there is effectively a tissue neutropenia. This is due to the underlying adhesion defect that prevents the directed movement of these phagocytic cells to sites of infection. In contrast, patients with chronic granulomatous disease (CGD) have significant problems with liver and bone abscesses as well as pneumonias with unique organisms, including *Staphylococcus aureus*, *Serratia marcesens*, *Burkholderia cepacia*, *Nocardia*, and *Aspergillus*. Furthermore, they tend to have a lower frequency of β-strep and *Escherichia coli* infections than do patients with neutropenia.

Screening studies directed at the evaluation of neutrophil function should start with the leukocyte count, differential, and morphologic review. If neutropenia (cyclic neutropenia requires multiple evaluations over time) and morphologic abnormalities are ruled out, the evaluation should be directed at assays that provide functional information about neutrophils. Included are the flow cytometric assessment of neutrophil adhesion molecules to assess for the expression of CD11a,b,c and CD18 surface antigens, which are absent or depressed in LAD-1 patients. The neutrophil oxidative burst pathway can be screened using either the nitroblue tetrazolium (NBT) test or a flow cytometric assay, both of which are abnormal in patients with CGD. Finally, evaluation of neutrophil-directed movement (chemotaxis) can be performed in vivo using the Rebuck skin window technique as well as in vitro with a Boyden chamber or a soft agar

system. Abnormalities of chemotaxis have been observed secondary to certain pharmacologic agents as well as the leukocyte adhesion deficiency, Chédiak-Higashi syndrome, Pelger-Huet anomaly, and juvenile periodontitis. A hallmark clinical feature of signficantly abnormal chemotaxis is diminished neutrophil infiltration and decreased inflammation.

Functional testing of neutrophils has its greatest yield when evaluating patients with recurrent infections associated with a genetic neutrophil abnormality. Many patients with histories of recurrent cutaneous abscesses fail to demonstrate abnormalities in the above tests. This likely is related to the relative insensitivity of the available tests in discerning more subtle functional abnormalities.

EVALUATING THE COMPLEMENT SYSTEM

The clinical setting in which complement defects should be suspected varies depending on the type of defect. Abnormalities in the early components of the complement pathway may have recurrent sinopulmonary infections but typically also have a history of autoimmunity. Defects in the later components of complement affecting the membrane attack complex (MAC, C5–C9) have increased susceptibility to infections with *Neisseria* organisms with meningitis and/or sepsis. There are rare defects in components of a second complement pathway, the alternate pathway, that may also present with recurrent infections (Table 83.4).

The best screening test for the classical complement pathway is the total hemolytic complement activity (CH50) assay (with the AP50 test used to screen for defects in the alternate complement pathway). Assuming correct handling of the serum sample (complement components are very labile), a markedly depressed CH50 result strongly suggests a classical complement component deficiency. Selected component immunoassays are available in larger laboratories, and component functional testing may be available in very specialized complement laboratories.

RECOMMENDATIONS

The clinical pattern of recurrent infections remains the single most useful clue in determining the likelihood of immune deficiency and identifying the best approach for evaluation. HIV infection has become the most likely cause of immune deficiency, and appropriate

Table 83.4 Evaluation of Suspected Complement Abnormality

Screening Tests
CH50 assay
AP50 assay

Secondary Tests
Component immunoassays
Component functional assays

diagnostic testing for HIV is critical, particularly in the setting of recurrent opportunistic infection. When the history identifies repeated bacterial infections involving the sinopulmonary tract, abnormalities in antibody production (and very rarely complement component deficiency) should be considered. Opportunistic infections suggest T-cell dysfunction, and bacterial and fungal infections of the skin, lungs, and bone strongly suggest defective neutrophil function. The current area of intense investigation is focused on recurrent/chronic infections involving a more limited range of microorganisms with much of this focused on the innate immune system or the interface between the innate and adaptive immune systems. It is important to keep in mind that the frequency of infections between individuals can vary significantly, and the line distinguishing normal from abnormal is not always clear. However, infections that are recurrent and difficult to treat or those that involve unusual organisms should definitely raise suspicion of an underlying immunodeficiency.

Laboratory studies are essential for evaluating the status of immune function. However, the prudent use of these tests requires that they be applied in an orderly fashion, starting with the simpler screening tests selected according to the clinical clues provided particularly from the patient history. The results of these tests are relatively easy to interpret when either clearly normal or absolutely abnormal. The difficulty arises in determining the actual degree of immune dysfunction when the results fall more in a gray zone. To address this, combinations of tests often help to clarify the status of immune function or dysfunction, and involvement of a specialist with extensive knowledge of the clinical presentation and evaluation of immunodeficiencies can also be crucial.

SUGGESTED READING

Ballow M. Primary immunodeficiency disorders: antibody deficiency. *J Allergy Clin Immunol*. 2002;109:581–591.

Buckley RH. Primary cellular immunodeficiencies. *J Allergy Clin Immunol*. 2002;109:747–757.

Casanova JL, Fieschi C, Bustamante J, et al. From idiopathic infectious diseases to novel primary immunodeficiencies. *J Allergy Clin Immunol*. 2005;116:423–425.

Casrouge A, Zhang SY, Eidenschenk C, et al. Herpes simplex encephalitis in human UNC-93B deficiency. *Science*. 2006;314:308–312.

Figueroa JE, Densen P. Infectious diseases associated with complement deficiencies. *Clin Microbiol Rev*. 1991;4:359–395.

Filipe-Santos O, Bustamante J, Chapgier A, et al. Inborn errors of IL-12/23 and IFN-gamma-mediated immunity: molecular, cellular and clinical features. *Semin Immunol*. 2006;18:347–361.

Fleisher TA, Oliveira JB. Functional and molecular evaluation of lymphocytes. *J Allergy Clin Immunol*. 2004;114:227–234.

Ku CL, Yang K Bustamante J, et al. Inherited disorders of human Toll-like receptor signaling: immunological implications. *Immunol Rev*. 2005;203:10–20.

Orange JR. Human natural killer cell deficiencies. *Curr Opin Allergy Clin Immunol*. 2006;6:399–409.

Rosenzweig SD, Holland SM. Phagocyte immunodeficiencies and their infections. *J Allergy Clin Immunol*. 2004;113:620–626.

84. Infections in the Neutropenic Patient

Rafik Samuel

Patients receiving cancer chemotherapy are at high risk for developing neutropenia and severe infections when their neutrophil count is depressed. There is no strict definition of neutropenia, but this term is used to define an absolute neutrophil count ≤1500 cells down to an absolute neutrophil count ≤500 cells/mL. Fever in the neutropenic patient is defined as a single temperature of >38.3°C or a temperature of >38.0°C over at least 30 minutes to 1 hour. However, some neutropenic patients do not mount a fever, and the presence of hypotension and hypothermia may be the presenting feature of infection.

Over the years, different approaches have been developed to address the clinical entity of fever and neutropenia. Some research has looked at preventing neutropenia with the use of colony-stimulating factors. Other research has focused on preventing infection in the neutropenic patient; still others have looked at the empiric use of antimicrobials to treat infections when fever occurs. In this chapter, I focus on these three approaches as well as the main causes of infections in these severely immunocompromised individuals.

CAUSES OF INFECTION IN THE NEUTROPENIC PATIENT

Gram-Negative Organisms

Enteric gram-negative organisms play a significant role in the morbidity and mortality due to infection in our neutropenic patients. These include *Escherichia coli*, *Klebsiella* spp., and *Enterobacter* spp. among others. These organisms can gain entry into the bloodstream and lead to serious infections as a result of mucosal damage and the ability of the organism to disseminate. Other organisms that can lead to significant disease include *Pseudomonas* spp., which may colonize the neutropenic patient and gain entry through skin damage or catheters. These organisms may cause a variety of infectious processes ranging from primary bacteremia due to an indwelling catheter to infections of the gastrointestinal, genitourinary, and respiratory tracts.

One infection unique to neutropenic patients is typhlitis. In patients with prolonged neutropenia, an inflammatory process of the cecum and ascending colon can develop. The exact etiology of this infectious process is not known. It may be due to increased growth of enteric organisms that leads to inflammation of the colon. Patients develop fever and right-sided abdominal pain and are at high risk for intestinal perforation. Computed tomography demonstrates the right-sided colitis and in severe cases can show pneumatosis coli or evidence of perforated bowel. In cases where perforation has not occurred, broad-spectrum antibiotics that cover enteric gram-negative rods, anaerobes, and enterococcus such as β-lactam/β-lactamase inhibitors or carbapenems should be adequate therapy. Surgery is technically difficult in these patients and not usually needed, as studies have demonstrated that antibiotics alone are usually able to keep the infection in check until the neutrophils return.

Because infections due to gram-negative organisms can be life threatening, patients with neutropenic fever should be started on an agent that targets these bacteria. There have been significant increases in the number of antibiotic-resistant gram-negative rods containing plasmid-mediated extended-spectrum β-lactamases in the Enterobacteriaciae family. These enzymes inactivate most penicillins, cephalosporins, and monobactams; therefore, the knowledge of the local resistance patterns is crucial in choosing the proper antibiotics. *Pseudomonas* resistance patterns are also important because carbapenemases and other resistance mechanisms can render *Pseudomonas* resistant to many previously effective antibiotics. Because resistance patterns vary significantly from patient to patient and over time, sensitivity from the culture is quite important to assure adequate therapy once the etiology of the infection is found. Even after the antibiotics are started, the origin of the infection should be ascertained so that appropriate procedures can be taken if necessary (eg, removal of indwelling catheter).

Gram-Positive Organisms

Among patients with neutropenia, there has been an increase in both severity and numbers of gram-positive infections due to more indwelling catheters and damage to mucosal surfaces. The bloodstream is the most common site of gram-positive infections. The three most common organisms causing bacteremia from indwelling catheters are coagulase-negative staphylococci, *Staphylococcus aureus*, and *Enterococcus* spp. In addition to indwelling catheters, mucosal and skin damage from chemotherapy can be a portal of entry for gram-positive organisms. Cellulitis is most commonly due to β-hemolytic streptococci and *S. aureus*. Over the years, infections due to viridans streptococci resulting in a sepsis picture have been noted in patients with severe mucositis (Table 84.1).

In patients with possible gram-positive infections, vancomycin is effective in treatment. It will be adequate coverage for the most common organisms such as staphylococci, streptococci, and most enterococci. *Enterococcus* spp., especially *E. faecium*, can be resistant to vancomycin. The rate of this resistance varies from one institution to another, but may be as high as 90% in some institutions. However, *E. faecalis* is much less likely to have vancomycin resistance. For patients with vancomycin-resistant organisms or an allergy to vancomycin, alternative agents include daptomycin, linezolid, and quinupristin–dalfopristin. Daptomycin has recently been shown to be effective in staphylococcal bacteremia and serious skin and soft-tissue infection. Its main side effect is elevation of creatinine phosphokinase (CPK) and muscle damage. When using daptomycin, monitoring of CPK is warranted. Linezolid is approved for skin and soft-tissue infections. Its advantage is that it is available orally; however, its main side effect is bone marrow suppression. Quinupristin–dalfopristin is active against staphylococci and *Enterococcus faecium* but not other enterococci. The use of quinupristin–dalfopristin is limited due to arthralgia and myalgia side effects of this agent.

Duration of treatment for the gram-positive organisms varies based on the type of infection. In general these organisms do not result in the sepsis syndrome and early mortality but may lead to significant complications of infection if not treated appropriately. Infections of the skin and soft-tissue require at least 7 days of therapy with adequate debridement when indicated. Bacteremia due to *S. aureus* may require up to 4 weeks of therapy if the source is not located or if the bacteremia does not resolve quickly, whereas enterococcal and coagulase-negative staphylococcal infections can be treated for shorter durations, especially if infected catheters are removed.

Anaerobes

Anaerobes can play an important role in the neutropenic patient as a result of mucosal damage. Anaerobic antibiotic coverage is warranted in patients with significant abdominal complaints while awaiting cultures. This includes coverage for *Bacteroides* spp. and *Prevotella* spp. Acceptable coverage can include a β-lactam/β-lactamase combination, carbapenem, or addition of metronidazole to other regimens.

Clostridium difficile colitis is always a concern in someone who develops diarrhea while on antibiotics. In addition, some cancer chemotherapeutics have antimicrobial activity and *C. difficile* has been reported in patients who have not received an antibiotic. Any antibiotic can result in *C. difficile* diarrhea. What complicates the picture is that chemotherapeutic agents can lead to diarrhea because of mucositis. When a patient develops significant diarrhea and abdominal pain while receiving antibiotics, empiric metronidazole or oral vancomycin is warranted while awaiting the toxin assay results. An important part of *C. difficile* diarrhea treatment includes stopping the agent that led to the diarrhea in the first place; unfortunately, that is not likely to be feasible in these patients because of the concern for other infections. Since the early 2000s there has been an increase in severe *C. difficile* diarrhea. There are epidemic strains of *C. difficile* that can lead to severe colitis resulting in colon perforation and emergent surgical intervention. This change in severity is believed to be due to increased production of *C. difficile* toxin. Therapy still includes metronidazole or oral vancomycin; however, close monitoring of complications is necessary.

Fungi

Fungal infections are increasingly common among patients with neutropenia and underlying acute leukemia or lymphoma. Some of the reasons for increased risk of infection include longer survival in patients with bacterial infections, indwelling catheters, parenteral nutrition, and prolonged antibiotic therapy (Table 84.2).

Candida spp. are the most common cause of fungal infections in these patients and one of the leading causes of catheter-associated

Table 84.1 Common Gram-Positive Bacteria Causing Infection in the Neutropenic Patient

Bacteria	Form of Infection	Antibiotic of Choice
Staphylococcus aureus	Bacteremia, skin, and skin structure infection	Vancomycin
Coagulase-negative staphylococci	Bacteremia	Vancomycin
Enterococcus spp.	Bacteremia	Vancomycin[a]
β-hemolytic streptococci	Skin and skin structure infection	Penicillin
α-hemolytic streptococci	Bacteremia, endovascular infection	Ceftriaxone[b]
Streptococcus pneumoniae	Respiratory	Ceftriaxone[c]
Diptheroids	Bacteremia	Vancomycin

[a] If vancomycin resistant, choices include daptomycin, linezolid, or quinupristin–dalfopristin (for *Enterococcus faecium*).
[b] Variable resistance to penicillin, macrolides, and clindamycin.
[c] Penicillin resistance varies; local resistance rates should be reviewed.

Table 84.2 Common Fungi Causing Infection in the Neutropenic Patient

Organism	Azole of Choice	Echinocandin Activiy	Amphotericin Activity
C. *albicans*	Fluconazole	Yes	Yes
C. *tropicalis*	Fluconazole	Yes	Yes
C. *parapsilosis*	Fluconazole	Yes[a]	Yes
C. *glabrata*	Voriconazole[b]	Yes	Yes
C. *krusei*	Voriconazole	Yes	Yes
Cryptococcus neoformans	Fluconazole	No	Yes
Aspergillus spp.	Voriconazole	Yes	Yes
Zygomycetes	Posaconazole	No	Yes
Histoplasma capsulatum	Itraconazole	No	Yes
Coccidioides immitis	Fluconazole	No	Yes
Blastomyces dermatitidis	Itraconazole	No	Yes

[a] C. *parapsilosis* tend to have higher minimal inhibitory concentration (MIC) to echinocandins, but are usually susceptible.
[b] C. *glabrata* tend to have higher MIC to voriconazole, but are usually susceptible.

infections. *Candida* can also be associated with disseminated disease involving organs such as the liver and spleen. Disseminated candidiasis may be difficult to diagnose by blood cultures alone because they are only 70% sensitive. In patients with prolonged neutropenia and fever, imaging of the abdomen, particularly of the liver and spleen, to look for disseminated fungal

The Susceptible Host

disease is necessary. Because the risk of *Candida* infections is high in patients with prolonged neutropenia, it is recommended to empirically start an antifungal agent to treat disease that may yet be undiagnosed if they remain febrile despite broad-spectrum antimicrobial therapy.

Therapy for *Candida* includes removal of the indwelling catheter if present to help clear the organism from the bloodstream. In addition, eye exam is necessary after completion of therapy to make sure the patient did not develop endophthalmitis, a rare complication of candidemia. *Candida* spp. have variable resistance to available agents, and appropriate choice in antifungals is critical. Multiple agents are available for treatment of *Candida* and include the azoles, echinocandins, and polyenes. The traditional therapy with amphotericin B is uncommonly used because of adverse events such as infusion reactions and nephrotoxicity. The lipid formulations of amphotericin are also not used frequently for *Candida* infections because of cost and the availability of good alternative agents.

The triazole fluconazole has activity against most *Candida* spp., including *Candida albicans*, *Candida tropicalis*, and *Candida parapsilosis*. Fluconazole has variable activity against *Candida glabrata* and no activity against *Candida krusei*. One advantage in the use of fluconazole is that it has recently become available as a generic agent and is significantly less expensive than the other antifungal agents. Another azole, voriconazole, has good activity against all the *Candida* spp.; however, interactions with other agents metabolized through the hepatic cytochrome P450 enzymes must be taken into account. Caution should be taken when considering voriconazole in patients who may have been previously on a different azole such as fluconazole because the *Candida* spp. isolated may have higher minimal inhibitory concentration (MICs) and may not be susceptible to voriconazole. The newest medications in the antifungal armamentarium are the echinocandins. They target the β-1,3 synthase enzyme in the cell wall of *Candida* spp. These agents include caspofungin, micafungin, and anidulafungin. These agents are active against all *Candida* spp. and may be more active than azoles in the setting of prosthetic infections. Because these agents have good activity against *Candida* spp., they are usually given in the setting of neutropenia and fever until the identity of the candida is determined, especially in the very ill.

Molds may cause significant disease in neutropenic patients that have underlying leukemia, lymphoma, myeloma, myelodysplastic syndromes, or prolonged neutropenia. The most common pathogen in this setting is aspergillus; however, other molds such as the zygomycetes have been increasing in frequency. *Aspergillus* spp. can cause a variety of different diseases; however, the most common forms of infection include rhinosinusitis and pulmonary disease.

Therefore, any patient with neutropenia who complains of sinus congestion or pain should be evaluated for possible fungal sinusitis. Typical findings include mucosal thickening on radiography, whereas direct visualization demonstrates necrosis or an eschar. Immediate therapy with a lipid formulation of amphotericin B (until zygomycetes are excluded) should be administered along with rapid surgical debridement. Pulmonary aspergillus may present as nodular disease, pulmonary infiltrate, infarction, or cavity. In both of these settings a biopsy demonstrating the organism on pathology in addition to a positive culture makes the diagnosis. Because many filamentous fungi may look like aspergillus on stain, microbiology is important to distinguish it from the others. Once the cultures grow aspergillus, therapy can be changed to voriconazole or can be continued with amphotericin B. A comparison of voriconazole and amphotericin B demonstrated superior efficacy with voriconazole compared to amphotericin B in aspergillus infections. Other agents with activity against aspergillus include itraconazole and the echinocandins. Combination therapy with 2 of the 3 classes is occasionally used. Many case series demonstrate that combinations of voriconazole and an echinocandin may be beneficial; however, results from prospective studies are pending. Duration of therapy should be prolonged, with radiologic evaluation to demonstrate improvement or cure. One unanswered question is how to adjust antifungal therapy if further courses of chemotherapy or stem cell transplantation are required in the future.

Reports of increased incidence of zygomycete infections in neutropenic patients is of concern. This trend has been noted since the early 2000s and may reflect increased use of an agent such as voriconazole, which has no activity against zygomycetes but excellent activity against other invasive molds and may select for this infection. There may be other reasons as well such as changes in immunosuppression or variability in the epidemiology of the organism. Either way, these organisms can present similarly to aspergillus. As with aspergillus, surgical debridement is a necessary adjunct to antifungal chemotherapy for therapeutic and diagnostic purposes. While awaiting the diagnostic test results, it may be prudent to use amphotericin B or one of its lipid formulations. If rhinosinusitis or pulmonary disease consistent with fungal infection occurs while the patient is on voriconazole or an echinocandin, zygomycete infection should be considered. The only agents currently active against these organisms are amphotericin B and a newer triazole, posaconazole. Posaconazole is available only as an oral agent. As with itraconazole, it requires a low pH to be absorbed, resulting in variable absorption. Multiple studies looking at posaconazole in the salvage setting for treatment of zygomycete infections have demonstrated its efficacy. As with aspergillus, prolonged therapy and evaluation with radiography to demonstrate improvement or cure is necessary.

Pneumocystis jiroveci (formerly *Pneomocystis carinii*) is seen in patients with leukemia or lymphoma—especially those who have been on steroids long term. *Pneumocystis jiroveci* is the cause of *P. carinii* pneumonia (PCP), which may present insidiously with progressive dyspnea, dry cough, and fever. When this presentation is noted, bronchoscopy with appropriate staining for the organism can be diagnostic. The yield of bronchoscopy for the diagnosis of PCP is lower in cancer patients than human immunodeficiency virus (HIV)-1–infected patients. Therapy including high-dose trimethoprim–sulfamethoxazole (and steroids if significant hypoxia is present) should be adequate for a duration of up to 3 weeks. In certain patients known to be at high risk for PCP, for example, preventative antibiotics are useful.

Other Organisms

Other organisms such as viruses may cause fever in the neutropenic patient, but they are not very common. Suspicion of viral infection requires understanding the correct epidemiological setting and obtaining appropriate serology or cultures. Atypical bacteria such as legionella, mycoplasma, or chlamydophila can cause pneumonia similarly as in those without neutropenia. Other gram-negative rods or gram-positive bacteria not mentioned earlier can be identified by appropriate cultures and treated based on their susceptibilities. Mycobacterial infections are not very common in the neutropenic but adequate cultures with acid-fast stains can usually establish the diagnosis. Appropriate therapy is determined by the organism and the site of infection but is similar to what is given to the non-neutropenic patient. The endemic fungi such as histoplasma or coccidioidomyces should be considered in the appropriate epidemiologic setting and treated similarly to the non-neutropenic patient. Finally, parasites should be considered where the epidemiology is appropriate and the symptoms are consistent with their diseases.

APPROACHES TO THE NEUTROPENIC PATIENT WITH FEVER

Prophylaxis

Granulocyte and granulocyte/monocyte colony-stimulating factors (CSFs) have been used in patients receiving chemotherapy to prevent neutropenia. The likelihood of developing neutropenia and subsequent fever is the driving factor for this approach. In controlled trials, human colony-stimulating factors have been shown to decrease the risk of febrile neutropenia and infection associated with intensive cancer chemotherapy. In one meta-analysis that reviewed patients who received cancer chemotherapy for either solid tumors or lymphoma, it was shown that rates of developing fever in those who received granulocyte colony-stimulating factor (G-CSF) was significantly lower than placebo. The use of G-CSF resulted in half the infections. In addition, they demonstrated that fewer patients needed a decrease in chemotherapy or delay of treatment. The major complication of G-CSF was bone pain. The policy on the use of CSFs in patients to prevent fever in patients with neutropenia is usually institution dependent.

Although not recommended by guidelines, there have been studies trying to answer the question of prophylactic antibiotics in the neutropenic patient. When blinded trials were analyzed, there was no reduction in the incidence of fever. When looking strictly at fluoroquinolones, there was a decrease in the incidence of fever. A recent study looking at >1500 patients with solid tumors or lymphoma showed that the use of levofloxacin decreased the incidence of febrile neutropenia from 85% to 65%. It also demonstrated a decreased rate of infection in the levofloxacin group. There was no difference in mortality.

There have been studies looking at antifungals as prophylaxis for invasive fungal infections. Fluconazole has been studied and has been shown to be effective in reducing fungal infections in stem cell recipients; however, the data are not as clear for individuals who have neutropenia due to cancer chemotherapy.

Itraconazole has been shown to be more effective than fluconazole; however, poor bioavailability and tolerability issues limit itraconazole. A recent study compared the use of posaconazole to either itraconazole or fluconazole in leukemic patients who had neutropenia. Posaconazole was shown to decrease infection with filamentous molds 10-fold and also decreased mortality. Side effects, mainly gastrointestinal in nature, were greater in the posaconazole group. At this point fungal prophylaxis is not universally recommended, but may be warranted in certain high-risk groups as these broader spectrum antifungals are more widely evaluated.

Empiric Therapy in the Neutropenic Patient with Fever

Historically, patients with neutropenia and fever were treated similarly to non-neutropenic patients. Some of these patients developed sepsis and increased morbidity and mortality before an infection was identified. Therefore, empiric therapy, especially for gram-negative infections, is recommended when they develop fever. However, over 50% of patients with neutropenia and fever have no identifiable cause. With better antibiotics and oral bioavailability, some neutropenic patients may be treated as outpatients and not require inpatient hospitalization; others need to be treated with intravenous antibiotics and monitored closely. Several risk prediction rules have been developed to identify low-risk patients. These are usually patients who have solid tumors receiving outpatient chemotherapy, those with no significant medical comorbidities, and expected neutropenia duration of about 7 days. These patients may be treated with oral agents or outpatient parenteral antibiotics. In randomized studies comparing ciprofloxacin + amoxicillin/clavulanate to ceftriaxone + amikacin, the outcomes were similar. Similar results were seen in this population when compared to ceftazidime. Careful attention to susceptibility patterns in the local area should be made, especially community-acquired methicillin-resistant *S. aureus* (MRSA) and gram-negative rods resistant to fluoroquinolones.

In patients who do not fit the criteria above, or have evidence of severe infection, hospital admission and empiric treatment with intravenous antibiotics is critical. Antibiotics should include gram-negative coverage. Potent single agents can be as effective as combination therapy. Acceptable empiric antibiotics are listed in Table 84.3.

Table 84.3 Antimicrobial Agents for Empiric Therapy in the Febrile Neutropenic Patient

Antibiotic[a],[b]
Ceftazadime
Cefepime
Imipenem
Meropenem
Piperacillin/tazobactam + aminoglycoside
Aztreonam + aminoglycoside

[a] If gram-positive infection is suspected, vancomycin can be added.
[b] If vancomycin allergic or suspect vancomycin-resistant enterococcus, alternative would be daptomycin, linezolid, or quinupristin/dalfopristin.

The role of empiric glycopeptides (eg, vancomycin) has been studied. In general this agent does not alter mortality in neutropenic patients and therefore is not required in all patients with neutropenia. Patients with significant risk for gram-positive infections should, however, receive vancomycin. These include patients with hypotension, significant oral mucositis, obvious skin or catheter site infections, or patients with a history of MRSA colonization. With increases in community-acquired MRSA, the use of vancomycin may be needed more frequently.

After patients have been started on empiric agents, reassessment of antibiotics at 3 to 5 days is necessary. By this time, results of cultures are available. If an infectious agent is identified, antibiotics can be tailored to that organism. If cultures are negative and the patient is still febrile, adjustment of antibiotics may be needed. Patients who are not on a glycopeptide could have vancomycin or a similar agent added. In those who are already on a glycopeptide, the glycopeptide could be stopped. In patients with continued fever at 5 days or in high-risk patients, an antifungal agent should be added to prevent or treat an indolent fungal infection.

The mainstay for empiric fungal therapy is amphotericin. There have been many studies comparing the newer azoles and echinocandins to amphotericin or one of its lipid formulations to empirically treat patients. These studies had composite endpoints including tolerability, time to fever resolution, prevention of fungal infections, and death. The azoles fluconazole and itraconazole have indications for empiric

Table 84.4 Antifungal Agents for Empiric Therapy in the Febrile Neutropenic Patient

Antifungal Agent
Amphotericin B
Liposomal amphotericin B
Amphotericin B lipid complex
Caspofungin
Itraconazole
Fluconazole
Voriconazole[a]

[a] Voriconazole is not approved for empiric therapy, but some experts prefer this agent.

antifungal therapy in the neutropenic patient with fever, whereas the newer agent, voriconazole, does not. Intuitively, there are concerns for the empiric use of fluconazole in this setting because it does not have activity against the molds or some *Candida* spp. A study comparing voriconazole to liposomal amphotericin B demonstrated that voriconazole was inferior to liposomal amphotericin B when looking at the composite score; however, there were significantly more fungal infections emerging in the amphotericin arm (21 vs 8). Many experts consider the balance of tolerability and efficacy to favor initiating voriconazole over amphotericin B. The echinocandin caspofungin was compared to liposomal amphotericin B with the results showing noninferiority of caspofungin (Table 84.4).

Adjunctive Agents

CSFs have been studied in febrile neutropenic patients. The results demonstrate decreased days of neutropenia in the patients who receive the CSFs. They have not been shown to decrease duration of fever, use of anti-infective agents, or cost. Importantly there has been no decrease in mortality. Therefore, the routine use of CSFs is not recommended.

White blood cell transfusions are not currently recommended as an adjunctive therapy for patients with neutropenia and fever. Transfusions have significant risk and toxicity. Some of the toxicities noted include transmission of viral infections such as cytomegalovirus, graft-versus-host reactions, and fever associated with transfusion reactions. Despite these risks, some centers do give transfusions to patients with refractory neutropenia and severe uncontrollable infections. At this point in time, this approach should be considered experimental and is best done in a clinical trial framework.

SUGGESTED READING

Bucaneve G, Micozzi A, Menichetti F, et al. Levofloxacin to prevent bacterial infection in patients with cancer and neutropenia. *N Engl J Med*. 2005;353:977–987.

Cornerly OA, Maertens J, Winston, DJ, et al. Posaconazole vs. fluconazole or itraconazole prophylaxis in patients with neutropenia. *N Engl J Med*. 2007;356:348–359.

Hughes WT, Armstrong D, Bodey GP, et al. 2002 Guidelines for the use of antimicrobial agents in neutropenic patients with cancer. *Clin Infect Dis*. 2002;34:730–751.

Kamana M, Escalante C, Mullen CA, et al. Bacterial infections in low-risk, febrile neutropenic patients: over a decade of experience at a comprehensive cancer center. *Cancer*. 2005;104:422–426.

Lyman GH, Kuderer NM, Djulbegovic B, et al. Prophylactic granulocyte colony-stimulating factor in patients receiving dose intensive cancer chemotherapy: a meta-analysis. *Am J Med*. 2002;112:406–411.

Walsh TJ, Pappas P, Winston DJ, et al. Voriconazole compared with liposomal amphotericin B for empirical antifungal therapy in patients with neutropenia and persistent fever. *N Engl J Med*. 2002;346:225–234.

85. Infections in Patients with Neoplastic Disease

Amar Safdar and Donald Armstrong

Patients with neoplastic disease and suspected infection come to the physician with the following main factors to be considered in their evaluation: (1) their epidemiologic background and (2) their known and unrecognized immune defect or defects including history of recurrent infections and familial/genetic predisposition to certain infections (Table 85.1). The febrile cancer patient raises the question whether the fever is caused by the neoplasm. After evaluation, the next question is whether to treat empirically. In this chapter, an approach to these patients is outlined, stressing the individuality of each patient along with the complexity of the evaluation.

EPIDEMIOLOGY

People may be exposed to a variety of organisms through travel, work, habits, or hobbies; in the home; or in other hospitals, outpatient clinics, and infusion centers. The right questions must be asked about their background. A person with children at home is likely to be exposed to a number of infectious agents such as influenza, parainfluenza, respiratory syncytial virus, varicella-zoster virus (VZV), human herpesvirus 6 (HHV6), and cytomegalovirus (CMV). Hospitals are a rich source of antibiotic-resistant microorganisms, including multidrug-resistant *Staphylococcus aureus* (MRSA), vancomycin-resistant and/or vancomycin-tolerant *Enterococcus* species, multidrug-resistant *Pseudomonas*, *Stenotrophomonas*, and extended-spectrum β-lactamase–producing *Enterobacteriaceae* such as *Escherichia coli* and *Klebsiella* species. It is important to know where an individual has been hospitalized and what resistance patterns are known to inhabit that hospital. Furthermore, as the spectrum of infection continues to change, it is imperative to follow these trends; just as community-acquired MRSA has recently surpassed hospitalization as a more common source of these resistant bacteria, other traditional risk factors for acquiring an infection may also change. In this regard, recent observations document life-threatening pulmonary infections due to *Stenotrophomonas*

maltophilia even in the absence of severe neutropenia or mechanical ventilation.

Systemic infections due to multiple organisms have been largely underrecognized, and the current paucity of published data regarding polymicrobial infections probably represents underreporting due to a lack of well-established definition and guidelines. Polymicrobial infections, including bloodstream, pulmonary, and urinary tract, account for ~15% of all infections in cancer patients. It is not uncommon to have gram-positive and gram-negative bacteremia along with *Candida* spp. bloodstream infection in severely immunosuppressed patients with orointestinal tract mucosal ulceration resulting from chemotherapy and/or radiation therapy.

With a thorough knowledge of the epidemiologic background of the patient, and therefore clues to possible causes of fever, the physician can direct investigation or start empiric antimicrobial therapy accordingly. The next step is to turn to the patient's underlying immune defect or defects to direct further evaluation and targets-specific empiric therapy. The immune dysfunction may result from the underlying cancer, antineoplastic therapy, including now-common use of monoclonal antibodies directed to interrupt immune pathways and hematopoietic stem cell transplantation. The organisms that must be considered in empiric therapy with reference to the host's immune dysfunction are listed in Table 85.1. In hospitalized patients, the organisms may be specific to the hospital and, therefore, an empiric regimen appropriate for one hospital may not be appropriate for another. The infectious complication also depends on the nature of the underlying neoplasm: In patients with a hematologic malignancy such as acute leukemia and lymphoma, the overall frequency is high (75% to 80%), whereas patients with solid tumors have substantially lower frequency of infection (≤30%) during the course of their disease.

NEUTROPHIL DEFECT

The most common neutrophil defect encountered in patients with malignancy is an absolute

Table 85.1 Infections Causing Pneumonia in Cancer Patients Based on the Underlying Immune Defect

Immune Defect (Associated Neoplastic Diseases)	Bacteria	Fungi	Parasites	Viruses
Granulocytopenia	*Staphylococcus aureus* *Streptococcus pneumoniae* *Streptococcus* spp. *Pseudomonas aeruginosa* Enterobacteriaceae *Escherichia coli* *Klebsiella* spp. *Stenotrophomonas maltophilia* *Acinetobacter* spp.	*Aspergillus fumigatus*; non-*fumigatus Aspergillus* Non-*Aspergillus* species hyalohyphomycosis such as *Pseudallescheria boydii*, *Fusarium solani*. *Mucorales* (zygomycoses) Dematiaceous (Black) fungi such as *Alternaria*, *Bipolaris, Curvularia*, *Scedosporium apiospermum* *Scedosporium prolificans*		Herpes simplex virus I and II VZV
Cellular immune dysfunction	*Nocardia asteroides* complex *Salmonella typhimurium* *Salmonella enteritidis* *Rhodococcus equi* *Rhodococcus bronchialis* *Listeria monocytogenes* *Mycobacterium tuberculosis* Nontuberculous mycobacteria *Legionella* spp.	*Aspergillus* and non-*Aspergillus* filamentous molds *Pneumocystis jiroveci* (*P. carinii*) *Cryptococcus neoformans* Endemic mycoses due to *Histoplasma capsulatum*, *Coccidioides immitis*, *Blastomyces dermatitidis*	*Toxoplasma gondii* *Microsporidium* spp. *Leishmania donovani* *Leishmania infantum* *Strongyloides stercoralis* *Cryptosporidium* *Cyclospora* spp.	Human cytomegalovirus Respiratory viruses Influenza A and Influenza B Parainfluenza type-3 Respiratory syncytial virus Adenovirus VZV HHV6 SARS-associated coronavirus? Parvovirus B19 Paramyxovirus? Hantavirus?
Humoral immune dysfunction and Splenectomy	*S. pneumoniae* *Haemophilus influenzae* *Neisseria meningitidis* *Capnocytophaga canimorsus* *Campylobacter*	*P. jiroveci* (*P. carinii*)?	*Giardia lamblia* *Babesia microti*	VZV Echovirus Enterovirus
Mixed defects	*S. pneumoniae* *S. aureus* *H. influenzae* *Klebsiella pneumonia*	*P. jiroveci* (*P. carinii*) *Aspergillus* spp *Candida* spp *C. neoformans*	*Toxoplasma gondii* *Strongyloides stercoralis*	Respiratory viruses Influenza Parainfluenza Respiratory syncytial virus
	P. aeruginosa *Acinetobacter* spp *Enterobacter* spp *S. maltophilia* *Nocardia asteroides* complex *L. monocytogenes* *Legionella* spp	*Mucorales* (zygomycoses) Endemic mycoses (severe systemic dissemination)		Adenovirus VZV

Abbreviation: HHV6 = human herpesvirus 6; SARS = severe acute respiratory syndrome; VZV = varicella-zoster virus.
Note: Patients with mixed immune defects includes recipients of allogeneic hematopoietic stem cell transplant; acute or chronic graft versus host disease; myelodysplastic syndrome; adult T-cell leukemia lymphoma, antineoplastic agents such as cyclophosphamide, fludarabine, *L. donovani*, and *L. infantum* may lead to serious visceral leishmaniasis. *L. donovani* is seen in Africa and Asia, *L. infantum* is seen in Africa, Europe, Mediterranean, Central and South America. VZV is rarely associated with systemic dissemination in patients with humoral immune defects, or even those with mixed immune dysfunctions. *Strongyloides stercoralis* may lead to serious, life-threatening hyperinfection syndrome in patients with marked cellular immune defects.

The Susceptible Host

neutropenia following cytotoxic chemotherapy. Patients with acute myelogenous leukemia, aplastic anemia, or myelodysplastic syndrome may present with severe neutropenia (≤500 cells/μL) due to the underlying disease. When doing the history and physical examination and evaluating laboratory and radiographic results, it should be remembered that neutropenic patients do not make pus. Physical signs may be absent or altered, as may x-ray findings. After careful evaluation, if there is no obvious site of infection, such as cellulitis or pneumonia, the source of infection is often the gastrointestinal tract, and empiric therapy should be directed against the organisms anticipated to be in that patient's intestinal flora at that time. These flora will vary according to the hospital the patient is in or has been in, previous courses of antibiotics, and other epidemiologic factors (see Chapter 84, Infections in the Neutropenic Patient). Recently, despite an overall increase in bloodstream infections due to gram-positive bacteria such as *Staphylococcus* spp., *Pseudomonas* spp. have remained an important cause of serious systemic infection in patients with febrile neutropenia. However, *Viridans streptococci* can lead to rapidly fulminant sepsis, disseminated intravascular coagulation, multiorgan failure, and shock in neutropenic patients with treatment-induced disruption of orointestinal mucosa.

Patients with prolonged neutropenia (>2 weeks) are at increased risk of invasive fungal infections (IFI). With the frequent use of fluconazole prophylaxis in high-risk neutropenic patients, a decline in systemic candidiasis has been encouraging, although this has led to a risk in infections due to drug-resistant *Candida* spp. such as *Candida glabrata* and *Candida krusei*. *Aspergillus* spp. account for most IFIs, although in the past decade a risk in nonamphotericin B–susceptible mold infections has raised serious concern regarding the emergence of these difficult-to-treat IFIs. Furthermore, increased use of *Aspergillus* active azole-based drugs such as voriconazole has resulted in a higher number of cases of sinupulmonary zygomycosis.

HELPER T-LYMPHOCYTE DEFECTS

$CD4^+$ lymphocyte–mononuclear phagocyte defects are seen regularly in patients with underlying lymphomas, such as Hodgkin's disease, peripheral T-cell lymphoma, and those with leukemia, such as acute lymphoblastic, hairy cell leukemia, human T-lymphotrophic virus 1–associated adult T-cell leukemia lymphoma, recipients of allogeneic hematopoietic stem cell transplantation (HSCT), and patients receiving treatment for graft-versus-host disease (GVHD). Antineoplastic therapy that disrupts the adaptive cellular immune response includes high-dose systemic corticosteroids given for extended duration; irradiation therapy; treatment with fludarabine and other purine analogs; and cyclosporine, tacrolimus, and antithymocyte globulins used in the treatment of GVHD. These patients are prey to an entirely different group of opportunistic pathogens than are patients with neutrophil defects as shown in the Table 85.1. Some of these, such as *Mycobacterium tuberculosis, Nocardia asteroides,* and CMV, produce subacute as well as acute disease, and immediate empiric therapy may not be necessary. In other instances, however, optimal specimens should be collected and empiric therapy instituted for a subacute infection that can become acute and produce rapidly fatal disease in the severely immunosuppressed individual. Examples are tuberculosis, histoplasmosis, and pneumocystosis. If a patient with a severe T-cell defect does have fever and looks toxic without specific signs or symptoms and if there is any question about a B-lymphocyte defect, empiric therapy that covers pneumocystosis (even with negative chest radiographic findings), salmonellosis, and pneumococcus should be initiated. A reasonable regimen for this is ceftriaxone plus trimethoprim–sulfamethoxazole.

In patients with complex cellular immune defects such as those with GVHD receiving corticosteroids, infections due to filamentous fungi such as *Aspergillus* species and nonamphotericin B–susceptible *Pseudallescheria boydii, Scedosporium* species, and other black (dematiaceous) fungi may present with asymptomatic pulmonary, sinus, and/or skin lesions. If appropriate therapy with an effective antifungal agent such as voriconazole is delayed, the progressive invasive fungal disease may extend locally and disseminate to the brain. These infections at that stage are often refractory to therapy. However, there are indications that immune enhancement strategies with recombinant growth factors such as granulocyte macrophage colony-stimulating factor and a proinflammatory cytokine such as interferon-γ may be beneficial in select groups of cancer patients with difficult-to-treat invasive fungal infections. Because voriconazole is often preferred to amphotericin B as the drug of choice for the treatment of systemic aspergillosis, a rise in invasive zygomycosis is concerning. Patients who are at a higher risk include patients with refractory leukemia, prolonged neutropenia, corticosteroid therapy, diabetes mellitus, and involvement of paranasal sinuses. In these patients treatment should include lipid formulations of amphotericin B (AmBisome or Abelcet), although recent experience with posaconazole has led to favorable outcomes in cancer and stem cell transplant recipients with life-threatening zygomycosis. Because the outcome is so poor in these patients when treated wth conventional therapy, other modalities have been tried, including combination antifungals (posaconazole plus Abelcet), hyperbaric oxygen therapy, granulocyte colony-stimulating factor–mobilized donor granulocyte transfusions, and recombinant cytokine therapy.

SPLENIC AND B-CELL DEFECTS

Patients without a spleen develop extraordinarily severe infections caused by *Streptococcus pneumoniae* (see Chapter 95, Overwhelming Postsplenectomy Infection). They may also develop generally less severe infections caused by *Haemophilus influenzae* and *Neisseria meningitidis*. These must be treated early and intensively. With the emergence of penicillin-resistant pneumococci, an empiric regimen should contain ceftriaxone and vancomycin. Infections with these same organisms are seen in patients with B-cell defects, especially those caused by multiple myeloma and chronic lymphocytic leukemia in whom hypogammaglobulinemia may be severe and prolonged. In all of these patients, the disease resulting from these encapsulated organisms can be especially severe, with accompanying bacteremias, often with no obvious source. The defect may last for years, and, because of humoral immune dysfunction, these patients may respond poorly to conventional vaccines. Methods to improve vaccine response in patients with B-cell defects are currently being explored. Therefore, at present, antibiotic prophylaxis is recommended in cancer patients who are at increased risk of serious pneumococcal disease.

SUMMARY

Evaluation of infections in the patient with neoplastic disease depends on multiple fac-

tors, which include (1) the epidemiologic background of the patient, (2) the immune defect or defects, (3) the resident organisms in a given hospital that could be responsible, and (4) clinical judgment. The first three can be estimated easily. The last requires considerable bedside experience, and, in general, it is prudent to err on the side of treatment rather than observation.

SUGGESTED READING

Aisenberg G, Rolston KV, Dickey BF, Kontoyiannis DP, Raad II, Safdar A. *Stenotrophomonas maltophilia* pneumonia in cancer patients without traditional risk factors for infection, 1997–2004. *Eur J Clin Microbiol Infect Dis.* 2007;26:13–20.

Armstrong D. Empiric therapy for the immunocompromised host. *Rev Infect Dis.* 1991;13: S763–S769.

Freifeld AC. Infectious complication in the immunocompromised host: the antimicrobial armamentarium. *Hematol Oncol Clin North Am.* 1993;7:813–839.

Kumashi P, Girgawy E, Tarrand JJ, Rolston KV, Raad II, Safdar A. *Streptococcus pneumoniae* bacteremia in patients with cancer: disease characteristics and outcomes in the era of escalating drug resistance (1998–2002). *Medicine (Baltimore).* 2005;84:303–312.

Quie PG, Solberg CO. Infections in the immunocompromised host. In: Armstrong D, Cohen J, eds. *Infectious Diseases.* London: Mosby; 1999.

Roden MM, Zaoutis TE, Buchanan WL, et al. Epidemiology and outcome of zygomycosis: a review of 929 reported cases. *Clin Infect Dis.* 2005;41:634–653.

Roslton KV, Bodey GP, Safdar A. Polymicrobial infections in cancer patients: an underappreciated and underreported entity. *Clin Infect Dis.* 2007;45:228.

Safdar A, Armstrong D. Infectious morbidity in critically ill patients with cancer. *Crit Care Clin.* 2001;17:531–570, vii–viii.

Safdar A. Strategies to enhance immune function in hematopoietic transplantation recipients who have fungal infections. *Bone Marrow Transplant.* 2006;38:327–337.

86. Corticosteroids, Cytotoxic Agents, and Infection

Babafemi O. Taiwo and Robert L. Murphy

Iatrogenic immunosuppression can be achieved using corticosteroids or noncorticosteroid agents. Although there is considerable overlap, noncorticosteroid immunosuppressants can be broadly divided into those that are primarily cytotoxic antineoplastic drugs and those that are used primarily in transplantation. Advances in immunosuppressive therapy have greatly decreased morbidity and mortality attributable to transplantation rejection and autoimmune diseases, but the cellular targets of immunosuppressive agents are frequently the cornerstones of the body's defenses against pathogenic microorganisms. As a result of this double-edged action, the use of immunosuppressants involves walking a fine line between therapy and iatrogenic harm. Indeed, with the advent of powerful immunosuppressive agents, there has been an emergence of a wider spectrum of infections.

The specific type of agent, the dosage used, the length of therapy, and the underlying disease process all affect the incidence and type of infectious complication likely to occur with immunosuppressive therapy. Understanding the mechanism of action of these agents will aid in determining the appropriate immunization/prophylaxis, and in choosing the appropriate empiric therapy in patients with signs of infection.

CORTICOSTEROIDS

Mechanisms of Action

Corticosteroids are powerful anti-inflammatory agents capable of quantitative and qualitative suppression of the immune system. In the case of an overaggressive immune response to antigenic stimuli, corticosteroids may benefit patients by decreasing the inflammatory response.

Corticosteroids suppress immunity by blocking lymphocyte proliferation through inhibition of the production of interleukins 1 and 6 (IL-1 and IL-6) in macrophages. They also reduce the formation of other cytokines such as IL-2, IL-4, interferon-γ, leukotrienes,

tumor necrosis factor (TNF), and prostaglandins. In addition, corticosteroids reduce adhesion molecules on endothelial cells and inhibit the migration of granulocytes to the sites of infection. Indirectly, corticosteroids cause defective phagocytosis due to their effect on glucose homeostasis. Antibody formation and turnover are also affected especially at high dosages and with prolonged use, and there may be reversible lymphopenia and monocytopenia. Collectively, these effects lead to inhibition of T-cell proliferation, cytotoxic T-cell response, and antigen-specific immune responses.

The clinical consequences of corticosteroid administration include increased susceptibility to intracellular pathogens, decrease in the response to delayed skin test hypersensitivity, and blockage of the normal febrile response. There is essentially no bone marrow suppression.

Corticosteroid Use in Infectious Diseases

The immunologic and/or inflammatory response to a pathogen may be excessive and deleterious to the host. Because the inflammatory mediators of tissue damage such as TNF, IL-1, and interferon-γ commonly cause significant injury at sites distant from the initiating infection, the systemic anti-inflammatory properties of corticosteroids may provide clinical benefit. The effectiveness of corticosteroid therapy in a variety of infections such as herpes zoster is controversial, but its beneficial role is established for infections such as hypoxemic *Pneumocystis jirovecii* (formerly *Pneumocystis carinii*) pneumonia (PCP). Table 86.1 outlines disease processes for which there is moderate to good evidence that corticosteroids are useful.

Corticosteroids and Risk of Infection

Myriad pathogens are associated with impaired cellular immunity and corticosteroid use (Table 86.2). Most of the organisms listed rarely cause significant or life-threatening infections in the immunocompetent patient. Some, such

Table 86.1 Infections/Complications of Infections with Moderate to Good Evidence That Adjuvant Corticosteroid Use Has Benefit

Infection	Corticosteroid Therapy
Acute bacterial meningitis caused by *Hemophilus influenzae* type B in children or *Streptococcus pneumoniae* in adults	Dexamethasone 0.15 mg/kg q6h × 4 d
Pneumocystis jirovecii pneumonia, $PO_2 \leq 70$ mm Hg in HIV-infected patients	Prednisone 40 mg BID × 5 d, then 40 mg qd × 5 d, then 20 mg qd for 11 d
Acute severe laryngotracheobronchitis (croup)	Dexamethasone >0.3 mg/kg qd × 3–4 d
Allergic bronchopulmonary Aspergillosis	Prednisone 45–60 mg qd until infiltrate clears then taper
Typhoid fever, critically ill with mental status changes or shock	High-dose dexamethasone × 2–3 d
Tuberculous pericarditis and meningitis	Prednisone 60–80 mg qd for several weeks followed by taper

Abbreviations: HIV = human immunodeficiency virus.

as *P. jirovecii,* cause disease only in immuno-compromised individuals.

Patients with severe opportunistic infections often have concurrent underlying impairment of cellular immunity separate from the iatrogenic impairment secondary to steroid use. Thus, the risk of infection varies by underlying disease process. For instance, patients with acquired immunodeficiency syndrome (AIDS) or childhood acute lymphocytic leukemia have higher rates of PCP than patients without these diseases but receiving chronic corticosteroid therapy. For patients requiring chronic corticosteroid therapy, the infection rate for many of the pathogens listed in Table 86.2 is actually quite low. Overall, the risk increases with the dose and duration of use and may be increased by concomitant administration of other immunosuppressants.

CYTOTOXIC ANTINEOPLASTIC AGENTS

Mechanisms of Action

Cancer itself is an immunocompromised state, but clinically significant infections in cancer patients are often related to the effects of cytotoxic antineoplastic agents. Although these agents are primarily cancer chemotherapeutic drugs, they are also used in hematopoietic stem cell transplantation and severe autoimmune disorders. In general, cytotoxic antineoplastic agents are antiproliferative, inhibit DNA and/or RNA synthesis, and are bone marrow suppressive. They act against both B and T

lymphocytes. The oldest class of these drugs is the alkylating agents, such as cyclophosphamide, busulphan, melphalan, and chlorambucil. The purine analogs fludarabine, pentostatin (2′-deoxycoformycin), and cladribine (2-chloro-2′-deoxyadenosine) constitute another important class.

Cytotoxic Antineoplastic Agents and Risk of Infection

Inhibition of proliferative cell types by cytotoxic antineoplastic agents is important for their immunosuppressive effect, but the associated decrease in the number of lymphocytes, monocytes, and granulocytes increases the risk of a variety of infections. One of the most common infectious complications of antineoplastic agents is bacterial infection from neutropenia. Because leukocytes are continuously replenished, this effect is typically reversible. When granulocytopenia is prolonged, patients become at risk for fungal pathogens such as *Aspergillus* and *Candida* species. Cytotoxic agents also cause variable decline in the level of serum immunoglobulins, numerical reduction in lymphocytes, changes in the ratio of B lymphocytes to T lymphocytes, or changes in ratio of CD4+ T lymphocytes to CD8+ T lymphocytes. The latter effects predispose patients to the intracellular pathogens listed in Table 86.2. Importantly, antineoplastic agents are different in their propensity for immunosuppression. For example, vincristine appears less likely to cause

Table 86.2 Pathogens Associated with Corticosteroid Use or Other Causes of Cellular Immunodeficiency

Bacteria

Legionella pneumophilia
Listeria monocytogenes
Mycobacterium tuberculosis
Nocardia species
Salmonella species
Rhodococcus equi

Fungi

Blastomyces dermatitidis
Candida species
Coccidioides immitis
Histoplasma capsulatum
Cryptococcus neoformans
Aspergillus species

Helminths

Strongyloides stercoralis
Protozoa
Cryptosporidium parvum
Pneumocystis jirovecii
Toxoplasma gondii
Plasmodia species

Viruses

Cytomegalovirus
Epstein–Barr
Herpes simplex
Varicella-zoster
Influenza

Table 86.3 Noncorticosteroid Immunosuppressive Agents in Transplantation

Immunobinding Agents Mechanism

Cyclosporine inhibition of calcineurin
Tacrolimus inhibition of calcineurin
Sirolimus (rapamycin) inhibition of target of rapamycin and IL-2–dependent T-cell proliferation

Antimetabolites

Azathioprine inhibition of purine metabolism and DNA synthesis
Mycophenolate mofetil inhibition of purine metabolism and DNA synthesis
Mycophenolic acid inhibition of purine metabolism and DNA synthesis

Biologic Products

OKT3 (muromanab-CD3 antibody) depletion of T cells
Polyclonal antithymocyte globulin (ATG): dysfunction and depletion of T cells
Alemtuzumab (monoclonal anti-CD52 antibody): depletion of T cells, B cells, thymocytes, monocytes
Rituximab (monoclonal anti-CD20 antibody): depletion of B cells
Daclizimab (monoclonal anti-CD25 antibody): inhibition of T-cell proliferation to IL-2
Basiliximab (monoclonal anti-CD25 antibody): inhibition of T-cell proliferation to IL-2

Abbreviation: IL = interleukin.

infectious complications compared to more toxic agents.

The infectious complications of purine analogs deserve special mention because these agents cause profound lymphopenia plus selective suppression (delayed recovery) of CD4+ T lymphocytes that may last several years after administration. Thus, patients have infection risks not dissimilar to what occurs in patients with AIDS. Infections caused by cytomegalovirus. *Pneumocystis jirovecii*, and *Listeria monocytogenes* are particular risks when corticosteroids are used concomitantly.

TRANSPLANT IMMUNOSUPPRESSANTS
Mechanisms of Action

Two of the most commonly used antirejection agents in transplantation (Table 86.3) are the calcineurin inhibitors cyclosporine and tacrolimus. Other agents include antimetabolites and biologic agents.

Cyclosporine is a cyclic polypeptide that binds to cytoplasmic immunophilin (cyclophilin), creating a cyclosporine–cyclophilin complex capable of inhibiting the action of the enzyme calcineurin. Because calcineurin is essential for the transcriptional process through which IL-2 and other cytokines are activated, cyclosporine inhibits growth and proliferation of T lymphocytes. There is relative sparing of B-cell function and absence of bone marrow suppression. Cyclosporine alone is associated with relatively low rates of infectious complications; however, it is commonly combined with other immunosuppressive agents such as prednisone to derive synergistic immunosuppression.

Tacrolimus is a macrolide produced by the fungus *Streptomyces tsukubaensis*. It binds to another immunophilin FKBP 12, forming tacrolimus–FKBP 12 complex that inhibits the action of calcineurin and the production of IL-2 in T lymphocytes. Overall, tacrolimus is a more potent immunosuppressant than cyclosporine, but these agents appear to result in comparable rates of patient and graft survival posttransplantation.

Rapamycin (sirolimus) is another macrolide antibiotic. Derived from *Streptomyces hygroscopicus*, it also binds to FKBP 12. However, its mechanism of action is different: It blocks

T-lymphocyte proliferation that is dependent on "target of rapamycin" and IL-2.

The antimetabolites azathioprine and mycophenolate mofetil (metabolized to active mycophenolic acid) are used in solid organ transplantation, often as adjuncts to calcineurin inhibitors. Azathioprine is a purine antagonist that inhibits DNA and RNA synthesis. Mycophenolate mofetil and mycophenolic acid also inhibit the synthesis of purine and block DNA synthesis in B and T lymphocytes. Antimetabolites are bone marrow suppressive when administered in large doses. A newer agent, leflunomide, is a pyrimidine synthesis inhibitor that is used also in rheumatoid arthritis.

Biologic transplant immunosuppressants include monoclonal or polyclonal antibodies that target and destroy T lymphocytes and/or B lymphocytes. They can be subclassified as depleting or nondepleting proteins. The more commonly used depleting proteins are antithymocyte globulin (ATG), OKT3 (muromonab-CD3), alemtuzimab, and rituximab. ATG is a preparation of polyclonal antibodies derived when horses or rabbits are immunized with human thymus lymphocytes. It targets different epitopes on T lymphocytes, resulting in depletion of T lymphocytes and a decrease in proliferation of newly formed lymphocytes. OKT3 is a mouse monoclonal antibody that binds to CD3 receptors on the surface of T lymphocytes. Within minutes of infusion, circulating T lymphocytes become virtually undetectable. There are uncommon reports of drug-induced meningitis during or after infusion of OKT3. Alemtuzimab (anti-CD52) is also associated with profound impairment of cellular immunity. The immunosuppressive effects of depleting proteins can persist for months or years. For example, proliferative response of lymphocytes may remain impaired after infused antibodies are no longer detectable and the quantity of circulating T lymphocytes has returned to normal. Therefore, it is always essential to know all the immunosuppressive agents to which a patient had been previously exposed when assessing the specific immunodeficiency state.

Nondepleting proteins reduce immune responsiveness without depleting T cells or B cells. Thus, they carry much lower infection risks compared with depleting antibodies. Daclizimab and basiliximab are examples of nondepleting monoclonal anti-CD 25 antibodies that block the IL-2 receptors on T lymphocytes. These agents have not been associated with an increased risk of infection conclusively, although clinical experience is still very limited.

Table 86.4 Some of the Pathogens Encountered in Patients with Deficiencies in Humoral Immunity and/or Granulocytopenia

Gram-negative Bacilli

Escherichia coli
Klebsiella species
Pseudomonas aeruginosa
Enterobacter cloacae
Hemophilus influenzae
Serratia species
Proteus species
Salmonella species

Gram-positive Cocci

Staphylococcus aureus
Staphylococcus epidermidis
Streptococcus pneumoniae
Streptococcus pyogenes
Enterococcus species

Anaerobes

Bacteroides species
Clostridium species
Fusobacterium species

Parasites

Giardia lamblia

Fungi

Candida species
Aspergillus species

TRANSPLANT IMMUNOSUPPRESSANTS AND RISK OF INFECTION (SEE CHAPTER 87, INFECTIONS IN TRANSPLANT PATIENTS)

The infectious disease complication is dictated by the induced immunosuppression. Because the immune defect usually involves T cells, intracellular pathogens (Table 86.2) are the primary culprit. Thus, cyclosporine therapy, which blocks T-lymphocyte activation and inhibits cell-mediated immunity, is likely to result in infection with an intracellular pathogen. Likewise, treatment with OKT3, ALG, tacrolimus, methotrexate, and azathioprine are also likely to inhibit cell-mediated immunity and increase the risk of infection with an intracellular pathogen. Special consideration should be made for *Mycobacterium tuberculosis*, endemic fungi, *Cryptococcus*, PCP, and herpesviridae.

In situations where the main defect involves B lymphocytes and primary antibody responses, infections with extracellular bacteria (Table 86.4) are more likely. Other factors that are predictive of the infectious complication posttransplant include the time elapsed since transplantation, underlying disease, and the presence of active or latent infections in the transplant recipient or donor. In general, infections in the first month posttransplant are caused by bacteria or *Candida* and often are related to the hospitalization and the surgical procedure. With the exception of herpes simplex virus reactivation, opportunistic infections due to transplant immunosuppressants occur after 1 month posttransplant. Epstein–Barr virus is unique in that it can cause posttransplant lymphoproliferative disorder, typically after 6 months posttransplant. Appropriate prophylaxis or empiric therapy is necessary to minimize the infectious complications of transplant immunosuppression.

Organ transplantation of human immunodeficiency virus (HIV)-infected patients is a promising new frontier with emerging challenges. For example, some immunosuppressants cause profound decline in CD4+ T-cell counts, and coadministration of protease inhibitors and some immunosuppressants (such as calcineurin inhibitors) can predispose to toxic levels of the immunosuppressant. Preliminary reports have suggested a higher risk of rejection among HIV-infected solid organ recipients compared to those who are not HIV-infected. The effect of organ transplantation and transplant immunosuppression on the morbidity and mortality gains attributable to highly active antiretroviral therapy (HAART) is currently unknown.

SUGGESTED READING

Dummer JS. Risk factors and approaches to infections in transplant recipients. In: Mandell GL, Bennett JE, Dolin R, eds. *Principles and Practice of Infectious Diseases*, 6th ed. Philadelphia, PA: Churchill Livingstone; 2005:3476–3486.

Lake DF, Briggs AD, Akporiaye ET. Immunopharmacology. In: Katzung BG, ed. *Basic and Clinical Pharmacology*, 9th ed. New York, NY: McGraw-Hill; 2004:931–957.

Renoult E, Buteau C, Lamarre V, Turgeon N, Tapiero B. Infectious risk in pediatric organ transplant recipients: is it increased with the new immunosuppressive agents? *Pediatr Transplant*. 2005;9(4):470–479.

Simon DM, Levin S. Infectious complications of solid organ transplantations. *Infect Dis Clin North Am*. 2001;15(2):521–549.

Van Burik J, Weisdorf D. Infections in recipients of hematopoietic stem cell transplantation. In: Mandell, Bennett, and Dolin, ed. *Principles and Practice of Infectious Diseases*, 6th ed. Philadelphia, PA: Churchill Livingstone; 2005:3486–3501.

Corticosteroids, Cytotoxic Agents, and Infection

Raymund R. Razonable and Carlos V. Paya

INTRODUCTION

Collectively, infections are the single most common complication of organ and tissue transplantation. Virtually any bacterial, fungal, viral, and parasitic pathogen can cause clinical disease in a transplant recipient. Several factors inherent to the transplant recipient or related to the donor, the environment, and the circumstances surrounding the transplant procedure (such as surgical techniques and immunosuppressive drugs) remarkably increase the risk of infectious complications. Generally, the overall infection risk is determined by (1) epidemiologic exposures and (2) the net state of immunosuppression.

RISK FACTORS OF INFECTION AFTER TRANSPLANTATION

Epidemiologic Exposures

The major sources of pathogens are (1) the transplant recipient who may harbor latent, active, or subclinical infection prior to transplantation; (2) the donor who may harbor latent, active, or subclinical infection that could be transmitted through the allograft; and (3) the environment surrounding the immunocompromised transplant patient. Table 87.1 lists some risk factors for acquiring infection after solid organ transplantation.

THE TRANSPLANT RECIPIENT

The epidemiologic exposures of potential transplant recipients should be assessed to determine the risk of infection and guide preventive measures. Table 87.2 lists the recommended screening tests in the evaluation of potential recipients (and their donors) prior to transplantation; these include screening for herpes simplex virus (HSV) 1 and 2, varicella-zoster virus (VZV), Epstein–Barr virus (EBV), cytomegalovirus (CMV), human T-cell lymphotrophic virus (HTLV) I/II, hepatitis viruses, *Mycobacterium tuberculosis*, *Toxoplasma gondii*, and *Treponema pallidum*. A more detailed history will often reveal the need for specialized screening in some patients. For example, patients from endemic areas should be screened for infections with human herpesvirus 8 (HHV8), *Coccidioides immitis*, *Strongyloides stercoralis*, and *Trypanosoma cruzi*. In some cases, the evaluation will reveal active infection in the transplant candidate. For example, bacterial cholangitis and spontaneous bacterial peritonitis are not uncommon prior to liver transplantation, although pacemaker device–associated infections or infections related to vascular catheters may be observed in patients awaiting heart and kidney transplantation, respectively. Pulmonary infections are not uncommon in lung transplant candidates. Although these infections do not generally preclude transplantation, they should be adequately controlled prior to and after the transplant procedure.

THE TRANSPLANT DONOR

The epidemiologic exposures of transplant donors should be determined so that the potential for allograft-transmitted infections is reduced. Screening for CMV, EBV, *T. gondii*, hepatitis B and C viruses, and human immunodeficiency virus (HIV) are routinely performed (Table 87.2). Routine screening may not always be possible, particularly for unusual and rare infections. For example, cases of allograft-transmitted *Histoplasma capsulatum*, *Cryptococcus neoformans*, lymphocytic choriomeningitis virus, rabies virus, and West Nile virus (WNV) have been observed rarely. In some areas, screening for pathogens that are endemic to the region may also be performed, including tests for HHV8 and *C. immitis*.

THE ENVIRONMENT

The health care environment is a major source of pathogens that cause disease in immunocompromised transplant recipients. Invasive procedures, such as the insertion of indwelling urinary catheters, intravascular catheters, and endotracheal tubes often provide avenues to which pathogens gain entry into the host. Blood products have also classically served as vehicles for pathogen transmission. For example, WNV has been transmitted through blood

Table 87.1 Some of the Risk Factors for Acquiring Infection Following Solid Organ Transplantation

Preoperative Period	Intraoperative Period	Postoperative Period
Lack of pathogen-specific immunity	Presence of pathogens in the transplant allograft	Prolonged hospitalization
Severity of underlying clinical illness	Prolonged operative time	Prolonged duration of stay in intensive care unit
Fulminant hepatic failure	Complicated surgical procedure	Prolonged antibiotic use
Renal insufficiency	Profound blood loss and infusion of large volume of blood products	Renal insufficiency
Anemia	Choleduchojejunostomy	Gastrointestinal and biliary complications
Prior fungal infection (ie, endemic mycoses)		Vascular complications
		Steroid use and treatment of allograft rejection
		Immunosuppresive drugs
		CMV and HHV6 reactivation
		Reoperation within 1 mo posttransplantation
		Retransplantation

Abbreviations: HHV = human herpesvirus; CMV = cytomegalovirus.

transfusion. The surgical procedure, which causes breaks in skin and mucous membranes, increases the infection risk, especially when it is prolonged or complicated and if it involves areas of high microbial content (gastrointestinal tract). Hospital construction is classically associated with increased risk of *Aspergillus* spp. infections. Numerous gram-positive and gram-negative bacteria may be acquired in the nosocomial setting, including *Legionella pneumophila,* multidrug-resistant *Pseudomonas aeruginosa*, vancomycin-resistant enterococci, and methicillin-resistant *Staphylococcus aureus*.

Many infections are acquired from the community where natural transmission of pathogens continually occurs. Influenza, parainfluenza, metapneumovirus, and respiratory syncytial virus (RSV) cause seasonal respiratory diseases in transplant patients. Pneumonia due to *Streptococcus pneumoniae, Haemophilus influenza, Mycoplasma pneumonia*, and *Chlamydia* spp. are commonly acquired in the community. Pneumonia and bacteremia due to encapsulated organisms are especially common in transplant patients with severe pharmacologically induced hypogammaglobulinemia. Community-acquired skin and soft tissue infections are most often due to *Staphylococcus* spp. and *Streptococcus* spp. although atypical mycobacteria and fungal pathogens such as *Cryptococcus neoformans* should also be considered. Opportunistic pathogens should be considered especially during periods of highest risk; these include *Pneumocystis jiroveci, Listeria monocytogenes, Toxoplasma gondii,* and *Cryptococcus neoformans*. Table 87.3 lists the epidemiologic exposures and the pathogens associated with the specific exposure.

Table 87.2 Recommended Infectious Disease Screening Tools in the Evaluation of Donors and Recipients Prior to Transplantation

Human immunodeficiency virus (HIV) antibody
Herpes simplex virus (HSV) 1 and 2 antibody
Cytomegalovirus (CMV) antibody
Epstein–Barr virus (EBV) antibody panel
Varicella-zoster virus (VZV) antibody
Toxoplasma antibody (in heart recipients)
Rapid plasma reagin test for syphilis
Human T-cell lymphotrophic virus (HTLV) I and II antibody
Hepatitis C virus (HCV) antibody
Hepatitis B virus (HBV) surface antigen
HBV surface antibody
HBV core immunoglobulin (IgM) and IgG antibody
PPD skin testing
Strongyloides serology (with stool ova and parasites for candidates from endemic areas)
Coccidioides serology (for candidates from endemic areas)
Trypanozoma cruzi (for donors and recipients from endemic areas)
West Nile virus (nucleic acid testing for living donors)

Net State of Immunosuppression

Two major factors influence the overall net state of immunosuppression: (1) pharmacologic immunosuppression and (2) the reactivation of

Table 87.3 Epidemiologic Exposures and Various Examples of Associated Pathogens in the Evaluation of Transplant Patients with Infectious Syndromes

Community-acquired Infections	
Residence in endemic areas	*Mycobacterium tuberculosis, Strongyloides stercoralis, Blastomyces dermatitidis, Histoplasma capsulatum, Coccidiodes immitis, Trypanozoma cruzi,* human herpesvirus 8
Exposure to index cases	*Mycobacterium tuberculosis,* respiratory viruses (influenza, parainfluenza, respiratory syncitial virus, adenoviruses)
Ingestion of contaminated water and food	*Salmonella* species, *Campylobacter jejuni, Listeria monocytogenes, Giardia lamblia*
Environmental source	*Aspergillus fumigatus, Nocardia asteroides, Sporothrix schenkii*
Vector-borne	West Nile virus
Nosocomial Infections	
Contaminated air	*Aspergillus fumigatus*
Contaminated water	*Legionella pneumophila*
Hand contact	Methicillin-resistant *Staphylococcus aureus,* vancomycin-resistant enterococci, drug-resistant gram-negative bacilli

immunomodulating viruses. The use of immunosuppressive drugs is essential to maintain allograft survival (for solid organ transplant [SOT] recipients) and to prevent graft-versus-host disease (in allogeneic hematopoietic stem cell transplant [HSCT] recipients). The degree of immunosuppression is particularly intense during the first 3 months after transplantation and could result in the impairment of cellular and humoral immunity. Although defect in cell-mediated immunity is a well-recognized effect of the immunosuppressive drugs, impairment in humoral immunity, as indicated by severe hypogammaglobulinemia, may also occur. Unfortunately, the use of immunosuppressive drugs (eg, mycophenolate mofetil [MMF], prednisone, tacrolimus, cyclosporine, alemtuzumab, among others) places the patients at very high risk of infectious complications. For example, OKT3 monoclonal antibody and antithymocyte globulin increases the risk of CMV disease and other opportunistic infections such as HHV6, *Aspergillus* spp., and *Pneumocystis jiroveci* and could accelerate the clinical course of posttransplant hepatitis C virus (HCV) infection. Severe hypogammaglobulinemia after transplantation may increase the risk of infections with encapsulated organisms. The reactivation of viruses with immunomodulating properties, such as CMV and HHV6, during periods of intense drug-induced immunosuppression may paradoxically further enhance the overall state of immunosuppression. CMV and HHV6 have been

described to increase the risk of superimposed bacterial and fungal opportunistic infections. The negative effect of CMV and HHV6 on the course of posttransplant HCV infection is also well described.

TIME COURSE OF INFECTIONS AFTER TRANSPLANTATION

In the absence of specific antimicrobial prophylaxis, infections after transplantation follow a stereotyped temporal pattern. Figures 87.1 and 87.2 depict the timing of infections after SOT (Figure 87.1) and allogeneic HSCT (Figure 87.2). It is emphasized that the natural history of these infections is changing, as influenced by various factors, most notably the use of antimicrobial prophylaxis. For example, CMV disease traditionally occurs during months 2 to 3 after transplantation, but this has been delayed to 3 to 6 months in some patients who received 100 days of antiviral prophylaxis. In addition, antimicrobial prophylaxis has also modified drug susceptibilities, as exemplified by the emergence of fluconazole-resistant *Candida* spp. infections in centers utilizing fluconazole prophylaxis.

Timetable of Infections after Solid Organ Transplantation

Infections after SOT follow a characteristic time frame that reflects the net state of

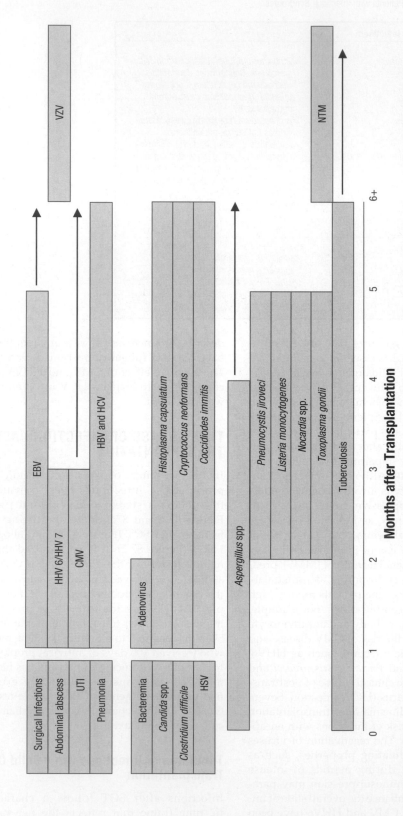

Figure 87.1 Natural history timeline of infections following solid organ transplantation in the absence of antimicrobial prophylaxis. Abbreviations: HSV = herpes simplex virus; CMV = cytomegalovirus; EBV = Epstein–Barr virus; HHV = human herpesvirus; VZV = varicella–zoster virus; HBV = hepatitis B virus; HCV = hepatitis C virus; UTI = urinary tract infection; NTM = nontuberculous mycobacteria.

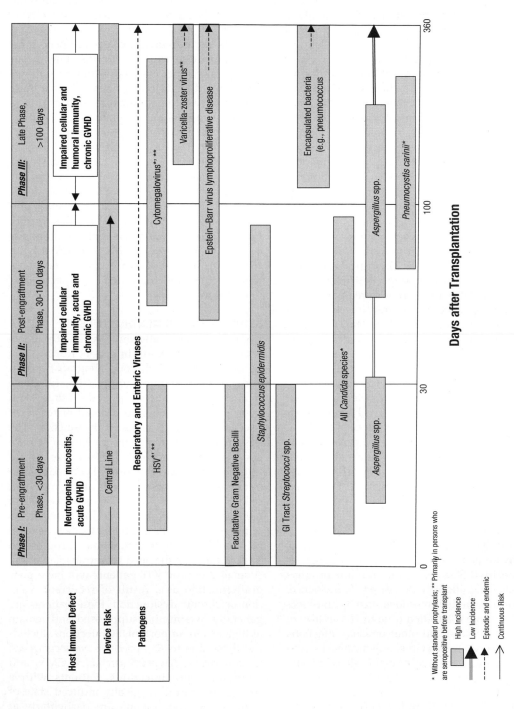

Figure 87.2 Natural history timeline of infections following allogeneic hematopoietic stem cell transplantation in the absence of antimicrobial prophylaxis. HSV = herpes simplex virus; CMV = cytomegalovirus; GVHD = graft-versus-host disease.

immunosuppression. These time frames are important to remember in considering the etiologic agents of various clinical syndromes. In this regard, although clinical syndromes such as pneumonia and cellulitis may occur at any time, the offending pathogen may be different at various time points.

THE FIRST MONTH AFTER SOT

The three major sources of infections during this period are (1) infection that is present in the recipient prior to transplantation (ie, bacterial peritonitis in liver recipients, catheter-related bacteremia in kidney recipients, bacterial pneumonia in lung recipients, and infected cardiac device in heart transplant recipients); (2) infection transmitted in the allograft (unrecognized bacterial infection prior to organ harvest); and (3) infections related to surgery and hospitalization.

The majority of infections that occur during this period are related to surgical procedures and hospitalization (Figure 87.1): surgical site infections due to *Staphylococcus* spp. and *Streptococcus* spp. or other nosocomially acquired pathogens; catheter-associated urinary tract infections with gram-negative bacteria such as *Escherichia coli*, gram-positive bacteria such as enterococcus, and fungi such as *Candida albicans*; nosocomial and ventilator-associated pneumonia due to drug-resistant *P. aeruginosa*, *Acinetobacter* spp., *S. aureus*, and others; and catheter-associated bacteremia with gram-positive bacteria such as coagulase-negative staphylococcus are seen. Intra-abdominal infections are especially common among patients who require abdominal re-exploration (for hepatic artery thrombosis, biliary leakage, or retransplantation). Prolonged hospitalization further increases the risk of nosocomial pneumonia, urinary infections, and antibiotic-related *Clostridium difficile* diarrhea.

During this period, HSV types 1 and 2 reactivate and may cause disease in the HSV-seropositive SOT recipient; antiviral prophylaxis has significantly decreased its incidence. Donor-transmitted infections such as an unrecognized fungal infection (due to *H. capsulatum* or *C. neoformans*) and other unusual infections such as WNV, rabies virus, or lymphocytic choriomeningitis virus may be manifested clinically during this period.

SECOND TO THE SIXTH MONTH AFTER SOT

This is the period when most opportunistic infections classically occur. During this period, infections due to immunomodulating viruses such as CMV, EBV, and HHV6 and infections that result from impaired cell-mediated immunity occur. Opportunistic infections with *L. monocytogenes*, *Aspergillus fumigatus*, and *P. jirovecii* are a reflection of this impaired immune function. In the absence of antiviral prophylaxis, the β-herpesviruses (CMV, HHV6, and HHV7) reactivate and cause disease during this period. Invasive aspergillosis, most commonly due to *A. fumigatus*, may occur during this time, especially among patients transplanted for fulminant hepatitis and those with epidemiologic exposure and profound immunosuppression. Pneumonia is the most common clinical presentation, but the clinical illness may go on to reflect the vasculotrophic nature of *Aspergillus* spp. and, hence, abscesses in many organs, including the liver and the brain, may be observed. Infection with endemic fungi (eg, *H. capsulatum* and *C. immitis*) and *C. neoformans* may occur during this period. *Pneumocystis jirovecii* pneumonia traditionally occurs during this period but prophylaxis with trimethoprim–sulfamethoxazole has made this infection, and those due to *Nocardia* spp., uncommon.

BEYOND THE SIXTH MONTH AFTER SOT

There are generally three types of patients with varying risk of infection during this period: (1) those with good allograft function and minimal immunosuppression, (2) those with chronic viral hepatitis, and (3) those with poor allograft function as a result of recurrent rejection or chronic allograft dysfunction. The vast majority of transplant patients will have good allograft function, and their level of immunosuppression has already been reduced to minimal levels. These patients are primarily at risk of infections similar to those observed in nonimmunocompromised populations. Patients with underlying chronic hepatitis may develop an accelerated course that may progress to graft failure and the need for retransplantation. A small group of SOT patients will have poor graft function as a result of recurrent rejection or chronic dysfunction; these patients are generally overimmunosuppressed and remain at high risk of opportunistic infections, including those due to *P. jirovecii*, *L. monocytogenes*, *C. neoformans*, *Nocardia asteroides*, CMV, and *Aspergillus* spp. infections. Patients with a persistent pharmacologically induced state of hypogammaglobulinemia are particularly at risk of pneumonia and bacteremia due to encapsulated organisms.

Infection with endemic mycoses such as *H. capsulatum* and *C. immitis*, and the reactivation of VZV occurs during this period. In endemic areas, HHV8 may reactivate to cause Kaposi's sarcoma (KS). EBV-related posttransplant lymphoproliferative disorder may occur at any time following transplantation. A few cases of CMV disease may occur during this time, especially in those who received prolonged antiviral prophylaxis.

Timetable of Infections after Hematopoietic Stem Cell Transplantation

Infections after HSCT also follow a traditional pattern (Figure 87.2) that reflects the different phases of immune recovery after transplantation.

PHASE 1: THE PRE-ENGRAFTMENT PERIOD (0 TO 30 DAYS AFTER HSCT)

The two major risk factors for infection during this period are (1) prolonged neutropenia and (2) disruption of mucocutaneous barrier, such as mucositis and use of vascular access catheters. *Candida* species is the most prevalent fungal infection during this period, and, hence, fluconazole is commonly used for prevention. As the neutropenia is prolonged, the risk for *Aspergillus* spp. is increased. HSV infections may occur and complicate mucositis. Breaks in mucocutaneous barrier, such as mucositis, predisposes to severe systemic infection and septic shock due to viridans streptococcus. Gram-positive bacteria such as *S. aureus* and coagulase-negative staphylococcus, gram-negative bacteria such as *E. coli* and *P. aeruginosa*, and fungi such as *C. albicans* may gain entry into the bloodstream through indwelling vascular catheters.

PHASE 2: POSTENGRAFTMENT PERIOD (DAYS 30–100 AFTER HSCT)

This period is characterized by an impaired cell-mediated immunity. Following engraftment, the risk of graft-versus-host disease is increased and immunosuppressive drugs to prevent this complication increase the risk of infections. This period is classically associated with the occurrence of CMV disease, which could manifest as severe pneumonia. The use of anti-CMV prophylaxis during this period may delay the onset of CMV disease to beyond 100 days after HSCT. HHV6 and adenovirus infections may occur during this period and cause febrile illness, rash, and hepatitis. Other pathogens that cause disease during this period include *Aspergillus* species,

Fusarium species, *Mucor* and *Rhizopus* species, and *P. jirovecii*.

PHASE 3: LATE-PHASE (BEYOND 100 DAYS AFTER HSCT)

In some patients, such as those with chronic graft-versus-host disease, the period beyond 100 days after transplantation is characterized by persistent impairment in cell-mediated and humoral immunity. In these patients, infections with CMV, VZV, EBV, *Aspergillus* species, and *P. jirovecii* may occur. Among patients who have adequate immune reconstitution, infections with community-acquired respiratory viruses such as influenza, parainfluenza, and respiratory viruses may occur and so are infections with encapsulated bacteria such as *S. pneumonia* and *H. influenza*. These latter infections are particularly common in patients with persistent low levels of immunoglobulins.

SELECTED PATHOGENS AND SYNDROMES

Bacterial Infections

Any bacterial pathogen can cause disease in transplant patients. In SOT patients, the standard practice of antibacterial prophylaxis such as cefazolin or cefotaxime during the perioperative period remarkably reduces the risk of surgical site infections. In some liver transplant centers, oral selective bowel decontamination (consisting of colistin, gentamicin, and nystatin) are administered to apply selective pressure to the intestinal flora (ie, to decrease colonization with gram-negative bacilli and fungi, while sparing the anaerobic organisms) and decrease the incidence of bacterial (and fungal) infections. Table 87.4 lists the most common strategies for the prevention of bacterial and other infections after transplantation.

In HSCT patients, some have advocated the use of intravenous immunoglobulins (IVIG) to prevent bacterial infections, such as sinopulmonary infections with *S. pneumoniae*, in patients with severe hypogammaglobulinemia. Antibacterial prophylaxis with penicillin and fluoroquinolones are often given to reduce the incidence of bacterial infections during periods of severe mucositis and neutropenia. However, fluoroquinolone use may increase the risk of sepsis due to viridans group streptococci. Empiric treatment with intravenous vancomycin and broad-spectrum cephalosporins or carbapenems is often used during periods of febrile neutropenia.

Table 87.4 Suggested Prophylactic Strategies in Transplantation

Indication	Prophylaxis	Dose and Duration	Comments
Perioperative prophylaxis	Cefotaxime	1 g q8h IV for 48 h	Should be adjusted based on resistance patterns
Perioperative prophylaxis	Cefazolin	1 g q8h IV for 48 h	Should be adjusted based on resistance patterns
Pneumocystis jirovecii	Trimethoprim–sulfamethoxazole	80 or 160 mg of trimethoprim component PO once daily	May protect against *Nocardia* spp., *Listeria* spp., and other bacteria
Herpes simplex virus	Acyclovir	200 mg PO tid for 28 d	Should be withheld when ganciclovir or valganciclovir is used; valacyclovir may be used if available
Cytomegalovirus	Valganciclovir	900 mg 1× daily; duration variable	Used as prophylaxis or preemptive therapy; may protect against HHV6, HSV, VZV
Cytomegalovirus	Ganciclovir	1 g PO tid; duration variable	Used as prophylaxis or preemptive therapy; may protect against HHV6, HSV, VZV
Candida spp.	Fluconazole	400 mg PO daily for 28 d	Targeted to patients with complicated and prolonged surgery or profound blood loss
Gram-negative bacilli and fungi	OBDS	Variable	Selective pressure favoring anaerobic environment, with goal of decreasing risk of fungal and bacterial infection
Hepatitis B virus	Hepatitis B immunoglobulin	10,000 IU d for first week then every 4 wk	Maintain serum HBIg level >100 IU; may be used in combination with lamivudine; role of other agents such as adefovir not yet defined
Aspergillus spp.	Amphotericin B	0.2 mg/kg/d	Administered to patients with fulminant hepatic failure

Abbreviations: HBIg = hepatitis B immunoglobulin; PO = orally; IV = intravenous; tid = 3 times daily; HHV = human herpesvirus; OBDS = oral bowel decontamination solution.

MYCOBACTERIUM SPECIES

In some patients, *M. tuberculosis* can cause disease particularly if the patient is from an endemic region and had inadequate prophylaxis or treatment. Pulmonary disease is the most common presentation, although dissemination may occur. *M. tuberculosis* has a higher propensity for dissemination and a lower response rate to treatment in transplant patients compared with the general population. Cavitary lung lesions and exudative pleural effusions are often seen. Patients often present with fever, night sweats, and weight loss. The diagnosis is established by culture, acid-fast smear, and molecular testing such as polymerase chain reaction (PCR) assays.

In the transplant patient, atypical mycobacteria, such as *Mycobacterium abscessus*, *Mycobacterium fortuitum*, and others, should be considered as potential causes of skin lesions, tenosynovitis, or joint infection. Typically, a painful, erythematous subcutaneous nodule may develop insidiously, and often after a local injury and may evolve into an abscess. Medical treatment accompanied by surgical debridement is often necessary.

NOCARDIA SPECIES

Nocardia spp. typically causes pneumonia but can involve the joints, skin, and brain. Risk factors include the degree of immunosuppression, as influenced by immunosuppressive drugs, graft rejection, and neutropenia. The use of trimethoprim–sulfamethoxazole prophylaxis during the first 3 to 6 months after transplantation, although intended to prevent *P. jirovecii* pneumonia, has lowered the incidence of nocardia (as well as listeria and other bacterial infections). Invariably, nocardia infections occur mainly among patients who are not receiving trimethoprim–sulfamethoxazole prophylaxis. Once the diagnosis is established, prolonged treatment with trimethoprim–sulfamethoxazole is the treatment of choice.

Viral Infections

CYTOMEGALOVIRUS

CMV is arguably the major infection that causes significant morbidity and mortality after transplantation. CMV infection occurs traditionally during the first 3 months after transplantation, although prophylaxis has delayed its onset. CMV causes direct and indirect effects. The direct effects, otherwise known as CMV disease, can be manifested as CMV syndrome (febrile illness with myelosuppression) or tissue-invasive disease (pneumonitis, gastrointestinal disease, hepatitis, retinitis, encephalitis). The indirect effects of CMV infection include its association with acute allograft rejection, other opportunistic infections such as invasive fungal disease and EBV-posttransplant lymphoproliferative disorder, and chronic allograft dysfunction such as transplant vascular sclerosis, bronchiolitis obliterans. The risk factors for developing CMV disease include a CMV-mismatch status; a CMV-seronegative patient who receives solid organ allograft from a CMV-seropositive donor (CMV D+/R) is a highest risk of CMV infection after SOT. In contrast, a CMV-seropositive patient who receives hematopoietic stem cells from a CMV-seronegative donor (CMV D–/R+) represents a high risk after allogeneic HSCT. Immunosuppressive regimens such as OKT3 monoclonal antibody, ATG, ALG, alemtuzumab, and mycophenolate mofetil increase the risk of CMV. The diagnos-

tic tests for CMV after transplantation include culture, histopathology, pp65 antigenemia, and molecular tests such as PCR to detect viral nucleic acid. Serology is not useful for diagnosis of acute disease after transplantation, but is used to assess the risk of disease prior to transplantation. PCR assays and pp65 antigenemia offer the most rapid methods for diagnosis of disease after transplantation.

Prevention is a key in the management of CMV. There are two methods of prevention: (1) antiviral prophylaxis, the administration of antiviral drugs, most commonly with valganciclovir, to all patients at risk of CMV disease; and (2) pre-emptive therapy, the administration of antiviral drugs, most commonly with IV ganciclovir or valganciclovir, to transplant patients with asymptomatic CMV pp65 antigenemia or CMV DNAemia. Treatment of CMV disease is with IV ganciclovir. Oral valganciclovir has been used for mildly symptomatic patients. Because of adverse effects such as nephrotoxicity and electrolyte imbalances, cidofovir and foscarnet are reserved only for the treatment of ganciclovir-resistant CMV disease. Viral load monitoring to detect the response to antiviral treatment is recommended; antiviral treatment is continued until clearance of the virus is demonstrated.

HERPES SIMPLEX VIRUS

The vast majority of HSV infections after transplantation represent reactivation of endogenous latent virus. Most commonly, the clinical presentation is that of orolabial and genital ulcers, although systemic or disseminated disease may occur in the form of hepatitis, pneumonitis, and esophageal disease. Most of these infections occur during the first month after transplantation, but preventive antiviral prophylaxis with acyclovir (or ganciclovir, which is intended primarily against CMV) has remarkably reduced its incidence. The diagnosis of mucocutaneous HSV disease is based mainly on clinical findings of typical herpetic lesions. PCR testing to demonstrate the viral DNA may confirm the diagnosis. Treatment is with oral acyclovir, valacyclovir, and famciclovir.

VARICELLA-ZOSTER VIRUS

Because over 90% of the adult population have antibodies against VZV, almost all cases of VZV disease after SOT and HSCT represent reactivation disease. Most commonly, this is in the form of mono- or multidermatomal zoster. Disseminated VZV disease may occur in severely immunocompromised individuals.

The incidence of VZV disease is approximately 10% of transplant patients. The median onset of disease is around 9 months after transplantation. The diagnosis is based mainly on clinical grounds with typical vesicular lesions in a dermatomal distribution (for typical localized disease) or in a widespread distribution (for disseminated disease). Treatment is with intravenous acyclovir for serious disease and with oral acyclovir, famciclovir, or valacyclovir for limited disease.

EPSTEIN–BARR VIRUS AND POSTTRANSPLANT LYMPHOPROLIFERATIVE DISEASE

EBV–posttransplant lymphoproliferative disease (PTLD) consists of all clinical syndromes associated with EBV-driven lymphoproliferation, whether this is nodal or extranodal, symptomatic or subclinical, localized or disseminated, monoclonal or polyclonal, or true malignancies containing chromosomal malignancies. Primary EBV infection is the most clearly defined risk factor for developing EBV–PTLD; CMV and OKT3 use further enhances the risk. The incidence varies among organ transplant types; it is highest in small bowel and lowest in kidney transplant recipients. The diagnosis of EBV–PTLD is confirmed by histopathology of specimens obtained by excisional biopsy. Surveillance measures such as PCR assays to quantitate EBV viral load is commonly utilized, although studies that demonstrate its utility is limited. Although low or absent EBV viral load has a very good negative predictive value, the specificity of higher EBV load is only modest. There is no reliable strategy for the treatment of EBV–PTLD. Hence, the optimal method of management is prevention. Reduction in immunosuppression is the main strategy for prevention and treatment. Antiviral prophylaxis with acyclovir and ganciclovir are of theoretical value but has not been proven to be effective for treatment. Pre-emptive therapy with the use of immunoglobulins, antiviral drugs, rituximab, and EBV-specific T cells has been used for preemptive treatment.

HUMAN HERPESVIRUSES 6 AND 7

The lymphotrophic β-herpesviruses, HHV6 and HHV7, infect >95% of humans. Hence, in adult transplant recipients, most of the cases are due to reactivation disease. Like CMV, the consequences of viral reactivation can be classified as direct and indirect effects. HHV6 can cause febrile illness, bone marrow suppression, hepatitis, pneumonitis, and encephalitis. The indirect effects of HHV6 and HHV7 appear to relate to their interaction with CMV and through their immune modulating properties. The diagnostic tests include serology, culture methods, immunohistochemistry, and nucleic acid testing. Insufficient data exist with regard to treatment, although HHV6 appears to be susceptible to ganciclovir, cidofovir, and foscarnet, whereas HHV7 may be resistant to ganciclovir in vitro.

HUMAN HERPESVIRUS 8

Infections with HHV8 may occur after transplantation to cause KS. Although most cases represent reactivation of the virus, primary HHV8 infection may also occur. The incidence of posttransplant KS parallels the geographic seroprevalence of HHV8, so that it occurs at a range of <1% in the United States to as high as 5% in endemic regions such as Saudi Arabia and South Africa. The median time to onset of KS is 22 months after transplantation. Skin involvement is the most common manifestation, and visceral lesions such as gastrointestinal and pulmonary KS may also be observed. Reduction or withdrawal of immunosuppression is the mainstay of treatment. Chemotherapy with doxorubicin, vincristine, and bleomycin has been used for treatment.

POLYOMAVIRUSES BK AND JC

Infection with the BK polyomavirus is mainly reported in kidney transplant recipients, where it causes tubulointerstitial nephritis; this is often manifested as an unexplained rise in serum creatinine and impairment in renal function. Ureteral stenosis may also be observed. In HSCT recipients, BK may manifest as hemorrhagic cystitis. The other human polyomavirus, JC virus, causes the rarely encountered but often fatal progressive multifocal leukoencephalopathy. The definitive diagnosis of BK virus–associated nephropathy is made by histopathologic examination of kidney biopsy specimens. Reduction in immunosuppression is the mainstay of treatment. Cidofovir and leflunomide are used as experimental therapies but are of no proven benefit. Surveillance testing, with the use of PCR or decoy cell testing, is used to identify BK infection early in efforts to prevent progression into allograft failure.

PARVOVIRUS B19

Parvovirus B19 primarily infects and lyses erythroid precursor cells and thus manifests mainly as refractory anemia. Organ-invasive manifestations in the form of pneumonitis, hepatitis, and myocarditis have been observed.

The diagnosis is based on serology, bone marrow examination to demonstrate pure red cell aplasia, and PCR tests to demonstrate the presence of parvovirus B19 DNA in clinical specimens. Use of serology is limited due to failure to mount immune reponse in some patients. The treatment is with IVIG, although the dose and duration remain undefined.

HEPATITIS C VIRUS

Chronic hepatitis C is currently the leading indication for liver transplantation. With immunosuppression after liver transplantation, the clinical course of HCV may be accelerated. There is currently no optimal strategy for preventing HCV recurrence following liver transplantation, although interferon-α or PEG-interferon, alone or in combination with ribavirin, are the currently suggested therapies for recurrent hepatitis C. The use of interferon-α and ribavirin has been shown to reduce HCV replication following liver transplantation. Because of intolerance to adverse effects and high treatment failure rates, the current practice is not to give anti-HCV therapy unless histologic recurrence is demonstrated.

Fungal Infections

Colonization with yeasts and fungi is common in transplant recipients. It is therefore essential to differentiate whether the isolation of fungi represents colonization or true infection. Factors that could indicate true infection include (1) the presence of compatible symptoms and (2) clinical and radiographic signs. Confirmation of true infection is often made by the demonstration of the fungal pathogen on biopsy specimens. The use of PCR assays and the detection of galactomannan may facilitate early detection.

The most common fungal infections in transplant patients are *Candida* spp., *Aspergillus* spp., and *Cryptococcus neoformans*. The majority of invasive fungal infections during the early posttransplant period are due to *Candida* spp., and these are often related to surgical procedures, indwelling urinary and intravascular catheters, and prolonged antibiotic use. *Aspergillus* spp. may also occur during the early period after transplantation, especially among patients with prior colonization, fulminant hepatitis, prolonged neutropenia, and severe immunocompromise. *Cryptococcus neoformans*, endemic mycoses, zygomycosis, dermatophytes, hyalohyphomycoses, and phaeohyphomycosis occur much later after transplantation

and traditionally beyond the sixth month after transplantation.

Liver transplant patients are at especially high risk of fungal infection with *Candida* spp. and *Aspergillus* spp. Antifungal prophylaxis, usually with relatively low-dose amphotericin B or fluconazole, is often given to patients with fulminant hepatitis and those who require retransplantation. Lung transplant recipients with certain identifiable risk factors (hyperacute rejection, ischemic bronchial segments, *Aspergillus* spp. colonization, CMV, anastomotic dehiscence, and retransplantation) are also at higher risk of developing invasive fungal disease, especially with *Aspergillus* spp. Heart transplant patients may infrequently develop invasive fungal infection. Kidney transplant patients have a risk of fungal infection that is comparable to that of liver transplant patients. Pancreas transplant patients are at notoriously high risk of invasive *Candida* spp. infections. Risk factors include anastomotic leaks and microbial translocation through the gastrointestinal wall. Allogeneic HSCT patients are particularly at risk of *Candida* spp. infections during periods of neutropenia. Graft-versus-host disease increases the risk for mycelial infections such as *Aspergillus* spp. Autologous HSCT patients often do not suffer from prolonged neutropenia and have a generally lower risk of invasive fungal infections. Hospital construction and renovations have been notoriously associated with increased incidence of invasive fungal infections, particularly aspergillosis, in severely immunocompromised patients.

There are three different antifungal strategies: (1) therapeutic, the treatment of established infection; (2) pre-emptive, the administration of antifungal drug to transplant patients at high risk of invasive fungal disease as suggested by clinical and laboratory features; and (3) prophylactic, the administration of antifungal drug to all patients to prevent infection. The treatment of established fungal infection should be based on the pathogen isolated.

PNEUMOCYSTIS JIROVECI

Pneumocystis jiroveci remains an important pathogen that causes pneumonia in SOT and HSCT patients. The clinical presentation is often subacute with low-grade fever, progressive dyspnea, hypoxemia, and nonproductive cough. Extrapulmonary disease may occur rarely. Co-infection with CMV and *Aspergillus* spp. is not uncommon. The overall incidence has decreased significantly with the use of prophylaxis, either trimethoprim–sulfamethoxazole or aerosolized pentamidine. The current guidelines recommend the use of *P. jiroveci* prophylaxis during the periods of immuno-compromise in all allogeneic HSCT and SOT recipients. The duration of prophylaxis is often between 3 and 6 months after transplantation. It may be prolonged in patients whose immunosuppression is prolonged, such as those with chronic graft-versus-host disease. The diagnosis of *P. jiroveci* pneumonia requires the demonstration of the organism in lung tissue and respiratory secretions. The diagnosis is often suggested by compatible clinical symptoms and radiographic signs. The treatment of choice is with trimethoprim–sulfamethoxazole with or without corticosteroids in patients with significant hypoxemia. Alternative therapies include pentamidine, atovaquone–dapsone–trimethoprim, primaquine–clindamycin, and pyrimethamine–sulfadiazine.

Parasitic Infections

Parasitic infections are becoming more common after transplantation, as a result of international travel and immigration. In the transplant recipient, parasitic infections usually represent reactivation of latent endogenous infection. Allograft-transmitted disease may also occur, as illustrated by the occurrence of donor-derived primary toxoplasma infection after heart transplantation.

TOXOPLASMA GONDII

Toxoplasma gondii infection after transplantation may manifest with fever and lymphadenopathy and could progress to cause tissue-invasive infection, including pneumonia, heart failure, and neurologic manifestations. Parasitism is often extensive in the brain, heart, lungs, and lymphoid organs. The diagnosis may be demonstrated by serology, and the demonstration of the organism in biopsy specimens. Molecular testing with the use of PCR may also be utilized if available. The prevention of toxoplasmosis is recommended mainly in heart transplant recipients, especially when there is a *Toxoplasma* D+/R– serologic mismatch. In this regard, the suggested prophylaxis is pyrimethamine and sulfadiazine for 3 months followed by lifelong trimethoprim–sulfamethoxazole prophylaxis. Alternative regimens include dapsone with pyrimethamine, and atovaquone. The treatment of established toxoplasmosis after transplantation includes the synergistic combination of pyrimethamine and sulfonamide or clindamycin.

TRYPANOSOMA CRUZI

Trypanosoma cruzi may cause Chagas disease (or American trypanosomiasis) and may be manifested as heart failure and brain abscesses in transplant recipients. Treatment is with benznidazole, reduction of the immunosuppression, and long-term administration of nifurtimox. Treatment often fails to eradicate the parasite.

STRONGYLOIDES STERCORALIS

Strongyloides stercoralis is a nematode the larvae of which has the tendency to disseminate in the setting of immune compromise, with larval accumulation in the lungs to cause Loeffler's syndrome or eosinophilic pneumonia. Peripheral eosinophila is often present. The gut penetration by the larva may also cause the translocation of bacteria and fungi and leads to systemic bacterial and fungal infections. This hyperinfection syndrome may be associated with pneumonitis, abdominal crisis, eosinophilic meningitis, and septic shock. Polymicrobial bloodstream infection, including *Candida* spp., gram-negative organisms such as *E. coli*, and other gut-derived bacteria, may occur and clue in for the diagnosis. Death is often due to gram-negative bacterial septic shock. The treatment options for *S. stercoralis* infection are thiabendazole, ivermectin, and albendazole. Treatment of the other superimposed infections should complement parasite-directed therapy.

CONCLUSIONS

Infections continue to cause significant morbidity and preventable mortality after transplantation. In general, the risk of infection is the net effect of epidemiological exposures and the overall state of immune dysfunction. The occurrence of infection is generally highest during periods of severe immunocompromise. The use of pharmacologic drugs for immunosuppression, which is essential to maintain the survival of the transplanted allograft, unfortunately impairs the ability of transplant recipients to surmount an adequate immune response and as a result, infections in transplant recipients are generally more severe and at times, the classic clinical manifestations of these infections may not be clearly evident. Hence, a high degree of suspicion is necessary for prompt and proper diagnosis of these infections.

Infections portend a worse outcome after transplantation. Hence, the major goal is prevention, prompt diagnosis, and aggressive treatment. An assessment of the risk of infection prior to transplantation is essential so that proper preventive measures, such as vaccination and use of antimicrobial prophylaxis, are administered. Surveillance procedures with use of culture and molecular surveillance tests are utilized. Empiric therapy is often administered as soon as the diagnosis of infection is suspected. Pathogen-specific therapy should be given as soon as the etiologic diagnosis is established. In addition, drainage of infected fluid (infected hematoma and abdominal abscesses), debridement of surgical infections, and removal of infected intravascular and urinary catheters are essential components of therapy. More importantly, reduction of the degree of pharmacologic immunosuppression should complement antimicrobial therapy.

SUGGESTED READING

American Journal of Transplantation Infections Disease Community of Practice. *American Journal of Transplantation*, 2004;4(s10):5–166.

Bowden R, Ljungman P, Paya CV, eds. *Transplant Infections*, 2nd ed. Philadelphia, PA: Lippincott Williams & Wilkins; 2003: 298–325.

Centers for Disease Control and Prevention, Infectious Disease Society of America, and the American Society of Blood and Marrow Transplantation. Guidelines for preventing opportunistic infections among hematopoietic stem cell transplant recipients. *Mortal Morbid Weekly Rep.* 2000;49(RR-10):1–125.

88. Diabetes and Infection

Stefan Bughi and Sylvia J. Shaw

Diabetes mellitus is a very prevalent disorder, affecting more than 21 million Americans, with a larger population having prediabetes, such as abnormal glucose tolerance test (~22 million). More than 90% of diabetic patients have type 2 diabetes. Microvascular and macrovascular complications are related to blood glucose control and disease duration and are more commonly seen in the elderly.

Diabetic patients are also at risk for infections (Table 88.1); approximately 50% of diabetic patients will have at least one hospital admission or outpatient visit for infection. Certain infections (ie, respiratory and foot infections) are overrepresented in the diabetic population and are associated with a higher risk of infection-related mortality.

PREDISPOSING FACTORS TO INFECTION

The abnormalities in host defense mechanisms in diabetic patients are related to uncontrolled diabetes. Hyperglycemia alters host immune response and has been implicated in disorders of immune function by alteration of polymorphonuclear leukocyte (PML) chemotaxis, phagocytosis, and decreased intracellular bactericidal activities. The effect of hyperglycemia on phagocytic activity is associated with an increase in cytosolic calcium and is reversible with the improvement of blood glucose level. There are other metabolic imbalances, which impair the immune system, such as presence of acidemia, reported to be reversed with the normalization of the pH. In addition, presence of chronic inflammatory changes may contribute to the metabolic imbalances (ie, via increased cytokines).

Defects in humoral immunity have been described with decreased opsonization of certain organisms and deficiency in the fourth component of complement. Defective cellular immunity has also been shown, with decreased response to phytohemaglutinins and poor skin test reactivity. Poor granuloma formation has also been reported in diabetic patients. All these changes are aggravated by microcirculatory failure, which alters the diffusion of both cellular and humoral factors to the affected site. Development of peripheral and autonomic neuropathy and progression of peripheral arterial disease further increase the diabetic patient's risk of infection.

RESPIRATORY INFECTIONS

Respiratory infections in the diabetic population are associated with increased mortality. For example, patients with diabetes are 4 times more likely to die from pneumonia or influenza compared to those in the nondiabetic population. They are also at risk to develop staphylococcal pneumonia, particularly because 30% of diabetics are nasal carriers of *Staphylococcus aureus* as compared to the healthy population. Patients with diabetes mellitus have a higher risk of developing *Klebsiella*, *Legionella* pneumonia, and pneumonitis following influenza. For this reason routine immunization against pneumococcus and influenza is recommended for all patients. Diabetic patients are also prone to aspiration pneumonia, especially in the presence of gastroparesis, a complication that occurs in 40% to 60% of those with diabetes. The risk of aspiration also increases with impairment of consciousness associated with hypoglycemia or the hyperosmolar state.

Diabetic patients are known to more frequently develop clinical tuberculosis (TB) and to have atypical locations and appearance of the disease. The incidence of TB is 16 times higher in the diabetic population than in the nondiabetic population. For this reason, the presence of a positive purified protein derivative (PPD) skin test, even with a normal chest radiograph, requires isoniazid (INH) prophylaxis for a minimum of 6 months, regardless of age.

MUCORMYCOSIS

More than three fourths of cases of rhinocerebral mucormycosis occur in diabetics, particularly in the presence of diabetic ketoacidosis. Mucormycosis is caused by a group of fungi known as *Mucorales*, the most common genera

Table 88.1 Common Infections Associated with Diabetes Mellitus

Organ System	Type of Infections
Respiratory	Pneumonia Aspiration pneumonia Pulmonary TB
Head and neck	Mucormycosis Invasive otitis externa
Gastrointestinal	Candida esophagitis Emphysematous cholecystitis
Genitourinary	Upper and lower urinary tract infections Emphysematous cystitis Emphysematous pyelonephritis Papillary necrosis Perinephric abscess Fungal UTI
Skin and soft tissue	Superficial infections Superficial necrotizing infections Deep necrotizing infections Diabetic foot infections (mild/moderate/severe)
Nosocomial	Soft tissue UTI Respiratory tract infections

Abbreviations: TB = tuberculosis; UTI = urinary tract infection.

being *Rhizopus*, *Absidia*, and *Rhizomucor*. These fungi invade nasal and paranasal membranes, as well as blood vessels, resulting in thrombosis and tissue infarction. Local spread of infection results in ophthalmoplegia, blindness, cavernous sinus thrombosis, meningoencephalitis, and brain abscesses, leading to rapid death in untreated cases. Patients with mucormycosis may present with facial or ocular pain, nasal stuffiness, generalized malaise, and fever. Many patients will develop periorbital edema, chemosis, and nasal black eschars or necrotic turbinates. Diagnosis is made by biopsy of the necrotic eschars and demonstration of nonseptate thick-walled hyphae with special staining. Computed tomography (CT) scan or magnetic resonance imaging (MRI) can be helpful in assessing the extent of disease and can aid the surgeon in debridement. Treatment with intravenous amphotericin B, 1 mg/kg/day, or liposomal amphotericin B, 5 mg/kg/day, should be started as soon as possible and should be given up to a total of 2 to 5.4 g of regular amphotericin B. Even with early diagnosis and

treatment, mortality with mucormycosis can be as high 50%. Those who survive may require reconstructive surgery and long-term psychologic counseling due to facial disfiguration. Untreated, this form of infection is 100% fatal.

INVASIVE OTITIS EXTERNA

Invasive otitis externa is an aggressive infection usually caused by *Pseudomonas aeruginosa*. It starts in the external auditory canal and progresses to the surrounding subcutaneous tissue. Rarely, the etiologic agent is *Aspergillus*, *Klebsiella pneumoniae*, or other organisms. More than 90% of patients have diabetes, often with poor metabolic control. Characteristically, the disease begins with periauricular cellulitis and granulation tissue at the junction of the cartilaginous and osseous portions of the external auditory canal. Infection spreads along the cartilage cleft, resulting in parotitis, mastoiditis, septic thrombophlebitis, cranial nerve palsy, and meningitis. Osteomyelitis of the temporomandibular joint, skull base, and cervical vertebrae can also occur. Facial nerve (VII) palsy occurs in 30% to 40% of cases and does not necessarily carry a poor prognosis. However, development of palsies of cranial nerves IX and XII implies deep infection. This can be complicated by sinus thrombosis and central nervous system (CNS) infection, which results in death in 30% of patients. The extent of tissue involvement can be determined accurately with the use of CT scan or MRI, which also helps the surgeon in performing extensive debridement.

Four weeks of parenteral antipseudomonal antibiotic therapy is generally recommended. Frequently, combination therapy of β-lactam agents (piperacillin, ceftazidime, cefipime, or aztreonam) with an aminoglycoside is used. Other regimens use a combination of two antipseudomonal β-lactams or even a single agent such as ciprofloxacin. If oral quinolones are used, longer therapy (3 months) is recommended by some authorities.

GASTROINTESTINAL INFECTIONS

Candida esophagitis has been reported to occur with increased frequency in diabetic patients and more often in those who receive broad-spectrum antibiotics. The most common presentation is retrosternal pain or dysphagia after the ingestion of cold or hot drinks. Oral thrush can be absent. Endoscopic examination and biopsy are the preferred diagnostic procedures. Treatment with oral fluconazole (400 mg initial dose, followed by 200 mg/day) is necessary for a minimum of 3 weeks or at least for 2 weeks after resolution of symptoms. An alternative therapy is itraconazole, 100 mg swished in mouth daily for 3 weeks. Oropharyngeal infection can be treated with itraconazole, 200 mg swished in mouth daily for 1 to 2 weeks. Infections with *Candida* species also respond to voriconazole intravenously or orally or caspofungin intravenously. Success of treatment may depend on normalization of blood sugar.

Emphysematous cholecystitis is a surgical emergency, characterized by gas production in or around the gallbladder. The infection is highly virulent and often induced by multiple pathogens; among the most common are *Clostridia* (50% to 70%) and gram-negative bacilli such as *Escherichia coli* and *Klebsiella*. This infection is predominantly seen in diabetic male patients (70%) and is associated with gallbladder gangrene (74%) and perforation (21%). There is high mortality even with early diagnosis (15% to 25%). Gallstones are present in half of these patients. Diagnosis requires serial x-ray examinations or CT scan.

Treatment requires high-dose parenteral broad-spectrum antibiotics aimed at both anaerobic and gram-negative bacteria (imipenem or piperacillin–tazobactam), together with prompt surgical intervention.

URINARY TRACT INFECTIONS

Diabetic female patients have a 2-fold to 4-fold higher incidence of bacteriuria. Diabetic women are at risk to develop recurrent asymptomatic bacteriuria, which in general is benign and seldom permanently eradicable. Treatment of asymptomatic bacteriuria is not beneficial. Diabetic patients have a higher prevalence of developing nosocomial urinary tract infection (UTI) and a higher risk of developing upper UTI (pyelonephritis). Predisposing factors are the presence of neurogenic bladder, uncontrolled diabetes and glycosuria, recurrent vaginitis, renal disease, and urologic instrumentation. Neurogenic bladder makes single-dose or a 3-day course of antibiotic treatment less effective, and patients may require a longer course of therapy for cystitis (ie, 5 to 7 days). If the infection occurs, 10 to 14 days of therapy may be necessary.

Emphysematous cystitis is often the result of infection with *E. coli* or other Enterobacteriaceae. More than 80% of cases are in diabetic patients, who may present with pneumaturia. Gas in the urinary bladder wall and the collection system may be seen on either plain x-ray or CT scan studies. The disease usually responds to antibiotics targeting the Enterobacteriaceae.

Emphysematous pyelonephritis is a life-threatening suppurative infection of the renal and perirenal tissue. It occurs predominantly in diabetic patients (70% to 90%), more often in women than in men. The disease is usually unilateral, more often affecting the left kidney. More than 40% of cases have underlying urinary tract obstruction; *E. coli* is the predominant isolated organism (70%). Patients present with fever, chills, flank pain, confusion, and often sepsis. Occasionally, patients present with fever of unknown origin. The diagnosis is made by demonstration of gas on plain x-ray film or CT scan of the abdomen. Treatment usually requires a combination of surgical intervention, removal of urologic obstruction when present, and frequently unilateral nephrectomy and antibiotic therapy. Survival rate is more than 90% in patients who have both surgical and antibiotic treatment versus 25% in cases treated with antibiotics alone.

Papillary necrosis can occur as a complication of emphysematous pyelonephritis or as an isolated entity. More than 50% of cases are described in diabetic patients, with other cases being seen in patients with analgesic abuse, sickle cell disease, and urinary tract obstruction. Many patients present acutely with fever, ureteral colic, microscopic or macroscopic hematuria, and pyuria. Half of the patients develop renal failure. Some patients have an indolent presentation and may pass sloughed papillary tissue in the urine. Diagnosis can be made by renal ultrasound. However, the test of choice is retrograde pyelography. For patients who present with obstruction and do not pass the detached papilla spontaneously, surgical removal is indicated through cystoscopy with ureteral instrumentation. Antibiotic therapy for a minimum of 2 weeks may be required, as in pyelonephritis.

Perinephric abscess should be suspected in patients who present with "pyelonephritis" but who have a poor response to 4 or 5 days of intravenous antibiotic therapy. One third of cases are described in diabetic patients who present with pyuria, moderate fever, and a mass over the affected kidney (50% of cases). Among the gram-negative organisms, *E. coli* is the most common isolate, and ascending infection is the usual route of spread. The diagnosis requires use of renal ultrasound, CT, or MRI studies, which also can help exclude ureteral obstruction. Surgical drainage is mandatory (open surgery or percutaneous catheter placement) in combination with 4 weeks of parenteral antibiotic therapy, such as cephalosporins, piperacillin/tazobactam, or ticarcillin/clavulanate.

Fungal UTIs occur with increased frequency in the diabetic population, especially after long-term broad-spectrum antibiotics or Foley catheter placement. Most of the patients have asymptomatic candiduria and are afebrile. However, severe infections complicated with fungus ball formation, obstruction, and sepsis have been seen. For this reason, all asymptomatic (presumably colonized) patients should be carefully observed for any signs of deterioration. Development of fever or azotemia must be investigated for possible ureteral obstruction, renal involvement, or disseminated fungal disease. Quantitative colony counts of only 10 000/mL of yeast in the urine may be sufficient to cause disease. Among the most common isolates are *Candida albicans*, *Candida tropicalis*, and *Candida glabrata*. Because fluconazole is excreted in the urine, either intravenous or oral route of administration are effective forms of therapy. Usual dose ranges from 50 to 200 mg/day, which can be increased to 400 mg/day for systemic infection. As an alternative therapy, amphotericin B can be used intravenously in patients with renal involvement or as bladder irrigations in patients with cystitis. Patients who have evidence of obstruction will require surgical intervention.

SKIN AND SOFT-TISSUE INFECTIONS

Superficial infections are often caused by *S. aureus*, which commonly colonizes the nasal mucosa and the skin of diabetic patients. Recurrent abscesses require drainage and antibiotic therapy. Elimination of the *S. aureus* carrier state can be achieved by application of bacitracin ointment to the nares and oral administration of rifampin, bactrim, or minocycline (two drugs in combination for 10 to 14 days). Diabetic patients also have a higher incidence of postoperative wound infections.

SUPERFICIAL NECROTIZING INFECTIONS

Crepitant (anaerobic) cellulitis is a superficial process. It is produced by multiple organisms, most often anaerobes. Infection is seen more frequently in diabetic patients with chronic, nonhealing lower-extremity ulcers or in other immunocompromised hosts, such as patients with chronic liver disease. Crepitus is present on palpation because of subdermal and subcutaneous gas dissection. Treatment of this infection requires appropriate parenteral antibiotics and surgical debridement. Necrotizing fasciitis occurs when infection spreads along the superficial fascial planes without muscle involvement. This is a mixed infection (type I) caused by both aerobes and anaerobes (eg, *Bacteriodes* species, *Enterococcus* species, *Peptostreptococcus*, *E. coli*, *Proteus*). However, it occasionally can be induced by group A streptococci either alone or in combination with *S. aureus* (type II). Recently, reports of group B streptococci–induced necrotizing fasciitis have been reported. This potentially lethal infection frequently presents with cutaneous necrosis, suppurative fasciitis, vascular thrombosis, and extreme systemic toxicity. In the later stages of the infection, destruction of the small nerve fibers results in patchy area of skin anesthesia. Necrotizing fasciitis early in its evolution is clinically indistinguishable from other soft-tissue infection. Therefore, if misdiagnosed or diagnosis is delayed, it has a mortality rate as high as 30% to 70%. Management requires broad-spectrum coverage antibiotics to cover both aerobic and anaerobic flora (eg, Zosyn, imipenem) and thorough debridement and drainage, using the "filleting procedure." The subcutaneous tissue is left open, and irrigation with normal saline or Ringer's lactate solution is performed. Many patients require repeated debridement followed later by reconstructive surgery. Infection produced by *S. pyogenes* is often complicated by toxic shock syndrome (see Chapter 18, Staphylococcal and Streptococcal Toxic Shock and Kawasaki Syndromes).

DEEP NECROTIZING INFECTIONS

Necrotizing cellulitis (nonclostridial myonecrosis) is produced by the same bacteria responsible for necrotizing fasciitis; however, infection progresses to deeper layers and involves the muscle. This form of infection occurs most commonly in diabetic patients (75%) and often involves the lower extremities. Infection can also affect the abdominal wall or perineum, especially after surgery, penetrating trauma, or instrumentation. Treatment requires coverage of both aerobic and anaerobic pathogens and should cover *S. aureus*, gram-negative enteric organisms, *E. coli*, *Proteus*, *Bacteroides fragilis*, and *Enterococcus* species. All patients need to have aggressive debridement, resection of the necrotic muscle, and supportive therapy. Hyperbaric oxygen therapy may be considered, if available.

Table 88.2 Suggested Empirical Antibiotic Regimens, Based on Clinical Severity, for Diabetic Foot Infections

Route and Agent(s)	Mild	Moderate	Severe
Advised route	Oral for most	Oral or parenteral, based on clinical situation and agent(s) selected	Intravenous, at least initially
Dicloxacillin	Yes	—	—
Clindamycin	Yes	—	—
Cephalexin	Yes	—	—
Trimethoprim–sulfamethoxazole	Yes	Yes	—
Amoxicillin/clavulanate	Yes	Yes	—
Levofloxacin	Yes	Yes	—
Cefoxitin	—	Yes	—
Ceftriaxone	—	Yes	—
Ampicillin/sulbactam	—	Yes	—
Linezolid[a] (with or without aztreonam)	—	Yes	—
Daptomycin[a] (with or without aztreonam)	—	Yes	—
Ertapenem	—,	Yes	—
Cefuroxime with or without metronidazole	—	Yes	—
Ticarcillin/clavulanate	—	Yes	—
Piperacillini/tazobactam	—	Yes	Yes
Levofloxacin or ciprofloxacin with clindamycin	—	Yes	Yes
Imipenem–cilastatin	—	—	Yes
Vancomycin[a] and ceftazidime (with or without metronidazole)	—	—	Yes

Note: Definitive regimens should consider results of culture and susceptibility tests, as well as the clinical response to the empirical regimen. Similar agents of the same drug class may be substituted. Some of these regimens may not have U.S. Food and Drug Administration approval for complicated skin and skin-structure infections, and only linezolid is currently specifically approved for diabetic foot infections.

[a] For patients in whom methicillin-resistant *Staphylococcus aureus* infection is proven or likely.

From Lipsky BA, Berendt AR, Deery HG, et al. Diagnosis and treatment of diabetic foot infections. *Plastic Reconstruct Surg.* 2006;117:212S–238S. Reprinted with permission.

Diabetic patients are also at risk for clostridial myonecrosis, including *Clostridium septicum*. Aggressive surgical removal of the affected muscles (or amputation) with appropriate antimicrobial therapy, as well as hyperbaric oxygen therapy, may be administered.

Foot infections in diabetic patients are responsible for 20% of their hospital admissions and a frequent precursor to amputations. The most important predisposing factors are peripheral neuropathy, vascular disease, immunopathy, and history of a previous ulcer. The severity of diabetic foot infection can vary from mild and superficial (often monobacterial, caused by *S. aureus* or *Staphylococcus epidermidis*) to moderate or severe deep infection. Tissue gangrene is usually induced by polymicrobial (mixed aerobic and anaerobic) infections. The presence of deep tissue abscess or bone involvement can be determined by use of MRI. The MRI study is used to make the diagnosis of bone involvement and also to delineate the extent of bone resection necessary to treat osteomyelitis. Evaluation of vascular supply in any patient with diminished or absent peripheral pulses requires arterial Doppler (with both pressure and wave form studies) and measurement of transcutaneous oxygen tension. Presence of dysvascular foot (ankle brachial index of <0.80 mm Hg or transcutaneous oxygen tension of <40 mm Hg) requires vascular evaluation and possible revascularization.

Mild infections without systemic symptoms can be treated with oral antibiotics (Augmentin, quinolones, or first-generation cephalosporins) and require close follow-up at 48 to 72 hours. If parenteral therapy is considered, cefazolin or cefuroxime may be used for presumed monobacterial infection. Moderate non-limbthreatening infections can be managed with local debridement and parenteral antibiotic therapy with a broader coverage. The empiric therapy can be altered based on culture results (Table 88.2). For soft-tissue infection, duration of therapy should be 10 to 14 days based on the clinical outcome. Limb-threatening infections (extensive cellulitis, deep ulcer, plus lymphangitis and/or osteomyelitis) may require broad coverage (piperacillin–tazobactam, imipenem, or meropenem) empirically, which should be altered based on culture results. Surgical debridement, drainage of any abscess collection, and excision of necrotic tissue should be done promptly. Bone infection may require extirpation of the affected bone or amputation, dictated by the extent of bone involvement, the status of vascular supply, and the extent of soft-tissue infection. Preservation of the ambulatory capacity should be considered. Postoperatively, the intraoperative culture should be used to guide choice of antibiotic therapy. Presence of residual soft-tissue infection should be treated for 2 to 4 weeks and residual infected bone for 4 to 6 weeks. If no surgery or residual dead bone is left postoperatively, >3 months of antibiotic therapy is recommended. When cultures are not available, empiric therapy with intravenous levofloxacin plus oral metronidazole, intravenous cefepime plus oral metronidazole, or imipenem, for a total of 10 weeks may be given. For patients with complicating factors such as extensive osteomyelitis, multiple recurrent infections, and poor vascular supply whose infected bone cannot be surgically removed, indefinite oral suppressive therapy may be considered.

The diabetic population is also at risk for nosocomial infections, particularly affecting skin and soft tissue, followed by UTI and respiratory tract infections. In patients with diabetic foot ulcers, 50% of isolates are methicillin-resistant *S. aureus* (MRSA). In addition to MRSA, vancomycin-resistant enterococci (VRE), diphtheroids (group JK), and *Pseudomonas* are the most common pathogens. Management of these infections requires use of newer antibiotics such as linezolid (MRSA, VRE), quinupristir/dalfoprisitin (VRE), tigecycline (MRSA, VRE), daptomycin (MRSA, VRE), and others. The newer antibiotics replace combination therapy, such as novobiocin plus ciprofloxacin or doxycycline plus rifampin for VRE, or more toxic or bacteriostatic antibiotics, such as chloramphenicol, gentamicin, rifampin, or bactrim.

Overall, because patients with diabetes mellitus have high incidence of chronic kidney disease, adjustment of the antibiotic dose based on renal function is imperative. Drug interaction and toxicity should be always considered prior to therapy since these patients are frequently on multiple medications.

SUGGESTED READING

Bertoni AG, Saydah S, Brancati FL. Diabetes and the risk of infection-related mortality in the United States. *Diabetes Care.* 2001;24:1044–1049.

Fridkin SK, Hageman JC, Morrison M, et al. Active bacterial core surveillance program of the emerging infections program network: methicillin-resistant Staphylococcus aureus disease in three communities. *New Engl J Med.* 2005;352:1436–1444.

Lipsky BA, Berendt AR, Deery HG, et al. Diagnosis and treatment of diabetic foot infections. *Plastic Reconstruct Surg.* 2006;117:212S–238S.

Sapico FL, Bessman AN. Infections in the diabetic patient. *Infect Dis Clin Prac.* 1992;1:339.

Shah BR, Hux JE. Quantifying the risk of infectious disease for people with diabetes. *Diabetes Care.* 2003;26:510–513.

Tan JS. Infectious complications in patients with diabetes mellitus. *Int Diabetes Monitor.* 2000;12:1–7.

89. Infectious Complications in the Injection Drug User

John Schmittner and Carlo Contoreggi

Intravenous drug abuse is a widespread public health problem because many of its medical complications (Table 89.1) are infectious due to the transmission of bloodborne infectious agents.

ENDOCARDITIS

Endocarditis, a life-threatening infection of the heart valves and/or endocardium, is associated with septic parenteral injections. Right-sided valvular infections are very frequent in injection drug users (IDU) because of septic inoculations. Intravenous injection with low-pressure venous return increases the susceptibility of right-sided structures to endocarditis. Concurrent pulmonary hypertension from drug adulterants, such as talc, may also predispose to right-sided valvular disease.

Despite the high prevalence of endocarditis, the offending pathogens are not specific to injectors. *Staphylococcus aureus* is the most commonly identified organism, but other pathogens are seen. These include *Pseudomonas*, Serratia, *Streptococcus* groups A and B, and *Streptococcus viridans*. Increasingly, fungal pathogens are seen with immunodeficiency.

Clinical diagnosis of endocarditis in the drug abuser can be difficult. The hallmark symptom is fever. Other constitutional symptoms such as chills, sweats, and arthralgia are less specific, but they are commonly observed in opiate-dependent patients during withdrawal. The physical signs associated with left-sided endocarditis are seldom present. Coexistent immunodeficiency appears to predispose to more severe systemic infections among human immunodeficiency virus (HIV-1)-infected IDU. Blood cultures may identify the offending pathogen and antimicrobial sensitivities.

Because clinical diagnosis alone presents challenges, echocardiographic findings have developed into the primary mechanism to diagnose and treat endocarditis. Both transthoracic echocardiography (TTE) and transesophageal echocardiography (TEE) are used to evaluate settings in which endocarditis is suspected (eg, high clinical suspicion but negative blood cultures), detection of vegetations on valves, detection of valve disease with assessment of hemodynamic severity, detection of associated shunts or abscesses, and re-evalation of patients with persistent fever, continued bacteremia, or clinical deterioration.

Initial antimicrobial therapy should cover penicillinase-resistant staphylococci. Antibiotic coverage with nafcillin or oxacillin plus gentamicin is usually begun to cover both gram-postive as well as gram-negative organisms. Once the organism is identified and sensitivities are available, medication choices may be modified. If methicillin-resistant staphylococcus is suspected, change nafcillin or oxacillin to vancomycin (see Chapter 36, Endocarditis of Natural and Prosthetic Valves: Treatment and Prophylaxis, for specifics of therapy).

The IDU is frequently not compliant with prolonged hospitalization. A recent preliminary study has shown efficacy of a 7-day course of oral ciprofloxacin and rifampin as combination therapy for uncomplicated right-sided endocarditis. Ciprofloxacin, 750 mg twice a day, and rifampin, 300 mg every 12 hours, were used in this trial; however, IDU compliance with the regimen is a key issue for any unmonitored antimicrobial treatment plan. Home delivery of antibiotics is an option only for patients who are deemed to be compliant and whose care is not complicated by developments such as emboli or cardiac compromise.

Right-sided endocarditis generally carries a good prognosis when a full course of antibiotic therapy sterilizes pathogens. Serious complications are not common, but septic pulmonary emboli may result in clinically evident ventilatory and perfusion mismatch and pneumonia. Inflammatory myocarditis seen with endocarditis is often multifactorial in substance abusers with cocaine, HIV-1 infection, and injection drug use.

PULMONARY INFECTIONS

Complications due to intravenous drug use include pneumonia, aspiration pneumonitis, lung abscess, and septic pulmonary emboli.

Table 89.1 Infectious Complications in the Injection Drug User

Endocarditis
Pulmonary infections
Bone and joint infection
Skin and soft-tissue infection
Viral hepatitis
Human T-cell leukemia/lymphoma virus
Immunologic abnormalities
Tuberculosis
Pneumocystis carinii pneumonia
Toxoplasmosis
Fungal infections
Opportunistic viral infections

Talc contamination of the injected drugs may flow through the bloodstream until they lodge in the pulmonary capillary bed, causing foreign-body granulomatosis, which can lead to pulmonary fibrosis. Chronic opiate addiction may result in decreased vital capacity and a decrease in diffusion capacity. IDUs also have a 10-fold increased risk of community-acquired pneumonia compared to the general population, most likely due to the destructive action of tobacco abuse and bacteremia.

BONE AND JOINT INFECTIONS

Gram-positive organisms and *Pseudomonas aeruginosa* are the most commonly implicated organisms. Osteomyelitis most commonly affects the fibrocartilaginous joints such as the vertebral, sternoarticular, and sacroiliac joints. In addition to bacterial infections, fungal infections are increasingly described in both immunodeficient and immunocompetent hosts. Treatment protocols do not differ; however, given the wide susceptibility of immunosuppressed patients, bone or joint cultures are necessary for accurate diagnosis.

SKIN AND SOFT-TISSUE INFECTIONS

Septic parenteral injections frequently lead to skin and soft-tissue infections. Infectious and chemical thrombophlebitis, abscesses, and cellulitis are all common venous insults.

Life-threatening cutaneous infections seen in this population include fasciitis, myonecrosis, and gangrene. Tissue crepitance, extensive cellulitis, evidence of systemic toxicity, and severe pain are highly suggestive of deep infection. Plain radiographs may be helpful in identification of extensive tissue destruction and gas production associated with gangrene.

Injected drugs and their adulterants are often damaging to veins. Progressive sclerosis of the veins is common. With the failure of easier peripheral access, often the IDU attempts more dangerous injection sites such as the femoral, axillary, jugular, penile, and mammary veins. Serious infections and thrombotic events such as jugular and axillary thrombosis, penile gangrene, and mammary and inguinal fasciitis can result from injections at these sites.

Once easy intravenous access is not available, many substance abusers will administer drugs subcutaneously; this is known as skin popping. Staphylococci and streptococci are the most frequent pathogens. However, with increasing immunosuppression, other bacterial pathogens are encountered. *Escherichia coli*, *Klebsiella*, *Bacteroides*, clostridia, and mixed flora consisting of both aerobic and anaerobic organisms are also seen, as are fungal organisms such as *Candida*.

Small localized infections can usually be treated locally with or without systemic antibiotics. Severe infections should be managed with surgical debridement and inpatient antibiotic therapy.

VIRAL HEPATITIS

The epidemiology of hepatitis A has changed dramatically in the past decade, with drug abuse being recognized as a significant risk for its transmission. Hepatitis A is associated with fecal-oral transmission. Contaminated marijuana has been reported as a transmission agent for hepatitis A.

Hepatitis B, C, and D (HBV, HCV, and HDV, respectively) are associated with parenteral transmission. The incidence of HBV and HCV in IDU populations is very high worldwide, with a significant proportion infected with both HBV and HCV.

Chronic HBV infection is associated with persistent hepatitis B surface antigen (HBsAg) and hepatitis Be antigen (HBeAg), although hepatic inflammation varies widely. HBeAg is associated with increased infectivity, more severe disease, and eventual cirrhosis. The HBV virion is not cytotoxic but mediates a host cytotoxic T-cell response that causes hepatocellular inflammation and necrosis. Coinfection with HIV-1 with its associated cellular immune deficiency reduces the severity of the host cytopathic response. Progressive HIV-1-associated cellular immunodeficiency manifests with reduced hepatic inflammation and lower serum transaminase concentrations. Other serologic measures of HBV infection in HIV-1 are not diminished.

HDV, or delta particle infection, is common in IDU. This infection, which requires co-infection with HBV, imparts a more severe course than HBV alone. Coinfection with HBV and HDV is associated with increased incidence of fulminant hepatic failure. Vaccination with HBV vaccine will also prevent HDV infection.

Though less well characterized than HBV, HCV appears to be heterogenous, with significant genetic and immunologic variability. Parenteral transmission is better established than other routes of HCV transmission (ie, familial, sexual, or maternal-fetal). Most cases are traced to parenteral exposures, either through blood or blood-product transfusion or injection drug use.

In IDU populations there is evidence that HBV and HCV co-infection increases the severity of clinical hepatitis and the persistence of transaminase elevation. The development of progressive hepatitis and end-stage liver failure in the IDU population is likely to increase as this population ages. Effective therapy for chronic HBV and HCV remains limited, but initial studies have shown efficacy of interferon-α treatment.

Despite improvements in therapy of patients with hepatitis C, substance abuse, depression, and alcohol abuse have major barriers to achieving successful clinical improvement and disease remission. Treatment with interferon requires considerable compliance and medication adherence and is challenging in non-substance-abusing patients. Patients who continue to abuse drugs and alcohol have limited economic and social support and often experience suboptimal outcomes. Interferon therapy is independently associated with neuropsychiatric complications and side effects, and data suggest patients with existing comorbid psychiatric disorders prior to institution of immune therapy fare worse overall. In IDU patients, overall poorer outcomes are not likely because of changes in the HCV during therapy but are more likely because of overall poorer treatment adherence. As with most other medical conditions that affect the IDU, integration of medical treatment with effective substance abuse and psychiatric care improves efficacy while improving the overall quality of life.

There remains considerable debate on the ethics of performing liver transplants in patients with alcohol and drug abuse. When organ recipients significantly outnumber available organs, many transplant groups routinely disqualify patients with substance abuse from consideration. The principal reasons for disqualification are history of abuse relapse, poor social support, and noncompliance with medical management. The availability of adequate alcohol and substance abuse treatment with patient compliance appears to contribute to better long-term outcomes.

HUMAN T-CELL LEUKEMIA/ LYMPHOMA VIRUS

The incidence of non-HIV retroviral infections is lower than that of HBV, HCV, or HDV among IDU in Europe, North America, and Australia. Human T-cell leukemia/lymphoma virus HTLV-2 infection is more frequently reported than HTLV-1 in IDU. Viral transmission occurs primarily parenterally and sexually, and maternal-fetal transmission is less frequent than with HIV. Endemic pockets of HTLV-2 infection exist in Asia and the Caribbean basin. With increased injection drug use and high-risk sexual exposures, we expect the prevalence of HTLV-2 infection to increase.

The clinical sequelae of HTLV-2 infection are less well defined than those of HIV-1. It appears that the incidence of disease from HTLV-2 infection alone is low, about 0.5%. HTLV-2 infection causes T-cell leukemia and lymphoma in both immunocompetent and immunodeficient patients. Tropical spastic paraparesis has also been associated with HTLV-2 infection.

HTLV-2 infection causes subtle immune dysfunction that is mild compared with that of HIV-1 infection. Co-infection with HIV-1 and HTLV-2 causes a more severe immune dysfunction than HIV-1 infection alone. Co-infection with HIV-1 has also been associated with acquired T-cell depletion ichthyosis in the IDU. The long-term clinical effects of HTLV-2 infection and the pace of its continued penetration into drug-abusing populations remains to be seen.

IMMUNOLOGIC ABNORMALITIES

IDUs have subtle abnormalities in immune function independent of HIV and other retroviral infections. Abnormal circulating immune factors include elevated plasma immunoglobulins, especially the immunoglobulins IgM and

IgG; false-positive rheumatoid factor and syphilis serology; and febrile agglutinins and complement fixation tests. Cellular immunity has also been demonstrated to be abnormal in the IDU. HIV-1 antibody-negative parenteral opiate abusers may have elevated total T-lymphocyte counts as well as increases in both T-helper and T-suppressor cells. Measures of cellular immunity show diminished function. Natural killer (NK) cell function is diminished, and cytotoxic T-cell (CTL) function may also be impaired.

Cellular immune functions are essential for host recognition of pathogens and for immune stimulants such as those in vaccines. It is likely that without intact cellular immunity, future HIV-1 vaccine effectiveness may be compromised in the active IDU.

Effective substance abuse treatment with discontinuation of septic injections may restore immunocompetence. Immune studies of patients maintained on methadone show that immune dysfunction improves after discontinuation of intravenous injecting.

TUBERCULOSIS

Mycobacterium tuberculosis, which is endemic in drug abusers, is a highly virulent pathogen that infects both immunocompetent and immunodeficient individuals. Co-infection of tuberculosis (TB) and HIV-1 is present in a significant number of new TB cases. In those infected with HIV-1, TB primarily shows pulmonary involvement early, whereas with progressive immunosuppression, disseminated extrapulmonary TB is common.

All HIV-1-infected patients should be tested for TB as early in the course of their disease as possible and every 6 months or if clinical symptoms suggest infection. Untreated individuals with exposure to TB as evidenced by positive purified protein derivative (PPD) are at high risk for recurrence of latent infection with progressive immunodeficiency. Immunocompromised hosts recently exposed to TB should receive prophylaxis, as should anergic individuals with known environmental exposure or patients who are at high risk. This includes IDUs.

PNEUMOCYSTIS CARINII PNEUMONIA

Pneumocystis carinii is a ubiquitous organism that colonizes the respiratory tract early in life and becomes a pathogen in the setting of moderate to severe immunodeficiency. In a recent study, *P. carinii* pneumonia (PCP) occurred in nearly 90% of New York City's IDU population

and was the most frequent acquired immunodeficiency syndrome (AIDS)-defining diagnosis.

TOXOPLASMOSIS

Toxoplasma gondii, a ubiquitous protozoal parasite found in soil, may be ingested in raw meat. Activation of infection usually occurs with severe immunosuppression, CD4 counts in the $100/mm^3$ range. Serologic testing early in the course of HIV-1 infection to determine exposure is indicated, with prophylaxis necessary only for seropositive patients with CD4 counts below $100/mm^3$.

FUNGAL INFECTIONS

These pathogens are seen in the setting of profound immunosuppression, with CD4 counts in the $50/mm^3$ to $100/mm^3$ range. Invasive *Candida* infections are commonly seen as vaginitis in mild to moderate immunosuppression, oropharyngeal candidiasis is seen in moderate disease with invasive esophageal candidiasis, and other fungal central nervous system and systemic disease is seen with profound immunodeficiency.

OPPORTUNISTIC VIRAL INFECTIONS

Herpes simplex virus, varicella-zoster virus, cytomegalovirus, and Epstein–Barr virus are common viral pathogens seen in the setting of severe to profound immunosuppression.

COMMENTS

The integration of substance abuse treatment with primary care for immunodeficiency is most effective for both clinical outcome and cost of care. It is essential for the health care provider to realize that this population is notoriously noncompliant and difficult to reach. Such constraints can influence treatment options, such as prescribing oral instead of intravenous antibiotics. Access to clearly identifiable care providers who can coordinate complex social services for patients will greatly aid in the management of the medically ill substance abuser. Compliance, though difficult to manage, may be aided through the use of specific contingencies for continued illicit drug use, medical noncompliance, and failure to keep scheduled appointments. However, due to the infectious nature of many of the complications of intravenous drug use, initiatives to decrease morbidity may have a profound public health impact.

SUGGESTED READING

Baddour LM, Wilson WR, Bayer AS, et al. Infective endocarditis: diagnosis, antimicrobial therapy, and management of complications: a statement for healthcare professionals from the Committee on Rheumatic Fever, Endocarditis, and Kawasaki Disease, Council on Cardiovascular Disease in the Young, and the Councils on Clinical Cardiology, Stroke, and Cardiovascular Surgery and Anesthesia, American Heart Association; endorsed by the Infectious Diseases Society of America. *Circulation.* 2005;111(23):394–434.

Bennett CL, Pascal A, Cvitanic M, et al. Medical care costs of intravenous drug users with AIDS in Brooklyn. *J Acquir Immune Defic Syndr.* 1992;5:1–6.

Brown SM, Stimmel B, Taub RN, et al. Immunologic dysfunction in heroin addicts. *Arch Intern Med.* 1974;134:1001–1006.

Chambers HE, Morris DL, Tauber MG, et al. Cocaine use and the risk for endocarditis in intravenous drug users. *Ann Intern Med.* 1987;104:833–836.

Darke S, Ward J, Zador D, et al. A scale for estimating the health status of opioid users. *Br J Addict.* 1991;86:1317–1322.

Dupont B, Drouhet E. Cutaneous, ocular and osteoarticular candidiasis in heroin addicts: new clinical and therapeutic aspects in 38 patients. *J Infect Dis.* 1985;152:577–591.

Hind CR. Pulmonary complications of intravenous drug misuse. 1. Epidemiology and non-infective complications. *Thorax.* 1990;45(11):891–898.

Lee HH, Weiss SH, Brown LS, et al. Patterns of HIV-1 and HTLV-1/11 in intravenous drug abusers from the middle Atlantic and central regions of the USA. *J Infect Dis.* 1990;162:347–352.

Levine DP. Infectious endocarditis in intravenous drug abusers. In: Levine DP, Sobel JD, eds. *Infections in Intravenous Drug Abusers.* New York, NY: Oxford University Press; 1991:251.

Loftis JM, Matthews AM, Hauser P. Psychiatric and substance use disorders in individuals with hepatitis C: epidemiology and management. *Drugs.* 2006;66(2):155–174.

Merck Manual of Diagnosis and Therapy: Drug Use and Dependence. Section 15. Chapter 195.

Nunes D, Saitz R, Libman H, et al. Barriers to treatment of hepatitis C in HIV/HCV-coinfected adults with alcohol problems. *Alcohol Clin Exp Res.* 2006;30(9):1520–1526.

Selwyn PA, Hand D, Lewis VA, et al. A prospective study of the risk of tuberculosis among intravenous drug users with human immunodeficiency virus infection. *N Engl J Med.* 1989;320:545–550.

90. Infections in the Alcoholic

Laurel C. Preheim and Ahmad R. Nusair

Acute and chronic alcohol ingestion exert direct and indirect effects on host defenses against infection (Table 90.1). Recent studies suggest that the immunotoxic effects of ethanol are due to direct cytotoxicity and to a shift in the balance of cytokines produced from the proinflammatory to more immunoinhibitory products. However, the adverse effects of ethanol itself may be indistinguishable from those due to concomitant cirrhosis, malnutrition, poor hygiene, adverse living conditions, and abuse of tobacco and other drugs. This discussion includes infections associated with increased frequency or severity in patients who abuse alcohol (Table 90.2). The suggested antibiotic dosages are for adult patients with normal renal function. Therapeutic decisions always should be made with the knowledge that alcoholic liver disease can interfere with the metabolism and excretion of certain anti-infective agents and that some antimicrobials can cause or exacerbate hepatic dysfunction.

PNEUMONIA

Bacterial pneumonia usually follows aspiration of oropharyngeal flora into the lungs. Severe intoxication is associated with altered consciousness and a diminished cough reflex. Elevated ethanol levels can interfere with cilial function on the surface of respiratory epithelial cells. Most alcoholics also smoke cigarettes, which further impairs mucociliary defenses against infection of the respiratory tract. The most frequent bacterial causes of pneumonia in ethanol abusers include *Streptococcus pneumoniae*, anaerobes, aerobic gram-negative bacilli, and *Haemophilus influenzae*. Standard diagnostic approaches are used to evaluate alcoholic patients who exhibit signs or symptoms of pneumonia. Organisms seen on sputum Gram stain often can help guide empiric antibiotic therapy. In addition to obtaining sputum and blood cultures, any significant pleural fluid visible on chest roentgenogram should be sampled for appropriate stains as well as cultured for aerobic and anaerobic organisms. Because the severity of bacterial pneumonia

Table 90.1 Immunodefects and Alcoholism

Mechanical Defects
Diminished cough reflex
Impaired glottal closure
Lung atelectasis due to ascites
Decreased ciliary function

Humoral Immunity
Increased serum immunoglobulins
Decreased alveolar IgG subclasses
Decreased complement activity
Decreased serum bactericidal activity

Cell-Mediated Immunity
Decreased skin test reactions
Decreased numbers of T lymphocytes
Alterations in T lymphocyte subsets
Altered cytokine production
Decreased suppressor cell activity
Decreased lymphocyte mitogenic response
Decreased natural killer cell function
Altered antigen presentation by macrophages and dendritic cells

Phagocytes
Granulocytopenia (rare)
Decreased granulocyte chemotaxis
Decreased granulocyte bactericidal activity
Decreased macrophage phagocytosis
Decreased macrophage bactericidal activity

Abbreviation: IgG = Immunoglobulin G.

is increased in alcoholics, hospitalization for parenteral antibiotic therapy is usually indicated. The length of hospital stay and the need for intensive care units are likely to be higher, and the expected mortality rate is greater than twice that for nonalcoholics.

Pneumococcal Pneumonia

Streptococcus pneumoniae, or the pneumococcus, remains the most common cause of both community-acquired bacterial pneumonia and bacterial meningitis in adults. Outbreaks of pneumococcal pneumonia have occurred among residents of men's shelters and prisons, where close proximity enhances the risk of transmission for oropharyngeal organisms.

Alcoholics have the usual signs and symptoms of pneumococcal pneumonia, including sudden onset, often with a single shaking chill, fever, and subsequent productive cough. Secondary complications, including acute respiratory distress syndrome, empyema, and bacteremia, are common in ethanol abusers, particularly those with liver disease. Despite appropriate therapy, the reported overall mortality for adult bacteremic pneumococcal pneumonia increases from approximately 20% to >50% in patients with cirrhosis. The Advisory Committee on Immunization Practices recommends pneumococcal polysaccharide vaccine for all alcoholics. However, the antibody responses may be blunted, and the efficacy of the vaccine has been questioned in this high-risk population.

Alcoholism, a comorbidity for community-acquired pneumonia, is a risk factor for infection with β-lactam–resistant *S. pneumoniae*. Current Infectious Diseases Society of America/American Thoracic Society consensus guidelines on the management of community-acquired pneumonia in adults recommend the empiric use of a respiratory fluoroquinolone such as moxifloxacin, gemifloxacin, or levofloxacin (750 mg daily) or combination therapy with a β-lactam effective against *S. pneumoniae* plus either a macrolide (azithromycin or clarithromycin) or doxycycline. The preferred β-lactam is high-dose amoxicillin (1 g 3 times daily) or amoxicillin/clavulanate (2 g 2 times daily). For hospitalized patients with suspected or confirmed pneumococcal pneumonia, third-generation cephalosporins such as ceftriaxone or cefotaxime are commonly used interchangeably with respiratory fluoroquinolones.

Anaerobic Pneumonia

Anaerobic oropharyngeal bacteria, including peptostreptococci, *Fusobacterium* sp., and *Prevotella melaninogenicus*, are commonly involved in aspiration pneumonia and can cause lung abscess and empyema. Intoxication interferes with several host defenses against aspiration of oropharyngeal contents. Elevated circulating ethanol levels can disrupt the coordinated beating of cilia on respiratory epithelium and thus impair mucociliary clearance of inhaled or aspirated organisms. Inebriation also can be associated with diminished gag and cough reflexes. Alcoholics frequently have severe periodontal disease, which can increase the number of anaerobic organisms in the aspirated inoculum. Clinical signs and

Table 90.2 Infections in Alcoholics

Bacterial pneumonia
Streptococcus pneumoniae
Anaerobes
Klebsiella pneumoniae
Haemophilus influenzae
Tuberculosis
Spontaneous bacterial peritonitis
Escherichia coli
K. pneumoniae
S. pneumoniae
Bacteremia
E. coli
S. pneumoniae
Group A streptococcus
Clostridium perfringens
Non-01 *Vibrio cholerae*
Vibrio vulnificus
Salmonella
Bartonella quintana
Endocarditis
Gram-negative bacilli
S. pneumoniae
Diphtheria
Pancreatic abscess
Hepatitis B and C
HIV infection and AIDS
Abbreviations: HIV = human immunodeficiency virus; AIDS = acquired immunodeficiency syndrome.

symptoms of anaerobic pneumonia commonly progress slowly over weeks or months before patients present with malaise, low-grade fever, cough producing foul-smelling sputum, and/or weight loss. Recommended therapy includes a β-lactam/β-lactamase inhibitor (piperacillin–tazobactam for gram-negative bacilli, ticarcillin–clavulanate, ampicillin–sulbactam, or amoxicillin–clavulanate). Clindamycin, 600 to 900 mg intravenously (IV) every 8 hours, is indicated for anaerobic pleuropulmonary infections in patients who are allergic to penicillin. A carbapenem (ertapenem, meropenem, or imipenem–cilastatin) can be used as an alternative antimicrobial.

Gram-Negative Pneumonia

Gram-negative bacilli such as *Klebsiella pneumoniae* and *Enterobacter* sp. are more likely to colonize the oropharynx and cause pneumonia in alcoholics than in nonalcoholics. The combination of bloody sputum and an upper lobe infiltrate with a bulging fissure that has been classically associated with *Klebsiella* pneumonia is rarely seen today. Mortality with gram-negative bacillary pneumonia exceeds that of pneumococcal pneumonia and increases further if neutropenia is also present. For pneumonia due to Enterobacteriaceae, a third-generation cephalosporin (ceftriaxone or cefotaxime) or a carbapenem is preferred therapy. A carbapenem should be used if the pathogen is an extended-spectrum β-lactamase producer. Alternative antimicrobials would include β-lactam/β-lactamase inhibitor combinations or a fluoroquinolone. When *Pseudomonas* is suspected or identified as the causative agent, an antipseudomonal β-lactam (ticarcillin, piperacillin, ceftazidime, cefepime, aztreonam, imipenem, meropenem) should be used in combination with ciprofloxacin or levofloxacin (750 mg daily) or an aminoglycoside. An alternative regimen would be an aminoglycoside plus ciprofloxacin or levofloxacin.

The coccobacillus *H. influenzae* frequently causes pneumonia in alcoholics. Amoxicillin is effective for infections caused by non-β-lactamase–producing strains. For pneumonia caused by β-lactamase–producing *H. influenzae*, a second- or third-generation cephalosporin or amoxicillin–clavulanate is preferred. A fluoroquinolone, doxycycline, azithromycin, and clarithromycin are alternative antimicrobials for infections caused by either β-lactamase–producing or non-β-lactamase–producing strains. Azithromycin is more active in vitro than clarithromcin for *H. influenzae*.

TUBERCULOSIS

Historically, tuberculosis has been strongly associated with ethanol abuse, and alcoholics have 15 to 200 times the tuberculosis incidence rates of control populations. After decades of steady decline, the number of new cases of tuberculosis in the United States rose in 1985 and continued to climb into the early 1990s. Due to renewed control efforts, the number of new cases has again declined annually since 1992. Most cases occur in urban areas, where the incidence is especially high among the homeless and patients with acquired immunodeficiency syndrome (AIDS). Outbreaks of tuberculosis have occurred among indigent alcoholics housed in shelters. Most individuals remain asymptomatic early in the disease. Later they may note malaise, fatigue, anorexia, weight loss, afternoon fevers, or night sweats. Cough is frequent, generally producing mucopurulent sputum that may be blood tinged. The most common abnormality on chest roentgenogram is a multinodular cavitary infiltrate in the apical or subapical posterior areas of the upper lobes or in the superior segment of a lower lobe. Pleural effusions may be present. Roentgenographic findings of tuberculosis are confined to the lower lung fields in up to 18% of patients.

Hospitalized patients suspected of having active pulmonary tuberculosis should be placed in respiratory isolation. Tuberculin skin testing is useful, but false-negative reactions occur in up to 20% of persons with known tuberculosis on first testing.

The diagnosis of tuberculosis depends on isolation of *Mycobacterium tuberculosis* from clinical specimens. Sputum smears reveal acid-fast bacilli in 50% to 80% of patients with pulmonary tuberculosis. Susceptibility testing should be performed on *M. tuberculosis* isolates from any clinical specimen. Although there is no convincing evidence that alcohol abuse is associated with increased risks of extrapulmonary infection, miliary tuberculosis should remain in the differential diagnosis of fever of unknown origin in an alcoholic patient.

Alcoholic patients are less likely than nonalcoholics to be compliant with therapy for tuberculosis and thus are more likely to relapse. Current treatment guidelines with special emphasis on directly observed therapy should be followed to reduce risks of both therapeutic failure and emergence of drug-resistant strains (see Chapter 155, Tuberculosis).

PERITONITIS

Up to 30% of patients with alcoholic liver disease and ascites develop spontaneous bacterial peritonitis (SBP). In this condition bacterial cultures of ascitic fluid are positive, the fluid contains more than 250 neutrophils/mm^3, and there is no evident intra-abdominal source of infection. Aerobic gram-negative bacilli, especially *Escherichia coli*, cause approximately 75% of SBP infections. Aerobic gram-positive cocci, including *Streptococcus pneumoniae*, *Enterococcus faecalis*, other streptococci, and *Staphylococcus aureus*, are responsible for most other SBP cases. Anaerobes cause only 6% of SBP cases, presumably because of the relatively high pO$_2$ of ascitic fluid.

Because enteric bacteria predominate in SBP it is thought that the gut is the major source of organisms for this infection. Several mechanisms have been proposed to explain the movement of organisms from the intestinal lumen to the systemic circulation. Cirrhosis-induced depression of the hepatic reticuloendothelial system impairs the liver's filtering function, allowing bacteria to pass from the bowel lumen to the bloodstream via the portal vein. Cirrhosis also is associated with a relative increase in aerobic gram-negative bacilli in the jejunum. A decrease in mucosal blood flow due to acute hypovolemia or drug-induced splanchnic vasoconstriction may compromise the intestinal barrier to enteric flora, thereby increasing the risk of bacteremia. Finally, bacterial translocation may occur with movement of enteric organisms from the gut lumen through the mucosa to the intestinal lymphatics. From there bacteria can travel through the lymphatic system and enter the bloodstream via the thoracic duct. It is assumed that SBP caused by nonenteric organisms also is due to bacteremia secondary to another site of infection with subsequent seeding of the peritoneum and ascitic fluid.

Patients with severe acute or chronic liver disease have decreased serum complement levels, diminished serum bactericidal activity, and reduced bacterial clearance by macrophages of the reticuloendothelial system. Because the ability of ascitic fluid to opsonize bacteria and thus facilitate phagocytosis correlates closely with total protein concentration, patients with low ascitic fluid protein levels are at particular risk for SBP. Other risk factors have been associated with SBP, including gastrointestinal bleeding, fulminant hepatic failure, and invasive procedures such as the placement of peritoneovenous shunts for the treatment of ascites. An elevated bilirubin level also is correlated with a high risk of peritonitis in patients with cirrhosis.

Many patients exhibit other findings of end-stage liver disease such as hepatorenal syndrome, encephalopathy, and variceal bleeding. Other clinical features include fever, vomiting, abdominal pain, and physical signs of peritonitis. However, signs or symptoms of infection are absent in approximately one third of patients with SBP, so diagnostic paracentesis is indicated for all alcoholic patients with ascites. Fluid should be submitted to the laboratory for chemistry tests, cell count and differential, and microbiologic stains and cultures. Centrifugation of ascitic fluid and Gram stain of the sediment will reveal organisms in 25% to 68% of patients with SBP. Some authorities recommend that a portion of ascitic fluid be inoculated directly into blood culture bottles at the bedside. Peripheral blood cultures should be performed if SBP is suspected.

Empiric therapy should be directed against the most likely gram-negative and gram-positive pathogens discussed above. Suitable choices include a third-generation cephalosporin (cefotaxime or certriaxone), β-lactam/β-lactamase inhibitor combinations, or a carbapenem (see Chapter 56, Peritonitis).

Tuberculous peritonitis can occur in patients with alcoholic liver disease. Clinical findings resemble those of bacterial peritonitis, and acid-fast stains of ascitic fluid are usually negative. The diagnosis is best made with stains and cultures of peritoneal tissue, especially when obtained by peritoneoscope-directed biopsy. The treatment regimen is the same as for pulmonary tuberculosis.

BACTEREMIA AND SEPSIS

The liver plays a major role in clearing bacteria from the bloodstream. Alcoholic cirrhosis adversely affects hepatic reticuloendothelial system function. Both intrahepatic and extrahepatic arteriovenous shunts divert blood from macrophages that line liver capillary beds. In addition, both acute intoxication and cirrhosis interfere with bactericidal activity of these tissue phagocytes. Hypocomplementemia, neutropenia, and reduced serum bactericidal activity also may contribute to bacteremia in these patients. Neutropenia is strongly associated with increased mortality, and treatment with granulocyte colony-stimulating factor may be warranted for neutropenic patients.

Escherichia coli is the most common cause of spontaneous bacteremia in alcoholic and cirrhotic patients. Additional organisms causing bacteremia or sepsis include other gram-negative bacilli, *S. pneumoniae*, group A streptococci, and *Clostridium perfringens*. Alcoholics with cirrhosis are particularly susceptible to sepsis caused by non-01 *Vibrio cholerae* and *Vibrio vulnificus*, an opportunistic pathogen found in marine waters. Bacteremia can follow ingestion of contaminated shellfish, or exposure to seawater can result in a cutaneous infection. The latter may progress from erythematous or ecchymotic patches to bullae formation, subcutaneous necrosis, and bacteremia. *Vibrio vulnificus* infections are associated with high mortality rates. Appropriate antibiotic therapy would include ceftazidime, 2 g IV every 8 hours, plus doxycycline, 100 mg IV or orally (PO) every 12 hours, cefotaxime, 2 g IV every 8 hours, or ciprofloxacin, 400 mg IV or 750 mg PO every 12 hours. Nontyphoidal salmonella septicemia, especially due to *Salmonella typhimurium* and *Salmonella choleraesuis*, also has been associated with alcoholic liver disease. Homeless people and alcoholics also are at increased risk for bacteremia due to *Bartonella quintana*, and the seroprevalance for this organism is high among homeless people in both the United States and Europe.

Bacteremia with or without sepsis syndrome is associated with increased mortality among alcoholics. A Danish study of patients with community-acquired bacteremia found that a digestive tract or respiratory tract source of infection was particularly deleterious in alcoholics without cirrhosis. In contrast, the mortality for alcoholic patients with cirrhosis was highest if the focus of infection was unknown or in the urinary tract. A multicenter study conducted in four U.S. urban university hospitals confirmed that a history of chronic alcohol abuse substantially increased the risk of acute respiratory distress syndrome for critically ill patients with septic shock. These patients also experienced greater frequency and severity of nonpulmonary organ dysfunction and, for survivors, an increased length of hospital stay. Chronic alcoholic patients also have a 3-fold or greater increased risk for developing a severe infection or septic shock after surgery. A German study evaluated patients with and without a history of chronic ethanol abuse who developed severe sepsis. At the onset of infection and during early septic shock, chronic alcoholic patients had lower plasma levels of proinflammatory cytokines, including interleukin (IL)-1β, IL-6, and IL-8. The authors concluded that ethanol abuse altered proinflammatory cytokine production and thus the host's immune defenses to infection.

ENDOCARDITIS

Alcoholism is one of the strongest risk factors for pneumococcal endocarditis, and a few reports link cirrhosis with increased frequency and severity of endocarditis due to other bacteria. It remains an uncommon complication of cirrhosis, however, seen in only 1% to 14% of cirrhotic patients. The aortic valve is most likely to be involved. Many patients have no demonstrable underlying cardiac valvular abnormalities. Compared with that in nonalcoholics, endocarditis in cirrhotic patients is more likely to involve gram-negative bacilli such as *E. coli* and less likely to be caused by α-hemolytic streptococci.

OTHER INFECTIONS

Diphtheria

The lifestyle and poor hygiene of many alcoholics can predispose them to *Corynebacterium diphtheriae* infection. Cutaneous rather than pharyngeal diphtheria was reported in most cases from three outbreaks from the Skid Row district of Seattle. Many skin lesions were secondarily infected with group A streptococci. A macrolide (clarithromycin, azithromycin, or erythromycin) remains the treatment of choice. Routine immunization with combined tetanus and diphtheria toxoid is highly recommended for all patients in high-risk groups.

Pancreatic Abscess

Alcohol abuse is a common cause of acute pancreatitis, and pancreatic abscess is a rare but potentially catastrophic complication. Primary abscesses characteristically evolve rapidly and culminate in severe sepsis. Secondary abscesses, which may present weeks after the acute inflammation, commonly involve infection of a pancreatic pseudocyst. The cardinal signs of abscess are high fever, septicemia, a rapidly enlarging abdominal mass, and multisystem organ failure in severe cases. Early surgical drainage is important. Initial empiric antibiotic therapy should be aimed at the most common pathogens, including *E. coli*, other enteric aerobes, and anaerobic gram-negative bacilli.

VIRAL HEPATITIS

Hepatitis viruses and alcohol abuse are the two main causes of liver cirrhosis. Alcoholics have a higher rate of unresponsiveness to the hepatitis B virus (HBV) envelope vaccine compared with nonalcoholics, and ethanol may adversely affect the cellular immune responses to the virus. In patients with chronic hepatitis B, the prevalence of e antigen tends to be higher, and levels decrease more slowly in heavy drinkers versus nondrinkers. Current evidence also suggests that alcohol use is associated with increased risks of cirrhosis and hepatocellular carcinoma in chronic HBV infection. Hepatitis C virus (HCV) also is found at a high incidence in alcoholic patients, and 20% to 30% of patients infected with hepatitis C will progress to cirrhosis. Some studies suggest that even moderate alcohol consumption may accelerate liver damage and hasten the clinical progression of hepatitis C infection. Abstinence from alcohol also has been shown to result in a reduction of viremia. The effect of alcohol on the interaction between HCV viral proteins and the immune system is poorly understood. Indirect evidence suggests that alcohol contributes to suppression of T-cell function, which may lead to persistence of HCV infection after exposure to the virus. Alcohol abuse is considered a contraindication to interferon-based therapy of hepatitis C due to concerns regarding patient compliance. Alcohol may interfere with the efficacy of interferon by other mechanisms as well. Response rates to interferon therapy are diminished by alcohol use, and the effectiveness is further reduced if alcohol consumption is increased.

HUMAN IMMUNODEFICIENCY VIRUS INFECTION

Individuals with human immunodeficiency virus (HIV) infection have significantly higher rates of alcohol use than the general population. Studies have reported the prevalence of alcohol abuse or dependence to range from 20% to 40% among HIV-infected primary care patients. It is unclear whether alcohol abuse predisposes to HIV infection at the time of exposure, although intoxication does have a disinhibiting effect on risk-taking behavior. It also is not certain whether alcohol consumption increases the rate of HIV replication within the host, although ethanol intake has been shown in some studies to increase HIV replication in isolated human blood mononuclear cells. It is likely that the well-described adverse effects of ethanol on cell-mediated immune function may reduce host defenses against HIV infection. Finally, the effect of ethanol ingestion on progression from asymptomatic HIV infection to AIDS-defining opportunistic infections has not been clearly established. In a retrospective human study, progression to AIDS was not abbreviated by the use of ethanol, but chronic alcohol ingestion by CD4-depleted mice enhanced persistence of *Pneumocystis carinii*. Aside from the direct

effects of acute alcohol ingestion, the concomitant malnutrition and liver disease seen with chronic alcoholism may amplify the immunosuppressive effects of ethanol and hasten the progression from asymptomatic HIV infection to manifestations of AIDS. There is good evidence that any alcohol use among HIV-infected patients is associated with diminished compliance with highly active antiretroviral therapy (HAART). Heavy alcohol users receiving antiretroviral therapy are twice as likely to have CD4 counts <500 than light or nondrinkers, and HAART-treated heavy alcohol users are 4 times less likely to achieve a positive virologic response.

SUGGESTED READING

Balasubramanian S, Kowdley KV. Effect of alcohol on viral hepatitis and other forms of liver dysfunction. *Clin Liver Dis*. 2005;9:83–101.

Friedman H, Newton C, Klein TW. Microbial infections, immunomodulation, and drugs of abuse. *Clin Microbiol Rev*. 2003;16:209–219.

Gentry-Nielsen MJ, Vander Top E, Snitily MU, et al. A rat model to determine the biomedical consequences of concurrent ethanol ingestion and cigarette smoke exposure. *Alcoholism Clin Exp Res*. 2004;28:1120–1128.

Mandell LA, Wunderink RG, Anzueto A, et al. Infectious Diseases Society of America/ American Thoracic Society consensus guidelines on the management of community-acquired pneumonia in adults. *Clin Infect Dis*. 2007;44:S27–S72.

Samet JH, Horton NJ, Meli S, et al. Alcohol consumption and antiretroviral adherence among HIV-infected persons with alcohol problems. *Alcohol Clin Ext Res*. 2004;28:572–577.

von Dossow V, Schilling C, Beller S, et al. Altered immune parameters in chronic alcoholic patients at the onset of infection and of septic shock. *Critical Care*. 2004;8:R312–R321.

91. Infections in the Elderly

Kent Crossley

Although virtually all significant types of infections that occur in the elderly are discussed elsewhere in this book, certain aspects of infectious diseases in older individuals need to be emphasized. This chapter stresses the unique aspects of the etiology and therapy of infections in the elderly (defined here as older than 65 years of age). Infections that occur in long-term care institutions are briefly discussed.

For several reasons, infections in the elderly are an important area of concern for medicine. The number of individuals who are older than 65 is increasing dramatically. Although representing only 13% of the U.S. population at present, the elderly consume 25% of all prescription medications and a similarly disproportionate amount of other health care services. Moreover, with few exceptions (some viral infections and venereal diseases), most common infections occur more often in older individuals.

Although the mortality associated with many infections is increased in the elderly, age alone is now seen as a relatively unimportant risk factor for infection-related death or serious morbidity. Rather, it is the variety of comorbid conditions that are increasingly common with advancing age that appear to be closely associated with greater morbidity and mortality from infection.

Since the early 1990s it has become clear that there is a general hyporesponsiveness of the immune system in elderly individuals. This is the most likely explanation for the muted symptoms and signs that are a common denominator of infections in the aged. It is well documented in a number of types of infectious illnesses that maximum temperatures, white blood cell count elevations, and the overtness of clinical signs and symptoms are all less pronounced in older individuals than in younger adults. In clinical terms, this means that an elderly patient may have a serious bacteremic infection without chills, fever, or leukocytosis. This is one of the most important things to remember about infections in the aged.

PRINCIPLES OF ANTIBIOTIC USE

Table 91.1 summarizes current recommendations for treatment of common infections in the elderly. Important points to note include the following:

1) Aminoglycoside antibiotics are best avoided in older individuals because of their potential toxicity. Although probably appropriate in neutropenic, immunocompromised elderly or in the presence of documented *Pseudomonas* infection, try to use other agents when possible. With careful monitoring, once-daily administration of these drugs for at least 10 days does not appear to be associated with more side effects in the elderly.

2) Because most antibiotics (quinolones, aminoglycosides, and most penicillins are examples) are excreted by renal routes and because of the decline in renal function with increasing age, higher dosages may be potentially more toxic in the elderly.

3) Broad-spectrum therapy is appropriate initially in the treatment of serious infection if the cause is unclear. Older individuals lack much of the physiologic reserve of younger adults and usually have one or more comorbid diseases. In the presence of a serious infection, the elderly can rapidly become very unstable. Using drugs that are active against most of the likely causes of the infection (with the least possible toxicity) is usually the best approach.

URINARY TRACT INFECTION

Urinary tract infection (UTI) is increasingly common with increasing age. This reflects obstruction as a result of prostatic enlargement in men and a variety of changes in the defense mechanisms of the female urinary system. The risk of instrumentation and catheterization, procedures often associated with development of infection, also increases in the elderly population.

Asymptomatic bacteriuria is more common in both elderly men and women than in younger subjects. Multiple studies have demonstrated that treatment of bacteriuria is without value, primarily because it usually rapidly recurs after therapy.

Escherichia coli accounts for the bulk of UTIs in young women. In older individuals,

Table 91.1 Antibiotics Recommended for Initial (Empiric) Therapy for the Elderly

Infection	Antibiotics	Comments
Acute fever, unidentified source	Imipenem, 0.5 g q6h IV, or meropenem, 0.5–1.0 q8h IV	Broad spectrum, limited toxicity
Urinary tract infection	*Gram-negative organisms:* Third-generation cephalosporin (eg, ceftazadime, 1.0 g q8–12h), broad-spectrum penicillin with β-lactamase inhibitor (eg, ticarcillin clavulanate, 3.1 g IV q4–6h), imipenem, meropenem, or quinolone (eg, ciprofloxacin, 400 mg IV q12h)	Consider imipenem or meropenem if in LTCF or a recurrent infection; use in combination with low-dose aminoglycoside (eg, gentamicin, 40–60 mg/d) if resistant organisms are probable Oral quinolone (eg, ciprofloxacin, 250 mg BID) appropriate if not seriously ill
	Gram-positive organisms: Vancomycin, 10–15 mg/kg q12h IV	Active against enterococci, staphylococci, and streptococci
Pneumonia	Third-generation cephalosporin (cefotaxime, 1.0–2.0 g q8–12h IV, or ceftriaxone, 1 g IM or IV q12h) plus a macrolide (eg, azithromycin, 0.5 g/d IV)	Consider using ceftazidime or imipenem for nosocomial pneumonia Macrolide (preferably azithromycin, 500 mg on day 1, then 250 mg on days 2–4), quinolone with antipneumococcal activity (eg, levofloxacin, 500 mg/d) for oral therapy in less seriously ill patients
Pressure sores	Broad-spectrum β-lactam agent with β-lactamase inhibitor (eg, ticarcillin–clavulanate)	Other treatment regimens active against Bacteroides, enteric gram-negative organisms, and staphylococci may be used
Infective endocarditis	Vancomycin with gentamicin	Modify as appropriate after results of cultures and antibiotic susceptibility testing are available
Infectious (bacterial) diarrhea	Ciprofloxacin (500 mg PO BID) or other quinolone	
Meningitis	Third-generation cephalosporin (eg, ceftriaxone, 2 g IV q12h) plus ampicillin, 50 mg/kg q8h IV	*Listeria monocytogenes* is not susceptible to cephalosporins
Septic arthritis	Nafcillin (2.0 g IV q4–6 h) or vancomycin	Consider addition of ceftazidime pending Gram stain results

Abbreviation: LTCF = long-term care facility.
Note: Therapy should be modified as appropriate after results of Gram stain, culture, and antibiotic susceptibility testing are available.

the bacteriology is more complex. Infecting organisms are usually from other genera (eg, *Serratia* and *Pseudomonas*) and are often resistant to multiple antibiotics. For this reason, urine culture and sensitivity should always be done before initiating therapy in an elderly individual.

A 10-day course of treatment is most appropriate for the clinical lower UTI (ie, cystitis) in elderly women. Although 1- or 3-day therapy with trimethoprim–sulfamethoxazole (TMP-SMX) or a quinolone antibiotic is well studied in younger women, there is relatively little information on the effectiveness of this regimen in older women. In men, because the focus of infection may be within the prostate, a minimum of 14 days of treatment is recommended. TMP-SMX or a quinolone would be an appropriate initial choice for a lower UTI. Because of the convenience of twice-daily dosing and the need to use only a small dose (because these antibiotics concentrate in the urine), ciprofloxacin (250 mg twice daily) or another quinolone is preferred.

For patients thought to have upper tract infection and for those who are seriously ill, therapy should be initially parenteral. Selection should be guided by Gram stain of the urine.

If gram-negative organisms are present, a broad-spectrum β-lactam agent with activity against *Pseudomonas aeruginosa* (eg, imipenem, ticarcillin–clavulanate, or ceftazidime) or a quinolone would be an appropriate initial choice. If a gram-positive organism is present in the Gram stain (nearly always representing staphylococci or enterococci), vancomycin would be the most appropriate antibiotic to start, pending culture and susceptibility results. Multiply-resistant gram-negative organisms may cause infection in patients with previous UTIs, those who have recently taken antibiotics, and immunosuppressed patients. In these situations (and in documented *Pseudomonas* infections), an agent such as imipenem, meropenem, or another broad-spectrum β-lactam should be given with an aminoglycoside.

Infections in individuals with chronic indwelling urinary catheters should be treated only when symptomatic. Virtually all catheterized patients will have asymptomatic bacteriuria. Treatment of catheterized patients with symptomatic infection needs to be based on culture and sensitivity results. Although there is not good evidence that catheter removal is important, it is often done before initial therapy for these infections.

PNEUMONIA

Pneumonia is an increasingly common problem with increasing age. *Streptococcus pneumoniae* is the single most common cause in the elderly. The effectiveness of administering pneumococcal polysaccharide vaccine (which is protective against most all of the penicillin-resistant strains identified to date) in the elderly is a topic of continuing controversy. Gram-negative organisms (eg, *Haemophilus influenzae, Moraxella,* and, less often, enteric organisms such as *E. coli*) are also causal. In contrast to traditional teaching, nonbacterial organisms such as *Mycoplasma pneumoniae* and *Chlamydia pneumoniae* are now recognized as important causes of pneumonia in older adults. *Mycoplasma pneumoniae* and *C. pneumoniae* may each account for up to 10% of episodes of acute pneumonia in the elderly. Respiratory syncytial virus (RSV) is also recently recognized as a significant cause of pneumonia in the aged. Although RSV-associated illness is similar to clinical influenza, bronchospasm appears to be more common. Rhinoviruses can also occasionally cause pneumonia in older individuals.

Because of the variety of agents that may cause pneumonia in the elderly, attempts to document the etiology of the infection by sputum cultures (and blood cultures if the patient is seriously ill) need to be made. Sputum cultures after initiation of treatment are usually of no value; appropriate cultures need to be obtained before starting therapy. The cost/benefit of blood cultures in the diagnosis of pneumonia has recently been questioned.

In an otherwise healthy elderly adult living in the community, initial therapy for pneumonia could be with either a macrolide or one of the newer quinolones. The newer quinolones (eg, levofloxacin) have activity against many gram-negative organisms, atypical agents such as *Mycoplasma* and *S. pneumoniae* (including those strains resistant to penicillin). Because of this, and their broad-spectrum and once-daily dosing, these agents have become increasingly popular in the outpatient therapy of pneumonia in elderly individuals.

For patients with community-acquired pneumonia who are hospitalized, empiric treatment should be broad spectrum and effective against gram-positive and gram-negative bacteria as well as atypical agents. Broad-spectrum parenteral β-lactams such as a third-generation cephalosporin (eg, ceftriaxone), a penicillin and β-lactamase inhibitor combination (eg, ticarcillin–clavulanate) in conjunction with a parenteral macrolide (eg, azithromycin) probably represents optimal therapy. Although only limited data are available, in a patient with a functioning gastrointestinal tract, oral therapy with a newer quinolone (such as levofloxacin) may be a possible option. Although parenteral therapy is most often appropriate in patients who are ill enough to be hospitalized, the nearly complete absorption of the quinolones after oral dosing and their broad spectrum suggest this may become a convenient and cost-effective approach.

TUBERCULOSIS

About one quarter of tuberculosis cases in the United States occur in individuals older than 65. This is a special problem for nursing homes because the incidence in long-term care is about 4 times that in the community. Older individuals with a positive tuberculin skin test who have one of a number of additional risk factors (eg, gastrectomy or steroid therapy) or who have recently converted their skin test need to be treated with isoniazid, 300 mg/day for 6 or 9 months, or rifampin for 4 months. Managing clinical tuberculosis in an elderly individual is similar to that in a younger patient, except that the drugs that are potentially ototoxic and nephrotoxic (eg, streptomycin) should be avoided. Monitoring for hepatic toxicity when using isoniazid is needed.

PRESSURE ULCERS

Efforts to attempt to prevent pressure-associated ischemia are extremely important. Once an ulcer develops, infection often follows. Topical antimicrobials are ineffective in the management of these lesions. Systemic antimicrobials should be used if clinical cellulitis is evident at the margin of a pressure ulcer or if there is evidence of deep infection or osteomyelitis. Therapy needs to be effective against anaerobic bacteria and both gram-negative and gram-positive organisms. Oral therapy might include a combination of an oral cephalosporin and metronidazole or amoxicillin–clavulanate. Appropriate parenteral therapy might include imipenem, ticarcillin–clavulanate, or one of the broader spectrum cephalosporins (eg, ceftriaxone and cefotaxime) or a quinolone combined with metronidazole or clindamycin for anaerobic coverage. If material can be obtained for culture (usually best done by needle aspiration), therapy can be modified when results are available.

Most of the other skin and soft-tissue infections in the aged, as in younger individuals, are caused by group A β-hemolytic streptococci or *Staphylococcus aureus*. Treatment of these infections is not significantly different in older individuals. Community-acquired methicillin-resistant *S. aureus* (MRSA) is of concern in all patients with skin and soft-tissue infection. For seriously ill patients, vancomycin is appropriate. In outpatient treatment, TMP-SMX should be used.

BACTEREMIA

In one recent study, nearly 15% of the cases of community-acquired bacteremia were in individuals older than 84 years. Usual primary sites of infection include the urinary tract, intra-abdominal sites, the lower respiratory tract, and skin and soft tissue. Appropriate empirical therapy would be that for the underlying infection. Especially in patients with bacteremia that does not promptly resolve, evaluation should rule out presence of an abscess or obstruction.

MENINGITIS

Streptococcus pneumoniae remains the most common cause of meningitis in older adults. The second most common cause is *Listeria monocytogenes*. This is important to know when selecting therapy, because this organism is not killed by cephalosporin antibiotics. Initial therapy of meningitis of unknown cause in an elderly individual must include ampicillin, which is active against *L. monocytogenes*.

INFECTIONS IN RESIDENTS OF LONG-TERM CARE FACILITIES

All of the types of infections that may occur in older individuals may develop in residents of long-term care facilities (LTCFs). MRSA and, in some areas of the United States, vancomycin-resistant enterococci (VRE) have a strong association with LTCF residency. Residents are also especially prone to epidemic respiratory or gastrointestinal diseases, which are particularly common in winter months. Selecting antibiotic therapy for patients who reside in LTCFs requires an awareness that resistant gram-negative organisms, MRSA, and VRE are all possible causes of serious infection.

SUGGESTED READING

Crossley KB, Peterson PK. Infections in the elderly. In: Mandell GL, Bennett JE, Dolin R, eds. *Principles and Practice of Infectious Diseases*. 6th ed. New York, NY: Churchill Livingstone; 2005:3517–3524.

Fernandez-Sabe N, Carratala J, Roson B, et al. Community-acquired pneumonia in very elderly patients: causative organisms, clinical characteristics, and outcomes. *Medicine (Baltimore)*. 2003;82:159–169.

Loeb MB. Pneumonia in nursing homes and long-term care facilities. *Semin Respir Crit Care Med*. 2005;26:650–655.

92. Neonatal Infection

Patrick G. Gallagher and Robert S. Baltimore

BACTERIAL INFECTIONS

Epidemiology

Neonatal infections are usually classified according to time and mode of onset in 3 categories: (1) prenatal, (2) perinatal, (early onset), and (3) nursery-acquired (late onset). The division in time between early and late onset is usually 2 to 5 days of age (Table 92.1). Infections that begin within the first month of life are considered neonatal, but many intensive care units for neonates provide continuing care for infants several months of age with complex problems that are the result of prematurity and complications of neonatal disorders. Therefore, neonatal nursery-associated infections may occur in infants up to a year of age. Bacterial infections due to rapidly dividing high-grade pathogens that set in substantially before birth usually result in a stillbirth. Generally it is not possible to distinguish infections acquired shortly prior to birth from those acquired as a result of contact with maternal vaginal, fecal, or skin flora during delivery.

Neonatal sepsis occurs in approximately 2 to 4 per 1000 live births in the United States. Worldwide reports vary from 1 to 10/1000 live births. Risk factors noted in Table 92.1 have a very strong predictive influence on infection rates. Full-term infants born without incident have a very low incidence of infection, lower than any other population of hospitalized patients. Infants susceptible to early-onset postnatal infections are primarily those born prematurely. Those premature infants born to mothers with an infection or whose membranes rupture more than 18 hours before delivery may have an infection rate of 20% or more. In extremely premature infants extra vigilance is required for early recognition and treatment of infection. Premature infants are much more likely to develop sepsis as a consequence of the amnionitis caused by ascending infection than are full-term infants. Similarly, premature infants are at a greater risk for developing an invasive infection if born to a mother with peripartum infection than are full-term infants.

Hospital-acquired infection in the nursery is an important and growing problem, and now represents most of the infections seen in neonatal units. As the technology for treating very premature and very sick infants has increased, so too has the population of surviving immunocompromised infants who require therapy with ventilators, intravascular catheters, total parenteral nutrition, and various surgical interventions, each of which carries a substantial risk of infection (see Table 92.1). The liberal use of broad-spectrum antibiotics in neonatal care units increases the risk of acquisition of pathogens by interfering with the development of normal flora in these infants, who have no flora at birth. In contrast, the risk of acquiring hospital-acquired viral infections appears to depend mostly on the chances of contact with the virus and not pre-existing disease in the infant. Infants with lung disease or cardiac conditions are particularly susceptible to severe infection with respiratory syncytial virus and human metapneumovirus. Therefore, community activity of respiratory and gastrointestinal viruses and defects in the barriers to prevent spread, especially handwashing, within the unit appear to be the most important risk factors for viral infection.

Microbiology

Table 92.1 lists the major bacterial organisms responsible for early and late postnatal sepsis. The organisms that cause meningitis in the neonate are the same. *Escherichia coli* and group B streptococci have accounted for about 80% of early-onset sepsis and meningitis in the past. The rate of group B streptococcal infection has been declining since the widespread adoption of intrapartum antibiotic prophylaxis to prevent early-onset group B streptococcal disease.

Since the early 1990s the microbiology of late-onset sepsis has shifted, with an increase in commensal organisms, particularly coagulase-negative and -positive staphylococci and *Candida* spp. This shift appears to be due to the increased survival of extremely premature

Table 92.1 Characteristics of Prenatal, Early-onset, and Late-onset Neonatal Infections

	Prenatal Onset	Early-onset Infections	Late-onset Infections
Age at Onset	Prior to birth	Birth to 2–5 days	2–5 to 30 days
Primary Route of Transmission	Transplacental or ascending	Maternal flora transmitted peripartum	Hospital-acquired
Risk Factors	Maternal infection Prolonged premature rupture of membranes	Prolonged premature rupture of membranes Septic or traumatic delivery Maternal infection, especially urogenital Fetal anoxia Male sex Maternal factors (poverty, pre-eclampsia, cardiac disease, diabetes)	Extreme prematurity Mechanical ventilation Contact with hands of colonized personnel Contact with aerosols of bacteria Contaminated equipment (e.g., isolettes, ventilators, IV lines) Debilitating illness, including bronchopulmonary dysplasia and short gut syndrome Congenital anomalies Surgery (including necrotizing enterocolitis) Prior exposure to broad-spectrum antibiotics
Most Common Pathogens	Cytomegalovirus Syphilis *Toxoplasma* Maternal vaginal flora Human immunodeficiency virus	*Escherichia coli* Group B streptococci *Klebsiella* spp. *Enterococcus* spp. *Listeria monocytogenes* Other Enterobacteriacae (*Proteus, Citrobacter, Enterobacter*)	Those causing early-onset infections *Staphylococcus aureus* Coagulase-negative staphylococci *Pseudomonas aeruginosa* *Candida* spp.

Abbreviation: IV = intravenous.

infants with increased utilization of mechanical ventilation, central venous catheters, parenteral alimentation, and broad-spectrum antibiotics. Empiric therapy is guided by this information on the microbiology of neonatal infections.

ANTIMICROBIAL THERAPY

Empiric Therapy for Early-Onset Sepsis

Antibiotics for early-onset infections are generally commenced prior to the identification of the infecting organism. Neonates, especially premature ones, typically fail to manifest classic signs and symptoms of infection. Thus, many schemata have been developed for empiric antibiotic treatment of infants with multiple epidemiologic risks alone or nonspecific signs and laboratory test abnormalities plus epidemiologic risk factors. The common features of these schemata are recognition of the risk factors listed in Table 92.1; the possibility that severe infection may present as temperature instability

or other vital sign changes, unexplained hyperbilirubinemia, vomiting, or changes in feeding; and the recognition that a very short delay in treatment may result in overwhelming sepsis and death. Such schemata vary from hospital to hospital according to the population served, the type of hospital, and resources for screening. Screening tests may also include hematologic findings such as white blood cell count, the ratio of immature to mature cells of the granulocyte series, and acute phase reactants such as erythrocyte sedimentation rate, C-reactive protein, concentrations of certain lymphokines such as interleukin-6 (IL-6), and each has been reported to have moderate positive and negative predictive values.

Treatment is designed to provide adequate antimicrobial activity against the organisms listed in Table 92.1. Often the focus of infection is unknown initially but therapy is directed against bacteremia and meningitis because experience demonstrates that these are the most likely foci. Approximately one fourth of infants

Table 92.2 Empiric Antibiotic Treatment for Presumed Neonatal Sepsis (With or Without Meningitis)

Age and Location of Infant at Onset	Antibiotic Regimen	Alternative Regimens
Early-onset sepsis	Ampicillin *plus* gentamicin[a]	Ampicillin *plus* cefotaxime
Late-onset sepsis (up to 1 month)		
Readmission from the community	Ampicillin *plus* cefotaxime (or ceftriaxone[b])	Ampicillin *plus* gentamicin[a] *with or without* cefotaxime (or ceftriaxone[†])
In the hospital, with no intravenous catheter(s)	Ampicllin *plus* gentamicin[a]	Ampicillin *plus* cefotaxime (or ceftriaxone[b])
In the hospital, with intravenous catheter(s)	Oxacillin *or* vancomycin[a] *plus* gentamicin*	Vancomycin[a] *plus* cefotaxime (or ceftriaxone[b])

[a] Adjust dose according to concentration of the antibiotic in the blood once a steady state has been achieved.
[b] Ceftriaxone can displace bilirubin from albumin thus intensifying hyperbilirubinemia and may also cause deposition of sludge in the gallbladder so it should be used with caution in newborns.

with bacterial sepsis also have meningitis. If pneumonia or a urinary tract infection is present, physical exam or screening tests, chest radiograph, and urinalysis will demonstrate these foci. Tables 92.2 and 93.3 list the antibiotics found to be safe, effective, and commonly used for neonatal infections. The recommended dosing (Table 92.3) takes into consideration the absorption, metabolism, distribution, and excretion, which differ from those of older children and change rapidly during early life.

Empiric treatment is generally a broad-spectrum penicillin with an aminoglycoside antibiotic or with an extended-spectrum (third-generation) cephalosporin (Table 92.2). A majority of pediatric infectious disease practitioners continue to use an extended-spectrum penicillin, usually ampicillin, with an aminoglycoside, usually gentamicin. The advantages of this combination are low cost, considerable experience, and known low toxicity. The advantages of the extended-spectrum cephalosporins are greater activity on a weight basis against many of the pathogens and excellent central nervous system penetration in the presence of inflammation. There is concern, however, about the development of resistant flora if these agents are used routinely in a large number of infants in a hospital unit, and rapid development of resistance to these agents has been reported. Recent studies suggest that prior treatment with third-generation cephalosporins increases the risk for invasive infections due to *Candida* species. Also *Listeria* and *Enterococcus* species are resistant to the cephalosporins. If gram-negative bacillary meningitis is diagnosed on the basis of examination of the cerebrospinal fluid, it is reasonable to use ampicillin plus an extended-spectrum cephalosporin as a first choice.

If *Pseudomonas aeruginosa* is a likely pathogen, tobramycin is a better aminoglycoside choice than gentamicin, because it has higher activity against this species. Extended-spectrum β-lactam agents such as ceftazidime and piperacillin are also used for *Pseudomonas* species. If infections due to gentamicin-resistant gram-negative bacilli have recently been encountered in the unit, amikacin or netilmicin are the aminoglycosides of choice.

Empiric Therapy for Late-Onset Sepsis

The infants most likely to have late-onset infections are ill residents of an intensive care nursery. Ideal empiric antibiotic therapy takes into consideration the resident flora of the nursery, especially isolates from previously infected neonates, and the particular risk factors of the patient. If intravascular cannulae have not been used, if the infant has not been treated for a previous infection, and if there have not been isolates of gentamicin-resistant gram-negative aerobic bacilli, it is appropriate to use the same empiric treatment as for early-onset sepsis (see Table 92.2). In fact, this is usually not the case, and another regimen is often more appropriate. Ill infants frequently have one or more intravascular catheters in place, and these may be the focus of infection. The most common bacterial species causing catheter-associated infections are coagulase-negative staphylococci and *Staphylococcus aureus*. Although penicillinase-resistant semisynthetic penicillins (oxacillin, nafcillin, methicillin) are usually the agents of choice against staphylococci, resistance to this class, commonly called methicillin-resistant *S. aureus* (MRSA), is rising in many institutions. Some institutions report high endemic rates of MRSA in neonatal

Table 92.3 Dose Schedules of Frequently Used Parenteral Antibiotics for Neonatal Infections[a]

Antibiotic Agent	<7 days of age		>7days of age	
	Dose (mg/kg/day)	Doses/day	Dose (mg/kg/day)	Doses/day
Penicillins				
Penicillin G	50,000–100,000 units[b]	2–3[<<]	100,000–200,000 units	3–4
Ticarcillin, ticarcillin/clavulanate	150–225 mg	2–3	225–300 mg	3–4
Piperacillin, piperacillin/tazobactam	150–225 mg	2–3	225–300 mg	3–4
Penicillinase-resistant penicillins (oxacillin, nafcillin)	50–100 mg	2	100–200 mg	3–4
Ampicillin	50–150 mg	2–3	100–200 mg	3–4
Aminoglycosides				
Amikacin[f]	7.5–20 mg	1–2	22.5–30 mg	3
Gentamicin[f]	5 mg	2	7.5 mg	3
Tobramycin[f]	5 mg	2	7.5 mg	3
Cephalosporins				
Cefotaxime	100 mg	2	100–200 mg	3
Ceftazidime	100–150 mg	2–3	100–150 mg	3
Ceftriaxone	50 mg	1	50–75 mg	1
Miscellaneous Antibiotics				
Clindamycin	10–15 mg	2–3	15–20 mg	3–4
Vancomycin[f]	20–30 mg	2	30–45 mg	3
Chloramphenicol[f]	25 mg	1	25–50 mg	1–2
Aztreonam	60–90 mg	2–3	90–120	3–4
Metronidazole	7.5–15	1–2	15–30	2
Antifungal Agents				
Amphotericin B	0.25–1.0 mg	1	0.25–1.0 mg	1
Amphotericin B lipid complex or liposomal	1–5	1	1–5	1
Flucytosine[d]	150 mg	4	150 mg	4
Fluconazole[e]	3–6 mg	1	3–6 mg	1
Antiviral Agents				
Acyclovir	45–60 mg	2–3	45–60 mg	2–3

[a] Dosing of very small premature infants (<1200 grams birth weight) may require longer dose intervals, and specialized literature or a pharmacy specialist should be consulted.

[b] Where there is a dose range the higher figure is used for treatment when meningitis is present. For sepsis without meningitis the higher end of the dose range is recommended for more severe infections or when the measured serum antibiotic concentration is lower than the therapeutic range.

[c] Where there is a range of number of doses/day the greater number and higher dose is used for neonates with a birth weight over 2 kilograms and the lower number doses with lower daily dose is for neonates with a birth weight under 2 kilograms.

[d] Limited data on dosing neonates. Dose indicated is from cases in the literature.

[e] Limited data in neonates. Child dose is listed.

[f] Dosing should be guided by laboratory determination of serum antibiotic concentrations once a steady state has been reached.

The Susceptible Host

intensive care units (NICUs). In addition, co-agulase-negative staphylococci appear to have a higher incidence in very low-birth-weight infants, and these pathogens are more likely to show methicillin resistance. Therefore, in institutions with substantial methicillin resistance of staphylococci it is reasonable to use vancomycin for empiric treatment of late-onset catheter-associated infections until the laboratory reports the antibiotic susceptibility of significant isolates. Generally an aminoglycoside is added. If an infant develops new symptoms of infection while receiving gentamicin, either amikacin or third-generation cephalosporin is substituted.

Once the results of culture and susceptibility test are available, empiric treatment is changed to definitive treatment. Penicillin is used for group B streptococci, ampicillin or ampicillin plus gentamicin is used for *Enterococcus* species or *Listeria*. Oxacillin, nafcillin, or vancomycin is used for staphylococci depending on susceptibility of the isolate. For gram-negative bacillary infections ampicillin or ampicillin plus an aminoglycoside or third-generation cephalosporin (depending on susceptibility) is continued for 7 to 10 days unless there is a focal infection in addition that requires a longer duration of treatment. When there is peritonitis due to necrotizing enterocolitis, the addition of clindamycin to the regimens recommended for sepsis may be of value for treatment of staphylococci and gram-negative anaerobes.

Adjunctive Therapy of Sepsis

In addition to antibiotic therapy, infants with sepsis require intensive medical management. Care should be provided to address fluid and electrolyte, metabolic, nutritional, respiratory, cardiovascular, renal, and hematologic needs. Extracorporeal therapies, including continuous renal replacement therapy (CRRT), plasma-based removal techniques, and extracorporeal membrane oxygenation (ECMO), have been explored in the treatment of neonatal sepsis. The most experience is with ECMO, which has been used successfully for the treatment of refractory septic shock in neonates. The use of agents to support or enhance the neonate's immune response has been studied but continues to be controversial. A number of small studies suggest that exchange transfusion, transfusion of concentrated white blood cells when there is severe neutropenia and bone marrow failure, commercial intravenous immunoglobulin preparations, and

organism-specific immunoglobulin preparations reduce mortality due to neonatal sepsis. These modalities have been shown to be either ineffective or only slightly better than placebo. Recent meta-analyses suggest intravenous immunoglobulin, 500 to 750 mg/kg as a single dose, may be beneficial in the treatment of neonatal sepsis. Hematopoietic growth factors, such as granulocyte colony-stimulating factor (G-CSF) and granulocyte–macrophage colony-stimulating factor (GM-CSF), have been studied in septic neonates with neutropenia, but results are inconclusive, and their use is not currently recommended. Activated protein C has shown benefit in adults and children with septic shock, but it has not been shown to be beneficial and may actually be deleterious in septic neonates. Steroids have not been proven to be of benefit in neonatal sepsis or meningitis.

Therapy and Management of Other Focal Infections

MENINGITIS

The doses of some antibiotics are increased when treating meningitis. This is to allow for the lower antibiotic concentrations in central nervous system tissue and cerebrospinal fluid (CSF) than in blood. Antibiotics that are bactericidal are preferred over those that are bacteriostatic as the latter work less well in the central nervous system. Intrathecal or intraventricular administration of antibiotics has not been associated with improvement in outcome. Intraventricular instillation may occasionally be warranted when treating resistant organisms if they have not been eradicated using conventional antibiotic dosing.

Ampicillin plus gentamicin or cefotaxime are recommended for empiric treatment of neonatal meningitis. Complications and delayed sterilization are more common with gram-negative bacillary meningitis in the newborn than with childhood meningitis beyond the neonatal period caused by the usual organisms for that age group. In evaluating the infant being treated for bacillary meningitis, repeat the lumbar puncture every 48 hours until the CSF is sterile and at the end of therapy to monitor antibiotic efficacy. Continued positive cultures may signal the need to change antibiotics or look for a focus such as a brain abscess with cranial imaging. Assuming no complications, antibiotics are usually continued for 3 weeks. For group B streptococcal meningitis repeat lumbar puncture has little value when there is a good clinical response and no late complications. Length of treatment is 2 to 3 weeks. Hydrocephalus is an unfortunately common complication of neonatal meningitis, usually associated with severe ventriculitis, and it is important to monitor the head circumference and serial head ultrasounds, if indicated, throughout therapy. Infants who develop an increase in ventricular size should be evaluated by a neurosurgeon. At this time there are no data to suggest that adjunctive steroid treatment is either safe or beneficial for neonatal meningitis.

PNEUMONIA

Neonatal pneumonia can occur prenatally, in association with early-onset sepsis, as a complication of a noninfectious respiratory condition such as respiratory distress syndrome or meconium aspiration, or as a nosocomial pneumonia associated with mechanical ventilation. Rarely is diagnostic lower-lung tissue or sputum of good quality available for microbiologic diagnosis. Thus there is little information on optimal therapy for pneumonia as an isolated infection. In general, the bacterial pathogens are the same as those for early- and late-onset sepsis, and empiric antimicrobial treatment is the same. Antibiotic therapy is usually for 10 to 14 days and extended to 21 days for the rare cases of staphylococcal pneumonia. In addition, organisms of maternal origin such as *Chlamydia trachomatis*, which can be treated with erythromycin or sulfisoxazole and genital mycoplasmas such as *Mycoplasma hominis* and *Ureaplama urealyticum,* for which there is no proven treatment, may be encountered. There are reports of treatment of *U. urealyticum* with erythromycin but little convincing evidence of efficacy.

URINARY TRACT INFECTION

Percutaneous bladder puncture is the best method of culture to avoid contamination. Bladder catheterization is acceptable but is more likely to result in contamination of the urinary tract. If the same organism is recovered from the urine and the blood, it may not be clear whether the urinary tract was the initial focus of infection or was seeded from blood unless there is an obvious urinary tract anatomic abnormality. Late-onset urinary tract infections may be associated either with a congenital malformation or urinary tract instrumentation or be spontaneous, with no discoverable underlying cause. Initial antibiotic treatment should be similar to the approach to the neonate with sepsis according to Table 92.2 and, following identification of the pathogen continued with one of the agents listed in Table 92.3, according to the susceptibility of the isolate. Due to unpredictable absorption of oral antibiotics the treatment is generally with parenterally administered drug. Although treatment for 10 to 14 days with an agent that has renal concentration and excretion is conventional, the neonate, like older individuals, may have a poor response or relapse in the presence of obstruction, a foreign body, or incomplete voiding. Due to the high rate of congenital malformations in neonates with urinary tract infections or vesico-ureteral reflux, imaging studies should be part of the evaluation and management.

SKELETAL INFECTIONS

Septic arthritis and osteomyelitis in the neonate are generally secondary to bacteremia. Although neonatal osteomyelitis is not common, *S. aureus* is the most frequently isolated organism, and group B streptococci and gram-negative aerobes, especially *E. coli,* are also encountered. *Staphylococcus aureus* skeletal infections in the neonate are often severely destructive and associated with later disabilities, and they have a tendency to be associated with multiple foci and rupture through the incompletely formed epiphyseal plate. Magnetic resonance imaging is a very useful adjunct in evaluating arthritis and osteomyelitis in this population, because metabolic bone disease of prematurity may make interpretation of radiographs difficult. Empiric therapy is similar to sepsis, but an agent active against *S. aureus* such as oxacillin or nafcillin should be added. Management includes aspiration of infected bone or septic joint, with open drainage considered if aspiration is insufficient to drain the focus. Length of treatment is generally at least 3 weeks for septic arthritis and at least 4 weeks for osteomyelitis. A longer course may be necessary if there is delayed sterilization, late appearance of a second focus, or other complications. There is too little experience with oral agents for skeletal infections in the neonate to recommend this route.

VIRAL INFECTIONS

Herpes Simplex Infections

Herpes infections of the newborn are transmitted from the mother's genital tract to the infant, usually at delivery but, rarely, ascending infection may occur in utero. The incidence is approximately 1 in 4000 to 5000 deliveries. The infants of mothers with primary genital herpes lesions at the time of delivery rather than recurrent herpes are at highest risk, but mothers of infants with herpes infection are often unaware of ever having had genital herpes. The incubation period is generally from 3 or 4 days to a month after birth. Most neonatal herpes infections are due to herpes simplex virus type 2. The presentation of neonatal herpes may include (1) only cutaneous, eye, and mucous membrane manifestations (vesicles); (2) only central nervous system infection; or (3) disseminated visceral infection. Combinations of the three may also occur. Severity and prognosis are worst for disseminated visceral disease and best for cutaneous disease.

Acyclovir is the antiviral agent of choice although vidarabine was used successfully in the past. Moderately ill infants who are treated early in the course of manifest infection appear to benefit the most from treatment. The recommended dose is now higher than that previously recommended. The usual dose in a term infant is 60 mg/kg/day divided every 8 hours. The optimal duration of treatment is unknown, but although early studies used a duration of 10 days, most practitioners extend the course to 14 to 21 days (the latter when the infection is disseminated or the central nervous system is involved) because of reports of recurrences with the shorter regimen, and employment of even longer courses are currently being investigated. Some experts recommend repeating the lumbar puncture to follow the polymerase chain reaction (PCR) results and to continue treatment for a longer time if the PCR is still positive at the end of planned treatment. Treatment would continue until the CSF PCR is negative.

Cytomegalovirus Infection

Cytomegalovirus (CMV) infection of the neonate usually is a consequence of infection spread from mother to infant during gestation, but CMV may also be acquired by the infant at the time of delivery or postnatally. The diagnosis of congenital CMV infection is established by detecting the virus by culture or other techniques in urine, blood, or other tissues obtained during the first 3 weeks of life. Many laboratories utilize rapid culture techniques combined with direct immunofluorescence detection using antibodies against intermediate early or early CMV antigens. The use of PCR and quantitative antigenemia in the blood, which have been useful in following older immunocompromised

individuals, has not yet proved useful in management of neonates.

There are antiviral agents available to treat CMV infection, including ganciclovir, its valine ester valganciclovir, foscarnet, cidofovir, and CMV immunoglobulin. There is limited experience in treating congenital infection with these agents. However, one study showed that infants with symptomatic congenital CMV infection and evidence of central nervous system involvement treated for 6 weeks with ganciclovir (6 mg/kg intravenously every 12 hours) have less hearing loss at 6 months and fewer developmental delays at 12 months compared to untreated controls. Concerns of marrow suppression and other potential long-term effects, such as germ cell toxicity and carcinogenicity, have led many to restrict the use of ganciclovir to treatment of congenital CMV with central nervous system involvement until its safety and efficacy have been rigorously demonstrated.

Varicella-Zoster Virus

Infants born of mothers who have active varicella are in danger of developing overwhelming infection due to varicella-zoster virus (VZV) if the mother's lesions appear in the period between 5 days before delivery and 2 days after delivery. The rationale is that infants exposed during this period may have received a large dose of VZV intravenously by transplacental exposure. Infants exposed earlier in utero receive antibody transplacentally from the mother and generally develop a mild infection. Infants exposed after birth also develop mild varicella. If an infant is exposed to VZV during the critical perinatal period described above, treatment with varicella-zoster immunoglobulin (VariZIG) 125 units (one vial) or immune globulin, intravenous given as soon as possible after delivery or exposure is recommended. VariZIG is investigational. VariZIG is produced by Cangene Corporation (Winnipeg, Canada) and is distributed by FFF Enterprises, Temecula, California. Neonates who develop severe perinatal VZV infections can be treated with acyclovir at a dose of 45 mg/kg/day in 3 divided doses for 5 to 7 days.

Viral Pneumonia

Respiratory syncytial virus, influenza viruses, parainfluenza viruses, and adenoviruses can cause severe respiratory disease in neonates, and the diagnosis is made by viral culture or rapid antigen tests. In general, antimicrobial treatment is not available. Ribavirin by aerosol, which in earlier studies appeared to shorten the course of respiratory syncytial virus–associated bronchiolitis in infants, is no longer recommended for routine use because subsequent studies cast doubt on the efficacy of ribavirin even for older infants.

SUGGESTED READING

Baltimore RS. Neonatal sepsis: epidemiology and management. *Pediatric Drugs.* 2003;5:723–740.

Bizzarro MJ, Raskind C, Baltimore RS, Gallagher PG. Seventy-five years of neonatal sepsis at Yale: 1928-2003. *Pediatrics.* 2005; 116:595–602.

Gallagher PG, Baltimore, RS: Sepsis neonatorum. In: McMillan JA, Feigin RD, DeAngelis C, Jones MD, eds. *Oski's Pediatrics: Principles and Practice.* 4th ed. Philadelphia: Lippincott Williams & Wilkins; 2006.

Kimberlin DW. Herpes simplex virus infections in neonates and early childhood. *Semin Pediatr Infect Dis.* 2005;16:271–281.

Kimberlin DW, Lin CY, Sanchez PJ, et al. National Institute of Allergy and Infectious Diseases Collaborative Antiviral Study Group: effect of ganciclovir therapy on hearing in symptomatic congenital cytomegalovirus disease involving the central nervous system: a randomized, controlled trial. *J Pediatr.* 2003;143:16–25.

Pickering L, et al, ed. *Red Book: Report of the Committee on Infectious Diseases.* 27th ed. Elk Grove Village, IL: American Academy of Pediatrics; 2006.

Remington JS, Klein JO, Baker C, Wilson CB. *Infectious Diseases of the Fetus and Newborn Infant.* 6th ed. Philadelphia, PA: Saunders; 2006.

Schrag S, Schuchat A. Prevention of neonatal sepsis. *Clin Perinatol.* 2005;32:601–615.

93. Pregnancy and the Puerperium: Infectious Risks

Raul E. Isturiz and Jorge Murillo

Infectious diseases that occur during pregnancy and the puerperium pose special risks to the mother, fetus, and infant. Furthermore, preventive and therapeutic measures often must be modified because of the potential for adverse events that may occur during these normally healthy periods to mother and developing child.

With the premise that the efficacy of any diagnostic, prophylactic, or therapeutic intervention must be individually weighted against possible side effects, this chapter discusses problems that are common or severe.

URINARY TRACT INFECTIONS

Asymptomatic bacteriuria and symptomatic infection of the upper and lower urinary tract are associated with significant risks to the mother and the fetus. A positive urine culture in an asymptomatic person makes a diagnosis of asymptomatic bacteriuria. For pregnant women it is recommended to routine culture a properly collected urine specimen at the first prenatal visit. Treatment should be provided if the urine culture is positive. Screening for recurrent or persistent bacteriuria should be done following therapy.

Suppressive therapy until delivery is recommended for women who have persistent bacteriuria after two or more courses of therapy. Short courses (3 days) of antimicrobial therapy are usually effective in eradicating asymptomatic bacteriuria in pregnancy. In general, penicillins and cephalosphorins are considered safe in pregnancy. Only drugs to which the microorganism is susceptible should be used.

The following regimens are recommended: amoxicillin, 500 mg orally (PO) 3 times a day; amoxicillin–clavulanate, 875 mg PO twice a day; nitrofurantoin, 50 mg PO 4 times a day; sulfisoxazole, 500 mg PO 3 times a day; cephalosporins, such as cefuroxime–axetil, 250 to 500 mg PO every 12 hours, or cefpodoxime, 100 mg PO every 12 hours, can also be used. Fosfomycin, 3 g PO as a single dose, was shown to be effective when compared to other drugs administered for a longer time.

A urine culture should be performed 1 week after completing therapy and monthly until the end of pregnancy.

Acute cystitis may be complicated by pyelonephritis. Pyuria is found in most patients, and urine culture should always be performed. Patients should be treated for 3 to 7 days if symptoms suggesting pyelonephritis are absent. There appears to be no difference between short courses and long courses of therapy although the data are limited. Patients can be empirically treated pending results of the urine culture and then adjusted accordingly to the susceptibilities of the bacteria isolated. The same antibiotic regimens suggested for asymptomatic bacteriuria can be utilized. Trimethoprim–sulfamethoxazole (one double strength tablet PO every 2 hours) can be used only in the second trimester. Quinolones are contraindicated in pregnancy. Follow-up urine culture should be obtained 1 week after the end of therapy. For recurrent infections, antimicrobial prophylaxis should be considered for the duration of therapy.

When acute pyelonephritis is the presumptive diagnoses, we prefer to admit pregnant patients to the hospital, maintain hydration with intravenous fluids, if vomiting is present, perform urine and blood cultures, and treat with intravenous antibiotics until the patient is afebrile for 24 hours. Once afebrile for 24 to 48 hours the woman can be switched to oral therapy (adjusted to susceptibly results from the culture) and can be discharged to complete 10 to 14 days of antimicrobial therapy. If fever and symptoms persist >48 hours after treatment, initiation-imaging studies of the urinary tract and repeat urine culture should be obtained. Antibiotic prophylaxis should be seriously considered in patients with recurrent pyelonephritis. Periodic urine cultures are also recommended for the remainder of the gestation.

Parenteral regimens for empiric initial treatment of acute pyelonephritis include the following: ceftriaxone, 1 g intravenously (IV) every 24 hours, ceftazidime, 2 g IV every 8 hours, cefepime, 2 g IV every 12 hours, piperacillin–tazobactam, 4.5 g IV every 8 hours, imipenem–cilastatin, 500 mg IV every 6 hours, and aztreonam, 1 to 2 g IV every 8 hours. In general we try to avoid aminoglycosides whenever possible.

PREMATURE RUPTURE OF FETAL MEMBRANES AND INTRA-AMNIOTIC INFECTION

Premature rupture of fetal membranes (PROM) can occur at any time before uterine contractions and labor start. Subclinical infection or inflammation of the chorioamniotic membranes causes an important proportion of cases. Intra-amniotic infection (IAI), present in 40% to 75% of women with PROM, is the infection of the membranes, the amniotic fluid, the placenta, and/or the uterus. IAI occurs in 0.5% to 10.5% of deliveries and causes 10% to 40% of total peripartum maternal febrile morbidity and 20% to 40% of early neonatal infection (mainly sepsis and pneumonia). It is also associated with a 50% rate of preterm deliveries before gestation week 30.

Maternal fever (≥38°C or 100.4°F) and tachycardia (≥100/min) and fetal tachycardia (≥160/min) are common initial manifestations of IAI. Uterine tenderness and foulness of amniotic fluid are late and less commonly present. Maternal leukocytosis (≥15 000/mm^3) is common. Maternal bacteremia occurs in up to 10% of cases but is more common when virulent organisms (*Eschenchia coli* 15%, group B streptococcus 18%) are causing the infection. Abnormal labor, necessity for C-section, hemorrhage, wound infection, and endometritis are maternal complications. Fetal and neonatal complications are more frequent in preterm IAI and include sepsis, pneumonia, respiratory distress, intraventricular hemorrhage, and low apgar score. Perinatal death rises to about 2% in term babies and 25% in preterm.

When IAI is suspected and, when febrile, other sources of fever can be excluded, especially when membranes are ruptured, an amniocentesis is performed. Amniotic fluid is obtained for aerobic (group B streptococcus, *E. coli*, enterococci), anaerobic (*Peptostreptococcus, Bacteroides*, and *Fusobacterium* species, *Gardnerella vaginalis*, and *Mobiluncus* species). Samples for Gram stain (48% sensitivity, 99% specificity), glucose level (sensible when below 15 mg/dL), white blood cell count (above 30/mm^3), and leukocyte esterase activity (trace or greater) and measurement of amniotic fluid cytokines (interleukin (IL)-1a, IL-6, IL-8, and tumor necrosis factor (TNF)) can be obtained at the same time. Combined, rapid tests can be helpful when used with caution and should not replace cultures.

Because antibiotics can halt the spread of this infection to mother, fetus, and newborn, preventing severe sepsis and mortality and shortening hospital stay, they are used immediately afterward. Ampicillin, 2 g IV every 6 hours, plus gentamicin, 5.1 mg/kg once daily, continued for 1 dose after delivery; clindamicin, 900 mg IV every 8 hours, can be added after cord clamping in cesarean deliveries to reduce endometritis. Alternatives include ampicillin–sulbactam, 1.5 to 3 g every 6 hours; ticarcillin–clavulanate, 3.1 g every 6 hours; or piperacillin–tazobactam, 3.375 g to 4.5 g every 6 hours. For serious infections due to resistant bacteria, such as β-lactamase–producing gram negatives, carbapenems can be substituted.

MYCOBACTERIAL INFECTION IN PREGNANCY

Untreated tuberculosis (TB) in pregnant women increases the risk for prematurity, fetal growth retardation, low birth weight, and perinatal mortality. Because TB can be transmitted to others, and because the disease often follows an unfavorable course during pregnancy and the puerperium, diagnosis, isolation, and treatment of the pregnant woman with active TB should never be postponed after expert counseling that must include human immunodeficiency virus (HIV) testing. PPD is safe and accurate during pregnancy. Provided no multidrug resistance (MDR) is suspected, the initial regimen consists of isoniazid (isonicotinyl hydrazine, INH), 5 mg/kg/day, maximum 300 mg/day (with pyridoxine 50 mg/day), rifampin, 600 mg/day, and ethambutol, 15 mg/kg/day for 9 months minimum. INH may exhibit increased maternal liver toxicity during pregnancy. Para-aminosalicylic acid has been used with INH. Pyrazinamide is not currently recommended in the United States for routine use, but might be needed for MDR or in acquired immunodeficiency syndrome (AIDS) patients. Steptomycin and the other aminoglycosides may adversely affect the fetal eight nerves at any age of gestation. The safety of cycloserine is untested; one report suggests teratogenicity from ethionamide. The fluoroquinolones are avoided in pregnancy but may need to be used for treatment of MDR TB unresponsive to other drugs.

Therapy for latent TB infection (LTBI) can be given with INH for 9 months after the first trimester for high-risk women (for example, those who are HIV positive) with documented recent infection or deferred until after delivery. The diagnosis of maternal TB at delivery requires rapid and thorough evaluation of mother and child. Mothers with LTBI are not separated from their infants, and babies do not require special evaluation or treatment. Breast-feeding is not discouraged.

In pregnant AIDS patients, the treatment of disseminated disease due to *Mycobacterium avium* complex (MAC) is difficult because agents such as ciprofloxacin, clofazimine, and amikacin may not be suitable. Azithromycin (Food and Drug Administration [FDA] category B) is the preferred macrolide for MAC prophylaxis and treatment (see Chapters 155, Tuberculosis, and 156, Nontuberculous Mycobacteria).

MALARIA AND PREGNANCY

In the United States, where malaria is uncommon and immunity is rare, pregnant women, especially primi and secundigravidas, are more vulnerable to very high parasitemia, severe infection, and mortality; fetuses are more vulnerable to low birth weight (LBW), prematurity, stillbirth congenital disease, and death. Hence, efforts should be directed at preventing exposure to malarial parasites and diagnosing and treating episodes promptly. The geographic distribution of drug-resistant malaria parasites, the clinical features in obstetric patients, and the laboratory diagnosis are the same as described in Chapter 198, Malaria: Treatment and Prophylaxis. We recommend hospitalization and treatment with antiparasitic drugs for all pregnant women with suspected malaria, but each antimalarial agent has some potential for untoward effects on the fetus. Chloroquine phosphate, the blood schizonticide of choice for oral prophylaxis (500 mg, 300 mg base once a week beginning a week prior to potential exposure and continued for 4 weeks afterwards) and therapy (1 g, 600 mg base stat, and then 500 mg in 6 hours and 500 mg daily for 2 doses) is generally considered safe and is effective for treatment of plasmodial species other than chloroquine-resistant *Plasmodium falciparum*. Mefloquine appears safer than other drugs, but concerns remain about stillbirth, LBW, and neuropsychiatric and cardiac side effects. Tetracyclines and doxycycline are contraindicated during pregnancy, but IV clindamycin (10 mg/kg followed by 5 mg/kg every 8 hours) is an alternative. Atovaquone (250 mg) combined with proguanil (100 mg) is highly effective against chloroquine and mefloquine-resistant *P. falciparum* malaria, but data in pregnancy are scarce. Rescue has been successful with atovaquone–proguanil combined with artesunate in multidrug-resistant *P. falciparum* infections without recorded toxicity. Small studies suggest that artemisin-derived antimalarials are well tolerated. Quinine sulfate or quinidine gluconate with or without clindamycin are alternative regimens that require continuous monitoring of vital signs, blood glucose, and electrocardiogram (EKG). Exchange transfusions might be added in severe complicated malaria during pregnancy.

During pregnancy, chloroquine alone or with proguanil remains preferred for chemoprophylaxis where still effective; mefloquine may be used instead. Pregnant women should not visit malarial zones; when unavoidable, antivector strategies are paramount.

TOXOPLASMOSIS

The rationale for early treatment of toxoplasmosis acquired during gestation is to decrease the incidence and severity of fetal infection. When the maternal diagnosis is established during pregnancy, spiramycin, a macrolide antibiotic with an antibacterial spectrum similar to erythromycin, 1 g orally 3 times a day, reduces the rate of transmission of infection to the fetus by approximately 60%. The drug, available in the United States through the FDA (1-301-827-2335), is continued until delivery, assuming fetal infection has been excluded. If fetal infection is confirmed (the diagnostic method of choice is amniotic fluid polymerase chain reaction [PCR] examination at 18 weeks of gestation), oral pyrimethamine, 25 mg/day, plus sulfadiazine, 4 g/day, is superior and therefore should be started together with folinic acid, 10 mg/day, as soon as the diagnosis is established.

Serologic screening is to be performed before pregnancy or at the first prenatal visit, before gestational week 22, and finally near term in previously seronegative women. If the tests are or become positive, acute immunoglobulin M (IgM) (requires confirmation in a reference laboratory; ie, Palo Alto Medical Foundation Research Institute, 650-853-4828), IgA, or IgE can prove recent infection and mandate therapy. HIV-infected women are treated with pyrimethamine–sulfadiazine, 100 mg twice a day on day 1, followed by 50 to 75 mg daily (pyrimehomine) and 8 to 4 g daily (sulfadiazine) and suppressed for life with 50 mg daily and 2 g daily. Maintenance trimethoprim–sulfamethoxazole (TMP-SMX) for *Pneumocystis carinii* pneumonia (PCP) prophylaxis may prevent toxoplasmosis.

HERPES SIMPLEX VIRUS INFECTION OF THE GENITAL TRACT

Maternal fetal transmission occurs by direct contact of the fetus with infected vaginal secretions during vaginal delivery. Ascending or transplacental infection rarely occurs. Acyclovir is an antiviral drug with an excellent safety profile, where used in pregnancy including the first trimester. The same experience is accumulating with the use of valacyclovir and famciclovir.

For primary genital infection, acyclovir is recommended at a dose of 400 mg PO 3 times a day for 10 to 14 days. For one or more recurrences of genital herpes simplex virus during pregnancy, acyclovir, 400 mg PO 3 times a day, given at 36 weeks through delivery is beneficial. In preterm premature rupture of membranes at less than or equal to 31 weeks in women with active genital herpetic lesions, expectant management is warranted, and acyclovir therapy may shorten the duration of the lesions, but no further data are available.

The greatest risk for neonatal herpes is in women who shed virus during delivery, which is most common in those who acquired herpes in the third trimester. Additional risk factors include mothers younger than 21 and the use of fetal scalp electrodes. Although cesarean section does not prevent all neonatal lesions, for women with active genital lesions or with history of genital herpes and vulvar pain or burning at the time of delivery, cesarean section should be offered.

Prophylactic cesarean delivery is not indicated for women with a history of recurrent herpetic lesions and no evidence of active lesions at the time of delivery.

The use of antiviral therapy during delivery is controversial; antiviral therapy can reduce the need for C-section and rates of viral shedding (and thereby reduce newborn exposure) during delivery; however, data are incomplete to make generalized recommendations, and the approach should be individualized with each patient. The benefit of treating asymptomatic mothers at delivery is unknown. After delivery, a high index of suspicion and immediate isolation and treatment of infants with early infections are warranted.

VARICELLA

Uncomplicated varicella in a pregnant female may be treated with acyclovir (800 mg PO 5 times a day) when started within 24 hours of the onset of the rash. Shorter duration of fever, and reduction in the number of lesions, reduces time to crusting of lesions, and less severe symptoms are noted.

Pneumonia is manifested by fever, dyspnea, cough, and tachypnea within 1 week of the rash. Chest x-rays show a diffused nodular infiltrate. Patients may rapidly progress to respiratory failure. Mortality in nontreated pregnant women may be as high as 40%. Supportive care and acyclovir, 10 mg/kg IV every 8 hours, is the treatment of choice.

Neonatal varicella is a serious disease with a 25% mortality rate. The greater mortality rate is observed when maternal infection occurs in fewer than 5 days prior to delivery. Varicella zoster immunoglobulin administered within 1 day of life to infants born to women with active varicella at delivery may reduce the severity of the disease.

VariZig is a purified human immunoglobulin made from plasma containing high levels of antivaricella antibodies. Pregnant women without immunity to varicella who have been exposed are eligible for VariZig if administered within 96 hours.

HEPATITIS

Acute hepatitis B occurs in 1 to 2 per 1000 pregnancies and does not seem to pose special risks to the mother. Perinatal exposure, however, poses a great risk (up to 20%) for acquisition of hepatitis B virus (HBV) by infants born to hepatitis B surface antigen (HbsAg)-seropositive mothers, an event that may take place well over 20 000 times each year in the United States. Transmission is higher if the mother is also hepatitis B e antigen (HbeAg) positive, and infants born to such mothers have up to a 90% chance of becoming chronically infected if untreated. Transmission is most efficient during delivery, but intrauterine infection has been documented. The diagnosis and treatment of hepatitis B during pregnancy is similar to that of nonpregnant patients. Hepatitis B vaccination is not contraindicated during pregnancy or lactation. Women of unknown HbsAg status at labor should be considered potentially infected. Screening of all pregnant women, as well as administration of vaccine and specific immunoglobulin prophylaxis to infants of mothers with positive serology, is recommended.

Hepatitis D co-infection during pregnancy during pregnancy is managed as described for hepatitis B.

The risk of transmission of hepatitis C virus (HCV) from mother to infant is approximately

5% but increases with high maternal viral loads, HIV co-infection, and gestational age. Recommendation for treatment strategies, C-section delivery, and avoidance of breast-feeding may decrease transmission, but no conclusive data exist. Screening is usually performed in high-risk women, their offspring, and potential adoptees.

Infection with hepatitis E virus (HEV) can be associated with higher maternal mortality during pregnancy, and infant mortality may be also increased. Immunoglobulin pooled from immune patients may prove beneficial.

Children born to hepatitis G virus (HGV) RNA-positive women co-infected with HIV are also likely to be HGV infected probably by antenatal transmission and remain infected for long periods.

PARVOVIRUS B19 INFECTION

Infections with parvovirus B19 (Erythrovirus) during pregnancy are associated with hydrops fetalis and fetal loss.

All pregnant women exposed to or with symptoms suggestive of parvovirus infection should have serologic testing for IgM and IgG antibodies. Women with positive IgM who are beyond 20 weeks of gestation should have weekly ultrasounds for at least 8 weeks after the acute infection to look for signs of fetal hydrops.

Hand washing and avoiding sharing food or drinks may partially prevent the spread of parvovirus B19.

HIV INFECTION

Antiretroviral therapy during gestation includes two separate issues: treatment of maternal HIV infection and prevention of perinatal transmission. Antiretroviral therapy should not be delayed by pregnancy if there is a clear indication for its use. The choice of a regimen should be individualized in each case. Several points should be addressed with the patient and include the following: risk for disease progression, current or prior antiretroviral therapy, drug toxicities and interactions, adherence, and use of zidovudine to reduce the risk of perinatal transmission. Current HIV RNA level is of utmost importance, because antiretroviral therapy (combination) is recommended for pregnant infected women with RNA levels greater than a 1000 copies/mL to prevent perinatal transmission.

Certain antiretroviral drugs should be avoided in pregnancy. These include efavirenz,

which has been linked to teratogenic effects; amprenavir liquid formulation since it has potential toxicity because it contains large amounts of propylene glycol; didanosine and stavudine because the combination has been associated to lactic acidosis, which was occasional fatal; and nevirapine, which has caused potentially fatal hepatotoxicity in woman with CD4 counts >250 cell/mm^3 (see Chapter 97, HIV-1 Infection: Antiretroviral Therapy).

The appropriate intrapartum management of the HIV-infected female aims to reduce the perinatal transmission.

The recommendation for the use of antiretroviral drugs to prevent or reduce perinatal transmission of HIV considers several clinical scenarios. Recommendations are updated regularly, and the reader is encouraged to consult the Web site http://AIDSinfo.nih.gov for the most current guidelines.

Intrapartum zidovudine prophylaxis is recommended regardless of the mode of delivery; the available information suggests that zidovudine adds an additional protective effect against perinatal transmission. Ideally zidovudine should be started 3 hours prior to the scheduled cesarean section or during labor (2 mg/kg IV in 1 hour, followed by 1 mg/kg/hour until delivery). The use of a single dose of nevirapine to prevent mother–child transmission should be reserved to countries with limited resources and without the proper infrastructure. To provide maximal antiviral activity, other antiretrovirals should be continued on schedule during labor. The duration between rupture of membranes and delivery should be minimized through stimulating labor. All procedures that may cause a break in the infant skin and artificial rupture of membranes should be avoided. In the case of vaginal delivery, the episiotomy may increase the exposure of the infant to maternal blood.

Elective cesarean delivery at 38 weeks of gestation is recommended to all if the viral loads are above 1000 copies/mL. Pregnant females with very low or undetectable viral loads have a marginal benefit from elective cesarean section.

POSTPARTUM ENDOMETRITIS

Infection of the uterine cavity remains a significant cause of postpartum fever. Predisposing factors include PROM, prolonged labor, numerous vaginal examinations, internal fetal monitoring, poor nutrition, lack of prenatal care, presence of sexually transmitted diseases (STDs), and cesarean section. Fever and tachycardia, foul lochia, uterine tenderness, and purulent cervical drainage are characteristic findings. Appropriate tests include a complete blood cell (CBC) count with differential, urinalysis, urine culture, and blood cultures. A biopsy of the decidual lining and a specimen of the fundus can be obtained. Cultures should target aerobic gram-negative bacilli, anaerobic gram-negative bacilli, aerobic streptococci, and anaerobic gram-positive cocci. Very early onset suggests group A streptococci; onset on postpartum day 3 or 4 suggests enteric bacteria, most commonly *E. coli*, enterococcus species or anaerobes, and onset after 7 days suggests *C. trachomatis*. Cesarean delivery is likely to be complicated by infection due to anaerobic gram-negative bacilli, such as *Bacteroides* species. When a mass is palpated, ultrasound and computed tomography (CT) can establish its characteristics and guide decisions about aspiration and/or further procedures.

Therapy includes draining the uterus and administering empiric, broad-spectrum intravenous antibiotics. Antibiotic therapy should be directed against *Bacteroides*, streptococci, enterobaacteriaceae, and chlamydia; useful regimens include the combinations of clindamycin plus a third-generation cephalosporin, or doxycycline plus ticarcillin/clavulanate, piperacillin/tazobactam, a carbapenem (imipenem, ertapenem, meropenem) or ampicillin/sulbactam. We continue treatment for 48 hours after the patient is afebrile and rarely prescribe oral antibiotics.

Lack of defervescence, or pulmonary embolization, should raise the possibility of septic pelvic thrombophlebitis, for which heparin is added to the antimicrobial regimen.

PUERPERAL MASTITIS

Acute breast infections, although not life-threatening, may produce significant discomfort and serious sequelae. High fever followed by localized symptoms or signs is the common clinical sequence. Blood cultures are useful; ultrasonography and needle aspiration may help establish the diagnosis in selected patients. *Staphylococcus aureus* and *Staphylococcus epidermidis* account for most cases. Many patients with mild to moderate infection can be treated as outpatients with oral or parenteral antibiotics. Oral cloxacillin and dicloxacillin, 250 to 500 mg every 6 hours, cephalexin or cephradine, 500 mg every 6 hours, or cefadroxil, 0.5 to 1 g every 12 hours, has been used with success and minimal side effects. Women with severe infections are treated with

IV therapy with oxacillin or nafcillin, 1 to 2 g every 4 to 6 hours, cefazolin, 2 g every 8 hours, cefuroxime, 750 to 1500 mg every 8 hours, or vancomycin, 1 g every 12 hours, depending on the penicillin allergy status. Breast abscesses occur in 4% to 10% of women despite antimicrobial therapy, and when they are present, surgical drainage is indicated. Antianaerobic coverage can be added pending microbiologic findings. Continuation of lactation is encouraged during therapy.

CESAREAN SECTION AND EPISIOTOMY WOUND INFECTIONS

The rate of infection after cesarean section is higher than after episiotomy, and the risk factors are different; however, both are polymicrobic, and both carry the potential for severe complications. Early recognition of simple infection, necrotizing fasciitis, synergistic gangrene, and clostridial myonecrosis can be lifesaving. Antibiotic regimens such as vancomycin plus piperacillin/tazobactam or vancomycin plus a carbapenem, with guidance from Gram stain and culture, are used in conjunction with drainage and excision of all necrotic and pale tissue. High-dose penicillin is used for *Clostridium perfingens* myonecrosis with radical surgery. Adjunctive hyperbaric oxygen is used when available.

SUGGESTED READING

Baker DA. Consequences of herpes simplex virus in pregnancy and their prevention. *Curr Opin Infect Dis*. 2007;20(1):73–76.

Brown, ZA, Gardella, C, Wald, A, et al. Genital herpes complicating pregnancy. *Obstet Gynecol*. 2005;106:845–856.

Faro S. Postpartum endometritis. *Clin Perinatol*. 2005;32(3):803–814.

French LM, Smaill FM. Antibiotic regimens for endometritis after delivery. *Cochrane Database Syst Rev*. 2004; CD001067.

Gardella C, Brown ZA. Managing genital herpes infections in pregnancy. *Cleve Clin J Med*. 2007;74(3):217–224.

Isturiz RE, Gotuzzo E. Tropical infectious disease concerns in pregnancy. In: Guerrant RL, Walker DH, Weller PE, eds. *Tropical Infectious Diseases: Principles, Pathogens and Practice*. 2nd ed. Philadelphia, PA: Elsevier; 2006:1708.

Muller AE, Oostvogel PM, Steegers EA, et al. Morbidity related to maternal group B streptococcal infections. *Acta Obstet Gynecol Scand*. 2006;85(9):1027–1037.

National Institutes of Health. Recommendations for use of antiretroviral drugs in pregnant HIV-1-infected women for maternal health and interventions to reduce perinatal HIV-1 transmission in the United States. http://AIDSinfo.nih.gov. October 12, 2006. Accessed January 3, 2006.

Newman J. Blocked ducts and mastitis. http://www.bflrc.com/newman/breastfeeding/mastitis.html. Accessed September 26, 2006.

Nicolle LE, Bradley S, Colgan R, et al. IDSA Guidelines for the diagnosis and treatment of asymptomatic bacteriuria in adults. *Clin Infect Dis.* 2005;40:643–654.

A new product (VariZig) for post-exposure prophylaxis of varicella available under an investigational new drug application expanded access protocol. *Morbid Mortal Weekly Rep.* 2006;55:209–210.

Yagi H, Fukushima K, Satoh S, et al. Postpartum retroperitoneal fasciitis: a case report and review of literature. *Am J Perinatol.* 2005;22(2):109–113.

94. Dialysis-Related Infection

Peter Mariuz and Roy T. Steigbigel

The incidence and prevalence of patients treated for end-stage renal disease (ESRD) continually increases in the United States. Data from the U.S. Renal Data System (USRDS) 2006 Annual Report show that for 2004, 335 034 patients were treated for ESRD with either hemodialysis (309 269) or peritoneal dialysis (25 765), and 102 104 patients started dialysis. The total number of patients on dialysis is higher as the USRDS does not include data on non-Medicare patients. After cardiovascular disease, infections are the second most common cause of death of patients receiving long-term dialysis (12% to 22%), and a leading cause of hospitalization. Data on the mortality of patients on dialysis followed for 16 years, a longer period than in the USRDS, show that infections account for 36% of deaths versus 14.4% for cardiovascular disease. Sepsis is responsible for more than 75% of deaths caused by infection. Abnormalities of cellular immunity, neutrophil function, and complement activation are associated with chronic renal failure and cited as risk factors for the increased susceptibility to infection. Most dialysis-related infections are caused by common microorganisms rather than by opportunistic pathogens and are primarily related to vascular and peritoneal dialysis access. This chapter focuses on the treatment of infections related to dialysis access devices.

TYPES OF ACCESS DEVICES FOR DIALYSIS

The wide variety of catheters available for hemodialysis (Table 94.1) differ according to the duration of use (acute versus chronic) and intraperitoneal versus extraperitoneal designs. The peritoneal catheters for acute use (≤3 days) have the same basic design, a relatively stiff length of straight or slightly curved nylon or polyethylene tubing with side holes at the distal portion. This is placed at the bedside over a guidewire. These catheters lack cuffs that may protect against bacterial migration from the skin along the outer surface of the catheter, so they have a high infection rate when used for longer than 3 days. Peritoneal access devices

for chronic use are made of silicone rubber or polyurethane, usually with 1 or 2 Dacron cuffs and side holes at the distal end. They can be placed by use of guidewire and dilators, peritoneoscopy, or, less frequently, laparoscopy. The silicone rubber or polyurethane surface elicits growth of squamous epithelium in the subcutaneous tunnel and at the catheter's entry and exit sites. The Dacron cuffs provoke a local inflammatory response resulting in the formation of fibrous and granulation tissues within 4 weeks. Both epithelial and fibrous tissues make bacterial migration along the tunnel more difficult. In addition, the fibrous tissue anchors the catheter. Examples of peritoneal catheters for chronic use include the straight or curled Tenckoff catheter widely used in the United States, Oreopoulos–Zellerman, Lifecath, and Toronto Western II. It is not known whether these newer catheters provide any advantage over the Tenckoff design.

INFECTIOUS COMPLICATIONS OF VASCULAR ACCESS DEVICES

In 2004, 28% of long-term hemo-dialysis (HD) patients used a catheter for permanent intravenous access. Each dialysis session requires four tubing connections, thus the high risk for introduction of microbes through the hub and lumen of catheters. The reported frequency of catheter-related bloodstream infections (CR-BSI) ranges from 0.9 to 2.0 episodes per patient-year. This is markedly higher compared to fistulas and grafts. The relative risk for infection-related hospitalization and death is increased 2- to 3-fold for catheter-dependent HD patients. Local infections occur at the exit site or in the tunnel of percutaneously inserted silicone catheters. The clinical presentations of exit-site infection include pain, erythema, tenderness, induration, and purulent discharge within 2 cm of the site. Tunnel infections are associated with pain, erythema, tenderness, or induration involving the subcutaneous tract of the catheter. Infection of autologous arteriovenous (AV) fistulas and prosthetic polytetrafluoroethylene (PTFE) grafts can manifest as cellulitis, perifistular abscess, false aneurysm, draining sinus,

Table 94.1 Vascular Access Devices for Hemodialysis

Temporary Venous Access (Usually Less Than 2–3 Weeks)	Permanent Access for ESRD
Single- or double-lumen (Mahurkar type) catheter into the subclavian vein	Arteriovenous fistula using autogenous saphenous vein or PTFE, Teflon
Silastin-Teflon shunt for CAVH or CAVHD	Dacron-cuffed double-lumen silicon catheter (Permcath); rarely used; surgically inserted into the subclavian or internal jugular vein through a subcutaneous tunnel
Twin wide-bore femoral catheter for CAVH or CAVHD	Scribner arteriovenous shunt, now used infrequently
Temporary venous access in ESRD: single- or double-lumen venous catheter inserted over guidewire into the subclavian, femoral,[a] or internal jugular vein	

Abbreviations: ESRD = end-stage renal disease; PTFE = polytetrafluoroethylene; CAVH = continuous arteriovenous hemofiltration; CAVHD = continuous arteriovenous hemodialysis.
[a] Femoral vein placement is associated with high rate of infection, so it is usually removed by 72 hours.

and in PTFE shunts, bleeding when the grafts' suture lines are involved. Fever, leukocytosis, or left shift in the differential leukocyte count may be present.

All local access device infections may be complicated by concomitant bacteremia, sepsis, and suppurative thrombophlebitis. Bacteremia may lead to metastatic foci of infection, including septic arthritis, septic pulmonary emboli, endocarditis, osteomyelitis, brain abscess, and splenic abscess. Bacteremia and sepsis most often present without signs or symptoms of infection at the access site. Most CR-BSI arise in the lumen following bacterial colonization and biofilm formation. Eradication of bacteria in endoluminal biofilm requires very high concentrations of antibiotics (up to 1000 times the concentrations needed to kill bacteria in solution). Systemic antibiotic therapy alone without catheter removal yields cure only in one third of these catheter-related bloodstream infections.

Microbiology

A specific microbiologic diagnosis of access-related infection can frequently be made by Gram stain and culture of purulent material from the cannula exit site or with AV fistulas from needle exit sites, fistulas, or abscess fluid. In addition, blood cultures drawn from the access device and other peripheral sites should be obtained to aid in identification of access site as origin of infection. Quantitative blood cultures (indicating colony counts from catheter blood that are 5-fold greater than from peripheral blood) or earlier time (at least 2 hours) to positivity of culture of blood from catheter compared to blood from another site indicates access site origin

of infection. The organisms responsible for access device infection are shown in Table 94.2. Catheter-related colonization without clinical manifestations of infection has been reported in up to 55% of hemodialysis catheters.

Therapy

Therapy is ultimately based on the results of cultures from infected sites and blood. Initial management plans are shown in Table 94.3. Indications for removal of the access device include tunnel infections, suppurative thrombophlebitis, septicemia, bacteremia with metastatic foci of infection, infections caused by *Staphylococcus aureus* and fungi, lack of response to medical therapy within 24 to 48 hours, recurrent infection in a catheter with the same pathogen, and involvement of the suture lines of PTFE grafts. Any associated fluid collections should be drained. In the absence of exit-site and tunnel infection, sepsis, or metastatic foci of infection, exchange of the catheter over a guidewire may be attempted. If there is no clinical improvement within 24 to 48 hours the catheter should be removed. CR-BSI caused by coagulase-negative staphylococci (not *S. aureus*) seem very amenable to this technique. Intravenous (IV) vancomycin is often used in initial therapy for access device infections because staphylococci are the most common pathogens. Depending on the type of dialyzer used, therapeutic blood levels of vancomycin may be achieved for 5 to 10 days. After a 1-g IV dose of vancomycin, serum levels should be monitored after 5 to 7 days to ensure adequate trough levels. To avoid overuse of vancomycin with induction of vancomycin-resistant bacteria, methicillin-sensitive

Table 94.2 Microbiology of Access Device Infections

Hemodialysis	Peritoneal Dialysis
Staphylococcus aureus (50%–80%) Other gram-positive bacteria (*S. epidermidis*, streptococci, including enterococci, diphtheroides), gram-negative organisms (*Escherichia coli, Pseudomonas aeruginosa, Acinetobacter* spp., and other enteric gram-negative bacteria) (15%–30%) Occasionally fungi	*Staphylococcus epidermidis* and *S. aureus* (50%) Other gram-positive bacteria (streptococci, including enterococci, diphtheroides) Gram-negative organisms (*E. coli, P. aeruginosa, Acinetobacter* spp., and other enteric gram-negative bacteria) Occasionally fungi
Percentages in parentheses are approximate proportional incidence from numerous references.	

Table 94.3 Treatment of Hemodialysis Access-Site Infections

Type of Infection	Therapy
Exit-site infection in a temporary access device with or without bacteremia	Catheter removal and vancomycin,[a] 1 g IV; subsequent doses based on serum levels; aminoglycosides or broad-spectrum β-lactam antibiotics if gram-negative organisms suspected
Tunnel infection	Catheter removal and antibiotics as above
Catheter-related sepsis	Catheter removal; empiric broad-spectrum antimicrobial therapy with vancomycin and gentamicin, 1.5 mg/kg IV in a single dose; subsequent antimicrobial therapy based on pathogen and sensitivity pattern
Suppurative thrombophlebitis	Catheter removal, antimicrobial therapy based on pathogen and sensitivity pattern; surgical consultation for possible exploratory venotomy
Arteriovenous fistula infection	Vancomycin and gentamicin as above; incision and drainage of abscess; ligation or removal of prosthetic arteriovenous fistulas for occlusion or tunnel infection or if response to treatment is not prompt; surgical repair of a malfunctioning infected shunt may be possible 10–14 days of therapy commonly used for exit and tunnel infections with catheter removal; if the catheter remains in place, 2–3 weeks of antimicrobials

[a] Alternatives to vancomycin include daptomycin and linezolid (see text).
Abbreviation: IV = intravenously.

staphylococci should be treated with nafcillin, 1 to 2 g IV every 4 to 6 hours. Newer antimicrobials with good activity against staphylococci are alternatives to vancomycin. They would be used in patients with allergy to vancomycin or for organisms with reduced sensitivity to vancomycin. These include daptomycin, 4 mg/kg or 6 mg/kg if bacteremia present every 48 hours (preferably after dialysis), and linezolid, 600 mg IV every 12 hours. Fifteen to thirty percent of infections are caused by gram-negative bacilli. If gram-negative organisms are suspected, an aminoglycoside, cefepime, or aztreonam should be used in combination with the antibiotic noted above for infection caused by gram-positive organisms. Vancomycin-resistant enterococci (VRE) resistant to ampicillin should be treated with linezolid or daptomycin. The initial choice of antimicrobials should be influenced by the sensitivity of organisms prevalent in the patient's geographic region.

When catheter salvage is attempted, antibiotic lock therapy (ALT) has been recommended in addition to parenteral antibiotics for uncomplicated catheter infections. The rationale is the known difficulty to eradicate bacteria in endoluminal biofilm with parenteral therapy. With ALT the catheter lumen is filled with several milliliters of antimicrobial solution at concentrations severalfold higher than the MIC of the antibiotic for the infecting organism with 50 to 100 U of heparin. Vancomycin (1 to 5 mg/mL), gentamicin, or amikacin (1 to 2 mg/mL); ciprofloxin (1 to 2 mg/mL); and cefazolin

(5 mg/mL) have been used most often. The solution is allowed to remain (lock) in the catheter for as long as possible. The same volume of solution is removed before the next dose of antibiotic or other medications or solutions are administered. The optimal duration of ALT is not known but it has been used most frequently for 2 weeks. Well designed, appropriately powered, randomized, controlled trials that show efficacy of ALT are lacking.

Lock therapy rather than catheter removal should not be used when the patient is septic or considered to have septic thrombophlebitis, endocarditis, osteomyelitis, neutropenia, fungal infection exit-site, or tunnel infections.

INFECTIONS ASSOCIATED WITH PERITONEAL DIALYSIS CATHETERS

There are several types of chronic peritoneal dialysis: continuous ambulatory peritoneal dialysis (CAPD), continuous cycling (CCPD), and nightly PD with a dry day. CAPD has a relatively high incidence of exit-site and tunnel infections (0.6 to 0.7 per dialysis-year). Whether PD catheter infections are less frequent with CCPD or nightly PD with a dry day remains controversial. Thirty percent of patient transfers from peritoneal to hemodialysis are a consequence of catheter complications and peritonitis. PD catheter exit-site and particularly tunnel infections may result in peritonitis and catheter loss. Peritonitis accounts for 15% to 35% of hospital admissions for patients on PD.

Exit-site infections present with erythema, tenderness, induration, and/or purulent discharge from the exit site. Pericatheter erythema without purulent drainage may be an early sign of infection. Crusting caused by a small amount of exudate at the exit site may not be indicative of infection. Erythema, tenderness, induration, pain, and abscess in the area between the catheter cuffs suggests tunnel infection. This can be confirmed by ultrasonography, which will reveal an area of hypoechogenicity (fluid collection) between the tube or the cuff of the catheter and surrounding tissues. Indications for tunnel sonography include presence of exit-site infection, recurrent peritonitis and for assessment of the efficacy of therapy and prognosis of tunnel infections. Computed tomography scans are also used to evaluate tunnel infections. A specific microbiologic diagnosis can be made by performing a Gram stain and culture of purulent exudate. The organisms responsible for PD catheter infections are shown in Table 94.2. *Staphylococcus aureus* and *Pseudomonas aeruginosa* exit-site infections are frequently associated with concomitant tunnel infections.

Therapy

Therapy is ultimately based on the results of microbiologic culture data. Initial management plans are shown in Table 94.4. Therapy should be continued until the exit site appears normal. Indications for catheter removal, shown in Table 94.5, include peritonitis, bacteremia, and sepsis. Relative indications for catheter removal are tunnel infections (particularly if there is no response to therapy noted on serial ultrasound examinations), involvement of the deep cuff (which often leads to peritonitis), chronic exit-site infections (no cure after 2 to 4 weeks of therapy), and exit-site infections associated with involvement of the superficial cuff as noted on ultrasound. Ultrasonographic evidence of tunnel involvement is associated with frequent catheter loss (50%) because of refractory or recurrent peritonitis. The use of serial ultrasound examinations may also be useful to monitor the efficacy of antimicrobial therapy of tunnel infections. A 30% or greater decrease in the size of the fluid collection after 2 weeks of therapy is often associated with catheter salvage. Prolonged courses of antimicrobial therapy, although sometimes necessary, should be avoided given the problem of antimicrobial resistance. Infections with VRE and, more ominously, vancomycin-resistant strains of *S. aureus* and *S. epidermidis* reported in dialysis patients receiving prolonged (months) treatment make the judicious use of this drug imperative. In chronic exit-site infections, adjunctive surgical therapy may help control infection and result in catheter salvage. Surgical procedures that have been used include cuff shaving (removal of the external cuff), debridement and curettage of the exit-site and sinus tract, incision, and debridement along the subcutaneous tunnel with exteriorization of the superficial cuff and relocation of the exit site. It is not known which of these is most effective. Among gram-positive organisms, *S. aureus* is more commonly associated with poor response to medical therapy, tunnel infections, and catheter loss.

PERITONITIS ASSOCIATED WITH CAPD INFECTIONS

Peritonitis is a common complication of PD. Although the incidence varies from center to

Table 94.4 Treatment of Peritoneal Dialysis Access Device Infections

Type of Infection	Therapy
Exit-site infection with minimal erythema without purulent discharge	Topical mupirocin, chlorhexidine, hydrogen peroxide, or povidone iodine bid; avoid mupirocin with polyurethane catheter.
Gram-positive exit-site infection	Dicloxacillin, 250–500 mg PO q6h, or cephalexin, 250–500 mg PO q6h, or trimethoprim-sulfamethoxazole, 160/800 mg PO bid. Clindamycin may also be used. IV or IP route can be used. For methicillin-resistant staphylococci: vancomycin, 1 g/wk IV. Rifampin, 600 mg PO qd, can be added for possible synergistic effect. Ultrasound to rule out tunnel or cuff involvement; 2–3 weeks of therapy generally recommended; shave external cuff and explore tunnel if infection persists; if this fails, catheter removal.
Gram-negative exit-site infection	*Pseudomonas aeruginosa* should be suspected pending culture results. Ciprofloxacin, 500 mg PO bid; not to be taken concomitantly with phosphate binders or antacids; alteration of therapy based on culture results. Therapy should be continued for 2–3 weeks. Catheter removal if infection persists beyond 2–3 weeks; early catheter removal should be considered if *Pseudomonas* or *Stenotrophomonas* isolated.
Tunnel infection	Antimicrobials as for exit-side infections with removal of catheter.

Abbreviations: BID = twice a day; PO = orally; IV = intravenously; IP = intraperitoneally.

Table 94.5 Indications for Peritoneal Dialysis Catheter Removal

Peritonitis
Bacteremia
Sepsis
Recurrent peritonitis (same pathogen)
Tunnel infections
Chronic exit-site infections
Infections caused by fungi

center, the overall incidence is 1.3 episodes per patient per year. Peritonitis may be less common in continuous cycle-assisted peritoneal dialysis (CCPD) and nocturnal intermittent peritoneal dialysis (NIPD) than in other forms of CAPD. An additional, modest reduction in the incidence of peritonitis has been achieved with use of Y-set transfer kit and "flush before fill" (particularly infections from skin flora). Bacteria gain entry to the peritoneum through the lumen of the catheter, often after improper technique in connecting the transfer set to the dialysate bag or the catheter to the transfer set from the outside surface of the catheter; complications from an exit-site or tunnel infection;

or by hematogenous spread from the bowel or pelvis. Clinical manifestations include abdominal pain, fever, chills, malaise, nausea, vomiting, constipation, or diarrhea with abdominal tenderness, rebound tenderness, and leukocytosis. The peritoneal fluid may appear cloudy and will almost always contain >100 polymorphonuclear leukocytes per cubic millimeter of fluid. In any suspected CAPD infection, including those that appear to be localized to the exit site, a Gram stain and culture of the peritoneal fluid should be obtained with cell count and differential.

Microbiology

A single pathogen is usually involved. Polymicrobial infection suggests a perforated viscus or other intra-abdominal or pelvic pathologic process. Most cases of peritonitis (70%) are caused by gram-positive bacteria. Collectively, *S. aureus* and *S. epidermidis* account for almost 50% of infections. *Pseudomonas aeruginosa* and enteric gram-negative bacilli constitute 20% to 30%, and fungi, mostly *Candida albicans,* <1% to 10%. Some 5% to 20% of cases are culture negative. Though infrequent, fungal peritonitis is associated with significant morbidity and mortality: Death rates are as high as 25%, and up to 40% of patients cannot resume PD.

Therapy

No clinical trials establishing the optimal anti-biotic drugs and route of administration have been done. Antibiotics may be given by the IV, oral (PO), or intraperitoneal (IP) route. The IP route is preferred because of its convenience. There is no therapeutic advantage to IV therapy. Helpful information for the initial choice of anti-microbials includes peritoneal fluid Gram stain results, history of microbe-specific peritonitis, coexistent exit-site infection, and intra-abdominal pathology. Given the increasing prevalence of vancomycin-resistant gram-positive bacteria, the routine use of this drug for empiric therapy can no longer be justified unless the dialysis center is known to have a high rate of infections with methicillin-resistant organisms. If the Gram stain suggests gram-positive bacteria or gram-negative bacteria or is negative or un-available, empiric therapy should be initiated; IP cefazolin or cephalothin, 500 mg/L loading dose and then 125 mg/L, in each exchange with an aminoglycoside, such as gentamicin, 0.6 mg/kg body weight, in one daily exchange. Alternatives to cefazolin or cephalothin include nafcillin, clindamycin, vancomycin, and cipro-floxacin, in order of preference.

Fluconazole, 200 mg PO or IP daily, should be used for yeast infections. The catheter should be promptly removed and treatment continued for at least 10 more days. Voriconazole, an echinocandin inhibitor, and amphotericin B are alternatives to fluconazole for patients who do not respond or who have organisms insensitive or less sensitive to fluconazole such as *Candida krusei* and *Candida glabrata*. After catheter removal, infections with filamentous fungi should be treated with amphotericin B or voriconazole.

After 24 to 48 hours, 70% to 90% of dialysate fluid cultures will yield a specific pathogen, and therapy should be modified accordingly. For *S. aureus* or *S. epidermidis* sensitive to nafcillin, it should be given at 125 mg/L in each exchange or the first-generation cephalosporin may be continued. The aminoglycoside should be stopped. Rifampin, 600 mg/day PO, may be added for patients responding slowly to the initial regimen but should not be used for more than a week as resistance to this drug often develops with prolonged use. In areas where tuberculosis is endemic, the use of rifampin to treat *S. aureus* peritonitis should be avoided. If the patient does not improve, there should be evaluation for tunnel infection. For staphylo-cocci resistant to methicillin (MRSA), nafcillin or

the cephalosporin and aminoglycoside should be discontinued. Vancomycin, 2 g (30 mg/kg) IP every 7 days, or, if the organism is sensitive, clindamycin, 300 mg/L loading dose and then 150 mg/L maintenance, can be used. Rifampin should be added as stated previously. For entero-cocci sensitive to ampicillin, the cephalosporin should be discontinued and ampicillin started at 125 mg/L in each exchange, and consider continuing the aminoglycoside. In penicillin-allergic patients, vancomycin, 2 g IP per week, should be used. Treatment of VRE depends on the antimicrobial sensitivities of the specific organism. If VRE is ampicillin susceptible, this is the drug of choice. Linezolid, 600 mg IV every 12 hours, or daptomycin, 4 mg/kg (6 mg/kg if bacteremia present) every 48 hours, preferably after dialysis, are useful for VRE resistant to ampicillin and for the penicillin-allergic patient. Because enterococci are part of the intestinal flora, intra-abdominal pathology must be considered. For other gram-positive organisms, therapy should be based on antibiotic sensitivity results. For gram-negative organisms other than *Pseudomonas* and *Stenotrophomonas maltophilia*, a first-generation cephalosporin may suffice, and the aminoglycoside can be discontinued. If the microbe is resistant to cefazolin, the choice of another cephalosporin should be based on sensitivity testing.

Fourteen days of therapy are usually ad-equate. If multiple gram-negative organisms are isolated, evaluation for intra-abdominal pa-thology should be undertaken. For *P. aeruginosa* or *S. maltophilia,* consider use of two agents (one being an aminoglycoside) chosen based on sen-sitivity testing results and continue for at least 3 weeks. However, eighth nerve toxicity may complicate aminoglycoside use, particularly after 2 to 3 weeks of therapy. If the infection is catheter related, the catheter should be removed with continued administration of antibiotics for 1 week.

For polymicrobial or anaerobic infections, consider surgical intervention, continue the aminoglycoside, continue or change the cepha-losporin based on sensitivity testing, and add metronidazole, 500 mg IV or PO every 8 hours.

Most patients with peritonitis demonstrate significant clinical improvement within 2 to 4 days. Patients who do not respond to therapy should be reevaluated. Peritoneal fluid should be obtained for cell counts, Gram stain, and culture. In addition, intra-abdominal or gyneco-logic pathology requiring surgical intervention and unusual pathogens (fungi, mycobacteria) must be considered. The catheter should be removed and cultures obtained for patients whose original cultures are negative and remain symptomatic after 2 to 4 days.

LESS COMMON PATHOGENS

There are conflicting data regarding the intrinsic risk of dialysis patients for developing tuberculosis. It is likely that any predisposition of these patients to tuberculosis is related more to the prevalence of tuberculosis in the community than to host factors. However, there is a higher incidence of extrapulmonary tuberculosis in this population than in those not receiving PD. Treatment is the same as for patients without ESRD except dosing of some agents must be adjusted for renal failure and others should be avoided. Isoniazid is given at 150 mg/day PO with a supplemental dose after dialysis. Rifampin requires no dosage adjustment. The dosage of ethambutol is 5 mg/kg/day PO with a supplemental dose after dialysis. Some authorities believe that pyrazinamide use should be avoided if possible; ethionamide is given at 250 to 500 mg/day PO.

Listeria monocytogenes septicemia, meningitis, and endocarditis have been rarely described in patients with ESRD, usually as a complication of iron overload or during immunosuppressive therapy. Yersiniosis complicating iron overload has also been reported. Disseminated or rhinocerebral phycomycosis in nondiabetic patients receiving hemodialysis may be related to deferoxamine use. Treatment for it includes amphotericin B, posaconazole, and surgical debridement of infected sites.

SUGGESTED READING

Allon M. Dialysis catheter-related bacteremia: treatment and prophylaxis. *Am J Kidney Dis.* 2004;44:779–791.

Goldman M, Vanherweghem JL. Bacterial infections in chronic hemodialysis patients: epidemiologic and pathophysiologic aspects. *Adv Nephrol.* 1990;19:315–332.

Mermel LA, Farr MB, Sherertz RJ, et al. Guidelines for the management of intravascular catheter-related infections. *Clin Infect Dis.* 2001;32:1249–1272.

Piraino B, Bailie GR, Bernardini J, et al. Peritoneal dialysis-related infections recommendations: 2005 update. *Perit Dial Int.* 2005;25:107–131.

Steigbigel RT, Cross AS. Infections associated with hemodialysis and chronic peritoneal dialysis. In Remington JS, Swartz MN, eds. *Current Clinical Topics in Infectious Diseases.* Vol 5. New York, NY: McGraw-Hill; 1984.

U.S. Renal Data System. *USRDS 2006 Annual Data Report.* Bethesda, MD: National Institutes of Health, National Institute of Diabetes and Digestive and Kidney Diseases; 2006.

Vychytil A, Lorenz M, Schneider B, et al. New criteria for management of catheter infections in peritoneal dialysis patients using ultrasonography. *J Am Soc Nephrol.* 1998;9:290–296.

95. Overwhelming Postsplenectomy Infection

Larry I. Lutwick, Amy Wecker, and Monica Panwar

What more thou didst deserve than in thy name,
And free thee from the scandal of such senses
　　As in the rancor of unhappy spleen
Measure thy course of life, with false pretenses
Comparing by thy death what thou hast been.
　　–"A Funeral Elegy," W. Shakespeare, 1612

INTRODUCTION

The human spleen (Figure 95.1) (in German: *milz*; *ohnemilz*: without a spleen), an organ that at one point had been deemed as nonessential as the appendix, has been associated in history as the source of melancholy thoughts. This concept brought forth the expression of "venting one's spleen" as a way of improving a person's overall situation. A similar therapeutic process, laughter ("If you desire the spleen, and will laugh yourself into stitches, follow me," Shakespeare [Figure 95.2A], *Twelfth Night*, Act III, Scene 2), is also linked to the spleen.

It seems ironic, therefore, that these concepts reflect that this collection of immune cells in the left upper quadrant of the abdomen appeared to function as a way of cleansing the body. Indeed, Shakespeare's "unhappy spleen," one that has been removed from residence (by splenectomy) or whose function is embarrassed by one or another disease (hyposplenism), predisposes (by not appropriately performing its cleansing function) its former owner to an infectious disease process with substantial morbidity and mortality by becoming *ohnemilz*.

This disease, overwhelming postsplenectomy infection (OPSI), also referred to as postsplenectomy sepsis (PSS), is one of a group of infectious disease processes, such as bacterial meningitis and meningococcemia, for which diagnosis and therapeutic intervention are required immediately to minimize the disease impact. Using Ben Franklin's (Figure 95.2B) "ounce of prevention is worth a pound of cure" concept, prevention as well as therapeutic intervention is an important part of any discussion of OPSI.

RISKS AND TIMING OF OPSI

The individual risk of OPSI is dependent on the cause of splenectomy as well as the time

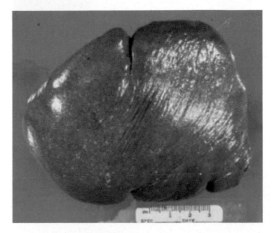

Figure 95.1 The spleen.

after the procedure. Overall, the lifetime risk of 1% to 2% is estimated related to trauma or idiopathic thrombocytopenic purpura (ITP), 3% for spherocytosis, 6% for Hodgkin's disease and portal hypertension, and as high as 11% for thalassemia. Although some asplenic conditions clearly have a lower risk of OPSI, if OPSI develops the morbidity and mortality are not lower in these cohorts. About 5% to 6% of total OPSI cases occur in individuals with poorly functioning spleens. A partial list of diseases associated with hyposplenism can be found in Table 95.1.

No ideal assay is available to measure adequate splenic function. The presence of Howell–Jolly bodies (nuclear remnants in circulating red blood cells [RBCs]) is too insensitive. Quantification of red cells containing "pocks" (actually vacuoles containing hemoglobin found in older RBCs) as seen by interference microscopy, however, appears to be a valuable tool.

About 50% of cases of OPSI following a splenectomy occur within 2 years of the event and about 75% within 5 years. It is important to know, however, that 2% to 3% of cases occur 20 years or longer after the event and reports of OPSI 4 decades after the onset of *ohnemilz*.

PRESENTATION AND DIAGNOSIS

The classical presentation of OPSI is one that begins often with an alert, relatively nontoxic

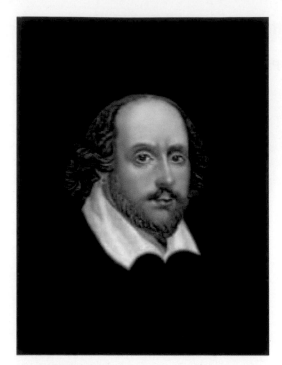

Figure 95.2A Shakespeare.

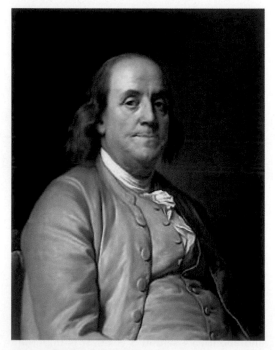

Figure 95.2B Ben Franklin.

Table 95.1 Common Causes of Hyposplenism

Blood Diseases
Primary thrombocytosis
Sickle cell hemoglobinopathies
Gastrointestinal Diseases
Celiac disease
Ulcerative colitis
Splenic Infiltration
Amyloidosis
Sarcoidosis
Malignant infiltration
Vasculitic Diseases
Autoimmune thyroiditis
Lupus erythematosis
Rheumatoid disease
Others
Ethanolism
Long-term parenteral nutrition
Spleen irradiation
Splenic vein thrombosis

patient who might walk into an emergency department complaining of fever and chills associated with myalgias and diarrhea. Often the individual deteriorates quickly, developing lactic acidosis due to organ hypoperfusion, disseminated intravascular coagulation (DIC), and multiorgan failure. This gastroenteritis-like presentation can, but should not, divert attention away from OPSI in the at-risk individual.

The progression to septic shock and death in these individuals can happen within hours of initial presentation. Overall mortality rates are 50% to 60%, with a majority of the deaths within 24 hours. Encouragingly, relatively recent pediatric data suggest that increased survival rates can result from prompt recognition and overall incidence can decrease with preventative measures. Purpura fulminans (Figure 95.3) has been associated with OPSI as well as with meningococcemia. It causes considerable endothelial injury, resulting in arterial thrombosis and gangrene of one or multiple extremities. If the affected individual survives, multiple extremity amputations can result.

Prompt diagnosis requires knowledge of the issue with spleen function or absence in an appropriately ill patient. Confirmation awaits finding positive blood cultures for the bacterial etiology or finding intraerythrocytic protozoa. Blood cultures are often positive within 6 to 8 hours due to the high initial bacteremia, which is as much as 10 000 times the organism load of a more routine bacteremia. Because of this massive bacteremia, organisms can be found in the buffy coat of the peripheral blood and sometimes on a standard peripheral smear. It should be noted that Wright stain is routinely used on peripheral blood smears and will stain

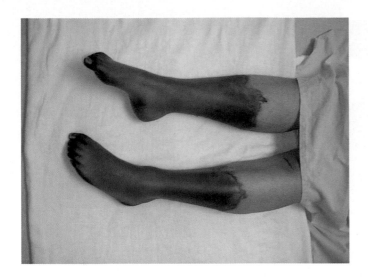

Figure 95.3 Purpura fulminans.

all bacteria blue, even the usual "red" organisms on Gram stain of gram-negative bacteria.

PATHOGENS

Streptococcus pneumoniae (the pneumococcus)

The pneumococcus is without question the most common cause of OPSI. This α-hemolytic, polysaccharide-encapsulated, gram-positive coccoid bacterium has a distinctive morphology on staining, a so-called lancet shape (Figure 95.4). Its capsule is a well-recognized virulence factor, interfering with phagocytosis by preventing effective C3b opsonization of the bacterial cells. Overall, *S. pneumoniae* is involved in 50% to 90% of OPSI cases, with the percentage of pneumococcal OPSI cases tending to increase with age. In series that include single case reports, pneumococci are often underrepresented because many case reports relate to less common causes of infection in asplenic hosts.

No single type or group of the 90 different capsular types appears to be more associated with OPSI than other forms of invasive pneumococcal disease. With the use of pneumococcal polysaccharide vaccination, however, especially in places with universal immunization using the newer heptavalent conjugated product, a shift of serotypes can occur.

It is important to note that antimicrobial drug resistance has become increasingly prevalent. Some isolates are only less sensitive to penicillin (particularly relevant in bacterial meningitis), some are fully resistant to penicillin, and some may be resistant to both penicillin as well as the extended-spectrum cephalosporins such as

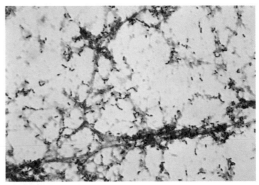

Figure 95.4 Pneumococcus.

ceftriaxone. The local epidemiology of pneumococcal resistance must be considered in the empiric treatment of OPSI. High levels of penicillin resistance are reported in Spain, parts of eastern Europe, and South Africa (Figure 95.5). In the United States, resistance is more prevalent in Alaska and the South but can be found anywhere. It is yet to be determined whether changes in serotypes in the postheptavalent conjugate vaccine era will in the long run increase or decrease antimicrobial resistance.

Haemophilus influenzae type b

Although studies report the frequency of *Haemophilus influenzae* type b (Hib)-associated OPSI to be about 10 times lower than that of the pneumococcus type b, the organism is classically the second most common cause of OPSI. It has primarily affected children younger than 15 years. *Haemophilus influenzae* is a small polysaccharide-encapsulated pleomorphic gram-negative coccobacillus (Figure 95.6) that can be confused with pneumococcus if the Gram stain

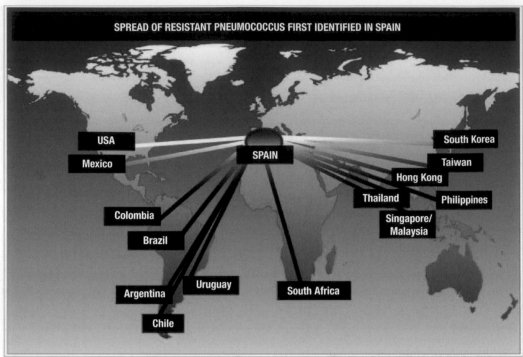

SPREAD OF RESISTANT PNEUMOCOCCUS FIRST IDENTIFIED IN SPAIN

USA

Mexico

SPAIN

South Korea

Taiwan

Hong Kong

Thailand

Philippines

Colombia

Singapore/
Malaysia

Brazil

Uruguay

South Africa

Argentina

Chile

Source: K. Klugmann. South African Institute of Medical Research

Figure 95.5 Spread of resistant pneumococcus.

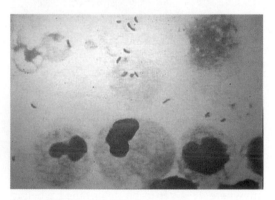

Figure 95.6 *Haemophilus influenzae.*

technique is poor (over- or underdecolorized). Like pneumococcus, the type b capsule is a major virulence factor for invasive disease.

The incidence of invasive Hib disease (and correspondingly of Hib-related OPSI) has dramatically decreased because of the use of the conjugated Hib vaccine. Neither nontypable strains nor non-b capsular organisms have been found to be significant causes of OPSI, although nontypable organisms may cause usually noninvasive infection in the human respiratory tract. When choosing antimicrobial therapy, it is important to know that many *H. influenzae* strains produce β-lactamases.

OTHER BACTERIAL ORGANISMS

Capnocytophaga canimorsus, a fastidious gram-negative rod formerly referred to as CDC group DF-2, is usually transmitted to humans from dog bites. Human infection with this normal part of canine and feline oral flora is relatively mild when occurring in the eusplenic host. Of reported severe cases, however, predisposing conditions can be identified in 80%, primarily asplenia or a hyposplenic condition. The presence of an eschar at the bite site 1 to 7 days after the bite, or observation of gram-negative bacilli in the blood buffy coat or peripheral smear, is highly suggestive of *C. canimorsus* infection.

The organism does not have a capsule as the pneumococcus and Hib do but appears to escape from immune surveillance by blocking the typical proinflammatory response of human macrophages perhaps related to the inability of Toll-like receptor 4 to respond to the organism. β-lactamase activity can be seen in 30% of strains.

Although *Neisseria meningitidis* (the meningococcus) is often cited as the third most common cause of OPSI and does occur in the asplenic host, it does not appear that meningococcemia is either more severe or more frequent than in asplenic individuals. Because meningococci are encapsulated and can cause quite severe invasive infection, most authorities include preventative strategies for it in dealing with the noneusplenic person.

Salmonellosis has been associated with, but does not play a large role in, OPSI. Most reports are associated with illnesses where cell-mediated immunity defects from either the illness or its treatment predispose to salmonellosis, such as in children with sickle cell anemia. Sickle cell disease, however, does cause hyposplenism as previously noted.

INTRAERYTHROCYTIC PARASITEMIAS

The human spleen plays a key role in malarial parasite clearance by removal of the intraerythrocytic parasites from the RBC without red cell destruction (pitting). Because pitting is absent or much diminished in the splenectomized or hyposplenic person, removal of malarial parasites (either killed by medication or viable) is delayed and disease may be more severe. During antimalarial therapy, delayed clearance in the noneusplenic does not, therefore, necessarily reflect antimalarial resistance. In partially malaria-immune individuals, the course of *P. falciparum* infection is not much changed by asplenia, but more fever and higher levels of parasitemia occur and there seems to be a risk for more symptomatic malaria episodes. How this relates to the nonimmune splenectomized person traveling into a malarious area is not clear but appropriate prophylaxis is indicated, regardless of splenic function.

In babesiosis, however, splenectomized patients are clearly at higher risk for illness with much higher levels of parasitemia (Figure 95.7) due to the lack of a spleen. This high parasitemia is associated with significant hemolysis. In the United States, infections have been reported from many states, but the most endemic areas are the islands off the coast of Massachusetts (including Nantucket and Martha's Vineyard) and New York (including eastern and south-central Long Island, Shelter Island, and Fire Island) and in Connecticut. Many of the initial individuals diagnosed with babesiosis were asplenics prior to the recognition that mild and even asymptomatic infections with babesiosis may occur in areas of endemicity for this tickborne organism. These noneusplenic individuals are responsible for most cases of morbidity and mortality related to babesiosis. These individuals may also acquire the infection by blood transfusion without travel into a highly endemic area because their underlying

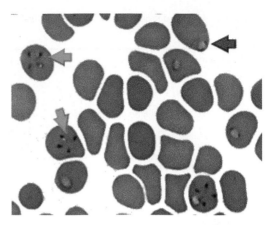

Figure 95.7 Babesiosis.

diseases associated with noneusplenism may cause the need for transfusion.

THERAPEUTIC INTERVENTIONS

Active intervention early on in the form of antimicrobial therapy administration is crucial to patient survival. For this reason, two modalities should be utilized in the prehospital stage of this process aimed at shortening the time to first dose of antimicrobial treatment. For these to be relevant, the asplenic or hyposplenic person has to be aware of the condition and communicate this knowledge to the physician involved. One modality often mentioned in reviews of this infection is having the asplenic person fill and keep current and carry with him/her a prescription for an appropriate orally administered antimicrobial agent (Table 95.2). The drug should be taken, ideally after talking with a physician by telephone, if a febrile illness develops, especially with prostration and without clear etiology while the person is coming to seek health care. It is not a substitute for medical care. The second prehospital modality comes into play when a potential OPSI case presents at a physician's office. Similar to suggestions for a patient with suspected bacterial meningitis, if available, a dose of an antimicrobial such as ceftriaxone should be given intravenously or intramuscularly. This should be done even if blood cultures cannot be performed. For obvious reasons, no controlled trials of these methods of early treatment have or will be done.

On emergency department arrival, it is imperative for the patient to impart the appropriate information regarding the spleen and the new symptoms at once for immediate triage. Specific therapy (Table 95.3) could consist of an extended cephalosporin such as

Table 95.2 Suggested Regimens for Initial Extramural Oral Therapy[a]

Ampicillin or Amoxicillin
Dose: 2 g Contraindicated in β-lactam hypersensitivity Not active against β-lactamase–producing organisms Not active against penicillin-resistant pneumococci
Amoxicillin/Clavulanate
Dose: Two 875 mg amoxicillin/125 mg clavanate tablets Contraindicated in β-lactam hypersensitivity
Trimethoprim/Sulfamethoxazole
Dose: Two 800 mg sulfamethoxazole/160 mg   trimethoprim tablets Contraindicated in sulfonamide hypersensitivity Inconsistent activity for pencillin-resistant pneumococci
Clarithromycin or Azithromycin
Dose: 2 g Inconsistent activity for pencillin-resistant pneumococci
Moxifloxacin
Dose: 800 mg
[a] Minimal to no data on any of any these regimens in overwhelming postsplenectomy infection.

Table 95.3 Treatment Options for Suspected Bacterial OPSI

Rationale: Adequate coverage for *S. pneumoniae* and *H. influenzae*

Ceftriaxone 2 g IV q12h
  Alternative in severe β-lactam allergy
    Moxifloxacin 400 mg IV q24h

Plus

Vancomycin 1 g IV a12h
  Alternatives in vancomycin intolerant patients
    Moxifloxacin 400 mg intravenously q24h

Abbreviations: OPSI = overwhelming postsplenectomy infection; IV = intravenously.

Table 95.4 Treatment Options for Intraerythrocytic Protozoa in OPSI

Babesiosis
(The usual adult dose treatment is for 1 week, but consideration is needed for longer lengths of treatment in asplenics with significant hemolysis. Exchange transfusions have been used as an adjunct in severe cases.)
Atovaquone 750 mg PO q12h plus Azithromycin 500 mg PO on day 1 then 250 mg PO per day OR Clindamycin 600 mg PO q8h plus Quinine 650 mg PO q8h
Falciparum malaria
(Most strains except from parts of Central America, the Caribbean, and the Middle East should be considered to be chloroquine-resistant and that antimalarial should not be used except with cases from known "sensitive" areas.)
Usual adult dose oral therapies (for parenteral treatment of severe falciparum malaria, consult WHO reference)

Atovaquone/Proguanil fixed combination
    4 tablets daily for 3 d
 	
OR
 	
Artemether/lumefantrine fixed combination[a]
    4 tablets 2× daily for 3 d
 	
OR
 	
Quinine 650 mg q8h for 7 d
plus
Doxycycline 200 mg daily for 7 d
or
Clindamycin 600 mg 2× daily for 7 d

[a] Not U.S. Food and Drug Administration approved. Abbreviations: OPSI = overwhelming postsplenectomy infection; PO = orally; WHO = World Health Organization.

ceftriaxone, a β-lactam/β-lactamase inhibitor, a newer fluoroquinolone, and/or vancomycin. The therapy must afford adequate activity against the encapsulated pathogens commonly implicated in OPSI. Choice of initial antimicrobial therapy should be guided by the community antimicrobial resistance profile.

In addition to antimicrobial therapy, aggressive cardiovascular and hemodynamic support is given as needed. Whether adjuvant immunological interventions decrease morbidity and/or mortality is not known but, in animal models, granulocyte-stimulating factor and intravenous immunoglobulin have been studied.

If an intraerythrocytic protozoan is involved, therapy should be directed in that direction. Table 95.4 lists some of the current therapies for falciparum malaria and babesiosis. Response to therapy for babesiosis in the noneusplenic person, however, clinically appears to be much slower independent of the delayed clearance of parasitized erythrocytes.

PREVENTION

Education

The importance of patient (and the respective family) education cannot be overemphasized. A philosopher once reflected that the half-life of truth is 8 months, underscoring the importance of physicians to continue to remind asplenic or hyposplenic patients and/or their families to tell any physician involved in their medical care of the splenic defect. A medical alert bracelet or necklace could also assist in this task. Early knowledge of asplenia can cause early treatment of presumptive OPSI.

The widespread knowledge of OPSI has also changed the landscape of surgical splenectomy. Whenever possible, the organ or part of it is retained in an effort to retain adequate organ function. In trauma situations, repair instead of removal is preferred. Splenectomy, however, is still required in the management of a variety of disease states.

Vaccination

The current Centers for Disease Control and Prevention (CDC) guidelines recommend administering the 23 valent unconjugated pneumococcal polysaccharide vaccine to all adult individuals with functional asplenia. The vaccine is to be administered as 2 doses only, 5 years apart. Because unconjugated polysaccharide vaccines are T lymphocyte independent, they do not prime the immune system to produce immunologic memory, so the second dose is not a booster in the true sense of the word but just another dose. Antibody titers wane over time and seemingly faster in the noneusplenic. It is not unreasonable to consider revaccination with the 23-valent vaccine every 5 years or even sooner. Repeated immunizations with this vaccine are not recommended by CDC, probably due to the lack of adequate safety studies (Table 95.5).

A number of case reports have surfaced documenting occurrence of OPSI with vaccine-related strains of pneumococci sepsis despite administration of the pneumococcal polysaccharide vaccine. This may be related to lack of an adequate response to the polysaccharide of the infecting type. The now-released heptavalent conjugated pneumococcal vaccine has shown promise related to the 7 capsular types in the biologic. Conjugation to a protein backbone makes the antigenic epitopes become T lymphocyte dependent, and it will produce immunologic memory and allow its use in infants. Information exists to suggest that the use of this vaccine may produce an antibody with more opsonophagocytic utility and with more avid binding to its target. Although not licensed for use in adults, consideration for the use of a series of this product followed by its unconjugated cousin is reasonable.

Table 95.5 Bacterial Vaccines to Consider in Patients with Asplenia/Hyposplenia

23 valent unconjugated pneumococcal vaccine
    Contains types 1, 2, 3, 4, 5, 6B, 7F, 8, 9N, 9V, 10A, 11A,
    12F, 14, 15B, 17F, 18C, 19A, 19F, 20, 22F, 23F, and 33F

Heptavalent conjugated pneumococcal vaccine[a]   Contains types 4, 6B, 9V, 14, 18C, 19F, and 23F
Conjugated *H. influenzae* vaccine   Contains type b
Quadrivalent meningococcal vaccine   Contains types A, C, Y, and W-135
[a] Not U.S. Food and Drug Administration approved for adults.

Both meningococcal polysaccharide and the *H. influenzae* type b conjugated vaccines are also part of CDC recommendations for asplenics. No booster doses of either vaccine have been endorsed but may be considered. The meningococcal vaccination is now available as a quadrivalent conjugated polysaccharide product for types A, C, Y, and W-135. To this point, there is no licensed vaccine for type B due to issues of immunogenicity of the antigen, and trials of outer membrane protein vaccines are in progress.

Hyposplenia or functional asplenia is not a contraindication to receiving any otherwise indicated live, attenuated vaccines such as MMR (measles, mumps and rubella), varicella-zoster virus (either for varicella or zoster), or yellow fever. Influenza vaccine should be administered yearly.

Antimicrobial Prophylaxis

Prophylactic antimicrobial therapy after splenectomy has been advised by some experts, but this has primarily been advocated in the pediatric population. Children are usually started on penicillin prophylaxis for the first 2 years, and studies conducted in sickle cell disease patients have demonstrated significant reduction in the incidence of pneumococcal sepsis. Sustained lifelong prophylaxis has been advocated by some authorities, but the issues of noncompliance and selection of resistant strains along with adverse drug reactions have prevented this from becoming the rule. There are no controlled trials to recommend lifelong antimicrobial prophylaxis in asplenic adults; however, the practice should be strongly considered if a patient has had an episode of OPSI.

SUGGESTED READING

Appelbaum PC, Shaikh BS, Widome MD, et al. Fatal pneumococcal bacteremia in a vaccinated, splenectomized child. *N Engl J Med.* 1979;300:203–204.

Bach O, Baier M, Pullwitt A, et al. Falciparum malaria after splenectomy: a prospective controlled study of 33 previously splenectomized Malawian adults. *Trans R Soc Trop Med Hyg.* 2005;99:861–867.

Buchanan GR, Holtkamp CA, Horton JA. Formation and disappearance of pocked erythrocytes: studies in human subjects and laboratory animals. *Am J Hematol.* 1987;25:243–251.

Centers for Disease Control and Prevention. Recommended immunization schedules for persons aged 0–18 years – United States, 2007. *MMWR.* 2006;55:(51&52):Q1–Q4.

Centers for Disease Control and Prevention. Recommended adult immunization schedule – United States, October 2006–September 2007. *MMWR.* 2006;55:Q1–Q4.

Childers BJ, Cobanov B. Acute infectious purpura fulminans: a 15-year review of 28 consecutive cases. *Am Surg.* 2003;69:86–90.

Evans DIK. Fatal post-splenectomy sepsis despite prophylaxis with penicillin and pneumococcal vaccine. *Lancet.* 1984;1:1124.

Gaston MH, Verter JI, Woods G, et al. Prophylaxis with oral penicillin in children with sickle cell anemia: a randomized trial. *N Engl J Med.* 1986; 314:1593–1599.

Hanage WP, Huang SS, Lipsitch M, et al. Diversity and antibiotic resistance among nonvaccine serotypes of Streptococcus pneumoniae carriage isolates in the post-heptavalent conjugate vaccine era. *J Infect Dis.* 2007;195:347–352.

Holdsworth RJ, Irving AD, Cuschieri A. Postsplenectomy sepsis and its mortality rate: actual versus perceived risks. *Br J Surg.* 1991;78:1031–1038.

Jackson LA, Neuzil KM, Whitney CG, et al. Safety of varying dosages of 7-valent pneumococcal protein conjugate vaccine in seniors previously vaccinated with 23-valent pneumococcal polysaccharide vaccine. *Vaccine.* 2005;23:3697–3703.

Jugenburg M, Haddock G, Freedman MH, et al. The morbidity and mortality of pediatric splenectomy: does prophylaxis make a difference? *J Pediatr Surg.* 1999;34: 1064–1067.

Molrine DC, Silber GR, Samra Y, et al. Normal IgG and impaired IgM responses to polysaccharide vaccines in asplenic patients. *J Infect Dis.* 1999;179:513–517.

Shin H, Mally M, Kuhn M, et al. Escape from immune surveillance by Capnocytophaga canimorsus. *J Infect Dis.* 2007;195: 375–386.

Styrt B. Infection associated with asplenia: risks, mechanisms, and prevention. *Am J Med.* 1990;88(5N):33N–42N.

Vernacchio L, Neufeld EJ, MacDonald K, et al. Combined schedule of 7-valent pneumococcal conjugate vaccine followed by 23-valent pneumococcal vaccine in children and young adults with sickle cell anemia. *J Pediatr.* 1998; 133:275–278.

Waghorn DJ. Overwhelming infection in asplenic patients: current best practice preventive measures are not being followed. *J Clin Pathol.* 2001;54:214–218.

Whitney CG, Farley MM, Hadler J, et al. Decline in invasive pneumococcal disease after the introduction of protein-polysaccharide conjugate vaccine. *N Engl J Med.* 2003;348:1737–1746.

World Health Organization. *Guidelines for the Treatment of Malaria.* Geneva, Switzerland: World Health Organization; 2006.

Zumla A, Lipscomb G, Corbett M, et al. Dysgonic fermenter-type 2: a zoonosis. Report of two cases and review. *Q J Med.* 1988;68:741–752.

PART XII

HIV

Fouad Bou Harb and Aaron E. Glatt

Even though infection with human immunodeficiency virus (HIV) can be devastating and depressing news to a patient, the early recognition of the infection, the monitoring of immune deficiency both clinically and quantitatively, the prophylaxis and treatment of opportunistic infections and highly active antiretroviral therapy (HAART) have made HIV infection a chronic disease with an increasing survival rate. At the end of 2003, an estimated 1 039 000 to 1 185 000 persons were living with HIV/acquired immunodeficiency syndrome (AIDS) in the United States; 24% to 27% were undiagnosed and unaware of their HIV infection. It is estimated that between 35 and 42 million people are living with HIV/AIDS worldwide. Primary care physicians need to be familiar with the history, clinical presentation, and complications of HIV infection, mostly during the early stages of the infection, when they are expected to care for these patients. This chapter will help clinicians in suspecting, counseling, screening, diagnosing, and evaluating immune deficiency, as well as implementing antiretroviral therapy and other therapies as indicated.

HIV CLINICAL PRESENTATION

Patients can present with different complaints ranging from an acute nonspecific retroviral syndrome (mononucleosis type) lasting 1 to 4 weeks after HIV-1/HIV-2 viral aqcuisition with an incubation period as long as 6 weeks to an AIDS-defining illness suggesting advanced immunocompromission, most commonly *Pneumocystis carinii* pneumonia, esophageal candidiasis, wasting, and Kaposi's sarcoma. During this initial presentation, it is important for clinicians to establish the route and risks for acquisition of HIV with open, nonjudgmental questions because this is important for reducing further transmission and recognizing complications.

HISTORY AND PHYSICAL EXAMINATION

HIV disease causes and predisposes to multiple organ disease. Evaluation should be systematic and comprehensive. After a detailed chief complaint and history of present illness are obtained, a thorough review of past medical, surgical, and social histories; medications; allergies; and systems on all patients is necessary. Detailed physical examination, with careful documentation of baseline observations, is essential for early recognition of new problems. It is important to recognize that HAART may significantly alter the natural history of HIV infection. In addition, HAART may be associated with side effects such as lipodystrophy, lipoatrophy, and other signs and symptoms.

General

Fever, weight loss, malaise, fatigue, shaking chills, night sweats, and loss of appetite can be initial findings of significant illness. They are less common in early HIV infection. They may signify worsening immunosuppression. Weight and nutritional assessment should be recorded at each visit.

Skin

The skin of nearly all HIV-infected persons will eventually be affected secondary to infectious and noninfectious dermatologic disorders. Skin or nail pigmentation and rashes of all varieties can occur in disseminated or sporadic fashion. They may be clues to underlying serious illness, co-infection, or worsening immunosuppression. Needle tracks or skin popping will be an indication of drug abuse and an opportune time to discuss prevention of transmission by not sharing needles (Table 96.1).

Lymph Nodes

Nonspecific small, symmetric, mobile nodes, commonly seen in patients with HIV infection, often reflect nonspecific reactive hyperplasia. Acute generalized lymphadenopathy can be seen during seroconversion. Non-Hodgkin's lymphoma (NHL) and infectious pathogens can present as single or multiple nodes.

At each visit lymph node groups should be assessed for size, quantity, texture, and tenderness. Biopsy is not helpful unless nodes

Table 96.1 Commonly Seen Cutaneous Manifestations in HIV Patients

Etiology	Clinical Features
Bacterial Infection	
Bacillary angiomatosis	Fleshy, friable, protuberant papules-to-nodules that tend to bleed very easily (numerous angiomatous, associated with fever, chills, and weight loss)
Staphylococcus aureus	Folliculitis, ecthyma, impetigo, bullous impetigo, furuncles, and carbuncles
Syphilis	May occur in different forms (primary, secondary, or tertiary); chancre may become painful due to secondary infection
Fungal Infection	
Candidiasis	Mucous membranes (oral, vulvovaginal), less commonly *Candida intertrigo* or *paronychia*
Cryptococcoses	Most common on the head and neck; they typically present as pearly 2- to 5-mm translucent papules that resemble molluscum contagiosum papules; other forms include pustules, purpuric papules, and vegetating plaques
Seborrheic dermatitis	Poorly defined, faint pink patches, with mild-to-profuse fine, loose, waxy scales in the hair-bearing areas such as the eyebrows, scalp, chest, and pubic area
Arthropod Infestations	
Scabies	Pruritus with or without rash; usually generalized but can be limited to a single digit
Viral Infection	
Herpes simplex	Painful vesicular lesion in clusters; perianal, genital, orofacial, or digital; can be disseminated
Herpes zoster	Painful dermatomal vesicles that may ulcerate or disseminate
HIV	Discrete erythematous macules and papules on the upper trunk, palms, and soles are the most characteristic cutaneous finding of acute HIV infection
Human papilloma virus	Genital warts (may become unusually extensive)
Kaposi's sarcoma (herpesvirus)	Erythematous macule or papule, enlarge at varying rates, violaceous nodules or plaques, occasionally painful
Molluscum contagiosum	Discrete umbilicated papules commonly on the face, neck, and intertriginous site (axilla, groin, or buttocks)
Noninfectious	
Drug reactions	More common and severe in HIV patients
Nutritional deficiencies	Mainly seen in children and patients with chronic diarrhea; diffuse skin manifestations, depending on the deficiency
Psoriasis	Scaly lesions; diffuse or localized; can be associated with arthritis
Vasculitis	Palpable purpuric eruption (can resemble septic emboli)

Abbreviation: HIV = human immunodeficiency virus.

are rapidly enlarging or are associated with fever and weight loss.

Head, Eyes, Ear, Nose, and Throat

Candida and herpes simplex virus often cause painful cheilitis, stomatitis, or pharyngitis and can manifest at any stage of HIV infection. *Candida* (oral thrush), cytomegalovirus (CMV) (oral ulcers), Epstein–Barr virus (EBV; oral hairy leukoplakia), varicella-zoster virus, mycobacterial infection, *Cryptococcus neoformans, Histoplasma capsulatum,* Kaposi's sarcoma, squamous cell carcinoma, and NHL may be visible on oral examination, and idiopathic aphthous ulcers are a significant cause of troublesome oral pain. Toothache and dental tenderness may indicate periodontal disease or abscess and may cause both fever and headache. Gingival and periodontal infection are particularly aggressive in patients with HIV infection. Facial pain, nasal obstruction, postnasal drip, and headache can be caused by sinusitis, which occurs frequently in HIV infection. Atopy may coexist.

Blurred vision, scotoma, floaters, or decreased visual acuity suggests CMV retinitis. Complete eye examinations at baseline and when retinitis is a consideration is essential, especially in hosts with CD4 cell count below 50/mL and if HAART is not successful. Headache of new onset or changing character may be an early manifestation of a central nervous system opportunistic process.

Cardiopulmonary

Precise baseline pulmonary and cardiovascular examinations are important because of increasing pulmonary and cardiac complications in advancing HIV disease. Shortness of breath at rest or with exertion, its duration and progression, whether a cough is dry or productive, and sputum color, amount, and odor may help with the differential diagnosis. Hemoptysis can be caused by tuberculosis, thrombocytopenia, bacterial pneumonia, or other lung pathology. Chest pain can be caused by pneumonia, spontaneous pneumothorax (often *Pneumocystis*-related), pericarditis, herpes zoster, or HIV-related cardiomyopathy. Palpitation and postural hypotension suggest symptomatic anemia.

Gastrointestinal

Gastrointestinal diseases are increasingly frequent as HIV disease progresses. Odynophagia, dysphagia, retrosternal chest pain, nausea,

anorexia, and weight loss are commonly associated with esophagitis due to *Candida,* herpes simplex, CMV, or, more rarely, lymphoma. Hepatic or splenic enlargement may be an early manifestation of HIV-related complications. Baseline size of spleen and liver should be documented.

Right upper quadrant pain associated with fever and elevated alkaline phosphatase may indicate viral or drug-induced hepatitis, cholelithiasis, or acalculous cholecystitis related to *Mycobacterium avium* complex (MAC), cryptosporidiosis, microsporidia, or CMV.

Epigastric or left upper quadrant pain may indicate drug-induced pancreatitis. Abdominal distension, tenderness, masses, constipation, or fecal incontinence may be caused by Kaposi's sarcoma, lymphoma, carcinoma, gastrointestinal opportunistic infections (CMV, histoplasmosis, tuberculosis), or parasitic infestation. Diarrhea occurs in 30% to 66% of adults with HIV. *Salmonella, Cryptosporidium, Isospora*, CMV, microsporidia, and other enteric pathogens commonly occur. Constipation is commonly seen in patients taking methadone, heroin, or opioids, as well as other medicines.

Painful defecation or rectal pain can be caused by trauma, perirectal abscess, herpes, squamous cell carcinoma, or other sexually transmitted diseases (eg, *Lymphogranuloma venereum* in people who engage in rectal intercourse). Careful sexual and social histories may help identify the pathogens. Perirectal areas should be carefully examined for lesions, abscess, fissures, proctitis, and ulcerations. Stools should be tested for occult blood.

Genitourinary, Obstetric, and Gynecologic Manifestations

Painful, frequent urination may indicate urinary tract infection, sexually transmitted disease, or vulvovaginitis. The latter are more common and possibly more difficult to treat in HIV infection. Recurrent or severe vaginitis, vaginal discharge, and pruritus are common and may not be related solely to sexual practices. Prompt evaluation of all genital discharges, ulcers, and lesions will allow correct identification of any sexually transmitted disease.

Women should be queried regarding menstrual history, fertility, method of birth control, and numbers and dates of pregnancies and abortions. Menstruation may become irregular in worsening HIV infection, and fertility declines as well. Prior tubal scarring from salpingitis or pelvic inflammatory disease predisposes to ectopic pregnancy and infertility. An external genital, rectal, and complete pelvic examination (speculum and bimanual), including Pap tests and appropriate cultures and stains, should be performed initially and at least annually even if exams are normal.

Neurologic

Neuropsychiatric complications eventually occur in up to 80% of patients, yet symptoms may go unrecognized because of coping strategies and the large reserve available until significant deterioration is noted. Subtle neurologic deterioration, memory loss, and poor concentration may be the only early signs of HIV dementia. Central and peripheral neurologic complications may be caused by HIV infection, opportunistic infections, medications, or malignancy. Illness can occur at any stage of HIV infection, albeit with different manifestations. Symptoms depend greatly on the location of the abnormality and the pathophysiology involved. Progressive multifocal encephalopathy or peripheral neuropathy can occur years or even decades after seroconversion; intracranial mass lesions are usually a late complication of HIV disease.

Distal predominantly sensory polyneuropathy, chronic inflammatory demyelinating polyneuropathy, mononeuropathy, herpesvirus and CMV radiculitis, and neuropathies of vitamin deficiency are commonly seen. Neurologic evaluation and appropriate diagnostic testing may differentiate treatable from less responsive pathology. A carefully documented baseline neurologic examination, including mental status assessment, cranial nerve testing, and evaluation of sensation, strength, coordination, and reflexes, should be part of an initial and yearly comprehensive evaluation. Mini-Mental Status Examination results should be clearly documented.

Musculoskeletal

Myalgia and proximal muscle weakness, tenderness, and wasting may be manifestations of primary HIV or drug-related myositis. Severe, persistent oligoarthritis, primarily affecting the large lower limb joints with exquisite pain, psoriatic arthritis with erosive changes and crippling deformities, and septic arthritis caused by *Staphylococcus aureus*, especially in substance abusers, are not uncommon. Changes in fat distribution secondary to HAART may also be present.

Medical History

A clear history of prior HIV-related events, CD4 cell counts, viral load, complications, opportunistic infections, and malignancies will help stage HIV infection, provide prognostic information, and clarify therapeutic options. Opportunistic infections signify marked immunocompromise and are discussed at length in a subsequent chapter.

HIV infection significantly increases the risk of tuberculosis (TB) and increases the yearly rate of conversion from latent to active TB to 7% to 8% yearly, whereas it is around 10% lifetime conversion rate in non-HIV patients. Tuberculosis seems to make HIV infection worse, with a more rapid progression to AIDS. Purified protein derivative (PPD) status, previous exposure to TB, and previous prophylaxis or treatment (date, duration, and medications) are critical. Noncompliance, prior hospitalizations, and geographic and social factors play major roles in development of drug resistance and empiric management. Syphilis may increase the rate of HIV acquisition as other sexually transmitted diseases (STDs) and initial presentation can be varied in co-infected patients.

Medications

Polypharmacy, with prescription agents and vitamin, mineral, and herbal supplements and alternative medications, is very common. They can cause or change disease manifestations and be associated with adverse effects and toxicity, which can be confused with symptoms of HIV-related disease. For example, vitamin overdosing may cause diarrhea, abdominal cramps, peripheral neuropathy, increased intracranial pressure, headache, anorexia, nausea, and vomiting. Drug interactions, sometimes leading to HAART failure, are also common and must be diligently sought for both prescription and nonprescription medicines.

Allergy

The physician should differentiate between allergic reaction and intolerance, which is commonly misinterpreted as allergy. The specific reaction, duration, and resolution of toxicity for each medication should be noted. Rash and fevers are the most common type of adverse drug manifestations thus should be differentiated from infectious etiologies common in HIV.

Social History

Particular attention must be given to all aspects of the psychosocial history, especially residence status, occupational history, substance abuse, and sexual history. A complete sexual history should be obtained, including orientation, practices, lifetime number of partners, prostitution, and any previous STDs. Dietary habits and water sources are important for certain pathogens.

Travel History

Because certain opportunistic infections occur predominantly in particular geographic regions, place of birth and travel history are particularly useful in formulating a differential diagnosis (eg, southwestern United States for coccidiomycosis and Ohio River Valley for histoplasmosis). History of travel to developing or tropical countries may raise suspicion of, eg, travelers' diarrhea, malaria, leishmania, kala-azar, strongyloidiasis, *Penicillium* infection (southeast Asia), and HIV-2.

Pets

Certain opportunistic infections have been associated with particular animals. Patients should be queried regarding exposure to animals and advised about methods of avoiding zoonoses. *Bartonella* (formerly *Rochalimea*) species have been associated with cat scratch disease and bacillary angiomatosis, and exposure to cats may be associated with toxoplasmosis.

LABORATORY STUDIES

Laboratory testing, although invasive, uncomfortable, and expensive, is often the only way to establish or confirm a diagnosis. Laboratory studies should be individualized, but several general principles apply (Tables 96.2 and 96.3).

A complete blood count may reveal mild normocytic, normochromic anemia, which often develops as HIV progresses. Macrocytosis develops on zidovudine and can help assess compliance. Pancytopenia may suggest bone marrow involvement or infiltration, isolated thrombocytopenia may be an early finding of HIV infection, and leukopenia and/or a blunted neutrophil response to infection is a common finding. Neutropenia often becomes more pronounced with various drug therapies (eg, zidovudine, trimethoprim–sulfamethoxazole, and pentamidine) and may require treatment with colony-stimulating factors.

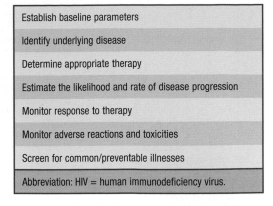

Table 96.2 Purposes of Laboratory Testing in HIV Infection

Establish baseline parameters
Identify underlying disease
Determine appropriate therapy
Estimate the likelihood and rate of disease progression
Monitor response to therapy
Monitor adverse reactions and toxicities
Screen for common/preventable illnesses
Abbreviation: HIV = human immunodeficiency virus.

Assessment of chemistries and liver function and hepatitis tests are useful in diagnosing concurrent illness and as a guide to monitoring drug toxicities and development of new illness, and choosing initial HAART mainly in hepatitis B co-infected patients.

A nonspecific syphilis test (RPR) or the Venereal Disease Research Laboratory (VDRL) tests, with confirmatory fluorescent treponemal antibody absorbed (FTA-abs) tests, should be performed initially and repeated annually in patients at risk. Lumbar puncture may be indicated for patients with reactive serologies, especially if the RPR is 1:16 or above or is of uncertain duration. This is more pressing if symptoms are present.

A PPD should be placed on initial evaluation and at least annually except in patients with a history of TB or reactive PPD. Any positive reaction should be carefully recorded in millimeters of induration. The new Quantiferon-TB Gold test adds no advantage over PPD in HIV patients. Baseline chest radiography is recommended regardless of PPD status.

Baseline antitoxoplasma immunoglobulin G (IgG) antibodies may influence prophylaxis decisions and help with the evaluation and empiric treatment of central nervous system mass lesions. CMV and EBV serologies, and baseline cryptococcal antigen testing, have no value. A Pap smear should be performed initially at 6 months and then annually if normal. Prompt referral to a gynecologist for any atypia is essential. Routine cholesterol, lipid, and blood sugar evaluations are important to monitor for metabolic abnormalities frequently seen in HIV-positive patients, especially those on HAART.

CD4 lymphocyte counts and viral load counts, the most useful markers of immunosuppression and response to therapy, should be obtained every 3 months as a guide for

Table 96.3 Routine Laboratory Studies Guidelines for HIV-Infected Adults

Test	Indication	Interval

Antitoxoplasma antibody (IgG)	Screening for previous exposure
	Guide diagnostic and empiric
	  management
		Baseline
		? Yearly in patients with negative
		  results

Chemistry and liver functions	Evaluation of baseline renal and liver
	  function, and nutritional status
	Diagnosis of concurrent hepatitis
	Monitoring of drug toxicities
	Monitoring of efficacy of therapy
		Baseline
		Every 6–12 mo
		More frequently in patients with
		  advanced disease, baseline
		  abnormalities, or with drug toxicity

Chest radiograph	Screening for disease Diagnosis of active disease	Baseline If pulmonary disease suspected

Complete blood count	Evaluation of anemia, leukopenia,
	  or thrombocytopenia
	Monitoring of drug toxicities
	Monitoring of efficacy of therapy
	Assessment of compliance
		Baseline
		Every 6 mo
		More frequently in patients with
		  abnormalities or those taking
		  marrow-suppressing agents

Hepatitis profile	Diagnosis of viral hepatitis Evaluation for vaccination Response to vaccination	Baseline During potential acute infection Postvaccination
Lymphocyte subset testing (CD4 cells)	Guiding initiation of prophylactic and/or antiretroviral therapy Prognostic information Monitoring of efficacy of therapy	Baseline Every 6 mo if >500 Every 3 mo if ≤500 Discontinue when ≤50

HIV viral load	Diagnostic in acute infection before
	  seroconversion (>10 000/mL)
	Monitoring of HIV activity
	Monitoring of efficacy of therapy
		Baseline
		Every month until antiretroviral therapy
		  efficacy is established
		Every 3 mo if truly stable clinically

RPR or VDRL	Screening for syphilis
	Monitoring of response to therapy
	Use of specific test (ie, FTA) for
	  confirmation and/or false-negative
	  specimen
		Baseline
		Yearly (at least) in patients at
		  risk/prior infection
		Monthly for 6 mo, and at 9 and
		  12 mo after therapy
		During new symptoms

Tuberculosis skin test (purified protein derivative)	Screening for infection or previous exposure Identification of new converters	Baseline, if negative history Yearly, if negative history More frequently if at greater risk

Abbreviation: HIV = human immunodeficiency virus; IgG = immunoglobulin G

treatment and prophylactic interventions. Six-month intervals may be appropriate in selected patients with high CD4 cell counts and a low viral load who are not candidates for therapy. Monitoring can be discontinued when clinical decisions are no longer based on the results. There is significant variability in CD4 cell counts; the aggregate picture over weeks or months is more useful than a single reading for major therapy decisions.

Viral load testing is essential for monitoring the efficacy of HAART and the most ultrasensitive assay available, capable of detecting as low a viral particle per milliliter as possible, should be used. Viral genotyping and phenotyping are commonly used to detect for resistance and to guide the choice of individual HAART regimens.

VACCINATIONS

Patients should receive immunizations as early as possible in the course of HIV infection to optimize response when the CD4 count is still high (preferably more then 500) (Table 96.4). Clinical efficacy is difficult to assess.

Pneumococcal vaccine should similarly be given when the patient is at an optimal level

Table 96.4 Vaccination Guidelines for HIV-Infected Adults

Vaccine	Frequency
Pneumococcal vaccine	Once (booster at 5 y)
Hepatitis B vaccine series	Series of three (0, 1, and 6 mo) (booster in 5 y)
Influenza	Yearly (in autumn)
Inactivated polio vaccine	As per standard published guidelines
Diphtheria/tetanus	As per standard published guidelines
Measles (MMR), VZV	As per standard published guidelines If not severely compromised
Haemophilus influenzae vaccine	Once
Travel-related vaccinations	Refer to CDC for guidelines for routinely recommended travel vaccinations As possible, vaccinate when CD4 >200

Abbreviations: HIV = human immunodeficiency virus; MMR = measles, mumps, and rubella vaccine; VZV = varicella-zoster virus; CDC = Centers for Disease Control and Prevention.

A vaccine is indicated among selected at-risk populations.

GUIDELINES FOR FOLLOW-UP

Patients receiving HAART need to be followed closely to ensure compliance, efficacy, and optimal management. Once fully stable, symptomatic HIV patients should be examined and re-evaluated every 1 to 3 months, and usually much more frequently if immunocompromise worsens. Follow-up of asymptomatic patients should be individualized. Most patients have numerous psychosocial needs that also must be addressed; referral to the appropriate staff is essential for complete and compassionate care.

SUGGESTED READING

Beck JM, Rosen MJ, Peavy HH. Pulmonary complications of HIV infection. Report of the 4th NHLBI workshop. *Am J Respr Crit Care Med.* 2001;164:2120–2126.

Centers for Disease Control and Prevention. 1993 Revised classification system for HIV infection and expanded surveillance case definition for AIDS among adolescents and adults. *Morbid Mortal Weekly Rep.* 1992;41:1.

Centers for Disease Control and Prevention. Guidelines for using the Quantiferon-TB Gold test for detecting Mycobacterium Tuberculosis infection. *Morbid Mortal Weekly Rep.* 2005;54(RR-15):49–55.

Centers for Disease Control and Prevention. Committee on immunization practices. Recommended adult immunization schedule–United States, October 2006–September 2007. *Morbid Mortal Weekly Rep.* 2006;55(40):Q1–Q4.

Ong K, Iftikhar S, Glatt A. Medical evaluation of the adult with HIV infection. *Infect Dis Clin North Am.* 1994;8:289.

Schacter T, Collier AC, Hughes J, et al. Clinical and epidemiologic features of primary HIV infection. *Ann Intern Med.* 1996;125:257–264.

USPHS/IDSA Prevention of opportunistic infection working Group. 1997 USPHS/IDSA guidelines for the prevention of opportunistic infections in persons infected with human immunodeficiency virus. *Morbid Mortal Weekly Rep.* 1997;46(RR-12):1.

of health. The merit of a booster in 5 years is controversial. Efficacy is doubtful if the CD4 cell count is less then 200. Consider revaccinating patients when the CD4 improves to above 200 on HAART. It is unknown if *Haemophilus influenzae* vaccination is indicated for HIV-infected adults.

Patients without serologic evidence of hepatitis B exposure or immunity should be given hepatitis B vaccine. It is unknown when and if a booster is necessary, but a single booster is often given to health care workers and others between 5 and 10 years after initial vaccination.

Influenza vaccine (only inactivated) is recommended annually. MMR and VZV are contraindicated in severely immunocompromised patients. Inactivated polio vaccine, standard childhood vaccinations, booster diphtheria, and tetanus immunizations can be given as per published guidelines. Hepatitis

97. HIV-1 Infection: Antiretroviral Therapy

Dionissios Neofytos and Kathleen E. Squires

Significant progress has been made in the management of HIV-1 disease since 1987, when the first antiretroviral agent, zidovudine, was released. Four classes of antiretrovirals are currently used for the treatment of HIV-1: nucleoside/nucleotide reverse transcriptase inhibitors (NRTIs), nonnucleoside reverse transcriptase inhibitors (NNRTIs), protease inhibitors (PIs), and fusion inhibitors (FIs). A combination of two NRTIs with one NNRTI or PI comprises the standard antiretroviral treatment regimen, also known as highly active antiretroviral therapy (HAART). As of the beginning of 2007, 22 agents have been approved by the U.S. Food and Drug Administration (FDA) for the treatment of HIV-1 (Table 97.1). The goal of antiretroviral treatment is to achieve maximal viral suppression and thus preserve the immune function of the patient and delay the clinical progression of HIV-1 disease. Treating HIV-infected patients requires commitment from both the caregiver and the patient, perpetual counseling and support, and judicial use of the available diagnostic and therapeutic tools by the clinician. Measurement of plasma HIV-1 RNA levels (viral load, VL) and CD4+ cell count is routinely used to monitor therapy. With the new ultrasensitive polymerase chain reaction (PCR) methods, reliable detection of 50 viral copies/mL or more can be accomplished. Failure to achieve undetectable levels of plasma HIV-1 RNA may suggest incomplete compliance, drug resistance, or unfavorable pharmacokinetics.

In this chapter the following topics are discussed: treatment initiation, antiretroviral drugs, recommended first-line antiretroviral regimens, and management of HIV infection during pregnancy. Emphasis will be given to the treatment of antiretroviral-naïve patients infected with HIV-1. Management of antiretroviral treatment-experienced patients is complex and should optimally include a clinician with expertise in resistance testing and interpretation and novel agents and treatment strategies.

TIMING OF INITIATION OF HAART

Initiating antiretroviral treatment in an HIV-1–infected patient is a challenging decision.

Table 97.1 Antiretroviral Drugs Approved in 2007

Nucleoside/tide Reverse Transcriptase Inhibitors (NRTIs)	Nonnucleoside Reverse Transcriptase Inhibitors (NNRTIs)
Zidovudine (Retrovir, ZDV)	Nevirapine (Viramune, NVP)
Didanosine (Videx, ddI)	Delaviridine (Rescriptor, DLV)
Zalcitabine (Hivid, ddC)	
Stavudine (Zerit, d4T)	Efavirenz (Sustiva, EFV)
Lamivudine (Epivir, 3TC)	**Protease inhibitors (PIs)**
Abacavir (Ziagen, ABC)	Saquinavir (Invirase, SQV)
Emtricitabine (Emtriva, FTC)	Ritonavir (Norvir, RTV)
Tenofovir (Viread, TDF)	Indinavir (Crixivan, IDV)
Fixed-dose Combinations	Nelfinavir (Viracept, NFV)
ZDV/3TC (Combivir)	Amprenavir (Agenerase, APV)
ZDV/3TC/ABC (Trizivir)	Lopinavir/r (Kaletra, LPV/r)
ABC/3TC (Epzicom)	Atazanavir (Reyataz, ATV)
TDF/FTC (Truvada)	Fosamprenavir (Lexiva, FPV)
EFV/TDF/FTC (Atripla)	Tipranavir (Aptivus, TPV)
	Darunavir (Prezista, TMC114)
	Fusion inhibitor (FI)
	Enfuvirtide (Fuzeon, T-20)

Multiple parameters need to be considered: early versus chronic and symptomatic versus asymptomatic HIV-1 infection, baseline resistance, CD4+ cell count and VL, and short- and long-term adverse effects of antiretroviral drugs (Table 97.2). Patient counseling and education prior to treatment initiation should be a significant part of the treatment plan. The patient should be thoroughly informed about the disease, its complications, and existing treatment options, and express interest in being treated. Likelihood of adherence should be assessed and taken into consideration before the final decision is made.

Recent evidence suggests that 8% to 25% of HIV-1–infected patients are infected with a virus resistant to at least one antiretroviral drug. Baseline resistance to NRTIs and NNRTIs has been associated with virologic failure and reduced treatment response. Moreover, pretreatment resistance testing in a modeling study was found to be cost-effective and prolonged life in patients infected with resistant virus. Based on the above, pretreatment baseline genotype is now strongly recommended by the Department of Health and Human Services (DHHS) for patients with acute HIV-1 (regardless of treatment initiation) and those with chronic HIV-1 infection prior to initiation of treatment (http://www.aidsinfo.nih.gov). Even though an indirect measure of resistance, a genotype is faster, cheaper, widely available, and thus preferred to a phenotype in this setting.

A number of well-documented reasons favor early treatment initiation. Coformulations of different antiretrovirals and once-daily regimens have facilitated HIV-1 treatment and increased compliance. Antiretroviral drugs are now better tolerated and less toxic, which will potentially optimize compliance to a specific regimen. Cohort data are showing a benefit to earlier therapy, whereas deferral of therapy may increase the risk of some HIV-1–associated complications. Finally, earlier therapy may decrease transmission of HIV-1, in particular, in the acute infection setting. However, long-term adverse effects (ie, cardiovascular complications) associated with most of the currently recommended regimens and the anticipation of new, safer, and more potent regimens may justify treatment deferral in some patient groups. Moreover, delaying treatment initiation will give the patient more time to understand the disease and treatment options and also help to avoid treatment fatigue.

Current guidelines for the treatment of adult and adolescent patients infected with HIV-1 are summarized in Tables 97.3 and 97.4. Specific recommendations for pregnant women are discussed in Pregnancy and HIV-1. The CD4+ cell count is the major determinant of treatment initiation, whereas the level of VL is a minor factor with the possible exception of preinitiation levels of >100 000 copies/mL. Briefly, initiation of antiretroviral treatment is recommended for patients with either of the following: symptoms related to HIV-1 regardless of CD4+ cell count and CD4+ cell count ≤200 cells/mm^3. Specific recommendations for initiation of HAART in patients with CD4+ cell count >200 cells/mm^3 remain to be finalized. In a retrospective analysis of 13 cohort studies from Europe and North America, including 12 574 adult HIV-1–infected patients who received antiretroviral treatment, no significant differences in outcome were noted in patients with CD4+ cell counts between 201 and 350 and >350 cells/mm^3. However, recent observational data from cohort studies suggest that there may be a potential benefit from initiating treatment in chronic asymptomatic

Table 97.2 Side Effects of the Most Commonly Prescribed Antiretroviral Agents

NRTIs	Lactic acidosis, hepatic steatosis, lipodystrophy[a]
ZDV	Anemia, neutropenia, macrocytosis, nausea, vomiting, fatigue
ddl, ddC, d4T[b]	Peripheral neuropathy, pancreatitis
d4T	Lipoatrophy[a], macrocytosis
ABC	Hypersensitivity reaction
FTC	Skin discoloration
TDF	Renal impairment/Fanconi syndrome
NNRTIs	Rash
NVP	Stevens–Johnson syndrome, hepatic failure
EFV	CNS and psychiatric symptoms, hepatitis, teratogenicity
PIs	Diarrhea, hyperlipidemia[c], insulin resistance, lipodystrophy
RTV	Diarrhea, liver toxicity
IDV	Nephrolithiasis, hyperbilirubinemia
NFV	Diarrhea
LPV/r	Diarrhea, asthenia
ATV	Hyperbilirubinemia, PR prolongation
FPV	Diarrhea, skin rash
SQV	Diarrhea, headache
DRV	Diarrhea, headache, skin rash[d]
TPV	Liver toxicity, intracranial hemorrhage
Fusion Inhibitors	
T-20	Injection site reactions, high risk for bacterial pneumonia

Abbreviation: CNS = central nervous system.
[a] Stavudine is the NRTI most commonly associated with lipodystrophy.
[b] Concomitant use of ddl, ddC, or d4T can lead to additive peripheral neuropathy, lactic acidosis, and pancreatitis.
[c] Atazanavir is not associated with hyperlipidemia.
[d] Darunavir has a sulfonamide component and may cause a skin rash in patients allergic to sulfonamides.

HIV-1–infected patients with CD4+ cell counts >350 cells/mm^3. Until more information from randomized studies is available, most clinicians would defer treatment in this group of patients, unless the VL is >100 000 copies/mL. Data from a British Columbia cohort suggest that CD4+ cell count percentage may be used as an adjunct in deciding to initiate HAART in patients with CD4+ cell counts between 200 and 350 cells/mm^3.

HAART initiation during acute HIV-1 infection is still controversial. CD4+ cell preservation, lower cell-associated HIV infectivity, and reduction of HIV-1 transmission have been cited as reasons for early treatment initiation. Until

Table 97.3 Current Guidelines for Initiating HAART (as of January 2007)

Disease type	DHHS	IAS-USA
Symptomatic HIV	HAART recommended	HAART recommended
Asymptomatic HIV		
CD4+ count ≤200 cells/mm³	HAART recommended	HAART recommended
CD4+ count: 201–350 cells/mm³	HAART should be offered	HAART should be considered[a]
CD4+ count >350 cells/mm³	HAART not recommended[b]	HAART not recommended[c]
CD4+ count >500 cells/mm³	Not applicable	HAART not recommended

Note: Adapted from DHHS (www.aidsinfo.nih.gov) and IAS-USA (Hammer S, 2006, *JAMA* 296:827–843.)
Abbreviations: DHHS = Department of Health and Human Services; IAS-USA = International AIDS Society-USA Panel;
HAART = highly active antiretroviral therapy.
[a] Consider treatment for CD4+ cell counts closer to 200 cells/ mm³, and/or for viral load >100 000 copies/mL or CD4+ cell count rapidly declines.
[b] For viral load ≤100 000 copies/mL: HAART should be deferred; for viral load >100 000 copies/mL: decision should be based on individual case.
[c] Consider treatment if viral load >100 000 copies/mL or CD4+ cell count rapidly declines.

more data from prospective, randomized trials are available, DHHS recommends considering treatment of primary infection, whereas the British HIV Association (BHIVA) recommends treatment only in the setting of a clinical trial (*HIV Medicine* 2006; 7:487–503.)

ANTIRETROVIRAL AGENTS

All of the antiretrovirals that are currently approved by the FDA and their most common adverse effects are listed in Tables 97.1 and 97.2, respectively. Figure 97.1 illustrates the viral life cycle and the sites where the different classes of antiretroviral agents exert their action. NRTIs are the most commonly prescribed antiretrovirals and represent the backbone of most antiretroviral regimens. As outlined in the 2006 DHHS guidelines for the treatment of HIV-1, each HAART regimen should contain 2 NRTIs (Table 97.4). The most popular NRTIs in clinical practice are zidovudine (ZDV; Retrovir), lamivudine (3TC, Epivir), emtricitabine (FTC, Emtriva), and tenofovir (TDF; Viread). These agents are available in coformulation tablets, namely Combivir (ZDV/3TC) and Truvada (TDF/FTC). Zidovudine/lamivudine coformulation is one of the most extensively studied and used dual nucleoside combinations, with proven efficacy and durability. It is administered as one tablet twice daily, and its use has been associated with bone marrow suppression. Tenofovir/emtricitabine has been tested in a head-to-head trial against zidovudine/lamivudine (both combinations coadministered with efavirenz) and showed comparable to superior

potency. The fixed-dose combination is administered as one tablet once daily, but tenofovir may cause renal impairment and acute tubular necrosis. Lamivudine and emtricitabine are potent and well-tolerated drugs and can be used interchangeably. There is compelling evidence that M184V, the signature mutation for lamivudine and emtricitabine, decreases the fitness of the virus and confers increased activity for zidovudine, stavudine (d4T; Zerit), and tenofovir.

It should be noted that stavudine is antagonistic to zidovudine and these agents should not be coadministered. For treatment-naïve patients, the combination of didanosine (ddI; Videx) and tenofovir in an NNRTI-based regimen has been associated with early virologic failure and CD4+ cell count decline. Moreover, when coadministered, tenofovir increases didanosine levels, thereby potentiating didanosine-related toxicities, and thus the didanosine dose should be decreased. Abacavir (ABC; Ziagen) has been associated with a hypersensitivity reaction that can occur in 2% to 9% of patients, mostly within the first 4 to 6 weeks of treatment. This is more commonly reported in whites, especially those positive for human leukocyte antigen (HLA)-B*5701, HLA-DR7, and HLA-DQ3. Symptoms are nonspecific and may include fever, malaise, rash, nausea, vomiting, and diarrhea. Abacavir should be discontinued and not restarted, because rechallenge reactions can be fatal. It should be noted that abacavir is part of two commonly used coformulations, namely Epzicom (3TC/ABC) and Trizivir (ZDV/3TC/ABC),

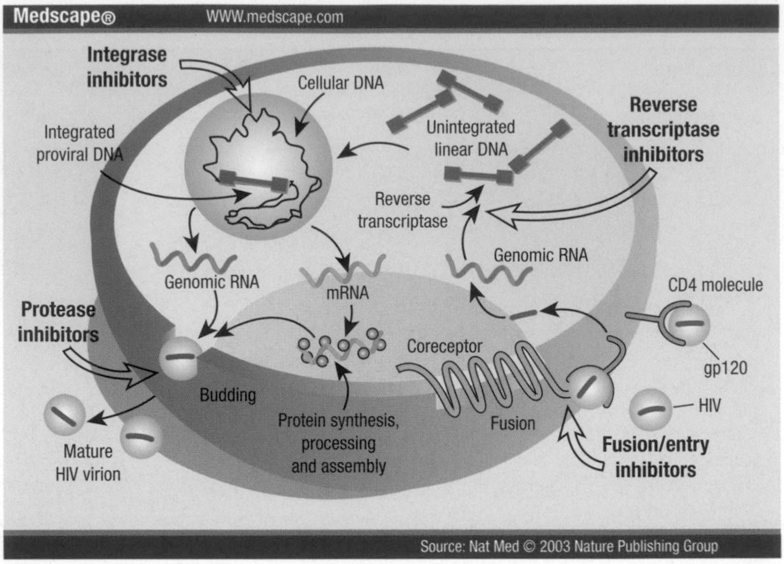

Figure 97.1. HIV-1 life cycle and most common targets of antiretroviral agents.

and any reactions to these preparations should alert the clinician to the possibility of abacavir hypersensitivity.

Efavirenz (EFV; Sustiva) is the preferred NNRTI in the 2006 DHHS and IAS-USA guidelines and one of the most commonly prescribed antiretroviral agents. Patients treated with efavirenz may experience significant neurologic adverse reactions on treatment initiation, including dizziness, impaired thinking and concentration, confusion, and vivid dreams. These symptoms commonly subside spontaneously within 2 to 4 weeks. Efavirenz may also cause a rash and mild transaminase elevation and is contraindicated in women who are considering pregnancy and/or not practicing safe sex during the first trimester of their pregnancy. Nevirapine (NVP; Viramune) is equally potent to efavirenz, based on the results of the 2NN trial. However, women infected with HIV-1 with CD4+ cell count >250 cells/mm^3 treated with nevirapine are at a 12-fold higher risk for nevirapine-associated symptomatic hepatic events, whereas men with CD4+ cell count >400 cells/mm^3 are 4 times more likely to develop serious hepatotoxicity. Most cases occur within the first 18 weeks of treatment, a rash may be present, and cases of fulminant hepatic failure and death have been reported. A 2-week lead-in period with a lower dose, baseline liver function tests, and regular follow-up are recommended when prescribing this agent. Etravirine (TMC 125) is an investigational NNRTI, active against most isolates with NNRTI resistance mutations, with a favorable pharmacological profile thus

far. It is currently available through expanded access programs in the United States.

Protease inhibitors remain a cornerstone in the treatment of HIV-1–infected patients. These agents have unique pharmacokinetic profiles that lead to differences in absorption in association with food and other medications, frequent daily dosing, high pill burden, and drug interactions that need to be considered prior to prescribing. All PIs are either metabolized or are substrates of the hepatic cytochrome P450 system. As a result, significant interactions with many medications exist, and careful review of the patient's medication list should be undertaken prior to initiating a PI. A list with the drugs that most commonly interact with PIs is provided in Table 97.5. More information about the specific drug interactions and dose modifications can be found elsewhere (http://www.aidsinfo.nih.gov). Ritonavir (RTV, r; Norvir) is one of the most potent inhibitors of cytochrome P450 CYP 3A4 and is used in low doses for "boosting" the levels of other protease inhibitors. This leads to increased bioavailability and less complex regimens, ensures more predictable efficacy, decreases resistance, and may increase tolerability and adherence. Boosting with ritonavir may lead to more drug interactions and metabolic adverse events in patients treated with PIs.

Three FDA-approved PIs—lopinavir (LPV/r; Kaletra), atazanavir (ATV; Reyataz), and fosamprenavir (FPV; Lexiva)—are listed as the preferred agents in the most recent DHHS guidelines (Table 97.4). Based on these guidelines, the preferred combination

Table 97.4 Recommended HAART Regimens for Treatment-Naïve Patients (DHHS 2006)

NNRTI Based	PI Based	NRTI
Preferred Regimens (1 NNRTI or 1 PI and 2 NRTIs)		
Efavirenz[a]	Atazanavir/ritonavir Fosamprenavir/ritonavir[b] Lopinavir/ritonavir[b, c]	Tenofovir/emtricitabine[c] Zidovudine/lamivudine[c]
Alternative Regimens (1 NNRTI or 1 PI and 2 NRTIs)		
Nevirapine[d]	Atazanavir +/- ritonavir[e] Fosamprenavir[b] Fosamprenavir/ritonavir[f] Lopinavir/ritonavir[c,f]	Abacavir/lamivudine[c] Didanosine/emtricitabine or lamivudine

Adapted from DHHS (www.aidsinfo.nih.gov).
Abbreviations: DHHS = Department of Health and Human Services; NRTI = nucleoside/tide reverse transcriptase inhibitor; NNRTI = nonnucleoside reverse transcriptase inhibitor; PI = protease inhibitor.
[a] Efavirenz is not recommended in women with high pregnancy potential and during the first trimester of pregnancy.
[b] Administered 2× daily.
[c] Administered as coformulation pills.
[d] Nevirapine should not be used in women and men with CD4+ counts >250 and 400 cells/mm^3, respectively.
[e] Atazanavir + ritonavir should be used when coadministered with tenofovir or efavirenz.
[f] Administered once daily.

regimen should include one of the three PIs listed above administered with low-dose ritonavir ("boosted PI" regimen). Atazanavir, administered with 100 mg of ritonavir, is the only boosted PI on the preferred list that is recommended to be administered once daily. It may be used without ritonavir in an alternative HAART regimen, unless coadministered with tenofovir or efavirenz. Although recent evidence suggests that both lopinavir/ritonavir and fosamprenavir/ritonavir can be administered once daily in treatment-naïve patients, the DHHS guidelines endorse twice-daily administration of these preferred boosted PIs. Lopinavir/ritonavir can be administered as 4 tablets once daily in treatment-naïve patients, but this dosing may lead to higher incidence of diarrhea and lower trough concentration levels. Similarly, fosamprenavir may be administered boosted or unboosted with ritonavir once or twice daily, respectively.

Lopinavir/ritonavir is now available in tablet formulation, which has decreased the pill burden and risk of food interactions and eliminated the need for refrigeration. Atazanavir has the lowest pill burden (2 pills) and fewer gastrointestinal and metabolic adverse effects. It should be noted that coadministration with proton pump inhibitors significantly reduces the serum level of atazanavir and is absolutely contraindicated.

Moreover, atazanavir should not be coadministered with indinavir, because of potential additive hyperbilirubinemia. Fosamprenavir is well tolerated with a low pill burden and lack of food restrictions. Saquinavir (SQV; Invirase) is available in a hard-gel formulation and may be administered once daily when boosted with ritonavir but has a higher pill burden. Saquinavir should not be used alone because of its poor oral bioavailability. Nelfinavir (NFV; Viracept) and boosted saquinavir may be included in the initial HAART regimen if none of the preferred or alternative PIs can be used. It should be noted that amprenavir (APV; Agenerase) has now been withdrawn from the market and largely replaced by fosamprenavir. Tipranavir (TPV; Aptivus) is approved for use in treatment-experienced patients but has been associated with liver toxicity and intracranial hemorrhage. Darunavir (DRV; Prezista) was licensed in 2006 for salvage treatment and is currently being studied in treatment-naïve patients in a once-daily dosing regimen. Depending on the results of this trial, the increasing experience with this agent and its side-effect profile, darunavir may be used earlier in the treatment of HIV–1 infected patients in the future.

Enfuvirtide (T-20; Fuzeon) is the only FI that is currently approved for use in treatment-experienced patients as salvage therapy. When

Table 97.5 Drugs That Interact with Protease Inhibitors

Gastrointestinal Drugs	Ergot Alcaloids
Over the counter antacids	**Cardiac agents**
H$_2$ blockers	Bepridil, Diltiazem[c]
Proton pump inhibitors	Amiodarone
Cisapride	Flecainide
Lipid-lowering agents[a]	Propafenone
Lovastatin, simvastatin	Quinidine
(Pravastatin)	**Antihistamines**
Oral contraceptives (OC)[b]	Astemizole
Ethinyl estradiol	Terfenadine
Psychiatric agents	**Erectile dysfunction**
Selective serotonin	**agents**
reuptake inhibitors	Sildenafil, tadalafil,
Serotonin norepinephrine	vardenafil
reuptake inhibitors	**Steroids**
Bupropion	Fluticasone
Nefazodone, mirtazapine,	**St. John's wort**
venlafaxine	(*Hypericum perforatum*)
Tricyclic antidepressants	**Recreational drugs**
Benzodiazepines	Heroin, marijuana, ecstasy,
Anticonvulsants (phenytoin,	methamphetamines
carbamazepine)	**Methadone**
Antipsychotics	**Antibiotics**
Pimozide	Rifampin, rifabutin,
Pain management drugs	rifapentine
Codeine, hydrocodone,	Macrolides[d] (erythromycin,
fentanyl, meperidine,	clarithromycin)
morphine	Azoles[d] (itraconazole,
	ketoconazole,
	voriconazole)

[a] Atazanavir may lead to a 2-fold increase of diltiazem levels.
[b] Atorvastatin and fluvastatin may be used with protease inhibitors at lower doses. Pravastatin should not be used with darunavir.
[c] Lopinavir/r, nelfinavir, and ritonavir may decrease the levels of OC. Atazanavir may increase the OC levels.
[d] Azithromycin does not interact with P450. Fluconazole minimally interacts with P450.

coadministered with tipranavir or darunavir in multiclass-resistant antiretroviral-experienced patients, significantly better virologic response was noted in the enfuvirtide-treated arms. Enfuvirtide is administered twice daily with subcutaneous injections, which may lead to injection site reactions.

In 2007, three new categories of antiretrovirals were being studied, most of them in phase II and III trials (Table 97.6). These include integrase inhibitors elvitegravir (GS-9137, raltegravir MK-0518), entry inhibitors (maraviroc, vicriviroc, AMD 070, TNX-355), and maturation inhibitors (bevirimat; PA-457). Preliminary results suggest that some of these agents are quite potent and well tolerated and may eventually be incorporated in combination regimens and/or

replace current components of a HAART-based regimen.

REGIMEN SELECTION

The recommended DHHS HAART regimens for treatment-naïve patients are summarized in Table 97.4. Thorough knowledge and careful review of the guidelines prior to designing a regimen are highly recommended. Moreover, the patient's commitment to initiate treatment, baseline resistance profile, ability to comply with a regimen, and social history should be assessed, and the antiretroviral regimen be constructed on a case-by-case basis. The use of coformulation pills has become more popular and facilitated more convenient, once-daily regimens and higher compliance rates.

The 2006 DHHS guidelines recommend the use of 2 NRTIs and 1 NNRTI or PI. Except for the coformulation tablets zidovudine/lamivudine and tenofovir/emtricitabine, as discussed earlier, the current DHHS guidelines suggest that abacavir/lamivudine and didanosine/lamivudine or didonosine/emtricitabine may be used as alternative NRTIs. The DHHS-preferred NNRTI and PIs for treatment-naïve HIV-1–infected patients include efavirenz and lopinavir, atazanavir, and fosamprenavir boosted with ritonavir. There is no distinction between choosing an NNRTI- and a PI-based regimen in these guidelines. Efavirenz has been compared to lopinavir/ritonavir in a head-to-head multicenter prospective, open-label, randomized trial. The NNRTI-based regimen was superior in virologic response, whereas the CD4+ cell count increase was significantly higher in the PI arm.

Parameters to be considered prior to treatment selection should include potency, tolerability, toxicity, and convenience (dosing frequency, pill burden, food and drug interactions). NNRTI-based regimens are well tolerated after the first couple of weeks of treatment, have relatively few long-term side effects, and are convenient. The FDA recently approved the coformulation pill Atripla (Gilead and Bristol-Myers Squibb), which combines efavirenz with emtricitabine and tenofovir and is administered as one pill once daily. Moreover, using an NNRTI-based regimen will preserve the PIs for later use and avoid PI-related adverse events. However, NNRTIs have a low genetic barrier to resistance; virus isolated from patients with detectable viral loads on an NNRTI-based regimen is likely to demonstrate mutations conferring resistance to

Table 97.6 Novel Antiretroviral Agents in Phase I–III Clinical Trials (as of January 2007)

Antiretroviral Category	Stage	Administration	Suggested Dosing
Entry Inhibitors			
Anti-CD4 monoclonal antibodies			
TNX-355	Phase II	Intravenous	Every 1–2 weeks
CCR5 Inhibitors			
Maraviroc[b]	Phase III	Oral	Once[c] or twice daily
Vicriviroc	Phase IIb	Oral	Once daily
CXCR4 Inhibitor			
AMD 070	Phase IIa	Oral	Once daily
Integrase Inhibitors			
Raltegravir MK-0518[b]	Phase III	Oral	Twice daily
Elvitegravir GS-9137	Phase III	Oral	Once daily[c]
Maturation Inhibitors			
Bevirimat (PA-457)	Phase IIa	Oral	Once daily

[a] Once-daily administration was stopped in treatment-naïve patients.
[b] Available through expanded access programs (EAP); TMC-125 (etravirine) is a second generation nonnucleoside reverse transcriptase inhibitor available through an EAP as well.
[c] Boosted with ritonavir.

both NNRTIs and NRTIs. In contrast, multiple mutations in the protease gene are required for high-level resistance, thus conferring a high genetic barrier to resistance. This is substantiated by the fact that NRTI-associated but not PI-associated mutations are seen in patients failing ritonavir-boosted PI-based regimens. Both clinical trials and experience have demonstrated long-term efficacy but there are disadvantages to the use of these regimens, including the relatively high pill burden, and the lipid and other metabolic abnormalities.

Alternative treatment strategies have been and continue to be explored. However, at the time of writing, none of the strategies to be discussed are to be recommended for management of HIV-1 infection outside of the setting of a clinical trial. Structured treatment interruption (STI) is one of the most commonly studied alternative therapeutic approaches for acute or chronic HIV-1 infection. Early data from the Border Asthma and Allergies Study (BASTA) study suggested that treatment interruption in patients with high pretreatment CD4+ counts may be a safe and cost-effective approach. However, the Strategies for Management of Antiretroviral Therapy (SMART) study was stopped prematurely in January 2006 because of a 6- and 2-fold risk of clinical progression and death, respectively, in the CD4+ cell-guided treatment interruption arm. Thus, STI is not currently recommended in the United States but continues to be studied in resource-poor settings. Monotherapy with ritonavir-boosted lopinavir or atazanavir as initial or maintenance therapy has been studied in small trials showing sustained virologic suppression. Until more data from bigger, randomized studies are available, boosted PI monotherapy is not currently recommended. Similarly, dual-, triple-NRTI, or NRTI-sparing regimens should not be routinely recommended. Other therapeutic approaches, including induction/maintenance therapy, quadruple therapy, or boosted double PI therapy, need to be investigated further.

HEPATITIS B, TUBERCULOSIS, AND HIV

For patients coinfected with HIV-1 and chronic active hepatitis B (HBV), two agents with anti-HBV activity (lamivudine, emtricitabine, and/or tenofovir) should be included in the NRTI backbone. Severe, acute exacerbations

Table 97.7 Recommended HAART Regimens in Pregnancy (as of January 2007)

	Recommended	Alternative	Not Recommended	Insufficient Data
NRTI	Zidovudine Lamivudine	Didanosine[a] Stavudine[a] Emtricitabine Abacavir	Zalcitabine[b]	Tenofovir
NNRTI	Nevirapine[c]	—	Efavirenz[b] Delavirdine[b]	—
PI	Nelfinavir Lopinavir/ritonavir[d]	Indinavir Saquinavir/ritonavir Ritonavir	—	Fosamprenavir Atazanavir Tipranavir Darunavir
FI	—	—	—	T-20

[a] Concomitant use of didanosine and stavudine has been associated with serious lactic acidosis, pancreatitis, and hepatic steatosis, especially during the third trimester.
[b] Potential teratogenicity.
[c] Nevirapine should not be used in women with CD4+ counts >250 cells/mm^3.
[d] Lopinavir/ritonavir capsules have been associated with lower levels during the third trimester; results from studies of the tablet formulations during pregnancy are pending.

of HBV infection have been reported in patients after abrupt discontinuation of therapy or development of resistance to any of these agents with HBV activities. Thus, in settings in which HAART needs to be changed, close monitoring and switching to another antiretroviral agent with anti-HBV activity or using adefovir or entecavir is recommended.

Special consideration should be given to HIV-1–infected patients treated for tuberculosis or other mycobacterial infections. When possible, antituberculosis therapy should be started 1 to 2 months before initiating antiretroviral therapy to avoid an immune reconstitution inflammatory response (see Chapter 98, Immune Reconstitution Inflammatory Syndrome). Drug interactions need to be carefully reviewed, and an optimized antiretroviral and antimycobacterial regimen should be selected. If an efavirenz-based regimen is used, rifabutin dose should be increased to 450 mg, or efavirenz should be dosed at 800 mg if administered with rifampin. For PI-based regimens, use of rifabutin is recommended, most commonly dosed at 150 mg once daily. Under special circumstances the combination pill zidovudine/abacavir/lamivudine (Trizivir) may be of some benefit in HIV-positive patients with tuberculosis, in an effort to decrease possible drug interactions.

PREGNANCY AND HIV

Management of pregnant women infected with HIV-1 requires consideration of three overlapping goals: (1) treatment of maternal HIV-1 infection, (2) reduction of transmission of HIV-1 to the fetus, and (3) minimization of toxicity of the treatment for the fetus. A multidisciplinary approach incorporating obstetric and HIV-1 clinical expertise will ensure optimal results. HAART is recommended for all HIV-1–infected pregnant women and should be initiated ultimately before a planned pregnancy or as soon as pregnancy is diagnosed. Zidovudine should always be included in the initial regimen, assuming the virus is not resistant. The goal of HAART in this setting is rapid and maximal viral suppression prior to delivery. In cases where the maternal plasma VL is ≤1000 copies/mL and there is concern about adherence, the DHHS guidelines suggest that zidovudine alone may be administered based on the Pediatric AIDS Clinical Trials Group (PACTG) 076 trial. Regardless of the antiretroviral regimen or viral status of the mother, the infant should receive prophylactic treatment with zidovudine for 6 weeks after delivery (See also Chapter 93, Pregnancy and the Puerperium: Infectious Risks). Table 97.7 summarizes the recommended antiretroviral regimens to be utilized during pregnancy. Notably, efavirenz is the only antiretroviral agent that is pregnancy category D and thus should be avoided, especially during the first trimester. The DHHS guidelines indicate that nelfinavir and lopinavir/ritonavir are the PIs of choice for the pregnant woman infected with HIV-1 due to the availability of study data.

Lower levels of lopinavir/ritonavir during the third trimester have been observed with the capsule formulation. Until results from ongoing trials using the tablet formulation of lopinavir/ritonavir during pregnancy are available, consultation with an HIV-1 expert and monitoring lopinavir levels are recommended.

SUMMARY

The management of HIV-1 disease remains complex, and the treating physician is challenged to consider many factors prior to initiating treatment in an HIV-1–infected patient. As new antiretroviral agents are introduced, resistance emerges, and additional data on HIV-1 accumulate, consultation with an HIV-1 expert may be warranted to optimize the management of patients infected with HIV-1. (For prophylaxis of HIV infection after occupational exposure, see Chapter 102, Percutaneous Injury: Risks and Management, and for prophylaxis following nonoccupational exposure, see Chapter 111, Nonsurgical Antimicrobial Prophylaxis.)

SUGGESTED READING

DHHS. Guidelines for the Use of Antiretroviral Agents in HIV-1-Infected Adults and Adolescents. http://www.aidsinfo.nih.gov.

Egger M, May M, Chene G, et al. Prognosis of HIV-1-infected patients starting highly active antiretroviral therapy: a collaborative analysis of prospective studies. *Lancet*. 2002;360: 119–129.

El-Sadr WM, Lundgren JD, Neaton JD, et al. CD4+ count-guided interruption of antiretroviral treatment. *N Engl J Med*. 2006;355:2283–2296.

Gallant JE. The M184V mutation: what it does, how to prevent it, and what to do with it when it's there. *AIDS*. 2006;16:556–559.

Gallant JE, DeJesus E, Arribas JR, et al. Tenofovir DF, emtricitabine, and efavirenz vs. zidovudine, lamivudine, and efavirenz for HIV. *N Engl J Med*. 2006;354:251–260.

Gazzard B, *HIV Med*. 2006;7:487–503.

Hammer SM, Saag MS, Schechter M, et al. Treatment for adult HIV infection: 2006 recommendations of the International AIDS Society—USA panel. *Top HIV Med*. 2006;14:827–843.

Harrigan PR, Hogg RS, Dong WW, et al. Predictors of HIV drug-resistance mutations in a large antiretroviral-naive cohort initiating triple antiretroviral therapy. *J Infect Dis*. 2005;191:339–347.

Weinstock HS, Zaidi I, Heneine W, et al. The epidemiology of antiretroviral drug resistance among drug-naive HIV-1-infected persons in 10 US cities. *J Infect Dis*. 2004;189: 2174–2180.

98. Immune Reconstitution Inflammatory Syndrome

Samuel A. Shelburne III

Research since the early 1970s has generated significant support for the concept that clinical manifestations of infectious diseases are often due more to the host immune response rather than to direct effects of a particular microbe. Perhaps the longest recognized example of the dominance of an immune response in determining a clinical presentation occurs in *Mycobacterium leprae* infection. However, the introduction of highly active antiretroviral therapy (HAART) for the treatment of human immunodeficiency virus (HIV) infection has markedly increased the appreciation for the dramatic interaction that can occur between microbes and a recovering immune system. The immune restoration mediated by HAART has markedly decreased the rates of opportunistic infections among HIV-infected patients, leading to dramatically lower mortality rates. However, in some patients, the recovery of immune function can lead to an inflammatory reaction aimed at either previously recognized or subclinical microbes or even autoimmune disorders. Multiple names have been given to this syndrome, including immune recovery disease, immune restoration disease, and immunoreconstitution disease. For the purposes of this chapter, we will utilize the term immune reconstitution inflammatory syndrome (IRIS) as it includes one of the defining features of these patients' presentations, i.e., inflammation.

IMMUNOLOGY OF IMMUNE RECOVERY WITH HAART

Although the pathologic basis of IRIS remains unclear, as its name implies there is no doubt that immune recovery is a vital component of IRIS. Thus, any systematic examination of IRIS must start with some insights into the effects of HAART on the immune system. The hallmark of HIV infection is the progressive loss of CD4+ T lymphocytes that results in immune deficiency, opportunistic infections, and death. The initiation of effective HAART leads to a >90% reduction in HIV-1 viral load within 1 to 2 weeks. A biphasic recovery of T lymphocytes

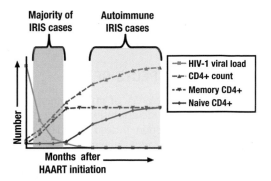

Figure 98.1 Relationship between immune recovery and development of immune reconstitution inflammatory syndrome (IRIS). Following initiation of highly active antiretroviral therapy (HAART) there is a rapid decrease in human immunodeficiency virus (HIV)-1 RNA levels accompanied by an increase in total CD4+ T-lymphocyte count mainly due to a rise in memory CD4+ cells. Most IRIS cases occur during this initial rise in CD4+ counts. Later increases in CD4+ counts are due to production of naïve CD4+ cells. Autoimmune IRIS disorders tend to occur during this phase of immune recovery.

then occurs. Initially there is a rapid increase in CD45RO+ memory T lymphocytes, presumably due to a reduction in apoptosis and redistribution from peripheral lymphoid tissues into the general circulation (Figure 98.1). Over the next several months to years a steady rise in naïve CD45+CD62L+ T lymphocytes is observed, most likely due to production of new CD4+ cells by the thymus. The numerical recovery of immune cells engendered by HAART is accompanied by an increase in measurable functional immune responses, such as delayed-type hypersensitivity (DTH) and in vitro lymphocyte proliferative assays. Moreover, the increase in CD4+ cells is usually accompanied by a decrease in proinflammatory cytokines such as interleukin (IL-18) and soluble tumor necrosis factor receptor interleukin (II). Thus, for the majority of patients responding to HAART, immune recovery is associated with an increase in the ability to respond to antigenic stimuli but an overall decrease in systemic inflammatory markers.

Table 98.1 Typical Serologic and Viral DNA Findings in a Patient Co-infected with Hepatitis B Who Develops IRIS after Starting HAART

Time from Starting HAART	Hepatitic Transaminases	Hepatitis B Surface Antibody	Hepatitis B Viral DNA
Before	Normal to minimally elevated	Negative	Positive
3–12 weeks after	Markedly elevated	Positive	Positive
12–24 weeks	Normal	Positive	Negative
Abbreviations: IRIS = immune reconstitution inflammatory syndrome; HAART = highly active antiretroviral therapy.			

HISTORICAL ASPECTS OF IRIS

The notion that recovery of immune response can lead to clinical deterioration did not originate with HIV infection. Indeed, clinicians have long noted that "paradoxical worsenings" occur during treatment of *Mycobacterium tuberculosis* infections and that such worsenings are temporally related to recovery of DTH to tuberculin antigens. Similarly, infection with *M. leprae* or treatment of such infection is often accompanied by inflammatory reactions.

The first recognition that treatment of HIV might lead to altered presentations of opportunistic infections occurred when zidovudine monotherapy was accompanied by atypical localized infections with *Mycobacterium avium* complex (MAC) infection. The introduction of HAART in the mid-1990s was quickly followed by numerous reports of unusual clinical deteriorations accompanying immune recovery. Serial evaluation of hepatitis B virus serology clearly demonstrated that appearance of anti-hepatitis B surface antibody in HAART-treated patients correlated with severe hepatitis (Table 98.1). Within a few years of HAART introduction, nearly all HIV-related opportunistic pathogens had been associated with IRIS, and autoimmune disorders began to be recognized as part of the syndrome.

DEFINITION OF IRIS

On review of the IRIS literature, one is quickly struck by the difficulties in defining the syndrome. There is no single physical finding, blood test, microbiologic culture, or imaging examination that is definitive for the diagnosis. In fact, IRIS remains, and is likely to remain, a diagnosis of exclusion. An IRIS definition must take into account the associated etiologic agent or autoimmune disorder, and thus only broad guidelines can be generally applied. Most investigators agree that the patients should have

Table 98.2 Criteria for Diagnosis of Immune Reconstitution Inflammatory Syndrome (IRIS)

HIV positive, usually with initial CD4+ ≤200

Decrease in HIV-1 RNA at least 1-$\log_{10}$ from baseline

Clinical presentation consistent with an inflammatory process

Presentation not consistent with:
    Typical course of newly diagnosed OI
    Expected course of previously diagnosed OI
    Adverse drug event

Abbreviations: HIV = human immunodeficiency virus; OI = Opportunistic infections.

an inflammatory condition that is temporally related to a response to antiretroviral therapy and that cannot be explained by the expected clinical course of either a previously or newly diagnosed opportunistic infection (Table 98.2). Clearly, these are broad guidelines that can be differentially applied by various physicians, but, at present, such an approach is the best that has been devised. Further efforts to more precisely delineate the syndrome are ongoing.

PATHOGEN-SPECIFIC IRIS

Mycobacterium avium Complex

Disseminated infection with *M. avium* complex (MAC) was a common opportunistic infection occurring in patients with advanced acquired immunodeficiency syndrome (AIDS). Blood and bone marrow cultures are usually positive in disseminated MAC, and minimal immune response is generally present. MAC was the first organism to be described in association with IRIS, when investigators described localized inflammatory MAC infections following treatment with zidovudine. In addition to those initial descriptions, MAC-related IRIS has been

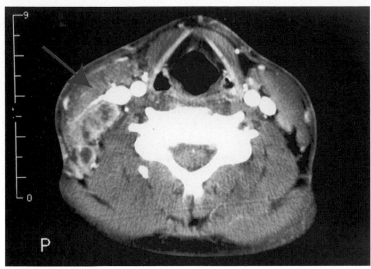

Figure 98.2 Necrotizing cervical lymphadenitis in a patient with previously diagnosed disseminated *M. avium* complex infection that was initiated on combination antiretroviral therapy. Six weeks later the patient presented with fever and tenderness of the right neck. Computed tomography scan showed necrotizing cervical lymphadenitis (red arrow). Biopsy showed well-formed granulomas with few acid-fast organisms consistent with *M. avium*. Cultures were negative.

well described by numerous investigators. MAC-related IRIS can occur either in patients who were previously known to be infected with MAC or as "unmasking phenomenon," in which the initiation of HAART results in clinical manifestations of a previously subclinical infection. MAC-related IRIS usually presents as fever in combination with lymphadenitis that may be subcutaneous, intrathoracic, or intra-abdominal, and stands in marked contrast to the blood and bone marrow culture-positive disseminated form (see Figure 98.2). Another well-described component of MAC-related IRIS is the formation of endobronchial lesions that can lead to airway obstruction. Finally, a granulomatous hepatitis form of MAC-related IRIS has been described as leading to hypercalcemia, presumably through increased production of $1,25(OH)_2$ vitamin D. The vast majority of MAC-related IRIS cases have occurred within 8 weeks of initiating antiretroviral therapy, although cases occurring as long as 18 months later have been described. The latter raise the question of whether some patients fail to completely reconstitute their immune response to MAC, thereby remaining at risk of infection despite numerical improvement in some parameters (Table 98.3).

Mycobacterium tuberculosis

IRIS related to *M. tuberculosis* (MTB) infection is particularly problematic in that paradoxical inflammatory responses are well known to occur during MTB treatment in non-HIV–infected individuals. Therefore, determining the degree to which HAART-treated patients are at increased risk for an inflammatory response during treatment for MTB is an area of active research. The morbidity or mortality of MTB-related IRIS are important to discern because of the tremendous numbers of patients co-infected with HIV and MTB and the increasing availability of HAART in countries where MTB is widespread.

Similar to MAC-related IRIS, MTB-related IRIS usually occurs within a few weeks to months after initiating HAART, although longer intervals have been described. When TB is limited to pulmonary infection, MTB-related IRIS generally consists of worsening pulmonary infiltrates, pleural effusions, and mediastinal lymphadenopathy (Figure 98.3). Patients with extrapulmonary MTB appear to have a higher incidence of IRIS and more IRIS-related symptoms compared to patients with pulmonary MTB infection. Lymphadenitis, either subcutaneous or intracavitary, is the most common presentation, but expansion of intracranial tuberculomas or an inflammatory meningitis carries the highest morbidity and mortality. Examination of clinical specimens from MTB-related IRIS patients usually reveals a brisk inflammatory response with few or no acid-fast organisms and negative cultures.

Cryptococcus neoformans

Cryptococcus neoformans infection in patients with AIDS usually presents as a disseminated infection with the central nervous system and lungs being most commonly involved. *Cryptococcus neoformans*–related IRIS tends to involve the central nervous system with

Table 98.3 Infection and Autoimmune Diseases Associated with IRIS in HIV-Infected Individuals

Organism/Autoimmune Disorder	Typical Manifestation(s)	Timing from Starting HAART	Comments
Mycobacterium avium complex	Lymphadenitis, endobronchial mass	Weeks to months	Localized process
Mycobacterium tuberculosis	Lymphadenitis, pneumonitis, tuberculoma	Weeks to months	Usually with extra-pulmonary *M. tuberculosis* infection
Cryptococcus neoformans	Meningitis, lymphadenitis	Weeks to few years	Intracranial hypertension common
Cytomegalovirus	Uveitis	Weeks to months	Often causes vision loss
Herpes simplex/varicella zoster viruses	Inflammatory skin lesions	Weeks to months	Very common
Hepatitis B and C viruses	Hepatitis	Weeks to months	Must rule out drug toxicity
JC virus	Inflammatory PML	Weeks to months	Can be fatal
Human herpes virus-8	Inflammatory Kaposi's sarcoma	Weeks to months	Especially problematic in lungs
Pneumocystis jiroveci	Pneumonitis	Days to weeks	Uncommon
Graves' disease	Thyrotoxicosis	Months to years	
Sarcoidosis	Lymphadenitis	Months to years	

Abbreviations: IRIS = immune reconstitution inflammatory syndrome; HIV = human immunodeficiency virus; HAART = highly active antiretroviral therapy; PML = progressive multifocal leukoencephalopathy.

an inflammatory meningitis predominating (Figure 98.4). The *C. neoformans* meningitis associated with IRIS tends to have higher cerebrospinal fluid (CSF) white blood cell counts and higher opening pressure compared with typical AIDS-associated *C. neoformans* meningitis. Although not an absolute rule, patients with IRIS-related *C. neoformans* meningitis tend to have lower CSF cryptococcal polysaccharide antigen compared to their initial treatment values. Conversely, patients with relapsing *C. meningitis* tend to have similar or higher CSF cryptococcal antigen levels compared to their original treatment values. Therefore, comparison of serial CSF, but not serum, cryptococcal antigen levels may be useful in differentiating IRIS-related *C. neoformans* meningitis from relapsing disease. Similar to the situation with MAC, *C. neoformans*–related IRIS may present as an apparent relapse or worsening of a previously recognized *C. neoformans* infection or as unmasking of a previously subclinical *C. neoformans* infection. In the latter situation, CSF cultures are negative but *C. neoformans* antigen is present in the CSF, possibly indicating inflammation against nonviable organisms. *Cryptococcus neoformans*–related IRIS meningitis is potentially fatal, presumably because of marked elevations in intracranial pressure. An underappreciated but vital component of therapy is relief of increased intracranial pressure through either repeated lumbar punctures or indwelling drainage devices.

A remarkable component of *C. neoformans*–related IRIS is the potential for complications several months or even years after starting therapy, including necrotizing pneumonia, lymphadenitis, and intracranial cryptococcomas. Lymphadenitis in association with *C. neoformans* rarely occurs in HIV-infected individuals except as a part of IRIS. Pathologic specimens show an intense inflammatory response surrounding yeastlike organisms, but cultures are negative. Steroids have been used anecdotally with impressive results.

Cytomegalovirus

Retinal disease due to cytomegalovirus (CMV) was a common complication of AIDS in the

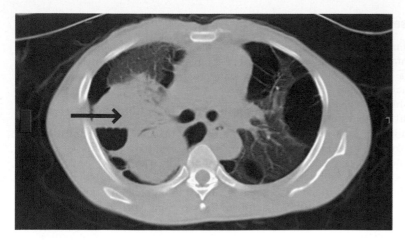

Figure 98.3 Necrotizing pneumonia in a patient with previously diagnosed *M. tuberculosis* infection who presented with shortness of breath and hemoptysis three weeks after starting HAART. Computed tomography scan of the thorax showed consolidation with necrosis (red arrow). Transbronchial biopsy showed necrotic tissue with all stains and cultures negative.

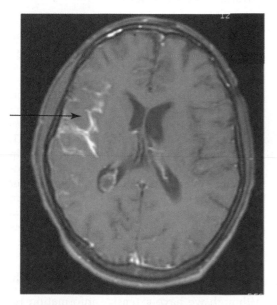

Figure 98.4 Contrast enhancement of the leptomeninges (red arrow) in patient with previously diagnosed *C. neoformans* meningitis who developed recurrent headache and fever 4 weeks after starting HAART. Cerebrospinal fluid examination showed an increased white blood cell count with elevated intracranial pressures. All stains and cultures were negative, and *C. neoformans* antigen was decreased compared to previous admission.

pre-HAART era. Similarly, some of the largest case series and pathogenesis investigations of IRIS have involved CMV disease. Various names have been applied to CMV-related IRIS, including immune recovery uveitis or immune recovery vitritis. The terms specifically highlight the observation that CMV-related IRIS is not limited to the retina but often involves other parts of the eye. CMV-related IRIS remains a major cause of vision loss in patients

with advanced AIDS. Eye examination of CMV-related IRIS is notable for an intense inflammatory response, far beyond that typically associated with typical AIDS-related CMV retinitis. Macular edema, proliferative retinopathy, and spontaneous vitreous hemorrhage may all occur. Given the disseminated nature of CMV infection, it is not surprising that CMV-related IRIS has been reported to involve organs other than the eye, producing colitis, pancreatitis, and dermatologic manifestations.

Herpes Simplex and Varicella-Zoster Viruses

Although rarely a cause of serious morbidity or mortality, the majority of opportunistic infections that occur following the initiation of antiretroviral therapy involve herpes simplex and varicella-zoster viruses (HSV, VZV). Whether such infections are a manifestation of IRIS is debatable, although some investigators have found that dermatologic manifestations of HSV and VZV disease are more common in patients who receive antiretroviral therapy compared with untreated controls. There are clearly some patients who develop an inflammatory form of HSV or VZV disease following initiation of HAART, but sorting out the exact incidence of such presentations is difficult. However, the incidence of either HSV or VZV flares following initiation of antiretroviral therapy is common enough that many practitioners routinely warn their patients about such presentations when commencing therapy. Systemic inflammatory syndromes related to HSV or VZV such an angiitis of the central nervous system can also occur as part of IRIS, although such cases are rare.

Hepatitis B and C Viruses

The role of immune reconstitution in determining the clinical presentation of hepatitis B and C virus infections is a highly problematic area of IRIS research. A major difficulty in understanding the relationship between an immune response and hepatitis is that the drugs that comprise HAART can induce liver inflammation themselves. Moreover, a liver biopsy, which is an invasive and not always available procedure, is usually needed to definitively determine the cause of a hepatic flare in such cases. Therefore, determining the role of IRIS in a patient infected with hepatitis B and/or C virus who develops hepatic inflammation after starting HAART is difficult. Nevertheless, there clearly is an increased risk of hepatitis after starting antiretroviral therapy in patients co-infected with hepatitis B or C virus, and immune reconstitution against virus-infected hepatocytes is highly suspected to play a contributing role (Table 98.2). Most cases of hepatitis after starting antiretroviral therapy result in only mild to moderate elevation of liver enzymes. For those co-infected patients with symptomatic hepatitis or in whom marked elevations of transaminases occur, a liver biopsy may help determine the pathogenetic basis of the inflammation.

JC Virus

Patients with advanced AIDS may suffer from progressive multifocal leukoencephalopathy (PML), a brain demyelinating disease characterized by a lack of inflammation. The primary treatment for PML is HAART. However, it is well recognized that a subset of patients with PML who initiate HAART have a rapid and often fatal inflammatory process in their central nervous system. The imaging and histopathologic findings of these patients stand in stark contrast to typical PML cases. IRIS related to PML is particularly problematic because of the exquisite sensitivity of the brain to inflammation and to the need to continue HAART as the primary PML treatment.

Human Herpes Virus-8

Human herpes virus-8 (HHV-8) is the etiologic agent of Kaposi's sarcoma (KS), a common AIDS-related malignancy. As with PML, HAART is a mainstay of treatment of patients with KS, but initiation of HAART can also result in a rapidly progressive, sometimes fatal, form of KS. Patients with visceral KS, especially those with pulmonary involvement, seem to be at highest risk for morbidity and mortality from KS-related IRIS. Augmented responses to HHV-8 have been demonstrated in some of these patients.

Miscellaneous Infectious Agents

Nearly all agents that cause opportunistic infections in AIDS patients have been described as contributing to IRIS. As HAART becomes more widely available in developing countries, IRIS is likely to shift to involve infectious agents endemic in these regions, such as parasites, mycobacteria, and endemic fungi.

Autoimmune Disorders

In addition to infectious agents, autoimmune disorders have been implicated as underlying IRIS. Autoimmune thyroiditis (Graves's disease) is increased in patients receiving HAART. Serial exams of stored sera have clearly demonstrated the relationship between initiating HAART and the development of anti–thyroid-stimulating hormone receptor antibody. Sarcoidosis has also been associated with response to HAART, a relationship that makes pathogenetic sense, in that sarcoidosis is driven by CD4+ T lymphocytes. Interestingly, there appears to be a greater period between antiretroviral therapy initiation and the development of autoimmune disorders as compared to IRIS related to infectious agents (Figure 98.1).

RISK FACTORS FOR DEVELOPING IRIS

Although we have extensive information regarding clinical manifestations and outcomes of patients with IRIS, we have very few data detailing which patients are likely to experience IRIS (Table 98.4). Several groups of investigators have attempted to define risk factors for developing IRIS, but the numbers of patients involved have been relatively small and the findings often discordant. One consistent finding is that patients with lower CD4+ T-lymphocyte counts at the time of initiating HAART are at higher risk for developing IRIS. This was originally thought to be due to more advanced immune suppression seen in such patients, allowing for establishment of subclinical infectious processes. However, more recent data suggest that patients with advanced immunodeficiency also have dysfunctional immune regulation. Therefore, patients with low CD4+ counts may be more likely to mount an

Table 98.4 Proposed Risk Factors for Developing IRIS

Proposed Risk Factors for Developing IRIS	Comments
Low CD4+ T-lymphocyte count or percentage prior to initiating HAART	Strongest predictor of IRIS development in many studies
Disseminated opportunistic infection	Strong predictor of developing IRIS in patients with *M. tuberculosis*
Initiating HAART in close proximity to starting therapy for an opportunistic infections	Found in some but not all studies
Rapid decline in HIV-1 RNA after starting HAART	Found in some but not all studies
High CD8+ T-lymphocyte count prior to starting HAART	Likely linked to low CD4+ counts
Genetic factors (HLA type, etc.)	Not systematically investigated to date
Antiretroviral naïve	Conflicting results from various studies
Rise in CD4+ T-lymphocyte count on antiretroviral therapy	Unlikely to be a risk factor

Abbreviations: IRIS = immune reconstitution inflammatory syndrome; HAART = highly active antiretroviral therapy; HIV = human immunodeficiency virus; HLA = human leukocyte antigen.

unrestrained inflammatory response against microbial or even self-antigens.

Other risk factors that have been proposed to underlie IRIS include genetic predispositions such as HLA type, a rapid decline in HIV-1 viral load, rapid increases in CD4+ T lymphocytes, and close timing between the initiation of antiretroviral therapy and starting therapy for an opportunistic infection (Table 98.4). The issue of timing influencing the possibility of developing IRIS has led some investigators to wait one to two months after initiating treatment for a severe opportunistic infection before starting HAART. Others have questioned such an approach, in light of the possibility of developing new HIV-related complications while waiting to initiate antiretroviral therapy.

TREATMENT OF PATIENTS WITH IRIS

There are no systematic studies comparing treatment options for patients with IRIS; therefore, no firm recommendations can be made at present. There are three major treatment options: stopping antiretroviral therapy, initiating immunomodulating therapy, and mechanical measures.

There is little information to support stopping HAART for a limited period of time, although some practitioners would do so if an

IRIS-related complication were life threatening. Steroids or nonsteroidal anti-inflammatory agents have been used on many patients with IRIS, with few descriptions of adverse events. Most published reports have used about 1 mg/kg of prednisone per day tapered over several weeks for severe IRIS cases, with anecdotal success. Finally, mechanical measures often form a key component of IRIS therapy, especially in cases where inflammation threatens vital structures such as the central nervous system. The utility of drainage procedures to relieve increased intracranial pressure in cases of *C. neoformans*–related IRIS meningitis cannot be overstated. Similarly, inflammatory lymph nodes, fluid collections, or masses that arise may be amenable to drainage procedures that can relieve morbidity and prevent mortality.

FUTURE DIRECTIONS IN IRIS RESEARCH

Although much has been learned in the decade since IRIS first became well recognized, there are a multitude of outstanding questions. There is a pressing need for a consensus definition that can be easily and systematically applied to future investigations. Risk factors for developing IRIS need to be clarified in a multicenter investigation so that preventive strategies can be rationally investigated. Finally, therapeutic regimens should be tested in a controlled fashion to allow for more definitive treatment recommendations. As antiretroviral therapy becomes more widely available, such investigations are taking on a new sense of urgency.

SUGGESTED READING

Battegay M, Nuesch R, Hirschel B, Kaufmann GR. Immunological recovery and antiretroviral therapy in HIV-1 infection. *Lancet Infect Dis*. 2006;6:280–287.

Chen F, Day SL, Metcalfe RA, et al. Characteristics of autoimmune thyroid disease occurring as a late complication of immune reconstitution in patients with advanced human immunodeficiency virus (HIV) disease. *Medicine*. 2005;84:98–106.

Connick E, Kane MA, White IE, Ryder J, Campbell TB. Immune reconstitution inflammatory syndrome associated with Kaposi sarcoma during potent antiretroviral therapy. *Clin Infect Dis*. 2004;39:1852–1855.

DeSimone JA, Pomerantz RJ, Babinchak TJ. Inflammatory reactions in HIV-1-infected persons after initiation of highly active antiretroviral therapy. *Ann Intern Med*. 2000;133:447–454.

French MA, Price P, Stone SF. Immune restoration disease after antiretroviral therapy. *AIDS*. 2004;18:1615–1627.

Lawn SD, Bekker LG, Miller RF. Immune reconstitution disease associated with mycobacterial infections in HIV-infected individuals receiving antiretrovirals. *Lancet Infect Dis*. 2005;5:361–373.

Ratnam I, Chiu C, Kandala NB, Easterbrook PJ. Incidence and risk factors for immune reconstitution inflammatory syndrome in an ethnically diverse HIV type 1-infected cohort. *Clin Infect Dis*. 2006;42:418–427.

Robertson J, Meier M, Wall J, Ying J, Fichtenbaum CJ. Immune reconstitution syndrome in HIV: validating a case definition and identifying clinical predictors in persons initiating antiretroviral therapy. *Clin Infect Dis*. 2006;42:1639–1646.

Shelburne SA III, Hamill RJ, Rodriguez-Barradas MC, et al. Immune reconstitution inflammatory syndrome: emergence of a unique syndrome during highly active antiretroviral therapy. *Medicine*. 2002;81:213–227.

Shelburne SA, Visnegarwala F, Darcourt J, et al. Incidence and risk factors for immune reconstitution inflammatory syndrome during highly active antiretroviral therapy. *AIDS*. 2005;19:399–406.

99. Differential Diagnosis and Management of Opportunistic Infections Complicating HIV Infection

Anthony Ogedegbe and Marshall J. Glesby

Even in the era of highly active antiretroviral therapy (HAART), the preponderance of HIV-associated morbidity and mortality stems from opportunistic infections. And despite broad access to HIV screening tests in developed countries, opportunistic infections remain the first indication of HIV infection in a significant proportion of patients.

Barring a few exceptions, HIV-associated opportunistic infections (OIs) predictably manifest at discrete CD4 T-cell count boundaries below which the risk of symptomatic disease rises sharply (Figure 99.1). This enables physicians to calibrate clinical suspicions for specific OIs based on contemporaneous CD4 T-cell measurements. Current clinical approaches to the evaluation and management of HOIs are discussed in this chapter.

MUCOCUTANEOUS INFECTIONS

Candidal infections of the mouth manifest as thrush and, to a lesser extent, angular cheilitis. Thrush appears as white, loosely adherent deposits on the tongue, palate, or oropharynx. Most cases are asymptomatic; however, individuals with moderate-to-severe disease may report oropharyngeal discomfort, nausea, or dysgeusia. Treatment consists of topical or oral azoles (Table 99.1).

Seborrhea dermatitis is a greasy, flaky, faintly erythematous rash. Facial involvement shows a predilection for the hairline of the forehead, eyebrows, bridge of the nose, and nasolabial folds. The role of *Malazesia furfur* infection in seborrhea dermatitis remains uncertain. Nonetheless, topical antifungal agents are effective in treating lesions, as are steroid creams (Table 99.1).

Recurrent or multidermatomal herpes zoster infection in an otherwise young, healthy adult may connote underlying HIV infection. Premonitory pain and paresthesias in the soon-to-be involved dermatome are followed days later by the sudden outcropping of clear vesicles on an erythematous base. Use of oral acyclovir or related agents, valacyclovir or famciclovir, within 72 hours improves symptoms, speeds up crusting of the lesions, and lessens postherpetic neuralgia (Table 99.1).

Orolabial and urogenital herpes simplex virus (HSV) infections become more frequent at CD4 counts ≤500 cells/μL. Characteristically, these appear as painful, clear vesicles. Oral acyclovir, valacyclovir, and famciclovir are all effective in abrogating both symptom severity and duration, as well as reducing the risk of recurrence when used prophylactically (Table 99.1).

Molluscum contagiosum is a poxvirus that causes characteristically firm, umbilicated and sometimes pedunculated skin nodules (Figure 99.2). The virus is particularly tropic for moist areas of the body, namely the axillae, perineum, antecubital, and popliteal fossae. Transmission requires intimate physical contact with an infected person. No specific chemotherapy exists; however, HAART can hasten regression of lesions. Alternatively, nodules can be physically removed by cryotherapy, curettage or laser-based modalities (Table 99.1).

Oral hairy leukoplakia results from Epstein-Barr virus infection of the lingual squamous epithelium. It presents as a series of white, painless, tightly adherent vertical ridges characteristically on the lateral aspect of the tongue. The most effective treatment is HAART (Table 99.1).

PULMONARY INFECTIONS

Critical aspects of the initial evaluation and management of pneumonia in HIV-infected patients include (1) immediate respiratory isolation of individuals with risk factors for active pulmonary tuberculosis; (2) *early* administration of empiric *pneumocystis jiroveci* (formerly pneumocystis carinii) pneumonia therapy where appropriate; and (3) devising empiric antibiotic regimens that reflect key elements of the history (eg, duration of symptoms; recent travel), degree of immunodeficiency, and radiographic findings (Table 99.2, Figure 99.3).

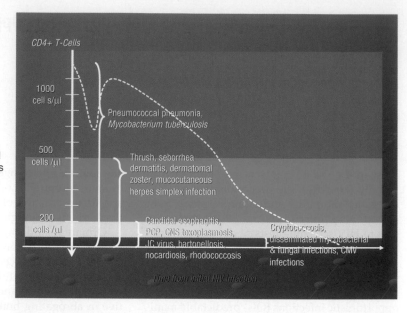

Figure 99.1 Spectrum of opportunistic infections in untreated HIV infection and the CD4 T-cell count ranges within which they manifest.

Although more expensive, computed tomography (CT) scans, given their increased sensitivity and superior image resolution over chest roentgenograms (CXR), are frequently necessary in evaluating patients with CD4 counts ≤200 cells/μL. This is particularly true in cases where the CXR suggests nodular, cavitary infiltrates, or intrathoracic lymphadenopathy. Here the etiologic possibilities are vast and chemotherapeutic options highly divergent. Thus additional CT evaluation may improve the accuracy of empiric antibiotic choices pending definitive results from bronchoalveolar lavage or lung biopsy (Figure 99.3). Barring the ubiquitous threat of pulmonary tuberculosis in HIV-positive patients (discussed below), standard empiric approaches for managing pneumonia in HIV-seronegative, immunocompetent individuals can usually be safely adopted in HIV-positive patients with CD4 counts >200 cells/μL and CD4 percentage >14 (Figure 99.3).

PNEUMOCYSTIS JIROVECI PNEUMONIA

Pneumocystis jiroveci pneumonia (PCP) presents as a subacute pneumonia characterized by fever, progressive dyspnea, and dry cough. Risk factors include CD4 counts ≤200 cells/μL, CD4 percentage ≤14, prior PCP, and thrush. Radiographically, PCP classically manifests as symmetric, perihilar interstitial, or alveolar infiltrates (Figure 99.4). However, caution should be exercised when attempting to eliminate PCP from the differential diagnosis solely on the basis of CXR findings. In our

experience, it is not uncommon to discover infiltrates compatible with PCP on CT in cases where the CXR had been read as "clear" or revealing "focal consolidations." Furthermore, a number of atypical radiographic findings have rarely been described in PCP, including upper lobe disease and cystic, nodular, and cavitating infiltrates. All this makes it critical that empiric PCP chemotherapy be included in the initial empiric antibiotic regimen administered to any HIV-positive individual, *irrespective of CXR findings*, presenting in respiratory failure (Figure 99.3). Exceptions to the rule include cases where contemporaneous CD4 count *and* percentage measurements are >200 cells/μL and >14% and rare instances where adherence specifically to *trimethoprim-sulfamethoxazole–based* PCP chemoprophylaxis—up until the time of presentation—is certain. Breakthrough PCP in either case is extremely rare (Figure 99.3).

Intravenous trimethoprim-sulfamethoxazole (TMP-SMX) is the preferred agent for treating *severe* PCP (Table 99.3). In patients with sulfa allergies, intravenous pentamidine should be used instead. Pentamidine-related toxicities—acute pancreatitis, hypoglycemia, and renal failure—are, however, common and should be aggressively sought when using this drug. Adjunctive steroids have been shown to improve survival in individuals presenting with a PaO_2 ≤70 mm Hg or alveolar-arterial (A-a) gradients >30 mm Hg. Nonetheless, mortality rates, even in the post-HAART era, approach 30% and remain as high as 60%–80% in ventilated patients.

In mild-to-moderate PCP, *oral* double strength TMP-SMX is the drug of choice.

Table 99.1 Management of Mucocutaneous Opportunistic Infections

Condition/Pathogen	First-Line Treatment	Notes
Thrush or candidal angular cheilitis	Clotrimazole troches, 10 mg PO 5 × daily; nystatin solution, 4–6 swish and swallow QID; or fluconazole, 100–200 mg PO qd for 7 days	In the event of azole resistance: amphotericin B suspension, 100 mg/mL PO QID; amphotericin B deoxycholate, 0.3–0.7 mg/kg IV qd; liposomal or lipid complex amphotericin, 3–5 mg/kg; voriconazole, 200 mg PO qd; or caspofungin 50 mg IV qd all for 7 days
Seborrhea dermatitis	Face: Imidazole cream (ketoconazole 2% or clotrimazole 1%) plus hydrocortisone 1.0%–2.5% or desonide 0.05% cream BID Scalp/body: Antidandruff shampoo (eg, Selsun Blue or Head and Shoulders) plus triamcinolone 0.1% cream (body) or solution (scalp)	Severe cases may require addition of oral ketoconazole, 200–400 mg qd for 2–4 weeks.
Varicella–zoster virus	Acyclovir, 800 mg PO 5 × daily; famciclovir, 500 mg PO TID; or valacyclovir, 1000 mg PO TID for 7–10 days	(1) Trigeminal or disseminated cutaneous zoster; attendant meningoencephalitis; or evidence of visceral involvement (ie, elevated transaminases and/or pancreatic enzymes) all merit IV acyclovir, 10 mg/kg q8h, until clinical resolution (minimum 14–21 days). (2) In the event of acyclovir resistance: foscarnet, 40–60 mg/kg IV q8h, or cidofovir plus IV hydration and oral probenecid to mitigate renal toxicity
Herpes simplex virus	Acyclovir, 400 mg PO TID; famciclovir, 500 mg PO BID; or valacyclovir, 1000 mg PO BID for 7–14 days	In the event of acyclovir resistance: foscarnet, 40–60 mg/kg IV q8h, or cidofovir plus IV hydration and oral probenecid to mitigate renal toxicity.
Molluscum contagiosum	Laser, cryotherapy, and curettage plus HAART	
Oral hairy leukoplakia	HAART	(1) OHL is pathognomonic of underlying HIV infection. (2) Rarely warrants specific therapy; but oral acyclovir 800 mg PO 5 × daily and POdophyllin have been used with variable success in severe cases.

Abbreviations: PO = orally; QID = four times per day; qd = every day; BID = twice per day; TID = three times per day; HAART = highly active antiretroviral treatment; IV = intravenously.

However, other effective chemotherapeutic agents are available and are particularly convenient for outpatient management when oral, non-sulfa-based therapies are desired; these include clindamycin–primaquine, dapsone–trimethoprim, and atovaquone (Table 99.3).

Clinical improvement in severe cases of PCP is typically protracted and can take as long as 5–7 days. Only cases failing to show improvement beyond this time period are deemed treatment failures. The following steps are then indicated where relevant: (1) instituting steroid therapy in cases where the initial PaO_2 or A-a gradient had suggested otherwise, (2) switching either to intravenous TMP-SMX or pentamidine (patients initially on the former should be switched to pentamidine), and/or (3) repeating sputum and/or bronchoalveolar lavage tests in hopes of identifying copathogens that would also warrant treatment. These include any credible bacterial, fungal, viral, or parasitic pulmonary pathogens. Most cases of treatment failure are, however, indicative of the severity of pneumocystis infection at the outset of treatment rather than treatment failure *per se*.

Mycobacterial Infections

Unlike PCP and most other acquired immunodeficiency syndrome (AIDs)-defining opportunistic infections, the relative risk of active *Mycobacterium tuberculosis* (MTB) infection in HIV-infected individuals compared to the general population is significantly >1 irrespective of CD4 count. The clinical presentation of MTB pneumonia, however, varies with CD4

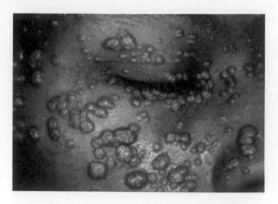

Figure 99.2 Molluscum contagiosum. Numerous flesh-colored umbilicated papules appeared on the face of a 33-year-old man with a 3-year history of acquired immunodeficiency syndrome and a CD4 cell count of 60 cells/µL. Prominent lesions along the margin of the eyelids prevented him from closing his eyes completely. Reproduced with permission from Stephanie Cotell. Cotell SL, Roholt NS. *N Engl J Med.* 1998;338(13):888.

count, with lower lobe, noncavitary, and extrapulmonary disease becoming increasingly more frequent at CD4 counts ≤350 cells/µL. Chemotherapy recommendations are, however, identical to seronegative patients with pulmonary MTB except clinicians have to be mindful of higher rates of treatment failure and drug resistance, as well as adverse pharmacokinetic interactions between some antituberculous medications and antiretroviral agents (Table 99.3).

The leading nontuberculous mycobacterial pulmonary pathogen in HIV-positive patients is *Mycobacterium* avium complex (MAC). Such cases are distinct from *disseminated* MAC (discussed below) in which severe CD4 lymphopenia and mycobacteremia are the *sine qua non* and concurrent MAC pneumonia rare. In the post-HAART era, the majority of cases manifest within weeks of initiating HAART, leading some to posit an immune reconstitution mechanism. Management comprises use of a second-generation oral macrolide, ethambutol, plus a third agent, typically rifabutin (Table 99.3).

Pneumonia due to *Mycobacterium kansasii* and, to a lesser extent, so-called rapid-grower mycobacteria, such as *Mycobacterium abscessus*, *Mycobacterium fortuitum*, and *Mycobacterium chelonae*, has also been reported in HIV-positive patients—usually with CD4 counts ≤200 cells/µL. Unlike the latter, which are often commensals in the lung, pulmonary specimens containing *M. kansasii* are more often indicative of active infection (see Table 99.3 for treatment recommendations).

Filamentous Bacteria

Pulmonary nocardiosis and rhodococcosis are particularly rare complications of AIDS in the post-HAART era. These microorganisms share a number of features that have contributed to their classification as actinomycetes—both are gram-positive, weakly acid-fast, and form multicellular filaments under certain laboratory conditions. Clinically, both are associated with nodular pulmonary infiltrates and/or abscesses that sometimes cavitate. Concurrent mediastinal lymphadenopathy is also common. Disseminated disease, with a predilection for brain and, to a lesser extent, skin lesions, can also occur. Unlike nocardia where positive blood cultures are rare, rhodococcal infections are frequently associated with bacteremia (up to 50% of cases in HIV-positive patients) that can be detected in routine blood cultures. Detection of nocardia requires that cultures be held for a minimum of 28 days and subcultured to selective media at 14 days. However, more timely diagnosis can be accomplished by detecting gram-positive, branching, multicellular filaments in tissue specimens. Chemotherapy is protracted in both cases and relapse common in the absence of durable immune recovery through HAART (Table 99.3).

Endemic Mycoses

Pneumonia due to any of the three major endemic mycoses in the United States—coccidioidomycosis, histoplasmosis, and blastomycosis—primarily affects individuals with CD4 counts ≤250 cells/µL. Mediastinal lymphadenopathy can also be observed. Rates of infection are higher in endemic areas, namely the San Joaquin valley and Ohio/Mississippi river basins, respectively. Individuals who have previously spent time in these areas, no matter how remotely, are also at higher risk because primary infection, once established, is immunologically contained rather than eradicated. In patients with higher CD4 counts, focal alveolar or nodular infiltrates, sometimes cavitating, are more common. In more immunodeficient individuals (ie, CD4 counts ≤100 cells/µL), diffuse, reticulonodular infiltrates, reflective of disseminated pulmonary disease, are more frequent. Disseminated infection may also present as fever, rash, marrow failure, and/or meningitis (see below). Life-threatening infections require induction chemotherapy with amphotericin-B-based drugs followed by maintenance treatment with oral triazoles (Table 99.3).

Table 99.2 Etiologic Correlates of Clinical and Radiologic Findings in HIV-Infected Patients with Pneumonia

Clinical Paradigms of Pneumonia in HIV	Typical Pathogens
(1) *Acute Pneumonia:* Abrupt onset of symptoms; high fever often with prominent chills or rigors; focal pleurisy; and marked elevations (or depressions) in white blood cell count plus bandemia	*Streptococcus pneumoniae, Staphylococcus aureus, Pseudomonas aeruginosa,* and *Legionella pneumophila*
(2) *Subacute Pneumonia:* Patients rarely present during the first week of illness; fever is low-grade; normal or slight deviations in the white blood cell count	*Pneumocystis jiroveci, Mycoplasma pneumoniae, Nocardia asteroides,* and *Rhodococcus equi*
(3) *Indolent Pneumonia:* Prominent constitutional symptoms such as fever, chills, night sweats, anorexia, and weight loss; respiratory symptoms lag behind by weeks: normal or slight deviations in the white blood cell count	*Mycobacterium tuberculosis, Mycobacteria avium complex, Nocardia asteroides,* and *Pneumocystis jiroveci*

Chest X-Ray or Computed Tomography Categories of Pneumonia	Typical Pathogens
(1) Focal/lobar asymmetric infiltrates *without* intrathoracic lymphadenopathy	*Streptococcus pneumoniae, Moraxella catarrhalis, Hemophilus influenzae* and *Mycobacterium tuberculosis* in individuals with primary infection or CD4 counts >350 cells/μL
(2) Diffuse interstitial or alveolar infiltrates *without* intrathoracic lymphadenopathy	*Pneumocystis jiroveci,* influenza virus, respiratory syncytial virus and *Mycoplasma pneumoniae*
(3) Nodular and/or cavitating infiltrates *without* intrathoracic lymphadenopathy *(acute presentations)*	*Staphylococcus aureus* (particularly with concurrent bacteremia or right-sided endocarditis); and rarely *Pseudomonas aeruginosa, Mycoplasma pneumoniae*
Nodular and/or cavitating infiltrates *plus* intrathoracic lymphadenopathy *(indolent presentations)*	*Mycobacterium tuberculosis, Aspergillus fumigatus,* and *Rhodococcus equi*

Pulmonary Aspergillosis

Severe CD4 lymphopenia is one of several risk factors that have been associated with pulmonary aspergillosis; other predisposing conditions include neutropenia, recent exposure to corticosteroids, and marijuana use. Two distinct clinical syndromes have been described: an isolated tracheobronchitis, which may be invasive, and parenchymal infection. Symptoms in both cases include fever, productive cough, chest pain, and hemoptysis. Wheezing is, however, specific to tracheobronchial involvement. On bronchoscopy, airway-obstructing mycelia and mucous balls are observed; pseudomembranes and/or ulcerations are reflective of airway invasion. Aspergillus pneumonitis presents either as pleural-based alveolar lesions, reticulonodular disease, or cavitating apical infiltrates. Treatment includes use of voriconazole and/or amphotericin B–based treatments (Table 99.3).

GASTROINTESTINAL INFECTIONS
Infections of the Esophagus

Candidal esophagitis is an AIDS-defining illness that manifests at CD4 counts ≤200 cells/μL. Typical symptoms include dysphagia, odynophagia, and sometimes chest pain or fever. In rare instances, esophageal perforation can occur either because of delayed or ineffectual treatment. Triazoles are the mainstay of therapy (Table 99.4); however, azole resistance is common particularly in patients with advanced

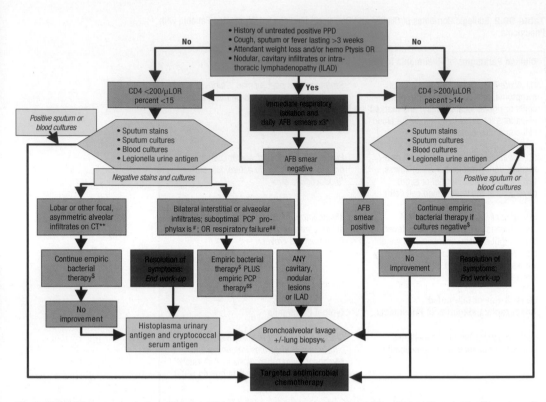

Figure 99.3 Management algorithm for HIV-positive patients presenting with community-acquired pneumonia

*Respiratory isolation and procurement of sputa for AFB smear do not preclude initiation of empiric therapy for nonmycobacterial pulmonary pathogens. In fact, the latter (including empiric PCP therapy where appropriate) should be started concurrently with AFB evaluation in patients at risk for rapid clinical deterioration.

**The inferior sensitivity and image resolution of chest x-rays relative to computed tomography may occasionally cause bilateral interstitial pulmonary infiltrates to appear focal or asymmetric. This, in turn, may result in serious errors in management; most significantly, inappropriate omission of empiric PCP therapy.

"Suboptimal PCP prophylaxis" is defined as either poor adherence to PCP prophylactic drugs or *use of non-trimethoprim-sulfamethoxazole* chemoprophylactic agents; the latter have been associated with breakthrough PCP despite good adherence.

##Irrespective of radiographic findings, any case of respiratory failure in a patient with risk factors for PCP merits immediate empiric PCP therapy plus adjunctive steroids pending results of sputum, blood, bronchoalveolaor, and/or lung biopsy evaluation.

$Empiric bacterial therapy should cover standard community-acquired organisms, including legionella species.

$$Where ever possible, the decision whether to continue or abort PCP therapy, once started empirically, should rest on results of microscopic evaluations of bronchoalveolar lavage or lung biopsy specimens. The latter remain sensitive for pneumocystis organisms up to a week after commencing therapy. Thus, negative tests for PCP within this time window should prompt searches for other causes of pneumonia and argues strongly for switching from PCP therapy to chemoprophylaxis.

%Open lung biopsy should be pursued in cases where transbronchial or fine-needle biopsies are nondiagnostic.

immunodeficiency. In such cases, amphotericin-B-based therapies or caspofungin are usually effective (Table 99.4).

Rarely, herpes simplex virus (HSV) or cytomegalovirus (CMV) may infect the esophagus, causing symptoms indistinguishable from those encountered in esophageal candidiasis. Patients with the former are, however, usually more immunodeficient—CD4 counts ≤100 cells/µL. In patients presenting with esophageal symptoms in the absence of thrush, it is customary to institute empiric candidal treatment and only pursue alternate causes (through endoscopically guided biopsy) in treatment failures (Table 99.4).

Diarrheal Illness

Patients taking protease inhibitor–based HAART often experience treatment-related diarrhea. However, absence of the requisite temporal relationship to HAART (ie, within *days* of starting therapy) or evidence of intestinal inflammation or invasion (ie, attendant fever, hematochezia, or severe abdominal pain) suggests an infectious cause. At CD4 counts >200 cells/µL, a differential diagnosis including the usual community-acquired pathogens—rotavirus, Norwalk virus, salmonella, campylobacter, shigella, yersinia, and giardia—applies. Invasive salmonellosis,

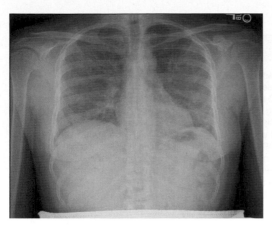

Figure 99.4 *Pneumocystis jiroveci* pneumonia. Bilateral interstitial infiltrates on chest x-ray in a 39-year-old woman with AIDS and CD4 count of 55 cells/μL who presented with 2 weeks of fever, dry cough, and shortness of breath.

campylobacteriosis, and shigellosis are, however, more frequent in HIV-infected individuals. Consequently, antibiotic treatment for these infections, whereas discretionary in immunocompetent, HIV-seronegative persons, is universally warranted in this population (Table 99.4).

Patients with CD4 ≤100 cells/μL may experience severe, protracted cryptosporidium, microsporidia, cyclospora, or isospora infection. Although much less frequent in the post-HAART era, effective chemotherapeutic agents against these organisms, with the exception of isospora and cyclospora, are sorely lacking. Antispasmodics and immune reconstitution via HAART are, therefore, the mainstays of management (Table 99.4).

Symptomatic CMV gastrointestinal disease most often develops in the colon. CMV colitis manifests at CD4 counts ≤100 cells/μL and presents as fever, bloody diarrhea, and abdominal pain. Treatment comprises 2 to 3 weeks of induction therapy with IV ganciclovir or oral valganciclovir with half the induction dose as maintenance therapy thereafter (Table 99.4).

HIV Cholangiopathy

Some intestinal pathogens—primarily *Microsporidia parvum* but also cryptosporidium, CMV, and cyclospora—are also able to infect and scar the biliary tract giving rise to a syndrome known as HIV cholangiopathy. Typically a complication of advanced HIV disease (CD4 counts ≤100 cells/μL), HIV cholangiopathy manifests as right upper quadrant discomfort

(rarely fever or jaundice) and serum alkaline phosphatase elevation. Radiographically, endoscopic retrograde cholangiopancreotography (ERCP) reveals an intra- as well as extrahepatic sclerosing cholangitis with or without papillary stenosis. Symptoms are typically refractory to chemotherapeutic agents directed at the culprit pathogen. However, cases marked by papillary stenosis or a dominant extrahepatic biliary stricture can be ameliorated endoscopically through sphincterotomy or stenting, respectively. Ursodeoxycholic acid (300 mg orally 3 times daily) is effective for symptom relief in patients with lesions not amenable to endoscopic intervention.

NEUROLOGICAL INFECTIONS
Meningitis

Cryptococcus neoformans is the most commonly identified cause of meningitis among HIV-infected patients. Patients present with a subacute meningitis manifesting as headache, fever, and lethargy. Progressive elevations in intracranial pressure manifesting as nausea, emesis, and blindness (from pressure on the optic nerve), sometimes culminating in coma, is characteristic of advanced illness. Serial spinal taps are sometimes necessary to alleviate severe headache. However, antifungal treatment is the mainstay of management and comprises an initial 2 weeks of induction therapy with amphotericin-B-based therapies and 5-flucytosine followed by oral fluconazole monotherapy (Table 99.5).

Similar presentations, including a proclivity for elevated intracranial pressure, are seen with MTB, histoplasma, and coccidioides meningitis, all of which are associated with lymphocytic pleocytoses, mildly reduced CSF glucose, and elevated CSF protein (see Table 99.5 for treatment recommendations).

Encephalitis

JC virus central nervous system (CNS) infection, although much less frequent in the post-HAART era, remains a dispiriting diagnosis owing to the dearth of effective chemotherapeutic agents. HAART is, therefore, the only recourse but may be associated with paradoxical worsening. Patients typically, but not exclusively, present with nonenhancing periventricular subcortical white matter lesions devoid of mass effect or surrounding edema. Involvement of the basal ganglia and/or

Table 99.3 Management of Pulmonary Opportunistic Infections

Pathogen	First-Line Treatment	Notes
Pneumocystis jiroveci	Mild to moderate disease: TMP-SMX-DS, 2 tabs PO TID; dapsone, 100 mg PO qd, plus TMP, 5 mg/kg PO q8h; clindamycin, 450 mg PO or 600 mg IV q8h, plus primaquine, 15 mg qd; or atovaquone, 1500 mg qd for 21 days Severe disease: TMP-SMX, 15 mg/kg IV (TMP component) qd in 3–4 divided doses, or, in patients with sulfa allergy, pentamidine, 4 mg/kg IV qd, plus prednisone (40 mg BID × 5 days; 20 mg BID × 5 days; 20 mg qd × 11 days) for 21 days	(1) Caution must be taken with the use of primaquine or dapsone in patients at risk for G6PD deficiency because of the risk of hemolytic anemia. Such individuals should be tested for the latter in anticipation of exposure to these drugs. (2) May discontinue *secondary* prophylaxis after CD4 >200 cells/μL for >3 months.
M. tuberculosis	Isoniazid, 5 mg/kg/d, plus rifampin, 600 mg PO qd, plus pyrazinamide, 15–30 mg/kg PO qd, plus ethambutol, 15–25 mg/kg/d as initial therapy	If patient is taking a protease inhibitor, replace rifampin with rifabutin, 150–300 mg PO qd, because rifampin significantly lowers serum levels of protease inhibitors.
M. avium complex	Clarithromycin, 500 mg PO BID, or azithromycin, 600 mg qd, plus ethambutol, 15–25 mg/kg/d, plus rifabutin, 300 mg PO qd for a minimum of 12 months	In patients on efavirenz, azithromycin is preferred over clarithromycin as part of the 3–drug regimen because efavirenz lowers the serum levels of the latter.
M. kansasii	Isoniazid, 5 mg/kg/d, plus rifampin, 600 mg PO qd, plus ethambutol, 25 mg/kg/d (× 2 months then 15 mg/kg) for 15–18 mo	(1) *M. kansasii* is intrinsically resistant to pyrazinamide. (2) If patient is taking a protease inhibitor, replace rifampin with rifabutin, 150–300 mg PO qd, because rifampin significantly lowers serum levels of protease inhibitors.
M. abscessus or M. chelonae	Clarithromycin, 500 mg PO BID for 6 mo	Add tobramycin and imipenem for first 2–6 wk in severe or disseminated infection.
M. fortuitum	Amikacin plus cefoxitin plus probenecid for the first 2–6 wk followed by doxycycline or TMP-SMX for 2–6 mo	
Histoplasma capsulatum (pulmonary and non-CNS disseminated disease)	Mild-to-moderate disease: Itraconazole, 200 mg PO TID for 3 d, followed by itraconazole, 200 mg BID for 12 wk Severe illness: Amphotericin B deoxycholate, 0.7 mg/kg IV qd, or liposomal or lipid complex amphotericin, 3–5 mg/kg, until clinically improved followed by itraconazole, 200 mg q12h for 12 wk	
Coccidioides immitis (pulmonary and non-CNS disseminated disease)	Mild-to-moderate disease: fluconazole, 400–800 mg PO qd Severe illness: Amphotericin B deoxycholate, 0.5–1.0 mg/kg IV qd, followed by fluconazole, 400–800 mg PO qd	Lifelong suppression with fluconazole, 400 mg PO qd, is recommended, even with CD4 >200 cells/μL HAART.
Blastomycosis dermatitidis (pulmonary and non-CNS disseminated disease)	Amphotericin B deoxycholate, 0.7–1.0 mg/kg IV qd, until clinically improved (minimum cumulative 1 g) followed by itraconazole, 200 mg for 12 wk	

Pathogen	First-Line Treatment	Notes
Aspergillus fumigatus (pulmonary and non-CNS disseminated disease)	Voriconazole, 6 mg/kg IV × 1, followed by either 4 mg/kg IV or 100–200 mg PO BID for 2–3 wk; oral voriconazole for suppression	(1) Alternatives to voriconazole: amphotericin B deoxycholate; liposomal or lipid complex amphotericin 3–5 mg/kg; or caspofungin +/– voriconazole. (2) Also note: voriconazole should not be used with either efavirenz or ritonavir; both significantly lower voriconazole serum levels.
Nocardia asteroides (pulmonary and non-CNS disseminated disease)	TMP-SMX (15 mg/kg/d TMP; 75 mg/kg/d SMX) × 3 weeks followed by 10 mg/kg/day TMP component PO	In severe cases: add amikacin or imipenem or third-generation cephalosporin when limited by aminoglycoside toxicity.
Rhodococcus equi (pulmonary and *non-CNS* disseminated disease)	Erythromycin or imipenem, 0.5 g IV q6h, plus rifampin, 600 mg PO qd for 2 wk, followed by oral clarithromycin or azithromycin plus rifampin for suppression	Alternative agents: ciprofloxacin or linezolid

Abbreviations: TMP-smx = trimethropim-sulfamethoxazole; DS = double strength; PO = orally; TID = three times a day; IV = intravenously; qd = every day; BID = twice a day; CNS = central nervous system; G6PD = Glucose-6-Phosphate Dehydrogenase Deficiency; HAART = highly active antiretroviral therapy.

thalamus is seen in only a small minority of patients. Lesions are more likely to enhance in patients who develop symptoms in the context of HAART. Symptoms in either case include progressive encephalopathy, amnesia, ataxia, vertigo, seizures, and motor deficits.

CMV meningoencphalitis is a marker of very advanced HIV immunodeficiency (≤100 cells/μL). Rapid cognitive deterioration marked by fever and headache is the usual presentation. Radiographically, the classic, almost pathognomonic, finding is a symmetric, T2-bright ependymitis with extension to the periventricular white matter on magnetic resonance imaging. However, nonspecific white matter changes are more common. Progressive cognitive decline, often culminating in death, is common despite use of intravenous ganciclovir. Dual therapy with foscarnet may improve outcomes (Table 99.5). Of note, CMV infection of the nervous system in individuals with ≤100 cells/μL may alternatively involve the lumbosacral roots. Patients present with rapidly progressive lower extremity flaccid weakness and sometimes urinary retention. CSF pleocytoses are characteristically neutrophilic.

Varicella zoster virus (VZV) CNS infection manifests as an acute meningoencphalitis. The temporal relationship to outbreaks of zoster is highly variable. Histopathologic lesions include acute white matter demyelination and a granulomatous vasculopathy that may culminate in stroke. Patients present with fever, encephalopathy, and acute motor-sensory deficits that typically follow, but may also precede, a dermatomal zoster outbreak. Treatment comprises intravenous acyclovir for a minimum of 2 to 3 weeks (Table 99.5). Clinicians should also be cognizant of acute transverse myelitis as a potential sequela of CNS CMV, VZV, and HSV infections. Unlike CMV lumbosacral polyradiculopathies, limb weakness in this case is spastic and reflexes brisk. Symptoms variably respond to prolonged courses of corticosteroid therapy, intravenous immunoglobulin, or plasmapheresis.

Brain Abscess

Space occupying brain lesions in patients with CD4 counts ≤200 cells/μL are most often caused by recrudescent CNS toxoplasma infection (Figure 99.5). Patients present with seizure, headache, altered sensorium, and fever. CNS toxoplasmosis is rare, but not unheard of, in patients *without* a positive toxoplasma immunoglobulin G (IgG) (≤10%). Where primary CNS lymphoma is unlikely (see Table 99.5), an empiric trial of antitoxoplasma antibiotics (Table 99.5) is usually instituted in lieu of more definitive, but invasive, stereotactic brain biopsy. Individuals failing to improve radiographically within 10–14 days of therapy are then subjected to biopsy for a histopathologic diagnosis. Rarer causes of brain abscess include MTB, cryptococcus, aspergillus, the endemic mycoses, nocardia,

Table 99.4 Management of Opportunistic Infections of the Digestive Tract

Condition/Pathogen	First-Line Treatment	Notes
Candidal esophagitis	Fluconazole, 100–400 mg PO qd for 14 d	In the event of azole resistance: amphotericin B suspension, 100 mg/mL PO QID; amphotericin B deoxycholate, 0.3–0.7 mg/kg IV qd; liposomal or lipid complex amphotericin, 3–5 mg/kg; voriconazole, 200 mg PO BID; or caspofungin, 50 mg IV qd, all for 14 d
Herpes simplex esophagitis	Acyclovir, 5 mg/kg IV, followed by acyclovir, 400 mg PO TID; famciclovir, 500 mg PO BID; or valacyclovir, 1000 mg PO BID for 7–14 days once patient is tolerating oral therapy	In the event of acyclovir resistance: foscarnet, 40–60 mg/kg IV q8h, or cidofovir, IV plus IV hydration, and oral probenecid to mitigate renal toxicity.
Cytomegalovirus Esophagitis	Ganciclovir, 5–6 mg/kg/day IV, or valganciclovir, 900 mg PO BID, once patient tolerating oral therapy, for 2–3 wk followed by half-dose valganciclovir for chronic suppression	In the event of ganciclovir resistance: foscarnet, 90 mg/kg IV q12h, or cidofovir, IV plus IV hydration, and oral probenecid to mitigate renal toxicity.
Salmonellosis	Ciprofloxacin, 500–750 mg BID, or levofloxacin, 500 mg qd for 7–14 d	(1) Relapse is common and may necessitate chronic suppression; therefore, treat for 4–6 weeks in patients with CD4 count ≤200 cells/μL or bacteremia. (2) Fluoroquinolone resistance is increasing, in which case azithromycin should be used.
Shigellosis	Ciprofloxacin, 500 mg BID, or levofloxacin, 500 mg qd for 3 d	(1) Treat for up to 14 days in patients with CD4 count ≤200 cells/μL or bacteremia. (2) Alternative agent: azithromycin.
Campylobacteriosis	Ciprofloxacin, 500 mg BID, or azithromycin, 500 mg qd for 3 d	(1) Treat for up to 14 d in patients with CD4 count ≤200 cells/μL or bacteremia. (2) Fluoroquinolone resistance is increasing rapidly, particularly in southeast Asia.
Cryptosporidiosis	HAART *plus* antispasmodic +/− nitazoxanide 500 mg PO q12 hours for 14 days	
Microsporidiosis	Albendazole, 400 mg q12h for 3 wk	The most common cause of diarrheal illness, *E. bieneusi*, is the least susceptible species to albendazole.
Cyclosporidiosis	TMP-SMX-DS q6h for 10 d then 1 tab 3×/wk	Alternative agent: ciprofloxacin.
Isosporiosis	TMP-SMX-DS q6h for 10 d then 1 tab 3×/wk	Alternative agents: ciprofloxacin, pyrimethamine plus folinic acid.

Abreviations: PO = orally; qd = every day; QID = four times a day; IV = intravenously; BID = twice a day; TID = three times a day; HAART = highly active antiretroviral therapy; TMP-SMX-DS = Trimethropim-Sulfamethoxazole-double strength.

and rhodococcus (see Table 99.5 for treatment recommendations). Unlike toxoplasmosis, however, these rarer cerebritides are often associated with concomitant pneumonia.

Retinitis

New blurred vision, photopsia, and/or scotomata in a patient with ≤100 cells/μL merits emergent evaluation for CMV retinitis. Left unaddressed, symptoms quickly progress and may result in blindness within days to weeks; the latter occurs either as a result of retinal detachment (a consequence of large, peripheral lesions), lesions over the macula, or involvement of the optic nerve. Fundoscopically, the diagnosis is confirmed by the presence of pale yellowish retinal exudates that enlarge over time. Ganciclovir-impregnated retinal implants combined with oral valganciclovir is first-line therapy (Table 99.5).

VZV is a less common cause of acute retinal necrosis. Like CMV retinitis, rapid, permanent visual loss may also ensue if untreated. Both

Table 99.5 Management of Neurological Opportunistic Infections

Pathogen/Condition	First-Line Treatment	Notes
Cryptococcus neoformans	Amphotericin B, 0.7 mg/kg IV qd, plus 5-flucytosine, 25 mg/kg q6h, or liposomal or lipid complex amphotericin, 4 mg/kg, plus 5-flucytosine, 25 mg/kg q6h for 2 wk, followed by 10 wk of fluconazole, 400 mg PO qd, followed by chronic suppression with fluconazole, 200 mg PO qd	Note: monitor 5-FC serum levels – peak and trough levels >80 mg/L and 40 mg/L, respectively, are associated with significant bone marrow toxicity.
M. tuberculosis	Isoniazid. 5 mg/kg/d, plus rifampin, 600 mg PO qd, plus pyrazinamide, 15–30 mg/kg PO qd, plus ethambutol 15–25 mg/kg/d for a minimum of 12 mo	If patient is taking a protease inhibitor, replace rifampin with rifabutin, 150–300 mg PO qd, because rifampin significantly lowers serum levels of protease inhibitors.
Histoplasma capsulatum Meningoencphalitis	Amphotericin B deoxycholate, 0.7 mg/kg IV qd; liposomal or lipid complex amphotericin, 3–5 mg/kg, until clinically improved followed by itraconazole, 200 mg for 12–16 wk. Chronic suppression with 200 mg qd thereafter.	Blood cultures, and even *DuPont* fungal isolators, are often negative in systemic histoplasma infections. However, a urinary histoplasma antigen-based test is >90% sensitive in patients with AIDS.
Coccidioides immitis Meningoencphalitis	Fluconazole 400–800 mg IV or PO qd	Lifelong suppression with fluconazole, 400 mg PO qd, is recommended, even with CD4 >200 cells/μL on HAART.
Blastomycosis dermatitidis Meningoencphalitis	Amphotericin B deoxycholate, 0.7–1.0 mg/kg IV qd, until clinically improved (minimum cumulative 1 gm) followed by itraconazole, 200 mg for 12 wk	
JC Virus (Progressive Multifocal Leukoencephalopathy)	HAART	
Varicella zoster virus	Meningoencephalitis: Acyclovir, 10 mg/kg IV for 14–21 d Retinitis: as above *plus* foscarnet, 60 mg/kg IV q8h, followed by chronic suppression with valacyclovir or famciclovir	In the event of acyclovir resistance: foscarnet 40–60 mg/kg IV q8h or cidofovir IV plus IV hydration and oral probenecid to mitigate renal toxicity.
Cytomegalovirus	Meningoencephalitis/polyradiculitis: Ganciclovir, 5–6 mg/kg/d IV, or valganciclovir, 900 mg PO BID, +/– IV foscarnet, 90–120 mg/kg/d, until clinical improvement Retinitis: As above plus sustained-release ganciclovir intraocular implant q6–9 mo	(1) Lifelong chronic suppression with valganciclovir is recommended. (2) Under supervision of a qualified ophthalmologist, may discontinue maintenance therapy after maximal improvement and CD4 count has been >150 cells/μL for >6 months.
T. gondii brain abscess	Pyrimethamine, 200 mg PO 1×, then 50–75 mg qd plus sulfadiazine, 1.0–1.5 g PO QID, plus folinic acid, 10–20 mg PO qd for 6 wk, followed by half-dose of all 3 drugs as chronic suppression	(1) Primary CNS lymphoma is the other leading cause of brain mass in this population but is more often unifocal, >4 cm, and distinguishable from cerebral toxoplasmosis on single photon emission computed tomography and positron emission tomography. (2) In patients with sulfa allergy: replace sulfadiazine with clindamycin, dapsone, or atovaquone.
Aspergillus fumigatus	Voriconazole, 6 mg/kg IV 1×, followed by either 4 mg/kg IV or 100–200 mg PO BID for 2–3 wk; oral voriconazole for suppression	Less preferred agents: (1) amphotericin B deoxycholate; (2) liposomal or lipid complex amphotericin, 3–5 mg/kg; or (3) caspofungin +/– voriconazole.
Nocardia asteroides	TMP-SMX (15 mg/kg/d TMP; 75 mg/kg/d SMX) plus ceftriaxone, 2 g IV qd × 6 wk, followed by reduced doses of both drugs IV for 6–12 mo	In sulfa-allergic patients: substitute TMP-SMX with amikacin
Rhodococcus equi	Erythromycin, 0.5 g IV q6h, plus imipenem, 0.5 g IV q6h, plus rifampin, 600 mg PO qd for 2 wk, followed by oral clarithromycin or azithromycin plus rifampin for suppression	Alternative agents: ciprofloxacin and linezolid

Table 99.6 Management of Disseminated Infections

Pathogen/Condition	First-Line Treatment	Notes
M. avium complex	Clarithromycin, 500 mg PO BID, or azithromycin, 600 mg qd, plus ethambutol, 15–25 mg/kg/day, plus rifampin, 600 mg PO qd, for a minimum of 12 mo	(1) In patients on efavirenz, azithromycin is preferred over clarithromycin as part of the 3-drug regimen; because efavirenz lowers drug levels of the latter. (2) If patient is taking a protease inhibitor, replace rifampin with rifabutin, 150–300 mg PO qd, because rifampin significantly lowers serum levels of protease inhibitors.
Histoplasma capsulatum	Mild-to-moderate disease: itraconazole, 200 mg PO TID for 3 days, followed by itraconazole, 200 mg BID for 12 wk Severe illness: Amphotericin B deoxycholate, 0.7 mg/kg IV qd; amphotericin liposomal or lipid complex, 3–5 mg/kg, until clinically improved followed by itraconazole, 200 mg for 12 wk	
Penicilliosis	Amphotericin B deoxycholate, 0.6 mg/kg IV qd for 2 wk, followed by itraconazole, 200 mg q12h for 10 wk and then 100 mg PO q12h for suppression	
Bartonellosis	Erythromycin, 500 mg PO q6h for 12 wk minimum and until CD4 count >200 cells/µL	(1) Doxycycline is preferred for CNS involvement. (2) Alternative agents for non-CNS disease: clarithromycin, 500 mg PO BID; azithromycin, 600 mg PO qd; or ciprofloxacin, 500 mg PO BID

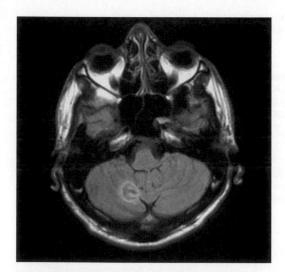

Figure 99.5 Cerebral toxoplasmosis in a 38-year-old HIV-positive man with CD4 count of 55 cells/mL who presented with headache and fever. Magnetic resonance imaging of the brain shows a 1.5 cm × 1.5 cm × 1.6 cm ring-enhancing lesion in the right cerebellar hemisphere.

immunodeficient and immunocompetent HIV-seropositive patients can be affected; however, *progressive outer retinal necrosis* (PORN) is almost exclusively observed in individuals with CD4 ≤50 cells/µL. Other hallmarks of PORN include a temporal association with episodes of dermatomal zoster and multifocal retinal opacities in the absence of ocular inflammation. Intravenous acyclovir for 2–3 weeks followed by oral valacyclovir has been successful in promoting lesion regression and forestalling blindness (Table 99.5).

DISSEMINATED INFECTIONS

Mycobacterium avium Complex

Patients with disseminated MAC present with characteristically high, spiking fevers, progressive weight loss, and sometimes diarrhea. Elevated alkaline phosphatase levels—present in approximately 50% of cases—and enlarged para-aortic lymph nodes are also observed. Treatment consists of clarithromycin (or azithromycin), weight-based ethambutol, and rifabutin (Table 99.6).

Histoplasmosis

Disseminated histoplasmosis is rare but is often more consequential than disseminated MAC. Presentations vary from indolent (progressive fever, weight loss, and pancytopenia) to fulminant. The latter is marked by fever, septic shock, acute respiratory distress syndrome,

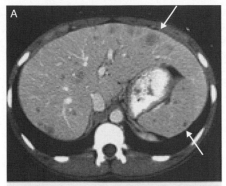

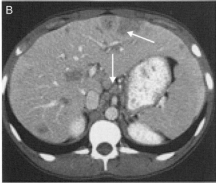

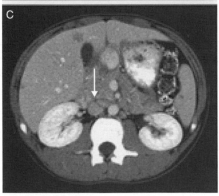

Figure 99.6 *Bartonella henselae* hepatosplenic peliosis. Computed tomography of the abdomen with intravenous contrast reveals multiple low-density lesions with central septations and surrounding halos (*arrows*) in the liver and spleen. An image obtained slightly below the image shown in A (B) shows larger lesions, as well as lymphadenopathy around the celiac axis (*arrows*). An image obtained below the image shown in B (C) shows additional lymphadenopathy in the peripancreatic and periportal regions (*arrow*). Reproduced with permission from Stephen Pelton, MD. Pelton SI, Kim JY, Kradin RL. Case records of the Massachusetts General Hospital. Case 27–2006. Department of Pediatric Infectious Disease, Boston Medical Center, Massachusetts General Hospital and Harvard Medical School, Boston, Massachusetts, USA.

and a high incidence of Addisonian crisis. Treatment includes use of amphotericin B-based chemotherapy followed by chronic suppression with oral itraconazole (Table 99.6).

Penicilliosis

Disseminated *penicillium marneffei*, a dimorphic fungus that converts to a yeast at body temperature, is the third most common HOI among patients residing in southeast Asia after cryptococcal and MTB infection. Patients at highest risk have CD4 counts ≤50 cells/μL. Usual symptoms include fever, weight loss, dry cough, rash (similar to the umbilicated lesions of molluscum), lymphadenopathy, hepatosplenomegaly, and elevated alkaline phosphatase. Blood cultures are positive within 5 to 7 days. Chemotherapy is similar to that of disseminated histoplasmosis (Table 99.6).

Bartonellosis

Patients present with fever, rash, abdominal, and/or bone pain. Risk factors include CD4 count ≤200 cells/μL and prior cat scratches or bites (*B. henselae*) or louse infestation (*B. quintana*). Mucocutaneous manifestations, known as bacillary angiomatosis, are variable in appearance but classically present as enlarging violaceous plaques or nodules that mimic Kaposi sarcoma. Bartonella osteomyelitis, a complication of *B. quintana* infection, is rare and involves the long bones and sometimes underlies cellulitic plaques.

Bartonella henselae infections are uniquely associated with hepatosplenic peliosis, cystic blood-filled, endothelium-lined spaces that appear as focal hypodense lesions on CT (Figure 99.6). Application of Warthin-Starry stain to tissue specimens reveals pleomorphic microorganisms. In the absence of diagnostic tissue samples, confirmation of bartonellosis rests on culture and serology. Blood cultures and subsequent chocolate or heart infusion agar subcultures, however, have to be held for a minimum of 21 days. Prolonged treatment with an oral macrolide is the treatment of choice (Table 99.6).

SUGGESTED READING

U.S. Department of Health and Human Services. Guidelines documents for treating opportunistic infections among HIV-infected adults and adolescents. http://aidsinfo.nih.gov/Guidelines/Guidelinedetail.aspx?Men

ultem=Guidelines&Search=off&Guideline ID=14&classID=4. Accessed January 2007.

Mandell GL, Bennet JE, Dolin R, eds. *Mandell, Douglas, and Bennett's Principles and Practice of Infectious Diseases*. 6th ed. Philadelphia, PA: Elsevier Churchill Livingstone; 2005.

Palella FJ Jr, Delaney KM, Moorman AC, et al. Declining morbidity among patients with advanced human immunodeficiency virus infection. HIV Outpatient Study Investigators. *N Engl J Med*. 1998;338:853–860.

100. Prophylaxis of Opportunistic Infections in HIV Infection

Judith A. Aberg

The use of infection prophylaxis has been a major advance in human immunodeficiency virus (HIV) disease. Even prior to the introduction of potent antiretroviral therapies, the morbidity and mortality rates were decreasing presumably due to recognition of pathogens and use of prophylaxis for opportunistic infections. The Centers for Disease Control and Prevention (CDC) published the 2002 update of the United States Public Health Service/Infectious Diseases Society of America guidelines for opportunistic infection prophylaxis in HIV disease. The major update pertains to the data generated since the 1999 edition regarding the safety of discontinuing both primary and secondary prophylaxis for several opportunistic infections. There are some minor differences with regard to duration of time the CD4 count increases above a set threshold before stopping prophylaxis and the duration of treatment for pathogen-specific diseases, most of which can be attributed to the study designs of the prophylaxis discontinuation trials for that specific pathogen.

Primary prophylaxis is that given before development of an infection. The best known and most effective is trimethoprim–sulfamethoxazole (TMP-SMX) prophylaxis against *Pneumocystis jiroveci* pneumonia, formerly known as *Pneumocytis carinii* (PCP). TMP-SMX is 90% or more effective and is estimated to add a year to survival in late HIV disease. Other prophylaxes that are highly effective (≥70% efficacy) have now become standard of care in HIV disease: prophylaxis against tuberculosis (TB) if there has been exposure or a positive tuberculin skin test and against disseminated *Mycobacterium avium* complex (MAC) infection and toxoplasmosis.

Secondary prophylaxis is that given after acute treatment of an opportunistic infection to prevent or reduce the incidence of relapse. For some difficult-to-treat infections, this is more accurately called *maintenance* or *chronic suppressive therapy*. A common error of clinicians not experienced in HIV is to omit secondary prophylaxis or to not restart prophylaxis should the CD4 count decline to thresholds at which patients would be at risk again. Unfortunately, there are limited data on when to reinitiate secondary prophylaxis, and the guidelines suggest using the same indications as one does for primary prophylaxis. Secondary prophylaxis is optional only if (1) the infection is nonlife-threatening, such as mucocutaneous herpes simplex or *Candida* esophagitis; (2) the patient refuses it; or (3) the patient cannot tolerate any prophylaxis regimen.

An outline of major primary prophylaxis decision points is presented in Table 100.1. Tables 100.2 and 100.3 list major primary and secondary prophylactic drugs and their indications, efficacy status, and dosages. Table 100.4 presents the major toxicities, drug interactions, and status of use in pregnancy.

PNEUMOCYSTIS JIROVECI PNEUMONIA
Primary and Secondary Prophylaxis

Patients with CD4 cells <200/μL or a history of oral candidiasis should be offered prophylaxis for PCP. Persons with a CD4% <14 or a history of an acquired immunodeficiency syndrome (AIDS)-defining illness should also be considered for initiation of PCP prophylaxis. TMP-SMX is the drug of choice. TMP-SMX also is effective prophylaxis for toxoplasma and certain bacterial infections, particularly pneumonia. Dose-limiting toxicity (mainly rash or fever) occurs in 25% of patients taking one double-strength (DS) tablet daily, and in 10% of those taking one DS tablet 3 times weekly. Patients having mild reactions to TMP-SMX may sometimes be treated through the reaction with antihistamines. Patients who have had mild to moderate (nonlife-threatening) reactions to higher dosages of TMP-SMX can be rechallenged with a lower dosage—one single-strength (SS) tablet daily or one DS tablet 3 times per week—after the reaction has resolved; less than 70% will tolerate the lower dosage. Because TMP-SMX is significantly more effective than the alternative PCP prophylaxes, oral desensitization to TMP-SMX may be considered (see Suggested Reading).

Efficacy is approximately equal for dapsone and atovaquone as an alternative PCP prophylaxis agent but is less effective than

Table 100.1 Outline of Major Primary Prophylaxis Decision Points

All patients	TB prophylaxis if indicated (see Table 100.2 and text) Pneumococcal vaccine q5yr Hepatitis A (HAV) vaccine if HAV susceptible Hepatitis B (HBV) vaccine if HBV susceptible PCP prophylaxis if indicated (see indications 2–5 in Table 100.2)
CD4 ≤200	Above plus add: PCP prophylaxis for all patients
CD4 ≤100	Toxoplasma prophylaxis if indicated (see Table 100.2)
CD4 ≤50	MAC prophylaxis Fundoscopic monitoring for CMV

Abbreviations: CD4 = CD4+ T lymphocytes/μL; TB = tuberculosis; PCP = *Pneumocystis jiroveci* pneumonia; MAC = disseminated *Mycobacterium avium* complex; CMV = cytomegalovirus.

that of TMP-SMX. Dapsone (a sulfone used in leprosy treatment) is significantly cheaper than atovaquone. Adverse effects include rash, anemia, methemoglobinemia, agranulocytosis, and hepatic dysfunction. It is tolerated by up to two thirds of those allergic to TMP-SMX. It should be avoided, however, if the patient has had a severe TMP-SMX reaction (exfoliation or erythema multiforme). Ideally, the clinician should test for glucose-6-phosphate dehydrogenase (G6PD) deficiency before dapsone use, although severe hemolysis is uncommon in North American populations. Nevertheless, given the diversity in our populations, G6PD testing is strongly recommended. The value of attempting to increase the efficacy of dapsone by adding a second drug (particularly if breakthrough PCP has occurred) is as yet unproved but may be tried. Second drugs being added to dapsone include atovaquone, pyrimethamine, trimethoprim, or aerosolized pentamidine.

Atovaquone suspension has the advantages of a lack of cross-reactivity with sulfas and dapsone, and efficacy for toxoplasmosis prophylaxis. Disadvantages include the inconvenience of a liquid, gastrointestinal side effects, taste aversion, and high cost.

Aerosolized pentamidine is occasionally used these days in patients who cannot tolerate any of the oral drugs. Its efficacy is similar to that of dapsone and atovaquone but its disadvantages, including expense, inconvenience, lack of prevention of toxoplasmosis or extrapulmonary pneumocystis, and atypical pulmonary manifestations, make this choice less attractive. About half of patients require pretreatment and sometimes posttreatment bronchodilator therapy (eg, inhaled albuterol) to prevent bronchospasm and cough.

Discontinuation of primary PCP prophylaxis may be considered for patients whose CD4+ cell count has risen to >200 cells/μL and remained in that range for ≥3 months. Resumption of prophylaxis is currently recommended when the CD4+ cell count falls to <200 cells/μL.

Discontinuation of secondary prophylaxis once the CD4 cell count has risen to >200 cells/μL on highly active antiretroviral therapy (HAART) has been shown to be safe in multiple studies. Prophylaxis should be reinitiated should the CD4 decline as for primary prophylaxis. In patients who developed PCP at a time with CD4 counts >200 cells/ μL, it is recommended that these patients be considered for PCP prophylaxis for life.

TOXOPLASMA (TOXO)

Primary Prophylaxis

Patients with CD4 cells <100/μL and immunoglobulin G (IgG) toxo antibodies run a one-third risk of developing cerebral toxoplasmosis. Patients who are IgG negative for toxo should be counseled regarding sources of infection, specifically undercooked meats and cat feces. Patients should be advised to change the cat litter box daily and to feed their cat(s) commercial cat food products. About 15% to 30% of HIV-infected persons in North America are toxo seropositive, and all those with CD4 counts <100 cells/μL should be offered toxo prophylaxis. TMP-SMX DS, one tablet daily, has been shown to be effective; the efficacy of TMP-SMX DS 3 times per week or once SS daily is likely. Alternatives to TMP-SMX include (1) dapsone plus pyrimethamine with leucovorin and (2) atovaquone. Although the guidelines recommend that pyrimethamine be added to dapsone, in a head-to-head comparison of dapsone versus aerosolized pentamidine, no cases of toxo were reported in the dapsone arm. Although this study was not powered to determine dapsone's efficacy in preventing toxo, most likely dapsone alone is adequate to prevent disease. Dapsone should be avoided after life-threatening sulfa reactions. If toxo-seropositive patients are receiving aerosolized pentamidine, toxo coverage must be added. It has been shown to be safe to discontinue toxo

Table 100.2 Primary Prophylaxis

Infection	Indication	Efficacy Status	Regimen Drug/Dosage
Pneumocystis jiroveci pneumonia (PCP)	1. CD4 ≤200 µL 2. Thrush 3. Chemotherapy 4. Consider for CD4 percentage ≤14% 5. Consider if prior AIDS-defining illness	Proved—standard of care	Trimethoprim-sulfamethoxazole (TMP-SMX) DS 160/800 mg/d or 3×/wk TMP-SMX SS, 80/400 mg/d
		Proved	Dapsone, 100 mg/d Atovaquone suspension, 1500 mg/d Aerosolized pentamidine, 300 mg q1mo
		Possible	IV pentamidine, 4 mg/kg q2 – 4 wk
Tuberculosis (TB)	1. Positive tuberculin skin test (TST) 2. History of positive PPD without prior prophylaxis 3. Recent exposure to active TB	Proved – standard of care	Isoniazid (INH), 300 mg, with pyridoxine, 50 mg/d for 9 mo (or for directly observed prophylaxis: INH, 900 mg with pyridoxine, 100 mg 2× per wk)
	Alternative for INH intolerance, or exposure to INH-resistant, but rifampin-sensitive, TB	Probable	Rifampin suspension, 600 mg/d for 4 mo
		Unknown	Rifabutin, 300 mg/d for 4 mo
	Alternative for exposure to TB resistant to both INH and rifampin	Unknown	Two- or three-drug regimen for 6 mo: Pyrazinamide (PZA), 1.5 g/d, plus ethambutol, 15–25 mg/kg/d, ± either ofloxacin, 400 mg BID *or* ciprofloxacin, 750 mg BID
Disseminated *Mycobacterium avium complex* (MAC)	CD4 ≤50/µL	Proved – standard of care	Azithromycin, 1200 mg qwk Clarithromycin, 500 mg PO BID
		Proved	Rifabutin, 300 mg/d
Toxoplasma	CD4 ≤100/µL and *Toxoplasma* IgG antibody positive	Proved – standard of care	TMP-SMX DS, 160/800 mg/d
		Probable	TMP-SMX SS, 80/400 mg/d or TMP-SMX DS 3× /wk Dapsone, 50–100 mg/d plus pyrimethamine, 50 mg weekly, with leuckovorin, 25 mg/wk
		Probable	Atovaquone suspension, 1500 mg/d, with or without pyrimethamine, 25 mg/d with leuckovorin, 10 mg/d
Cytomegalovirus (CMV)	CD4 ≤50/µL and CMV IgG antibody positive	All patients	Fundoscopic monitoring
		Unproven – not routinely recommended	Valganciclovir 900 mg BID 2× daily

Abbreviations: CD4 = CD4+ cell count; DS = double-strength; SS = single-strength; AIDS = acquired immunodeficiency syndrome; IV = intravenously; BID = twice a day; PO = orally; IgG = immunoglobulin G.

[a] Do not use rifampin if patient is using a protease inhibitor or nonnucleoside reverse transcriptase inhibitor; substitute a rifabutin-containing regimen, with appropriate rifabutin dosage modification (see footnote to Table 100.4).

Table 100.3 Secondary Prophylaxis = Chronic Maintenance/Suppression

Infection		Efficacy	Drug/Dosage
PCP		Proved	Same as primary
Disseminated *Mycobacterium avium* complex (MAC)		Proved	Continue acute treatment for at least 12 mo until CD4 increase, eg,clarithromycin, 500 mg PO BID, plus ethambutol, 15–25 mg/kg/d, with or without rifabutin, 300 mg/d, or fluoroquinolone
Toxoplasma		Proved	Sulfadiazine, 500 mg q6h, plus pyrimethamine, 50 mg/d, with leucovorin, 10 mg/d (also covers PCP prophylaxis)
		Probable, somewhat less effective	Clindamycin, 300–450 mg QID, *plus* pyrimethamine, 50 mg/d, with leucovorin, 10 mg/d
		Probable	Atovaquone, 750 mg BID-QID, with or without pyrimethamine, 50 mg/d, with leucovorin, 10 mg/d
Herpes simplex	Only if frequent/severe recurrences	Proved	Acyclovir, 400 mg BID, or famciclovir, 500 mg BID
		Probable	Valacyclovir, 500 mg BID
Candida esophagitis	Only if frequent/severe recurrences	Proved	Fluconazole, 100–200 mg/d Voriconazole 200 mg BID
		Probable	Itraconazole oral solution, 200 mg/d; itraconazole capsule, 200–400 mg/d; or ketoconazole, 200–400 mg/d
Cryptococcus		Proved	Fluconazole, 200–400 mg/d
		Proved, but less effective	Itraconazole, 200 mg BID
Cytomegalovirus (CMV)		Proved	Valganciclovir 900 mg qd Ganciclovir IV, 5 mg/kg/d; foscarnet IV, 90–120 mg/kg/d;
		Proved for retinitis	Ganciclovir eye implant intravitreally q6-9 mo with oral ganciclovir, 1–1.5 g TID
		Alternative for retinitis	Cidofovir, 5 mg/kg IV q2wk, with probenecid, 2 g 2 h before dose and 1 g at 2 h and 8 h after the dose. Oral ganciclovir, 1–1.5 g TID no longer recommended
Histoplasma		Proved	Itraconazole capsule, 200 mg BID
Coccidioides		Probable	Fluconazole, 400 mg/d
Salmonella bacteremia	Often—use for at least several months	Probable, drug of choice	Ciprofloxacin, 500 mg BID
		Alternative	Trimethoprim-sulfamethoxazole DS, 160/180 mg PO BID

Abbreviations: PCP = *Pneumocystis jirovecl* pneumonia; DS = double-strength; PO = orally; BID = twice a day; QID = four times a day; IV = intravenously; TID = three times a day.
Note. All drugs are oral unless otherwise stated.
[a] See text for discussion of discontinuation during period of CD4+ cell rebound.

Table 100.4 Major Toxicities, Drug Interactions, and Use in Pregnancy

Antimicrobial Agent	Major Adverse Reactions	Major Drug Interactions: Effect on Drug Activity	Use in Pregnancy[a]
Acyclovir	GI + renal at high dosage		Yes (C)
Atovaquone	Rash, often clearing on treatment, diarrhea	Decreased by rifampin and metoclopramide	No data (C)
Azithromycin	GI upset, rarely hepatitis	See clarithromycin (azithromycin interacts less than clarithromycin)	Yes, preferred over clarithromycin (B)
Cidofovir (given with probenecid)	Major nephrotoxicity; neutropenia, metabolic acidosis, ocular hypotony Probenecid: rash, nausea, fever	Cidofovir: Increased nephrotoxicity with other drugs causing same Probenecid: Increases AZT, ACE inhibitors, acetaminophen, NSAIDs, benzodiazepines, theophylline, and others	Avoid if possible, teratogenic at low dosages in animals (C)
Ciprofloxacin	GI upset, photosensitivity	Increases theophyllin Absorption decreased by antacids, ddI, sucralfate, iron, magnesium, zinc	Arthropathy warnings (C)
Clarithromycin	GI upset, rarely hepatitis	Increases cisapride (potential cardiac arrhythmias), rifabutin (increased uveitis), and carbamazepine	No data, animal teratogen (C)
Clindamycin	GI upset, *Clostridium difficile* colitis, rash in 20% of HIV patients (often can treat through)		Yes (B)
Dapsone	Rash, fever, hepatitis, anemia, especially with G6PD deficiency; methemoglobinemia	Decreased by rifampin and antacid drugs (H$_2$ blockers)	Yes (C)
Ethambutol	GI upset, optic neuritis, elevated uric acid	Decreased by aluminum antacids – give 2 h apart	Yes (B)
Famciclovir	Nausea, headache		Yes, but acyclovir preferred because of greater experience (B)
Fluconazole	GI upset, rash, rarely hepatitis	Decreased by rifampin, increases cisapride (cardiac arrhythmias), rifabutin (uveitis), carbamazepine, phenytoin, sulfonylurea hypoglycemics, warfarin	Avoid if possible: A few cases of fetal abnormalities reported after prolonged use at dosages ≥400 mg/d (C)
Foscarnet	Nephrotoxicity; decreased calcium, potassium, magnesium; nausea, anemia; rarely mucosal ulcers	Increased nephrotoxicity with other drugs causing same; increased hypocalcemia with pentamidine	If absolutely necessary (C)
Ganciclovir	Neutropenia, fatigue, some decrease in renal function	Increased neutropenia with other drugs causing same; increases ddI levels	No (marked embryo toxicity in animals) (C)
INH	Peripheral neuropathy, hepatitis, CNS effects	Increases carbamazepine (and vice versa), disulfiram, phenytoin, absorption decreased by aluminum antacids	Yes (N/A)

(continued)

Table 100.4 *(continued)*

Antimicrobial Agent	Major Adverse Reactions	Major Drug Interactions: Effect on Drug Activity	Use in Pregnancy[a]
Itraconazole	GI upset, rash, rarely hepatitis; occasional hypertension and hyperkalemia with high dosages	Absorption decreased by antacids, ddl, and sucralfate; see fluconazole for other important interactions	Avoid if possible, based on fluconazole data (C)
Ketoconazole Ofloxacin: See *Ciprofloxacin*	Adrenocortical and sex hormone suppression, with high dosages; rarely hepatitis	Absorption decreased by antacids, ddl, and sucralfate; see fluconazole for other interactions	Avoid if possible, based on fluconazole data (C)
Pentamidine, aerosol	Bronchospasm, cough		Yes: no data, but systemic absorption minimal
Pentamidine IV	Hypoglycemia, nephrotoxicity, hypotension, pancreatitis, hypocalcemia	Increased nephrotoxicity with other drugs causing same; increased hypocalcemia with foscarnet	No animal data (C)
Pyrazinamide (PZA)	Hepatitis, elevated uric acid	Decreased markedly by AZT	Avoid if possible: no animal data (C)
Pyrimethamine	GI upset, neutropenia, anemia, hemolysis with G6PD deficiency	Increased bone marrow suppression when used with other antifolates	Yes[c] (C)
Rifabutin	Uveitis, neutropenia, orange urine	Increased by protease inhibitors (PIs), clarithromycin and fluconazole (leading to more uveitis) – reduce dosage with PI[b]; decreased by certain NNRTI – may need to increase dosage[b]; decreases NNRTI delavirdine – avoid concomitant use	Yes (B)
Rifampin	Hepatitis, rash, orange urine	Markedly decreases protease inhibitor, NNRTI, and atovaquone—avoid rifampin, substitute rifabutin; decreases oral azoles, contraceptives, hypoglycemics, dapsone, methadone, phenytoin, warfarin	Yes (C)
Trimethoprim-sulfamethoxazole (TMP-SMX) and sulfadiazine	Nausea, rash, fever, hepatitis, neutropenia, photosensitivity, nephrotoxicity; hemolysis with G6PD deficiency	TMP-SMX increases warfarin	Yes (C)

Abbreviations: GI = Gastrointestinal; ACE = angiotensin-converting enzyme; NSAIDs = nonsteroidal anti-inflammatory drugs; ddl = didanosine; HIV = human immunodeficiency virus; G6PD = glucose-6-phosphate dehydrogenase; CNS = central nervous system; NNRTI = nonnucleoside reverse transcriptase inhibitor (nevirapine, efavirenz, delavirdine); INH = ; AZT = zidovudine.

Key: N/A = Not available (drug approved before requirement for such testing). Yes = Category B; or Category C where there has been sufficient experience to say that if fetal risk exists, it must be very low. If necessary = insufficient experience, but drug is theoretically safer than alternative. No data = insufficient experience; may need to be used if disease is serious.

[a] FDA Pregnancy categories: B = animal studies indicate no fetal risk but there are no human studies, *or* animal studies show fetal risk, but adequate studies in pregnant women have shown no adverse effects, including in the first trimester; C = animal studies demonstrate fetal risk but there are no human trials, *or* neither human nor animal studies are available; D = evidence exists for fetal risk in humans, but benefit may outweigh risk.

[b] Reduce rifabutin dosage to 150 mg/d for use with the protease inhibitors (PIs) amprenavir, indinavir, nelfinavir, or saquinavir; use rifabutin 150 mg qod with the PI ritonavir. Rifabutin dosage is increased to 450 mg/d when used with the NNRTI efavirenz, and possibly also with the NNRTI nevirapine.

[c] Consider deferral of pyrimethamine for primary toxoplasma patients until after pregnancy.

prophylaxis once the CD4 count has risen >200 cells/μL for at least 3 months.

Secondary Prophylaxis

About half of the full treatment dose of sulfadiazine and pyrimethamine with leucovorin is most commonly used, and this regimen also provides PCP prophylaxis. Most non-U.S. countries use TMP-SMX as sulfadiazine is unavailable, and TMP-SMX may be considered as an alternative. For sulfa-intolerant patients, clindamycin at higher dosages plus pyrimethamine with leucovorin is usually effective but does not cover PCP. Atovaquone with or without pyrimethamine and leucovorin may also be used and has the advantage of providing protection against PCP. Patients who have completed a 6-week course of initial therapy, remain asymptomatic, and have had a sustained increase of their CD4 counts >200 cells/μL for at least 6 months on HAART may be considered for discontinuation of secondary prophylaxis. Both primary and secondary prophylaxis should be reinitiated should the CD4 count decline to <200 cells/μL.

FUNGAL INFECTIONS
Primary Prophylaxis

Primary prophylaxis of *Candida* esophagitis and systemic fungal infections is not recommended, despite efficacy, because of the effectiveness of treating acute disease and concerns for drug resistance, drug interactions, lack of survival benefit, and cost. In areas highly endemic for histoplasma or coccidioides, disseminated disease resulting from these soil fungi may account for 25% of opportunistic infections. In such areas, the use of primary prophylaxis may be discussed with patients whose CD4 cell counts are <100 cells/μL. Itraconazole is used for histoplasma, and fluconazole is used for coccidioides.

Secondary Prophylaxis

Candida suppression may be considered if recurrences are very frequent or severe. A large randomized study comparing continuous fluconazole prophylaxis versus episodic treatment for acute candidiasis failed to demonstrate an increased risk of azole resistance. Continuous azole, echinocandin, or amphotericin B prophylaxis should be considered only for those with severe recurrent candidiasis. For cryptococcus suppression, fluconazole is the antifungal of choice. For patients intolerant to fluconazole, itraconazole, 400 mg/day, can be used, although it is less effective. For histoplasma suppression, itraconazole, 200-mg capsule twice daily, is used; for coccidioides suppression, fluconazole, 400 mg/day.

Discontinuation of secondary prophylaxis for cryptococcosis and histoplasmosis has been shown to be safe and effective in patients whose CD4 counts remain >100 to 200 cells/μL for at least 6 months. Prophylaxis should be reinitiated should the CD4 decline to 100 to 200 cells/μL. There are insufficient data to recommend discontinuation of secondary prophylaxis against coccidioidomycosis.

MYCOBACTERIUM AVIUM COMPLEX
Primary Prophylaxis

Disseminated MAC occured in 30% or more of persons with AIDS in the pre-HAART era, almost always when the CD4+ cell count is <50/μL. It causes extreme fever, rigors, drenching night sweats, anemia, and severe wasting. Weekly azithromycin is most commonly used because of the low pill burden and lower likelihood of drug interactions compared with clarithromycin. Clarithromycin is the second choice; rifabutin is generally used only if the azalides cannot be used. It is important to rule out active MAC or TB infection before starting these drugs in symptomatic individuals due to potential for development of macrolide resistance.

Multiple studies have demonstrated that it is safe to discontinue primary prophylaxis when the CD4 count is >100 cells/μL for at least 3 months. There have been reports of atypical localized MAC infections in patients with high CD4 counts so it is important to consider MAC in the differential diagnosis in patients whose nadir CD4 counts were <50 cells/μL. Prophylaxis should be reinitiated should the CD4 count decline to <50 to 100 cells/μL.

Secondary Prophylaxis

Patients should remain on the antimycobacterial regimen that controlled their infection for at least 1 year. There are data to suggest that a 3-drug combination of clarithromycin, ethambutal, and rifabutin may provide a survival benefit in persons not starting HAART. It is safe to discontinue secondary prophylaxis among those who have completed at least 12 months antimycobacterial therapy, are asymptomatic, and have had a CD4 count >100 cells/µL for at least 6 months on HAART. Prophylaxis should be reinitiated should the CD4 count decline to <100 cells/µL.

TUBERCULOSIS

Primary Prophylaxis

There is no other medical condition that so predisposes to the development of active TB as does HIV infection. In tuberculin skin test (TST)-positive patients, the risk of active TB is 5% to 10% per year for HIV-positive patients versus 5% to 10% per lifetime for HIV-negative persons.

Indications for prophylaxis include the following: (1) positive TST ≥5 mm, (2) history of positive TST and never completed prophylaxis, and (3) recent contact with active TB case (social or nosocomial) (note: prophylaxis must be given after any significant exposure, even if patient has previously received TB prophylaxis, because TB reinfection can occur).

Nine months of isoniazid (INH) with pyridoxine to prevent peripheral neuropathy is the treatment of choice. Alternatives include 4 months of either rifabutin or rifampin. Two months of two drugs (rifampin or rifabutin plus pyrazinamide) is not recommended because of potential hepatotoxicity. Rifampin cannot be used with protease inhibitors; the rifabutin dosage must be altered with these drugs. Clinicians should consider repeating the TST in individuals whose TST was negative and now have increased CD4 count >200 cells/µL.

It is critical to rule out active TB before starting prophylaxis. Chest radiographs are sufficient for asymptomatic patients. If chest x-ray results show parenchymal infiltrate, intrathoracic nodes, or fibrotic scarring, three sputum cultures should be obtained. If there is no other explanation for infiltrate, the clinician should start the patient on full 4-drug treatment for TB. After 2 months of treatment, if cultures are negative and chest radiographic findings are unchanged, the drugs may be discontinued. If the patient has received rifampin (or rifabutin) plus pyrazinamide for 2 months, the patient will have completed the short-course prophylaxis regimen and needs no further prophylaxis.

Secondary Prophylaxis

After a full course of therapy for TB, no chronic suppressive therapy is needed. Treatment of TB in HIV patients results in very high cure rates *if* the organism is drug sensitive and the patient compliant. However, when TB treatment is suboptimal, relapse rates are significantly higher in HIV than non-HIV patients. Therefore, it is critical that all HIV-infected persons receive directly observed therapy for TB.

VARICELLA-ZOSTER

No prophylaxis has been shown effective for zoster. For varicella-zoster virus (VZV), susceptible persons (those who have not had chickenpox or shingles or who lack VZV antibodies) should receive VZV immunoglobulin (VZIG) within 4 days after close contact with a person who has chickenpox or shingles. There are no data on the use of acyclovir for prevention of VZV after exposure in HIV-infected persons. Although the VZV vaccine has been shown to be effective in preventing shingles in an elderly population, it is not recommended to vaccinate HIV-infected adults with VZV given it is a live vaccine and its safety/effectiveness are unknown.

HERPES SIMPLEX VIRUS

Primary Prophylaxis

HIV-infected persons should use condoms during every sexual contact to reduce the risk of acquiring sexually transmitted infections including herpes simplex virus (HSV). Primary prophylaxis is not recommended.

Secondary Prophylaxis

The options for secondary prophylaxis are suppression versus retreating each episode. Acyclovir is preferable because of its relatively low cost. Famciclovir and valacyclovir offer no dosing advantage in the usual twice-daily prophylaxis regimens. Valacyclovir at very high dosages in a trial of cytomegalovirus (CMV) prophylaxis was associated with an unexplained trend to increased mortality and thrombotic thrombocytopenic purpura. Intravenous foscarnet or cidofovir may be used for acyclovir-resistant HSV infections.

CYTOMEGALOVIRUS

Primary Prophylaxis

CMV disease, mainly retinitis and gastrointestinal, is diagnosed in about 10% to 25% of

AIDS patients, almost always when the CD4+ cell count is <50/μL. Those with CMV IgG antibodies are at risk. Prophylaxis with oral ganciclovir or valganciclovir is not routinely recommended for several reasons, including conflicting reports of efficacy, drug toxicity, pill burden, and cost. Patients should receive fundoscopic monitoring when CD4 counts are ≤50 cells/μL. CMV IgG-negative persons should receive CMV-negative or leukocyte-poor blood products.

Secondary Prophylaxis

Anti-CMV drugs can reduce the progression of CMV retinitis, although they will not reverse damage already done to the retina. Ganciclovir (GCV) implants with oral valganciclovir are now the first line of therapy for CMV retinitis. Valganciclovir has better oral bioavailability than oral GCV and has largely replaced intravenous GCV. For intravenous GCV, maintenance dosages of up to 7.5 mg/kg/day, or 5 to 7.5 mg/kg every 12 hours, have been used and may require granulocyte colony-stimulating factor support. With foscarnet, single daily maintenance doses of >120 mg/kg/day cannot be used, but the induction doses of 90 mg/kg every 12 hours can be maintained if tolerated. The combination of GCV and foscarnet is synergistic and recommended for neurologic disease. Dosages of both these drugs must be altered if renal function is abnormal. In other forms of CMV disease, such as gastrointestinal, "CMV wasting syndrome" (viremia, fever, and weight loss), hepatitis, and pneumonia, some clinicians discontinue suppression if there has been a good response to acute treatment because apparent spontaneous remissions may occur. Cidofovir is less often used because of nephrotoxicity.

Discontinuation of secondary prophylaxis (chronic suppression) for CMV retinitis is safe to consider when the CD4 cell count is >100 to 150/μL for longer than 6 months and there was a nonsight-threatening lesion, there is adequate vision in the other eye, and the patient is able to undergo regular ophthalmologic examinations. All patients discontinuing prophylaxis should have regular fundoscopic monitoring to detect early recurrence and immune reconstitution uveitis. Reinitiation of prophylaxis should be started when the CD4 declines to <100 to 150 cells/μL.

BACTERIAL INFECTIONS
Primary and Secondary Prophylaxis

The administration of pneumococcal vaccine is recommended. Revaccination every 5 years is currently suggested. Because vaccine efficacy is less when CD4 cells are low, revaccination may be given to patients initially vaccinated when CD4 cells were <200/μL who are now experiencing a CD4 count >200 cells/μL. Some experts recommend waiting until CD4 count is >200 cells/μL to vaccinate. Although the use of TMP-SMX (for PCP prophylaxis) and azithromycin or clarithromycin (for MAC prophylaxis) may reduce bacterial respiratory infections, they are not used solely for such purposes because of concerns about drug resistance. HIV-infected persons with *Salmonella* infection may require long-term therapy with a fluoroquinolone; however, the duration of prophylaxis is unknown, and decisions are individually based.

SUGGESTED READING

Aberg JA, Gallant JE, Anderson J, et al. Primary Care Guidelines for the Management of Persons Infected with Human Immunodeficiency Virus: Recommendations of the HIV Medicine Association of the Infectious Disease Society of America. *Clin Infect Dis.* 2004;39:609–629.

Centers for Disease Control and Prevention. 2002 USPHS/IDSA guidelines for the prevention of opportunistic infections in persons infected with human immunodeficiency virus: U.S. Public Health Service (USPHS) and Infectious Diseases Society of America (IDSA). *Morb Mortal Weekly Rep.* 2002;51(RR-8). http://www.cdc.gov/mmwr/preview/mmwrhtml/rr5108a1.htm. 2002;51(RR08):1–46. Treating opportunistic infections among HIV-exposed and infected children: recommendations from CDC, the National Institutes of Health, and the Infectious D iseases Society of America. *MMWR Recomm Rep.* 2004;53(RR-15):1–112. Erratum in: *Morb Mortal Weekly Rep.* 2005;54(12):311.

Primary care guidelines for the management of persons infected with human immunodeficiency virus: recommendations of the HIV Medicine Association of the Infectious Disease Society of America. *Clin Infect Dis.* 2004;39:609–629.

PART XIII

Nosocomial Infection

101. Prevention of Nosocomial Infection in Staff and Patients

Nimalie D. Stone and John E. McGowan, Jr.

Healthcare-associated infections (HAIs), also known as nosocomial infections, are those infections acquired in the hospital or other health care facility (HCF). They affect more than 2 million patients annually (Table 101.1). Adverse consequences of these infections are formidable, resulting in an estimated 900 000 deaths and an overall cost of about $4.5 billion annually in the United States. Since the 1999 report from the Institute of Medicine, *To Err Is Human: Building a Safer Health System,* reports from several other groups have led to heightened attention to the development of safer health care environments. Leading regulatory, accreditation, and quality-monitoring organizations, including the Joint Commission on Accreditation of Healthcare Organizations (JCAHO), have targeted some HAIs as preventable adverse events and an issue of patient safety. Increased public awareness of the cost and seriousness of HAIs has led to the promotion of public disclosure of HAI rates and motivated several states to develop legislation mandating disclosure of HAIs by hospitals and other health care organizations.

To address the growing concerns, cost, and adverse impact of these infections, HCFs must focus on minimizing the risk of acquiring HAIs within the health care environment. Preventive efforts are especially important in the integrated health care systems that characterize many areas of the United States. In January of 2005, the Institute for Healthcare Improvement (IHI) launched the 100 000 Lives Campaign to target preventable health care-associated errors and deaths. Three of the six interventions in this campaign focused on HAIs (central line infections, surgical site infections, and ventilator-associated pneumonias). Several professional and governmental organizations have provided guidelines to minimize these infections, and groups of interventions ("bundles") that can be implemented to minimize these and other HAI. This chapter describes strategies and resources to decrease such infections.

The main focus of efforts to minimize these infections are early recognition and description of the pattern of infection in the HCF, analysis

Table 101.1 Impact of Healthcare-associated Infections[a]

	Year	
	1975	**1995**
Hospital admissions	38 000 000	36 000 000
Hospital patient days	299 000 000	190 000 000
Average length of stay	7.9 days	5.3 days
Nosocomial infections	2 100 000	1 900 000

[a] Adapted from Weinstein RW, *Emerging Infect Dis.* 1998;4:416.

of the epidemiologic features, and action to control and prevent these infections by interventions targeted to the epidemiologic features. Attention must be directed to all aspects of care provided by the integrated health care system. This requires strategies for preventing infection in acute care hospitals, extended care facilities, and ambulatory care settings such as same-day surgery and home care settings.

Spread of infection within an HCF traditionally requires three elements: a source of infecting organisms, a susceptible host, and a mode of transmission. These factors interact with each other. For example, the classic way a patient and organism meet is by exogenous transfer; here, the infected person acquires organisms in the HCF. After transfer of an organism, the likelihood that it will cause HAI is determined in part by the potential victim's ability to resist infection. This in turn is influenced by pre-existing illness, such as diabetes or acquired immunodeficiency syndrome (AIDS); treatments, such as corticosteroids; and use of instruments and procedures (eg, catheters and surgery). These factors all are more prominent in today's HCF than ever before. As a result, resistance of the patient may be reduced to such a degree that infection can develop from organisms of the patient's own flora, and transfer from an exogenous source no longer is required. Even so, transfers from other persons or the hospital environment remain the most important current sources of infecting organisms in the HCF setting.

When exogenous HAI occurs, pathogens are transmitted by several routes, and the same organism may be spread by more than one of these pathways. The most important today is contact transmission by a direct exchange between the body surfaces of an infected or colonized person (the source) to the body surface of one who is not (for example, from the hands of a health care worker, patient, visitor, or volunteer to the skin or wound of a patient). Contact transmission through indirect transfer occurs via an intermediate object (eg, food, water, medication, instrument, dressing, glove). Less common is spread by airborne transmission of infecting organisms in droplets, droplet nuclei, or dust. Transmission by vectors such as mosquitoes, flies, rats, and other vermin is significant in some parts of the world but virtually absent in the United States.

Knowing the infecting organism, the likely victim (patient, health care worker, volunteer, visitor), the source (reservoir) of the organism, and the mode of transmission is essential to design of control measures. These efforts focus on eliminating the organism, removing the reservoir, blocking spread from reservoir to victim, or strengthening the potential victim against the organism's weapons. A study by the Centers for Disease Control and Prevention (CDC) in 1983 suggested that only about 9% were being prevented. More recently it has been estimated that 20% to 30% of all HAIs are preventable with available techniques.

Minimizing HAIs depends on two crucial activities: (1) recognizing and analyzing new problems as they arise so that appropriate control measures can be instituted and (2) maintaining continuous attention to a series of measures that have been proved to minimize the occurrence of endemic infections. Each is considered in turn.

NEW AND CONTINUING PROBLEMS

Addressing a new HAI in an HCF, whether epidemic or endemic, requires several steps (Table 101.2). Perhaps the most important phase in the investigation is the initial step, realizing that a problem exists and defining its features. Epidemics are rare today, so in most HCFs a rise in endemic infection will be the problem. Often the patient's physician or the laboratory may provide the first report of a problem. Regular monitoring of HAIs within an HCF can provide a baseline rate, deviations

Table 101.2 Steps in Investigation of a Health Care Institution Outbreak

Recognize the problem (surveillance, early warning from patient's physician)   Case definition

Complete case finding
    Reliability of reporting (search database for other
        cases; review lab methods)
    Completeness of reporting
    Obtain additional data

Define occurrence
Characterize the outbreak (demography, location, time)
Form hypotheses about causes (mode of acquisition, reservoirs, vectors)
Initiate control activities, with procedural changes as required
Do follow-up surveillance to make sure control measures work
Adapted in part from McGowan JE Jr, Metchock B. Infection control epidemiology and clinical microbiology. In: Murray PR, Baron EJ, Pfaller MA, et al., eds. *Manual of Clinical Microbiology.* 7th ed. Washington, DC: American Society for Microbiology; 1999:107–115.

from which can alert providers to a new problem. On occasion, infection control personnel may become aware of the problem through their contact with, and surveillance of, clinical services, follow-up clinics, or associated extended care facilities, or through another HCF in the region. That initial recognition should lead to careful description of the problem under consideration. Even a rough case definition will allow initial control measures to be taken and enable all persons involved to agree on the nature of the problem.

Once a definition has been made, attempts to identify all possible cases begin. This effort at complete case finding is crucial because the more cases that are available for analysis, the better the chance of determining the process involved. Case finding has three major aspects. The first activity is ascertaining the reliability of clinical and laboratory information. For example, can a case of the entity under investigation be identified by its clinical characteristics? Are laboratory methods and facilities available to make the diagnosis? Next, the completeness of reporting must be considered. Most HAIs manifest themselves while the afflicted patient is still in the HCF, but some appear only after the patient has been discharged. For example, in today's world of rapid discharge from acute care facilities, more than half of all surgical wound infections become manifest after the patient has left the hospital. Other infections may involve a clinical setting where microbiologic testing is rarely employed. Thus, laboratory results cannot be used as the sole basis for surveillance, and this is likely to remain true as integrated health care systems continue to evolve. A caution is appropriate: Infections with onset during HCF stay sometimes have been acquired in the community and have been incubating since HCF admission. Thus, not all infections with onset during HCF stay are health care associated.

When as many cases as possible have been identified, whether this episode is an important deviation from usual occurrence can be considered. Certain situations or types of infection are so dramatic or uncommon that even a single case may be recognized as a problem requiring immediate attention; for example, the first emergence of a pan-drug–resistant organism in a facility (eg, an XDR strain of *M. tuberculosis*). However, in some situations the cost to deal with some infection problems may be higher than the gain from eliminating the problem. Assuming the decision is made to continue the evaluation, the next step is framing the problem in terms of its location, time course, persons involved, common procedures and instruments employed, and other features. Confirming the identity of the responsible organism often is important in this characterization.

Forming postulates about the reasons for the outbreak, defining the reservoir of the organisms, and identifying the mode of acquisition by the victim (eg, patient, health care worker, visitor) comes next. These features usually point to specific control measures to halt the progress of the problem. Usually several control measures will be considered, so it is appropriate to decide which factor or factors will be most practical to alter. When one or more actions are taken, follow-up data must be collected to make sure the control measures achieved the desired effect.

SPECIFIC MEASURES AND PROGRAMS

Infection control faces many challenges today. Increasing populations of immunocompromised patients and the growing presence of antimicrobial-resistant bacteria are prominent features of HAI. To combat these changes, infection control requires a structured management process staffed by dedicated personnel to influence behavior of doctors, nurses, and other health care workers. This is similar to quality control in industry, and infection control in HCFs is one of the best examples of quality management in action. A consensus panel report recommended three principal goals for infection control programs in health care institutions. These are as follows: (1) protect the patient; (2) protect the health care worker, visitors, and others in the health care environment; and (3) accomplish the previous two goals in a cost-effective manner, whenever possible. These goals are relevant to patient care activities in any health care setting, including acute care hospitals, skilled nursing facilities, long-term care facilities, rehabilitation units, urgent care centers, same-day surgery facilities, ambulatory care centers, and home care programs. The success or failure of the infection control program is defined by its effectiveness in achieving these goals.

To deal with endemic HAIs, the HCF must have a defined intervention system with clear goals for changing behavior and practice and for maintaining these improvements. Both *direct* actions to change behavior (eg, choosing a handwashing agent that minimizes skin drying) and *indirect* methods (eg, education to tell why handwashing is important) are essential. Because it is not clear how to deal with most patient and organism factors, the major focus must be on HAIs that are preventable. Thus, major attention is given to proper patient care practices aimed at reducing microbial reservoirs and limiting spread of organisms from person to person (Table 101.3). The CDC, through its Hospital Infection Control Practices Advisory Committee (HICPAC), has published several *Infection Control Guidelines* dividing between those which protect the patient and those which protect the health care worker. Recent examples include (1) *Guideline for Hand Hygiene in Health Care Settings*, (2) *Guideline for Environmental Infection Control in Health Care Facilities*, (3) *Guideline for Prevention of Intravascular Device-Related Infections*, (4) *Guideline for Prevention of Health Care-Associated Pneumonia*, and (5) *Guideline for Influenza Vaccination of Health Care Personnel*. These and others are available on the HICPAC Web site (see Suggested Reading). In addition, the CDC, independent of HICPAC, has produced other recommendations such as those for management of multidrug-resistant organisms in health care settings, prevention and control of specific infections such as mumps and viral hemorrhagic fevers in health care settings, and guidance on public reporting of health care–associated infections. These and

Table 101.3 Patient Care Practices to Reduce Healthcare-associated Infection in Patients and Health Care Workers

Hand hygiene

Barrier precautions (isolation)
    Standard precautions (universal precautions, body
      substance isolation)
    Transmission-based precautions (airborne, droplet,
      contact)

Control and prevention of device- and procedure-related
infections in patients
    Surgery (asepsis, perioperative antimicrobial
      prophylaxis)
    Disinfection and sterilization of supplies and
      equipment
    Closed drainage systems for indwelling urinary
      catheters
    Intravascular catheters and their delivery systems
      (eg, bottles, tubings)
    Ventilators, nebulizers, other respiratory therapy
      equipment

Immunization
    Patients and potential patients (eg, pneumococcal
      vaccine)
    Health care workers (eg, hepatitis B vaccine)

others are available on the CDC Web site (see Suggested Reading).

Hand hygiene addresses the most frequent mode of spread of many health care–associated pathogens, carriage on the hands of health care workers. Most of the microorganisms that cause hospital infections are present only transiently on the hands and are easily removed by a brief handwashing. Although simple, handwashing before and after each patient contact is time-consuming and often not performed. Therefore, in the current CDC guidelines, alcohol-based hand rubs are recommended as an effective alternative to soap and water. They significantly reduce the number of bacterial organisms on the hands, act quickly, and are less irritating than repetitive washes with soap and water. Dispensers for these agents can be placed in every patient room and in common areas around a hospital unit to facilitate their use by patients, health care workers, and visitors.

Barrier precautions (isolation) are intended to prevent organisms present on one patient from reaching another. Published guidelines by the CDC for isolation in hospitals are based on two levels of performance. First are standard precautions, designed for care of all patients in the hospital regardless of diagnosis or whether they are thought to have an infection. This includes universal blood and body fluid precautions and procedures to reduce risk of transmission of pathogens from moist body substances. Second-level, transmission-based precautions are used for patients documented or suspected to be infected or colonized with highly transmissible or epidemiologically difficult pathogens. This latter group contains measures that vary according to the way the target organism spreads: airborne, droplet, or contact. Of particular use are lists of specific clinical syndromes that are highly suspicious for infection, with the appropriate transmission-based empiric precautions for each, until a diagnosis can be made.

Control of device- and procedure-related infections is a major focus because the four most frequent types of HAI—urinary tract infections, surgical site infections, bloodstream infections, and pneumonia—all are closely associated with procedures and instruments. Several guidelines, bundles, and critical pathways have been developed to minimize infections associated with them. Among the most important are those for surgery. Avoiding long preoperative hospital stays, preoperative treatment of active infections, appropriate hair removal (avoidance of shaving) at the operative site, limitation of traffic in the operating room, proper airflow in the operating room, appropriate time and selection of perioperative antimicrobials, and maintenance of perioperative normothermia and glucose control can all help reduce infections. The most important determinant of infection risk after surgery is the technical skill of the surgeon and operative team. Length of surgery, amount of trauma to tissues, degree of contamination of surgical fields, and several other factors contribute to the likelihood of postoperative infection. It is perhaps for this reason that feeding individual infection rates back to surgeons has been found to lead to decreased rates of surgical wound infection.

Invasive devices penetrate anatomic barriers of the patient. The physician must be especially careful in the use of urinary catheters, intravascular devices, and ventilators, as these invasive devices are key risk factors for urinary tract, bloodstream, and respiratory infections that arise in an HCF. Fortunately, guidelines and critical pathways for proper use have been developed for each of these devices, and infection control plans for most HCFs include measures to ensure proper implementation. Individual physicians contribute best to reducing the infection risk from these devices by considering and reconsidering whether the devices are needed for their patients. "When in doubt, leave it out" is still a good philosophy when it comes to using these implements, as their use carries an increased risk of infection in all cases.

A final way to minimize infections in HCFs is strengthening those in the institution against infection. For patients, proper nutrition, control of underlying diseases that predispose to infection, and proper immunization are all important elements. For example, the rise of strains of *Streptococcus pneumoniae* that are resistant to penicillin and, in some cases, to the newer cephalosporins make treatment of infections due to this organism much more difficult. This means that the role of immunization against this organism must be advanced for adults. Likewise, immunization against hepatitis B virus is crucial for protection of the health care worker, and immunization against viral agents that may be transmitted in the HCF, such as influenza virus, should be promoted as well.

MAINTAINING CONTROL MEASURES

Design and implementation of infection control practices is important but perhaps easier than maintaining these practices after they are introduced. As control of HAIs is linked to patient safety initiatives, more focus and newer ideas for promoting these practices are being developed. For example, the IHI 100 000 Lives Campaign developed a group of interventions, compiled together into a bundle, to address specific HAIs like ventilator-associated pneumonia or central-line associated bloodstream infection. Implementation of all the components in the bundle maximally reduces the risk of an infection. This kind of packaged and evidence-based approach helps caregivers insure that they are carrying out all the necessary measures to prevent HAI. Such approaches are strongly encouraged by third-party payers and regulators. For practicing physicians, enthusiasm for these strategies can be easily generated by remembering that each control measure is a proven way to avoid an HAI and provide the best care for their patients.

SUGGESTED READING

Centers for Disease Control and Prevention. The CDC Infection Control Guidelines. CDC Web site: http://www.cdc.gov/ncidod/dhqp/guidelines. htm.html. Accessed November 26, 2007.

Coffin SE, Zaoutis TE. Infection control, hospital epidemiology, and patient safety. *Infect Dis Clinics N Am*. 2005;19:647–665.

Gastmeier P, Stamm-Balderjahn S, Hansen S, et al. How outbreaks can contribute to prevention of nosocomial infection: analysis of 1,022 outbreaks. *Infect Control Hosp Epidemiol*. 2005;26:357–361.

Healthcare Infection Control Practices Advisory Committee (HICPAC). CDC Web site. http://www.cdc.gov/ncidod/dhqp/hicpac_charter. html. Accessed November 26, 2007.

Kohn L, Corrigan J, Donaldson M. *To Err Is Human: Building a Safer Health System*. Institute of Medicine report. Washington, DC: National Academy Press; 1999.

Lautenbach E, Woeltje K, eds. *Practical Handbook for Healthcare Epidemiologists*. 2nd ed. Thorofare, NJ: Slack; 2004.

Mayhall CG, ed. *Hospital Epidemiology and Infection Control*. 3rd ed. Philadelphia, PA: Lippincott, Williams & Wilkins; 2004.

Scheckler WE, Brimhall D, Buck AS, et al. Requirements for infrastructure and essential activities of infection control and epidemiology in hospitals: a consensus panel report. *Infect Control Hosp Epidemiol*. 1998;19:114–124.

Weinstein RA. Nosocomial infection update. *Emerg Infect Dis*. 1998;4:416–420.

Wenzel RP, ed. *Prevention and Control of Nosocomial Infections*. 4th ed. Philadelphia, PA: Lippincott Williams & Wilkins; 2003.

102. Percutaneous Injury: Risks and Management

Elise M. Beltrami and Denise M. Cardo

Health care personnel (HCP) are at increased risk of occupational exposure to bloodborne pathogens such as hepatitis B virus (HBV), hepatitis C virus (HCV), and the human immunodeficiency virus (HIV) from needlesticks and injuries from other sharp objects. Risk factors for transmission of bloodborne pathogens as a result of occupational exposure are likely related to the source patient (eg, titer of virus in his/her blood or body fluid), the injury (eg, quantity of blood or body fluid transferred during the exposure), and the recipient individual (eg, immunologic status).

Percutaneous exposures are the most common mechanism for transmission of bloodborne pathogens. It has been estimated that hospital-based HCP in the United States sustain an average of 384 325 (range: 311 091 to 463 922) percutaneous injuries annually. Data from several surveillance systems have demonstrated that the majority of reported injuries occur in the acute care setting, particularly medical floors, operating rooms, and intensive care units.

Prevention of contact with blood, percutaneous injuries, and the occupational transmission of bloodborne pathogens requires a diversified approach, including the development of improved engineering controls (eg, safer medical devices), work practices (eg, technique changes to reduce handling of sharp objects), and infection control measures, including personal protective equipment. Another important strategy to prevent infection includes HBV immunization.

Although preventing exposures is the primary means of preventing bloodborne pathogen infection, appropriate postexposure management is an important element of workplace safety. Health care organizations should have a system that includes written protocols for prompt confidential reporting, evaluation, counseling, treatment, and follow-up of any occupational exposures that may place HCP at risk for acquiring bloodborne infection. Each incident of occupational exposure to blood or body fluid that may contain HBV, HCV, or HIV should be evaluated as rapidly as possible and should include the testing of the blood of the source patient for the appropriate bloodborne pathogens, testing of the exposed person for prior infection, and prompt administration of prophylactic agents when indicated.

EVALUATION OF THE EXPOSURE AND THE EXPOSURE SOURCE

Wounds should be washed with soap and water. There is no evidence that the use of antiseptics for wound care or expressing fluid by squeezing the wound further reduces the risk of bloodborne pathogen transmission. However, the use of antiseptics is not contraindicated. The exposure should be evaluated for potential to transmit HBV, HCV, and HIV based on the type of body substance involved and the route and severity of the exposure. Blood, fluid containing visible blood, or other potentially infectious fluid (including semen; vaginal secretions; and cerebrospinal, synovial, pleural, peritoneal, pericardial, and amniotic fluids) or tissue can be infectious for bloodborne viruses.

The person whose blood or body fluid is the source of a percutaneous injury should be evaluated for HBV, HCV, and HIV infection. Information available in the medical record at the time of exposure (eg, laboratory test results, admitting diagnosis, or past medical history) or from the source individual may confirm or exclude possible bloodborne virus infection. If the HBV, HCV, and/or HIV infection status of the source is unknown, the source person should be informed of the incident and tested for serologic evidence of bloodborne virus infection as soon as possible. Procedures should be followed for testing source persons, including obtaining informed consent, in accordance with applicable state and local laws. Confidentiality of the source person should be maintained at all times. If the exposure source is unknown or cannot be tested, decisions about postexposure management should be made on a case-by-case basis, after considering the type of exposure and the clinical and/or epidemiologic likelihood of transmission of HBV, HCV, or HIV.

BLOODBORNE PATHOGENS

Hepatitis B Virus Infection

HBV infection is a well-recognized occupational risk for HCP. The risk of HBV infection is primarily related to the degree of contact with blood and also to the hepatitis B e antigen (HBeAg) status of the source patient. In studies of HCP who sustained injuries from needles contaminated with blood containing HBV, the risk of developing clinical hepatitis if the blood was both hepatitis B surface antigen (HBsAg) and HBeAg positive was 22% to 31%, and the risk of developing serologic evidence of HBV infection, 37% to 62%. By comparison, the risk of developing clinical hepatitis from a needle contaminated with HBsAg-positive, HBeAg-negative blood was 1% to 6%, and the risk of developing serologic evidence of HBV infection, 23% to 37%.

Any person who performs tasks involving contact with blood, blood-contaminated body fluids, other body fluids, or sharp objects should be vaccinated against HBV. Prevaccination serologic screening for previous infection is not indicated for persons being vaccinated because of occupational risk unless the hospital or health care organization considers screening cost-effective. Hepatitis B vaccine can be administered at the same time as other vaccines with no interference with antibody response to the other vaccines. If the vaccination series of three doses, recommended to be given at time zero, 1 month, and 6 months, is interrupted after the first dose, the second dose should be administered as soon as possible. The second and third doses should be separated by an interval of at least 2 months. If only the third dose is delayed, it should be administered when convenient. HCP who have contact with patients or blood and are at ongoing risk for percutaneous injuries should be tested 1 to 2 months after completion of the three-dose vaccination series for anti-HBs. Persons who do not respond to the primary vaccine series (ie, serum anti-HBs ≤10 mIU/mL) should complete a second three-dose vaccine series or be evaluated to determine if they are HBsAg positive. Revaccinated persons should be retested at the completion of the second vaccine series. Primary nonresponders to vaccination who are HBsAg negative should be considered susceptible to HBV infection and should be counseled regarding the need to obtain hepatitis B immunoglobulin (HBIG) prophylaxis for any known or probable parenteral exposure to HBsAg-positive blood (Table 102.1). Booster doses of hepatitis B vaccine are not necessary, and periodic serologic testing to monitor antibody concentrations after completion of the vaccine series is not recommended. Any blood or body fluid exposure of an unvaccinated susceptible person should lead to initiation of the hepatitis B vaccine series.

For percutaneous exposures to HBV-infected blood, the decision to provide prophylaxis must take into account several factors, including the HBsAg status of the source and the hepatitis B vaccination and vaccine-response status of the exposed person. The hepatitis B vaccination status and the vaccine-response status (if known) of the exposed person should be reviewed. Table 102.1 summarizes prophylaxis recommendations for percutaneous or mucosal exposure to blood according to the HBsAg status of the exposure source and the vaccination and vaccine-response status of the exposed person. When HBIG is indicated, it should be administered as soon as possible after exposure (preferably within 24 hours). The effectiveness of HBIG when administered >7 days after exposure is unknown. Hepatitis B vaccine, when indicated, should also be given as soon as possible (preferably within 24 hours) and can be given simultaneously with HBIG. If hepatitis B vaccine is given simultaneously with HBIG, it should be administered intramuscularly at a separate site (vaccine should always be given in the deltoid muscle). For exposed persons who are in the process of being vaccinated, but have not completed the vaccination series, vaccination should be completed as scheduled and HBIG added as indicated in Table 102.1. Persons exposed to HBsAg-positive blood or body fluids who are known not to have responded to the primary vaccine series and have not completed a second three-dose vaccine series should receive a single dose of HBIG and the first dose of the hepatitis B vaccine as soon as possible after exposure. For those who previously completed a second vaccine series but failed to respond, two doses of HBIG should be given, one as soon as possible after exposure and the second 1 month later. HBV testing should be performed on any exposed person who has an illness compatible with hepatitis.

Hepatitis C Virus Infection

HCV is not transmitted efficiently through occupational exposures to blood. The average

Table 102.1 Recommended Postexposure Prophylaxis for Percutaneous or Permucosal Exposure to Hepatitis B Virus (HBV), United States

Vaccination and Antibody Response Status of Exposed Worker[a]	Treatment When Source is Found to be:		
	HBsAg[b] Positive	HBsAg Negative	Source Unknown or not Available for Testing
Unvaccinated	HBIG[c] × 1; and initiate HB vaccine series[d]	Initiate HB vaccine series	Initiate HB vaccine series
Previously Vaccinated			
Known responder[e]	No treatment	No treatment	No treatment
Known nonresponder[e]	HBIG × 1 and initiate revaccination or HBIG × 2[f]	No treatment	If known high risk source, treat as if source were HBsAg positive
Antibody response unknown	Test exposed person for anti-HBs[g] 1. If adequate,[e] no treatment 2. If inadequate,[e] HBIG × 1 and vaccine booster	No treatment	Test exposed for anti-HBs: 1. If adequate, no treatment 2. If inadequate, vaccine booster and recheck titer in 1–2 months

[a] Persons who have previously been infected with HBV are immune to reinfection and do not require postexposure prophylaxis.
[b] Hepatitis B surface antigen.
[c] Hepatitis B immunoglobulin; dose 0.06 mL/kg intramuscularly.
[d] Hepatitis B vaccine series. Healthcare personnel should be tested 1–2 months after completion of the vaccination series for anti-HBs.
[e] A responder is a person with adequate levels of serum antibody to HBsAg (ie, anti-HBs ≥10 mIU/mL); a nonresponder is a person with inadequate response to vaccination (ie, serum anti-HBS ≤10 mIU/mL).
[f] The option of giving one dose of HBIG and reinitiating the vaccine series is preferred for nonresponders who have not completed a second three-dose vaccine series. For those who previously completed a second vaccine series but failed to respond, two doses of HBIG are preferred.
[g] Antibody to HBsAg.

incidence of anti-HCV seroconversion after accidental percutaneous exposure from an HCV-positive source is 1.8% (range, 0% to 7%). The risk for transmission after exposure to fluids or tissues other than HCV-infected blood has not been quantified but is thought to be low.

Health care professionals who provide care to persons exposed to HCV in the occupational setting should be knowledgeable regarding the risk for HCV infection and appropriate counseling, testing, and medical follow-up. For the person exposed to an HCV-positive source, testing for anti-HCV and alanine aminotransferase (ALT) activity should be performed at baseline, and follow-up testing for anti-HCV and ALT activity should be performed at 4 to 6 months (testing for HCV RNA may be performed at 4 to 6 weeks if earlier diagnosis of HCV infection is desired). Immunoglobulin and antiviral agents are not recommended for postexposure prophylaxis (PEP) after exposure to HCV-contaminated blood.

No guidelines exist for administration of therapy during the acute phase of HCV infection. One strategy that has been advocated by some authorities involves the periodic monitoring (eg, at 2-week intervals) of exposed HCP by polymerase chain reaction (PCR) for HCV RNA and then implementing therapy (eg, with pegylated interferon and ribavirin) if HCV infection is documented to have occurred, as measured by repeated positive RNA assays for HCV in the serum of the exposed person. Other authorities advocate a "watchful waiting" strategy where clinicians monitor exposed HCP biweekly by PCR, follow those who develop viremia over time to see if chronic infection develops, and then treat only individuals who remain positive for HCV RNA by PCR and have elevated ALT levels 2 to 4 months into the course of their infections. Under this strategy, individuals who spontaneously clear their infections would be spared the toxicities and expense of interferon therapy. Both strategies represent reasonable approaches to the management of occupational HCV exposures based on the currently available information.

Human Immunodeficiency Virus Infection

Prospective studies of HCP have estimated that the average risk of HIV transmission

Table 102.2 Recommended HIV PEP for Percutaneous Injuries

	Infection Status of Source				
Exposure Type	HIV-Positive, Class 1[a] Asymptomatic HIV infection or known low viral load (eg, ≤1500)	HIV-Positive, Class 2[a] Symptomatic HIV infection, AIDS, acute seroconversion, or known high viral load	Source of Unknown HIV Status (eg, deceased source person with no samples available for HIV testing)	Unknown Source (eg, a needle from a sharps disposal container)	HIV-Negative
Less severe, eg, solid needle or superficial injury	Recommend basic two-drug PEP	Recommend expanded three-drug PEP	Generally, no PEP warranted; however, consider basic two-drug PEP[b] for source with HIV risk factors[c]	Generally, no PEP warranted; however, consider basic two-drug PEP[b] in settings where exposure to HIV-infected persons is likely	No PEP warranted
More severe, eg, large-bore hollow needle, deep puncture, visible blood on device, or needle used in patient's artery or vein	Recommend expanded three-drug PEP	Recommend expanded three-drug PEP	Generally, no PEP warranted; however, consider basic two-drug PEP[b] for source with HIV risk factors[c]	Generally, no PEP warranted; however, consider basic two-drug PEP[b] in settings where exposure to HIV-infected persons is likely	No PEP warranted

[a] If drug resistance is a concern, obtain expert consultation. Initiation of PEP should not be delayed pending expert consultation, and, because expert consultation alone cannot substitute for face-to-face counseling, resources should be available to provide immediate evaluation and follow-up care for all exposures.
[b] The designation "consider PEP" indicates that PEP is optional and should be based on an individualized decision made by the exposed person and the treating clinician.
[c] If PEP is offered and taken, and the source is later determined to be HIV negative, PEP should be discontinued.
Abbreviations: HIV = human immunodeficiency virus; AIDS = acquired human immunodeficiency syndrome; PEP = postexposure prophylaxis.

after a percutaneous exposure to HIV-infected blood is approximately 0.3% (95% confidence interval [CI] = 0.2%–0.5%). Epidemiologic and laboratory studies suggest that a variety of factors may affect the risk of HIV transmission after an occupational exposure. In a retrospective case–control study of HCP who had percutaneous exposure to HIV, the risk for HIV infection was found to be increased with exposure to a larger quantity of blood from the source patient as indicated by (1) a device visibly contaminated with the patient's blood, (2) a procedure that involved a needle placed directly in a vein or artery, or (3) a deep injury. The risk also was increased for exposure to blood from source patients with terminal illness, probably reflecting either the higher titer of HIV in blood late in the course of acquired immunodeficiency syndrome (AIDS) or other factors.

HCP exposed to HIV should be evaluated within hours (rather than days) after their exposure and should be tested for HIV at baseline (ie, to establish infection status at the time of exposure). The recommendations found in Table 102.2 apply to situations where an exposed person had an exposure to a source person with HIV infection or where information suggests that there is a likelihood that the source person is HIV infected. These recommendations are based on the risk for HIV infection after different types of exposure and limited data regarding efficacy and toxicity of postexposure prophylaxis (PEP). Because most occupational HIV exposures do not result in the transmission of HIV, potential toxicity must be carefully considered when prescribing PEP. When recommended, PEP should be initiated as soon as possible. PEP probably should be administered for 4 weeks, if tolerated. If the source person's HIV infection status is unknown at the time of exposure, use of PEP should be decided on a case-by-case basis, after considering the type of exposure and the clinical and/or epidemiologic likelihood of HIV infection in the source. The selection of a drug regimen for HIV PEP must strive to balance the risk for infection against the potential toxicity of the PEP agent(s) used. When possible, the regimens should be implemented in consultation with health care professionals having expertise in antiretroviral treatment and HIV transmission. The majority of HIV exposures will warrant a two-drug regimen, using two nucleoside reverse transcriptase inhibitors (NRTIs) or one NRTI and one

Table 102.3 Practice Recommendations for Health Care Facilities (HCFs) Implementing Guidance for Management of Occupational Exposures to Bloodborne Pathogens (BBPs)

Practice Recommendation	Implementation Checklist
Establish a BBP management policy	All institutions where HCP may experience exposures should have a written policy for management of exposures The policy should be based on the U.S. Public Health Service (PHS) guidelines The policy should be reviewed periodically to ensure it is consistent with current PHS recommendations
Implement management policies	HCFs should provide appropriate training to all personnel on the prevention of and response to occupational exposures HCFs should establish hepatitis B vaccination programs HCFs should establish exposure-reporting systems HCFs should have personnel available at all times of the day who can manage an exposure readily HCFs should have ready access to PEP for use by exposed personnel as necessary
Establish laboratory capacity for BBP testing	HCFs should provide prompt processing of specimens from exposed and source persons to guide management of occupational exposures Testing should be performed with appropriate counseling and consent
Select and use appropriate postexposure prophylaxis (PEP) regimens	HCFs should develop a policy for the selection and use of PEP antiretroviral regimens for HIV exposures within their institution Hepatitis B vaccine and hepatitis B immunoglobulin (HBIG) should be available for timely administration HCFs should have access to resources with expertise in the selection and use of PEP
Provide access to counseling for exposed health care personnel (HCP)	HCFs should provide counseling for HCP who may need help to deal with the emotional impact of an exposure and who should be instructed to use precautions to prevent secondary transmission during the follow-up period HCFs should provide medication adherence counseling to assist HCP complete human immunodeficiency virus (HIV) PEP as necessary
Monitor for adverse effects of PEP	HCP taking antiretroviral PEP should be monitored periodically for adverse events through clinical evaluation, including blood testing, at baseline and 2 weeks postexposure
Monitor for seroconversion	HCF should develop a system to encourage exposed HCP to return for follow-up testing Exposed HCP should be tested for hepatitis C virus (HCV) and HIV

Monitor exposure management programs	HCFs should develop a system to monitor reporting and management of occupational exposures to ensure timely and appropriate response
	Evaluate:
	  Exposure reports for completeness and accuracy
	  Access to care (ie, the time of exposure to the time of evaluation)
	  Laboratory result reporting time
	Review:
	  Exposures to ensure that HCP exposed to sources not infected with BBPs do not receive PEP or PEP is stopped
	Monitor:
	  Completion rates of HBV vaccination and HIV PEP
	  Completion of exposure follow-up

nucleotide reverse transcriptase inhibitor (NtRTI) (Table 102.2). Combinations that can be considered for PEP include zidovudine (ZDV) and lamivudine (3TC) or emtricitabine (FTC), stavudine (d4 T) and 3TC or FTC, and tenofovir (TDF) and 3TC or FTC. The addition of a third (or even a fourth) drug should be considered for exposures that pose an increased risk for transmission or that involve a source in whom antiretroviral drug resistance is likely. Expanded PEP regimens should be protease inhibitor (PI) based. The PI preferred for use in expanded PEP regimens is lopinavir/ritonavir (LPV/RTV). Other PIs acceptable for use in expanded PEP regimens include atazanavir, fosamprenavir, RTV-boosted indinavir, RTV-boosted saquinavir, or nelfinavir. Reevaluation of the exposed person should be considered within 72 hours postexposure, especially as additional information about the exposure or source person becomes available. HCP with occupational exposure to HIV should receive follow-up counseling to use precautions to prevent secondary transmission during the follow-up period, postexposure testing, and medical evaluation regardless of whether they receive PEP. HIV-antibody testing should be performed for at least 6 months postexposure (eg, at 6 weeks, 12 weeks, and 6 months). HIV-antibody testing using enzyme immunoassay should be used to monitor for seroconversion. If PEP is used, the HCP should be monitored for drug toxicity by medical evaluation at baseline and again 2 weeks after starting PEP. The scope of postexposure blood testing should be based on medical conditions in the exposed person and the toxicity of the drugs included in the PEP regimen.

GUIDANCE FOR HEALTH CARE FACILITIES

In Table 102.3, specific practice recommendations for the management of occupational bloodborne pathogen exposures are outlined to assist health care institutions with the implementation of established exposure management guidelines. All recommendations given are valid as of March 2007. Please see http://www.cdc.gov/ncidod/dhqp/gl_occupational.html for any updates.

SUGGESTED READING

Beltrami EM, Williams IT, Shapiro CN, Chamberland ME. Risk and management of blood-borne infections in health care workers. *Clin Micro Rev.* 2000;13:385–407.

Cardo DM, Culver DH, Ciesielski CA, et al. A case-control study of HIV seroconversion in health care workers after percutaneous exposure. *N Engl J Med.* 1997;337:1485–1490.

Centers for Disease Control and Prevention. Updated U. S. Public Health Service guidelines for the management of occupational exposures to HIV and recommendations for postexposure prophylaxis. *Morbid Mortal Weekly Rep.* 2005;54(RR-9):1–17.

Centers for Disease Control and Prevention. Updated U. S. Public Health Service guidelines for the management of occupational exposures to HBV, HCV, and HIV and recommendations for postexposure prophylaxis. *Morbid Mortal Weekly Rep.* 2001;50(RR-11):1–52.

Department of Labor Occupational Safety and Health Administration. Occupational exposure to blood-borne pathogens: final rule. *Fed Reg.* 1991;56:C29-CFR Part 1910.1030:64175.

Henderson DK. Managing occupational risks for hepatitis C transmission in the health care setting. *Clin Micro Rev.* 2003;16:546–568.

Hospital Infection Control Practices Advisory Committee (HICPAC). Guidelines for infection control in healthcare personnel, 1998, Centers for Disease Control and Prevention. *Infect Control Hosp Epidemiol.* 1998;19:407–463.

Panlilio AL, Orelien JG, Srivastava PU, et al. Estimate of the annual number of percutaneous injuries among hospital-based healthcare workers in the United States, 1997—1998. *Infect Control Hosp Epidemiol.* 2004;25:556–562.

103. Hospital-Acquired Fever

Susan K. Seo and Arthur E. Brown

Fever is a common clinical problem in hospitalized patients. Although the development of fever in a hospitalized patient may be the clinical expression of a community-acquired infection that has completed its incubation period, this chapter focuses on the possible causes of new-onset fever occurring after hospital admission. The reader, however, should keep other diagnoses in mind and inquire about the patient's history of travel, pet and animal exposure, hobbies, sexual activity, dietary preferences and exposures, occupational exposures, recent immunizations, drug (including corticosteroids) and herbal ingestion within the past month, recent exposure to febrile or ill individuals, and other epidemiologic factors such as season of the year.

Hospital-acquired fever may be due to an infectious and/or noninfectious cause, either happening alone or concurrently. An etiology can be identified after appropriate work-up in 72% to 88% of patients. It is not uncommon for length-of-stay and resource utilization to be increased due to the management of the febrile episode.

Not surprisingly, nosocomial infections account for 70% to 75% of causes of fever in hospitalized patients and include bloodstream infections, lower respiratory tract infections, surgical site infections, and urinary tract infections (Table 103.1). Noninfectious causes comprise 25% to 30%. These are usually related to some form of vascular disruption (eg, myocardial infarction, pulmonary embolism), inflammatory (eg, gout) or collagen vascular disease (eg, lupus), endocrine disorder (eg, adrenal insufficiency), malignancy, or drug (Table 103.2). In some instances, the only identifiable factor may be a procedure (eg, surgery, respiratory intubation) performed within 24 hours of fever onset.

A comprehensive review of the patient's history and a full physical exam should be performed to find clues to the source(s) of fever. Disorders of immune function, valvular heart disease, history of previous placement of prosthetic devices (eg, orthopedic), prior illness and treatment, drug allergies, and history of transplantation should be reviewed with the

Table 103.1 Infectious Causes of Hospital-Acquired Fever

Bloodstream
  Intravascular device-related (eg, triple-lumen central venous catheter, Hickman, Broviac, Port)
  Sepsis due to bacterial or fungal organisms

Central Nervous System
  Epidural abscess
  Meningitis

Gastrointestinal
  Cholangitis
  Diverticulitis
  Intra-abdominal abscess
  Pseudomembranous colitis

Respiratory Tract
  Aspiration pneumonia
  Empyema
  Hospital-acquired pneumonia
  Sinusitis
  Ventilator-associated pneumonia

Skin and Soft Tissue
  Cellulitis
  Myonecrosis
  Necrotizing fasciitis

Surgical Site (incisional, deep space, or abscess)

Urinary Tract
  Catheter-related
  Postinstrumentation (eg, cystoscopy)

Other
  Endocarditis
  Prosthetic-device infection
  Suppurative thrombophlebitis
  Transfusion-related (bacterial, fungal, viral, parasitic)

patient. Attention should also be paid to risk factors for hospital-acquired fever such as recent surgical, endoscopic, or interventional radiologic procedures, recent urinary and respiratory tract instrumentation, intravascular devices, drug therapy, and immobilization. The physical examination should be complete but focus on vital signs; general appearance; signs of toxicity; skin rash; presence of genital, mucosal, and/or conjunctival lesions; presence of cardiac murmur or rub; new crackles; decreased breath sounds; egophony and/or pleural friction rub on lung auscultation; abdominal tenderness;

Table 103.2 Examples of Noninfectious Causes of Hospital-Acquired Fever

Biologic Agents (eg, vaccines, cytokines) / Drugs
Alcohol or drug withdrawal
Drug fever
Drug overdose (eg, anticholinergic agents)
Neuroleptic malignant syndrome

Cardiac Causes
Myocardial infarction
Pericarditis

Collagen Vascular Diseases
Vasculitis

Endocrine Disorders
Adrenal insufficiency
Thyroid storm

Factitious Fever

Inflammatory Diseases
Gout, Pseudogout
Nonviral hepatitis

Intra-abdominal Conditions
Acalculous cholecystitis
Acute pancreatitis
Mesenteric ischemia
Upper or lower gastrointestinal bleeding

Malignancy
Tumor fever

Neurologic Conditions
Intracranial or subarachnoid hemorrhage
Seizures
Stroke
Subdural hematoma

Procedure Related
Benign postoperative fever
Endobronchial intubation
Transfusion reaction

Thromboembolic Disease
Deep venous thrombosis
Pulmonary embolus
Superficial thrombophlebitis

Vascular Conditions
Sickle cell crisis

hepatosplenomegaly; costovertebral angle tenderness; arthritis; spinal tenderness; meningismus; and/or neurologic dysfunction.

Obviously, the postoperative patient will have special attention given to the operative site and wounds. Consultation with the surgeon regarding the operative findings, technical difficulties, and complications is essential. Similarly, conferring with the endoscopist after bronchoscopy, endoscopic retrograde cholangiopancreatography, colonoscopy, or cystoscopy

may reveal information regarding the etiology of postendoscopic fever in such a patient. The patient with cancer may receive a significant amount of blood products over time and may develop transfusion-related infections (see Chapter 104, Transfusion-Related Infection). Infections found in the alcoholic, drug abusing, thermally injured, diabetic, elderly, or immunocompromised patient require special consideration (see chapters covering these topics). The immunocompromised patient with cancer in particular may have a variety of possible infectious etiologies to consider (see Chapter 85, Infections in Patients with Neoplastic Disease).

The investigation of hospital-acquired fever should take into consideration possible foci of infection. The initial evaluation typically includes a complete blood count, urinalysis, chest radiograph, and cultures of blood, urine, and, if indicated, sputum. Adequate sputum for microbiologic evaluation should contain few epithelial cells and numerous polymorphonuclear neutrophils if the patient is not neutropenic. However, obtaining a good specimen, particularly in critically ill and/or neutropenic patients, might be difficult. Appropriate cultures of wound sites and drainage are also important. It is essential to obtain fresh material from the drainage site rather than the material that has been dwelling in the collection apparatus. In the patient with diarrhea, stool specimens should be obtained and tested for *Clostridium difficile* toxin. When a rash is present, a biopsy of the skin should be obtained for both histologic and microbiologic examination. Vascular access devices are suspect. If possible, these should be removed, and the tips sent for culture.

It is important that the specimens are obtained correctly and are transported to the microbiology laboratory quickly. This aids in the recovery of fastidious organisms, particularly anaerobic bacteria. Examination of the Gram-stained specimen is useful in judging the adequacy of the specimen and aids in the presumptive etiologic diagnosis. This information is invaluable as the clinician can better tailor empiric antimicrobial therapy until final culture results are available.

Further radiographic studies may be needed, depending on the clinical situation. Appropriate computed tomography scans should be conducted to locate a deep (ie, pelvic) source of fever in a postoperative patient who underwent abdominal surgery. Ultrasonographic studies help in evaluating the liver and spleen and the vascular system. Sometimes, gallium scans or indium-labeled white blood cell scans may assist in locating occult foci of infection. Once located, radiographically guided drainage or open drainage of the abscess can be achieved.

In summary, determining the cause of fever in hospitalized patients can be very challenging. Although infection is common, the clinician needs to be aware that hospital-acquired fever may constitute a variety of other conditions.

SUGGESTED READING

Arbo MJ, Fine MJ, Hanusa BH, Sefcik T, Kapoor WN. Fever of nosocomial origin: etiology, risk factors, and outcomes. *Am J Med*. 1993;95:505–512.

Bor DH, Makadon HJ, Friedland G, et al. Fever in hospitalized medical patients: characteristics and significance. *J Gen Intern Med*. 1988;3:119–125.

Filice GA, Weiler MD, Hughes RA, Gerding DN. Nosocomial febrile illnesses in patients on an internal medicine service. *Arch Intern Med*. 1989;149:319–324.

Hedrick TL, Sawyer RG. Health-care-associated infections and prevention. *Surg Clin N Am*. 2005;85:1137–1152.

McGowan Jr JE, Rose RC, Jacobs NF, Schaberg DR, Haley RW. Fever in hospitalized patients with special reference to the medical service. *Am J Med*. 1987;82:580–586.

Richards MJ, Edwards JR, Culver DH, Gaynes RP. Nosocomial infections in medical intensive care units in the United States. National Nosocomial Infections Surveillance System. *Crit Care Med*. 1999;27:887–892.

104. Transfusion-Related Infection

William R. Jarvis and Virginia R. Roth

The transfusion of blood and blood components is associated with a very low but ever-present risk of infection. It is estimated that 1 in every 2000 units of blood may carry an infectious agent and that about 4 in 10 000 recipients develop a chronic disease or die as a result of receiving contaminated blood. A wide variety of viral, bacterial, and parasitic agents have been associated with blood transfusion (Table 104.1). Concerns have also been raised about the potential for transmission of Creutzfeldt–Jakob disease (CJD) and its new variant (nv-CJD) through blood products. However, no human episodes of CJD or nv-CJD have been causally liked to blood transfusion, and case–control studies have not found blood transfusion to be a risk factor for CJD. The risk of viral transmission has been markedly reduced with improved screening, particularly using nucleic acid testing (NAT). The risk is now estimated to be 1 in 2 million units for human immunodeficiency virus (HIV) or hepatitis C virus (HCV) and approximately 1 in 200 000 units for hepatitis B virus (HBV). Because the risk of viral or parasitic infection is very low and blood is screened for HCV, HBV, HIV, and human T-cell lymphoma/leukemia virus (HTLV) 1, the remainder of this chapter focuses on bacterial complications of blood transfusion, which can be diagnosed and treated.

Although the rate of bacterial contamination of blood products is unknown, the rate of bacterial infection associated with blood products is estimated to be similar to that of viral infection. The Bacterial Contamination of Blood Products (BaCON) study, a collaboration among the Centers for Disease Control and Prevention, American Red Cross, American Association of Blood Banks (AABB), and Department of Defense, conducted active surveillance for transfusion-transmitted bacteremia between 1998 and 2000. There were 34 bacteremic episodes and 9 deaths. The rate of transfusion-transmitted bacteremia (events per 10^6 units) was 9.98 for single donor platelets, 10.64 for pooled platelets, and 0.21 for red blood cell units; for fatal reactions, the rates

Table 104.1 Infections Transmissible by Blood Transfusion

Viruses
Hepatitis
Hepatitis A virus (HAV)
Hepatitis B virus (HBV)
Hepatitis C virus (HCV)
Hepatitis D virus (HDV)
Hepatitis G virus (HGV)
Cytomegalovirus (CMV)
Epstein–Barr virus (EBV)
Nonhepatitis
HIV-1 and 2
HTLV-1 and 2
Human herpes virus 8 (HHV-8)[a]
Parvovirus B19
Colorado tick fever virus
West Nile virus
Dengue virus
Avian Influenza virus[a]
Bacteria
Yersinia
Pseudomonas
Staphylococcus
Other gram-positive or gram-negative bacteria
Rickettsia
Spirochetes
Syphilis
Recurrent fever
Lyme disease[a]
Ehrlichia[a]
Protozoa
Plasmodium spp. (malaria)
Babesia spp.
Trypanosoma cruzi (Chaga's disease)
Toxoplasma spp.
Leishmania spp.
Nematode (loasis, other microfilaria)

Abbreviations: HIV = human immunodeficiency virus; HTLV = human T-cell lymphoma/leukemia virus.
[a] Potential risk only, no reported case.

were 1.94, 2.22, and 0.13, respectively. The fatality rate associated with transfusion-related sepsis has been estimated to be 1 in 6 million transfused units. Transfusion-transmitted bacterial sepsis is the second most common cause of transfusion-related fatality (after clerical error). Between October 1995 and September 2004, 85 (13%) of 665 transfusion fatalities

Table 104.2 Blood Component Storage Conditions and Estimated Bacterial Contamination Rates

Component	Storage Conditions	Estimated Contamination Rate
Whole blood CPDA–1 CPD plus AS	≤8 h at room temp ≤35 d at 1°C–6°C ≤45 d at 1°C–6°C	0.03%
Packed red blood cells CPDA–1 CPD plus AS	 ≤35 d at 1°C–6°C ≤45 d at 1°C–6°C	≤0.5%
Platelets	≤5 d at 20°C–24°C	Single donor, ≤2.5% Pooled, ≤10%
Plasma	Frozen, stored ≤18°C For use, thawed and stored ≤24 h at 1°–6°C	≤0.1%

Abbreviations: CPDA = citrate-phosphate-dextrose-adenine (additives); CPD = citrate-phosphate-dextrose; AS = adenine saline (additives).

reported to the Food and Drug Administration were due to bacteria; 58/85 (63%) were due to gram-negative bacteria. However, more common nonfatal episodes of transfusion reaction, which may result from bacterial contamination of blood or blood components, often are assumed to be an immune response to transfused leukocytes and are not fully investigated for contamination.

WHOLE BLOOD AND ERYTHROCYTES

After collection, whole blood may be maintained at room temperature for ≤8 hours before being stored at 1°C to 6°C (33.8°F to 42.8°F) up to 35 to 42 days, depending on the additives used (Table 104.2). Erythrocytes may be prepared from whole blood at any point during the normal storage period of the whole blood. Then, the erythrocytes may be stored at 1°C to 6°C up to the expiration date of the whole blood unit from which they were prepared. The growth of psychrophilic organisms, such as *Yersinia enterocolitica* or *Pseudomonas* species, is favored by these storage conditions, accounting for most erythrocyte transfusion-related sepsis episodes (Table 104.3). These episodes tend to occur with units that have been stored for >14 to 25 days, which reflects a growth lag of about 7 to 14 days followed by exponential growth of the organism; levels of 10^9 organisms/mL are reached by 38 days, and 315 ng of endotoxin/mL (approximately 4,000 EU/mL) by 28 to 34 days. Transfusion of such units can lead to both septic and endotoxic shock.

PLATELETS

Each year, approximately 9 million platelet-unit concentrates are transfused in the United States. Platelets are stored in oxygen-permeable containers with agitation at 20°C to 24°C (68°F to 75.2°F) for ≤5 days. The most common transfusion-associated infection reported in the United States is bacterial contamination of platelet components. Bacterial contamination is estimated to occur at the incidence rate of 1:1000 to 1:3000 platelet units. Platelet transfusion-related sepsis usually involves common skin organisms, eg, *Staphylococcus epidermidis*, *Staphylococcus aureus*, or other aerobic bacteria that can grow rapidly at room temperature (Table 104.3). Sepsis episodes related to platelet transfusion also tend to occur with units that are late in the storage period (around 4 to 5 days), when there may be a higher titer of organisms than early in the storage period. In addition, sepsis episodes occur more frequently with pooled platelet units than with single-donor apheresis units. A pooled platelet unit is prepared by combining 6 to 10 random donor platelet concentrates up to 4 hours before transfusion. In contrast, an apheresis unit is prepared by separating platelets from the whole blood of a single donor and returning other blood components to the donor. The higher rate of sepsis associated with pooled platelets primarily is seen because, on average, pooled platelets are stored longer than apheresis platelets. With pooled platelets, there also is a higher risk of contamination associated

Table 104.3 Reported Episodes of Transfusion-Associated Sepsis

Pathogen	Percentage	Duration in Days from Collection to Transfusion	
		Median	Range
Erythrocytes			
Yersinia enterocolitica	49.0	24	7–41
Pseudomonas fluorescens	23.5	24	16–32
Serratia liquefaciens	7.8	21	17–26
Treponema pallidum	2.0	≤1	—
Pseudomonas putida	2.0	—	—
Other species	15.7	23	20–26
Platelets			
Staphylococcus epidermidis	33.3	4	3–5
Salmonella cholerasuis	11.7	≤1	—
Serratia marcescens	8.3	2	1–3
Staphylococcus aureus	5.0	5	3–6
Bacillus cereus	5.0	—	—
Streptococcus viridans group	3.3	3	1–6
Salmonella enteriditis	3.3	5	3–5
Other species	23.3	4	2–6

with the exposure to multiple donors or with the manipulation of the concentrates. In March 2004, an AABB standard was introduced that required routine quality control testing for bacterial contamination of apheresis platelet products. These were implemented in many U.S. and Canadian blood centers and have reduced the risk of platelet-associated bacterial infection.

PLASMA AND PLASMA-DERIVED PRODUCTS

Plasma is either collected by apheresis or prepared from whole blood and is stored at below −18°C (−0.4°F) within 6 hours of collection. It can be thawed in a water bath using a plastic overwrap or in a microwave and subsequently stored at 1°C to 6°C up to 24 hours before transfusion. The survival of bacteria is not supported by these storage conditions. However, equipment may carry contamination; for example, one reported episode of sepsis associated with a plasma transfusion was attributed to a contaminated water bath used for thawing the unit.

Contamination of plasma-derived products also is thought to be rare. They are prepared from plasma stored under very stringent conditions, and many of the products also undergo viral inactivation procedures. However, contamination may still occur, as demonstrated by outbreaks of hepatitis C virus infections associated with the administration of contaminated intravenous immunoglobulin or hepatitis A virus associated with plasma-derived products.

SOURCES OF CONTAMINATION

Contamination of blood or blood components may occur intrinsically if a donor is bacteremic or viremic at the time of donation; it also may occur extrinsically from the skin during phlebotomy or from containers and other equipment used during processing and storage. The infecting organism may reflect the

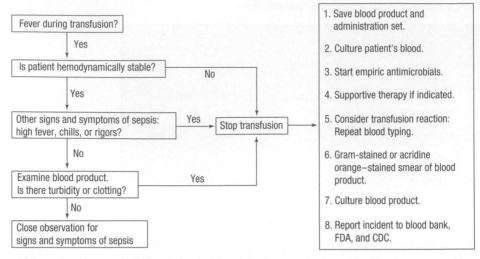

Figure 104.1 Algorithm for the evaluation of fever associated with transfusion.

source of contamination. With *Y. enterocolitica*–contaminated erythrocytes, the implicated source often is an asymptomatic episode of gastrointestinal (GI) illness within the previous month. Because the GI illness usually is mild, the donor may not recall or may neglect to report the episode during prescreening.

CLINICAL MANAGEMENT

Although these contamination episodes are rare, it is important to consider the possibility of blood and blood component contamination when a patient develops a fever during or soon after a transfusion (Figure 104.1). If bacteremia cannot be ruled out, the transfusion should be stopped immediately. Any residual blood product or administration set should immediately be quarantined and refrigerated. A Gram-stain and/or acridine orange-stain smear of the blood product should be performed. Stain and/or culture of blood component segments usually are negative, even when the unit itself is positive; this may reflect low-level contamination of the unit at the time of donation. Cultures of the blood product in the bag, the patient's blood before antimicrobials are begun, and any intravenous solution used during transfusion should be obtained promptly. Information about the donor should be reviewed completely. If organisms are recovered from the recipient and blood product, molecular typing of patient and donor isolates may prove causality.

After appropriate cultures are obtained, broad-spectrum empiric antimicrobial therapy should be started. Empiric treatment of sus-

pected sepsis associated with blood products must be based on the component. Because most reported sepsis episodes associated with erythrocyte transfusion have been caused by *Y. enterocolitica* or *Pseudomonas* species, particularly *Pseudomonas fluorescens*, initial therapy may include trimethoprim–sulfamethoxazole or an antipseudomonal β-lactam plus an aminoglycoside. Because infectious complications associated with platelets usually are caused by aerobic bacteria, eg, coagulase-negative staphylococci or *S. aureus* and occasionally gram-negative organisms, initial empiric therapy may include a penicillinase-resistant penicillin and an aminoglycoside. Empiric therapy should be narrowed as soon as an infecting pathogen is identified and antimicrobial susceptibility results are available.

PREVENTION

Sensitive, rapid diagnostic tests for detecting bacterial contamination are not yet available. Therefore, minimizing the risk of transfusion-associated sepsis depends on appropriate donor screening, donor site inspection and preparation, and proper handling of the blood components (Table 104.4). Detection of infectious complications associated with blood products may be increased by educating the medical and blood bank staff about the signs and symptoms of patients with transfusion reactions, the importance of immediately reporting transfusion reactions to the blood bank, promptly culturing the blood of the recipient, promptly performing stains and culture of the blood component, and ensuring

Table 104.4 Prevention of Transfusion-Associated Sepsis

Donors
Screen for infectious diseases (health questionnaire); inquire about travel, behaviors, dental work, signs and symptoms of recent illness.

Phlebotomy
Inspect site; avoid dimpled areas of the skin. Prepare site properly. Use aseptic techniques.

Bag and Component Preparation
Use aseptic techniques. Perform proper cleaning and disinfection of processing equipment; use plastic overwraps in water baths for thawing. Use appropriate storage conditions. Visually inspect contents before transfusion.

quarantined refrigerated storage of the unit and administration set until contamination has been excluded.

SUGGESTED READING

Blajchman MA. Bacterial contamination and proliferation during the storage of cellular blood products. *Vox Sang.* 1998;74(suppl 2): 155–159.

Fang CT, Chambers LA, Kennedy J, et al. Detection of bacterial contamination in apheresis platelet products: American Red Cross experience, 2004. *Transfusion.* 2005;45:1845–1852.

Goodnough LT, Brecher ME, Kanter MH, et al. Transfusion medicine: blood transfusion. *N Engl J Med.* 1999;340:438–447.

Kuehnert MJ, Roth VR, Haley NR, et al. Transfusion-transmitted bacterial infection in the United States, 1998 through 2000. *Transfusion.* 2001;41:1493–1499.

Niu MT, Knippen M, Simmons L, et al. Transfusion-transmitted *Klebsiella pneumoniae* fatalities, 1995 to 2004. *Transfus Med Rev.* 2006;20:149–157.

Pealer LN, Marfin AA, Petersen LR, et al. Transmission of West Nile virus through blood transfusion in the United States in 2002. *N Engl J Med.* 2003;349:1236–1245.

Ramirez-Arcos S, Jenkins C, Dion J, et al. Canadian experience with detection of bacterial contamination in apheresis platelets. *Transfusion.* 2007;47: 421–429.

Roth VR, Kuehnert MJ, Haley NR, et al. Evaluation of a reporting system for bacterial contamination of blood components in the United States. *Transfusion.* 2001;41:1486–1492.

Schreiber GB, Busch MP, Kleinmann SH, et al. The risk of transfusion-transmitted viral infections. The Retrovirus Epidemiology Donor Study. *N Engl J Med.* 1996;334:1685–1690.

Wagner SJ, Friedman LI, Dodd RY. Transfusion-associated bacterial sepsis. *Clin Microbiol Rev.* 1994;7:290–302.

105. Intravascular Catheter-Related Infections

Dany Ghannam and Issam Raad

Central venous catheter (CVC) use is primarily directed to secure a vascular access for fluids, medications, blood products, total parenteral nutrition (TPN), and hemodialysis. Their use is not limited only to inpatients but also to the outpatient settings. The national nosocomial infection surveillance system reported that the rate of catheter-related bloodstream infection (CRBSI) ranges from 2.1 to 30.2 BSIs per 1000 vascular catheter days. More than 80 000 CRBSIs are estimated to occur annually in the intensive care units (ICUs) in the United States with an attributable mortality ranging from 12% to 25%. In the initially ill patient, the direct implication of CRBSI is an extension of hospital stay by an average of 6 to 7 days; the added cost ranges from $28 690 to $56 167 per each individual episode in ICU patients.

PATHOGENESIS

Colonization is universal after insertion of a CVC, can occur as early as 1 day after insertion, and is quantitatively independent of a catheter-related infection. Electron microscopy studies of catheter surfaces show that adherent microorganisms can be found in either a free-floating form or sessile form embedded in a biofilm.

The dynamic process of adherence is the result of the interaction of three factors: the intrinsic properties of the catheter, microbial factors, and host-derived proteins. The physical characteristics of the catheter, such as surface irregularities and charge difference, facilitate bacterial adherence. Furthermore, some microorganisms adhere better to polyvinyl chloride, silicone, and polyethylene surfaces than to Teflon polymers and polyurethane. Concomitantly, in reaction to the foreign nature of the catheter, a thrombin sheath forms on the internal and external surfaces of the catheter. This newly formed sheath results from the deposition of host-derived proteins such as fibrinogen, fibronectin, laminin, and thrombospondin during the process of insertion.

Microorganisms colonize vascular catheters through different sources: For short-term catheters, the skin of the site of insertion is the major source for colonization; bacterial skin flora migrate along the external surface of the catheter. The hub of the vascular device is the most common source of colonization for long-term catheters. Microorganisms are introduced from the hands of medical personnel. In this case, colonizing bacteria migrate along the internal surface of the catheter. Hematogenous seeding and contamination of the infusate or additives such as contaminated heparin flush (such as in the nationwide outbreaks in 1971 of *Enterobacter agglomerans* and *Enterobacter cloacae*) are rare causes of colonization and infection of vascular devices.

Colonizing microorganisms enhance their adherence by producing a microbial biofilm of extracellular, polysaccharide-rich slimy material, or glycocalyx. Biofilms form on the external surface of short-term catheters and internal surface of long-term catheters (dwell time of at least 30 days). This biofilm enables bacteria not only to adhere to the surface of the catheter but also to resist antibiotics whereby "chronic" biofilm eradication becomes a difficult task.

Other factors could also potentiate the risk for a CRBSI; femoral catheterization was associated with higher rate of infections and thrombotic complications than was subclavian catheterization; transparent occlusive dressing was also associated with significantly increased rates of insertion site colonization, local catheter-related infection, and CRBSI when CVCs remain for more than 3 days compared to gauze dressing.

Skin flora such as *Staphylococcus epidermidis*, *Staphylococcus aureus*, *Bacillus* species, and *Corynebacterium* species remain the predominant source of CRBSI, followed by microorganisms that contaminate the hands of medical personnel, such as *Pseudomonas*, *Acinetobacter*, *S. maltophilia*, and *Candida*. Emerging pathogens such as *Achromobacter*, rapidly growing mycobacteria (*M. chelonae* and *M. fortuitum*), and fungal elements such as *Fusarium*, *Malassezia furfur*, and *Rhodotorula* species have been described in specific conditions (ie, hyperalimentation, interleukin-2 therapy).

CLINICAL MANIFESTATIONS

The clinical presentation of CRBSI consists of nonspecific systemic manifestations and local manifestations at the skin insertion site.

The systemic features of CRBSI are generally indistinguishable from those of bloodstream infection arising from other foci of infection and include fever and chills, which may be accompanied by hypotension, hyperventilation, altered mental status, and nonspecific gastrointestinal manifestations such as nausea, vomiting, abdominal pain, and diarrhea. Deep-seated infections such as endocarditis, osteomyelitis, retinitis, and organ abscess may complicate CRBSI caused by some virulent organisms like *Staphylococcus aureus, Pseudomonas aeruginosa,* and *Candida albicans.*

The local manifestations are neither sensitive nor specific and cannot be relied on to identify catheter colonization or CVC-related BSI. On one hand, they could be completely absent especially in immunocompromised and neutropenic patients. On the other hand, peripherally inserted central catheter (PICC) lines (inserted in the basilic or cephalic veins) can be associated with sterile local exit site inflammation (26%) secondary to irritation of small veins (ie, cephalic vein) by insertion of a large catheter.

The suggested definitions of catheter infections by the Centers for Disease Control and Prevention (CDC) are as follows:

1. Catheter colonization
   The isolation of 15 or more colony-forming units (CFU) of any microorganism by semiquantitative culture (roll-plate method) or 3 or more CFU by quantitative culture (eg, sonication technique), from a catheter tip or subcutaneous segment in the absence of simultaneous clinical symptoms
2. Local catheter-related infection
   Exit-site infection: purulent drainage from the catheter exit site or erythema, tenderness, and swelling within 2 cm of the catheter exit site, and colonization of the catheter if removed
   Port-pocket infection: erythema and/or necrosis of the skin or subcutaneous tissues either over or around the reservoir of an implanted catheter, and colonization of the catheter if removed
   Tunnel infection: erythema, tenderness, and induration of the tissues above the catheter and >2 cm from the exit site and colonization of the catheter if removed

CRBSI is defined as bacteremia or fungemia in a patient who has an intravascular device and ≥ 1 positive result of culture of blood samples obtained from the peripheral vein, clinical manifestations of infection (eg, fever, chills, and/or hypotension), and no apparent source for bloodstream infection (with the exception of the catheter). One of the following should be present: a positive result of semiquantitative (≥ 15 CFU per catheter segment) or quantitative ($\geq 10^2$ CFU per catheter segment) catheter culture, whereby the same organism (species and antibiogram) is isolated from a catheter segment and a peripheral blood sample; simultaneous quantitative cultures of blood samples with a ratio of $\geq 5:1$ (CVC vs peripheral); differential time to positivity (ie, a positive result of culture from a CVC is obtained at least 2 hours earlier than is a positive result of culture from peripheral blood).

DIAGNOSIS

The diagnosis of catheter-related infection is challenging and often difficult to perform. A definite diagnosis often requires catheter removal and culture and is thus retrospective. The current available laboratory diagnostic techniques are noted in Table 105.1.

PREVENTIVE STRATEGIES

Central venous catheters should only be used when medically necessary and should be removed as soon as possible to prevent the potential complications.

Several preventive measures have shown efficacy in decreasing the risk of catheter-related infection. Risk factors and beneficial preventive interventions are listed in Tables 105.2 and 105.3, respectively.

The CDC does not recommend routine guidewire-assisted catheter exchange. However, the guidewire may be used to (1) replace a malfunctioning catheter, (2) convert an existing catheter to a different type, and (3) determine the source of the bloodstream infection, allowing culture of the exchanged catheter.

Recent developments in catheter coating with antiseptics and antimicrobials seem promising. A meta-analysis of 12 clinical trials showed better efficacy of antiseptic impregnated vascular catheters with chlorhexidine and sulfadiazine in preventing CRBSI when compared with nonimpregnated catheters.

More recent studies of catheters coated with minocycline and rifampin demonstrated

Table 105.1 Current Available Laboratory Diagnostic Techniques

After Catheter Removal
- Semiquantitative culture of catheter tip: Catheter colonization is defined by a growth of 15 colony-forming units (CFU) or greater of a catheter tip culture by the roll-plate technique. Although commonly used, this method is limited by recovering microorganisms only from the external surface of the catheter.
- Quantitative culture of catheter segments: This method consists of culturing both external and internal surfaces of the catheter by sonication, centrifugation, and vortexing of two segments: the subcutaneous tunneled segment and the catheter tip. A growth of ≥1000 CFU correlated best with colonization; CRBSI would be defined by the same cutoff accompanied by a high clinical suspicion and absence of evidence of other sites' infection.
- Catheter staining: Consists of Gram or acridine orange staining of the catheter tip, with identification of the microorganisms under direct microscopy. However, this technique is time-consuming and operator dependent, which limits its usefulness.

Before Catheter Removal
- Endoluminal brush technique: A wire brush is used to culture the endoluminal surface in situ, then Gram or acridine orange staining of the blood drawn through the catheter. Counts of >100 CFU/mL are considered positive with a sensitivity of 95% and specificity of 84%; however, this method is associated with a 6% risk of transient bacteremia.
- Paired quantitative blood cultures: This method consists of obtaining paired QBC simultaneously or within 10 minutes with the same amount of blood from the CVC and a peripheral vein. The hypothesis is that higher load of organisms on the internal lumen of the CVC signifying CRBSI would translate into a colony count from the CVC greater by many folds than the peripheral stick. A CVC/peripheral ratio of CFU/mL of 5/1 has been chosen by the IDSA to represent true infection. A meta-analysis found that quantitative blood culture is the most accurate for diagnosing a CRBSI with a pooled sensitivity of 75%–93% and specificity of 97%–100%.
- Differential time to positivity (DTP): The DTP of qualitative paired simultaneous CVC and peripheral blood culture has been a more practical test for centers that lack the logistics for QBC, especially with the introduction of automated radiometric blood culture systems that record the time at which a culture turns positive. The technique involves measuring the difference between the time required for culture positivity. A meta-analysis showed that the DTP of 120 minutes predicts CRBSI, with a pooled sensitivity and specificity for short term catheters of 89% and 87%, respectively, and 90% and 72% for long-term catheters.
- Catheter drawn QBC: This method includes a single quantitative blood culture drawn through the CVC. The cutoff of 100 CFU/mL establishes the diagnosis with a pooled sensitivity of 81%–86% and pooled specificity of 85%–96%. One major drawback to this technique is that it cannot distinguish between CRBSI and high-grade bacteremia, especially in immunocompetent patients.

Acridine orange leukocyte cytospin technique (AOLC): This test involves 1 mL of EDTA blood aspirated through the CVC and then centrifuged, stained, and viewed by ultraviolet light. A positive test is indicated by the presence of any bacteria. This method is expensive but takes 30 minutes, with a sensitivity of 87% and specificity of 94%. Note that this technique has only been tested by a small group of investigators.

Table 105.2 Risk Factors Associated with Infections of Intravascular Catheters

Definite	Possible
1. Violation of aseptic technique during catheter insertion and maintenance	1. Site of catheter insertion
2. Contaminated antiseptic skin solutions	2. Triple-lumen catheters skin solutions catheters thrombosis
3. Frequent manipulation of catheters	3. Transparent occlusive plastic dressing
4. Cut downs to insert catheters	4. Neutropenia
5. Prolonged placement of catheters	5. Catheter-related thrombosis
6. Total parenteral nutrition through catheter	
7. Interleukin-2 therapy	

a lower rate of catheter colonization and CRBSI when compared with uncoated catheters. Furthermore, when compared with antiseptic impregnated catheters, antibiotic-coated catheters lowered the rate of infection 12-fold.

Catheter lock solution technique consists of flushing the catheter lumen and then filling it with 2 to 3 mL of a combination of an anticoagulant plus an antimicrobial agent. The solution would remain locked preferably for 24 hours daily depending on the study.

A recent meta-analysis concluded that the use of a vancomycin plus heparin lock solution in high-risk patient populations being treated with long-term central intravenous devices (IVDs) reduces the risk of BSI with a risk ratio of 0.34. Minocycline and EDTA solution was superior in an in vitro biofilm model and an animal model

Table 105.3 Measures to Decrease Risk of Colonization of Central Venous Catheters

---

Short-Term Placement (≤10 d)

To prevent colonization of external surface of catheter:
    Maximum sterile barrier (handwashing, sterile gloves, large drape, sterile gown, mask, cap)
    Infusion therapy team
    Cutaneous antimicrobial or antiseptic agents (mupirocin, chlorhexidine)
    Silver-impregnated catheters
    Antimicrobial coating of catheter

Long-Term Placement (>10 d)

To prevent colonization of catheter lumen:
    Maximum sterile barrier (handwashing, sterile gloves, large drape, sterile gown, mask, cap)
    Infusion therapy team
    Antimicrobial flush or lock
    Tunneling
    Antimicrobial coating of catheter

---

to vancomycin–heparin lock solution. Ethanol as a lock solution has demonstrated reduction in risk of relapse of CRBSI in a prospective study of tunneled CVCs in a pediatric cancer population. More prospective studies are needed to better assess the efficacy of this technique.

THERAPY

The management of catheter-related infections involves confirming the source of infection, the choice of antimicrobials and duration of therapy, and the decision regarding the need for catheter removal. To confirm the infection, microorganisms recovered from different cultures (ie, blood through a venous catheter, a peripheral vein, catheter tip, and, if applicable, skin insertion site) must be the same. The duration of therapy is extended if the CRBSI is judged to be complicated (ie, associated with septic thrombophlebitis, endocarditis, or metastatic infection). Most of the CRBSIs will be treated for a period of 7 to 14 days, depending on the isolated microorganisms. However, in cases of complicated CRBSI, the vascular catheter should be removed and the infection treated with parenteral antibiotics for at least 4 weeks.

Coagulase-Negative Staphylococci

The optimal duration of therapy of CRBSI with coagulase-negative staphylococci (CNS) has not been defined. The Infectious Diseases Society of America (IDSA) guidelines recommend removing the CVC and treating for 5 to 7 days; otherwise, if the CVC is to be retained, duration of treatment should be 10 to 14 days. Because most CNS are nosocomially acquired and are resistant to penicillinase-resistant penicillins, the choice of a glycopeptide (ie, vancomycin) is recommended pending susceptibility results. Dalbavancin, a long-acting once-weekly new glycopeptide was superior to vancomycin for adult patients with CRBSIs caused by CNS and *S. aureus*, including methicillin-resistant *S. aureus* (MRSA) in a phase 2, open-label, randomized, multicenter study with comparable side effects. Linezolid and daptomycin were also used successfully.

Staphylococcus aureus

Staphylococcus aureus CRBSI is associated with high rates of deep-seated infection like osteomyelitis, septic phlebitis, and endocarditis. Failure to remove the catheter is associated with persistent bacteremia, relapses, and increased mortality. For methicillin-sensitive *S. aureus*, nafcillin or first-generation cephalosporin is the first choice. Vancomycin, linezolid, daptomycin, and dalbavincin are options for MRSA. Ten to fourteen days of intravenous therapy is enough if the CVC is removed and no deep-seated infection is present. If fever or bacteremia persists for more than 72 hours after catheter removal, transesophageal echocardiography should be considered to rule out infective endocarditis, and the intravenous therapy duration should be expanded to at least 4 weeks.

Candida

IDSA guidelines recommend removing the CVC and treating for 14 days after the last positive blood culture in uncomplicated cases. Endophthalmitis (15% of untreated cases) merits 6 weeks of therapy. Fluconazole and caspofungin were equivalent to amphotericin B in candidemia with a better safety profile; therefore, fluconazole or caspofungin should be considered in documented cases of catheter-related candidemia; if the rates of fluconazole-resistant *Candida glabrata* and *Candida krusei* in the hospital is high, caspofungin is the best alternative to amphotericin B.

Gram-Positive Bacilli

Vancomycin remains the antibiotic of choice in the treatment of CRBSI caused by gram-positive bacilli such as *Bacillus* and *Corynebacterium* species. Removal of the catheter is recommended.

Table 105.4 Management of Catheter-Related Infections

Microorganism	Duration of Therapy	Catheter Removal Advisable
Coagulase-negative staphylococci		Consider
CVC removed	5–7 d	
CVC retained	10–14 d	
Staphylococcus aureus		
Uncomplicated	10–14 d	Yes
Complicated	4 wk	Yes
Gram-positive bacilli	7 d	Yes
Gram-negative rods	10–14 d	Yes
Candida species		Yes
Uncomplicated	14 d	
Complicated	6 wk	
Mycobacterium	14 d	Yes

Abbreviation: CVC = central venous catheter.

Gram-Negative Bacilli

Enteric gram-negative bacilli are rare causes of CRBSI. However, *Klebsiella pneumoniae*, *Enterobacter* spp., *P. aeruginosa*, *Acinetobacter* spp., and *Stenotrophomonas maltophilia* were reported to be involved in CRBSI. Catheter removal is recommended in addition to therapy with an appropriate antimicrobial for 10 to 14 days.

Mycobacterial Disease

Catheter removal is recommended, and surgical intervention may be needed in long-term catheters infected with *M. chelonae* or *M. fortuitum*. A 14-day course of antimicrobials is suggested. However, a longer duration of therapy is required in complicated cases.

SUGGESTED READING

Darouiche RO, et al. A comparison of two antimicrobial-impregnated central venous catheters. *N Engl J Med.* 1999;340:1–8.

Fraenkel D, Rickard C, Thomas P, et al. A prospective, randomized trial of rifampicin-minocycline-coated and silver platinum-carbon-impregnated central venous catheters. *Crit Care Med.* 2006;34(3):668–675.

Mermel LA, Farr BM, Sherertz RJ, et al. Infectious Diseases Society of America; American College of Critical Care Medicine; Society for Healthcare Epidemiology of America. Guidelines for the management of intravascular catheter-related infections. *Clin Infect Dis.* 2001;32(9):1249–1272.

Pearson ML. Guideline for prevention of intravascular device-related infections. Part I. Intravascular device related infections: an overview. Part II: recommendations for the prevention of nosocomial intravascular device related infections. Hospital Infection Control Practices Advisory Committee. *Am J Infect Control.* 1996;24:262.

Raad I. Intravascular-catheter-related infections. *Lancet.* 1998;351:893–898.

Raad I, Hanna H, Dvorak T, et al. Optimal antimicrobial catheter lock solution, using different combinations of minocycline, EDTA, and 25 percent ethanol, rapidly eradicates organisms embedded in biofilm. *Antimicrob Agents Chemother.* 2007 Jan;51(1):78–83.

Safdar N, Fine JP, Maki DG. Meta-analysis: methods for diagnosing intravascular device-related bloodstream infection. *Ann Intern Med.* 2005;142(6):451–466.

Veenstra DL, et al. Efficacy of antiseptic-impregnated central venous catheters in preventing catheter-related bloodstream infection: a meta-analysis. *JAMA.* 1999; 281:261–267.

106. Infections Associated with Urinary Catheters

Lindsay E. Nicolle

Urinary tract infections (UTIs) are a common and clinically important outcome of the use of urinary catheters. Urinary catheters may be (1) short-term indwelling urethral catheters, (2) long-term indwelling urethral catheters, or (3) intermittent catheterization.

A patient has a short-term indwelling catheter when the duration of catheterization is less than 30 days and a long-term indwelling catheter when the catheter remains in situ more than 30 days. Considerations for indwelling suprapubic catheters are similar to those for indwelling urethral catheters. Different types of catheterization are indicated in different populations and have different risks for the occurrence of infection (Table 106.1).

PATHOGENESIS

Acquisition of urinary infection with catheter use is virtually always through ascending infection (Table 106.2). For indwelling urethral catheters, bacteria usually ascend into the bladder on the mucous sheath on the external surface of the catheter, up the drainage tubing in the urine column, or with bacterial biofilm on the inner surface of the tubing. Organisms colonizing the periurethral area ascending on the external surface of the catheter are a more common source of bacteriuria for women, and organisms gaining access through the tubing occurs more often in men. Disruption of the closed drainage system from the bladder to the drainage bag also may introduce bacteria, and there is a high incidence of urinary infection within 24 hours following such a break in the system. Bacteria introduced at the time of catheterization account for less than 5% of infections.

With intermittent catheterization, organisms are repeatedly introduced into the bladder at catheterization. Individuals managed with intermittent catheterization usually have a neurogenic bladder with incomplete bladder emptying, so organisms, once introduced, may persist in the bladder. The infecting organisms are usually present as colonizing bacteria in the periurethral area but may also be introduced by contamination of the hands of the individual performing catheterization or the catheter itself.

BACTERIOLOGY

Urinary infection identified in the setting of urethral catheterization is considered complicated UTI. *Escherichia coli* remains an important pathogen in these infections, but other organisms are also frequently isolated. These include other Enterobacteriaceae such as *Klebsiella pneumoniae, Citrobacter* species, *Enterobacter* species, and *Serratia marcesens*. For long-term indwelling catheters, in particular, infections with urease-producing organisms such as *Proteus mirabilis, Morganella morganii,* or *Providencia stuartii* are common. *Pseudomonas aeruginosa* and other gram-negative nonfermenters such as *Acinetobacter* species are frequently isolated, as are gram-positive organisms, particularly enterococci and coagulase-negative staphylococci. *Candida albicans* and other yeast species also occur, usually isolated from subjects receiving antimicrobials. The high frequency of recurrent infection requiring repeated courses of antimicrobials promotes acquisition of more resistant organisms.

Polymicrobial bacteriuria is a characteristic of infection in subjects with long-term indwelling catheters but may also occur with other types of catheterization. Long-term indwelling catheters or short-term catheters in situ for more than a few days are covered with a bacterial biofilm, usually greater on the inner surface of the catheter. This biofilm is composed of microorganisms, extracellular bacterial substances, and protein and minerals from urine. There is a complex microbial flora with multiple organisms growing in the biofilm. These organisms are relatively protected from both antimicrobials and the host inflammatory and immune response. Infection is usually present with 2 to 5 organisms at any time. Urine specimens obtained for culture through the biofilm-laden catheter may differ in number, type, and quantity of organisms isolated compared to culture of simultaneous bladder urine.

MORBIDITY AND MORTALITY

Most catheter-acquired urinary infections are asymptomatic. However, symptomatic

Table 106.1 Types of Catheter Use and Frequency of Urinary Infection in Catheterized Populations

Catheter	Usual Population	Infection Rate
Indwelling Urethral		
Short term	Acute-care facility Output monitoring Postsurgical Acute retention	5% per day Women > men
Long term	Long-term care: 5%–10% of residents Chronic retention – men Incontinence – women	100% prevalence
Intermittent catheter	Neurogenic bladder Spinal cord injury Multiple sclerosis Other impaired bladder emptying	1%–3% per catheterization

Table 106.2 Methods by Which Organisms Gain Access to the Bladder in Catheter-Acquired Urinary Infection

Ascending Infection
Introduced at catheterization
Ascending from periurethral area on mucous sheath on external catheter surface
Ascending from interior drainage bag or tubing on biofilm
Intraluminal from drainage bag with urine reflux or bacterial biofilm
Introduced with breaks in closed drainage
Other (uncommon)
Hematogenous from another body site

infection does occur frequently in catheterized subjects and may be associated with significant morbidity. Pyelonephritis, fever, and bacteremia may require hospitalization or result in extended hospitalization when nosocomially acquired. Local symptoms may include prostatitis and epididymitis, purulent urethritis, and urethral abscesses. Bacteriuria with urease-producing organisms is also a cause of catheter obstruction. Acute urinary infection in subjects with spinal cord injury or other neurologic diseases may further impair function through increased lower-limb spasticity or autonomic hyperreflexia. Urinary infection in residents with chronic indwelling urethral catheters is the most frequent cause of bacteremia in long-term care facilities. Occasionally, acute urosepsis associated with catheterization may lead to death. Mortality is uncommon, however, relative to the high frequency of urinary infection and catheter use.

DIAGNOSIS

The diagnosis of urinary infection in a catheterized patient requires microbiologic

documentation. Clinical findings will then determine whether infection is symptomatic or asymptomatic. Culture of an appropriately collected urine specimen is essential. The specimen must be collected before antimicrobial treatment is initiated. It may be obtained directly at the time of catheterization for intermittent catheter use, from a newly placed catheter in subjects with long-term indwelling urethral catheters, or by aspiration from the catheter port of a short-term indwelling catheter. Quantitative criteria for the microbiologic diagnosis of urinary infection are shown in Table 106.3. For short-term indwelling urethral catheters, lower quantitative counts of 10^3 colony-forming units (CFU)/mL or more usually progress to $\geq 10^5$ CFU/mL or more over 24 to 48 hours, unless the catheter is removed or antimicrobial therapy is given.

A diagnosis of symptomatic urinary infection requires a positive urine culture. However, a positive urine culture is common in catheterized patients at any time. Patients with short-term indwelling catheters have an increasing prevalence of bacteriuria the longer the catheter remains in situ; those maintained on intermittent catheterization have a prevalence of about 50% at any time. Virtually all individuals with chronic long-term indwelling catheters are persistently bacteriuric. Thus, although a positive urine culture is necessary for diagnosis of urinary infection, it is not sufficient to identify symptomatic infection—clinical symptoms must also be present.

Clinical presentations consistent with urinary infection are listed in Table 106.4. Although the occurrence of acute pyelonephritis with fever, flank pain and tenderness, or fever with an obstructed catheter may allow a diagnosis of symptomatic urinary infection with a high

Table 106.3 Microbiologic Diagnosis of Urinary Infection in Subjects with Catheter

Clinical Presentation	Quantitative Count of Bacteria
Asymptomatic	$\geq 10^5$ CFU/mL single specimen
Symptomatic Lower tract symptoms[a] Systemic symptoms	 $\geq 10^2$ CFU/mL $\geq 10^4$ CFU/mL

[a] Usually subjects with intermittent catheterization.
Abbreviation: CFU = colony-forming unit.

Table 106.4 Clinical Presentations of Acute Urinary Infection in Subjects with Bladder Catheters

Asymptomatic
Symptomatic
Systemic
Acute pyelonephritis Fever with catheter obstruction Fever with acute hematuria Bacteremia with urinary isolate Increased lower leg spasms or autonomic hyperreflexia in spinal cord injury Fever with no genitourinary localizing findings ($\leq 50\%$ urinary source)
Local[a]
Urethritis Epididymitis Urethral abscess Bladder stones Catheter obstruction Prostatitis Scrotal abscess

[a] Local complications are primarily seen with long-term indwelling urethral catheters.

degree of confidence, there are other presentations where determining a urinary source for symptoms is problematic. A frequent clinical scenario is fever and a positive urine culture, without localizing findings to the genitourinary tract or another potential site of infection. Catheterized patients may present with fever alone as a manifestation of urinary infection. In one study of subjects with long-term indwelling catheters, however, only 33% of such episodes were due to a urinary source. Thus, in the absence of localizing genitourinary findings or bacteremia with the urinary isolate, symptomatic urinary infection is a possible but not definite diagnosis, and alternative diagnoses should also be considered.

Pyuria is a universal accompaniment of bacteriuria in individuals with indwelling catheters and is also present in most bacteriuric patients who use intermittent catheterization. Pyuria may also be present in the absence of bacteriuria due to irritation of the bladder by the catheter. The presence of pyuria or level of pyuria associated with bacteriuria has not been shown to have any prognostic clinical significance. Thus, pyuria is insufficient to make a diagnosis of urinary infection, and the presence of bacteriuria is not, by itself, an indication of symptomatic infection. The absence of pyuria may be helpful in excluding urinary infection in a catheterized subject.

TREATMENT

Treatment of asymptomatic bacteriuria is not indicated for subjects managed by intermittent catheterization or with an indwelling urethral catheter. As previously noted, pyuria is not an indication for treatment in an individual who is asymptomatic. For women, if bacteriuria persists for 48 hours after removing a short-term indwelling catheter, treatment may be indicated.

This clinical question has not been addressed for men, and no definitive recommendation can be given.

When symptomatic infection is clinically diagnosed, a urine specimen for culture should be obtained in every case before initiation of antimicrobial therapy. For individuals with long-term indwelling catheters, the catheter should be replaced immediately before initiating antimicrobial therapy and a specimen for culture obtained from the newly placed catheter. This allows collection of a urine specimen that is representative of bladder rather than biofilm microbiology. Replacing the catheter immediately prior to antimicrobial therapy has also been shown to shorten the time to defervescence and decrease the likelihood of symptomatic relapse in short-term follow-up. It is assumed these beneficial effects result from removal of the biofilm with its high concentration of organisms in a relatively protected environment. For short-term indwelling catheters, where biofilm formation is less likely, routine catheter replacement is not recommended.

Oral antimicrobials appropriate for treatment of urinary infection are listed in Table 106.5, and parenteral antimicrobials are listed in Table 106.6. The decision to initiate oral or parenteral therapy is determined by the patient's clinical status and the likelihood of resistant organisms. Parenteral therapy should

Table 106.5 Oral Antimicrobials for Treatment of Urinary Tract Infection in Catheterized Patients with Normal Renal Function

Antimicrobial	Dosage
Penicillins	
Amoxicillin	500 mg TID
Amoxicillin–clavulanic acid	500/125 mg TID or 875/125 mg BID
Cephalosporins	
Cephalexin	500 mg QID
Cefaclor	500 mg QID
Cefadroxil	1 g OD or BID
Cefuroxime axetil	250 mg BID
Cefixime	400 mg OD
Cefpodoxime proxetil	100–400 mg BID
Fluoroquinolones[a]	
Norfloxacin	400 mg BID
Ciprofloxacin	250–500 mg BID
Ofloxacin	200–400 mg BID
Fleroxacin	400 mg OD
Lomefloxacin	400 mg OD
Levofloxacin	250–500 mg OD
Other	
Nitrofurantoin	50–100 mg QID
Trimethoprim	100 mg BID
Trimethoprim–sulfamethoxazole	160/800 mg BID

[a] Recommended for oral empiric therapy.

Table 106.6 Parenteral Antimicrobials for Treatment of Urinary Tract Infection in Individuals with Normal Renal Function

Antimicrobial	Dosage
Aminoglycoside	
Amikacin	5 mg/kg q8h or 15 mg/kg q24h
Gentamicin[a]	1–1.5 mg/kg q8h or 4–5 mg/kg q24h
Tobramycin[a]	1–1.5 mg/kg q8h or 4–5 mg/kg q24h
Penicillin	
Ampicillin	1–2 g q6h
Piperacillin	3 g q4h
Piperacillin/tazobactam	4 g/500 mg q8h
Ticarcillin/clavulanic acid	50 mg/kg q6h
Cephalosporins	
Cefazolin	1–2 g q8h
Cefoxitin	1 g q8h
Cefotetan	1 g q12h
Cefotaxime	1–2 g BID or TID
Cefepime	2 g q12h
Ceftazidime	0.5–2 g q8h
Other	
Aztreonam	1 g q6h
Imipenem/cilastatin	500 mg q6h
Vancomycin	500 mg q6h or 1 g q12h

[a] Recommended for initial empiric therapy with ampicillin if renal function is normal.

be initiated in patients who are hemodynamically unstable, are vomiting, have impaired gastrointestinal absorption, or have a high likelihood of being infected with an organism resistant to oral agents.

If symptoms are mild, antimicrobial therapy should not be initiated until the urine culture results are available. This allows for selection of antimicrobial therapy specific for the infecting organism. Empiric antimicrobial therapy should be initiated pending urine culture results when a patient is significantly ill with fever or other systemic symptoms or when the patient has severe irritative symptoms. The selection of initial empiric therapy may be assisted by knowledge of bacteriology of previous urine cultures in the patient when available or by resistance patterns of endemic flora in an institution. An aminoglycoside, with or without ampicillin for enterococci, is usually appropriate for initial empiric parenteral therapy. In the presence of moderate to severe renal failure, an extended-spectrum β-lactam antimicrobial or fluoroquinolone may be preferred rather than an aminoglycoside. When there is a concern about resistant organisms, alternative empiric therapy with coverage specific for expected susceptibilities should be selected. Once urine culture and susceptibility results from the pretherapy urine specimen are available, usually 48 to 72 hours after initiation of therapy, antimicrobial therapy can be reassessed and, if appropriate, changed to alternative specific therapy. This will often include a change to oral therapy for patients in whom parenteral therapy was initiated.

If the patient continues to require an indwelling catheter, the treatment duration should be for as short a period as possible (5 to 7 days). Longer courses of therapy will promote the emergence of organisms of increasing resistance, potentially increasing the difficulty in treating future episodes of symptomatic infection. If the catheter is removed, 7 to 14 days of therapy should be given. For subjects managed with intermittent catheterization, 7 days is recommended for lower tract symptoms and 10 to 14 days for systemic infection.

PREVENTION

The most effective means of preventing catheter-associated infection is not to use a catheter or, if there is a compelling clinical indication for use, to limit the duration of catheterization to as short a period as possible (Table 106.7). For short-term indwelling catheters, the maintenance of a closed drainage system is important in delaying acquisition of infection. Antimicrobial therapy given during the first 3 days of catheterization or at the time of catheter removal is associated with a decreased frequency of infection. However, these antimicrobial strategies are not recommended because they are associated with an increased frequency of infection with more resistant organisms. Other interventions that have been systematically evaluated, such as daily periurethral cleaning with either soap or a disinfectant, addition of disinfectants to the drainage bag, and the coating of the catheter with antibacterial substances, are not effective in decreasing the frequency of infection.

It is not clear that any interventions will decrease the frequency of urinary infection with chronic indwelling urethral catheters. Preventive strategies in these patients must focus on preventing symptomatic infection through early identification of catheter obstruction and prevention of catheter trauma to the genitourinary mucosa.

For spinal cord–injured patients managed with intermittent catheterization, use of prophylactic antimicrobials may decrease the frequency of infection in the early postinjury period but

Table 106.7 Prevention of Catheter-Acquired Urinary Tract Infection

Effective
Limit duration of catheter use
Aseptic insertion (for indwelling catheter)
Maintain closed drainage system
Antibiotics first 4 days (not recommended)[a]
Antibiotics at removal (not recommended)[a]

Not Effective
Bladder irrigation with antimicrobial
Periurethral care with soap or disinfectant
Disinfectant in drainage bag
Coating of catheter with antimicrobial substances[b]

[a] Not recommended because of emerging antimicrobial resistance.
[b] Nitrofurazone or silver alloy coating may decrease bacteriuria with short-term catheters but have not been shown to decrease symptomatic infection.

are not effective in the long term. Infection with organisms of increased antimicrobial resistance occurs. Thus, prophylactic antimicrobials are not recommended in patients using intermittent catheterization. Maintenance of bladder volumes of less than 500 mL in these subjects likely decreases the frequency of infection. For nursing home patients, rates of infection with intermittent catheterization are similar if either a clean or sterile catheter technique is used. Thus, clean technique is recommended because it is less costly.

Antimicrobial therapy should be given to subjects with asymptomatic bacteriuria before an invasive genitourinary procedure such as transurethral prostatic resection or stone extraction where there is a high likelihood of mucosal trauma. Antimicrobial therapy is initiated before the surgical procedure and is conceptually "prophylaxis" to prevent bacteremia and sepsis rather than treatment of asymptomatic bacteriuria. Antimicrobial therapy is not indicated before a chronic indwelling urethral catheter change because this is not a high-risk procedure.

Urinary tract infection in catheterized patients is primarily a technological problem of biofilm formation on inert devices. Thus, substantive progress in preventing infections will require technological development of devices resistant to biofilm formation. Many antimicrobial-coated or -impregnated urinary catheters have been developed, and some of these are widely used. Nitrofurazone-coated or silver alloy–coated catheters may result in a small decrease in the incidence of bacteriuria in hospitalized patients with short-term catheters, but there is no evidence that they decrease the frequency of symptomatic infection. Antibiotic-coated catheters would not be anticipated to have any efficacy for long-term catheters. Catheters developed using other biomaterials or coatings are under further investigation, but none have yet been documented to decrease morbidity.

SUGGESTED READING

Cardenas DD, Hooton TM. Urinary tract infection in persons with spinal cord injury. *Arch Phys Med Rehabil.* 1995;76:272–280.

Johnson JR, Kuskowski MA, Wilt TJ. Systematic review: antimicrobial urinary catheters to prevent catheter-associated urinary tract infection in hospitalized patients. *Ann Intern Med.* 2006;144:116–126.

Nicolle LE. Catheter-related urinary tract infection. *Drugs Aging.* 2005;22:627–639.

Trautner BW, Darouiche RO. Role of biofilm in catheter-associated urinary tract infection. *Am J Infect Control.* 2004;32:177–183.

Warren JW. Catheter-associated urinary tract infections. *Infect Dis Clin North Am.* 1997;11:609–622.

Infections Related to Surgery and Trauma

107. Postoperative Wound Infections

E. Patchen Dellinger

Postoperative wound infection is the archetypal surgical infection because it follows a surgical procedure and requires surgical intervention for resolution. As with many infections, best results are obtained by prompt diagnosis and treatment, which is facilitated by understanding the risk factors. The most obvious factor influencing risk of infection is the density of bacterial contamination of the incision. This was recognized several decades ago in the wound classification system that divides all surgical wounds into the following 4 categories: clean, clean-contaminated, contaminated, and dirty. Clean wounds result from an elective procedure without break in technique that does not involve any area of the body other than skin normally colonized by resident bacteria. Clean-contaminated wounds result from a procedure such as elective bowel resection that intentionally opens the gastrointestinal (GI) tract or other colonized region such as the female genital tract but does not result in grossly visible spill of contents during the procedure. Contaminated procedures are those with gross spill from the GI tract or trauma and emergency procedures in which a wound has been created without normal antisepsis and sterile technique. A dirty wound is one that results from an operation in an area of active infection or previous bowel injury and leak. Among these categories, infection risk ranges historically, before modern understanding and practice of perioperative antibiotic prophylaxis, from 2% for clean wounds to 30% to 40% for dirty wounds when the skin is closed primarily.

Studies done many decades ago demonstrate that essentially all surgical incisions, even in clean operations, have some bacteria in the wound at the end of the procedure. Clinicians have recognized that the nature of host defenses and the extent to which the operative procedure or pre-existing disease impairs these defenses also influences the risk of wound infection. Modern wound classifications that include underlying risk as well as the risk of bacterial contamination predict infection more accurately. The most widely used system now assigns 1 point each for wound classification of contaminated or dirty, an operation lasting longer than the 75th percentile for that procedure, and an American Society of Anesthesiology (ASA) physical status classification of 3 or 4. In this system, the risk of postoperative wound infection for patients with risk points of 0, 1, 2, or 3 is 1.5%, 2.9%, 6.8%, and 13.0%, respectively (Table 107.1). These data reflect modern use of perioperative prophylactic antibiotics, as discussed in Chapter 112, Surgical Prophylaxis.

DIAGNOSIS

The diagnosis of postoperative wound infection is obvious when the wound opens and discharges pus. However, the diagnosis is ideally made earlier and prompt therapeutic intervention undertaken. It is rare for a postoperative wound infection to be clinically evident before the fourth or fifth postoperative day. The sole exceptions to this are infections caused by β-hemolytic streptococci and by histotoxic *Clostridium* species and, more rarely, wound toxic shock. These infections can be clinically evident within fewer than 24 hours, and although they are rare, they tend to be devastating. The wound of any patient with severe systemic signs of infection during the first few days after an operation should be inspected for signs of infection (Figure 107.1). Streptococcal infections are marked by local signs of inflammation and at times an exudate containing white blood cells (WBCs) and gram-positive cocci. Clostridial infections lack signs of inflammation and produce a thin exudate lacking WBCs because of the action of the exotoxins, but gram-positive rods without spore formation are evident on Gram smear. Thirteen cases of wound toxic shock were confirmed by the Centers for Disease Control and Prevention (CDC) during an 18-month period, representing less than 1% of all cases of toxic shock reported during that period. More than half of these cases presented within 48 hours of an operation. The earliest signs were fever, diarrhea, and vomiting. Profuse watery diarrhea, erythroderma, and hypotension were also characteristic. Initially, local signs of

Table 107.1 Comparison of National Research Council (NRC) Wound Classification with National Nosocomial Infectious Surveillance (NNIS) Risk Index for Prediction of Surgical-Site Infections (SSI) Risk

| NRC Class | NNIS Risk Index | | | | | Maximum Ratio (NRC)[a] |
	0	1	2	3	All	
Clean	1.0	2.3	5.4	—	2.1	5.4
Clean-contaminated	2.1	4.0	9.5	—	3.3	4.5
Contaminated	—	3.4	6.8	13.2	6.4	3.9
Dirty	—	3.1	8.1	12.8	7.1	4.1
All	1.5	2.9	6.8	13.0	2.8	—
Maximum ratio (NNIS)[a]	2.1	1.7	1.8	1.0	—	—

Modified from Dellinger EP, Ehrenkranz NJ. Surgical infections. In: Bennett JV, Brachman PS, eds. *Hospital Infections*. 4th ed. Philadelphia, PA: Lippincott-Raven; 1998, .

[a] Ratio of the lowest to the highest infection rate in wound class or risk index. Note that the highest maximum ratio for any of the NNIS indices is 2.1, whereas the lowest maximum ratio for any of the NRC wound classes is 3.9. Clearly, the NNIS index more accurately describes the infection risk of operative procedures.

Wound Infection Algorithm

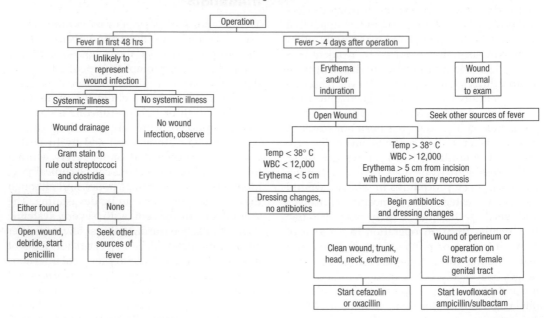

Figure 107.1 Wound infection algorithm.

wound infection were often absent. Drainage and irrigation of the wound in combination with a systemic antistaphylococcal antibiotic is recommended. Although most wound infections are diagnosed between 5 and 15 days after the procedure, in some cases, diagnosis may be delayed considerably. This is more likely with wounds with a significant amount of tissue overlying the area such as abdominal wounds in morbidly obese patients and wound infections under chest wall musculature following a posterolateral thoracotomy.

Because most patients have some fever in the first several days after a major operative procedure such as abdominal exploration or thoracotomy, fever is not a specific sign of postoperative infection (Figure 107.2). It is tempting for the surgeon to continue prophylactic antibiotics or to restart antibiotics if the patient shows early postoperative fever, but this impulse should be resisted because these infections cannot be resolved without opening the wound. When antibiotics are given early without a commitment to open the wound, the most likely results are

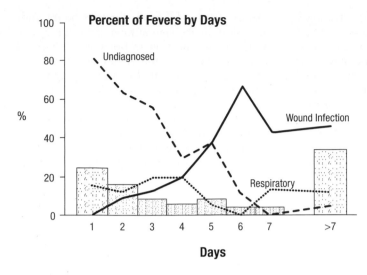

Figure 107.2 Bars represent the percent of all postoperative fevers occurring on the indicated day following an operative procedure. Lines indicate the percentage of fevers occurring on each day attributable to the cause indicated. (From Dellinger EP. Approach to the patient with postoperative fever. In: Gorbach SL, Bartlett JG, Blacklow NR, eds. *Infectious Diseases*. 3rd ed. Philadelphia, PA: Lippincott Williams & Wilkins; 2004:817–823.)

a delay in diagnosis and definitive treatment, a consequent increase in morbidity, and risk of additional complication such as wound dehiscence or herniation. A few surgical wounds exhibit erythema adjacent to the incision, either concentrated around skin sutures or staples or diffusely. In the absence of marked induration and/or drainage, this erythema usually does not indicate wound infection. The average clinician will be sorely tempted to prescribe antibiotics for a patient with such a wound, but most resolve without any specific treatment, and no data suggest that administration of antibiotics in such a situation will prevent the need to open the wound.

THERAPY

Incisional Drainage

The primary treatment for a wound infection is to open the wound and evacuate the infected material. Antibiotics are used as adjunctive treatment only for patients who exhibit signs of significant systemic response to the infection or in whom there is evidence of invasive soft-tissue infection beyond the boundaries of the surgical incision. The evidence for infection may be most prominent in a portion of the incision, but in most cases, the entire incision will be involved under the skin and will have to be opened. If necrotic tissue is found in the wound, some preliminary debridement may be helpful, but the small shreds of involved tissue will separate by themselves over time if the wound is left open and subjected to gauze dressing changes 2 to 3 times daily, decreasing in frequency as the wound clears.

The importance of dressing changes is greater if the wound is deep, as in patients with severe obesity or in posterolateral thoracotomy wounds in muscular patients. If the wound is undermined, it is important to place the dressing so that gauze is in contact with all areas of the wound, but the dressings should not be put in forcefully or under pressure because this causes pain, inhibits drainage of exudate, and stimulates excess scar formation and slows wound closure, which occurs through the normal mechanism of contracture of granulation tissue.

When an incision is opened initially, it should be inspected by a physician who understands the procedure and the underlying anatomy. If the procedure was a celiotomy or a thoracotomy, the integrity of the closure of the abdominal or chest wall should be verified and evidence sought for purulent fluids originating deep to the abdominal or chest wall. In some cases, the incisional infection is not the primary event but is a signal of more severe and more extensive infection at a deeper level (see Chapters 54 and 56, Abdominal Abscess and Peritonitis, respectively).

Antibiotics

Antibiotics should be administered empirically at the time of diagnosis, and opening of the wound should occur only when there are signs of a significant systemic reaction with temperature above 38°C (100.4°F), elevated pulse rate, or absolute WBC count above 12 000; when inspection of the wound reveals invasive infection in the subcutaneous space or at the fascial level; or when surrounding erythema and induration extend >5 cm from the line of incision. The agent chosen should be guided by Gram smear of the wound exudate and the nature of the procedure. Infections following clean operations that have not entered the GI tract and that involve the head and neck, trunk, or extremities tend to be caused by *Staphylococcus aureus* or, less commonly, streptococcal species. If Gram smear confirms gram-positive cocci and if antibiotics will be given, treatment is appropriate with an initial parenteral dose of cefazolin or oxacillin, 1 g intravenously (IV). For patients allergic to penicillin and cephalosporins, clindamycin, 900 mg, or vancomycin, 1 g IV, is acceptable. If the patient can take oral fluids and is not thought to have bacteremia, subsequent treatment can be with oral cephalexin or cephradine, 500 mg, or clindamycin, 450 mg 4 times daily. As community-acquired methicillin-resistent *S. aureus* (CA-MRSA) increase in frequency, consideration should be given to initiating treatment with sulfamethoxazole/trimethroprim, 800/160 mg orally (PO) every 12 hours, doxycycline, 100 mg PO every 12 hours, or vancomycin, 1 g IV every 12 hours, until susceptibility data are available. Antibiotic treatment should be continued only as long as systemic signs of infection or local cellulitis continue to be present, usually 3 days or less.

For infections that follow operations in the axilla, gram-negative enteric bacilli are more commonly causative, and after operations on the perineum or involving the GI tract or the female genital tract both facultative and obligate anaerobic bacilli and cocci are often involved. In these cases, if antibiotic treatment is thought necessary, initial treatment can be ampicillin-sulbactam, 3 g IV every 6 hours, or levofloxacin, 500 mg IV/PO every 24 hours, with or without clindamycin. Patients allergic to penicillin and cephalosporins can receive levofloxacin, 500 mg IV every 12 hours, combined with either clindamycin, 900 mg IV every 8 hours, or metronidazole, 1 g IV every 12 hours, or they can take aztreonam, 1 g IV every 8 hours, plus clindamycin, 900 mg IV every 8 hours. Again, the treatment should usually be 3 days or less. If the patient is able to take oral agents, switching to an oral regimen of amoxicillin-clavulanate, 500 mg every 6 hours, or levofloxacin, 500 mg every 24 hours, combined with either clindamycin, 450 mg, or metronidazole, 500 mg every 6 hours, should be considered.

In the rare patient who has an invasive wound infection caused either by β-hemolytic streptococci or by a histotoxic *Clostridium* species diagnosed in the first 48 hours after operation, aggressive antimicrobial therapy is necessary in addition to opening the wound and inspecting it in the operating room under general anesthesia, with the option of aggressive soft-tissue debridement if evidence of spreading soft-tissue invasion and necrosis is found. Penicillin G, 4 million units IV every 4 hours, is appropriate if the diagnosis of streptococcal or clostridial infection is firm. If in doubt, cefazolin or vancomycin provides treatment for staphylococcal infections in addition to streptococcal and clostridial infections, but the addition of metronidazole for anaerobic coverage may be prudent. CA-MRSA have recently been reported to cause necrotizing soft-tissue infections, so initial treatment of these infections with gram-postive cocci should include the use of vancomycin, 1 g IV every 12 hours.

WOUND CLOSURE

The most reliable method for handling an infected wound that has been opened is to continue dressing changes and allow the wound to close spontaneously by secondary intention. In straightforward wound infections, this results in a very satisfactory result in most cases. In a minority of wounds, the incision can be reclosed, usually with tapes, after the incision has cleared up and is lined by healthy granulation tissue. The failures that occur at this time are as often caused by the geometry of the wound as they are by the bacterial content.

SUGGESTED READING

Culver, DH, Horan TC, Gaynes RP, et al. Surgical wound infection rates by wound class, operative procedure, and patient risk index. National Nosocomial Infections Surveillance System. *Am J Med.* 1991;91(3B):152S–157S.

Dellinger EP. Surgical infections. In: Mulholland MW, Lillemoe KD, Doherty GM, Maier RV, Upchurch GR Jr, eds. *Greenfield's Surgery: Scientific Principles and Practice.* 4th ed. Philadelphia, PA: Lippincott Williams & Wilkins; 2005:163–177.

Dellinger EP. Approach to the patient with postoperative fever. In: Gorbach SL, Bartlett JG, Blacklow NR, eds. *Infectious Diseases.* 3rd ed. Philadelphia, PA: Lippincott Williams & Wilkins; 2004:817–823.

Garibaldi, RA, Brodine S, Matsumiya S, et al. Evidence for the non-infectious etiology of early postoperative fever. *Infect Control.* 1985;6:273–277.

Horan, TC, Gaynes RP, Martone WJ, et al. CDC definitions of nosocomial surgical site infections, 1992: a modification of CDC definitions of surgical wound infections. *Am J Infect Control.* 1992;20:271–274.

Miller LG, Perdreau-Remington F, Rieg G, et al. Necrotizing fasciitis caused by community-associated methicillin-resistant Staphylococcus aureus in Los Angeles. *N Engl J Med.* 2005;352:1445–1453.

National Academy of Sciences, National Research Council, et al. Postoperative wound infections: the influence of ultraviolet irradiation on the operating room and of various other factors. *Ann Surg.* 1964;160 (suppl 2):1.

Stevens DL, Bisno AL, Chambers HF, et al. Practice guidelines for the diagnosis and management of skin and soft-tissue infections. *Clin Infect Dis.* 2005;41:1373–1406.

Paydar KZ, Hansen SL, Charlebois ED, Harris HW, Young DM. Inappropriate antibiotic use in soft tissue infections. *Arch Surg.* 2006; 141:850–854; discussion 855–856.

108. Trauma-Related Infection

Mark A. Malangoni

Infection is a relatively common complication of trauma, particularly among patients with a greater severity of injury. Although exsanguinating hemorrhage and central nervous system injury are the most common causes of early mortality, patients who die more than 48 hours after injury often succumb to infectious complications or their consequences.

Trauma-related infection represents either infection at an original site of injury or infection that occurs as a direct result of the injury. Examples of the former are an infected soft-tissue laceration or osteomyelitis at the site of an open fracture. The latter include empyema after a penetrating wound to the chest and an intra-abdominal abscess that follows a gunshot wound to the colon. Infection also may occur at sites remote from the area of injury; however, these infections usually are related to the use of invasive monitoring devices or lifesaving treatments such as mechanical ventilation, and will not be discussed further.

Injury can lead to infection by (1) direct contamination of a sterile site with exogenous microorganisms; (2) disruption of the natural epithelial barrier of the gastrointestinal, respiratory, or gynecologic tract, with contamination from endogenous microorganisms; (3) impairment of local antimicrobial clearance mechanisms by direct damage to tissue and the introduction of substances such as foreign bodies or hematomas that act as adjuvants to promote infection; and (4) impairment of systemic antimicrobial defenses through secondary effects related to the consequences of injury.

Various pre-existing conditions also may contribute directly to the development of trauma-related infections. Examples include diabetes mellitus, obesity, malnutrition, advanced age, alcoholism, and renal failure. Lack of strict control of hyperglycemia, hypoxemia, and hypothermia may also contribute to the likelihood of developing a trauma-related infection. These pre-existing diseases and perturbations due to the injury per se act by impairing local or systemic defense mechanisms. Invasive and diagnostic interventions such as the placement of endotracheal tubes, intravascular catheters, and urinary catheters provide direct access to sterile body sites, bypassing the normal defenses to infection and providing a portal of entry for pathogens. These microorganisms may cause infection at the site of entry or may cause a distant infection following hematogenous dissemination.

Trauma-related infection occurs either from the introduction of small numbers of highly pathogenic bacteria or following contamination from a large inoculum of less pathogenic organisms. Several potential pathogens are found consistently throughout the body (Table 108.1). Improper treatment can predispose to infection by impairing the clearance of subpathologic concentrations of bacteria. Importantly, the adequacy of the blood supply to the area of injury can affect the propensity to develop infection, and impairments of perfusion because of pre-existing disease or the injury per se will increase the risk of developing a trauma-related infection. Similar to other infections, trauma-related infections occur when there is a disturbance in the normal relationship among microorganisms, the local environment, and innate or acquired host defenses.

Efforts to prevent infection should begin immediately after injury. Initial management includes examination of external wounds to determine the extent and severity of injury and to identify foreign bodies, hematomas, devitalized tissue, and associated fractures. These wounds should be covered with a sterile dressing, preferably moistened with 0.9% normal saline, as soon as possible to prevent further contamination. Bleeding should be controlled by the application of direct pressure or by identification and ligation of bleeding points. Hematomas should be evacuated and injury to specialized tissues such as muscle, tendon, nerve, and vascular structures assessed. Debridement of all devitalized soft tissues is essential to proper wound management. The injury site should be irrigated with a physiologic solution such as 0.9% normal saline as soon as possible; however, this process should not impede transfer of the patient to a trauma center for definitive care.

In traumatic wounds associated with fractures, there is a direct relationship between the

Table 108.1 Potential Pathogens and Their Anatomic Locations

Staphylococcus epidermidis	Skin, oropharynx
Staphylococcus aureus	Skin, oropharynx, upper gastrointestinal tract
Enterococci	Gastrointestinal tract
β-hemolytic streptococci	Oropharynx
Streptococcus pneumoniae	Oropharynx
Anaerobic streptococci	Oropharynx, vagina
Enterobacteriaceae (eg, *Escherichia coli*, *Klebsiella*, *Enterobacter*)	Gastrointestinal tract, vagina, perineum
Candida albicans	Oropharynx, gastrointestinal tract
Clostridium perfringens	Skin, perineum
Bacteroides fragilis	Distal gastrointestinal tract
Bacteroides species (non-*fragilis*)	Oropharynx, gastrointestinal tract

risk of infection and the severity of soft-tissue injury. Early immobilization of the fracture helps reduce additional soft-tissue damage and can help decrease the risk of infection by preventing dissemination of contaminating bacteria. Foreign material must be removed manually or by irrigation.

After appropriate cleansing, debridement, and hemostasis are completed, the type and technique of wound closure can be addressed. In general, simpler techniques are preferred over more elaborate ones. Clean wounds with a low risk for infection should undergo primary closure. Clean wounds at increased risk for infection include those that have devitalized or ischemic tissue, are located near areas of heavy colonization (groin or perineum), have a delay of 6 hours or more to definitive care, and are complicated by the presence of associated diseases that compromise clearance of contaminating organisms. Crush injury, high-velocity and shotgun injuries, coexisting thermal injury, and irregular or stellate configurations are other indicators of wounds at risk for infection. Heavily contaminated wounds or wounds that are at high risk for infection should not be closed initially. In this situation, it is more prudent to repeat cleansing and debridement of the site of injury and delay closure until the wound is cleaned and can be sutured safely. Unless the wound environment can be treated sufficiently to allow for closure with a low risk of infection, wounds should be allowed to heal by secondary intention. Although this may seem

inconvenient for the patient, it often avoids the risks associated with infection.

Stab wounds and low-velocity gunshot wounds can usually be irrigated and closed primarily as long as there has not been significant exogenous or endogenous contamination. With intestinal injury the concentration of microorganisms contaminating the site of injury is increased, and they should not be closed primarily. High-velocity missile track wounds are best managed by debridement and irrigation of entrance and exit sites, followed by coverage with sterile dressings. They should be left open, cleansed 2 to 3 times daily, and allowed to heal by secondary intention. Complex wounds with extensive areas of soft-tissue devitalization are best managed by debridement and irrigation with loose approximation of the skin. Any remaining areas of exposed soft tissue can be managed with wet-to-dry dressing changes using 0.9% normal saline to promote a healthy granulating bed that can be covered later with a split-thickness skin graft or full-thickness skin or can be allowed to heal by secondary intention. Although it may be tempting to use antiseptic or antimicrobial-containing agents for irrigation, these substances offer no advantage in the early treatment of wounds and can impair healing. When wounds that are healing by secondary intention begin to granulate and contract, it may be appropriate to switch to hydrocolloid gels or alginates, which are associated with less discomfort and a less frequent need for dressing changes (usually once daily).

Table 108.2 Antibiotic Therapy for Traumatic Wounds[a]

Clean lacerations	No antibiotics recommended
Heavily contaminated lacerations or lacerations at risk for infection	Cefazolin, 1–2 g IV q8h Amoxicillin–clavulanate, 500 mg PO q12h, or 250 mg PO q8h, or cephalexin, 500 mg PO q6h For penicillin-allergic patients, use Ciprofloxacin 400 mg IV or 500 mg PO q12h plus metronidazole 500 mg IV or PO q6h or Moxifloxacin 400 mg IV or PO q24h
Farm injuries and human bites; soil contamination; delays in care of heavily contaminated wounds	Piperacillin–tazobactam, 3.375 g IV q6h, or Amoxicillin–clavulanate, 500 mg PO q12h, or 250 mg q8h (see Chapter 23, Human and Animal Bites) For penicillin-allergic patients, use Ciprofloxacin 400 mg IV or 500 mg PO q12h plus metronidazole 500 mg IV or PO q6h, or Moxifloxacin 400 mg IV or PO q24h
Penetrating abdominal wounds	Cefotetan, 2 g IV q12h, or Cefoxitin, 2 g IV q6h, or Piperacillin–tazobactam, 3.375 g IV q6h (≤24-h duration); For penicillin-allergic patients, use Ciprofloxacin 400 mg IV q12h plus metronidazole 500 mg IV q6h, or Moxifloxacin 400 mg IV q24h (≤24-h duration)

[a] Local infection data and resistance patterns may require coverage for methicillin-resistant *Staphylococcus aureus* (MRSA), also (v. text)
Abbreviations: IV = intravenously; PO = orally; q8h = every 8 hours.

Negative pressure wound therapy is also useful to reduce the time to healing after contamination has been reduced. It also has the advantage of requiring less frequent dressing changes.

Antibiotic therapy is not a substitute for sound clinical judgment, excellent local wound care, aseptic technique, and careful handling of tissues. For uncomplicated minor wounds with minimal contamination and a low risk of infection, antibiotic therapy is unnecessary. Empiric antibiotic therapy may be beneficial when there is heavy bacterial contamination, an open fracture, involvement of a joint space, major soft-tissue injury, or delay of initial management for greater than 6 hours and for patients who are predisposed to infections. Cultures of contaminated wound sites usually add little to treatment decisions. Tetanus toxoid and tetanus immunoglobulin should be administered in accordance with established guidelines for contaminated wounds. Empiric antibiotic therapy should be directed against gram-positive bacteria in most wounds. When contamination with anaerobes and gram-negative enteric bacteria has occurred, such as with a farm injury or a human bite, the antimicrobial spectrum must include agents effective against these organisms. Treatment should be continued only for 24 hours in wounds with a minor or moderate degree of contamination because longer periods of drug use are not associated with better results. Recommended antibiotic choices are listed in Table 108.2.

There has been a recent increase in the incidence of community-acquired methicillin-resistant *Staphylococcus aureus* (CA-MRSA) infections. The high prevalence of these strains and the continued spread of methicillin-resistant strains in hospitalized patients require a reassessment of the approach to the treatment of patients with infections potentially due to these organisms. It is mandatory that cultures be done at the time of surgical drainage and debridement. When MRSA is suspected, empirical therapy should be chosen based on whether this is a community-acquired or hospital-acquired strain. Hospital-acquired strains usually require treatment with vancomycin, linezolid, or daptomycin, whereas CA-MRSA, in addition to the preceding agents, is often susceptible to trimethoprim–sulfamethoxazole, clindamycin, and tetracyclines.

Intra-abdominal infection after penetrating abdominal trauma is an important paradigm that defines risk factors for trauma-related infection in a single body cavity. Increased patient age, number and degree of organ injuries, units of blood products transfused, and presence of severe contamination, such as with a colon injury, define a group of patients at high risk for infection after penetrating abdominal trauma. These factors are indicators of decreased physiologic reserve, impairments as a result of the systemic effects of injury, the harmful effects of hemorrhagic shock, and the contribution of heavy bacterial contamination to the risk of infection. Because these risk factors cannot be completely defined before operation, empiric treatment with a broad-spectrum cephalosporin effective against gram-negative anaerobes is indicated (Table 108.2). Patients with a low risk of infection need only a single dose of antibiotic, but those with a high risk of infection, such as colon injury, should be treated for 24 hours. Treatment longer than 24 hours is of no added value.

Traditionally, antibiotic therapy for established intra-abdominal infection after penetrating trauma included an aminoglycoside combined with either clindamycin or metronidazole. Because of the risks of nephrotoxicity and difficulty achieving appropriate serum concentrations using aminoglycosides, single-agent regimens such as imipenem–cilastatin or meropenem are preferred. For patients who are allergic to these drugs, ciprofloxacin plus metronidazole or moxifloxacin are useful alternatives.

Bullets or pellets that penetrate the gastrointestinal tract and lodge in soft tissues can result in soft-tissue infections. This usually occurs because of the concomitant consequences of direct tissue injury and bacterial contamination. In this situation, the contaminating foreign body should be removed, debridement done, and the area drained.

SUGGESTED READING

Bozorgzadeh A, Pizzi WF, Barie PS, et al. The duration of antibiotic administration in penetrating abdominal trauma. *Am J Surg.* 1999;177:125–131.

Fridkin SK, Hageman JC, Morrison M, et al. Methicillin-resistant Staphylococcus aureus disease in three communities. *N Engl J Med.* 2005;352:1436–1444.

Stewart RM, Myers JG, Dent DL. Wounds, bites, and stings. In: Moore EE, Feliciano DV, Mattox KL, eds. *Trauma.* 5th ed. New York, NY: McGraw-Hill; 2004:1059–1077.

109. Infected Implants

Isabella Rosa-Cunha and Gordon Dickinson

This chapter addresses infections associated with artificial devices of a specialized nature. Optimal treatment requires participation of surgical specialists experienced in the management of these difficult infections. This is especially the case for pseudophakic endophthalmitis, in which therapy includes intraocular injections.

INTRAOCULAR LENS-ASSOCIATED INFECTIONS (PSEUDOPHAKIC ENDOPHTHALMITIS)

Cataract surgery is one of the most commonly performed operations in the United States. More than 1 million intraocular lenses are implanted each year. Pseudophakic endophthalmitis is a serious complication after cataract surgery, and despite modern pharmacological and surgical methods, its treatment is still difficult and may threaten visual acuity. Fortunately, the incidence of pseudophakic endophthalmitis is very low. Pseudophakic endophthalmitis is thought to occur as a consequence of contamination with flora of the conjunctival sac or lid margin at the time of surgery. There also have been reports of infections arising from contamination of lenses and neutralizing and storage solutions.

The differential diagnosis of endophthalmitis following cataract extraction includes sterile inflammation as well as bacterial and fungal infection. The most common presenting signs and symptoms include pain in the involved eye, decreased visual acuity, red eye, lid edema, hypopyon, and absent or poor red reflex. A single bacterial strain is usually isolated; the most common pathogen is a coagulase-negative staphylococcus (approximately 50% in one large series) followed by *Staphylococcus aureus*. Virtually any microorganism can be implicated. Delayed-onset pseudophakic endophthalmitis has been reported after uncomplicated initial cataract surgery. This entity presents one or more months after surgery and is manifest by waxing and waning ocular inflammation. The leading cause of delayed-onset pseudophakic endophthalmitis is *Propionibacterium acnes*. Diagnostic evaluation requires aqueous and vitreous samples for Gram stain and culture.

Vitrectomy may have therapeutic as well as diagnostic value.

Patients should be seen by an ophthalmologist immediately. Antimicrobials administered intraocularly and topically are the mainstay of treatment for this localized infection. Because of unpredictable antibiotic penetration, systemic antibiotics are of secondary importance and generally unnecessary (see Chapter 15, Endophthalmitis).

BREAST IMPLANT–ASSOCIATED INFECTIONS

Breast implants are used in reconstruction of the breast following mastectomy or for cosmetic purposes. It is estimated that in the United States >130000 breast implants are inserted annually. The implants typically consist of silicone shells filled with silicone gel or saline (silicone gel implants have recently been reapproved for use in the United States). They are implanted in a subglandular or submuscular pocket through inframammary, transaxillary, periareolar, or transareolar approaches. Breast implant–related infection is not common; however, it is the leading complication following breast implant placement, with an average incidence rate of 2% to 2.5%. Endogenous flora of human breast tissue is similar to skin flora and accounts for most infections. Contaminated implants, contaminated saline, the surgery itself, or hematogenous seeding of the implant may also be a source of breast implant–associated infection. The most common pathogen is *S. aureus*, followed by coagulase-negative staphylococcus and *Propionibacterium* sp. Other less common organisms include *Lactobacillus*, diphtheroids, *Bacillus*, and α-streptococcus. Fungal infection has been reported but is rare. The patient's underlying condition and surgical technique are the major infection risk determinants. The signs and symptoms are variable, but common findings are fever, tenderness, induration, breast erythema, and ultrasonographic evidence of fluid around the prosthesis. Severe sepsis can develop, and there are case reports of toxic shock syndrome.

Clusters as well as sporadic infections caused by *Mycobacterium fortuitum* complex have been reported. The source of the pathogen is usually not identified, and the route of infection is unknown. Local signs and symptoms are similar to other breast implant infection and usually are accompanied by a history of lack of improvement on standard antibiotic therapy. Systemic symptoms are usually absent. The onset of infection is more subtle than those caused by other pathogens and may range from 1 week to 2 years after implantation. Gram stain of the fluid usually reveals no organisms but many polymorphonuclear leukocytes. Stain for acid-fast bacilli is sometimes positive. A definitive diagnosis is established by culture of the organism.

Breast implant–associated infections are treated with systemic antibiotics. Empiric therapy should target the most common pathogens. Because methicillin-resistant *S. aureus* and methicillin-resistant coagulase-negative staphylococci have become increasingly common, empiric regimens should include vancomycin or another agent active against such resistant strains. Subsequent adjustment should be made according to culture results. Agents with potential activity for most organisms of the *M. fortuitum* complex include amikacin, cefoxitin, fluoroquinolones, clarithromycin, azithromycin, doxycycline, and imipenem, but susceptibility studies should be obtained, and combination of two or more effective agents is recommended to prevent development of resistance. Duration of the therapy will depend on the causative organism, severity of infection, and clinical response, but it usually ranges from 10 to 14 days. Infections caused by mycobacteria require months of therapy. Removal of the implant is mandatory in most cases with debridement of the capsule surrounding it, and postsurgical drainage is advocated. The preferred practice of surgical replacement entails a 2-stage procedure. Whether the contralateral implant should also be removed is a matter of debate.

PENILE IMPLANT–ASSOCIATED INFECTION

The first artificial penile prosthesis was implanted in the early 1970s. Since then, several penile prostheses have been developed and, despite the advent of effective oral agents for the treatment of erectile dysfunction, penile prosthesis implantation remains an effective and acceptable treatment for the group of men who fail conservative therapy. Annually in the United States, approximately 15 000 inflatable penile implants are inserted. Infection of the penile prosthesis represents the major complication of this type of prosthesis and is estimated to occur in 3% of cases. Many risk factors for infections have been mentioned, including diabetes mellitus, duration of surgery, immunosuppression, reoperation for technical failures, and inadequate prophylactic antibiotic coverage. The use of antimicrobial coating on the prosthesis has been shown to reduce the infection rate significantly. Most penile prosthesis–associated infections likely originate in the operating room at the time of the implantation. Common sources of infection include skin, colorectal and perianal flora, urine, and operating room environment. Infection can present within days after surgery to several weeks or months postimplantation. *Staphylococcus epidemidis* is isolated in more than 50% of cases; other bacteria include *S. aureus* and gram-negative enteric bacteria such as *Escherichia coli, Pseudomonas aeruginosa, Klebsiella* sp., and *Proteus sp*. Gonococcal and fungal infections have been reported. Signs and symptoms of infections include new-onset pain, swelling, tenderness, erythema, induration, fluctuance, erosion, and extrusion of prosthesis. Infections caused by *S. epidermidis* are often subtle and may present with dysfunction of the prosthesis or pain upon manipulation of the device.

Empiric antibiotic therapy treatment should be directed at both gram-positive bacteria and gram-negative coliform bacteria, pending isolation of the causative pathogen. There is universal consensus that if a penile implant–associated infection occurs, the implant and all associated foreign material should be removed. There are, however, diverging views about surgical management. The preferred approach is a 2-stage operation with the infection-associated device removed and the wound allowed to heal, followed by replacement 4 to 6 months later. For selected patients, surgeons may elect to remove the infection-associated device, debride the wound, and implant a new device in a single-stage operation. For uncomplicated infections, a 10- to 14-day course of systemic antibiotics is given, whereas for complicated infections, antibiotic therapy should be continued for a week or more after all signs of infection have resolved.

SUGGESTED READING

Clegg HW, Foster MT, Sanders WE Jr, Baine WB. Infection due to organisms of the mycobacterium fortuitum complex after augmentation mammoplasty: clinical and epidemiologic features. *J Infect Dis*. 1983;147:427–433.

Darouiche RO. Treatment of infections associated with surgical implants. *N Engl J Med*. 2004;350:1422–1429.

Results of the Endophthalmitis Vitrectomy Study. A randomized trial of immediate vitrectomy and of intravenous antibiotics for the treatment of postoperative bacterial endophthalmitis. Endophthalmitis Vitrectomy Study Group. *Arch Ophthalmol*. 1995;113:1479–1496.

Pittet B, Montandon D, Pittet D. Infection in breast implants. *Lancet Infect Dis*. 2005;5:94–106.

110. Infection in the Burn-Injured Patient

Roger W. Yurt and Rafael Gerardo Magaña

The diagnosis of infection in the patient with major burn injury is especially problematic because the signs of infection are the same as those of the response to injury.

The tissue injury that occurs with a major burn and the associated inflammatory response to it cause one of the greatest perturbations of homeostasis that occurs in any disease state. Thus the greatest challenge in developing a differential diagnosis in the burn-injured patient is to distinguish between the injury state and infection. That the manifestation of infection may be blunted by diminished immune response further complicates evaluation of the patient while also contributing to an increased susceptibility to infection.

The challenge posed in the clinical and laboratory evaluation of the burn-injured patient is summarized in the outline of injury-related changes in Table 110.1.

INJURY PATHOPHYSIOLOGY AND SUCEPTIBILITY TO INFECTION

The initial approach to the burn-injured patient is oriented toward limiting the progression of the injury by stabilization of the patient and maintenance of blood flow to the wound. The zone of coagulative necrosis consists of tissue that has been irreversibly damaged, whereas the surrounding zone of stasis contains areas of potentially reversible injury. Adjacent areas, known as the hyperemic zone, may also evolve to become necrotic if the blood flow is not maintained. For this reason, the primary goal of early burn therapy is to ensure adequate delivery of oxygen, nutrients, and circulating cells to the wound. In addition to prevention of progression of the injury, immediate burn care focuses on maintenance of a viable tissue interface at which both specific and nonspecific defenses against infection can be mounted.

The depth of burn injury is categorized as partial or full thickness. Full-thickness injuries will heal only by contraction, ingrowth of surrounding epidermis, or grafting of tissue because all epidermis in the wound has been destroyed. These wounds are leathery and dry,

Table 110.1 Clinical and Laboratory Signs Related to Injury That Complicate the Evaluation of the Patient with Burn Injury

Sign	Abnormality
General condition	Lethargy-Electrolyte imbalance Analgesic effects Hyperventilation Pain, topical agents Tachycardia Pain, volume depletion, hypermetabolism
Fluid balance	Hypovolemia Initial injury Delayed-evaporative loss
Fluid composition	Hypernatremia Free water loss Inadequate fluid replacement Hyponatremia Excessive free water Effects of topical silver nitrate Hyperglycemia Stress
Temperature	Hypothermia Heat loss to the environment Large fluid requirement Hyperthermia Hypermetabolism Endotoxin from the wound
Neutrophil response	Neutrophilia Acute 5–7 days after injury Neutropenia 2–3 days after injury

contain thrombosed vessels, and are insensate. Partial thickness wounds contain residual epidermis, which can close the wound if blood flow is maintained and infection does not supervene.

Burn wounds are erythematous and moist, and pain is elicited by touch. Deep partial-thickness wounds contain only epithelial elements associated with organelles of the skin. They take longer to heal (2 to 3 weeks) than superficial partial-thickness wounds, and there is a greater functional and cosmetic deformity if they are allowed to heal primarily. These wounds are difficult to differentiate by clinical evaluation from superficial partial-thickness injuries, which usually heal within 10 days to 2 weeks.

The dynamic aspect of burn wounds is dramatically seen when partial-thickness wounds convert to full-thickness wounds during a difficult resuscitation of a patient. Although this is rarely seen with current methods of resuscitation, resuscitation that is delayed or performed on patients at extremes of age occasionally will show this progression.

Any agent that causes cellular death can lead to a deeper wound. With this in mind, caustic topical agents and vasopressors are avoided, the wound is not allowed to desiccate, and the patient is kept warm.

Both mortality and susceptibility to infection correlate directly with the extent of the surface area injury. Distribution of surface area varies with age, so a chart is used to plot accurately the extent and depth of surface area burned. The rule of nines may be used to estimate the extent of injury as follows: torso, back and front, each 18%; each leg 18%; each arm 9%; and head 9%. Calculation of the extent of injury is helpful in estimating fluid requirements and prognosis. Patients with greater than 25% to 30% total body surface area burn exhibit the pathophysiologic features already described.

PREVENTION OF INFECTION

Current data do not support the general use of prophylactic systemic antibiotics in the inpatient population. Frequent evaluation of the wound and surrounding tissue allows early and appropriate therapy of cellulitis while sparing a majority of patients exposure to unnecessary antibiotics. However, it is common practice to give systemic antibiotics (penicillin) to outpatients with burns because it is not possible to observe closely and ensure appropriate care of the wound. The use of systemic antibiotics in these patients is individualized such that those who are likely to follow up with their care and recognize changes in their wounds are not given antibiotics. The one time that prophylactic systemic antibiotics are used in inpatients is at the time of surgical manipulation because this may cause bacteremia. Antibiotics are administered immediately before and during burn wound excision. The choice of antibiotics is dictated by knowledge of the current flora in the burn center or, more specifically, by the burn wound flora of the individual patient.

The mainstay of prevention of burn wound infection is aggressive removal of the necrotic tissue and closure of the wound with autograft. In the interim, topical antimicrobial prophylaxis will decrease the incidence of conversion of partial-thickness to full-thickness wound by local infection, and these agents may prolong the sterility of the full-thickness burn wound. Silver sulfadiazine is the most commonly used topical agent and is a soothing cream with good activity against gram-negative organisms. Because it does not penetrate the wound, it is used only as a prophylactic antimicrobial. Bacterial resistance to silver sulfadiazine has been reported, and it has been reported to cause neutropenia. Silver nitrate in a 0.5% solution is an effective topical agent when used before wound colonization. This agent does not penetrate the eschar, and therefore its broad-spectrum gram-negative effectiveness is diminished once bacterial proliferation has occurred in the eschar. Additional disadvantages of this agent include the need for continuous occlusive dressings, which limits the evaluation of wounds and restricts range of motion. The black discoloration of the wound, as well as the environment, contributes to the decrease in the use of silver nitrate. Mafenide acetate (Sulfamylon) cream has a broad spectrum of activity against staphylococci. A significant advantage of this agent is that it penetrates burn eschar and therefore is effective in the colonized wound. The disadvantages of Sulfamylon are a transient burning sensation, an accentuation of postinjury hyperventilation, and inhibition of carbonic anhydrase activity.

Recent experience with a new silver-impregnated dressing that does not have to be changed daily suggests that this agent is a good alternative for prophylaxis against infection in partial-thickness wounds.

The goal of burn therapy is to prevent burn wound infection by permanent closure of the wound as rapidly as possible. Early removal of necrotic tissue and wound closure has the advantages of removal of eschar before colonization, which typically occurs 5 to 7 days after injury, and of reduction of the overall extent of injury. A drawback of early excisional therapy is the possibility that burned tissue that may heal if left alone over a 2- to 3-week period may be unnecessarily excised.

Advances in resuscitation have led to the ability to salvage an increasing number of patients from the shock phase immediately after injury and have resulted in a greater number of patients surviving to the time (2 to 3 days after the injury) when the effects of inhalation injury become clinically prominent. In patients without inhalation injury but with large burns, postinjury hyperventilation and subsequent decreases in tidal volume may lead to atelectasis and subsequent pneumonia. Diminished mucociliary function and destruction of the airways by inhalation of products of combustion lead to airway obstruction and infection.

Frequent diagnostic and therapeutic bronchoscopies are necessary in this group of patients. Attempts at specific prophylaxis of the sequelae of inhalation injury, such as nebulization of antibiotics and treatment with steroids, have failed to show any benefit.

Nosocomial infections are of even greater concern in the burn intensive care setting than other units because of the large open colonized wounds. Cross-contamination is avoided by use of gowns, gloves, and masks by nurses, medical staff, and visitors. The patient is not touched except with a gloved hand, and each patient is restricted to his or her own monitoring and diagnostic equipment. If adequate nursing care can be provided, it is preferable to isolate patients who have large open wounds in individual rooms. Cohort patient care has been shown to be effective in reducing endemic infections.

DIAGNOSIS AND TREATMENT OF INFECTIONS

Wound Infection

Because the full-thickness burn wound is at high risk for infection, routine clinical and laboratory surveillance of the wound is an absolute necessity. Daily observation of the wound for discoloration, softening or maceration of the eschar, or the development of cellulitis provides early detection of wound-associated infection. Although surface cultures of the burn wound provide insight into the organisms that are colonizing the wound, evaluation of a biopsy of the burn wound is the only way to obtain accurate assessment of the status of the wound. Systematic evaluation of burn wounds with quantitative culture of biopsies of all areas of wound change documents the clinical diagnosis of wound infection and provides identification and antimicrobial sensitivity of the involved organism. Routine biopsy of full-thickness burn wounds on an every-other-day schedule provides evidence of advancing wound infection and serves as a basis for initiating therapy. A rapid fixation technique allows histologic diagnosis of invasive infection within 3 hours, whereas quantitative counts and identification of the organism is available in 24 hours.

This combined use of histologic and culture techniques provides early diagnosis as well as the identity of the organism and its sensitivity to antimicrobials. When the findings are consistent with invasive infection (greater than or equal to 10^5 organisms/g of tissue), aggressive surgical therapy is instituted to excise the involved wound. In preparation for surgery or in patients who require stabilization before general anesthesia is given, a penetrating topical agent is used (Sulfamylon). The choice of antibiotic is based on previous biopsy sensitivity data or data accumulated on sensitivities of the current flora in the patient population.

A growing number of patients present with primary nonsuppurative gram-positive infections. These infections are often caused by methicillin-resistant *Staphylococcus aureus* (personal observation), and whether diminished neutrophil response or a change in the nature or the virulence of such organisms may explain this phenomenon is unknown.

Pulmonary Infection

From a practical standpoint, inhalation injury is diagnosed by history, physical examination, and bronchoscopy. A history of exposure to fire in a closed space along with findings of carbonaceous sputum, singed nasal vibrissae, and facial burns are associated with a high incidence of inhalation injury. In the burn patient, pulmonary complications after injury are not uncommon and may increase the mortality rate of ventilator-associated pneumonia (VAP), which may increase from 40% to 60%–77% in the presence of significant inhalation injury. Bronchoscopy reveals upper airway edema and erythema, whereas bronchorrhea, carbon in the bronchi, and mucosal slough suggest lower airway and parenchymal injury.

Carboxyhemoglobin levels may be elevated, but with a half-life of 45 minutes on 100% oxygen the level may be normal. Chest x-ray studies are of little value in making the diagnosis of inhalation injury because they are often normal for the first 72 hours after injury. Xenon ventilation–perfusion lung scan reveals trapping of xenon in the ventilation phase and is supportive of a diagnosis of small airway obstruction secondary to injury of the distal airways and parenchyma. Although hematogenous pneumonia is less common than in the past, it remains a significant problem in the patient with burns. When it occurs, the source (most commonly the wound or suppurative vein) must be defined and eradicated.

Prophylactic antibiotics are not used for either bronchopneumonia or hematogenous pneumonia; specific therapy is based on knowledge of previous endobronchial culture, and sensitivity is substantiated by repeat cultures at the time of diagnosis. Diagnosing pneumonia in this population may be difficult. Different clinical scores have been developed to this end; however, they are of little value because they have low specificity and sensitivity when compared to specimens obtained via bronchoalveolar lavage. A culture with 10^4 organisms/mL is generally considered to be significant enough to warrant antibiotic therapy. Bronchoalveolar lavage with negative results also reduces the usage of unnecessary antibiotics.

Suppurative Thrombophlebitis

Suppurative thrombophlebitis is mentioned in particular in relation to the patient with burn injury because it is the most common cause of repeatedly positive blood cultures in the presence of appropriate antibiotics in this population. These findings alone should lead to a presumptive diagnosis of a suppurative process in a previously cannulated vein. The process may be insidious, with only minimal clinical findings. Because this complication is common, venous cannulation should be minimized, but when it is necessary catheters should be exchanged every 3 days. Treatment consists of surgical excision of the entire involved vein to the level of normal bleeding vessel. In this setting the differential diagnosis should include endocarditis.

Chondritis/Suppurative Chondritis

Burn wounds that involve the ear are of particular concern, because its cartilage has no intrinsic blood supply and thus has the potential to develop chondritis and subsequent suppurative chondritis. Because the ear is covered only by skin and has no subcutaneous tissue, the cartilage is at risk for infection when there is a full-thickness burn causing local necrosis. This often leads to loss of tissue and permanent deformity and, in some cases, loss of the ear.

Damaged skin acts as a portal of entry. In addition, local edema may predispose to thrombosis of central vessels. *Pseudomonas* and *Staphylococcus* are the most common pathogens involved in this pathology.

Sulfamylon is of benefit in this condition because it can penetrate eschar to the level of cartilage and prevent bacterial invasion.

Pressure-related damage to the ear must be avoided. Therefore, the ear should be dressed in topical only or topical and one layer of nonadherent gauze. To avoid pressure on the ear, a pillow for the head should not be allowed.

Once suppurative chondritis ensues, surgical intervention is mandatory and consists of drainage and debridement of all nonviable tissue. This can be accomplished by making an incision on the helical rim of the ear (bivalving), with subsequent drainage and excision of nonviable tissue. The ear is then dressed with an antibacterial solution, changed on a twice-daily schedule, and allowed to heal by secondary intention. Special attention should be given to avoid any form of compression to keep the dressings in place, because this may increase the extent of necrosis.

SUGGESTED READING

Andrews CP, Coalson JJ, Smith JD, Johanson WG Jr. Diagnosis of nosocomial bacterial pneumonia in acute, diffuse lung injury. *Chest*. 1981;80:254.

Corce MA, Swanson JM. *The Futility of the Clinical Pulmonary Infection Score in Trauma Patients*.

Darling GE, Keresteci MA, Ibanes D, et al. Pulmonary complications in inhalation injuries with associated cutaneous burn. *J Trauma*. 1996;40:83–89.

Dowling JA, Foly FD, Moncrief JA. Chondritis in the burned ear. *Plast Reconstr Surg*. 1968;42:115–122.

Fagon JY, Chastre J, Hance AJ, et al. Evaluation of clinical judgment in the identification and treatment of nosocomial pneumonia in ventilated patients. *Chest*. 1993;103:547.

Jordan MH, Gallagher JM, Allely RR, Leman CJ. A pressure prevention device for burned ears. *J Burn Care Rehabil*. 1992;13:673–677.

Johnson WG, Seidenfeld JJ, Gomez P, et al. Bacteriologic diagnosis of nosocomial pneumonia following prolonged mechanical ventilation. *Am Rev Respir Dis*. 1988;137:259–264.

Kamal A, Kamel AH, El Oteify M. *Annals of Burns and Fire Disasters: Early Management of the Burned Auricle*. Vol. XVII. Assiut University Hospital, Assiut, Egypt: Burns Unit, Plastic and Reconstructive Surgery Department; 2004.

Meduri GU. Diagnosis and differential diagnosis of ventilator-associated pneumonia. *Clin Chest Med*. 1995;16:61.

Polk HC Jr. Quantitative tracheal cultures in surgical patients requiring mechanical ventilatory assistance. *Surgery*. 1975;78:485–491.

Shirani KZ, Pruitt BA, Mason AD. The influence of inhalation injury and pneumonia on burn mortality. *Ann Surg.* 1987;205:82–87.

Wahl WL, Ahrns KS, Brandt MM, et al. Bronchioalveolar lavage in diagnosis of ventilator-associated pneumonia in patients with burns. *J Burn Care Rehabil.* 2005;26:57–61.

Yurt RW. Burns. In: Polk HC, Gardner V, Stone HH, eds. *Basic Surgery.* St. Louis, MO: Quality Medical; 1993.

Yurt RW. Burns. In: Mandell GL, Gennett JE, Dolin R, eds. *Mandell, Douglas, and Bennett's Principles and Practices of Infectious Diseases.* 6th ed. New York, 2005, Churchill Livingstone.

PART XV

Prevention of Infection

111. Nonsurgical Antimicrobial Prophylaxis

James P. Steinberg and Nadine G. Rouphael

PREVENTION

Chemoprophylaxis is the use of an antimicrobial agent to prevent infection. Chemoprophylaxis is often administered after exposure to a virulent pathogen or before a procedure associated with risk of infection. Chronic chemoprophylaxis is sometimes administered to persons with underlying conditions that predispose to recurrent or severe infection. Antibiotics can also be used to prevent clinical disease in persons infected with a microorganism such as *Mycobacterium tuberculosis*. This strategy has been called secondary prophylaxis but is now referred to as pre-emptive therapy. Immunization, another excellent means of preventing infection, is discussed in Chapter 113, Immunizations. This chapter discusses the specific areas where antimicrobial prophylaxis is generally accepted. For information on prophylaxis of bacterial endocarditis, see Chapter 36, Endocarditis of Natural and Prosthetic Valves: Treatment and Prophylaxis; for information on prophylaxis in persons infected with the human immunodeficiency virus (HIV), see Chapter 100, Prophylaxis of Opportunistic Infections in HIV Disease; for malaria prophylaxis, see Chapter 198, Malaria: Treatment and Prophylaxis; for prophylaxis related to transplant recipients and neutropenic patients, see Chapter 87, Infections in Transplant Patients, and Chapter 84, Infections in the Neutropenic Patient; and for surgical prophylaxis, see Chapter 112, Surgical Prophylaxis.

Several concepts are important in determining whether chemoprophylaxis is appropriate for a particular situation. In general, prophylaxis is recommended when the risk of infection is high or the consequences significant. The nature of the pathogen, type of exposure, and immunocompetence of the host are important determinants of the need for prophylaxis. The antimicrobial agent should eliminate or reduce the probability of infection or, if infection occurs, reduce the associated morbidity. The ideal agent is inexpensive, orally administered in most circumstances and has few adverse effects. The ability to alter the normal microbial flora and select for antimicrobial resistance should be limited, so duration of prophylaxis as well as choice of agents is critical. The emerging crisis of antibiotic-resistant bacteria underscores the importance of rational and not indiscriminate use of antimicrobial agents. In addition, the development of antibiotic-resistant pathogens necessitates reassessment of many of the established prophylactic regimens.

The efficacy of chemoprophylaxis is well established in situations such as perioperative antibiotic administration, exposure to invasive meningococcal disease, prevention of recurrent rheumatic fever, and prevention of tuberculosis. Chemoprophylaxis is accepted in other situations without supporting data. When the risk of infection is low, such as with bacterial endocarditis following dental procedures, randomized clinical trials of prophylaxis are not feasible. However, the consequences of infection may be catastrophic, providing a compelling argument for chemoprophylaxis despite the low risk of infection. When prophylaxis is advocated without data confirming efficacy, there should be a scientific rationale to support the use of a particular antimicrobial agent.

Table 111.1 lists the situations in which antimicrobial prophylaxis is indicated after exposure to certain pathogens. Because the duration of exposure is usually brief, the duration of chemoprophylaxis is short, which helps limit adverse reactions, minimizes the potential for resistance, and limits cost. Some of these pathogens are virulent and can produce serious disease in normal hosts. With exposure to pathogens that cause meningitis, the decision whether to use prophylaxis can be complicated. Because of fear and anxiety provoked by these illnesses there is a tendency to provide prophylaxis to persons outside the high-risk populations. Table 111.1 includes chemoprophylaxis for human, dog, and cat bites. It is important to remember that, aside from antibiotics, immunization (rabies and tetanus vaccines), irrigation, and debridement are crucial in the management of both animal and human bites. Table 111.1 also includes microorganisms that have gained notoriety as possible agents of

Table 111.1 Prophylaxis Following Selected Exposures

Exposure	Pathogen	Prophylaxis[a]	Comments
Meningitis and meningococcal bacteremia	*Neisseria meningitidis* (see Chapters 141, Meningococcus and Miscellaneous Neisseriae, and 73, Bacterial Meningitis)	Rifampin, 600 mg (5 mg/kg for children ≤1 mo and 10 mg/kg for children >1 mo) q12h for 4 doses Ciprofloxacin, 500 mg (single dose) (adults only) Ceftriaxone, 250 mg IM 1 dose (125 mg for children ≤15 y)	Recommended for close contacts only (eg, household contacts, roommates, day-care contacts); prophylaxis not recommended for health care workers unless very close contact such as mouth-to-mouth resuscitation or intubation: secondary cases reported with meningococcal pneumonia, but role of prophylaxis is uncertain; sulfonamide resistance precludes routine use of sulfadiazine
Meningitis	*Haemophilus influenzae*	Rifampin, 600 mg (20 mg/kg for children) daily for 4 d	Recommended for unvaccinated children ≤4 years after exposure at home or day care: when such a child is present, prophylaxis should be given to all household contacts (except pregnant women) regardless of age: index case should receive prophylaxis to eradicate nasopharyngeal colonization
Perinatal group B streptococcus (GBS)	Group B streptococcus	Penicillin G, 5 million units IV initial dose then 2.5 million q4h, or ampicillin, 2 g IV initial dose then 1 g IV q4h, until delivery If penicillin allergic use clindamycin, 900 mg IV q8h, or cefazolin, 2 g loading dose then 1g IV q8h, or erythromycin, 500 mg IV q6h, or vancomycin, 1g IV q12h until delivery	Women should be screened with vaginal and rectal swabs at 35–37 wk of gestation and intrapartum prophylaxis given if GBS isolated. Prophylaxis should also be given if (1) history of GBS bacteriuria, (2) GBS disease during previous pregnancy, or (3) with unknown GBS status and either intrapartum temperature >38°C or >18 h of ruptured membranes or delivery ≤37 wk of gestation
Human bite	*Streptococcus viridans,* other streptococci, oral anaerobes, *Staphylococcus aureus, Eikenella corrodens*	Amoxicillin–clavulanic acid, 875/125 mg BID or 500/125 mg TID for 3–5 d For penicillin allergy, consider clindamycin, 300 mg QID, plus either ciprofloxacin, 500 mg BID, or TMP–SMX, 1 double-strength tablet BID	Risk of infection depends on the depth of the wound, extent of tissue damage, and the etiologic pathogen: *Eikenella* is resistant to clindamycin, first-generation cephalosporins, and erythromycin Clenched-fist injuries often require parenteral antibiotics
Cat bite	*Pasteurella multocida, S. aureus,* streptococci	Amoxicillin–clavulanic acid, 875/125 mg BID or 500/125 mg TID for 3–5 d For penicillin allergy, consider doxycycline, 100 mg BID, or cefuroxime axetil, 500 mg BID	A high percentage of cat bites become infected without prophylaxis Clindamycin and first-generation cephalosporins are not as active as penicillin against *P. multocida,* which is present in oral flora of 50% to 70% of cats
Dog bite	*S. viridans,* oral anaerobes, *S. aureus, P. multocida, Capnocytophaga canimorsus* (formerly DF-2)	Amoxicillin–clavulanic acid, 875/125 mg BID or 500/125 mg TID for 3–5 d For penicillin allergy, consider doxycycline, 100 mg BID, or clindamycin, 300 mg QID, plus either ciprofloxacin, 500 mg BID, or TMP–SMX, 1 double-strength tablet BID	Infection less common than with cat or human bites; need for routine prophylaxis for all bites uncertain; persons without spleens at risk of overwhelming *Capnocytophaga* sepsis, should receive prophylaxis following any dog bite
Sexual assault	*Trichomonas vaginalis, Chlamydia trachomatis, Treponema pallidum, Neisseria gonorrhoeae,* HIV	Ceftriaxone, 125 mg IM single dose, plus metronidazole, 2 g single dose, plus doxycycline, 100 mg BID for 7 d, or azithromycin, 1 g single dose Nonoccupational HIV postexposure prophylaxis (nPEP) may be given to the exposed person within 72 h of unprotected sexual contact with a known HIV-positive source and often consists of the following regimens: (1) Efavirenz + lamivudine or emtricitabine + zidovudine or tenofovir (2) Lopinavir/ritonavir + zidovudine + lamivudine or emtricitabine. However, the regimen should be individualized if the source patient's antiviral regimen, viral load, or genotype is known. This should be done by an experienced HIV practitioner.	Consider use of antiretroviral agents following selected high-risk exposures Efavirenz should not be used in pregant women

Exposure	Pathogen	Prophylaxis[a]	Comments
Sexual assault, cont.		HIV nPEP is typically given for 28 days. For prophylaxis following occupational HIV exposure, see Chapter 102, Percutaneous Injury: Risks and Management	
Sexual contacts	T. pallidum	Benzathine penicillin G, 2.4 million units IM	Treat if exposed within the previous 90 days
	N. gonorrhoeae	Single dose of ceftriaxone, 125 mg IM, or cefixime, 400 mg	Because of possibility of concomitant chlamydial infection, contacts of persons with gonorrhea should also receive azithromycin or doxycycline. Cefixime availability in the United States is limited; cefpodixime is being evaluated as a possible replacement. Resistance to quinolones, first observed in men who have sex with men (MSM) and in certain geographic locations, is now sufficiently widespread to preclude routine use of ciprofloxacin or levofloxacin
	C. trachomatis	Azithromycin, 1 g single dose, or doxycycline, 100 mg BID for 7 d	Use azithromycin in pregnant women
	T. vaginalis	Metronidazole, 2 g single dose Tinidazole, 2 g single dose	No satisfactory alternatives are available in the United States
Influenza	Influenza A and B	Oseltamivir, 75 mg, or zanamivir, 10 mg (or 2 inhalations) once daily used after exposure to influenza or for the duration of the influenza outbreak in the community in high-risk population	Chemoprophylaxis should not be a substitute for vaccination. Oseltamivir approved for chemoprophylaxis in children >1 y and zanamivir in children >5 y. Historically, amantadine and rimantadine have been used for prophylaxis for influenza A. However, high levels of resistance (>80%) occurred during the 2005–2006 influenza season. Consequently, these agents should not be used unless the circulating strain of influenza is known to be susceptible
Whooping cough	Bordetella pertussis	Azithromycin, 500 mg single dose on day 1 then 250 mg per day on days 2–5, or erythromycin, 500 mg QID for 14 d, or clarithromycin, 500 mg BID for 7 d. TMP–SMX, 160/800 mg BID for 14 d, used as an alternate regimen	Use pediatric dosing for children
Lyme disease	Borrelia burgdorferi	Antimicrobial prophylaxis following tick bite is not recommended in most situations. However, single-dose doxycycline, 200 mg, is now recommended (1) within 72 h of the removal of an adult or nymph Ixodes scapularis tick and (2) if the tick has been attached more than 36 h and (3) if the exposure occurred in a region where prevalence of Borrelia burgdorferi in ticks is greater than 20%.	
Anthrax	Bacillus anthracis	Ciprofloxacin, 500 mg BID, or levofloxacin, 500 mg daily for 60 d; alternatives include doxycycline, 100 mg BID, and amoxicillin, 500 mg TID	Inhalational anthrax is considered one of the major threats associated with bioterrorism
Plague	Yersinia pestis	Doxycycline, 100 mg BID for 7 d or for duration of exposure, or tetracycline, 500 mg QID, or ciprofloxacin, 500 mg BID	Incubation period for pneumonic plague is short (2–3 d); for established infection, streptomycin IM or gentamicin remains the agent of choice
Tularemia	Francisella tularensis	Doxycycline, 100 mg BID for 14 d, or ciprofloxacin, 500 mg BID	Can produce disease following inhalation or percutaneous exposure

Abbreviation: TMP–SMX = trimethoprim-sulfamethoxazole.

[a] All regimens are administered orally unless otherwise specified.

Table 111.2 Chronic Prophylaxis in Specific Clinical Settings

Underlying Condition or Recurrent Infections	Pathogens	Prophylaxis[a]	Comments
Acute rheumatic fever (prevention of recurrences)	Streptococcus pyogenes	Penicillin G, 1.2 million units IM every 3-4 wk; alternatives include penicillin V, 250 mg BID; erythromycin, 250 mg BID; sulfadiazine, 1 g daily (0.5 g if weight ≤60 lb)	Risk diminishes with increasing age and time since initial attack; optimal duration unknown but continue prophylaxis at least until the early 20s or for 5 y after most recent attack; some authorities advocate lifelong prophylaxis, especially after rheumatic carditis; risk of prophylaxis failure may be greater with 4-wk dosing of penicillin compared to 3-wk dosing
Recurrent urinary tract infection (UTI)	Gram-negative bacilli	TMP–SMX, 1/2 single-strength tablet (40 mg, 200 mg) daily or 3 times/wk, or trimethoprim, 100 mg, or norfloxacin, 200 mg, or ciprofloxacin, 250 mg, or nitrofurantoin, 50–100 mg, or cephalexin, 125–250 mg daily	For selected patients with more than three infections yearly; consider prophylaxis for 6–12 mo; alternative strategy is postcoital TMP-SMX, 1 tablet or ciprofloxacin, 500 mg, or cephalexin, 125-250, or nitrofurantoin 50–100 mg
Recurrent otitis media	Streptococcus pneumoniae, Haemophilus influenzae, Moraxella catarrhalis	Sulfisoxazole, 50 mg/kg, or amoxicillin, 20 mg/kg daily, or azithromycin, 10 mg/kg qwk	Recommended for children with more than three infections in 6 mo; increasing antibiotic resistance has decreased the efficacy of this strategy and has led some experts to abandon it
Chronic bronchitis, bronchiectasis	S. pneumoniae, H. influenzae, M. catarrhalis	Amoxicillin, 500 mg TID, or TMP–SMX, 1 double-strength tablet BID, or erythromycin, 250 mg QID, or tetracycline, 500 mg QID	May be useful in selected patients with frequent exacerbations (>4/y); some authorities prefer antibiotics at first sign of infection
Asplenia, including sickle cell disease	Predominantly S. pneumoniae; also H. influenzae Neisseria meningitidis	Penicillin V, 250 mg BID (125 mg BID for children ≤5 y), or benzathine penicillin G, 1.2 million units IM every 4 wk; prophylaxis generally continued 2 y after splenectomy; for children with sickle cell disease, prophylaxis continued at least until aged 5 y	Efficacy of chemoprophylaxis clearly established for children with sickle cell disease; some authorities recommend amoxicillin or TMP–SMX for children aged ≤5 y because of risk of H. influenzae infection; however, this risk has been dramatically reduced because of immunization; chemoprophylaxis generally not recommended for adults (lower risk); penicillin-resistant pneumococcus diminishes attractiveness of antibiotic prophylaxis and increases the importance of vaccination
Lymphedema with recurrent cellulitis	S. pyogenes	Benzathine penicillin G, 1.2 million units IM monthly, or penicillin, 250–500 mg BID In penicillin-allergic patients, use macrolides	Given only to patients with frequent episodes of cellulitis; efficacy is limited in patients with significant underlying disease
Spontaneous bacterial peritonitis	Escherichia coli, S. pneumoniae, Klebsiella pneumoniae	Norfloxacin, 400 mg daily, or ciprofloxacin, 750 mg weekly, or TMP–SMX, 1 double-strength tablet 5 d/wk	Used in persons with ascites protein concentration of ≤1 g/dL and in persons with previous SBP (secondary prophylaxis)

Abbreviation: TMP–SMX = trimethoprim-sulfamethoxazole.
[a] All regimens are administered orally unless otherwise specified.

biologic warfare or terrorism and infections that are sexually transmitted.

Persons with an underlying predisposition to infection may benefit from prophylactic antimicrobial agents (Table 111.2). In contrast to short-term prophylaxis administered after exposures, chronic prophylaxis is often required. Because of the duration of antibiotic administration, the complications of chemoprophylaxis, including alteration of the microbial flora and antibiotic resistance, are major

considerations. The emergence of antibiotic-resistant *Streptococcus pneumoniae* may force reassessment of the standard chemoprophylactic recommendations when pneumococcus is a prominent pathogen, as with anatomic or functional asplenia and recurrent otitis.

Chemoprophylaxis for tuberculosis is generally administered to those already infected with *Mycobacterium tuberculosis* (ie, have a positive tuberculin or purified protein derivative [PPD] skin test), in an attempt to

Table 111.3 Criteria for Preventive Therapy for Persons with Positive PPD Skin Tests

Situation	PPD size (5 TU)
HIV infection, organ transplant recipients, patients receiving immunosuppressive regimen or tumor necrosis factor-α inhibitors, recent TB contact, chest radiograph showing fibrotic changes suggestive of prior TB	PPD $\geq$5 mm
Normal hosts from high-incidence groups: residents or employees of extended-care facilities, hospitals, or jail/prison, immigrants from endemic areas, intravenous drug users, mycobacterial laboratory personnel, person $\leq$18 years exposed to TB. High-risk conditions: silicosis, diabetes mellitus, chronic renal failure, some hematologic disorders (ie, leukemia, lymphoma), some malignancies (ie, carcinoma of head and neck, lung) weight loss >10% of ideal body weight, gastrectomy, jejunoileal bypass	PPD $\geq$10 mm
Normal hosts from low-incidence groups	PPD $\geq$15 mm
Abbreviations: PPD = purified protein derivative (tuberculin test); TB = tuberculosis; HIV = human immunodeficiency virus.	

Table 111.4 Controversial Areas Regarding the Use of Prophylactic Antibiotics[a]

Condition	Comments
Prosthetic device infections	Routine chemoprophylaxis before dental work, or other procedures that cause transient bacteremia in patients with prosthetic joints or vascular prostheses, may not be warranted although it is commonly used; prosthetic joint infections caused by oral flora, including α-streptococci, are uncommon, with a rate approaching that of endocarditis in patients with mitral valve prolapse without regurgitation, for which chemoprophylaxis is not recommended; coronary stents do not appear to be prone to infection
Catheter associated UTI	Systemic antibiotics reduce incidence of UTI during initial 4 to 5 days after Foley catheter insertion; with prolonged catheterization antibiotic-resistant bacteria appear in urine with increasing frequency, dissuading most authorities from routine use of prophylaxis; prophylactic antibiotics possibly useful in selected high-risk patients during short-term catheterization
IV catheter–associated infections	Flushing central venous catheters with an antibiotic solution, usually vancomycin (antibiotic lock) proposed to reduce catheter-associated bacteremia; however, Centers for Disease Control and Prevention opposes this strategy except in special circumstances
Pancreatitis	In severe pancreatitis with necrosis, antibacterial (as well as antifungal) prophylaxis has been suggested. However, even if antimicrobials might seem to decrease mortality, in pancreatic necrosis they do not prevent infections
Abbreviation: UTI = urinary tract infection; IV = intravenous. [a] See also Chapter 67, Infection of Native and Prosthetic Joints.	

prevent the development of active tuberculosis (TB). The criteria for administering chemoprophylaxis are listed in Table 111.3 and take into account the underlying illness (immunosuppression, chronic medical conditions) and recent exposure to TB. PPD results can sometimes lead to false-positive (ie, prior bacille Calmette-Guérin [BCG] vaccination) or false-negative (ie, anergy) testing; therefore, newer diagnsotic tests for latent TB are being evaluated (QuantiFERON TB Gold, T SPOT-TB). Prior to initiating prophylaxis for latent TB, the clinician should rule out active TB with a chest radiograph. Current recommendations for treatment of latent TB are 9 months of izoniazid (isonicotinyl hydrazine, INH), 300 mg daily (10 mg/kg/day in children) with pyridoxine, 50 mg/day, usually given with INH to prevent peripheral neuropathy. Six months of INH can be considered in HIV-negative patients. Short-course (4 months) chemoprophylaxis with rifampin, 600 mg/day, can be used as an alternative regimen and should also be used to treat contacts of patients with INH-resistant TB. In the setting of suspected infection with multidrug-resistant *M. tuberculosis,* the decision to provide chemoprophylaxis and the choice of regimen should be made by experienced health care professionals.

Chemoprophylaxis has been advocated for other situations, but at this time, it cannot be considered standard practice (Table 111.4). Although data are limited, it is likely that cost-benefit analyses would not favor routine prophylaxis in these settings or that the benefits of prophylaxis in the short term would be outweighed by long-term consequences such as the development of antibiotic-resistant organisms.

SUGGESTED READING

Blumberg HM, Leonard MK Jr, Jasmer RM. Update on the treatment of tuberculosis and latent tuberculosis infection. *JAMA.* 2005;293(22):2776–2784.

Centers for Disease Control and Prevention. Prevention and control of influenza: recommendations of the Advisory Committee on Immunization Practices (ACIP). *MMWR Recomm Rep.* 2006;55(RR-10):1–42.

Centers for Disease Control and Prevention. Recommended antimicrobial agents for the treatment and postexposure prophylaxis of pertussis. *Morbid Mortal Weekly Rep.* 2005;54(RR14):1–16.

Centers for Disease Control and Prevention. Sexually transmitted diseases treatment guidelines. *Morbid Mortal Weekly Rep.* 2006;55(RR-11):1–94.

Franz DR, Jahrling PB, Friedlander AM, et al. Clinical recognition and management of patients exposed to biological warfare agents. *JAMA.* 1997;278:399–411.

Osmon DR. Antimicrobial prophylaxis in adults. *Mayo Clin Proc.* 2000;75(1):98–109.

Smith DK, Grohskopf LA, Black RJ, et al. Antiretroviral postexposure prophylaxis after sexual, injection-drug use, or other non-occupational exposure to HIV in the United States: recommendations from the U.S. Department of Health and Human Services. *MMWR Recomm Rep.* 2005;54(RR-2):1–20.

Villatoro E, Bassi C, Larvin M. Antibiotic therapy for prophylaxis against infection of pancreatic necrosis in acute pancreatitis. *Cochrane Database Syst Rev.* 2006;18(4):CD002941.

Wormser GP, Dattwyler RJ, Shapiro ED, et al. The clinical assessment, treatment, and prevention of lyme disease, human granulocytic anaplasmosis, and babesiosis: clinical practice guidelines by the Infectious Diseases Society of America. *Clin Infect Dis.* 2006;43(9):1089–1134.

112. Surgical Prophylaxis

Thomas L. Husted and Joseph S. Solomkin

The prevention of surgical site infection (SSI) remains a focus of attention because wound infections continue to be a major source of expense, morbidity, and even mortality. A patient who develops a wound infection while still hospitalized has an approximately 60% greater risk of being admitted to the intensive care unit, and an attributable extra hospital stay of 6.5 days, at an additional direct cost of $3000. Risk of readmission within 30 days is 5 times more likely for infected patients, at a cost of more than $5000.

The epidemiologic data testifying to the significance of SSI are overwhelming. SSIs are the third most frequently reported nosocomial infection, accounting for 14% to 16% of nosocomial infections in hospitalized patients. Approximately 40% of nosocomial infections occurring among surgical patients are SSIs, two thirds of which affect the incision and one third involve organ/space infection. Three quarters of deaths of surgical patients with SSI are attributed to that infection, nearly all of which are organ/space infections. Because of the importance of these infections following operation, considerable effort has been expended to identify other potentially controllable variables that influence infection rates. A major review of this subject and an extensive list of recommendations for preoperative patient preparation and operating room environment have recently been published by the Hospital Infection Control Practices Advisory Committee (HICPAC) of the Centers for Disease Control and Prevention (CDC).

This chapter describes current notions of risk factors for SSIs and discusses problems relating to knowing what infection rates really are. Next, we provide recommendations for practices and describe the data supporting those practices. Guidelines published by several expert groups have created a near-uniform approach to antibiotic usage for prophylaxis. Nonetheless, it is important to note that administration of systemic anti-infectives is only part of a broad program of infection control involving adequate operating room ventilation, sterilization, barrier usage, and delicate surgical technique.

RISK FACTORS FOR SURGICAL SITE INFECTION

Information on appropriate antimicrobial prophylaxis is of considerable significance. Factors to be considered are the cost of infection that *might* have been prevented had prophylaxis been given and the cost of providing antimicrobial therapy to a large number of patients, especially if the yield is the prevention of a relatively small number of infections or even failure of prevention. The costs of providing therapy extend far beyond the acquisition and administration charges to include the costs of treating adverse reactions and the more ominous potential cost of dealing in future times with drug-resistant bacteria. Therefore, enormous effort has been expended to identify factors that increase the risk of infection and would, at least potentially, suggest providing antimicrobial prophylaxis.

Whether surgical prophylaxis has any substantial impact on bacterial resistance patterns is unknown but unlikely. In comparison to the substantial quantity of antibiotics prescribed in the community for upper respiratory infections, the number of antimicrobials provided to surgical patients for prophylaxis is quite small. Furthermore, *within the hospital*, antimicrobial resistance is principally engendered in the intensive care units, not the postoperative ward. The intensive care unit is home to patients at great risk of infection by virtue of acute and chronic disease and by the insertion of a range of monitoring and infusion catheters. These elements lower the inoculum needed to initiate infection and provide portals of entry.

HISTORICAL ASPECTS

Administration of antibiotics to decrease the incidence of postoperative wound infection is a surprisingly recent strategy. The investigational background for the use of anti-infectives for this purpose was developed in the 1950s and 1960s, considerably later than the initial availability of anti-infectives. In fact, early studies of anti-infective prophylaxis, performed in the 1950s, reported either no decrease in infection rates or even higher infection rates than control. These results are explained by the fact that anti-infectives were begun only in the postoperative period. During this time, important developments were made to rationalize antimicrobial prophylaxis. The most fundamental was definition of the decisive period, the time following wound contamination that antibiotics would still reduce the incidence of infection.

WOUND CLASSIFICATION SYSTEMS FOR IDENTIFYING RISK OF INFECTION

It is assumed that at least three categories of variables serve as predictors of SSI risk: (1) those that estimate the intrinsic degree of microbial contamination of the surgical site, (2) those that measure the duration of the operation and other less easily quantifiable elements of the procedure, and (3) those that serve as markers for host susceptibility.

In 1964, the National Research Council sponsored an examination of the efficacy of ultraviolet irradiation and provided the data to validate a wound classification scheme describing risk of infection in relation to the extent of wound contamination (13). That document is a landmark in this area, and the classification scheme has remained useful to the present day (Table 112.1). A clear connection between the contaminating flora at various surgical sites and subsequent infecting pathogens was established. This microbiologic correlation included recognition of the role of anaerobes in postoperative wound infection and abscess formation.

Two subsequent CDC efforts, the SENIC project (Study of the Efficacy of Nosocomial Infection Control) and NNIS (National Nosocomial Infection Surveillance), sought to examine other variables as predictors of infection. These showed that, even within the category of clean wounds, the SSI risk varied from 1.1% to 15.8% (SENIC) or from 1.0% to 5.4% (NNIS), depending on the presence of other risk factors.

The size of these studies is truly phenomenal. Information was collected on 58 498 patients undergoing operations in 1970 to develop a simple multivariate risk index. Analyzing 10 risk factors with stepwise multiple logistic regression techniques, they developed a model that combined information on four of the risk factors to predict a patient's probability of getting a wound infection. Information was then collected on another sample of 59 352 surgical patients seen in 1975–1976 to validate the proposed index.

The variables that were significantly and independently associated with subsequent SSI included: (1) an abdominal operation, (2) an operation lasting >2 hours, (3) a surgical site with a wound classification of either contaminated or dirty-infected, and (4) an operation performed on a patient having three or more discharge diagnoses. Each of these variables contributes one point when present, and the risk index varies from 0 to 4. This means that each variable has the same significance as any other. By the inclusion of factors measuring the risk due to the patient's susceptibility as well as that due to the level of wound contamination, the simplified index predicts surgical wound infection risk about twice as well as the traditional classification of wound contamination.

The problem with this system is that it is not operation specific and depends on variables collected after the operation (at discharge). To further refine the risk-scoring system, a second study was then performed through the NNIS system from 44 hospitals from January 1987 to the end of December 1990. A risk index was developed to predict a surgical patient's risk of acquiring an SSI. The risk index score, ranging from 0 to 3, is the number of risk factors present among the following: (1) a patient with an American Society of Anesthesiologists preoperative assessment score of 3, 4, or 5; (2) an operation classified as contaminated or dirty-infected; and (3) an operation lasting over T hours, where T depends on the operative procedure being performed. The SSI rates for patients with scores of 0, 1, 2, and 3 were 1.5, 2.9, 6.8, and 13.0, respectively. It is important to note that this system provides little insight into risk of infection in clean or clean-contaminated wounds other than identifying a correlation with length of operation.

TECHNIQUES FOR IDENTIFYING SURGICAL SITE INFECTIONS

Given the clinical and economic importance of SSIs, all hospitals are required to have a program to monitor the incidence of postoperative infections. The methods for monitoring such infections were developed at a time when most surgical procedures were occurring in the hospital and patients were generally hospitalized for the procedure and remained in hospital for several days postoperatively. One of the weak points, in fact, of the SENIC and NNIS data presented above is that they relied on in-hospital patient monitoring. Identification and reporting schemes for infections occurring

Table 112.1 Surgical Wound Classification

Class I/Clean: An uninfected operative wound in which no inflammation is encountered and the respiratory; alimentary, genital, or uninfected urinary tract is not entered. In addition, clean wounds are primarily closed and, if necessary, drained with closed drainage. Operative incisional wounds that follow nonpenetrating (blunt) trauma should be included in this category if they meet the criteria.

Class II/Clean-Contaminated: An operative wound in which the respiratory, alimentary, genital, or urinary tracts are entered under controlled conditions and without unusual contamination. Specifically, operations involving the biliary tract, appendix, vagina, and oropharynx are included in this category, provided no evidence of infection or major break in technique is encountered.

Class III/Contaminated: Open, fresh, accidental wounds. In addition, operations with major breaks in sterile technique (eg, open cardiac massage) or gross spillage from the gastrointestinal tract, and incisions in which acute, nonpurulent inflammation is encountered are included in this category.

Class IV/Dirty-Infected: Old traumatic wounds with retained devitalized tissue and those that involve existing clinical infection or perforated viscera. This definition suggests that the organisms causing postoperative infection were present in the operative field before the operation.

outside the hospital were not well developed or tested. This means that the available data primarily address major surgical procedures, primarily done for intra-abdominal or intra-thoracic pathology, for which patients were confined in hospital.

It is known that approximately half of surgical site infections develop after discharge, with most occurring within 21 days after operation. Although SSIs occurring after hospital discharge cause substantial morbidity, their epidemiology is not well understood, and methods for routine postdischarge surveillance have not been validated. A postdischarge surveillance program, including self-reporting of infections by patients and return of questionnaires by patients and surgeons, is labor and resource intensive. A variety of techniques have been tested, including physician questionnaires, direct patient contacts, and computer screens of pharmacy, outpatient, microbiologic, and readmission databases. None have been found superior to others; however, it is likely that as more elements of patients' medical care are computerized, automated surveillance systems will become increasingly effective.

ACCEPTED INDICATIONS FOR ANTI-INFECTIVE PROPHYLAXIS

There is a wide consensus on specific procedures that warrant antimicrobial prophylaxis. Consensus statements by the Surgical Infection Society, the Infectious Diseases Society of America, the American Society of Hospital Pharmacists, the Canadian Infectious Diseases Society, and the French Society of Anesthesia and Intensive Care all agree on a number of indications. There is also considerable

agreement as to which procedures do not warrant prophylaxis.

What follows in this section are recommendations for class II, III, and IV surgical procedures; class I procedures are addressed separately in a following section. Controlled trials of antimicrobial prophylaxis in minimally invasive procedures have recently been reported. In low-risk laparoscopic cholecystectomy and arthroscopic surgery, routine prophylaxis is not indicated. In contaminated laparoscopic procedures, such as high-risk cholecystectomy and bowel surgery, it is best to apply the standards for similar open procedures.

In many areas of antibiotic administration sufficient numbers of studies have been done to allow synthesis of the data. Although there is some skepticism regarding these meta-analyses, anti-infective prophylaxis lends itself well to this type of review in that much of the literature is of good quality, the response to therapy is uniform, and the outcome parameter (SSI) is a specific and well-defined event.

It is worthwhile to note that one benefit of meta-analysis is the identification of benefit early in the evolution of a practice concept, thereby sparing many patients either the extra risk that their procedure might carry if prophylaxis is not given or the extra risk of an adverse event from receiving a medication that would not benefit them.

CHOICE OF ANTI-INFECTIVES FOR PROPHYLAXIS

It is certainly not necessary to cover the entire spectrum of contaminants of a surgical wound. The anticipated pathogens from various operative sites are detailed in Table 112.2.

Table 112.2 Pathogens Causing Surgical Site Infections and Antimicrobial Drugs of Choice for Prophylaxis

Procedure	Likely Pathogen(s)[a]	Drug/Dosing	For History of Penicillin Anaphylactoid Reactions
Clean procedures for which prophylaxis is accepted	S. aureus and epidermidis	Cefazolin, 1 g preoperatively	Clindamycin, 600 mg, or vancomycin, 1 g
Head and neck procedures entering the oropharynx; esophageal procedures	Streptococci; oropharyngeal anaerobes (eg, peptostreptococci)	Cefazolin, 1 g preoperatively	Clindamycin, 600 mg, or vancomycin, 1 g
High-risk gastroduodenal and biliary	Enterobacteriaceae and streptococci	Cefazolin, 1 g preoperatively	Ciprofloxacin, 400 mg
Placement of all grafts, prostheses, or implants	S. aureus; coagulase-negative staphylococci	Cefazolin, 1 g preoperatively	Clindamycin, 600 mg, or vancomycin, 1 g
Cardiac	S. aureus; coagulase-negative staphylococci	Cefazolin, 1 g preoperatively	Clindamycin, 600 mg, or vancomycin, 1 g
Neurosurgery	S. aureus; coagulase-negative staphylococci	Cefazolin, 1 g preoperatively	Clindamycin, 600 mg, or vancomycin, 1 g
Breast	S. aureus; coagulase-negative staphylococci	Cefazolin, 1 g preoperatively	Clindamycin, 600 mg, or vancomycin, 1 g

Orthopedic
  Total joint replacement
  Closed fractures/use of nails, bone plates, other internal fixation devices
  Functional repair without implant/device
  Trauma
	S. aureus; coagulase-negative staphylococci; gram-negative bacilli	Cefazolin, 1 g q8h 3×	Gentamicin, 2 mg/kg, + clindamycin, 600 mg q12h 2×

Noncardiac thoracic
  Thoracic (lobectomy, pneumonectomy, wedge resection, other noncardiac mediastinal procedures)
  Closed tube thoracostomy
	S. aureus; coagulase-negative staphylococci; Streptococcus pneumoniae; gram-negative bacilli	Cefazolin 1 g 1×	Clindamycin, 600 mg

Vascular	S. aureus; coagulase-negative staphylococci	Cefazolin 1 g 1×	Clindamycin, 600 mg
Appendectomy[b]	Gram-negative bacilli; anaerobes	Cefazolin, 1 g, + metronidazole, 500 mg q8h 3×, or cefotetan, 1 g 1×, or cefoxitin, 1 g 4×	Ciprofloxacin, 400 mg, + metronidazole, 500 mg q12h 2×
Colorectal	Gram-negative bacilli; anaerobes	Cefazolin, 1 g, + metronidazole, 500 mg preoperatively, or cefotetan, 1 g preoperatively or cefoxitin 1 g[c]	Ciprofloxacin, 400 mg, + metronidazole, 500 mg preoperatively
Obstetric and gynecologic	Gram-negative bacilli; enterococci; group B streptococci; anaerobes	Cefazolin, 1 g preoperatively	Ciprofloxacin, 400 mg, + metronidazole, 500 mg preoperatively
Urologic (May not be beneficial if urine is sterile)	Gram-negative bacilli	Cefazolin, 1 g preoperatively	Ciprofloxacin, 400 mg preoperatively

[a] In selected patients at risk for S. aureus infection, methicillin-resistant S. aureus (MRSA) should also be considered and coverage expanded accordingly; see text under Specific Prophylactic Concerns.
[b] For nonperforated appendicitis. If perforated, treatment is therapeutic.
[c] Redose if procedure last >4 h.

Little investigational work has been done on appropriate dosing. In general, doses of the selected agent that would be used for treatment of established infection are recommended. The more important issue for prophylaxis concerns the need to maintain effective antibiotic levels throughout the procedure. This is typically accomplished by providing repetitive dosing for lengthy procedures. This is in part a function of the half-life of the agent selected and is an additional argument in favor of agents such as cefazolin that have half-lives approaching 2 hours. A current recommendation is to readminister the anti-infective at intervals of twice the half-life of the agent provided. It is important to note that increasing the dose of an agent provides less benefit than shortening the dosing interval because of drug clearance. There are now a large number of studies that document effective prophylaxis with no further dosing after the patient leaves the operating room.

Gastroduodenal Procedures

Prophylaxis is recommended for most gastrointestinal (GI) procedures. The density of organisms and proportion of anaerobic organisms progressively increase along the GI, so the recommendation depends on the segment of GI tract entered during the procedure. The intrinsic risk of infection associated with procedures entering the stomach, duodenum, and proximal small bowel is quite low and does not support a routine recommendation for prophylaxis. However, any disease or therapeutic intervention that decreases gastric acidity causes a marked increase in the number of bacteria and the risk of wound infection. Therefore, previous or current use of antacids, histamine blockers, or proton pump inhibitors qualifies the patient for prophylaxis. Prophylaxis is also indicated for procedures treating upper GI bleeding. Gastrointestinal stasis also leads to an increase in bacterial counts, so prophylaxis is warranted in procedures to correct obstruction. Additionally, the intrinsic risk of infection in patients with morbid obesity and advanced malignancy is sufficiently high to warrant prophylaxis in these patients. Although the local flora is altered in these circumstances, cefazolin provides adequate prophylaxis and is the recommended agent.

Generally, elective surgery on the stomach or duodenum for ulcer disease is often not included in those procedures requiring prophylaxis. The highly acidic environment results in a very low endogeneous bacterial density, and rates of postoperative infection without prophylaxis are low. High-risk gastroduodenal procedures include operations for cancer, bleeding, obstruction, and perforation, as well as operation in the presence of acid-reducing medical or surgical therapy. Prophylaxis is also recommended for gastric procedures for morbid obesity.

Colorectal Procedures

Colorectal procedures have a very high intrinsic risk of infection and warrant a strong recommendation for prophylaxis. Several studies have demonstrated efficacy with rates of infection decreasing from greater than 50% to less than 9%. Antibiotics are directed at gram-negative aerobes and anaerobic bacteria.

MECHANICAL CLEANSING

Commonly used colon preparation routines have changed substantially in that most patients self-administer these regimens at home and are admitted to hospital the morning of surgery. All prophylactic regimens begin with a mechanical bowel preparation, intended to greatly reduce the amount of feces present. Most commonly, polyethylene glycol regimens are used. It is worth noting that the true value of these preparative activities is primarily to facilitate the operative procedure. Several trials have recently documented that mechanical cleansing does not alter wound infection rates if systemic antibiotic prophylaxis is used.

A current standard is a 4-L polyethylene glycol preparation. These are available either as Colyte, NuLYTE, or GoLYTELY. Bowel preparation with bisacodyl and 2 L of polyethylene glycol is reportedly more acceptable to patients than a 4-L regimen and is equally effective in cleansing the colon.

Although not directly related to postoperative SSI, it is important to be aware of the fluid losses that occur following polyethylene glycol preparations. Patients receiving outpatient preparation compared to those with inpatient preparation require significantly more intraoperative fluid and colloid administration, greater amounts of fluid in the first 24 hours postoperatively, and significantly more postoperative fluid challenges. Patients with multiple medical problems may not tolerate extensive fluid shifts; therefore, other preoperative arrangements, such as inpatient or outpatient intravenous fluid therapy, need to be considered to minimize complications that may outweigh potential cost savings.

These regimens decrease fecal bulk but do not decrease the concentration of bacteria in the stool. In fact, the risk of infection with mechanical preparation alone is still 25% to 30%. The GI side effects of the osmotic mechanical preparations now used complicate oral administration of antibiotics.

INTESTINAL DECONTAMINATION AND SYSTEMIC ANTI-INFECTIVES

In North America, it is common to use a regimen of erythromycin base and neomycin given at 1 PM, 2 PM, and 11 PM (1 g of each drug per dose) the day before a procedure. Times of administration are shifted according to the anticipated time of starting the procedure, with the first dose given 19 hours before operation. Metronidazole can be substituted for erythromycin, which also fulfills the role of parenteral prophylaxis.

Outside North America, however, oral non-absorbable antibiotic preparation has largely been abandoned in favor of parenteral treatment. A major systematic review has recently been reported for colorectal prophylaxis. This review examined 147 trials published between 1984 and 1995, including over 23 000 patients, and 70 different regimens were tested. The results confirmed that the use of antimicrobial prophylaxis is effective for the prevention of surgical wound infection after colorectal surgery. There was no significant difference in the rate of surgical wound infections between many different regimens. However, certain regimens were found to be inadequate. Inadequate regimens included metronidazole alone (which lacks activity against facultative and aerobic gram-negative organisms), doxycycline alone, piperacillin alone (which lacks activity against anaerobes), and oral neomycin plus erythromycin on the day before operation.

The addition of an effective parenteral agent reduced infection rates seen with neomycin/erythromycin to the same level as that seen with the parenteral agent alone. Several trials showed extra benefit of oral antibiotics if inadequate parenteral antibiotics (such as metronidazole alone or piperacillin alone) were employed. These authors found that a single dose administered immediately before the operation (or short-term use) is as effective as long-term postoperative antimicrobial prophylaxis. This study also found no evidence to suggest that the new-generation cephalosporins are more effective than first-generation cephalosporins. Antibiotics selected for prophylaxis in colorectal surgery should be active against both aerobic and anaerobic bacteria.

Oral or topical application of antibiotics in addition to the parenteral administration of appropriate anti-infectives is of no benefit. Administration should be timed to make sure that the tissue concentration of antibiotics around the wound area is sufficiently high when bacterial contamination occurs. Guidelines should be developed locally to achieve a more cost-effective use of antimicrobial prophylaxis in colorectal surgery.

Prophylaxis is also recommended for appendectomy. Although the intrinsic risk of infection is low for uncomplicated appendicitis, the preoperative status of the patient's appendix is typically not known. Cefotetan and cefoxitin are acceptable agents. Metronidazole combined with an aminoglycoside or a quinolone is also an acceptable regimen. For uncomplicated appendicitis, coverage need not be extended to the postoperative period.

Complicated appendicitis (eg, with accompanying perforation or gangrene) is an indication for antibiotic *therapy*, thereby rendering any consideration of prophylaxis irrelevant.

Biliary Tract Procedures

The recommendations for antibiotic prophylaxis for procedures of the biliary tract depend on the presence of specific risk factors. In general, prophylaxis for elective cholecystectomy (either open or laparoscopic) may be regarded as optional. Risk factors associated with an increased incidence of bacteria in bile and thus of increased risk for postoperative infection include age over 60 years, disease of the common duct, diagnosis of cholecystitis, presence of jaundice, and previous history of biliary tract surgery. Only one factor is necessary to establish the patient as high risk. In most cases of symptomatic cholelithiasis meeting high-risk criteria, cefazolin is an acceptable agent. Agents with theoretically superior antimicrobial activity have not been shown to produce a lower postoperative infection rate.

Neurosurgical Procedures

Studies evaluating the efficacy of antibiotic prophylaxis in neurosurgical procedures have shown variable results. Nonetheless, prophylaxis is currently recommended for craniotomy, laminectomy, and shunt procedures. Coverage targets *S. aureus* or *Staphylococcus epidermidis*.

Head and Neck Procedures

For procedures necessitating entry into the oropharynx or esophagus, coverage of aerobic bacteria is indicated. Prophylaxis has been shown to reduce the incidence of severe wound infection by approximately 50%. Either penicillin or cephalosporin-based prophylaxis is effective; cefazolin is commonly used. Prophylaxis is not indicated for dentoalveolar procedures, although prophylaxis is warranted in immunocompromised patients undergoing these procedures or in patients with suspected valvular heart disease.

General Thoracic Procedures

Prophylaxis is routinely used for nearly all thoracic procedures. This is particularly true with a significant likelihood of encountering high numbers of microorganisms during the procedure. Pulmonary resection in cases of partial or complete obstruction of an airway is a procedure in which prophylaxis is clearly warranted. Likewise, prophylaxis is strongly recommended for procedures entailing entry into the esophagus. Although the range of microorganisms encountered in thoracic procedures is extensive, most are sensitive to cefazolin, which is the recommended agent.

Cardiac Procedures

Prophylaxis against *S. aureus* and *S. epidermidis* is indicated for patients undergoing cardiac procedures. Although the risk of infection is low, the morbidity of mediastinitis or a sternal wound infection is great. Numerous studies have evaluated antibiotic regimens based on penicillin, first- and second-generation cephalosporins, or vancomycin. Cardiopulmonary bypass reduces the elimination of drugs, so additional intraoperative doses typically are not necessary.

Antistaphylococcal penicillins and first-generation cephalosporins have traditionally been the prophylactic antibiotics of choice for patients undergoing cardiothoracic operations. Recently published studies have claimed improved outcomes with respect to postoperative wound infection when second-generation cephalosporins were used for prophylaxis.

A meta-analysis of placebo-controlled trials of cardiothoracic prophylaxis demonstrated a consistent benefit to the administration of antibiotic prophylaxis, with an approximate 5-fold reduction in wound infection rate. The second-generation cephalosporins (cefamandole and cefuroxime) performed better than cefazolin, with an approximate 1.5-fold reduction in wound infection rate. Administration of prophylaxis beyond 48 hours was not associated with decreased wound infection rates.

Obstetric and Gynecologic Procedures

Prophylaxis is indicated for cesarean section and abdominal and vaginal hysterectomy. Numerous clinical trials have demonstrated a reduction in risk of wound infection or endometritis by as much as 70% in patients undergoing cesarean section. For cesarean section, the antibiotic is administered immediately after the cord is clamped to avoid exposing the newborn to antibiotics. Despite the theoretic need to cover gram-negative and anaerobic organisms, studies have not demonstrated a superior result with broad-spectrum antibiotics compared with cefazolin. Therefore, cefazolin is the recommended agent.

Twenty-five randomized controlled trials of antibiotic prophylaxis that used rigorous protocols were analyzed. Overall, 21.1% of the patients who did not receive antibiotic prophylaxis had serious infections after abdominal hysterectomy. Among patients who received any antibiotics, only 9.0% had serious postoperative infections. The authors concluded that preoperative antibiotics are highly effective in the prevention of serious infections associated with total abdominal hysterectomy and that they should be used routinely. They also noted that the use of controls who receive no treatment is no longer justified in trials of antibiotic prophylaxis for total abdominal hysterectomy.

Urologic Procedures

The range of potential urologic procedures and intrinsic risk of infection varies widely. In general, it is recommended to achieve preoperative sterilization of the urine if clinically feasible. For procedures entailing the creation of urinary conduits, recommendations are similar to those for procedures pertaining to the specific segment of the intestinal tract being used for the conduit. Procedures not requiring entry into the intestinal tract and performed in the context of sterile urine are regarded as clean procedures. It should be recognized, however, that prophylaxis for specific urologic procedures has not been fully evaluated.

Orthopedic Procedures

Antibiotic prophylaxis is clearly recommended for certain orthopedic procedures. These include the insertion of a prosthetic joint, ankle fusion, revision of a prosthetic joint, reduction of hip fractures, reduction of high-energy closed fractures, and reduction of open fractures. Such procedures are associated with a risk of infection of 5% to 15%, reduced to less than 3% by the use of prophylactic antibiotics. Cefazolin provides adequate coverage. The additional use of aminoglycosides and extension of coverage beyond the operative period is common but lacks supportive evidence.

Noncardiac Vascular Procedures

Available data support the recommendation for anti-infective coverage for vascular procedures using synthetic material, those requiring groin incisions, and those affecting the aorta. Cefazolin is the recommended agent, because most infections are caused by *S. aureus* or *S. epidermidis*. Prophylaxis is not recommended for patients undergoing carotid endarterectomy.

ANTI-INFECTIVE PROPHYLAXIS FOR CLEAN PROCEDURES

The biggest controversy regarding antibiotic prophylaxis centers on prophylaxis for clean surgery. Prophylaxis has prevented postoperative wound infection after clean surgery in a majority of clinical trials with sufficient power to identify a 50% reduction in risk. The low control rates of infection means that very large studies must be done to see a significant effect; studies of greater than than 1000 procedures are needed to detect such reductions reliably.

The major study on this subject was a randomized, double-blind trial of 1218 patients undergoing herniorrhaphy or surgery involving the breast, including excision of a breast mass, mastectomy, reduction mammoplasty, and axillary-node dissection. The prophylactic regimen was a single dose of cefonicid administered approximately half an hour before surgery. The patients were followed up for 4 to 6 weeks after surgery. The patients who received prophylaxis had 48% fewer probable or definite infections than those who did not. For patients undergoing a procedure involving the breast, infection occurred in 6.6% of the cefonicid recipients and 12.2% of the placebo recipients; for those undergoing herniorrhaphy, infection occurred in 2.3% of the cefonicid recipients and 4.2% of the placebo recipients. There were comparable reductions in the numbers of definite wound infections, wounds that drained pus, and *Staphylococcus aureus* wounds as well as the need for postoperative antibiotic therapy, nonroutine visits to a physician for problems involving wound healing, incision and drainage procedures, and readmission because of problems with wound healing.

An observational study was then done on the effects of antibiotic prophylaxis on definite wound infections in 3202 patients undergoing herniorrhaphy or selected breast surgery procedures identified preoperatively and monitored for 4 or more weeks. Thirty-four percent of patients received prophylaxis at the discretion of the surgeon; 86 definite wound infections (2.7%) were identified. Prophylaxis recipients were at higher risk for infection, with a higher proportion of mastectomies, longer procedures, and other factors. Patients who received prophylaxis experienced 41% fewer definite wound infections and 65% fewer definite wound infections requiring parenteral antibiotic therapy after adjustment for duration of surgery and type of procedure. Additional adjustment for age, body mass index, the presence of drains, diabetes, and exposure to corticosteroids did not change the magnitude of this effect.

The argument then is not whether such therapy lowers infection rates but rather whether it is worth the cost. Additionally, the control infection rate is so low that physicians will not be aware of a decreased infection rate unless very careful surveillance is performed, and then only for patients from several practices. Comparing one effective regimen with another, as has been done with colorectal surgical prophylaxis, is simply not going to happen.

To justify use of prophylaxis for clean procedures at a single institution, an accurate assessment of infection rates must be available. This requires a considered effort at postdischarge follow-up. When these data are available, the risk/benefit ratio can be more knowledgeably assessed. Without accurate information on infection rates by procedure, known risk factors described above may serve as guides. Extremes of age, poor nutritional status, diabetes, and obesity are recognized as significant additional risk factors.

The use of systemic prophylaxis for hernia repair entailing the insertion of mesh is considered desirable because the morbidity of infected mesh in the groin is substantial. However, no prospective trials demonstrate the effectiveness or necessity of this practice. Modified radical mastectomy and axillary-node dissection also warrant prophylaxis, because wounds near or in the axilla have an intrinsic risk of infection. If prophylaxis is desired or indicated for any of these procedures, cefazolin is the agent of choice.

Laparoscopic and Thoracoscopic Procedures

Specific data supporting recommendation of antibiotic prophylaxis for laparoscopic or thoracoscopic procedures are lacking. Therefore, pending the availability of new data, recommendations for the same procedure performed using the "open technique" should be followed.

SPECIFIC PROPHYLACTIC CONCERNS

The emergence of methicillin-resistant *S. aureus* (MRSA) in postoperative surgical infections has become an increasing problem for in-hospital patients and those discharged home. Although the cause of an increasing presence of MRSA in the community is hotly debated, it is futile to ignore this pathogen as a cause of SSIs. Several studies have demonstrated increased 90-day mortality, greater length of stay, and increased costs associated with MRSA postoperative infection compared to methicillin-sensitive *S. aureus* (MSSA). Significantly, MRSA has been demonstrated to be the leading pathogen in cardiac surgery and an independent risk factor for increased mortality in these patients.

Although MRSA has long been considered a health care–associated infection, increasingly MRSA is brought into the hospital by patients who are carriers of the pathogen. Therefore, specific recommendations can be made to limit the spread of MRSA and the occurrence of SSIs due to MRSA. Patients who are known or suspected to be colonized with MRSA (which may include institutionalized patients from nursing homes or long-term acute care facilities) should have perioperative anti-infective prophylaxis targeted to the usual pathogens and MRSA.

Traditionally vancomycin has fulfilled this requirement; however, newer boutique agents are being marketed to fill this need, eg, daptomycin. In addition to institutionalized patients and known carriers, cardiac surgery patients should also be screened for colonization with MRSA. Nasal swabs are usually sufficient to determine colonization and initiate therapy (intranasal mupirocin) for these patients while modifying operative anti-infective prophylaxis. Prospective randomized studies will need to be developed and performed to establish absolute recommendations. Meanwhile, MRSA prophylaxis is not necessary for every surgical patient, but those patients meeting risk factors for increased incidence (eg, institutionalized, recent antimicrobial therapy, known colonization) and for increased morbidity from MRSA infection (cardiac surgery patients) should have MRSA prophylaxis strongly considered.

SUGGESTED READING

American Society of Health-System Pharmacists. ASHP therapeutic guidelines on antimicrobial prophylaxis in surgery. *Am J Health Syst Pharm.* 1999;56:1839–1888.

Bratzler DW, Houck PM, Richards C, et al. Use of antimicrobial prophylaxis for major surgery: baseline results from the National Surgical Infection Prevention Project. *Arch Surg.* 2005;140:174–182.

Culver DH, Horan TC, Gaynes RP, et al. Surgical wound infection rates by wound class, operative procedure, and patient risk index. National Nosocomial Infections Surveillance System. *Am J Med.* 1991; 91:152S–157S.

Fields CL. Outcomes of a postdischarge surveillance system for surgical site infections at a Midwestern regional referral center hospital. *Am J Infect Control.* 1999;27:158–164.

Mangram AJ, Horan TC, Pearson ML, et al. Guideline for prevention of surgical site infection, 1999. Hospital Infection Control Practices Advisory Committee. *Infect Control Hosp Epidemiol.* 1999;20:250–278.

NNIS. CDC. National Nosocomial Infections Surveillance (NNIS) System report, data summary from January 1992-October 2004, issued 2005. *Am J Infect Control.* 2004;32:470–485.

Napolitano LM. Surgical site and complicated skin and soft tissue infections: epidemiology, prevention, and emerging treatment guidelines. *Surg Rounds.* 2006; supp Sept: S11–S19.

Platt R, Zucker JR, Zaleznik DF, et al. Prophylaxis against wound infection following herniorrhaphy or breast surgery. *J Infect Dis.* 1992;166:556–560.

113. Immunizations

Elaine C. Jong

Long-lasting immunity against many serious infectious diseases can be elicited through active immunization, the administration of specific antigens (killed or attenuated microorganisms; purified polysaccharides, proteins, or other components; or recombinant antigens produced by genetic engineering) that stimulate the recipient host's production of protective antibodies. Vaccine doses may be given orally, administered as mucosal vaccines, or given by injection using intradermal, subcutaneous, or intramuscular routes. Passive immunization is the process by which protective immunity is obtained through transfer of preformed antibodies from an immune host to a nonimmune recipient, either as immunoglobulin or antibody-specific immunoglobulin.

Protective efficacy resulting from active immunization with a vaccine depends on several factors: the age of the host, with decreased efficacy of certain vaccines observed in the very young and very old; the immune status of the host, with decreased efficacy observed in persons with compromised immune status because of disease or therapy; and the characteristics of the vaccine product itself.

In active immunization, protective levels of specific antibodies usually develop within 2 to 4 weeks on completion of the primary immunization regimen. With the exception of purified polysaccharide vaccines, the antibody response can be recalled and boosted when the immune system is challenged by additional "booster" doses of the vaccine antigen(s) or by exposure to the naturally occurring pathogen. Passive immunization can confer rapid protection, but serum levels of protective antibodies in recipients are highest immediately after receipt, decreasing with the passage of time, and there is no immune recall on challenge.

Active or passive immunization may be used for pre-exposure protection against certain diseases, and in some cases, the two forms may be administered simultaneously at different sites. Tetanus, hepatitis A, hepatitis B, and rabies are examples of infections for which active and passive immunizations might be administered at the same time, usually after a high-risk exposure, to invoke rapid immunity as well as the longer-lasting antibody response.

Several different vaccines may be administered concomitantly at separate sites without decreased efficacy, although the timing and sequence of vaccines have to be taken into account. For example, when immunoglobulin is given for passive immunization against hepatitis A, antibodies against several common infections may be present in sufficient amounts to interfere with the response to the corresponding vaccines. Vaccines against measles, mumps, and rubella (MMR) and varicella may be given on the same day, but immunoglobulin should not be given for 3 months before or 3 weeks after MMR vaccine and not for 2 months after varicella vaccine (chickenpox). However, vaccines against tetanus, diphtheria, yellow fever, typhoid fever, hepatitis B, rabies, and meningococcal meningitis can be given on the same day as immunoglobulin. If immunoglobulin is given on the same day as hepatitis A vaccine, the vaccine is still efficacious, although the resulting peak antibody titer is lower than when the vaccine is given alone.

The current standard of practice requires that potential vaccine recipients be informed of the potential benefits and adverse side effects of each vaccine. The Vaccine Information Statements (VISs) prepared by the national Immunization Action Coalition (IAC) can be downloaded and copies made for use in patient education from the Web site (http://www.cdc.gov/vaccines/pubs/vis/default.htm). All VISs are available in English and up to 17 additional languages. Tolerance to minor adverse effects associated with each vaccine and the potential for more serious vaccine-associated symptoms must also be taken into account in the person who is a candidate for multiple vaccine doses on the same day.

CHILDHOOD AND ADOLESCENT IMMUNIZATIONS

The routine immunizations recommended during childhood and adolescence cover communicable diseases of traditional public health importance: diphtheria, pertussis (whooping cough), tetanus, polio, *Haemophilus influenzae* type b, hepatitis B, measles, mumps, and rubella. New recommendations have been made regarding the recently licensed rotavirus vaccine for infants and regarding the use of influenza vaccine in infants 6 to 59 months of age. Recommendations on pneumococcal conjugate vaccine have been renewed, and recommendations on hepatitis A vaccine and varicella vaccine in children have been updated. The 11- to 12-year-old age group has been targeted for routine administration of quadrivalent meningococcal conjugate vaccine, tetanus/diphtheria/acellular pertussis vaccine, and quadrivalent human papillomavirus vaccine. Figure 113.1 shows the immunization schedules for these vaccines according to recommendations from the Centers for Disease Control and Prevention (CDC) Advisory Committee on Immunization Practices (ACIP) and endorsed by the American Academy of Pediatrics (AAP). This information is available on the CDC Web site (http://www.cdc.gov/vaccines/) and is updated on an annual basis.

In 2006, a new vaccine was licensed to protect infants and young children from severe gastroenteritis caused by rotavirus. The new rotavirus vaccine (RotaTeq, Merck) is administered as a series of three oral doses given at 2, 4, and 6 months of age. The first dose of vaccine should be received by 12 weeks of age, and all doses of the vaccine should be received by 32 weeks of age. The new rotavirus vaccine is different than an earlier rotavirus vaccine (RotaShield) that was withdrawn from the market in 1999 after reports of that vaccine's association with intussusception.

Efforts to implement pneumococcal conjugate vaccine (Prevnar, Wyeth) as part of the pediatric immunization schedule were hampered by product supply shortages in the past, but this vaccine is once again available and included in the national childhood vaccine coverage goals.

New recommendations have emerged for the use of varicella (chickenpox) vaccine (Varivax, Merck) and hepatitis A virus vaccine (Havrix, GlaxoSmithKline; VAQTA, Merck), both vaccines having been licensed in the United States in the 1990s. Varicella vaccine is given at 12 months of age or older and may be administered at the same time as the MMR vaccine (M-M-R II, Merck). Both varicella–zoster virus (VZV) and MMR are live virus vaccines administered by injection. If the two vaccines are not given simultaneously at different sites,

the ACIP recommends that the vaccine doses be separated by 28 days if possible to reduce or eliminate possible interference of the vaccine given first with the vaccine given second. A second dose of varicella vaccine is now recommended for children, between 4 and 6 years old, on entry into school to boost waning immunity from the first dose received in infancy.

In 1999, ACIP recommended hepatitis A vaccine for children 24 months of age or older residing in 11 western states in the United States, where a high incidence of hepatitis A transmission was reported. In addition, children aged 2 through 18 years in the following groups were considered at high risk and were prioritized for hepatitis A immunization: foster children, Native American and Alaskan Native, homeless, street teens, male teens who have sex with males, illicit drug users, and those with clotting factor disorders or chronic liver disease. In 2005, the licensure for hepatitis A vaccine (Havrix; VAQTA) was changed to lower the minimum age of use to 12 months, and hepatitis A vaccine was recommended in the CDC National Immunization Program (NIP) Vaccines for Children (VFC) Program. The VFC Program recommendation incorporates hepatitis A vaccine into the standard immunization schedule for infants between 12 and 23 months of age and leaves the pre-existing programs in place for administering hepatitis A vaccine to children between 2 and 18 years of age in the targeted risk groups described above.

Quadrivalent meningococcal conjugate vaccine (MCV4) (Menactra, SanofiPasteur) is now recommended by the ACIP and AAP as a routine vaccine for children 11 to 12 years of age. This recommendation augments the 1999 ACIP recommendation for immunization against meningococcal disease for college-bound students. CDC data and published studies had shown that freshman dormitory residents appear to be at 3-fold increased risk for meningococcal disease, relative to other persons their age. A single dose of either MCV4 or meningococcal polysaccharide vaccine (MPV4) (Menomune, SanofiPasteur) offers protection against serogroups A, C, Y, and W-135. Although the currently available vaccines do not cover serogroup B, approximately 70% of cases among college students in 1998 to 1999 in the United States were caused by serogroups C and Y. Primary immunization consists of a single dose given by injection, intramuscular for meningococcal conjugate vaccine, and subcutaneously for meningococcal polysaccharide vaccine. Meningococcal conjugate vaccine may be boosted after approximately 5 years (although the official booster interval has not yet been determined) if the risk of exposure is still present, compared with meningococcal polysaccharide vaccine that is not considered boostable because of the suboptimal immune response to when subsequent doses are given after the primary immunization. If both vaccines are available, the meningococcal conjugate vaccine should be selected, because the vaccine elicits a protective antibody response sufficient to eradicate asymptomatic oropharyngeal meningococcal carriage of the vaccine serogroups.

DEPARTMENT OF HEALTH AND HUMAN SERVICES • CENTERS FOR DISEASE CONTROL AND PREVENTION

Recommended Immunization Schedule for Persons Aged 0–6 Years—UNITED STATES • 2007

Vaccine ▼ Age ►	Birth	1 month	2 months	4 months	6 months	12 months	15 months	18 months	19–23 months	2–3 years	4–6 years
Hepatitis B[1]	HepB	HepB		see footnote 1		HepB				HepB Series	
Rotavirus[2]			Rota	Rota	Rota						
Diphtheria, Tetanus, Pertussis[3]			DTaP	DTaP	DTaP		DTaP				DTaP
Haemophilus influenzae type b[4]			Hib	Hib	Hib[4]	Hib		Hib			
Pneumococcal[5]			PCV	PCV	PCV	PCV				PCV / PPV	
Inactivated Poliovirus			IPV	IPV		IPV					IPV
Influenza[6]						Influenza (Yearly)					
Measles, Mumps, Rubella[7]						MMR					MMR
Varicella[8]						Varicella					Varicella
Hepatitis A[9]						HepA (2 doses)				HepA Series	
Meningococcal[10]										MPSV4	

Range of recommended ages

Catch-up immunization

Certain high-risk groups

This schedule indicates the recommended ages for routine administration of currently licensed childhood vaccines, as of December 1, 2006, for children aged 0–6 years. Additional information is available at http://www.cdc.gov/nip/recs/child-schedule.htm. Any dose not administered at the recommended age should be administered at any subsequent visit, when indicated and feasible. Additional vaccines may be licensed and recommended during the year. Licensed combination vaccines may be used whenever any components of the combination are indicated and other components of the vaccine are not contraindicated and if approved by the Food and Drug Administration for that dose of the series. Providers should consult the respective Advisory Committee on Immunization Practices statement for detailed recommendations. Clinically significant adverse events that follow immunization should be reported to the Vaccine Adverse Event Reporting System (VAERS). Guidance about how to obtain and complete a VAERS form is available at http://www.vaers.hhs.gov or by telephone, 800-822-7967.

1. Hepatitis B vaccine (HepB). (Minimum age: birth)
At birth:
• Administer monovalent HepB to all newborns before hospital discharge.
• If mother is hepatitis surface antigen (HBsAg)-positive, administer HepB and 0.5 mL of hepatitis B immune globulin (HBIG) within 12 hours of birth.
• If mother's HBsAg status is unknown, administer HepB within 12 hours of birth. Determine the HBsAg status as soon as possible and if HBsAg-positive, administer HBIG (no later than age 1 week).
• If mother is HBsAg-negative, the birth dose can only be delayed with physician's order and mother's negative HBsAg laboratory report documented in the infant's medical record.
After the birth dose:
• The HepB series should be completed with either monovalent HepB or a combination vaccine containing HepB. The second dose should be administered at age 1–2 months. The final dose should be administered at age ≥24 weeks. Infants born to HBsAg-positive mothers should be tested for HBsAg and antibody to HBsAg after completion of ≥3 doses of a licensed HepB series, at age 9–18 months (generally at the next well-child visit).
4-month dose:
• It is permissible to administer 4 doses of HepB when combination vaccines are administered after the birth dose. If monovalent HepB is used for doses after the birth dose, a dose at age 4 months is not needed.

2. Rotavirus vaccine (Rota). (Minimum age: 6 weeks)
• Administer the first dose at age 6–12 weeks. Do not start the series later than age 12 weeks.
• Administer the final dose in the series by age 32 weeks. Do not administer a dose later than age 32 weeks.
• Data on safety and efficacy outside of these age ranges are insufficient.

3. Diphtheria and tetanus toxoids and acellular pertussis vaccine (DTaP). (Minimum age: 6 weeks)
• The fourth dose of DTaP may be administered as early as age 12 months, provided 6 months have elapsed since the third dose.
• Administer the final dose in the series at age 4–6 years.

4. Haemophilus influenzae type b conjugate vaccine (Hib).
(Minimum age: 6 weeks)
• If PRP-OMP (PedvaxHIB® or ComVax® [Merck]) is administered at ages 2 and 4 months, a dose at age 6 months is not required.
• TriHiBit® (DTaP/Hib) combination products should not be used for primary immunization but can be used as boosters following any Hib vaccine in children aged ≥12 months.

5. Pneumococcal vaccine. (Minimum age: 6 weeks for pneumococcal conjugate vaccine [PCV]; 2 years for pneumococcal polysaccharide vaccine [PPV])
• Administer PCV at ages 24–59 months in certain high-risk groups. Administer PPV to children aged ≥2 years in certain high-risk groups. See MMWR 2000;49(No. RR-9):1–35.

6. Influenza vaccine. (Minimum age: 6 months for trivalent inactivated influenza vaccine [TIV]; 5 years for live, attenuated influenza vaccine [LAIV])
• All children aged 6–59 months and close contacts of all children aged 0–59 months are recommended to receive influenza vaccine.
• Influenza vaccine is recommended annually for children aged ≥59 months with certain risk factors, health-care workers, and other persons (including household members) in close contact with persons in groups at high risk. See MMWR 2006;55(No. RR-10):1–41.
• For healthy persons aged 5–49 years, LAIV may be used as an alternative to TIV.
• Children receiving TIV should receive 0.25 mL if aged 6–35 months or 0.5 mL if aged ≥3 years.
• Children aged <9 years who are receiving influenza vaccine for the first time should receive 2 doses (separated by ≥4 weeks for TIV and ≥6 weeks for LAIV).

7. Measles, mumps, and rubella vaccine (MMR). (Minimum age: 12 months)
• Administer the second dose of MMR at age 4–6 years. MMR may be administered before age 4–6 years, provided ≥4 weeks have elapsed since the first dose and both doses are administered at age ≥12 months.

8. Varicella vaccine. (Minimum age: 12 months)
• Administer the second dose of varicella vaccine at age 4–6 years. Varicella vaccine may be administered before age 4–6 years, provided that ≥3 months have elapsed since the first dose and both doses are administered at age ≥12 months. If second dose was administered ≥28 days following the first dose, the second dose does not need to be repeated.

9. Hepatitis A vaccine (HepA). (Minimum age: 12 months)
• HepA is recommended for all children aged 1 year (i.e., aged 12–23 months). The 2 doses in the series should be administered at least 6 months apart.
• Children not fully vaccinated by age 2 years can be vaccinated at subsequent visits.
• HepA is recommended for certain other groups of children, including in areas where vaccination programs target older children. See MMWR 2006;55(No. RR-7):1–23.

10. Meningococcal polysaccharide vaccine (MPSV4). (Minimum age: 2 years)
• Administer MPSV4 to children aged 2–10 years with terminal complement deficiencies or anatomic or functional asplenia and certain other high-risk groups. See MMWR 2005;54(No. RR-7):1–21.

The Recommended Immunization Schedules for Persons Aged 0–18 Years are approved by the Advisory Committee on Immunization Practices (http://www.cdc.gov/nip/acip), the American Academy of Pediatrics (http://www.aap.org), and the American Academy of Family Physicians (http://www.aafp.org).
SAFER • HEALTHIER • PEOPLE™

CS103164

(continued)

DEPARTMENT OF HEALTH AND HUMAN SERVICES • CENTERS FOR DISEASE CONTROL AND PREVENTION

Recommended Immunization Schedule for Persons Aged 7–18 Years—UNITED STATES • 2007

Vaccine ▼ Age ▶	7–10 years	11–12 YEARS	13–14 years	15 years	16–18 years
Tetanus, Diphtheria, Pertussis[1]	see footnote 1	Tdap	Tdap		
Human Papillomavirus[2]	see footnote 2	HPV (3 doses)	HPV Series		
Meningococcal[3]	MPSV4	MCV4	MCV4[3] / MCV4		
Pneumococcal[4]		PPV			
Influenza[5]		Influenza (Yearly)			
Hepatitis A[6]		HepA Series			
Hepatitis B[7]		HepB Series			
Inactivated Poliovirus[8]		IPV Series			
Measles, Mumps, Rubella[9]		MMR Series			
Varicella[10]		Varicella Series			

Range of recommended ages

Catch-up immunization

Certain high-risk groups

This schedule indicates the recommended ages for routine administration of currently licensed childhood vaccines, as of December 1, 2006, for children aged 7–18 years. Additional information is available at **http://www.cdc.gov/nip/recs/child-schedule.htm.** Any dose not administered at the recommended age should be administered at any subsequent visit, when indicated and feasible. Additional vaccines may be licensed and recommended during the year. Licensed combination vaccines may be used whenever any components of the combination are indicated and other components of the vaccine are not contraindicated and if approved by the Food and Drug Administration for that dose of the series. Providers should consult the respective Advisory Committee on Immunization Practices statement for detailed recommendations. Clinically significant adverse events that follow immunization should be reported to the Vaccine Adverse Event Reporting System (VAERS). Guidance about how to obtain and complete a VAERS form is available at **http://www.vaers.hhs.gov** or by telephone, **800-822-7967.**

1. **Tetanus and diphtheria toxoids and acellular pertussis vaccine (Tdap).**
   (Minimum age: 10 years for BOOSTRIX® and 11 years for ADACEL™)
   • Administer at age 11–12 years for those who have completed the recommended childhood DTP/DTaP vaccination series and have not received a tetanus and diphtheria toxoids vaccine (Td) booster dose.
   • Adolescents aged 13–18 years who missed the 11–12 year Td/Tdap booster dose should also receive a single dose of Tdap if they have completed the recommended childhood DTP/DTaP vaccination series.

2. **Human papillomavirus vaccine (HPV).** *(Minimum age: 9 years)*
   • Administer the first dose of the HPV vaccine series to females at age 11–12 years.
   • Administer the second dose 2 months after the first dose and the third dose 6 months after the first dose.
   • Administer the HPV vaccine series to females at age 13–18 years if not previously vaccinated.

3. **Meningococcal vaccine.** *(Minimum age: 11 years for meningococcal conjugate vaccine [MCV4]; 2 years for meningococcal polysaccharide vaccine [MPSV4])*
   • Administer MCV4 at age 11–12 years and to previously unvaccinated adolescents at high school entry (at approximately age 15 years).
   • Administer MCV4 to previously unvaccinated college freshmen living in dormitories; MPSV4 is an acceptable alternative.
   • Vaccination against invasive meningococcal disease is recommended for children and adolescents aged ≥2 years with terminal complement deficiencies or anatomic or functional asplenia and certain other high-risk groups. See *MMWR* 2005;54(No. RR-7):1–21. Use MPSV4 for children aged 2–10 years and MCV4 or MPSV4 for older children.

4. **Pneumococcal polysaccharide vaccine (PPV).** *(Minimum age: 2 years)*
   • Administer for certain high-risk groups. See *MMWR* 1997;46(No. RR-8):1–24, and *MMWR* 2000;49(No. RR-9):1–35.

5. **Influenza vaccine.** *(Minimum age: 6 months for trivalent inactivated influenza vaccine [TIV]; 5 years for live, attenuated influenza vaccine [LAIV])*
   • Influenza vaccine is recommended annually for persons with certain risk factors, health-care workers, and other persons (including household members) in close contact with persons in groups at high risk. See *MMWR* 2006;55 (No. RR-10):1–41.
   • For healthy persons aged 5–49 years, LAIV may be used as an alternative to TIV.
   • Children aged <9 years who are receiving influenza vaccine for the first time should receive 2 doses (separated by ≥4 weeks for TIV and ≥6 weeks for LAIV).

6. **Hepatitis A vaccine (HepA).** *(Minimum age: 12 months)*
   • The 2 doses in the series should be administered at least 6 months apart.
   • HepA is recommended for certain other groups of children, including in areas where vaccination programs target older children. See *MMWR* 2006;55 (No. RR-7):1–23.

7. **Hepatitis B vaccine (HepB).** *(Minimum age: birth)*
   • Administer the 3-dose series to those who were not previously vaccinated.
   • A 2-dose series of Recombivax HB® is licensed for children aged 11–15 years.

8. **Inactivated poliovirus vaccine (IPV).** *(Minimum age: 6 weeks)*
   • For children who received an all-IPV or all-oral poliovirus (OPV) series, a fourth dose is not necessary if the third dose was administered at age ≥4 years.
   • If both OPV and IPV were administered as part of a series, a total of 4 doses should be administered, regardless of the child's current age.

9. **Measles, mumps, and rubella vaccine (MMR).** *(Minimum age: 12 months)*
   • If not previously vaccinated, administer 2 doses of MMR during any visit, with ≥4 weeks between the doses.

10. **Varicella vaccine.** *(Minimum age: 12 months)*
    • Administer 2 doses of varicella vaccine to persons without evidence of immunity.
    • Administer 2 doses of varicella vaccine to persons aged <13 years at least 3 months apart. Do not repeat the second dose, if administered ≥28 days after the first dose.
    • Administer 2 doses of varicella vaccine to persons aged ≥13 years at least 4 weeks apart.

The Recommended Immunization Schedules for Persons Aged 0–18 Years are approved by the Advisory Committee on Immunization Practices (http://www.cdc.gov/nip/acip), the American Academy of Pediatrics (http://www.aap.org), and the American Academy of Family Physicians (http://www.aafp.org).

SAFER • HEALTHIER • PEOPLE™

CS100131

MCV4 is FDA-approved for use in children aged 2 to 10 years, in addition to its prior approval for use in persons aged 11 to 55 years. The ACIP recommends that MCV4 is preferable to MPSV4 for vaccination of children aged 2 to 10 years who are at increased risk for meningococcal disease, including travelers or residents of countries in which meningococcal disease is hyperendemic or epidemic, and certain other high-risk groups. See MMWR 2007;56(48);1265–1266.

Since the late 1990s, a substantial increase in the number of confirmed pertussis cases in the United States among persons 10 to 19 years

Catch-up Immunization Schedule
for Persons Aged 4 Months–18 Years Who Start Late or Who Are More Than 1 Month Behind

UNITED STATES • 2007

The table below provides catch-up schedules and minimum intervals between doses for children whose vaccinations have been delayed. A vaccine series does not need to be restarted, regardless of the time that has elapsed between doses. Use the section appropriate for the child's age.

CATCH-UP SCHEDULE FOR PERSONS AGED 4 MONTHS–6 YEARS					
Vaccine	Minimum Age for Dose 1	Minimum Interval Between Doses			
		Dose 1 to Dose 2	Dose 2 to Dose 3	Dose 3 to Dose 4	Dose 4 to Dose 5
Hepatitis B[1]	Birth	4 weeks	8 weeks (and 16 weeks after first dose)		
Rotavirus[2]	6 wks	4 weeks	4 weeks		
Diphtheria, Tetanus, Pertussis[3]	6 wks	4 weeks	4 weeks	6 months	6 months[3]
Haemophilus influenzae type b[4]	6 wks	4 weeks if first dose administered at age <12 months / 8 weeks (as final dose) if first dose administered at age 12-14 months / No further doses needed if first dose administered at age ≥15 months	4 weeks[4] if current age <12 months / 8 weeks (as final dose)[4] if current age ≥12 months and second dose administered at age <15 months / No further doses needed if previous dose administered at age ≥15 months	8 weeks (as final dose) This dose only necessary for children aged 12 months–5 years who received 3 doses before age 12 months	
Pneumococcal[5]	6 wks	4 weeks if first dose administered at age <12 months and current age <24 months / 8 weeks (as final dose) if first dose administered at age ≥12 months or current age 24–59 months / No further doses needed for healthy children if first dose administered at age ≥24 months	4 weeks if current age <12 months / 8 weeks (as final dose) if current age ≥12 months / No further doses needed for healthy children if previous dose administered at age ≥24 months	8 weeks (as final dose) This dose only necessary for children aged 12 months–5 years who received 3 doses before age 12 months	
Inactivated Poliovirus[6]	6 wks	4 weeks	4 weeks	4 weeks[6]	
Measles, Mumps, Rubella[7]	12 mos	4 weeks			
Varicella[8]	12 mos	3 months			
Hepatitis A[9]	12 mos	6 months			
CATCH-UP SCHEDULE FOR PERSONS AGED 7–18 YEARS					
Tetanus, Diphtheria/ Tetanus, Diphtheria, Pertussis[10]	7 yrs[10]	4 weeks	8 weeks if first dose administered at age <12 months / 6 months if first dose administered at age ≥12 months	6 months if first dose administered at age <12 months	
Human Papillomavirus[11]	9 yrs	12 weeks			
Hepatitis A[9]	12 mos	6 months			
Hepatitis B[1]	Birth	4 weeks	8 weeks (and 16 weeks after first dose)		
Inactivated Poliovirus[6]	6 wks	4 weeks	4 weeks	4 weeks[6]	
Measles, Mumps, Rubella[7]	12 mos	4 weeks			
Varicella[8]	12 mos	4 weeks if first dose administered at age ≥13 years / 3 months if first dose administered at age <13 years			

1. Hepatitis B vaccine (HepB). *(Minimum age: birth)*
- Administer the 3-dose series to those who were not previously vaccinated.
- A 2-dose series of Recombivax HB® is licensed for children aged 11–15 years.

2. Rotavirus vaccine (Rota). *(Minimum age: 6 weeks)*
- Do not start the series later than age 12 weeks.
- Administer the final dose in the series by age 32 weeks. Do not administer a dose later than age 32 weeks.
- Data on safety and efficacy outside of these age ranges are insufficient.

3. Diphtheria and tetanus toxoids and acellular pertussis vaccine (DTaP). *(Minimum age: 6 weeks)*
- The fifth dose is not necessary if the fourth dose was administered at age ≥4 years.
- DTaP is not indicated for persons aged ≥7 years.

4. *Haemophilus influenzae* type b conjugate vaccine (Hib). *(Minimum age: 6 weeks)*
- Vaccine is not generally recommended for children aged ≥5 years.
- If current age <12 months and the first 2 doses were PRP-OMP (PedvaxHIB® or ComVax® [Merck]), the third (and final) dose should be administered at age 12– 15 months and at least 8 weeks after the second dose.
- If first dose was administered at age 7–11 months, administer 2 doses separated by 4 weeks plus a booster at age 12–15 months.

5. Pneumococcal conjugate vaccine (PCV). *(Minimum age: 6 weeks)*
- Vaccine is not generally recommended for children aged ≥5 years.

6. Inactivated poliovirus vaccine (IPV). *(Minimum age: 6 weeks)*
- For children who received all-IPV or all-oral poliovirus (OPV) series, a fourth dose is not necessary if third dose was administered at age ≥4 years.
- If both OPV and IPV were administered as part of a series, a total of 4 doses should be administered, regardless of the child's current age.

7. Measles, mumps, and rubella vaccine (MMR). *(Minimum age: 12 months)*
- The second dose of MMR is recommended routinely at age 4–6 years but may be administered earlier if desired.
- If not previously vaccinated, administer 2 doses of MMR during any visit with ≥4 weeks between the doses.

8. Varicella vaccine. *(Minimum age: 12 months)*
- The second dose of varicella vaccine is recommended routinely at age 4–6 years but may be administered earlier if desired.
- Do not repeat the second dose in persons aged <13 years if administered ≥28 days after the first dose.

9. Hepatitis A vaccine (HepA). *(Minimum age: 12 months)*
- HepA is recommended for certain groups of children, including in areas where vaccination programs target older children. See *MMWR* 2006;55(No. RR-7):1–23.

10. Tetanus and diphtheria toxoids vaccine (Td) and tetanus and diphtheria toxoids and acellular pertussis vaccine (Tdap). *(Minimum ages: 7 years for Td, 10 years for BOOSTRIX®, and 11 years for ADACEL™)*
- Tdap should be substituted for a single dose of Td in the primary catch-up series or as a booster if age appropriate; use Td for other doses.
- A 5-year interval from the last Td dose is encouraged when Tdap is used as a booster dose. A booster (fourth) dose is needed if any of the previous doses were administered at age <12 months. Refer to ACIP recommendations for further information. See *MMWR* 2006;55(No. RR-3).

11. Human papillomavirus vaccine (HPV). *(Minimum age: 9 years)*
- Administer the HPV vaccine series to females at age 13–18 years if not previously vaccinated.

Information about reporting reactions after immunization is available online at **http://www.vaers.hhs.gov** or by telephone via the 24-hour national toll-free information line 800-822-7967. Suspected cases of vaccine-preventable diseases should be reported to the state or local health department. Additional information, including precautions and contraindications for immunization, is available from the National Center for Immunization and Respiratory Diseases at **http://www.cdc.gov/nip/default.htm** or telephone, **800-CDC-INFO (800-232-4636)**.

DEPARTMENT OF HEALTH AND HUMAN SERVICES • CENTERS FOR DISEASE CONTROL AND PREVENTION • SAFER • HEALTHIER • PEOPLE

CS103164

Figure 113.1 Recommended immunization schedule for persons 0 to 18 years.

of age was reported to the CDC. In 2005, the ACIP and AAP recommended that a booster dose of tetanus/diphtheria vaccine combined with acellular pertussis vaccine (TDaP) formulated for adolescent and adult populations be administered routinely to children at 11 to 12 years of age (Boostrix, GlaxoSmithKline, approved for 10 to 18 years old; Adacel, SanofiPasteur, approved for 11 to 64 years old).

The quadrivalent human papillomavirus (HPV) vaccine (Gardasil, Merck) was licensed in 2006 and provides immunity against HPV types 6, 11, 16, and 18, highly associated with cervical cancer in women. The vaccine is administered as an intramuscular injection at 0, 2, and 6 months. ACIP recommends HPV vaccine for routine immunization of young women aged 11 to 12 years, although the vaccine is licensed for use in females 9 to 26 years old and may be administered as early as 9 years old if the girl is at risk of exposure. Catch-up HPV vaccination is recommended for females aged 13 to 26 years who have not been previously vaccinated. Although clinical trials of concomitant administration of HPV vaccine with the other vaccines recommended for adolescents have not been performed, there are no theoretical reasons not to administer the first dose of HPV during the same clinic visit as MCV4 and TDaP vaccines, with the vaccines being administered at different anatomic sites. HPV vaccine is contraindicated in pregnancy.

Figure 113.2 provides a summary of vaccine products available for use in the United States adapted from the 2007 CDC NIP Pink Book. Consult the CDC Web site (http://www.cdc.gov) and vaccine package inserts for additional details on the vaccines, indications, and dosing.

COMBINATION VACCINES

The number of recommended early childhood immunizations creates issues of compliance and scheduling for parents, patients, and health care providers. Depending on the use of existing combination vaccines and new vaccines presently under development, the number of immunization injections per clinic visit can be decreased. The approved use of vaccine combinations (different vaccines combined and administered through the same syringe) depends on efficacy and safety data from clinical trials. Several commercially prepared combination vaccines are available for pediatric use (Figure 113.2), and in some cases, compatible vaccines from a single vaccine manufacturer supplier are available and may be combined according to package insert instructions.

ADULT IMMUNIZATIONS

Recommendations for adult immunizations are based on the history of immunizations received in the past and on the need to give booster doses of certain vaccine series where immunity has been shown to wane over a given period. A detailed review of immunizations is indicated for international travelers, health care workers, and others who have risks of exposure related to occupational activities, individuals 65 years of age and older, and persons with compromised immune status due to disease (human immunodeficiency virus [HIV]), medications, cancer, or other chronic medical conditions.

The adult immunization history should be updated and documented at the time of initial intake into a primary care practice, during interim health maintenance visits, on employment in one of the health care or social services professions, and/or prior to international travel. Travel immunizations will be covered in Chapter 114, Advice for Travelers. If the immunization history of the person is uncertain or unknown, a conceptual framework of the prevalent practices pertaining to childhood, school, military service, and occupational immunization programs and standards will be helpful for assessing the current immunization status.

The ACIP recommendations on adult immunizations is given in Figure 113.3. The ACIP recommendations for adults have been endorsed by the American Academy of Family Practitioners (AAFP) and the American College of Obstetrics and Gynecology (ACOG).

ROUTINE IMMUNIZATIONS FOR ADULTS

Tetanus/Diphtheria Vaccine and Pertussis Vaccine

The primary series of tetanus and diphtheria vaccines are given in childhood as a part of the diphtheria/tetanus/acellular pertussis (DTaP) vaccine series. A booster dose of the adult formulation of the tetanus/diphtheria (Td) vaccine is used to boost immunity in persons 7 years of age or older, and booster doses of Td are recommended every 10 years throughout adult life. Epidemiologic studies show that immunity to pertussis wanes over time after childhood DTaP immunization and that adolescents and adults susceptible to pertussis transmit the infection to infants at highest risk of serious complications from the infection. In partially immune adolescents and adults, pertussis often causes a prolonged respiratory illness without the characteristic "whooping cough" and thus may not be recognized as such.

ACIP now recommends that a single dose of TDaP vaccine be used to replace the next booster dose of Td vaccine among persons 19 to 64 years of age to boost levels of pertussis immunity in the adult population. The TDaP vaccine (Adacel, SanofiPasteur, 11 to 64 years old) can be administered to adults at an interval shorter than 10 years from the last Td vaccine

U.S. Vaccines

Vaccine	Name	Manufacturer	Type	Route	Comments
Anthrax	BioThrax	BioPort	Inactivated Bacterial	SC	
DTaP	Daptacel	sanofi	Inactivated Bacterial	IM	Tetanus & diphtheria toxoids and pertussis vaccine. Not licensed for 5th dose.
	Infanrix	GlaxoSmithKline	Inactivated Bacterial	IM	Tetanus & diphtheria toxoids and pertussis vaccine.
	Tripedia	sanofi	Inactivated Bacterial	IM	Tetanus & diphtheria toxoids and pertussis vaccine.
DT	(Generic)	sanofi	Inactivated Bacterial Toxoids	IM	Pediatric formulation
DTaP/Hib	TriHIBit	sanofi	Inactivated Bacterial	IM	ActHIB reconstituted with Tripedia. Licensed for 4th dose of DTaP & Hib series (not primary series).
DTaP/IPV/HepB	Pediarix	GlaxoSmithKline	Inactivated Bacterial & Viral	IM	Approved for doses at 2, 4, 6 months (through 6 years of age). Not licensed for boosters.
Haemophilus influenzae type b (Hib)	HibTITER	Wyeth	Inactivated Bacterial	IM	**HbOC.** Polysaccharide conjugate (diphtheria protein carrier). 3-dose schedule.
	PedvaxHIB	Merck	Inactivated Bacterial	IM	**PRP-OMP.** Polysaccharide conjugate (mening. protein carrier). 2-dose schedule.
	ActHIB	sanofi	Inactivated Bacterial	IM	**PRP-T.** Polysaccharide conjugate (tetanus toxoid carrier). 3-dose schedule.
Hepatitis A	Havrix	GlaxoSmithKline	Inactivated Viral	IM	Pediatric ($\leq$18) and adult formulations. Pediatric = 720 EL.U., 0.5mL Adult = 1,140 EL.U., 1.0mL Minimum age = 1 year.
	Vaqta	Merck	Inactivated Viral	IM	Pediatric ($\leq$18) and adult formulations. Pediatric = 25 U, 0.5mL Adult = 50 U, 1.0mL Minimum age = 1 year.
Hepatitis B	Engerix-B	GlaxoSmithKline	Inactivated Viral (recombinant)	IM	Pediatric ($\leq$19) and adult formulations. Pediatric formulation is not licensed for adults.
	Recombivax HB	Merck	Inactivated Viral (recombinant)	IM	Pediatric ($\leq$19), adult, and dialysis formulations. Two pediatric doses may be substituted for an adult dose.

(continued)

dose. Depending on community outbreaks of pertussis, occupational exposures, and/or personal health risks, TDaP vaccine may be administered at a minimal interval of 2 years from the last Td vaccine dose based on current vaccine safety data.

HEALTH CARE WORKERS

Health care workers exposed to patients with confirmed pertussis infections may warrant antimicrobial prophylaxis and should consult the facility's infection control or occupational health consultant. ACIP recommends the use of TDaP vaccine as a one-time substitute for a Td vaccine booster among health care workers, especially for those providing care to pediatric patients.

Measles, Mumps, and Rubella

The measles, mumps, and rubella vaccines are usually given as a combination vaccine (MMR) in early childhood, at 12 to 15 months of age. However, up to 5% of vaccine recipients may fail to respond to primary immunization and

Vaccine	Name	Manufacturer	Type	Route	Comments
HepA/HepB	Twinrix	GlaxoSmithKline	Inactivated Viral	IM	Pediatric dose of HepA + adult dose of HepB. Minimum age = 18 years. 3-dose series.
HepB/Hib	Comvax	Merck	Inactivated Bacterial & Viral	IM	Should not be used for HepB birth dose.
Human Papillomavirus (HPV)	Gardasil	Merck	Inactivated Viral (recombinant)	IM	Quadrivalent, Types 6, 11, 16 & 18. Licensed for females 9-26 years.
Influenza	Fluarix	GlaxoSmithKline	Inactivated Viral	IM	Trivalent Types A & B. Minimum age = 18 years.
	Fluvirin	Chiron	Inactivated Viral	IM	Trivalent Types A & B Purified surface antigen. Minimum age = 4 years.
	Fluzone	sanofi	Inactivated Viral	IM	Trivalent Types A & B Subvirion. Minimum age multidose vial = 6 months. Age range 0.25ml prefilled syringe = 6-35 months. Minimum age 0.5ml prefilled syringe = 3 years.
	FluLaval	GlaxoSmithKline	Inactivated Viral	IM	Trivalent Types A & B. Minimum age = 18 years.
	FluMist	Medimmune	Live attenuated viral	Intra-nasal	Trivalent Types A & B. Age range 5-49 years.
Japanese Encephalitis	JE-Vax	sanofi	Inactivated viral	SC	
MMR	M-M-R II	Merck	Live attenuated viral	SC	Measles, mumps, rubella.
MMRV	ProQuad	Merck	Live attenuated viral	SC	Measles, mumps, rubella, varicella.
Measles	Attenuvax	Merck	Live attenuated viral	SC	Edmonston-Enders strain
Mumps	Mumpsvax	Merck	Live attenuated viral	SC	Jeryl Lynn strain
Rubella	Meruvax II	Merck	Live attenuated viral	SC	RA 27/3 strain
Meningococcal	Menomune	sanofi	Inactivated bacterial	SC	Polysaccharide, containing serogroups A, C, Y, & W-135.
	Menactra	sanofi	Inactivated bacterial	IM	Polysaccharide conjugate (diphtheria toxoid carrier), containing serogroups A, C, Y, & W-135. Age range 11-49.
Pneumococcal	Pneumovax 23	Merck	Inactivated bacterial	SC or IM	Polysaccharide. Contains 23 strains. Minimum age = 2 yrs.
	Prevnar	Wyeth	Inactivated bacterial	IM	Polysaccharide conjugate (diphtheria protein carrier). Contains 7 strains. Routine age range = 2-59 months.

have inadequate or waning immunity to measles by adulthood. For this reason, the ACIP and AAP recommend that a second dose of measles vaccine (as a component of MMR) be given in childhood on school entry. In many American colleges and universities, documentation of receipt of a second dose of measles vaccine or of immunity as evidenced by serum testing for measles antibodies is required for registration. There is no contraindication to using the MMR vaccine to boost measles immunity, even if the recipient is already immune to mumps and rubella. Monovalent measles, mumps, and rubella vaccines are commercially available (Figure 113.2) but are not commonly recommended, stocked, and/or used in vaccine immunization programs.

Potential vaccine adverse reactions include the rare occurrence of usually transient, but occasionally prolonged, arthralgias and arthritis

Vaccine	Name	Manufacturer	Type	Route	Comments
Polio	Ipol	Sanofi	Inactivated viral	SC or IM	Trivalent, Types 1, 2, & 3.
Rabies	BioRab	BioPort	Inactivated viral	IM	
	Imovax Rabies	Sanofi	Inactivated viral	IM	
	RabAvert	Chiron	Inactivated viral	IM	
Rotavirus	RotaTeq	Merck	Live viral	Oral	Pentavalent. Age range 6-32 weeks. First dose between 6 & 12 weeks; complete 3-dose series by 32 weeks.
Td	Decavac	Sanofi	Inactivated bacterial toxoids	IM	Tetanus/diphtheria toxoids. Adult formulation
	(Generic)	Massachusetts Biological Labs	Inactivated bacterial toxoids	IM	Tetanus/diphtheria toxoids. Adult formulation
TDap	Boostrix	GlaxoSmithKline	Inactivated bacterial	IM	Tetanus & diphtheria toxoids & pertussis vaccine. Licensed for ages 10-18.
	Adacel	Sanofi	Inactivated bacterial	IM	Tetanus & diphtheria toxoids & pertussis vaccine. Licensed for ages 11-64.
TT	(Generic)	Sanofi	Inactivated bacterial toxoid	IM	Tetanus toxoid. May be used for adults or children.
Typhoid	Typhim Vi	Sanofi	Inactivated bacterial	IM	Polysaccharide.
	Vivotif Berna	Berna	Live bacterial	Oral	Ty21a strain.
Varicella	Varivax	Merck	Live viral	SC	
Vaccinia (Smallpox)	Dryvax	Wyeth	Live viral	Percutaneous	
Yellow fever	YF-Vax	Sanofi	Live viral	SC	
Zoster (Shingles)	Zostavax	Merck	Live viral	SC	Licensed for age 60 and older.

December 2006

Figure 113.2 U. S. vaccines. SC = subcutaneously; IM = intramuscularly; MMR = measles, mumps, and rubella vaccine; MMRV = measles, mumps, rubella, and varicella vaccine; Hep = hepatitis.

attributed to the rubella component of the MMR vaccine in nonimmune women of reproductive age – the very group most likely to benefit from immunization against rubella. As with any vaccine, the potential risks versus benefits of immunization with MMR vaccine should be discussed with potential vaccine recipients, along with the VIS statements.

CONTRAINDICATIONS

MMR vaccine is a live virus combination vaccine. Women of childbearing age should not be pregnant at the time of receiving MMR vaccine and should defer pregnancy for 3 months after MMR immunization.

HIV-INFECTED PERSONS

MMR immunization is recommended for use in susceptible persons with asymptomatic HIV infection, as the potential benefits of immunization appear to outweigh the serious course of natural measles infections in this population.

HEALTH CARE WORKERS

People born before 1957 are generally considered immune to measles, mumps, and rubella by virtue of having had the natural infectious diseases in the pre-MMR vaccine era. However, because a small percentage in this group did not acquire lasting immunity from historical accounts of diagnosed/presumed infections, and because health care workers may be at increased risk of acquiring measles and mumps infections and transmitting them to other patients/clients, health care workers should provide proof of prior receipt of two doses of MMR vaccine or serological immunity to measles and mumps.

Varicella Vaccine and Zoster (Shingles) Vaccine

Varicella (chickenpox) infections are more likely to result in severe disease among adults

Recommended Adult Immunization Schedule
United States, October 2006–September 2007

Recommended adult immunization schedule, by vaccine and age group

Age group (yrs) ▶ Vaccine ▼	19–49 years	50–64 years	≥65 years
Tetanus, diphtheria, pertussis (Td/Tdap)[1]*	1-dose Td booster every 10 yrs Substitute 1 dose of Tdap for Td		
Human papillomavirus (HPV)[2]*	3 doses (females)		
Measles, mumps, rubella (MMR)[3]*	1 or 2 doses	1 dose	
Varicella[4]*	2 doses (0, 4–8 wks)	2 doses (0, 4–8 wks)	
Influenza[5]*	1 dose annually	1 dose annually	
Pneumococcal (polysaccharide)[6,7]	1–2 doses		1 dose
Hepatitis A[8]*	2 doses (0, 6–12 mos, or 0, 6–18 mos)		
Hepatitis B[9]*	3 doses (0, 1–2, 4–6 mos)		
Meningococcal[10]	1 or more doses		

Recommended adult immunization schedule, by vaccine and medical and other indications

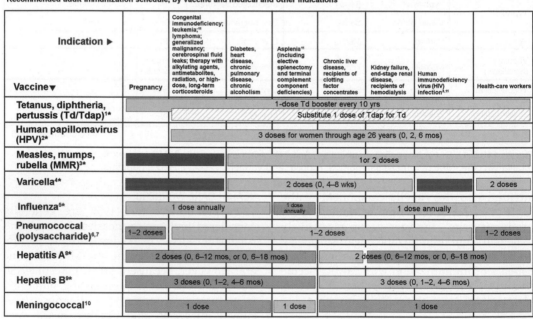

Indication ▶ Vaccine ▼	Pregnancy	Congenital immunodeficiency;[11] leukemia;[11] lymphoma; generalized malignancy; cerebrospinal fluid leaks; therapy with alkylating agents, antimetabolites, radiation, or high-dose, long-term corticosteroids	Diabetes, heart disease, chronic pulmonary disease, chronic alcoholism	Asplenia[11] (including elective splenectomy and terminal complement component deficiencies)	Chronic liver disease, recipients of clotting factor concentrates	Kidney failure, end-stage renal disease, recipients of hemodialysis	Human immunodeficiency virus (HIV) infection[3,11]	Health-care workers
Tetanus, diphtheria, pertussis (Td/Tdap)[1]*	1-dose Td booster every 10 yrs Substitute 1 dose of Tdap for Td							
Human papillomavirus (HPV)[2]*		3 doses for women through age 26 years (0, 2, 6 mos)						
Measles, mumps, rubella (MMR)[3]*	(contraindicated)	1 or 2 doses						
Varicella[4]*	(contraindicated)	2 doses (0, 4–8 wks)					(contraindicated)	2 doses
Influenza[5]*	1 dose annually			1 dose annually	1 dose annually			
Pneumococcal (polysaccharide)[6,7]	1–2 doses	1–2 doses						1–2 doses
Hepatitis A[8]*	2 doses (0, 6–12 mos, or 0, 6–18 mos)			2 doses (0, 6–12 mos, or 0, 6–18 mos)				
Hepatitis B[9]*	3 doses (0, 1–2, 4–6 mos)			3 doses (0, 1–2, 4–6 mos)				
Meningococcal[10]	1 dose		1 dose		1 dose			

* Covered by the Vaccine Injury Compensation Program

These recommendations must be read along with the footnotes, which can be found on the next 2 pages of this schedule.

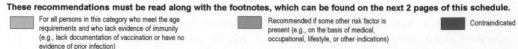

For all persons in this category who meet the age requirements and who lack evidence of immunity (e.g., lack documentation of vaccination or have no evidence of prior infection)

Recommended if some other risk factor is present (e.g., on the basis of medical, occupational, lifestyle, or other indications)

Contraindicated

compared to children, often accompanied by complications such as varicella pneumonia. A live attenuated viral vaccine against varicella (Varivax, Merck) was released in the mid-1990s. The primary series for young people 12 years of age or older and adults consists of two doses given by injection 1 month apart.

VZV causes varicella and becomes dormant within the nerves following exposure but can reactivate later in life, usually around 50 years old. The risk of reactivation increases with age, causing herpes zoster or "shingles," a condition characterized by a vesicular rash that follows a dermatomal distribution that often leads to

Footnotes

1. Tetanus, diphtheria, and acellular pertussis (Td/Tdap) vaccination. Adults with uncertain histories of a complete primary vaccination series with diphtheria and tetanus toxoid–containing vaccines should begin or complete a primary vaccination series. A primary series for adults is 3 doses; administer the first 2 doses at least 4 weeks apart and the third dose 6–12 months after the second. Administer a booster dose to adults who have completed a primary series and if the last vaccination was received ≥ 10 years previously. Tdap or tetanus and diphtheria (Td) vaccine may be used; Tdap should replace a single dose of Td for adults aged <65 years who have not previously received a dose of Tdap (either in the primary series, as a booster, or for wound management). Only one of two Tdap products (Adacel® [sanofi pasteur, Swiftwater, Pennsylvania]) is licensed for use in adults. If the person is pregnant and received the last Td vaccination ≥10 years previously, administer Td during the second or third trimester; if the person received the last Td vaccination in <10 years, administer Tdap during the immediate postpartum period. A one-time administration of 1-dose of Tdap with an interval as short as 2 years from a previous Td vaccination is recommended for postpartum women, close contacts of infants aged <12 months, and all health-care workers with direct patient contact. In certain situations, Td can be deferred during pregnancy and Tdap substituted in the immediate postpartum period, or Tdap can be given instead of Td to a pregnant woman after an informed discussion with the woman (see http://www.cdc.gov/nip/publications/acip-list.htm). Consult the ACIP statement for recommendations for administering Td as prophylaxis in wound management (http://www.cdc.gov/mmwr/preview/mmwrhtml/00041645.htm).

2. Human Papillomavirus (HPV) vaccination. HPV vaccination is recommended for all women aged ≤26 years who have not completed the vaccine series. Ideally, vaccine should be administered before potential exposure to HPV through sexual activity; however, women who are sexually active should still be vaccinated. Sexually active women who have not been infected with any of the HPV vaccine types receive the full benefit of the vaccination. Vaccination is less beneficial for women who have already been infected with one or more of the four HPV vaccine types. A complete series consists of 3 doses. The second dose should be administered 2 months after the first dose; the third dose should be administered 6 months after the first dose. Vaccination is not recommended during pregnancy. If a woman is found to be pregnant after initiating the vaccination series, the remainder of the 3-dose regimen should be delayed until after completion of the pregnancy.

3. Measles, Mumps, Rubella (MMR) vaccination. *Measles component:* adults born before 1957 can be considered immune to measles. Adults born during or after 1957 should receive ≥1 dose of MMR unless they have a medical contraindication, documentation of ≥ 1 dose, history of measles based on health-care provider diagnosis, or laboratory evidence of immunity. A second dose of MMR is recommended for adults who 1) have been recently exposed to measles or in an outbreak setting; 2) were previously vaccinated with killed measles vaccine; 3) have been vaccinated with an unknown type of measles vaccine during 1963–1967; 4) are students in postsecondary educational institutions; 5) work in a health-care facility, or 6) plan to travel internationally. Withhold MMR or other measles-containing vaccines from HIV-infected persons with severe immunosuppression. *Mumps component:* adults born before 1957 can generally be considered immune to mumps. Adults born during or after 1957 should receive 1 dose of MMR unless they have a medical contraindication, history of mumps based on health-care provider diagnosis, or laboratory evidence of immunity. A second dose of MMR is recommended for adults who 1) are in an age group that is affected during a mumps outbreak; 2) are students in postsecondary educational institutions; 3) work in a health-care facility; or 4) plan to travel internationally. For unvaccinated health-care workers born before 1957 who do not have other evidence of mumps immunity, consider giving 1 dose on a routine basis and strongly consider giving a second dose during an outbreak. *Rubella component:* administer 1 dose of MMR vaccine to women whose rubella vaccination history is unreliable or who lack laboratory evidence of immunity. For women of childbearing age, regardless of birth year, routinely determine rubella immunity and counsel women regarding congenital rubella syndrome. Do not vaccinate women who are pregnant or who might become pregnant within 4 weeks of receiving vaccine. Women who do not have evidence of immunity should receive MMR vaccine upon completion or termination of pregnancy and before discharge from the health-care facility.

4. Varicella vaccination. All adults without evidence of immunity to varicella should receive 2 doses of varicella vaccine. Special consideration should be given to those who 1) have close contact with persons at high risk for severe disease (e.g., health-care workers and family contacts of immunocompromised persons) or 2) are at high risk for exposure or transmission (e.g., teachers of young children; child care employees; residents and staff members of institutional settings, including correctional institutions; college students; military personnel; adolescents and adults living in households with children; non-pregnant women of childbearing age; and international travelers). Evidence of immunity to varicella in adults includes any of the following: 1) documentation of 2 doses of varicella vaccine at least 4 weeks apart; 2) U.S.–born before 1980 (although for health-care workers and pregnant women, birth before 1980 should not be considered evidence of immunity); 3) history of varicella based on diagnosis or verification of varicella by a health-care provider (for a patient reporting a history of or presenting with an atypical case, a mild case, or both, health-care providers should seek either an epidemiologic link with a typical varicella case or evidence of laboratory confirmation, if it was performed at the time of acute disease); 4) history of herpes zoster based on health-care provider diagnosis; or 5) laboratory evidence of immunity or laboratory confirmation of disease. Do not vaccinate women who are pregnant or might become pregnant within 4 weeks of receiving the vaccine. Assess pregnant women for evidence of varicella immunity. Women who do not have evidence of immunity should receive dose 1 of varicella vaccine upon completion or termination of pregnancy and before discharge from the health-care facility. Dose 2 should be administered 4–8 weeks after dose 1.

5. Influenza vaccination: *Medical indications:* chronic disorders of the cardiovascular or pulmonary systems, including asthma; chronic metabolic diseases, including diabetes mellitus, renal dysfunction, hemoglobinopathies, or immunosuppression (including immunosuppression caused by medications or HIV); any condition that compromises respiratory function or the handling of respiratory secretions or that can increase the risk of aspiration (e.g., cognitive dysfunction, spinal cord injury, or seizure disorder or other neuromuscular disorder); and pregnancy during the influenza season. No data exist on the risk for severe or complicated influenza disease among persons with asplenia; however, influenza is a risk factor for secondary bacterial infections that can cause severe disease among persons with asplenia. *Occupational indications:* health-care workers and employees of long-term–care and assisted living facilities. *Other indications:* residents of nursing homes and other long-term–care and assisted living facilities; persons likely to transmit influenza to persons at high risk (i.e., in-home household contacts and caregivers of children aged 0–59 months, or persons of all ages with high-risk conditions); and anyone who would like to be vaccinated. Healthy, nonpregnant persons aged 5–49 years without high-risk medical conditions who are not contacts of severely immunocompromised persons in special care units can receive either intranasally administered influenza vaccine (FluMist®) or inactivated vaccine. Other persons should receive the inactivated vaccine.

(continued)

debilitating chronic pain. The ACIP recommends that the newly licensed zoster vaccine (Zostavax, Merck) be given to all people 60 years of age and older, including those who have had a previous episode of shingles. The zoster vaccine is a live attenuated virus vaccine and should be used with caution in adults younger than 60 years of age and in adults with immunocompromised status.

CONTRAINDICATIONS

Varicella vaccine and zoster vaccine are live virus vaccines and contraindicated in pregnant women. Women of childbearing age should not be pregnant at the time of receiving varicella vaccine and should defer pregnancy for 3 months after varicella immunization. Varicella vaccine and zoster vaccine are contraindicated in persons with compromised immunity, including

Footnotes

6. Pneumococcal polysaccharide vaccination. *Medical indications:* chronic disorders of the pulmonary system (excluding asthma); cardiovascular diseases; diabetes mellitus; chronic liver diseases, including liver disease as a result of alcohol abuse (e.g.,cirrhosis); chronic renal failure or nephrotic syndrome; functional or anatomic asplenia (e.g., sickle cell disease or splenectomy [if elective splenectomy is planned, vaccinate at least 2 weeks before surgery]); immunosuppressive conditions (e.g., congenital immunodeficiency, HIV infection [vaccinate as close to diagnosis as possible when CD4 cell counts are highest], leukemia, lymphoma, multiple myeloma, Hodgkin disease, generalized malignancy, organ or bone marrow transplantation); chemotherapy with alkylating agents, antimetabolites, or high-dose, long-term corticosteroids; and cochlear implants. *Other indications:* Alaska Natives and certain American Indian populations and residents of nursing homes or other long-term–care facilities.

7. Revaccination with pneumococcal polysaccharide vaccine. One-time revaccination after 5 years for persons with chronic renal failure or nephrotic syndrome; functional or anatomic asplenia (e.g., sickle cell disease or splenectomy); immunosuppressive conditions (e.g., congenital immunodeficiency, HIV infection, leukemia, lymphoma, multiple myeloma, Hodgkin disease, generalized malignancy, or organ or bone marrow transplantation); or chemotherapy with alkylating agents, antimetabolites, or high-dose, long-term corticosteroids. For persons aged ≥65 years, one-time revaccination if they were vaccinated ≥5 years previously and were aged <65 years at the time of primary vaccination.

8. Hepatitis A vaccination. *Medical indications:* persons with chronic liver disease and persons who receive clotting factor concentrates. *Behavioral indications:* men who have sex with men and persons who use illegal drugs. *Occupational indications:* persons working with hepatitis A virus (HAV)–infected primates or with HAV in a research laboratory setting. *Other indications:* persons traveling to or working in countries that have high or intermediate endemicity of hepatitis A (a list of countries is available at http://www.cdc.gov/travel/diseases.htm) and any person who would like to obtain immunity. Current vaccines should be administered in a 2-dose schedule at either 0 and 6–12 months, or 0 and 6–18 months. If the combined hepatitis A and hepatitis B vaccine is used, administer 3 doses at 0, 1, and 6 months .

9. Hepatitis B vaccination. *Medical indications:* Persons with end-stage renal disease, including patients receiving hemodialysis; persons seeking evaluation or treatment for a sexually transmitted disease (STD); persons with HIV infection; persons with chronic liver disease; and persons who receive clotting factor concentrates. *Occupational indications:* health-care workers and public-safety workers who are exposed to blood or other potentially infectious body fluids. *Behavioral indications:* sexually active persons who are not in a long-term, mutually monogamous relationship (i.e., persons with >1 sex partner during the previous 6 months); current or recent injection-drug users; and men who have sex with men. *Other indications:* household contacts and sex partners of persons with chronic hepatitis B virus (HBV) infection; clients and staff members of institutions for persons with developmental disabilities; all clients of STD clinics; international travelers to countries with high or intermediate prevalence of chronic HBV infection (a list of countries is available at http://www.cdc.gov/travel/diseases.htm); and any adult seeking protection from HBV infection. Settings where hepatitis B vaccination is recommended for all adults: STD treatment facilities; HIV testing and treatment facilities; facilities providing drug-abuse treatment and prevention services; health-care settings providing services for injection-drug users or men who have sex with men; correctional facilities; end-stage renal disease programs and facilities for chronic hemodialysis patients; and institutions and nonresidential daycare facilities for persons with developmental disabilities. *Special formulation indications:* for adult patients receiving hemodialysis and other immunocompromised adults, 1 dose of 40 μg/mL (Recombivax HB®) or 2 doses of 20 μg/mL (Engerix-B®).

10. Meningococcal vaccination. *Medical indications:* adults with anatomic or functional asplenia, or terminal complement component deficiencies. *Other indications:* first-year college students living in dormitories; microbiologists who are routinely exposed to isolates of *Neisseria meningitidis*; military recruits; and persons who travel to or live in countries in which meningococcal disease is hyperendemic or epidemic (e.g., the "meningitis belt" of Sub-Saharan Africa during the dry season [December–June]), particularly if contact with local populations will be prolonged. Vaccination is required by the government of Saudi Arabia for all travelers to Mecca during the annual Hajj. Meningococcal conjugate vaccine is preferred for adults with any of the preceeding indications who are aged ≤55 years, although meningococcal polysaccharide vaccine (MPSV4) is an acceptable alternative. Revaccination after 5 years might be indicated for adults previously vaccinated with MPSV4 who remain at high risk for infection (e.g., persons residing in areas in which disease is epidemic).

11. Selected conditions for which *Haemophilus influenzae* type b (Hib) vaccination may be used. Hib conjugate vaccines are licensed for children aged 6 weeks–71 months. No efficacy data are available on which to base a recommendation concerning use of Hib vaccine for older children and adults with the chronic conditions associated with an increased risk for Hib disease. However, studies suggest good immunogenicity in patients who have sickle cell disease, leukemia, or HIV infection or have had splenectomies; administering vaccine to these patients is not contraindicated.

This schedule indicates the recommended age groups and medical indications for routine administration of currently licensed vaccines for persons aged ≥19 years, as of October 1, 2006. Licensed combination vaccines may be used whenever any components of the combination are indicated and when the vaccine's other components are not contraindicated. For detailed recommendations on all vaccines, including those used primarily for travelers or that are issued during the year, consult the manufacturers' package inserts and the complete statements from the Advisory Committee on Immunization Practices (http://www.cdc.gov/nip/publications/acip-list.htm).

Report all clinically significant postvaccination reactions to the Vaccine Adverse Event Reporting System (VAERS). Reporting forms and instructions on filing a VAERS report are available at http://www.vaers.hhs.gov or by telephone, 800-822-7967.

Information on how to file a Vaccine Injury Compensation Program claim is available at http://www.hrsa.gov/vaccinecompensation or by telephone, 800-338-2382.To file a claim for vaccine injury, contact the U.S. Court of Federal Claims, 717 Madison Place, N.W., Washington, D.C. 20005; telephone, 202-357-6400.

Additional information about the vaccines in this schedule and contraindications for vaccination is also available at http://www.cdc.gov/nip or from the CDC-INFO Contact Center at 800-CDC-INFO (800-232-4636) in English and Spanish, 24 hours a day, 7 days a week.

Approved by the Advisory Committee on Immunization Practices, the American College of Obstetricians and Gynecologists, the American Academy of Family Physicians, and the American College of Physicians

Figure 113.3 Recommended adult immunization schedule.

individuals with HIV infection. Some experts suggest that zoster vaccine may be considered for off-label use in immune-competent persons of any age who anticipate treatments or advancing illness that will result in immunocompromised status and in HIV-infected persons with CD4 lymphocytes ≥15% (CD4 ≥200 mm³) ≥3 months on a stable antiretroviral drug regimen for ≥3 months, because the potential benefit would outweigh the potential risks.

HEALTH CARE WORKERS

Current occupational health recommendations for health care workers include documentation of varicella immunity or varicella immunization as a condition for working in certain clinics and hospitals.

Polio Vaccine

Immunization against polio is a part of the childhood immunization program, and booster doses are not given routinely in adulthood in the Western Hemisphere (North and South America) and Western Europe, where polio is considered eradicated. Current pediatric regimens use the enhanced inactivated polio vaccine (IPV) (Ipol, SanofiPasteur) administered by injection for primary immunization. A single dose of IPV is recommended as a booster in adults when there is imminent risk of exposure, such as travel to certain regions of Africa and Asia where polio is still transmitted, or for occupational exposure (eg, work in certain research laboratories).

Hepatitis B Vaccine

Hepatitis B immunization has been included as one of the regular immunizations covered by childhood immunization programs in the United States since 1991. Hepatitis B vaccine should be considered a "catch-up" immunization among young adults born before the hepatitis B vaccine was incorporated into the routine childhood immunization programs. Hepatitis B immunization should also be recommended to individuals at risk of exposure to hepatitis B virus through occupational risk; treatment with blood products; contact with infected family, friends, or others; or international travel.

The primary series for hepatitis B immunization consists of three doses given by intramuscular injection into the deltoid muscle at 0, 1, and 6 months (Recombivax B, Merck; Engerix B, GlaxoSmithKline). An accelerated schedule consisting of three doses of hepatitis B vaccine given at 0, 1, and 2 months, with a booster dose at 12 months, has FDA approval (Engerix B).

A combination vaccine against hepatitis A plus hepatitis B (Twinrix, GlaxoSmithKline) has been licensed for 18 years of age and older and is given on a standard schedule of 0, 1, and 6 months. Recently, an accelerated schedule for hepatitis A plus B vaccine has received FDA approval. The accelerated dosing schedule of three doses given on 0, 7, and 21 to 28 days, followed by a fourth dose at 12 months, produces protective immunity against hepatitis A and hepatitis B following the first three doses. The fourth dose is given to assure long-lasting immunity. The accelerated schedule will be most useful for international travelers seeking immunizations with <1 month's time before trip departure, and also will be useful for susceptible health care workers who need rapid protection before duty assignments.

An ancillary observation on hepatitis B vaccine immunogenicity was that the antibody response to hepatitis B is enhanced when A and B antigens are given simultaneously in the same syringe or concomitantly when monovalent hepatitis A and hepatitis B vaccines are given at the same time but at separate sites of injection. The adjuvant effect of hepatitis A has possible implications for hepatitis B–susceptible adults aged 30 years or older, who tend to respond with lower antibody levels to monovalent hepatitis B vaccine compared with younger hepatitis B vaccine recipients. The utility of combination hepatitis A plus hepatitis B immunization in other groups of hepatitis B vaccine low responders or nonresponders (eg, obese, cigarette smokers, male) needs further investigation.

HEALTH CARE WORKERS

Hepatitis B immunization or immunity is required for work in certain occupations, including health care workers, policemen, firemen, morticians, and others who are likely to have work-related contact with human blood and other bodily substances.

Pneumococcal Vaccine

Pneumococcal polysaccharide vaccine (Pneumovax 23, SanofiPasteur) is recommended for all adults 65 years of age and older and for younger persons aged 2 to 64 years with chronic cardiopulmonary conditions or chronic diseases. A single dose given by injection of the purified polysaccharide 23-valent pneumococcal vaccine results in protective immunity. A booster dose after a 5-year interval may be recommended in geriatric populations. A conjugate pneumococcal vaccine for adults is under development.

Viral Influenza Vaccine

The vaccine against viral influenza is reformulated annually based on the current worldwide epidemiology of influenza viruses according to the World Health Organization (WHO). Thus annual immunization with the "flu" vaccine is recommended for adults aged 50 years and older (as well as infants aged 6 to 59 months), persons with cardiopulmonary conditions and debilitating diseases, and international travelers.

Because the flu vaccine distributed for a given season may not be totally protective against all strains of influenza viruses in circulation in the months following the annual flu vaccine formulation, medications against the flu may be considered in certain high-risk persons. Prophylaxis with or prompt initiation of treatment after onset of symptoms with oseltamivir (Tamiflu) during outbreaks of influenza A, or treatment with zanamivir (Relenza) during outbreaks of influenza A or B, may prevent or ameliorate a breakthrough attack of the flu.

In addition to the traditional inactivated influenza virus vaccines administered by injection (Fluarix, GlaxoSmithKline; Fluvirin, Chiron; Fluzone, SanofiPasteur), a live attenuated influenza vaccine (LAIV) (FluMist, Medimmune) administered by intranasal application is approved for recipients aged 5 to 49 years and has been recently licensed.

Hepatitis A Vaccine

The conditions allowing transmission of hepatitis A are ubiquitous, although the relative risk appears to be highest in countries where sanitation and hygiene are suboptimal and there is widespread fecal contamination of food and water supplies. In areas of low endemicity for hepatitis A virus (HAV), outbreaks of the disease are related to contamination of food during preparation by infected food handlers and to ingestion of fresh or frozen fruits and vegetables imported from areas highly endemic for hepatitis A, contaminated during cultivation or processing. Shellfish from sewage-contaminated beds are another source of foodborne transmission.

In the United States, adults identified by the CDC as being at increased risk for hepatitis A or severe outcomes include travelers, men who have sex with men, users of injecting and noninjecting drugs, persons who have clotting-factor disorders, persons working with nonhuman primates, and persons with chronic liver disease.

Children can serve as a significant reservoir of HAV in outbreaks and in endemic communities. Hepatitis A infections are mild and often anicteric in young children, so infected children are not detected. Fecal–oral transmission to other children and family members, as well as adult teachers or caretakers, can easily occur in household, day care, and institutional settings, especially if children in diapers are present. It is important to note that HAV case fatality rates in healthy individuals rise with age, so although the rate is 0.1% from younger than 1 to 14 years of age, it is 0.4% in those from 15 to 39 years of age, 1.1% in those older than 40 years, and 2.7% in persons older than 49 years.

Several safe and highly efficacious inactivated hepatitis A vaccines have become available commercially since the 1994 release of Havrix (Smithkline Beecham, Philadelphia, PA; Rixensart, Belgium), the first inactivated HAV vaccine, derived from the HM-175 viral strain, and given by injection. The others include VAQTA (Merck Vaccine Division, West Point, NJ), an inactivated parenteral HAV vaccine derived from the CR-326 F strain; AVAXIM (Pasteur Merieux MSD, Paris), an inactivated parenteral HAV vaccine derived from the GBM viral strain; and Epaxal Berna (Swiss Serum Research Institute, Bern), an inactivated parenteral virosomal HAV vaccine derived from the RG-SB viral strain. Havrix and VAQTA are available in the United States and Canada, as well as worldwide. The other vaccines are distributed mostly in western Europe.

The immunization schedules for all the hepatitis A vaccines listed above consist of a single primary dose given by intramuscular (IM) injection into the deltoid muscle, resulting in protective antibody titers within 4 weeks that confer protection for 6 months up to 1 year. The first vaccine dose is followed by a booster dose 6 to 12 months later, producing levels of antibody predicted to give protection up to 10 years or more by mathematical modeling.

Vaccine interchangeability, that is, when one of the inactivated hepatitis A vaccines is used for the primary dose and then a hepatitis A vaccine made by a different manufacturer is used for the booster dose, has been studied among several of the vaccines listed previously. Although not a recommended or officially approved practice at the time of writing, it appears from the preliminary results of clinical studies that Havrix and VAQTA may be used interchangeably without significant loss of protective antibody levels elicited (data on file, Merck Vaccine Division, West Point, NJ).

Immunoglobulin

Immunoglobulin (IG) is purified human immunoglobulin used to provide protection against HAV infection through the passive transfer of preformed antibodies against HAV present in the IG (at least 100 IU/μL). Immunoglobulin is recommended for prevention of hepatitis A following known exposure to a confirmed case of HAV (0.02 mL/kg) and in nonimmune travelers going to HAV-endemic areas when there is <2 weeks remaining before departure (0.02 mL/kg to 0.06 mL/kg).

SPECIAL CONSIDERATIONS

Attenuated live viral or bacterial vaccines are generally contraindicated for pregnant women and patients with compromised immunity. Exceptions are the recommendations for giving the MMR vaccine to children with HIV infection and giving the yellow fever vaccine and oral polio vaccines to a pregnant woman traveler with imminent departure to a high-risk destination in a foreign country. In these cases, the theoretical risk of serious adverse vaccine complications may be outweighed by the anticipated benefits of vaccine-elicited protection.

Limited data suggest that administration of toxoid, killed virus, and purified derivative vaccines to HIV patients as appropriate may elicit protective immunity in the vaccine recipient if the CD4 count is greater than 200/mm^3. An observed rise in viral loads in some HIV patients following vaccination has been of some concern, but the phenomenon is thought to be frequently transient. The current consensus is that a severe infection with a given vaccine-preventable pathogen is more likely to be associated with a more detrimental rise in viral load than that seen secondary to the corresponding immunization.

Annual doses of influenza vaccines are recommended for persons aged 50 years or older and for persons of all ages with cardiovascular or pulmonary disease. The vaccines against encapsulated bacteria (*H. influenzae* type b, pneumococcal, and meningococcal vaccines) are recommended for persons who have a history of functional asplenia or of splenectomy because of the risk of overwhelming sepsis associated with infections from these agents.

Vaccine efficacy can be affected by various conditions and therapies that lead to compromise of the immune system. In patients receiving hemodialysis, the suboptimal immune response to hepatitis A and B vaccines may necessitate higher-than-standard antigen doses,

given as a special vaccine formulation or as additional doses after the standard series has been administered.

TRAVEL IMMUNIZATIONS

The patient seeking vaccine advice for international travel presents an opportunity to review and update routine immunizations as well as assess the risk of exposure to exotic diseases during the trip (see Chapter 114, Advice for Travelers).

SUGGESTED READING

American College of Physicians. *Guide for Adult Immunization.* 3rd ed. Philadelphia, PA: American College of Physicians; 1994.

Centers for Disease Control and Prevention. Recommended immunization schedules for persons aged 0–18 years – United States, 2007. *Morbid Mortal Weekly Rep.* 2007;55(51&52): Q1–Q4.

Centers for Disease Control and Prevention. Hepatitis B virus: a comprehensive strategy for eliminating transmission in the United States through universal childhood vaccination: recommendations of the Immunization Practices Advisory Committee (ACIP). *Morbid Mortal Weekly Rep.* 1991;40:1.

Centers for Disease Control and Prevention. Pertussis vaccination: acellular pertussis vaccine for reinforcing and booster use – supplementary ACIP statement. Recommendations of the Immunization Practices Advisory Committee (ACIP). *Morbid Mortal Weekly Rep.* 1992;41(RR-1):1.

Centers for Disease Control and Prevention. Committee on Immunization Practices. Use of vaccines and immune globulins in persons with altered immunocompetence. *Morbid Mortal Weekly Rep.* 1993;42(RR-4):1.

Centers for Disease Control and Prevention. Standards for pediatric immunization practices recommended by the National Vaccine Advisory Committee, approved by the U. S. Public Health Service. *Morbid Mortal Weekly Rep.* 1993;42(RR-5):1.

Centers for Disease Control and Prevention. Prevention of hepatitis A through active or passive immunization. Recommendations of the Advisory Committee on Immunization Practices (ACIP). *Morbid Mortal Weekly Rep.* 1999;48(RR-12):1.

Centers for Disease Control and Prevention. Pertussis – United Sates, 2001–2003. *Morbid Mortal Weekly Rep.* 2005;54:1283–1286.

Immunizations

PART XVI

Travel and Recreation

Phyllis E. Kozarsky and Jay S. Keystone

There are more than 700 million international travelers annually and despite tragic events such as 9/11 or emerging disease epidemics such as severe acute respiratory syndrome (SARS), it appears that travel will continue to grow as one of the major "businesses" of the world. Indeed, travel is becoming more exotic and adventuresome, leaving no space on Earth untouched. However, studies continue to show that 50% to 75% of short-term travelers, particularly to the tropics or subtropics, develop some health impairment. Fortunately, most problems are minor, with only 5% requiring medical attention and fewer than 1% requiring hospitalization. Valuable sources of information for travel health advisors are found in Table 114.1.

All travelers should be encouraged to carry a travel health kit, which should always remain with the traveler and never be stowed with baggage (except for those items that can not be taken in the carry-on luggage) (Table 114.2). In addition, travelers should make sure that they are aware of a health care provider at home should they develop illness. Those with more serious chronic diseases will want to make sure they have additional health insurance to cover them in the event of illness abroad and should consider purchasing medical evacuation insurance (as well as trip cancellation insurance). All primary care providers should make it a habit of asking their patients who see them for routine examinations whether they will be traveling. Should travel be on their agendas, it is wise to refer them to a travel health clinic that can give them comprehensive advice as well as appropriate immunizations and medications as necessary.

IMMUNIZATIONS

Immunizations may be divided into those of worldwide importance and those of special importance to certain travelers. Those of worldwide importance should be considered by physicians not only for travelers but also for the general public who are at risk. Examples of those having worldwide importance include diphtheria; tetanus; polio; measles, mumps, and rubella (MMR); influenza; pneumococcus; and hepatitis B vaccines (see Chapter 113, Immunizations). Immunizations of special importance for certain travelers include yellow fever, typhoid, rabies, meningococcal meningitis, Japanese B encephalitis, and hepatitis A. Two vaccines rarely indicated are bacille Calmette-Guérin and cholera, of which the latter is not available in the United States. Immunizations should always be recommended according to risk of disease and not according to the country visited. For example, two travelers may be visiting Thailand; however, one is a business traveler staying in a deluxe hotel in Bangkok, whereas the other is staying in a refugee camp along the Thai-Cambodian border. Their travel health needs, including immunizations and antimalarials, will be quite different although their country of destination is the same.

Most vaccines may be administered simultaneously. A notable exception is measles vaccine, which should be administered at least 2 weeks before or 6 weeks after the receipt of immunoglobulin if used for hepatitis A protection. In addition, the immune response to an injected live-virus vaccine (eg, MMR, varicella, or yellow fever) might be impaired if administered within 28 days of another live virus vaccine; however, it is acceptable to administer them on the same day. Table 114.3 lists the immunizations of special importance and their schedules.

Immunizations of Worldwide Importance

DIPHTHERIA, TETANUS, AND PERTUSSIS

Diphtheria continues to be a problem worldwide, with outbreaks since the mid-1990s affecting areas in eastern and northern Europe. Serosurveys have shown that tetanus titers are lacking in many Americans, particularly in women and in adults older than 50 years. A diphtheria–tetanus booster should be administered at 10-year intervals. Physicians may encourage frequent high-risk travelers to receive a tetanus booster alone every 5 years because a tetanus-prone wound does not necessitate a booster or tetanus immunoglobulin if tetanus toxoid has been given within 5 years.

Table 114.1 Sources of Information for Travel Health Advisers

1. *Health Information for International Travel*. Published by Elsevier and the U.S. Department of Health and Human Services Centers for Disease Control and Prevention (CDC) 2008. Available to health care professionals and the public through the CDC Travelers' Health Web site (www.cdc.gov/travel). An updated book reviewing malaria chemoprophylaxis, immunization requirements, and recommendations for international travel.

2. Centers for Disease Control and Prevention Voice Information System, Atlanta, GA. A computer-assisted telephone information hotline for worldwide travel health advice. Telephone: 877-FYI-TRIP

3. International Association for Medical Assistance to Travelers (IAMAT) Web site: www.Iamat.org. Provides information on tropical diseases, climate charts, list of English-speaking physicians.

4. Travel Medicine Advisor. Published by American Health Consultants, Atlanta, GA. This comprehensive looseleaf text, continually revised, provides bimonthly updates and alerts. Telephone: 404-262-7436. Web site: www.travelmedicineadvisor.com

5. *Health Hints for the Tropics*. 13th ed. 2005. Published by the American Society of Tropical Medicine and Hygiene (ASTM&H) and written by several of its members. Authoritative source of information for the travel health adviser and for the traveler. Available from ASTM&H Headquarters, 60 Revere Drive, Suite 500, Northbrook, IL 60062. Telephone: 847-480-9592; fax: 847-480-9282.

6. International Society of Travel Medicine (ISTM). An association of travel health advisers. The ISTM sponsors biennial meetings. Members receive a quarterly journal and newsletter. For information visit their Web site: www.istm.org.

7. Shoreland, Inc. Company providing multimedia tools for travel health advisors and for corporations. Telephone: 800-433-5256; Web site: www.shoreland.com.

8. SOS International. Company providing multimedia tools for travel health advisors and for corporations. Also provides medical evacuation and health insurance for travel. Web site: www. Internationalsos.com.

9. Rose S and Keystone JS. *International Travel Health Guide*. 13th ed. Travel Medicine, Inc. Telephone: 800-872-8633; Web site: www.travmed. com. Annually updated travel health book for health care workers and the public.

However, all travelers (as well as all non-traveler adults) should receive one dose of the new combined tetanus/diphtheria/acellular pertussis vaccine as immunity to pertussis has waned in the adult population and rates of pertussis have increased. Indeed, pertussis has become the least controlled bacterial vaccine–preventable disease in the United States, with >25 000 cases reported in 2005.

POLIO

Studies in the United States have found varying levels of immunity to polio in the general population, with data revealing 12% of adult American travelers unprotected against at least one serogroup. The Centers for Disease Control and Prevention (CDC) recommends that all adults complete a primary series if they have never received one and also receive a booster dose of the enhanced injectable polio vaccine once only before travel to an endemic area. (The oral polio vaccine is no longer available in the United States.) If time permits, infants and children younger than 2 years should receive at least three doses of polio vaccine. Intervals between doses may be reduced to 4 weeks to optimize immunization status before departure.

Countries considered free of endemic wild poliovirus circulation are the United States, Canada, Japan, Australia, New Zealand, and most of eastern and western Europe. The Western Hemisphere has been declared polio free; there have been no reported cases of paralytic disease caused by wild poliovirus in the Americas in several years. The last cases of indigenously acquired polio in the United States occurred in 1979. Unfortunately, outbreaks of vaccine-derived poliovirus have occurred in the Dominican Republic and Haiti since 2000. Eradication of polio worldwide is still a challenge as outbreaks continue to occur in West and Central Africa.

MEASLES, MUMPS, AND RUBELLA

Measles continues to be a major cause of morbidity and mortality in the developing world. Outbreaks of measles in the United States continue to be epidemiologically linked to cases of imported measles. International adoptees, who often have been inadequately immunized, have been the origin of some outbreaks.

Because the rate of primary failure with the vaccine was somewhat greater in persons born after 1956 and vaccinated before 1980, the CDC recommends that travelers in this group be revaccinated. Immunization may be given at 6 months of age if necessary for travel, followed by a booster injection at 15 months.

Table 114.2 Travel Health Kit

Usual prescription drugs
Aspirin (Tylenol, NSAID)
Bismuth subsalicylate
Sunscreen
Antihistamine, decongestant
Insect repellent
Rehydration solution packets
Steroid cream
Loperamide
Codeine tablets
Mild sedative
High-altitude sickness prophylaxis
Antimalarial chemoprophylaxis
Digital thermometer
Bandages, gauze, adhesive
Antiseptic solution
Antacid
Anti–motion sickness medication
Laxative
Cough preparation
Topical antifugal, antibacterial cream or ointment
Antibiotic for self-treatment of travelers' diarrhea
Abbreviation: NSAID = nonsteroidal anti-inflammatory drug.

Mumps and rubella are less of a health threat to travelers, although both diseases may have serious complications.

PNEUMOCOCCUS AND INFLUENZA

The vaccine against *Streptococcus pneumoniae* should be administered to those at risk for severe illness from this infection, including those older than 65 years. Influenza is the most common vaccine-preventable illness seen in travelers. Influenza vaccine is recommended for travelers of all ages, including all pregnant women. The largest documented travel-related outbreak of influenza occurred in the "nonflu" season of late summer in Alaska and the Canadian Yukon in 1998. Many travelers and travel health advisors alike do not recognize the importance of immunizing travelers against influenza. Influenza occurs year-round in the tropics and from May through November in the southern hemisphere. Thus vaccine should be administered in the United States to all travelers until the vaccine expiration date (usually in June of the year following its availability). The Southern Hemisphere vaccine is not available in the United States.

HEPATITIS B

Hepatitis B vaccine has typically been reserved for persons such as health care workers in contact with blood or body fluid secretions in developing countries and for long-term travelers to countries with a high prevalence of infection. Ideally, however, everyone should be immunized against this most important cause of acute and chronic liver disease. Although the vaccine is often recommended primarily for those who may have casual sex during international travel, injuries and illness may be equally important risk factors. A recent study showed that 17% of U.S. international travelers who sought medical assistance received an injection, which is particularly significant in light of the fact that up to 75% of injections in the developing world are given with unsterile equipment. In Asia and Africa, up to 20% of children and adults are hepatitis B carriers. The vaccine is recommended in the United States for all infants, children, and adolescents. A combined hepatitis A and B vaccine has been available in the United States since 2000, and an accelerated regimen (0, 7, 21 days) was approved by the Food and Drug Administration in 2007.

Immunizations of Special Importance for the Traveler

YELLOW FEVER

Yellow fever is a viral illness transmitted by mosquitoes in tropical Africa and South America. It is rare in travelers, but because of its high mortality, individuals journeying to endemic areas require protection. Some countries require evidence of vaccination from all entering travelers and even from individuals whose destination is a noninfected area but who will be crossing the yellow fever zone or landing on an aircraft temporarily in the zone. The vaccine can be administered only at an approved yellow fever vaccination center. State and local health departments may administer the vaccine, or one can find a yellow

Table 114.3 Immunizations for Foreign Travel

Vaccine	Adult Dosage	Duration of Efficacy
Live Attenuated		
Yellow fever	1 (0.5 mL) SC 10 days to 10 yr before travel	Booster q10yr
Typhoid	1 enteric-coated capsule taken on alternate days for 4 doses with cool liquid 1 h before a meal	Booster series q5yr
Inactivated		
Typhoid	1 dose (0.5 mL) IM	Booster q2yr
Rabies pre-exposure	3 doses (1.0 mL) IM on days 0, 7, and 21 or 28	No serologic testing and no boosters for most travelers (seek advice from CDC)
Meningococcal (quadrivalent A/C/Y/W-135) (conjugate or polysaccharide)	1 dose (0.5 mL) SC	Reimmunization recommended q5yr for polysaccharide; unknown for conjugate
Japanese B encephalitis	3 doses (1 mL) SC days 0, 7, 30	Duration of immunity unknown; booster recommended at 3 yr
Hepatitis A	2 doses, at 0 and 6–12 mo HAVRIX (6–18 mo VAQTA)	Probable lifelong immunity
Passive Prophylaxis		
Immunoglobulin for protection against hepatitis A	0.02 mL/kg for travel ≤3 mo 0.04 mL/kg for travel 4–6 mo	Repeat dose q4-6mo

Abbreviations: SC = subcutaneous; IM = intramuscular; CDC = Centers for Disease Control and Prevention.
[a] If traveler is taking chloroquine or mefloquine for malaria chemoprophylaxis, the series must be completed before initiation of antimalarial treatment.
[b] If risk is high and continuous, serology should be checked every 6 mo. Acceptable antibody level is ≥1.5 titer by rapid fluorescent focus inhibition test.

fever vaccine administration site location by accessing the CDC travelers' health Web site at www.cdc.gov/travel and searching the yellow fever clinic registry. Documentation of yellow fever vaccination should be placed on the International Certificate of Vaccination card, which may be obtained from the clinic where the vaccine is administered and which should be carried with the passport. Individuals for whom the vaccine is contraindicated must carry a waiver on a physician's letterhead to prevent health officials from requiring an injection at a border crossing.

Since 1992, rare cases of encephalitis or autoimmune neurologic disease have been reported in recipients of yellow fever vaccine. In addition, a multiorgan system illness similar to yellow fever and termed *yellow fever vaccine–associated viscerotropic disease* has also been reported following vaccination. Viscerotropic illness has a high mortality, and such episodes are being tracked by the CDC.

Both these syndromes have occurred only in primary vaccinees, and severe viscerotropic illness occurs more freqently in the older age population. Although such events occur with a frequency of only several per million doses, health care providers are advised to administer the vaccine only to persons truly at risk for exposure to yellow fever.

TYPHOID

Although *Salmonella enterica* Typhi is prevalent in many countries in Africa, Asia, and Central and South America, typhoid fever is not common in travelers. The oral Ty21a oral capsular vaccine or the injectible Vi polysaccharide vaccine should be used by travelers to endemic areas who are going off tourist routes or who are particularly adventuresome with regard to their food and beverage intake. In addition, long-term and frequent short-term travelers to developing countries should receive vaccine. The highest rate of typhoid is seen in those returning from the Indian subcontinent, particularly those who visited friends and relatives (VFRs) in those areas. VFRs are high-risk travelers for a number of other travel-related illnesses (eg, malaria, tuberculosis [TB], and sexually transmitted infections [STIs]), and special efforts should be made to educate such travelers regarding their risk of typhoid and other infections, as well as preventive measures that may be taken.

RABIES

The pre-exposure rabies vaccine series should be administered to those spending >30 days where rabies is a constant threat or to those whose travel involves working with or around animals that may be infected. The risk is highest where dog rabies is highly endemic, such as Mexico, El Salvador, Guatemala, Peru, Colombia, Ecuador, India, Nepal, the Philippines, Sri Lanka, Thailand, and Vietnam. Most cases reported to the CDC were acquired outside the United States. Travelers should avoid contact with domestic animals and, if bitten, should wash the wound immediately with soap and water and seek medical care. Even if a pre-exposure rabies series has been administered, postexposure prophylaxis must be given. Those who have received pre-exposure vaccinations have a much simplified postexposure series and do not require rabies immunoglobulin (RIG), which is often very difficult to find in many countries. For assistance with problems or questions, one should contact the local or state health department or the CDC rabies team in the Division of Viral and Rickettsial Diseases at 404-639-1050.

MENINGOCOCCAL MENINGITIS

The meningococcal meningitis vaccines are very protective against disease due to *Neisseria meningitis* serogroups A, C, Y, and W-135. Vaccination is routinely recommended for college students who will be living in dormitories, as well as for travelers. Long-term travelers to the meningitis belt in sub-Saharan Africa and short-term travelers during the dry season should be protected. Vaccination is also recommended for travelers to areas where outbreaks have occurred in the past decade and is required for those attending the Haj. There are two vaccines in the United States; age of the individual and availability typically determine which is used. The new conjugate vaccine has the advantage of longer protection and prevention of nasal carriage in those who are exposed to infection.

JAPANESE ENCEPHALITIS

Japanese encephalitis (JE) occurs in Asia during the summer, autumn in temperate regions, and primarily during the rainy season in the tropics. It is transmitted by night-biting mosquitoes in rural rice-growing, pig-farming areas. Most infections are asymptomatic, but those who do develop clinical illness have a high mortality and 50% or greater likelihood of neurologic sequelae. Between 1978 and 1993, 11 U.S. residents developed clinical JE, 8 of whom were military personnel or their dependents. There were no cases in U.S. travelers between 1993 and 2003, after which a college-age student developed illness after exposure in rural Thailand. The risk of JE is about 1 per 5000 per month of rural travel in endemic areas. The risk to short-term urban travelers is quite low. Adventuresome travelers to rural areas and long-term travelers are at greatest risk and should therefore consider immunization.

HEPATITIS A AND IMMUNOGLOBULIN

Hepatitis A is one of the most common immunizable infection in travelers. In contrast to other serious foodborne illnesses, many travel-related cases have occurred with standard tourist itineraries. In fact, the estimated incidence of symptomatic hepatitis A in travelers to the developing world per month of stay abroad is as high as 20 per 1000 in some destinations. The hepatitis A vaccine is available in the United States and is strongly recommended for all travelers. It is also currently administered to children in the United States. Immunoglobulin (Ig) is less available and protects travelers immediately but only for a short duration. Most clinics in the United States no longer carry Ig, and the CDC has recently changed its recommendations so that providers can administer the hepatitis A vaccine to imminent travelers without Ig. Immunoglobulin is still recommended in addition to the vaccine for imminent travelers who are older or who are immunocompromised. It is important to recognize that mortality from hepatitis A increases with age and approaches 3% in those older than 50 years.

MALARIA

For prevention of malaria, see Chapter 198, Malaria: Treatment and Prophylaxis.

TRAVELERS' DIARRHEA

Prevention of diarrhea requires careful selection of food and beverages while traveling in the developing world. Foods that are well cooked and still hot or steaming are safest. Fruits peeled by the traveler are safe. Because vegetables such as lettuce and tomatoes grow in areas where human fertilizer may be used and because they cannot be peeled, salads should be avoided unless washed carefully with purified water. Commercially bottled carbonated beverages, alcohol, hot tea, and coffee are also safe. The purity of plain bottled water is not regulated, so this is best avoided. Ice cubes should also be avoided because they are often made with tap water. Milk and dairy products should be pasteurized, cooked, or avoided. Disinfection requires brief boiling or the use of halogens (eg, chlorine, iodine), although the protozoan cysts of *Giardia lamblia* and *Entamoeba histolytica* are more resistant to the latter as are *Cyclospora* sp. and *Cryptosporidia* sp. Many inexpensive portable purifiers that contain halogenation are available from camping stores.

Without exception, every traveler should carry an antibiotic for self-treatment of travelers' diarrhea. However, prophylaxis of diarrhea with a daily dose of an appropriate antibiotic (eg, 500 mg ciprofloxacin) may be wise for few short-term travelers who are at very high risk of illness or of serious complications of diarrhea. For more detail, see Chapter 119, Travelers' Diarrhea.

SCHISTOSOMIASIS

Schistosomiasis is caused by infection with a blood fluke, *Schistosoma mansoni, Schistosoma haematobium,* or *Schistosoma japonicum,* which in one part of its life cycle can penetrate the human skin without causing symptoms. A subacute illness similar to serum sickness (Katayama fever) may occur about 6 weeks after exposure, and chronic problems such as portal hypertension, urinary obstruction, and bladder cancer may result. Reports of American travelers contracting schistosomiasis and developing unusual central nervous system findings such as transverse myelitis from aberrant egg deposition have heightened the awareness of this disease. Travelers to endemic areas put themselves at risk when they wade, swim, or bathe in freshwater lakes, streams, or rivers containing the reservoir snails.

If exposure to possibly infected water sources is unavoidable, towel-drying the skin immediately after contact may be protective. Screening for exposure involves a serologic test best performed by the Division of Parasitic Diseases at the CDC.

MISCELLANEOUS CONSIDERATIONS

The traveler infected with human immunodeficiency virus (HIV) confronts several potential problems. They typically have greater susceptibility to a variety of infections, including travelers' diarrhea, and more chronic and serious consequences from such problems. A physician may give a waiver if the yellow fever vaccine is required by the destination, but if the traveler will be in an area of high endemicity and if he or she is asymptomatic with a CD4 lymphocyte count above 200/mm^3, it may be reasonable to give the vaccine. When it was inadvertently administered to HIV-infected military personnel and to pregnant travelers, no adverse events occurred. However, at times it may be more appropriate to counsel the traveler regarding the wisdom of altering his or her itinerary if the risk of yellow fever is high and the vaccine is contraindicated. Protection against measles is important, thus immunization with MMR should be considered, although complications have been reported. Some countries have regulations preventing the entry of HIV-infected individuals.

Even the most experienced travelers suffer jet lag. It is estimated that the body takes about 1 day to adjust for each time zone crossed. Adequate hydration while traveling, resting after arrival, and judicious use of short-acting benzodiazepines assist the adjustment. Many other maneuvers may be helpful as well. Bright light can reset the internal clock. For travel eastward, it is recommended that travelers seek bright light in the early morning, and for westward travel, they should be in bright light in the late afternoon. Artificial light sources with the appropriate lux intensity may also be used. The use of melatonin is controversial. Melatonin tablets available in health food stores may not contain standardized amount of hormone, may contain contaminants, and thus cannot be recommended.

With more children, senior citizens, and disabled persons traveling, it is becoming more important to consider the ability of the traveler to withstand the environment and special challenges that destinations offer. For example, travel involving high altitude, difficult terrain, scuba diving, and even commercial flying may be inappropriate for those who have certain underlying medical problems or who may not be fully prepared for hardships they could encounter. For in-depth counseling and/or evaluation, a travel health specialist should be consulted. The International Society of Travel

Medicine Web site (www.istm.org) has a listing of travel clinics worldwide that health care providers and the public may access. It is becoming more important, as travel becomes more exotic and adventuresome, that travelers access these clinics for counseling. As well, many of these clinics see travelers who return with illness, although the Web site of the American Society of Tropical Medicine and Hygiene also contains a clinic listing, focusing on those specialists who treat diseases in travelers.

SUGGESTED READING

Centers for Disease Control and Prevention. *Health Information for International Travel 2008*. Atlanta, GA: U.S. Department of Health and Human Services, Public Health Service; 2007.

Keystone JS, Kozarsky PE, Freedman DO, Nothdurft HD, Connor BA, eds. *Travel Medicine*. Edinburgh: Elsevier Ltd; 2004.

115. Fever in the Returning Traveler

Martin S. Wolfe

A common problem of travelers, either on the trip or after they return, is a febrile illness, usually caused by infection. Fever in a traveler is often caused by disease not specifically related to travel and just as likely to occur at home. These include, among others, such cosmopolitan causes as common cold, sinusitus, influenza, tonsillitis, pyelonephritis, and bacterial or mycoplasmal pneumonia. However, the subject of this chapter is more exotic diseases acquired in developing countries (See Table 115.1). With the great increase in volume and speed of travel between developed and developing countries, physicians in the United States and other developed countries are seeing more patients with exotic tropical infections. Some of these infections are widespread in developing countries, and others are limited to small areas. Thus knowledge of geographic distribution may be essential to the correct diagnosis.

The most common tropical fevers in travelers are malaria, enteric fever, hepatitis, amebic liver abscess, and rickettsial and arboviral infections.

MALARIA

A febrile traveler returning from an area of endemic malaria must first and foremost be evaluated for malaria. Most malarial infections occur in travelers who have had inappropriate, irregular, or no chemoprophylaxis. However, all febrile travelers from a malarious area must be examined for malaria because no chemoprophylactic regimen can be considered fully protective. Potentially lethal falciparum malaria usually occurs within 4 weeks after leaving a malarious area. *Plasmodium vivax* and *Plasmodium ovale* malaria may occur up to 3 years after exposure if primaquine has not been taken to eliminate persistent latent parasites in the liver. *Plasmodium malariae*, which does not have a latent liver phase, is the least common species seen in travelers, but may present 20 years or more after exposure. Typical symptoms are high fever, shaking, chills, sweats, headache, and myalgias. Symptoms may be modified or masked according to the immune status, as in an im-

Table 115.1 Causes of Tropical Fevers in Travelers

Most Common

Cosmopolitan infections (common cold, sinusitis, pyelonephritis, etc.)
Malaria
Enteric fever
Hepatitis
Rickettsial infections
Arboviral infections (dengue, chikungunya, and others)
Bacterial diarrhea or dysentery
Viral gastroenteritis
Early Giardia or *Entamoeba histolytica* diarrhea
Amebic liver abscess

Less Common

African trypanosomiasis
Tuberculosis
Brucellosis
Leptospirosis
Histoplasmosis
Legionnaire's disease
Human immunodeficiency virus
Acute schistosomiasis
Drug fevers

Uncommon

Visceral leishmaniasis (kala-azar)
Lyme disease
Relapsing fever
Melioidosis
Viral hemorrhagic fevers

mune native of an endemic area, or by the use of prophylactic antimalarial drugs. Severe *Plasmodium falciparum* infections can rapidly lead to such lethal complications as cerebral malaria, renal failure, severe hemolysis, and adult respiratory distress syndrome.

Diagnosis is by appropriately prepared and carefully examined Giemsa-stained thin and thick malaria smears. A single negative set of smears cannot rule out malaria; smears should be repeated at 6-hour intervals for at least 24 hours. Specific prophylaxis and therapy for malaria is discussed in Chapter 198, Malaria: Treatment and Prophylaxis.

ENTERIC FEVER

Typhoid and paratyphoid fevers can be contracted from contaminated food or water where the prevalence of these bacteria is high. Typhoid vaccines offer protection to no more than 70% of recipients. Enteric fever should be suspected in travelers returning from an endemic area with fever, headaches, abdominal pain, diarrhea, or cough. Symptoms may not develop until several weeks after return. Diagnosis is confirmed by positive blood, stool, or urine culture. Febrile agglutinin (Widal) or salmonella antibody tests may be useful. *Salmonella typhi* organisms worldwide have developed multiple antibiotic resistance, and a fluoroquinoline is the drug of choice. See Chapter 148, Salmonella, for specific therapy details.

HEPATITIS

Travelers to the developing world who have not received hepatitis A vaccine or immune serum globulin (ISG) run a significant risk of contracting hepatitis A from ubiquitously contaminated water or food. Rare cases of hepatitis E have been contracted in South Asia and elsewhere, and this type of hepatitis may not be prevented by ISG. Hepatitis B is usually contracted from sexual contact and is uncommon in travelers. In the preicteric phase of acute hepatitis, fever, chills, myalgias, and fatigue may occur, and this syndrome can mimic malaria and other acute tropical fevers. Hepatitis serologic testing can confirm the type of infection, but when these tests are negative in a patient with apparent hepatitis, cytomegalovirus or mononucleosis infection should be considered.

AMEBIC LIVER ABSCESS

A period of acute diarrhea often precedes development of an amebic liver abscess. A returned traveler with fever and right upper quadrant pain should be suspected of this infection. Stools will be positive for *Entamoeba histolytica* in only 10% to 15% of liver abscess cases. Sonography or computed tomography (CT) of the liver will show a filling defect, and an amebic serology test will confirm infection. Needle aspiration is seldom required for diagnosis or treatment. There is very rapid clinical response to metronidazole, 750 mg 3 times daily for 10 days, followed by a luminal drug such as paromomycin (Humatin), 500 mg 3 times daily for 7 days.

RICKETTSIAL INFECTIONS

Tick typhus can be contracted in West, East, and South Africa and in the Mediterranean littoral.

Infection typically begins with a skin eschar at the tick-bite site; fever, chills, and headache; and in a few days, a diffuse papular rash can develop. Epidemic, scrub, and murine typhus and Q fever are much less commonly contracted by travelers. The Weil–Felix agglutination battery can be used for initial screening, and confirmation can be obtained from indirect fluorescent antibody tests for specific rickettsial organisms. Tetracycline is highly effective, and response is generally rapid. A single 200-mg dose of doxycycline may be adequate, but 100 mg twice a day for 5 to 7 days may be required for some *Rickettsia* species.

VIRAL FEVERS

Dengue fever, endemic in most parts of the tropical world, is the most commonly imported arbovirus infection. Symptoms include fever, headache, body and bone ache, and eye pain. Typically, a diffuse rash appears on the third to fifth day as other symptoms abate. Chikungunya virus has similar clinical symptoms to dengue but differs in causing severe joint pains rather than deep bone pain. A recent outbreak of Chikungunya in islands of the Indian Ocean has led to numerous imported cases into Europe, North America, and parts of Asia. Japanese B encephalitis is a rare infection of travelers to rural areas of the Far East. A number of other rarer acute viral illnesses have been imported from endemic areas, including lethal Lassa and Marburg fever viruses from West and Central Africa. Diagnosis is usually confirmed serologically, and treatment is generally supportive. See Chapters 181, Dengue and Denguelike Illness, and 192, Viral Hemorrhagic Fevers.

LESS COMMON FEBRILE ILLNESSES IN TRAVELERS

African trypanosomiasis was contracted by 31 American travelers from 1967 to 2001, almost all in travelers to East Africa. Although the risk is low, even short-term travelers to game parks of East and Central Africa should take precautions against tsetse fly bites. Travelers should inform their physician of exposure history if symptoms such as trypanosomal chancre at a bite site, fever, evanescent rash, headache, and lethargy develop up to 4 weeks after returning home. See Chapter 200, Trypanosomiases and Leishmaniases.

Tuberculosis remains a threat worldwide. Although travelers uncommonly are infected, any returnee with fever, cough, and chest radiography evidence suggestive of pulmonary disease should be evaluated for tuberculosis. Tuberculin skin testing before and after travel is recommended.

Brucellosis is contracted from contaminated raw goat or cow milk or soft cheese. Presentation can be with fever, chills, sweats, body aches, headache, monarticular arthritis, weight loss, fatigue, or depression. Diagnosis is by blood culture and/or specific agglutination tests. Treatment is with a tetracycline plus streptomycin or rifampin.

Leptospirosis is common in the tropics but is rarely contracted by travelers. Infection is acquired through direct or indirect contact (such as contaminated water) with infected animals. Recreational activities, such as water sports and adventure travel, are emerging as important risk factors for this infection. Most infections are anicteric and mild. Initial symptoms may include high remittent fever, chills, headache, myalgias, nausea, and vomiting. No more than 10% of patients develop jaundice. Diagnosis is usually made with serology. Early therapy with penicillin or tetracycline is usually beneficial.

Histoplasmosis, a cosmopolitan disease, has rarely infected travelers to Latin America. Visitors to caves contaminated with bat droppings are at particular risk. Consideration should be given to histoplasmosis in a returned traveler with fever and pulmonary or, less likely, disseminated disease. Ketoconazole or itraconazole given for 3 to 6 weeks is effective treatment for acute symptomatic cases.

Visceral leishmaniasis (kala-azar) is extremely rare in American tourists, although European travelers have been infected around the Mediterranean littoral. Symptoms include fever, hepatosplenomegaly, and wasting. Diagnosis is confirmed by demonstrating leishmanial organisms in a biopsy specimen of liver, spleen, or bone marrow. Pentavalent antimonial compounds are the drug of choice for initial treatment.

Lyme disease occurs in Europe and the United States and may also be present in other parts of the world. Hikers in particular should take precautions against tick bites in any recognized endemic area.

Relapsing fever is caused by a spirochetal organism and occurs in a louseborne, primarily epidemic form and in a more widely scattered tick-borne endemic form. The latter form is present in the western United States and has been diagnosed in returnees from that area

to the eastern United States. Imported relapsing fever is uncommon, but cases have been contracted in West Africa, Spain, and Central America. Diagnosis is by finding the spirochetes in a thick or thin Giemsa-stained blood smear. Treatment is with a tetracycline.

Legionnaire's disease cases in travelers have continued to rise since 1995, and it is believed that travel-related cases are underestimated. Most cases (80%) are associated with travel within Europe. Diagnosis in suspected cases is made from culture, seroconversion, and urinary antigen detection. Initial treatment is with azithromycin or a fluoroquinolone plus rifampin.

Melioidosis is endemic primarily in southeast Asia and sporadically occurs in other areas. The majority of imported cases are seen in refugees from southeast Asia, in returned servicemen from that area, and occasionally in tourists. An asymptomatic form of infection is most common, but acute pneumonic and septicemic forms may occur. Chronic suppurative forms may also develop in various organs. These forms can lie dormant for many years and have the capacity to flare into acute fulminant symptoms. Any patient with a pneumonic process who is returning from rural areas of southeast Asia should be considered to have possible melioidosis. Diagnosis is by special culture techniques or by serology. The most effective treatment is with ceftazidime or imipenem.

Human immunodeficiency virus (HIV) infection is a particular hazard from sexual contact, blood transfusion, or contaminated needle or syringe contact in highly endemic areas of the tropical world. A number of disposable syringes and needles should be carried by the traveler who may need injection while traveling in areas where only nondisposable products are used. HIV serology screening should be done on any traveler with such exposure.

Most viral and bacterial causes of diarrhea, amebic dysentery, and occasionally *Giardia lamblia* may also cause fever, which may precede diarrhea by some hours or days. Acute schistosomiasis, acute fascioliasis, and acute bancroftian filariasis are uncommon causes of fever in travelers.

Drugs used for prophylaxis or treatment of travel-related infections may themselves be a cause of fever. These include sulfonamide-containing drugs such as trimethoprim–sulfamethoxazole and pyrimethamine with sulfadoxine (Fansidar) (used for malaria treatment). Quinine and doxycycline may rarely cause fever. Drugs obtained abroad, often in combinations and without prescription, may cause a cryptic fever. It is worthwhile to stop all nonessential medications pending an etiologic diagnosis in febrile travelers.

SUGGESTED READING

Aronson NE, Sander JW, Moran KA. In harm's way: infections in deployed American military forces. *Clin Infect Dis.* 2006;43: 1045–1051.

Bottieau E, Clerinx J, Van den Enden E, et al. Infectious mononucleosis syndromes in febrile travelers returning from the tropics. *J Travel Med.* 2006;13:191–197.

Centers for Disease Control and Prevention. Chikungunya fever diagnosed among international travelers—United States, 2005–2006. *Morbid Mortal Weekly Rep.* 2006;55:1040–1042.

Drugs for parasitic infections. *The Medical Letter on Drugs and Therapeutics.* Vol. 5 (Suppl.) 2007. http://www.medicalletter.org. Accessed October 4, 2007.

Liu LX, Weller PF. Approach to the febrile traveler returning from Southeast Asia and Oceania. *Curr Clin Top Infect Dis.* 1992;12: 138–164.

Magill AJ. Fever in the returned traveler. *Med Clin North Am.* 1998;12:445–469.

Strickland GT. Fever in the returned traveler. *Med Clin North Am.* 1992;76:1375–1392.

Suh KN, Kozarsky PE, Keystone JS. Evaluation of fever in the returned traveler. *Med Clin North Am.* 1999;83:997–1017.

Weinberg M, Weeks J, Lance-Parker S, et al. Severe histoplasmosis in travelers to Nicaragua. *Emerg Infect Dis.* 2003; 9:1322–1325.

Wilson ME. *A World Guide to Infections.* New York, NY: Oxford University Press; 1991.

116. Systemic Infection from Animals

David J. Weber, George S. Ghneim, and William A. Rutala

INTRODUCTION

Zoonoses are defined as diseases and infections that are naturally transmitted between vertebrate animals and humans. Currently there are more than 200 recognized zoonotic diseases, and 75% of emerging infectious diseases fit into this category. Zoonotic diseases can be transmitted to humans through bites and scratches, direct contact, aerosols, arthropod vectors, or contamination of food or water. There are many reasons for the increased impact of zoonotics in current times. Contact with domestic animals continues to be frequent, even in urban centers. Pets are a major reservoir and source of zoonoses, especially for children. In 2004, 39% of households owned a dog, 34% owned a cat, and 6% owned a pet bird. The total number of animals owned was 73 million dogs, 90 million cats, and 17 million birds. Other common pets include fish, reptiles, rabbits, hamsters, gerbils, mice, and farm animals such as horses.

Recent factors that have had a significant impact on emergence of zoonotics are human encroachment on wildlife habitat, wildlife trade and translocation, the ownership of exotic pets, petting zoos, and ecotourism. The recent epidemics of West Nile virus and monkeypox in North America have demonstrated the role of wildlife and exotic pets in the emergence of zoonotic diseases in industrialized nations. Traditional leisure pursuits such as hunting, camping, and hiking are increasingly common and continue to bring people into close contact with wild animals, arthropods, and sometimes contaminated water. Occupational exposures to domestic animals or animal products, especially in backyard operations, remain a leading cause of zoonotic disease exposure.

For all of the reasons described above, it is increasingly important for physicians, veterinarians, and public health professionals to work together in recognizing and controlling zoonotic diseases. The Centers for Disease Control and Prevention (CDC) has recently become a World Organization for Animal Health (OIE) Collaborating Center for Emerging and Remerging Zoonoses and now dedicates an entire issue of the Emerging Infectious Disease journal to zoonotics. The key to such efforts continues to lie with the astute clinician diagnosing and reporting these diseases, and the goal of this chapter is to assist in these efforts.

CLINICAL APPROACH

Zoonoses are caused by a diverse group of microorganisms. Infectious syndromes caused by zoonotic pathogens are equally diverse. Hence, classification of zoonoses is difficult for the clinician. Diseases may be classified by the nature of the pathogen, animal host, mode of transmission from animal to human, geographic range of host, or clinical syndrome (ie, systemic disease or specific organ system of infection). Although most zoonoses are relatively unusual, they must be included in the differential diagnosis of many clinical syndromes. All patients with an infectious syndrome whose cause is not apparent after a standard history and physical examination should be questioned to assess the possibility of a zoonosis. First, the clinician should question patients about exposure to pets and ask whether they own or have had recent contact with a dog, cat, bird, fish, reptile, or rodent. If contact may have occurred, the clinician should ask about a history of bites or scratches. Second, the patient should be asked about exposure to farm animals (which may also be pets) such as horses, pigs, cattle, and fowl (ie, chickens and turkeys). The clinician should determine the amount and degree of exposure. Third, patients should be asked about leisure pursuits such as hunting, fishing, hiking, and camping. The clinician should assess specific animal contacts such as dressing or skinning animals, ingestion of water from streams and lakes, and bites by arthropods such as ticks (see also Chapter 117, Tick-Borne Disease). Fourth, the clinician should obtain a careful travel history. Ascertaining whether a patient has had an animal bite or scratch while visiting an area endemic for rabies is particularly important. Because the incubation period for rabies may extend for years, persons bitten or scratched by dogs or other possible rabid hosts should be considered for postinjury prophylaxis. In general, evaluation for specific zoonoses should be based on the possibility of exposure (Table 116.1).

A brief description of the approach to possible systemic infections caused by animals is provided in subsequent paragraphs. More detailed information may be found in specific chapters in this book or in the Suggested Reading at the end of this chapter.

ZOONOTIC DISEASES ACQUIRED BY ANIMAL BITE OR SCRATCH

Dog bites account for 70% to 90% of animal bites and cat bites account for 3% to 15%. Bites from wild animals constitute <1% of bite wounds. The infection rate from penetrating dog bites is approximately 5% to 15%. Cat bites are much more likely to become infected. Most dog and cat bites occur on the extremities. Males are more likely to be bitten by a dog than are females, whereas the opposite is true for cat scratches and bites. Approximately 1% of rodent bites become infected.

Although infections following animal bites may be caused by various flora, some generalizations can be made. The most common pathogen to cause infection following feline bites is *Pasteurella multocida* (see Chapter 23, Human and Animal Bites), which generally results in rapid progressive cellulitis similar to that caused by *Streptococcus pyogenes*. Occasionally sepsis may result, especially in the immunocomprised host. The agents of rat bite fever, *Streptobacillus moniliformis* and *Spirillum minus*, may be transmitted by several small rodents, including the rat, mouse, and gerbil. Both agents cause a systemic illness. Infections with *Aeromonas hydrophila* may follow bites inflicted in fresh or brackish water or by aquatic animals such as snakes and alligators. Severe local infection progressing to crepitant cellulitis with systemic toxicity may occur. Although most cases of tularemia follow the handling of rabbits, infection may be transmitted by animal bites or scratches, especially domestic cats (other animals include the coyote, pig, and squirrel). *Capnocytophaga canimorsus* is an unusual systemic infection strongly associated with dog bites. More than 50% of patients have reported dog bites before clinical infection, although infection has also been reported following scratches from dogs, cat bites or scratches, and contact with wild animals. Approximately 80% of patients reported in the literature have a predisposing condition, most

commonly splenectomy. Other predisposing conditions have included Hodgkin's disease, trauma, idiopathic thrombocytopenia purpura, alcohol abuse, steroid therapy, and chronic lung disease. Bites from seals, whales, and walruses may transmit a murine mycoplasma. *Erysipelothrix rhusiopathiae* is carried most commonly by swine but is also found in sheep, horses, cattle, chickens, crabs, fish, dogs, and cats. A local infection, erysipeloid, may result from bites or injury with these animals usually during occupational exposure. Thus, abattoir workers, butchers, fishermen, farmers, and veterinarians are at risk for infection with *E. rhusiopathiae*. Sepsis and endocarditis may result from local infection.

ZOONOTIC DISEASES ACQUIRED BY ARTHROPOD BITES

Due to major changes in the environment and how humans interact with this environment, the incidence of zoonotic diseases vectored by arthropods has increased dramatically in recent years. The most significant of these diseases are vectored by ticks and include Rocky Mountain spotted fever (RMSF), Lyme disease, and ehrlichiosis/anaplasmosis. RMSF is caused by the rickettsial agent *Rickettsia rickettsii* and is the most severe rickettsial disease occurring in the United States. This disease is characterized with an acute onset of fever, malaise, headaches, chills, and in most cases a maculopapular rash. The rash of RMSF typically appears between the third and fifth days of illness but is absent in 5% to 15% of patients. Initially maculopapular, it begins on extremities, often around the wrist and ankles. As the rash progresses, it spreads centripetally to the trunk and characteristically involves the palms and/or soles. As it evolves, it becomes more clearly defined and more petechial and may rarely progress to skin necrosis and gangrene. RMSF has a case fatality rate of 13% to 25% when untreated. Lyme disease has been reportable since 1992, and almost 10000 cases were reported that year. In 2004 there were approximately 23000 cases of Lyme disease reported in the United States. Lyme disease is characterized by a distinctive circular rash, called an erythema migrans (EM). Erythema migrans is characteristically an expanding annular erythematous plaque with central clearing, most commonly seen in the axilla, thigh, and groin. Color varies from pink to violaceous. Erythema migrans may last up to 4 weeks and may recur during the secondary stage of infection. Two

Table 116.1 Infectious Diseases Acquired from Animals

Disease	Persons at Risk[a]	Birds, Fowl	Cats, Dogs	Farm Animals	Fish, Reptiles,[b] Water	Rabbits	Rodents	Arthropod Vectors	Wild Animals
Viral									
Avian influenza (H5N)	I, V, VI	+++							
Bovine papular stomatitis	I, II			+					
California encephalitis	III, rural, public							+++	
Colorado tick fever	III							+++	
Eastern equine encephalitis	III, public							+++	
Hantavirus pulmonary syndrome	I, III, public						+++		
B virus (*Herpesvirus simiae*)	IV, V								Macaca monkeys
Lymphocytic choriomeningitis	III, IV, V, public						+++		
Milker nodule (pseudocowpox)	I, II			+					
Newcastle disease	I, II, IV, V	++							
Orf (contagious ecthyma)	I, II			+					
Powassan encephalitis	I, III, public							+++	
Rabies	III, VI, public		++	+					+++
Rotavirus	I, III, IV, public			++					
SARS-coV	I, II, IV, V								+
St. Louis encephalitis	I, III, public							+++	
Venezuelan encephalitis	I, III, public							+++	
Western equine encephalitis	I, III, public							+++	
Yellow fever	III, VI							+++	
Bacterial									
Aeromonas	III, IV, VIII, public				+++				
Anthrax (wool sorter disease)	I, II, IV, X		+	+++					
Brucellosis	I, II, III, V		+	+++					
Campylobacteriosis	I, II, III, IV	+	++	+++	++		++		
Capnocytophaga canimorsus sepsis	III, IV, IX, public		+++						

(continued)

Table 116.1 *(continued)*

Disease	Persons at Risk[a]	Birds, Fowl	Cats, Dogs	Farm Animals	Fish, Reptiles,[b] Water	Rabbits	Rodents	Arthropod Vectors	Wild Animals
Cat scratch fever	III, IV, IX, public		+++						
Edwardsiella tarda infection	IV, VIII				++				
Ehrlichiosis	I, III, IV, VI, IX, public							+++	
Erysipeloid	I, II, III, VIII	++	+	+	++		++		
Leptospirosis	I, III, IV, V	++	+	++	+		++		
Listeriosis	IX, public	+	+	+++			+		
Lyme disease	I, III, IV, VI, public							+++	+
Murine typhus	I, III, VI						(Vector)	+++	
Mycobacteriosis (*M. marinum*)	VIII				+++				
Pasteurellosis	III, IV, public	+++	+++			++			++
Plague	III, IV, V, VII, X		+				++		
Plesiomonas infection	VIII				+++				
Psittacosis	I, II, III, IV, V, VI	+++							
Q fever	I, II, V		++	+++					++
Rat-bite fever	I, III, IV						++		
Relapsing fever	I, III, IV							+++	(Vector)
Rocky Mountain spotted fever	I, III, IV, IX, public		(Vector)					+++	
Salmonellosis	I, II, III, IV, VIII, IX	+++	+	+++	+++	+++	+++	+	+++
Staphylococcus aureus infection	I, II, IV, V, IX		+	++					
Group A streptococcal infection	I, II, IV, public		+	+					
Tuberculosis	I, V, IX	+	+			+			
Tularemia	I, III, IV, X		++	++		+++	++	+++	++
Vibriosis	III, VIII					++			
Vibrio vulnificus infection	VIII, IX					+++			
Yersiniosis	I, II, III, IV, VIII	+	+	++	+		++	++	

Disease	Persons at Risk[a]	Birds, Fowl	Cats, Dogs	Farm Animals	Fish, Reptiles,[b] Water	Rabbits	Rodents	Arthropod Vectors	Wild Animals
Fungi									
Ringworm	I, II, III, IV, V, VI		++						
Parasites									
Babesiosis	III, IV, IX							+++	
Cryptosporidiosis	I, II, III, IV, VI, IX	+	++	+++	++	+	+		
Cystircercosis	Public		++						
Dipylidiasis	IV		++						
Dirofilariasis	III		(Vector)					+++	
Echinococcosis	I		+	++					
Giardiasis	I, III, IV	+			++		+		+++
Toxocariasis	IV		++						
Toxoplasmosis	IV, IX		+++	+					
Trichinosis	Public			+					++

Abbreviation: SARS-coV = severe acute respiratory syndrome-coronavirus.

+, Rare source; ++, occasional source; +++, most-common source; (vector), not spread directly by animal but always via vector.

[a] Persons at risk: Group I (agriculture), farmers and other people in close contact with livestock and their products; group II (animal-product processing and manufacture), all personnel of abattoirs and of plants processing animal products or by-products; group III (forestry, outdoors), persons frequenting wild habitats for professional or recreational reasons; group IV (recreation), persons in contact with pets or wild animals in the urban environment; group V (clinics, laboratories), health care personnel who attend patients and health care workers, including laboratory personnel, who handle specimens, corpses, or organs; group VI (epidemiology), public health professionals who do field research; group VII (emergency), public affected by catastrophes, refuges, or people temporarily living in crowded or highly stressful situations; group VIII (fisherman), people catching or cleaning fish or engaging in recreational activities in the water; group IX (immunocompromised hosts), people who are immunocompromised because of immunodeficiency, cancer chemotherapy, organ transplants, immunosuppressive medications, liver and/or renal disease; group X (disaster responders, public), potential bioterrorist agent.

[b] Reptiles include lizards, snakes, and turtles.

[c] Rodents include hamsters, mice, and rats.

other important diseases vectored by ticks are human granulocytic ehrlichiosis (HGE), caused by *Ehrlichia chaffeensis*, and human granulocytic anaplasmosis (HGA), caused by *Anaplasma phagocytophilium*.

Mosquito-borne zoonotic diseases are common and significant throughout much of the world but play only a minor role domestically. The most common in the United States is West Nile virus, a viral disease that first appeared in North America in 1999. The vast majority of infected have subclinical or mild disease, whereas 1 in 150 infected will develop an encephalitis. A unique feature of this mosquito-borne disease is the presentation of ascending paralysis ("West Nile polio"). Other mosquito-borne zoonotics that occur in the United States are western equine encephalitis (WEE), eastern equine encephalitis (EEE), St. Louis encephalitis, Lacrosse encephalitis, and California encephalitis. Other than EEE, these agents generally cause mild disease but can occasionally cause severe encephalitis in immunocompromised patients. EEE is rare but does have a case fatality rate of about 33%.

Plague, caused by *Yerisinia pestis*, still persists in wild rodents in the western half of the United States and is vectored by rodent fleas. Although tularemia, caused by *Francisella tularensis*, occurs throughout the entire United States and is vectored by ticks, deerflies, and other insects. Tularemia also has several reservoirs such as rabbits, voles, and badgers. Both plague and tularemia may cause local skin and soft tissue infection and serious systemic illness.

ZOONOTIC DISEASES ACQUIRED BY INHALATION

Although community-acquired pneumonia (CAP) is a common disease, few cases of pneumonia are due to zoonotic agents. Lower respiratory infection due to zoonotic agents generally causes an "atypical" pneumonia and may be mistaken for infection caused by *Legionella* spp., *Mycoplasma pneumoniae*, or *Chlamydophila pneumoniae*. Zoonotic diseases that may be acquired in the home include *Pasteurella multocida* infection (cats and dogs), psittacosis (birds), and Q fever (parturient cats). Hunting or hiking in the United States may bring people into contact with animals capable of transmitting brucellosis (farm animals), plague (rodents, ground squirrels, prairie dogs), Q fever (farm animals, cats), Rocky Mountain spotted fever (ticks), and tularemia (rabbits). Persons engaged in processing animal products such as hides are at risk for brucellosis and anthrax. The hantavirus cardiopulmonary syndrome (HCPS) due to Sin nombre virus (SNV) results from inhalation of aerosols of excreta from infected rodents and is a systemic illness characterized by fever, headache, myalgias, and respiratory failure.

Few zoonotic pneumonias are capable of being transmitted from person to person. However, person-to-person transmission has been reported of avian influenza (H5N1 strain), *Chamydophila psittaci* (psittacosis), *Coxiella burnetii* (Q fever), and *Mycobacterium bovis* and *Yersinia pestis* (plague). Avian influenza (H5N1) and pneumonic plague represent potentially serious nosocomial pathogens, and patients with these diseases should be placed on CDC-recommended isolation precautions. Several zoonotic agents acquired via the respiratory route are potential agents of bioterrorism, including anthrax, brucellosis, plague, Q fever, and tularemia. A worldwide epidemic of pneumonia, the severe respiratory disease syndrome (SARS), occurred in 2003 due to a novel coronovirus (SARS-coV). Molecular epidemiology suggested transmission from the palm civet and that the ultimate reservoir for the virus was bats.

ZOONOTIC DISEASES ACQUIRED VIA INGESTION

Zoonotic diseases acquired through ingestion as a group are the most commonly acquired zoonotic diseases in the world. The main category in this group is bacterial disease that causes diarrhea, along with fever and abdominal cramps. *Campylobacter* is the most common agent and is normally found in the intestines of birds. Birds are also the primary reservoir of *Salmonella*, but it can also be found in many reptiles and some mammals. The main reservoir of *Escherichia coli* O157:H7 are cattle and similar ungulates. One possible consequence of infection with *E. coli* O157:H7, especially in children and the elderly is hemolytic uremic syndrome (HUS). In these individuals the infection leads to the destruction of red blood cells and renal failure. Brucellosis and listeriosis are also bacterial foodborne zoonotic diseases of increasing importance in the United States due to the consumption of unpasteurized dairy products, but both cause a generalized febrile illness. Pregnant women are at higher risk for severe listeriosis.

There are also zoonotic agents that are transmitted via contaminated water. The most common is cryptosporidiosis, a protozoal disease that can be found in drinking and recreational water throughout the entire United States. Cryptosporidiosis generally causes a self-limited mild diarrheal illness. Giardiasis is also a protozoal waterborne zoonotic disease that is common and causes a mild diarrheal illness. Leptospirosis due to a spirochete bacteria is a disease that is generally transmitted through contaminated water. Although not common in the United States, there are sporadic outbreaks. Most cases are initially a vague febrile illness that may progress to severe hepatic, renal, or neurological disease. The reservoirs for leptospirosis are generally rodents, cattle, pigs, and small mammals (eg, raccoons, opossums).

SYSTEMIC INFECTIONS RESULT FROM ZOONOTIC DISEASES

Many zoonoses cause severe systemic symptoms. The range of possible pathogens can often be narrowed if the patient manifests specific organ involvement. Diseases to consider in patients with fever without focal signs on initial history and physical examination include *Aeromonas* sepsis, babesiosis, brucellosis, *Capnocytophaga canimorsus* sepsis, ehrlichiosis, cat scratch disease, leptospirosis, listeriosis, plague, Q fever, rat-bite fevers, relapsing fever, RMSF and other rickettsial infections, salmonellosis, tularemia, and viral hemorrhagic fevers.

Zoonoses may be associated with skin lesions. A generalized maculopapular rash may occur with cat scratch fever, Colorado tick fever, ehrlichiosis, leptospirosis, lymphocytic choriomeningitis, psittacosis, RMSF and other rickettsial infections (exceptions include Q fever and trench fever), rat-bite fever resulting from *Spirillum minus*, relapsing fever, and salmonellosis. Most rashes associated with zoonoses are too nonspecific to be of significant clinical utility. Crepitant or gangrenous lesions may be associated with *Aeromonas, C. canimorsus,* or *Vibrio vulnificus* and related species. Petechial and purpuric lesions may occur with viral hemorrhagic fevers (eg, dengue, yellow fever, Ebola, Lassa), RMSF, *Rickettsia prowazekii* infection, rat-bite fever resulting from *Streptobacillus moniliformis,* relapsing fever, and *C. canimorsus* sepsis. A local eschar often occurs with rickettsial infections due to *Rickettsia conorii, Rickettsia australis, Rickettsia sibirica, Rickettsia akari,* and *Rickettsia tsutsugamushi.* Local skin lesions with or without lymphangitis may occur with cat scratch fever, rat-bite fever resulting from *Spirillum minus,* and tularemia.

SUGGESTED READING

Acha PN, Szyfres B. *Zoonoses and Communicable Diseases Common to Man and Animals.* 3rd ed., Scientific Publication No. 580, Washington, DC: Pan American Health Organization; 2003.

Chomel BB. Zoonoses of house pets other than dogs, cats, and birds. *Pediatr Infect Dis J.* 1992;11:479–487.

Cunha BA. The atypical pneumonias: clinical diagnosis and importance. *Clin Microbiol Infect.* 2006;12(suppl 3):12–24.

Kotton CN. Zoonoses in solid-organ and hematopoietic stem cell transplant recipients. *Clin Infect Dis.* 2007;44:857–866.

Krauss H, Weber A, Appel M, et al. *Zoonoses.* 3rd ed. Washington, DC: American Society of Microbiology; 2003.

Kruse H, Kirkemo AM, Handerland K. Wildlife as source of zoonotic infections. *Emerg Infect Dis.* 2004;10:2067–2072.

Litwin CM. Pet-transmitted infections: diagnosis by microbiologic and immunologic methods. *Pediatr Infect Dis J.* 2003;22:768–777.

Mushatt DM, Hyslop NE. Neurologic aspects of North American zoonoses. *Infect Dis Clin North Am.* 1991;5:703–731.

Palmer SR, Soulsby L, Simpson DIH. *Zoonoses.* Oxford, UK: Oxford University Press; 1998.

Swartz MN. Cellulitis. *New Engl J Med.* 2004;350:904–912.

Taplitz RA. Managing bite wounds: currently recommended antibitoics for treatment and prophylaxis. *Postgrad Med.* 2004;116:49–52, 55–56, 59.

Weber DJ, Rutala WA. Zoonotic infections. *Occup Med.* 1999;14:247–284.

Weinberg AN. Respiratory infections transmitted from animals. *Infect Dis Clin North Am.* 1991;5:649–661.

Weinberg AN, Weber DJ. Animal-associated human infections. *Infect Dis Clin North Am.* 1991;5:1–6.

117. Tick-Borne Disease

Steven C. Buckingham

Ticks can transmit numerous bacterial, parasitic, and viral pathogens to humans, and the secretions of some species can induce allergic reactions or cause paralysis. This chapter aims to provide a broad overview of tick-borne infections endemic to North America and to discuss general principles regarding their epidemiology, therapy, and prevention. Details about each of these infections are provided in their respective chapters.

EPIDEMIOLOGY

Tick-borne infections occur most often in the spring and summer, when ticks are most active, but are reported in colder months as well. In general, males are affected more often than females. Some patients with tick-borne infections will recall a recent tick bite, and many, but not all, report having spent time in a rural or wooded area within 2 to 4 weeks before the onset of illness. Frequently, however, patients are unaware of their recent tick exposure, for several reasons: Tick bites are usually painless, ticks may attach in sites covered by hair or clothing, and ticks in their larval and nymphal stages are very small but still capable of transmitting infection. Tick-borne infections have been reported in urban areas and, in endemic areas, among patients whose only outdoor exposures occurred in their own backyards. Thus the historical findings of tick bite or outdoor exposure may provide useful diagnostic clues, but their absence never excludes the possibility of a tick-borne illness.

Clinicians must understand the epidemiology of tick-borne infections to make presumptive diagnoses. The geographic distributions of tick-borne infections (listed in Table 117.1) correspond to the distributions of their associated tick vectors; thus, patients' geographic residence and travel history are keys to deciding which tick-borne illnesses are possible or likely.

CLINICAL MANIFESTATIONS

Most tick-borne infections present with non-specific signs and symptoms, similar to those observed in viral syndromes (eg, fever, malaise, headache, and myalgias). Sometimes, certain constellations of symptoms suggest a specific diagnosis. For example, the combination of erythema migrans, arthritis, and neurologic abnormalities suggests Lyme disease, whereas a cutaneous ulcer with associated regional adenopathy suggests tularemia.

Some of the typical physical and laboratory findings associated with specific tick-borne infections endemic to the United States are listed in Table 117.1. It must be emphasized, however, that not all patients with these illnesses will have all of their typical findings; for example, fewer than two thirds of patients with Rocky Mountain spotted fever (RMSF) have the "classic triad" of fever, rash, and headache. Moreover, these illnesses have broad differential diagnoses; for example, the symptoms and signs of RMSF overlap considerably with those of ehrlichiosis, brucellosis, salmonellosis, Q fever, numerous viral infections (eg, Epstein–Barr virus, cytomegalovirus, and enterovirus) and many other illnesses.

THERAPY

Tick-borne infections should, in general, be diagnosed presumptively, based on clinical findings and epidemiologic history. Because most specific tests yield negative results in early disease or must be sent out to a reference laboratory, the clinician often must prescribe antibiotics empirically (ie, before a diagnosis is confirmed by laboratory testing). This is particularly true with regard to RMSF, in which mortality rates are significantly higher among patients who receive antirickettsial therapy on the fifth day of illness or later.

Details regarding the treatment of specific tick-borne infections are provided in the respective chapters. Generally speaking, doxycycline is appropriate for treatment of most tick-borne infections endemic to North America. At one time, chloramphenicol was advocated for use in children younger than 8 years, owing to concerns over doxycycline's perceived potential to stain permanent teeth.

Table 117.1 Tick-Borne Diseases of the United States

Disease	Organism	Vector	Geographic Distribution	Typical Clinical Findings[a]
Rocky Mountain spotted fever (RMSF)	*Rickettsia rickettsii*	*Dermacentor variabilis* (dog tick) *Dermacentor andersoni* (wood tick) *Ambylomma americanum* (Lone Star tick)	Eastern United States Western United States Southeastern and southcentral United States	Fever, headache, petechial rash, hyponatremia, thrombocytopenia
Human monocytotropic ehrlichiosis (HME)	*Ehrlichia chaffeensis*	*A. americanum*	Southeastern and southcentral United States	Similar to RMSF, but rash less common; leukopenia, thrombocytopenia, elevated transaminases
Human granulocytotropic anaplasmosis (HGA)[b]	*Anaplasma phagocytophilum*	*Ixodes scapularis* (blacklegged tick)	Northeastern and upper midwestern United States	Similar to HME, but rash is rarely present
		Ixodes pacificus	Pacific coast states	
Ehrlichia ewingii infection	*Ehrlichia ewingii*	*A. americanum*	Southeastern and southcentral United States	Same as HGA
Lyme disease	*Borrelia burgdorferi*	*I. scapularis*	Northeastern and upper midwestern United States	First stage: fever, erythema migrans
		I. pacificus	Pacific coast states	Second stage: multiple skin lesions, conjunctivitis, arthralgias, myalgias, headache, cranial nerve palsies Third stage: arthritis; encephalopathy, dementia, peripheral neuropathy
Southern tick-associated rash illness	*Borrelia lonestari*	*A. americanum*	Southeastern and southcentral United States	Rash similar to erythema migrans
Endemic relapsing fever	*Borrelia hermsii* *B. turicatae* *B. parkeri*	*Ornithodoros* species	Western mountains and deserts	Fever, chills, relapsing course
Tularemia	*Francisella tularensis*	*D. variabilis* *D. andersoni* *A. americanum*	Eastern United States Western United States Southeastern and southcentral United States	Fever, cutaneous eschar, lymphadenopathy, pulse–temperature dissociation
Babesiosis	*Babesia microti*	*Ixodes scapularis*	Northeast, Midwest, and West Coast	Fever, malaise, headache, hepatosplenomegaly, thrombocytopenia, hemolytic anemia
Colorado tick fever	Coltivirus	*D. andersoni*	Rocky Mountain states	Fever, headache, leukopenia, thrombocytopenia; biphasic course
Tick paralysis[c]	Neurotoxin	*Dermacentor* spp.; others	Worldwide; most United States cases in western states	Ascending flaccid paralysis

[a] Not all patients will have all of the "typical" findings for these diseases. All the above diseases (except tick paralysis) may present simply with fever and vague constitutional symptoms.
[b] Formerly termed *human granulocytic ehrlichiosis*.
[c] Tick paralysis is not caused by an infection, but its epidemiology is similar to that of tick-borne infections.

Travel and Recreation

Now, however, doxycycline is recognized as the drug of choice for the treatment of all suspected rickettsioses or ehrlichioses in North America, regardless of the patient's age. The principal reason for this change is that doxycycline treatment achieves superior outcomes in patients with RMSF or human monocytic ehrlichiosis, compared to chloramphenicol. Moreover, doxycycline does not penetrate teeth as well as tetracycline does; whereas repeated administrations of tetracycline to young children certainly can cause unsightly tooth discoloration, there is no evidence that a single course of doxycycline will do so.

PREVENTION OF TICK-BORNE DISEASES

Prevention of tick-borne diseases consists of avoidance of tick bites and prompt removal of attached ticks. During spring and summer months, it is prudent to examine persons and pets that have been outdoors at least daily for attached ticks. Wearing light-colored clothing will facilitate the identification of ticks. Nymphs and larvae are very small and may hide in areas such as the head, neck, axillae, belt line, or scrotum; thus, these areas must be scrutinized closely.

Attached ticks should be removed by grasping with tweezers close to the skin and pulling gently with steady pressure; the bite site should then be washed with soap and water. Attempts to detach ticks by applying petroleum jelly, fingernail polish, isopropyl alcohol, or a hot, extinguished kitchen match are discouraged, as these methods are both ineffective and potentially dangerous.

The repellant N,N-diethyl-meta-toluamide (DEET) is very effective for preventing tick, mosquito, chigger, and fly bites. Because protection increases with increasing concentrations, repellants containing 20% to 30% DEET are currently recommended for adults and children. When used appropriately, DEET is quite safe; concerns over its toxicity have been vastly overstated. Nevertheless, a few cautionary statements are in order. DEET must not be ingested and should be applied only to exposed, intact skin, or to clothing. It should not be introduced to the mouth, eyes, or other mucous membranes (and thus should not be applied to the hands of children). Children should not apply DEET-containing products to themselves, and DEET is not recommended for use on children younger than 2 months. DEET should not be overused; in most cases, one application per day is adequate. Treated skin should be washed with soap and water after coming indoors.

Permethrin is an insecticide that may be sprayed on clothing, providing an additional layer of protection against tick bites (and those of other arthropods). Clothes should be sprayed on each side of the fabric for 30 to 45 seconds and allowed to dry for 2 to 4 hours before wearing. Permethrin maintains potency for at least 2 weeks after application, even if clothes are washed. Although permethrin is occasionally associated with skin erythema or edema, systemic adverse effects have not been noted.

SUGGESTED READING

Buckingham SC. Tick-borne diseases in children: epidemiology, clinical manifestations and optimal treatment strategies. *Paediatr Drugs.* 2005;7:163–176.

Centers for Disease Control and Prevention. Diagnosis and management of tick-borne rickettsial diseases in the United States—Rocky Mountain spotted fever, ehrlichioses, and anaplasmosis: a practical guide for physicians and other health care and public health professionals. Mortal Morbid Weekly Rep. 2006;55(No. RR-4):1.

Holman RC, Paddock CD, Curns AT, Krebs JW, McQuiston JH, Childs JE. Analysis of risk factors for fatal Rocky Mountain spotted fever: evidence for superiority of tetracyclines for therapy. *J Infect Dis.* 2001;184:1437–1444.

Insect repellants. *Med Lett Drugs Ther.* 2003; 45:41–42.

Needham GR. Evaluation of five popular methods for tick removal. *Pediatrics.* 1985;75:997–1002.

Parola P, Raoult D. Ticks and tickborne bacterial diseases in humans: an emerging infectious threat. [published erratum appears in Clin Infect Dis 33:749, 2001]. *Clin Infect Dis.* 2001;32:897–928.

Raoult D, Roux V. Rickettsioses as paradigms of new or emerging infectious diseases. *Clin Microbiol Rev.* 1997;10:694–719.

Smith M, Unkel JH, Fenton SJ, DeVincenzo JP. The use of tetracyclines in pediatric patients. *J Pediatr Pharmacol Ther.* 2001;6:66.

Spach DH, Liles WC, Campbell GL, et al. Tickborne diseases in the United States. *N Engl J Med.* 1993;329:936–947.

118. Recreational Water Exposure

Andrea K. Boggild and Mary Elizabeth Wilson

Many common forms of recreation involve water exposure. Pathogens in water infect susceptible humans by multiple routes: through skin and mucous membranes, via inhalation of aerosols, aspiration, and ingestion. Clinical manifestations of these infections range from superficial skin lesions to fatal, systemic infections. The survival of many water-associated pathogens is influenced by climate, season, other environmental conditions, and the level of sanitation. The types and abundance of organisms vary depending on the salinity, pH, temperature, and other characteristics of the water. Hence, many are found only or primarily in certain geographic regions or during some seasons of the year. The risk of infection by waterborne pathogens is a function of the duration and type of exposure, concentration density of organisms in water, and host immunity. This chapter describes the types of pathogens, geographic distribution, sources and routes of transmission, clinical presentations, and management of water-associated infections. Water can also be a source of toxins, including heavy metals. Oceans and beaches are the sites of marine envenomations. These topics are beyond the scope of this chapter.

United States residents make approximately 360 million visits to recreational water venues annually. Thus, outbreaks of infections related to recreational water exposures are common. In the United States in 2003–2004, for example, 62 waterborne disease outbreaks in 26 states were reported to the Centers for Disease Control and Prevention (CDC). More than 2600 persons were affected by these outbreaks, 58 of whom required hospitalization and 1 of whom died. Over the past 20 years, the number of reported diarrheal illnesses following recreational water exposure has steadily increased. Of the 62 outbreaks reported in 2003–2004, almost half (*n* = 30) were outbreaks of gastroenteritis, whereas dermatitis, acute respiratory illness, meningoencephalitis, and mixed infections accounted for smaller respective percentages. Cryptosporidiosis, giardiasis, *E. coli* O157: H7 gastroenteritis, norovirus, shigellosis, leptospirosis, and *Pseudomonas* dermatitis have been the most commonly reported infections related to recreational water exposures in the United States in recent years. Outbreaks of adenovirus 3 (causing pharyngitis), cercarial dermatitis, and hepatitis A (public swimming pool) have also been reported. Chlorinated swimming pools, water parks, lakes, ponds, and whirlpools have been common sources. Although outbreaks related to recreational water use can occur throughout the calendar year, most occur in the summer months between May and August.

Patients typically do not volunteer specific descriptions of water exposures, as they may not recognize their relevance. Table 118.1 lists several sources of water exposures that have been associated with infections and can be used as a checklist to help the clinician obtain relevant history. Most water-associated infections will become apparent within hours to days (usually ≤14 days) of exposure. An important exception is schistosomiasis, which may first manifest months or longer after exposure. Relevant history includes types of exposures; dates, duration, and location of exposures; and type of water (eg, mountain stream, lake, hot tub, chlorinated pool, salt water). During participation in water sports, people commonly ingest water and inhale aerosols.

Ingestion of contaminated water, whether during swimming, showering, or drinking often causes infections manifested by diarrhea. Some pathogens have the capacity to cause systemic infection after ingestion. Fecally contaminated water may contain a potpourri of microbes – bacteria, viruses, protozoa, and helminths – causing a variety of illnesses with differing manifestations and incubation periods. Swimming at beaches near a sewage outlet, for example, leads to increased rates of conjunctivitis, otitis externa, skin and soft-tissue infections, as well as gastrointestinal infections.

Recreational water activities are often group activities, so contaminated water may be associated with outbreaks, sometimes involving dozens or even hundreds of people. In addition to caring for the acutely ill patient, the clinician must consider the public

Table 118.1 Types of Activities Associated with Water Exposures

Swimming, wading, diving
Near-drowning events
Fishing, hunting
Rafting, boating, sailing, surfing, windsurfing, water-skiing
Water parks (wave pools and water slides)
Sitting in hot tubs, whirlpools
Showering and bathing, ritual washing
Drinking water and water-containing beverages (untreated surface water consumed during hiking, camping)
Care of fish tanks, aquaria

Table 118.2 Clinical Manifestations of Infections Related to Water Exposures

Skin and Mucosal Surface Exposures
Conjunctivitis
Keratitis
Otitis externa
Dermatitis (including folliculitis)
Mastitis
Cellulitis
Fasciitis
Endometritis (reported after intercourse in water)
Systemic infection

Aspiration, Inhalation, Ingestion
Pharyngitis
Sinusitis
Meningoencephalitis
Pneumonitis
Gastroenteritis, colitis
Systemic infection

health implications and alert the appropriate authorities. Early interventions may slow or halt an outbreak and allow early recognition of other cases. In many instances, outbreaks are the result of inadequate operation or maintenance procedures. For example, in a recent U.S.-wide inspection of >5000 spas, nearly 3000 were found to be in violation of water quality and other maintenance parameters, resulting in the immediate closure of 11% of those inspected. As further illustration of this point, in August 2003, inadequate disinfection of an athletic facility spa resulted in an outbreak of methicillin-resistant *Staphylococcus aureus* (MRSA) skin infections among college football players, thus establishing this emerging pathogen as one with potential for waterborne transmission.

The route of entry may influence the clinical findings for several of the water-associated pathogens, with skin penetration causing local wound infections and ingestion causing diarrheal infections. Table 118.2 lists the range of clinical manifestations of infections that follow water exposure. With some of the more virulent organisms or in the setting of immune compromise, infection may enter the bloodstream after any one of several entry points. Minor trauma, cuts, bites, and breaks in the skin can provide the portal of entry for many water-dwelling microbes. Table 118.3 summarizes infections and infestations that enter through the skin. Table 118.4 lists specific infections acquired via aspiration, inhalation, and ingestion.

Several water-associated infections can be rapidly progressive or can lead to serious complications. Because some of these are infrequent or rare, they may be unfamiliar to

most physicians. The following section provides a brief summary of each. More common infections, such as shigellosis, campylobacteriosis, salmonellosis, and *E. coli* O157:H7 that can be acquired through water exposure are covered in more detail in other chapters of this book. Table 118.5 lists the recommended treatment for the less familiar water-associated infections and ones that are not covered in other chapters of the text.

ACQUIRED BY PENETRATION THROUGH SKIN

Pseudomonas Dermatitis or Folliculitis

Use of hot tubs and whirlpools (spas), and occasionally swimming pools and water slides, has been associated with development of a characteristic diffuse rash caused by the aerobic, gram-negative organism *Pseudomonas aeruginosa*. The rash, which is maculopapular or vesiculopustular and usually pruritic, develops within 48 hours of exposure and typically resolves within a week. Lesions are more prominent in areas covered by a bathing suit or clothing. Associated findings may include otitis externa, mastitis (in men and women), conjunctivitis, and lymphadenopathy. Infection is typically self-limited in healthy hosts; immunocompromised persons may develop hemorrhagic bullae, pneumonia, and bacteremia. Outbreaks can be large, involving hundreds of persons. Eight of thirteen outbreaks of dermatitis affecting 274 people in 2003–2004 were caused by *Pseudomonas aeruginosa*. In

Table 118.3 Infections and Infestations Acquired via Percutaneous and Permucosal Water Exposures

Pathogen or Disease	Source
Bacteria	
Aeromonas hydrophila[a,b]	Freshwater streams, lakes, soil
Burkholderia pseudomallei (Melioidosis)[a,b]	Fresh water, soil (tropics, subtropics)
Chromobacterium violaceum[a,b]	Freshwater rivers, soil (tropics, subtropics)
Leptospirosis[b]	Fresh water contaminated with animal urine (especially tropics, subtropics)
Mycobacterium marinum[a]	Fish tanks, swimming pools
Pseudomonas aeruginosa[a]	Hot tubs, whirlpools, swimming pools
Vibrio vulnificus, other vibrios[a,b]	Seawater
Tularemia[a,b,c] (*Francisella tularensis*)	Fresh water contaminated by infected animal; inoculation of skin, conjunctiva, oropharyngeal mucosa
Helminths	
Schistosomiasis[a,b]	Freshwater streams, lakes (focal in Asia, Africa, South America, parts of Caribbean)
Cercarial dermatitis (avian schistosomes)[a]	Fresh and salt water (worldwide)
Protozoa	
Acanthamoeba species[a,b] (keratitis)	Fresh water, especially stagnant ponds during hot summers; hot tubs, swimming pools, thermal springs
Viruses	
Adenovirus[a,b] (swimming pool conjunctivitis)	Swimming pools; likely other freshwater sites
Coxsackieviruses[a,b]	Fresh water
Other	
Seabather's eruption[a]	Seawater

Note. *Pseudomonas* dermatitis and *M. marinum* are rarely associated with systemic infection, primarily in compromised hosts.
[a] Skin and soft tissue.
[b] Systemic infection.
[c] Conjunctivitis.

each outbreak, use of a pool or spa was implicated. Infections can be prevented if water is maintained at a pH of 7.2 to 7.8 with adequate chlorination (free, residual chlorine levels should be in the range of 2.0 to 5.0 mg/L).

OTITIS EXTERNA (SWIMMER'S EAR)

Infection of the external ear canal, otitis externa, is common in swimmers. Usual symptoms are mild pain and pruritus around the ear. Pain may become more severe if infection progresses to involve deep tissues and bone, as is more commonly the case with underlying medical conditions, such as diabetes mellitus. Common organisms are *S. aureus* and *P. aeruginosa*; multiple bacterial species are often recovered from cultures. Purulent drainage and local lymphadenopathy may develop. Occasionally infections progress to cellulitis that requires systemic antibiotic therapy. Topical therapy can be effective in early infections. See Chapter 06, Otitis Media and Externa, for treatment.

Cercarial (Schistosome) Dermatitis

Cercarial dermatitis, also known as swimmer's or clam digger's itch, is caused by an allergic response to penetration of skin by cercariae

Table 118.4 Specific Infections Acquired via Inhalation, Aspiration, or Ingestion

Disease or Pathogen	Main Clinical Finding
Acanthamoeba (especially *Naegleria fowleri*)	Meningoencephalitis
Adenovirus 3	Pharyngitis, fever, conjunctivitis
Amebiasis (*Entamoeba histolytica*)	Colitis, liver abscess
Balantidiasis (*Balantidium coli*)	Diarrhea or dysentery
Campylobacteriosis	Diarrhea
Cholera (*Vibrio cholerae*)	Diarrhea, dehydration
Coxsackieviruses	Diarrhea
Cryptosporidiosis	Diarrhea
Cyclospora	Diarrhea
E. coli O157:H7	Bloody diarrhea
Giardiasis	Subacute diarrhea
Hepatitis A virus	Acute hepatitis
Hepatitis E virus	Acute hepatitis (severe and potentially fatal in pregnancy)
Legionnaire's disease	Pneumonia
Leptospirosis	Fever, severe myalgia, conjunctival suffusion; can be hemorrhagic
Melioidosis	Pneumonia, sepsis, skin lesions; protean manifestations
Norovirus ("Norwalk-like viruses")	Diarrhea, vomiting
Poliovirus	Nonspecific febrile illness; flaccid paralysis ≤1%
Pontiac fever	Fever (self-limited)
Primary amebic meningoencephalitis (PAM)	See *Acanthamoeba*
Rotavirus	Watery diarrhea
Salmonellosis	Diarrhea; extraintestinal manifestations if bacteremic diarrhea; dysentery
Shigellosis	Diarrhea, dysentery
Toxoplasmosis	Fever, lymphadenopathy, lymphocytosis
Tularemia	Fever, lymphadenopathy, pneumonia; manifestations depend on route of transmission
Typhoid/paratyphoid fever (enteric fever)	Fever, systemic infection, gastrointestinal sequelae
Vibrio parahemolyticus	Watery diarrhea; occasionally dysentery
Vibrio vulnificus	Sepsis, bullous skin lesions
Yersinia enterocolitica	Fever, diarrhea, acute mesenteric lymphadenitis

Table 118.5 Diagnosis and Treatment of Selected Infections

Pathogen or Disease	Diagnosis[a]	Treatment
Aeromonas hydrophila	C	TMP/SMX or FQ[b,c]; (third-generation cephalosporins; AG; imipenem)
Burkholderia pseudomallei	C	Ceftazidime[b,c] (imipenem[b,c] or meropenem; TMP/SMX + doxycycline[c])
Chromobacterium violaceum	C	Limited clinical data; may be sensitive to FQ, TMP/SMX, tetracyclines, AG, extended spectrum penicillins
Francisella tularensis (tularemia)	S, C	Gentamicin,[b] streptomycin,[b] or tobramycin[b] (doxycycline or ciprofloxacin; chloramphenicol)
Leptospirosis	S, C	Penicillin G[b,c] or doxycycline[b]
Mycobacterium marinum	C (at 30°C)	Minocycline or clarithromycin (TMP/SMX; rifampin + ethambutol; doxycycline)
Primary amebic meningoencephalitis	Visualization of trophozoites in CSF; C	*Naegleria*[d]: amphotericin B IV and IT *Acanthamoeba*: Itraconazole, TMP/SMX, rifampin; pentamidine *Balamuthia:* Pentamidine + fluconazole + sulfadiazine + flucytosine ± clarithromycin
Schistosomiasis	Eggs in tissue, urine, or stool; S	Praziquantel[b,c]
Vibrio vulnificus	C	Doxycycline + ceftazidime[b] (cefotaxime; ciprofloxacin; doxycycline + AG [FQ])

Abbreviations: AG = aminoglycoside; FQ = fluoroquinolone; IT = intrathecal; TMP/SMX = trimethoprim-sulfamethoxazole.
[a] Method of diagnosis: C = culture, S = serology.
[b] Considered first-line therapy at time of printing.
[c] Randomized controlled trial level of evidence for therapy.
[d] Reports of treatment success are scant.

of nonhuman larval trematodes of the genus *Schistosoma* (often avian schistosomes). A pruritic, maculopapular rash develops in water-exposed areas of the body (Figure 118.1). Both total duration of exposure and duration of exposure to shallow water correlate with increased likelihood of developing cercarial dermatitis. Shallow water exposure is a particular risk factor as this is where snail beds are most dense and cercarial accumulation is greatest.

Lesions appear hours to a day or more after water exposure and are often less prominent in areas covered by a bathing suit or other protective clothing. Papules may become vesicular. Secondary bacterial infection may result from scratching-related skin abrasions. Lesions peak in 2 to 3 days and typically resolve over 1 to 2 weeks without specific therapy. In persons with previous exposures lesions may develop sooner and may be more severe. Treatment is symptomatic and may include antihistamines and topical steroids. Systemic steroids have been used in severe cases. Nonhuman schistosomes are widely distributed, including in temperate

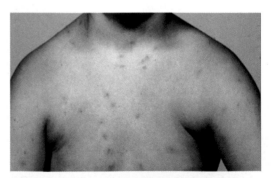

Figure 118.1 Skin lesions of cercarial dermatitis (Courtesy of Jay Keystone, MD).

areas, and may contaminate fresh, brackish, and seawater.

Schistosomiasis

Penetration of the skin by human schistosomes (eg, most often *Schistosoma mansoni*, *Schistosoma haematobium*, *Schistosoma japonicum*) may cause redness, urticaria, and pruritic papules, typically less severe than the cercarial dermatitis described above. Systemic manifestations

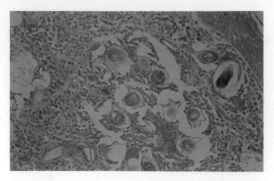

Figure 118.2 Granulomatous inflammation surrounding eggs of *Schistosoma haematobium* in the bladder wall.

of schistosomiasis may develop months or years later. Among 28 travelers who developed schistosomiasis after water exposures in Mali, 36% gave a history of schistosomal dermatitis. Infection can follow even brief water exposures, including river rafting. Attack rates have often been high in travelers who swim, wade, or bathe in infested water. An acute illness characterized by fever, malaise, and eosinophilia (Katayama fever) may develop 2 to 6 weeks after exposure and corresponds to larval migration following initial skin penetration. Neurologic complications (including transverse myelitis) can occur early or late. Clinical findings vary with the species of schistosome and are related to granulomatous reactions to eggs in tissue (Figure 118.2). Maps showing the geographic distribution of schistosomiasis are included in the text by Wilson.

SEABATHER'S ERUPTION (ALSO MARINE DERMATITIS OR SEA LICE)

Seabather's eruption is caused by penetration of the skin by *Linuche unguiculata*, *Edwardsiella lineata*, and other larvae of the phylum Cnidaria. Characteristic findings include an intensely pruritic, papular rash that begins 4 to 24 hours after swimming in the ocean. The lesions are found in areas covered by a bathing suit and at points of contact (eg, flexural areas, wristbands of diving suits) (Figure 118.3). The tiny larvae are entrapped by the bathing suit, which acts as a mechanical stimulus for the release of nematocysts and injection of toxin by the larvae. Outbreaks are sporadic. Persons with extensive involvement may have systemic symptoms, including fever. Lesions usually clear within 10 days. Antihistamines and topical steroids may provide symptomatic relief. Systemic steroids have been used in severe cases.

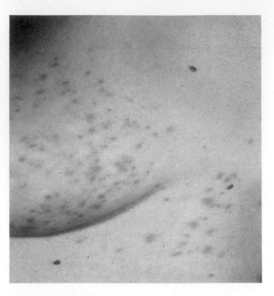

Figure 118.3 Skin lesions of seabather's eruption (image from Ryan ET, Wilson ME, Kain KC. Illness after international travel. *N Engl J Med* 2002;347:505–516. Copyright © Massachusetts Medical Society. All rights reserved. Adapted with permission, 2007).

Vibrio Soft-Tissue Infections

As resident marine flora, *Vibrio vulnificus*, *Vibrio parahemolyticus*, *Vibrio alginolyticus*, and other vibrio species can cause soft-tissue infections through recreational water exposure. In 2003–2004, 142 *Vibrio* cases following recreational water exposure were reported from 16 states. Organisms can be introduced by injuries (often on the lower extremity) that break the skin during swimming in the ocean or walking on beaches or can enter via pre-existing open skin lesions. After trauma, *V. vulnificus* can cause pustular lesions, lymphangitis, and cellulitis, which may be mild or rapidly progressive, causing pain, myositis, skin necrosis, and gangrene. Surgical debridement (or amputation) in addition to antibiotic therapy and general support may be necessary. Of all *Vibrio*-associated illnesses secondary to recreational water exposure reported to the CDC in 2003–2004, *V. vulnificus* carried the highest rate of hospitalization and mortality.

Vibrio soft-tissue infections, including necrotizing fasciitis, can also follow ingestion of contaminated food (commonly raw shellfish). Many vibrios, in addition to *V. cholerae*, can cause diarrheal illness, and gastroenteritis may be associated with high-grade bacteremia and high mortality. Large bullous skin lesions may occur with primary *Vibrio* bacteremia (especially *V. vulnificus*). Severe infections are more common in persons with chronic liver disease or other underlying diseases that compromise immune function.

Vibrios are found in seawater or brackish water and are part of the usual bacterial flora of coastal waters in the United States and elsewhere. They are more abundant in warmer months, and most reported infections occur in the summer. Unseasonally warm temperatures throughout Europe in the summer of 2006 led to an increase in the number of cases of skin and ear infections due to *V. alginolyticus* and *V. parahemolyticus* in countries such as Denmark and the Netherlands, which have been historically protected from these organisms due to their cooler climate.

Treatment of soft-tissue and systemic infections following seawater exposure should include coverage for *Vibrio* species.

Aeromonas hydrophila

Aeromonas hydrophila is a nonspore-forming, motile, facultatively anaerobic gram-negative organism found in freshwater lakes, streams, and soil. Puncture wounds or soft-tissue injury in contaminated water may lead to cellulitis that can resemble acute streptococcal infection with lymphangitis and fever. If not treated with effective drugs, it can progress to bullae formation and necrotizing myositis with gas in soft tissues. Findings can mimic gas gangrene. Soft-tissue infections may require local debridement along with systemic antibiotic therapy.

Ingestion of *Aeromonas* may cause diarrhea. Although *Aeromonas* is frequently isolated from environmental waters, evidence of clearly defined outbreaks of diarrhea attributable to aeromonads is lacking. Aspiration of *Aeromonas*-contaminated water may lead to *Aeromonas* pneumonia and bacteremia.

Melioidosis (*Burkholderia pseudomallei*)

This water- and soil-associated gram-negative organism found especially in tropical and subtropical areas is a common cause of pneumonia, skin lesions, and sepsis in parts of southeast Asia and Australia. The organism can be acquired through minor skin wounds or via aspiration or ingestion. Infection can be acute, subacute, or chronic and has protean manifestations, including cavitary lung disease, splenic abscesses, and osteomyelitis. The organism can persist silently in the human host and reactivate decades after acquisition,

thus making the clinical distinction from tuberculosis difficult.

Acanthamoeba Infections, Including Primary Amebic Meningoencephalitis

Free-living amebae of the genus *Acanthamoeba*, found in soil and fresh water, can enter human tissues and cause local or disseminated infection. Several species of *Acanthamoeba* have been reported to cause keratitis and granulomatous inflammation, which may be acute or subacute. Soft-tissue infections have also been reported, although are more likely to result from infection with the related free-living ameba *Balamuthia mandrillaris*. Minor trauma to the cornea, as may occur in persons who wear contact lenses, predisposes to infection. The diagnosis is confirmed by finding *Acanthamoeba* on biopsy, corneal scrapings, or culture (Figure 118.4). Treatment typically requires both debridement and topical therapy (several agents have been tried: combination of miconazole nitrate, propamidine isethionate, and Neosporin; propamidine isethionate and dibromopropamidine; among others, although level of evidence is case series only).

Free-living ameba, including *Acanthamoeba* species, though, usually *Naegleria fowleri*, cause primary amebic meningoencephalitis (PAM), typically in young healthy persons. Trophozoites enter the nasal passages during swimming or diving, penetrate the cribriform plate and invade the central nervous system via olfactory neuroepithelium, causing rapid destruction of gray and white matter. Symptoms usually begin 3 to 7 days after exposure to water. Infection causes high fever, headache, and stiff neck, resembling bacterial

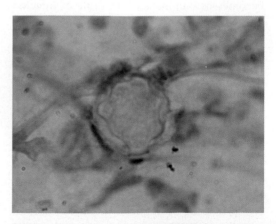

Figure 118.4 Cyst of *Acanthamoeba* from corneal specimen, iron–hematoxylin stain.

meningitis, which rapidly progresses to coma and, usually, death. Diagnosis is made by finding trophozoites in the cerebrospinal fluid (CSF) (wet mount, Giemsa staining after fixation, or by culture), although in most cases of PAM, diagnosis is postmortem. Infections have followed exposures in lakes, rivers, stagnant ponds, thermal springs, canals, and hot tubs and are more common during very warm periods, due to the thermophilic nature of these free-living protozoa. Disruption of lake or riverbed sediment by deep swimming or digging is a particular risk factor for PAM and may therefore serve as an important historical clue for clinicians. Ritualistic washing before prayers, which involves sniffing water to cleanse the nose, has also emerged as a risk factor for PAM in rural Nigeria.

Chromobacterium violaceum

This gram-negative organism is found in abundance in tropical and subtropical freshwater rivers and soils. The rarely reported infections have usually followed penetrating skin injury and are typically bacteremic. Persons with chronic granulomatous disease are at risk for severe infection. Clinical data are limited, and evidence to guide management decisions is lacking.

Leptospirosis

Spirochetes of the genus *Leptospira* cause leptospirosis, a zoonosis of global significance. Leptospirosis has caused outbreaks in swimmers (lake, creek, other fresh water), kayakers, white-water rafters (eg, in Costa Rica), and, more recently, among the Year 2000 Eco-Challenge participants in Borneo. Fresh water becomes contaminated with urine of infected domestic and wild animals. Humans become infected when organisms enter through skin (especially if abraded) or mucous membranes, or after ingestion of contaminated water or food. Infections are more common in tropical and subtropical areas and during warm seasons in temperate regions. In the United States, infections have been especially common in Hawaii, although sporadic infections and occasional clusters occur in other areas, primarily in warmer months. In July 1998, an outbreak of leptospirosis occurred in Springfield, Illinois, primarily affecting triathletes who swam in Lake Springfield. Imported cases in travelers, however, can be seen throughout the year in North America. The single outbreak of leptospirosis reported to the CDC in 2003–2004 affected three military personnel who swam near a waterfall in Guam.

Infected persons can develop a systemic infection with protean manifestations, commonly including fever, headache, severe myalgia, and conjunctival suffusion. The spectrum of clinical disease can range from asymptomatic or mild infection to the most serious form, Weil's disease, characterized by an icterohemorrhagic fever. A biphasic course is classic, and complications such as aseptic meningitis, pneumonia, and acute renal failure are seen in one quarter to one third of all cases of leptospirosis.

Mycobacterium marinum

Mycobacterium marinum usually invades only superficial tissue after local inoculation. Infection manifests as red plaques, papules, or nodules (sometimes with sporotrichoid or lymphocuticular spread) (Figure 118.5). The infection is referred to as "swimming pool granuloma" and "fish tank granuloma" because of the associations with fish and water. This subacute infection, most often on the hand or arm, can occur after exposure to fresh or salt water in aquariums and in swimming pools. Because the organism is relatively chlorine resistant, infection can follow exposures in chlorinated pools.

Tularemia

Tularemia, caused by *Francisella tularensis*, an organism that sometimes contaminates water (from infected animals), can infect via multiple routes, including through conjunctivae, skin, oropharynx, and gastrointestinal (GI) tract. Ticks and other arthropods can transmit infection. It is mentioned in this chapter because infection can be severe, even fatal, but does respond to appropriate therapy.

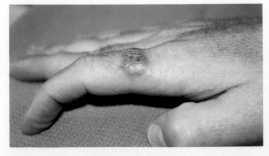

Figure 118.5 Cutaneous nodule of *Mycobacterium marinum* 4 months after swimming pool exposure.

ACQUIRED BY INHALATION, ASPIRATION, OR INGESTION

Legionnaire's Disease

Legionella can infect susceptible hosts through inhalation of aerosols generated by showers, whirlpools/spas, and sinks. Temperature is the most important abiotic factor influencing survival and growth of *Legionella*, which proliferates in hot-water tanks and heat-exchanging systems. Several outbreaks of legionnaire's disease, an acute pneumonic process, have been traced to exposures in resort hotels and to whirlpools on cruise ships. Hence, this is an infection to consider in persons with febrile illness and pneumonia after travel. In 1994 an outbreak occurred in cruise ship passengers exposed to a contaminated whirlpool spa. Fifty cases were identified from nine cruises. In addition, several outbreaks of Pontiac fever have been traced to exposures in hot tubs or whirlpools. More recently, an outbreak of Pontiac fever affecting 101 people occurred following exposure to a hotel spa in Oklahoma in 2004. In August 2006, 116 cases of Pontiac fever occurred in members exposed to a whirlpool at an English leisure club. Pontiac fever results from the aerosolized antigens of *Legionella pneumophila* and is characterized by a self-limited febrile illness. Randomized controlled trials support the use of either macrolides (clarithromycin, azithromycin) or fluoroquinolones (levofloxacin) for the management of legionnaire's disease or for empiric coverage of *L. pneumophila* in cases of community-acquired pneumonia.

Cryptosporidiosis

Cryptosporidium, an apicomplexan protozoan, has eclipsed *Giardia* as the most common parasitic cause of gastroenteritis outbreaks following recreational water exposure in the United States. Of 30 gastroenteritis outbreaks reported in the United States in 2003–2004, 11 were caused by *Cryptosporidium*, resulting in 1206 cases of illness. In the same reporting period, *Cryptosporidium hominis* was responsible for the single largest outbreak following recreational water exposure, causing 617 cases of gastroenteritis in a Kansas state community exposed to contaminated pool water. Most cases of *Cryptosporidium* occur following exposures at treated water venues, such as swimming pools. A number of factors contribute to the spread and transmission of *Cryptosporidium*, notably the wide range of animal reservoirs, the large number of fully infectious oocysts excreted

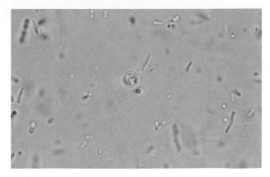

Figure 118.6 Oocyst of *Cryptosporidium hominis*, iron–hematoxylin stain (Courtesy of Donald Martin, MD).

by human and animal hosts (Figure 118.6), the relative resistance of oocysts to standard disinfection practices, and a low minimum infective dose.

Although the clinical course is usually self-limited, severe and prolonged diarrhea may occur in young children and in those who are immunocompromised. Nitazoxanide has recently emerged through randomized controlled trials as an effective agent for the treatment of cryptosporidiosis in both healthy adults and children and in those who are immunocompromised.

Giardiasis

Since the first documented outbreak in 1965, 122 waterborne outbreaks affecting 27 000 individuals have been attributable to the flagellated protozoan *Giardia*. Outbreaks of giardiasis have frequently been traced to ingesting unfiltered, unchlorinated, or inadequately chlorinated surface waters. Many infections in campers and hikers have followed drinking from mountain streams, even in remote wilderness areas. Like *Cryptosporidium*, *Giardia* has a broad mammalian host range, and cysts are excreted in fully infectious form (Figure 118.7). There are a number of

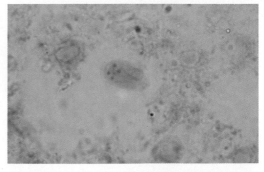

Figure 118.7 Cyst of *Giardia intestinalis*, iron–hematoxylin stain (Courtesy of Donald Martin, MD).

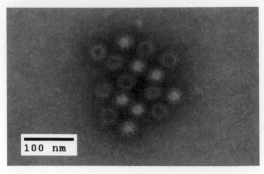

Figure 118.8 Electron micrograph of norovirus isolated from stool of a child with gastroenteritis (Courtesy of Susan Richardson and John Nishikawa, MD).

effective therapeutic options for giardiasis that have been evaluated in randomized controlled trials, including metronidazole, nitazoxanide, tinidazole, mebendazole, albendazole, and furazolidone.

NOROVIRUS ("NORWALK-LIKE VIRUSES")

In the 2003–2004 reporting period, norovirus was responsible for five waterborne disease outbreaks, which caused 300 cases of gastroenteritis, rendering it second only to *Cryptosporidium* in the number of individuals who were sickened by a specific etiologic agent. The majority of individuals were sickened by norovirus following exposure at treated water venues, notably swimming pools. Although community outbreaks of norovirus are often linked to transmission via doorknobs, toilets, and shared utensils, recreational water exposure significantly contributes to the overall case burden. The increasing number of cases reported over the past few years has been attributed to improved awareness and availability of viral detection methods, although diagnostic test underutilization is still likely to result in underreporting of viral agents of gastroenteritis. Visualization of norovirus in stool via electron microscopy is definitive (Figure 118.8). Management is supportive.

SUGGESTED READING

American Public Health Association. *Control of Communicable Diseases Manual*. In: Heymann DL, ed. 18th ed. Washington DC: American Public Health Association; 2004.

Dziuban EJ, Liang JL, Craun GF, et al. Surveillance for waterborne-disease outbreaks associated with recreational water use—United States, 2003–2004. *Morbid Mortal Weekly Rep*. 2006;55 (No. SS-12):1–24.

Henrickson SE, Wong T, Allen P, Ford T, Epstein PR. Marine swimming-related illness: implications for monitoring and environmental policy. *Env Health Perspect*. 2001;109(7):645–650.

Leclerc H, Schwartzbrod L, Dei-Cas E. Microbial agents associated with waterborne diseases. *Crit Rev Microbiol*. 2002;28(4):371–409.

Theron J, Cloete TE. Emerging waterborne infections: contributing factors, agents, and detection tools. *Crit Rev Microbiol*. 2002;28(1):1–26.

Wilson ME. *A World Guide to Infections: Diseases, Distribution, Diagnosis*. New York, NY: Oxford University Press; 1991.

119. Travelers' Diarrhea

Karen J. Vigil and Herbert L. DuPont

Diarrhea is the most frequent health problem encountered by persons going from industrialized to developing countries. From the 50 million people traveling annually, approximately 40% will suffer from so-called travelers' diarrhea (TD) at least once.

Classically, TD is defined as the passage of three or more unformed stools within 24 hours in association with at least one of the following symptoms of enteric infection: nausea, vomiting, abdominal pain or cramps, fever, fecal urgency, tenesmus, or the passage of bloody/mucoid (dysenteric) stools. This definition includes illness occurring up to 10 days after travelers return to their home countries.

Cases of TD can be categorized by severity as being mild (no disturbance in normal activities), moderate (modified travel activities required), or severe (illness requires confinement to bed). Fewer than 1% of patients are admitted to a hospital, but almost 40% are required to change their travel schedule.

Acute TD lasts for less than 2 weeks. Illness lasting more than 2 weeks is considered "persistent" and is seen in 2% to 10% of travelers. Possible etiologies of persistent diarrhea include intestinal infection by protozoal parasites, for example, giardiasis or cryptosporidiosis, and occasionally bacterial enteropathogens can cause a more protracted diarrhea. Unmasked gastrointestinal disease is seen in this setting occasionally, including celiac sprue, inflammatory bowel disease, and malabsorptive syndromes. Postinfectious irritable bowel syndrome has been shown to occur in as many as 10% of people after an episode of TD.

Food is the most important source of bacterial enteropathogens, which explains a majority of cases of TD. Water, which becomes more contaminated during rainy seasons, is often the source of viral gastroenteritis. Genetic factors contribute significantly to susceptibility to enteric infections. Fecal levels of inflammatory cytokines, including interleukin (IL)-8, are elevated in people who developed bacterial diarrhea. Host polymorphisms in the promoter (-251 position) region of the IL-8 gene was shown to be associated with increased rates of diarrhea due to one of the common causes of TD, enteroaggregative *Escherichia coli* (EAEC).

ETIOLOGY

Bacterial enteropathogens cause up to 80% of TD cases. There is some relationship between geographic areas and the enteropathogens responsible for illness. For example, the diarrheagenic *E. coli*, particularly enterotoxigenic *E. coli* (ETEC) and EAEC, are the major etiologic organisms in most areas of the developing world, responsible for ~50% to 60% of cases. Invasive pathogens, such as *Shigella*, *Salmonella*, and *Campylobacter*, represent 10% to 15% of cases but may account for up to 30% of cases in Asia, of which ciprofloxacin-resistant *Campylobacter* is of the greatest concern as it may not respond to customary self-treatment. Noncholera *Vibrios* are found to cause TD in coastal areas of the world in a small number of cases. *Vibrios cholerae*, the causative agent of cholera, is a rare but serious cause of TD.

Other than bacterial pathogens, parasites and viruses also cause TD. *Giardia* is an important pathogen in mountainous areas of North America and Russia. *Cryptosporidium* species is an important cause of diarrhea in travelers to Russia. *Cyclospora cayetanensis* has been found to be a causative organism of TD in Nepal, Haiti, and Peru. Noroviruses cause almost 20% of TD cases and remain a special problem on cruise ships. There is a strong association between norovirus gastroenteritis and a clinical presentation of TD with nausea and vomiting.

The causes of TD in some areas of the world are also affected by the regional climate. ETEC was shown to be the major pathogen in the rainy, summer season in Mexico, with emergence of *Campylobacter jejuni* in the dry wintertime. In semitropical Morocco, *C. jejuni* was also found to be the most important pathogen in the dry winter season.

PREVENTION AND CHEMOPROPHYLAXIS

Disease prevention is important to facilitate the purpose of the leisure or business trip and to prevent chronic enteric complications. Prevention measures consist of education for the future traveler on usually safe and occasionally unsafe foods and chemoprophylaxis.

Travelers should be instructed to avoid consuming moist foods served at room temperature and tap water (including ice). Food served steaming hot (>59°C), dry foods (eg, bread), fruits that can be peeled, and foods with high sugar content (eg, syrup, honey, or jelly) generally are safe.

Chemoprophylaxis may be used for short-term travel (≤3 weeks) in persons on a tight schedule (musicians, athletes, business persons, tourists, and politicians), in those who have experienced TD before (possibly related to genetic susceptibility), and for those who request it. Additional persons who might routinely employ chemoprophylaxis include those with underlying illness that might predispose them to increased risk of diarrhea or complications of illness, including persons with achlorhydria (from prior gastric surgery or regular use of proton pump inhibitors), inflammatory bowel diseases, human immunodeficiency virus (HIV) infection or other immunosuppression (eg, malignancy), insulin-dependent diabetes, or congestive heart failure.

Bismuth subsalicylate (BSS) is modestly effective in the prevention of TD, with protection rates of approximately 65%. The dosage recommended for prophylaxis is 2 tablets (262 mg/tablet) orally with meals and at bedtime (8 tablets/day). Rifaximin was shown to have a protection rate of 72% to 77% in a study in Mexico where diarrheagenic *E. coli* were the major pathogens. The drug was free of side effects when given for 2 weeks and was associated with minimal changes in fecal flora. We recommend rifaximin as the routine approach when chemoprophylaxis is desired because of its convenience and safety. It should not be given for trips longer than 3 weeks. The recommended dose is 200 mg (1 tablet) with each of the major daily meals (usually 2 tablets a day) for as long as the person remains in the high-risk region.

Immunologic protection against ETEC diarrhea is feasible. An oral vaccine consisting of cholera toxin B subunit and inactivated whole-cell cholera strains has become available in some parts of the world. This vaccine protects against ETEC diarrhea and probably cholera. A novel transcutaneous patch ETEC vaccine is also in development. Vaccination for TD with an anti-ETEC preparation can offer important protection from the major cause of the illness but cannot be completely protective because TD is a syndrome caused by multiple organisms.

TREATMENT

Hydration and Dietary Recommendations

Travelers' diarrhea can cause dehydration in infants, the elderly, or persons who have underlying medical illness, such as HIV infection, diabetes, or malnutrition. Fluids combined with electrolytes are the most important form of therapy. In the nondehydrated person without important underlying medical illness, commercially available sports drinks, diluted fruit juices, and other flavored soft drinks taken with saltine crackers and/or soups are usually enough to meet the fluid and salt needs during TD. Oral rehydration powders or solutions are also commercially available (eg, CeraLyte).

During the early hours of diarrheal illness, it may be helpful to temporarily withhold solid foods that are complicated to absorb and that act as a stimulant of intestinal motility. In most cases of diarrhea, carbohydrates (noodles, rice, potatoes, oat, wheat, banana) and steamed or baked white meats (fish and chicken) can be ingested. As illness improves and stools become formed, the diet can return to normal. In general, dairy products should be avoided in adults for the first day or two. It is important to feed patients with diarrhea to facilitate enterocyte renewal.

Nonantimicrobial Therapy

Symptomatic therapy can be used in cases of mild TD. Bismuth subsalicylate (BSS) is a commonly used antidiarrheal drug. This agent has antimicrobial, antisecretory, and anti-inflammatory properties. BSS can decrease the number of unformed stools passed in cases of TD by approximately 40%. BSS rarely causes mild tinnitus, and it commonly produces blackening of the tongue and stools from bismuth sulfide, a harmless salt of the nonabsorbed bismuth moiety. If a person is taking antimalarials for malaria prophylaxis, BSS should not be used concomitantly, because it can prevent absorption of the antimalarial drug.

Antimotility agents such as loperamide (Imodium) and diphenoxylate with atropine (Lomotil) are synthetic opioids that have selective effects on the intestine. These agents can improve diarrhea by slowing intestinal transit, leading to greater absorption of fluids and electrolytes. Loperamide is a drug of choice for symptomatic treatment of subjects

Table 119.1 Recommended Empiric Treatment of Travelers' Diarrhea in Adults

Agent	Dosages	Comments
Loperamide	4 mg initially, then 2 mg after each stool, not to exceed 8 mg/d[a]	Should not be used in patients with fever and dysentery
Bismuth subsalicyte	30 mL or 2 tablets (262 mg/tablet) PO q 30 min up to 8 doses/d[a]	Should not be used with doxycycline when used for malaria prophylaxis
Ciprofloxacin	500 mg PO BID or 750mg PO qd for 1-3 d	Treatment failures most common because of resistant strains of *Campylobacter*
Rifaximin	200 mg PO TID for 3 d	Not recommended for febrile dysenteric diarrhea
Azithromycin	1000 mg single dose or 500 mg PO 1× and then 250 mg qd for 1 or 2 more d	Treatment of choice for febrile dysentery when *Campylobacter* is known to be the causative agent

[a] To be used for no more than 48 h.

without fever and not passing bloody stools. This agent will reduce the number of stools passed during a diarrhea episode by approximately 60%.

Antisecretory agents are being developed that work through a variety of pathways including calmodulin inhibition, chloride channel inhibition, and enkephalinase inhibition.

Antimicrobial Therapy

Antimicrobial therapy in patients with TD shortens the duration of diarrhea and cures the disease. Clinical trials use time from initiation of therapy to passage of the last unformed stool (TLUS) as a primary parameter of efficacy. Antibiotic therapy is indicated in patients with moderate to severe disease because it has been shown to reduce TLUS by 1 to 3 days compared with placebo.

A variety of effective treatments for TD are available (Table 119.1). Rifaximin, 200 mg three times a day (TID) for 3 days, has a TLUS of 25.7 hours and a treatment failure of 10%, similar to ciprofloxacin, 500 mg twice a day (BID) for 3 days (25 hours and 6%, respectively), for treatment of noninvasive forms of the disease. Poorly absorbed (≤0.4%) rifaximin has an advantage for uncomplicated watery diarrhea in its safety profile. Rifaximin is not effective in the treatment of invasive forms of TD, particularly those associated with fever or dysentery.

For febrile dysenteric diarrhea, a systemic antibiotic, including the fluoroquinolones (ciprofloxacin, levofloxacin) or azithromycin, is preferred. Fluoroquinolones should not be used in children and pregnant women because they have been shown to damage articular cartilage in growing animals. These agents may interfere with xanthine metabolism, so patients taking theophylline may need to adjust their dosage of the drug. Fluoroquinolone resistance has become a problem with *Campylobacter* strains seen worldwide, which is a limitation of ciprofloxacin or levofloxacin.

Azithromycin is an azalide antibiotic related to macrolides and is more active than erythromycin against ETEC, *Salmonella* species, *Shigella* species, *Vibrio cholerae,* and *C. jejuni*. In a clinical trial in Thailand, where *Campylobacter* has become resistant to ciprofloxacin, azithromycin was more effective than ciprofloxacin against *Campylobacter*. Azithromycin is effective against most forms of bacterial diarrhea and can be given as a single 1000-mg dose or daily in a lower dose for 3 days (see Table 119.1). Azithromycin may be the drug of choice for some regions of Asia where invasive pathogens are most common and is also the drug of choice for rescue therapy when rifaximin chemoprophylaxis is employed.

Travelers to high-risk areas should be encouraged to take with them an antibiotic for self-treatment of diarrhea that develops. It takes approximately 24 hours for a drug to cure the diarrhea. The antibiotic can be started after passage of the third unformed stool, to avoid unnecessary exposure to antibiotics for milder self-limiting syndromes. Some travel medicine experts prefer to begin the treatment with passage of the first unformed stool in a diarrheal episode to help reduce the duration of illness.

Combination Therapy

Perhaps the optimal approach for empiric treatment of nondysenteric travelers' diarrhea is to give the combination of loperamide with an antibiotic to combine a near-immediate effect of the loperamide with a curative effect of the antibiotic. This approach is not appropriate for patients with febrile, dysenteric diarrhea where a systemically absorbed antimicrobial agent alone should be used.

SUGGESTED READING

Adachi JA, Ericsson CD, Jiang ZD, et al. Azithromycin found to be comparable to levofloxacin for the treatment of US travelers with acute diarrhea acquired in Mexico. *Clin Infect Dis*. 2003;37(9):1165–1171.

Adachi JA, Jiang ZD, Mathewson JJ, et al. Enteroaggregative Escherichia coli as a major etiologic agent in traveler's diarrhea in 3 regions of the world. *Clin Infect Dis*. 2001;32(12):1706–1709.

DuPont HL. Azithromycin for the self-treatment of traveler's diarrhea. *Clin Infect Dis*. 2007;44(3):347–349.

DuPont HL, Ericsson CD. Prevention and treatment of traveler's diarrhea. *N Engl J Med*. 1993;328(25):1821–1827.

DuPont HL, Jiang ZD, Belkind-Gerson J, et al. Treatment of Traveler's diarrhea: randomized trial comparing rifaximin, rifaximin plus loperamide, and loperamide alone. *Clin Gastroenterol Hepatol*. 2007;5(4):451–456.

DuPont HL, Jiang ZD, Okhuysen PC, et al. A randomized, double-blind, placebo-controlled trial of rifaximin to prevent travelers' diarrhea. *Ann Intern Med*. 2005;142(10):805–812.

Ericsson CD, DuPont HL, Mathewson JJ. Optimal dosing of ofloxacin with loperamide in the treatment of non-dysenteric travelers' diarrhea. *J Travel Med*. 2001;8(4):207–209.

Gorbach SL. How to hit the runs for fifty million travelers at risk. *Ann Intern Med*. 2005;142(10):861–862.

Ko G, Garcia C, Jiang ZD, et al. Noroviruses as a cause of traveler's diarrhea among students from the United States visiting Mexico. *J Clin Microbiol*. 2005;43 (12):6126–6129.

Kuschner RA, Trofa AF, Thomas RJ, et al. Use of azithromycin for the treatment of Campylobacter enteritis in travelers to Thailand, an area where ciprofloxacin resistance is prevalent. *Clin Infect Dis*. 1995;21(3):536–541.

Okhuysen PC, Jiang ZD, Carlin L, Forbes C, DuPont HL. Post-diarrhea chronic intestinal symptoms and irritable bowel syndrome in North American travelers to Mexico. *Am J Gastroenterol*. 2004;99(9):1774–1778.

Steffen R. Epidemiologic studies of travelers' diarrhea, severe gastrointestinal infections, and cholera. *Rev Infect Dis*. 1986;8(Suppl 2): S122–S130.

Tribble DR, Sanders JW, Pang LW, et al. Traveler's diarrhea in Thailand: randomized, double-blind trial comparing single-dose and 3-day azithromycin-based regimens with a 3-day levofloxacin regimen. *Clin Infect Dis*. 2007;44(3)338–346.

PART XVII

Bioterrorism

120. Bioterrorism

Eleni Patrozou and Andrew W. Artenstein

INTRODUCTION

Bioterrorism (BT), the deliberate use of microbial agents or their toxins as weapons for political gain, continues to represent a persistent global threat due to the apparent availability of these substances and the potential willingness of terrorists to deploy them against civilian targets. An actual calculation of "risk" as it relates to BT is not possible; whereas the negative consequences associated with exposure to biological agents may be quite high, the probability of exposure to these hazards is truly unknown — it remains in the unpredictable and malicious minds of terrorists. Because of the potential for catastrophic sequelae, it is important for clinicians to understand the diagnostic and therapeutic approach to illnesses caused by agents of BT to mitigate the effects of an attack.

Bioterrorism agents are considered weapons of mass terror because of their potential for large-scale morbidity and mortality; one early model postulated nearly 200 000 casualties from a release of 50 kg of aerosolized anthrax spores upwind of a population center of 500 000. Yet they possess unique properties among such weapons because, unlike conventional, chemical, and nuclear weapons, BT agents have a clinical latency period during which transmission may occur and detection is difficult. The Centers for Disease Control and Prevention (CDC) has classified BT threats into priority groupings, based on their feasibility for deployment and their potential for mortality and public health impact; this categorization (Table 120.1) has informed current biodefense strategies.

CLINICAL PRESENTATION

The clinical pictures of diseases caused by agents of bioterrorism are varied but, with few exceptions among the CDC category A and B threats, can be categorized into a limited number of syndromic presentations (Table 120.2). Unfortunately, there are suggestive but essentially no pathognomonic features of BT-related illness. For this reason a high index of suspicion

among clinicians is necessary to capitalize on subtle clues, many of which may be epidemiologic in nature. Nonetheless, many of these agents demonstrate suggestive clinical and laboratory findings (Table 120.2) that in the appropriate clinical context should prompt further, targeted evaluations and warrant appropriate management. More detailed clinical information on each agent is covered in organism-specific chapters of this book.

DIAGNOSIS

Rapid detection and accurate identification of BT agents are important not only for confirming that a BT event has occurred but also for treating individual patients and implementing appropriate public health measures. By definition BT is insidious; in the absence of credible advance warning, it is likely that clinical illness will be the initial manifestation of a BT attack. Early recognition, although critical, is problematic for a variety of reasons: (1) targets of BT, especially in a free society, are diverse and unpredictable; (2) the clinical latency of BT agents, discussed above, makes it likely that clusters of symptomatic individuals will present for medical care days to weeks after an "event" and at geographically diverse locations; (3) initial clinical manifestations of many BT-related illnesses are nondiagnostic and may be mistaken for other, more common diagnoses; (4) clinicians are inexperienced with the clinical manifestations of these infections; and (5) even if the classic clinical findings are known, because BT agents are manipulated in the laboratory, they may not present in the same manner as naturally occurring infection. Conversely, in the setting of a high level of suspicion, early recognition may be aided by a number of epidemiological and clinical clues: case clustering, which because of the clinical latency of BT requires attention to surveillance and communications; unusual clinical presentations; or unusual disease patterns, such as rare diseases occurring in nonendemic areas or concurrent disease in humans and animal populations.

Table 120.1 Agents of Concern for Use in Bioterrorism

HIGHEST PRIORITY—CATEGORY A
Based Upon Potential Mortality, Morbidity, Virulence, Transmissibility, Aerosol Feasibility, and Psychosocial Implications of an Attack

Microbe/Toxin	Disease
Bacillus anthracis	Anthrax – Inhalational, cutaneous
Variola virus	Smallpox and its variants
Yersinia pestis	Plague – Pneumonic, bubonic, septicemic
Clostridium botulinum	Botulism
Francisella tularensis	Tularemia – Pneumonic, typhoidal
Viral hemorrhagic fevers	
Filoviruses	Ebola, Marburg
Arenaviruses	Lassa fever, South American hemorrhagic fevers
Bunyaviruses	Rift Valley fever, Congo–Crimean hemorrhagic fever

MODERATELY HIGH PRIORITY – CATEGORY B
Based Upon Potential Morbidity, Aerosol Feasibility, Dissemination Characteristics, and Diagnostic Difficulty

Microbe/Toxin	Disease
Coxiella burnetti	Q fever
Brucella species	Brucellosis
Burkholderia mallei	Glanders
Alphaviruses	Viral encephalitides
Ricin	Ricin intoxication
Staphylococcus enterotoxin B	Staphylococcal toxin illness
Salmonella species, *Shigella dysenteriae*, *E.coli* 0157;H7, *Vibrio cholerae*, *C. parvum*	Food- and waterborne gastroenteritis

EMERGING THREAT AGENTS – CATEGORY C
Based Upon Potential for Production and Dissemination, Availability, Morbidity/Mortality

Microbe/Toxin	Disease
Hantaviruses	Viral hemorrhagic fevers
Flaviviruses	Yellow fever
Mycobacterium tuberculosis	Multidrug-resistant tuberculosis

MISCELLANEOUS
Other Examples of Candidate Threat Agents That Possess Some Elements of Bioterrorism Concern

Genetically engineered vaccine- and/or antimicrobial-resistant Category A or B agents
Human immunodeficiency virus 1
Adenoviruses
Influenza
Rotaviruses
Hybrid pathogens – e. g., smallpox/plague, smallpox/ebola

The CDC has developed a national laboratory response network (LRN) for BT that integrates selected microbiological laboratories across the United States into a network and mandates uniform practices for specimen collection, processing, shipping, security, and testing. Laboratories within the LRN consortium are designated as having screening, confirmatory, or reference functions. The network of laboratories is connected by a secure communications system, thus ensuring the timely flow of information among the CDC, other governmental agencies, state health authorities, and other laboratories. The mission of the LRN is to enable a rapid and organized response to BT; the CDC routinely audits the performance of network members using panels of unknown pathogens.

Although diagnostic tests are available for most BT agents, many are not readily available in clinical laboratories, are time-consuming, have less than optimal sensitivity and specificity, or cannot test for multiple agents simultaneously. Diagnostic platforms that can assess for the presence of multiple pathogens concurrently, so-called multiplex strategies, offer attractive advantages, especially in the arenas of environmental surveillance and in screening either patients presenting with nonspecific symptoms or asymptomatic individuals who have possible exposure to an unknown agent.

The preferred methods for the laboratory diagnosis of BT agents differ depending on the agent in question. For most bacterial agents the gold standard diagnostic assay remains standard culture; other supporting assays include modified staining with light microscopy, motility testing, lysis by gamma phage, capsule production staining, hemolysis, wet mounts, staining for spores, slide agglutination, direct fluorescent antibody, enzyme-linked immunosorbent assay (ELISA), and rapid immunochromatography. Routine assays for viral agents include virus isolation through tissue culture or growth in eggs, direct and indirect immunofluorescence, immunodiffusion in agar, electron microscopy, modified staining and light microscopy, plaque reduction neutralization, hemagglutination inhibition, neuraminidase activity, complement fixation, and ELISA. Pathologic examination of tissues and immunohistochemistry also play an important role in diagnosing BT agents.

Molecular assays are becoming the new gold standard for BT detection, with sensitivities and specificities close to 100% when compared with culture or serologic assays. These assays detect infectious agents in humans through target nucleic acid isolation and amplification followed by specific pathogen identification. Several technologies and methods have been used for multiplex detection of different BT agents. Although still in the developmental stages, it is likely that DNA microfluidic devices will be commonly used diagnostic platforms in the future. These methods are sensitive and specific and theoretically can be used on unprocessed specimens in field settings, thus obviating laborious microbial isolation steps. However, several challenges, including sampling issues, data analysis, development of specific probes, quality control, cost containment, automation, performance, and integration, must be addressed before such methods replace the standard ones.

Laboratory Diagnosis of Specific Category A Agents

BACILLUS ANTHRACIS

Presumptive laboratory identification of *Bacillus anthracis* is based on the presence of large gram-positive bacilli in either gram- or immunohistochemical-stained material from

Table 120.2 Syndromic Differential Diagnoses and Clinical Clues for Category A Agents of Bioterrorism (BT)

Syndrome	Clinical Presentation	Differential Diagnosis	BT-Associated Disease	Disease-Specific Clues
Influenzalike illness	Nonspecific constitutional and upper respiratory symptoms: malaise, myalgias, nausea, emesis, dyspnea, cough +/− chest discomfort, without coryza or rhinorrhea → abrupt onset of respiratory distress +/− shock +/− mental status changes, with CXR abnormalities (wide mediastinum or infiltrates or pleural effusions)	Influenza, community-acquired bacterial pneumonia, viral pneumonia, Legionella, Q fever, psittacosis, mycoplasma, Pneumocystis pneumonia, tularemia, dissecting aortic aneurysm, bacterial mediastinitis, SVC syndrome, histoplasmosis, coccidioidomycosis, sarcoidosis, ricin and Staphylococcus enterotoxin B (pulmonary edema/ARDS)	Inhalational anthrax	• 3-day average symptom duration before presentation • Abdominal pain, headache, mental status abnormalities, hypoxemia common • Mediastinal adenopathy: ~90% (Fig. 120.1a) • Hemorrhagic pleural effusions: ~70% • CT more sensitive than CXR in early hemorrhagic mediastinal adenopathy • Meningoencephalitis: possibly ~50% • Blood cultures positive in untreated; pleural fluid cultures or antigen-specific immunohistochemical stain usually positive
Skin lesions(s)	Pruritic, painless papule on exposed areas→vesicle(s)→ ulcer→edematous black eschar +/− massive local edema and regional adenopathy, +/− fever, evolving over 3–7 days	Recluse spider bite, staphylococcal lesion, atypical Lyme disease, Orf, glanders, tularemia, plague, rat-bite fever, ecthyma gangrenosum, rickettsialpox, atypical mycobacteria, cutaneous diphtheria, cutaneous leishmaniasis	Cutaneous anthrax	• Painless; spider bite is painful lesion • Nonpitting local edema may be massive (Fig. 120.1b) • If untreated, may progress to systemic involvement • Blood cultures, skin biopsy (from vesicular edge or erythema at edge of eschar)
Fulminant pneumonia	Abrupt-onset constitutional symptoms and rapidly progressive respiratory illness with cough, fever, rigors, headache, sore throat, myalgias, dyspnea, pleuritic chest pain, GI symptoms, lung consolidation, +/−hemoptysis, +/−shock; variable progression to respiratory failure	Severe community-acquired bacterial or viral pneumonia, inhalational anthrax, pulmonary infarct, pulmonary hemorrhage, influenza, mycoplasma pneumonia, Legionella, Q fever, SARS, tuberculosis	• Pneumonic plague • Pulmonary tularemia	• Lobar or multilobar involvement +/− buboes • Hemoptysis common • Characteristic sputum Gram stain • Cough generally nonproductive • Pulse–temperature dissociation in 40% • Hilar adenopathy, pleural effusions • Ulceroglandular form most common after natural or cutaneous exposures • Erythema multiforme or nodosum in significant minority of systemic disease
Sepsis with bleeding diathesis and capillary leak	Sepsis syndrome, GI symptoms, mucosal hemorrhage, altered vascular permeability, DIC, purpura, acral gangrene, hepatitis, hypotension, +/− CNS findings, multiorgan system failure	Meningococcemia; gram-negative sepsis, streptococcal, pneumococcal, or staphylococcal bacteremia with shock; malaria, leptospirosis, typhoid fever, borrelioses, typhoidal tularemia; overwhelming postsplenectomy sepsis; acute leukemia; Rocky Mountain spotted fever; fulminant hepatitis, TTP, hemolytic uremic syndrome, SLE , hemorrhagic smallpox; hemorrhagic varicella (in immunocompromised)	• Septicemic plague • Viral hemorrhagic fever	• Occurs in minority of aerosol exposures • Cutaneous findings as late sequelae +/−buboes • High-density bacteremia • Maculopapular rash in Ebola, Marburg • Certain organ systems preferentially involved with specific VHF etiologies

Syndrome	Clinical Presentation	Differential Diagnosis	BT-Associated Disease	Disease-Specific Clues
Febrile prodrome with generalized exanthem	Fever, malaise, prostration, headache, myalgias and enanthema followed by development of synchronous, progressive, centrifugal papular→ vesicular→pustular rash on face, mucous membranes, extremities>>trunk→generalization +/– hemorrhagic component, with systemic toxicity	Varicella, drug eruption, Stevens–Johnson syndrome, measles, secondary syphilis, erythema multiforme, severe acne, disseminated herpes zoster or simplex, meningococcemia, monkeypox, generalized vaccinia related to smallpox vaccination, insect bites, Coxsackievirus, vaccine reaction	Smallpox	• Palms and soles involved • Rash is denser peripherally even after fully evolved (Figs. 120.2, 120.3) • Lesions are well circumscribed, firm, and almost nodular (Fig. 120.4) • Secondary bacterial infection common • Hemorrhagic variant in pregnant and immunocompromised patients associated with severe systemic toxicity, bleeding diathesis, and early mortality
Progressive weakness	Acute onset of afebrile, symmetric, descending flaccid paralysis that begins in bulbar muscles, dilated pupils, diplopia or blurred vision, dysphagia, dysarthria, ptosis, dry mucous membranes→airway obstruction + respiratory muscle paralysis, clear sensorium and absence of sensory changes	Myasthenia gravis, brain stem CVA, polio, Guillain–Barré syndrome variant, tick paralysis, chemical intoxication	Botulism	• Expect dearth of GI symptoms in aerosol attack as opposed to foodborne botulism • Low-dose inhalation exposure may delay symptom onset • Prominent anticholinergic effects

Abbreviations: CXR = chest x-ray; SVC = ; ARDS = acute respiratory disease syndrome; CT = computed tomography; GI = gastrointestinal; SARS = severe acute respiratory syndrome; DIC = disseminated intravascular coagulation; CNS = central nervous system; TTP = ribothymidine 5-triphosphate; SLE = systemic lupus erythematosus; VHF = viral hemorrhagic fever; CVA = cerebrovascular accident.

skin lesions, cerebrospinal fluid, pleural fluid, or blood in an appropriate clinical setting or on the growth of aerobic, nonhemolytic, large, catalase positive, gray-white colonies on sheep-blood-agar cultures containing nonmotile, nonencapsulated, gram-positive, spore-forming rods. Although the diagnosis may be suspected at the screening laboratory level, confirmatory diagnostic tests must be performed in containment facilities of the LRN. Such tests include susceptibility to lysis by gamma phage and polymerase chain reaction (PCR). Although there are no assays that have been rigorously and prospectively validated for the rapid diagnosis of inhalational anthrax during its early, nonspecific clinical stages, the development of assays that detect cell-wall and capsular antibodies and antiprotective antigen responses should improve the outlook for early diagnosis of anthrax.

Serologic testing is of little value in the diagnosis of acute disease but may have some use in undiagnosed survivors who demonstrate seroconversion. The use of nasal cultures for detecting B. anthracis early after potential exposure may be of some use in defining the epidemiological parameters of exposure but are not useful in making individual decisions about the use of treatment or prophylaxis.

YERSINIA PESTIS

The gold standard for Y. pestis diagnosis remains standard microbiologic techniques such as microscopy of stained specimens and culture applied to expectorated sputum, bronchial washings, blood, or lymph node aspirates. The organism is suggested by its characteristic appearance as small gram-negative coccobacillary forms with bipolar, "safety-pin," uptake of Wright–Giemsa stain. Yersinia pestis grows slowly at routine incubation temperatures and may be misidentified by automated identification systems. Confirmation of the diagnosis requires the deployment of specialized testing: direct fluorescent antibody tests to detect the presence of F1 envelope antigen or PCR. Rapid tests to detect the F1 antigen are under investigation for potential field applicability on direct clinical specimens.

FRANCISELLA TULARENSIS

Francisella tularensis appear as small, intra- and extracellular gram-negative coccobacilli in stains of clinical specimens. Because the organism does not grow readily in standard laboratory media and because it is highly infectious to laboratory personnel, specialized microbiologic and safety procedures must be instituted for this pathogen. For this reason, the diagnosis is usually based on clinical features, and cultures should be pursued in higher-level laboratories of the LRN. Serology is generally useful only in retrospect, as it takes longer than 2 weeks to develop a serologic response in most individuals. Although rapid diagnostics for tularemia are not commercially available, several PCR-based platforms, immunochromatography, and ELISAs for rapid testing in field settings are in development.

CLOSTRIDIUM BOTULINUM

The diagnosis of botulism is largely based on epidemiological and clinical features and

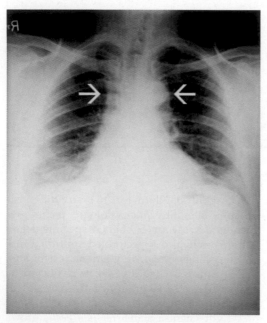

Figure 120.1a Inhalational anthrax. Note widened mediastinum (arrows). (Courtesy of Centers for Disease Control and Prevention.)

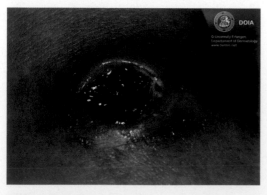

Figure 120.1b Cutaneous anthrax. (Courtesy of University of Heidelberg.)

the exclusion of other possible differential diagnoses. If laboratory diagnosis is necessary, the gold standard currently remains a mouse bioassay at a reference laboratory; PCR may have some utility in detecting *C. botulinum* nucleic acids in environmental samples.

SMALLPOX

The majority of smallpox cases present with a vesicular, centrifugal rash (Figures 120.2, 120.3, and 120.4) that in the appropriate clinical and epidemiological context should prompt immediate notification of state or local public health authorities; specimens from suspected smallpox patients must be collected and transported under the direction of health authorities and in collaboration with the facilities of the LRN. Laboratory confirmation of the clinical diagnosis, especially in early or atypical cases in a suspected outbreak, is important; clinical diagnosis is probably sufficient in a confirmed outbreak. Infection control measures should be implemented prior to the acquisition of specimens in suspected cases.

Diagnostic assays in smallpox are typically performed on lesion scrapings, vesicular fluid, crusts, blood, or tonsilar swabs. A presumptive poxvirus diagnosis may be obtained by observing brick-shaped virions on electron microscopy of vesicular scrapings or by noting aggregations of virus particles, Guarnieri bodies, on histopathologic examination of tissue specimens. Isolation of variola virus in live cell cultures, followed by nucleic acid identification of specific orthopoxvirus species, is confirmatory but only performed in national reference laboratories with the highest level of biocontainment. The development of standard and multiplexed PCR platforms promises a reliable and less cumbersome way to discriminate between variola and other orthopoxviruses in clinical specimens.

VIRAL HEMORRHAGIC FEVERS

Clinical microbiology and public health laboratories are not currently equipped to make a rapid diagnosis of any of the implicated viruses, and clinical specimens would need to be sent to the CDC or the U.S. Army Medical Research Institute of Infectious Diseases (USAMRIID), the highest-level laboratories in the LRN. Definitive diagnosis depends on identification of a specific viral etiology. Methods of early diagnosis at specialized laboratories include rapid enzyme immunoassays for antigen detection or viral immunoglobulin M (IgM), reverse transcriptase-PCR, and viral isolation in a biosafety level-4 facility. In general, serology is of limited

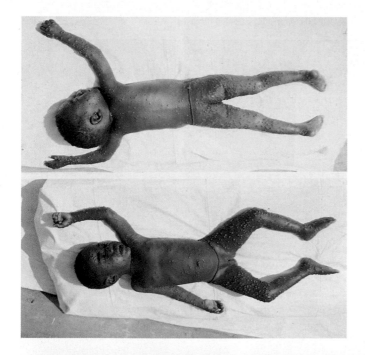

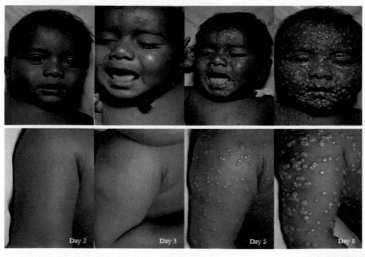

Figure 120.2 Smallpox. Note heavy concentration of lesions on face and extremities compared to trunk. Compare also to the truncal concentration seen in varicella. (Courtesy of World Health Organization.)

Figure 120.3 Progression of smallpox exanthem over the first eight days of illness. (Courtesy of World Health Organization.)

value in early diagnosis because antibodies to these viruses usually do not appear until after the second week of illness.

MANAGEMENT

Once the diagnosis of bioterrorism-associated illness is considered, the initial step in the evaluation and management of an individual or group of patients is the immediate implementation of appropriate infection control measures according to the suspected agents (Table 120.3). This will ensure the maximal protection of health care workers as well as other patients in the environment. Empiric

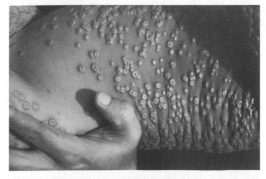

Figure 120.4 Smallpox. Lesions are characteristically round, uniform in size, and at same stage of development. (Courtesy of Centers for Disease Control and Prevention.)

Table 120.3 Epidemiological Characteristics for Selected Bioterrorism-Associated Diseases

Disease	Incubation Period Range (days)	Person-to-Person Transmission	Infection Control Precautions for Patients	Case-Fatality Rate
Inhalational anthrax	2–43*	No	Standard	Untreated – 100% Treated – 45%
Cutaneous anthrax	1–12	No	Standard	Untreated – 20% Treated – <1%
Botulism	12–72 hours	No	Standard	6%
Primary pneumonic plague	1–6	Yes	Droplet	Untreated – 100% Treated – ~50%
Bubonic plague	2–8	No	Standard	Untreated – 60% Treated – <5%
Smallpox	7–19	Yes	Contact + Airborne	Unvaccinated – 30% Vaccinated – 3%
Tularemia pneumonia	1–21	No	Standard	Untreated – 60% Treated – <4%
Viral hemorrhagic fevers	2–21	Yes	Contact + Airborne	Marburg – 25% Ebola – 80% Other forms – 2–30%
Viral encephalitides	1–14	No	Standard	10 – 35%
Q fever	2–41	No	Standard	3%
Brucellosis	5–60	No	Standard	Untreated – 5%
Glanders	1–21	Yes	Contact + Droplet	Untreated – Approaches 100% Treated – Low

* Based on limited data from human outbreaks; experimental animal data support clinical latency periods of up to 100 days.

antimicrobial therapy of BT-associated illness should be initiated once the diagnosis is seriously considered, as the early institution of appropriate therapy will not only potentially confer outcome advantages but will also favorably affect the spread of transmissible pathogens. The use of prophylactic antimicrobials is warranted for some agents. Recommendations for specific antimicrobial strategies for diseases caused by category A agents of BT are provided in Table 120.4.

Anthrax

Given the rapid clinical progression and attendant high mortality of inhalational anthrax, the early administration of appropriate antimicrobials is essential and is likely to confer a survival advantage, as patients appear to quickly reach a clinical threshold beyond which survival is unlikely. There have been no controlled clinical studies for the treatment of inhalational anthrax in humans because of its rare and sporadic occurrence in nature. During the anthrax attacks in the United States in 2001, the CDC promulgated treatment protocols recommending combination antimicrobials for the initial management of suspected inhalational anthrax using either intravenous ciprofloxacin or doxycycline as essential components and a variety of options to complete the regimen (Table 120.4). Reasons to empirically treat with multiple drugs include heightened concerns regarding the deployment of antimicrobial-resistant pathogens by terrorists, the potential for meningeal involvement in victims of inhalational anthrax, and the need to employ an antimicrobial that will achieve adequate drug levels in the central nervous system and the potential for additive or synergistic effects using multiple therapies with different targets.

Once the antimicrobial susceptibility profile of the organism has been determined and clinical improvement is evident, therapy may

Table 120.4 Treatment Recommendations for Bioterrorism Category A Agents

ANTHRAX-INHALATIONAL

	Adults	Children
Treatment	• Initial IV therapy: Ciprofloxacin 400mg every 12h **or** doxycycline 100mg every 12h **and** 1 or 2 additional antimicrobials (rifampin, vancomycin, penicillin, ampicillin, chloramphenicol, imipenem, clindamycin, and clarithromycin) • If meningitis is suspected, choose agents with optimal CNS penetration	• Initial IV therapy: Ciprofloxacin 10–15mg/kg every 12h **or** doxycycline for those: >8y and weight >45Kg, 100mg every 12h; >8y and weight ≤45kg, 2.2mg/kg every 12h; ≤8y, 2.2 mg/kg every 12h **and** 1 or 2 additional antimicrobials as above
Postexposure Prophylaxis	• Ciprofloxacin 500mg orally every 12h **or** doxycyxline 100mg orally every 12h **plus** anthrax vaccine (unlicensed indication) • Amoxicillin 500mg orally every 8h for pregnant women	• Ciprofloxacin 20–30 mg/kg per day orally taken in 2 daily doses, not to exceed 1g/dl **or** if weight ≥20kg, amoxicillin 500mg orally every 8h **and** if weight <20kg, amoxicillin 40mg/kg taken orally in 3 doses every 8h
Comments	• IV treatment initially before switching to oral antimicrobial therapy when clinically appropriate • Continue oral and IV treatment to complete total of 60–100 days • Treatment for immunocompromised individuals and pregnant women as above; recommendation based on life-threatening nature of illness • Levofloxacin may be used as an alternative flouroquinolone for postexposure prophylaxis	• IV treatment initially before switching to oral antimicrobial therapy when clinically appropriate • Continue IV and oral treatment for 60–100 days

ANTHRAX - CUTANEOUS

	Adults	Children
Treatment	• Oral therapy: Ciprofloxacin 500mg, twice daily **or** doxycycline 100mg twice daily	• Oral therapy: Ciprofloxacin 10–15mg/kg every 12h (not to exceed 1g/d) **or** doxycycline for those: >8y and weight >45kg, 100mg every 12h; >8y and weight ≤45kg, 2.2mg/kg every 12h; ≤8y, 2.2 mg/kg every 12h
Postexposure Prophylaxis	• Prophylaxis for possible exposure to weaponized forms of anthrax should be as noted for inhalational anthrax above	
Comments	• Duration: 60 days	

BOTULISM

	Adults	Children
Treatment	• Early administration of antitoxin • Supportive treatment (hydration, nasogastric suctioning for ileus, mechanical ventilation for respiratory failure)	
Postexposure Prophylaxis	• Antitoxin administration	

(continued)

Table 120.4 *(continued)*

PLAGUE

	Adults	Children
Treatment	• Preferred: Streptomycin 1g intra-muscular twice daily *or* gentamicin 5mg/kg intra-muscular or IV once daily or 2mg/kg loading dose followed by 1.7mg/ kg intra-muscular or IV 3 times daily • Alternative: Doxycycline100mg IV twice daily *or* ciprofloxacin 400mg IV twice daily *or* chloramphenicol 25mg/kg IV 4 times daily	• Preferred: Streptomycin 15mg/kg intra-muscular twice daily (maximum daily dose 2g) *or* gentamicin 2.5mg/kg intra-muscular or IV 3 times daily • Alternative: Doxycycline for those: Weight ≥45kg, give adult dosage; weight <45kg, give 2.2 mg/kg IV twice daily (maximum 200mg/d) *or* ciprofloxacin 15mg/kg IV twice daily (should not exceed 1g/d) *or* chloramphenicol 25mg/kg IV 4 times daily
Postexposure Prophylaxis	• Preferred: Doxycycline 100mg orally twice daily *or* ciprofloxacin 500mg orally twice daily • Alternative: Chloramphenicol 25mg/kg orally 4 times daily	• Preferred: Doxycycline for those: Weight ≥45kg, give adult dosage; weight <45kg, give 2.2mg/kg orally twice daily *or* ciprofloxacin 20mg/kg orally twice daily • Alternative: Chloramphenicol 25mg/kg orally 4 times daily
Comments	• 10 days for treatment regimens • 7 days for postexposure prophylaxis	

SMALLPOX

	Adults	Children
Treatment	• There is no treatment approved by the Food and Drug Administration for orthopoxviruses, although there are multiple promising agents in animal studies • Treatment is supportive • Antimicrobial agents effective against *Staphylococcus aureus* and streptococci should be used if smallpox lesions are secondarily infected, if bacterial infection endangers the eyes, or if the eruption is very dense and widespread • Adequate hydration and nutrition for substantial fluid and protein losses • Topical idoxuridine should be considered for the treatment of corneal lesions, although its efficacy is unproved for smallpox	
Postexposure Prophylaxis	• Vaccination within 7 days of exposure unless contraindicated	

TULAREMIA

	Adults	Children
Treatment	• Preferred: Streptomycin 1g intra-muscular twice daily *or* gentamicin 5mg/kg intra-muscular or IV once daily • Alternative: Doxycycline100 mg IV twice daily *or* ciprofloxacin 400mg IV twice daily *or* chloramphenicol 15mg/kg IV 4 times daily (not to be used in pregnancy)	• Preferred: Streptomycin 15mg/kg intra-muscular twice daily (should not exceed 2g/ d) *or* gentamicin 2.5mg/kg intra-musuclar or IV 3 times daily • Alternative: Doxycycline for those: Weight ≥45kg, give 100mg IV twice daily; weight <45 kg, give 2.2 mg/kg IV twice daily *or* ciprofloxacin 15 mg/kg IV twice daily (should not exceed 1g/d) *or* chloramphenicol 15mg/kg IV 4 times daily
Postexposure Prophylaxis	• Doxycycline 100mg orally twice daily *or* ciprofloxacin 500mg orally twice daily	• Doxycycline for those: Weight ≥45kg, 100mg orally twice daily; weight <45kg, 2.2 mg/kg orally twice daily *or* ciprofloxacin 15mg/kg orally twice daily (should not exceed1g/d in children)
Comments	• Treatment: 10 days for streptomycin, gentamicin, and ciprofloxacin; 14–21 days for doxycycline or chloramphenicol • Postexposure prophylaxis: 14 days	

	Adults		Children	
Treatment	• Intensive supportive care • Ribavirin • For confirmed or suspected Bunyaviridae (Old World Hantavirus, Crimean–Congo hemorrhagic fever, Rift Valley fever) and Arenaviridae (Lassa virus) infections under an Investigational New Drug (IND) protocol • Not useful for Ebola or Marburg viral hemorrhagic fevers			

	Adults		Children	
Ribavirin	**Loading Dose**	**Maintenance Dose**	**Loading Dose**	**Maintenance Dose**
Intravenous	• 30mg/kg IV (maximum 2g) once	• 16 mg/kg IV (maximum 1g per dose) q 6h for 4 days followed by 8mg/kg IV (maximum 500 mg per dose) every 8h for 6 days	• Same as for adults (weight based)	
Oral	• 2,000mg orally once	• Weight >75kg: 600mg orally bid for 10 days • Weight ≤75kg: 400mg orally in a.m., 600mg orally in p.m. for 10 days	• 30mg/kg orally once	• 7.5mg/kg orally twice daily for 10 days

	• Convalescent plasma in Argentinian and Bolivian hemorrhagic fevers
Postexposure Prophylaxis	• Prophylactic ribavirin for Bunyaviridae and Arenaviridae infections, under IND status, may be useful

be tailored. Isolated cutaneous disease may be managed with single, oral antimicrobials but, as in other forms of anthrax, β-lactam agents as monotherapy are contraindicated due to resistance concerns. The recommended duration of therapy is 60 days for all BT-associated forms of anthrax due to presumed concomitant inhalational exposure to the primary aerosol and experimental animal data supporting a persistent risk of latent infection from delayed germination of spores.

Because anthrax is a toxin-mediated illness, some advocate the use of clindamycin as part of combination therapy despite the dearth of clinical data, citing the drug's theoretical benefit of diminishing bacterial toxin production, a strategy employed in some toxin-mediated streptococcal infections. Central nervous system penetration is another consideration in therapy selection and drives the preferential use of ciprofloxacin over doxycycline, plus augmentation with chloramphenicol, rifampin, or penicillin when meningitis is suspected. Corticosteroids have been used as adjunctive therapy in the setting of meningitis or severe mediastinal edema, but there are no data to definitively support their use. In the future it is likely that novel therapies, such as toxin inhibitors or receptor antagonists, will be available, in concert with antimicrobials, to treat systemic anthrax. Anthrax vaccine has been proven to be effective in preventing cutaneous anthrax in human clinical trials and in preventing inhalational disease after aerosol challenge in nonhuman primates. The vaccine, which acts by generating an immune response to protective antigen, a key component of anthrax toxin, has been generally found to be safe but requires six doses over the course of 18 months with the need for annual boosting. It is hoped that second-generation anthrax vaccines will prove effective and more robust. Passive immunotherapy with anthrax immunoglobulin may serve an adjunct role to antimicrobials and may provide additional benefit in illness caused by multidrug-resistant pathogens. A recently approved monoclonal antibody targeted against anthrax-protective antigen blocks the formation of anthrax toxins and may have use in advanced disease, drug-resistant cases, or a part of a combination, multifocal approach to therapy.

Plague

Yersinia pestis is typically susceptible in vitro to penicillins, many cephalosporins, carbapenems, aminoglycosides, quinolones, and tetracyclines. It is variably susceptible to trimethoprim, chloramphenicol, and rifampin and is commonly resistant to macrolides and clindamycin. Recommended therapeutic approaches to plague in the BT setting are detailed in Table 120.4.

Naturally occurring antibiotic-resistant strains of *Y. pestis* have been reported in endemic areas of the world and are extremely concerning with respect to the development of biologic weapons.

Production of the currently licensed formalin-inactivated vaccine was discontinued by its manufacturers in 1999; this product had demonstrated efficacy in preventing or ameliorating bubonic disease but not primary pneumonic plague. A subunit vaccine using a bacterial capsular protein has demonstrated protective efficacy in an animal model of pneumonic plague.

Tularemia

Francisella tularensis is generally susceptible in vitro to aminoglycosides, tetracyclines, rifampin, and chloramphenicol; however, many strains are resistant to β-lactams. Similar to the treatment of plague and lacking contraindications, therapy with streptomycin or gentamicin is preferred although alternatives, such as ciprofloxacin, are effective. Because the use of drug-resistant organisms is possible in a bioterrorist event, empiric therapy should account for this, and antimicrobial susceptibility testing of isolates should be expeditiously accomplished. A live attenuated vaccine derived from the avirulent live vaccine strain has been used to protect laboratorians working with *F. tularensis* but is not approved for commercial use.

Botulism

Supportive medical care, airway protection, and mechanical ventilation represent the primary modes of therapy for botulism. Advancements in these modalities account for the improvements in clinical outcomes observed since the mid-1950s; the mortality rate from foodborne botulism in the United States has decreased from 60% to 6%. Passive immunization with equine antitoxin, early in the course of clinical illness, remains the specific treatment of choice to neutralize circulating toxin. Timely administration of this product may be neuroprotective and mitigate severity of disease but will not reverse extant paralysis. Antitoxin should be given to patients with neurologic symptoms as soon as possible after the diagnosis of botulism is suspected; treatment should not be delayed for definitive diagnosis. In the United States, antitoxin is available only from the CDC via state and local health departments. As with any equine-based antisera, anaphylaxis is a potential risk in allergic individuals. To screen for hypersensitivity, skin testing with escalating challenge doses may be necessary before proceeding to a full dose. Patients responding to intradermal challenge with systemic symptoms or signs of hypersensitivity may be desensitized with expert guidance and ready access to epinephrine and airway protection in the event of an adverse reaction.

Smallpox

A suspected case of smallpox warrants immediate implementation of stringent contact and airborne precautions, in a negative-pressure, respiratory isolation setting, and immediate engagement of public health authorities for diagnostic, forensic, and epidemiologic purposes. Vaccination of potential exposures, so-called ring vaccination and containment, must be expeditiously performed; vaccination of symptomatic individuals is indicated if in the early stages of illness, as this is known to be effective in controlling the spread of disease, may mitigate the individual course of disease, and/or may prevent death. There are no currently approved antiviral treatments for smallpox, although cidofovir, licensed for the treatment of cytomegalovirus, has shown promise in vitro and in animal studies for the prevention of orthopoxvirus infection if given proximate to exposure. Topical idoxuridine may be useful in the setting of ocular involvement. Bacterial superinfection is a common complication of smallpox and a frequent cause of death in infected individuals. Aggressive deployment of penicillinase-resistant antimicrobial agents should be used to manage secondary infections with additional consideration given to the institutional and community prevalence of methicillin-resistant *Staphylococcus aureus* (MRSA) in specific areas. Vaccinia immune globulin (VIG) is indicated for the management of specific, severe complications of smallpox vaccine; there is no evidence to support the use of VIG in either the treatment or prophylaxis of smallpox infections.

Viral Hemorrhagic Fevers

The mainstay of treatment for all etiologies of viral hemorrhagic fevers (VHF) is supportive medical care, with special attention paid to hemodynamics, volume status, and respiratory parameters. As many of these agents cause systemic hypotension while at the same time causing capillary leak syndromes, careful monitoring of fluid and electrolyte balance is an important component of patient management. Invasive hemodynamic monitoring, mechanical ventilation, blood product support, dialysis, and neurologic support are often needed.

Although there are no approved antiviral therapies for VHF, the nucleoside analog ribavirin has in vitro and in vivo activity against some arenaviral and bunyaviral etiologies of VHF, such as Rift Valley fever, Lassa fever, and Congo–Crimean hemorrhagic fever. The drug has been shown to reduce morbidity from hemorrhagic fever with renal syndrome, caused by Old World hantaviruses, and to probably reduce morbidity and mortality from Lassa fever. Intravenous ribavirin given within the first 6 days of fever to patients with Lassa fever who had high levels of viremia decreased mortality from 76% to 9%. The drug is available under IND status from the CDC and USAMRIID and is associated with significant hemolysis, cytopenias from marrow suppression, and is teratogenic in animals. Ribavirin appears to have no clinical utility in infections caused by filoviruses, such as Marburg or Ebola, or flaviviruses.

SUGGESTED READING

Arnon SS, Schechter R, Inglesby TV, et al. Botulinum toxin as a biological weapon: medical and public health management. *JAMA*. 2001;285:1059–1070.

Artenstein AW. Bioterrorism and biodefense. In: Cohen J, Powderly WG, eds. *Infectious Diseases*. 2nd ed. London: Mosby; 2003: 99–107.

Artenstein AW. Initial management of a suspected outbreak of smallpox. In: Cohen J, Powderly WG, eds. *Infectious Diseases*. 2nd ed. London: Mosby; 2003;1022–1025.

Artenstein AW. Anthrax: from antiquity to answers. *J Infect Dis*. 2007;195:471–473.

Borio L, Inglesby TV, Peters CJ, et al. Hemorrhagic fever viruses as biological weapons: medical and public health management. *JAMA*. 2002;287:2391–2405.

Dennis DT, Inglesby TV, Henderson DA, et al. Tularemia as a biological weapon: medical and public health management. *JAMA*. 2001;285:2763–2773.

Fan J, Kraft AJ, Henrickson KJ. Current methods for the rapid diagnosis of bioterrorism-related infectious agents. *Pediatr Clin N Am*. 2006;53:817–842.

Henderson DA, Dennis DT, Inglesby TV, et al. Smallpox as a biological weapon: medical and public health management. *JAMA*. 1999;281:2127–2137.

Inglesby TV, Dennis DT, Henderson DA, et al. Plague as a biological weapon: medical and public health management. *JAMA*. 2000;83:2281–2290.

Inglesby TV, O'Toole T, Henderson DA, et al. Anthrax as a biological weapon, 2002: updated recommendations for management. *JAMA*. 2002;287:2236–2252.

Pien BC, Royden Saah J, Miller SE, et al. Use of sentinel laboratories by clinicians to evaluate potential bioterrorism and emerging infections. *Clin Infect Dis*. 2006;42: 1311–1324.

Woods B, 2005. *USAMRID's Medical Management of Biological Casualties Handbook*. 6th ed. Frederick, MD: U.S Army Medical Research Institute of Infectious Diseases; April 2005.

Specific Organisms – Bacteria

121. Actinomycosis

Thomas A. Russo

ETIOLOGIC AGENTS

Actinomycosis is an infectious syndrome caused by anaerobic or microaerophilic bacteria, primarily from the genus *Actinomyces*. It is most commonly caused by *Actinomyces israelii*; however, *Actinomyces naeslundii*, *Actinomyces odontolyticus*, *Actinomyces viscosus*, *Actinomyces meyeri*, *Actinomyces gerencseriae*, and *Propionibacterium propionicum* are less common causes of infection. Nearly all of actinomycotic infections are polymicrobial in nature. *Actinobacillus actinomycetemcomitans*, *Eikenella corrodens*, *Fusobacterium*, *Bacteroides*, *Capnocytopaga*, *Staphylococcus*, *Streptococcus*, and Enterobacteriaceae are commonly coisolated ("companion organisms") with the agents of actinomycosis in various combinations depending on the site of the infection. Recently a variety of bacterial species isolated from human clinical specimens have been reclassified as *Actinomyces*. Increasing data support that *Actinomyces europaeus*, *Actinomyces neuii*, *Actinomyces radingae*, *Actinomyces graevenitzii*, *Actinomyces turicensis*, *Actinomyces cardiffensis*, *Actinomyces houstonensis*, *Actinomyces hongkongensis*, and *Actinomyces funkei* also cause human actinomycosis.

EPIDEMIOLOGY AND PATHOGENESIS

The etiologic agents of actinomycosis are members of the normal oral flora and are often present in bronchi and the gastrointestinal and female genital tracts. Although males have a higher incidence of infection (perhaps due to more frequent trauma and poorer dental hygiene), actinomycosis occurs in all age groups and geographic locations. Disruption of the mucosal barrier is the critical step for the development of actinomycosis. Subsequently, local infection may ensue and once established, if untreated, spreads contiguously ignoring tissue planes in a slow, progressive manner. Although acute inflammation may initially occur at the site of infection, the hallmark of actinomycosis is the characteristic chronic, indolent phase. This stage is manifested by lesions that usually appear as single or multiple indurations. Central necrosis develops that consists of neutrophils and sulfur granules (a finding virtually diagnostic of this disease). The walls of the mass are fibrotic and characteristically described as "wooden." Over time sinus tracts to the skin, adjacent organs, or bone may develop. Rarely distant hematogenous seeding occurs. Foreign bodies appear to facilitate infection. This occurs most frequently with intrauterine contraceptive devices (IUCDs). The contribution of the non-*Actinomyces* coisolates or companion organisms to the pathogenesis of actinomycosis is uncertain.

INFECTIOUS SYNDROMES

Clinical presentations are myriad. Once common in the preantibiotic era, today the incidence of actinomycosis is diminished and, as a result, so is its timely recognition. It has been called "the most misdiagnosed disease" and stated that "no disease is so often missed by experienced clinicians." Actinomycosis remains a diagnostic challenge. An awareness of the full spectrum of disease will expedite diagnosis and treatment and minimize the unnecessary surgical interventions, morbidity, and mortality that all too often occur with this disease. Three clinical presentations, in particular, warrant consideration of this unique infection. First, the combination of chronicity, progression across tissue boundaries, and masslike features mimics malignancy, with which it is often confused. Second, cure of established actinomycosis requires prolonged treatment. Short courses of therapy with active agents usually result in only transient improvement. Therefore, actinomycosis should be thought of with refractory or relapsing infections. Last, development of a sinus tract, which may spontaneously resolve and recur, should prompt consideration of this disease.

Oral–Cervicofacial Disease

This is the most frequent site for infection. The usual presentation is a soft-tissue swelling, abscess, or mass lesion that is often mistaken for a neoplasm. The angle of the jaw is the most common location, but actinomycosis should be considered with any mass lesion or relapsing infection in the head and neck. Rarely, otitis, sinusitis, and canniculitis can also occur. Pain, fever, and leukocytosis are variably present. Contiguous spread to the cranium, cervical spine, or the thorax and the attendant complications are potential sequelae.

Thoracic Disease

The usual presentation is an indolent, progressive course that involves the pulmonary parenchyma and/or the pleural space. Chest pain, fever, and weight loss are common. A cough, when present, is variably productive. The most common radiographic appearance is either a mass lesion or pneumonia. Cavitary disease or hilar adenopathy may develop. Many cases have pleural thickening, effusion, or empyema. Pulmonary disease that crosses fissures or pleura; involves the mediastinum, contiguous bone, or the chest wall; or is associated with a sinus tract should suggest actinomycosis. Mediastinal infection is uncommon. The structures within the mediastinum and the heart, including heart valves, can be involved in various combinations, resulting in a variety of presentations. Isolated disease of the breast occurs rarely.

Abdominal Disease

Abdominal actinomycosis is often unrecognized. Months to years usually pass from the inciting event (eg, appendicitis, diverticulitis, peptic ulcer disease, foreign body perforation, bowel surgery, or ascension from IUCD-associated pelvic disease) to diagnosis. Because of the flow of peritoneal fluid and/or direct extension of primary disease, virtually any abdominal organ, region, or space can be involved. The usual presentation is either an abscess or a mass lesion that is often fixed to underlying tissue and mistaken for a tumor. Sinus tracts to the abdominal wall or perianal region may develop. Hepatic infection usually presents as single or multiple abscesses or masses. Isolated disease is presumably via hematogenous seeding from cryptic foci. All levels of the urogenital tract can be infected. Bladder involvement, usually due to extension of pelvic disease, may result in obstruction or fistulas to bowel, skin, or uterus. Renal disease usually presents as pyelonephritis and/or renal and perinephric abscess.

Pelvic Disease

Actinomycotic involvement of the pelvis is strongly associated with IUCDs. Although the magnitude of risk is unclear, it would appear to be small. Disease rarely occurs when an IUCD has been in place for less than 1 year; however, the risk of infection increases with time and is often seen in the setting of the "forgotten" IUCD. Symptoms are typically indolent with fever, weight loss, abdominal pain, and abnormal vaginal bleeding or discharge being most common. An endometritis, if untreated, may progress to a pelvic mass or a tubo-ovarian abscess. Unfortunately, diagnosis is often delayed, and a "frozen pelvis" mimicking malignancy or endometriosis will develop by the time of recognition.

Central Nervous System

Central nervous system (CNS) infection is rare. Single or multiple brain abscesses are most common, usually appearing on computed tomography (CT) as a ring enhancing lesion with a thick wall that may be irregular or nodular.

Musculoskeletal Infection

Osteomyelitis is usually due to adjacent soft-tissue infection but may be associated with trauma (eg, fracture of the mandible) or hematogenous spread. The uncommon infection of the extremities is usually a result of trauma. Skin, subcutaneous tissue, muscle, and bone are involved alone or in various combinations. Cutaneous sinus tracts frequently develop.

Disseminated Disease

Hematogenous spread of infection from any location may rarely result in multiorgan involvement with the lungs and liver most commonly affected. The presentation of multiple nodules may mimic disseminated malignancy.

DIAGNOSIS

The diagnosis of actinomycosis is rarely considered. Most often the first mention of actinomycosis is from the pathologist after extensive surgery. Because medical therapy alone is often sufficient for cure, the challenge for the clinician is to consider actinomycosis so that this uncommon and unusual infection can be diagnosed in the least invasive fashion and unnecessary surgery can be avoided. CT- or ultrasound-guided aspirations or biopsies are successfully used to obtain clinical material for diagnosis, although surgery may be required. The diagnosis is most commonly made by microscopic identification of sulfur granules (an in vivo matrix of bacteria and host material) in pus or tissues, although occasionally sulfur granules can be grossly identified from draining sinus tracts or pus. Microbiologic identification is less frequent, due to either prior antimicrobial therapy or omission. To optimize yield, the avoidance of even a single dose of antibiotics is mandatory. Because these organisms are normal oral and genital tract flora, their identification in the absence of sulfur granules from sputum, bronchial washings, and cervicovaginal secretions is of little significance. Although not routinely utilized, 16S rRNA gene amplification and sequencing has been successfully used to increase diagnostic sensitivity.

TREATMENT

Antimicrobial Therapy

Controlled trials evaluating either antimicrobials or studies designed to define duration of therapy in the treatment of actinomycosis have not been performed and will never be done. Therefore, treatment decisions are based primarily on the collective clinical experience since the mid-1950s. Two principles of therapy have evolved. It is necessary to treat this disease both with high doses and for a prolonged period of time. Presumably, this is because of the difficulties of antimicrobials penetrating the thick-walled masses that commonly occur with this infection and/or the sulfur granules themselves.

Although therapy should always be individualized, 18 to 24 million units of penicillin intravenously (IV) for 2 to 6 weeks, followed by oral therapy with penicillin or amoxicillin for 6 to 12 months is a reasonable guideline for serious infections and bulky disease. Cases with less extensive disease, particularly in the head and neck region, may require a shorter course of therapy. If the duration of therapy is extended beyond the resolution of measurable disease, then relapses, one of the clinical hallmarks of this infection, will be minimized. Computed tomography and magnetic resonance imaging (MRI) studies are generally the most objective modalities to accomplish this goal. MRI scans are often more sensitive than CT scans for detecting residual infection and

Table 121.1 Antibiotic Therapy for Actinomycosis[a]

Group 1: Extensive Successful Clinical Experience[b]

Penicillin (18–24 million units/d IV q4h), (1–2 g/day PO q6h)
Erythromycin (2–4 g/d IV q6h), (1–2 gm/day PO q6h)
Tetracycline (1–2 g/d PO q6h)
Doxycycline (200 mg/d IV or PO q12-24h)
Minocycline (200 mg/d IV or PO q12h)
Clindamycin (2.7 gm/d IV q8h), (1.2–1.8 gm/d PO q6-8h)

Group 2: Anecdotal Successful Clinical Experience

Ceftriaxone
Ceftizoxime
Imipenam
Piperacillin–tazobactam

Group 3: Agents Predicted to be Efficacious Based on in Vitro Activity

Moxifloxacin
Vancomycin
Linezolid
Quinupristin–dalfopristine

Abbreviations: IV = intravenously; PO = orally.
[a] Additional coverage for concomitant "companion" bacteria may be required.
[b] Controlled evaluations have not been performed. Dose and duration require individualization depending on the host, site, and extent of infection. As a general rule, a maximum antimicrobial dose for 2–6 weeks of parenteral therapy followed by oral therapy for a total duration (6–12 months) is required for serious infections and bulky disease; whereas a shorter duration may suffice for less extensive disease, particularly in the oral-cervicofacial region.

should be employed if possible, particularly in areas where the consequences of relapse are particularly significant (eg, CNS). For penicillin-allergic patients, tetracycline has been used most extensively with success. Erythromycin, doxycycline, and clindamycin are other suitable alternatives (Table 121.1). In the pregnant, penicillin-sensitive patient erythromycin is a safe alternative. Remarkably, little clinical information is available on the newer antimicrobial agents. Anecdotal successes have been reported with imipenem, ceftriaxone, ceftizoxime, and piperacillin–tazobactam (Table 121.1). Available data suggest that oxacillin, dicloxacillin, cephalexin, metronidazole, and aminoglycosides should be avoided.

Home Therapy

For home IV therapy, the ease of once-a-day dosing makes ceftriaxone appealing in certain circumstances; however, a greater body of literature supporting its efficacy would be desirable. The availability of portable infusion pumps for home therapy allows for both the appropriate dosing and practical administration of IV penicillin. For infections in critical sites (eg, CNS) this approach remains the safest until more information is available on other agents. The pharmacokinetic properties, availability of oral and parenteral formulations, and potential efficacy of azithromycin also make this agent appealing. Unfortunately few in vitro and no clinical data exist on its use to treat actinomycosis.

Treatment of Coisolates

It is unclear whether other bacteria frequently coisolated with the etiologic agents of actinomycosis require treatment; however, many of them are pathogens in their own right. Designing a therapeutic regimen that includes coverage for these organisms during the initial treatment course is reasonable. If microbiology is not available, it is important to consider the site of infection when designing empiric coverage. For example, *Actinobacillus actinomycetemcomitans*, *Eikenella corrodens*, *Fusobacterium*, and *Capnocytopaga* are more likely to be coisolates in head and neck infection, whereas the Enterobacteriaceae are more commonly coisolated in abdominal infection.

Surgery or Percutaneous Drainage

In the preantibiotic era, surgical removal of infected tissue was the only beneficial treatment. Despite the availability of effective antimicrobial therapy, combined surgical therapy is still advocated by some authorities. However, an increasing body of literature now supports the approach of initially attempting a cure with medical therapy alone. Successes have been reported in cases of extensive disease, which initially appeared to be incurable using antibiotics alone. Computed tomography and MRI should be used to monitor the response to therapy. In most cases either surgery can be avoided or a less extensive procedure will be necessary. This approach is particularly important when the possibility of sparing critical organs is involved, such as the bladder or reproductive organs in women of childbearing age. In a patient with disease in a critical location (eg, epidural space, selected CNS disease), or if suitable medical therapy fails, surgical intervention may be appropriate.

In the setting of actinomycosis presenting as a well-defined abscess, percutaneous drainage in combination with medical therapy is a reasonable approach.

Treatment of the Immunocompromised Host

It is unclear which host defense components are most critical in affording protection against actinomycosis and whether certain hosts are more susceptible to infection. Actinomycosis has been described in association with human immunodeficiency virus (HIV) infection, steroid use, and lymphoproliferative tumors. Whether these infections were because of disease-associated disruptions of mucosa (eg, cytomegalovirus [CMV] infection with HIV infection), host defense abnormalities, immunosuppressive therapy, or some combination of these is unclear. From a treatment perspective it is reasonable to initially use the same approach as that for noncompromised hosts. Aggressive treatment directly against HIV (eg, highly active antiretroviral therapy) and minimizing immunosuppressive therapy is also desirable if possible. There are no data on the use of immunomodulatory therapy (eg, interferon-γ or immunoglobulins).

REFRACTORY DISEASE

Usually actinomycosis responds well to medical therapy. However, refractory or perceived refractory disease has been described in HIV-infected individuals as well as apparently normal hosts. In this setting basic principles of infectious disease apply. Exclude infection elsewhere (eg, line-related, *Clostridium difficile* colitis) and/or noninfectious causes (eg, drug fever, unrelated disease) as being responsible. Confirm that high-dose parenteral therapy is being utilized for initial treatment. Identify and drain significant purulent collections associated with the actinomycotic infection. Consider the possibility that untreated coisolates (companion organisms) may be responsible. Although penicillin-resistant strains or evolution of resistance during therapy has not yet been clearly documented in vivo, this possibility should be considered when other more likely scenarios are excluded. Finally, surgery should be considered when infection is refractory to medical therapy, although as stated above, this usually can be avoided, at least initially.

ACTINOMYCES-LIKE ORGANISMS

An unresolved issue is whether screening cervical or endometrial specimens for *Actinomyces*-like organisms (ALO) or their detection by immunofluorescence (IF) can predict/ prevent IUCD-associated disease. Furthermore, a Papanicolaou smear may fail to detect ALOs even in the presence of active actinomycosis. Although the risk appears to be small, the consequences of infection are significant. Therefore, until more quantitative data become available, in the presence of symptoms that cannot be accounted for, regardless of whether ALOs or IF-positive organisms are detected, it would appear prudent to remove the IUCD and, if advanced disease is excluded, empirically treat for 14 days for possible early pelvic actinomycosis. The detection of ALOs or IF-positive organisms in the absence of symptoms warrants patient education and close follow-up, but not removal of the IUCD, unless an equally suitable means of contraception can be agreed upon.

SUGGESTED READING

Clarridge JE III, Zhang Q. Genotypic diversity of clinical Actinomyces species: phenotype, source, and disease correlation among genospecies. *J Clin Microbiol*. 2002;40:3442–3448.

Colmegna I, Rodriguez-Barradas M, Rauch R, et al. Disseminated Actinomyces meyeri infection resembling lung cancer with brain metastases. *Am J Med Sci*. 2003;326:152–155.

Goldstein EJ, Citron DM, Merriam CV, et al. In vitro activities of the new semisynthetic glycopeptide telavancin (TD-6424), vancomycin, daptomycin, linezolid, and four comparator agents against anaerobic gram-positive species and Corynebacterium spp. *Antimicrob Agents Chemother*. 2004; 48:2149–2152.

Kayikcioglu F, Akif Akgul M, Haberal A, et al. Actinomyces infection in the female genital tract. *Eur J Obstet Gynecol Reprod Biol*. 2005;118:77–180.

Lecouvet F, Trenge L, Vandercam B, et al. The etiologic diagnosis of infectious discitis is improved by amplification-based DNA analysis. *Arthritis Rheum*. 2004;50:2985–2994.

Milazzo I, Blandino G, Musumeci R, et al. Antimicrobial activity of moxifloxacin against periodontal anaerobic pathogens involved in systemic infections. *Int J Antimicrob Agents*. 2002;20:451–456.

Pulverer G, Schütt-Gerowitt H, Schaal KP. Human cervicofacial actinomycoses: microbiologic data for 1997 cases. *Clin Infect Dis*. 2003;37:490–497.

Russo TA. Actinomycosis. In: Mandell GL, et al., eds. *Principles and Practice of Infectious Diseases*. 6th ed. New York: Churchill Livingstone; 2005:2924–2934.

Smith AJ, Hall V, Thakker B, et al. Antimicrobial susceptibility testing of Actinomyces species with 12 antimicrobial agents. *J Antimicrob Chemother*. 2005;56:407–409.

Sudhakar SS, Ross JJ. Short-term treatment of actinomycosis: two cases and a review. *Clin Infect Dis*. 2004;38:444–447.

122. Anaerobic Infections

Sydney M. Finegold

Anaerobic infections are common and some are serious, with a high mortality rate. They are easily overlooked because special precautions are needed for specimen collection and transport to do good bacteriologic studies and because some clinical laboratories fail to grow many or most anaerobes (a number of laboratories do not even do anaerobic cultures).

Treatment of anaerobic infections may be difficult. Failure to treat for anaerobes in mixed infections may lead to poor or no response. Many antibacterial agents have poor activity against many or most anaerobes, particularly aminoglycosides, the older quinolones, trimethoprim–sulfamethoxazole, and monobactams. Resistance of anaerobes to antimicrobials is increasing.

The most important anaerobes clinically are various genera of gram-negative rods. *Bacteroides*, especially the *Bacteroides fragilis* group, made up of several species (including *B. fragilis*), is particularly important. The other principal gram-negative genera are *Prevotella, Porphyromonas, Fusobacterium, Bilophila*, and *Sutterella*. Among the gram-positive anaerobes are cocci (formerly in *Peptostreptococcus*, now in several genera) spore-forming (*Clostridium*), and non–spore-forming bacilli (especially *Actinomyces* and *Propionibacterium*) (Table 122.1).

SOURCE OF ANAEROBIC INFECTION

Virtually the only source of anaerobes causing infection is the indigenous flora of mucosal surfaces and, to a much lesser extent, the skin (Table 122.2). The major exception is *Clostridium difficile*, the principal cause of antimicrobial agent–associated colitis, which has caused nosocomial infections. Anaerobes outnumber aerobes by 10:1 in the oral and vaginal flora and by 1000:1 in the colon. Factors predisposing to anaerobic infection include disruption of normal mucosal or cutaneous barriers by disease, surgery, or trauma; tissue injury (which reduces oxidation-reduction potential, favoring growth of anaerobes); impaired blood supply; obstruction of a hollow viscus; and foreign body. Other important factors include the numbers of

Table 122.1 Anaerobes Most Commonly Encountered in Infection[a]

Bacteroides fragilis group, especially *B. fragilis*
Pigmented and nonpigmented *Prevotella*
Fusobacterium nucleatum
Anaerobic gram-positive cocci
Clostridium perfringens, Clostridium ramosum

[a] These five groups together account for about two thirds of anaerobes from clinically significant infections involving anaerobes.

Table 122.2 Incidence of Various Anaerobes as Normal Flora in the Human[a]

	Anaerobic Cocci	Anaerobic Gram-Negative Bacilli	Clostridia	NSF-GPR
Mouth	++++[b]	++++	Rare	+ to ++
Intestine	++++	++++	++++	++++
Genitourinary Tract[c]	+++	++	+	+ to ++

[a] Skin and upper respiratory tract are less important.
[b] The ranking + to ++++ reflects both consistency of occurrence and density of numbers.
[c] Includes vagina, external genitalia and urethra.

organisms that get into deeper tissues (the inoculum size), various virulence factors (toxins, enzymes, and other substances) produced by anaerobes, and whether the host's defense system is intact.

TYPES OF INFECTION INVOLVING ANAEROBES

In terms of overall frequency, there are four major sites of anaerobic infection: pleuropulmonary, intra-abdominal, female genital tract, and skin and soft tissue with or without involvement of underlying bone. Other infections that primarily involve anaerobic bacteria but are seen less commonly include brain abscess and bite-wound infections. Virtually all types of infection occurring in humans may involve anaerobic bacteria, and no organ or tissue of the body is immune to infection with these organisms. Table 122.3 lists infections commonly involving anaerobic bacteria. Abscess formation and tissue destruction are common characteristics of anaerobic infection. Synergy between various anaerobes or between anaerobes and aerobes is often important in mixed anaerobic infections.

Some anaerobic infections are unique (eg, lung abscess, actinomycosis) and are readily suspected clinically. Major clues to anaerobic infection are listed in Table 122.4. Only the foul or putrid odor of a lesion or its discharge is specific; the other clues nonetheless may be highly suggestive. The Gram stain is useful because many anaerobes are unique morphologically. Information as to the relative numbers of various organisms may be extremely useful in directing empiric therapy.

Relatively recently, a number of serious infections involving various clostridia have been documented. Included are a more serious form of *Clostridium difficile*–associated diarrheal disease or colitis involved in a number of hospital-acquired outbreaks, endometritis and toxic shock syndrome due to *Clostridium sordelli* following abortions, and serious soft-tissue infections (including necrotizing fasciitis and anaerobic myonecrosis) due to *C. sordellii* and *C. novyi* in "skin-popping" drug addicts.

COLLECTION AND TRANSPORT OF SPECIMENS

Proper collection and transport of specimens is crucial for recovery of anaerobes in the laboratory. Because anaerobes are normal flora, the clinician should be certain not to contaminate the specimens with such flora; this may be difficult at times. A good example of the problem is the patient with suspected aspiration pneumonia. Expectorated sputum is unsuitable because of the large numbers of anaerobes and other organisms present in saliva as indigenous flora; it is necessary to bypass the normal flora. If an empyema is present, thoracentesis provides a good specimen and is indicated therapeutically. In the absence of pleural fluid, bronchoalveolar lavage or use of a plugged double-lumen catheter with a protected bronchial brush, with quantitative culture, should be used.

Proper transport requires placing the specimen under anaerobic conditions in a nonnutritive holding medium (in an oxygen-free glass tube or vial) for the trip to the laboratory.

Table 122.3 Infections Commonly Involving Anaerobic Bacteria

Brain abscess
Subdural empyema
Endophthalmitis, panophthalmitis
Periodontal disease
Root canal infection
Odontogenic infections
Chronic sinusitis
Chronic otitis media, mastoiditis
Peritonsillar abscess
Neck space infections
Aspiration pneumonia
Lung abscess
Pleural empyema
Pyogenic liver abscess
Peritonitis
Intra-abdominal abscess
Appendicitis
Wound infection after bowel or female genital tract surgery or trauma
Endometritis
Salpingitis, tuboovarian abscess
Pelvic abscess
Human and animal bite infection
Infected decubitus ulcer
Anaerobic cellulitis
Clostridial myonecrosis (gas gangrene)
Synergistic nonclostridial myonecrosis
Anaerobic streptococcal myositis
Necrotizing fasciitis
Chronic osteomyelitis
Actinomycosis
Antimicrobial-induced colitis and pseudomembranous colitis

Table 122.4 Major Clues to Anaerobic Infection

Foul-smelling discharge
Infection close to mucosal surface
Tissue necrosis, gangrene
Gas in tissues or discharges
Infection associated with malignancy
Infection secondary to human or animal bite
Infection related to the use of aminoglycosides, quinolones, trimethoprim–sulfamethoxazole, monobactams, or other drugs with poor activity against anaerobes
Classic clinical picture such as gas gangrene, actinomycosis
Infections that are classically of anaerobic origin (eg, brain abscess, lung abscess)
Septic thrombophlebitis
Unique morphology on Gram stain of exudate
No growth on routine culture; sterile pus

Table 122.5 Usual Flora in Anaerobic Pleuropulmonary Infections[a]

Anaerobes
Anaerobic gram-positive cocci
Pigmented *Prevotella* (*P. denticola, P. melaninogenica, P. intermedia, P. nigrescens, P. loescheii*)
Nonpigmented *Prevotella* (*P. oris, P. buccae, P. oralis*)
Fusobacterium nucleatum
Bacteroides fragilis group
Non–spore-forming gram-positive rods (*Actinomyces, Eubacterium, Lactobacillus*)
Viridans streptococci

[a] In hospital-acquired infections (eg, aspiration pneumonia), various nosocomial pathogens, such as *Staphylococcus aureus*, Enterobacteriaceae, and *Pseudomonas*, may be involved in addition to the indigenous flora listed above.

Table 122.6 Usual Flora in Intra-Abdominal Infection[a]

Predominant Anaerobes
Bacteroides fragilis
Bacteroides thetaiotaomicron
Bilophila wadsworthia
Anaerobic gram-positive cocci
Clostridium
Predominant Aerobes and Facultatives
Escherichia coli
Streptococcus (viridans group)
Pseudomonas aeruginosa
Enterococcus
Biliary Tract Infection
Uncomplicated
E. coli, Klebsiella, Enterococcus, and *Clostridium perfringens*
Complicated (eg, prior surgery, malignancy)
B. fragilis group may also be involved

[a] In hospital-acquired infections, nosocomial pathogens, such as *Staphylococcus aureus* and various Enterobacteriaceae, may also be involved.

THERAPY

The two key approaches to treatment are surgery and antimicrobial therapy. Debridement and drainage usually are essential. Failure to carry out prompt and thorough surgical therapy may lead to lack of response to appropriate antimicrobial agents. Some abscesses are amenable to percutaneous drainage under guidance of ultrasound or computed tomography.

Hyperbaric oxygen (HBO) may have value in selected circumstances, such as gas gangrene, to help demarcate the infection; for example, it may indicate where amputation should be done in the case of an extremity infection. There has never been clear-cut clinical evidence of significant benefit from HBO; however, surgical therapy should never be delayed to administer HBO.

Initial antimicrobial therapy is necessarily empiric; it takes some time to get definitive information on the infecting flora because it is usually complex. Rational empiric therapy is based on the clinician's assessment of the nature of the infectious process, knowledge of the usual infecting flora in such infections (Tables 122.5–122.9), and patterns of resistance of anaerobic bacteria to antimicrobial drugs in the particular hospital. Also, the clinician must take into account how the usual flora may have been modified by pathophysiology or disease and by prior antimicrobial therapy. Careful analysis of the Gram stain of the specimen may also suggest the need to modify the empiric approach. In certain situations, the pharmacologic properties of the drugs and whether they are bactericidal or not are important considerations. In central nervous system infections, for example, the drug must cross the blood–brain barrier well. In such infections and in endocarditis, bactericidal activity is important. A good clinician will be in close contact with the microbiology laboratory, particularly in the case of a very sick patient. Ideally, such contact begins before the specimen is submitted and is maintained until full

Table 122.7 Usual Flora in Female Genital Tract Infections

Anaerobes

Anaerobic gram-positive cocci
Bacteroides fragilis group
Prevotella (especially *P. bivia, P. disiens*)
Clostridium (especially *C. perfringens*)
Actinomyces, Eubacterium (in intrauterine
    contraceptive device–associated infections)

Aerobes

Streptococcus (groups A, B, others)
Escherichia coli
Klebsiella
Gonococcus (in sexually active patients)
Chlamydia (in sexually active patients)
Mycoplasma hominis (in postpartum patients)

Table 122.8 Usual Flora in Diabetic Foot Ulcers

Anaerobes

Anaerobic gram-positive cocci
Bacteroides fragilis group (especially *B. fragilis* and
    B. thetaiotaomicron)
Other *Bacteroides*
Pigmented *Prevotella*

Aerobes

Enterococcus
Staphylococcus aureus
Streptococci (especially group B)
Proteus mirabilis
Escherichia coli
Other Enterobacteriaceae
Pseudomonas aeruginosa

Table 122.9 Predominant Flora of Skin and Soft-Tissue Abscess

In Intravenous Drug Abusers

Anaerobes

Fusobacterium nucleatum
Anaerobic gram-positive cocci
Actinomyces odontolyticus
Pigmented *Prevotella*

Aerobes

Staphylococcus aureus
Streptococcus (*S. anginosus* group, viridans group,
    group A)

In Nonintravenous Drug Abusers

Anaerobes

Anaerobic gram-positive cocci
Pigmented *Prevotella*
Actinomyces
Fusobacterium nucleatum

Aerobes

Staphylococcus aureus
Streptococcus (*S. anginosus* group, group A,
    viridans group)

Table 122.10 Principal β-Lactamase–Producing Anaerobes

Bacteroides fragilis group

Bacteroides splanchnicus, B. capillosus

Pigmented *Prevotella, Porphyromonas*

Prevotella oralis group

Prevotella: P. oris, P. buccae

Prevotella: P. bivia, P. disiens

Bilophila wadsworthia

Fusobacterium nucleatum

Fusobacterium: F. mortiferum, F. varium

Clostridium ramosum

Clostridium clostridioforme group (*C. clostridioforme,
C. bolteae, C. hathewayi*)

Clostridium butyricum

culture results are available. The microbiologist may take advantage of information from the clinician to use special selective or other media in setting up the culture and can often look at cultures more often than is done with routine cultures, using an anaerobic chamber or other device to examine the culture without exposing it to oxygen. Preliminary culture information may dictate modification of the initial empiric antimicrobial regimen. The use of molecular techniques may lead to much more rapid identification than with conventional procedures.

Antimicrobial resistance is an increasing problem with anaerobic bacteria. Various mechanisms for such resistance are known; they are the same as are seen with aerobes. β-lactamase production is one of the most common mechanisms of such resistance; fortunately, this can be overcome to some extent by combinations of β-lactam drugs with β-lactamase inhibitors such as clavulanic acid, sulbactam, or tazobactam. Table 122.10 lists the more common β-lactamase–producing anaerobes. Unfortunately, hyperproduction of β-lactamases and production of metalloenzyme β-lactamases may render some of our better drugs inactive.

Tables 122.11 and 122.12 summarize the activity of various antimicrobials against

Specific Organisms – Bacteria

Table 122.11 Susceptibility of Gram-Positive Anaerobic Bacteria

Percentage Susceptible[a],[b]	Anaerobic Gram-Positive Cocci (Formerly Peptostreptococcus)	C. difficile[c]	C. ramosum	C. perfringens	Other Clostridium Species	NSF-GPR[d]
>95	Penicillin G; Piperacillin; Amoxicillin + clavulanate; Ampicillin + sulbactam; Piperacillin + tazobactam; Ticarcillin + clavulanate; Cefoperazone; Ceftriaxone; Cefoxitin; Ceftazidime; Ceftizoxime; Tigecycline; Imipenem; Meropenem; Ertapenem; Chloramphenicol; Linezolid; Metronidazole; Gatifloxacin	Ampicillin; Piperacillin; Ticarcillin; Amoxicillin + clavulanate; Ampicillin + sulbactam; Piperacillin + tazobactam; Ticarcillin + clavulanate; Imipenem; Meropenem; Vancomycin; Tigecycline; Metronidazole	Amoxicillin + clavulanate; Piperacillin + tazobactam; Ticarcillin + clavulanate; Ceftizoxime; Imipenem; Ertapenem; Metronidazole; Vancomycin	Ampicillin; Piperacillin; Ticarcillin; Ampicillin + sulbactam; Amoxicillin + clavulanate; Piperacillin + tazobactam; Ticarcillin + clavulanate; Ceftizoxime; Imipenem; Ertapenem; Chloramphenicol; Ciprofloxacin; Gatifloxacin; Tigecycline; Linezolid; Vancomycin; Metronidazole; Azithromycin; Clarithromycin; Erythromycin	Amoxicillin; Ampicillin; Carbenicillin; Piperacillin; Ticarcillin; Ampicillin + sulbactam; Amoxicillin + clavulanate; Imipenem; Ertapenem; Chloramphenicol; Metronidazole	Piperacillin; Amoxicillin + clavulanate; Ampicillin + sulbactam; Piperacillin + tazobactam; Ticarcillin + clavulanate; Cefotaxime; Ceftizoxime; Imipenem; Meropenem; Ertapenem; Chloramphenical; Clindamycin; Tigecycline; Levofloxacin
85–95	Levofloxacin; Clindamycin; Vancomycin	Ceftriaxone; Chloramphenicol	Ampicillin; Piperacillin; Ampicillin + sulbactam; Chloramphenicol; Clindamycin	Clindamycin	Moxalactam; Penicillin G	Cefoxitin; Ceftriaxone; Penicillin G; Gatifloxacin; Azithromycin; Clarithromycin; Erythromycin; Cefoperazone
70–84	Ciprofloxacin; Moxifloxacin; Azithromycin; Clarithromycin; Erythromycin	Ertapenem; Linezolid	Cefoxitin; Clindamycin		Levofloxacin; Vancomycin; Linezolid; Clindamycin; Tetracycline	Moxalactam; Moxifloxacin; Linezolid; Tetracycline; Vancomycin
50–69	Tetracycline	Clindamycin; Tetracycline; Azithromycin; Clarithromycin; Erythromycin	Tetracycline	Tetracycline	Cefoperazone; Cefotaxime; Cefoxitin; Ceftizoxime; Ceftriaxone; Ciprofloxacin; Azithromycin; Clarithromycin; Erythromycin	Ciprofloxacin; Metronidazole
<50		Cefoxitin; Ceftizoxime; Ciprofloxacin[c]	Ciprofloxacin; Moxifloxacin; Azithromycin; Clarithromycin; Erythromycin; Linezolid		Ceftazidime	

[a] The order of listing of drugs within percent susceptible categories is not significant.
[b] According to the NCCLS-approved breakpoints (M11-A3), using the intermediate category as susceptible.
[c] Breakpoint is used only as a reference point. *Clostridium difficile* is primarily of interest in relation to antimicrobial-induced pseudomembranous colitis. These data must be interpreted in the context of level of drug achieved in the colon and impact of agent on indigenous colonic flora. Fluoroquinolones may be an important factor in hospital outbreaks of *C. difficile*–associated disease.
[d] Non–spore-forming, gram-positive rods.

Table 122.12 Susceptibility of Gram-Negative Anaerobic Bacteria

Percentage Susceptible[a,b]	B. fragilis	Other B. fragilis Group[c]	Other Bacteroides	C. gracilis	Prevotella
>95	Piperacillin Amoxicillin + clavulanate Piperacillin + tazobactam Ticarcillin + clavulanate Ampicillin + sulbactam Cefoxitin Meropenem Ertapenem Imipenem Chloramphenicol Levofloxacin Metronidazole	Ampicillin + sulbactam Piperacillin + tazobactam Ticarcillin + clavulanate Ertapenem Imipenem Meropenem Chloramphenicol Gatifloxacin Metronidazole	Cefoperazone Piperacillin Amoxicillin + clavulanate Ampicillin + sulbactam Ticarcillin + clavulanate Cefoxitin Ceftizoxime Cefotaxime Imipenem Chloramphenicol Levofloxacin Metronidazole Clindamycin	Piperacillin Ticarcillin + clavulanate Amoxicillin + clavulanate Piperacillin + tazobactam Cefoxitin Ceftizoxime Ceftriaxone Imipenem Meropenem Ertapenem Chloramphenicol Ciprofloxacin Metronidazole Azithromycin Clindamycin Erythromycin Tetracycline	Ticarcillin + clavulanate Cefoxitin Piperacillin Ceftizoxime Amoxicillin + clavulanate Ampicillin + sulbactam Piperacillin + tazobactam Imipenem Meropenem Ertapenem Tigecycline Chloramphenicol Metronidazole Clindamycin Gatifloxacin
85–95	Ceftizoxime Clindamycin Moxifloxacin Gatifloxacin	Amoxicillin + clavulanate Piperacillin Cefoxitin Ceftizoxime	Ceftazidime Ceftriaxone Clarithromycin Erythromycin Linezolid	Gatifloxacin Moxifloxacin	Ceftriaxone Azithromycin Clarithromycin Erythromycin Linezolid
70–84	Moxalactam Ceftriaxone Clarithromycin Tigecycline Linezolid	Levofloxacin Moxifloxacin Clarithromycin Clindamycin Tigecycline Linezolid	Moxalactam Ofloxacin Azithromycin		Ciprofloxacin Oflaxacin Moxifloxacin
50–69	Cefoperazone Cefotaxime Ceftazidime	Cefoperazone Moxalactam Ofloxacin	Ciprofloxacin Tetracycline Tigecycline		Tetracycline
<50	Vancomycin Ciprofloxacin Azithromycin Erythromycin Tetracycline	Vancomycin Cefotaxime Ceftazidime Ceftriaxone Ciprofloxacin Azithromycin Erythromycin			

[a] The order of listing of drugs within percentage susceptible categories is not significant.
[b] According to the NCCLS-approved breakpoints (M11-A3), using the intermediate category as susceptible.
[c] Excluding B. fragilis

Specific Organisms – Bacteria

Porphyromonas	Sutterella wadsworthensis	F. nucleatum	F. mortiferum and F. varium	Other Fusobacterium	B. wadsworthia
Ceftriaxone	Amoxicillin + clavulanate	Piperacillin	Piperacillin	Ampicillin + sulbactam	Ampicillin + sulbactam
Piperacillin	Ticarcillin + clavulanate	Amoxicillin + clavulanate	Piperacillin + tazobactam	Piperacillin + tazobactam	
Amoxicillin + clavulanate	Cefoxitin	Piperacillin + tazobactam	Ticarcillin + clavulanate	Cefoxitin	
Cefoxitin	Ceftriaxone	Ticarcillin + clavulanate	Cefoxitin	Imipenem	Cefoxitin
Ceftizoxiime	Ciprofloxacin	Cefoxitin	Imipenem	Meropenem	Ceftizoxime
		Ceftizoxime	Meropenem	Chloramphenicol	Piperacillin
Ertapenem	Imipenem	Ceftriaxone	Chloramphenicol	Linezolid	Ticarcillin
Imipenem	Meropenem	Imipenem	Linezolid		Amoxicillin + clavulanate
Meropenem	Ertapenem	Meropenem			Ampicillin + sulbactam
Chloramphenicol		Ertapenem		Metronidazole	Cefoxitin
Tigecycline		Chloramphenicol	Metronidazole	Clindamycin	Ceftizoxime
Linezolid		Tigecycline			Imipenem
Metronidazole		Linezolid		Tetracycline	Chloramphenicol
Azithromycin					
Moxifloxacin		Levofloxacin			Ciprofloxacin
		Gatifloxacin			Metronidazole
		Moxifloxacin			
		Metronidazole			
		Clindamycin			
		Tetracycline			Tetracycline
Ciprofloxacin	Piperacillin		Amoxicillin + clavulanate	Piperacillin	Clindamycin
Clarithromycin	Piperacillin + tazobactam	Azithromycin	Ceftizoxime	Amoxicillin + clavulanate	
Clindamycin	Ceftizoxime		Ceftriaxone	Ticarcillin + clavulanate	
Erythromycin			Moxifloxacin	Cefotaxime	
				Ceftizoxime	
				Ceftriaxone	
	Metronidazole	Ciprofloxacin	Clindamycin	Ceftazidime	Linezolid
			Tetracycline	Moxalactam	
				Ciprofloxacin	
				Azithromycin	
Tetracycline	Clindamycin		Ciprofloxacin		Ertapenem
	Linezolid		Vancomycin		Amoxicillin
	Vancomycin				Ampicillin
		Clarithromycin	Azithromycin	Clarithromycin	Vancomycin
		Erythromycin	Clarithromycin	Erythromycin	
			Erythromycin		

the major anaerobes encountered clinically, as found in the Wadsworth Anaerobic Bacteriology Laboratory experience. Testing was done by the Wadsworth agar dilution method. Antimicrobials not listed in the table are not approved by the Food and Drug Administration or are generally not recommended for therapy of anaerobic infections. In most cases, clinical data support the use of these agents for management of infection with the organisms indicated. Patterns of susceptibility vary among geographic locations and even among hospitals in the same city, primarily because of the patterns of usage of antimicrobial agents. Four drugs or groups of drugs are active against most clinically significant anaerobic bacteria. These are metronidazole; carbapenems, such as imipenem; chloramphenicol; and combinations of β-lactam drugs with a β-lactamase inhibitor. Non–spore-forming anaerobic gram-positive bacilli (eg, *Actinomyces* and *Propionibacterium*) are commonly resistant to metronidazole. There are disturbing reports of resistance in small numbers of strains of the *B. fragilis* group to all of the above agents. Three other drugs or groups of drugs have good activity but are less active than the four groups just mentioned. These are cefoxitin, clindamycin, and broad-spectrum penicillins such as ticarcillin and piperacillin. Some 15% to 25% of strains of the *B. fragilis* group are resistant to these latter compounds in many hospitals in the United States and elsewhere. Cefoxitin and clindamycin are relatively weak in activity against clostridia other than *Clostridium perfringens* (20% to 35% of such strains are resistant), and some anaerobic cocci are resistant to clindamycin.

Some cephalosporins, such as ceftizoxime and ceftriaxone, have sufficient antianaerobic activity to be useful in treating certain anaerobic infections and are comparable with cefoxitin and clindamycin plus gentamicin in double-blind comparative studies. These cephalosporins clearly have been shown to be effective in three types of infections: appendicitis with no more than localized complications, female genital tract infections such as pelvic inflammatory disease and endometritis, and infected foot ulcers or similar soft-tissue infection with or without underlying bone infection. One may save on drug costs with these cephalosporins; this also saves the more potent drugs for serious infections. However, they should not be prescribed for severely ill patients.

Because most anaerobic infections are mixed, involving aerobic or facultative bacteria in addition to anaerobes, antimicrobial therapy must cover the key pathogens of all types. Some of the drugs discussed earlier have significant activity against certain aerobes as well, but it may be necessary to add another agent to cover the other flora.

In general, for therapy of serious anaerobic infections, antimicrobials should be given parenterally in the maximum approved dosages, taking into account the weight and renal and hepatic function of the patient. This is because penetration of drugs into abscesses, necrotic tissue, and poorly perfused tissue, all common in serious anaerobic infections, is less than optimal.

Relatively prolonged therapy is also an important consideration in anaerobic infections to avoid relapse; for example, lung abscess usually requires therapy for several weeks, empyema for 2 to 3 months, and actinomycosis for 6 to 12 months or longer. Duration of therapy must be individualized, taking into account the site, type, extent, and severity of the infection, the nature of the infecting organisms, whether or not the host is immunocompromised or in poor condition because of associated or underlying illness, the speed of response to treatment, and other such factors.

SUGGESTED READING

Ackermann G, Schaumann R, Pless B, Claros MC, Goldstein EJ, Rodloff AC. Comparative activity of moxifloxacin in vitro against obligately anaerobic bacteria. *Eur J Clin Microbiol Infect Dis.* 2000;19:228–232.

Bangsberg DR, Rosen JI, Aragon T, Campbell A, Weir L, Perdreau-Remington F. Clostridial myonecrosis cluster among injection drug users: a molecular epidemiology investigation. *Arch Int Med.* 2002; 162:517–522.

Brook I. *Pediatric Anaerobic Infections.* 3rd ed. New York, NY: Marcel Dekker; 2002.

Duerden BI, Drasar BS, eds. *Anaerobes in Human Disease.* Chichester, UK: Wiley-Liss; 1991.

Finegold SM. Anaerobic infections in humans: an overview. *Anaerobe.* 1995;1:3–9.

Finegold SM, George WL, eds. *Anaerobic Infections in Humans.* San Diego, CA: Academic Press.

Fischer M, Bhatnagar J, Guarner J, et al. Fatal toxic shock syndrome associated with Clostridium sordellii after medical abortion. *New Engl J Med.* 2005;353:2352–2360.

Jousimies-Somer HR, Summanen P, Citron DM, Baron EJ, Wexler HM, Finegold SM. *Wadsworth-KTL Anaerobic Bacteriology Manual*. 6th ed. Belmont, CA: Star; 2002.

Pepin J, Alary M-E, Valiquette L, et al. Increasing risk of relapse after treatment of *Clostridium difficile* colitis in Quebec, Canada. *Clin Infect Dis*. 2005;40:1591–1597.

Styrt B, Gorbach SL. Recent developments in the understanding of the pathogenesis and treatment of anaerobic infections. *New Engl J Med*. 1989;321:240–246, 298–302.

123. Anthrax and Other Bacillus Species

Boris Velimirovic

Anthrax is primarily a disease of grazing domestic animals. It is an acute disease caused by the spore-forming, gram-positive, nonmotile, toxin-producing aerobic rod *Bacillus anthracis*. It is the oldest known zoonosis with worldwide distribution: rare and sporadic and almost disappearing in the United States and in central and northern Europe, moderately common in southern Europe, and common in the former Soviet Union, in tropical and subtropical Africa, Asia, the Caribbean, and South America. The most affected countries are Turkey, Afghanistan, Iran, Pakistan, the Central Asian republics of the former Soviet Union, and sub-Saharan and South Africa. The incidence of human anthrax has decreased considerably in all countries since the introduction of an effective vaccine for use in animals. The frequency of infections in humans depends on the prevalence of the disease in livestock, which increases in years of drought.

EPIDEMIOLOGY

The ability to form spores permits the organism to survive environmental and disinfective measures that destroy most other bacteria. Public health problems largely arise from its long persistence in the soil (up to 90 years). In the Anglo-American biologic warfare experiments conducted in 1942 to 1943 on the uninhabited island of Gruinard off the western coast of Scotland, an estimated 4×10^{14} spores were exploded over the surface. Animal tests for more than 20 years demonstrated the persistence of virulent spores, eventually eliminated by disinfection of the area with a mixture of formaldehyde and sea water. Concern about the military use of anthrax during the 1991 Persian Gulf War resulted in vaccination of U.S. troops. It was estimated that 100 L of spores sprayed over a city could kill 3 million people. In August 1991, Iraq admitted to a United Nations inspection team that it had conducted research on the offensive use of *B. anthracis* before the Persian Gulf War and, in 1995, admitted to "weaponizing" anthrax.

Anthrax bacteria are easy to cultivate and mass produce, and about 30 countries have the capacity to do so. Accidents are also possible, such as the one that occurred in 1979 after an explosion in a Soviet biologic laboratory in former Sverdlovsk (now Ekaterinburg), which generated an aerosol causing at least 42 deaths from anthrax pneumonia. The largest recorded outbreak of cutaneous anthrax in humans occurred in Zimbabwe during the civil war in 1979 to 1980, affecting 6 of the 8 provinces. More than 10 000 human cases and 1832 deaths were documented secondary to an unprecedented outbreak in cattle. It was alleged that this was a deliberately produced enzootic by aerial spread as part of the war efforts.

Infection of the skin comes about by direct occupational contact with contaminated goat hair, wool, hides, bone meal, and other similar products during processing, spinning, and weaving or by direct contact such as with infected carcasses, tissues, and meat.

Inhalation anthrax results from aspiration of *B. anthracis* or spores via small aerosolized *bacillus*-bearing particles. If they are less than 5 µm in size, the spores germinate in the alveoli and multiply. They can also be ingested and absorbed through intestinal mucosa. Vegetative forms multiply in the regional lymph nodes, producing toxin. If transported through oral mucosa, they can produce a cervical form. There is no evidence that milk from infected animals transmits the disease. Biting flies and other insects may perhaps be the mechanical vectors. Incubation is usually 48 hours but may be longer.

For epidemiologic purposes, the disease is divided into agricultural and industrial anthrax; the occupational history is important. At particular risk are veterinarians, veterinary assistants, herders, agricultural and ranch workers, slaughterhouse employees, tannery and textile industry workers, home craftsmen using imported yarn from endemic areas (24 cases in Switzerland in 1978 to 1981), and people handling bone-meal fertilizer. The statement that approximately 90% of human cases reported in recent years occurred in mill workers handling imported goat hair is perhaps valid for inhalation anthrax in a few Western industrialized countries but definitely not true for the world as a whole.

PATHOGENESIS

Anthrax bacilli proliferate at the site of entry and are numerous beneath the central necrotic area of the skin lesion. They are transported to the regional lymph nodes, producing a hemorrhagic lymphadenitis. If they penetrate the bloodstream, septicemia can cause metastatic lesions practically everywhere, with hemorrhagic edema and necrosis.

The virulence of the organism is variable, determined by at least two factors: an extracellular toxin and the capsular polypeptide. The number of organisms in the initial inoculum also plays a role. The toxin causes vascular permeability, edema and fluid loss, and oligemic shock, which is the mechanism of death. The toxin consists of at least three components— edema factor, protective antigen, and lethal factor—each of which is nontoxic but acts synergistically. Differing concentrations of individual toxins in any given strain of *B. anthracis* lead to varying pathogenicity and virulence. Systemic shock and death from anthrax primarily result from the effects of cytokines produced by macrophages stimulated by the lethal toxin.

CLINICAL PICTURE

Infection occurs in three distinct forms: cutaneous, pulmonary, and intestinal.

Cutaneous Infection

The most common form accounts for up to 98% of all cases. There are two types: dry and edematous (see Chapter 120, Bioterrorism, Figure 120.1b). After an incubation period of 1 to 7 days, a small red papule develops at the entry points on the exposed parts of the skin—a minor injury, cut, or abrasion—or after active rubbing on the skin with the fingers, usually on the hand or other parts of the upper extremities, on the face (about half of all cases), lips, eyebrows, or neck but also eyelids, feet, upper chest or back, breast, penis, and scrotum. This papule progresses within 12 to 48 hours to a fluid-filled blister. The fluid in the vesicle is initially clear, but soon it becomes dark and bluish black. The blister is surrounded by inflammation, extensive hard induration, edema in the adjacent deeper tissues, lymphadenitis, and lymphadenopathy. There is no carbuncle. Fever is mild, the lesion is not painful, and double lesions occur. Satellite vesicles can develop near the initial lesion. The vesicle ruptures and develops into a pustule (*pustula maligna*); the tissue necrotizes and progresses to a lesion that is relatively painless, and then it becomes a dark or black eschar (*anthrax* is the Greek word for coal) of about 1 to 3 cm in diameter or larger. This heals and the scab falls off, leaving a scar. The differential diagnosis includes plague and leishmaniasis in endemic areas.

In untreated cases, there may be hematogenous spread via regional lymph nodes, fever, and bacteremia, which may be fatal in 5% to 20% of cases. Localization on the head or neck has a more serious prognosis. Up to 80% of cases of cutaneous anthrax heal spontaneously without treatment.

Pulmonary Infection

Pulmonary (inhalation) anthrax is a rare disease; only two cases were reported between 1920 and 1990 in the United States. It is almost invariably fatal. The illness is biphasic; the initial phase lasts about 4 days and is manifested by a "flulike" illness with a nonproductive cough suggestive of mild bronchopneumonia, atypical pneumonia, influenza, psittacosis, tularemia, legionnaire's disease, *hantavirus* pulmonary syndrome, and pneumonic plague. Radiographs may show mediastinal widening (see Chapter 120, Bioterrorism, Figure 120.1a). The victim may die within 24 hours.

After several days and often after an apparent improvement from the primary phase (in which the patient is well oriented, alert, and unagitated), there is a sudden onset of rapidly progressive respiratory failure, acute dyspnea, circulatory collapse, cyanosis, stridor, signs of pleural effusion, and an elevated temperature. The patient usually dies of toxemia and suffocation within 24 hours of the onset of this second stage. Postmortem findings are of massive pulmonary edema, hemorrhagic mediastinitis, and hydrothorax. Not all persons who inhale the spores develop clinical disease. Subclinical infection, as assumed on the basis of serologic tests, may provide some protection against a new challenge. The pulmonary form of anthrax worries authorities most because of its potential for mass casualties.

Intestinal Infection

The intestinal form is difficult to diagnose. It appears 2 to 5 days after ingestion of meat contaminated with spores of *B. anthracis*, which penetrate the intestinal mucosa. The local ulcerative lesions, most often in the ileocecal region but also in the jejunum, are similar to those of the cutaneous form and are accompanied by nonspecific symptoms such as nausea, vomiting, dizziness, anorexia, fever, abdominal pain, splenomegaly, bloody diarrhea, and hemorrhagic ascites in the absence of liver damage. This may progress to shock and renal failure. About half the patients die. Local lesions, hemorrhagic spots in the serosa, and a typical small, soft, necrotic spleen are characteristic postmortem findings. A gastric form is extremely rare.

Other Clinical Forms

Meningeal anthrax follows cutaneous disease in up to 3% to 5% of cases; it rarely results from inhalation. The hemorrhagic meningitis produced is almost invariably fatal in 2 to 4 days, but successful treatment is documented. Renal, oropharyngeal, and ophthalmic forms have been described.

The incidence of milder or subclinical cases in cutaneous and pulmonary forms, and of chronic cases in the intestinal form, is unknown. The differential diagnosis of anthrax must consider staphylococcal pustular dermatitis, streptococcal lesions, cutaneous diphtheria and plague, any pneumonia in the respiratory form, and various enteric infections in the intestinal form. It is assumed that the clinical disease provides permanent immunity.

LABORATORY DIAGNOSIS

Diagnosis is made by visualization and culture of *B. anthracis* from pus, blood, exudates, or cerebrospinal fluid. *B. anthracis* measures 3 to 8 μm by 1 to 1.5 μm and is surrounded by a large capsule. It is strongly gram positive and non-acid fast. Methylene blue, Wright–Giemsa, and toluidine blue stains are commonly used to demonstrate anthrax bacilli in blood smears. Giemsa or Malachite green stain is best to stain spores. In the gastrointestinal form, the organism can be demonstrated in vomitus or feces and in the pulmonary form in sputum or hemoptysized specimens. Bacilli are usually not present in the bloodstream in large numbers except in septicemia just before death.

The bacillus can be identified by specific fluorescent antibody techniques in tissue sections. Examination of paired sera by indirect microhemagglutination or enzyme-linked immunosorbent assay (ELISA) may be helpful.

Unfortunately, the diagnosis of inhalation and intestinal anthrax is usually made postmortem.

THERAPY

The general approach to management of cutaneous and pulmonary anthrax is presented in Figures 123.1 and 123.2. For specific antibiotic regimens for treatment and prophylaxis please see Chapter 120, Bioterrorism, Table 120.4. Treatment should be started on clinical suspicion, without waiting for laboratory confirmation. In cutaneous anthrax, complete sterilization of the wound is achieved within 24 hours. The edema resolves within about 5 days, although it may increase in the first 24 to 48 hours because of the release of toxin from disintegrating bacilli.

PREVENTION

Prevention of cutaneous anthrax is possible by immunization of persons at high risk (eg, veterinarians in endemic areas, workers in imported wool–processing plants and textile factories) with a cell-free vaccine prepared from a culture filtrate of a nonvirulent, nonencapsulated strain containing the protective antigen (PA) absorbed to aluminum hydroxide gel. The vaccine is given parenterally, three doses at 2-week intervals followed by three booster inoculations at 6-month intervals and then annual booster inoculations. Little is known about the protective effect of vaccine in inhalation anthrax in humans. In experiments, rhesus monkeys survived exposure to a lethal dose only when vaccine and antibiotics (penicillin, ciprofloxacin, and doxycycline) were given simultaneously.

The human live vaccine has been licensed for use in certain endemic areas and reserved as an emergency method to be applied in a critical situation. In addition, scarification and subcutaneous administration and aerosol were used in the former USSR. In 1996, the State Research Institute of Applied Microbiology of Obolensk, Russia, claimed that it had developed a novel vaccine against anthrax in humans, supposed to have not only antitoxic but also antispore activity. The best measure to eliminate human anthrax is control in domestic animals by effective surveillance and the immunization of animals in endemic areas.

A licensed vaccine, currently given to American military personnel, is an aluminum hydroxide–adsorbed preparation (Michigan Biological Product Institute) derived from culture fluid supernatant taken from an attenuated strain. It raises strong humoral

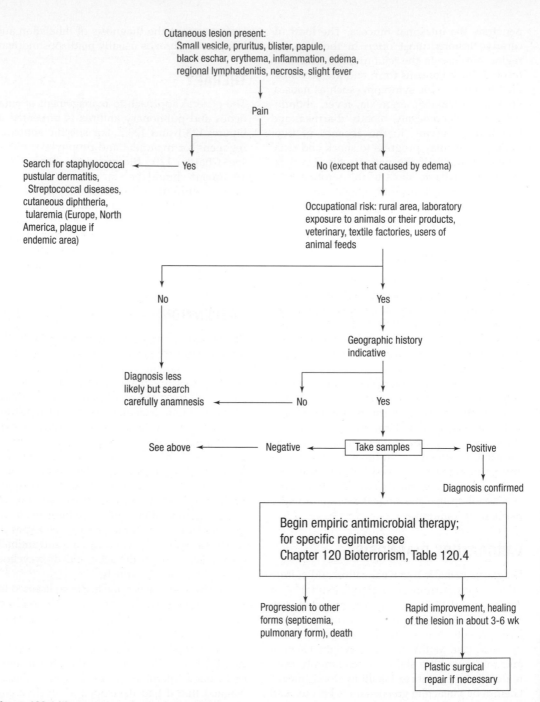

Figure 123.1 Management of cutaneous anthrax.

immunity specifically to lethal toxin. The vaccination series consists of six subcutaneous doses at 0, 2, and 4 weeks, and then at 6, 12, and 18 months, followed by annual boosters. If a biologic warfare attack is threatened or may have occurred, prophylaxis of unimmunized persons with ciprofloxacin (500 mg orally twice a day), or doxycycline (100 mg orally twice a day) is recommended. Should an anthrax attack be confirmed, chemoprophylaxis should be continued for 60 to 100 days and until at least three doses of vaccine have been received by all those exposed.

BACILLACEAE INFECTIONS

Non-*anthracis* bacilli are ubiquitous gram-positive, spore-forming organisms that were

SIGNS OF PNEUMONIA:

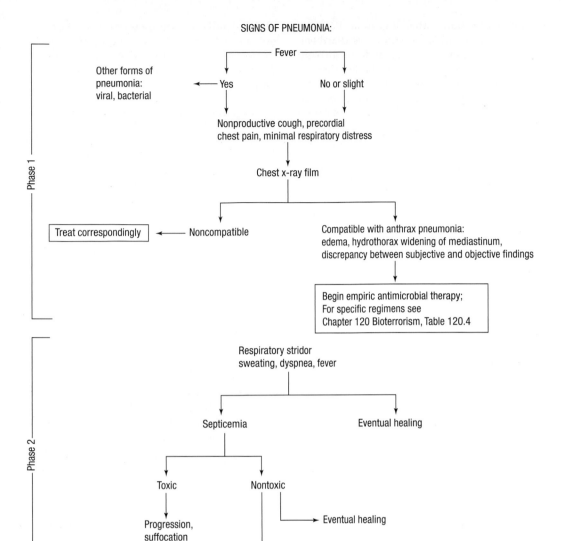

Figure 123.2 Management of pulmonary anthrax.

once believed to be nonpathogenic but are now recognized as causing a variety of infections, injuries, and skin abrasions from road contact in motor vehicle accidents.

Many ubiquitous saprophytic species of aerobic spore-forming bacilli are hard to classify or to distinguish from *B. anthracis* except on the basis of pathogenicity. The *Bacillus* species most commonly encountered are *Bacillus cereus, Bacillus subtilis,* and *Bacillus licheniformis.* Bacilli more or less closely resembling the anthrax bacillus have been isolated from soil, water, meat, fish, bone meal, wool, dust, oil cake, and, less often, from animals and humans. These organisms have been termed *Bacillus pseudoanthracis*

or *Bacillus anthracoides.* Other *Bacillus* species have occasionally been responsible for disseminated infections in immunocompromised hosts.

Bacillus cereus is a gram-positive aerobic or facultatively anaerobic spore-forming rod. It is ubiquitous and is present in soil, dust, water, and on vegetation, food, and spices. It is part of the normal fecal flora. *Bacillus cereus* food poisoning is a toxin-mediated disease rather than infection. It causes a short-incubation emetic illness and a long-incubation diarrheal illness, both by production of enterotoxins. The emetic illness often results from eating poorly preserved or nonrefrigerated fried or boiled rice. The symptoms develop 1 to 6 hours after ingestion. Patients usually recover within 24 hours. The diarrheal syndrome is characterized by abdominal pain and watery stools. It has an incubation time of 10 to 12 hours. Other toxins may contribute to the pathogenicity of *B. cereus* in nongastrointestinal disease. Ten other *Bacillus* species isolated from clinical material other than feces or vomitus were commonly dismissed as saprophytes or opportunistic pathogen contaminants. They are presently recognized as an infrequent cause of serious systemic infection, transient bacteremia, and bronchopneumonia, particularly in neonates and drug addicts, the immunosuppressed, hemodialysis and postsurgical patients, and those with prosthetic implants such as ventricular shunts. The most common severe infections are ocular, including endophthalmitis, panophthalmitis, and keratitis, usually with the characteristic corneal ring abscesses. Even with prompt surgical and antimicrobial treatment, enucleation of the eye and blindness can often result. Simultaneous therapy via more than one route may be required in ocular infection.

Septicemia, meningitis, endocarditis, necrotizing pneumonia, lung abscess, fasciitis, osteomyelitis, and surgical and traumatic wound infections are other manifestations of severe disease. *Bacillus cereus* and most other nonanthrax *Bacillus* species are considered resistant to older penicillins and cephalosporins, including the third generation. They are usually susceptible to treatment with clindamycin, vancomycin, chloramphenicol, and erythromycin. They are also susceptible to aminoglycosides. Vancomycin is considered by some authors as the drug of choice for serious *Bacillus* infections. An addition of fosfomycin to the antibiotic regimen is reported to have resulted in complete cure in the cerebrospinal fluid when vancomycin alone failed. Many strains of *B. cereus* isolated from milk in Nairobi, Kenya, in 1996 showed resistance to eight commonly used antimicrobial agents.

In India, filarial lymphedema is complicated by frequent episodes of dermatolymphadenitis, which do not depend on the presence or absence of microfilariae. *Bacillus cereus* and various cocci have been isolated by biopsies and from the blood. Antibiotic therapy is effective in prevention and treatment. *Bacillus* spores may survive treatment with common disinfectants (except 2% glutaraldehyde, soaking for 10 hours), and they may resist boiling.

SUGGESTED READING

Abramova FA, Grinberg LM, Yampolskaya OV, et al. Pathology of inhalation anthrax in 42 cases from the Sverdlovsk outbreak, 1979. *Proc Natl Acad Sci U S A*. 1993;90:2291–2294.

Bastian L, Weber S, Regel G. Bacillus cereus pneumonia after thoracic trauma. *Anaestesiol Intensivmed Notfallmed Schmerztherap*. 1997;32:124–129.

Drobniewski FA. Bacillus cereus and related species. *Clin Microbiol Rev*. 1993;6:324–338.

Franz DR, Jahrling PB, Friedlander AM, et al. Clinical recognition and management of patients exposed to biological warfare agents. *JAMA*. 1997;278:399–411.

Frazier AA, Franks TJ, Galvin JR. Inhalational anthrax. *JRC Thorac Imag*. 2006;21(4):252–258.

Hanna P. How anthrax kills. *Science*. 1998;280:1671, 1673–1674.

Holty JE, Bravata DM, Liu H, et al. Systematic review: a century of inhalational anthrax cases from 1900 to 2005. *Ann Intern Med*. 2006;144(4):270–280.

Holty JE, Kim RY, Bravate DM. Anthrax: a systematic review of atypical presentations. *Ann Emerg Med*. 2006;48(2):200–211.

Koneman E, et al. *Diagnostic Microbiology*. 5th ed. Philadelphia, PA; Lippincott-Raven; 1997.

Little SF. Anthrax vaccines: a development update. *BioDrugs*. 2005;19(4):233–245.

Velimirovic B. Anthrax. In: Standards Commission of the International Committee of the Office International des Epizooties: *Manual of Recommended Diagnostic Techniques and Requirements for Biological Products*. 15:1, 1989, Paris.

World Health Organization. *Health Aspects of Chemical and Biological Weapons: Report of a WHO Working Group of Consultants*. Geneva, Switzerland: World Health Organization; 1999.

124. Bartonellosis (Carrión's Disease)

Craig J. Hoesley

Bartonellosis is a bacterial disorder with a striking geographic distribution: the western slope of the Peruvian, Ecuadorian, and Colombian Andes 2000 to 8000 feet (725 to 2900 meters) above sea level. The causative microorganism, *Bartonella bacilliformis*, is a small, motile, gram-negative bacillus. Other members of the *Bartonella* genus causing human disease include *Bartonella henselae* (cat scratch disease, bacillary angiomatosis, infective endocarditis), *Bartonella quintana* (trench fever, bacillary angiomatosis, infective endocarditis), *Bartonella clarridgeiae* (cat scratch disease), *Bartonella elizabethae* (infective endocarditis), *Bartonella vinsonii* subsp. *berkhoffii* (infective endocarditis), *Bartonella koehlerae* (infective endocarditis), and *Bartonella grahamii* (neuroretinitis). Bartonellosis, also known as Carrión's disease, is restricted to the Andes region of South America because its vector, a sandfly, *Phlebotomus verrucarum*, is confined to this geographic area.

The clinical manifestations of this unique biphasic illness have been studied extensively. After inoculation by the bite of an infected sandfly, the bacteria enter the endothelial cells of blood vessels and replicate during the incubation period. Within 2 to 6 weeks after infection, the nonimmune host develops Oroya fever (erythrocytic invasive phase), which is characterized by anorexia, headache, malaise, and a potentially striking hemolytic anemia (Figure 124.1). Most commonly, only a few red blood cells are parasitized, and the disease is subclinical or mild without anemia. Less commonly severe disease may occur with up to 100% of erythrocytes parasitized resulting in profound hemolytic anemia and a high mortality.

Historically, mortality in untreated Oroya fever approached 50% as a result of both acute hemolytic anemia and secondary infections. In a report of 68 persons with Oroya fever, the most common symptoms were fever, malaise, anorexia, and headache, whereas the most common signs were pallor, hepatomegaly, cardiac murmur, and jaundice. The mortality rate in this case series was only 9%, suggesting the timely provision of appropriate antibacterial therapy is beneficial. In addition to the anemia, leukopenia with decreased absolute CD4 cell counts produces transient immunosuppression. This initial phase of infection ends with the sudden disappearance of bacteria from the erythrocytes. During the acute or convalescent stage of Oroya fever, secondary infections with *Salmonella*, *Mycobacterium tuberculosis*, amebae, and malaria are possible and contribute significantly to the overall mortality of this disorder.

Individuals who survive the acute phase of infection may or may not develop the cutaneous stage of the disease. Within weeks to months after resolution of the acute phase, superficial and/or subcutaneous nodules evolve in crops on exposed skin. These skin lesions, known as *verruga peruana*, resemble Kaposi's sarcoma or bacillary angiomatosis. Verruga may persist for several months to 1 year and can resolve spontaneously with little or no residua. Individuals who recover from either of the clinical forms of bartonellosis are immune; recurrent Oroya fever does not occur, and recurrent cutaneous manifestations are rare. In 1885, Daniel Carrión, a Peruvian medical student, proved that Oroya fever and verruga peruana were different manifestations of the same infectious agent. He inoculated himself with blood taken from a verruga of an infected patient and, approximately 3 weeks later, developed fever and severe hemolytic anemia that ultimately resulted in his death. In honor of these contributions, bartonellosis is also commonly termed *Carrión's disease*.

The diagnosis is suggested by the clinical picture and by the examination of the peripheral blood film. Bacilli may be seen within red blood cells, either singly or in pairs or clusters. *Bartonella* species are slow growing and fastidious, but they can be cultivated on blood-enriched media (optimally incubated at 25°C to 30°C) or in the presence of endothelial cells. Formation of colonies on an agar surface directly from an infected clinical specimen may require more than 21 days of incubation and subculturing on freshly prepared media. Acridine orange staining procedures and lysis centrifugation

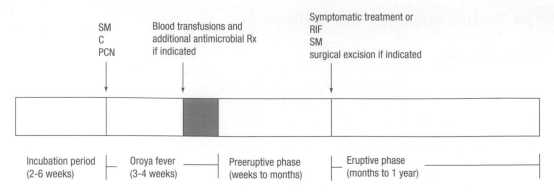

Figure 124.1 Bartonellosis (Carrión's disease); clinical course and treatment. SM = streptomycin; C = chloramphenicol: PCN = penicillin; RIF = rifampin.

Table 124.1 Therapy of *Bartonella* Disease

Oroya Fever Phase	
Agent of choice	Chloramphenicol
Alternative agents	Penicillins
	Streptomycin
	Erythromycin
	Quinolones
	Tetracycline
Verruga Phase	
Agent of choice	Rifampin
	Streptomycin
Alternative agents	Erythromycin and
	sulfonamides

culture methods enhance the detection and recovery, respectively, of *Bartonella* species from blood specimens. Serologic methods may aid in the diagnosis of bartonellosis, including an immunoglobulin M (IgM) fluorescence antibody test, an IgG fluorescence antibody test, an IgG enzyme-linked immunosorbent assay, and an indirect hemagglutination antibody test. The reported sensitivity of serologic assays has ranged from 70% to 82% in the acute phase of the illness and greater than 90% in the chronic cutaneous stage.

THERAPY

Table 124.1 lists therapeutic options for *Bartonella bacilliformis* disease. In patients with Oroya fever, clinical observations suggest that penicillin, chloramphenicol, tetracycline, and streptomycin are effective. Chloramphenicol at a dose of 2 to 4 g/day for 7 or more days is the therapy of choice because of the frequent association of *Salmonella* infection in endemic regions. After the institution of therapy, fever generally disappears within 2 to 3 days,

although blood smears may remain positive for some time. Blood transfusions may be indicated as supportive therapy in patients experiencing massive parasitism and severe anemia during the Oroya fever phase of the disorder.

In the cutaneous phase, verruga lesions do not respond consistently to antimicrobial agents, but a recent review of 77 patients with the eruptive phase of bartonellosis reported a good response to rifampin (46 [84%] of 55 patients) and a modest response to streptomycin (5 [56%] of 9 patients). Verruga lesions refractory to antimicrobial therapy may require surgical resection.

Prevention of infection requires control of the vector with insecticides and the use of insect repellant and bed netting by nonimmune individuals visiting endemic areas.

SUGGESTED READING

Alexander B. A review of bartonellosis in Equador and Columbia. *Am J Trop Med Hyg*. 1995;52:354–359.

Garcia-Caseres U, Garcia F. Bartonellosis: an immunodepressive disease and the life of Daniel Alcides Carrion. *Am J Clin Pathol*. 1991;95:S58–S66.

Ihler G. Bartonella bacilliformis: dangerous pathogen slowly emerging from deep background. *FEMS Microbiol Lett*. 1996;144:1–11.

Maguina C, Garcia PJ, Gotuzzo E, et al. Bartonellosis (Carrión's disease) in the modern era. *Clin Infect Dis*. 2001;33:772–779.

Rolain JM, Brouqui P, Koehler JE, et al. Recommendations of treatment of human infections caused by *Bartonella* species. *Antimicrob Agent Chemother*. 2004;48:1921–1933.

Specific Organisms – Bacteria

125. Cat Scratch Disease and Other Bartonella Infections

William A. Schwartzman

INTRODUCTION

Cat scratch disease (CSD) (La Maladie de Griffe de Chat) was first described in 1950 by Rene Debré. Its cause remained a mystery until the late 20th century, when the polymerase chain reaction (PCR) was applied to amplification and sequencing of 16SRNA genes as a method of identifying organisms that had not been successfully cultured. In 1992, David Relman and co-workers used this technique to identify the agent of CSD, bacillary angiomatosis and parenchymal bacillary peliosis (BAP). The causative organism, a small gram-negative bacillus, belongs to the α_2 subdivision of proteobacteria and is closely related to the agent of trench fever and to *Brucella* sp.

First named *Rochalimaea henselae*, the organism was subsequently grouped within the family Bartonellaceae, along with a number of other mammalian bacterial parasites, including the agents of trench fever, *Bartonella quintana* (formerly *Rochalimaea quintana*) and Carrión's disease, *Bartonella bacilliformis*. These organisms, and probably others of the genus, share the ability to invade vascular endothelial cells, bone marrow erythroblasts, and mature erythrocytes. *Bartonella henselae, B. quintana, and B. bacilliformis* also share the ability to induce macrophage-mediated secretion of proinflammatory cytokines and vascular endothelial cell growth factor (VEGF) and to suppress apoptosis of vascular endothelial cells. These virulence factors are implicated in the proliferative vascular lesions seen with bartonella infections in immunocompromised patients and in the ability of these organisms to cause prolonged bacteremia in nonhuman reservoir species and humans.

Since the identification of *B. henselae*, there has been an explosion of knowledge about the manifestations of CSD and those of the expanding roster of *Bartonella* species that populate a variety of mammalian reservoirs from small rodents to horses, cows, and, in one report, the blood of porpoises (Table 125.1).

The clinical spectrum of CSD in the immunocompetent host includes classic CSD as well as ophthalmologic, neurological, cardiovascular, parenchymal, musculoskeletal, and immune complex–mediated glomerulonephritis as well as prolonged fever without adenopathy or focal lesions. Parenchymal masses associated with CSD have been mistaken for malignancies such as breast cancer or lymphoma.

In hosts with severely compromised cell-mediated immunity, including patients with acquired immunodeficiency syndrome (AIDS), organ transplant recipients, and those with hematological malignancies, *B. henselae* and *B. quintana* cause vascular tumors called bacillary angiomas (BA) and blood-filled cavities of liver and spleen called BAP. We will address the clinical features, diagnosis, and treatment of CSD in its classic form as well as the less common syndromes associated with bartonella infections.

CLASSIC CAT SCRATCH DISEASE

CSD is the most common cause of regional lymphadenitis in children and young adults. Approximately 24 000 cases occur each year with a prevalence of roughly 9.3/10 000 ambulatory patients per year and a seroprevalence ranging from 3% to 6%. CSD tends to occur in late summer or fall and to vary in frequency with the geographic distribution of the cat flea, *Ctenotophyledes felis*.

The first clinical manifestations of CSD appear 5 to 7 days after the scratch or bite from an infected cat (rarely, a dog) or the bite of an infected cat flea, with the appearance of a small erythematous nodule at the site of bacterial entry. Although this inoculation papule may go unnoticed, it is said to be present in 70% of CSD cases. This nodule represents the initial host response to *Bartonella* and is characterized by palisading macrophages, acute and chronic inflammatory cell infiltration, as well as activation and invasion of vascular endothelial cells. Painful swelling of the proximal lymph nodes follows the appearance of the inoculation papule by 7 to 14 days and may be accompanied by constitutional symptoms and fever. The histopathology of the lymph node

Table 125.1 Bartonella Species Currently Reported to Have Caused Zoonotic Infections

Species	Reservoir	Vector	Human Disease
B. henselae	Cat, dog	Cat flea (*Ctenotophylides felis*) other?	CSD, retinitis, IE, myocarditis, encephopathy, aseptic meningitis, myelitis, neuropathy, osteomyelitis, BAP, glomerulonephritis, purpura, pseudomalignancy, prolonged asymptomatic bacteremia
B. quintana	Rat, human?	Louse	CSD, IE, trench fever, encephalopathy, BAP, osteomyelitis, prolonged asymptomatic bacteremia
B. vinsonii subsp. *berkhoffii*	Coyote, dog	Unknown	IE
B. vinsonii subsp. *arupensis*	White-footed mouse	Unknown	IE, neurological disorders
B. koehlerae	Cat	Flea, *C. felis*	IE
B. elizabethae	Rat	Oriental rat flea *Xenopsylla cheopsis*	IE
B. washoensis	California ground squirrel (*Spermophilus beecheyii*)	Unknown	Fever, myocarditis
B. alsatica	Rabbit	Unknown	IE
B. grahamii	Wild mice	Unknown	Neuroretinitis
B. clarridgeae	Cat	Flea, *C. felis*	Possible CSD

is highly characteristic of CSD, involving both acute and chronic inflammatory cells and the presence of microabscesses that are described as "stellate" or star-shaped. Aggregates of small coccobacilli may be identified in these abscesses using either silver impregnation stains such as Warthin–Starry and Steiner stains or by immunofluorescent staining with commercially available monoclonal antibodies specific for *B. henselae* or *B. quintana*. The clinical diagnosis of classic CSD can be confirmed by histopathology, PCR of tissue, or the demonstration of elevated immunoglobulin G (IgG) and IgM antibodies to *B. henselae or B. quintana* by enzyme-linked immunofluorescent assay or direct fluorescent antibody (DFA). Needle aspiration for cytology, special stains, and cultures may be helpful in ruling out malignant, mycobacterial, bacterial, or fungal causes of regional lymphadenopathy. Classic CSD usually resolves over several weeks to months without treatment. Although one prospective randomized controlled trial indicated that a 5-day course of azithromycin hastened the resolution of lymph node swelling, most experts do not recommend antimicrobial

therapy for mild to moderately severe classic CSD. Where lymph nodes become fluctuant and painful, needle aspiration may be all that is required to relieve discomfort and hasten resolution. The syndrome of classic CSD in immunocompetent hosts is thought to be due to an exuberant host response to relatively few organisms, which is one possible explanation for the relatively minor impact of antimicrobials in this setting (Table 125.2).

OPHTHALMOLOGIC CSD

Approximately 3% of CSD patients develop ocular pathology. These manifestations may be unilateral or bilateral and include conjunctivitis, retinitis, choroiditis, iridocyclitis, endophthalmitis, or orbital abscess with osteomyelitis.

Most frequently patients present with retinitis and vision loss in the context of classic CSD; however, ocular infections may present with vision loss unassociated with adenopathy. CSD retinitis may be indicated by the presence of characteristic exudates radiating from the macula, so-called macular star or stellate retinitis.

Table 125.2 Treatment Recommendations for *Bartonella* Infections[a]

Clinical Presentation	Adult Treatment Recommendations
Mild to moderate classic CSD	No antimicrobials recommended
Severe CSD with large painful lymphadenopathy	Azithromycin, 500 mg PO, d 1, 250 mg d 2–5, aspiration if fluctuant
Retinitis	Doxycycline, 100 mg PO BID for 4–6 wk, + rifampin, 300 mg PO BID for 4–6 wk; consider topical corticosteroids
Encephalopathy	Doxycycline, 100 mg PO or IV for 6 wk, + rifampin, 300 mg PO BID for 4–6 wk; duration is not a matter of consensus at this time
Suspected *Bartonella* BCNE	Gentamicin, 3 mg/kg/d × 14 d, + ceftriaxone, 2 g/d IV or IM × 6 wk
Confirmed *Bartonella* BCNE	Gentamicin, 3 mg/kg/d IV × 14 d, + doxycycline, 100 mg BID × 6 wk
Trench fever, prolonged *B. quintana* bacteremia	Gentamicin, 3 mg/kg/d IV × 14 d, + doxycycline, 200 mg/d PO × 4 wk
BA	Erythromycin, 500 mg PO QID × 3 mo, or doxycycline, PO QID 100 mg BID × 3 mo
PH	Erythromycin, 500 mg PO QID × 4 mo, or doxycycline, PO QID 100 mg BID × 4 mo

[a] Adapted from Rolain JM, Brouqui P, Koehler JE, Maguina C, Dolan MJ, Raoult D. Recommendations for treatment of human infections caused by Bartonella species. *Antimicrob Agents Chemother.* 2004;48:1921–1933.

The diagnosis may be confirmed by demonstrating elevated IgG or IgM antibodies to *B. henselae* or PCR of tissue biopsy specimens.

Parinaud oculoglandular syndrome is a nodular, or "cobblestone," conjunctivitis accompanied by enlargement of the preauricular lymph nodes on the side of the conjunctivitis. This is thought to represent conjunctival inoculation of *B. henselae*, with subsequent regional adenopathy, the ocular equivalent of classic CSD.

Resolution of ocular CSD may be spontaneous; however, treatment with 4 to 6 weeks of doxycycline, with rifampin, with or without topical corticosteroids is recommended.

NEUROLOGICAL CSD

Neurological manifestations of CSD are relatively rare, accounting for 0.17% to 2% of cases. These include encephalopathy involving cortex, internal capsule or midbrain, myelopathy, granulomatous cerebral angiitis, vertebral osteomyelitis, and peripheral neuropathy.

This encephalopathy may present with agitation, delirium, or new onset of seizures, including status epilepticus, coma, cerebellar ataxia, and disruptions of basal ganglia or midbrain. Anecdotal reports of successful treatment have included supportive measures with antiepileptic medication, usually accompanied by intravenous antibiotics with or without high-dose corticosteroids. A combination of intravenous or oral doxycycline with rifampin for at least 14 days is recommended; however, the most appropriate choice of antimicrobials, optimum duration of therapy, and the role of corticosteroids in these cases have not been resolved.

A number of mechanisms have been proposed for CSD encephalopathy, including direct bacterial involvement of neurons, host inflammatory response, autoimmune disease, and toxin production.

In immunocompromised patients, an acute psychiatric syndrome similar to acute mania has also been described, which improves rapidly with antimicrobial therapy directed against *B. henselae*, and an association has been noted between intrathecal synthesis of *B. henselae* antibodies and worsening of human immunodeficiency virus (HIV)-associated encephalopathy.

CARDIOVASCULAR INFECTIONS

Bartonella quintana and *B. henselae* are significant causes of blood culture-negative infectious endocarditis (BCNE). Estimates of the relative contributions of bartonella species to these infections are based on several large case series from reference centers equipped to diagnose these relatively fastidious organisms, including the agent of Q fever, *Coxiella burnettii*, *Legionella pneumophila*, *Brucella* species, *Chlamydia psittaci*, *Tropherema whipplei*, *Mycoplasma hominis*, nutritionally deficient streptococci, and the fungal causes of BCNE.

In a series of 349 cases of BCNE reported by Houpikian and Raoult in 2005, *Bartonella* species accounted for 29% of all cases. *Bartonella quintana* represented 75% of these and *B. henselae* 25%. As reported in previous series, *B. quintana* endocarditis was associated with body louse infestation, immunodeficiency, and chronic alcoholism, whereas *B. henselae* endocarditis was associated with cat contact and pre-existing valvular disease. The overall mortality was 7% with no difference between the two species. The aortic valve was the predominant site for both species, and valve replacement was performed in 75% of cases. Several cases of renal failure secondary to necrotizing crescentic glomerulonephritis have been reported in the context of both *B. henselae* and *B. quintana* endocarditis.

To date, four additional *Bartonella* species have been reported to cause infective endocarditis (IE) in humans, *Bartonella vinsonii*, *Bartonella* subsp. *berkhoffii*, *Bartonella elizabethae*, *Bartonella koehlerae*, and *Bartonella alsatica*. The diagnosis of bartonella endocarditis was made by culture in roughly 30% of cases, whereas PCR of valvular tissue yielded 67%. Serological demonstration of anti-*Bartonella* antibody titers ≤1:800 by DFA provided an acceptable noninvasive method of diagnosis in this series.

Suspected *Bartonella* BCNE should be treated with gentamicin for 2 weeks, combined with 6 weeks of intravenous or intramuscular ceftriaxone, to cover other possible causes of BCNE, with or without oral or intravenous doxycycline for 6 weeks. For proven bartonella endocarditis, a combination of gentamicin for 2 weeks plus intravenous or oral doxycycline for 6 weeks is recommended.

Although rare, myocarditis has been associated with *Bartonella* infections. *Bartonella washoensis*-associated myocarditis was reported in a 70-year-old immunocompetent man, presumably associated with the presence of a large reservoir of the organism in the California ground squirrels (*Spermophilus beecheyii*) in recreational areas near Reno, Nevada. *Bartonella henselae* has been associated with a case of chronic active myocarditis in a 43-year-old immunocompetent man with classic CSD. An autoimmune reaction triggered by the *B. henselae* infection was postulated.

PROLONGED BACTEREMIA WITHOUT ENDOCARDITIS

Prolonged symptomatic or asymptomatic bacteremia is more frequently caused by *B. quintana* but may also be caused by *B. henselae* as well as other less common members of the genus. When accompanied by fever and constitutional symptoms, prolonged, relapsing *B. quintana* bacteremia was called trench fever in World War I and was at first thought to be a variant of endemic typhus, until Dr. Henrique da Rocha Lima determined it to be a distinct louseborne infection. Following World War II, trench fever was considered to be an historical relic, until its resurrection in the late 20th century as a significant cause of illness among the world's growing population of urban homeless, so-called urban trench fever.

Although the relation of prolonged bacteremia to infectious endocarditis has not been established, it is assumed that antimicrobial treatment of *B. henselae* and *B. quintana* bacteremia may have a role in preventing endocarditis. The currently recommended therapy for *B. henselae* and *B. quintana* bacteremia is intravenous gentamicin for 14 days with oral or intravenous doxycycline for 28 days. A thorough search for evidence of endocarditis should accompany the treatment of bartonella bacteremia.

PARENCHYMAL CSD

CSD with or without regional lymphadenopathy may be accompanied by hepatic or splenic foci of infection. The clinical presentation of hepatosplenic bartonellosis includes chronic or subacute course characterized by fever and abdominal pain that may be accompanied by nausea and vomiting. Hepatic transaminases may be elevated and may demonstrate disproportionate elevations of hepatic alkaline phosphatase over aspartate aminotransferase (AST) and alanine aminotransferase (ALT). Abdominal ultrasound or computerized axial tomography may demonstrate radiolucencies in liver and spleen. Histopathology of these lesions frequently demonstrates either necrotizing granulomas or stellate microabscesses similar

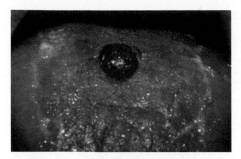

Figure 125.1 Lingual bacillary angiomatosis in acquired immunodeficiency syndrome.

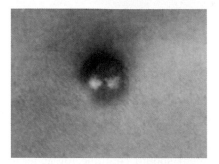

Figure 125.2 Cutaneous bacillary angiomatosis in acquired immunodeficiency syndrome.

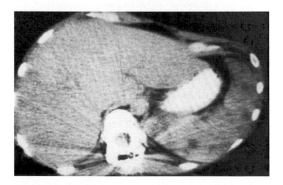

Figure 125.3 Computed tomography scan of splenic bacillary angiomatosis and peliosis.

to those described in the lymph nodes of classic CSD. Anecdotal reports suggest that doxycycline plus rifampin for periods of from 7 to 14 days may be effective in these cases, but spontaneous resolution has also been documented and there is currently no consensus favoring antimicrobial treatment.

MUSCULOSKELETAL

Bartonella henselae is a rare cause of osteomyelitis. Small case series describe typical presentations, including fever and bone pain in children or young adults with cat or kitten exposure, with or without associated lymph-adenopathy. These may involve single or multiple foci of infection and frequently involve the axial skeleton or pelvic bones. The etiologic diagnosis in these cases was made by serology, histopathology, or PCR of bone biopsy specimens. There is no evidence that antimicrobial therapy is effective.

BARTONELLA IN IMMUNOCOMPROMISED PATIENTS

Infections in immunocompetent hosts are characterized by an exuberant inflammatory response to relatively few organisms and a poor response to antimicrobial agents. However, in those with compromised cell-mediated immunity, such as individuals with AIDS or hematological malignancies, organ transplant recipients, those receiving immunomodulating agents for treatment of hepatitis C, or those with rheumatologic diseases, the same organisms commonly cause systemic infections characterized by vasoproliferative lesions teeming with organisms. These respond dramatically to antimicrobial therapy.

The proliferative vascular lesions seen in these patients (BA) may develop in practically any anatomical site or organ, including skin, mucosa of the nasopharynx, gastrointestinal tract, central nervous system, bone, or lymph nodes. Cutaneous BA is a 1-cm to 2-cm erythematous nodule with a surrounding collar of scaling skin (Figures 125.1 to 125.2). These are friable and bleed easily and may itch.

Microscopically, they are formed by the growth of disorganized vascular channels, with prominent, rounded endothelial cells projecting into irregular vascular lumens. These lesions are easily distinguished from the more organized spindle cells of Kaposi's sarcoma. When stained with hematoxylin and eosin, azurophilic granular material can be seen representing clumps of bartonella. Although they may also be seen with Brown–Brenn tissue Gram stain or silver impregnation stains such as Steiner or Warthin–Starry, they are more easily visualized by immunohistochemical or immunofluorescent methods.

A second type of vascular lesion, bacillary parenchymal peliosis or peliosis hepatitis (PH), may involve liver or spleen. Computerized tomography (CT) or magnetic resonance imaging may demonstrate hypodense nodular lesions (Figure 125.3). Histologically, PH lesions are blood-filled areas that appear to arise where normal sinusoidal endothelial cells

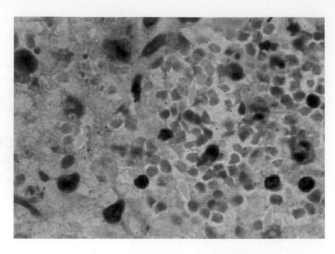

Figure 125.4 *Bartonella henselae*, peliosis hepatitis in acquired immunodeficiency syndrome immunohistochemical stain with rabbit anti-*B. henselae* GroEL. Erythrocytes with dark red stain (eg, those indicated with green arrows) are infected with *B. henselae*.

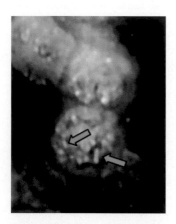

Figure 125.5 Immunofluorescent image (100×) of erythrocytes in Fig. 125.4, optical section at the miderythrocyte level, image deconvolved to eliminate haze. Numerous small bacilli are seen within the erythrocytes (green arrows).

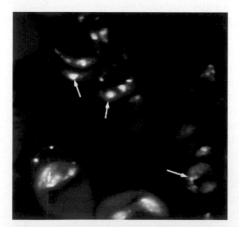

Figure 125.6 Confocal laser image of same specimen with superimposed phase contrast image of erythrocytes (red pseudo color, fluorescent bacteria are indicated by white arrows).

have become disrupted by *Bartonella* infection. The endothelial cells and erythrocytes of these lesions contain intracellular bacteria (Figures 125.4–125.6).

Treatment of patients with BAP usually results in a rapid clinical improvement; however, treatment should continue for at least 3 months to avoid relapses. Although erythromycin is recommended, doxycycline appears to be as effective, with fewer gastrointestinal side effects.

SUGGESTED READING

Bhatti Z, Berenson CS. Adult systemic cat scratch disease associated with therapy for hepatitis C. *BMC Infect Dis*. 2007;7:8.

Foucault C, Brouqui P, Raoult D. Bartonella quintana characteristics and clinical management. *Emerg Infect Dis*. 2006;12: 217–223.

Houpikian P, Raoult D. Blood culture-negative endocarditis in a reference center: etiologic diagnosis of 348 cases. *Medicine (Baltimore)*. 2005;84:162–173.

Koehler JE, Sanchez MA, Tye S, et al. Prevalence of Bartonella infection among human immunodeficiency virus-infected patients with fever. *Clin Infect Dis*. 2003;37:559–566.

Martinez-Osorio H, Calonge M, Torres J, et al. Cat-scratch disease (ocular bartonellosis) presenting as bilateral recurrent iridocyclitis. *Clin Infect Dis*. 2005;40:e43–e45.

Mathieu S, Vellin JF, Poujol D, et al. Cat scratch disease during etanercept therapy. *Joint Bone Spine*. 2007; Mar;74(2):184–186. Epub 2007 Feb 5.

Ohl ME, Spach DH. Bartonella quintana and urban trench fever. *Clin Infect Dis*. 2000;31:131–135.

Specific Organisms – Bacteria

Relman DA, Loutit JS, Schmidt TM, et al. The agent of bacillary angiomatosis. An approach to the identification of uncultured pathogens. *N Engl J Med*. 1990;323:1573–1580.

Rolain JM, Brouqui P, Koehler JE, et al. Recommendations for treatment of human infections caused by Bartonella species. *Antimicrob Agents Chemother*. 2004;48:1921–1933.

Wheeler SW, Wolf SM, Steinberg EA. Cat-scratch encephalopathy. *Neurology*. 1997;49:876–878.

126. Bordetella

Sarah S. Long

Bordetellae are fastidious, non–carbohydrate-fermenting, tiny, gram-negative coccobacilli that grow aerobically on starch blood agar or synthetic medium supplemented with nicotin-amide and amino acids for growth and char-coal or cyclodextrin resin for protection from fatty acids and other inhibitory substances. Bordetellae have multiple attachment proteins, including a 69-kd outer membrane protein (pertactin), filamentous hemagglutinin, and fimbriae. *Bordetella pertussis* is the only species that expresses the major virulence protein, per-tussis toxin. *Bordetella pertussis* is an exclusive human pathogen that is the sole cause of epi-demic pertussis and the usual cause of sporadic pertussis. *Bordetella parapertussis* is an infrequent cause of pertussis and is genetically more closely aligned with *Bordetella bronchiseptica*, a common veterinary pathogen causing upper respira-tory tract illnesses in animals. Other *Bordetella* species do not cause pertussislike illnesses. Occasional case reports of *B. bronchiseptica* in humans include upper and lower respiratory tract illnesses, endocarditis, septicemia, post-traumatic meningitis, and peritonitis. *Bordetella holmesii* and *B. holmesii*-like organisms have oc-casionally caused bronchitis, endocarditis, sep-ticemia, and respiratory failure. *Bordetella hinzii* has caused bloodstream infection in a handful of cases, associated usually with pulmonary symptoms. Asplenia or immunosuppression has been present in many adults infected with *Bordetella* non-*pertussis* and non-*parapertussis* species. Exposure to pets is also a factor.

EPIDEMIOLOGY AND CLINICAL MANIFESTATIONS

Pertussis is the only vaccine-preventable dis-ease for which universal immunization is given and the incidence of which continues to rise. The >25 000 cases reported in the United States in 2004 were the highest number reported since 1959. The actual number of cases is likely to be exponentially greater than that reported, because pertussis is undersuspected, under-diagnosed, and underreported. Age-related incidence of pertussis is highest in infants ≤2 months of age (~200 per 100 000), but the great-est number of cases and the reservoir for *B. pertussis* occur in adolescents, adults, and the elderly who have waned immunity following preschool vaccination and lack natural subclini-cal reinfections that boosted immunity in a pre-vious era. It was estimated during a prospective vaccine trial in adults that there are possibly 1 million cough illnesses due to *B. pertussis* in the United States annually.

Classic pertussis illness occurs almost ex-clusively in unimmunized older infants and children. It includes 2-week stages: an afebrile, upper respiratory tract illness with escalating cough (catarrhal stage) followed by paroxysms of machine-gun bursts of coughing, frequently with whoops and posttussive vomiting (parox-ysmal stage), fading into fewer and less severe paroxysms (convalescent stage). Young infants have rapid onset of "fits" of gagging, gasping, and cyanotic or apneic episodes, with parox-ysmal cough and whoop occurring only later, sometimes in convalescence. Adults do not have distinct stages, and at least one third have only a prolonged nonspecific cough illness. Clues to pertussis in adolescents and adults are (1) pure or predominant cough illness that is escalating after 1 week, (2) cough illness in which there are sudden paroxysms (repeated bursts of cough on one breath, bulging watery eyes, red face), or (3) cough illness associated with posttussive emesis. Patients are afebrile, have few upper or lower respiratory tract signs or symptoms, do not have myalgia or malaise, and are well between paroxysms. Adults with pertussis describe a typical paroxysm as begin-ning with an aura of anxiety and fear to take a breath, followed by strangulating cough, feel-ing of suffocation, and posttussive exhaustion. Whoop is uncommon.

DIAGNOSIS

Differential diagnosis predominantly includes other infectious agents such as *Mycoplasma pneu-moniae*, *Chlamydophila pneumoniae*, adenovirus, influenza, and parainfluenza. History of illness onset is most helpful. These other infections typically begin abruptly and include fever, systemic symptoms, multiple mucous membrane involvement, or rash—none of which is part of pertussis. Simple laboratory tests generally are not helpful in differentiating causes, as only unimmunized persons with pertussis have remarkable lymphocytosis.

Culture is still considered the gold standard for laboratory diagnosis of pertussis. Culture requires (1) collection of a posterior nasopharyngeal specimen obtained either by aspiration or with Dacron or calcium alginate swab, (2) use of Regan–Lowe transport medium, and (3) inoculation of specialized agar medium and incubation for up to 10 days. Polymerase chain reaction (PCR) assay is being used increasingly because of possible improved sensitivity and rapid result. The PCR test requires similar collection of a posterior nasopharyngeal specimen using a Dacron swab (not a calcium alginate) or nasal wash technique. No U.S. Food and Drug Administration (FDA)-licensed PCR test is available, and there are no standardized protocols, reagents, or reporting formats. Unacceptably high rates of false-positive results are reported from some laboratories and have led to misidentification of outbreaks. Direct fluorescent antibody (DFA) testing offers rapid identification on direct smears of nasopharyngeal specimens, using monoclonal antibodies. DFA is performed reliably only by experienced technologists. Serologic testing for increase/seroconversion of immunoglobulin G (IgG) antibody to pertussis toxin (PT-IgG) in acute and convalescent serum in a previously unimmunized individual, or a single level in the second to third week of cough illness that is >2 standard deviations above the expected resting level in distantly immunized individuals is diagnostic. Standardization of testing, reporting, and diagnostic cutoff levels is under development. Generally, PT-IgG levels >2 years after immunization of >90 EU/mL is highly suggestive, and levels > 50 EU/mL are suggestive of pertussis.

In unimmunized individuals, pertussis usually is confirmed easily by positive DFA, PCR, and culture. However, these tests are positive in ≤10% of cough illnesses due to *B. pertussis* in adolescents and adults. A single elevated serum PT-IgG antibody level is the best diagnostic test in adolescents and adults.

TREATMENT

An antimicrobial agent is given when pertussis is suspected or confirmed, for potential clinical benefit and to limit the spread of infection to others (Table 126.1). In vitro, *B. pertussis* is susceptible to erythromycin, newer macrolides, quinolones, and third-generation cephalosporins. A macrolide is the preferred agent for treatment. Ampicillin, rifampin, and trimethoprim–sulfamethoxazole have modest activity, but first- and second-generation cephalosporin do not. In clinical studies, erythromycin is superior to amoxicillin for eradication of *B. pertussis*. Rare isolates resistant to erythromycin have been reported. *B. parapertussis* is less susceptible in vitro to all agents except erythromycin. *Bordetella bronchiseptica* is susceptible in vitro to antipseudomonal penicillins, aminoglycosides, and quinolones but generally is not susceptible to cephalosporins; clinical failure has occurred with agents effective in vitro. *Bordetella holmesii* has in vitro susceptibilities similar to *B. bronchiseptica*, but isolates have been susceptible to third-generation cephalosporins.

Secondary sinusitis, otitis media, bronchitis, or pneumonia can complicate *B. pertussis* infection, which denudes ciliated epithelium and inhibits local phagocytic function. Pathogens of secondary infections are *Streptococcus pneumoniae*, *Staphylococcus aureus*, *Haemophilus influenzae*, and *Moraxella catarrhalis*. Convalescence is protracted, with exacerbations of cough with subsequent respiratory illnesses; these are not caused by reinfection or reactivation of *B. pertussis*.

Control Measures

Postexposure prophylaxis (PEP) using the same agents, doses, and duration as for treatment (Table 126.1) should be given promptly to all household contacts and other close contacts regardless of their age or history of immunization. Studies have repeatedly shown efficacy of chemoprophylaxis in maternal–neonatal exposure, in households, and in residential facilities. PEP of contact has little effect if instituted ≥2 weeks after exposure to the index case. Health care workers (HCWs) not wearing a mask who were exposed at close range to an individual with pertussis before the fifth day of treatment should be given PEP promptly. Cases and contacts with any respiratory tract illness should be excluded from high-risk settings (eg, school, health care facilities) until the fifth day of treatment.

Five doses of Tdap vaccine should be given on the recommended schedule before 7 years of age. In 2006, universal immunization of adolescents was recommended at 11 to 12 years

Table 126.1 Recommended Antimicrobial Agents for Treatment and Postexposure Prophylaxis of Pertussis[a]

Agents	Age Group			
	≤1 month	1–5 months	≥6 months and children	Adults
Primary Agents				
Azithromycin	Recommended agent 10 mg/kg/d, once daily ×5 d	10 mg/kg once daily ×5 d	10 mg/kg (max 500 mg) once on d 1; then 5 mg/kg (max 250 mg) once on d 2–5	500 mg once on d 1; then 250 mg once on d 2–5
Clarithromycin	Not recommended	15 mg/kg/d divided BID ×7 d	15 mg/kg/d (Max 1 g/d) divided BID ×7 d	1 g/d divided BID ×7 d
Erythromycin	Not preferred	40–50 mg/kg/d divided QID ×14 d	40–50 mg/kg/d (Max 2 g/d) divided QID × 14 d	2 g/d divided QID × 14 d
Alternate Agent				
TMP-SMX	Contraindicated	Contraindicated at age ≤2 mo. At ≥2 mo, TMP 8 mg/kg/d-SMX 40 mg/kg/d divided BID ×14 d	TMP 8 mg/kg/d-SMX 40 mg/kg/d (max TMP 320 mg/d) divided BID ×14 d	TMP 320 mg-SMX 1600 mg/d divided BID ×14 d

Abbreviations: TMP-SMX = trimethoprim-sulfamethoxazole; BID = twice a day; QID = four times a day.
[a] Recommendations of the Centers for Disease Control and Prevention and the American Academy of Pediatrics.

of age (with catch-up of older adolescents) using Tdap vaccine, which has reduced content of diphtheria toxoid and acellular pertussis antigens compared with pediatric DTaP. Tdap also is recommended by the Centers for Disease Control and Prevention (CDC) for adults who have not previously received Tdap, to replace Td with emphasis on earlier implementation in HCWs with direct patient contact and in family members and other close contacts of newborn babies. When pertussis is suspected or confirmed, immunization status of contacts should be evaluated, and DTaP (for children ≤7 years) or Tdap (for individuals aged 11 to 64 years) should be given promptly if recommended doses were not received previously.

SUGGESTED READING

American Academy of Pediatrics. Pertussis. In: Pickering LK, ed. *2006 Red Book: Report of the Committee on Infectious Diseases*. 27th ed. Elk Grove Village, IL: American Academy of Pediatrics; 2006:498–520.

Baughman AL, Bisgard KM, Edwards KM, et al. Establishment of diagnostic cutoff points for levels of serum antibodies to pertussis toxin, filamentous hemagglutinin, and fimbriae in adolescents and adults in the United States. *Clin Diagn Lab Immunol.* 2004;11:1045–1053.

Calugar A, Ortega-Sanchez IR, Tiwari T, et al. Nosocomial pertussis: costs of an outbreak and benefits of vaccinating healthcare workers. *Clin Infect Dis.* 2006;42:981–988.

Centers for Disease Control and Prevention. Preventing pertussis among adults: recommendations for use of tetanus and diphtheria toxoids and acellular pertussis (Tdap) vaccine. *Morbid Mortal Weekly Rep.* 2006;55(RR17):1–33.

Centers for Disease Control and Prevention. Preventing tetanus, diphtheria and pertussis among adolescents: use of tetanus toxoid, reduced diphtheria toxoid and acellular pertussis vaccines: Recommendations of the Advisory Committee on Immunization Practices (ACIP). *Morbid Mortal Weekly Rep.* 2006;55(RR-2):1–35.

Committee on Infectious Diseases, American Academy of Pediatrics. Prevention of pertussis among adolescents: recommendations for use of tetanus toxoid, reduced diphtheria toxoid, and acellular pertussis (Tdap) vaccine. *Pediatrics.* 2006;117:965–978.

Lee GM, Lett S, Schauer S, et al. Societal costs and morbidity of pertussis in adolescents and adults. *Clin Infect Dis.* 2004;39:1572–1580.

Senzilet LD, Halperin SA, Spika JS, et al. Pertussis is a frequent cause of prolonged cough illness in adults and adolescents. *Clin Infect Dis.* 2001;32:1691–1697.

Tiwari T, Murphy TV, Moran J, et al. National Immunization Program. Centers for Disease Control and Prevention. Recommended antimicrobial agents for treatment and postexposure prophylaxis of pertussis. *Morbid Mortal Weekly Rep*. 2005;54 (RR-14):1–13.

Ward JI, Cherry JD, Chang S-J, et al. Efficacy of an acellular pertussis vaccine among adolescents and adults. *N Engl J Med*. 2005;353:1–9.

Specific Organisms – Bacteria

127. *Moraxella (Branhamella) catarrhalis*

Lisa S. Hodges and Joseph A. Bocchini, Jr.

Once thought a nonpathogenic inhabitant of the human respiratory tract, *Moraxella catarrhalis* is now recognized as an important etiologic agent of otitis media in children, sinusitis in children and adults, and pneumonia in adults with chronic obstructive pulmonary disease (COPD).

Moraxella catarrhalis is a gram-negative kidney-shaped diplococcus similar in morphology to the *Neisseria*. The bacterium was first described by Ghon and Pfeiffer as *Micrococcus catarrhalis* in 1902 and has since undergone several reclassifications. In 1970 it was placed into the genus *Branhamella* based on fatty acid content and DNA homology. In 1979 the name *Moraxella (Branhamella) catarrhalis* was proposed, and this is the most widely accepted nomenclature at this time.

EPIDEMIOLOGY

Moraxella catarrhalis has been recovered exclusively from humans and is a normal inhabitant of the upper respiratory tract. Colonization rates are highest in infants and young children (40%–70%), decreasing into adulthood (1%–5%). The organism is recovered with increased frequency in children with recurrent otitis media and in adults with chronic lung disease.

Infection with *M. catarrhalis* is seasonal with an increase in prevalence during winter and spring months.

PATHOGENESIS

The pathogenesis of infection is complex with both host and bacterial factors determining the evolution from colonization to clinical disease. *Moraxella catarrhalis* expresses adhesion factors and several outer membrane proteins that facilitate preferential binding to human pharyngeal and middle ear epithelial cells. Some strains of *M. catarrhalis* demonstrate an ability to form biofilms in sequestered sites such as the middle ear.

Prior colonization of the nasopharynx by *M. catarrhalis* appears to enhance the adherence and invasion of human epithelial cells by *S. pyogenes*. *Moraxella catarrhalis* has been seen in association with group A β-hemolytic streptococcus in acute pharyngotonsilitis.

Risk factors that allow *M. catarrhalis* to proceed from oropharyngeal to tracheobronchial colonization in adults include smoking, cardiopulmonary disease, corticosteroids, immunosuppressive agents, malignancy, underlying lung disease, and immunoglobulin G deficiency.

CLINICAL SYNDROMES

Moraxella catarrhalis is the third most common etiologic cause of acute otitis media in infants and children after *S. pneumoniae* and *Haemophilus influenzae*. Cultures of middle ear fluid reveal that 15% to 20% of infections are caused by *M. catarrhalis*. Infections are clinically indistinguishable from those caused by nontypeable *H. influenzae* and *S. pneumoniae* and can be polymicrobial.

Moraxella catarrhalis is a common cause of acute sinusitis in children and adults. It is isolated alone or in combination with other bacteria, from the sinus aspirates of 15% to 20% of children with clinical and radiographic evidence of acute sinusitis and is exceeded only by *S. pneumoniae* and nontypeable *H. influenzae* as a causative agent.

Moraxella catarrhalis is a well-recognized cause of lower respiratory tract infection in adults, particularly in the setting of COPD and other chronic lung diseases. Acute exacerbation of chronic bronchitis is the most common lower respiratory tract infection caused by this organism.

Moraxella catarrhalis is the second most common bacterial cause of acute exacerbations of COPD after nontypeable *H. influenzae*. One study estimated that this organism was responsible for 30% of acute exacerbations. Exacerbations are characterized by cough, purulent sputum production, shortness of breath, and occasionally low-grade fever. Pneumonia occurs predominantly in persons over the age of 50 but can be seen in younger individuals. It is usually mild to moderate in severity with either patchy or lobar alveolar infiltrates on chest radiograph. Bacteremia is rare, and pleural effusion and empyema are uncommon. A presumptive diagnosis can be made from a sputum smear that demonstrates many poly-morphonuclear leukocytes with intracellular and extracellular gram-negative diplococci. Because *M. catarrhalis* is somewhat resistant to decolorization, this step in the Gram-stain procedure requires special attention.

Nosocomial outbreaks with a single strain of *M. catarrhalis* have been reported, implicating person-to-person transmission in a susceptible population such as seen in respiratory units and health care facilities.

Less common clinical syndromes associated with *M. catarrhalis* include conjunctivitis in infants that mimics the opthalmia neonatorum of *Neisseria gonorrhoeae*. Meningitis, especially in children, has occurred as a result of hema-togenous spread from the nasopharynx or as a consequence of ventriculoperitoneal shunt placement or surgery. Bacteremia in children may present like occult pneumococcal bacteremia but has also been associated with petechial and purpuric rashes resembling meningococcemia. Bacteremia in adults has been reported in patients with chronic lung disease secondary to lower respiratory tract infection and in normal hosts, usually without an evident portal of entry. Other infections include tracheitis, endocarditis, pericarditis, septic arthritis, osteomyelitis, and peritonitis.

THERAPY

In many cases of otitis media and mild-to-moderate exacerbations of COPD, spontaneous resolution of *M. catarrhalis* infection occurs with the development of strain-specific immunity, an important consideration in determining the need for antimicrobial therapy in an individual patient.

Virtually all strains of *M. catarrhalis* now produce β-lactamase, making them resistant to penicillin, amoxicillin, and ampicillin. Three β-lactamases (BRO-1, BRO-2, and BRO-3) are found in *M. catarrhalis* and are chromosomal in origin, possibly acquired by interspecies gene transfer from a gram-positive organism. The addition of a β-lactamase inhibitor (clavulanate, sulbactam, or tazobactam) to a penicillin restores its bactericidal activity against *M. catarrhalis*.

Moraxella catarrhalis is susceptible to amoxicillin–clavulanate, ampicillin–sulbactam, piperacillin–tazobactam, second- and third-generation cephalosporins (including the oral agents), aminoglycosides, aztreonam, and carbapenems. It is also sensitive to macrolides, tetracyclines, trimethoprim–sulfamethoxizole (TMP-SMX), and fluoroquinolones.

Most infections caused by *M. catarrhalis* can be treated with oral antibiotics. For acute otitis media or sinusitis documented by tympanocentesis or sinus aspiration, respectively, to be caused by *M. catarrhalis*, amoxicillin–clavulanate administered for 10 days (otitis media) or 2 weeks (sinusitis) is the drug of choice. In patients with known penicillin allergy, macrolides, TMP-SMX, or fluoroquinolones may be used where appropriate.

Acute exacerbations of chronic bronchitis caused by *M. catarrhalis* can also be treated with a variety of oral antibiotics, including amoxicillin–clavulanate, second- or third-generation cephalosporins, TMP-SMX, macrolides, doxycycline, or fluoroquinolones.

For more serious infections, such as pneumonia, parenteral antibiotics are generally preferred. The drug of choice for *M. catarrhalis* pneumonia is ampicillin–sulbactam; however, ceftriaxone could also be used. In patients with known penicillin allergy, a macrolide or a fluoroquinolone is an acceptable alternative.

In most patients with otitis, sinusitis, or an acute exacerbation of chronic bronchitis, the etiologic agent will not be known. The decision to treat and the choice of empiric therapy should consider *M. catarrhalis* but include all common pathogens associated with the specific infection syndrome.

SUGGESTED READING

Deshpande LM, Sader HS, Fritsche TR, Jones RN. Contemporary prevalence of BRO β-lactamases in Moraxella catarrhalis: report from the SENTRY antimicrobial surveillance program (North America, 1997 to 2004). *J Clin Microbiol.* 2006;44:3775–3777.

Hall-Stoodley L, Hu FZ, Gieseke A. Direct detection of bacterial biofilms on middle-ear mucosa of children with chronic otitis media. *JAMA.* 2006;296:202–211.

Hendley JO, Hayden FG, Winther B. Weekly point prevalence of Streptococcus pneumoniae, Haemophilus influenzae and Moraxella catarrhalis in the upper airways of normal young children: effect of respiratory illness and season. *Acta Pathol Microbiol Immunol Scand.* 2005;113:213–220.

Lafontaine ER, Wall D, Vanlerberg SL, Donabedian H, Sledjeski DD. Moraxella catarrhalis coaggregates with Streptococcus pyogenes and modulates interactions of

S. pyogenes with human epithelial cells. *Infect Immun.* 2004;72:6689–6693.

Murphy TF, Brauer AL, Grant BJ, Sethi S. Moraxella catarrhalis in chronic obstructive pulmonary disease. *Am J Respir Crit Care Med.* 2005;172:195–199.

Murphy TF. Moraxella (Branhamella) catarrhalis and other gram-negative cocci. In *Principles and Practice of Infectious Diseases.* 6th ed. Philadelphia, PA: Elsevier; 2005.

Yokota S, Harimaya A, Sato K, Somekawa Y, Himi T, Fujii N. Colonization and turnover of Streptococcus pneumoniae, Haemophilus influenzae, and Moraxella catarrhalis in otitis-prone children. *Microbiol Immunol.* 2007;51:223–230.

Moraxella (Branhamella) Catarrhalis

128. Brucellosis

Carlos Carrillo and Eduardo Gotuzzo

Brucellosis is a zoonotic disease found in Latin America, Mediterranean countries (Spain, Italy, Greece), and Arabian countries (Iraq, Kuwait). According to the Centers for Disease Control and Prevention (CDC), the number of cases dropped from 6147 in 1947 to 104 in 1991 with modern bovine brucellosis eradication, mainly by pasteurization of milk or dairy products.

Most cases of brucellosis in the United States are related to occupational exposure to *Brucella abortus*. The affected are mainly men and occasionally laboratory and technical personnel. However, in Texas and Florida, the ingestion of unpasteurized dairy products is the common mechanism, and the pathogen responsible is *Brucella melitensis*, attacking men and women in equal proportion and sometimes children. *Brucella melitensis* produces a more severe clinical pattern and can even produce a chronic form. The attack rate is higher, especially in family outbreaks, with rare subclinical infections. *Brucella abortus* produces a mild disease with low attack rates (≤10%) and more subclinical cases.

CLINICAL MANIFESTATIONS

Brucellosis is one of the most protean diseases because any system can be involved. We prefer to divide it into three forms: acute, subacute, and chronic.

Acute Brucellosis

Usually, there is high fever, mainly in the evening, with malaise, headache, perspiration, arthralgias, and myalgias. In most cases, constipation, back pain, and loss of weight (as much as 20 pounds in 2 months) are found. Generally, granulomatous hepatitis, hematologic disorders, and articular compromise (especially peripheral arthritis and sacroiliitis) are seen.

In this form of the disease, any of the routine agglutination assays produce an appropriate diagnosis (immunofluorescence [IF], enzyme-linked immunosorbent assay [ELISA], counterimmunoelectrophoresis [CIE], and Bengal rose test) with high specificity and sensitivity.

Rarely, false-positive results may be caused by *Francisella tularensis* and *Yersinia enterocolitica*. With the epidemic of cholera in Latin America, the cross-reaction between *Vibrio cholerae* and *Brucella* is significant, producing false-positive serology to *Brucella* in patients with cholera. Even vaccines against cholera produce false-positive reactions transiently.

The medium Ruiz-Castañeda with Carrillo's modification (addition of 0.025% sodium phosphate sulfonate [SPS] and 0.05% cysteine) increased the yield of *Brucella*. In the acute form, two blood cultures are as efficient as one bone marrow culture.

Subacute Brucellosis

Subacute form (undulant fever or Malta fever) is the typical and classic form described in endemic areas. There is intermittent low fever, often with articular compromise (peripheral arthritis, sacroiliitis, and/or spondylitis), hematologic changes (eg, pancytopenia, thrombocytopenia, hemolytic anemia), or hepatic damage (granulomatous hepatitis). Patients with incomplete treatment are also included in this form of brucellosis (Figure 128.1). In this form of the disease, the 2-mercaptoethanol test detects immunoglobulin G, and titer above 1:80 defines active infection. *Brucella* is isolated in 40% to 70% of serial blood cultures; the bone marrow culture (0.5 to 1 mL of aspirate from the iliac crest) permits isolation in 90% of these patients.

Chronic Brucellosis

In the chronic form with >1 year of illness, there usually is an afebrile pattern with myalgia, fatigue, depression, arthralgias, and so on. The most important differential diagnosis is chronic fatigue syndrome. Other localized forms are granulomatous or recurrent uveitis and spondylitis. Peripheral arthritis and sacroiliitis are rare.

This form of disease is produced mainly by *B. melitensis*. It is found mainly in adults older than 30 years, especially older than 50 years, and is rare in children. The routine serologic

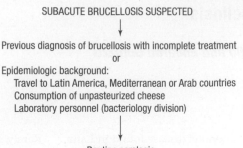

SUBACUTE BRUCELLOSIS SUSPECTED

Previous diagnosis of brucellosis with incomplete treatment

or

Epidemiologic background:
  Travel to Latin America, Mediterranean or Arab countries
  Consumption of unpasteurized cheese
  Laboratory personnel (bacteriology division)

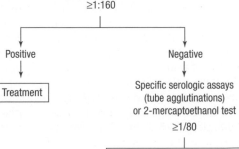

Routine seralogic
assays against *Brucella*
≥1:160

Positive → Treatment

Negative → Specific serologic assays
(tube agglutinations)
or 2-mercaptoethanol test
≥1/80

Figure 128.1 Algorithm for the evaluation and treatment of subacute brucellosis.

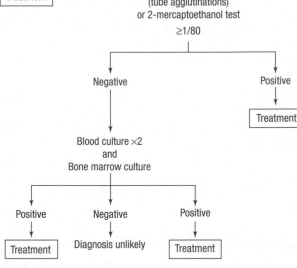

Negative

Positive → Treatment

Blood culture ×2
and
Bone marrow culture

Positive → Treatment

Negative → Diagnosis unlikely

Positive → Treatment

tests and blood cultures give a diagnosis only 10% to 20% of the time. We recommend Coombs test specific for *Brucella* or blocking antibodies. The bone marrow in our experience produces a positive culture in 50% to 75% of patients (Figure 128.2).

THERAPY

The intracellular character of *Brucella* results in an important therapeutic challenge, especially in subacute and chronic forms. Antibiotics should have in vitro activity, but the intracellular concentration must be adequate.

Tetracyclines have shown excellent in vitro activity throughout the world. The MIC90 (minimum inhibitory concentration) was 2 μg/mL for tetracycline and 0.125 μg/mL for

doxycycline in our surveillance in Peru. During the past 25 years, the antibiotic activity pattern of tetracycline against *B. melitensis* has not changed, which is remarkable because these are still our drugs of choice.

In addition, oxytetracycline and doxycycline showed that the minimal bactericidal concentration (MBC) was equal to MIC. All these features in conjunction with worldwide experience point to tetracyclines as the keystone of treatment.

The differences among tetracyclines are tolerance, dosage, and safety profile; however, the new ones have better tolerance and fewer side effects and can be used with meals without reducing efficacy. We prefer to use doxycycline or minocycline.

The other important aspect is the need to combine antibiotics to reduce the rate of relapse.

Specific Organisms – Bacteria

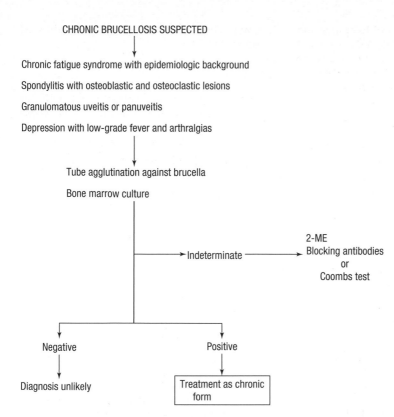

CHRONIC BRUCELLOSIS SUSPECTED

Chronic fatigue syndrome with epidemiologic background

Spondylitis with osteoblastic and osteoclastic lesions

Granulomatous uveitis or panuveitis

Depression with low-grade fever and arthralgias

Tube agglutination against brucella

Bone marrow culture

Indeterminate → 2-ME Blocking antibodies or Coombs test

Negative → Diagnosis unlikely

Positive → Treatment as chronic form

Figure 128.2 Algorithm for the evaluation and treatment of chronic brucellosis. 2-ME = 2-mercaptoethanol.

Most antibiotics can reduce the fever, but recurrence is high.

Rifampin has been introduced as a preferential agent because of its excellent in vitro activity and intracellular concentration. The possibility of rapid resistance was shown in our strains when 5 of 10 strains exposed in vitro to rifampin developed resistance by the seventh day.

The third effective group of drugs against *Brucella* is the aminoglycosides, with good in vitro activity and good clinical response. The largest study was done with streptomycin; however, gentamicin, netilmicin, and amikacin showed the same and even better results in open trials.

Comparative studies have been done of doxycycline plus rifampin versus doxycycline plus streptomycin (D-S). Both schedules had a high cure rate (more than 95%); however, D-S had a lower relapse rate. The doxycycline levels in the plasma of patients treated with rifampin were significantly lower than those of patients treated with D-S. Patients who were rapid acetylators had lower levels because they had higher clearance rates. In addition, the half-life and the area under the curve were significantly lower in these patients. These new data suggest that relapses may result from this interaction.

Adults

Our standard treatment for adult patients is oral doxycycline, 100 mg twice a day for 45 days, plus streptomycin, 1 g intramuscularly per day for 2 weeks (prolonging treatment with streptomycin for more than 2 weeks has not proved to be more effective); or gentamycin 160 mg per day for 7 days; or doxycycline, 100 mg twice a day, plus rifampin, 600 mg once a day, both for 45 days. Only in a case of spondylitis, endocarditis, or brain abscess do we prolong treatment for 3 months. In chronic brucellosis we prefer to use standard treatment for 45 days and then 3 months of doxycycline only. Some experts recommend adding levamisole for this special form during 3 months.

Children

In children younger than 8 years, tetracyclines cannot be used. The combination of rifampin, 15 to 20 mg/kg once a day for 4 weeks, and aminoglycosides at standard dose for 5 to 10 days is highly effective in children. The use of cotrimoxazole has also been recommended in children. Cotrimoxazole may be used 240 mg for 4 weeks plus rifampin 20 mg/kg once a day for 4 weeks.

This schedule has a high level of tolerance and few adverse effects; however, the efficacy is not as acceptable as with other schedules. Some report excellent results of cotrimoxazole for 4 weeks plus gentamicin for 5 to 10 days.

Pregnancy and Brucellosis

Brucellosis during pregnancy is a special problem because the best drug should be avoided and the clinical course and fetal prognosis are poor. In our experience with more than 70% women with brucellosis, early and adequate treatment showed excellent evolution of pregnancy, and the babies were normal. However, when antibiotic treatment is begun late, the prognosis is worse. A good schedule is cotrimoxazole plus rifampin for 6 weeks. Folic acid supplements should be given. Another option is aminoglycoside for 10 days plus rifampin or cotrimoxazole for 6 weeks; we have a review of our experience and this looks as a good option.

Other Antibiotics

Some drugs, such as chloramphenicol, erythromycin, ampicillin, and cephalosporins, showed moderate in vitro activity, but the clinical experience is not as good as with the other drugs. Recently, the fluoroquinolones showed better in vitro activity, and they have good intracellular penetration. However, some trials showed that norfloxacin and ciprofloxacin had less clinical efficacy. Only ofloxacin in one trial showed good efficacy.

Steroids

We recommend to add corticosteroids only for 3 to 6 weeks for uveitis and for 2 to 10 weeks for severe thrombocytopenic purpura. If there is no response, we maintain steroids for 2 to 4 months. After this time, if the thrombocytopenia is still evident, we recommend splenectomy.

SUGGESTED READING

Colmenero JD, Fernández-Gallardo LC, Agundez JA, et al. Possible implication of doxycycline-rifampin interaction for treatment of brucellosis. *Antimicrob Agent Chemother.* 1994;38:2798–2802.

Miguel PS, Fernandez G, Vasallo FJ, et al. Neurobrucellosis mimicking cerebral tumor: case report and literature review. *Clin Neurol Neurosurg.* 2006;108(4):404–406.

Pappas G, Akritidis N, Bosilkovski M, Tsianos E. Brucellosis. *N Engl J Med.* 2005;352(22): 2325–2336.

Pappas G, Papadimitriou P, Akritidis N, Christou L, Tsianos EV. The new global map of human brucellosis. *Lancet Infect Dis.* 2006;6(2):91–99.

Young EJ. Human brucellosis. *Rev Infect Dis.* 1983;15:821–842.

Trujillo IZ, Zavala AN, Caceres JG, Miranda CQ. Brucellosis. *Infect Dis Clin North Am.* 1994;8:225–241.

129. *Campylobacter*

David W. K. Acheson

Campylobacter (Greek *campylo,* curved; *bacter,* rod) are motile, non–spore-forming gram-negative rods. They are a very common cause of gastrointestinal (GI) infection in humans in many parts of the world. *Campylobacter* organisms were first isolated in the early 1900s from aborted sheep fetuses. However, it was many years later and not until the 1970s that *Campylobacter* were isolated from stool. There are many members of the genus *Campylobacter;* the major enteric pathogen for humans is *Campylobacter jejuni,* although *Campylobacter coli, Campylobacter fetus, Campylobacter upsaliensis,* and *Campylobacter lari* are also pathogenic to humans. *Campylobacter jejuni* is most frequently associated with GI disease, and *C. fetus* usually causes systemic infection, often in debilitated patients. *Campylobacter* is microaerophilic, and although all will grow at 37°C (98.6°F), *C. jejuni* grows best at 42°C (107.6°F). A number of selective media are in use, including Skirrows, Butzler's, and Campy-BAP. Although several serotypes of *C. jejuni* have been reported, there are few data regarding the relative virulence of these different types, although some appear to be more closely associated with the development of Guillain–Barré syndrome (GBS) than others.

EPIDEMIOLOGY

Campylobacter is one of the most commonly diagnosed enteric bacterial infection in many parts of the United States and Europe. It is estimated that there are more than 2 million cases per year in the United States. It is especially common in children younger than 1 year of age and in young adults, and it occurs most often in the summer. *Campylobacter* species are found in fowl and many wild and domestic animals, and most human infections probably result from contamination of milk and other animal food sources, especially poultry. The recent increase in consumption of raw milk has led to illness associated with *Camplylobacter.* The organisms can also be transmitted by direct contact with infected animals and contaminated water, and cross-contamination between infected poultry

and other foods is probably one of the most frequent modes of transmission. Small numbers of organisms may cause disease; as few as 800 have been shown to cause infection in volunteer studies, but the infecting dose is usually about 10^4. Although asymptomatic carriage of *Campylobacter* is thought to be uncommon in developed countries, in less developed nations carriage rates as high as 37% have been reported among children.

CLINICAL FEATURES

The incubation period for *C. jejuni* infection varies and is typically between 1 and 7 days, with most cases occurring 2 to 4 days after exposure. Very short incubation periods of fewer than 12 hours have been reported. *Campylobacter jejuni* illness typically presents with a prodrome of fever, headache, myalgia, and malaise for up to 24 hours before intestinal symptoms develop. The fever may be as high as 40°C (104°F), and the diarrhea varies from a few loose stools to copious watery discharge. Blood is often present in the stool but varies in amount. The illness usually lasts less than a week, but patients untreated with antibiotics often continue to excrete the organisms for several weeks. Documented bacteremia is rare in *C. jejuni* infections; however, studies from the United Kingdom have indicated that it may be more common than previously thought. Routine surveillance of infection in England and Wales detected 394 cases of *Campylobacter* bacteraemia in 11 years that inceased with age, with a range of 0.3/1000 in children aged 1 to 4 years to 5.9/1000 in patients aged 65 years or more. Overall 89% of the identified isolates were *C. jejuni* or *C. coli.* This may explain why focal infections such as endocarditis, meningitis, septic abortion, acute cholecystitis, pancreatitis, and cystitis have all been documented. Postinfectious reactive arthritis may also occur, especially in human leukocyte antigen (HLA)-B27–positive individuals. One of the most serious consequences of infection with *C. jejuni* is the development of GBS. This is an autoimmune disorder of the peripheral nervous system resulting in an ascending flaccid paralysis that carries a mortality rate of up to 5%. GBS is thought to be caused by molecular mimicry between polysaccharides on the outer surface of *C. jejuni* and gangliosides in the myelin sheaths of peripheral nerves.

In contrast to *C. jejuni, C. fetus* commonly produces systemic disease, often in vascular sites: endocarditis, pericarditis, and mycotic aneurysms of the abdominal aorta. Central nervous system infections such as meningoencephalitis also occur with *C. fetus,* as do other localized infections, including septic arthritis, spontaneous bacterial peritonitis, salpingitis, lung abscess, empyema, cellulitis, urinary tract infection, vertebral osteomyelitis, and cholecystitis. In patients with acquired immunodeficiency syndrome (AIDS), *Campylobacter* species other than *C. fetus* and *C. jejuni* may also cause bacteremia.

DIAGNOSIS

Campylobacter have a characteristic darting motility, and a presumptive diagnosis of *Campylobacter* infection may be made by examination of stool passed within 2 hours using direct dark-field or phase-contrast microscopy. Leukocytes and red cells are also often seen in stool samples, with 75% of patients having polymorphonuclear leukocytes in their stool. Confirmation of the diagnosis of *C. jejuni* infection is based on a positive stool or blood culture, although *Campylobacter* is fastidious and may die during transport to the laboratory. DNA probes, polymerase chain reaction, and serologic testing all have been used to confirm diagnosis but are not routinely available. Direct detection of *Campylobacter* antigens in stool using enzyme immunoassays is a relatively new approach that is now commercially available. This method has the attraction of not requiring live organisms but has the detraction of not producing an isolate that will be available for antimicrobial sensitivity testing. *Campylobacter fetus* may be isolated from blood held in culture up to 14 days. The fastidious nature of the organisms means that failure to culture *Campylobacter* does not rule them out as the cause of significant clinical disease.

THERAPY

As with many diarrheal diseases, fluid replacement is the most important therapy in *Campylobacter* diarrhea. Oral rehydration is usually adequate, but patients with severe dehydration should be given volume replacement with intravenous solutions of electrolytes and water.

Most *Campylobacter* infections are mild and self-limited and do not result in a visit to a physician. These mild infections do not usually require antimicrobial therapy. Antimicrobial therapy should be reserved for patients who are severely ill, elderly, pregnant, or immunocompromised but may on occasion also be indicated in patients with bloody stools, high fever, extraintestinal infection, worsening symptoms or relapses, and those with symptoms lasting longer than 1 week. Treating patients later in the course of the disease (after several days of symptoms) will remove *Campylobacter* from the stool, but it is not likely to have a dramatic effect on the duration of symptoms. Person-to-person spread generally is not considered a major concern with *Campylobacter,* so treating to prevent this is not generally recommended (except in the case of food handlers). However, there may be exceptions to this, for example, the reduction of spread in day-care settings. Antibiotic therapy can have a dramatic positive effect on symptoms of *C. jejuni* infection, justifying a trial of therapy in severe or persistent illness.

Campylobacter jejuni is usually susceptible to many antimicrobial agents in vitro, including macrolides, tetracyclines, aminoglycosides, chloramphenicol, quinolones, and nitrofurans (Table 129.1). They are inherently resistant to trimethoprim and most cephalosporins except cefotaxime, ceftazidime, and cefpirone. Erythromycin has consistently been the drug most widely used in the treatment of *C. jejuni* because it is inexpensive, safe, and time tested and remains the treatment of choice. Erythromycin treatment will terminate GI shedding of *Campylobacter* within 24 to 72 hours, which should be kept in mind when treating infections in day-care or preschool settings to avoid spread of the disease. Resistance to erythromycin has been reported but is generally low in *C. jejuni*; it is higher in *C. coli*. Erythromycin stearate is resistant to acid and poorly absorbed, so it is the preparation of choice for treating *Campylobacter*. In children, erythromycin ethylsuccinate should be used. Of the other macrolides, clindamycin, azithromycin, and clarithromycin are all active but offer little advantage over erythromycin and are more expensive. Fluoroquinolones are generally very active against *Campylobacter* when they are susceptible, and there was a period when it appeared that these would be the drugs of choice. However, the increasing problems with fluoroquinolone resistance now make fluoroquinolones much less desirable and

Table 129.1 Recommended Antimicrobial Agents for *Campylobacter*

	Drug	Dosage and Duration
Preferred	Erythromycin	Adults: 500 mg PO BID × 5 d Children: 30–50 mg/kg/d QID × 5 d
Alternative after checking senstivitiy	Ciprofloxacin	Adults: 500 mg PO BID × 7 d
Other agents	Nitrofurans (furazolidone) Aminoglycosides Chloramphenicol	

not a first-line therapy. In Sweden, quinolone resistance in clinical isolates of *C. jejuni* increased more than 20-fold in the early 1990s. There has also been a documented rise in the incidence of resistance to quinolones in other parts of Europe since 1992, with up to 57% of *C. jejuni* and 43% of *C. coli* isolates being resistant (determined by disk diffusion using naladixic acid and ciprofloxacin). Other studies from Spain have confirmed this trend, with 30% to 40% of *C. jejuni* strains being resistant to three fluoroquinolones. Similar trends of increasing fluoroquinolone resistance are occurring in the United States. A report from Minnesota of almost 5000 isolates of *Campylobacter* in humans indicated that the frequency of fluoroquinolone-resistant *C. jejuni* isolates increased from 1.3% in 1992 to 10.2% in 1998. *Campylobacter jejuni* was also isolated from 74% of the domestic chicken products tested, and ciprofloxacin resistance was documented in 14%. Despite the initial enthusiasm for this group of drugs, they are expensive, they are not recommended for children in the United States, and the increasing resistance problems make them an unsuitable first choice of therapy. Serious systemic *Campylobacter* infections should be treated with an aminoglycoside or a carbapenem (resistance to these antimicrobials has remained under 1%). Extraintestinal infection with *C. jejuni* needs at least 10 days of treatment, and systemic infection with *C. fetus* warrants 2 to 3 weeks of therapy.

PROGNOSIS AND PREVENTION

Most patients recover totally following infection with *C. jejuni*. Complications such as reactive arthritis and GBS are unusual. Systemic *C. fetus* infections have a significant mortality, especially in patients with underlying disease such as diabetes mellitus or cirrhosis or who are immunocompromised. Transmission of *Campylobacter* infection can be reduced by careful food handling, with special attention to cross-contamination from poultry products. Proper cooking of food, pasteurization of milk, and protection of water supplies are all critical in preventing infection with *Campylobacter*.

SUGGESTED READING

Allos, BM. Clinical features and treatment of Campylobacter infection. In: UpToDate 2007; UpToDate. http://www.uptodate.com/ Accessed November 14, 2007.

Giesendorf BAJ, et al. Development of species-specific DNA probes for Campylobacter jejuni, Campylobacter coli, and Campylobacter lari by polymerase chain reaction fingerprinting. *J Clin Microbiol.* 1993; 31:1541–1546.

Nachamkin I, Allos B, Ho T. Campylobacter species and Guillain-Barré syndrome. *Clin Microbiol Rev.* 1998;11:555–567.

Skirrow MB. Campylobacter enteritis: a "new" disease. *Br Med J.* 1977 July 2;2(6078)9–11.

Skirrow MB, Blaser MJ. Campylobacter jejuni. In: Blaser MJ, et al., eds. *Infections of the Gastrointestinal Tract.* New York: Raven Press; 1995.

Skirrow MB, Jones DM, Sutcliffe E, Benjamin J. Campylobacter bacteraemia in England and Wales, 1981–1991. *Epidemiol Infect.* 1993;110:567–573.

130. Clostridia

Richard Quintiliani, Jr., and Richard Quintiliani, Sr.

Clostridia include bacterial species that are responsible for generating some of the most potent toxins known to humans. They are obligate, anaerobic, spore-forming bacilli that live in soil and the intestinal tract of animals and man. Of the 83 clostridia strains, approximately 30 are clearly or potentially pathogenic. Distinctive types of infection have been associated with certain species of *Clostridium*: gastrointestinal illness with *Clostridium perfringens* and *Clostridium difficile*; neurologic syndromes with *Clostridium botulinum* and *Clostridium tetani*; focal suppurative infections, myonecrosis, and gas gangrene with *Clostridium perfringens*, *Clostridium novyi*, *Clostridium septicum*, *Clostridium histolyticum*, *Clostridium bifermentans*, and *Clostridium fallax*; and bacteremia with *Clostridium perfringens*, *Clostridium septicum*, *Clostridium sordellii*, and *Clostridium tertium*.

BOTULISM

Pathogenesis

Botulism is a neuroparalytic illness caused by a neurotoxin produced from the anaerobic, spore-forming bacterium *C. botulinum*. The disease can be categorized as (1) foodborne, (2) wound, (3) intestinal (infant botulism), and (4) inhalational botulism, a human-made form from the inhalation of aerosolized botulism toxin. Fewer than 200 cases of all forms of botulism are reported annually in the United States.

The eight strains (A, B, C1, C2, D, E, F, and G) of *C. botulinum* have separated on the antigenic specificities of their toxins. Of these antigenic types, type A is the most common cause of foodborne botulism. Only types A, B, E, and F cause illness in humans. On a weight basis, botulism toxins are the most potent poisons known. Its incredible toxicity relates to the ability of the toxin to cleave one or more of the proteins by which neuronal vesicles release acetylcholine into the neuromuscular junction. All forms of botulism result from absorption of the toxin into the circulation from either a mucosal surface (gut, lung) or a wound. The toxin cannot penetrate the intact skin. The toxin is resistant to degradation by gastric acidity and human gastrointestinal enzymes but can be inactivated in chlorinated water in 20 minutes and in fresh water after 3 to 6 days.

In the United States, it has become the first biological toxin to be licensed for the treatment of a variety of human diseases such as cervical torticollis, strabismus, and blepharospasm associated with dystonia. However, it is commonly used "off label" for such conditions as headache, chronic low back pain, stroke, traumatic brain injury, cerebral palsy, achalasia, and various dystonias and for cosmetic purposes to decrease wrinkling.

Foodborne Botulism

Foodborne botulism is caused by ingestion of preformed toxin in contaminated foods, with home-canned or prepared foods being the most often implicated vehicle. Because the toxin is rapidly inactivated by heat ($\geq 85°C$ for 5 minutes), it is always transmitted by the ingestion of foods that are not properly heated. The most commonly implicated foods in the United States are vegetables with low acid content such as asparagus, green beans, beets, peppers, carrots and corn. It is now known that even foil-wrapped baked potatoes can cause foodborne botulism if held at room temperature after baking, and then served plain as in a potato salad. Other notable examples of commercial foods that have caused botulism outbreaks include inadequately eviscerated fish, yogurt, cream cheese, chopped garlic in oil, chili peppers, tomatoes, and jarred peanuts. Because honey can contain spores of *C. botulinum*, cases of botulism have been caused by ingesting raw honey and have been a particular problem in infants, which is discussed later. In fact, feeding honey to children younger than 12 months is no longer recommended.

Botulism typically begins as neuromuscular blockade resulting in symmetric weakness, usually beginning 12 to 72 hours after ingestion of contaminated food. Patients are usually alert and afebrile. The most common complaints include double vision, blurred vision, drooping eyelids, slurred speech, difficulty swallowing, dry mouth, and muscle weakness. Along with these symptoms, patients often note lassitude, dizziness, ileus, bladder distension, and constipation. It should be stressed that it is not possible to have botulism without having multiple cranial nerve palsies. Because the toxin does not penetrate brain parenchyma, patients are not confused or obtunded. Yet, they often complain of lethargy and have communication problems, probably because of the bulbar palsies. In brief, the classic triad of botulism includes the following: (1) symmetric, descending flaccid paralysis with prominent bulbar palsies; (2) an afebrile patient; and (3) a clear sensorium. Another useful clinical observation is that the bulbar palsies can be characterized as 4 D's: diplopia, dysarthria, dysphonia, and dysphasia.

Botulism is often misdiagnosed because many clinicians are unfamiliar with the disease. Many cases are initially misdiagnosed as a polyradiculoneuropathy (eg, Guillain–Barré syndrome), a cerebrovascular accident, intoxication, hysterical paralysis, poliomyelitis, tick paralysis, heavy metal intoxication, or myasthenia gravis. It should be remembered that botulism differs from other flaccid paralysis in its prominent cranial nerve palsies disproportionate to milder weakness and hypotonia below the neck and in its absence of sensory nerve damage.

Initial testing may include brain imaging, lumbar puncture, electromyography, or edrophonium chloride testing. The diagnosis of botulism is confirmed by (1) demonstration of botulinum toxin in serum by intraperitoneal injection into mice; (2) isolation of *C. botulinum* in stool; or (3) identification of toxin, the organism, or both in food.

The mouse bioassay can detect as little as 0.03 ng of botulinum toxin and usually yields results in 1 to 2 days. Fecal and gastric specimens require anaerobic culture with results usually available in 5 to 21 days. Toxin production by culture isolates is confirmed by bioassay.

A test dose of edrophonium chloride (tensilon test) briefly reverses paralytic symptoms in many patients with myasthenia gravis and occasionally in some patients with botulism. The classic electromyographic findings of botulism include normal nerve conduction velocity, normal sensory nerve function, a pattern of brief, small-amplitude motor potentials, and, most characteristic, an incremental response to repetitive stimulator often seen only at 50 Hz. In botulism the cerebrospinal fluid (CSF) is normal, whereas in Guillain–Barré, the CSF protein level is usually elevated.

Patients with botulism should be monitored initially in an intensive care unit (ICU) setting. The mainstay of treatment is supportive therapy with mechanical ventilation and passive immunization with equine antitoxin. If food exposure was recent, gastric lavage should be attempted. Cathartics and enemas are given to remove unabsorbed toxin from the colon. Cathartic agents containing magnesium should be avoided because of the theoretical concern that increased magnesium levels may enhance the action of botulinum toxin. The administration of antitoxin is the only specific pharmacologic treatment available. In the United States, botulinum antitoxin is available from the Centers for Disease Control and Prevention (CDC) via state and local health departments. The licensed trivalent antitoxin contains neutralizing antibodies against botulinum toxin types A, B, and E, the most common causes of human botulism. A single vial (7500 IU of type A, 5500 IU of type B, and 8500 IU of type E antitoxin) per patient is administered intravenously and one vial intramuscularly. Although the package insert recommends repeating the dose in 4 hours, most experts feel this is unnecessary. Because of a rather high incidence of hypersensitivity reactions (9% to 20%), skin testing should be performed prior to administering the antitoxin. A recommendation for desensitization is also included in the package insert. In the absence of infectious complications, antibiotic treatment has no value.

Often patients with botulism exhibit inadequate gag and cough reflexes. Airway obstruction or aspiration usually precedes hypoventilation. The proportion of patients with botulism who require mechanical ventilation has varied from 20% in foodborne outbreaks to more than 60% in infant botulism. When death occurs in botulism, it is usually caused by airway obstruction (pharyngeal and upper airway muscle paralysis) and inadequate tidal volume (diaphragmatic and accessory respiratory muscle paralysis). Although only about 5% to 10% patients with botulism die in the United States, the paralysis of botulism can persist for weeks to months with requirements for fluid and nutritional support and assisted ventilation. Like tetanus, botulism does not result in long-term immunity.

Wound Botulism

First recognized in 1943, wound botulism usually results from severe trauma and open fractures contaminated by soil. Recently, intravenous drug abuse has been implicated. It has been particularly a problem in those addicts using so-called black tar heroin by the subcutaneous and intramuscular route. The clinical manifestations are similar to foodborne botulism except for the absence of gastrointestinal symptoms. The median incubation period is longer (7 days with a range of 4 to 14 days). Fever may be present because of wound infection.

As in foodborne botulism, botulinum antitoxin is administered together with debridement of contaminated wounds. Anaerobic cultures of the wound should be obtained. Although its efficacy has not been proved, intravenous penicillin, 10 to 20 million units per day, should be given. In general, aminoglycosides, polymixins, and clindamycin are contraindicated because of their ability to exacerbate neuromuscular blockade.

Infant Botulism

First described in 1976, infant botulism is the most common cause of botulism in the United States. The disease most commonly occurs during the second month of life. Infant botulism usually presents with constipation that is then often followed by feeding difficulties, hypotonia, increased drooling, and a weak cry. The usual source of the organism is soil where the density of spores may be high. However, as mentioned above, raw honey has often been implicated as a cause of infant botulism owing to the high concentration of *C. botulinum* spores in this food, which is often given to infants for nutritional purposes.

Unlike foodborne botulism, infant botulism is not acquired through the ingestion of toxin but rather through the ingestion of spores, which then germinate in the intestinal tract and then elaborate toxin. It appears that an infant's gastrointestinal tract is permissive to the germination of spores, which is not true in adults. Of all the forms of botulism, infant botulism carries the highest mortality of about 50%.

Supportive care remains the mainstay of treatment, with intubation or tube feeding sometimes becoming necessary. There is no evidence to support the use of antibiotics or botulinum antitoxin. It is believed that the antitoxin might result in lysis of intraintestinal organisms, thus liberating more neurotoxin into the gut. The safety and efficacy of human botulism immunoglobulin is being determined. This product is available in the United States solely for the treatment of infant botulism. For information on obtaining human botulism immunoglobulin, contact local and state health departments or the CDC at 404-639-2206, 404-639-2888, or 770-488-7100.

Inhalational Botulism

Unfortunately, botulinum toxin has been considered by some countries, as well as terrorist groups, as a potential biologic weapon against a civilian population. Considerable concern for its use in this manner relates to the observation that a single gram of crystalline toxin, evenly dispersed and inhaled has the capability of killing more than a million people. Effective response to a deliberate release of botulinum toxin will depend on timely clinical diagnosis, case reporting, and epidemiological investigation. Interestingly, a variant of inhalational botulism has been reported in patients who have snuffed cocaine where the spores gain entry to sinuses, where they can germinate producing toxin and causing botulism.

TETANUS

Clostridium tetani is commonly found in soil all over the world. It is a strict anaerobe and often possesses terminal endospores that give the organism a drumstick appearance. About 1 million cases of tetanus occur annually worldwide, mostly in developing countries. About 50 to 100 cases of tetanus are reported each year in the United States, mostly in patients older than 60 years.

Two toxins are generated by *C. tetani*, of which one is tetanospasmin, which is responsible for the clinical manifestations associated with tetanus, whereas the other is tetanolysin, the role of which in human tetanus is unclear. Common portals of entry are wounds, burns, tympanic membrane perforation from otitis media, and skin ulcers. Infection of the umbilical stump can cause neonatal tetanus.

Generalized Tetanus

Diagnosis is based primarily on the history and clinical presentation. A complete immunization history should be obtained if possible. A serum antitoxin level of 0.01 IU/mL or higher or a history of immunization makes the diagnosis unlikely. Cerebrospinal fluid studies are generally within normal limits. Isolation of *C. tetani* from the wound does not prove the diagnosis because it can be part of normal skin flora.

In generalized tetanus the incubation period is usually 7 to 21 days but ranges from 2 days to months. A shorter incubation period correlates with severe disease and frequent complications. The most common presenting complaints are trismus (lockjaw), generalized weakness, stiffness, cramping, difficulty swallowing, and difficulty in urination. Increasing muscle rigidity with reflex spasms ensues. Contraction of facial muscles results in a characteristic expression, risus sardonicus. Other entities that can mimic trismus include strychnine poisoning, hypocalcemia, subarachnoid hemorrhage, hysterical trismus, and dystonic reactions to neuroleptic drugs or other central dopamine antagonists. Typically, in theses dystonic reactions, the spasms almost always involve lateral head turning, which can be promptly corrected with anticholinergic agents, like benztropine or diphenhydramine. Differential diagnosis also includes hypocalcemia, subarachnoid hemorrhage, and hysterical trismus. An important clinical observation is that patients with hysterical trismus usually have no difficulty in voiding, whereas in patients with trismus caused by tetanus usually the periurethral muscles are involved, resulting in the inability to void. The general muscle spasms in tetanus can result in hypoxia from laryngospasm or tonic contraction of respiratory muscles.

Therapy depends on when the patient is first diagnosed. Within the first hours after presentation, the most important thing is to assess airway and ventilation to ascertain whether the patient warrants endotracheal intubation using benzodiazine sedation and neuromuscular blockade (eg, vecuronium, 0.1 mg/kg). To control spasm and decrease rigidity, a benzodiazepine, such as diazepam, in 5-mg increments, or lorazepam, in 2-mg increments, should be given intravenously. The dose should produce sedation and minimize reflex spasms but not compromise the airway or ventilation. If airway or ventilation problems occur, the patient usually requires intubation using a short-acting neuromuscular blocking agent. The patient should be placed in the ICU in a quiet, darkened area. In addition, within the first 24 hours, the patient should receive human tetanus immunoglobulin (HTIG), 500 units, intramuscularly. At a different site, absorbed tetanus toxoid such as tetanus–diphtheria vaccine (0.5 mL) should be administered intramuscularly. Antibiotic therapy should also be given with metronidazole at a dose of 500 mg, intravenously, every 6 hours for 7 to 10 days.

Over the next 2 to 3 weeks, the benzodiazepine dose should be tapered depending on the clinical response. Before discharge, which usually takes 2 to 6 weeks, another dose of tetanus–diphtheria vaccine should be given.

Local Tetanus

Local tetanus is manifested by fixed rigidity of muscles at or near the site of injury, probably resulting from partial immunity to tetanospasmin. It can progress to generalized tetanus but often resolves spontaneously. Occasionally, patients may develop boardlike abdomen that mimics an acute surgical abdomen.

Cephalic Tetanus

A rare manifestation of tetanus is so-called cephalic tetanus, which usually results from otitis media or head wounds. It is manifested by dysfunction of one or more cranial nerves, usually the facial nerve, and trismus. It can subsequently change to generalized tetanus.

Neonatal Tetanus

Although rare in the United States, it has been estimated that it is the cause of death in 200 000 to 500 000 neonates in developing countries. In developing countries, ghee, or clarified butter, and cow dung are often applied to the umbilical stump as a cultural practice. Neonatal tetanus usually presents within the first 2 weeks of life, usually the result of an infected umbilical stump. Usually, the infant presents with general weakness and failure to nurse, which subsequently leads to generalized rigidity and spasms. Children of nonimmunized mothers are at a particular risk for developing neonatal tetanus.

Vaccination against Tetanus

For immunization against tetanus, tetanus toxoid is available in two forms, of which one is an adsorbed (aluminum salt precipitated), whereas the other is a fluid toxoid. Of these two choices, the adsorbed toxoid is preferred because the antitoxin response reaches higher titers and is longer lasting as compared with the fluid toxoid. Tetanus toxoid is available as a single preparation, combined with diphtheria toxoid as pediatric DT or adult Td, and with both diphtheria toxoid and acellular pertussis vaccine as DTaP or Tdap. It is also available as a combined DTaP-IPV-hepatitis B combination. Pediatric formulations (DT and DTaP) contain a similar amount ot tetanus toxoid but 3 to 4 times as much diphtheria toxoid.

Children youger than 7 years should receive either DTaP or pediatric DT. The first, second, and third doses should be separated by a minimum of 4 weeks, and the fourth dose should follow the third dose by no less than 6 months.

Typical routine vaccination schedules in children include four doses of DTaP administered at 2, 4, 6, and 15 to 18 months. If a child has a contraindication to pertussis vaccine, pediatric DT should be used to complete the vaccination. Because immunity typically lasts for about 10 years, routine boosters are recommended every 10 years. However, persons who sustain a wound that is other than clean and minor should receive a tetanus booster if more than 5 years have elapsed since the last dose (Table 130.1).

Unvaccinated persons ≥7 years of age or older should receive the adult formulation (adult Td), even if they have not completed a series of DTaP or pediatric DT. The primary series is three doses. The first two doses should be separated by at least 4 weeks, and the third dose should be given 6 to 12 months after the second dose. The use of single-antigen tetanus is usually not recommended because periodic boosting of both diphtheria toxoid and tetanus toxoid are needed.

For more detailed information on tetanus vaccination in unusual situations (adults who have contact with infants aged ≤12 months, or health care personnel), one should contact the following Web sites: www.cdc.gov/vaccines/pubs/pinkbook/downloads/tetanus.pdf or www.cdc.gov./mmwr/pdf/rr/rr5517.pdf.

GAS GANGRENE (CLOSTRIDIAL MYONECROSIS)

Clostridia gas gangrene or myonecrosis is usually a fulminate infection characterized by muscle necrosis and systemic toxicity. The most common organism isolated is *C. perfringens* (formerly *Clostridium welchii*), which accounts for >80% of cases. *Clostridium novyi*, *C. septicum*, *C. sordellii*, *C. histolyticum*, *C. fallax*, and *C. bifermentans* are sometimes implicated. The major sources of these organisms are soil and the intestines of humans and animals. Gas gangrene can occur in a variety of clinical settings, can be posttraumatic or postoperative, or may occur spontaneously, usually in patients with diabetes, peripheral vascular disease, or an underlying malignancy.

The incubation period averages 4 days, with the patient initially presenting with severe, persistent pain at the site of the wound.

Table 130.1 Tetanus Wound Management

Vaccination History	Clean, Minor Wounds		All Other Wounds	
	Td	TIG	Td	TIG
Unknown of <3 doses	Yes	No	Yes	Yes
3+ doses	No*	No	No**	No

* Yes, if >10 years since last dose
** Yes, if >5 years since last dose

Tachycardia, mental changes, hypertension, and renal failure can be seen in its acute phase. The skin is edematous, with gas sometimes noted on palpation, often along with hemorrhagic bullae. Approximately 15% have associated bacteremia. Gram stain of the wound discharge usually shows gram-positive or gram-variable rods with few or no white cells.

Immediate surgical debridement is the cornerstone of treatment. Intravenous penicillin, 24 million units divided every 4 to 6 hours per day, with the use of intravenous clindamycin, 900 mg every 8 hours, for synergistic purposes. The addition of an aminoglycoside or a third-generation cephalosporin (eg, ceftriaxone, cefotaxime) should be used in mixed infections that include gram-negative organisms. Other antibiotics that can be used include metronidazole, chloramphenicol, tetracycline, and β-lactam/β-lactamase inhibitor combinations (eg, ampicillin–sulbactam, piperacillin–tazobactam). The use of hyperbaric oxygen remains controversial.

Owing to the high density of anaerobes in the colon, it comes as no surprise that colonic surgery ranks as the most common surgical procedure associated with gas gangrene. The clinician should also be aware that 10% to 20% of all diseased gall bladders grow *Clostridium* spp. from bile and, hence, gas gangrene from this source becomes the next most common abdominal surgical procedure complicated by gas gangrene. It usually presents as emphysematous cholecystitis or gas gangrene of the abdominal wall. The finding of gas in the biliary tract on radiography or computed tomography requires prompt surgical intervention and antimicrobial therapy. Other causes of *Clostridial myonecrosis* include criminal abortion, retained placenta, prolonged rupture of the membranes, intrauterine fetal demise, missed abortion in postpartum women, intramuscular injection of epinephrine, black tar heroine injection (skin popping), and acupuncture.

CLOSTRIDIA BACTEREMIA

Bacteremia caused by clostridia species can have a fulminate course. *Clostridium perfringens* accounts for >60% of isolates. Many patients, however, may have no symptoms attributable to the bacteremia and have been admitted to the hospital for another medical condition, often for an intra-abdominal problem. These patients with so-called benign clostridia bacteremia do not require antibiotic therapy. This has been observed most commonly after delivery of a baby. The second most common *Clostridium* species isolated from blood is *C. septicum*, which is usually associated with underlying hematologic malignancy, colonic carcinoma, or cyclic neutropenia. In fact, when *C. septicum* bacteremia occurs, 70% to 80% are associated with malignancies, most frequently leukemia in relapse or colon carcinoma.

Virtually all *C. perfringens* species are susceptible to penicillin although some resistance to low levels of penicillin has been encountered. Metronidazole, clindamycin, and chloramphenicol are alternatives in a penicillin-allergic patient. *Clostridium septicum* is also extremely susceptible to penicillin as well as to other antibiotics. *Clostridium tertium* is unusual in that it is resistant to β-lactam antibiotics as well as to clindamycin and metronidazole. The organism is uniformly susceptible to vancomycin, trimethoprim–sulfamethoxazole, ciprofloxacin, and levofloxacin. Recently, overwhelming infections from *C. sordelli* have been described, particularly in previously healthy young women after an obstetric event; in fact, the cases reported after childbirth, miscarriage, and abortion have been almost uniformly fatal.

FOOD POISONING FROM *CLOSTRIDIUM PERFRINGENS*

One of the most common and dangerous causes of food poisoning in humans is caused by enterotoxin-producing strains of *Clostridium perfringens*. Of the five strains of *C. perfringens* (A through E), type A causes most cases of foodborne illness and infectious diarrhea. The usual sources are meat and meat products in which the toxin survives cooking. In this situation, the spores can germinate with vegetative cells multiplying, which can produce a large amount of enterotoxin in the process. To avoid disease, cooked meat should be refrigerated if not served immediately, and rewarmed meat should be heated to an internal temperature of ≥75°C (167°F) before serving.

Criteria used to establish the diagnosis of *C. perfringens* food poisoning include (1) more than 10^5 *C. perfringens* organisms per gram of incriminated food, (2) median spore count of more than 10^6 per gram of stool from ill persons, and (3) isolation of the same serotype of *C. perfringens* from stool and suspected food. Molecular methods for detection of *C. perfringens* include enzyme immunoassay for detection of toxins as well as gene probe or polymerase chain reaction assays for detection of toxin gene.

Clostridium perfringens food poisoning should be suspected in any outbreak of diarrhea occurring 7 to 15 hours after ingestion of a common food source. After an incubation period of 8 to 12 hours, the patient develops diarrhea (>90% of cases), midepigastric pain (>80%), nausea (25%), fever (>24%), and vomiting (>9%). The disease is typically self-limited and resolves in less than 24 hours. Therapy is supportive, with fluid replacement playing a major role. Antibiotics and drugs that inhibit intestinal peristalsis are not indicated and may even prolong the illness. Almost all patients have spontaneous improvement in 6 to 24 hours. Fatalities are rare.

On rare occasions, however, type C causes foodborne infections that result in a fulminating necrotizing enteritis with a high morbidity and fatality rate. First reported in Germany between 1946 and 1949, it is now found only in the highlands of Papua, New Guinea, where it is known as pig belly because of its association with pig feasts. It is believed that the disease results from deficiency or absence of intestinal proteolytic enzymes specific for the type C toxin, which is usually caused by nutritional factors, inhibitors in the diet, or both. A pig-belly vaccine for children (2, 4, and 6 months of age) has been used by the Papua, New Guinea, Health Services with significant success by reducing the incidence to one fifth within 2 years.

CLOSTRIDIUM DIFFICILE COLITIS

Clostridium difficile, the agent that causes pseudomembranous colitis associated with antibiotic therapy, is discussed in Chapter 50, Antibiotic-Associated Diarrhea.

SUGGESTED READING

Allen SD, Emery CL, Lyerly DM. Clostridium. In: Murray PR, Baron EJ, Jorgensen JH, et al., eds. *Manual of Clinical Microbiology*. 8th ed. Washington, DC: ASM Press; 2003:461.

Arnon S, Schechter R, Inglesby TV, et al. Botulinum toxin as a biological weapon. *JAMA*. 2001;285(No. 8):1059–1070.

Bodey GP, Rodriguez S, Fainstein V, et al. Clostridial bacteremia in cancer patients. *Cancer*. 1991;67:1928–1942.

Ernst ME, Klepser ME, Marangos MN. Tetanus: pathophysiology and management. *Ann Pharmacother*. 1997;31:1507–1513.

Pascual FB, McGinley EL, Zanardi LR, et al. Tetanus surveillance – United States, 1998–2000. Centers for Disease Control and Prevention Summaries, June 20, 2003. *Morbid Mortal Weekly Rep*. 2003;52.

Shapiro RL, Hatheway C, Swerdlow DL. Botulism in the United States: clinical and epidemiologic review. *Ann Intern Med*. 1998;129:221–228.

131. Corynebacteria

Carlos H. Ramírez-Ronda and Carlos R. Ramírez-Ramírez

CORYNEBACTERIUM DIPHTHERIAE (DIPHTHERIA)

Diphtheria is an acute, infectious, preventable, and sometimes fatal disease caused by *Corynebacterium diphtheriae*. The infection is usually localized to the upper part of the respiratory tract and the skin; from here it gives rise to local and systemic signs or it can be asymptomatic. These signs are the result of a toxin produced by the microorganisms multiplying at the site of infection. The systemic complications particularly affect the heart and the peripheral nerves.

Cause

Diphtheria is distributed worldwide, with the highest incidence in temperate climates. It occurs predominantly under poor socioeconomic conditions, where crowding is common and where many persons are either not immunized or inadequately immunized. There have been reports of diphtheria outbreaks in the newly independent states of the former Soviet Union. Diphtheria is seen in developed countries in people that return and travel to endemic areas as well as in immigrants from endemic areas.

The only significant reservoir of *C. diphtheriae* is the human host. The organism is transmitted directly from one person to another, and intimate contact is required. Transmission is usually by way of infected droplets of nasopharyngeal secretions. Infective skin exudate has been involved in human-to-human transmission. Transmission may also occur via animals, fomites, or milk. The infectious period is usually 2 weeks from onset of symptoms, as long as 6 weeks, and, if treated with antibiotics, to less than 4 days.

Immunity depends on antitoxin in the host's blood. Antitoxin is formed by immunization or by clinical or subclinical infection, including skin infections. The Schick test consists of an intradermal injection of 0.1 mL of purified diphtheria toxin dissolved in buffered human serum albumin. This is injected into the volar surface of one arm, and 0.1 mL of purified diphtheria toxoid is used as a control in the other arm. The test can be used to assess the immune status of the subject. Reaction to toxin but not to toxoid indicates that the patient is immune and that levels of antitoxin exceed 0.03 U/mL. This test provides only an estimate of immunity, and the inability to perform it should not delay treatment of asymptomatic contacts of diphtheria. The Schick test is not to be used before adult immunization. Immunity does not prevent carriage.

Clinical Features

Diphtheria may be symptomless or rapidly fatal. The incubation period varies from 1 to 7 days but is most commonly 2 to 4 days.

ANTERIOR NARES DIPHTHERIA

The infection is localized to the anterior nasal area and is manifested by unilateral or bilateral serous or serosanguineous discharge that erodes the adjacent skin, resulting in small crusted lesions. The membrane may be seen in the nose.

TONSILLAR (FAUCIAL) DIPHTHERIA

Tonsillar diphtheria is the most common presentation and the most toxic form. The onset is usually sudden, with fever rarely exceeding 38°C (100.4°F), malaise, and mild sore throat. The pharynx is moderately infected, and a thick, whitish-gray tonsillar exudate is often seen. The tonsillar and cervical lymph nodes are enlarged. The exudate may extend to other areas and result in nasopharyngeal diphtheria and massive cervical lymphadenopathy (bull neck appearance also called malignant diphtheria). The most common complaints are sore throat (85%), pain on swallowing (23%), nausea and vomiting (25%), and headache (18%).

PHARYNGEAL DIPHTHERIA

Pharyngeal diphtheria is diagnosed when the membrane extends from the tonsillar area to the pharynx.

LARYNGEAL AND BRONCHIAL DIPHTHERIA

Laryngeal and bronchial diphtheria involves the larynx. The voice becomes hoarse, and inspiratory and expiratory stridor may appear; dyspnea and cyanosis occur, and the accessory muscles of respiration are used. Tracheostomy or intubation is needed.

CUTANEOUS DIPHTHERIA

Classically described as diphtheria in tropical areas, cutaneous diphtheria now is seen in nontropical areas as well. It takes the form of a chronic nonhealing ulcer, sometimes covered with a grayish membranous exudate. Another form is secondary infection of a pre-existing wound. Finally, superinfection with *C. diphtheriae* may occur in a variety of primary skin lesions, such as impetigo, insect bites, ectyma, and eczema.

Complications of Diphtheria

MYOCARDITIS

Although electrocardiographic (ECG) changes have been described in up to 66% of cases, overt clinical myocarditis is less common (10%–15%). The onset is insidious, occurring in the second or third week of the infection. The patient exhibits a weak, rising pulse; distant heart sounds; and profound weakness and lethargy. Overt signs of heart failure can occur. The most common ECG changes are flattening or inversion of T waves, bundle branch block or intraventricular block, and disorders of rhythm. Serial determination of cardiac enzyme concentrations identifies most patients with myocarditis. The prognosis is poor, especially when heart block supervenes.

PERIPHERAL NEURITIS

Neurologic toxicity has been described in about 5% of patients with diphtheria, but in severe diphtheria up to 75% of patients develop neurologic complications. The most common form of cranial nerve palsy is paralysis of the soft palate. There may be nasal regurgitation and/or nasal speech. This condition is usually mild, and recovery occurs within 2 weeks. Ciliary paralysis and oculomotor paralysis are the next most common forms. Peripheral neuritis affecting the limbs may appear during the fourth to eighth week. It is usually manifested by weakness of the dorsiflexors and decreased or absent deep-tendon reflexes. Diphtheritic polyneuritis has been described after cutaneous diphtheria.

Diagnosis

Diagnosis is made on clinical grounds and can be confirmed by laboratory tests (Figure 131.1).

The clinical features of a fully developed diphtheritic membrane, especially in the pharynx, are sufficiently characteristic to suggest diphtheria and for treatment to be started immediately.

Specific diagnosis of diphtheria depends completely on demonstration of the organism in stained smears and its recovery by culture. In experienced hands, methylene blue–stained preparations are positive in 75% to 85% of cases. The bacilli can be recovered by culture in Loeffler's or Tindale's medium within 8 to 12 hours if patients have not been receiving antimicrobial agents. *Corynebacterium diphtheriae* can be seen as gram-positive bacilli in a "Chinese letter" distribution pattern on Gram or methylene blue stain (Figure 131.2); one can find metachromatic granules on Loeffler's stain and black colonies with halos with growth on Tinsdale's medium. The presence of β-hemolytic streptococci does not rule out diphtheria because such streptococci are recovered in up to 20% to 30% of patients with diphtheria.

The differential diagnosis of tonsillar-pharyngeal diphtheria should include streptococcal pharyngitis, adenoviral exudative pharyngitis, infectious mononucleosis, and Vincent's angina, among others (Table 131.1).

Therapy

The best and most effective treatment of diphtheria is prevention by immunization with diphtheria toxoid. The most important aspect of treatment is to administer the antitoxin as soon as diphtheria is clinically suspected, without awaiting laboratory confirmation. The patient should be hospitalized, isolated, and kept in bed for 10 to 14 days (see Figures 131.1 and 131.3).

USE OF ANTITOXIN

The antitoxin is equine, and the minimal effective dose remains undefined; therefore, dosage is based on empiric judgment. It is usually accepted that for patients with mild or moderate cases, including those with tonsillar and pharyngeal membrane, 50 000 U intramuscularly is enough (for a child, 20 000 to 30 000 U recommended by the American Academy of Pediatrics). In severe cases, such as with a more extensive membrane and/or thrombocytopenia, 60 000 to 120 000 U depending on severity is the recommended dose; critically ill patients should receive at least half of it by slow intravenous infusion.

Before administration of the antitoxin, any history of allergy or reactions to horse serum or horse dander must be determined. All patients

Diphtheria
Corynebacterium diphtheriae

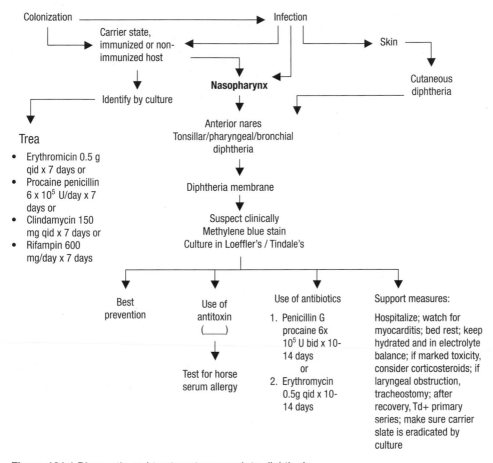

Trea

- Erythromycin 0.5 g qid x 7 days or
- Procaine penicillin 6 x 10^5 U/day x 7 days or
- Clindamycin 150 mg qid x 7 days or
- Rifampin 600 mg/day x 7 days

Colonization ———————→ Infection

Carrier state, immunized or non-immunized host

Skin

Nasopharynx

Cutaneous diphtheria

Identify by culture

Anterior nares
Tonsillar/pharyngeal/bronchial diphtheria

Diphtheria membrane

Suspect clinically
Methylene blue stain
Culture in Loeffler's / Tindale's

Best prevention	Use of antitoxin (___)	Use of antibiotics	Support measures:
	Test for horse serum allergy	1. Penicillin G procaine 6x 10^5 U bid x 10-14 days or 2. Erythromycin 0.5g qid x 10-14 days	Hospitalize; watch for myocarditis; bed rest; keep hydrated and in electrolyte balance; if marked toxicity, consider corticosteroids; if laryngeal obstruction, tracheostomy; after recovery, Td+ primary series; make sure carrier slate is eradicated by culture

Figure 131.1 Diagnostic and treatment approach to diphtheria.

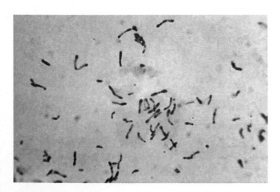

Figure 131.2 Gram-positive bacilli in a "Chinese letter" distribution pattern on Gram stain.

must be tested for antitoxin sensitivity with dilute horse antitoxin in saline 1:10 and an eye test. This is followed by a scratch test with a 1:100 dilution; if negative in half an hour, the scratch test is followed by an intradermal test, 1:100 dilution. If all tests are negative, antitoxin can be given. The intravenous route is recommended. A slow intravenous infusion of 0.5 mL antitoxin in 10 mL saline is followed in half an hour by the balance of the dose in a dilution of 1:20 with saline, infused at a rate not to exceed 1 mL/min. Others give the antitoxin dose intramuscularly in mild to moderate cases only.

If the patient is sensitive to horse serum, desensitization should be carried out with care, preferably in an intensive care unit. Epinephrine, intubation equipment, and respiratory assistance should be available. The following doses of horse serum antitoxin should be injected at 15-minute intervals if no reaction occurs:

1) 0.05 mL of 1:20 dilution subcutaneously
2) 0.10 mL of 1:10 dilution subcutaneously
3) 0.3 mL of 1:10 dilution subcutaneously

Table 131.1 Differential Diagnosis of Diphtheria

Affected Area	Other Conditions
Nose	Sinusitis, foreign body, snuffles of congenital syphilis, rhinitis
Fauces and pharynx	Streptococcal or adenoviral exudative pharyngitis, ulcerative pharyngitis (herpetic, coxsackie-viral), infectious mononucleosis, oral thrush, peritonsillar abscess, retropharyngeal abscess, Vincent's angina, lesions associated with agranulocytosis or leukemia
Larynx	Laryngotracheobronchitis, epiglottitis
Skin	Impetigo, pyogenic ulcers, herpes simplex infection

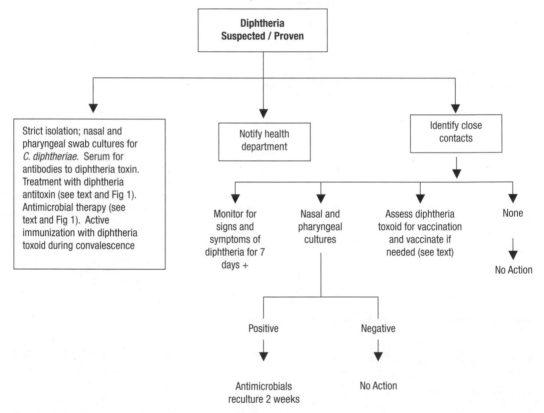

Figure 131.3 Public health management of diphtheria.

4) 0.1 mL of undiluted antitoxin subcutaneously
5) 0.2 mL of undiluted antitoxin subcutaneously
6) 0.5 mL of undiluted antitoxin subcutaneously
7) Remaining estimated therapeutic dose intramuscularly

During all tests and on injection of antitoxin, a syringe containing epinephrine 1:1000 dilution in saline should be at hand to be used immediately in a dose of 0.01 mL/kg subcutaneously or intramuscularly at any sign of anaphylaxis. A good precaution is to have open venous access with normal saline prior to the test. If needed, a similar amount of epinephrine diluted to a final concentration of 1:10 000 in saline may be given slowly intravenously and repeated in 5 to 15 minutes. Other information and instructions in the package insert accompanying the antitoxin should be observed.

ANTIBIOTICS

Corynebacterium diphtheriae is susceptible to several antimicrobial agents. After cultures have been performed, antibiotics should be administered to prevent multiplication of the microorganism at the site of infection and to eliminate the carrier state. Penicillin G, the drug of choice, is usually given as procaine penicillin, 600 000 U intramuscularly every 12 hours for 10 to 14 days. Erythromycin, also very active against the diphtheria bacillus, is given at 2 g/day divided in four doses for the same period.

SUPPORTIVE MEASURES

Complications such as dehydration, malnutrition, and congestive heart failure should be diagnosed promptly and properly treated. In cases of severe laryngeal involvement, marked toxicity, or shock, corticosteroids (prednisone 3 to 5 mg/kg/day) have been advocated, but there are no hard data on their effectiveness. For laryngeal obstruction with respiratory stridor, a tracheotomy must be performed promptly.

Before the patient is discharged, specimens from throat and nose or suspected lesions should be cultured. At least two and preferably three consecutive negative cultures should be obtained.

After recovery, toxoid administration against tetanus and diphtheria (Td) should be administered to complete a primary immunization series if the patient has not been immunized.

Carriers

The chronic carrier state may occur despite immunity derived either from clinical disease or from immunization. The carrier state occasionally persists in the absence of antecedent disease. Erythromycin, 0.5 g orally 4 times a day for 7 days in adults, is the treatment of choice for the carrier state. Alternative antibiotics are procaine penicillin G, 600 000 U intramuscularly daily for 14 days, clindamycin, 150 mg orally four times a day for 7 days, or rifampin, 600 mg/day orally for 7 days.

Epidemics

The approach to epidemic disease is as follows:

1) Identify all primary cases, hospitalize, and treat.
2) Use toxoid in all the population at risk.
3) Culture all contacts for diphtheria, and treat all persons with C. diphtheriae in throat, nose, or skin lesions with erythromycin for 7 days to eliminate carrier state (Figure 131.3).
4) Watch primary contacts closely during the first week of exposure and treat at first signs or symptoms. Alternatively, all susceptible primary contacts can be given 1500 to 3000 U of diphtheria antitoxin, administered as previously described, in addition to toxoid. This low-level dose will boost them while they are forming their antibody.

Prevention

Children who have had a complete course of primary immunization with diphtheria-tetanus-pertussis (DTaP) vaccine may be given a booster injection on exposure to diphtheria. This is done in case of outbreaks but is not routine. Antibiotic prophylaxis is highly effective.

Household and other close contacts of a patient with diphtheria should be observed attentively for 7 days. They should receive either an intramuscular injection of 1.2 million units of benzathine penicillin or a 7-day course of erythromycin taken orally. Cultures should be performed before and after treatment. An injection of toxoid appropriate for age and immunization status can also be given. Susceptible close contacts who have had no (or only one) prior injections of toxoid should promptly be given 3000 to 10 000 units (depending on body size) of antitoxin, with the usual precautions being followed. When indicated, active immunization with toxoid should be continued to completion. Routine immunization for diphtheria is discussed in Chapter 113, Immunizations.

NONDIPHTHERIC CORYNEBACTERIA

Nondiphtheric corynebacteria were once considered commensals. They are present in the skin and often are recovered from blood cultures. The presence of the microorganism in the blood has been considered contaminant, but there are many instances in which nondiphtheric corynebacteria are associated with bacteremias, sepsis, pneumonias, endocarditis, central nervous system infections, and intraocular infections, especially in immunocompromised patients and patients with vascular and central nervous system catheters and prosthetic devices. A common predisposing factor is neutropenia.

The diagnosis of infections with nondiphtheric corynebacteria usually involves their recovery from blood or other sterile body fluid. Corynebacteria can be identified by conventional methods; since 2000, a new system, the Rapid CORYNE System, was found to be excellent and an alternative to conventional methods.

Clinically, there are no specific findings that suggest nondiphtheric corynebacteria, but their association with central lines, skin, and subcutaneous infections in immunocompromised patients leads the clinician to

Table 131.2 Epidemiology and Clinical Features of Selected Nondiphtheric Corynebacteria

Corynebacterium	Epidemiology	Clinical Features
C. group JK	Skin, systemic	Soft-tissue, pneumonias, shunt infections; skin rash; endocarditis
C. minutissimum	Skin	Erythrasma, reddish-brown macular lesions, fluoresce under Wood's lamp
C. ulcerans	Skin, systemic	Cardiac and central nervous system involvement; diseases in horses and cattle
C. pseudotuberculosis	Skin exposure, farm animals, raw milk	Dermonecrotic toxin, suppurative granulomas, lymphadenitis, disease in farm animals
C. bovis	Shunts, skin	Meningitis, spinal epidural; abscess; ventriculoperitoneal or jugular shunts
C. pseudodiphtericum	Systemic	Pneumonia endocarditis, tracheitis, urinary tract
C. striatum	Immunosuppressed	Pneumonias, meningitis, abscesses, bacteremias

associate a given infection with a gram-positive rod. Table 131.2 lists the epidemiology and clinical features of selected nondiphtheric corynebacteria.

CORYNEBACTERIUM GROUP JK

Corynebacterium group JK is gram-positive coccobacillus or coccus resembling the streptococcus. Characteristically, it shows high-grade antibiotic resistance, being susceptible only to vancomycin in vitro and in vivo.

Clinical Features

Diseases associated with *Corynebacterium* group JK include soft-tissue infections, pneumonitis with or without cavitation, continuous ambulatory peritoneal dialysis-related peritonitis, neurosurgical shunt infections, skin rash, catheter-related epicardial abscess, and endocarditis. It should always be considered a possible cause of sepsis in the neutropenic patient and in patients with prosthetic devices in place.

Therapy

Despite their high antibiotic resistance, these corynebacteria remain susceptible to vancomycin. Total effective duration of treatment has not been established. Clinical response must be followed, usually treating for 4 to 6 weeks. Newer fluoroquinolones, mainly ciprofloxacin, have also shown good results. Infected prosthetic material often requires removal.

CORYNEBACTERIUM MINUTISSIMUM

Infection with *C. minutissimum* usually involves the skin, and the classical disease entity is erythrasma. Erythrasma is a skin infection characterized by brownish-reddish macules that itch and when exposed to a Wood's lamp fluoresce. The most frequent location is the intertriginous areas.

Bacteremia with *C. minutissimum* has been described in patients with leukemia in blast crisis. There are also reports of trichomycosis axillaris associated with this corynebacterium.

CORYNEBACTERIUM ULCERANS

Corynebacterium ulcerans, like *C. diphtheriae*, produces diphtheria toxin by lysogeny but without apparent clinical consequences. However, there are documented reports of *C. ulcerans* bacteremias with cardiac and central nervous system involvement as well as pneumonia.

CORYNEBACTERIUM PSEUDOTUBERCULOSIS

Infection with *C. pseudotuberculosis* is associated with exposure to farm animals or consumption of raw milk. Clinically, it presents as a suppurative granulomatous lymphadenitis most likely related to the dermonecrotic toxin it produces. This organism responds to long-term treatment with erythromycin or tetracycline.

CORYNEBACTERIUM BOVIS

Most infections reported with *C. bovis* are associated with central nervous system processes. There have been cases of meningitis, epidural abscesses, and shunt infections.

CORYNEBACTERIUM PSEUDODIPHTHERICUM

Sites of infection caused by *C. pseudodiphthericum* include heart valves, wounds, urinary tract, and lungs, with pneumonia and necrotizing tracheitis. The susceptibilities of this microorganism are varied, with both susceptibility and resistance to erythromycin, clindamycin, and penicillin. There is a case of response to penicillin intravenously (12 million units daily for 14 days).

CORYNEBACTERIUM STRIATUM

Persons with an underlying immunosuppressive process are usually victims of *C. striatum*. There are reports of pneumonias, pulmonary abscesses, meningitis, and bacteremias with *C. striatum*. Most patients were treated with vancomycin.

OTHERS

There have been reports of *Corynebacterium* CDC group A-4 associated with native valve endocarditis in immunocompetent patients as well as sepsis in immunocompromised hosts with infected Hickman catheters. *Corynebacterium aquaticum,* an environmental organism of fresh water, has been associated with septicemia in a neutropenic patient with an indwelling central venous catheter who used untreated stored rainwater to shower. *Corynebacterium afermentans* (CDC group ANF-1) was reported to cause endocarditis in a prosthetic valve.

Therapy

Some corynebacteria are susceptible to erythromycin, sulfonamides, chloramphenicol, gentamicin, imipenem, some of the newer fluoroquinolones, and vancomycin. For most serious and systemic infections, we prefer to use vancomycin at 1 g every 12 hours for at least 2 weeks in adults with normal renal function. In some patients, especially immunocompromised patients, combination therapy can be used with vancomycin plus imipenem at 500 mg intravenously every 6 hours, vancomycin plus rifampin at 600 mg daily orally, or vancomycin plus ciprofloxacin at 750 mg orally every 12 hours for 2 to 4 weeks. Erythromycin at a dosage of 2 to 4 g in divided doses can be used as an alternative regimen. The optimal effective therapy for these infections has not been determined, but 8 weeks of treatment are often required. For unresponsive cases, surgical consultation is recommended.

SUGGESTED READING

Brooks GF, Bennett JV, Feldman RA. Diphtheria in the United States 1959–1970. *J Infect Dis.* 1974;129:172–178.

Brown A. Other corynebacteria. In Mandell GL, Bennett JE, Dolin R, eds. *Mandell, Douglas and Bennett's Principles and Practice of Infectious Diseases.* 6th ed. Philadelphia, PA: Churchill Livingstone; 2004.

Clarridge JE, Popovic T, Inzana TJ. Diphtheria and other corynebacterial and coryneform infections. Vol 3. In: Hausler WJ, Sussman M, eds. *Topley and Wilson's Microbiology and Microbial Infections.* New York: Oxford University Press; 1998.

Efstratiou A, Engler KH, Mazurova IK, et al. Current approaches to the laboratory diagnosis of diphtheria. *J Infect Dis.* 2000;181(Suppl 1):S138–S145.

Galazka AM, Robertson SE, Oblapenko GP. Resurgence of diphtheria. *Eur J Epidemiol.* 1995;11:95–105.

Halsey N, Bartlett JG. Corynebacteria. In: Gorbach SL, Barlett JG, Blacklow NR, eds. *Infectious Diseases.* Philadelphia, PA: Lippincott, Williams & Wilkins; 2004.

Kneen R, Pham NG, Solomon T, et al. Penicillin vs. erythromycin in the treatment of diphtheria. *Clin Infect Dis.* 1998;27:845–850.

Koopman JS, Campbell J. The role of cutaneous diphtheria infections in a diphtheric epidemic. *J Infect Dis.* 1975;131:239–244.

Lipsky BA, Goldberg AC, Tompkins LS, et al. Infections caused by nondiptheria corynebacteria. *Rev Infect Dis.* 1982;4:1220–1235.

MacGregor RR. Corynebacterium diphtheriae. In: Mandell GL, Bennett JE, Dolin R, eds. *Mandell, Douglas and Bennett's Principles and Practice of Infectious Diseases.* 6th ed. Philadelphia, PA: Churchill Livingstone; 2004.

132. Enterobacteriaceae

L. W. Preston Church

The Enterobacteriaceae comprise several genera commonly referred to as the enteric gram-negative bacilli and several species less commonly encountered in clinical practice (Table 132.1). The unique features of *Salmonella*, *Shigella*, and *Yersinia* are considered in separate chapters. These organisms are ubiquitous in the environment and are readily recovered from water and soil. The human reservoir for most species is the colon, although other mucosal sites may become colonized, particularly in health care–related settings. Members of the Enterobacteriaceae are important causes of community-acquired and hospital-acquired infections of almost any organ system, with hospital-acquired strains increasingly demonstrating resistance to multiple classes of antibiotics through a variety of resistance mechanisms. This growing dilemma underscores the need for accurate diagnoses and intelligent use of a diminishing antimicrobial arsenal.

URINARY TRACT INFECTION

The Enterobacteriaceae are the most important etiology of both community-acquired and nosocomial urinary tract infection, with *E. coli* the most frequently encountered pathogen. The success of *E. coli*, in part, may be attributed to the adaptation of specialized adherence fimbriae that facilitate attachment to normal uroepithelium.

The symptoms of urinary tract infection are common to all uropathogens but may assist in defining the location and extent of infection. In women the three principle manifestations are urethritis, characterized primarily by dysuria; cystitis, characterized by frequency, urgency, dysuria, suprapubic tenderness with or without fever; or pyelonephritis, characterized by nausea and vomiting, fever, chills, flank pain and costovertebral angle tenderness. In the male urinary tract additional structures may be involved as seen in epydidimitis and acute or chronic prostatitis. In the elderly or the patient with an indwelling urinary catheter or a spinal cord injury, many of the signs and symptoms may be absent and the lines separating infection from asymptomatic bacteruria may be blurred.

Presenting features rarely distinguish the infecting agent with the exception of urinary tract infection with alkaline urine (pH8), often in the presence of staghorn renal calculi, which is strongly suggestive of *Proteus* species.

An important corollary of urinary tract infection is asymptomatic bacteruria—the presence of a uropathogen in significant quantity, usually defined as $>10^5$ organisms/mL, with or without pyuria in the absence of symptoms. Although asymptomatic bacteruria infrequently progresses to symptomatic infection, treatment is indicated only in pregnancy (done for the increased risk for pyelonephritis), young children, or prior to instrumentation of the urinary tract, as with insertion of a Foley catheter. Bacteruria in the presence of symptoms defines urinary tract infection. Although $>10^5$ organisms/mL is often used as the cutoff for significant bacteruria in defining a urinary tract infection, for a properly obtained sample yielding a likely pathogen in the presence of appropriate symptoms, $>10^4$ organisms/mL is a more sensitive measure. For samples obtained by suprapubic tap or other means of percutaneous drainage, a lower threshold of $>10^3$ organisms/mL may be appropriate.

GASTROINTESTINAL AND INTRA-ABDOMINAL INFECTION

Although many of the Enterobacteriaceae are part of the normal gut flora, this group is the principle cause of intra-abdominal infections through a variety of mechanisms. Several strains of *E. coli* are associated with diarrheal disease of the small and large intestine (Table 132.2). Most, if not all, of those infections are self-limited illnesses although the severity varies. Enterotoxigenic *E. coli* (ETEC) is the most common cause of travelers' diarrhea and enjoys a long list of colorful synonyms such as Montezuma's revenge. Disease is the result of choleralike toxins that result in excess secretion of water by the small bowel into the gut lumen, overwhelming the capacity of the colon to resorb water. For most of the enteropathogenic *E. coli*, diagnostic testing is not routinely available although specific toxins or genes may

Table 132.1 Medically Important Enterobacteriaceae

Genus and Species	Comments
Citrobacter diversus, C. freundii	Usually nosocomial, most frequently involving urinary tract
Edwardsiella tarda	Associated with fresh water ingestion causing diarrhea
Enterobacter aerogenes, E. cloacae, E. sakasaki	Intestinal colonizer typically surfaces as a pathogen in hospitalized patients receiving antibiotics; antibiotic resistance common
Escherichia coli	Most common cause of urinary tract infection. Several diarrheal pathotypes. Pneumonia, particularly in alcoholics, diabetics, immunocompromised or nosocomial (HAP, VAP) Important in community and nosocomial infections of all types. High level antimicrobial resistance including ESBL increasing
Ewingella americana	Nosocomial infections, rare
Hafnia alvei	Rare
Klebsiella pneumoniae, K. oxytoca	Community and nosocomial pathogen. Common cause of urinary tract infection with bacteremia. Important cause of pneumonia as for *E. coli*. High level antimicrobial resistance including ESBL
Kluyvera species	Rare
Morganella morganii	Uncommon cause of nosocomial infections
Pantoea agglomerans	Environmental pathogen
Plesiomonas shigeloides	Associated with fresh water ingestion causing diarrhea
Proteus mirabilis, P. vulgaris	Urinary tract infections (frequently bacteremic), especially in presence of foreign body or urologic abnormalities
Providencia stuarti, P. retgeri	Catheter-associated urinary tract infections
Salmonella enterica	See Chapter 148, *Salmonella*
Serratia marcescens	Environmental pathogen, antibiotic resistance common
Shigella species	See Chapter 153, Shigella
Yersinia species	See Chapter 158, Yersinia

Abbreviations: HAP = hospital-acquired pneumonia; VAP = ventilator-associated pneumonia; ESBL = extended-spectrum beta-lactamase.

be detected by polymerase chain reaction (PCR) or DNA probes. The important exception is enterohemorrhagic *E. coli* (EHEC) and if suspected the stool should be cultured on sorbital–MacConkey agar to identify the 0157:H7 strain most commonly associated with this disease. EHEC typically manifests as acute bloody diarrhea accompanied by abdominal pain and cramping. Fever is notably absent. Most commonly associated with undercooked ground meat, outbreaks have been associated with unpasteurized apple cider and other uncooked or unpasteurized products. Hemolytic uremic syndrome, characterized by acute renal failure and thrombocytopenia, complicates 7% to 15% of cases of EHEC with the greater proportion of cases occurring in the very young and the elderly.

Obstruction of diverticuli or the appendix may be part of the mechanism behind diverticulitis and appendicitis, both polymicrobial infections in which the Enterobacteriaceae have an active role. Gut flora may, through perforation of a viscus, form an abscess anywhere within the abdominal or pelvic cavities or result in peritonitis. Introduction of these organisms into the biliary system, especially in the content of obstruction, may result in cholecystitis.

Specific Organisms – Bacteria

Table 132.2 Pathogenic *E. coli* of the Gastrointestinal Tract

Pathotype		Clinical Illness	Comments
ETEC	Enterotoxogenic *E. coli*	Acute watery diarrhea, usually self-limited	Most common cause of travelers' diarrhea and in children worldwide
EAEC	Enteroaggregative *E. coli*	Mucoid diarrhea	May cause chronic diarrhea, emerging in travelers
EPEC	Enteropathogenic *E. coli*	Acute diarrhea and vomiting	Common in children in developing countries
EIEC	Enteroinvasive *E. coli*	Watery diarrhea or dysentery (fever, abdominal pain, tenesmus, blood)	Occurs in outbreaks
EHEC	Enterohemorrhagic *E. coli*	Watery and bloody diarrhea	Hemolytic–uremic syndrome

Liver abscess may result from extension of an infectious process in the biliary system or may be seeded from the gut via the portal venous system. These infections may be characterized by fever and abdominal pain that may or may not be localizing. Leukocytosis with a left shift may be an important clue to the diagnosis. In cholecystitis and cholangitis the total bilirubin is usually elevated if the common bile duct is involved but is elevated only 25% of the time if not obstructed. Alkaline phosphatase is elevated in two thirds of liver abscess, usually with little to no elevation of bilirubin or aminotransferases. Infection of the pancreas or a pancreatic pseudocyst may be extremely troublesome to diagnose as the signs and symptoms of abdominal pain, nausea, vomiting, fever, and leukocytosis may all be manifestations of acute pancreatitis. Infection should be suspected with the appearance of a new febrile episode, especially after manipulation of the pancreas as during endoscopic retrograde cholangiapancreatography (ERCP).

Finally, the Enterobacteriaceae are the primary etiologic agent of spontaneous bacterial peritonitis (SBP). Despite the proximity to the gastrointestinal (GI) tract, SBP is a consequence of hematogenous seeding of pre-existing ascites, most commonly in the context of cirrhosis but occasionally complicating nephritic syndrome or severe right-sided heart failure. Clinical manifestations include presence of ascites by exam or imaging, which is usually new or clinically worse abdominal pain, tenderness, and fever.

PNEUMONIA AND PLEURAL SPACE INFECTIONS

The Enterobacteriaceae account for 5% to 15% of all pneumonias for which an etiologic agent can be identified, regardless of whether the pneumonia is community or nosocomially acquired. Clinical findings are rarely helpful in determining the etiology of a bacterial pneumonia although aspiration, older age, and comorbid conditions such as heart failure, renal disease, or diabetes may favor a gram-negative etiology. Production of dark-red mucoid or "currant jelly" sputum suggests pneumonia due to *Klebsiella pneumoniae* but the other hallmarks of "Friedlander's" pneumonia are nonspecific. No pattern on chest radiograph is pathognomonic of gram-negative pneumonia, but the diagnosis should be considered whenever necrotizing pneumonia, pneumatoceles, cavitation, or empyema are seen.

SKIN AND SOFT-TISSUE INFECTIONS

Enterobacteriaceae may be involved in a variety of skin and soft-tissue infections. Pure infections with one of these organisms may occur as surgical wound infections, especially in abdominal or pelvic locations or as a secondary infection of burns. More commonly these organisms are part of mixed infections, especially with anaerobic bacteria. In this context they may cause complicated and often destructive infections of decubitis ulcers or diabetic foot infections or present as part of a spectrum of rapidly progressive and destructive infections of soft tissue, including synergistic necrotizing cellulitis, gangrenous balanitis, perineal phlegmon (Fournier's gangrene), progressive bacterial synergistic gangrene, and necrotizing fasciitis. In general these infections complicate a pre-existing wound or trauma (which may be surprisingly trivial) or may arise from extension from an internal source such as a perforated viscus. Diabetes mellitus is a frequently encountered risk factor. All of these conditions, which differ primarily by location or depth of tissue involvement, are characterized by moderate to severe pain, swelling, crepitus on exam or radiologic evidence of tissue gas, malodorous wound discharge, and evidence of skin necrosis. Affected individuals are usually systemically ill appearing with fever and leukocytosis.

BONE AND JOINT INFECTIONS

Septic arthritis, osteomyelitis, and prosthetic joint infections may be seen with any of the Enterobacteriaceae. Overall they are considerably less frequent than infections of similar sites due to gram-positive cocci and account for 5% to 25% of these infections. Focal infections may result from extension of a localized soft-tissue infection, as in the diabetic foot, as early or late postoperative complications, particularly in the presence of orthopedic devices or by contamination from penetrating injuries. Local vascular and lymphatic seeding from the prostate may lead to lumbar vertebral osteomyelitis, and hematogenous seeding can affect any bone or joint. Clinical presentations will be the same as for any bacterial infection of these sites, varying from small draining sinuses with no associated symptoms to local pain, swelling, erythema, wound dehiscence, and fever. Vertebral infections may have pain in a localized or radicular pattern and may have associated focal neurologic abnormalities if concomitant epidural abscess is present.

Diagnosis rests on clinical suspicion and may be augmented by imaging studies including conventional x-rays, radionuclide scanning, computed tomography (CT), or magnetic resonance imaging (MRI); the latter two modalities may be particularly useful in the evaluation of suspected vertebral infections. Elevated erythrocyte sedimentation rates or C-reactive protein are not useful for diagnosis but may be useful markers to follow response to therapy. In the context of these organisms, surface swabs are unreliable in identifying the agents of deep infection, and sterilely obtained cultures of fluid, bone, or tissue are required for diagnosis.

CENTRAL NERVOUS SYSTEM INFECTIONS

Escherichia coli accounts for the majority of bacterial meningitis due to gram-negative bacilli, with the majority of cases occurring within the first few weeks of life or in the immunocompromised or elderly. Outside of these risk groups most infections are the result of trauma or other causes for bacteremia such as parenteral drug use. Hyperinfection with strongyloides may lead to bacteremia and meningitis as migrating larvae allow colonic bacteria to cross the gut lumen and possibly travel to different anatomic sites in association with larval invasion. Due to the nature of the host, classic signs of fever and nuchal rigidity may be absent and alteration of consciousness may be the only clue. Diagnosis hinges on analysis of the cerebrospinal fluid (CSF). Gram stains are positive in approximately 50% and may be misinterpreted as negative due to similar staining characteristics of the bacteria and the cellular and protein elements in the CSF. Latex agglutination for the *E. coli* K1 antigen, found on 75% of neonatal CSF isolates, may be a useful adjunctive test.

Focal suppurative infections of the central nervous system (CNS), including brain abscess, subdural empyema, and spinal epidural abscess, all occur to a limited extent with these organisms. As noted for vertebral osteomyelitis, chronic prostatitis may lead to seeding of the lower lumbar area with Enterobacteriaceae and produce both osteomyelitis and spinal epidural abscess in this location. One particularly problematic infection is ventriculitis due to ventricular shunt infections. *Enterobacter* species, which thrive in hospital environments, are frequently identified and may be difficult to treat due to intrinsic and acquired antimicrobial resistance.

BACTEREMIA, ENDOVASCULAR INFECTION, AND SEPSIS

A positive blood culture for one of the Enterobacteriaceae, when properly obtained in the evaluation of suspected infection, should always be regarded as a true-positive result and a source aggressively sought. Any of the previously described syndromes may include bacteremia, but the majority of gram-negative bacteremias without a clinically apparent source will have originated in the urinary tract or as an intra-abdominal infection. Intravascular catheters, particularly those used for parenteral nutrition or hemodialysis or those in a femoral vein location, are also important sources of gram-negative bacteremia. In this setting the line exit site and tunnel show no evidence of infection; the line as a source is suspected on the basis of positive blood cultures obtained through the line and ideally from the periphery as well. Some

Enterobacteriaceae

studies suggest that a differential time to positive culture of >2 hours in favor of the culture obtained through the line signifies the line as the source, assuming that equal volumes of blood were obtained for culture and the timing of the cultures was similar. Often the line as a source can be confirmed by culture of the catheter tip in a semiquantitative fashion by rolling it across an agar plate.

Other intravascular devices, including vascular stents, prosthetic vascular grafts, and implanted transvenous pacemakers and defibrillators (AICD) are all at risk for infection and may only manifest as fever, leukocytosis, and bacteremia. The specific risk for stent infections exists until the shunt has endothelialized, a period that may now take up to a year for drug-eluting coronary artery stents and probably never completely occurs with large vessel stents. Infections of these devices are often very difficult to demonstrate. Tagged white cell scans may identify a stent or graft infection, but negative scans do not preclude this diagnosis. Echocardiography, particularly by the transesophageal route, may identify abnormalities on the pacing wires or adjacent cardiac structures suggesting infection. Chest x-ray or chest CT findings of septic pulmonary embolism also support a diagnosis of infected pacemaker or AICD.

Despite the frequency of bacteremia due to the Enterobacteriaceae, they account for only 2% to 5% of both native valve and prosthetic valve endocarditis. Associated mortality of up to 50% is the norm. Injection drug use is a risk factor. Congestive heart failure and large valvular vegetations are typical findings.

Bacteremia with Enterobacteriaceae for any reason may progress rapidly to the complications of gram-negative sepsis or septic shock. Sepsis is defined as the presence of the systemic inflammatory response syndrome with a known pathogen; septic shock is sepsis plus hypotension that fails to respond to simple fluid administration and is usually accompanied by evidence of tissue hypoperfusion such as lactic acidosis, oliguria, or acute lung injury. Although the injection of purified lipopolysaccharides from Enterobacteriaceae produce a picture of septic shock with fever and refractory hypotension that may lead to organ failures, the role of endotoxin in the pathophysiology of sepsis and septic shock remains controversial, and how these organisms initiate the cytokine and neuroendocrine cascades that lead to the clinical picture of sepsis remains unclear.

PRINCIPLES OF ANTIMICROBIAL THERAPY

Suggested antibiotic regimens for the infections described in this chapter are outlined in Table 132.3. Under most circumstances, final antibiotic selection needs to be determined by results of culture and susceptibility and fine tuned on the basis of medication allergies and toxicities, penetration into target tissues, suspected or proven presence of copathogens, renal and hepatic function, possible drug–drug interactions, cost, convenience of dosing, and ease of administration.

Simple urinary tract infections respond well to short-course oral therapy; these choices can be made on the basis of local susceptibility patterns, and culture is generally unnecessary. Community-acquired complicated urinary tract infections, including pyelonephritis with or without bacteremia, also respond to oral antibiotics as long as nausea and vomiting do not preclude their administration. Infections in chronically catheterized patients or acquired in health care or extended care settings are often resistant to oral agents, and parenteral therapies are generally preferred for patients requiring hospitalization until culture results are available.

The antibiotic therapy of enteric infections is controversial. Most of these infections are self-limited and resolve without antibiotics. In my practice I try to wait until an etiologic diagnosis is made—by the time stool cultures are positive, most patients have improved. In travel settings, patients are frequently provided antibiotics to self-administer for the same syndromes, justified perhaps by limited access to medical care and the inconvenience of diarrhea on overseas journeys. In the case of EHEC, some observational studies suggest a significantly greater risk of hemolytic-uremic syndrome (HUS) with antibiotic administration.

Recent studies on the duration of therapy for hospital-associated pneumonia (HAP) have demonstrated equivalent results with 8 days of therapy compared with longer courses. Whether this can be applied to community-acquired gram-negative pneumonia, which has traditionally been treated for 3 weeks or longer, is unclear but would appear reasonable in the absence of postobstructive pneumonia, lung abscess, or empyema.

Gram-negative osteomyelitis and infections of orthopedic hardware generally require 6 weeks of antibiotics for acute infections and longer durations for chronic osteomyelitis.

Table 132.3 Suggested Antimicrobial Regimens for Selected Infections

Infection	Typical Pathogens	Recommended Antibiotics	Alternatives	Treatment Duration (days)
UTI, uncomplicated	E. coli, Klebsiella, Proteus	Oral TMP-SMX, FQ	Ampicillin, cephalexin, nitrofurantoin	3
Urinary tract infection, complicated (including pyelonephritis, male UTI)	E. coli, Klebsiella, Proteus	Ceftriaxone, FQ	Pip/tazo, aminoglycosides, carbapenams, aztreonam	7–14
UTI, recurrent catheter associated	All	Carbapenams, cefepime	Aminoglycosides	14
Diarrhea	E. coli	None	FQ, rifaximin, azithromycin	3–5
Spontaneous bacterial peritonitis	E. coli, Klebsiella	Cefotaxime	FQ, moxi, pip/tazo, ceph3, cefepime, carbapenams	10–14
Diverticulitis	E. coli + anaerobes	FQ or TMP-SMX + metronidazole, moxi	Pip/tazo, ceph3 + metronidazole	7–10
Cholangitis, cholecystitis, pancreatitis, other abdominal abscesses	All	Pip/tazo, cefepime + metronidazole, carbapenams	FQ + metronidazole, moxi, tigecycline	To resolution
Complicated skin/soft tissue	All	Pip/tazo, carbapenams	Tigecycline, FQ, moxi	To resolution + 2 days
Pneumonia, community acquired	E. coli, Klebsiella	Ceftriaxone, cefepime, FQ, moxi	Pip/tazo, carbapenams	≤21
Pneumonia, hospital or ventilator acquired	E. coli, Klebsiella, Enterobacter, Serratia	Carbapenams, cefepime, pip/tazo (usually with aminoglycoside or FQ as initial therapy)	Tigecycline	8
Meningitis	E. coli	Cefepime, ceftriaxone, meropenam		14
Meningitis/ventriculitis, shunt associated	Enterobacter	Cefepime or meropenam ± aminoglycoside	Ceph3	To normalization of CSF
Osteomyelitis, prosthetic joint infection	All	Ceftriaxone, cefepime	FQ, carbapenam, tigecycline	≥42
Bacteremia (line)	All	Cefepime	Carbapenam, pip/tazo, FQ, moxi	10–14
Endocarditis, intravascular device	All	Cefepime or ceftriaxone ± aminoglycoside	Pip/tazo ± aminoglycoside	42

Abbreviations: FQ = ciprofloxacin or levofloxacin; moxi = moxifloxacin; pip/tazo = piperacillin/tazobactam; ceph3 = ceftriaxone, cefotaxime, ceftazidime; TMP-SMX = trimethoprim-sulfamethoxazole; UTI = urinary tract infection; CSF = cerebrospinal fluid.

Fluoroquinolones have excellent bone penetration and work well against susceptible organisms, although concerns have been raised in animal models that suggest these agents may impede fracture healing and that long half-life parenteral cephalosporins may be preferable for an infected fracture nonunion. If hardware is retained in an infected site, prolonged oral suppressive therapy should be considered until hardware can be removed.

Suspected or proven severe infections, such as bacteremia or necrotizing soft-tissue infections, are best initially treated with two parenteral antibiotics, usually a cell wall–active agent (antipseudomonal penicillins, cephalosporins, or carbapenams) plus an aminoglycoside or fluoroquinolone. The rationale for this combination approach is not for synergy or demonstration of improved efficacy, as commonly believed, but rather to maximize the probabili-

Specific Organisms – Bacteria

ty that an antibiotic active against the infecting agent has been chosen. The choice of cell wall agent should depend on local susceptibility patterns; in particular, if there is risk of infection due to extended-spectrum β-lactamase (ESBL)-producing organisms, a carbapenam should be chosen. Once an organism has been identified and susceptibility determined, treatment can be reduced to a single effective agent, with the caveat that an aminoglycoside should not be used as a single agent for a gram-negative bacteremia due to demonstration of inferior outcomes.

Line-associated infections are most successfully managed if the line is removed, followed by 10 to 14 days of an appropriate antibiotic. Successful treatment with retention of the line can be achieved with parenteral administration of antibiotics through the line with or without antibiotic lock but risks recurrent bacteremia and additional risk of metastatic complications of bacteremia.

Aspiration of abscesses may be both diagnostic and therapeutic and should be pursued when possible. Aggressive debridement is critical to the successful management of necrotizing skin and soft-tissue infections. Infected decubitus ulcers and burns may respond to local debridement and penetrating topical agents such as mafenide acetate (Sulfamylon). Adjunctive use of hyperbaric oxygen in these infections is controversial and expensive.

Focal CNS infections should be drained when possible and ventricular shunts removed. Third- and fourth-generation cephalosporins and meropenam have sufficient CNS penetration to treat most gram-negative infections as single agents although pairing with an aminoglycoside is generally recommended; intrathecal administration of antibiotics should be reserved for resistant organisms without other adequate treatment options. The role of steroids in gram-negative meningitis has not been specifically studied but analogy to studies of meningitis due to *H. influenzae*, *S. pneumoniae*, and *S. typhi* suggest a benefit is possible when administered prior to or concurrent with the initial dose of antibiotics.

A discussion of adjunctive measures for treatment of sepsis and septic shock is beyond the scope of this chapter. It has been clearly established, however, that patients with more than one new organ failure due to sepsis realize a substantial survival benefit with the administration of dotrecogin-α, and provides encouragement that additional immunomodulators may further improve survival in an illness with 30% mortality.

CONCLUSION

The Enterobacteriaceae cause a broad array of infections and are prominent causes of urinary tract infection, pneumonia, skin and soft-tissue infection, and intra-abdominal infection. The complex resistance patterns emerging in nosocomial isolates creates a challenge in constructing appropriate initial treatment regimens. Aggressive pathogen identification and the appropriate modification of antibiotics to a targeted approach remain keys to successful management.

SUGGESTED READING

Derouiche RO. Treatment of infections associated with surgical implants. *New Engl J Med.* 2004;350:1422–1429.

Ericcson CD, DuPont HL. Rifaximin in the treatment of infectious diarrhea. *Chemotherapy.* 2005;51(Suppl 1):73–80.

Fung HB, Chang JY, Kuczynski S. A practical guide to the treatment of skin and soft tissue infections. *Drugs.* 2003;63:1459–1480.

Gaynes R, Edwards JR. Overview of nosocomial infections caused by the gram-negative bacilli. *Clin Infect Dis.* 2005;41:848–855.

Jacoby GA, Munoz-Price LS. The new β-lactamases. *New Engl J Med.* 2005;352:380–391.

Mandell LA, Wunderink RG, Anzueto A, et al. Infectious Diseases Society of America/American Thoracic Society Consensus guidelines on the management of community-acquired pneumonia in adults. *Clin Infect Dis.* 2007;44:S27–S72.

Mylotte JM. Nursing home-acquired bloodstream infection. *Infect Control Hosp Epidemiol.* 2005;26:833–837.

Mylonakis E, Calderwood SB. Infective endocarditis in adults. *New Engl J Med.* 2001;345:1318–1330.

Rose WE, Ryback MJ. Tigecycline: first of a new class of antimicrobial agents. *Pharmacotherapy.* 2006;26:1099–1110.

Safdar N, Handelsman J, Maki DG. Does combination antimicrobial therapy reduce mortality in gram-negative bacteremia? A meta-analysis. *Lancet Infect Dis.* 2004;4:519–527.

Wong CS, Jelacic S, Habeeb RL, et al. The risk of hemolytic-uremic syndrome after antibiotic treatment of *Escherichia coli* O157:H7 infections. *New Engl J Med.* 2000;342:1930–1936.

133. Enterococcus

Ronald N. Jones

Since the early 1970s, the enterococci have steadily emerged as major hospital-acquired (nosocomial) pathogens. In statistics from the National Nosocomial Infectious Surveillance System (NNISS), they are the second most common gram-positive cause of nosocomial bloodstream infection and the third most common cause of nosocomial wound infections. In fact, enterococci rank first among gram-positive cocci in producing urinary tract infections (17.4%, see Table 133.1). The significant increases in occurence of this genus since the early to mid-1970s is related to patterns of general antimicrobial use in the hospital and in particular to widespread use of extended-spectrum cephalosporins, β-lactamase inhibitor/penicillin combinations, fluoroquinolones, carbapenems, and aminoglycosides and the emergence of resistances in the genus.

Cephalosporins are not active or bactericidal against enterococci, and they may therefore result in a selective advantage for this genus. Fluoroquinolones are also only modestly active against these species. *Enterococcus faecalis* produce most human enterococcal infections (70% to 80%), and *Enterococcus faecium* accounts for most (10% to 16%) of the remainder. Antimicrobial resistance is a particular problem among *E. faecium* isolates. Other species of interest are *Enterococcus casseliflavus* and *Enterococcus gallinarum*, not because of the frequency with which they are isolated, but because of the intrinsic low-level resistance to vancomycin (eg, the *vanC* genotype and resultant generally intermediate phenotype; minimum inhibitory concentrations [MICs], 4–8 µg/mL).

In addition to the problems posed by the increasing frequency of enterococcal infection, the therapy of these infections has become challenging as resistance to ampicillin, high-level resistance to aminoglycosides (preventing bacteriocidal combination therapy), and, most recently, glycopeptide (vancomycin and teicoplanin) have occurred, but emerging linezolid (an oxazolidinone), daptomycin, tigecycline (a glycylcycline), and quinupristin/dalfopristin resistance have also narrowed the therapeutic regimens. In addition, the value (risk of failure) of trimethoprim–sulfamethoxazole (TMP–SMX) in therapy even for urinary tract infection has become controversial regardless of in vitro susceptibility. All enterococci are intrinsically resistant to achievable in vivo levels of aminoglycosides; however, synergic killing may occur when aminoglycosides are combined with a cell wall–active agent such as a penicillin or a glycopeptide. Strains resistant to high levels of aminoglycoside (>500 µg/mL of gentamicin or >1000 µg/mL of streptomycin) are not susceptible to the synergic codrug effects of the aminoglycosides. It is clinically significant that cross-resistance to the synergic activity of the aminoglycosides is incomplete between gentamicin (and the related compounds tobramycin, netilmicin, amikacin, kanamycin, and isepamicin) and streptomycin. Streptomycin may be used successfully in combination to treat some high-level gentamicin-resistant strains. The selection of the appropriate aminoglycoside codrug should be directed by validated in vitro susceptibility tests and the availability of streptomycin for clinical use.

Resistance to vancomycin is more common with *E. faecium* isolates than with *E. faecalis*, but it may occur with either species. Reports in the United States in the late 1990s suggest that the overall vancomycin-resistant rate for enterococci was at 20% among bloodstream infections, and higher resistance rates for some other drugs and species limit therapeutic choices. These resistance rates have escalated in 2005–2006 (Table 133.2). Acquired vancomycin resistance is often associated with resistance to teicoplanin (Van A phenotype or *vanA* gene) or may occur in the absence of cross-resistance to teicoplanin (Van B phenotype or *vanB* gene). This difference may be clinically significant in nations where teicoplanin is clinically available and could also be relevent in the United States when dalbavancin, a long-acting lipoglycopeptide, is marketed. Willems and colleagues have identified a hospital-adopted *E. faecium* clone (CC-17) that has evolved ampicillin-, vancomycin-, and fluoroquinolone-resistant patterns. This CC-17 has been documented

Table 133.1 Percentage of Various Gram-Positive Pathogens Causing Nosocomial Infections in the NNIS (CDC) Comparing 1975 to 2003

Pathogen	Percentage for 1975/2003 by Infection Site			
	Bloodstream	Wounds[a]	Pneumonia	Urine
Enterococci	8.1/14.5	11.9/13.9	3.0/1.3	14.2/17.4
S. aureus	16.5/14.3	18.5/22.5	13.4/27.8	1.9/3.6
CoNS	10.3/42.9	7.4/15.9	2.6/1.8	3.2/4.9
Other species	8.0/4.5	8.8/5.8	6.9/3.2	2.2/1.2

[a] Skin and skin structure infections (SSSI).
Abbreviations: CoNS = coagulase-negative staphylococci; NNIS = National Nosocomial Infections Surveillance System; CDC = Centers for Disease Control and Prevention.

Table 133.2 Susceptibility Rates of Enterococcal Strains Isolated from the SENTRY Antimicrobial Surveillance Program Hospital Patients in 2005–2006 (>30 Medical Centers in the United States)[a]

Antimicrobial Agent	Percentage Susceptible		
	All Enterococci (2941)	E. faecalis (1849)	E. faecium (956)
Ampicillin	68	>99	7
Chloramphenicol[b]	90	87	96
Ciprofloxacin	43	62	5
Daptomycin	>99	100	>99
Linezolid	99	>99	97
Quinupristin/Dalfopristin	31	2	90
Tetracycline	38	27	59
Teicoplanin	75	97	30
Tigecycline	>99	>99	>99
Vancomycin	73	95	28
Gentamicin (HL)	75	72	79
Streptomycin (HL)	67	76	46

Abbreviation: HL = high-level resistance.
[a] Data on file, SENTRY Antimicrobial Surveillance Program (JMI Laboratories, North Liberty, IA).
[b] Data from 2003 and 2005–2006.

in vancomycin-resistant enterococci (VRE) populations in the United States (Figure 133.1) and since 1999 has progressively increased at rates comparable to those in the United States. Vancomycin resistance in *E. faecium* bacteremic isolates (SENTRY Program, 1999–2006) now approaches 70%. Intrinsic low-level resistance to both glycopeptides has been observed in

E. casseliflavus and in *E. gallinarum*, the so-called Van C phenotype.

For the clinician, the problems posed by the emergence of resistance have been exacerbated by the technical difficulties in reliable detection of these resistances. In vitro resistance to TMP–SMX as a result of the ability of the most prevalent enterococci to use thymidine or

Specific Organisms – Bacteria

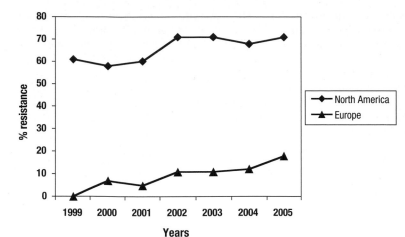

Figure 133.1 Progression of vancomycin resistance in *E. faecium* among bloodstream isolates studied in North America and Europe, including presence of isolates with antibiograms consistent with those of CC-17 (SENTRY Program, 1999–2005).

thymine in the susceptibility test medium (escapes bactericidal action) has been addressed by the use of media free of or low in concentration for these antagonists. However, there are significant amounts of antagonists in the urine, and therefore the meaning of in vitro test results performed in these "improved" test conditions is doubtful. Routine testing against ampicillin without testing for organism β-lactamase production may result in false-susceptible results. However, β-lactamase production is an exceedingly rare mechanism of resistance (≤0.1%) among *E. faecalis* isolates. A number of problems with the detection of high-level aminoglycoside resistance using the most prevalent automated and commercial broth microdilution susceptibility test systems (Vitek, Vitek 2, MicroScan, BD Phoenix) have been reported, although in some cases these now appear to have been resolved. Similarly, with vancomycin and other newer agent resistances from both automated susceptibility test systems and disk diffusion test interpretive criteria may require modifications over time to enable consistent, accurate detection of resistant strains.

Highly reliable, empiric therapy of enterococcal infection is not consistently satisfactory given the complexity of resistance patterns, and therefore, availability of prompt, reliable susceptibility test results is critical. At present, disk diffusion susceptibility testing, Etest (AB BIODISK, Solna, Sweden), Vitek Systems, and the reference broth microdilution or agar dilution methods are reliable methods for detection of important enterococcal resistances. However, recent reports of false resistance have been reported for some newer agents, including linezolid caused by fuzzy zone diameter edges and trailing end points by dilution test methods.

ENTEROCOCCAL BLOODSTREAM INFECTION

Isolation of enterococci from blood cultures may occur with or without endocarditis. In community-acquired enterococcal bloodstream infection approximately one third of cases are associated with endocarditis, compared with fewer than 5% of nosocomial enterococcal bacteremias. These nosocomial infections are usually associated with urinary tract disease or instrumentation, intra-abdominal infection, infected intravascular devices, neoplastic disease, and significant neutropenia.

Infective endocarditis, even when caused by more susceptible strains of enterococci, is more difficult to achieve cures for than endocarditis due to viridans group streptococci. Only two thirds of patients will be cured if a penicillin is used alone. A combination of a cell wall–active agent (a penicillin, usually ampicillin, or a glycopeptide) with an aminoglycoside for 4 to 6 weeks continues to be recommended. In general, ampicillin (2- or 4-fold more active) is used in preference to penicillin. High-dose penicillins (ampicillin, 2 g every 4 hours, or penicillin G, 18 to 30 million U/day) are appropriate, combined with gentamicin, 1 mg/kg every 8 hours or the use of the less toxic infusion pattern of once-daily dosing. However, limited clinical information supports the use of once-daily aminoglycosides for endocarditis. Monitoring of aminoglycoside serum concentrations is essential to ensure adequate therapeutic levels and to minimize toxicity during the extended therapeutic course, as well as vancomycin monitoring if used (see also Chapter 36, Endocarditis of Natural and Prosthetic Valves: Treatment and Prophylaxis).

The choice of an aminoglycoside for combination therapy is between gentamicin and streptomycin (limited availability). Gentamicin is generally preferred because synergic killing is more consistent (see Table 133.2), ototoxicity is less frequent, and facilities to measure serum levels are more easily available. Enterococcal strains resistant to high levels of aminoglycoside in vitro are not susceptible to enhanced (synergistic) killing with a penicillin or vancomycin-like agents, and in such patients use of aminoglycosides constitutes exposure to potential toxicity without apparent clinical benefit. Cross-resistance between gentamicin and streptomycin is not universal, and strains resistant to one should be tested against the other (Table 133.2). Optimal therapy is not well defined for strains resistant to high levels of both aminoglycosides. Prolonged therapy with high dosages of a penicillin or ampicillin, possibly by continuous infusion, may be successful in some cases. Combination therapy with vancomycin and a penicillin has also been reported successful, and daptomycin has received an indication for bacteremia and right-side infectious endocarditis. Linezolid, quinupristin/dalfopristin, or chloramphenicol could also be a therapeutic option.

Enterococcal resistance to penicillin or vancomycin and to high levels of aminoglycoside will be increasingly encountered in hospital practice and possibly in clinic patients, as well. There is no established therapy for this group of organisms although several newer agents appear promising. Vancomycin-resistant enterococci of the Van B phenotype remain susceptible to teicoplanin, which is not available in the United States. Teicoplanin is not bactericidal alone, and combinations with an aminoglycoside appear appropriate for strains for which the combination will show synergistic killing. It is important that teicoplanin be used in adequate doses, particularly if used alone (at least 6 mg/kg twice on the first day and once daily thereafter). Monitoring for adequacy of trough levels (at least 20 μg/mL) is important where feasible, although facilities for such monitoring may not be available. Similarly, close adherence to package insert recommendations is critical to success with daptomycin, linezolid, and quinupristin/dalfopristin. Serum inhibitory and bactericidal titers may be useful to follow therapy of serious infections (sepsis with or without endocarditis or osteomyelitis).

Therapy with dalbavancin or teicoplanin is not an option for Van A VRE strains, and this is the predominant pattern (>80% strains) of vancomycin resistance in the United States. Various therapeutic approaches have been suggested, but none are widely accepted. Older drugs such as chloramphenicol and doxycycline have demonstrated a variable degree of activity (>50% susceptible by Clinical Laboratory Standards Institute [CLSI] criteria; Tables 133.2 and 133.3) against the multidrug-resistant enterococci. Case reports indicate that these drugs used alone or with codrugs can be successful in an acceptable number of cases, but each agent is only bacteriostatic. Even with eradication of enterococci from the bloodstream, mortality remains high (30% to 50%). Fluoroquinolones (ciprofloxacin, levofloxacin, garenoxacin, and moxifloxacin) may have limited value for strains tested as susceptible (see Tables 133.2 and 133.3), although resistance may emerge rapidly when these drugs are used alone. Combinations of ampicillin and a fluoroquinolone have been found bactericidal for some strains in vitro. A pristinomycin combination agent (quinupristin–dalfopristin or Synercid) is a generally bacteriostatic option available for use in therapy of *E. faecium* infection only. This agent is not active against *E. faecalis* strains. A variety of other agents, some in development (see Table 133.3), are more active against enterococci and may have slightly expanded potential for future enterococcal treatment. Daptomycin (formerly LY-146032, a cyclic lipopeptide), oxazolidinones (linezolid), and glycylcyclines (tigecycline) are the most highly effective compounds of more recent interest (see Tables 133.2 and 133.3). However, most of these drugs (except daptomycin) demonstrate little bactericidal action against multidrug-resistant enterococci, and experience with their use awaits reports from structured clinical studies.

Therapy for enterococcal bloodstream infection in the absence of endocarditis follows the same general principles as for endocarditis except that bactericidal therapy may not be required. Bactericidal effect should be sought in the immunocompromised patient, and empiric therapy for such patients should be initiated with the broadest spectrum agents (vancomycin or daptomycin), because patients likely to develop nosocomial enterococcal infection are also at risk for infection with methicillin-resistant staphylococci. As with all other pathogens, removal of potential foci of infection, such as an indwelling vascular device, and drainage of an abscess, is essential for successful therapy.

Specific Organisms – Bacteria

Table 133.3 In Vitro Susceptibility of Alternative Antimicrobial Agents for U.S. Enterococcal Isolates with Resistance to Glycopeptides (797 Isolates in 2005–2006; SENTRY Program)[a]

Antimicrobial Agent	Percentage by Category[b]		
	Susceptible	Intermediate	Resistant
Glycopeptidelike			
Dalbavancin	14	—	—
Daptomycin	**>99**	—	—
Oxazolidinones			
Linezolid	**97**	1	2
Pristinomycins			
Quinupristin/Dalfopristin	84	3	13
Glycylcyclines			
Tigecycline	**>99**	—	—
Fluoroquinolones			
Garenoxacin	2	4	94
Levofloxacin	2	0	98
Moxifloxacin	2	1	97
Cephalosporins			
Ceftobiprole	11	1	88
Others			
Chloramphenicol	**94**	5	1
Clindamycin	4	1	95
Doxycycline	58	31	11
Erythromycin	3	0	97
Imipenem	12	0	88
Rifampin	22	4	74
Trimethoprim–sulfamethoxazole[c]	17	2	81

[a] Modified from results of the SENTRY Antimicrobial Surveillance Program (JMI Laboratories, North Liberty, IA).
[b] Categorical criteria per Clinical Laboratory Standards Institute (CLSI) M100-S17 (2007) or ≤4 μg/mL (susceptible) for ceftobiprole, garenoxacin at ≤1/≥4 μg/mL, and dalbavancin at ≤0.5 μg/mL (susceptible).
[c] Trimethoprim–sulfamethoxazole (1:19 ratio), susceptible results of in vitro tests may be misleading.

THERAPY OF NONSEVERE INFECTIONS AND URINARY TRACT DISEASE

In the absence of immediate susceptibility test results, ampicillin is a reasonable option for therapy of mild to moderate infections and particularly for urinary tract infections, given the high levels of ampicillin achieved in the urine. Nitrofurantoin is also active against most enterococci (>90%; data not shown) and is useful in therapy of urinary tract infection only.

Clearly, these approaches must be modified in the context of local epidemiology (antibiogram) and emergence of resistant strains. In centers with very high incidence of infection with ampicillin-resistant enterococci, usually *E. faecium,* this may not be appropriate therapy. For infection with drug-resistant organisms, the options are similar to those discussed for bloodstream infection, except that synergic combinations are usually not advised.

ENTEROCOCCAL CARRIAGE

There is no general acceptance that fecal carriage or colonization by multidrug-resistant enterococci is an indication for therapy; however, given the risk to the patient of subsequent disseminated infection, there is high epidemiologic interest in this issue. Studies of the intestinal tract reservoir/source of VRE have greatly increased our knowledge of colonization and factors leading to persisting carriage. The third-generation cephalosporins have clearly been implicated in promoting enterococcal colonization, but not all other cephalosporins or β-lactams present similar risks. Examples of low-risk agents that do not disrupt normal bowel flora via biliary excretion and/or possess an antianaerobic spectrum are aztreonam and cefepime, in contrast to cefoxitin and clindamycin that have promoted VRE colonization. Some antimicrobials like piperacillin/tazobactam inhibit establishment of VRE in the gut during therapy, but promote overgrowth when exposed to VRE in the period of posttherapy recovery of normal flora. If colonization of VRE was present before piperacillin/tazobactam therapy, the drug leads to persistence of the enterococcal colonization. Data from clinical trials continue to be necessary to more adequately understand these complex interactions of antimicrobials, indigenous bowel flora, and colonizing resistant enterococci.

It seems reasonable to review the patient's therapy with a view toward discontinuation of any nonessential antimicrobials that might confer a selective advantage for the enterococci. There have been reports of the successful use of oral bacitracin or investigation agents such as ramoplanin to eradicate fecal carriage of vancomycin- and ampicillin-resistant enterococci. However, relapses after discontinuation of selective intestinal tract decontamination remain high. The implications for infection control focus on (1) gastrointestinal selective decontamination; (2) antimicrobial use strategies (limit or restriction of selecting agents); (3) assuring persistence of the gastric acid barrier; (4) restoring indigenous colonic microflora; (5) assuring, where possible, de-

contamination of the hospital environment or patient's cutaneous surfaces; and (6) preventing patient-to-patient transmission via promoting handwashing/gloving by health care workers.

COMMENTS

Therapy of enterococcal infections is one of the most challenging areas in the contemporary treatment of infectious disease. Quality laboratory support is essential to the management of these infections in the most appropriate manner while minimizing toxicity. Given the emerging inadequacies of our therapeutic armamentarium (ampicillin and glycopeptides) and the clear evidence that nosocomial spread of this pathogen can occur, an aggressive position with respect to hospital environment surveillance and infection control remains of critical importance. Also, more study will be required to develop new, safe therapeutic agents and to focus our treatments on existing or newer antimicrobial agents (eg, daptomycin, linezolid) that produce acceptable enterococcus infection eradication.

SUGGESTED READING

Deshpande LM, et al. Antimicrobial resistance and molecular epidemiology of vancomycin-resistant enterococci from North America and Europe: a report from the SENTRY Antimicrobial Surveillance Program. *Diagn Microbiol Infect Dis.* 2007;58:163–170.

Donskey CJ. The role of the intestinal tract as a reservoir and source for transmission of nosocomial pathogens. *Clin Infect Dis.* 2004;39:219–226.

Eliopoulos GM. Quinupristin-dalfopristin and linezolid: evidence and opinion. *Clin Infect Dis.* 2003;36:473–481.

Frampton JE, Curran MP. Tigecycline. *Drugs.* 2005;65:2623–2625; discussion 2636–2637.

Gaynes R, Edwards JR. Overview of nosocomial infections caused by Gram-negative bacilli. *Clin Infect Dis.* 2005;41:848–854.

Jones RN. Global epidemiology of antimicrobial resistance among community-acquired and nosocomial pathogens: a five-year summary from the SENTRY Antimicrobial Surveillance Program (1997–2001). *Semin Respir Crit Care Med.* 2003;24:121–134.

Kerr KG, Reeves D. Vancomycin resistance in enterococci: a clinical challenge. *J Antimicrob Chemother.* 2003;51(suppl 3):iii1.

Leavis HL, Willems RJ, Top J, et al. High-level ciprofloxacin resistance from point mutations in *gyrA* and *parC* confined to global hospital-adapted clonal lineage CC17 of *Enterococcus faecium. J Clin Microbiol.* 2006;44:1059–1064.

Rice LB, Hutton-Thomas R, Lakticova V, et al. β-lactam antibiotics and gastrointestinal colonization with vancomycin-resistant enterococci. *J Infect Dis.* 2004;189:1113–1118.

Steenbergen JN, Alder J, Thorne GM, et al. Daptomycin: a lipopeptide antibiotic for the treatment of serious Gram-positive infections. *J Antimicrob Chemother.* 2005;55:283–288.

Willems RJ, Top J, van Santen M, et al. Global spread of vancomycin-resistant *Enterococcus faecium* from distinct nosocomial genetic complex. *Emerg Infect Dis.* 2005;11:821–828.

134. *Erysipelothrix*

W. Lee Hand

Erysipelothrix rhusiopathiae, a pleomorphic, gram-positive bacillus, is the only species of the genus *Erysipelothrix*. This organism causes both a self-limited soft-tissue infection (erysipeloid) and serious systemic disease. *Erysipelothrix rhusiopathiae* is widespread in nature and infects many domestic animals. Swine are probably the major reservoir of *E. rhusiopathiae*. The microorganism is also found in sheep, cattle, horses, chickens, and dogs, as well as in fish and crabs. Infection in humans is usually due to occupational exposure. Butchers, abattoir workers, fishermen, farmers, and veterinarians are at risk for *Erysipelothrix* infections. The clinical spectrum of human infection includes localized cutaneous infection, diffuse cutaneous disease, and systemic bloodstream infection.

LOCALIZED CUTANEOUS INFECTION

Erysipeloid of Rosenbach, the localized cutaneous form of illness, is the most common type of human infection caused by *E. rhusiopathiae* (Figure 134.1). Fingers and/or hands (sites of exposure) are almost always involved in this soft-tissue infection.

Mild pain may occur at the site of inoculation, followed by itching, throbbing pain, burning, and tingling. The characteristic skin lesion slowly progresses from a small red dot at the site of inoculation to a fully developed erysipeloid skin lesion, consisting of a well-developed purplish center with an elevated border. Patients often complain of joint stiffness and pain in the involved fingers, but swelling is minimal or absent. Small hemorrhagic, vesicular lesions may be present at the site of inoculation. Erysipeloid lesions do not resemble true cellulitis, as opposed to erysipelas, which is due to group A streptococcal infection. Thus, Rosenbach introduced the term *erysipeloid* for the human cutaneous disease caused by *Erysipelothrix*. Pain may be disproportionate to the degree of apparent involvement. Local lymphangitis and adenitis develop in 30% of patients. However, systemic symptoms such as high fever or chills are uncommon.

A provisional diagnosis is based on a history of contact with potentially contaminated

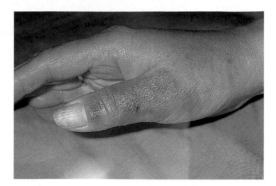

Figure 134.1 Erysipeloid. (From Gary M. White and Neil H. Cox, *Diseases of the Skin*, Philadelphia: WB Saunders, 1995.)

materials or occupational exposure, plus compatible physical findings. Gram-stained smears and cultures of aspirated material from skin lesions are often negative because the organism is deep within the dermis.

DIFFUSE CUTANEOUS DISEASE

Most erysipeloid skin lesions resolve even without specific treatment. However, erysipeloid occasionally will progress to the diffuse cutaneous form in untreated patients. Eating of contaminated meat has also been reported as a cause of this clinical entity. The characteristic purplish skin lesions expand with gradual clearing of the center. Bullous lesions may appear at the primary site or at distant locations. These patients often have systemic symptoms such as high fever, chills, and arthralgias. Blood cultures are invariably negative.

SYSTEMIC INFECTION (BACTEREMIA OR ENDOCARDITIS)

Bacteremic infection caused by *E. rhusiopathiae* is generally a primary infection and not the result of dissemination from localized cutaneous disease. Nevertheless, one third of patients with bloodstream infection have skin lesions suggestive of erysipeloid. Persistent bacteremia with *E. rhusiopathiae* has been reported after eating contaminated seafood. Cutaneous serpiginous lesions or multiple bullous lesions over the trunk and extremities may be seen. Most patients

Table 134.1 Antibiotic Therapy for *Erysipelothrix rhusiopathiae* Infection

Type of *Erysipelothryix* Infection	Antibiotics of Choice		
	Drug	Dose and Route	Duration
Localized Cutaneous			
Primary	Penicillin V	500 mg q6h PO	7 d
Alternatives	Ciprofloxacin (other fluoroquinolones may be used)	250 mg q12h PO	7 d
	Clindamycin	300 mg q8h PO	7 d
	Erythromycin (other macrolides may be used)	500 mg q6h PO	7 d
Severe Bacteremic or Endocarditis			
Primary	Penicillin G	2–4 million units q4h IV	4 wk
Alternatives	Ceftriaxone	2 g q24h IV	4 wk
	Imipenem	500 mg q6h IV	4 wk
	Ciprofloxacin (other IV fluoroquinolones may be used)	400 mg q12h IV	4 wk

have fever for 2 to 3 weeks before presentation. Fever and chills may resolve spontaneously, but relapse is to be expected.

Patients with severe underlying heart disease or liver disease may present with a clinical picture resembling gram-negative sepsis. More than one third of patients with disseminated infection are alcoholics, and chronic liver disease is a major predisposing factor. Bacteremia has also been reported in immunocompromised individuals, who often are receiving corticosteroid and/or cytotoxic drug treatment for collagen–vascular disease or malignancy.

Erysipelothrix rhusiopathiae bacteremia is usually associated with a severe clinical course and is frequently complicated by endocarditis. *Erysipelothrix* endocarditis often results in extensive destruction of cardiac valves, especially the aortic valve. Approximately one third of endocarditis patients die, and an additional one third require cardiac valve replacement. Absence of typical findings of endocarditis on initial physical examination or echocardiography does not exclude this diagnosis in patients with positive blood cultures. Reported complications of endocarditis have included proliferative glomerulonephritis with acute renal failure and visceral botryomycosis.

Earlier publications indicated that 90% of bacteremic infections were associated with endocarditis. This perceived high frequency

may, at least in part, be a result of reporting bias because a number of bacteremic cases without endocarditis have been reported more recently.

Unusual reported infections due to *Erysipelothrix* include necrotizing fasciitis (after local inoculation), septic arthritis (associated with bacteremia), and peritoneal dialysis-associated peritonitis.

The diagnosis of disseminated *E. rhusiopathiae* infection depends on identification of this organism in blood cultures. Commercial media are satisfactory for isolation from blood, and growth is usually recognized in 2 or 3 days. The organism may initially be misidentified as a *Lactobacillus* species.

Therapy

Erysipeloid may resolve spontaneously within 3 weeks, but treatment with appropriate antibiotic therapy hastens the healing process and prevents relapse. Local therapy with rest and heat is helpful for patients with painful, swollen lesions or arthritis. The involved hand or finger should be carried in a sling or splint. Surgical incision or debridement of local lesions is not necessary.

Penicillin and imipenem are the most active antibiotics against *Erysipelothrix* with in vitro testing. Penicillin is a time-tested, effective agent for treatment of all forms of *E. rhusiopathiae* infection. Other β-lactam antibiotics are also active against this organism. Fluoroquinolones and clindamycin demonstrate good in vitro activity. Macrolides, tetracyclines, and chloramphenicol have less predictable activity against *Erysipelothrix* and should not be used in the treatment of disseminated infection. *Erysipelothrix rhusiopathiae* is resistant to sulfonamides, trimethoprim–sulfamethoxazole, aminoglycosides, and vancomycin. Limited data indicated that daptomycin has good in vitro activity.

Antibiotic therapy should be based upon the clinical picture and results of blood cultures (Table 134.1). Oral antibiotic therapy is appropriate for localized cutaneous infection. Parenteral antibiotic treatment is indicated if patients have systemic infection or severe diffuse cutaneous disease. Penicillin G has been the historic drug of choice. Alternatives include ceftriaxone, imipenem, and fluoroquinolones. Patients with bacteremia or endocarditis should receive at least 4 weeks of intravenous antibiotic therapy.

SUGGESTED READING

Dunbar SA, Clarridge JE III. Potential errors in recognition of Erysipelothrix rhusiopathiae. *J Clin Microbiol*. 2000;38:1302–1304.

Garcia-Restoy E, Espejo E, Bella F, Llebot J. Bacteremia due to Erysipelothrix rhusiopathiae in immunocompromised hosts without endocarditis. *Rev Infect Dis*. 1991;13:1252–1253.

Gorby GL, Peacock JE Jr. Erysipelothrix rhusiopathiae endocarditis: microbiologic, epidemiologic, and clinical features of an occupational disease. *Rev Infect Dis*. 1988;10:317–325.

Klauder JV. Erysipeloid as an occupational disease. *JAMA*. 1938;111:1345.

McNamara DR, Zitterkopf NL, Baddour LM. Photoquiz: a woman with a lesion on her finger and bacteremia. *Clin Infect Dis*. 2005;41:1005–1006, 1057–1058.

Ognibene FP, Cunnion RE, Gill V, et al. Erysipelothrix rhusiopathiae bacteremia presenting as septic shock. *Am J Med*. 1985;78:861–864.

Reboli AC, Farrar WE. Erysipelothrix rhusiopathiae: an occupational pathogen. *Clin Microbiol Rev*. 1989;2:354–359.

Soriano F, Fernandez-Roblas R, Calvo R, et al. In vitro susceptibilities of aerobic and facultative non-spore-forming gram-positive bacilli to HMR 3647 (RU 66647) and 14 other antimicrobials. *Antimicrob Agents Chemother*. 1998;42:1028–1033.

Venditti M, Gelfusa V, Terasi A, et al. Antimicrobial susceptibilities of Erysipelothrix rhusiopathiae. *Antimicrob Agents Chemother*. 1990;34:2038–2040.

135. HACEK

Vivian H. Chu and Daniel J. Sexton

The acronym HACEK describes a heterogeneous group of organisms that share three major characteristics. First, they are small gram-negative rods that are commonly present as part of normal oral–pharyngeal or respiratory flora. Second, they are fastidious microorganisms that require special culture media. Third, they have a predilection to infect heart valves. The HACEK group includes *Haemophilus* species (except *Haemophilus influenzae*), *Actinobacillus actinomycetemcomitans*, *Cardiobacterium hominus*, *Eikenella corrodens*, and *Kingella* species. These organisms are infamous for their ability to cause endocarditis although, rarely, they can also cause a variety of other infections (Table 135.1). For example, human bites can result in cellulitis or abscess formation resulting from HACEK organisms, especially *Eikenella* species, and various *Haemophilus* species can cause epiglottitis or brain abscesses.

Members of the HACEK group are normal indigenous flora of the oral cavity. Systemic hematogenous spread may occur after dental manipulation or secondary to periodontal disease. Thereafter, individuals with underlying valvular heart disease are at risk of developing endocarditis. Antibiotic prophylaxis before dental manipulation does not ensure complete prevention against these fastidious organisms. However, the risk of endocarditis is very small after dental manipulation, even in patients with significant valvular disease. Millions of patients undergo dental procedures annually, yet the cases of infective endocarditis (IE) caused by HACEK group organisms are rare.

DIAGNOSIS

Bacteria in the HACEK group are commonly but often erroneously considered in the differential diagnosis for culture-negative endocarditis. In the past the traditional method of increasing the recovery of HACEK bacteria was to extend the incubation of blood culture bottles from 5 to 7 days to 2 to 3 weeks. However, with improvements in blood culture methods, this practice is no longer recommended. A recent multicenter study showed that the mean and median times to detection of HACEK isolates using current laboratory methods and media were 3 and 3.4 days, respectively. In addition, none of the cultures that were held for prolonged incubation and terminal subculturing yielded additional growth. Several other studies have demonstrated that isolation of HACEK organisms usually occurs within 5 days, suggesting that prolonged incubation is no longer needed to detect HACEK bacteria.

HACEK organisms typically grow on 5% sheep blood and chocolate agar but not on MacConkey's agar. Because growth is often poor or absent in an unenhanced atmosphere, incubation in 5% to 10% carbon dioxide (CO_2) is recommended. After growth is observed, standard biochemical tests will identify individual HACEK species. The use of 16S ribosomal RNA (rRNA) gene analysis may be useful for HACEK organisms that are not readily identified with standard biochemical tests.

CLINICAL FEATURES

Endocarditis caused by members of the HACEK group typically occurs in individuals with pre-existing valvular abnormalities and a recent history of oral/dental manipulation. However, some patients have no history of recent dental problems or procedures and in others a prior history of valvular disease may have been overlooked or unknown.

Endocarditis due to members of the HACEK group usually has a subacute course that may include frequent embolization due to the presence of large valvular vegetations. Other clinical features typical of endocarditis such as musculoskeletal symptoms, renal insufficiency, and weight loss may occur in a pattern clinically indistinguishable from endocarditis due to other organisms.

THERAPY

There have been no large trials to evaluate the best therapy for IE caused by HACEK group organisms. Currently available information on treatment is derived from in vitro susceptibility

Table 135.1 HACEK-Associated Infections

Haemophilus aphrophilus, Haemophilus haemolyticus, Haemophilus parahaemolyticus, Haemophilus parainfluenzae, Haemophilus paraphrophilus, Haemophilus segnis	Brain abscess, endocarditis, endophthalmitis, epiglottitis, hepatic abscess, intra-abdominal infection, meningitis, neonatal sepsis, necrotizing fasciitis, otitis media, pneumonia, sinusitis, septic arthritis, urinary tract infection
Actinobacillus actinomycetemcomitans	Brain abscess, cellulitis, empyema, endocarditis, endophthalmitis, osteomyelitis, periodontal infection, parotitis, pericarditis, pneumonia, synovitis, thyroid abscess, urinary tract infection
Cardiobacterium hominis	Endocarditis, meningitis
Eikenella corrodens	Abscessed tooth, Bartholin's gland abscess, brain abscess, cellulitis, conjunctivitis, dacryocystitis, empyema, endocarditis, endometritis, gingivitis, intra-abdominal abscess, intravascular space infections, keratitis, liver abscess, mediastinitis, meningitis, mycotic aneurysm, otitis externa, parotitis, pericarditis, pneumonia, septic pulmonary emboli, subdural empyema, thyroid abscess, thyroiditis
Kingella dentrificens, Kingella indologenes, Kingella kingae	Abscess, endocarditis, epiglottitis, intervertebral diskitis, meningitis, oropharyngeal infections, osteomyelitis, septic arthritis

testing and the results of small case series or individual case reports. In the past, ampicillin plus an aminoglycoside was widely recommended as the therapy of choice. This treatment was advocated because synergy between β-lactams and aminoglycosides could often be demonstrated in vitro, but such synergy has not been conclusively proven to occur in vivo. Moreover, a number of case reports have documented therapeutic failures of combined therapy with ampicillin and gentamicin in the treatment of infections caused by *A. actinomycetemcomitans* and *Haemophilus*. In addition, authors of several recent reports have described β-lactamase production by numerous strains of HACEK group organisms. Because of their fastidious growth requirements, susceptibility testing for many members of the HACEK group is sometimes difficult to obtain in routine microbiology laboratories. We and others believe that HACEK group organisms should be considered ampicillin resistant unless proved otherwise. In light of this, we do not advocate ampicillin as empiric or initial therapy for infections due to HACEK group organisms.

Most HACEK organisms, with the notable exceptions of *A. actinomycetemcomitans* and *E. corrodens*, are susceptible to first- and second-generation cephalosporins, and virtually all species are susceptible to third-generation cephalosporins. Therefore we believe the best therapy for IE caused by HACEK group bacteria is cefotaxime or ceftriaxone. We advocate using ceftriaxone, 2 g intravenously (IV) or intramuscularly (IM) once daily, because of its convenience and suitability for outpatient parenteral therapy (Table 135.2). The duration of therapy for native valve endocarditis should be at least 4 weeks; at least 6 weeks of therapy is recommended for prosthetic valve endocarditis.

HACEK group organisms are also susceptible in vitro to most fluoroquinolones, trimethoprim–sulfamethoxazole, and aztreonam. Thus one of these agents may be used in the β-lactam–intolerant patient. There is a growing body of evidence to support the use of ciprofloxacin as outpatient therapy for HACEK endocarditis.

A number of investigators advocate empirical therapy with either ceftriaxone along with an aminoglycoside or ciprofloxacin until sensitivities return. A fluoroquinolone such as ciprofloxacin is the preferred alternative for patients who are allergic to a β-lactam. Ciprofloxacin is an appropriate choice for the outpatient segment of therapy because of its high bioavailability after oral ingestion and excellent safety profile. However, because of the lack of published data about fluoroquinolone therapy for HACEK group bacterial infections, we prefer to use ceftriaxone as initial therapy. Despite the technical difficulties in obtaining in vitro susceptibility results, we advocate obtaining such results to confirm sensitivity to the agents being used or contemplated for use. Careful follow-up of all patients undergoing treatment is also recommended, including periodic assessment of clinical and microbiologic

Table 135.2 Antibiotics Recommended for Serious Infections

	Antibiotic	Dosage and Route	Length of Therapy
First choice	Ceftriaxone	2 g IV or IM qd	4–6 wk
Alternative	Ciprofloxacin	750 mg PO q12h	4–6 wk

response using careful examinations and follow-up blood cultures. Careful monitoring for compliance is advised for all patients treated with oral therapy.

HACEK group organisms are usually susceptible to tetracycline and chloramphenicol; however, both of these agents are bacteriostatic and thus are poor choices for endovascular infections. Most HACEK group members are resistant to metronidazole, vancomycin, erythromycin, and clindamycin.

PROGNOSIS

Most patients with endocarditis caused by HACEK group organisms have a favorable prognosis. Although surgical intervention may be needed for valvular insufficiency, most infections can be cured with medical therapy. Reported success rates with medical therapy have ranged from 82% to 87% in patients with both native valve and prosthetic valve endocarditis.

NONENDOCARDIAL INFECTIONS

Nonendocardial infections caused by HACEK group organisms are rare. Such infections are usually responsive to short courses of antibiotic therapy. Surgical drainage is indicated for abscesses. We and other authorities recommend 3 to 4 weeks of parenteral therapy followed by an additional 3 weeks of antibiotics by mouth for treatment of septic arthritis caused by *K. kingae* and other HACEK group organisms. Two to 4 weeks of parenteral therapy followed by 1 to 6 months of oral therapy is recommended for the treatment of osteomyelitis caused by HACEK organisms.

SUGGESTED READING

Babinchak TJ. Oral ciprofloxacin therapy for prosthetic valve endocarditis due to Actinobacillus actinomycetemcomitans. *Clin Infect Dis.* 1995;21:1517–1518.

Baron EJ, Scott JD, Tompkins LS. Prolonged incubation and extensive subculturing do not increase recovery of clinically significant microorganisms from standard automated blood cultures. *Clin Infect Dis.* 2005;41:1677–1680.

Das M, Badley AD, Cockerill FR, et al. Infective endocarditis caused by HACEK microorganisms. *Annu Rev Med.* 1997;48:25–33.

Kaplan AH, Weber DJ, Oddone EZ, et al. Infection due to Actinobacillus actinomycetemcomitans: 15 cases and review. *Rev Infect Dis.* 1989;11:46–63.

Petti CA, Bhally HS, Weinstein MP, et al. Utility of extended blood culture incubation for isolation of Haemophilus, Actinobacillus, Cardiobacterium, Eikenella, and Kingella organisms: a retrospective multicenter evaluation. *J Clin Microbiol.* 2006;44:257–259.

Wilson WR, Karchmer AW, Dajani AS, et al. Antibiotic treatment of adults with infective endocarditis due to streptococci, enterococci, staphylococci, and HACEK microorganisms. *JAMA.* 1995;274:1706–1713.

136. *Helicobacter Pylori*

Ping-I Hsu and David Y. Graham

INTRODUCTION

Helicobacter pylori are gram-negative spiral shaped bacteria that infect more than 50% of humans globally. *Helicobacter pylori* infection is a serious chronic transmissible infectious disease that causes damage to gastric structure and function and is a major cause of morbidity and mortality worldwide. The prevalence of *H. pylori* is inversely related to the general health and well-being of a society. However, as with other chronic infectious diseases, the infection remains clinically latent in most with about 20% of infected individuals developing clinically recognizable diseases. The natural niche for the organism is the human stomach, where it causes destructive inflammation (eg, gastritis). *Helicobacter pylori* is now accepted as the major cause of gastric and duodenal ulcer disease, gastric cancer, and primary B-cell gastric lymphoma. It is also responsible for some cases of nonulcer dyspepsia.

DISCOVERY OF *H. PYLORI*

In the early 1980s, Robin Warren, a pathologist in Perth, Western Australia, who had observed small curved bacteria in gastric biopsy specimens, teamed up with a young trainee in internal medicine, Barry Marshall, to further investigate the role of these bacteria in human disease. By 1982, with a bit of luck, Marshall successfully isolated the organism from biopsy specimens. The organism was initially named *Campylobacter pyloridis* based on the insight from Warren that the organism looked like a *Campylobacter*. That organism is now known as *H. pylori* and is a microaerophilic, gram-negative, spiral rod approximately 0.6 × 3.5 µ with approximately 7 unipolar flagellae. The biochemical features that help identify it include the presence of urease, oxidase, and catalase.

The initial report by Warren and Marshall led to many investigators becoming involved in studying the organism and its potential role in disease. There were many obstacles to overcome, including the need to develop accurate tests to identify where the infection was present, to identify effective therapies, and actually to do the studies to test the hypothesis that, if *H. pylori* were the cause of peptic ulcer, instead of a colonizer of inflamed gastric mucosa, eradication of the organism would cure the disease. By 1994 the data were unequivocal, leading to a consensus conference held by the National Institutes of Health that concluded that *H. pylori* was a major cause of peptic ulcer disease and recommended that ulcer patients with *H. pylori* infection receive treatment with antimicrobial agents. In the same year, the International Agency for Cancer Research declared that *H. pylori* is a class I carcinogen for gastric cancer. Subsequently, several studies demonstrated that *H. pylori* infection was also the prime cause of gastric mucosa-associated lymphoid tissue lymphoma (MALToma). In 2005, Warren and Marshall received the Nobel Prize for Physiology and Medicine for culture of the organism and proof of its relation to peptic ulcer disease.

EPIDEMIOLOGY AND TRANSMISSION

Helicobacter pylori infection is usually acquired in childhood. Three transmission routes have been proposed: fecal–oral, oral–oral, and gastro–oral. We consider *H. pylori* a "situational opportunist" as transmission may involve any route that allows bacteria from one person's stomach to gain access to another's. Fecal–oral transmission is perhaps most important. *Helicobacter pylori* has been cultured from stools of infected young children and adults. In countries with unclean water supplies there is also good evidence for waterborne transmission. Oral–oral transmission has also been shown, for example, by African women who premasticate foods given to their infants. *Helicobacter pylori* can be easily cultured from gastric contents obtained either by gastric aspiration or from vomit such that contact with gastric secretions is a definite risk factor. Gastro–oral transmission likely accounted for the disproportionately high prevalence of *H. pylori* among gastroenterologists from the era when endoscopy was typically done without gloves or universal precautions.

Iatrogenic transmission is also possible in situations where endoscopes or instruments in contact with the gastric mucosa are not adequately disinfected before use in another individual. The major risk factors for *H. pylori* infection include the following: birth in a developing country, low socioeconomic status, crowded living conditions, large family size, unsanitary living conditions, unclean food or water, presence of infants in the home, and exposure to gastric contents of infected individuals. The major associations can be summarized as examples of poor household hygiene.

The prevalence of *H. pylori* infections varies by geographic location, ethnic background, socioeconomic condition, and age. In developing countries, 70% to 90% of the populations are infected by *H. pylori* by age 20. In developed countries, the prevalence of infection is lower, ranging from 25% to 50%. The *H. pylori* prevalence among middle-class whites born in the United States and whose parents were also born in the United States is now less than 15% and is still falling. The prevalence of *H. pylori* in developed countries represents a birth cohort phenomenon reflecting the low rate of transmission among children. However, the infection is still common among the disadvantaged and among immigrants to developed countries. This fall in transmission rates among children is a common feature of developed countries and is also seen in developing countries as they improve their standards of living, sanitation, and household hygiene.

PATHOGENESIS OF INFECTION

After gaining access to the stomach, *H. pylori*, being motile, are able to "swim" to and enter into the mucus layer overlying the gastric mucosal epithelium. *Helicobacter pylori* possess the necessary battery of factors that allow the organism to colonize the gastric mucosa (flagella, urease, adhesions) and evade the host defense (urease, catalase, superoxide dismutase, and poorly reactive lipopolysaccharide). Flagellae allow the bacterium to burrow through the mucus to the mucosal surface, where it is protected from the acidic gastric contents. Although *H. pylori* can attach to superficial gastric mucus cells and resist clearance from the stomach, small numbers of *H. pylori* are also found within gastric epithelial cells that may serve as a sanctuary, allowing evasion of host defenses and may be in part responsible for the failure of topical antibiotic therapy. Attachment of *H. pylori* to the gastric mucosa is associated with

local production of proinflammatory cytokines (eg, interleukin 8), which induces infiltration of polymorphonuclear leukocytes and ultimately leads to the characteristic histological pattern of an acute inflammatory reaction superimposed on chronic inflammation with organized lymphoid follicles.

The clinical outcome of *H. pylori* infection is determined by a complex interaction of the host, bacterium, and environmental factors. A number of putative virulence factors have been described, including the presence of the *cag* pathogenicity island (PAI), the outer membrane inflammatory protein (OipA), the vacuolating cytotoxin (VacA), and the blood group binding adhesin (BabA). The *cag* PAI region encodes a type IV bacterial secretion apparatus, which translocates or injects the CagA protein and possibly other proteins into the host target cells. Phosphorylation of CagA may activate host signaling pathways and subsequently influence host cellular functions, including proliferation, apoptosis, cytokine release, and cell motility. VacA is present in nearly all *H. pylori* strains, but only about half of the *H. pylori* strains produce VacA toxin *in vitro*. VacA induces epithelial vacuolation *in vitro*, but its function *in vivo* remains unclear. *Helicobacter pylori* that differed in *vacA* genotype determined by variations in the signal sequence (s1a, s1b, s1c) and midregion of the *vacA* (m1, m2) gene have been described. Triple positive strains that express *cagA*, *vacA* s1, and *babA*2 or quadruple positive strains that, in addition, express *oipA* were initially considered more virulent, but more recent work has not confirmed that hypothesis. Nonetheless, organisms that contain an intact PAI are more likely to be associated with peptic ulcer or gastric cancer than those that do not. However, gastric cancer and peptic ulcers are also caused by *H. pylori* possessing none of these putative virulence factors, leading to the conclusion that all *H. pylori* infections cause destructive damage and should be eradicated.

PATTERN OF GASTRITIS AND CLINICAL OUTCOMES OF *H. PYLORI* INFECTION

The outcome of an *H. pylori* infection is closely related to the severity and pattern of the *H. pylori*–induced gastritis. The stomach can be considered as having two regions, the acid-secreting corpus and the non–acid-secreting antrum. Whereas *H. pylori* colonize the entire surface of the stomach, the acid-secreting corpus is relatively resistant to *H. pylori* colonization. It is thought that the highly acid contents (pH ≤1) ejected from the gastric pits impair the ability of the bacterium to associate with all but the most superficial mucosa. Inhibition of acid secretion associated with a highly selective vagotomy, use of antisecretory drugs, or a febrile illness releases this inhibition and allows the bacteria to interact with the mucosa in such a way as to produce more and deeper levels of inflammation. Interleukin 1β produced in response to the presence of the bacteria acts as a potent antisecretory agent and further reduces acid secretion allowing the infection to become established in the corpus leading to pangastritis.

Antral inflammation is associated with up-regulation of gastrin production and inhibition of the normal acid inhibitory effect of antral acidity that further increases the amount and duration of gastric acid secretion. In patients with antral predominant gastritis, acid secretion from the corpus is uninhibited, and these patients are at markedly increased risk of developing a duodenal ulcer. In contrast, in hosts with low acid secretory capacity due to a low number of parietal cells or inhibition of parietal cells, the organism is capable of colonizing a wider niche and presents with pangastritis or with corpus-predominant gastritis. Chronic active inflammation of the corpus mucosa may lead to oxyntic gland atrophy and replacement of the corpus mucosa with pseudopyloric metaplasia often containing islands of intestinal metaplasia. This low acid-secreting state is the phenotype associated with the development of gastric mucosal dysplasia and eventually gastric cancer.

The progression of *H. pylori*–related chronic gastritis to gastric cancer is modulated by bacterial, environmental, and host factors. For example, as noted above, the presence of the *cag* PAI signifies the presence of an infection with increased inflammation and an increased risk of cancer. Diets high in salt and low in fresh fruits and vegetables are associated with more rapid progression of damage and an earlier transformation to atrophic gastritis. A number of host genetic factors, especially polymorphisms in the genes regulating the intensity of the inflammatory response to the infection, have been shown to influence the outcome. For example, single-nucleotide polymorphisms in the genes encoding interleukin 1 that are associated with an increased inflammatory response are also associated with an increased risk of developing gastric atrophy and cancer. Importantly, *H. pylori* infection is the necessary but not sufficient

cause of gastric cancer such that eradication of the organism prevents the disease despite the presence of the other environmental and host risk factors.

In addition, gland atrophy in the corpus leading to hypochlorhydria or achlorhydria may be extremely important in the cancer sequence. This low acidity state not only allows gastric colonization by enteric bacteria but also may be responsible for the formulation of carcinogenic substances (eg, nitrosamines) from dietary and other sources.

DIAGNOSIS OF *H. PYLORI* INFECTION

Helicobacter pylori infection can be reliably diagnosed by a wide variety of tests including noninvasive assays (ie, those not requiring upper gastrointestinal endoscopy) and by those where it is necessary to obtain a sample of the gastric contents (invasive or minimally invasive tests) (Table 136.1). The noninvasive methods include detection of an immune response to the infection (eg, serologic tests), urea breath tests, and stool antigen assays. More invasive methods include rapid urease tests, histology, and culture. In addition, there are a number of tests available that are used for research purposes such as detection of the presence of *H. pylori* using the polymerase chain reaction.

The method of choice clinically depends on availability, cost, and whether endoscopy is otherwise indicated. Because the diagnosis of an active *H. pylori* infection should be followed by eradication therapy, the primary consideration for testing is the willingness to treat the infection. Currently, testing for *H. pylori* infection is indicated in patients with a wide variety of conditions, including active peptic ulcer disease, a past history of documented peptic ulcer, nonulcer dyspepsia, gastric mucosal-associated lymphoid tissue (MALToma), and adenocarcinoma (Table 136.2).

According to guidelines of the European *H. pylori* Study Group, urea breath tests and stool antigen assays are recommended in dyspeptic patients without alarm symptoms or under 45 years of age, at low risk of malignancy as part of a "test and treat strategy." Generally, the urea breath test is the test of choice but it is less widely available than stool antigen testing. The original stool antigen tests used polyclonal antibodies against *H. pylori* antigens and have been superseded by the more accurate tests using monoclonal antibodies. Stool antigen tests using polyclonal antibodies are still widely available, and if one decides on stool antigen

Table 136.1 Summary of Diagnostic Tests

Test	Sensitivity (%)	Specificity (%)	Cost
Noninvasive Tests			
Serology			
Laboratory, serum, ELISA	86–95	78–95	$$
In-office, serum	88–94	74–88	$
In-office, whole blood	67–88	75–91	$
Urea Breath Test			
^{13}C-urea breath test[a]	90–96	88–98	$$$
^{14}C-urea breath test[b]	90–95	90–95	$$
Stool antigen test	83–98	81–100	$$
Invasive Tests			
Rapid urease test	88–95	93–100	$
Histology	93–98	95–99	$$$
Culture	77–98	100	$$$

[a] No radiation exposure.
[b] Low radiation exposure.

Table 136.2 Indications for Testing for *Helicobacter pylori* Infection[a]

Duodenal or gastric ulcer (present or history of)
Evaluate success of eradication therapy
Gastric low-grade MALT lymphoma
Atrophic gastritis
After endoscopic resection of early gastric cancer
Uninvestigated dyspepsia
Nonulcer dyspepsia

Chronic NSAID/aspirin therapy[b]
Chronic antisecretory drug therapy
   (eg, gastroesophageal reflux disease)[c]
Relatives of gastric cancer patients
Relatives of patients with duodenal ulcer
Relatives of patients with *H. pylori* infection
Patient desires to be tested

[a] All proven to have an active *H. pylori* infection should be treated.
[b] When planning long-term therapy.
[c] When planning long-term antisecretory therapy.
Abbreviations: MALT = mucosa-associated lymphoid tissue; NSAID = nonsteroidal anti-inflammatory drug.

testing one should therefore specify a test with monoclonal antibodies. Serologic testing using laboratory enzyme-linked immunosorbent assay (ELISA) testing or an in-the-office rapid test is a less expensive alternative. However, the sensitivity and specificity of serologic tests, particularly in-the-office tests, is typically lower than that of the urea breath test or stool antigen test (using monoclonal antibodies). However, serologic testing remains useful in conditions of high and low pretest probability. For example, a positive test in a patient with a known high probability condition such as a peptic ulcer disease would be considered reliable as would a negative test in a low *H. pylori* prevalence region in a patient with a low-probability condition such as gastroesophageal reflux disease (GERD). In contrast, when one obtains an unexpected result (eg, a negative serologic test in a patient with duodenal ulcer disease), it is likely to be a false-negative test and a test for active infection should be ordered. Because antibody titers fall slowly they cannot be relied on to assess posteradication status of *H. pylori* infection.

When endoscopy is clinically indicated, the test of choice is a rapid urease test using an antral specimen or two specimens, one from the antrum and one the corpus. Biopsy urease testing provides both a high sensitivity and specificity for the diagnosis of *H. pylori* infection. If a biopsy urease test is negative, absence of an *H. pylori* infection should be confirmed by histology. Histology has the advantages of providing a permanent record and allowing identification of the pattern and severity of gastritis. Prospective studies have consistently shown that hematoxylin and eosin (H&E) staining of gastric mucosal biopsies has poor sensitivity and specificity for diagnosis of active *H. pylori*

Specific Organisms – Bacteria

infections and a special stain such as the Genta or El-Zimaity triple stains or the combination of H&E and the Diff-Quik stains should be requested. Culturing *H. pylori* is often impractical as most clinical laboratories have not established this as a routine test. However, culture to establish drug susceptibility of *H. pylori* isolates is useful to choose therapy and is clearly indicated in patients who fail to eradicate *H. pylori* by standard antimicrobial regimens. Cultures can also be obtained using minimally invasive methods using a brush or string test.

CAUTIONS ABOUT FALSE-NEGATIVE DIAGNOSTIC TESTS

False-negative results are possible and even likely if the patient has taken drugs that reduce the bacterial load such as antibiotics, bismuth, or proton pump inhibitors (PPI). In general, one should stop these drugs for 1 to 2 weeks before testing. H_2-receptor antagonists do not adversely affect any of these tests (although they apparently may adversely affect the ^{14}C-urea breath test) and can be used if needed to control symptoms. In clinical practice, post-eradication assessment for *H. pylori* infection should be conducted at least 4 weeks following the completion of eradication therapy to avoid false-negative results.

INDICATIONS FOR *H. PYLORI* ERADICATION

Current indications for *H. pylori* eradication are summarized in Table 136.2. The recommendation to eradicate *H. pylori* in patients with peptic ulcer disease includes active and inactive disease, complicated disease, and following gastric surgery for peptic ulcer. *Helicobacter pylori* eradication is also strongly recommended in gastric MALToma. Eradicating *H. pylori* results in complete regression of 60% to 83% of MALToma. Additionally, *H. pylori* infection is the prime cause of human chronic gastritis, a condition that initiates the pathogenic sequence of events leading to vitamin B12 deficiency, atrophic gastritis with metaplasia, dysplasia, and gastric cancer sequence. Several randomized trials have shown possible regression of precancerous lesions or, at least, a decrease of lesion progression following *H. pylori* eradication such that eradication therapy is indicated in all patients with atrophic gastritis. *Helicobacter pylori* eradication is also strongly recommended in infected patients who are first-degree relatives of gastric cancer patients.

Helicobacter pylori eradication is an advisable option in infected patients with nonulcer dyspepsia (Figure 136.1), and a Cochrane Systemic Review has confirmed that there is a benefit of eradicating *H. pylori* in patients with nonulcer dyspepsia.

GASTROESOPHAGEAL REFLUX DISEASE, BARRETT'S ESOPHAGUS, AND ADENOCARCINOMA OF THE ESOPHAGUS

One source of confusion and uncertainty has been the confusion concerning a possible link between *H. pylori* and reflux esophagitis, Barrett's esophagus, and adenocarcinoma of the esophagus. This confusion is the result of misunderstandings and mischaracterizations of the history of GERD, the pathophysiology of these diseases, and the misuse of the epidemiologic concept of "protection" and likely resulted in some patients receiving poor care. In reality, and as the Maastricht 2005 consensus stated, neither *H. pylori* infection nor *H. pylori* eradication causes GERD. *Helicobacter pylori* eradication also does not impede antisecretory drug therapy of GERD. Current evidence is consistent with the notion that *H. pylori* should be eliminated whenever the organism is found.

Routine testing for *H. pylori* is not recommended in GERD patients, but all GERD patients requiring long-term maintenance therapy with PPIs should undergo testing because, as noted above, acid suppression therapy in *H. pylori*–infected individuals leads to worsening of corpus gastritis and an acceleration of the rate of development of atrophic gastritis of the corpus. This is the precursor lesion for gastric carcinoma. Although there are no hard data that prolonged PPI therapy in patients with *H. pylori* infection will actually increase the rate of gastric cancer, few want to do that experiment, considering that *H. pylori* eradication has no untoward effects on treatment of GERD and also prevents the progression of atrophic gastritis in GERD patients requiring long-term PPI therapy.

CHRONIC NONSTEROIDAL ANTI-INFLAMMATORY DRUG AND ASPIRIN USE

The two most common causes of peptic ulcers are *H. pylori* infection and nonsteroidal anti-inflammatory drug (NSAID) use. Although they are independent risk factors for peptic

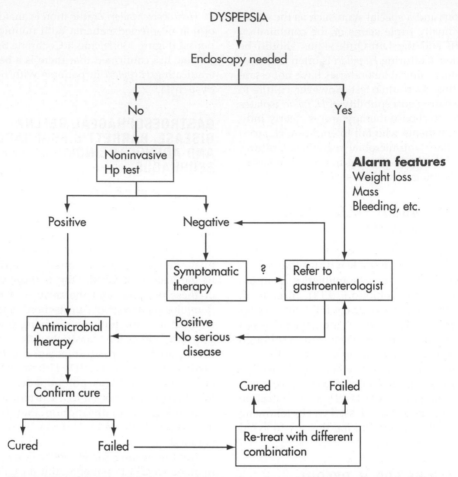

Figure 136.1 This algorithm shows one approach to the evaluation of patients presenting with dyspepsia. It has become apparent that in the United States, where the incidence of gastric cancer is very low, noninvasive testing with serology, urea breath testing, or fecal antigen testing is sufficient and endoscopy can be reserved for those with alarm symptoms. Referral to a gastroenterologist should be considered for those with alarm symptoms, those who have failure of symptoms to resolve after successful therapy, and those who fail one or more courses of therapy. The exception is those with clear-cut gastroesophageal reflux disease whose symptoms are not anticipated to resolve after successful cure of *H. pylori*. Those over the age of 50 with a long history of symptomatic gastroesophageal reflux would be one group in whom referral should be considered to exclude Barrett's esophagus.

ulcer and ulcer complications, there is evidence of synergy, as the presence of an *H. pylori* infection is associated with an approximate doubling of the risk of an ulcer complication. As such, eradication of *H. pylori* will significantly reduce the risk of ulcers among NSAID-aspirin users, and testing for *H. pylori* in patients in whom long-term NSAID or aspirin therapy is recommended.

Because *H. pylori* and NSAID use are independent causes of peptic ulcer, eradication of *H. pylori* alone will not prevent NSAID-associated ulcers or ulcer complications among NSAID users. Eradication of *H. pylori* can only prevent *H. pylori* ulcers and eliminate any synergy between

H. pylori and NSAIDs. Textbooks and review articles often state that the PPI maintenance therapy is superior to *H. pylori* eradication in preventing ulcer recurrence and/or bleeding for high-risk chronic NSAID users. Although this is often presented as an either/or question, it is not. Clearly gastroprotective therapy with an antisecretory drug or misoprostol can potentially affect NSAID ulcer pathogenesis in both *H. pylori*–infected and –uninfected individuals. In contrast, *H. pylori* eradication simply changes an *H. pylori*–positive patient into an *H. pylori*–negative patient. As noted above, although *H. pylori* eradication reduces the ulcer risk among NSAID users, uninfected

Table 136.3 Recommended Antibiotic Combinations for *H. pylori* Infections

Legacy Therapies
Triple therapy[a]: A PPI + 1 g of amoxicillin + 500 mg of clarithromycin or 500 mg of metronidazole–tinidazole BID for 14 days
Quadruple therapy: A bismuth salt, 500 mg of metronidazole, 500 mg of tetracycline all TID + a PPI BID for 14 days
Sequential therapy[b]: A PPI + 1 g of amoxicillin BID for 5 days. On day 6 stop amoxicillin and add clarithromycin, 250 or 500 mg BID, and metronidazole–tinidazole, 500 BID, to complete the 10-day course
Salvage therapy: Best if based on the results of susceptibility testing or uses drugs not previously given in the past (see text for details)
One option: A bismuth salt, 100 mg of furazolidone, tetracycline 500 mg all TID + a PPI BID for 14 days
[a] Should be replaced by concomitant quadruple therapies or sequential therapy. [b] See text for details regarding doses, duration, and whether the sequential administration of drugs is actually needed. In general, we recommend 14 days of therapy until it can be shown that an acceptable success rate (>95%) can be achieved with a shorter duration.

NSAID users still have a 4- to 5-fold increased risk compared to nonusers. The decision to use gastroprotectives is therefore independent of the decision to test for *H. pylori,* and the issue of "superior to" is not the answer to any clinically relevant question.

TREATMENT OF *H. PYLORI* INFECTION

As previously recommended initial therapy for *H. pylori* infection consists of an antisecretory drug (eg, a PPI) or ranitidine bismuth citrate (RBC) plus two antibiotics, such as clarithromycin (500 mg) and amoxicillin (1 g) administered twice daily for 7 to 14 days. Metronidazole (500 mg BID) can be used as an alternative to amoxicillin (Table 136.3). However, in most Western countries this recommendation is out of date as it is now difficult to achieve eradication rates of 80% or greater. The main reasons for eradication failure include poor patient compliance, antibiotic resistance, and short duration of therapy (7 instead of 14 days). Smoking also may play a role in failure of this triple therapy. Until recently, the successful rate of standard triple therapies could be improved by extending the duration of therapy to 14 days, but the rapid increase in clarithromycin resistance has dulled that benefit. Standard or traditional triple therapy should now probably be abandoned except in areas where clarithromycin resistance is low, and even then it should be administered for 14 days. Traditional quadruple therapy consisting of a bismuth (eg, bismuth subcitrate, 120 mg), tetracycline (500 mg), and metronidazole (500 mg) all given 3 or 4 times daily and an antisecretory agent

(eg, a PPI) given twice a day for a minimum of 7 (preferably 14) days should be the first choice therapy in areas where current triple therapies have proven clinically inadequate.

Recent comparative studies from Italy have shown a 10-day sequential regimen, including a PPI and amoxicillin dual therapy for 5 days, followed by a PPI, clarithromycin, and tinidazole–metronidazole triple therapy for a further 5 days achieved a higher eradication rate than standard triple therapy, and the benefit was present in both adults and children. The efficacy of sequential therapy appears very promising and should probably replace standard triple therapy. Studies are needed to test dose and duration of this therapy as well as whether similar results cannot be achieved by giving all four drugs together as concomitant rather than sequential therapy. The alternative is to use traditional quadruple therapy, which until recently was considered the preferred therapy for those who had failed initial eradication therapy (see below).

TREATMENT FOLLOWING ONE TREATMENT FAILURE

With regard to treatment failures, the approach is to use antibiotics not used in the original treatment program (bismuth and amoxicillin excepted). If both clarithromycin and metronidazole–tinidazole have been used (eg, in a sequential therapy) metronidazole–tinidazole can still be used in a quadruple therapy. A good choice is traditional quadruple therapy (see above or Table 136.2). Replacing the PPI and the bismuth compound in the quadruple therapy with RBC achieves similar results. If bismuth compounds are unavailable or the patient is allergic to amoxicillin, treatment choices become more difficult. The Maastricht group recommended the combination of PPI–amoxicillin or tetracycline and metronidazole, but that recommendation was based on studies treating very few patients. In reality, the problems of single and multiple treatment failures have tended to merge.

MULTIPLE TREATMENT FAILURES OR SALVAGE THERAPIES

Drug choices include a fluoroquinolone (eg, levofloxacin), amoxicillin, clarithromycin, metronidazole–tinidazole, tetracycline, furazolidone, rifabutin, bismuth compounds, and the different PPIs. One approach is to use the general formula for traditional quadruple therapy and substitute another antibiotic for metronidazole (eg, furazolidone, 100 mg). Another is to use the general formula for triple therapy and substitute a drug for clarithromycin (eg, levofloxacin or rifabutin). Learning from the success of sequential therapy, one might substitute drugs for clarithromycin in this therapy or for both clarithromycin and metronidazole. The choice of agents based on susceptibility testing is best, but the final choice will depend on availability and patient acceptability. Generally, therapy should be given for 14 days.

CONFIRMATION OF CURE

Therapy should be followed by confirmation of cure. The confirmatory test should be delayed until 4 to 6 weeks after the end of antimicrobial therapy to allow the bacteria, if present, an opportunity to repopulate the stomach. Drugs that inhibit *H. pylori* such as PPIs should not be allowed for 1 and preferably 2 weeks prior to testing. The urea breath test is the ideal method of evaluating the outcome of therapy for those in whom follow-up endoscopy is not needed. An alternate approach would be to use the stool antigen test, but in that case, testing should be delayed for 6 to 8 weeks.

SUGGESTED READING

Cianci R, Montalto M, Pandolfi F, Gasbarrini GB, Cammarota G. Third-line rescue therapy for Helicobacter pylori. *World J Gastroenterol*. 2006;12:2313–2319.

De Korwin JD. Advantages and limitations of diagnostic methods for H. pylori infection. *Gastroenterol Clin Biol*. 2003;27:380–390.

Graham DY. Helicobacter pylori infection in the pathogenesis of duodenal ulcer and gastric cancer: a model. *Gastroenterology*. 1997;113:1983–1991.

Graham DY. The changing epidemiology of GERD: geography and *Helicobacter pylori*. *Am J Gastroenterol*. 2003;98:1462–1470.

Lu H, Yamaoka Y, Graham DY. Helicobacter pylori virulence factors: facts and fantasies. *Curr Opin Gastroenterol*. 2005;21:653–659.

Malfertheiner P, Megraud F, O'Morain C, et al. Current concepts in the management of *Helicobacter pylori* infection: the Maastricht III Consensus Report. *Gut*. 2007;56:772–781.

Rustgi AK. Barry Marshall 2005 Nobel Laureate in Medicine and Physiology. *Gastroenterology*. 2005;129:1813–1814.

Shiotani A, Graham DY. Pathogenesis and therapy of gastric and duodenal ulcer disease. *Med Clin North Am*. 2002;86:1447–1466.

Vilaichone RK, Mahachai V, Graham DY. Helicobacter pylori diagnosis and treatment. *Gastroenterol Clin North Am*. 2006;35:229–247.

137. Gonococcus: *Neisseria Gonorrhoeae*

Michael F. Rein

Neisseria gonorrhoeae is the second most common sexually transmitted bacterial pathogen after *Chlamydia trachomatis*, resulting in an estimated 600 000 cases per year in the United States. The gonococcus causes disease by attaching primarily to columnar or cuboidal epithelial cells (Table 137.1) via pili and outer membrane proteins. It then penetrates between and through the cells to submucosal areas, where it elicits a neutrophilic host response. The clinical spectrum of primary infection with *Neisseria gonorrhoeae* mirrors that of *Chlamydia trachomatis*, which is the most important etiological differential diagnosis.

Acute urethritis, manifesting as some combination of urethral discharge and dysuria, is the most common presentation of disease in men, although some infected men are asymptomatic. Gram stain of urethral discharge may be used for presumptive diagnosis of gonococcal urethritis. Polymorphonuclear neutrophils (PMN) with gram-negative, intracellular diplococci (Figure 137.1) are observed in 95% of infected, symptomatic men, and the finding is 98% specific. Observing PMN without gram-negative intracellular diplococci (GNID) supports a diagnosis of nongonococcal urethritis (see Chapter 58, Urethritis and Dysuria), but the sensitivity of GNID in asymptomatic men is only about 75%, and Gram stain cannot be used to rule out gonorrhea in these patients.

In women, the primary site of infection is the endocervix, although the organism can be recovered from the urethra and periurethral (Skene's) and Bartholin's glands in adults and from the vagina itself in prepubescent girls. Asymptomatic infection is more common in women than men. Gram stains of cervical smears from infected women are 97% specific for the disease when GNID are observed but only 50% to 70% sensitive.

Anorectal gonorrhea occurs in up to 40% of women with endocervical disease and as an isolated finding in homosexual men who practice receptive anal intercourse. Most patients are asymptomatic, but acute proctitis may occur. Most patients with pharyngeal infection, acquired from fellatio, are also asymptomatic,

Table 137.1 Sites of Primary Infection by *Neisseria gonorrhoeae*

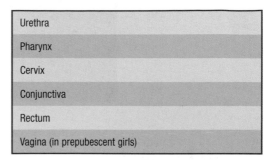

Urethra
Pharynx
Cervix
Conjunctiva
Rectum
Vagina (in prepubescent girls)

but pharyngitis may occur. Gonococcal conjunctivitis in adults, usually acquired by autoinoculation from a genital focus, produces varying degrees of inflammation.

Disseminated gonococcal infection is increasingly uncommon, occurring historically in perhaps 0.5% to 3% of infected patients. It usually presents as the arthritis–dermatitis syndrome, manifesting as asymmetric, migratory polyarthritis, arthralgias, or tenosynovitis and accompanied in 75% of cases by small papules or by vesicles or pustules with an erythematous base. Hereditary deficiency of the terminal components of complement or infection with organisms resistant to the bactericidal activity of serum predisposes to dissemination. Endocarditis and meningitis are very rare complications.

DIAGNOSIS

Definitive diagnosis requires demonstrating the presence of the organism. This is traditionally accomplished by culture of infected material, but culture has been largely supplanted by molecular techniques. Nucleic acid amplification tests (NAAT) are those most widely used clinically in the United States. The ligase chain reaction is highly specific and sensitive when used on a urethral, cervical, or vaginal specimen. However, studies on urine suggest an unacceptably low sensitivity of about 60% in women. Disadvantages of such molecular technology include the ability of the tests to

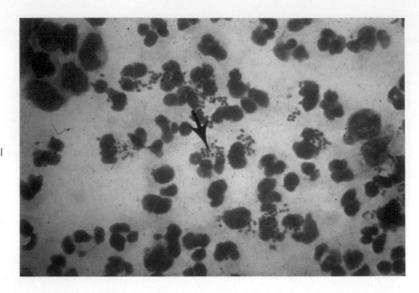

Figure 137.1 Gram stain of urethral discharge, showing gram-negative intracellular diplococci diagnostic of gonorrhea. Coincident nongonococcal urethritis cannot be ruled out. Courtesy of Centers for Disease Control and Prevention.

detect dead organisms for perhaps as long as 2 weeks after successful treatment, their not being licensed for use on anal or pharyngeal specimens, and their inability to provide a specimen for testing of antimicrobial sensitivity. New data are being developed, and the clinician should review the material provided with these tests as an indication of their appropriate use. It is important to obtain appropriate cultures and susceptibility testing on all patients who to do not improve on therapy, once reinfection and nonadherence to medication have been ruled out.

THERAPY

Uncomplicated anogenital infection with *N. gonorrhoeae* can be treated with a single dose of an appropriate medication. Treatment has been complicated by the emergence of resistance to many antimicrobials. Historically, one can follow the rapid appearance and dissemination of organisms resistant to penicillins, sulfonamides, tetracyclines, and, most recently, fluoroquinolones (FQ). None of these classes of agents should ever be used to treat gonorrhea. Resistance has been mediated by a series of chromosomal mutations and by plasmids that encode for resistance genes and for the ability to transfer between strains and even genera. Plasmid-mediated resistance (penicillins, tetracyclines) has spread particularly quickly.

Clinical failures with quinolone antibiotics have been described since 1990 and are felt to result from the widespread use of these drugs for many infections. The initial mechanism of resistance to quinolones is mutation in the *gyrA* gene coding for the A subunit of DNA gyrase, also known as topoisomerase II. Subsequent mutation in the *parC* gene of topoisomerase IV appears to be associated with higher minimum inhibitory concentrations (MICs) than mutations in *gyrA* alone, and strains with MICs ≥2.0 μg/mL are more likely to possess both mutations. Reduced permeability through the cytoplasmic membrane and increase in an efflux pump may also contribute to quinolone resistance. Failures of 500 mg of ciprofloxacin and 400 mg of ofloxacin have been reported worldwide. The prevalence of FQ resistance in southeast Asia is estimated at 90%. Resistant organisms were initially identified in Hawaii and California but have spread eastward, especially among men who have sex with men (MSM). In the first half of 2006, the Gonococcal Isolate Surveillance Project, which performs sensitivity testing on about 3% of male urethral isolates, noted that 13.3% of all U.S. strains were resistant to the FQs. The level of resistance was 8.6% even when isolates from Hawaii and California were excluded. FQ resistance was found in 29% of MSM and 6.7% of heterosexual men. Fluoroquinolones are no longer recommended for the treatment of gonorrhea in the United States.

Treatment of gonococcal disease is further complicated by frequent co-infection with *Chlamydia trachomatis* (see Chapter 58, Urethritis and Dysuria) in genital infections, proctitis, and conjunctivitis. Thus patients with gonorrhea should be treated as well for co-incident chlamydial infection unless the second infection has already been excluded by dual testing with NAAT. Dual therapy may also slow the

Specific Organisms – Bacteria

emergence of resistance if the gonococcal isolate is also susceptible to the antichlamydial agent. Management of sexual partners should probably extend back for 60 days prior to the onset of symptoms or date of diagnosis. All patients with gonorrhea should be advised to undergo testing for infection with human immunodeficiency virus. The recommended antigonococcal regimens are sufficiently effective that test of cure is not necessary, but retesting at 3 months should be encouraged to detect reinfection. In some settings, medication or prescriptions may be provided for patients to deliver to their sexual partners. Although this approach, so-called expedited treatment, increases the effectiveness of treating partners, its legality has not been well defined.

STANDARD THERAPY

Intramuscular ceftriaxone is highly effective, and a 125-mg regimen is recommended by the Centers for Disease Control and Prevention (CDC). The injection volume is 0.5 mL, and the drug is often diluted in 1% lidocaine to further reduce discomfort. The smallest vial of ceftriaxone available for clinical use contains 250 mg, and unless more than 1 patient is to be treated, the use of the lower dose does not result in cost savings. Other single-dose parenteral regimens (ceftizoxime or cefotaxime, 500 mg IM) offer no advantage over ceftriaxone. Resistance to cefoxitin, often in association with high-level tetracycline resistance, mandates that this drug should no longer be used in the treatment of uncomplicated gonorrhea.

Oral cephalosporins are effective. Cefixime is the best studied but has suffered from limited availability as a tablet. It is more readily available as a liquid, but this form is less convenient and has a short shelf life. Cefpodoxime, in a single oral dose of 200 mg, has Food and Drug Administration (FDA) approval but with limited data. This dose produced a cure rate of 96.5% but with a lower limit of the 95% confidence interval of 94.8%, falling just short of the 95% required for a CDC recommendation. Current studies of the 400-mg dose may correct this shortcoming, and this dose is already used in many clinical facilities.

Fluoroquinolones should no longer be used to treat uncomplicated gonorrhea (see above). Azithromycin, 2 g, has the putative advantage of treating coincident chlamydial infection, but it is expensive, elicits gastrointestinal intolerance, and is subject to increasing resistance; it is not recommended.

The aminocyclitol spectinomycin is listed by the CDC as an alternative for patients who are pregnant or for children who have a history of immediate hypersensitivity to ß-lactams. Resistance appeared rapidly after it was used heavily among military personnel in Korea, and the drug does not reach adequate concentrations in saliva, rendering it ineffective in the treatment of pharyngeal disease. It is intermittently and currently unavailable. Earlier data support the use of gentamicin (see Table 137.2), which may be effective in the same settings. Although this drug is again being used in some facilities, lack of current data and concern about rapid appearance of resistance make test of cure important.

NONSTANDARD THERAPY

The monobactam aztreonam and the carbapenems imipenem–cilastatin, meropenem, and ertapenem are uniformly effective against *N. gonorrhoeae* but are costly and available only in intravenous form. These drugs are never primary therapy for gonorrhea. Penicillins formulated with a β-lactamase inhibitor (ie, amoxicillin–clavulanate, ampicillin–sulbactam, ticarcillin–clavulanate, and piperacillin–tazobactam) are costly, and although they are active against pencillinase–producing *N. gonorrhoeae* strains, they are likely not effective in the setting of chromosomally mediated resistance, and they should not be used.

EXTRAGENITAL DISEASE

A single dose of ceftriaxone, 1 g IM, in adults apparently cures gonococcal conjunctivitis, but clinical data are extremely limited. A single saline flush of the conjunctiva should be considered, but topical antibiotics have no proven additional benefit.

No prospective studies on the treatment of disseminated gonococcal infection have been performed since 1976; hence, recommendations are empiric, because the worldwide spread of resistant gonococci occurred after that time. The gonococcal arthritis–dermatitis syndrome should be treated with ceftriaxone (Table 137.3). Regimens employing other third-generation cephalosporins should be equally effective. If frank septic arthritis is not present, the patient can be switched to an oral regimen (Table 137.4), preferably with a cephalosporin, to complete 7 to 10 days of therapy. The actual optimal duration of therapy is unknown. Spectinomycin, if available, is an

Table 137.2 Regimens for Uncomplicated Gonorrhea (Urethritis, Cervicitis, Proctitis)

Drug	Dose	CDC Recommended	Safe in Pregnancy	Effective in Pharynx	Comments
Ceftriaxone	125 mg IM	Yes	Yes	Yes	The gold standard
Ceftriaxone	250 mg IM	Formerly	Yes	Yes	Used in other countries, see text
Ceftizoxime	500 mg IM	Secondary	Yes	Yes	No advantage over ceftriaxone
Cefotaxime	500 mg IM	Secondary	Yes	Yes	No advantage over ceftriaxone
Cefixime	400 mg PO	Yes	Yes	Yes	Largely unavailable in tablet form, see text
Cefpodoxime	400 mg PO	No	Yes	Uncertain	Limited data, see text
Ciprofloxacin	500 mg PO	No	No	Yes	Significant resistance, not recommended, see text
Other fluoroquinolones	Various	No	No	Yes	No advantage over ciprofloxacin, not recommended
Azithromycin	2 g PO	No	Yes	Unknown	Expensive, nauseating, not recommended
Spectinomycin	2 g IM	Yes	Yes	No	Unavailable
Gentamicin	280 mg IM	No	Yes	No	Old regimen, test of cure required, see text

Table 137.3 Initial Regimens for Disseminated Gonococcal Infection[a]

Drug	Dose	CDC Recommended	Safe in Pregnancy	Comments
Ceftriaxone	125 mg IM or IV q24h	Yes	Yes	The gold standard
Ceftizoxime	500 mg IV q8h	Secondary	Yes	No advantage over ceftriaxone
Spectinomycin	2 g IM q12h	Yes	Unclear	Unavailable

[a] Intravenous therapy should be continued for 24 to 48 hours after improvement begins. Thereafter the patient can be switched to an oral regimen.

Table 137.4 Follow-up Regimens for Disseminated Gonococcal Infection

Drug	Dosage	CDC Recommended	Comments
Cefixime	400 mg PO, 2× daily	Yes	Largely unavailable in tablet form, see text
Cefpodoxime	400 mg PO, 2× daily	No	No data

alternative for pregnant women, children, and those who are allergic to β-lactams. Gonococcal endocarditis should be treated with 4 weeks of an appropriate parenteral regimen, preferably ceftriaxone or another third-generation cephalosporin. Meningitis should be treated for 10 to 14 days. There are no current studies of extended courses of fluoroquinolones as treatment for extragenital disease, and in the face of recent increases in resistance, these drugs should not be used.

SUGGESTED READING

Bauer HM, Mark KE, Samuel M, et al. Prevalence and associated risk factors for fluoroquinolone-resistant *Neisseria gonorrhoeae* in California 2000–2003. *Clin Infect Dis*. 2005;41:795–803.

Centers for Disease Control and Prevention. Sexually transmitted disease treatment guidelines, 2006. *Morbid Mortal Weekly Rep.* 2006;55(RR-11):42–49.

Centers for Disease Control and Prevention. Update to CDC's *Sexually Transmitted Diseases Treatment Guidelines*, 2006. Fluoroquinolones no longer recommended for treatment of gonococcal infections. *Morbid Mortal Weekly Rep.* 2007;56:332–336.

Cooke RL, Hutchinson SL, Ostergaard L, et al. Systematic review: noninvasive testing for *Chlamydia trachomatis* and *Neisseria gonorrhoeae*. *Ann Intern Med*. 2005;142:914–925.

DeMaria A Jr. Challenges of sexually transmitted disease prevention and control: no magic bullet, but some bullets would still be appreciated. *Clin Infect Dis*. 2005;41:804–807.

Gaydos CA. Nucleic acid amplification tests for gonorrhea and chlamydia: practice and applications. *Infect Dis Clin N Am*. 2005;19:367–386.

Goldman MR, Whittington WLH, Handsfield HH, et al. Effect of expedited treatment on sex partners on recurrent or persistent gonorrhea or chlamydial infections. *N Engl J Med*. 2005;352:676–685.

Rice P. Gonococcal arthritis (disseminated gonococcal infection). *Infect Dis Clin N Am*. 2005;19:853–861.

Tan NJ, Rajan VS, Pang R, Sng EH. Gentamicin in the treatment of infections with penicillinase-producing gonococci. *Br J Vener Dis*. 1980;56:394–396.

Tapsall JW. What management is there for gonorrhea in the postquinolone era? *Sex Transm Dis*. 2006;33:8–10.

Wang SA, Harvey AB, Conner SM, et al. Antimicrobial resistance for *Neisseria gonorrhoeae* in the United States, 1983–2003: the spread of fluoroquinolone resistance. *Ann Intern Med*. 2007;147:81–88.

138. Haemophilus

Timothy F. Murphy

HAEMOPHILUS INFLUENZAE

Haemophilus influenzae is an exclusively human pathogen whose ecological niche is the human respiratory tract. The species *H. influenzae* includes strains with six antigenically distinct polysaccharide capsules designated a through f. Serotype b strains cause serious invasive disease in infants, including meningitis and bacteremia. Polysaccharide–protein conjugate vaccines have virtually eliminated disease caused by type b strains in countries where the vaccine is widely used. However, invasive disease caused by *H. influenzae* type b is still a significant problem worldwide in countries where the vaccine is not used.

Strains of *H. influenzae* that lack a polysaccharide capsule are called nontypeable because they are nonreactive with the typing sera directed at each of the six capsular polysaccharides. Nontypeable strains of *H. influenzae* demonstrate enormous genetic diversity and are an important cause of human respiratory tract disease.

Because type b and nontypeable strains of *H. influenzae* differ from one another in epidemiology, clinical manifestations, and treatment, they are considered separately in each section of this chapter.

Epidemiology and Respiratory Tract Colonization

H. INFLUENZAE TYPE B

Prior to the widespread use of the *H. influenzae* conjugate vaccines, approximately 3% to 5% of infants were colonized in the nasopharynx by type b strains with higher rates observed in day-care centers. The conjugate vaccines have resulted in a marked decrease in the colonization rate, contributing to the dramatic decrease in invasive type b infections in this country.

NONTYPEABLE H. INFLUENZAE

Nontypeable strains of *H. influenzae* frequently colonize the nasopharynx of healthy children, with higher rates in day-care centers. When nasopharyngeal cultures are performed in children longitudinally, essentially every child is colonized at some time. The application of molecular typing methods is contributing new information regarding the dynamics of respiratory tract colonization: (1) Frequent transmission of strains occurs among children in day-care centers. (2) Colonization with nontypeable *H. influenzae* in the first several months of life is associated with recurrent otitis media. (3) Different antibiotics have different effects on the dynamics of colonization.

Nontypeable *H. influenzae* colonizes the upper respiratory tract of healthy adults and adults with chronic obstructive pulmonary disease (COPD). The airways below the vocal cords are sterile in healthy people. However, the airways of adults with COPD are colonized with bacteria, the most common isolate being *H. influenzae*. Colonization of the respiratory tract of adults with COPD by *H. influenzae* is a dynamic process with new strains being acquired and replacing old strains periodically. The acquisition of a new strain of nontypeable *H. influenzae* by an adult with COPD is associated with the occurrence of an exacerbation. Recent studies indicate that some strains of commensal *H. haemolyticus* are being misidentified as *H. influenzae*, so caution must be used in distinguishing these two species and in interpreting older studies.

Clinical Manifestations

H. INFLUENZAE TYPE B

Type b strains cause invasive infections predominantly in children under the age of 6 years. Meningitis is the most serious manifestation of infection by *H. influenzae* type b in children and occurs mostly under the age of 2 years. Fever and altered central nervous system function are the most common presenting symptoms. Nuchal rigidity may or may not be present. Epiglottitis is a life-threatening infection involving the epiglottis and supraglottic tissues. Cellulitis, pneumonia, and bacteremia are less common manifestations of *H. influenzae* type b infections. All forms of infection due to type b strains are uncommon in countries where the conjugate vaccines are used.

NONTYPEABLE *H. INFLUENZAE*

Based on cultures of middle ear fluid, non-typeable *H. influenzae* causes 25% to 35% of episodes of acute otitis media in children and is the most common bacterial cause of recurrent otitis media. Approximately three quarters of all children experience an episode of otitis media by the age of 3 years, and otitis media is the most common reason that children receive antibiotics. A significant subset of children who are called *otitis prone* have recurrent or persistent otitis media, which are associated with a delay in speech and language development.

Nontypeable *H. influenzae* is an important cause of lower respiratory tract infection in adults with COPD. The course of COPD is characterized by intermittent exacerbations of the disease, and many of these exacerbations are caused by bacterial infection. Nontypeable *H. influenzae* is the most common bacterial cause of exacerbations. Clinically, exacerbations are characterized by increased sputum production, increased sputum purulence, and increased dyspnea compared to baseline symptoms. Exacerbations result in missed work time, doctors office visits, emergency room visits, hospital admissions, and respiratory failure requiring mechanical ventilation and are thus associated with enormous morbidity, mortality, and health care costs.

In addition to exacerbations of COPD (which are characterized by an absence of infiltrate on chest x-ray), nontypeable *H. influenzae* causes community-acquired pneumonia, particularly in the elderly and in those with COPD.

A small proportion of sinusitis is caused by bacterial infection. Determining the etiology of sinusitis requires needle aspiration of the sinus, so little information on the relative proportion of etiologic agents is available. Based on studies in which sinus aspirates were cultured, non-typeable *H. influenzae* causes sinusitis in adults and children.

Nontypeable strains of *H. influenzae* are unusual causes of a variety of invasive infections that are documented primarily by small series and case reports.

Treatment

H. INFLUENZAE TYPE B

Meningitis due to *H. influenzae* type b can be rapidly fatal, so treatment should be initiated without delay. Initial treatment should be a third-generation cephalosporin, including either ceftriaxone or cefotaxime (Table 138.1). Administration of corticosteroids to patients

Table 138.1 Treatment of *H. influenzae* Type b Meningitis

Therapeutic Agent	Intravenous Dose	Duration
Ceftriaxone or	75 to 100 mg/kg daily in 2 divided doses	1 to 2 wk
Cefotaxime	200 mg/kg daily in 4 divided doses	1 to 2 wk
Alternative: Ampicillin plus	200 to 300 mg/kg daily in 4 divided doses	1 to 2 wk
Chloramphenicol	75 to 100 mg/kg daily in 4 divided doses	1 to 2 wk
Dexamethasone[a]	0.6 mg/kg daily in 4 divided doses	2 d

[a] Recommended for children >2 months of age.

with *H. influenzae* type b meningitis reduces the incidence of neurological sequelae. The mechanism appears to be a reduction in inflammation that results from release of bacterial cell wall fragments when bacteria are killed by antibiotics. Dexamethasone should be administered to children with meningitis due to *H. influenzae* type b (Table 138.1). In addition to antimicrobial and corticosteroid therapy, attention should be directed to providing supportive care, including treatment of hypotension, acidosis, and respiratory failure that can be associated with meningitis.

Other invasive infections caused by *H. influenzae*, including epiglottitis, are treated with the same antibiotics as meningitis, but the doses are somewhat lower. Maintaining an airway is critical in patients with epiglottitis.

NONTYPEABLE *H. INFLUENZAE*

Many infections caused by nontypeable *H. influenzae*, such as otitis media and exacerbations of COPD, can be treated with oral antimicrobial agents. Approximately 30% of strains of *H. influenzae* produce ß-lactamase and are therefore resistant to amoxicillin. Many episodes of otitis media and exacerbations of COPD are treated empirically without the advantage of culture results. In these circumstances, the antimicrobial agent should be active against *Streptococcus pneumoniae* and *Moraxella catarrhalis* because these bacteria also cause otitis media and exacerbations of COPD.

Oral antibiotics that are active against most strains of nontypeable *H. influenzae* include amoxicillin–clavulanic acid, fluoroquinolones, macrolides (eg, azithromycin, clarithromycin), various extended-spectrum cephalosporins, and telithromycin.

Parenteral antibiotic therapy is indicated for more serious infections caused by nontypeable *H. influenzae* such as bacteremia and pneumonia that require hospital admission. Parenteral antimicrobial agents that are active include third-generation cephalosporins, ampicillin–sulbactam, fluoroquinolones, and the newer macrolides (azithromycin, clarithromycin).

Prevention

H. INFLUENZAE TYPE B

Conjugate vaccines are highly effective in preventing invasive infections due to type b strains. Three vaccines are currently licensed and commercially available in the United States (Table 138.2). All children should receive a series of *H. influenzae* type b conjugate vaccines. The first dose is given at 2 months of age and the primary series is given between 2 and 6 months of age. A booster is administered between 12 and 15 months. Specific recommendations vary for the different vaccines. Details are outlined in the recommendations of the American Academy of Pediatrics (www.aap.org).

NONTYPEABLE *H. INFLUENZAE*

A recent study of pneumococcal polysaccharide conjugated to an outer membrane protein of nontypeable *H. influenzae* showed efficacy in preventing otitis media due to both *S. pneumoniae* and *H. influenzae*. Although no vaccines for nontypeable *H. influenzae* are currently licensed, such vaccines are likely to be available in the future.

HAEMOPHILUS DUCREYI

Haemophilus ducreyi is the etiologic agent of chancroid, which is a sexually transmitted disease characterized by genital ulcer and inguinal lymphadenopathy. Although uncommon in the United States, chancroid is a common cause of genital ulcers in developing countries and facilitates the transmission of human immunodeficiency virus (HIV). Transmission is primarily heterosexual with more males than females being affected in most studies. Many infections in males have been associated with contact with commercial sex workers.

The typical lesion begins as a papule and evolves into an ulcer that is painful and well circumscribed with ragged edges.

Table 138.2 Conjugate Vaccines for Prevention of *H. influenzae* Type b Infections

Generic Name	Trade Name	Manufacturer	Content
HbOC	HibTITER	Wyeth	Oligosaccharide conjugated to CRM$_{197}$, a mutant diphtheria toxin
PRP-OMPC	PedvaxHIB	Merck	Native PRP[a] conjugated to an outer membrane complex of *N. meningitidis*
PRP-T	ActHIB	Aventis Pasteur	Native PRP[a] conjugated to tetanus toxoid

[a] PRP: polyribitol ribose phosphate, the capsular polysaccharide of *H. influenzae* type b

Table 138.3 Treatment Regimens for Chancroid[a]

Antibiotic	Dose and Route	Duration
Azithromycin	1 g PO	Single dose
Ceftriaxone	250 mg IM	Single dose
Ciprofloxacin	500 mg PO 2× daily	3 d
Erythromycin base	500 mg PO 3× daily	7 d

[a] Recommendations of the Centers for Disease Control, August 4, 2006.

Approximately half of patients have inguinal lymphadenopathy. The primary differential diagnoses include primary syphilis and genital herpes. In the setting of HIV infection, chancroid can be more severe, including multiple ulcers and longer duration of ulcers. The diagnosis is best established by culturing the ulcer. However, because the organism is difficult to grow and requires selective media, the diagnosis is often made clinically in practice. Polymerase chain reaction (PCR)-based assays are under development and will facilitate making an etiological diagnosis of genital ulcers.

The preferred treatment of chancroid is a single 1-g oral dose of azithromycin. Alternative regimens are listed in Table 138.3. Contacts of patients with chancroid should be treated if sexual contact occurred within the 10 days preceding the onset of symptoms in the patient, whether or not symptoms are present in the contact.

SUGGESTED READING

Bong CT, Bauer ME, Spinola SM. *Haemophilus ducreyi*: clinical features, epidemiology, and prospects for disease control. *Microbes Infect.* 2002;4:1141–1148.

Heilmann KP, Rice CL, Miller AL, et al. Decreasing prevalence of beta-lactamase production among respiratory tract isolates of *Haemophilus influenzae* in the United States. *Antimicrob Agents Chemother.* 2005;49:2561–2564.

Leibovitz E, Jacobs MR, Dagan R. Haemophilus influenzae: a significant pathogen in acute otitis media. *Pediatr Infect Dis J.* 2004;23:1142–1152.

Murphy TF. Respiratory infections caused by non-typeable *Haemophilus influenzae. Curr Opin Infect Dis.* 2003;16:129–134.

Murphy TF, Brauer AL, Schiffmacher AT, Sethi S. Persistent colonization by *Haemophilus influenzae* in chronic obstructive pulmonary disease. *Am J Respir Crit Care Med.* 2004;170:266–272.

Murphy TF, Brauer AL, Sethi S, Kilian M, Cai X, Lesse AJ. *Haemophilus haemolyticus*: a human respiratory tract commensal to be distinguished from *Haemophilus influenzae. J Infect Dis.* 2007;195:81–89.

Prymula R, Peeters P, Chrobok V, et al. Pneumococcal capsular polysaccharides conjugated to protein D for prevention of acute otitis media caused by both *Streptococcus pneumoniae* and non-typable *Haemophilus influenzae*: a randomised double-blind efficacy study. *Lancet.* 2006;367: 740–748.

Sethi S, Evans N, Grant BJB, Murphy TF. New strains of bacteria and exacerbations of chronic obstructive pulmonary disease. *N Engl J Med.* 2002;347:465–471.

139. Legionellosis

Thomas J. Marrie

LEGIONELLOSIS

Etiologic Agents

The genus name *Legionella* was derived from the fact that the first recognized outbreak of infection due to these microorganisms affected members of the American Legion. *Pneumophila* ("lung loving") was the species designation for the first isolate. There are now 48 species in the family Legionellaceae and about half of these have caused disease in humans. *Legionella pneumophila* serogroup 1 accounts for 80% to 90% of cases of legionnaire's disease (LD) (Table 139.1). However, in Australia and New Zealand *Legionella longbeachae* accounts for 30% of the cases. Legionellaceae are gram-negative, aerobic, non–spore-forming bacilli that measure 0.3 to 0.9 μm wide and 2 to 20 μm long. These organisms require special media for growth. Charcoal yeast extract agar buffered to pH 6.9 and containing α-ketoglutarate along with cefamandole, polymyxin B, and anisomycin to prevent growth of other microorganisms is the primary medium used for isolation of these organisms. Addition of α-ketoglutaric acid to the medium promotes growth of *Legionella* likely by stimulation of oxygen-scavenging enzymes.

These organisms are visualized poorly if at all by Gram stain. In tissue, silver impregnation stains such as the Dieterle or Warthin–Starry method allow visualization of the organisms.

EPIDEMIOLOGY AND PATHOGENESIS

Legionellae are aquatic microorganisms and thus the epidemiology of infections due to these organisms is linked to water systems that are contaminated with these bacteria. The earliest known outbreak of LD occurred in 1965 at St. Elizabeth's Hospital in Washington, D.C. The outbreak that gave this illness its name and led to the isolation of the causative microorganism was associated with the 58th Annual Convention of the American Legion held at a hotel in Philadelphia from July 21 to July 24, 1976. One hundred eighty-two of the attendees at the convention developed pneumonia. One hundred forty-seven (81%) were hospitalized,

Table 139.1 Legionellaceae That Have Been Reported as Causing Pneumonia

Legionella pneumophila serogroups 1–15 (serogroup 1 most commonly; also 3, 4, 6, 13)
Legionella micdadei
Legionella bozemanii
Legionella dumoffi
Legionella sainthelensi
Legionella longbeachae
Legionella anisa
Legionella maceachernii
Legionella waltersii
Legionella feelei
Legionella wadsworthi
Legionella parisiensis
Legionella hackeliae
Legionella jordanis
Legionella lansingensis
Legionella cincinnatiensis

and twenty-nine (16%) died. This outbreak of pneumonia of apparent unknown cause triggered an extensive epidemiologic and microbiologic investigation by the Centers for Disease Control and Prevention (CDC), culminating in the isolation of a new microorganism, *Legionella pneumophila*, about 6 months later.

We now know that legionellosis can occur as sporadic (endemic) cases or as outbreaks in the community or in health care facilities. We have learned a lot about legionellosis by studying outbreaks. Outbreaks have varied in size from a few cases to the largest outbreak yet reported of 800 suspected and 449 confirmed cases in Murcia, Spain, in July 2001. A recent study from Europe from 2000 to 2002 indicated that there were 10 322 cases of LD with infection rates among the reporting countries from 0 to 34.1 cases per million population. Thirty-six outbreaks involving 211 persons were linked to hospitals; 38 outbreaks with 1059 cases occurred in community settings; 2 outbreaks were linked to private homes; and 113 outbreaks were travel-associated clusters involving 315 persons. Travel within Europe accounted for 88% of the cases. The remainder were associated with travel to the Americas, Caribbean, Far East, Africa, and Middle East.

When data on 3254 patients with LD reported to the CDC from 1980 through 1989 were analyzed, investigators found that disease rates did not vary by year but were higher in the northern states and during the summer. The mean age of patients with LD was 52.7 years compared with 34.7 years for the U.S. population. In contrast to earlier reports, persons with LD were now more likely to be black. They were also more likely to be smokers, have diabetes, cancer, acquired immunodeficiency syndrome (AIDS), or end-stage renal disease. Indeed, the observed number of cases among patients with AIDS was 42-fold higher than expected. Twenty-three percent of the cases were nosocomially acquired.

Some of the features that were noted in a review of the first 1000 cases of LD in the United States were that 71% of the cases were male and states with the highest attack rates were east of the Mississippi River. In addition, in the 2 weeks before onset of illness 37% of the patients had traveled overnight; 29% had been a hospital visitor, and 5% had been hospitalized for 2 days or fewer before onset of illness.

Other risk factors for LD in the setting of an outbreak are cigarette smoking (relative risk 1.7 to 3.4) and consumption of 3 or more drinks of alcohol per day (confers a relative risk of 3.5). More recently investigators have begun to combine studies of traditional risk factors with a dissection of host susceptibility using molecular biology tools. A mutation leading to a stop codon at position 392 results in a dysfunctional toll-like receptor (TLR) 5 protein unable to recognize flagellin and is a risk factor for Legionella pneumophila infection in nonsmokers. Reduced interferon-γ release has been noted in patients who have recovered from LD. More recently it has been observed that treatment with a tumor necrosis antagonist can predispose to LD. It is interesting in light of the above information about the role of cell-mediated immunity in LD that patients with human immunodeficiency virus (HIV) infection who have a defect in cell-mediated

immunity are relatively infrequently infected with Legionella spp. However, when they do develop Legionella infection, these patients take longer to become afebrile, have more respiratory symptoms, and have a higher rate of respiratory failure as well as mortality when compared with patients with Legionella but without HIV infection.

As with most infectious diseases, outbreaks provide an opportunity to learn about the mechanisms of transmission of LD. In most instances, Legionella is transmitted to humans by inhalation of aerosols containing the bacteria. Outbreaks have been associated with exposure to a variety of aerosol-producing devices, including showers, a grocery store mist machine, cooling towers, whirlpool spas, decorative fountains, and evaporative condensers. It is also likely that aspiration of contaminated potable water by immunosuppressed patients is a mechanism whereby infection with Legionella is acquired. Microaspiration of pathogens from a colonized nasopharynx is the mechanism for most cases of pneumonia in humans. We have demonstrated Legionella in the nasopharynx of patients with LD, but there are no studies showing colonization of the nasopharynx before the onset of LD.

Legionellosis is believed to occur worldwide, but data are limited or nonexistent for many countries. It is likely that legionellosis is uncommon in areas without hot-water heaters and complex water distribution systems. However, even in these areas, aspiration of contaminated natural water, as, for example, following boating accidents, can result in LD. Legionnaire's disease has been found throughout North America, Europe, the United Kingdom, Argentina and Brazil in South America, Singapore, Thailand, and Australia. A few cases of LD have been reported from India.

PATHOGENESIS

Our knowledge of the pathogenesis of Legionella infections in humans is still incomplete. The alveolar macrophage is the target cell for Legionellae in the lower airways. Only virulent strains of Legionella are capable of initiating parasite-directed endocytosis. Following phagocytosis or endocytosis, there is abrogation of phagosome–lysosome fusion, which is essential for the intracellular growth of this microorganism. The replicative phagosome becomes associated with the endoplasmic reticulum.

Following a latent period of about 12 hours, the bacteria start dividing. During this latent period, there is synthesis of up to 35 proteins and repression of 32 proteins. Iron must be available in the phagosome for growth. Virulent *L. pneumophila* strains are sensitive to sodium chloride.

Once the replicative phagosome has been established, the bacteria begin to multiply with a doubling time of 2 hours. Heat shock protein 60 (Hsp 60) is a dominant protein during this intracellular phase, suggesting that it has an essential role in the viability of the microorganism. Several morphologic changes occur as the number of bacteria increase: They become shorter and accumulate intracytoplasmic membranes and vesicles.

It is likely that *Legionellae* behave differently while multiplying in macrophages than they do while multiplying in amebae, their natural hosts. Because airborne amebae have been found in water aerosols, this finding may have implications for LD in humans.

INFECTIOUS SYNDROMES

Pneumonia is the most common manifestation of infection with *Legionella* spp. It may occur in the community as sporadic cases or as outbreaks. In addition, *Legionella* is one of the agents of nosocomial pneumonia. The pneumonia may have a variety of extrapulmonary manifestations and in some cases is dominated by these extrapulmonary manifestations. Pontiac fever is a syndrome related to inhalation of *Legionella* spp. lipopolysaccharide.

In the Philadelphia outbreak, fever was present in 97% of the patients, malaise in 89%, cough in 86%, chills in 74%, dyspnea in 59%, myalgias in 55%, headache in 53%, chest pain in 52%, sputum production in 50%, and diarrhea in 41% at presentation. Sixty percent had a white blood cell count >10 000/mm^3, and 34% had bilateral pulmonary infiltrates on chest radiograph.

When patients with LD are compared with those with community-acquired pneumonia due to other agents, the patients with LD are more likely to have myalgias, headache, diarrhea, and a higher mean oral temperature at the time of presentation. They also present to hospital sooner after the onset of symptoms—4.7 days vs. 7.7 days (*P* = .02). When patients with LD were compared with patients with bacteremic pneumococcal pneumonia, the following features were associated with *Legionella* pneumonia: male sex odds ratio (OR) 4.6, 95% confidence interval (CI) 1.48–14.5; heavy alcohol consumption 4.8 (1.39–16.42); previous β-lactam therapy 19.9 (3.47–114.2); axillary

temperature >39°C 10.3 (2.71–38.84); myalgias 8.5 (2.35–30.74); gastrointestinal symptoms 3.5 (1.01–12.18). Negative associations included pleuritic chest pain, previous upper respiratory tract infection, and purulent sputum.

In a study comparing the radiographic features of LD, pneumococcal pneumonia, mycoplasma pneumonia, and psittacosis it was noted that radiographic deterioration following diagnosis was a particular feature of LD occurring in 30/46 (65%) compared with 14/27 (51%) patients with bacteremic pneumococcal pneumonia. About half the patients with LD have unilateral pneumonic involvement throughout the course of their illness. The lower lobes are involved most commonly, and pleural effusions are seen in about 35%. The severity of the radiographic findings correlated significantly with the presence of *L. pneumophila* in sputum by direct fluorescent antibody. Lung abscess, empyema, and bulging fissure sign are other radiographic features that are occasionally seen in patients with LD.

Relative bradycardia is seen in about two thirds of patients with LD. Most patients appear acutely ill. Crackles are generally present on auscultation of the chest. Many experts feel that LD cannot be distinguished from other causes of pneumonia on the basis of clinical features.

One of the remarkable things about LD is the range of extrapulmonary manifestations. Although they occur in about 30% of patients, they can dominate the clinical picture and determine the outcome.

There can be a variety of central nervous system manifestations. These include lethargy, confusion, delirium, stupor, coma, seizures, hallucinations, slurred speech, fine or coarse tremors, hyperactive reflexes, absence of deep tendon reflexes, and signs of cerebellar dysfunction, including nystagmus and gait disturbance. Peripheral neuropathy and cranial nerve palsies, including incontinence or urinary retention, are other manifestations. Myocarditis, pericarditis, and endocarditis have all been reported, albeit uncommonly, as extrapulmonary manifestations of LD. Acute renal failure, tubulointerstitial nephritis, tubular necrosis, and rapidly progressive glomerulonephritis are the renal manifestations in LD. Reactive arthritis and osteomyelitis are uncommon rheumatologic manifestations. Legionnaire's disease usually worsens during the first week even when therapy with erythromycin has been instituted.

The clinical course of LD with currently available treatments seems to be different now than what it was when erythromycin was the treatment of choice. This is exemplified by a study of 25 patients with LD who were treated with azithromycin. These patients were all diagnosed by using an assay for *Legionella* urinary antigen and thus early diagnosis (results are available in a few hours in contrast to several days for culture of the microorganism or weeks for a serological diagnosis) may have accounted for the very favorable outcomes. Twenty-two of twenty-three evaluable patients were cured. At the 10-day follow-up, 45% had signs and symptoms, whereas at the 4- to 6-week follow-up period 35% had signs and symptoms. It is also apparent that different strains of *Legionella* may vary in virulence. Thus in the Murcia, Spain, outbreak involving 800 suspect and definite cases the mortality was 1.1% for definite and 0.9% for suspect cases.

Pontiac Fever

In July 1968, an explosive epidemic of acute febrile illness occurred at a county health department facility in Pontiac, Michigan. This self-limiting illness of 2 to 5 days' duration, was characterized principally by fever, headache, myalgia, and malaise. It affected at least 144 persons, including 95 of 100 persons employed in the health department building. The mean incubation period was approximately 36 hours. Later it was shown that Pontiac fever was due to *L. pneumophila* endotoxin. There has been speculation that Pontiac fever is due to inhalation of a free-living ameba that is commonly present in environmental sites containing *Legionella*. Subsequently many outbreaks of Pontiac fever have occurred. It has been associated with exposure to *L. pneumophila* serogroups 1, 6, and 7; *L. feelei*; *L. micdadei*; and *L. anisa*. Most commonly, exposure to contaminated whirlpools, cleaning evaporative condensers, and water fountains has resulted in Pontiac fever. The pathogenesis is still incompletely understood, although some investigators feel it is exposure to *Legionella* endotoxin that results in the symptoms. In support of this is the finding of high concentrations of *Legionella* endotoxin in contaminated water associated with Pontiac fever. One hundred seventy people who had visited a hotel and leisure complex in Lochgoilhead, a village on the west coast of Scotland, became ill with headache, fever, arthralgia, myalgia, cough, and breathlessness. This illness was initially labeled Lochgoilhead fever but because *L. micdadei* was isolated from the whirlpool spa and 60 of 72 persons with symptoms seroconverted to *L. micdadei*, this

was really Pontiac fever. An outbreak of Pontiac fever and legionellosis at a hotel in Oklahoma from March 15 to March 21, 2004, is instructive because the sensitivity and specificity of the *Legionella* urinary antigen test was 35.7% and 100%, respectively, and for serology 46.4% and 90%. Because the urinary antigen test detects *L. pneumophila* serogroup 1 lipopolysaccharide (endotoxin) this outbreak adds to the evidence that *Legionella* endotoxin is the cause of Pontiac fever. In the Oklahoma outbreak, 3 of 101 (2.9%) persons with Pontiac fever were hospitalized.

Nosocomial Legionnaire's Disease

The clinical features of nosocomial LD are not different from those of nosocomial pneumonia due to any bacterium. Immunocompromised patients, especially those receiving corticosteroid therapy, are most susceptible to *Legionella* if it is contaminating the hospital water supply. Indeed, nosocomial LD is all about contamination of the hospital's potable water: if there is no *Legionella* in the potable water there are usually no cases of nosocomial LD. This has led to a debate about whether to conduct routine surveillance for *Legionella* in the potable water and if it is found to eradicate it. However, there are those who maintain that if you do not have a problem with nosocomial LD you should not do routine surveillance. This is somewhat of a chicken-and-egg story. Having battled nosocomial LD for many years my opinion is that all hospitals should do routine surveillance of their water for *Legionella*. If it is present, all cases of nosocomial pneumonia should be investigated for *Legionella* and, if found, measures to control or eradicate *Legionella* from the hospital water supply should be taken (Table 139.2). Immunocompromised patients should not drink the hospital water (if it is contaminated with *Legionella*) nor should they shower in it. Only sterile water should be used to flush nasogastric tubes. Occasionally unusual sources of nosocomial LD such as contaminated esophageal probes are found. The CDC have issued guidelines for the prevention of health care–associated pneumonia but have not made any firm recommendations on the measures outlined in Table 139.2 for eradication or control of *Legionella* in potable water.

DIAGNOSIS

A high index of suspicion is necessary for the diagnosis of sporadic cases of LD. Outbreaks of pneumonia usually trigger a work-up for *Legionella* so these are easier to diagnose.

Specific Organisms – Bacteria

Table 139.2 Control of *Legionella* in Hot Water Systems

1. Physical Measures

Maintain water temperature above 55°C
Ultraviolet irradiation
Sonication
Terminal tap water filters

2. Chemical Measures

Prevent scale formation in the pipes
Biocides: Sodium hypochlorite, ozone
Charcoal filters
Copper–silver ionization

3. Maintain Good Plumbing Practices

Dead spaces in calorifiers should be removed
Dead legs should be removed
Regular flushing of outlets
Pumps and calorifiers should be in series not in parallel

Isolation of the organism from respiratory secretions or other specimens is the definitive diagnostic test. Detection of *Legionella* antigen in urine by enzyme-linked immunosorbent assay is about 80% sensitive and >95% specific. This test is readily available for *L. pneumophila* serogroup 1. Diagnostic kits are also available for detection of antigens of *L. pneumophila* 1 to 6. *Legionella* antigen is excreted in the urine for days to weeks (rarely up to 1 year) after the onset of pneumonia. It should be noted that the antigen test positivity rate varies with the severity of the disease, being positive in 40% to 53% of mild cases and 88% to 100% of severe cases.

Demonstration of a 4-fold rise in antibody titer between acute and convalescent serum samples using an indirect immunofluorescence whole-cell assay can also be used to diagnose LD. Up to 12 weeks may be required to demonstrate a 4-fold rise in antibody, so serology is not useful for the acute management of this disease. A single or static titer of 1:256 or greater is no longer considered satisfactory for the diagnosis of LD. Polymerase chain reaction applied to respiratory secretions, pulmonary tissue, or pleural fluid is also useful.

TREATMENT (TABLE 139.3)

In the original outbreak of LD it was observed that those who were treated with the macrolide erythromycin had a lower mortality rate than individuals who were treated with other antibiotics. Subsequently a newer macrolide, azithromycin, was shown to have a bactericidal effect in the guinea pig alveolar macrophage model and it had a 5-day postantibacterial effect when it was removed from the system, whereas erythromycin in the same model was bacteriostatic and had no postantibacterial effect. These observations have been confirmed in clinical trials wherein 20 of 21 patients treated with azithromycin were cured.

It is noteworthy that because β-lactam antibiotics do not penetrate into cells they are ineffective in LD even though they show activity in vitro. Data from a prospective, nonrandomized study indicate that levofloxacin is superior to macrolides for the treatment of severe LD. In this study carried out in Murcia, Spain, 3.4% of the patients receiving levofloxacin had complications compared with 27.2% of those receiving macrolides; the levofloxacin patients had a shorter length of stay: 5.5 vs 11.3 days. Addition of rifampin to levofloxacin provided no additional benefit. In a study of 139 cases of *L. pneumophila* pneumonia from a prospective series of 1934 consecutive cases of community-acquired pneumonia the overall mortality rate was 5%. Eighty patients received initial therapy with a macrolide and 40 with levofloxacin. Patients who received levofloxacin had a shorter time to defervescence, 2 vs 4.5 days, and to clinical stability, 3 vs 5 days. The complication rates were the same in both groups at 25%. The case fatality rate for those treated with levofloxacin was 2.5% vs 5% for those treated with macrolides (*P* = .906). The median length of stay was 8 days for the levofloxacin-treated group and 10 days for those who received macrolides (*P* = .014). In a study of 33 patients admitted to an intensive care unit with LD, fluoroquinolone administration within 8 hours of intensive care unit arrival was associated with decreased mortality. This is not surprising in that there are now several studies showing that administration of antibiotics to elderly patients with community-acquired pneumonia within 4 to 8 hours of presentation to an emergency room is associated with lower mortality than administration of the first dose of an antibiotic at a later time.

In a recent study from Spain the authors compared monotherapy, 11 patients treated with clarithromycin, to combination therapy with clarithromycin and rifampin, 21 patients. All patients were cured; however, the patients who received rifampin had a 50% longer length of stay and a trend toward higher bilirubin levels.

Many factors should be considered when deciding on the duration of therapy. Immune status and severity of the infection are probably the two most important factors. In mild to moderate cases in immunocompetent subjects

Table 139.3 Antibiotic Treatment of Legionnaire's Disease

1. Fluoroquinolones
Levofloxacin, 750 mg IV (PO for mild cases) once daily
Moxifloxacin, 400 mg IV or PO once daily (only available PO in most countries)
Ciprofloxacin, 750 mg IV or PO q12h
2. Macrolides
Azithromycin, 1 g IV or PO, as a loading dose and then 500 mg IV or PO (due to the long half-life) of azithromycin; only 5 days necessary for treatment of mild cases; 7–10 days for more severe cases
Erythromycin, 1 g q6h IV; phlebitis is problematic at this dosage (unless infused through a central line); transient deafness, especially in patients who are receiving treatment with diuretics, also occurs at this dosage level
Clarithromycin, 500 mg q12h IV or PO (IV formulation not available in all countries)
3. Doxycycline, 200 mg loading dose, and then 100 mg q12h IV or PO
4. Rifampin, 300 to 600 mg q12h PO (IV formulation available in some countries). Rifampin should only be used in combination with a macrolide. There are no data supporting a synergistic role when it is used with other classes of antimicrobials.

Note. For cases of mild to moderately severe disease in immunocompetent patients treatment for 7 days is usually sufficient. For immunocompromised patients, treatment for 21 days or longer may be necessary. In these instances individual decisions are necessary and are based on the underlying process that requires the immunosuppression, degree of immunosuppression, and response to therapy. Close follow-up is necessary once treatment is discontinued as relapse is not infrequent.

with a rapid response to therapy, a duration of 10 days is sufficient. Indeed in this setting a 5-day course of azithromycin, given its long half-life, is probably sufficient. In patients with severe disease and or immunocompromised state a 3-week course of treatment with either fluroquinolones or macrolides (other than azithromycin) is necessary to avoid relapse. One should also remember that in some patients with legionellosis polymicrobial infection may be present.

Patients who are seriously ill with legionnaires disease require management in an ICU. In this setting (sepsis and septic shock) there is evidence that low-dose corticosteroid therapy is beneficial to those who are relatively adrenal insufficient (≤9 mcg/mL response in cortisol level to a dose of adrenocorticotrophic hormone.

SUGGESTED READING

England AC, Fraser DW, Plikaytis BD, Tsai TF, Storch G, Broome CV. Sporadic legionellosis in the US: the first 1000 cases. *Ann Intern Med.* 1981;94:164–170.

Fraser DW, Tsai TR, Orenstein W, et al. Legionnaires' disease – description of an epidemic of pneumonia. *N Engl J Med.* 1977;297:1189–1197.

Guidelines for preventing health-care-associated pneumonia. *Morbid Mortal Weekly Rep.* 2004;53(RR03):1–36.

Mykietiuk A, Carratalia J, Fenandez-Sabe N, et al. Clinical outcomes for hospitalized patients with *Legionella* pneumonia in the antigenuria era: the influence of levofloxacin therapy. *Clin Infect Dis.* 2005;40: 794–799.

Pedro-Botet L, Yu VL. Legionella: macrolide or quinolones? *Clin Microbiol Infect Dis.* 2006;12(suppl 3):30–35.

Yu VL, Plouffe JF, Pastoris MC, et al. Distribution of Legionella species and serogroups isolated by culture in patients with sporadic community-acquired legionellosis: an international collaborative survey. *J Infect Dis.* 2002;186:127–128.

Specific Organisms – Bacteria

140. Leprosy

Fiona Larsen, Arlo Upton, J. B. Stricker, and Clay J. Cockerell

EPIDEMIOLOGY

Leprosy is an ancient disease that has been the cause of great morbidity and mortality for centuries. The causative agent, *Mycobacterium leprae*, is an unculturable, obligate intracellular, gram-positive, acid-fast bacillus. It multiplies very slowly in the host and grows best at 33°C (91.4°F), which accounts for its predilection for cooler parts of the body such as the skin, testis, anterior segment of eye, mucous membranes of nasal passages, and ear lobes and extremities.

Leprosy is endemic in a number of regions, mainly in Asia, Africa, South America, and the Pacific. It is especially prevalent in India and Brazil. Isolated pockets of disease are found in many parts of the world, and as a consequence of international travel, affected individuals may be encountered in any location. In the United States, infected patients may be found in any state, but most are in California, Hawaii, Florida, Texas, and Louisiana. Most cases are seen in immigrants born in endemic regions.

Worldwide, the overall number of registered cases (prevalence) of leprosy has fallen as a result of multidrug therapy (MDT), but the number of newly registered cases (incidence) remains relatively constant, suggesting that current therapy strategies have not had an appreciable impact on transmission. The primary mechanism of transmission is thought to be via nasal inhalation of aerosolized organisms. *Mycobacterium leprae* cannot breach intact skin. Armadillos are known to harbor *M. leprae*, and a number of cases have been traced to exposure to these animals, although direct transmission of the organism to humans has not been definitively demonstrated. Polymerase chain reaction (PCR) studies indicate that nasal carriage of *M. leprae* can occur in persons without clinical evidence of infection and is transient. Serological studies suggest that most people in endemic areas have been exposed to the organism, resulting in development of mucosal immunity that prevents progressive infection. However, transmission of the organism is likely to occur during subclinical infection—which may explain the undiminished incidence of clinical disease. Very few exposed persons go on to develop clinical disease; the incubation period ranges from 9 months to 20 years. Risk factors for the development of clinically apparent leprosy include high bacterial index of index case and close (household) contact with, and genetic relatedness to, the index cases. Genetic studies have identified abnormalities in innate and acquired immunity, increasing our knowledge of the genetic predisposition of some individuals to the disease. A locus within the gene PARK2/PACRG located on chromosome 6q25–q27 has been associated with susceptibility to leprosy, but the exact mechanism by which it exerts this influence is unclear.

PATHOPHYSIOLOGY

The clinical disorder recognized as leprosy develops as a consequence of both the host's immune reaction to *M. leprae* as well as from direct effects of bacillary spread and multiplication. Those susceptible to infection demonstrate an impaired cell-mediated immune response to the organism. This is thought to result from a genetic predisposition because cases cluster in families, and there is a high concordance rate in identical twins.

Mycobacterium leprae has a tropism for nerves that are damaged as a consequence of immune response to intraneural bacilli as well as physical effects induced by proliferation of bacilli within nerves. As a result, many of the clinical manifestations are due to peripheral nerve damage with loss of motor and sensory function leading to ulcers, contractures, and loss of tissue substance. Other tissues, such as the skin, may harbor innumerable organisms in some forms of the disease, and deforming cutaneous nodules may develop. Immune response to organisms in skin lead to severe forms of vasculitis with extensive cutaneous necrosis.

CLASSIFICATION AND CLINICAL PRESENTATION

There may be a number of different clinical presentations in patients with leprosy, depending on the level of immunity and the duration of the disease. Individuals with the early indeterminate form present with one or more scaly hypopigmented anesthetic macules of the skin appearing initially on the face, although the limbs, trunk, or buttocks may be involved. If untreated, this may progress to any form of the disease. Others present only with sensorimotor neuropathy with enlargement of the peripheral nerves without skin lesions. Nerves affected most commonly include the ulnar and median nerves, often resulting in a claw hand deformity; the common peroneal nerve, leading to foot drop; the posterior tibial nerve, which results in claw toes and plantar insensitivity; and the facial, radial cutaneous, and great auricular nerves. Other areas of the body, such as the nasopharynx, eyes, and testicles, may also be involved.

Classically, patients present with symptoms that can range from one pole (tuberculoid) to another (lepromatous) or anywhere in between (borderline tuberculoid, borderline, or borderline lepromatous). Tuberculoid leprosy is the form with a small number of asymmetric skin lesions that are hypopigmented, have sharp borders, and are associated with anesthesia. Commonly, cutaneous nerves are enlarged and few bacilli are present on biopsy (paucibacillary form). Lepromatous leprosy presents as widely distributed symmetric skin lesions that can manifest as macules, papules, plaques, or nodules, which are red to brown (Figure 140.1). Often, it can also present as diffuse thickening of the skin with loss of underlying adnexa. Biopsy shows many bacilli (multibacillary form). Borderline cases may present anywhere between these two extremes.

A number of different schemes have been developed to clinically classify patients so that treatment can be tailored appropriately. The World Health Organization (WHO) clas-

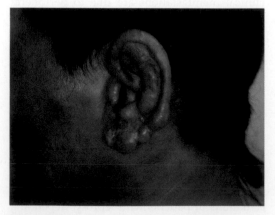

Figure 140.1 Lepromatous leprosy on the ear.

sification is the most commonly used system, although the Ridley–Jopling classification was the first to be developed and is based on clinical signs and symptoms. The WHO classification is based on the number of skin lesions and number of bacilli present in smears. Patients with five or fewer skin lesions without evidence of bacilli on skin smears are considered paucibacillary, whereas those with six or more skin lesions with or without bacilli on skin smears are considered to be multibacillary. The clinical forms in the Ridley–Jopling classification referred to as indeterminate, tuberculoid, and borderline tuberculoid correlate with paucibacillary disease, whereas those with borderline, borderline lepromatous, and polar lepromatous forms have multibacillary disease.

Leprosy in reaction refers to clinical disease produced when there is a change in the host's immune response to *M. leprae*. There are two forms of reactional leprosy. Type 1 reactions are induced by cell-mediated immunity and are referred to as *upgrading* and *downgrading* reactions. Upgrading reactions are characteristically seen in patients with borderline lepromatous disease who undergo a shift toward more tuberculoid (paucibacillary) forms. These may develop after induction of therapy. Downgrading reactions occur with transformation from a tuberculoid to a more lepromatous (multibacillary) form and often develop in the absence of treatment. Both may appear similar clinically and are manifest by erythema and edema of existing skin lesions associated with painful neuropathy and ulceration. Type 2 reactions are immune complex mediated and include erythema nodosum leprosum (ENL) and Lucio's phenomenon. Both of these are manifestations of immune complex–mediated vasculitis that lead to prominent inflammation and often ulceration with acute damage to nerves. Patients present with fever, multiple erythematous tender nodules, and varying degrees of neuritis, edema, arthralgias, leukocytosis, iridocyclitis, pretibial periostitis, orchitis, and nephritis.

Patients infected with human immunodeficiency virus (HIV) do not have an increased incidence of leprosy in regions where both diseases are endemic, unlike tuberculosis. Coinfection with *M. leprae* and HIV appears to have minimal effect on the course of either leprosy or HIV.

DIAGNOSIS

To make a diagnosis of leprosy, the disease must first be considered, particularly in anyone with

a history of travel to endemic areas, with unusual skin lesions or a sensorimotor neuropathy.
The diagnosis is primarily clinical and is based
on the presence of 1 of 3 cardinal findings: hypopigmented or reddish patches with definitive
loss of sensation, thickened peripheral nerves,
and demonstration of acid-fast bacilli.

Definitive diagnosis of *M. leprae* is sometimes
difficult, as the organism cannot be cultured
in vitro. The gold standard for the diagnosis
of leprosy is a skin biopsy specimen obtained
from the advancing edge of an active lesion
and detection of bacilli in tissue sections using
the Fite–Faraco staining method. The slit skin
smear has a high specificity but a low sensitivity (10%–50% of all leprosy patients are smear
negative). Therefore, its utility as an adjunctive
procedure to semiquantitate acid-fast organisms
in infected skin is useful for monitoring the response of patients during and after treatment.
No serological tests are available for routine
laboratory diagnosis of leprosy.

The major recent advance in the laboratory
diagnosis of leprosy is the development of PCR
assays that have reported specificity of 100%
and a sensitivity ranging from 34% to 80% in
patients with paucibacillary forms of the disease
to greater than 90% in patients with multibacillary forms of the disease.

TREATMENT

Treatment depends on whether the individual
has paucibacillary or multibacillary disease.
Virtually all patients are treated with MDT with
monthly supervision as first implemented by
the WHO in 1981 (Table 140.1), which has been
modified several times since then. Dapsone and
clofazimine are weakly bactericidal when used
alone, although they are mycobactericidal and
kill more than 99% of bacilli when used in combination. Rifampin is highly bactericidal alone.
No antileprosy drugs should be prescribed in
isolation because of the likelihood of developing resistance. Administration of antibiotics
renders the patient noninfectious in a matter
of weeks.

Paucibacillary patients (fewer than five lesions) receive a supervised dose of rifampin,
600 mg orally once per month for 3 months,
and a daily unsupervised dose of dapsone, 100
mg orally for 6 months. At the end of 6 months,
therapy is discontinued. Multibacillary patients
receive a supervised dose of rifampin, 600 mg
orally once monthly, a 300-mg dose of clofazimine, an unsupervised daily dose of dapsone,
100 mg orally, and a 50-mg daily oral dose of

Table 140.1 World Health Organization–Recommended Drug Therapy

	Paucibacillary	Multibacillary
Monthly, supervised	600 mg rifampin	600 mg rifampin and 300 mg clofazimine
Daily, unsupervised	100 mg dapsone	100 mg dapsone and 50 mg clofazimine
Duration of therapy	6 mo	12 mo
Follow-up	2 y	5 y

clofazimine for 12 months. Relapses should be
treated in the same manner as the initial disease, providing there is no drug resistance. The
WHO recommends that a single lesion should
be treated with a single oral dose combination of
rifampicin, 600 mg, ofloxacin, 400 mg, and minocycline, 100 mg. This regimen has demonstrated
similar bactericidal activity and relapse rates to
conventional treatment, but as long-term data
are not yet available it remains controversial.

All patients are evaluated monthly or more
frequently, depending on complications, for
at least 2 years for paucibacillary patients and
at least 5 years for multibacillary patients. Most
programs continue inspections for 5 to 10 years
in all patients. Relapse rates are approximately
1% in both paucibacillary and multibacillary
patients. The WHO recommends that all patients be instructed to recognize the signs and
symptoms of recurrent disease as well as adverse reactions to medications. It may take up
to 5 years for bacilli to be completely cleared in
patients with multibacillary disease. Although
many of the neurologic problems may be permanent, skin lesions usually disappear within
1 year of treatment, and reappearance of skin
lesions is highly suggestive of relapse.

Major drug side effects are relatively uncommon with present regimens. Clofazimine may
cause gastrointestinal symptoms and a purplish
skin discoloration, which clear with discontinuation of the drug. Dapsone often causes mild
anemia, although severe anemia may result in
patients with glucose-6-phosphate dehydrogenase deficiency, so all patients should be tested
for this enzyme before initiation of therapy.
Other side effects include agranulocytosis, cutaneous eruptions, peripheral neuropathy, gastrointestinal distress, and nephrotic syndrome.
It is of interest that, when given in combination

Leprosy

with rifampicin, dapsone is cleared from the plasma 7 to 10 times more quickly, although this has not been shown to affect clearance of bacilli. Rifampicin, in the doses advocated by the WHO, rarely causes adverse effects but may cause orange discoloration of the urine, stool, and other body fluids. Pregnant women have safely taken dapsone and clofazimine, but experience with rifampicin is limited.

TREATMENT OF REVERSAL REACTIONS

Reversal reactions occur in up to 25% of patients, usually during therapy. Early diagnosis and prompt treatment of reversal reactions is of great importance to prevent many of the deforming complications of leprosy (Table 140.2).

Mild reactions can be treated symptomatically; however, severe type 1 reactions with neuritis or silent neuropathy require prompt initiation of systemic glucocorticoid therapy, starting at a minimum dose of 40 to 60 mg of prednisolone, tapering once the reaction is controlled. In patients with nerve damage from reactional leprosy that is present for 3 to 6 months, the response to therapy is less than 67%. When present for longer than 6 months, the response to therapy is even poorer.

Mild to moderate type 2 reactions can be treated with nonsteroidal anti-inflammatory drugs and other symptomatic modalities. Severe ENL or the presence of neuritis requires prednisolone (as prescribed in type 1 reactions). Clofazimine is useful for chronic reactions, and its use has been credited with the overall decrease of ENL in leprosy. Patients are given 300 mg/day orally until lesions begin to resolve, following which the dose is tapered slowly to 100 mg over 12 months. Thalidomide, 300 to 400 mg orally, will supress ENL within 48 hours and is considered the drug of choice for young men with severe ENL. Its high teratogenic potential has prevented its widespread

Table 140.2 Recommended Treatment of Reversal Reactions

	Type I Reaction	Erythema Nodosum Leprosum
Mild	Symptomatic	NSAIDs, symptomatic
Severe	40–60 mg prednisolone	40–60 mg prednisolone or 300 mg clofazimine (chronic) or 300–400 mg thalidomide
Duration	Slowly taper as tolerated	Slowly taper prednisolone as tolerated Taper clofazimine to 100 mg in 12 months Taper thalidomide as tolerated to 100 mg, discontinue as soon as indicated

Note. All patients should receive prednisolone in the presence of neuritis.
Abbreviation: NSAIDs = nonsteroidal anti-inflammatory drugs.

use. Azathioprine and methotrexate may be useful when the type 2 reaction is not able to be controlled by steriods alone and may have a steroid sparing effect. Cyclosporin has been used to treat type 2 reactions; results have been mixed. More controlled studies are needed to evaluate efficacy of these medications.

SUGGESTED READING

Britton WJ, Lockwood DN. Leprosy. *Lancet.* 2004;363:1209–1219.

Moschella SL. An update on the diagnosis and treatment of leprosy. *J Am Acad Dermatol.* 2004;51:417–426.

Scollard DM, Adams LB, Gillis TP, et al. The continuing challenges of leprosy. *Clin Microbiol Rev.* 2006;19(2):338–381.

WHO Study Group. *Chemotherapy of Leprosy.* Geneva, Switzerland: World Health Organization; 1994.

141. Meningococcus and Miscellaneous Neisseriae

Edmund C. Tramont and Charles Davis

MENINGOCOCCAL INFECTION

Meningococcal infection, first recognized nearly 2 centuries ago as epidemic cerebrospinal fever, occurs worldwide as sporadic, endemic, and epidemic cases. Worldwide, most cases are caused by serogroups A and C, whereas in the United States, serogroups B and Y predominate (see "Culture and Laboratory Findings"). Humans are the only natural host for the bacteria. Transmission of the organism occurs from person to person by direct contact with contaminated respiratory secretions or airborne droplets with subsequent colonization of the nasopharynx. Nasopharyngeal carriage approximates 5% to 15% in nonepidemic periods but may approach 50% to 95% during epidemics, especially serogroup A epidemics. The carriage rate is also increased when there is crowding, such as in military barracks, dormitories, prisons, convocations, and sporting events. The oropharyngeal and nasopharyngeal carriage may persist for several weeks to several months. Sexual transmission of meningococci in women and homosexual men may result in anogenital carriage. Most cases of disease (eg, bacteremia, meningitis) occur in children between 6 months and 5 years of age. With few exceptions, invasive meningococci have a polysaccharide capsule that forms the basis for serogrouping of strains. Invasive disease occurs almost exclusively in persons who lack specific antimeningococcal antibody to the colonizing meningococcal strain. Individuals with complement component deficiencies are at an increased risk for developing invasive meningococcal infections because their serum loses the ability of complement-antibody mediated lysis of the bacteria. Hence, complement deficiency should be considered in persons with recurrent episodes of invasive meningococcal infection. Asplenic individuals are also at increased risk for acquiring invasive meningococcal disease because of decreased efficiency of clearing the encapsulated invading microorganisms. On rare occasions, persons may develop serum immunoglobulin A (IgA) antibodies that block the bactericidal action of immunoglobulin G (IgG) and immunoglobulin M (IgM) antibodies or possess genetic upper airway surfactant protein mutations resulting in an impaired local first line innate immune defense.

Clinical Features

As with most other invasive gram-negative bacteria, the clinical consequences of meningococcal infection are primarily the result of meningococcal endotoxin (lipopolysaccharide) release and subsequent activation of the procoagulation, anticoagulation, fibrinolysis, complement, and kallikrein–kinin cascades together with the release of various inflammatory mediators ("cytokine storm"). The clinical manifestation of meningococcal infection ranges from a mild transient bacteremia to fulminate meningococcemia, also referred to as Waterhouse–Friderichsen syndrome or purpura fulminans (Figure 141.1), with or without meningitis. Unless treated early, the mortality rate of the latter is high. Most commonly, *Neisseria meningitidis* acquisition results in asymptomatic colonization of the nasopharynx. The mildest form of invasive disease, a transient bacteremia, begins insidiously with fever, malaise, and symptoms of an upper respiratory tract infection. A few petechial skin lesions may appear, but neither signs nor symptoms of sepsis or meningitis develop. Symptoms usually resolve spontaneously within 24 to 48 hours. Acute meningococcemia, which often follows a few to several days of upper respiratory tract symptoms, is heralded by fever, chills, malaise, weakness, headache, myalgias, and nausea and/or vomiting. Skin manifestations, especially a petechial rash (Figure 141.2), raise the index of suspicion for meningococcal infection. They commonly appear in crops on the ankles, wrists, axilla, trunk, and mucous membranes, whereas the palms, soles, neck, and face are usually spared. The rash may also be urticarial, maculopapular, ecchymotic, or gangrenous depending on the degree of vascular pathology. In severe meningococcal disease,

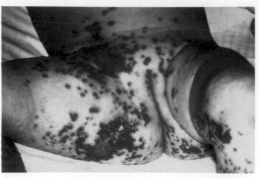

Figure 141.1 Purpura fulminans (Waterhouse–Friderichsen syndrome or severe ecchymotic rash).

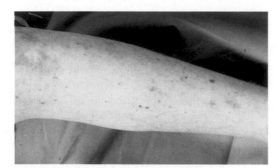

Figure 141.2 Petechiae lower extremity, meningococcemia.

Table 141.1 Differential Diagnosis of Rash and Meningitis

Neisseria meningitidis
Haemophilus influenzae type b
Streptococcus pneumoniae
Rickettsiae, especially Rocky Mountain spotted fever
Viruses, especially echovirus and coxsackie virus

Infections that May Be Associated with Petechial Rashes
 Bacterial
    N. meningitidis
    H. influenzae type b
    N. gonorrhea
    S. pneumoniae
    S. pyogenes
    E. coli
    Klebsiella species
    Pseudomonas species
    Streptobacillus moniliformis (rat-bite fever)

Viral
    Enteroviruses
    Rubella
    Atypical measles
    Epstein–Barr virus
    Cytomegalovirus, congenital
    Colorado tick fever
    Arboviruses
    Rickettsial
    Rickettsia rickettsii (RMSF)
    Rickettsia prowazekii (epidemic typhus)

Spirochetes   Leptospirosis
Parasites   *Plasmodium falciparum*
Endocarditis
Disseminated intravascular coagulopathy associated with septicemia

the rash rarely fails to develop (Table 141.1). Fulminate meningococcemia complicates acute meningococcemia in 5% to 15% of cases and is associated with the rash progressing into massive skin and mucosal hemorrhage, disseminated intravascular coagulopathy (DIC), and vascular collapse. Adrenal hemorrhage may occur despite appropriate therapy.

Meningitis may occur with or without any manifestations of meningococcemia. Clinically, meningococcal meningitis resembles acute meningitis of any cause, presenting with fever, headache, altered sensorium, and nuchal rigidity.

On rare occasions, a chronic meningococcemia develops. This is characterized by intermittent febrile episodes, lasting 2 to 10 or more days, accompanied by a variety of skin lesions (macular, maculopapular, petechial, ecchymotic, or pustular), arthralgias or arthritis, myalgias, and splenomegaly. The infection may last for months and can be fatal, but it usually resolves spontaneously.

Occasionally, *N. meningitidis* may produce oropharyngitis, sinusitis, pneumonia, conjunctivitis, endophthalmitis, proctitis, urethritis, cervicitis, immune-mediated

arthritis, endocarditis, myocarditis, pericarditis, and pelvic inflammatory disease (PID). Except in advanced cases, the response to appropriate antibiotic treatment is dramatic.

Culture and Laboratory Findings

Neisseria meningitidis is an aerobic, oxidase-positive, gram-negative diplococcus that grows best at 35°C to 37°C (95°F to 98.6°F) in a moist environment of 5% to 7% carbon dioxide, typically a candle jar. Oxidative metabolism of glucose and maltose but not sucrose, lactose, or fructose is the principle means in the laboratory for differentiating *N. meningitidis* from other *Neisseria* species. The organism is surrounded by a polysaccharide capsule that provides the basis for serogrouping. The meningococcus has been classified as serogroups A, B, C, D, 29E, H, I, J, K, L, W-135, X, Y, Z, and nontypable (indicates organism is noncapsulated). Serogroups A, B, C, W-135, and Y are responsible for the vast majority of cases of invasive disease. With rare exceptions, invasive meningococci are encapsulated, attesting to the virulence conveyed by the polysaccharide capsule. In contrast, meningococci colonizing mucous membranes are usually not encapsulated.

When possible, specimens should be cultured for *N. meningitidis* before antibiotic therapy is instituted. For culture of a normally sterile site, such as blood or cerebrospinal fluid (CSF), nonselective culture agar is preferred. A selective antibiotic containing culture media, such as Thayer–Martin, Martin–Lewis, or New York City culture medium, is necessary when the culture specimen is obtained from a nonsterile site, such as the oropharynx or urethra. If petechial or hemorrhagic lesions are present, meningococci may be demonstrated in up to 70% of cases on Gram staining, fluorescent staining, acridine orange staining, or methylene blue staining of tissue fluid extracted from these lesions. Organisms may also be demonstrated in the buffy coat of peripheral blood, typically when there are $\geq 10^5$ organisms/mL.

In patients with meningitis, the CSF is generally cloudy with a leukocytosis consisting predominantly of polymorphonuclear neutrophils associated with hypoglycorrhachia. The Gram stain of the CSF is positive in about 75% of cases (Figure 141.3). The CSF and blood are the most common sources of positive cultures. Rapid identification of *N. meningitides* capsular polysaccharide in CSF, serum, and urine by latex particle agglutination (LPA) is also available, but its sensitivity in the CSF is no better than that of a Gram stain. As with any laboratory test, a negative Gram stain or LPA does not rule out the diagnosis. LPA specificity may be hampered by the potential cross-reactivity of the group B test antiserum with the K1 antigen of *Escherichia coli*, an organism that has a predilection for causing meningitis in neonates. In contrast, the polymerase chain reaction (PCR) test is very sensitive and specific and it can also be used to rapidly serogroup strains. The PCR and LPA tests are particularly useful to establish the diagnosis in patients who have received prior antibiotics.

Therapy

Penicillin G remains the drug of choice for all forms of meningococcal disease. Penicillin G therapy should be administered intravenously (IV), at least initially. Adults should receive 300 000 U/kg IV daily divided every 4 hours. Infants should receive 250 000 U/kg/day IV in divided doses every 4 hours.

However, initial antimicrobial therapy is usually given empirically based on the clinical presentation, which is indistinguishable from that due to other bacteria, such as *Streptococcus pneumoniae, Staphylococcus aureus, Hemophilus influenzae,* and other gram-negative organisms. Thus, without a specific diagnosis, initial empirical therapy should be with a broad-spectrum cephalosporin antibiotic, especially ceftriaxone, but also cefuroxime, cefotaxime, and ceftazidime or ampicillin plus an aminoglycoside, such as gentamicin, netilmycin, or amikacin. However, the existence of ampicillin-resistant and penicillin-resistant strains of meningococcus is well documented and, over time, an increased prevalence is anticipated. Chloramphenicol is primarily of historical importance but it remains an effective substitute in patients allergic to other antibiotics. The dosage is 100 mg/kg/day in divided doses every 6 hours up to 4 g/day. Even though sulfonamides have been used with success in the past, they should not be used empirically because of unpredictable susceptibility of the organism (Table 141.2).

Seven to ten days of therapy is sufficient, with the antibiotic being given intravenously for at least the first 4 days. Supportive care is extremely important. Potential complications such as volume depletion, acidosis, hypoxemia, and adrenal insufficiency should be anticipated and

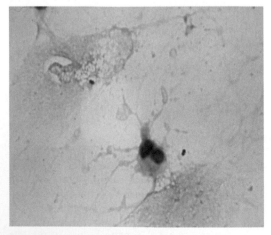

Figure 141.3 Meningococcal meningitis, Gram stain of CSF. Note gram-negative diplococci and polymorphonuclear leukocyte.

Table 141.2 Treatment of Meningococcal Meningitis

Antibiotic	Intravenous Dosage	Comment
Penicillin G	Adults: 300 000 U/kg/day divided q4h Children: 250 000 U/kg/day divided q4h	Remains drug of choice; exceeds usual MIC with meningeal inflammation; relatively resistant strains reported
Ampicillin	Adults: 12 g qd divided q4h Children: 50–75 mg/kg q6h	As effective as penicillin; exceeds MIC with meningeal inflammation; relatively resistant strains reported
Ciprofloxacin	Adults: 400–600 mg q12h Children: 10–15 mg/kg q12h	Appropriate spectrum and pharmacokinetics; few studies in children
Ceftriaxone	Adults: 1g q12h Children: 80–150 mg/kg/d divided q12h or qd	Good CNS penetration; exceeds usual MIC
Cefotaxime	Adults: 8–12g/d divided q4h Children: 200 mg/kg/d divided q6–8h	Exceeds usual MIC with meningeal inflammation
Ceftazidime	Adults: 1–2 g q8–12h Children: 125–150 mg/kg/d divided q8h	Exceeds usual MIC with meningeal inflammation
Chloramphenicol	Adults: 25 mg/kg q6h (maximum 4g/d) Children: 25 mg/kg q6h	Concentrates in CSF; because of potential to cause irreversible aplastic anemia (1:10 000 to 1:40 000); it is rarely used in the United States but is used more frequently in underdeveloped countries

Abbreviations: MIC = minimal inhibitory concentration; CNS = central nervous system; CSF = cerebrospinal fluid.
Note. In all instances treatment should extend 7 to 10 days.

managed appropriately. Long-term sequelae include hearing loss, other cranial palsies, and mental retardation. Adjunctive steroid therapy is indicated when acute adrenal insufficiency is a possibility, especially when the patient has progressed into the Waterhouse–Friderichsen syndrome or is obtunded. Dexamethasone, 0.15 mg/kg every 6 hours in infants and 8 to 12 mg every 12 hours in children and adults, is recommended. Some clinicians also use short-term steroids (1–3 days) in patients with meningitis. The management of DIC may also be prudent even though the use of heparin in such cases remains controversial. Immunoglobulin therapy with high titers of antibody to core antigen and/or to tumor necrosis factor have been of little benefit.

Prevention

ANTIMICROBIAL CHEMOPROPHYLAXIS

Most cases of *N. meningitidis* are sporadic. However, person to-person transmission has been a source of "household" or "close contact" outbreaks. *Neisseria meningitidis* is harbored in the nasopharynx of patients and as a commensal in asymptomatic carriers. The organism is spread through direct contact, especially respiratory droplets. The risk of contracting a symptomatic *N. meningitidis* infection is ap-

proximately 4 cases per 1000 among persons who have had "close contact" with a known carrier or patient with a virulent strain. Close contacts are defined as persons living in the same household, dormitory, or barracks; attending a day care center; handling clinical specimens or cultures; or anyone who has spent >4 hours with the index case 0 to 7 days prior to the onset of illness to cover the 1- to 10-day incubation period, for example, airline passengers, cruise shipmates, and nursing home residents and workers (Table 141.3).

This risk of developing secondary invasive disease after exposure to a close contact is greatly diminished by chemoprophylaxis: administering prophylactic antibiotics to individuals who have had close contact to an index case. Rifampin is considered the drug of choice for chemoprophylaxis even though rifampin-resistant strains have emerged. Rifampin, 600 mg orally every 12 hours for 4 doses for adults or 10 mg/kg every 12 hours for 4 doses for children, eradicates meningococci for 75% to 98% of carriers (Table 141.4). Effective alternatives include ceftriaxone, ciprofloxacin, ofloxacin, azithromycin, minocycline, and spectinomycin. A single intramuscular injection of ceftriaxone, 250 mg in adults and 125 mg in children, is 97% effective in eradicating the carrier state as well as being effective

Table 141.3 Considered Close Contact of an Index Case

All household members
Day-care and preschool classmates, attendees, and workers
Health care workers with contact with oral and/or respiratory secretions from the index case
Workers and classmates in boarding schools or camps
Workers and classmates if two or more cases occur in a 6-month period
The index case, if treated with penicillin or chloramphenicol
Living in a common military barrack
Sharing an aircraft cabin, especially if sitting next to the index case
Cruise shipmates with >4 hours contact with the index case
Laboratory workers handling culture from an index case

for treating meningitis. Ciprofloxacin, 500 mg as a single dose, has an efficacy rate of 89% to 97%; however, its use is contraindicated in pregnancy, and it is not licensed in the United States for use in children younger than 18 years. However, studies involving children younger than 12 years have found the drug to be highly efficacious and without any untoward sequelae. A single dose of ofloxacin, 400 mg, was found to be 97% effective in eradicating carriage; however, it has the same limitations as ciprofloxacin. A single 500-mg dose of azithromycin had a 93% efficacy rate at eradicating meningococcal carriage. Minocycline is effective, given at a dosage of 100 mg twice a day for 5 days, but an unacceptable incidence of vestibular side effects precludes its routine use. Spectinomycin (Spiramycin) is the primary prophylactic agent in many European countries, given at a dosage of 500 mg orally 4 times a day for 5 days to adults and 10 mg/kg orally 4 times a day for 5 days in children. Unfortunately, sulfonamide resistance is too highly prevalent and should be used only if the isolate from the index case is known to be sensitive. One must be aware that chemoprophylaxis with penicillin prevents invasive disease but does not predictably eradicate the carrier state and therefore transmission (Table 141.4).

VACCINE IMMUNOPROPHYLAXIS

Except for serogroup B, immunity to invasive meningococcal disease is correlated directly with naturally acquired bactericidal antibodies induced principally by the capsular polysaccharide (natural immunity develops in most individuals by age 5 years as a consequence of asymptomatic nasopharyngeal or gastrointestinal carriage of other cross-reacting microbial species). Hence, group-specific meningococcal polysaccharide vaccines have been developed. There are two U.S. Food and Drug Administration (FDA)-licensed meningococcal vaccines consisting of a mixture of purified high-molecular-weight capsular polysaccharides from serogroups A, C, Y, and W-135. The oldest (Menimmune or MPSV4), licensed in the early 1970s, consists only of the high-molecular-weight polysaccharides, whereas the newest (Menactra or MCV4), licensed in 2005, is conjugated with 48 µg of diphtheria toxoid.

The oldest polysaccharide tetravalent vaccine has virtually eliminated meningococcal disease caused by these serogroups in U.S. military recruits. The duration of immunity induced is not precisely known but it is estimated to be 2 to 3 years. Because this lack of induced long-lasting immunity is problematic and because this vaccine is poorly immunogenic in children younger than 2 years, the newer conjugated vaccine was developed. In older children and young adults, it elicits an initial antibody response that is similar to the polysaccharide-alone vaccine but it is more immunogenic in young children (≤4 years) and based on the results with other polysaccharide conjugate vaccines, the response is likely more durable. In fact, the effect in the United Kingdom with a conjugated serogroup C vaccine in children 1 to 17 years of age has been dramatic. Thus, childhood vaccination should be considered. It is likely that this vaccine will eventually replace the original nonconjugated vaccine. Unfortunately, there is as yet no vaccine to prevent serogroup B disease, a major cause of sporadic cases.

Vaccine immunoprophylaxis cannot be relied on to prevent meningococcal disease after exposure to an index case because of the 4- to 10-day lag time to develop antibodies. Therefore, it is recommended primarily for high-risk groups with an increased chance of future exposure, such as persons moving into a dormitory or military barracks, and high-risk individuals with an increased chance of developing invasive disease, such as persons with terminal complement component deficiencies and those who have anatomic or functional asplenia. Immunization is also recommended for travelers to areas in which *N. meningitidis* is hyperendemic (Nepal, India [New Delhi]),

Table 141.4 Antibiotics Used for Chemoprophylaxis of *Neisseria meningitides*

Antibiotic/Comment	Efficacy at Eradicating Nasopharyngeal Carriage	Dosage
Rifampin Drug of choice Safety in pregnancy not demonstrated Body fluid discoloration May render birth control pills ineffective	75%–98%	Adults: 600 mg PO q12h × 4 doses Children ≥1 mo: 10 mg/kg PO q12h × 4 doses Children ≤1 mo: 5mg/kg PO q12h × 4 doses
Ceftriaxone Can be given to young children and pregnant women	92%–97%	Adults: 250 mg IM × 1 dose Children ≤15: 125 mg IM × 1 dose
Ciprofloxacin Safety in pregnancy not established Not licensed in children under 18 years	89%–97%	Adults: 500 mg PO × 1 dose
Ofloxacin Same as for ciprofloxacin	97%	Adults: 400 mg PO × 1 dose Children: 200 mg PO × 1 dose
Spiramycin	90%–95%	Adults: 500 mg PO QID × 5 days Children: 10mg/kg PO QID × 5 days
Minocycline Proved effective but vestibular toxicity Not to be used in pregnant or lactating women	90%–95%	Adults: 100 mg PO q12h × 5 days Children: 1 mg/kg PO q12h × 5 days
Sulfadiazine Excellent CNS penetration Cannot be given to persons with G6PD deficiency Resistance limits its usefulness*	95%	Adults: 1g PO q8h × 3 days Children: 1g PO q12h × 3 days
Azithromycin	93%	Adults: 500 mg PO × 1 dose

Abbreviations: CNS = central nervous system; G6PD, glucose-6-phosphate dehydrogenase.
Note. Sulfadiazine sensitive = ≤0.1 mg/100 mL.

and the sub-Saharan Africa "meningitis belt," which stretches from Senegal in the west to Ethiopia in the east, particularly if their stay is prolonged.

As with the other polysaccharide-based vaccines, *Haemophilus influenzae* and *Streptococcus pneumoniae,* the concern that vaccination with these four serogroup vaccines would lead to replacement by other serogroups has not materialized.

INFECTIONS WITH OTHER *NEISSERIA* SPECIES

The nonpathogenic *Neisseria* species (*Neisseria lactamica, Neisseria sicca, Neisseria subflava, Neisseria mucosa, Neisseria flavescens, Neisseria cinerea, Neisseria kochii, Neisseria elongata,* and *Neisseria polysaccharea*) are usually commensals of the oropharynx and nasopharynx. Infections

caused by these organisms are extremely rare, occurring primarily in immunosuppressed hosts, especially those who are hypogammaglobulinemic or have defective antibody production (ie, chronic lymphocytic leukemia). The relative lack of virulence of these organisms is attributed to the lack of encapsulation, and hence they have no predilection to resist bacterial lysis by nonspecific components of the blood or to invade the meninges. Thus they are easily controlled by normal innate host defense mechanisms.

Because these organisms normally reside in the oropharynx, local extension of infection is most commonly to the ear, sinuses, and lung. Conjunctivitis, meningitis, endophthalmitis, endocarditis, and urethritis have also been reported, attesting to the common tissue tropism that these sites share with the nasoharynx. These nonpathogenic *Neisseria* are easily treated with penicillin, cephalosporins, or quinolone antibiotics.

SUGGESTED READING

Apicella MA. Neisseria meningitidis. In: Mandell GL, Bennet JE, Dolin R, eds. *Principles and Practice of Infectious Diseases*. New York, NY: Elsevier, Churchill, Livingstone; 2005.

Gardner Pearce. Prevention of meningococcal disease. *N Engl J Med*. 2006;355:1466–1473.

Prevention and control of meningococcal disease: recommendations of the Advisory Committee on Immunization Practices (ACIP). *MMWR Recomm Rep*. 2005;54:1–21.

142. *Listeria*

Bennett Lorber

INTRODUCTION

Listeria monocytogenes is an infrequent cause of illness in the general population, but, in certain groups, including neonates, pregnant women, elderly persons, and those with impaired cell-mediated immunity, whether due to underlying disease or immunosuppressive therapy, it is an important cause of life-threatening bacteremia and meningoencephalitis. Increasing interest in this organism has arisen from concerns about food safety following foodborne epidemics. Separate from its clinical relevance, the study of this bacterium has provided insights into bacterial pathogenesis and the role of cell-mediated immunity in resistance to intracellular pathogens.

MICROBIOLOGY

Listeria monocytogenes is a small, facultatively anaerobic, nonsporulating, catalase-positive, oxidase-negative, gram-positive rod that grows readily on blood agar, producing incomplete β-hemolysis. It possesses polar flagellae and exhibits a characteristic tumbling motility at room temperature (25°C). Optimal growth occurs at 30°C to 37°C, but, unlike most bacteria, *L. monocytogenes* also grows well at refrigerator temperature (4°C to 10°C), and, by so-called cold enrichment, it can be separated from other contaminating bacteria by long incubation in this temperature range. Selective media are available to isolate the organism from specimens containing multiple species (food, stool) and are superior to cold enrichment.

In clinical specimens, the organisms may be gram variable and may look like diphtheroids, cocci, or diplococci. Routine growth media are effective for growing *L. monocytogenes* from normally sterile specimens (cerebrospinal fluid [CSF], blood, joint fluid), but media typically used to isolate diarrhea-causing bacteria from stool cultures inhibit listerial growth. Laboratory misidentification as diphtheroids, streptococci, or enterococci occurs all too often, and the isolation of a "diphtheroid" from blood or CSF

should always alert one to the possibility that the organism is really *L. monocytogenes*.

Six listerial species are recognized (*Listeria monocytogenes, Listeria seeligeri, Listeria welshimeri, Listeria innocua, Listeria ivanovii,* and *Listeria grayi*), but only *L. monocytogenes* is pathogenic for humans. There are at least 13 serotypes of *L. monocytogenes*, based on cellular O and flagellar H antigens, but almost all disease is due to types 4b, 1/2a, and 1/2b, limiting the utility of serotyping for epidemiological investigations. A number of newer molecular techniques, including pulsed-field gel electrophoresis, ribotyping, and multilocus enzyme electrophoresis, have been employed to separate isolates into distinct groups and have proved useful for investigating epidemics.

EPIDEMIOLOGY

Listeria monocytogenes is an important cause of zoonoses, especially in herd animals. It is widespread in nature, being found commonly in soil and decaying vegetation and as part of the fecal flora of many mammals. The organism has been isolated from the stool of approximately 5% of healthy adults with higher rates of recovery reported from household contacts of patients with clinical infection. Many foods are contaminated with *L. monocytogenes*, and recovery rates of 15% to 70% or more are common from raw vegetables, raw milk, fish, poultry, and meats, including fresh or processed chicken and beef available at supermarkets or deli counters. Ingestion of *L. monocytogenes* must be a very common occurrence.

Two active surveillance studies performed between 1980 and 1986 by the Centers for Disease Control and Prevention (CDC) indicated annual infection rates of 7.4 per 1 million population, accounting for approximately 1850 cases a year in the United States, with 425 deaths. By 1993, after the institution of food industry regulations designed to minimize the risk of foodborne listeriosis, the annual incidence had declined to 4.4 cases per million, or 1092 cases, with 248 deaths. A similar decline in incidence of human listeriosis was seen in France following control measures to decrease food contamination. Following more recent risk assessment for *L. monocytogenes* in deli meats, regulatory and industry changes have been designed to prevent future contamination of ready-to-eat meat and poultry.

The highest infection rates are seen in infants ≤1 month and in adults >60 years of age. Pregnant women account for about 30% of all cases and 60% of cases in the 10- to 40-year age group. Almost 70% of nonperinatal infections occur in those with hematologic malignancy, acquired immunodeficiency syndrome (AIDS), bone marrow or solid organ transplants, or in those receiving corticosteroid therapy, but seemingly healthy persons may develop invasive disease, particularly those older than 60 years.

Subsequent to the 1983 report of an outbreak of foodborne human listeriosis due to contaminated coleslaw, a number of other foodborne outbreaks resulting in invasive disease (eg, bacteremia, meningitis) have been documented, with vehicles including milk, soft cheeses, butter, as well as smoked trout, ready-to-eat pork products, hot dogs, and deli-ready turkey. A 2002 outbreak due to contaminated turkey deli meat involved 54 patients in 9 states and resulted in the recall of more than 30 million pounds of food products, one of the largest meat recalls in U.S. history. Sporadic cases have been traced to contaminated cheese, turkey franks, and alfalfa tablets. The importance of food as a source of sporadic listeriosis was illuminated by two CDC studies in which 11% of all refrigerator food samples were contaminated, 64% of patients had at least one contaminated food, and, in 33% of instances, the patient and food isolates had identical strains. Delicatessen-style ready-to-eat meats, especially chicken, had the highest rates of contamination. Cases were more likely than were controls to have eaten soft cheeses or deli-counter meats, and 32% of sporadic cases could be attributed to these foods.

Human listeriosis is typically acquired through ingestion of contaminated food, but other modes of transmission occur. These include transmission from mother to child transplacentally or through an infected birth canal and cross-infection in neonatal nurseries. Contaminated mineral oil used for bathing infants was the source of one outbreak. Localized cutaneous infections have occurred in veterinarians and farmers after direct contact with aborted calves and infected poultry.

The CDC has established PulseNet (http://www.cdc.gov/pulsenet/), a network of public health and food regulatory laboratories that use pulsed-field gel electrophoresis to subtype foodborne pathogens to promptly detect disease clusters that may have a common source. This system has proved effective in the early detection of listeriosis outbreaks.

PATHOGENESIS

Except for vertical transmission from mother to fetus and rare instances of cross-contamination in the delivery suite or neonatal nursery, human-to-human infection has not been documented.

Infection most often begins after ingestion of contaminated food. The oral inoculum required to produce clinical infection is unknown; experiments in healthy mammals indicate that $\geq 10^9$ organisms are required. Alkalinization of the stomach by antacids, H_2 blockers, proton pump inhibitors, or ulcer surgery may promote infection. The incubation period for invasive infection is not well established, but evidence from a few cases related to specific ingestions points to a mean incubation period of ~30 days, with a range from 11 to 70 days. In one report, two pregnant women, whose only common exposure was attendance at a party, developed listerial bacteremia with the same uncommon enzyme type; incubation periods for illness were 19 and 23 days.

Listeria monocytogenes can cause disease without promoter organisms, but, on occasion, intercurrent gastrointestinal infection with another pathogen may enhance invasion in individuals colonized with *L. monocytogenes*. Evidence for this is found in the common history of antecedent gastrointestinal symptoms in patients and household contacts, the long incubation period from ingestion to clinical illness, and two instances in which clinical listeriosis closely followed shigellosis. Both listerial meningitis and bacteremia have occurred shortly after colonoscopy or sigmoidoscopy.

In the intestine, *L. monocytogenes* crosses the mucosal barrier aided by active endocytosis of organisms by endothelial cells. Once in the bloodstream, hematogenous dissemination may occur to any site; *L. monocytogenes* has a particular predilection for the central nervous system (CNS) and the placenta. It is generally believed that listeriae reach the CNS by a bacteremic route, but animal experiments suggest that brainstem infection may develop by intraaxonal spread of bacteria from peripheral sites to the CNS.

Several virulence factors have been identified that enable *L. monocytogenes* to function as an intracellular organism. The bacterium possesses the cell surface protein internalin, which interacts with E-cadherin, a receptor on macrophages and intestinal lining cells, to induce its own ingestion. A membrane lipoprotein appears to promote entry into nonmacrophage cells. The major virulence factor, listeriolysin O, along with phospholipases, enables listeriae to escape from the phagosome and avoid intracellular killing. Once free in the cytoplasm, the bacterium can divide and, by inducing host cell actin polymerization, propel itself to the cell membrane. Subsequently, by means of pseudopodlike projections, it can invade adjacent macrophages. The bacterial surface protein Act A is necessary for the induction of actin filament assembly and cell-to-cell spread and, therefore, is a major virulence factor. Through this novel life cycle, *L. monocytogenes* moves from cell to cell, evading exposure to antibodies, complement, or neutrophils.

Iron, which is essential for the life of virtually all bacteria, appears to be an important virulence factor of *L. monocytogenes*. Siderophores of the organism enable it to take iron from transferrin. In vitro, iron enhances organism growth, and, in animal models of listerial infection, iron overload is associated with enhanced susceptibility to infection and iron supplementation with enhanced lethality, whereas iron depletion results in prolonged survival. Attesting to the importance of iron acquisition as a virulence factor in humans are the clinical associations of sporadic listerial infection with hemochromatosis and of outbreaks with transfusion-induced iron overload in patients receiving hemodialysis.

IMMUNITY

Resistance to infection with the intracellular bacterium *L. monocytogenes* is predominantly cell mediated, as evidenced by experiments showing that immunity could be transferred by sensitized lymphocytes but not by antibodies. Further evidence is provided by the overwhelming clinical association between listerial infection and conditions of impaired cell-mediated immunity, including lymphoma, pregnancy, AIDS, and corticosteroid immunosuppression. Tumor necrosis factor-α (TNF-α) neutralizing agents (eg, infliximab) are increasingly used to treat rheumatoid arthritis and Crohn's disease; invasive listeriosis has complicated use of these immune modulating agents. The production of nitric oxide by activated macrophages may play a role in natural immunity to listeriosis independent of T-cell

function. The role of humoral immunity is unknown, although both immunoglobulin M (absent in neonates) and classical complement activity (low in neonates) have been shown to be necessary for efficient opsonization of *L. monocytogenes*.

Although listeriosis is 100 to 1000 times more common in patients with AIDS compared with the general population, it is somewhat surprising that it is not seen more commonly, given the ubiquity of the organism. The use of trimethoprim–sulfamethoxazole (TMP–SMX) for prophylaxis against *Pneumocystis jiroveci* (formerly *Pneumocystis carinii*) provides protection against listeriosis. Frequency of listeriosis is not increased in those with deficiencies in neutrophil numbers or function, splenectomy, complement deficiency, or immunoglobulin disorders.

CLINICAL MANIFESTATIONS

The species name derives from the fact that an extract of the *L. monocytogenes* cell membrane has potent monocytosis-producing activity in rabbits, but monocytosis is a very rare feature of human infection.

Infection in Pregnancy

Mild impairment of cell-mediated immunity occurs during gestation, and pregnant women are prone to developing listerial bacteremia with an estimated 17-fold increase in risk. Listeriae proliferate in the placenta in areas that appear to be unreachable by usual defense mechanisms, and cell-to-cell spread facilitates maternal–fetal transmission. For unexplained reasons, CNS infection is extremely rare during pregnancy in the absence of other risk factors. Bacteremia manifests clinically as an acute febrile illness, often accompanied by myalgia, arthralgia, headache, and backache. Illness may occur at any time during pregnancy but usually occurs in the third trimester, probably related to the major decline in cell-mediated immunity seen at 26 to 30 weeks of gestation. Twenty-two percent of perinatal infections result in stillbirth or neonatal death; premature labor is common. Untreated bacteremia is generally self-limited, although if there is a complicating amnionitis, fever may persist in the mother until the fetus is aborted. Early diagnosis and antimicrobial therapy can result in the birth of a healthy infant.

There is no convincing evidence that listeriosis is a cause of habitual abortion in humans.

Neonatal Infection

When in utero infection occurs, it can precipitate spontaneous abortion. The fetus may be stillborn or die within hours of a disseminated form of listerial infection known as granulomatosis infantiseptica and is characterized by widespread microabscesses and granulomas that are particularly prevalent in the liver and spleen. In this entity, abundant bacteria are often visible on Gram stain of meconium.

More commonly, neonatal infection manifests similar to group B streptococcal disease in one of two forms: (1) early-onset sepsis syndrome, usually associated with prematurity and probably acquired in utero, or (2) late-onset meningitis, occurring at about 2 weeks of age in term infants, who most likely acquired organisms from the maternal vagina at parturition. Cases have occurred after cesarean delivery, however, and nosocomial transmission has been suggested.

In early-onset disease, *L. monocytogenes* can be isolated from the conjunctivae, external ear, nose, throat, meconium, amniotic fluid, placenta, blood, and, sometimes, CSF; Gram stain of meconium may show gram-positive rods and provide early diagnosis. The highest concentrations of bacteria are found in the neonatal lung and gut, which suggests that infection is acquired in utero from infected amniotic fluid rather than via a hematogenous route. Purulent conjunctivitis and a disseminated papular rash have rarely been described in neonates with early-onset disease, but clinical infection is otherwise similar to that due to other bacterial pathogens.

Bacteremia

Bacteremia without an evident focus is the most common manifestation of listeriosis after the neonatal period. Clinical manifestations typically include fever and myalgias; a prodromal illness with nausea and diarrhea may occur. Because immunocompromised patients are more likely than healthy persons to have blood cultures during febrile illnesses, transient bacteremias in healthy persons may go undetected.

Central Nervous System Infection

Organisms that cause bacterial meningitis most frequently (*Streptococcus pneumoniae*, *Neisseria meningitidis*, and *Haemophilus influenzae*) rarely cause parenchymal brain infections such as cerebritis and brain abscess. By contrast, *L. monocytogenes* has tropism for the brain itself (particularly the brain stem), as well as for the meninges. Many patients with listerial meningitis experience altered consciousness, seizures, or movement disorders and truly have meningoencephalitis.

MENINGITIS

Active surveillance studies of bacterial meningitis conducted by the CDC indicate that *L. monocytogenes* accounts for 20% of bacterial meningitis cases in neonates as well as in those older than 60 years and carries a mortality of 22%. Worldwide, *L. monocytogenes* is one of the three major causes of neonatal meningitis, is second only to pneumococcus as a cause of bacterial meningitis in adults older than 50 years, and is the most common cause of bacterial meningitis in patients with lymphoma, patients with organ transplants, or those receiving corticosteroid immunosuppression for any reason. Twenty percent of bacterial meningitis in those older than 50 years is caused by *L. monocytogenes*; therefore, empiric therapy for bacterial meningitis in all adults older than 50 years with a negative CSF Gram stain should include an antilisterial agent (either ampicillin or TMP–SMX), especially in the absence of associated pneumonia, otitis, sinusitis, or endocarditis, which would suggest an alternative etiology.

Clinically, meningitis due to *L. monocytogenes* is usually similar to that due to more common causes; features particular to listerial meningitis are summarized in Table 142.1.

BRAIN STEM ENCEPHALITIS (RHOMBENCEPHALITIS)

An unusual form of listerial encephalitis involves the brain stem. In contrast to other listerial CNS infections, this illness usually occurs in healthy older children and adults; neonatal cases have not been reported. The typical clinical picture is one of a biphasic illness with a prodrome of fever, headache, nausea, and vomiting lasting about 4 days, followed by the abrupt onset of asymmetrical cranial nerve deficits, cerebellar signs, and hemiparesis or hemisensory deficits or both. Nuchal rigidity is present in about 50%, CSF is only mildly abnormal, and CSF culture is positive in about 40%; almost two thirds are bacteremic. Respiratory failure develops in about 4% of cases. Magnetic resonance imaging is superior to computed tomography for demonstrating rhombencephalitis. Mortality is high, and serious sequelae are common in survivors.

Table 142.1 Distinctive Features of Listerial Meningitis Compared with More Common Bacterial Etiologies

Feature	Frequency (%)
Presentation can be subacute (mimics tuberculous meningitis)	~10
Stiff neck is less common	15–20
Movement disorders (ataxia, tremors, myoclonus) are more common	15–20
Seizures are more common	~25
Fluctuating mental status is common	~75
Positive blood culture is more common	75
Cerebrospinal fluid (CSF)	
Positive Gram stain is less common	40
Normal CSF glucose is more common	>60
Mononuclear cell predominance is more common	~30

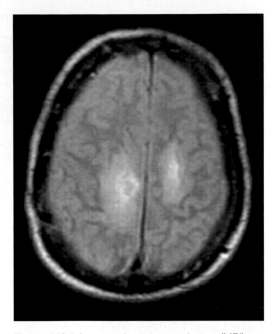

Figure 142.1 A magnetic resonance image (MRI) of the brain showing bilateral frontoparietal lesions with ring enhancement (abscess) on the right. The patient was a 70-year-old man with multiple myeloma who presented with difficulty walking followed by inability to stand and progressive quadriparesis. An aspirate of the abscess grew *Listeria monocytogenes*.

CEREBRITIS AND BRAIN ABSCESS

Parenchymal brain infection may occur without true abscess formation and is referred to as cerebritis; concomitant meningitis may or may not be present. Macroscopic brain abscesses account for about 10% of CNS listerial infections (Figure 142.1). Bacteremia is almost always present, and concomitant meningitis with isolation of *L. monocytogenes* from the CSF is found in 25%; both of these features are rare in other forms of bacterial brain abscess. About 50% of cases occur in known risk groups for listerial infection. Subcortical abscesses located in the thalamus, pons, and medulla are common; these sites are exceedingly rare when abscesses are due to other bacteria. Mortality is high, and survivors usually have serious sequelae.

Endocarditis

Listerial endocarditis may account for as much as 7.5% of adult listerial infections, produces both native valve and prosthetic valve disease, and has a high rate of septic complications and a mortality of 48%. Listerial endocarditis, but not bacteremia per se, may be an indicator of underlying gastrointestinal tract pathology, including cancer.

Localized Infection

Focal infections from which *L. monocytogenes* has been isolated include direct inoculation resulting in conjunctivitis, skin infection, and lymphadenitis. Bacteremia can lead to hepatic infection, cholecystitis, peritonitis, splenic abscess, pleuropulmonary infection, septic arthritis, osteomyelitis, pericarditis, myocarditis, arteritis, and endophthalmitis. Complications, including disseminated intravascular coagulation, adult respiratory distress syndrome, and rhabdomyolysis with acute renal failure, have been documented. There is nothing clinically unique about these localized infections; many, but not all, have occurred in those known to be at risk for listeriosis.

Febrile Gastroenteritis

Many patients with invasive listeriosis give a history of antecedent gastrointestinal illness, often accompanied by fever. Although isolated cases of gastrointestinal illness due to *L. monocytogenes* appear to be quite rare, at least 7 outbreaks of foodborne gastroenteritis due to *L. monocytogenes* have been documented. In the largest outbreak to date 1566 individuals, most of them children between the ages of 6 and 10, became ill after eating caterer-provided cafeteria food at two schools, and 19% were

Table 142.2 Intravenous Therapy for Invasive Listeriosis

Syndrome	Antibiotic[a]	Dosage[b]	Interval	Minimum Duration
Meningitis	Ampicillin plus gentamicin	200 mg/kg 5 mg/kg	q4h q8h	3 wk
Brain abscess or rhombencephalitis	Ampicillin plus gentamicin	200 mg/kg 5 mg/kg	q4h q8h	6 wk
Endocarditis	Ampicillin plus gentamicin	200 mg/kg 5 mg/kg	q6h q8h	6 wk
Bacteremia	Ampicillin	200 mg/kg	q6h	2 wk

[a] Penicillin-allergic patients without endocarditis can be treated with trimethoprim–sulfamethoxazole alone, using 15 mg/kg of trimethoprim daily at 6- to 8-hour intervals. Patients with endocarditis should be desensitized to ampicillin and treated as above.
[b] Maximum daily dose of ampicillin should not exceed 15 g.

hospitalized. Illness typically occurs 24 hours after ingestion of a large inoculum of bacteria (range 6 hours to 10 days) and usually lasts 1 to 3 days (range 1–7 days); attack rates have been quite high (52%–100%). Common symptoms include fever, watery diarrhea, nausea, headache, and pains in joints and muscles. Vehicles of infection have included chocolate milk, cold corn and tuna salad, cold smoked trout, and delicatessen meat. *Listeria monocytogenes* should be considered to be a possible etiology in outbreaks of febrile gastroenteritis when routine cultures fail to yield a pathogen.

DIAGNOSIS

Listeriosis should be a major consideration as part of the differential diagnosis in any of the following clinical settings:

1. Septicemia or meningitis in infants younger than 2 months.
2. Meningitis or parenchymal brain infection in: (a) patients with hematologic cancer, AIDS, organ transplantation, corticosteroid immunosuppression, or those receiving anti-TNF agents; (b) patients with subacute presentation; (c) adults >50 years; and (d) those in whom CSF shows gram-positive bacilli.
3. Simultaneous infection of the meninges and brain parenchyma.
4. Subcortical brain abscess.
5. Fever during pregnancy.
6. Blood, CSF, or other normally sterile specimen reported to have "diphtheroids" on Gram stain or culture.
7. Foodborne outbreak of febrile gastroenteritis when routine cultures fail to identify a pathogen.

Diagnosis requires isolation of *L. monocytogenes* from clinical specimens (eg, CSF, blood) and identification through standard microbiologic techniques. Antibodies to listeriolysin O have not proved useful in invasive disease, nor have polymerase chain reaction probes. Antibodies to listeriolysin O may be useful during investigation of outbreaks of febrile gastroenteritis. Magnetic resonance imaging is superior to computed tomography for demonstrating parenchymal brain involvement, especially in the brain stem.

TREATMENT

No controlled trials have established a drug of choice or duration of therapy for listerial infection. Recommendations for treatment of invasive infections are presented in Table 142.2.

Ampicillin is generally considered the preferred agent. Based on synergy in vitro and in animal models, most authorities suggest adding gentamicin to ampicillin for treatment of bacteremia in those with severely impaired cell-mediated immunity and in all cases of meningitis and endocarditis. In one uncontrolled study, the combination of TMP–SMX plus ampicillin was associated with a lower failure rate and fewer neurologic sequelae than ampicillin combined with an aminoglycoside.

For those intolerant of penicillins, TMP–SMX is believed to be the best alternative. Chloramphenicol, at one time regarded as the agent of choice for patients with penicillin allergy, should not be used to treat listerial infection because of unacceptable failure and relapse rates. No currently available cephalosporin should be used; none has adequate activity, and meningitis has developed in patients receiving cephalosporins. For this reason, ampicillin is always included in empirical therapy for septicemia or meningitis in infants ≤2 months of age.

Vancomycin has been used successfully in a few patients with penicillin allergy, but other patients have developed listerial meningitis while receiving the drug. Rifampin is active in vitro and is known to penetrate phagocytic cells; clinical experience is minimal, however, and in animal models the addition of rifampin to ampicillin was not more effective than was ampicillin used alone. Both imipenem and meropenem have been used successfully to treat listeriosis, but caution is advised because both drugs lower the seizure threshold, treatment failures have been reported, and imipenem was less effective than ampicillin in a mouse model.

Initial dosing of antibiotics as for meningitis is prudent for all patients, even in the absence of CNS or CSF abnormalities, because of the high affinity of this organism for the CNS. Patients with meningitis should be treated for no fewer than 3 weeks; bacteremic patients without CSF abnormalities can be treated for 2 weeks.

No data exist concerning antimicrobial efficacy in listerial gastroenteritis; the illness is self-limited, and treatment is not warranted. Clinically significant antimicrobial resistance has not been encountered, but vigilance is warranted because transfer of resistance from enterococci to *L. monocytogenes* has been reported. Because iron is a virulence factor for *L. monocytogenes*, it seems prudent to withhold iron replacement in patients with iron deficiency until the listerial infection is resolved.

PREVENTION

Table 142.3 contains recommendations developed by the CDC for prevention of foodborne listeriosis.

Except from infected mother to fetus, human-to-human transmission of listeriosis does not occur; therefore, patients do not require isolation. Neonatal listerial infection complicating successive pregnancies is virtually unheard of, and intrapartum antibiotics are not recommended for mothers with a history of perinatal listeriosis. There is no vaccine. Listerial infections are effectively prevented by TMP–SMX given as prophylaxis against *P. jiroveci* to recipients of organ transplants or to individuals with the human immunodeficiency virus. The utility, or even the feasibility, of eradicating gastrointestinal colonization as a means

Table 142.3 Dietary Recommendations for Preventing Foodborne Listeriosis

For All Persons
1. Cook raw food from animal sources (eg, beef, pork, and poultry) thoroughly.
2. Wash raw vegetables thoroughly before eating.
3. Keep uncooked meats separate from vegetables, cooked foods, and ready-to-eat foods.
4. Avoid consumption of raw (unpasteurized) milk or foods made from raw milk.
5. Wash hands, knives, and cutting boards after handling uncooked foods.
Additional Recommendations for Persons at High Risk[a]
1. Avoid soft cheeses (eg, Mexican-style, feta, Brie, Camembert) and blue-veined cheese; there is no need to avoid hard cheeses, cream cheese, cottage cheese, or yogurt.
2. Leftover foods or ready-to-eat foods (eg, hot dogs) should be reheated until steaming hot before eating.
3. Consider avoidance of foods in delicatessen counters.[b]

[a] Those immunocompromised by illness or medications, pregnant women, and the elderly.
[b] Although the risk for listeriosis associated with foods from delicatessen counters is relatively low, pregnant women and immunosuppressed persons may choose to avoid these foods or to thoroughly reheat cold cuts before consumption.

to prevent invasive listeriosis is unknown. However, asymptomatic persons at high risk for listeriosis, known to have ingested a food implicated in an outbreak, could reasonably be given several days of oral ampicillin or TMP–SMX.

SUGGESTED READING

Bakardjiev AI, Stacy BA, Portnoy DA. Growth of Listeria monocytogenes in the guinea pig placenta and role of cell-to-cell spread in fetal infection. *J Infect Dis*. 2005;191:1889–1897.

Gottlieb SL, Newbern EC, Griffin PM, et al. Multistate outbreak of listeriosis linked to turkey deli meat and subsequent changes in US regulatory policy. *Clin Infect Dis*. 2006;42:29–36.

Hamon M, Bierne H, Cossart P. Listeria monocytogenes: a multifaceted model. *Nat Rev Microbiol*. 2006;4:423–434.

MacDonald PDM, Whitwam RE, Boggs JD, et al. Outbreak of listeriosis among Mexican immigrants as a result of consumption of illicitly produced Mexican-style cheese. *Clin Infect Dis*. 2005;40:677–682.

Mylonakis E, Hohmann EL, Calderwood SB. Central nervous system infection with Listeria monocytogenes: 33 years' experience at a general hospital and review of 776 episodes from the literature. *Medicine*. 1998;77:313–336.

Mylonakis E, Paliou M, Hohmann EL, et al. Listeriosis during pregnancy: a case series and review of 222 cases. *Medicine*. 2002;81:260–269.

Ooi ST, Lorber B. Gastroenteritis due to Listeria monocytogenes. *Clin Infect Dis*. 2005;40:1327–1332.

Schlech WF III, Schlech WF IV, Haldane H, et al. Does sporadic Listeria gastroenteritis exist?: a 2-year population-based survey in Nova Scotia, Canada. *Clin Infect Dis*. 2005;41:778–778.

143. *Nocardia*

Lisa Haglund

Nocardia species are soilborne bacteria that are aerobic and slow-growing. In culture, they may require 2 to 4 weeks before colonies appear. *Nocardia* are gram-positive and weakly acid-fast filaments, 0.5 to 1.0 μm in diameter, that branch at right angles (Figure 143.1). Nine nocardial species pathogenic for humans were described between 1888 and 1996: *Nocardia farcinica*, *Nocardia asteroides*, *Nocardia carnae*, *Nocardia brasiliensis*, *Nocardia otitidiscaviarum* (formerly *Nocardia caviae*), *Nocardia transvalensis*, *Nocardia brevicatena*, *Nocardia nova*, and *Nocardia pseudobrasiliensis*. Since then, with availability of newer molecular techniques, 24 new nocardial species of human significance have been described, and taxonomy of the genus is in a state of flux. For example, *N. asteroides sensu stricto* is not currently defined in molecular terms, and reports of isolation of *N. asteroides* have actually represented several nocardial species. Further studies should provide taxonomic clarification and correlation with disease states. *Nocardia* are opportunistic pathogens; *N. brasiliensis* is more virulent, affecting normal hosts, and has a range geographically restricted to areas with warmer climates.

Nocardiosis is typically a suppurative infection with multiple abscesses. It is rarely granulomatous and not fibrotic. Acquisition of infection is by the respiratory tract or by traumatic inoculation. Although nocardia are ubiquitous, they rarely colonize the human respiratory tract. Accordingly, treatment should be initiated when nocardia are repeatedly isolated from pulmonary specimens, particularly from an immunocompromised host. Antimicrobial therapy (alone or in combination with surgical drainage) is recommended, and the duration of therapy must be prolonged to prevent relapse.

More than 75% of patients with systemic nocardiosis possess underlying risk factors. Predisposing conditions are listed in Table 143.1. As the number of solid organ and hematopoietic stem cell transplantations increased, the incidence of nocardiosis rose, although some transplantation centers

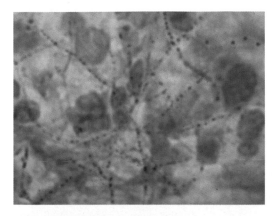

Figure 143.1 *Nocardia*, Gram stain. (Courtesy of David Schlossberg MD.)

have observed lower incidence since use of cyclosporine and newer immunosuppressants that permit lower corticosteroid dosages. There is a correlation with the level of immunosuppression following transplantation, with most cases of nocardiosis occurring >3 but <18 months after transplantation. Among human immunodeficiency virus (HIV)-infected persons, there is also a correlation with level of immunosuppression, as almost all cases of nocardiosis occur in individuals with CD4 lymphocyte count ≤100 cells/mm^3. In both of these severely immunocompromised populations, co-occurrence of other opportunistic infections, particularly aspergillosis, may be found and should be sought if expected clinical improvement fails to occur with therapy.

Nocardiosis remains an uncommon opportunistic complication of HIV infection and transplant recipients. One explanation is that the prophylactic use of trimethoprim–sulfamethoxazole (TMP–SMX), pyrimethamine or dapsone for *Pneumocystis jirovecii* (formerly *Pneumocystis carinii*) may also prevent nocardiosis. Ten to fifteen percent of HIV-infected persons and 20% of transplant recipients diagnosed with nocardiosis had been receiving these drugs prophylactically. The nocardia isolates causing these infections are seldom resistant to sulfa drugs in vitro.

Table 143.1 Risk Factors for Systemic Nocardiosis

Chronic pulmonary disease	Solid organ transplantation	Systemic lupus erythematosus	Renal failure
Alcoholism	Hematopoietic stem cell transplantation	Systemic vasculitis	Whipple disease
Cirrhosis		Ulcerative colitis	Hypogammaglobulinemia
Lymphoreticular malignancy	Chronic corticosteroid use	Sarcoidosis	Chronic granulomatous disease
Diabetes	Other drug-induced immunosuppression		Human immunodeficiency virus infection
	Cushing syndrome		

PATHOGENESIS OF SYSTEMIC NOCARDIOSIS

Neutrophils inhibit the growth of nocardia, but organisms are not killed until cell-mediated immunity is activated. If cellular immunity is impaired, the organism causes indolent abscesses and then slowly spreads to distant sites, such as the brain or cerebrospinal fluid. Illness is usually subacute to chronic but may be fulminant in an immunocompromised host. Weight loss, anorexia, and fatigue are common in systemic nocardiosis.

MYCETOMA, CUTANEOUS NOCARDIOSIS, TRAUMATIC NOCARDIOSIS

Nocardial species can cause mycetoma, which typically manifests as a swollen area with sinuses draining purulent material. Unlike other causes of mycetoma (botryomycosis and *Actinomyces israelii*), nocardial mycetoma may present without grain formation. Primary cutaneous nocardiosis manifests as nontender, red, irregularly shaped raised lesions. Occasionally, these form sinus tracts and drain purulent material. Regional lymphadenopathy is infrequently observed. *Nocardia* arthritis usually presents as a monoarthritis, commonly involving the knee. Disease is often inoculated through a puncture wound. Other inoculation nocardial infections described include postoperative wound infections (including mediastinitis after cardiac transplantation), osteomyelitis, and keratitis.

PULMONARY NOCARDIOSIS

Pulmonary disease is apparent in 65% to 85% of systemic nocardial infections. The roentgenographic features include infiltrates that may cavitate, sometimes accompanied by empyema, pericarditis, or mediastinitis. There is no specific radiographic appearance, thus a high degree of suspicion must be maintained to make the diagnosis. Sputum cultures may be overgrown with other organisms before *Nocardia* colonies appear. Therefore, it may be helpful to notify the microbiology lab to hold cultures for *Nocardia*. Respiratory samples submitted for fungal culture are more likely to grow *Nocardia* than those submitted for mycobacterial (acid-fast bacillus [AFB]) culture.

NOCARDIA MENINGITIS AND BRAIN ABSCESS

Central nervous system (CNS) nocardiosis is detected in 20% to 40% of systemic nocardial infections. Two thirds have clinical findings such as fever, headache, stiff neck, or altered mental status. Hypoglycorrhachia is found in two thirds of patients. Mildly elevated cerebrospinal fluid protein and a neutrophilic pleocytosis of approximately 1000 white blood cells are usually found. Nocardial brain abscess can be a complication of nocardial meningitis or can present in the absence of meningitis. Although meningitis without underlying brain abscess has been described, this is quite unusual, and an underlying abscess should always be suspected. Because of the high incidence of CNS infection, an imaging study of the brain should be performed if any personality or neurological changes are found during work-up of systemic nocardiosis.

THERAPY OF NOCARDIOSIS: SULFONAMIDE THERAPY

Sulfonamides are currently the first-line agents for nocardiosis, and sulfadiazine, 6 to 8 g intravenously (IV) or orally daily, is a typical adult regimen. Trimethoprim–sulfamethoxazole (TMP–SMX) is an alternative first-line treatment for nocardiosis, although it has never been shown to be superior to a sulfonamide alone. Table 143.2 summarizes typical dosages and durations of therapy for sulfonamide therapy of nocardiosis.

Sulfadiazine became a commonly used agent by 1940. As a short-acting sulfonamide

Table 143.2 Sulfonamide Dosage and Duration of Therapy for Treatment of *Nocardia*

Type of Nocardiosis	Dosage (divided BID-QID)	Duration	Comments
Cutaneous	5–10 mg/kg/d TMP–SMX[a]	2–4 mo	Longer for extensive disease or bony involvement as seen in mycetoma
Pulmonary	10 mg/kg/d TMP–SMX	6–12 mo	12-mo minimum duration for immunocompromised host
Central nervous system	15 mg/kg/d TMP–SMX 50–100 mg/kg/d sulfadiazine	12 mo	

[a] TMP–SMX dosage based on mg/kg of the trimethoprim (TMP) component.

Table 143.3 Other Regimens for Treatment of *Nocardia*

Drug	Dosage	Duration	Comments
Minocycline	100–200 mg PO BID	3–6 mo	Useful for pulmonary disease; poor CNS penetration
Imipenem–cilastatin	500 mg IV q6h	Until oral agent can be given	Dose must be adjusted for renal failure
Amikacin	5–7.5 mg/kg IV q12h	Until oral agent can be given	Nephrotoxic; dosage must be adjusted for renal failure
Ceftriaxone	2 g IV q12h	Until oral agent can be given	
Cefotaxime	2 g IV q8h	Until oral agent can be given	

with rapid absorption and prompt urinary excretion, it had to be given in large dosages for therapeutic effect. Unfortunately, with its low urinary solubility, there is a high incidence of crystalluria.

TMP–SMX is a well-absorbed combination agent with a long plasma half-life of 11 and 9 hours for TMP and SMX, respectively. It is available orally as single- or double-strength tablets (80 mg TMP plus 400 mg SMX and 160 mg TMP plus 800 mg SMX, respectively) and as a liquid suspension containing 40 mg TMP plus 200 mg SMX per 5 mL. It is also available IV (5 mL = 80 mg TMP plus 400 mg SMX).

The most frequent side effects of TMP–SMX are upper gastrointestinal symptoms and skin rashes (3%–4% each). Leukopenia, thrombocytopenia, and megaloblastic changes can develop rarely. Adverse effects of sulfonamide therapy include acute renal failure as a result of tubular damage from sulfa crystalluria. This effect may be prevented by adequate hydration and by alkalinizing the urine. Hepatitis, intrahepatic cholestasis, pancreatitis, and aseptic meningitis have been reported with TMP–SMX. Serious adverse reactions are rare and include anaphylaxis, Stevens–Johnson syndrome, and hematologic effects, including thrombocytopenia, leukopenia, and hemolytic anemia.

TMP–SMX and other sulfonamides should not be given to patients with a demonstrated deficiency of folic acid or glucose-6-phosphate dehydrogenase. In HIV-infected patients, there is an increased incidence of adverse reactions to TMP–SMX, including reversible hyperkalemia and a severe hypersensitivity reaction with fever, hypotension, and multiorgan involvement on rechallenge with the drug 2 to 3 weeks after previous course of therapy.

OTHER AGENTS WITH ANTINOCARDIAL ACTIVITY

In recent years *Nocardia farcinica*, among the most prevalent of nocardial species, *Nocardia otitidiscaviarum*, and *Nocardia transvalensis* have been reported to have resistance to sulfa drugs. Antimicrobial susceptibility testing of nocardia requires prolonged incubation and remains technically difficult. Susceptibility results are most reliable from an experienced laboratory. *In vitro* susceptibility does not uniformly correlate with clinical outcome in humans; therefore, clinical response should also guide selection of definitive antimicrobial therapy. The parenteral agents with greatest in vitro activity include imipenem–cilastatin (500 mg IV every 6 hours), amikacin (5–7.5 mg/kg IV every 12 hours), cefotaxime (2 g IV every 8 hours), or ceftriaxone (2 g IV every 12 hours) (Table 143.3). With susceptible organisms, these agents have been as efficacious as sulfonamides in animal models; in fact, they may be more rapidly bactericidal than sulfonamides. So far, no large human case series has been published establishing clinical superiority of these alternative parenteral regimens to sulfonamide therapy, but in the immunocompromised patient, strong consideration should be given to initial empiric use of amikacin and imipenem–cilastatin, while awaiting availability of *in vitro* susceptibilities. In CNS nocardiosis, it is worthwhile to recall that seizures are a potential side effect of imipenem–cilastatin therapy.

Tetracyclines manifest excellent activity against nocardial species. Minocycline has the best in vitro activity among the tetracyclines and is given 100–200 mg orally twice a day for 3 to 6 months (Table 143.3). Its drawbacks include poor cerebrospinal fluid penetration and side effects of vertigo, making it unsuitable for central nervous system nocardial disease.

Amoxicillin–clavulanate is an alternative to TMP–SMX or minocycline for treatment of cutaneous and lymphocutaneous disease caused by *N. brasiliensis*. Macrolides and the newer quinolones show some in vitro activity, but few patients with systemic nocardiosis have received these agents therapeutically. Linezolid 300 to 600 orally twice daily has been used with success in a few patients, but the long treatment course needed for nocardiosis may be complicated with bone marrow suppression and peripheral neuropathy.

SUGGESTED READING

Brown-Elliott BA, Brown JM, Conville PS, Wallace RJ Jr. Clinical and laboratory features of the Nocardia spp. based on current molecular taxonomy. *Clin Microbiol Rev*. 2006;19:259–282.

Filice GA. Nocardiosis in persons with human immunodeficiency virus infection, transplant recipients, and large, geographically defined populations. *J Lab Clin Med*. 2005;145:156–162.

Lederman ER, Crum NF. A case series and focused review of nocardiosis: clinical and microbiological aspects. *Medicine*. 2004;83:300–313.

Saubolle MA, Sussland D. Nocardiosis: review of clinical and laboratory experience. *J Clin Microbiol*. 2003;41:4497–4501.

Walensky RP, Moore RD. A case series of 59 patients with nocardiosis. *Infect Dis Clin Pract*. 2001;10:249–254.

144. *Pasteurella Multocida*

Naasha J. Talati and David S. Stephens

Pasteurella multocida ("killer of many species") is a gram-negative, pleomorphic coccobacillus best known for its association with soft-tissue infections after animal bites. However, this organism is also capable of causing invasive and life-threatening infections.

Pasteurella multocida is found worldwide. It commonly colonizes the upper respiratory tract of many animals, most notably cats (70% to 90%) and dogs (50% to 66%). Human infection is usually related to animal exposure. Direct inoculation by a bite or scratch is the most common mode of transmission of *P. multocida* to humans. Inoculation can also occur by nontraumatic animal contact, such as when a wound is licked by an animal. The second mode of transmission is by colonization of the human respiratory tract occurring with exposure to animals such as nuzzling or grooming of pets. The organism has been cultured from the respiratory tract of healthy veterinary workers and animal handlers as well as from ill patients. Infections can also occasionally occur with no history of animal contact.

There are several species and subspecies of *Pasteurella*, but the most common ones causing human disease are *P. multocida, Pasteurella dagmatis, Pasteurella canis*, and *Pasteurella stomatis*. These organisms are nonmotile, gram-negative facultative anaerobes that on Gram stain can resemble *Haemophilus* and *Neisseria* species. The organism grows well on sheep and chocolate agar and appears as watery mucoid blue colonies.

Most of the virulence factors have been studied in animals. Pathogenesis of *Pasteurella* depends on the ability of the bacteria to stick to the host's respiratory epithelium, typically the tonsils. Some of this adherence is mediated through fimbrae. Some *Pasteurella* species are capable of producing a leukotoxin that affects leukocytes and prevents a cellular immune response. In addition most virulent *Pasteurella* also have a capsule and can be classified according to their capsular antigens A to F that cause different animal diseases. Binding of transferrin is another mechanism by which *Pasteurella* can ensure a continuous supply of iron for its growth.

CLINICAL PRESENTATION

Infections caused by *P. multocida* can be divided into three groups: bite wound infections, infections of the respiratory tract, and invasive disease.

Bite Wound Infection

Infections of the skin and soft tissue most commonly occur after a bite or scratch but can occasionally occur after an animal licks an open wound. Bite wounds account for 60% to 86% of *P. multocida* infections. *Pasteurella multocida* is found as a pathogen in 75% of infected cat bites and in up to 50% of infected dog bites. Most bite wounds grow multiple organisms. Infection with *P. multocida* is characterized by extremely rapid onset. Local pain and inflammation often occur within 4 to 6 hours of the injury and almost always within 24 hours. Purulent drainage is present in 40% and lymphangitis in 20%, but fever and systemic symptoms are often absent. A rapid inflammatory reaction with no fever should prompt the clinician to suspect *P. multocida* in bite wound infections.

Bite wound infections with *P. multocida* can lead to serious sequelae, even with aggressive and appropriate antibiotic and surgical management. Tenosynovitis, abscess formation, and osteomyelitis often result, but bacteremia is rare. Cat bites are more commonly associated with osteomyelitis because of the deep puncture wounds that penetrate the periosteum. Poor functional outcome is common with these infections, especially when they involve the extremities. In patients with risk factors for invasive infections as discussed subsequently, an apparently insignificant and uninfected wound may be associated with serious sequelae weeks later.

Respiratory Tract Infection

The respiratory tract is the second most common site of infection. Patients colonized with *Pasteurella* usually suffer from chronic obstructive pulmonary disease (COPD) and bronchiectasis. The organism has been associated with sinusitis, otitis, epiglottitis, bronchitis, pneumonia, lung abscess, and empyema. The mode of acquisition into the lower respiratory tract includes inhalation of contaminated aerosols or direct innoculation of the oral cavity with animal secretions and subsequent aspiration. Bacteremia is seen in 55% of cases. Most patients are elderly and have some underlying respiratory illness, such as COPD, bronchiectasis, chronic sinusitis, or pulmonary neoplasm. The clinical presentation is indistinguishable from other forms of bacterial pneumonia.

Invasive or Disseminated Infection

Invasive or disseminated infection with *P. multocida* is rare. These infections spread hematogenously from wounds or from pulmonary colonization. Invasive infections generally occur in children, pregnant women, the elderly, cirrhotic patients, or patients with other immunocompromised states. Most cases are associated with a history of animal bites or scratches, some are associated with animal exposure without injury, and a small percentage of cases have no history of exposure to animals.

Infectious arthritis is a rare complication of *Pasteurella* and generally occurs in patients with underlying joint disease or steroid use. The arthritis is usually monoarticular, and the most common site is the knee. Fifteen percent of patients have a polyarticular arthritis, usually in association with bacteremia. In a series of 37 cases, 32% had a prosthetic joint infection. Osteomyelitis has usually been seen in the setting of an animal bite (9 of 13 cases) and usually involves the upper extremity.

Meningitis is a relatively rare manifestation of *P. multocida* infection. The largest series of adult patients in the literature reports 29 cases from 1989 to 1999. There are four mechanisms by which *P. multocida* can cause meningitis: (1) direct innoculation after an animal bite, (2) contamination from colonized site after trauma or neurosurgery (29%), (3) bacteremic seeding of meninges (25%), and (4) local spread from an infected site, such as otitis (28%). The clinical presentation and cerebrospinal fluid (CSF) findings are typical of bacterial meningitis. A useful clue to diagnosis is that 89% of patients report animal exposure (with only 15% reporting an animal bite). Patients are generally older than 55 years, about 60% have a concomitant

bacteremia, and 50% have a positive CSF Gram stain. Neurological complications such as cranial nerve palsies and seizures are seen in 17%, and mortality is 25%.

Bacteremia is documented in 20% to 30% of invasive infections. The main risk factors for bacteremia are cirrhosis, diabetes, and malignancy. However, up to 38% of patients have no underlying disease, 17% have no animal exposure, and 13% have no localized site of infection. Case reports of sepsis have recently been increasing in the literature: 47 cases were reported between 1984 and 2003. The mortality is 28%. Thirty one cases of endocarditis caused by *Pasteurella* species have been reported, including one case of prosthetic valve disease. The mitral and aortic valves are most commonly affected. Presentation is acute in 64% of cases. Mortality is 40%, but rises to 57% in immunocompromised individuals.

Pasteurella is also known to cause intraabdominal infections. Twelve cases of spontaneous bacterial peritonitis have been reported, mostly in patients with alchoholic cirrhosis; mortality is around 30%. Cases of peritoneal dialysis-associated infection have been reported in 15 patients, all of whom had a cat, and all patients improved with antibiotic therapy. Cases of appendicitis-associated peritonitis have also been reported.

Other serious infections caused by *P. multocida* for which there are case reports in the literature include pyelonephritis, thyroiditis, mycotic aneurysm, vascular graft infection, endophthalmitis, liver abscess, chorioamnionitis, neonatal sepsis, and chronic ulceration of the penis.

THERAPY
Antibiotics

In general, the antibiotic of choice for treatment of *P. multocida* infections is penicillin. Ampicillin and amoxicillin are effective, but antistaphylococcal penicillins such as oxacillin and nafcillin are not recommended. The second- and third-generation cephalosporins have good activity against *P. multocida*, but first-generation cephalosporins and cefaclor are not reliable. Twenty to thirty percent of bovine and porcine species are resistant to penicillin; however, to date only 5 human cases of β-lactamase–producing *P. multocida* have been reported in the literature. Interestingly, all cases had a respiratory

Table 144.1 Antibiotic Susceptibilities of *Pasteurella multocida*

Usually Susceptible	Variable	Usually Resistant
Penicillin and derivatives	Semisynthetic penicillins	Vancomycin
Ampicillin (± sulbactam)	Oxacillin	Clindamycin
Amoxicillin (± clavulanate)	Dicloxacillin	Erythromycin (oral)
Ticarcillin (± clavulanate)	Cloxacillin	
Piperacillin (± tazobactam)	Nafcillin	
Second- and third-generation cephalosporins[a]	Cefaclor	
Cefuroxime	First-generation	
Cefotetan	cephalosporins	
Cefoxitin	Cephalexin	
Cefixime[b]	Cefazolin	
Cefprozil[b]	Cephradine	
Loracarbel[b]	Cefadroxil	
Cefpodoxime[b]	Erythromycin (IV)	
Ceftriaxone	Aminoglycocides	
Ceftizoxime	Gentamicin	
Cefotaxime	Tobramycin	
Ceftazidime	Amikacin	
Ciprofloxacin[b]		
Chloramphenicol		
Trimethoprim–sulfamethoxazole[b]		
Aztreonam		
Imipenem		
Tetracycline		
Doxycycline		

[a] Cefaclor, an oral second-generation cephalosporin, is often not effective.
[b] There are few clinical data on the use of these agents but by in vitro testing they should be effective.

infection with *P. multocida*. The resistance to penicillin is thought to be plasmid mediated. Patients who were treated with amoxicillin–clavulanate did well. Antibiotic susceptibility testing should be routinely performed.

Pasteurella multocida is uniformly sensitive to tetracycline and chloramphenicol. Fluoroquinolones, azithromycin, clarithromycin, and trimethoprim–sulfamethoxazole (TMP–SMX) have good in vitro activity. Clinical experience with these agents is limited, but they are an option for patients with allergies to penicillin and cephalosporins who cannot take tetracycline. Tables 144.1 and 144.2 show appropriate antibiotics and doses.

Many strains are resistant to erythromycin, especially at levels achievable with oral dosing. Most strains are only moderately sensitive to aminoglycosides and are universally resistant to clindamycin and vancomycin.

Prophylactic Antibiotic Therapy for Bite Wounds

Although antimicrobial therapy is clearly indicated for infected bite wounds, its value in prophylaxis after an uninfected bite wound remains unclear. This is largely due to the fact that studies on this subject have enrolled small numbers of patients. The decision to prescribe antibiotics at the time of injury depends on the risk of infection, which can be assessed by the criteria in Table 144.3. In addition, specific risk factors for *P. multocida* are listed in Table 144.4. In general, if a wound shows no sign of infection after 24 hours, *P. multocida* infection is unlikely to develop. However, for individuals with underlying risk factors and bites at risk for *P. multocida* infection, prophylaxis is reasonable even if they present late. As bite wounds usually contain multiple organisms, including anaerobes, prophylaxis is

Table 144.2 Doses of the Most Efficacious Agents for Treatment of *Pasteurella multocida*

Agent	Oral	Parenteral
Penicillin V	500–750 mg q6h	
Penicillin G		10 million to 20 million units/day divided q4h
Amoxicillin (± clavulanate)	250–500 mg q6h	
Ampicillin	250–500 mg q6h	1–2 g q4–6h
Ampicillin–sulbactam		1.5–3 g q6h
Ticarcillin–clavulanate		3.1 g q4–8h
Piperacillin		3–4 g q4–6h
Cefuroxime	250–500 g q12h	750 mg–1.5 g q8h
Cefoxitin		1–2 g q4–8h
Cefotaxime		1–2 g q4–8h
Ceftriaxone		1–2 g q24h
Ciprofloxacin	500–750 mg q12h	400 mg q12h
TMP–SMX	160 mg TMP (1 DS tab) bid	10 mg/kg/day TMP divided q6–12h
Aztreonam		500 mg–2 g q6–12h
Imipenem		500 mg–1 g q6–8h
Tetracycline	250–500 mg q6h	500 mg–1 g q12h
Doxycycline	100–200 mg q12h	100–200 mg q12h
Chloramphenicol	12.5–25 mg/kg q6h	12.5–25 mg/kg q6h

Abbreviations: TMP–SMX = trimethoprim–sulfamethoxazole; DS = double strength.

usually with amoxicillin–clavulanate for 3 to 5 days. Alternatives include TMP–SMX or a quinolone, in addition to clindamycin or flagyl to cover anaerobes. For further discussion of the management of bite wounds, see Chapter 23, Human and Animal Bites.

Treatment of Infected Wounds

Infected wounds should be thoroughly cleaned and have deep cultures performed before the initiation of antibiotics. Surgical evaluation should be performed especially when joints or extremities are involved or when there is extensive tissue damage. If infection with intense local inflammation develops within 24 hours, *P. multocida* should be strongly suspected. Because the rate of serious sequelae is high, the clinician should have a low threshold for admission and surgical consultation. If infection develops only after 24 to 48

hours, gram-positive organisms are more likely to be the cause, and therapy should be directed toward *Staphylococcus, Streptococcus* species, and anaerobes. However, if the patient has underlying risk factors for *P. multocida* infection, coverage for this organism should be included in the regimen. Table 144.1 shows the antibiotics of choice for *P. multocida*. Uncomplicated cellulitis should be treated for 7 to 10 days, but more complicated wound infections may require longer treatment.

Therapy for Other *P. multocida* Infections

The most important factor in successful treatment of other *P. multocida* infections is suspicion of the organism. A history of animal contact should always be obtained and the patient examined carefully for signs of even minor trauma. Gram stains of wounds or purulent

Table 144.3 Risk Factors for Wound Infection

	High	Low
Type of wound	Puncture Crush injury Foreign material introduced Extends to bone or joint Requires surgical repair	Laceration No crushing of tissues No contamination Superficial No surgical repair
Site of wound	Extremity, especially hand	Trunk, buttocks, head, minor facial wounds
Species of animal	Cat, pig, bovine	Dog, rodent
Delay before presentation	>8 h	≤6 h, or >48–72 h without signs of infection
Management prior to presentation	Poor cleaning	Good cleaning
Patient characteristics	>55 y or ≤1 y of age Immune compromise, liver disease	No underlying disease

Table 144.4 Risk Factors for *Pasteurella multocida* Infection

Wound	Patient
Deep puncture	≤1 y or >55 y of age
Feline, porcine	Liver disease, especially cirrhosis HIV
Deep feline scratch	Solid tumors, leukemias Immune modulating medications Chronic respiratory disease Collagen-vascular disease Pregnancy Artificial heart valve History of cranial trauma or surgery

collections are positive in up to 50% of cases. If *P. multocida* infection is a possibility, therapy should be initiated with a penicillin or a third-generation cephalosporin. Tetracycline, fluoroquinolones, and TMP–SMX are alternatives if β-lactam allergy is present.

In patients with meningitis who are allergic to β-lactams, chloramphenicol can be used; one patient was also successfully treated with aztreonam. The optimal duration of treatment for respiratory infections is not known, but most series suggest 7 to 10 days. Joint infections, osteomyelitis, and abscesses require drainage and debridement in addition to antibiotic therapy. Attempts to save the prosthetic joint resulted in cure in only 20%; therefore, aggressive surgical debridement and removal of prosthetic material is advocated. Patients with endocarditis arc treated with a combination of medical and surgical therapy, and duration of antibiotics is generally 6 weeks.

SUGGESTED READING

Goldstein EJ. Bite wounds and infection. *Clin Infect Dis.* 1992;14:633–638.

Green BT, Ramsey KM, Nolan PE. Pasteurella multocida meningitis: case report and review of the last 11 y. *Scand J Infect Dis.* 2002;34(3):213–217.

McDonough JJ, Stern PJ, Alexander JW. Management of animal and human bites and resulting human infections. *Curr Clin Top Infect Dis.* 1987;8:11–36.

Nettles RE, Sexton DJ. Pasteurella multocida prosthetic valve endocarditis: case report and review. *Clin Infect Dis.* 1997;25(4):920–921.

Kanaan N, Gavage P, Janssens M, et al. Pasteurella multocida septicemia caused by close contact with a domestic cat: case report and literature review. *J Infect Chemother.* 2004;10:250–252.

Raffi F, et al. Pasteurella multocida bacteremia: report of 13 cases over 12 years and review of the literature. *Scand J Infect Dis.* 1987; 19:385–393.

Talan DA, et al. Bacteriologic analysis of infected dog and cat bites. *N Engl J Med.* 1999;340:85–92.

Tamaskar I, Ravakhah K. Spontaneous bacterial peritonitis with Pasteurella multocida in cirrhosis: case report and review of literature. *South Med J.* 2004 Nov;97(11):1113–1115.

Weber DJ, et al. Pasteurella multocida infections: report of 34 cases and review of the literature. *Medicine.* 1984;63:133–154.

Weber DJ, Hansen AR. Infections resulting from animal bites. *Infect Dis Clin North Am.* 1991;5:663–680.

145. Pneumococcus

Maurice A. Mufson

INTRODUCTION

Streptococcus pneumoniae (the pneumococcus) remains no less important today as a pathogen of community-acquired pneumonia, meningitis, and acute otitis media than it has for the past several decades for several important reasons: (1) pneumococcal diseases, especially pneumococcal pneumonia, occur commonly; (2) invasive (bacteremic) pneumococcal diseases carry high case fatality rates; and (3) penicillin-resistant and multidrug-resistant strains continue to spread increasingly worldwide. *Streptococcus pneumoniae* ranks first as a cause of community-acquired pneumonia and second as a cause of bacterial meningitis and as an important bacterial pathogen of otitis media among infants and children. The high incidence and often fatal outcome of invasive disease despite prompt and appropriate antibiotic treatment provided the rationale for development and subsequent licensure in the United States of two effective polysaccharide vaccines, namely a 23-valent vaccine comprising 23 polysaccharides of the most common serotypes that are associated with community-acquired pneumonia in adults and children older than 2 years and a 7-valent conjugate vaccine comprising 7 polysaccharides, each conjugated to a carrier protein, of the 7 most common serotypes associated with community-acquired pneumonia and otitis media in infants and children younger than 2 years. The 7-valent conjugate vaccine is included now in the routine immunization program of all infants and children.

The emergence and continued frequent occurrence of penicillin resistant and multidrug-resistant strains underlie the urgency for the prevention of *S. pneumoniae* infection, especially in persons at high risk of serious disease. The 23-valent polysaccharide vaccine induces anticapsular antibodies sufficient to provide an efficacy rate of about 75% in immunocompetent adults and it can protect high-risk persons, especially from invasive disease. The 7-valent conjugate polysaccharide vaccine induces high levels of anticapsular antibodies in infants and children younger than 5 years and it is highly efficacious. In the first years after its introduction, the occurrence of invasive disease in infants and children declined substantially.

DIAGNOSTIC PROCEDURES
Pneumonia

Usually the initial diagnosis of *S. pneumoniae* pneumonia represents a presumptive clinical judgment on the basis of symptoms, signs, epidemiological findings, and the results of rapid laboratory tests, when available. Antibiotic treatment is begun based on expert empiric guidelines for the treatment of community-acquired pneumonia. Indisputable evidence of the specific etiological diagnosis of pneumococcal infection requires isolation of the organism from the blood or another otherwise sterile site, such as pleural fluid, but usually the results of these cultures are not available until the next day. Blood cultures must be done to assess the invasive nature of the infection; a single set of cultures obtained before the start of antibiotic treatment is adequate to isolate the organism. It is important to obtain cultures early before antibiotic treatment is begun and to test all *S. pneumoniae* strains recovered from sputum and blood, cerebrospinal fluid, and pleural fluid for susceptibility to penicillin and other antibiotics commonly used in the treatment of pneumococcal disease because of the increasing emergence of intermediate and high resistant strains worldwide. *Streptococcus pneumoniae* can be isolated also from respiratory tract secretions after overnight incubation of the culture. The finding of pneumococci in sputum or a nasal swab must be interpreted in light of their frequent carriage in the upper respiratory tract, and it adds some confidence in establishing a specific etiological diagnosis.

Laboratory procedures for rapid identification of *S. pneumoniae* infection include (1) recognition of the organism on a Gram-stained smear of respiratory secretions by its characteristic diploid, gram-positive lancet shape, which provides a reasonable degree of confidence in establishing the diagnosis, and (2) detection of pneumococcal antigens in urine. The detection of pneumococcal C-polysaccharide cell wall antigen in a urine specimen by a commercial immunochromatographic procedure (NOW *Streptococcus pneumoniae* Test) provides a highly sensitive and specific test for establishing the diagnosis in adults who become blood culture positive. The test involves dipping a special swab into a urine specimen at room temperature and applying the swab to an immunochromatographic membrane in a bookletlike device that is closed after the swab is set up. A positive test result, which must be read 15 minutes later, appears as a pink-to-purple colored line in a window on the cover of the booklet. In invasive disease, the test is about 80% to 85% sensitive and about 90% to 95% specific. It is, however, much less sensitive and specific in children with pneumococcal pneumonia.

Meningitis

By contrast, a specific diagnosis of pneumococcal meningitis can be confirmed quickly during the initial examination of the patient by identification of the organism on a Gram stain of cerebrospinal fluid or by detection of pneumococcal C-polysaccharide cell wall antigen in a cerebrospinal fluid specimen using the immunochromatographic NOW *Streptococcus pneumoniae* Test. This test is performed and read in the same manner as described for testing a urine specimen from patients in whom a diagnosis of pneumococcal pneumonia is suspected. However, in patients with pneumococcal meningitis, the test shows a very high sensitivity (100% or nearly so) and very high specificity (100% or nearly so) in both children and adults.

The availability of rapid diagnostic tests for the diagnosis of *S. pneumoniae* meningitis facilitates prompt initiation of appropriate antibiotic therapy while waiting for the results of the culture of the cerebrospinal fluid. Culture is necessary not only to provide definitive confirmation of *S. pneumoniae* infection but also to test the strain to determine whether it is resistant to penicillin or other antibiotics usually used in the treatment of pneumococcal meningitis.

Antibiotic Susceptibility Testing

Streptococcus pneumoniae strains are routinely tested for antibiotic susceptibility against a panel of antibiotics specified by the Clinical and Laboratory Standards Institute (CLSI, Wayne, PA) that includes penicillin, cefaclor, cefuroxime, cefotaxime, imipenem, ofloxacin,

erythromycin, tetracycline, chloramphenicol, trimethoprim–sulfamethoxazole, and vancomycin. Automated procedures can be used to determine the minimum inhibitory concentration (MIC) of each strain to all of these antibiotics. The MIC of an *S. pneumoniae* strain can be determined readily by the E-test (AB Biodisk, Solna, Sweden) in which a penicillin-impregnated plastic-coated paper strip is placed on a blood agar plate inoculated with the strain to produce a semiconfluent growth (Figure 145.1). After incubation for 24 hours in a 5% CO_2 atmosphere, the MIC is read on the scale printed on the E-strip at the point that the ellipsoid zone of inhibition intersects the strip. The MIC level for penicillin-susceptible strains is ≤0.06 µg/mL, for intermediate resistant strains is 0.1 to 1 µg/mL, and for highly resistant strains is ≥2 µg/mL. All penicillin intermediate and highly resistant strains are tested for MIC to cefaclor, cefuroxime, cefotaxime, and imipenem using E-test strips for these antibiotics. Also, all *S. pneumoniae* strains are tested against the panel of antibiotics specified by the CLSI using the Kirby–Bauer disk diffusion method, including ofloxacin (5 µg), erythromycin (15 µg), tetracycline (30 µg), chloramphenicol (30 µg), trimethoprim–sulfamethoxazole (1.25 µg/23.75 µg), and vancomycin (30 µg).

INFECTIONS DUE TO THE PNEUMOCOCCUS

Pneumonia

IMPORTANCE

Streptococcus pneumoniae pneumonia accounts for about two thirds of the community-acquired pneumonias. Invasive infection develops in about one fifth of the pneumococcal pneumonias or about 500 000 cases annually. The incidence of invasive pneumococcal pneumonia is highest in children younger than 4 years and adults 60 years of age and older. In children younger than 4 years, the incidence of bacteremic pneumococcal pneumonia is about 45 to 60 cases per 100 000 population, and in adults 60 years of age and older it ranges from 30 to 75 cases per 100 000 population. The overall case fatality rate in invasive pneumococcal pneumonia is about 15% to 25%. It is higher in older adults and the elderly, varying between 20% and 35%. Underlying diseases that pose a special risk of serious pneumococcal pneumonia include immunodeficiency syndromes, splenic dysfunction, splenectomy, acute alcoholism,

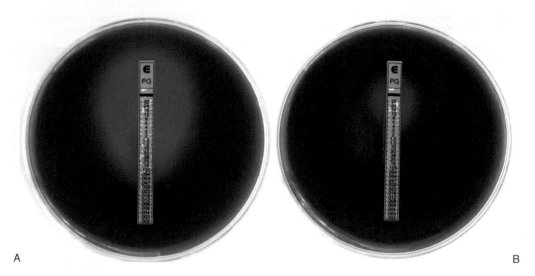

Figure 145.1 Blood agar plates with confluent growth of *S. pneumoniae*. (A) A susceptible strain; (B) an intermediate resistant strain.

delirium tremens, Lannaec cirrhosis, chronic obstructive pulmonary disease, congestive heart failure, and malignancy. Because of the high case fatality rate in invasive pneumococcal pneumonia, these cases need to be treated promptly and aggressively. In children, the case fatality rate in invasive pneumococcal pneumonia is less than 1%. Nonbacteremic pneumococcal pneumonia holds little risk of death, and overall in these cases the case fatality rate is less than about 4%.

Clinical and Laboratory Findings

Usually, pneumococcal pneumonia begins suddenly with a severe shaking chill or rigor in most persons, followed almost immediately by sustained fever of 102°F to 105°F. Cough, productive of rusty sputum, and pleuritic chest pain occur in three fourths of patients. Dyspnea is common, and patients may lie on the affected side to splint the involved lung. Malaise, weakness, anorexia, and prostration are common. Patients with pneumococcal pneumonia appear toxic and manifest fever, tachycardia, tachypnea, and shallow respirations. Auscultation of the chest reveals signs of bronchopneumonia or consolidation. A lower lobe pneumonia may give rise to abdominal pain. Extrapulmonary infection may occur, including meningitis, endocarditis, and arthritis.

Often leukocytosis is present with an increased number of neutrophils and band forms, although leukopenia may develop in overwhelming infections and in elderly patients. A chest roentgenogram shows the extent and character of the pneumonia and the presence of pleural fluid, especially very small accumulations.

Course and Treatment

With appropriate antibiotic treatment the earliest response is usually seen within 12 to 36 hours, but sometimes it takes up to 96 hours. Fever defervesces first followed by amelioration of the respiratory rate, cough, and chest pain. However, resolution of radiographic findings occurs during the ensuing 2 to 3 weeks and usually it is complete.

As *S. pneumoniae* is the dominant pathogen of community-acquired pneumonia, deciding on a treatment regimen for community-acquired pneumonia involves two key points: (1) judging the likelihood that *S. pneumoniae* is the pathogen and whether it is resistant to penicillin or other antibiotics, because as many as one third of the *S. pneumoniae* strains exhibit intermediate or high resistance to penicillin, depending on the individual community, and (2) applying a validated quantitative severity score for assessing the severity of the pneumonia, as an adjunct to clinical judgement.

Because *S. pneumoniae* is frequently suspected as the pathogen of community-acquired pneumonia on clinical grounds, sometimes aided by the results of rapid diagnostic procedures, the likelihood is that the physician will not know whether the strain is penicillin susceptible or resistant until cultures become

Table 145.1 Recommended Antibiotic Treatment Regimens for *S. pneumoniae*[a] Pneumonia When the Diagnosis Is Suspected on Clinical Findings or Confirmed by Laboratory Procedures or a Positive Blood Culture

Severity of Pneumonia	Recommended Antibiotic Choices	Recommended Antibiotic Dosages
Ambulatory; healthy young adult lacking comorbid conditions and no antibiotic treatment recently	1. A macrolide or 2. Doxycycline	1. Azithromycin, 500 mg on day 1, 250 mg PO days 2–5, clarithromycin, 500 mg PO q12h for 7–14 d, or erythromycin, 500 mg PO q12h for 7–14 d or 2. Doxycycline, 100 mg PO q12h for 7–14 d
Ambulatory, older adult (60 years of age and older), with comorbid conditions or recent treatment with antibiotics	1. A fluoroquinolone with antipneumococcal activity or 2. Amoxicillin–clavulanate, amoxicillin, or cefuroxime plus a macrolide	1. Levofloxacin, 750 mg PO q24h for 5 d; gatifloxacin, 400 mg PO q24h for 7–14 d; moxifloxacin, 400 mg PO q24h for 7–14 d; or gemifloxacin, 320 mg PO q24h for 7 d; or, 2. Amoxicillin–clavulanate 875 mg/125 mg PO q12h for 7–14 d; amoxicillin 875 mg PO q12h for 7–14 d; or cefuroxime axetil 500 mg PO q12h for 7–14 d, plus azithromycin or clarithromycin as described above.
In-hospital admission, adult with or without comorbid conditions, or with or without recent treatment with antibiotics	1. A fluoroquinolone with anti-pneumococcal activity or 2. A β-lactam, either ceftriaxone or cefotaxime; plus a macrolide	1. Levofloxacin, gatifloxacin, or moxifloxacin, PO or IV, dosed as described above; or, 2. Ceftriaxone, 1–2 g IV or IM q24h for 7–14 d, cefotaxime, 1–2 g IV q8h for 7–14 d, plus azithromycin, 500 mg IV, then PO, q24h for 7–10 d or clarithromycin, dosed as described above.

[a] Penicillin-susceptible *S. pneumoniae* and intermediate and highly penicillin-resistant *S. pneumoniae* with MICs 4 µg/mL or less can be treated with these regimens. Highly penicillin-resistant *S. pneumoniae* strains with MICs greater than 4 µg/mL occur uncommonly and require antibiotic treatment based on antibiotic susceptibility determinations.

positive. Consequently, appropriate antibiotic treatment must be started based on guidelines for the empiric antibiotic treatment of community-acquired pneumonia (Table 145.1). Importantly, invasive pneumococcal pneumonia caused by intermediate and resistant strains with MICs <4 µg/mL can be successfully treated with antibiotic regimens that are employed to treat penicillin-susceptible strains.

Quantitative measures for assessing severity of pneumonia facilitate determining the clinical approach to the patient with community-acquired pneumonia and can validate clinical judgment of severity. One such assessment is the CURB-65 score, which assigns 1 point to each of 5 measures, all of which are readily obtainable at the first examination, namely new onset confusion, blood urea nitrogen greater than 7 mmol/L, respiratory rate equal or greater than 30/min, systolic blood pressure less than 90 mm Hg or diastolic blood pressure equal to or less than 60 mm Hg, and age equal to or greater than 65 years. A score of 3, 4, or 5 represents severe pneumonia with

a high risk of death that must be managed in the hospital; a score of 2 represents less severe pneumonia, but one that carries an increased risk of death (these cases should be managed in the hospital); and a score of 0 or 1 represents mild pneumonia that can be managed on an ambulatory basis.

Adults with pneumonia judged to be mild, for example, those with a CURB-65 score of 0 or 1 and who are younger than 60 years and otherwise healthy, can be treated on an ambulatory basis, and the choice of an antibiotic regimen is a macrolide, such as azithromycin, clarithromycin or erythromycin, or doxycycline (Table 145.1). If the infecting pneumococcal strain is grown in culture and it is penicillin sensitive or intermediate resistant, the antibiotic can be changed to amoxicillin–clavulanate, 875 mg/125 mg orally every 12 hours for 7 to 14 days.

Adults, especially elderly adults, with more severe pneumonia, for example, with a CURB-65 score of 2, 3, 4, or 5, require hospitalization and need to be treated with combination antibiotic therapy, namely a third-generation cephalosporin, such as ceftriaxone or cefotaxime, plus a macrolide, such as azithromycin or clarithromycin (Table 145.1). However, until the strain of *S. pneumoniae* can be isolated and tested for antibiotic sensitivity, the physician must choose an appropriate antibiotic regimen on an empiric basis. Although pneumonia due to penicillin high-resistant strains with an MIC between 2 and 4 µg/mL might well respond to very high doses of penicillin G, the more appropriate approach to treatment is either a fluoroquinolone alone, such as levofloxacin, 750 mg IV or orally daily for 5 days, gatifloxacin, 400 mg IV every 24 hours or orally for 7 to 14 days, moxifloxacin, 400 mg IV or orally every 24 hours for 7 to 14 days, or combination therapy of ceftriaxone, 1 to 2 g IV or IM every 24 hours for 7 to 14 days, or cefotaxime, 1 to 2 g IV or orally every 8 hours for 7 to 14 days, plus a macrolide, such as azithromycin, 500 mg IV every 24 hours for 2 or more days and then orally for a total of 7 to 10 days, or clarithromycin, 500 mg orally every 12 hours for 7 to 14 days. When blood cultures become positive for *S. pneumoniae*, these patients are likely to be continued on empiric therapy. As the patient improves, cephalosporin antibiotics administered IV can be changed to an appropriate oral cephalosporin, such as cefuroxime–axetil. Highly penicillin-resistant *S. pneumoniae* strains with MICs greater than 4 µg/mL occur uncommonly and require antibiotic treatment based on antibiotic susceptibility determinations.

Analysis of data from several retrospective observational studies of the treatment of invasive pneumococcal pneumonia showed that combination antibiotic therapy initiated on an empiric basis with a macrolide plus a penicillin or cephalosporin appeared to result in fewer deaths than treatment with a penicillin or cephalosporin alone. This point of view has evoked controversy for several reasons: (1) penicillin-sensitive and penicillin intermediate and highly resistant strains of *S. pneumoniae* (MICs of 1 to 4 µg/mL) respond well to treatment with a penicillin or a third-generation cephalosporin; (2) observational studies contain inherent biases; and (3) the mechanisms by which such combination antibiotic therapy reduces the case fatality rate in invasive pneumococcal pneumonia remains unclear. Consequently, this issue is unsettled, and prospective randomized trials are needed to resolve this controversy. However, until such trials can be carried out, combination antibiotic therapy with a third-generation cephalosporin and a macrolide remains a reasonable choice for severely ill adults with community-acquired pneumococcal pneumonia and especially those with invasive disease (Table 145.1).

Meningitis

IMPORTANCE AND CLINICAL FINDINGS

Pneumococcal meningitis, the most common meningitis in adults and children, occurs in persons of all ages. It occurs mainly in older adults and it is fatal in about 20% to 30% of cases depending on the adult population studied. The highest case fatality rates occur in persons older than 50 years. Among children, the case fatality rate is about 10%, substantially higher than the case fatality rate in invasive pneumococcal pneumonia, but about one third of the children who survive meningitis develop neurological abnormalities. Because many patients have a bacteremia, it is important to search not only for a primary source of infection in these patients but also for metastatic localization. Among elderly persons, the symptoms of meningitis may be moderated and include confounding findings such as a stiff-feeling neck because of arthritic changes in the cervical vertebrae. The clinical symptoms of meningeal inflammation include fever, headache, and stiff neck and the presence of a Kernig or Brudzinski sign or both; elevated cerebrospinal fluid pressure, frequent neutrophils, glucose level <40 mg/mL and total protein about 100 mg/mL; and neurologic complications, including seizures and cranial nerve abnormalities. The disease can ensue as a complication of *S. pneumoniae* invasive pneumonia, purulent mastoiditis and sinusitis, endocarditis, asplenia, sickle cell disease, and alcoholism or a skull fracture with communication between the nasopharynx and the subarachnoid space. PCV 7 (7-valent protein-conjugated pneumococcal polysaccharide vaccine [Prevnar]) covers about 80% of the capsular serotypes that cause meningitis in children.

Pneumococcal meningitis is a medical emergency, and patients suspected of having this disease require immediate diagnosis and treatment. The clinical diagnosis of meningitis almost always seems apparent on the basis of clinical findings alone. However, a specific etiologic diagnosis of pneumococcal meningitis requires confirmation by laboratory procedures, and this can be done in almost all cases by recognition of the typical morphology of *S. pneumoniae* on a Gram smear of cerebrospinal fluid or by testing the fluid by the rapid immunochromatographic NOW *Streptococcus pneumoniae* Test or both. Nonetheless, the infecting strain needs to be

Table 145.2 Recommended Antibiotic Treatment Regimens for *S. pneumoniae* Meningitis

Age Group	Recommended Antibiotic Choices	Recommended Antibiotic Dosages
Child	Ceftriaxone, or cefotaxime* plus vancomycin**	Ceftriaxone, 50 mg/kg IV q12h, or cefotaxime[a], 50 mg/kg IV q6h plus vancomycin, 15 mg/kg IV q6h[b]
Child with penicillin allergy	Chloramphenicol plus vancomycin	Chloramphenicol, 1 g IV q6h plus vancomycin 15 mg/kg IV q6h
Adult	Ceftriaxone, or cefotaxime plus vancomycin plus dexamethasone[c] Maybe plus rifampin	Ceftriaxone, 2 g IV q12h, or cefotaxime, 2 g IV q4h plus vancomycin, 1 g IV q12h plus dexamethasone 10 mg IV q4h for 4 d[c] Maybe plus rifampin, 300 mg PO q12h
Adult with penicillin allergy	Chloramphenicol plus vancomycin Maybe plus rifampin	Chloramphenicol, 1 g IV q6h plus vancomycin, 500–750 mg IV q6h Maybe plus rifampin, 300 mg PO q12h

[a] *Streptococcus pneumoniae* isolated from cerebrospinal fluid must be tested for antibiotic susceptibility and changes in antibiotic treatment should be based on these results. Most intermediate and highly penicillin-resistant *S. pneumoniae* respond to these third-generation cephalosporins because they achieve levels in the cerebrospinal fluid above the MIC of most of these strains.
[b] One recent retrospective study found an association with increased risk of hearing loss in children treated with vancomycin early (median time less than 1 hour) and proposed starting vancomycin 2 hours or later after the first dose of ceftriaxone or cefotaxime.
[c] The European Dexamethasone in Acute Bacterial Meningitis Study recently reported that adults with pneumococcal meningitis treated with adjunctive dexamethasone, 10 mg IV q4h for 4 days, had significantly fewer deaths compared with the placebo-treated group. Its use as adjunctive therapy in children with pneumococcal meningitis remains unresolved.

isolated so that antibiotic susceptibility tests can be done.

Treatment

Adults and children need to be treated with combination therapy, including a third-generation cephalosporin and vancomycin (Table 145.2). Among adults with a suspected or proven penicillin resistant or multidrug-resistant meningitis, the treatment includes a third-generation cephalosporin, such as ceftriaxone, 2 g IV every 12 hours, plus vancomycin, 15 mg/kg every 24 hours (Table 145.2). Vancomycin should be used when a penicillin- or multidrug-resistant infection is suspected or proved; indiscriminate use of vancomycin can encourage the emergence of resistant isolates. The European Dexamethasone in Acute Bacterial Meningitis Study recently reported that adults with pneumococcal meningitis treated with adjunctive dexamethasone, 10 mg IV every 4 hours for 4 days, had significantly fewer deaths compared with the placebo-treated group. When a highly penicillin-resistant or multidrug-resistant infection is suspected or proven in children, the treatment includes a third-generation cephalosporin, such as ceftriaxone, 200 m/kg/day IV, plus vancomycin,

15 mg/kg/day IV every 6 hours. One recent retrospective study found an association with increased risk of hearing loss in children treated with vancomycin early (median time less than 1 hour) and proposed starting vancomycin 2 hours or later after the first dose of ceftriaxone or cefotaxime. Dexamethasone use as adjunctive therapy in children with pneumococcal meningitis remains unresolved.

Otitis Media

IMPORTANCE AND TREATMENT

Streptococcus penumoniae ranks among the top three common pathogens of acute otitis media (AOM) in children (the other pathogens are *Hemophilus influenzae* and *Moraxella catarrhalis*) and penicillin-resistant *S. pneumoniae* represents an increasing problem in the treatment of otitis media. In children with a penicillin-susceptible pneumococcal AOM, amoxicillin, 80 mg/kg/day, remains the first-line therapy; other treatment regimens (especially for children who fail this therapy) include amoxicillin–clavulanate, 45 mg/kg/day, oral cefuroxime–axetil, or ceftriaxone, 50 mg IM every 24 hours. When penicillin-resistant strains are suspected, treat with amoxicillin–clavulanate or intramuscular ceftriaxone.

In adults, AOM can be treated with amoxicillin–clavulanate, erythromycin, azithromycin, clarithromycin, or sulfamethoxazole–trimethoprim. When penicillin-resistant strains are the likely pathogen, treat with azithromycin or clarithromycin.

Pneumococcal Polysaccharide Vaccine

Currently, two pneumococcal vaccines are licensed for general use: the first is a 23-valent pneumococcal polysaccharide (Pneumovax 23) (PPV23) approved by the Food and Drug Administration (FDA) in 1983 for administration to persons at high risk of serious pneumococcal infection, including all adults 65 years of age and older, and the second is a PCV7 approved by the FDA in 2000 for administration to infants and children as a routine childhood immunization.

PPV23 is safe, cost-effective, and efficacious, with an overall efficacy rate of about 65% to 75% in immunocompetent adults for vaccine serotypes. The 23 serotypes included in PPV23 represent the most common serotypes that occur among children and adults and cause approximately 90% of the invasive disease in the United States. PPV23 should be offered to all persons age 65 years and older, all persons residing in nursing homes or other chronic care facilities, and all immunocompetent persons 2 years of age and older with underlying disease, including heart and lung diseases, renal disease, and diabetes mellitus, that place them at increased risk of serious pneumococcal pneumonia. It also should be offered to all immunocompromised persons, including persons with functional and anatomic asplenia, lymphoma, leukemia, and human immunodeficiency virus (HIV).

The dose of PPV23 is 0.5 mL injected subcutaneously or intramuscularly in the deltoid muscle or the lateral midthigh muscles. Injection site reactions occur infrequently, including soreness, erythema, swelling, and induration and an injection site cellulitislike reaction. Systemic reactions are uncommon. PPV23 can be administered at any time of the year (not exclusively in the fall when influenza vaccine is available) but most doses of PPV23 are administered at this time, and persons who need both vaccines often receive PPV23 together with influenza vaccine at a different injection site with equivalent antibody responses.

Routine revaccination with PPV23 is not recommended. However, a second dose of PPV23 is recommended for persons 65 years of age and older who received their first dose of vaccine before 65 years of age and at least 5 years earlier; for persons who received only the 14-valent vaccine; and for persons 2 years of age and older judged at highest risk of developing serious pneumococcal disease and most likely to exhibit a rapid decline in antibody, including those with functional and anatomic asplenia, lymphoma, leukemia, HIV, multiple myeloma, malignancy, or nephrotic syndrome and chronic renal failure, and persons undergoing chronic renal hemodialysis. Antibodies wane in time in all adults, and second doses of vaccine provide satisfactory booster responses. Injection site reactions occur somewhat more frequently after revaccination than after primary vaccination.

PCV7 is safe and highly efficacious (efficacy rate 100% for preventing invasive disease due vaccine serotypes and efficacy rate about 57% for preventing otitis media due to vaccine serotypes) in preventing AOM and invasive pneumococcal disease. PCV7 is routinely administered to all infants starting at 2 months of age. The vaccine contains purified capsular polysaccharide for 7 serotypes, namely 4, 6B, 9V, 14, 18C, 19F, and 23F, each conjugated to nontoxic diphtheria protein carrier CRM_{197} (the quantity of diphtheria toxin is insufficient to provide a booster effect). The recommended routine immunization schedule is 2, 4, 6, and 12 to 15 months of age, and the dose is 0.5 mL intramuscularly. PCV7 is associated with few injection site reactions (10% to 20%), including erythema, tenderness, and induration. However, systemic reactions occurred more frequently, including fever equal or greater than 38°C (100.4°F) (21%), irritability (45%), drowsiness (33%), restless sleep (21%), decreased appetite (18%), vomiting (13%), diarrhea (10%), and rash (0.6%).

The seven capsular serotypes comprising PCV7 account for about 50% to 60% of the invasive infections in children and about 75% of invasive infections in children 2 years of age and younger. Six of the vaccine serotypes/serogroups, namely 4, 6, 9, 14, 19, and 23, account for nearly all of the intermediate and high-resistant strains that infect children. PCV7 is not recommended for children 5 years of age and older.

SUGGESTED READING

Buckingham SC, McCullers JA, Lujan-Zilbermann J, et al. Early vancomycin therapy and adverse outcomes in children with pneumococcal meningitis. *Pediatrics.* 2006;117:1688–1694.

Clinical and Laboratory Standards Institute. Performance Standards for Antimicrobial Susceptibility Testing; Sixteenth Informational Supplement. M100–S16. CLSI, Wayne, Pennsylvania. Performance Standards for Antimicrobial Susceptibility Testing; Sixteenth Informational Supplement. M100–S16. CLSI, Wayne, Pennsylvania. 2006.

File TM, Garau J, Blasi F, et al. Guidelines for empiric antimicrobial prescribing in community-acquired pneumonia. *Chest*. 2004;125:1888–1901.

Lim WS, van der Eerden MM, Laing R, et al. Defining community acquired pneumonia severity on presentation to hospital: an international derivation and validation study. *Thorax*. 2003;58:377–382.

Mandell LA, Bartlett JG, Dowell SF, et al. Update of practice guidelines for the management of community-acquired pneumonia in immunocompetent adults. *Clin Infect Dis*. 2003;37:1405–1433.

Mufson MA, Stanek RJ. Bacteremic pneumococcal pneumonia in one American city: a 20-year longitudinal study, 1978-1997. *Am J Med*. 1999;107:34S–43S.

Saha SK, Darmstadt GL, Yamanaka N, et al. Rapid diagnosis of pneumococcal meningitis implications for treatment and measuring disease burden. *Ped Infect Dis J*. 2005;24:1093–1098.

Stanek RJ, Mufson MA. A 20-year epidemiological study of pneumococcal meningitis. *Clin Infect Dis*. 1999;28:1265–1272.

Waterer GW. Optimal antibiotic treatment in severe pneumococcal pneumonia - time for real answers. *Eur J Clin Microbiol Infect Dis*. 2005;24:691–692.

Weisfelt M, van de Beek D, de Gans J. Dexamethasone treatment in adults with pneumococcal meningitis: risk factors for death. *Eur J Clin Microbiol Infect Dis*. 2006;25:73–78.

146. *Pseudomonas, Stenotrophomonas,* and *Burkholderia*

Titus L. Daniels and David W. Gregory

Pseudomonas aeruginosa is an aerobic, gram-negative bacillus with a diversified ecologic niche. *Pseudomonas aeruginosa* is highly pathogenic among immunocompromised patients and is responsible for substantial morbidity and mortality. *Pseudomonas aeruginosa* is principally a health care–associated pathogen, although community-onset infection has been described among immunocompetent and immunocompromised patients (ie, neutropenia, human immunodeficiency virus [HIV], acquired immunodeficiency syndrome [AIDS]). Such patients may be encountered by primary care and subspecialty physicians alike, and diagnosis requires a high index of suspicion. Infections commonly associated with *P. aeruginosa* include pneumonias, bloodstream infections (BSI), urinary tract infections, and surgical site infections (Table 146.1). Two related species, *Stenotrophomonas maltophilia* and *Burkholderia cepacia*, are briefly discussed.

EPIDEMIOLOGY

The epidemiology of *P. aeruginosa* infections reflects its predilection for moist environments. In hospitals, *P. aeruginosa* has been isolated from respiratory devices, disinfectants, distilled and tap water, and sinks. *Pseudomonas aeruginosa* can readily colonize the upper respiratory tract of mechanically ventilated patients, the gastrointestinal tract of patients receiving chemotherapy or broad-spectrum antibiotics, and the wounds of burn patients. Colonization usually precedes invasive infection.

Among health care–associated infections occurring in intensive care units, *P. aeruginosa* is the most commonly identified gram-negative pathogen, and the second most commonly identified organism overall. Emergence and spread of antimicrobial resistance, especially multidrug resistance (MDR), among *P. aeruginosa* is frequent. The National Nosocomial Infections Surveillance System 2003 report revealed that 29.5% of intensive care unit isolates are resistant to quinolones and 31.9% are resistant to third-generation cephalosporins. Furthermore, 21.1% of the isolates are resistant

Table 146.1 Risk Factors for *P. aeruginosa* Infections

Type of Infection	Setting
Bacteremia	Neutropenia, pulmonary or urinary tract focus, burns
Pneumonia	Mechanical ventilation, neutropenia, chronic lung disease
Endocarditis	Injection drug use, prosthetic heart valve
Meningitis, brain abscess	Hematogenous or contiguous spread, neurosurgery, penetrating head trauma
Urinary tract infection	Bladder instrumentation
Osteomyelitis, septic arthritis (eg, sternoclavicular joint)	Contiguous or hematogenous spread, injection drug use
Osteochondritis	Puncture wounds of the feet
Malignant external otitis	Diabetes, advanced age
Green nail syndrome	Water immersion, wet skin

to imipenem, an agent once considered universally active against *P. aeruginosa*. The emergence and spread of MDR *P. aeruginosa* challenges the clinician when selecting appropriate antimicrobial therapy and underscores the importance of obtaining cultures with susceptibility testing in patients suspected to have bacterial infections. Knowledge of local antimicrobial resistance trends is essential to ensure optimal patient outcomes.

DIAGNOSIS

The clinical features of *P. aeruginosa* infections are indistinguishable from those of other bacterial organisms, and a definitive diagnosis requires specimen cultures from the suspected site of infection (ie, blood, sputum, urine) to identify the organism. Other clinically important gram-negative organisms that resemble *P. aeruginosa* come from the genera *Stenotrophomonas, Burkholderia,* and *Ralstonia.*

Table 146.2 Antimicrobial Agents for *P. aeruginosa*

Antimicrobial Agent	Dose[a]/Route /Interval	Comment
β-Lactams		
Ticarcillin–clavulanate	3.1 g IV q 4–6h	
Piperacillin	3–4 g IV q4–6h	
Piperacillin–tazobactam	4.5 g IV q6h	Recommended pneumonia dose
	3.375 g IV q6h	Recommended nonpneumonia dose
Ceftazidime	2 g IV q8h	Preferred agent for CNS infections
Cefepime	2 g IV q12h	
Meropenem	1 g IV q8h	
Imipenem–cilastatin	0.5 g IV q6h	
Aztreonam	2 g IV q8h	Frequently reserved for penicillin-allergic patients
Quinolones		
Ciprofloxacin	400 mg IV q12h 500–750 mg PO q12h	Most active antipseudomonal quinolone in vivo
Levofloxacin	750 mg IV/PO daily	
Aminoglycosides[b,c,d]		
Amikacin	15 mg/kg IV once daily or 7.5 mg/kg IV q12h	
Gentamicin	5 mg/kg IV once daily or 2 mg/kg loading dose, then 1.7 mg/kg IV q8h	
Tobramycin	5 mg/kg IV once daily or 2 mg/kg loading dose, then 1.7 mg/kg IV q8h	
Polymyxins		
Polymyxin E (colistin)	1.5 mg/kg IV q8h	
Polymyxin B	0.75–1.25 mg/kg IV q12h	

[a] Suggested dosing is for adult patients with normal renal and hepatic function.
[b] Aminoglycosides are not recommended for monotherapy against *P. aeruginosa*.
[c] Once-daily aminoglycoside dosing has been shown to be effective, less nephrotoxic and less ototoxic, and is the preferred dosing method.
[d] Aminoglycoside levels and renal function should also be closely monitored during therapy.
Abbreviation: CNS = central nervous system.

ANTIMICROBIAL THERAPY

Initial selection of an agent should be guided by the site of infection, the patient's allergic history, and the institutional antibiogram. Early, aggressive antimicrobial therapy, with modification when susceptibility results become available, imparts a survival advantage and minimizes the emergence of antimicrobial resistance. Although several antipseudomonal antibiotics exist (Table 146.2), intrinsic or acquired resistance and bacterial persistence at sites of infection complicate management and eradication.

β-lactam antibiotics active against *P. aeruginosa* include the extended-spectrum penicillins, some extended-spectrum cephalosporins, the carbapenems (except ertapenem), and the mono-bactam aztreonam. These agents form the basis for treatment of most *Pseudomonas* infections due to extensive clinical experience and patient tolerability. The high prevalence of reported penicillin allergy is the primary limitation.

The aminoglycosides tobramycin, amikacin, and gentamicin have excellent in vitro activity against *P. aeruginosa*. The concentration-dependent bactericidal activity and the postantibiotic effect of aminoglycosides provide the rationale for once-daily dosing. Aminoglycoside monotherapy should be avoided due to selection of resistant mutants and increased risk of clinical failure. Renal function and serum aminoglycoside levels should be monitored closely.

The quinolones have been frequently used for the treatment of *P. aeruginosa* and other bacteria. They possess excellent tissue penetration, good oral bioavailability, and a favorable safety profile. Ciprofloxacin and levofloxacin are the most active quinolones against *P. aeruginosa*, with ciprofloxacin considered the more active of the two. Increasing resistance to the quinolones, however, should temper heavy reliance on their use as the basis for empiric therapy against *P. aeruginosa*.

Use of polymyxin antibiotics has re-emerged due to MDR and pandrug-resistant gram-negative infections, including *P. aeruginosa*. The polymyxins possess activity against a variety of gram-negative organisms but have been limited in use due to their adverse effects, namely nephrotoxicity and neurotoxicity. Polymyxins are currently recommended only for isolates resistant to other antibiotics. Susceptibility testing should be performed as resistance to the polymyxins has been reported.

Much controversy exists over the use of combination therapy ("double-coverage") for the treatment of infections due to *P. aeruginosa*. Data from a Cochrane review of sepsis comparing β-lactam and aminoglycoside combination therapy versus β-lactam monotherapy found no advantage to combination therapy for all-cause mortality (RR 1.01; 95% CI 0.75–1.35) or clinical failure (RR 1.11; 95% CI 0.95–1.29). Empiric combination therapy for most serious infections may still be warranted when considering local resistance data and to ensure appropriate treatment of other possible infecting organisms. The guiding principle for selecting combination therapy should be that each agent has a unique mechanism of action to avoid a possible antagonistic effect; β-lactam and aminoglycoside combination therapies are the most studied and continue to be primarily recommended.

INFECTIONS CAUSED BY *P. AERUGINOSA*

Respiratory Infections

Pseudomonas aeruginosa pneumonia may follow colonization of patients in the setting of mechanical ventilation, antibiotic administration, neutropenia, AIDS, and chronic pulmonary disease, particularly in patients with cystic fibrosis (Table 146.3). Lower respiratory tract infection may be distinguished from airway colonization by an increase in quantity and purulence of respiratory secretions. Clinical manifestations may be fulminant with fever, chills, dyspnea, productive cough, and systemic toxicity. Diffuse bronchopneumonia with nodular infiltrates is commonly seen on chest radiograph. Cavitary lesions may occasionally be seen. Pneumonia may be accompanied by bacteremia, particularly in neutropenic patients. Empiric antimicrobial treatment in the hospitalized or neutropenic patient with fever and lung infiltrate should include coverage for *P. aeruginosa*. Conventional antimicrobial therapy for *P. aeruginosa* pneumonia includes an antipseudomonal β-lactam combined with an aminoglycoside or a quinolone. Inhaled tobramycin (300 mg every 12 hours) may be considered as adjunctive therapy.

Patients with cystic fibrosis are prone to chronic lower respiratory infections with mucoid strains of *P. aeruginosa*. These infections usually persist for a lifetime, with frequent acute exacerbations manifested by decreased exercise tolerance, increased cough and sputum, and weight loss. Therapy consists of an antipseudomonal penicillin containing ticarcillin or piperacillin plus an aminoglycoside. These patients may require large doses because of altered pharmacokinetics. Aggressive physiotherapy, nutrition, and hydration are essential.

Bloodstream Infections (BSI)

BSI may complicate *P. aeruginosa* infections at other sites. Predisposing factors include neutropenia, hematologic malignancy, organ transplantation, vascular and urinary tract catheterization, and antibiotic use. The lower respiratory tract is the most common source of *Pseudomonas* bacteremia, followed by skin, soft tissues, and the urinary tract. Evaluation

Table 146.3 Management of *Pseudomonas aeruginosa* Infections

Infection	Antibiotics[a]	Adjunctive
Meningitis	Ceftazidime[b] + AG	Intrathecal AG
Bacteremia	AP-BL + AG or FQ	Identify source
Endocarditis	AP-BL + AG or FQ	Valvulectomy for persistent bacteremia
Pneumonia	AP-BL + AG or FQ	Aggressive respiratory care
Malignant external otitis	AP-BL + AG or FQ	Surgical debridement may be necessary
Osteomyelitis	AP-BL + AG or FQ	Surgical debridement
Urinary tract	FQ alone or AP-BL ± AG	Remove catheter

Abbreviations: AP-BL = antipseudomonal β-lactam; AG = aminoglycoside; FQ = fluoroquinolone (ie, ciprofloxacin or levofloxacin).
[a] Recommended antibiotics for empiric coverage against *P. aeruginosa*. Therapy should be refined once susceptibility data are available.
[b] Aztreonam may be used for patients with penicillin or cephalosporin allergy. Other AP-BL do not achieve reliable cerebrospinal fluid concentrations.

should include an aggressive search for the source of the bacteremia.

No distinct clinical characteristics differentiate *P. aeruginosa* BSI from other gram-negative bacteremias. Most patients have fever, tachycardia, and tachypnea. Many have signs of systemic toxicity with hypotension, shock, disseminated intravascular coagulopathy, and altered mental status. Skin manifestations include papules, bullae, and, rarely, ecthyma gangrenosum (Figure 146.1), a focal skin lesion characterized by hemorrhage, necrosis, and vascular invasion by bacteria. Prompt initiation of combination antimicrobial therapy is crucial because there is a high mortality. Therapy should continue for 2 to 3 weeks in seriously ill patients.

Infective Endocarditis

Infective endocarditis caused by *P. aeruginosa* occurs primarily in the setting of injection drug use and occasionally with prosthetic heart valves. Injection drug users acquire this organism from nonsterile diluents such as tap water or nonsterile paraphernalia. Bacteremia with fever is invariable present. Tricuspid valve infection, which is typical, commonly presents with signs of septic pulmonary embolism. If treatment is early and aggressive with effective antibiotics, cure may be achieved without surgery. Tricuspid valvulectomy may be necessary in the event of bacteriologic failure or recurrence. Involvement of the aortic and mitral

valves may manifest as a severe acute illness with sepsis and large arterial emboli necessitating early surgical valve replacement in addition to antimicrobial treatment. Combination therapy with a β-lactam agent and an aminoglycoside in high doses (eg, tobramycin, 8 mg/kg/day) is recommended. Antibiotic therapy should be continued for at least 6 weeks.

Urinary Tract Infections

Pseudomonas aeruginosa is the third most common nosocomial urinary pathogen. These infections are most commonly associated with indwelling urinary catheters. Bacteremia, a common complication, may lead to metastatic infection (eg, vertebral osteomyelitis). Symptomatic urinary tract infections should be treated by removing the catheter when possible and by administering an antibiotic. Monotherapy with an antipseudomonal β-lactam or a quinolone suffices unless there is secondary bacteremia or upper urinary tract infection. Oral quinolones may be used successfully even in complicated urinary tract infections. A 7- to 10-day course of treatment is adequate for uncomplicated cases. Longer courses, at least 2 to 3 weeks, are necessary for pyelonephritis, renal abscess, or complicating bacteremia. Asymptomatic bacteriuria need not always require treatment. Eradication of the bacteriuria is often impossible if the patient has an anatomic abnormality or a foreign body,

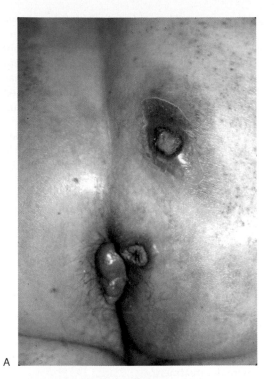

A

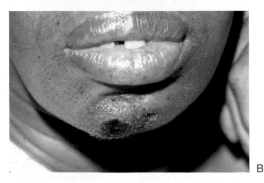

B

Figure 146.1 Ecthyma gangrenosum. (A) Lesions with ulceration and surrounding erythema. (B) A more classic lesion with necrosis and surrounding erythema.

and antibiotics in this setting may select only resistant organisms.

Meningitis

Pseudomonas aeruginosa is a rare cause of meningitis and brain abscess. Infection may occur by (1) extension from a contiguous structure such as mastoid or sinuses, (2) direct inoculation from penetrating trauma or neurosurgical procedures, or (3) metastatic spread from a distant site. Ceftazidime is the antimicrobial of choice because of its excellent in vitro activity and its ability to penetrate cerebrospinal fluid (CSF). Aztreonam and the carbapenems have good in vitro activity, but experience with these agents is limited. Addition of an aminoglycoside may be justified on the basis of possibly conferring synergy and preventing emergence of antibiotic resistance. Because of poor penetration of aminoglycosides into CSF, intrathecal or intraventricular doses may be required. There are anecdotal reports of successful therapy with parenteral ciprofloxacin, but quinolones should be used only when other antibiotics have failed or when organisms are resistant to β-lactam agents. Cure of *Pseudomonas* central nervous system infections may require surgical drainage of brain abscesses, debridement of infected tissues, and removal of prosthetic materials. A minimum of 2 weeks and as many as 6 weeks of antimicrobial therapy may be necessary.

Ear Infections

Otitis externa is most commonly caused by *P. aeruginosa* and is usually associated with immersion (swimmer's ear). Patients complain of pain and pruritus. Examination reveals edema, exudate, and erythema of the pinna and external canal. This infection is treated with topical agents such as antibiotic drops (polymyxin, neomycin, or a quinolone) plus hydrocortisone or dilute acetic acid (see Chapter 6, Otitis Media and Externa).

A more invasive and necrotizing process involving the bone and soft tissues of the external auditory canal and with potential to extend to the temporal bone and base of the skull is referred to as *malignant otitis externa* (Figure 146.2). This principally affects elderly persons and diabetics. Otalgia and purulent drainage from the external ear canal are present. Neurologic complications such as cranial nerve palsies may become manifest. Computed tomography (CT) or magnetic resonance imaging (MRI) is useful to delineate the extent of bone and soft-tissue destruction and to monitor treatment. Because debridement may be necessary, surgical consultation is advised. Combination antimicrobial treatment is recommended for a minimum of 4 weeks. The course of treatment should be extended to 6 to 8 weeks for more extensive disease.

Bone and Joint Infections

Pseudomonas aeruginosa causes osteomyelitis and septic arthritis as a result of hematogenous dissemination or contiguous spread. Vertebral

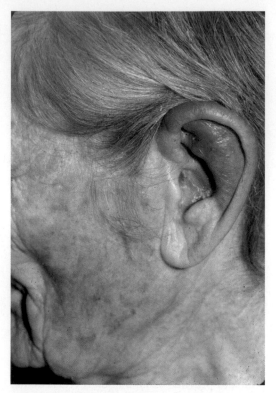

Figure 146.2 Malignant otitis externa. Edema and erythema of the helix, antihelix, and scapha of the ear are seen here. As infection progresses, the tragus often becomes involved. Visualization of the canal is frequently limited due to edema and pain.

osteomyelitis usually occurs in elderly patients with urinary tract infections associated with bladder instrumentation and in intravenous drug users. Neck or back pain with paraspinal tenderness is a common presentation. Computed tomography and MRI are sensitive diagnostic means of defining the extent of disease. The pathogen can be isolated by needle aspiration or biopsy under fluoroscopic or CT guidance. Occasionally, surgical exploration for biopsy, culture, and decompression is necessary. Removal of prosthetic material is usually necessary. Combination antibiotic therapy with an antipseudomonal β-lactam and either an aminoglycoside or quinolone should be used for a minimum of 4 to 6 weeks. Monotherapy has been used successfully, but treatment failures have occurred.

Contiguous osteomyelitis arises from direct extension of infected overlying skin and soft tissues or penetrating trauma. *Pseudomonas aeruginosa* may be implicated in this setting in patients with infected diabetic foot ulcers. Vascular insufficiency and the polymicrobial nature of this infection may complicate

management. The goal of therapy is to achieve effective levels of antimicrobials in bone and soft tissues. Prolonged antimicrobial treatment (up to 6 weeks), including a β-lactam antipseudomonal agent and an aminoglycoside, has been the current standard, but quinolones used either alone or in combination with a β-lactam have proved efficacious in open-label trials.

Osteochondritis of the foot involving bone and fibrocartilaginous joints is frequently seen following puncture wounds through the soles of footwear colonized by *P. aeruginosa* (Figure 146.3). Treatment consists of surgical debridement combined with an antimicrobial agent such as ceftazidime or ciprofloxacin for a minimum of 4 weeks.

Skin Infections

Exposure to contaminated whirlpools, hot tubs, and swimming pools may produce *P. aeruginosa* folliculitis, a diffuse red maculopapular or vesicopustular rash (Figure 146.4). The eruption is self-limited and does not require specific antimicrobial treatment.

Burn wounds may become colonized and subsequently infected with *P. aeruginosa*. Bloodstream invasion may thus occur, resulting in septicemia. Systemic antibiotic combinations should be administered. A topical agent such as mafenide acetate or silver sulfadiazine may be considered to reduce burn wound colonization. Avoidance of hydrotherapy also reduces the risk of *Pseudomonas* infections in burn patients.

Persons with a history of submersion of the hands may develop greenish discoloration of the nail plates and *Pseudomonas* nail bed infection. This condition has been called *green*

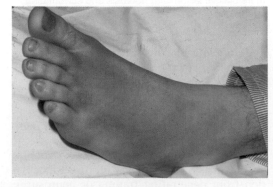

Figure 146.3 Osteochondritis following a nail puncture wound of the sole. Cellulitis is often a prominent feature in patients with acute osteochondritis due to *P. aeruginosa*, as evidenced in this photo. Edema is also a common finding.

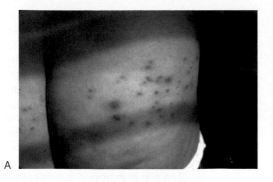

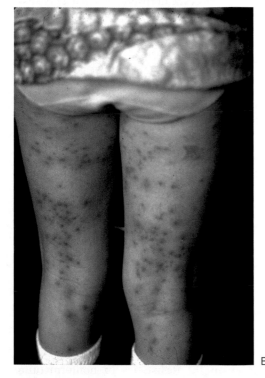

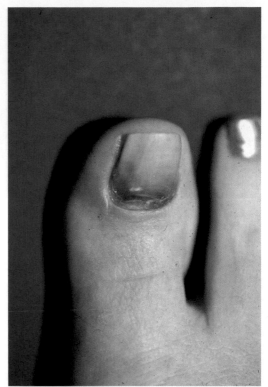

Figure 146.5 Green nail syndrome. Note the characteristic green appearance of the nail.

Figure 146.4 Folliculitis. The folliculitis of *P. aeruginosa* may appear similar to other common dermatologic conditions. The appearance of the lesions in **A** raises the possibility of shingles. The patient in **B** has a widespread infection that may be confused with *Staphylococcal* infection or steroid-induced folliculitis. Culturing the contents of the lesions will aid in obtaining an accurate diagnosis.

nail syndrome (Figure 146.5). Treatment requires elimination of the exposure; orally administered ciprofloxacin is a useful adjunct.

The warm, moist toe webs of the feet may become infected with *P. aeruginosa*. The spaces between the third, fourth, and fifth toes are the most common sites. Toe web infections have been most commonly associated with military recruits, athletes, and laborers. Tinea pedis is a common antecedent. The infected tissue is damp, boggy, macerated, and white. Adjacent skin and subcutaneous tissue may become inflamed. More severe infection can progress to ulceration (Figure 146.6).

Pseudomonas toe web infection may resemble tinea pedis but does not improve with topical antifungal agents. *Pseudomonas* should be suspected when green pigment is visible on the patient's socks, bandages, or on dried exudate. Green toenails strongly suggest the diagnosis, and further evidence is obtained if Wood's light shows green–white fluorescence (Figure 146.7).

Treatment of toe web infections includes an antipseudomonal antimicrobial and soaking with 2% acetic acid solution. Prevention of infection is best achieved by keeping feet and toes clean and dry and by wearing work boots or athletic shoes on alternate days to allow for the lining to fully dry.

INFECTIONS CAUSED BY RELATED SPECIES

Stenotrophomonas maltophilia is a health care–associated, gram-negative pathogen that may cause bacteremia, pneumonia, and

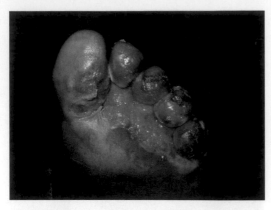

Figure 146.6 Toe web infection. As toe-web infections progress, a characteristic macerated appearance is seen.

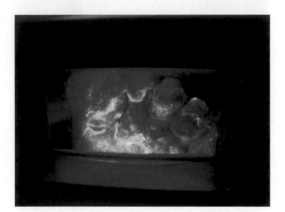

Figure 146.7 Use of a Wood's light reveals the typical luminescence classically described with *P. aeruginosa*.

wound infection. *Stenotrophomonas malto-philia* health care–associated pneumonia is associated with mechanical ventilation, tracheostomy, use of nebulizers, and previous exposure to broad-spectrum antibiotics. Patients usually have pre-existing lung conditions such as chronic obstructive pulmonary disease. Isolation of *S. maltophilia* from the respiratory tract in ventilator-associated pneumonia is an important predictor of mortality. Management of *S. maltophilia* pneumonia and other infections is often difficult because the organism is usually resistant to most antipseudomonal β-lactams, carbapenems, and

aminoglycosides. Trimethoprim–sulfamethoxazole (TMP–SMX) is the antibiotic of choice for therapy. Ceftazidime, ticarcillin–clavulanate, and the quinolones have variable activity among strains. Combination therapy with TMP–SMX and a β-lactam such as ticarcillin–clavulanate or ceftazidime (if susceptibility is documented) has been proposed based on in vitro synergy and anecdotal reports of clinical efficacy. The polymyxins retain activity against selected highly resistant isolates.

Burkholderia cepacia is an opportunistic pathogen that may colonize the respiratory tract of a patient with cystic fibrosis and lead to persistent disease with progressive respiratory failure. Therapy is thwarted by antibiotic resistance to many β-lactam agents and aminoglycosides. Susceptibility testing is essential as resistance to quinolones, TMP–SMX, and the carbapenems is common and variable. Chloramphenicol may retain activity, whereas the polymyxins are generally ineffective.

SUGGESTED READING

American Thoracic Society; Infectious Diseases Society of America. Guidelines for the management of adults with hospital-acquired, ventilator-associated, and healthcare-associated pneumonia. *Am J Respir Crit Care Med*. 2005;171:388–416.

Gaynes R, Edwards JR. Overview of nosocomial infections caused by Gram-negative bacilli. *Clin Infect Dis*. 2005;41:848–854.

Kollef MH, Sherman G, Ward S, et al. Inadequate antimicrobial treatment of infections: a risk factor for hospital mortality among critically ill patients. *Chest*. 1999;115:462–474.

McGowan JE. Resistance in nonfermenting Gram-negative bacteria: multidrug resistance to the maximum. *Am J Med*. 2006;119 (suppl 1):S29–S36.

Paterson DL. The epidemiological profile of infections with multidrug-resistant Pseudomonas aeruginosa and Acinetobacter species. *Clin Infect Dis*. 2006;43:S43–S48.

Waterer GW, Wunderink RG. Increasing threat of Gram-negative bacteria. *Crit Care Med*. 2001;29(suppl 4):N75–N81.

147. Rat-Bite Fevers

Neil S. Lipman

For 2300 years, illness associated with rat bites has been recognized in India, which is believed to be the country of origin for the disease. The first recorded description of rat-bite fever was in lectures by a physician at Yale in the early 19th century. It was not until 1902 that Japanese workers describing the clinical entity in a European journal coined the term *Rattenbisskrankheit*, or rat-bite fever. Rat-bite fever comprises two clinically similar but distinct bacterial diseases, caused by two unrelated agents, *Streptobacillus moniliformis* and *Spirillum minus*. The organisms are distributed worldwide, with *S. moniliformis* more common in the United States and Europe and *S. minus* more common in the Far East.

Rat-bite fevers are most frequently associated with the bite or, less frequently, a scratch from laboratory or wild rats. A number of reported cases were not associated with rat bites or contact, although all patients had a history of occupational exposure to rat-infested areas or contaminated materials. Disease caused by these agents has also followed contact with a variety of other species, including mice, gerbils, guinea pigs, squirrels, dogs, cats, ferrets, turkeys, and weasels, all of which presumably had contact with rats or contaminated materials. Estimates are that upward of 14 000 rat bites occur annually in the United States, most of them to individuals of low socioeconomic status in cities. Diagnosis is rare, likely the result of a low incidence of disease despite substantial potential exposure, a low index of suspicion of attending physicians, the routine postexposure use of effective antimicrobials, and the difficulty of isolating the organism in the laboratory. The true incidence in the United States is unknown, because the disease is not reportable. More than 50% of the reported cases in the United States are associated with children under the age of 12. Rat-bite fever is also an occupational disease of laboratory workers; it is the most commonly reported zoonosis associated with laboratory rats.

The rat is the natural reservoir and primary host of both *S. moniliformis* and *S. minus*, neither of which is routinely associated with natural disease in the species. Rarely, otitis media has been described with *S. moniliformis* in the laboratory rat. The organisms are nasopharyngeal commensals and may be found in other tissues, including the urine and the blood. Surveys of wild rats report carrier rates up to 50%. Estimates of infection rates in laboratory rats during the first half of this century were similar to those reported for wild populations, but modern production techniques and maintenance, in concert with frequent monitoring of commercial suppliers, has reduced this rate dramatically. The actual carrier rate in laboratory rats is unknown but is suspected to be extremely low. Although disease in humans has occasionally been associated with other species, these species are not believed to be commensal carriers.

PRESENTATION

Rat-bite fevers are acute, systemic illnesses with relapsing fever. Streptobacillary rat-bite fever, streptobacillary fever, or streptobacillosis follows infection with *S. moniliformis*. Haverhill fever and epidemic arthritic erythema are diseases caused by streptobacillosis acquired through ingestion of contaminated water, raw milk, or food. Sodoku, which derives from the Japanese word for rat (*so*) and poison (*doku*), spirillary rat-bite fever, and spirillosis are diseases that result from *S. minus* infection. Although similar, these diseases can be differentiated clinically (Table 147.1). Streptobacillary rat-bite fever has a shorter incubation period than the spirillary form and is often accompanied by rash and arthralgia. Haverhill fever is more frequently associated with vomiting, diarrhea, and sore throat. An indurating chancre develops at the site of inoculation and accompanies clinical signs in the spirillary form. Dual infections, albeit extremely rare, may occur. Most cases of streptobacillary disease spontaneously resolve within 2 weeks. If the patient goes untreated, 7% to 10% of cases are fatal. The clinical course of disease in infants may be particularly rapid and fatal. Recently, mortality has been reported in adults following a short (≤12 hour) presentation.

Table 147.1 Clinical Features of Rat-Bite Fevers

Clinical Features	Streptobacillary Form	Spirillary Form
Incubation period	2–10 d	7–21 d
Fever	+++	+++
Chills	+++	+++
Myalgia	+++	+++
Rash	++ Morbilliform/petechial	++ Maculopapular
Lymphadenitis	+	++
Arthralgia, arthritis	++	−
Indurated bite wound	−	+++
Recurrent fever/constitutional signs (untreated)	Irregular periodicity	Regular periodicity

The incubation period of streptobacillary rat-bite fever is 2 to 10 days; however, onset usually occurs within 3 days of exposure. Clinical signs develop despite rapid healing of the bite wound, presumably as a result of bacteremia and septicemia. Illness of sudden onset is characterized by remittent chills, fever, headache, and myalgia and results from direct infectious as well immune-mediated mechanisms. A morbilliform or petechial rash, which may be a result of leukocytoclastic vasculitis, develops in 75% of patients, frequently within days of onset, on either the lateral or the extensor surfaces of the extremities, occasionally involving the palms and the soles. Infrequently, the rash may be generalized and/or present with pustules, desquamation, and purpura. Simultaneous with rash development, approximately 50% of patients have severe arthralgia or frank arthritis of at least one, but frequently more than one, large joint. The arthritis may be suppurative or nonsuppurative and monoarticular or migrating and polyarticular and rarely occurs without other manifestations. Untreated, the course is biphasic, with fever and symptoms diminishing 2 to 5 days after onset and recurring several days later. Arthritis, endocarditis, myocarditis, pericarditis, hepatitis, pancreatitis, parotiditis, prostatitis, pneumonia, nephritis, meningitis, metastatic abscessation, septicemia, and chorioamnionitis are reported complications. Relapsing fever with return of constitutional symptoms of 1 to 6 days' duration is not uncommon. Afebrile cases have been described.

In the United States, the spirillary form is considerably less common than streptobacillary disease and is rarely associated with infection acquired from laboratory rats. Illness follows an incubation period, usually 7 to 21 days but sometimes as short as 2 days or as long as months. There is initial healing of the bite wound. Subsequently, an indurated chancre or eschar develops at the wound site and is accompanied by a regional lymphadenitis and lymphangitis, fever, rigors, myalgia, and, in about 50% of the cases, an erythematous maculopapular rash originating from the wound. Arthritis is uncommon. Untreated, fevers and other symptoms resolve but then recur regularly, and mortality is approximately 6.5%.

DIAGNOSIS

Diagnosis is suggested by a rat bite (or contact with rat-infested areas or contaminated materials) and clinical presentation. Patients may present without a history of rat bite or after a prolonged disease course. For infections caused by *S. moniliformis*, definitive diagnosis depends on isolation of the organism by microbiologic culture and/or identification of the bacterium in culture or tissue samples by amplifying part of the 16s RNA gene, followed by sequencing, using polymerase chain reaction. There are no reliable serologic tests currently available in humans for either organism. A high index of suspicion in the laboratory is frequently necessary, as these organisms are extremely difficult to isolate.

Specific Organisms – Bacteria

Streptobacillus moniliformis is a fastidious, facultatively anaerobic, highly pleomorphic, asporogenous, gram-negative rod measuring less than 1 × 1 to 5 µm long. Curved and looping, nonbranching filaments as long as 150 µm may be formed. Characteristic bulbous swellings may be observed in older cultures or in cytologic specimens, resulting in dismissal of the organism as proteinaceous debris. The bacterium has two variants, the bacillary and the cell wall–deficient, penicillin-resistant, apathogenic L-phase variant. Spontaneous conversion from one form to another, which alters the organism's sensitivity to antimicrobial agents, may be responsible for clinical relapses and resistance to therapy. *Streptobacillus moniliformis* is difficult to identify in most hospital laboratories because of its fastidious growth requirements and slow growth. The organism may be demonstrated by Giemsa, Gram, Wright, or silver stain in blood, synovial fluid, or other body fluids; samples should be mixed with 2.5% sodium citrate to prevent clotting before examination. Blood and joint fluid should be cultured in media enriched with 15% blood; 20% horse, calf, or rabbit serum; or 10% to 30% ascitic fluid. Media employed successfully include blood agar bases, chocolate agar, Schaedler agar, thioglycollate broth, meat-infusion broth, and tryptose-based media. Nalidixic acid can be added to the media to prevent overgrowth by gram-negative bacteria. Brain–heart infusion cysteine broth supplemented with Panmede, a papain digest of ox liver, has been advocated. The medium should not contain sodium polyanethol sulfonate, an anticoagulant and bacterial growth promoter used in blood culture media, as it inhibits the growth of the organism. Inoculated media are incubated at 37°C (98.6°F) in humidified 5% to 10% carbon dioxide atmosphere. Characteristic "puffballs" appear after 2 to 6 days in broth; on agar 1- to 2-mm round, gray, smooth, glistening colonies are observed. L-forms produce colonies with a typical fried-egg appearance. Identification is made by biochemical profile. The API ZYM system and fatty acid profiles may be valuable in rapid identification. The Centers for Disease Control and Prevention's Meningitis and Special Pathogens Branch or a state public health laboratory can be contacted for assistance with culture and/or diagnosis.

Spirillum minus is a gram-negative aerobic, motile, rigid spiral bacterium. It is 0.2 to 0.5 × 3 to 5 µm long and has 2 to 6 wide angular windings and pointed ends with one flagellum at each pole. *Spirillum minus* cannot be grown on any artificial medium. It may be demonstrated in dark-field microscopy in wet mounts of blood, exudate from the bite wound, cutaneous lesions, and lymph nodes or in Giemsa- or Wright-stained specimens from these sites. Isolation requires intraperitoneal inoculation of infected materials into guinea pigs or mice followed by dark-field examination of the animal's blood or peritoneal exudate 1 to 3 weeks later.

Differential diagnosis of rat-bite fevers can be broad and can include septic arthritides such as Lyme disease, gonococcal arthritis, and brucellosis and noninfectious inflammatory polyarthropathies such as rheumatoid arthritis. Presentation with fever and rash mimic systemic lupus erythematosus, viral exanthems, rickettsial infections, secondary syphilis, and drug reactions. A biologic false positive for syphilis occurs in up to 25% of patients with streptobacillary disease and in up to 50% of cases with the spirillary form.

THERAPY

Both streptobacillary and spirillary forms of rat-bite fever respond well to appropriate antimicrobial therapy. *Spirillum minus* is more sensitive to therapy. Penicillin is the drug of choice for both organisms, and a dramatic response to therapy may be expected. Dosage of 600 000 U of procaine penicillin G, administered intramuscularly (IM) twice daily for at least 7 days, is recommended for uncomplicated forms of the disease. Intravenous penicillin therapy should be initiated, until antimicrobial sensitivity is determined, in cases of severe disease. Endocarditis, if present, should be treated parenterally with 15 to 20 million units daily for 4 to 6 weeks. Tetracycline, 500 mg/kg orally every 6 hours, or streptomycin, 7.5 mg/kg IM twice daily, are effective alternatives in penicillin-allergic patients. Amoxicillin–clavulanate, doxycycline, second- and third-generation cephalosporins, ciprofloxacin, chloramphenicol, clindamycin, the macrolides erythromycin and clarithromycin, and vancomycin have been successfully employed. Treatment failures have been reported with erythromycin. Prophylactic administration of penicillin may be considered following a rat bite, although the risk of nascent infection is low. However, prophylaxis should be a high consideration in infants because of the possibility of rapid progression and severe outcomes.

SUGGESTED READING

Andre JM, Freydiere AM, Benito Y, et al. Rat bite fever caused by Streptobacillus moniliformis in a child: human infection and rat carriage diagnosed by PCR. *J Clin Pathol.* 2005;58:1215–1216.

Berger C, Altwegg M, Meyer A, Nadal D. Broad range polymerase chain reaction for diagnosis of rat-bite fever caused by Streptobacillus moniliformis. 2001; *Pediatr Infect Dis J.* 20:1181–1182.

CDC. Fatal rat-bite fever—Florida and Washington, 2003. *Morbid Mortal Weekly Rep.* 2006;53:1198–1202.

Cole JS, Stoll RW, Bulger RJ. Rat-bite fever: report of three cases. *Ann Intern Med.* 1969;71:979–981.

Edwards R, Fitch RG. Characterization and antibiotic susceptibilities of Streptobacillus moniliformis. *J Med Microbiol.* 1986;21:39–42.

Graves MH, Janda JM. Rat-bite fever (Streptobacillus moniliformis): a potential emerging disease. *Int J Infect Dis.* 2001;5:151–154.

Holroyd KJ, Reiner AP, Dick JD. Streptobacillus moniliformis polyarthritis mimicking rheumatoid arthritis: an urban case of rat-bite fever. *Am J Med.* 1988;85:711–714.

Pins MR, Holden JM, Yang JM, et al. Isolation of presumptive Streptobacillus moniliformis from abscesses associated with the female genital tract. *Clin Infect Dis.* 1996; 22:471–476.

von Graevenitz A, Zbinden R, Mutters R. Actinobacillus, Capnocytophaga, Eikenella, Kingella, Pasteurella, and other fastidious or rarely encountered gram-negative rods. In: Murray PR, Baron EJ, Jorgensen JH, Pfaller MA, Yolken RH, eds. *Manual of Clinical Microbiology.* 8th ed. Washington, DC: American Society for Microbiology; 2003:609–621.

Roughgarden JW. Antimicrobial therapy of rat-bite fever. *Arch Intern Med.* 1965;116:39–53.

Sens MA, Brown EW, Wilson LR, Crocker TP. Fatal Streptobacillus moniliformis infection in a two-month old infant. *Am J Clin Pathol.* 1989;91:612–616.

Wullenweber M. Stretobacillus moniliformis—a zoonotic pathogen. Taxonomic considerations, host species, diagnosis, therapy, geographical distribution. *Lab Anim.* 1995;29:1–15.

148. *Salmonella*

Bruce S. Ribner

The salmonellae are gram-negative, non–spore-forming, facultatively anaerobic bacteria in the family Enterobacteriaceae. More than 2500 different serotypes of *Salmonella* have been identified.

Salmonellae are widely distributed in nature. They are generally found in the gastrointestinal (GI) tracts of the hosts with which they are associated. Some salmonellae, such as *S. typhi* and *S. paratyphi*, are found to colonize only the human GI tract. Other *Salmonella* serotypes, such as *S. typhimurium*, have a wide range of hosts, including humans. Finally, some organisms, such as *S. dublin* and *S. arizona*, are rarely found in the GI tracts of humans. The specificity and range of the different serotypes help determine the epidemiology of infections caused by these bacteria.

Infections caused by the salmonellae are grouped into three major syndromes: gastroenteritis, typhoid or enteric fever, and localized infection outside of the GI tract. Although there is considerable overlap between these syndromes, their epidemiology and clinical presentations are distinct enough to make discussion by syndrome useful.

GASTROENTERITIS

Gastroenteritis accounts for most *Salmonella* infections in humans. The incidence of *Salmonella* gastroenteritis in the United States doubled during the 1980s and 1990s. Much of this increase was attributed to the widespread contamination of chickens and eggs as the industry became increasingly centralized. Since the mid-1990s the rate of *Salmonella* gastroenteritis has remained constant, probably due to increased public awareness and improved sanitation during commercial processing. It is estimated that there are 1.4 million episodes of *Salmonella* gastroenteritis annually in the United States. Most cases of *Salmonella* gastroenteritis are traced to the ingestion of inadequately cooked poultry or eggs, either directly or through the consumption of such foods as Caesar salad, sauces containing raw eggs, and inadequately cooked stuffing contaminated by salmonellae from raw poultry. A recent study detected salmonellae contamination in 15% of the chickens sold in the United States; 84% of these isolates were resistant to at least one antibiotic. Beef, milk, and, rarely, fruits and vegetables have also been responsible for salmonellae infections. Pet reptiles, such as turtles, snakes, and lizards, and baby ducklings and chicks often have asymptomatic colonization of the GI tract. Young children who play with these animals often forget to wash their hands before eating, resulting in *Salmonella* gastroenteritis. Individuals at greatest risk for acquiring disease are neonates, those with achlorhydria or who are taking antacids, transplant recipients, individuals with lymphoma, and patients with acquired immunodeficiency syndrome. Children under 5 years of age represent 27% of all patients with *Salmonella* gastroenteritis.

Salmonella Gastroenteritis

Salmonella gastroenteritis has an incubation period of 12 to 72 hours, with shorter incubation periods being associated with higher amounts of ingested bacteria. The typical illness is accompanied by fever, nausea, vomiting, abdominal cramping, and watery diarrhea; it lasts 4 to 7 days. The stool usually contains neutrophils, but dysentery, with gross blood and pus in the stool, is uncommon. Patients with *Salmonella* gastroenteritis occasionally have headaches and myalgias. Bacteremia, seen in approximately 5% of patients, is most common in those with underlying diseases and tends to occur early during the course of the illness. *Salmonella* gastroenteritis is typically a mild disease; it rarely leads to severe dehydration and cardiovascular collapse, although it is estimated that there are 500 fatalities a year in the United States from *Salmonella* gastroenteritis. Severe forms of the illness are most likely to be seen in infants, debilitated patients, and patients with immunologic impairment.

Approximately 50% of newborns with *Salmonella* gastroenteritis have GI carriage of the organism for longer than 6 months. This rate decreases with age; fewer than 10%

of adults remain colonized at 3 months. The administration of antibiotics during the early phase of illness is felt to increase the likelihood of carriage.

TYPHOID OR ENTERIC FEVER

Typhoid fever is caused by salmonellae serotypes such as *S. typhi* and *S. paratyphi*, which are almost exclusively associated with humans. Transmission is by ingestion of contaminated food and water; although person-to-person transmission is possible, it is uncommon, because of the large inoculum size required to cause illness in normal individuals. In contrast to *Salmonella* gastroenteritis, the incidence of typhoid fever in developed countries has markedly decreased over the past few decades as sanitation and the quality of the water supply have improved. Most typhoid fever in the United States is acquired during foreign travel. A high percentage of infections acquired in the United States results from the ingestion of food prepared by chronic carriers, many of whom initially became colonized in another country.

Typhoid fever has an incubation period that is usually 7 to 21 days (range of 3 to 60 days), depending on the size of the inoculum and the health of the host. Symptoms consist of fever, abdominal pain, hepatosplenomegaly, headache, and myalgias. Diarrhea is rare after the first few days. Although typhoid fever has classically been characterized as having a temperature–pulse dissociation with bradycardia in the face of a high fever, this phenomenon is uncommon. Rose spots, which are faint, maculopapular, salmon-colored blanching lesions found predominantly on the trunk, are seen in approximately one third of patients. Biopsy of these lesions reveals perivascular, mononuclear cell infiltration, and culture frequently yields the organism.

Ninety percent of patients with typhoid fever have bacteremia during the first week of illness. This percentage decreases as the illness progresses. Positive stool cultures do not appear before the second week of illness, and the rate increases until, by the third week, 75% of patients have positive stool cultures. The white blood cell count is usually low in relation to the degree of illness. Occasionally an absolute leukopenia is seen.

The patient with untreated typhoid fever will have 4 to 8 weeks of sustained fever. Mortality of those with untreated disease is estimated to be 15% worldwide but only 1% in the United States. Mortality is highest in the immunocompromised, especially those with hemoglobinopathies, malaria, schistosomiasis, and infection with human immunodeficiency virus (HIV). The major complication of untreated disease is hemorrhage from intestinal perforation secondary to ulceration and necrosis of the Peyer's patches in the ileum. Such hemorrhage may be seen during the third or fourth week of illness, often when the patient seems to be clinically improving. Other complications include pericarditis, endocarditis, splenic and hepatic abscesses, cholangitis, meningitis, and pneumonia. Ten percent of untreated patients relapse. Although one fourth of patients with typhoid fever will have positive urine cultures, actual infection of the urinary tract with *S. typhi* and *S. paratyphi* is rare.

The differential diagnosis in a patient presenting with enteric fever may include malaria, amebiasis, and viral illnesses such as dengue or Epstein–Barr virus infection, and infection with non-*Salmonella* bacterial pathogens such as *Yersinia*, *Campylobacter*, and *Pseudomonas*.

LOCALIZED INFECTIONS OUTSIDE OF THE GASTROINTESTINAL TRACT

On rare occasions, *Salmonella* infection may present as a localized infection at a site other than the GI tract. This is most likely in patients with underlying illnesses. Thus, sustained bacteremia with *S. choleraesuis* or *S. dublin* suggests an intravascular focus such as seeding of an atherosclerotic plaque or of the clot within a pre-existing aneurysm, especially if the patient is elderly. If infection is localized to the abdominal aorta, surgery is generally necessary, as medical management alone is associated with a high mortality rate. Rarely, sustained bacteremia may result from endocarditis with a valve ring or septal abscess. Localized infection may also present as a hepatic or splenic abscess, especially if the patient has biliary tract stones, cirrhosis, or cholangitis.

Salmonellae are the second most common cause of gram-negative meningitis in neonates. They are also a common cause of osteomyelitis in children with hemoglobinopathies such as sickle cell disease.

Historically, *Salmonella* infection of the urinary tract was rare in the absence of nephrolithiasis, renal schistosomiasis, or renal tuberculosis. However, recent studies have documented an increase in *Salmonella* cystitis in elderly women, most of whom lacked structural abnormalities. It is felt that *Salmonella* cystitis most likely represents ascending infection of strains with greater pathogenicity for the urinary tract.

Approximately 2% of individuals who have *Salmonella* gastroenteritis will develop Reiter's syndrome. This occurs within 2 weeks of the onset of diarrhea and is associated with human leukocyte antigen (HLA) B27.

CHRONIC CARRIAGE

Because *Salmonella* is excreted in the stool of a high percentage of those recovering from acute infection for several months, the chronic carrier state is not considered to be present unless the organism persists in the stool for more than 1 year. This occurs in approximately 1% to 4% of those with *S. typhi* infection and in fewer than 1% of those infected with other serotypes. Biliary tract carriage is most likely to occur in the elderly and those with chololithiasis. Urinary tract carriage is most likely in those with bladder schistosomiasis and nephrolithiasis. Many chronic carriers have no clear history of a preceding acute *Salmonella* infection.

DIAGNOSIS

Gastroenteritis

Although certain features may suggest *Salmonella* gastroenteritis in a patient, many other pathogens may produce an illness that is clinically indistinguishable. The diagnosis of *Salmonella* gastroenteritis depends on the isolation of the organism from a stool specimen. As many clinical laboratories report that only 1% to 3% of stool specimens submitted for culture yield an enteric pathogen, and as mild gastroenteritis caused by *Salmonella* should not be treated with antibiotics (see Therapy below), many authorities have devised algorithms for selecting patients with gastroenteritis who should have stool cultures. Epidemiologic factors that should be sought as indicators of possible infectious diarrhea include the following: (1) travel to a developing area; (2) day-care center attendance or employment; (3) consumption of unsafe foods (eg, raw meats, eggs, or shellfish; unpasteurized milk or juices) or swimming in or drinking untreated fresh surface water from, for example, a lake or stream; (4) visiting a farm or petting zoo or having contact with reptiles or with pets with diarrhea; (5) knowledge of other ill persons (such as in a dormitory or office or at a social function); (6) recent or regular medications (antibiotics, antacids, antimotility agents); (7) underlying medical conditions predisposing to infectious diarrhea (acquired immunodeficiency syndrome [AIDS], immunosuppressive medications, prior gastrectomy, extremes of age); (where appropriate) (8) receptive anal intercourse or oral–anal sexual contact; and (9) occupation as a food handler or caregiver. Signs and symptoms that suggest a bacterial etiology for gastroenteritis include fever, abdominal pain, and bloody stools. Some laboratories have also included a screen for the presence of fecal leukocytes or lactoferrin to select those stools that warrant further culture for enteric pathogens.

As mentioned previously, only 5% of patients with *Salmonella* gastroenteritis will have an accompanying bacteremia. This is most common in those with underlying diseases and tends to occur early during the course of the illness.

Typhoid or Enteric Fever

The patient with typhoid or enteric fever most commonly will present with symptoms of fever, abdominal pain, hepatosplenomegaly, headache, and myalgias. In endemic areas, the differential diagnosis is frequently between typhoid fever and malaria. Less commonly, rickettsial infection, dengue fever, plague, and tularemia may present with a similar syndrome. Systemic vasculitis may also present with a clinical picture similar to enteric fever. The definitive diagnosis of typhoid requires isolation of *S. typhi* or *S. paratyphi* or demonstration of the presence of antigens of these bacteria in body fluids. The body sites most likely to yield positive assays depend on the stage of illness. During the first week, blood cultures are most likely to be positive, whereas during the second and third week of illness stool cultures are usually positive. Cultures of rose spots, if present, and of bone marrow aspirate are also frequently positive.

Serology for antibody to *S. typhi* antigens has been used widely in the past for the diagnosis of typhoid fever. Such assays must be used with caution, as the antibodies persist for years after infection and may be elevated from vaccination. Although a 4-fold rise in antibody titers in the context of an appropriate clinical illness is strong support for the diagnosis of enteric fever, a very elevated single assay can also be highly suggestive.

Localized Infections Outside of the Gastrointestinal Tract

The diagnosis of localized *Salmonella* infection outside of the GI tract depends on the isolation of the organism. This is especially true of localized infections such as visceral abscesses or endothelial infections, as there are no features that distinguish localized infection by the salmonellae as compared with the more common bacterial pathogens.

Chronic Carriage

As mentioned previously, the chronic carrier state is not considered to be present unless the organism persists in the stool for more than 1 year. Although colonic colonization in the absence of biliary involvement has been reported, the overwhelming majority of patients with GI colonization have the gallbladder as the focus. To determine the site of colonization, a colonoscopy to detect mucosal abnormalities and a culture of the common bile duct drainage have been used. Imaging of the gallbladder can also be useful in determining underlying causes for colonization of the gallbladder.

Patients with urinary tract chronic colonization can be evaluated with imaging studies to determine whether anatomic abnormalities, such as strictures or stones, are present. Such abnormalities make medical management alone less likely to be successful.

THERAPY
Gastroenteritis

Salmonella gastroenteritis is usually a self-limited disease, and therapy should be primarily directed to the replacement of fluid and electrolyte losses. Widespread resistance to chloramphenicol, ampicillin, and trimethoprim–sulfamethoxazole (TMP–SMX) now exists among the salmonellae, and multi-drug-resistant salmonellae have been reported. Antimicrobial therapy for uncomplicated non-typhoidal *Salmonella* gastroenteritis, including short-course or single-dose regimens with oral fluoroquinolones, amoxicillin, or trim-ethoprim–sulfamethoxazole, does not significantly decrease the length of illness, including duration of fever or diarrhea, and is associated with an increased risk of relapse, positive cultures after 3 weeks, and adverse drug reactions. However, certain patients are at increased risk for invasive infection and may benefit from pre-emptive antimicrobial therapy. Such patients would include neonates, those older than 50 years, and persons with immunosuppression or cardiac valvular or endovascular abnormalities, including prosthetic vascular grafts.

Treatment in these patients should consist of an oral or intravenous antimicrobial administered for 48 to 72 hours or until the patient becomes afebrile. Specific recommendations are listed in Table 148.1.

Typhoid Fever

Fluoroquinolones are the agents of choice for treatment of typhoid fever. They are more rapidly effective and are associated with lower rates of relapse and stool carriage than chloramphenicol, ampicillin, and trimethoprim–sulfamethoxazole. They are also felt to be more effective than ceftriaxone. Strains sensitive to nalidixic acid can be treated with ciprofloxacin for 5 to 7 days. For uncomplicated disease, oral therapy is as effective as parenteral therapy. Patients infected by strains with intermediate resistance minimum inhibitory concentration (MIC) to ciprofloxacin of 0.125 to 1 µg/mL should be treated with higher doses of ciprofloxacin for 10 to 14 days. Patients with *S. typhi* strains with MIC values for ciprofloxacin of 2 µg/mL or greater should be treated with a third-generation cephalosporin or azithromycin.

Although the use of fluoroquinolones in children and pregnant women has been limited by concerns over toxicity, some studies have suggested that they may be superior to other agents in these populations as well. As additional studies document their safety in these populations, they may become first-line therapy. However, due to their toxicity in animal models, further studies are needed.

Most authorities recommend a short course of dexamethasone for severe disease with altered mental status or shock (see Table 148.1).

Chronic Carrier

Patients with positive stool or urine cultures for salmonellae >12 months after resolving their acute infection are considered carriers. Over 80% of these patients can have the carrier state eradicated with the administration of oral amoxicillin for 3 months, trimethoprim–sulfamethoxazole for 3 months, or ciprofloxacin for 1 month. The presence of anatomic abnormalities, such as biliary or kidney stones, makes eradication much more difficult and should be evaluated prior to initiating long-term therapy. In the presence of such abnormalities, surgery combined with antimicrobial therapy is often required for eradication. Patients with urinary carriage associated with *Schistosoma*

Table 148.1 Therapy of *Salmonella* Infections

Syndrome	Suggested Therapy
Gastroenteritis	
Normal host	Rehydration
Immunocompromised adult	Ciprofloxacin, 500 mg PO or IV BID for 2–3 d or TMP–SMZ, 160/ 800 mg PO or IV BID for 2–,3 d or Ceftriaxone, 2 g IV qd for 2–3 d
Neonate or immunocompromised child	Ceftriaxone, 100 mg/kg qd IV for 2–3 d or TMP–SMX, 5 mg/kg TMP BID for 2–3 d
Typhoid Fever	
Adult, sensitive strain	Ciprofloxacin, 500 mg PO or IV BID for 5–7 d
Adult, intermediate strains[a]	Ciprofloxacin, 750 mg PO or IV BID for 10–14 d
Adult, resistant strains[b]	Ceftriaxone, 2 g IV qd for 10–14 d or Azithromycin, 500 mg PO for 7 d
Children, pregnant women	Ceftriaxone, 60 mg/kg up to 2 g qd for 10–14 d; may switch to PO TMP–SMX once stable and susceptibility data available
All patients with severe typhoid fever (delirium, obtundation, stupor, coma, or shock) should receive dexamethasone, 3 mg/kg initially, followed by 1 mg/kg q6h for 48 h	
Chronic Carrier	
Adult	Amoxicillin, 1 g PO TID for 3 mo or TMP–SMX, 160/800 PO BID for 3 mo or Ciprofloxacin, 750 mg PO BID for 4 wk
Children	Amoxicillin, 40 mg/kg PO up to 1 g TID for 3 mo or TMP–SMX, 5 mg/kg TMP BID for 3 mo

Abbreviations: TMP–SMX = trimethoprim–sulfamethoxazole; MIC = minimum inhibitory concentration.
[a] MIC to ciprofloxacin of 0.125 to 1 μg/mL.
[b] MIC values to ciprofloxacin of 2 μg/mL or greater.

haematobium should be treated with praziquantel before attempting eradication of *S. typhi*.

PREVENTION

The prevention of *Salmonella* infection relies on proper food handling and sanitation. In developed countries, this involves careful attention to the separation of raw and cooked foods and an awareness of the multiple ways in which cross-contamination can occur in food preparation areas. Parents should also monitor their children to insure careful hand hygiene after contact with reptiles and fowl.

For travel to developing countries, there are currently two commercially available vaccines for the prevention of *S. typhi* infection. One is an oral live-attenuated vaccine, whereas the second is a parenteral capsular polysaccharide vaccine. These vaccines achieve approximately 50% to 80% efficacy, starting roughly 2 weeks after vaccination, and confer protection that lasts for several years. They are recommended for travelers to parts of the world where typhoid fever is endemic. However, as none of the available vaccines are completely protective, the first line of prevention for travelers to areas where typhoid is endemic is care in consumption of food and water. Travelers should avoid tap water, ice produced from local tap water, salads, uncooked vegetables, and unpasteurized milk and milk products such as cheese, and should eat only food that has been cooked and is still hot or fruit that has been washed in clean water and then peeled by the traveler personally.

SUGGESTED READING

CDC. Salmonellosis. Centers for Disease Control and Prevention Web site. http://www.cdc.gov/ncidod/dbmd/diseaseinfo/salmonellosis_g.htm. Accessed January 3, 2005.

CDC. Typhoid Fever. Centers for Disease Control and Prevention Web site. http://www.cdc.gov/ncidod/dbmd/diseaseinfo/typhoidfever_g.htm. Accessed January 4, 2006.

Guerrant RL, Gilder TV, Steiner TS. Practice guidelines for the management of infectious diarrhea. *Clin Infect Dis.* 2001;32(3): 331–351.

Parry CM, Hien TT, Dougan G, White NJ, Farrar JJ. Typhoid fever. *N Engl J Med.* 2002;347(22):1770–1782.

Pegues DA, Ohl ME, Miller SI. Salmonella species, including Salmonella typhi. In Mandell GL, Bennett JE, Dolin R, eds. *Mandell, Douglas, and Bennett's Principles and Practice of Infectious Diseases.* Orlando, FL: Churchill Livingstone; 2005:2636–2650.

Richens J. Typhoid fever. In: Cohen J, Powderly WG, eds. *Infectious Diseases.* 2nd ed. St. Louis, MO: Mosby; 2004:1561–1565.

149. *Staphylococcus*

Suzanne F. Bradley

Treatment of staphylococcal infection is dependent on the site involved, the severity of infection, and the antibiotic susceptibility pattern of the organism causing the infection. Although most serious staphylococcal infections are due to coagulase-positive staphylococci (*Staphylococcus aureus*), infections due to coagulase-negative staphylococci (eg, *Staphylococcus epidermidis*) are increasing and may also be life threatening. *Staphylococcus aureus* is a highly invasive pathogen, able to spread hematogenously to many organs, leading to metastatic foci of infection. Coagulase-negative staphylococci generally require the presence of prosthetic material to gain a foothold and cause infection.

SUSCEPTIBILITY TO ANTIBIOTICS

Staphylococci have a propensity to develop resistance to antibiotics relatively quickly. Virtually all staphylococci should be considered to be resistant to penicillins that are susceptible to penicillinase (eg, amoxicillin, ampicillin, piperacillin, mezlocillin, and ticarcillin). However, the addition of clavulanic acid, sulbactam, or tazobactam to several of the above penicillins renders them resistant to penicillinase and thus useful for treating staphylococcal infections. Examples are amoxicillin–clavulanic acid (Augmentin), ampicillin–sulbactam (Unasyn), pipercillin–tazobactam (Zosyn), and ticarcillin–clavulanic acid (Timentin).

Cephalosporins are useful for the treatment of staphylococcal infections. First-generation cephalosporins (cefazolin, cephalexin) are the most active, followed by second-generation agents (cefuroxime, cefotetan, cefoxitin). Third-generation (ceftriaxone, cefotaxime) and fourth-generation (cefipime) cephalosporins have less activity. Only first-generation cephalosporins should be used for serious staphylococcal infections.

Since the 1970s, both *S. aureus* and coagulase-negative staphylococci have become increasingly resistant to penicillinase-resistant penicillins (nafcillin, methicillin, oxacillin) and the penicillins that are combined with sulbactam, tazobactam, and clavulanic acid. These methicillin-resistant *S. aureus* (MRSA) and methicillin-resistant *S. epidermidis* (MRSE) are common in hospitals throughout the United States, Europe, and Australia, and in some medical centers account for as many as 50% of all *S. aureus* isolates causing nosocomial infections. These hospital strains are usually resistant to many other classes of antibiotics, including cephalosporins, macrolides, lincosamines (clindamycin), quinolones, and aminoglycosides, but some remain susceptible to sulfonamides and tetracyclines.

New community-associated MRSA (CA-MRSA) strains have emerged that are not related to hospital- or health care–associated MRSA strains (HA-MRSA). These CA-MRSA strains are resistant to β-lactam antibiotics, but, in contrast with HA-MRSA strains, often are susceptible to sulfonamides, quinolones, tetracyclines, and macrolides. Strains of CA-MRSA that are resistant to erythromycin but appear to be susceptible to clindamycin on initial screening should be further tested for inducible cross-resistance to clindamycin using a double disk diffusion test (D test). If inducible resistance is shown, the laboratory will report resistance to both erythromycin and clindamycin.

Until recently, vancomycin has been the primary treatment for serious MRSA infections. However, vancomycin treatment has been slow or ineffective in clearing MRSA infection, and vancomycin-resistant *S. aureus* (VRSA) has emerged with prolonged use. Minimum inhibitory concentrations (MICs) of vancomycin appear to be increasing for MRSA. Some experts now recommend using higher dosages of vancomycin to achieve a trough serum concentration of 15 to 20 µg/mL when treating serious MRSA infections. These higher serum vancomycin concentrations may be associated with more toxicity, however. Newer antibiotics with activity against MRSA, such as linezolid, quinupristin–dalfopristin, daptomycin, and tigecycline, have been developed. It is likely these agents will assume an increasing role for treatment of serious MRSA infections in the future. Currently, the most experience for treating MRSA infections has been with linezolid and daptomycin; quinupristin is difficult to administer and associated with many side effects, and experience with tigecycline is limited.

Although it may be tempting to treat both methicillin-susceptible *S. aureus* (MSSA) and MRSA infections with vancomycin or one of the newer agents, there are several reasons that this practice should be discouraged. One is that MSSA infections clear more slowly when treated with vancomycin than with a β-lactam antibiotic. The second is that the overuse of vancomycin has contributed to the increase in vancomycin resistance among enterococci (VRE) as well as *S. aureus*. Finally, resistance to the newer agents has already been reported in *S. aureus*. Thus, organisms that are identified as MSSA should be treated with a penicillinase-resistant β-lactam antibiotic; only if the infecting organism is MRSA should vancomycin or newer agents be used.

The situation with coagulase-negative staphylococci is more difficult, because the routine assays used by most laboratories to determine methicillin resistance are not as well established for coagulase-negative staphylococci as for *S. aureus*. Thus, some authorities recommend the use of vancomycin for serious coagulase-negative staphylococcal infections in spite of susceptibility patterns suggesting methicillin susceptibility. A polymerase chain reaction test that detects the presence of the *mec*A gene that encodes for methicillin resistance is used in some laboratories for both *S. aureus* and coagulase-negative staphylococci; however, this test is costly, labor intensive, and not readily available at most hospitals. Detection of methicillin resistance by latex agglutination testing for the presence of PBP2a is also available.

For patients allergic to β-lactam antibiotics, other antimicrobial agents for staphylococcal infections include (depending on susceptibility results) trimethoprim–sulfamethoxazole (TMP–SMX), quinolones, such as levofloxacin or moxifloxacin, clindamycin, and erythromycin. The use of these antistaphylococcal agents should generally be restricted to the treatment of localized, uncomplicated infections. Vancomycin, daptomycin, linezolid, quinupristin–dalfopristin, and tigecycline are also alternatives for serious *S. aureus* infections in allergic patients.

INFECTION CONTROL ISSUES

Because of the difficulty in treating MRSA infections and the propensity for *S. aureus* to spread among patients from the hands of health care workers, guidelines for the control of MRSA within acute care hospitals have been issued. Patients who have MRSA isolated should be placed in a private room in Contact Precautions, ensuring that health care workers wear gloves for general care of the patient, don gowns when performing tasks likely to result in contamination of clothing by secretions, and assiduously wash their hands before and after patient care. Special care should be taken with wounds from which MRSA has been isolated and with sputum in a patient with pneumonia due to MRSA.

Decolonization of patients who are infected or colonized with MRSA is generally not carried out, in part because the effect is transient and recolonization the rule. However, it has been known for some time that colonization of nares and skin prior to a surgical procedure is associated with an increased risk of postoperative staphylococcal wound infection. Recent data suggest that transient decolonization of the nares by application of mupirocin ointment can decrease the risk of postoperative wound infection. However, the drug is not approved for this indication, and treatment of all patients preoperatively is discouraged because resistance to mupirocin has been shown to develop rapidly in hospitals in which treatment is widespread. Many authorities advocate using this drug only for efforts designed to disrupt transmission during outbreaks.

INFECTIONS DUE TO *S. AUREUS*
Skin and Soft-Tissue Infections

The most common infections caused by *S. aureus* are skin and soft-tissue infections. Folliculitis, furuncles, abscesses, and wound infections are common and can often be treated with oral antibiotics. At the moment, β-lactam antibiotics (penicillinase-resistant penicillins and first-generation cephalosporins) remain the most effective drugs for treating mild to moderate infections (Table 149.1). For more severe infection, empiric treatment for CA-MRSA should be considered until culture results are available. For any skin lesion, incision, drainage, and culture of purulent material are important adjuncts to assure early identification of MRSA and resolution of infection.

Cellulitis is commonly due to *S. aureus* and may be difficult to differentiate from that due to β-hemolytic streptococci. Initial treatment of cellulitis should always include drugs effective against both *S. aureus* and β-hemolytic streptococci. In the clinically

Table 149.1 Treatment of Noncardiac Infections Due to *Staphylococcus aureus*

Infection	First-Line Drugs[a]	Second-Line Drugs[a,b]	Comments
Folliculitis, furunculosis, minor abscesses, and wound infections	Dicloxacillin, 250 mg, or Cephalexin, 250 mg PO q6h for 7–10 d	Clindamycin, 300 mg q6h TMP–SMZ,160/800 mg PO q12h, for 7–10 d	Community-acquired MRSA (CA-MRSA) increasing
Cellulitis	Nafcillin, 1 g q4h, or Cefazolin, 1 g IV q8h for 10–14 d	Vancomycin, 1 g IV q12h Linezolid, 600 mg PO q12h for 10–14 d	If CA-MRSA suspected, vancomycin until patient afebrile and nontoxic, then switch to oral agent
Moderate to severe wound infections			
MSSA	Nafcillin, 2 g q4h, or Cefazolin, 2 g IV q8h for 2 wk	Vancomycin, 1 g IV q12h for 2 wk	Drainage and culture of abscesses essential for resolution
MRSA	Vancomycin, 1 g IV q12h for 2 wk	Linezolid, 600 mg PO q12h Daptomycin, 4 mg/kg IV q24h	Monitor vancomycin troughs Aim for 10–15 μg/mL
Osteomyelitis			
MSSA	Nafcillin, 2 g IV q4h, or Cefazolin, 2 g IV q8h, for 6 wk Vancomycin, 1 g IV q12h 6 wk	Vancomycin, 1 g IV q12h for 6 wk	Vertebral osteomyelitis, with or without paraspinous or epidural abscess, often requires longer duration of therapy
MRSA		Linezolid, 600 mg PO q 12h Daptomycin, 4 mg/kg IV q24h	Monitor vancomycin troughs Aim for 15–20 μg/mL
Septic arthritis			
MSSA	Nafcillin, 2 g q4h, or Cefazolin, 2 g IV q8h for 4 wk	Vancomycin, 1 g IV q12h for 4 wk	Repeated needle aspiration, arthroscopic drainage, or operative drainage of joint fluid essential for resolution of infection
MRSA	Vancomycin, 1 g IV q12h for 4 wk	Linezolid, 600 mg PO q12h Daptomycin, 4 mg/kg IV q24h for 4 wk	
Pneumonia			
MSSA	Nafcillin, 2 g IV q4h for 2–4 wk	Vancomycin, 1 g IV q12h for 2–4 wk	Empyema, when present, must be drained
MRSA	Vancomycin 1 g IV q12h for 2–4 wk	Linezolid, 600 mg IV/PO q12h	Daptomycin not effective
Bacteremia			
MSSA	Nafcillin 2 g IV q4h (see text for discussion regarding length of therapy	Vancomycin, 1 g IV q12h (see text for discussion regarding length of therapy)	Length of therapy depends on source of bacteremia and whether visceral foci of infection, including endocarditis, are present.
MRSA	Vancomycin 1 g IV q12h (see text for discussion)	Daptomycin, 6 mg/kg IV q24h (see text)	Careful diagnostic work-up and clinical assessment of the patient is essential. regarding length of therapy

Abbreviations: MSSA = methicillin-susceptible *Staphylococcus aureus*; MRSA = methicillin-resistant *Staphylococcus aureus*; TMP–SMX = trimethoprim–sulfamethoxazole.
[a] Usual adult doses. Doses of cefazolin and vancomycin dependent on renal function.
 Linezolid, monitor complete blood count weekly.
 Daptomycin, monitor creatine phosphokinase 1×–2× weekly.
[b] Second-line drugs used mostly for patients allergic or intolerant to β-lactam antibiotics.

stable patient, penicillinase-resistant penicillins or first-generation cephalosporins can be used until the organism is identified and antimicrobial susceptibilities are reported. Many patients will require intravenous administration of antibiotics until the acute illness has improved, then therapy can be switched to oral agents. Initial therapy with nafcillin or cefazolin followed by dicloxacillin or cephalexin is preferred for MSSA infection. In the patient with MRSA infection or in whom there is a high likelihood of MRSA infection, vancomycin followed by an oral agent based on culture results is preferred.

Osteoarticular Infections

Staphylococcus aureus is the leading cause of osteoarticular infections. These infections are difficult to treat and frequently require long-term therapy with intravenous antibiotics. Most difficult to treat are those patients who have prosthetic joints or hardware in place. Nafcillin or vancomycin should be used until antibiotic susceptibilities are available. In the case of septic arthritis, drainage of infected synovial fluid is essential to preserve joint function and eradicate infection. Intravenous therapy should continue for at least 4 weeks. For treatment of osteomyelitis, intravenous antibiotics should be given for a minimum of 6 weeks. Patients with vertebral osteomyelitis, paraspinous abscess, and/or epidural abscess often require treatment beyond 6 weeks to prevent relapse. This can usually be accomplished by giving an appropriate oral agent following the course of intravenous antibiotics.

Pulmonary Infections

In the past, staphylococcal pneumonia was seen primarily in elderly patients with underlying illnesses. Recently, severe CA-MRSA staphylococcal pneumonia has been seen in children and young adults, sometimes following influenza infection. Abscesses and empyema commonly complicate staphylococcal pneumonia. Given the severity of this infection, empiric treatment against MRSA should be started. Vancomycin failures have been noted, but the benefit of primary or adjunctive use of linezolid in this setting remains controversial. Daptomycin should not be used because the drug does not achieve adequate lung tissue levels. Definitive treatment choices should be based on the organism's susceptibilities and should continue for 2 to 4 weeks depending on the patient's response. Drainage of loculated fluid in the pleural space is essential for resolution of infection.

Bacteremia

Bacteremia may reflect a transient event, often associated with a removable focus, most often an intravascular catheter, or it may be the first indication of deep-seated visceral infection, including endocarditis. If a catheter is the presumed source of the infection and it has been promptly removed and antibiotic treatment begun, the length of therapy can be guided by the patient's clinical response and the length of time that bacteremia persists. If immediate resolution of bacteremia and fever is documented, the patient can be treated with 14 days of antibiotic therapy with nafcillin or cefazolin for MSSA or vancomycin for MRSA bacteremia. Patients with persistent fever and/or bacteremia documented for >72 hours following removal of the catheter should have, in addition to routine clinical assessment for visceral foci of infection, echocardiography to help define whether endocarditis is present. If there is no clinical, laboratory, or echocardiographic evidence for endocarditis or other visceral infection, then treatment for a total of 2 weeks is appropriate. For patients in whom deep-seated infections are documented and for those in whom the clinical suspicion of endocarditis is high, longer courses of therapy (4–6 weeks) are required. Under no circumstances should patients simply have the catheter removed without antibiotic treatment because of the propensity of *S. aureus* to seed to multiple organs, including brain, spleen, kidney, joints, and bones.

Endocarditis

The most serious staphylococcal infection is endocarditis. Patients with left-sided cardiac lesions frequently have metastatic abscesses in spleen, brain, kidney, and myocardium, and the mortality rate varies from 25% to 70% depending on the host and the extent of infection. Transesophageal echocardiography has become an important tool for both diagnostic and therapeutic reasons. The patient must be monitored closely for symptoms and signs of septic complications that require surgical intervention. Right-sided endocarditis is most commonly found in intravenous drug users. In that population, the mortality rate is significantly lower, and shorter courses of therapy may be indicated.

For details of specific antibiotic regimens for endocarditis, see Chapter 36, Endocarditis of Natural and Prosthetic Valves: Treatment and Prophylaxis.

Toxic Shock Syndrome

Under certain conditions, such as those brought about by the use of tampons during menstruation and the packing of surgical wounds, *S. aureus* elaborates toxins that lead to multiorgan system disease in the absence of bacteremia. Treatment of shock and the removal of tampons or surgical packing are the primary goals of therapy. Antistaphylococcal therapy is secondary, initiated primarily to eradicate the carriage of toxin-producing *S. aureus* strains (see Chapter 18, Staphylococcal and Streptococcal Toxic Shock and Kawasaki Syndromes).

INFECTIONS DUE TO COAGULASE-NEGATIVE STAPHYLOCOCCI

Infections due to coagulase-negative staphylococci are often hospital acquired and are usually associated with prosthetic devices. Because coagulase-negative staphylococci are frequently resistant to many antibiotics, the most consistently reliable antibiotic for initial therapy is vancomycin. There are recent data noting the benefit of using rifampin as an adjunctive agent in the treatment of infected prosthetic devices. The recommended treatment regimen for prosthetic valve endocarditis is vancomycin or nafcillin combined with rifampin for 6 weeks and gentamicin for 2 weeks (see Chapter 36, Endocarditis of Natural and Prosthetic Valves: Treatment and Prophylaxis). For prosthetic joint infections, vancomycin or nafcillin, with rifampin, for 6 weeks is recommended. Antimicrobial therapy alone often fails in patients with prosthetic device infections, necessitating the removal of the device for cure. Infected intravenous devices that are easily removed, such as central venous catheters, peripherally inserted central catheters, and midline catheters, should be removed, and 7 to 10 days of antimicrobial therapy given. For those intravenous devices, such as Hickman or Groshong catheters and subcutaneous ports, that are more difficult to remove, a 2-week trial of vancomycin or nafcillin with or without rifampin may be adequate. However, if relapse occurs in this setting, or if tunnel infection or septic phlebitis is present, then the catheter or port should be removed (see Chapter 105, Intravascular Catheter-Related Infections).

SUGGESTED READING

Baddour LM, Wilson WR, Bayer AS, et al. Infective endocarditis: diagnosis, antimicrobial therapy, and management of complications. A statement for healthcare professionals from the Committee on Rheumatic Fever, Endocarditis, and Kawasaki Disease, Council on Cardiovascular Disease in the Young, and the Councils on Clinical Cardiology, Stroke, and Cardiovascular Surgery and Anes-thesia, American Heart Association– Executive Summary. *Circulation*. 2005;111:3167–3184.

Carpenter CF, Chambers HF. Daptomycin: another novel agent for treating infections due to drug-resistant gram-positive pathogens. *Clin Infect Dis*. 2004;38:994–1000.

Deresinski S. Methicillin-resistant Staphylococcus aureus: an evolutionary, epidemiologic, and therapeutic odyssey. *Clin Infect Dis*. 2005;40:562–573.

Eliopoulos GM. Quinupristin-dalfopristin and linezolid: evidence and opinion. *Clin Infect Dis*. 2003;36:473–481.

Fowler VG, Boucher HW, Corey GR, et al. Daptomycin versus standard therapy for bacteremia and endocarditis caused by Staphylococcus aureus. *N Engl J Med*. 2006;355:653–665.

Fowler VG Jr, Sanders, LL, Sexton DJ, et al. Outcome of Staphylococcus aureus bacteremia according to compliance with recommendations of infectious diseases specialists: experience with 244 patients. *Clin Infect Dis*. 1998;27:478–486.

Gorwitz RJ, Jernigan DB, Powers JH, et al. Strategies for clinical management of MRSA in the community: summary of an experts' meeting convened by the Centers for Disease Control and Prevention. 2006. http://www.cdc.gov/ncidod/dhqp/ar_mrsa_ca.html. Accessed January 3, 2006.

Hidayat LK, Hsu DI, Quist R, et al. High-dose vancomycin therapy for methicillin-resistant Staphylococcus aureus infections: efficacy and toxicity. *Arch Intern Med*. 2006;166:2138–2144.

Lewis JS, Jorgensen JH. Inducible clindamycin resistance in staphylococci: should clinicians and microbiologists be concerned? *Clin Infect Dis*. 2005;40:280–285.

Lowy FD. Staphylococcus aureus infections. *N Engl J Med*. 1998;339:520–532.

Moellering RC. Linezolid: The first oxazolidinone antimicrobial. *Ann Intern Med*. 2003;138:135–142.

Noskin GA. Tigecycline: a new glycylcycline for treatment of serious infections. *Clin Infect Dis*. 2005;41(suppl 5):S303–S314.

Raad II, Hanna HA. Intravascular catheter related infections: new horizons and recent advances. *Arch Intern Med*. 2002; 162:871–878.

Stevens DL. The role of vancomycin in the treatment paradigm. *Clin Infect Dis*. 2006;42: S51–S57.

Zetola N, Francis JS, Nueremberger EL, Bishai WR. Community-acquired methicillin-resistant Staphylococcus aureus: an emerging threat. *Lancet Infect Dis*. 2005;5:275–286.

150. Streptococcus Groups A, B, C, D, and G

Dennis L. Stevens, J. Anthony Mebane, and Karl Madaras-Kelly

CLASSIFICATION

In the early 1950s, Lancefield divided streptococci into groups based on carbohydrates present in the cell wall and designated the groups A through H and K through T. In addition, streptococci may be classified by their characteristics on culture on sheep blood agar. β-Hemolytic streptococci produce zones of clear hemolysis around each colony; α-hemolytic streptococci (*Strepococcus viridans*) produce a green discoloration characteristic of incomplete hemolysis; absence of hemolysis is characteristic of γ-streptococci.

GROUP A

Pharyngitis

The sole member of Lancefield group A is *Streptococcus pyogenes*. Group A streptococcus is ubiquitous in the environment but with rare exceptions is exclusively found in or on the human host. About 5% to 20% of the population harbor group A streptococcus in their pharynx, and some are colonized on their skin. This organism produces a variety of suppurative infections; however, streptococcal pharyngitis, the most common, is characterized by the onset of sore throat, fever, painful swallowing, and chilliness. These symptoms combined with submandibular adenopathy, pharyngeal erythema, and exudates correlate with positive throat cultures in 85% to 90% of cases. Sore throat without fever or any of the other signs and symptoms has a low predictive value for pharyngitis caused by group A streptococcus. Rapid strep tests correlate with positive cultures in 68% to 99% of cases, but results depend greatly on the individual performing the test as well as the bacterial colony count. Colony counts greater than 100 per plate correlated with positive rapid strep tests in 95% of patients, and counts less than 100 per plate correlated with positive rapid strep tests for only 68% of patients.

Therapy

Penicillin remains the drug of choice for group A streptococcal pharyngitis and tonsillitis (Table 150.1). In the past, the purpose of treatment of streptococcal pharyngitis was largely to prevent postinfectious immunologic sequelae. However, because some patients with pharyngitis have subsequently developed streptococcal toxic shock syndrome with or without necrotizing fasciitis, it seems prudent to diagnose and treat streptococcal pharyngitis aggressively in an attempt to prevent this complication as well. Antibiotic treatment of streptococcal pharyngitis reduces pharyngeal pain and fever by approximately 24 hours in children. Penicillin treatment within 10 days of the onset of pharyngitis is extremely effective in the prevention of rheumatic fever, although it is unclear whether it prevents poststreptococcal glomerulonephritis. Penicillin fails to eradicate group A streptococcus from the pharynx in 5% to 25% of patients with pharyngitis or tonsillitis, although penicillin resistance has never been documented. The most likely explanation for such failure, particularly in patients with tonsillitis, is the inactivation of penicillin by β-lactamases produced by co-colonizing organisms such as *Staphylococcus aureus*, *Haemophilus influenzae*, *Moraxella catarrhalis*, and *Bacteroides fragilis*. A second course of penicillin fails in >50% of patients, and treatment with dicloxacillin, a cephalosporin, Augmentin, erythromycin, or clindamycin will subsequently cure 90% to 95% of patients. Preparations containing procaine penicillin G plus benzathine penicillin are no more effective than benzathine alone but are less painful on injection. Ceftriaxone is under study for this indication. Resistance to erythromycin is about 5% in the United States, but in 1970, it reached a prevalence of 70% in Japan during a period of extensive erythromycin use in that country. In Finland and Sweden, emergence of erythromycin resistance has also paralleled erythromycin use.

Prophylactic treatment for populations at risk (eg, schools, military) is indicated during epidemics of streptococcal pharyngitis when rheumatic fever is prevalent. The incidence of rheumatic fever has declined in developed nations but flourishes in third world countries. Antistreptococcal prophylaxis should be

Table 150.1 Streptococcal Infections

Organism	Lancefield Group	Type of Infection	Therapy
Streptococcus pyogenes	A	Pharyngitis and impetigo	Benzathine penicillin IM, 1.2 million U for adults; 600 000 U for children ≤60 lb Penicillin G or V, 400 000 U PO QID for 10 days for adults; 200 000 U QID for children ≤60 lb Erythromycin ethyl succinate, PO 40 mg/kg/d
		Recurrent streptococcal pharyngitis, tonsillitis	Same as above or ampicillin + clavulanic acid, PO 20–40 mg/kg/d Oral cephalosporin Clindamycin, 10 mg/kg/d PO in 4 doses
		Cellulitis and erysipelas	Nafcillin, 8–12 g/d IV for 7–10 d Penicillin G or V, 200 000 U PO QID for 10 days Dicloxacillin, 500 mg PO QID for 10 days for adults
		Necrotizing fasciitis, myositis, and streptococcal toxic shock syndrome	Clindamycin, 900 mg IV q8h in adults and penicillin, 4 million U IV q4h for adults
		Prophylaxis of rheumatic fever	Benzathine penicillin, 1.2 million U IM q28d Penicillin G, 200 000 U PO bid for children ≤60 lb Sulfadiazine, 1 g/d for patients >27 kg; 500 mg/d for patients ≤27 kg Erythromycin, 250 mg PO BID
Streptococcus agalactiae	B	Neonatal sepsis	Penicillin, IV 100 000–150 000 U/kg/d in 2–3 divided doses for infants ≤7 days of age Penicillin, 200 000–250 000 U/kg/d IV in 4 divided doses for infants >7 days of age Ampicillin, 100 mg/kg/day IV in 2–3 divided doses for infants ≤7 d of age Ampicillin, 150–200 mg/kg/day IV in 4 divided doses for infants >7 d of age
		Postpartum sepsis	Ampicillin, 8–12 g IV in 4–6 divided doses or penicillin 12–24 million U/d for adults
		Septic arthritis	Penicillin or ampicillin as for neonatal sepsis or postpartum sepsis above
		Soft-tissue infection Osteomyelitis	Penicillin or ampicillin as for postpartum sepsis above
		Intrapartum prophylaxis	1. Acqueous penicillin G 5 million U IV loading dose followed by 2.5 million U q4h for 4 doses 2. Ampicillin 2 g IV loading dose followed by 1 g q4h for 4 doses
Streptococcus equi	C	Bacteremia Cellulitis Pharyngitis	Penicillin as for streptococcal toxic shock syndrome above
Enterococcus faecalis[a]	D	Endocarditis Bacteremia Urinary tract infection Gastrointestinal abscess	Ampicillin + gentamicin
Streptococcus bovis	D	Bacteremia Abscesses	Penicillin as for *Streptococcus equi* above
Streptococcus canis	G	Bacteremia Cellulitis Pharyngitis	Penicillin as for *Streptococcus equi* above

[a] Linezolid has activity against vancomycin-resistant enterococci (VRE). See Chapter 133, Enterococcus, for more details.

continuous in individuals with a history of rheumatic fever. Benzathine penicillin given intramuscularly once each month has the greatest efficacy, although oral agents such as phenoxymethyl penicillin are also effective. In recent years, the U.S. military has demonstrated that such prophylaxis, particularly benzathine penicillin, prevents epidemics of streptococcal infections among young soldiers living in crowded conditions. Routine follow-up culture to verify eradication is not recommended except in patients with a history of rheumatic fever. Following appropriate treatment for symptomatic pharyngitis, treatment is not needed for continued positive cultures unless symptoms recur.

Scarlet Fever

Severe cases of scarlet fever were prevalent in the United States, western Europe, and Scandanavia during the 19th century, and mortality rates of 25% to 35% were not uncommon. In contrast, scarlet fever today is rare and, when it occurs, is very mild. The primary site of infection is usually the pharynx, although surgical site infections have also been described. Classically, a diffuse, erythematous rash with sandpaper consistency appears 2 days after the onset of pharyngitis. Circumoral pallor and "strawberry" tongue are common findings, and desquamation occurs approximately 6 to 10 days later. The cause of the rash is uncertain, although most agree that extracellular toxins, likely the pyrogenic exotoxins formerly called "scarlatina toxins," are responsible. Treatment of the underlying infection with penicillin (see "Pharyngitis") and general supportive measures are indicated. Specifically, severe hyperpyrexia (fevers to 107°F to 110°F [41.7°C to 43.3°C]) have been described, and antipyretics may be necessary to prevent febrile seizures.

Pyoderma (Impetigo Contagiosa)

Impetigo is a superficial vesiculopustular skin infection. Although *S. aureus* is the most common organism isolated in modern times, group A streptococcus is likely the most significant pathogen. Impetigo is most common in patients with poor hygiene or malnutrition. Colonization of the unbroken skin occurs first; then minor abrasions, insect bites, and so on initiate intradermal inoculation. Single or multiple thick, crusted, golden-yellow lesions develop within 10 to 14 days. Penicillin orally or parenterally, or bacitracin or mupirocin topically, is effective treatment and will reduce transmission of streptococci to susceptible individuals. None of these treatments, including penicillin, prevent poststreptococcal glomerulonephritis. Although *S. aureus* may cause impetigo, it has never been implicated as a cause of glomerulonephritis.

Erysipelas

Erysipelas occurs most commonly in the elderly and very young. It is caused almost exclusively by group A streptococcus and is characterized by an abrupt onset of fiery red localized on the face or extremities (Figure 150.1). Distinctive features are well-defined margins, particularly along the nasolabial fold, scarlet or salmon red rash, rapid progression, and intense pain. Flaccid bullae may develop during the second to third day of illness, and desquamation of the involved skin occurs 5 to 10 days into the illness. In contrast, the rash of scarlet fever is generalized, has a diffuse pink or red hue that blanches on pressure, and has a sandpaper consistency. The organism is present in the lesion, although it is difficult to culture. Treatment with penicillin, a cephalosporin, or nafcillin is effective. Swelling may progress despite treatment, although fever, pain, and the intense redness usually diminish with 24 hours of treatment.

Cellulitis

Streptococcus pyogenes (group A streptococcus) is the most common cause of cellulitis, and although group A is the most common, β-hemolytic streptococci of groups B, C, and G also cause cellulitis in specific clinical settings. Patients with chronic venous stasis or lymphedema are predisposed to recurrent cellulitis caused by groups A, C, and G streptococci. Cellulitis in diabetic and elderly patients, particularly those with peripheral vascular disease, may also be caused by group

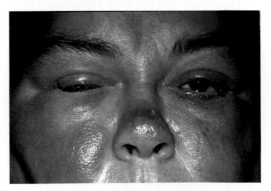

Figure 150.1 Erysipelas in a middle-aged woman. Note the brilliant red (salmon color) and the distinct demarcation along the nasolabial fold. The patient had a temperature of 39°C, tachycardia, normal blood pressure, and negative blood cultures. She responded well to intravenous penicillin G but developed superficial desquamation over the cheeks 10 days after admission.

B streptococci. Clinical clues to the category of cellulitis such as dog bite (*Capnocytophaga*), cat bite (*Pasteurella multocida*), human bite (mouth anaerobes and *Eikinella corrodens*), freshwater injury (*Aeromonas hydrophila*), seawater (*Vibrio vulnificus*), and furuncles (*S. aureus*) are extremely important. Definitive diagnosis in the absence of such factors rests on aspiration of the leading edge of the cellulitic lesion. At best, a bacterial cause is established in only 15% of cases. Cellulitis caused by groups A, B, C, and G streptococcus responds to penicillin, nafcillin, erythromycin, clindamycin, and a variety of cephalosporins. Ceftriaxone, cefpodoxime proxetil, and cefuroxime axetil have the greatest in vitro activity, and all have U.S. Food and Drug Administration (FDA)-approved indications for the treatment of streptococcal cellulitis. Although most quinolones have efficacy in the treatment of cellulitis, older quinolones such as ciprofloxacin should be avoided because of their poor in vitro activity against streptococci. Newer quinolones may be considered as second-line therapy.

Invasive Group A

In the past 10 years, there has been an increase in the number of severe group A streptococcal soft-tissue infections and bacteremia associated with shock and death in 30% to 70% of cases. Shock and organ failure early in the course of infection define streptococcal toxic shock syndrome, and the inciting infection may be necrotizing fasciitis, myositis, pneumonia, peritonitis, septic arthritis, uterine infection, and others. Predisposing factors include varicella virus infections, penetrating or blunt trauma, and nonsteroidal anti-inflammatory agents.

Therapy

When large numbers of streptococci accumulate, more organisms are in the stationary phase and are less affected by β-lactam antibiotics (the Eagle phenomenon). The decreased expression of critical penicillin-binding proteins in such slow-growing bacteria presumably explains the lack of efficacy of penicillin. In vitro, clindamycin—but not penicillin—prevents synthesis of toxins. Interestingly, in experimental necrotizing fasciitis and myositis, clindamycin has markedly better efficacy than penicillin. Thus some authorities recommend treatment with both penicillin and clindamycin (and debridement when appropriate). Uncontrolled observations suggest that intravenous immunoglobulin may be helpful as well.

GROUP B

Streptococcus agalactiae (the only species in Lancefield group B) colonize the vagina, gastrointestinal tract, and occasionally the upper respiratory tract of normal humans. Group B streptococci are the most common cause of neonatal pneumonia, sepsis, and meningitis in the United States and western Europe, with an incidence of 1.8 to 3.2 cases per 1000 live births. Preterm infants born to mothers who are colonized with group B streptococci in the third trimester and have premature rupture of the membranes are at highest risk for early-onset pneumonia and sepsis. The mean time of onset is 20 hours, and symptoms are respiratory distress, apnea, and fever or hypothermia. Ascent of the streptococcus from the vagina to the amniotic cavity causes amnionitis. Infants may aspirate streptococci either from the birth canal during parturition or from amniotic fluid in utero. Radiographic evidence of pneumonia and/or hyaline membrane disease is present in 40% of cases. Type III strains account for most cases of group B streptococcal meningitis.

Late-onset neonatal sepsis occurs 7 to 90 days postpartum. Symptoms are fever, poor feeding, lethargy, and irritability. Bacteremia is common, and meningitis occurs in 80% of cases.

The standards of modern-day prenatal care include swab culture of the lower vagina and anorectum for these organisms at 35 to 37 weeks of pregnancy. Women presenting in labor without such cultures can be screened with a rapid antigen-detecting kit, although the false-negative rate may be 10% to 30%. Both passive immunization with intravenous immunoglobulin and active immunization with multivalent polysaccharide vaccine show promise and in the future may become the best approach to prevention of neonatal sepsis as well as postpartum infection in the mother.

Adults with group B infections include postpartum women and patients with peripheral vascular disease, diabetes, or malignancy. Soft-tissue infection, septic arthritis, and osteomyelitis are the most common presentations.

Therapy

Penicillin is the treatment of choice, although in practice many neonates are empirically treated with ampicillin, 100 to 200 mg/kg/day, plus gentamicin. Once the diagnosis is established, penicillin or ampicillin should be given (Table 150.1). Adults should receive 12 million to 24 million units of penicillin per day for bacteremia, soft-tissue infection, or osteomyelitis; the dosage should be 8 to 12 g of ampicillin or 24 million units per day of penicillin for meningitis. Vancomycin or a first-generation cephalosporin is the alternative for patients allergic to penicillin. Intrapartum administration of ampicillin or aqueous penicillin G to women colonized with group B streptococcus during the third trimester, who had group B strep bacteriuria during the pregnancy, or who have premature labor or prolonged rupture of the membranes prevents group B neonatal sepsis. Infants should continue to receive ampicillin for 36 hours postpartum.

GROUPS C AND G

Groups C and G, which may be isolated from the throats of both humans and dogs, produce streptolysin O and resemble group A in colony morphology and spectrum of clinical disease. Before rapid identification tests were developed, many infections caused by groups C and G, such as pharyngitis, cellulitis, skin and wound infections, endocarditis, meningitis, osteomyelitis, and arthritis, were mistakenly attributed to group A. Rheumatic fever following group C or G streptococcal infection has not been described. These strains also cause recurrent cellulitis at the saphenous vein donor site in patients who have undergone coronary artery bypass surgery. Both organisms are susceptible to penicillin, erythromycin, vancomycin, and clindamycin.

GROUP D

Group D consists of gram-positive, facultatively anaerobic bacteria that are usually nonhemolytic but may demonstrate α- or β-hemolysis. *Streptococcus faecalis*, renamed *Enterococcus faecalis*, was previously classified as group D because it hydrolyzes bile esculin and possesses the group D antigen. *Streptococcus bovis* is also a cause of subacute bacterial endocarditis and bacteremia often in patients with underlying gastrointestinal malignancy. Enterococci are commonly isolated from stool, urine, and sites of intra-abdominal and lower-extremity infection. Enterococci cause subacute bacterial endocarditis and have become an important cause of nosocomial infection, not because of increased virulence, but because of antibiotic resistance. First, person-to-person transfer of

multidrug-resistant enterococci is a major concern to hospital epidemiologists. Second, superinfections and spontaneous bacteremia from endogenous sites of enterococcal colonization are described in patients receiving quinolone or moxalactam antibiotics. Last, conjugational transfer of plasmids and transposons between enterococci in the face of intense antibiotic pressure within the hospital milieu have created multidrug-resistant strains, including some with vancomycin and teicoplanin resistance.

Therapy

Serious infections with enterococci, such as endocarditis or bacteremia, require a synergistic combination of antimicrobials, that is, ampicillin or vancomycin together with an aminoglycoside (see Chapter 133, Enterococcus). Unlike enterococci, *S. bovis* remains highly sensitive to penicillin. Vancomycin-resistant enterococci (VRE) are being described with increasing frequency. Linezolid, an oxyzolidinone antibiotic, has excellent activity against VRE, although antibiotic resistance can develop during therapy.

SUGGESTED READING

American Academy of Pediatrics. *Report of the Committee on Infectious Diseases 1991*. Elk Grove Village, IL: American Academy of Pediatrics; 1991.

Baker CJ, Edwards MS. Group B streptococcal infections. In: Remington JS, Klein JO, eds. *Infectious Diseases of the Fetus and Newborn Infant*. 3rd ed. Philadelphia, PA: Saunders; 1991.

Bisno AL. Group A streptococcal infections and acute rheumatic fever. *N Engl J Med*. 1991;325:783–793.

Pfaller MA, Jones RN, Marshall SA, et al. Nosocomial streptococcal bloodstream infections in the SCOPE program: species and occurrence of resistance. The SCOPE hospital study group. *Diagn Microbiol Infec Dis*. 1997;29:259–263.

Stevens DL. Invasive group A streptococcus infections. *Clin Infect Dis*. 1992;14:2–11.

Stevens DL, Tanner MH, Winship J, et al. Severe group A streptococcal infections associated with a toxic shock like syndrome and scarlet fever toxin A. *N Engl J Med*. 1989;321:1–7.

Stevens DL, Bisno AL, Chambers HF, et al. Practice guidelines for the diagnosis and management of skin and soft-tissue infections. *Clin Infect Dis*. 2005;41:1373–1406.

151. Viridans Streptococci

Caroline C. Johnson

Viridans streptococci are a heterogeneous group of microorganisms that produce (partial) α-hemolysis or no hemolysis when grown on sheep blood agar. Various species can be distinguished according to their physiologic and biochemical characteristics, more than 20 of which have been associated with human infections. Typically, however, clinical laboratories speciate isolates only if they are recovered from blood or other usually sterile sites. Isolates recovered in mixed culture or from mucosal surfaces are normally reported only as nonhemolytic or α-hemolytic streptococci. Table 151.1 lists the most common species of viridans streptococci isolated from blood cultures.

Viridans streptococci are an important part of the normal microbial flora in humans. They are indigenous to the oral cavity, the upper respiratory tract, the female genital tract, and the gastrointestinal tract. Because these microorganisms lack traditional virulence factors, such as endo- and exotoxins, viridans streptococci are often considered to be of low virulence. However, a propensity to adhere to endovascular tissues accounts for their ability to produce endocarditis; extracellular dextran plays an important role in adherence and propagation of viridans streptococci on cardiac valves. Furthermore, some viridans streptococci are known to cause abscess formation, particularly the *Streptococcus milleri* group, composed of *Streptococcus intermedius*, *Streptococcus constellatus*, and *Streptococcus anginosus*.

INFECTIONS

Viridans streptococci are important causes of infective endocarditis. In addition, they are increasingly identified as causes of septicemia in immunocompromised hosts. With infection at other body sites, such as the central nervous system or lower respiratory tract, viridans streptococci may occur as sole pathogens but are more typically found as part of a mixed aerobic-anaerobic infection.

Infective Endocarditis

Viridans streptococci account for approximately 20% to 40% of cases of infective endocarditis.

Table 151.1 Most Common Species of Viridans Streptococci Isolated from Blood Cultures

Streptococcus sanguis
Streptococcus mitis
Streptococcus salivarius
Streptococcus intermedius
Streptococcus uberis
Streptococcus mutans
Streptococcus constellatus
Streptococcus (Gemella) morbillorum

Typically, patients have underlying cardiac valve abnormalities, such as mitral valve prolapse, degenerative valve disease, or rheumatic heart disease. Viridans streptococcal endocarditis develops insidiously and follows an indolent course. Fever, fatigue, and malaise are characteristic, but nonspecific, early clinical manifestations. In later stages of infection, cardiac murmurs may be detected in more than 90% of cases. Congestive heart failure and major embolic episodes are the most common complications of infective endocarditis, occurring in nearly one third of cases. The critical element for diagnosis of infective endocarditis is demonstration of continuous bacteremia. In the absence of recent antimicrobial therapy, two blood cultures will yield viridans streptococci in 95% of cases. Echocardiography, either transthoracic or transesophageal, may provide additional diagnostic and prognostic information in cases of endocarditis.

Bacteremia and Septicemia

Transient bacteremia due to viridans streptococci may occur in daily life, especially in individuals with poor dental hygiene or periodontal disease. It is rarely of clinical significance. In contrast, prolonged bacteremia has emerged as a genuine problem among patients undergoing cancer chemotherapy, especially among children. Viridans streptococci are now a leading cause of bacteremia in febrile, neutropenic patients in many cancer centers. Infection occurs in association with aggressive cyto-reductive therapy for acute leukemia or bone marrow transplantation, typically after high-dose cytosine arabinoside treatment. Other predisposing factors include oral mucositis, prophylactic administration of trimethoprim–sulfamethoxazole (TMP-SMX) or quinolone, presence of an indwelling central venous catheter, and use of antacids or histamine type 2 (H_2) antagonists. Although most immunocompromised patients with viridans streptococcal bacteremia present solely with fever, one fourth may also manifest organ dysfunction. A fulminant shock syndrome characterized by hypotension, rash with palmar desquamation, acute renal failure, adult respiratory distress syndrome, and death has also been described.

Meningitis and Brain Abscess

Viridans streptococci are an uncommon cause of meningitis, accounting for fewer than 5% of culture-proven cases. Infections occur in patients of all ages, including neonates. The source of infection for most cases is underlying ear, nose, or throat pathology, endocarditis, extracranial infection, or head trauma. Clinical manifestations are typical of acute pyogenic meningitis with signs of meningeal irritation, neurologic deficits, seizures, and altered sensorium. Although cerebrospinal fluid (CSF) pleocytosis is characteristically present with viridans streptococcal meningitis, the Gram stain of CSF is positive less than half of the time.

Viridans streptococci are also a cause of primary brain abscess, typically in association with anaerobic bacteria. Predisposing conditions include head and neck infection, lung abscess, and endocarditis. Clinical manifestations of brain abscess are primarily related to the size and location of the intracranial lesion, with headache being the most common presenting complaint. Fever is present in less than half of cases. Computed tomography or magnetic resonance imaging is useful both for diagnosis and to follow the course of antimicrobial therapy. Definitive microbiological diagnosis can be established from culture of brain abscess material obtained by excision or through stereotactic aspiration.

Pneumonia

Viridans streptococci are frequently identified in cultures of respiratory tract secretions. When recovered from expectorated sputum, viridans

streptococci are rarely considered significant, because of their presence as normal oral flora. However, they may also be found in lower respiratory tract specimens obtained from patients with pneumonia by transtracheal aspiration or protected bronchial brush. Typically, viridans streptococci cause lower respiratory tract infection in association with other oral organisms, especially anaerobes, following aspiration of oropharyngeal material. Predisposing conditions include periodontal disease, gingivitis, depressed cough and gag reflexes, dysphagia from esophageal disease, depressed consciousness, seizures, and ethanol abuse. Pneumonia usually develops in dependent lung segments and may lead to necrosis with abscess formation and/or empyema. The diagnosis of aspiration pneumonia should be suspected by the presence of purulent sputum and an abnormal radiograph in a patient at high risk of aspiration. Viridans streptococci are also occasionally identifed as sole pathogens in patients with lower respiratory tract infection.

THERAPY

Penicillin and related β-lactam antibiotics have long been considered the drugs of choice for therapy for infections due to viridans streptococci because of previously uniform susceptibility to these agents. However, resistance has now emerged as a significant problem, especially among nosocomial isolates and in those obtained from immunocompromised patients. Using a minimum inhibitory concentration (MIC) breakpoint criterion of ≤0.125 µg/mL for determining susceptibility, penicillin resistance has been reported in up to 50% of isolates recovered in some centers; up to 10% of all isolates are resistant to high concentrations of penicillin (MIC ≥ 4 ug/mL). In contrast, most community isolates of viridans group streptococci, including those associated with infective endocarditis, remain susceptible to penicillin. Other β-lactam antibiotics have in vitro activity similar to that of penicillin. Vancomycin has consistently excellent activity against viridans streptococci, whereas tetracycline, clindamycin, and erythromycin have variable activity, often with 25% to 50% of isolates reported resistant. Most strains of viridans streptococci are resistant to TMP–SMX.

Because of the unpredictable antibiotic susceptibility of viridans streptococci, in vitro testing should be performed on all clinically significant isolates recovered from normally sterile body sites, such as blood or CSF. Antibiotic

Table 151.2 Antibiotic Treatment of Specified Infection due to Viridans Streptococci

Infection Type	Antibiotic Regimen[a]	Duration
Septicemia	Penicillin G, 12–18 million units IV qd, in divided doses, and/or vancomycin,[b] 15 mg/kg (not to exceed 1 g) IV q12h	2 wk
Meningitis	Ceftriaxone, 2–4 g IV qd, in divided doses and/or vancomycin,[b] 15 mg/kg (not to exceed 1 g) IV q12h	2 wk
Brain abscess	Ceftriaxone, 2–4 g IV qd, in divided doses and/or vancomycin,[b] 15 mg/kg (not to exceed 1 g) IV q12h, plus metronidazole, 500 mg IV or PO q6h	≥6 wk
Pneumonia[c] (aspiration)	Clindamycin, 600 mg IV or PO q8h or penicillin G, 8–12 million units IV qd, in divided doses plus metronidazole, 500 mg IV or PO q6h or β-lactam/β-lactamase inhibitor combination	2–3 wk
Endocarditis	See Chapter 36, Endocarditis of Natural and Prosthetic Valves: Treatment and Prophylaxis, Table 36.3	

[a] Doses should be adjusted according to age, weight, and renal function.
[b] For suspected or confirmed infections due to β-lactam–resistant viridans streptococci.
[c] Presence of enteric gram-negative bacilli might require additional antimicrobial agents.

regimens that are currently recommended for treatment of infective endocarditis are summarized in Chapter 36, Endocarditis of Natural and Prosthetic Valves: Treatment and Prophylaxis, Table 36.3. Selection of the specific antimicrobial regimen for endocarditis is individualized for each patient; for streptococcal isolates that are moderately or highly resistant to β-lactam agents, penicillin should be given in combination with low doses of aminoglycoside.

Table 151.2 lists recommended antibiotic regimens for the treatment of septicemia, central nervous system infections, and lower respiratory tract infections due to viridans streptococci.

SUGGESTED READING

Bruckner L, Gigliotti F. Viridans group streptococcal infections among children with cancer and the importance of emerging antibiotic resistance. *Semin Pediatr Infect Dis.* 2006;17(3):153–160.

Claridge JE III, Attorri S, Musher DM, Hebert J, Dunbar S. Streptococcus intermedius, Streptococcus constellatus, and Streptococcus anginosus ("Streptococcus milleri group") are of different clinical importance and are not equally associated with abscess. *Clin Infect Dis.* 2001;32(10):1511–1515.

Doern GV, Ferraro MJ, Brueggemann AB, et al. Emergence of high rates of antimicrobial resistance among viridans group streptococci in the United States. *Antimicrob Agents Chemother.* 1996;40:891–894.

Enting RH, deGans J, Blankevoort JP, Spanjaard L. Meningitis due to viridans streptococci in adults. *J Neurol.* 1997;244:435–438.

Hoen B, Alla F, Selton-Suty C, et al. Changing profile of infective endocarditis: results of a 1-year survey in France. *JAMA.* 2002;288:75–81.

Prasad KN, Mishra AM, Gupta D, Husain N, Husain M, Gupta RK. Analysis of microbial etiology and mortality in patients with brain abscess. *J Infect.* 2006;53(4):221–227.

Richard P, Amador Del Valle G, Moreau P, et al. Viridans streptococcal bacteraemia in patients with neutropenia. *Lancet.* 1995;345:1607–1609.

Watanakunakorn C, Pantelakis J. Alpha-hemolytic streptococcal bacteremia: a review of 203 episodes during 1980–1991. *Scand J Infect Dis.* 1994;25:403–408.

152. Poststreptococcal Immunologic Complications

Barbara W. Stechenberg

Infections caused by group A β-hemolytic *Streptococcus* (*Streptococcus pyogenes*) are unusual in that they have been associated with nonsuppurative complications, acute rheumatic fever (ARF), and acute glomerulonephritis. These distinct clinical entities are not related to toxic effects of the organism and follow the infections by an interval during which immunologic mechanisms are triggered. Table 152.1 compares some features of two clinical syndromes. This chapter describes clinical manifestations and treatment for these sequelae.

ACUTE RHEUMATIC FEVER

ARF is a multisystem collagen-vascular disease that follows untreated or undetected group A streptococcal pharyngitis in 1% to 3% of persons. It is seen most commonly in children ages 5 to 17 and is associated with a genetic predisposition. There also appear to be strains of *S. pyogenes* more likely to be implicated in this condition (see Table 152.1).

The diagnosis of ARF is made clinically and is based on the modified Jones criteria (Table 152.2). The presence of two major or one major and at least two minor criteria suggests the diagnosis. Recent infection with *S. pyogenes* also must be suggested by either isolation of the organism from the throat or serologic evidence in the form of elevation of antistreptolysin-O, antihyaluronidase, or antideoxyribonuclease B titers. The exception to this rule is chorea, which becomes manifest 2 to 6 months after infection, by which time evidence of a recent streptococcal infection may be lacking.

The most common clinical manifestations of ARF are carditis and arthritis. The former usually presents as a significant murmur, most commonly mitral insufficiency. Both myocarditis and pericarditis may accompany this valvulitis. It is the only manifestation that may result in residual disease. The arthritis is a migratory polyarthritis that generally involves the medium-size joints (elbows, wrists, ankles, and knees). In adults, the clinical presentation may be purely migratory and not necessarily additive. Pain is often striking. Another characteristic finding is the dramatic response of the arthritis to salicylate therapy. Chorea known as Sydenham chorea or St. Vitus' dance usually occurs as an isolated, often subtle, neurologic disorder with behavioral aspects. Erythema marginatum and subcutaneous nodules are rarely seen. The strongest diagnoses of ARF are based on carditis or chorea. The weakest is based on arthritis as a single major manifestation with two minor criteria.

The term *PANDAS* (pediatric autoimmune neuropsychiatric disorder associated with group A *Streptococcus*) has been used to refer to a group of neuropsychiatric or behavioral disorders, particularly obsessive-compulsive disorder (OCD), Tourette's syndrome and tic disorder, with a possible relationship to group A streptococcal infections, and, perhaps, related pathologically to Sydenham chorea. Swedo and colleagues have proposed an autoimmune pathogenesis for these disorders. Suggested diagnostic criteria include the presence of OCD or a tic disorder; pediatric onset; abrupt onset of symptoms or a course characterized by dramatic exacerbations of symptoms; an association with group A streptococcal infection; and abnormal results of neurologic examination, such as choreiform movements, motor hyperactivity, and tics. Extensive investigation of its epidemiology, diagnosis, and treatment as well as its relationship to ARF are still underway.

Prevention

Primary prevention of ARF requires the proper diagnosis and treatment of *S. pyogenes* pharyngitis. The accepted standard of care is the performance of a throat culture or rapid streptococcal antigen detection test. If the latter is negative, a throat culture should be done because of the variable sensitivity of that test. Treatment of streptococcal pharyngitis should be undertaken, generally with oral phenoxymethyl penicillin (penicillin V) at 250 to 500 mg 2 or 3 times a day for 10 days; if compliance is an issue, benzathine penicillin G, 1.2 million units intramuscularly (IM) (if >60 lbs, 27 kg or 600 000 U if ≤27 kg), is acceptable. For patients

Table 152.1 Comparison of Acute Rheumatic Fever (ARF) and Acute Poststreptococcal Glomerulonephritis (AGN)

Feature	ARF	AGN
Prior infection	Pharyngitis	Pharyngitis or pyoderma
M-types	3, 5, 6, 14, 18, 19, 24	Pharynx: 1, 2, 3, 4, 12, 15 Skin: 4, 9, 52, 55, 59, 60, 61
Latency	2–4 wk	Throat: 10 d Skin: 3 wk
Recurrences	Common	Rare
Antibiotic prophylaxis	Useful	Not useful
Sequelae	Common (heart)	Rare

Table 152.2 Modified Duckett Jones Criteria for Acute Rheumatic Fever[a]

Major Criteria	Minor Criteria
Carditis	Previous rheumatic fever
Arthritis	Clinical
Chorea	Fever
	Arthralgia
Erythema marginatum	
Subcutaneous nodules	Laboratory
	Prolonged PR interval
	Elevated acute-phase
	reactants: erythrocyte
	sedimentation rate,
	C-reactive protein, white
	blood cell count

[a] Requirements: (1) evidence of antecedent group A streptococcal infection and (2) two major criteria or one major and at least two minor criteria.

allergic to penicillin, erythromycin, 50 mg/kg/day (maximum, 1 g/day) in 3 or 4 divided doses for 10 days, is the antibiotic of choice. Prompt treatment should prevent most cases of ARF after symptomatic pharyngitis. Initiation of therapy up to 8 days after infection begins is probably beneficial.

Therapy

Treatment of ARF involves three important areas: eradication of *S. pyogenes*, treatment of the acute manifestations, and prevention of both recurrences and infective endocarditis in those with residual carditis. The first is accomplished with the regimens for primary prevention. These regimens should be used even if the throat culture is negative at the time of diagnosis of ARF.

The mainstay of treatment of ARF is salicylates, both for arthritis and mild to moderate carditis. A dosage of 70 to 80 mg/kg/day should be initiated to produce a therapeutic blood level of 20 to 25 mg/dL. This is continued for at least 2 weeks, until acute inflammation has subsided, and then decreased gradually over the next 2 to 4 weeks. Patients with arthritis should be repeatedly evaluated for carditis during the initial 2 weeks. Persons with severe carditis and/or congestive heart failure should be treated with steroids, usually prednisone, at 2 mg/kg/day acutely for at least 2 weeks, with a gradual withdrawal over 4 to 6 weeks, with the introduction of salicylates to prevent rebound. Supportive care of carditis is important; digitalization should be done slowly starting with one quarter of the usual initial dose.

Sydenham chorea is usually self-limited over several weeks. If symptoms are debilitating, phenobarbital may be started at 15 to 30 mg every 6 to 8 hours. Haloperidol is an alternative. Bed rest must be used judiciously; it is more important in patients with acute carditis and chorea. It is used during the acute phase and then liberalized on an individual basis.

Secondary Prevention

Secondary prevention of infection with *S. pyogenes* is based on the fact that persons with ARF have at least 10% to 30% chance of recurrence of ARF when reinfected with this organism. Because of concerns about compliance, benzathine penicillin G, 1.2 million units IM every 4 weeks, is recommended, particularly in the first 5 years after clinical presentation and in persons with carditis. In areas of high prevalence of ARF, this regimen should be given every 3 weeks. Oral penicillin, 250 mg twice a day, is an acceptable alternative. Patients allergic to penicillin are treated with sulfadiazine, 500 mg twice a day. Erythromycin, 250 mg twice daily, should be reserved for persons allergic to both penicillin and sulfa. The duration of secondary prevention is controversial; many believe it should be lifelong, but there is evidence for discontinuing at age 21 or after 5 years (whichever is longer). Persons with residual carditis should be educated about the importance of oral hygiene. They should receive antibiotics for prophylaxis against infective endocarditis (see Chapter 36, Endocarditis of Natural and Prosthetic Valves: Treatment and Prophylaxis).

ACUTE POSTSTREPTOCOCCAL GLOMERULONEPHRITIS

Poststreptococcal acute glomerulonephritis (AGN) is an inflammatory disorder of the glomeruli. It occurs when soluble immunoglobulin G immune complexes are deposited at the glomerular basement membrane, causing complement activation and release of cytokines. This leads to infiltration of inflammatory cells. The streptococcal antigen involved has not been completely elucidated. It can follow either throat or skin infection with *S. pyogenes*. Table 152.1 lists the major strains associated with AGN and designated nephritogenic; since the early 1980s, the incidence of AGN has decreased remarkably, perhaps with a decrease in these M-types. AGN has rarely been associated with infection with group C streptococci.

The epidemiology of AGN reflects that of streptococcal pharyngitis (age 5 to 15 years; winter to spring) and pyoderma (younger age; summer months). Prompt therapy does not prevent AGN. The incubation period is about 10 days with pharyngeal strains and about 3 weeks following pyoderma.

Clinical manifestations include edema (85%), gross hematuria (25%), and hypertension (60% to 80%). A consequence of volume overload, the hypertension may lead to encephalopathic changes in a small number of patients. Symptoms referable to the cardiovascular system (cardiomegaly, congestive heart failure, pulmonary edema) are sometimes present. Fever is uncommon. Some patients have a mixed acute nephritis/nephrotic syndrome with ascites and anasarca. AGN is typically self-limited, with spontaneous diuresis and improvement in hypertension within 1 week. In fact, up to 50% have been asymptomatic during

outbreaks. In children, fewer than 2% of cases are complicated by acute renal failure. This number may be higher in adults. Progression to chronic renal failure is also very unlikely.

Freshly voided urine typically demonstrates mild proteinuria, red and white blood cells, and red and white blood cell casts. Gross hematuria (usually brown) disappears rapidly, although microscopic hematuria persists for months as does the proteinuria. Striking hypocomplementemia is seen in 90% of patients, primarily C3 and CH50 with a normal C4. Diagnosis is supported by the latter finding in association with evidence of preceding *S. pyogenes* infection. Following pharyngeal infection, antistreptolysin-O elevations are common. However, it is less useful following skin infections, after which anti-DNAase B or antihyaluronidase are more likely to be high. Attempts to culture the organism also should be undertaken.

Therapy

Therapy is supportive. Antibiotics should be given to eradicate any streptococcal carriage. However, no data have demonstrated that this therapy either prevents AGN or alters its natural history. As noted for ARF, penicillin is the agent of choice. Either benzathine penicillin G, 1.2 million units IM, or phenoxymethyl penicillin (Pen-V), 250 to 500 mg orally 2 to 3 times a day, are appropriate. Erythromycin, 250 mg 4 times a day, is an alternative for individuals allergic to penicillin. Oral therapy should be continued for 10 days. Patients with obvious edema, hypertension, or azotemia may require hospitalization, although most patients respond to careful restriction of fluid and salt intake. Diuretic therapy is usually successful in controlling hypertension. Prognosis is generally excellent. Relapses are rare.

There is no need for antibiotic prophylaxis to prevent future attacks because repeated episodes are rare.

SUGGESTED READING

Berrios X, del Campo E, Guzman B, et al. Discontinuing rheumatic fever prophylaxis in selected adolescents and young adults. *Ann Intern Med.* 1993;118:401.

Bisno AL. Group A streptococcal infections and acute rheumatic fever. *N Engl J Med.* 1991;325:783–793.

Ferrieri P. Proceedings of the Jones Criteria Workshop: Jones Criteria Workshop. *Circulation.* 2002;106:2521–2523.

Kurlan R, Kaplan EL: The pediatric autoimmune neuropsychiatric disorders associated with streptococcal infections (PANDAS) etiology for tics and obsessive-compulsive symptoms: hypothesis or entity? Practical considerations for the clinician. *Pediatrics.* 2004;113:883–886.

Popovic-Polovic M, Kostić M, Antić-Peco A, et al. Medium and long-term prognosis of patients with acute post-streptococcal glomerulonephritis. *Nephron.* 1991;58:393–399.

Special Writing Group of the Committee on Rheumatic Fever, Endocarditis and Kawasaki Disease. Guidelines for the diagnosis of acute rheumatic fever. *JAMA.* 1992;268:2069–2073.

Swedo SE, Leonard HL, Rapoport JL. The pediatric autoimmune neuropsychiatric disorders associated with streptococcal infections (PANDAS) subgroup: separating fact from fiction. *Pediatrics.* 2004;113:907–911.

Tejani A, Ingulli E. Post-streptococcal glomerulonephritis. *Nephron.* 1990;55:1–5.

Veasy GL, Hill HR. Immunologic and clinical correlations in rheumatic fever and rheumatic heart disease. *Pediatr Infect Dis J.* 1997;16:400–407.

153. Shigella

David W. K. Acheson

Shigella are a familiy of enteric pathogens consisting of four different species that are a common cause of diarrheal disease. *Shigella* are usually transmitted person to person but may also be transmitted via food, often from an infected food worker. The majority of illness from *Shigella* is short lived and does not require specific antibiotic therapy; however, some forms can be life threatening.

MICROBIOLOGY

Shigella belongs to the family Enterobacteriaceae and closely resembles *Escherichia coli* at the genetic level. Four species of *Shigella*—*Shigella dysenteriae, Shigella flexneri, Shigella boydii,* and *Shigella sonnei*—are differentiated by group-specific polysaccharide antigens of lipopolysaccharide, designated A, B, C, and D, respectively. *Shigella dysenteriae* consists of 10 antigenic types, of which type 1 produces a potent cytotoxin known as Shiga toxin. *Shigella flexneri* is divided into 6 types and 14 subtypes, and *S. boydii* into 18 serologic types. Although there is only 1 *S. sonnei* serotype, there are at least 20 colicin types. Shigellae are biochemically very similar, and differentiation among species is based primarily on serologic methods using group- and type-specific antisera.

EPIDEMIOLOGY

Shigellosis occurs throughout the world with varying species distribution. *Shigella dysenteriae* and *S. flexneri* are the predominant species in developing countries, whereas *S. sonnei* is the major isolate in developed countries, accounting for more than three quarters of the isolates in the United States. *Shigella flexneri* is being seen more frequently in the United States in homosexual men and is thought to be transmitted sexually in this group. *Shigella boydii* is uncommon except in the Indian subcontinent. Fecal–oral transmission is the typical way for these bacteria to spread. They will colonize only in humans and some nonhuman primates, so typically the route of spread is human to human and not via an animal vehicle. The spread is often person to person directly or via contaminated food (often salads) or water, and the disease is often associated with poor personal hygiene. Flies are also known to transmitt *Shigella*. One of the most striking features of shigellosis is the exceedingly small inoculum of organisms required to cause disease. As few as 10 to 100 *S. dysenteriae* have been shown to cause dysentery in adults. The other species may require 1000 to 10 000 bacteria, but this is still a small enough dose to be readily transmitted by fecal contamination of hands, water supply, or food.

CLINICAL FEATURES

Shigellosis characteristically begins with constitutional symptoms, including fever, fatigue, anorexia, and malaise with an incubation period of 1 to 4 days typically but may be as long as 8 days. Watery diarrhea usually develops and may become bloody and progress to dysentery within a few hours or days. The latter classically consists of a small amount of blood and mucus but may be grossly purulent. Progression to clinical dysentery is uncommon in *S. sonnei* infection, occurs more often in *S. boydii* infection, is common in *S. flexneri,* and occurs in most patients when *S. dysenteriae* is the cause. Although fluid loss is usually not a major problem in shigellosis (usually no more than 30 mL/kg/day), hyponatremia can be severe because of inappropriate secretion of antidiuretic hormone, especially in infants infected with *S. dysenteriae* type 1 or *S. flexneri.*

Shigellosis may cause both local and systemic complications. Intestinal obstruction and toxic megacolon during shigellosis are uncommon in the United States but occur regularly in developing countries and are associated with high mortality. *Shigella* bacteremia is considered to be uncommon; however, when routinely looked for, it is not rare and has been documented in 4% of a series of patients in Bangladesh. Bacteremic patients were more likely to die, and mortality in *Shigella* sepsis was 21% compared with 10% in the absence of bacteremia. Systemic complications are especially frequent during infection with *S. dysenteriae*, including toxic megacolon and leukemoid reactions with leukocyte counts in excess of 50000/dL. Hemolytic uremic syndrome (HUS) and neurologic complications, especially seizures, may occur. HUS is associated with the Shiga toxins produced by *S. dysenteriae* and may result in significant morbidity and mortality. Other complications include reactive arthritis, especially after infection with *S. flexneri* and may occur alone or as part of Reiter's syndrome. The pathogenesis of shigellosis is highly complex, involving multiple genes in both chromosomal and plasmid locations. Several reviews have been published on this topic (see the suggested reading at the end of this chapter).

DIAGNOSIS

Shigellosis may be diagnosed clinically, microbiologically, or serologically. Patients with the classical picture of dysentery, with frequent small-volume bloody stools, abdominal cramps, tenesmus, and large numbers of leukocytes in the stool, especially if febrile, can be given a presumptive diagnosis of shigellosis. However, in the early stages of shigellosis it may be difficult to differentiate clinically from other enteric infections. Studies in Bangladesh indicate that 85% of patients with shigellosis had >50 fecal leukocytes per high-power field. This level is higher than usual in other enteric infections. *Shigella* are especially fastidious and rapidly die off if stool samples are not properly handled. The best way to isolate *Shigella* is to obtain stool as opposed to rectal swabs, rapidly inoculate specimens onto selective culture plates, and quickly incubate them at 37°C (98.6°F). To optimize isolation, a variety of media such as MacConkey, deoxycholate, and eosinmethylene blue, and highly selective media such as Hektoen-enteric, salmonella-shigella, and xylose-lysinedeoxycholate should be used. Detection of antibodies to *Shigella* lipopolysaccharide is an alternative but is generally used for epidemiologic studies and not for routine diagnosis in the clinical microbiology laboratory. Molecular techniques, including DNA probes and polymerase chain reaction techniques, have also been described for the detection of *Shigella* but are not routinely used except in research.

THERAPY

Diarrhea from *Shigella* is generally not severely dehydrating; however, replacement of lost fluids and electrolytes is the most important therapy and can often be done orally and may be all that is required. Most infections in developed countries are caused by *S. sonnei* and are self-limiting within a few days. In more severe infections, usually those caused by *S. flexneri* or *S. dysenteriae*, hyponatremia with serum sodium below 120 mmol/L may be a significant problem requiring infusion of 3% hypertonic saline 12 mL/kg over 2 hours to raise the serum sodium by around 10 mmol/L. This therapy must be combined with restricted access to drinking water. Hypoglycemia, also a common problem in children with shigellosis in developing countries, may require intravenous replacement therapy. One way to do this is rapid infusion of glucose 1 g/kg body weight over 5 to 10 minutes, and then a continuous infusion of glucose, 50 g/L, until the infection is under control. Shigellosis involves major catabolic stress, and nutritional replacement is an important part of therapy.

Specific antimicrobial therapy in shigellosis requires the administration of agents that shorten the illness and reduce the mortality. There is a constantly changing landscape of resistance in *Shigella*, and many *Shigella* carry resistance for streptomycin, tetracycline, and chloramphenicol; more are now resistant to ampicillin and depending on locale, a varying proportion are also resistant to trimethoprim–sulfamethoxazole (TMP–SMX). In a study from Turkey published in 1998, of 289 *Shigella* strains isolated from children, 75% of the isolates were *S. sonnei* and 24.8% were *S. flexneri*; 79% of the isolates were resistant to streptomycin, 56% to tetracycline, 55.7% to TMP–SMX, 27.7% to ampicillin, and 19.7% to chloramphenicol. None of the isolates was resistant to ciprofloxacin, naladixic acid, cephalothin, ampicillin–sulbactam, and ceftriaxone. The authors concluded that TMP–SMX should not be used empirically in the treatment of shigellosis. In a second study undertaken between 1996 and 1997 at Kasturba Medical College Hospital, Manipal, 5 strains of *S. flexneri* and 1 strain of *S. dysenteriae* (of a total of 29 isolates found during the study period) were found to show resistance to naladixic acid and the newer fluoroquinolones (ciprofloxacin, norfloxacin, and ofloxacin). Since 1983 in England and Wales, the incidence of resistance to ampicillin in *S. dysenteriae*, *S. flexneri*, and *S. boydii* infections has increased from 42% to 65%, and the incidence of resistance to trimethoprim from 6% to 64%. For *S. sonnei*, almost 50% of isolates were resistant to ampicillin or trimethoprim, and 15% were resistant to both antimicrobials. However,

Table 153.1 Antimicrobial Therapy for Shigellosis in Adults

Drug	Dose	Comments
Ciprofloxacin	500 mg PO 2× daily for 5 d	1 g PO once for mild disease due to *Shigella* species other than *S. dysenteriae*
Other 4-quinolones	Variable	
Trimethoprim–sulfamethoxazole	160 mg TMP/800 mg SMX PO 2× daily for 5 d	Only when shown to be susceptible
Azithromycin	500 mg PO daily for one day, then 250 mg PO daily for 4 d	Alternative therapy
Abbreviation: PO = orally.		

Table 153.2 Antimicrobial Therapy for Shigellosis in Children

Drug	Dose	Comments
Azithromycin	12 mg/kg for the first day (maximum 500 mg) and then 6 mg/kg/dose (maximum 250 mg) for an additional 4 d	First-line oral therapy in areas of high resistance to TMP–SMX and ampicillin
Cefixime	8 mg/kg/day, single dose, (maximum 400 mg/d) for five days	Alternative first-line therapy
Ceftriaxone	50 mg/kg per day (maximum 1.5 g) in a single daily dose, for 5 d	First-line parenteral therapy when antimicrobial succeptiblity is unknown
Ciprofloxacin	10 mg/kg (maximum 500 mg/dose) every 12 h for 5 d	Alternative therapy for children >17 yr and for children with contraindications to ceftriaxone
Trimethoprim–sulfamethoxazole	10 mg/kg TMP and 50 mg/kg SMX per day (maximum 160 mg TMP and 600 mg SMX), in 2 divided doses for 5 d	Only when micobes shown to be susceptible

it is important to remember that many of these infections were likely imported from other countries. More recent studies published in 2006 from Eritrea, northeast Africa, indicate that high rates of resistance were observed against ampicillin, chloramphenicol, and TMP–SMX; 6% of the *S. flexneri* isolates were resistant to nalidixic acid. In Yemen, a study published in 2005 showed a statistically significant increase in resistance against tetracycline, cephradine, TMP–SMX, nalidixic acid, and aztreonam ($P \leq .05$) over a 10-year period of study. Almost 55.2% of the strains were resistant to four drugs. Significant resistance is also seen in the United States, with a 2005 outbreak of *S. sonnei* in Kansas, Kentucky, and Missouri reported to have shigellosis cases associated with day-care centers caused predominantly by multidrug-resistant (resistant to ampicillin and TMP–SMX) strains of *S. sonnei*.

Shigellosis, when mild, can be treated conservatively without antibiotic therapy. However, antibiotics will likely reduce the length of the illness and diminish the likelihood that the infected patient will spread the illness to others. There are circumstances in which the patient is toxic, bacteremic, elderly, immunocompromised, or otherwise at greater risk and requires antibiotic treatment. Currently the initial treatment of choice for adults in whom the antibiotic susceptibility is unknown is ciprofloxacin or some other fluoroquinolone (Table 153.1). Infections with *S. dysenteriae* require a 5-day course of therapy with a quinolone; however, other species of *Shigella* may require only 1 or 2 doses. If the isolate is known to be susceptible to TMP–SMX, then TMP–SMX (160/800 mg twice daily for 5 days) is appropriate. Another alternative is azithromycin (Table 153.1). Ampicillin and amoxicillin are not recommended due to the high rate of resistance, and third-generation cephalosporins are not recommended because of lack of efficacy.

In children the goals of antibiotic therapy are to improve symptoms (reduce the duration of fever, diarrhea, and fecal excretion) and decrease spread of infection to others. If illness is severe and parenteral therapy is required, the first-line treatment is ceftriaxone, 50 mg/kg/day, maximum 1.5 g, in a single daily dose for 5 days. Changes can then be made based on resistance studies of the bacterial isolates. Ciprofloxacin, 10 mg/kg, maximum 500 mg/dose, every 12 hours for 5 days, is an alternative therapy for older children (>17 years) and children with contraindications to ceftriaxone (Table 153.2). If oral therapy is to be used, azithromycin, 12 mg/kg for the first day, maximum 500 mg, and then 6 mg/kg/dose, maximum 250 mg, for an additional 4 days, is the suggested first-line oral treatment in areas of the world with high resistance to TMP–SMX and ampicillin when the antibiotic susceptibility of the organism is unknown. Alternative treatments for children younger than 18 years of age include nalidixic acid and cefixime.

SUGGESTED READING

Agha R, Goldberg, MB. Management of Shigella gastroenteritis in adults. UpToDate Web site. http://www.uptodate.com. Accessed November 14, 2007.

Amieva MR. Important bacterial gastrointestinal pathogens in children: a pathogenesis perspective. *Pediatr Clin North Am.* 2005;52:749–777.

Ashkenazi S. Treatment and prevention of Shigella infections in children. UpToDate Web site. http://www.uptodate.com. Accessed November 14, 2007.

Aysev AD, Guriz H. Drug resistance of *Shigella* strains isolated in Ankara, Turkey, 1993–1996. *Scand J Infect Dis.* 1998;30:351–353.

Cheasty T, Skinner JA, Rowe B, et al. Increasing incidence of antibiotic resistance in Shigellas from humans in England and Wales: recommendations for therapy. *Microb Drug Res.* 1998;4:57–60.

Keusch GT. *Shigella* and enteroinvasive *Escherichia coli.* In: Blaser MJ, et al, eds. *Infections of the Gastrointestinal Tract.* Philadephia, PA: Lippincott Williams & Wilkins; 2002.

Niyogi SW. Shigellosis. *J Microbiol.* 2005;43: 133–143.

154. Tularemia

Richard B. Hornick

Francisella tularensis is an unusual, gram-negative, rod-shaped bacteria that causes the disease tularemia. *Francisella tularensis* is unusual because of its virulence, the geographic distribution of the few known varieties, and the organism's unique preference for residing inside macrophages and neutrophils (it appears to prevent the oxidative burst and can escape the phagosome to persist in the neutrophil). Tularemia is acquired in most patients through contact with infected tissues of cottontail or jackrabbits or from bites of dogs, cats, snakes, and other animals that have become contaminated from biting or eating infected rabbits. Human infections can be induced by ticks, mosquitoes, and deer flies that have fed on an infected animal.

Tularemia has an American heritage. McCoy studied a plaguelike disease in ground squirrels in 1911 in Tulare County, California. Dr. Edward Francis subsequently selected the name tularemia (1921) for the disease because his investigations demonstrated that a bacteremia must occur and because of the first demonstration of infected animals in Tulare County. The organism was subsequently named *Francisella tularensis* to honor the extensive studies of Dr. Francis. Further studies have identified infection in more than 100 wild and domestic animals and the ectoparasites and biting insects that feed on them.

One of the two major strains is unique in the United States. Type A (biovar tularensis) is found often in cottontail rabbits. It is highly virulent (cottontails die within a week); very few organisms (50) injected subcutaneously or aerosolized and inhaled as small particles (5 μ) will induce disease. Type B strains (biovar holartica) are found in European and Asian countries, as well as in North America. This strain is less virulent in that mortality and morbidity are less in infected persons than that induced by type A. Volunteers were infected with doses 1000 times greater than with type A. Type B is found in rodents, woodchucks, and contaminated water. It does not kill cottontail rabbits. Subspecies of type A have been identified by pulse field gel electrophoresis (type A-east and type A-west). The former has the expected virulence potential of type A strains. Type A-west is less virulent than type B strains.

For many years the virulence of this organism, especially by aerosol disposal, has caused it to be studied as a potential biological weapon. The studies resulted in a very effective attenuated vaccine available to prevent disease (see below).

TYPES OF INFECTIONS

There are four types of disease, each related to the route of infection: ulceroglandular, pneumonitis, typhoidal, and oculoglandular. In nature the mechanisms of transmission are through minute cuts or pores in the skin, producing an ulcer; the organisms are often acquired when skinning or eviscerating an infected animal. In this process of eviscerating, large numbers of organisms can be aerosolized from the organs, especially the liver. Small numbers of these may reach the lower levels of the lung and cause pneumonitis. Ticks may deposit the organisms on the skin adjacent to the site of their bite. The organism will then be transmitted into the skin when the wound is scratched or rubbed.

The incubation period for the ulceroglandular form of tularemia is 2 to 6 days. Patients usually present with an ulceration of a finger, often around the edge of the nail bed. Regional draining lymph nodes enlarge and may become fluctuant if antibiotic therapy has not been administered. These nodes will heal without being drained when appropriate antibiotic therapy is given. Some nodes, when incised, resolve very slowly despite antibiotic therapy.

The incubation period for the most serious form of tularemia, pneumonitis, is 4 to 6 days. The affected areas of the lung may be difficult to interpret on chest radiographs. The pattern of several rounded opacities suggests tularemia. However, few patients demonstrate this radiographic picture. Various radiographic findings may be present, including lobar pneumonia, pleural effusions, abscess, mediastinal adenopathy, and tracheal compression. Oculoglandular tularemia presents with small yellowish granulomatous lesions on the palpebral conjunctivae. The preauricular lymph nodes enlarge and are tender. Untreated, the cornea may be perforated by the infectious process. Contaminated fingers rubbing an eye can initiate the infection. Spread from ulceroglandular disease can also induce pneumonitis.

Typhoidal tularemia occurs when the ingested organisms spread throughout the body from the oropharynx. Cervical lymph nodes are enlarged, and mesenteric nodes may also be involved and cause abdominal pain. Very large numbers of *F. tularensis* are required. The gastrointestinal tract appears to be resistant to infection or disease.

DIAGNOSIS

Each of these clinical presentations is difficult to diagnose, especially in patients remote from endemic areas. Historical facts regarding recent exposures to animals, ticks, and deer flies, among others, provide a significant assist and will direct therapeutic options. Fever and chills are common with each form of disease. The ulcer may have a black base, similar to that caused by *B. anthracis*. Very little pus is present in the ulcer.

Patients with pneumonia are quite ill, with chills, fever, substernal burning, and nonproductive cough. Headache, myalgia, photophobia, malaise, and extreme fatigue are common but not distinctive. Cervical lymph nodes may be enlarged, and these, plus the substernal burning in a patient with a sudden onset of pneumonitis and the history of direct or indirect animal exposure, should raise concerns about tularemia.

Laboratory findings are not helpful; the leukocyte count will be normal if no abscess is present, despite the obvious pneumonitis or ulceroglandular disease. Blood, sputum, and other culture specimens can be obtained, but the laboratory must be alerted to the possibility of tularemia. Laboratory personnel have become infected from laboratory accidents. Appropriate class 4 facilities are needed to prevent spread to humans or laboratory animals.

Serologic studies are the safest method to make a diagnosis. However, the agglutinating antibodies do not appear for 7 to 10 days and peak at 3 to 4 weeks. Paired specimens of serum obtained 2 weeks apart with a 4-fold rise in titer is confirmatory. A single specimen with a titer of 1:160 or greater without any prior known exposure to *F. tularensis* is diagnostic. Polymerase chain reaction is a quick method but available only in experimental laboratories.

Skin Tests

Although the skin test is a reliable diagnostic tool (the test can be positive in the first week of disease), the antigen is not readily available. The Centers for Disease Control and Prevention in Atlanta may be able to provide the test solution.

TREATMENT

Streptomycin therapy changed tularemia from a deadly disease to one that was readily controlled. It is very effective. Patients should receive 1 g every 12 hours for 10 days. Prompt defervescence will occur. Appropriate dosage adjustments are needed when renal insufficiency is present. Gentamicin also is effective (and more readily available), 5 mg/kg/day with normal renal function. Tetracyclines and chloramphenicol are effective but are second choices to the aminoglycosides; they are not bactericidal, and responses are slower with relapses possible. The fluoroquinolone group is effective in experimental animals and in in vitro tests. They have been evaluated in only a few patients, with good results. No antibiotic-resistant strains have been isolated from patients with tularemia.

Mortality from pneumonia caused by type A is less than 1% to 2% if treatment is instituted promptly. Without appropriate therapy, mortality approaches 50%. Type B pneumonitis is milder.

Ulceroglandular disease caused by type A has a 5% mortality if untreated; type B ulceroglandular infection is indolent and self-limited without antibiotic therapy.

Isolation of patients is unnecessary; no evidence of person-to-person spread has been documented.

An effective live attenuated vaccine is available for those with occupations that expose them to infected animals or ectoparasites. It is available from the U.S. Army Medical Research Institute of Infectious Diseases, Fort Detrick, Maryland, 21702.

SUGGESTED READING

Fulop M, Leslie D, Titball R. A rapid, highly sensitive method for the detection of *Francisella tularensis* in clinical samples using the polymerase chain reaction. *Am J Trop Med Hyg*. 1996;54:364–366.

Gill V, Cunha BA. Tularemia pneumonia. *Semin Respir Infect*. 1997;12:61–67.

Specific Organisms – Bacteria

Hornick RB. Tularemia revisited. *N Engl J Med.* 2001;345:1637–1639.

Jacobs RF. Tularemia. *Adv Pediatr Infect Dis.* 1996;12:55–69.

Staples JE, Kubota KA, Chalcraft LG, et al. Epidemiology and molecular analysis of human tularemia, United States, 1964–2004. *Emerg Infect Dis.* 2006;12:1113–1118.

Steinemann TL, Sheikholeslami MR, Brown HH, et al. Oculoglandular tularemia. *Arch Ophthalmol.* 1999;117:132–133.

Waag DM, Sandström G, England MJ, et al. Immunogenicity of a new lot of *Francisella tularensis* vaccine strain in human volunteers. *FEMS Immuno Med Microbiol.* 1996; 13:205–209.

155. Tuberculosis

Asim K. Dutt

In the United States, the epidemiology of tuberculosis (TB) has changed in recent years. Infection by human immunodeficiency virus (HIV) and the increase in homelessness, poverty, and drug abuse are major factors in this change. Tuberculosis occurs most commonly among ethnic minorities, African Americans, and Hispanics 25 to 44 years of age. Immigrants from developing countries with a high prevalence of TB and drug resistance have contracted almost one half of the new cases in this country for the past several years. Drug-resistant disease is a major concern.

DIAGNOSIS

The chest x-ray is frequently suggestive of TB (Figure 155.1). Whenever there is a suspicion of pulmonary TB, three spontaneously produced sputum specimens should be examined by microscopy and culture. If necessary, sputum production may be induced by inhalation of aerosol of warm saline (Figure 155.2). Methods such as early-morning gastric lavage and laryngeal swab on suction are less productive. When suspicion of TB is high and microscopy is negative on at least three specimens, a bronchial washing or transbronchial biopsy through a fiberoptic bronchoscope or postbronchoscopy sputum may be productive. In an unconscious patient, tracheal aspiration or transthoracic needle aspiration of the lung may be needed to obtain a specimen. On rare occasions diagnosis must be made by open lung biopsy.

Positive sputum microscopy suggests TB, but the only positive identification of *Mycobacterium tuberculosis* is by culture or DNA probe to distinguish it from less virulent mycobacteria. Drug susceptibility testing should be performed. Several new approaches with the development of new diagnostic tests are suggested for TB infection, active TB, and rapid detection of drug resistance.

Latent TB Infection

Tuberculosis skin test (TST) has been in use for many decades, but the results are flawed and unreliable in detecting TB infection. With

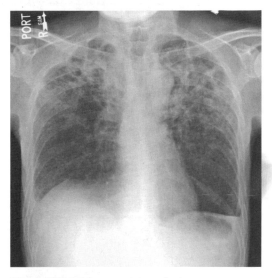

Figure 155.1 Pulmonary tuberculosis. Characteristic findings on chest x-ray (CXR) include upper lobe infiltrates, involvement of apical or posterior segments, and cavities with thick walls, smooth inner contours, and no air-fluid levels. Pleural reaction and distal infiltrates from endobronchial spread may be seen. Disease activity cannot be determined from the CXR alone and must be proven or excluded by sputum smear and culture. (Courtesy of David Schlossberg, MD.)

advancement in immunology and genomics, T-cell–based in vitro assays of interferon (IFN) released by T cells after stimulation with *Mycobacterium tuberculosis* antigens are developed to identify TB infection. Two IFN assays are available as commercial kits: the Quanti FERON-TB gold assay (Cellestis, Ltd) and the TB SPOT-TB (Oxford Immunotec). The former is approved by the U.S. Food and Drug Administration (FDA).

Studies indicate that IFN-γ detection has higher specificity for *M. tuberculosis* and less cross-reactivity with bacilli calmette–guérin (BCG) vaccination than TST. The test is unreliable in the subgroup of patients with immunosuppression (including HIV/ acquired immunodeficiency syndrome [AIDS]), extrapulmonary TB, children and populations in high-incidence countries. The test requires laboratory infrastructure and support. The Centers for Disease Control and Prevention (CDC) recommends

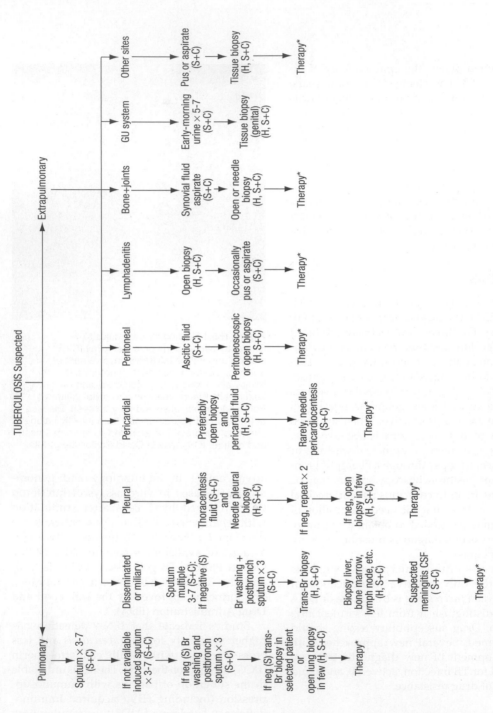

Figure 155.2 Diagnosis of suspected tuberculosis S, Smear; C, culture for mycobacteria; H, histology; Br, Bronchial; Bronch, bronchoscopy; CSF, cerebrospinal fluid; Bx, biopsy; neg, negative; GU, genitourinary. * Therapy started in suspected cases, awaiting culture results and/or clinical response.

the Quanti FERON-TB gold test for detection of latent infection, which has the advantage of a single test for patients. Cost-effectiveness of the use of the test in clinical settings needs further evaluation.

Diagnosis of Tuberculosis

Nucleic acid amplification (NAA) tests amplify nucleic acid regions and identify the M. tuberculosis complex. The NAA test can be directly used in clinical specimens (such as sputum) as "direct amplification tests." The Amplicor MTB test (Roche Diagnostic System), the Amplified Mycobacterium Direct test (MTD) (Gene-Probe, Inc.), and the BD Probe-Tec ET assay (Becton Dickinson Biosciences) are commercially available. The MTD and Amplicor tests are FDA approved. However, NAA tests cannot replace conventional tests (microscopy and culture) and should be interpreted along with conventional tests and clinical data. The tests should be performed only in reliable laboratories.

Rapid Detection Drug Resistance

Line Probe assays are novel DNA strip tests that use the polymerase chain reaction (PCR). Commercially available kits include the INNO-LiPA RIF TB kit (Immunogenetics) and Geno Type MTBDR assays (Hain Lifescience). These kits are not FDA approved. Although sensitivity on culture isolates may be over 95% in detecting rifampin resistance, the tests are expensive and require sophisticated laboratory support.

Also, phage-based assays are available as commercial kits but are not approved by the FDA. The test is performed in culture isolates and has high sensitivity but low specificity. This may be used for rifampin resistance in culture isolates. That increases turnaround time. The tests show promise but are not routinely used.

For the diagnosis of extrapulmonary TB secretions and/or biopsy, material must be obtained from the site (Figure 155.2). In the case of tuberculous meningitis it may be necessary to initiate therapy empirically because the disease may become irreversible before the diagnosis can be made.

THERAPY

Principles of Chemotherapy

Table 155.1 lists drugs, dosages, and major side effects. Several first-line bactericidal drugs are commonly combined initially because they reduce the bacterial population rapidly without the risk of resistance. Second-line drugs are most useful when resistance to 2 or more first-line drugs is found or they cannot be used because of life-threatening side effects or intolerance (Figure 155.3).

The bactericidal drugs in suitable combinations actually kill actively multiplying extracellular bacilli in TB lesions. Rapid elimination of these bacilli renders the sputum bacteriologically negative, leading to cure. No bactericidal drug should be used alone to treat active TB because this inevitably leads to resistance to that drug. When initial therapy fails at this stage, the sputum bacteriology does not become negative, as shown by persistence of positive sputum smears beyond 2 months. Failure of therapy is usually due to emergence of drug-resistant organisms, most often due to poor compliance, prescription of an inadequate regimen, or inadequate dosage of individual drugs.

In the continuation phase of therapy, the drugs slowly eliminate small populations of intermittently metabolizing persisters in the closed caseous lesion or within macrophages. Incomplete therapy may lead to relapse after discontinuation of treatment, often with drug-sensitive organisms.

Drug-Resistant Organisms

The inclusion of a number of drugs in a regimen should be based on the awareness of the circumstances under which drug-resistant bacilli are likely to be present (Table 155.2).

At the minimum, a 4-drug regimen should be initiated when drug resistance is likely, until susceptibility results are available. The number of drugs in the initial regimen may have to be increased to 5 to 7 if the organisms are resistant to 3 or more drugs and HIV infection is present, as often occurs in large cities in the United States and in many developing countries.

MANAGEMENT OF TUBERCULOSIS

Newer approaches are advocated for a better outcome. For the care of patients with TB, responsibility for completion and success now lies with the health care providers and not the patients. The duration of treatment in the continuation phase should be extended in specific situations. New anti-TB medications show promise; these are used when necessary. Directly observed therapy (DOT) is strongly recommended when the patient is

Table 155.1 Antituberculosis Drugs

Drug	Daily Dosage	Twice-Weekly Dosage	Side Effects	Mode of Action
First-line Drugs				
Isoniazid	5 mg/kg (usually 300 mg) PO or IM	15 mg/kg (usually 900 mg) PO	Peripheral neuritis, hepatotoxicity, allergic fever and rash, lupus erythematosus phenomenon	Acts strongly on rapidly dividing extracellular bacilli; acts weakly on slowly multiplying intracellular bacilli
Rifampin	10 mg/kg (usually 450–600 mg) PO	10 mg/kg (usually 450–600 mg) PO	Hepatotoxicity, nausea, vomiting, allergic fever and rash, flulike syndrome, petechiae with thrombocytopenia or acute renal failure during intermittent therapy	Acts on both rapidly and slowly multiplying extracellular and intracellular bacilli, particularly on slowly multiplying persisters
Rifabutin (Ansamycin)	300 mg PO daily, twice or thrice weekly	Used as RIF Substitute	Same as rifampin; Uveitis, arthralgia leukopenia	Same as above
Rifapentine	300–600 mg PO Once weekly in continuation phase.	Seronegative HIV, non cavitary TB	same as Rifampin; not used in HIV	
Rifamate (INH 150mg plus RIF300)	2 capsules PO qd	2 caps plus 2 tablets of INH (300mg)	Same as INH/RIF	Same as INH/RIF
Rifater (INH 50mg plus RIF 120mg plus PZA 300mg)	5-6 capsules PO qd		same as INH/RIF/PZA	Same as INH/RIF/PZA
pyrazinamide	25–30 mg/kg PO (usually 1.5–2.0g)	45–50 mg/kg PO (usually 3–3.5 mg)	Hyperuricemia, hepatotoxicity, allergic fever and rash	Active in acid pH 2.5 g) on intracellular bacilli
Ethambutol	15–25 mg/kg/d initially, followed after 2 months with 15 mg/kg/d	50 mg/kg PO	Optic neuritis, skin rash, hyperuricemia	Weakly active 800–1,600 against both extracellular and intracellular bacilli to inhibit the development of resistance
Second-line Drugs				
Streptomycin	10–15 mg/kg (usually 0.5–1 g) 5 days/week; IM or IV	20–25 mg/kg (usually 1–1.5 g)	Cranial nerve VIII damage (vestibular and auditory), nephrotoxicity, allergic fever, rash	Active against rapidly multiplying bacilli in neutral or slightly alkaline extracellular medium
Kanamycin	15–30mg/kg qd IM or IV	15–30mg/kg	same as streptomycin	same as streptomycin
Amikacin	15–30 mg/kg qd IM or IV	15–30mg/kg	same as streptomycin	same as streptomycin
Capreomycin	15–30 mg/kg/d IM or IV	15–30mg/kg	same as streptomycin	same as streptomycin

Drug	Daily Dosage	Twice-Weekly Dosage	Side Effects	Mode of Action
Ethionamide	10–15 mg/kg (usually 500–750 mg) in divided doses PO with 100 mg pyridoxine	Not used	Nausea, vomiting, anorexia, allergic fever and rash, hepatotoxicity, neurotoxicity, hypothyroidism	Same as streptomycin
Cycloserine	15–20 mg/kg (usually 0.75–1 g) in divided doses with 200 mg pyridoxine PO	Not Used	Personality changes, psychosis, convulsions, rash	Same as ethambutol
Paraminosalicylic acid	150 mg/kg (usually 12 g) in divided doses PO	Not Used	Nausea, vomiting, diarrhea, hepatotoxicity, allergic rash and fever, hypothyroidism	Weak action on extra-cellular bacilli; inhibits development of drug-resistant organisms
Thiocetazone*	150 mg PO	Used rarely	Allergic rash and fever Stevens-Johnson syndrome, blood disorders, nausea, vomiting	Same as paraminosalicylic acid
Clofazimine	200–300 mg PO qd	Not Used	Pigmentation of skin, abdominal pain	Not fully known
Newer Agents				
Ofloxacin	400 mg q12h	Not Used	Gastrointestinal: diarrhea, nausea, abdominal pain, anorexia; central nervous system: dizziness, restlessness, nightmares, ataxia, seizures	Rapidly multiplying bacilli at neutral or alkaline pH
Gatifloxacin	400 mg PO qd	Not Used	Same as ofloxacin	Same as ofloxacin
Levofloxacin	500 mg PO qd	Not Used	Same as ofloxacin	Same as ofloxacin
Moxifloxacin	400 mg PO qd	Not Used	Same as ofloxacin	Same as ofloxacin
Azithromycin	500 mg/day	Not Used	Diarrhea, nausea, abdominal pain, elevation of liver enzymes	Rapidly multiplying bacilli in macrophages
Clarithromycin	1 g q12h	Not Used	Same as azithromycin	Same as azithromycin

*Not available in the United States.

observed to ingest each dose of medication, for improving completion of therapy with a good outcome.

Drug Regimens

Any of several drug regimens with variable durations may be selected according to the local conditions.

NINE-MONTH REGIMEN

Since the mid-1970s, Arkansas Department of Health physicians have treated patients with isoniazid (INH) and rifampin (RIF) in a combination capsule (Rifamate) for 9 months. The Arkansas regimen consists of INH–RIF, 2 capsules daily for 1 month, followed by 2 INH–RIF capsules and 2 300-mg INH tablets twice weekly for another 8 months, with a

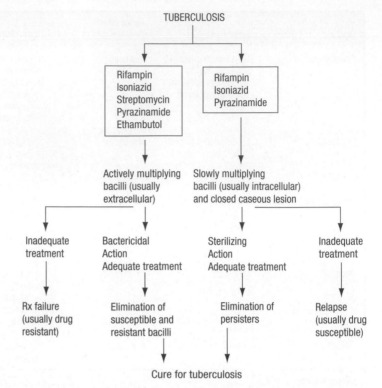

Figure 155.3 Principles of chemotherapy of tuberculosis.

TUBERCULOSIS

Rifampin
Isoniazid
Streptomycin
Pyrazinamide
Ethambutol

Rifampin
Isoniazid
Pyrazinamide

Actively multiplying bacilli (usually extracellular)

Slowly multiplying bacilli (usually intracellular) and closed caseous lesion

Inadequate treatment

Bactericidal Action
Adequate treatment

Sterilizing Action
Adequate treatment

Inadequate treatment

Rx failure (usually drug resistant)

Elimination of susceptible and resistant bacilli

Elimination of persisters

Relapse (usually drug susceptible)

Cure for tuberculosis

Table 155.2 Conditions and Patients with Increased Risk of Drug-Resistant TB

History of treatment with anti-TB drugs, including preventive therapy
Patients from areas with high prevalence of initial or primary drug resistance (>4%), eg, urban population in the northeastern United States, Florida, California, U.S.-Mexican border
Foreign-born persons from areas with high prevalence of drug-resistant TB, eg, southeast Asia, Mexico, South America, Africa
Contacts of persons with drug-resistant disease
Disease in persons who are homeless, drug abusers, and HIV infected
Persons with positive sputum smears and cultures after 2 mo of chemotherapy

success rate of over 95%. Development of drug resistance has not been a problem because the patient cannot take a single drug alone, and side effects are minimal.

The main objection to a 2-drug regimen is possible presence of drug-resistant bacilli during initial therapy. In Arkansas the incidence of initial or primary resistance is below 3%. Moreover, patients with risk factors (see Table 155.2) are excluded from this regimen. However, the regimen should never be prescribed in large cities, in places with high prevalence of primary drug resistance, or in certain areas of the United States such as the Mexican border and areas in which southeast Asians have settled.

Successful results were obtained by a regimen consisting of INH, RIF, and ethambutol (EMB) given daily for the initial 2 months followed by INH and RIF for 7 months, given either daily or twice weekly. The regimen is safer than 2-drug therapy until drug susceptibility is known.

It is recommended that the duration of treatment of any of the above regimens should be extended in drug-susceptible pulmonary TB patients who show cavitations in the initial chest x-ray or whose sputum culture had not converted to negative during the intensive phase of therapy (2 months). These clinical indicators may predict adverse outcome with regard to failure and relapse. The continuation phase of therapy should be extended for another 3 months. Sputum smears and cultures must be obtained at the end of the intensive phase of treatment.

SIX-MONTH REGIMEN

The addition of pyrazinamide (PZA), 25 to 30 mg/kg, to the INH, 300 mg, and RIF, 600 mg

Table 155.3 Regimens for the Initial Treatment of TB

	TB without HIV Infection			
Option 1	**Option 2**	**Option 3**	**TB with HIV Infection**
INH, RIF, PZA (if initial INH resistance is ≤4%) daily for 8 wks, followed by INH and RIF daily or twice weekly for 16 wks	INH, RIF, PZA, EMB, or SM daily for 2 wks, then 2× weekly for 6 wks (DOT), subsequently INH and RIF twice weekly for 16 wks (DOT)	INH, RIF, PZA, EMB, or SM. 3× a week for 6 months (DOT)	Option 1, 2, or 3 for a total of 9 mo, at least 6 mo beyond culture conversion
Add EMB or SM if resistance is >4%			
Total treatment 6 mo (at least 3 mo past culture conversion)	Total treatment 6 mo	Total treatment 6 mo	Total treatment 6–9 mo

Abbreviations: INH = isoniazid; RIF = rifampin; PZA = pyrazinamide; EMB = ethambutol; SM = streptomycin; DOT = directly observed therapy.
From Centers for Disease Control and Prevention Initial therapy for tuberculosis in the era of multidrug resistance Recommeodations of the Advisory Council for the Elimination *of* Tuberculosis. *Morbid Mortal Weekly Rep.* 1993;42(RR.7):I–8.

daily for the initial 2 months, followed by INH, 300 mg, and RIF, 600 mg daily, or INH, 900 mg, and RIF, 600 mg twice weekly for another 4 months (a total of 6 months), has proved to be highly successful. The CDC and American Thoracic Society guidelines recommend this regimen if the prevalence of primary drug resistance is below 4% (Table 155.3, option 1).

The 3-drug regimen reduces the duration of therapy to 6 months. Addition of PZA accelerates reduction of the bacterial population and adds little to the toxicity of the regimen, although its cost is greater. The addition of a third drug, PZA, ensures against failure in the event of initial resistance to either INH or RIF. In clinical studies, 6 months of therapy with these drugs has been less effective in RIF-resistant cases than in INH-resistant cases.

SIX-MONTH THERAPY WHEN RESISTANCE IS SUSPECTED

When drug resistance is suspected or likely, drug therapy consisting of at least 4 drugs, such as INH, 300 mg, RIF, 600 mg, PZA, 2 to 3 g/kg, and streptomycin (SM), 0.5 to 1 g intramuscularly (IM) 5 days a week, or ethambutol (EMB), 25 mg/kg, should be administered initially (option 1, Table 155.3). After drug susceptibility results are available, usually in 2 months, the regimen is modified accordingly. If the organisms are found to be susceptible to both drugs, therapy is completed with INH–RIF daily or twice weekly for another 4 months. In cases of INH resistance, therapy may consist of RIF, PZA, and EMB for another 6 to 7 months. INH should be included in the

regimen because of its action on persisters, which generally remain INH sensitive. In RIF-resistant cases other bactericidal drugs should be continued for at least 10 to 12 months to prevent relapse.

A 4-drug regimen for 6 months is generally recommended for all patients of TB due to uncertainty of drug-resistant organisms.

TREATMENT OF MULTIDRUG-RESISTANT DISEASE

Where the prevalence of multidrug resistance (MDR) and HIV infection are very high, it is necessary to initiate a 5- to 7-drug regimen, including second-line drugs. This is applicable to large urban populations such as in New York City, Miami, parts of New Jersey, and San Francisco, as well as for persons from developing countries.

In the treatment of MDR disease, ie, resistance to INH and RIF, some basic principles must be followed: (1) a single drug must not be added to a failing regimen, (2) at least 3 new drugs that the patient has not yet taken should replace the existing drug regimen until the susceptibility results are available, (3) the total duration of therapy must be prolonged to 24 months or more, (4) the regimen should include an injectable drug for at least 4 months after the culture is converted to negative, and (5) directly observed therapy (DOT) should be used to ensure compliance, because it is the patient's last chance at a cure.

Extensively drug-resistant TB (XDR-TB) has been reported recently from different parts of the world, first from South Africa. XDR-TB is defined as resistance to at least RIF and INH among the first line of anti-TB drugs (MDR-TB), in addition to resistance to any fluoroquinolone and to at least 1 of 3 injectable second-line anti-TB drugs used in TB treatment (capreomycin, kanamicin, amikacin). This development is a serious concern globally.

Most drugs used for MDR disease are second-line drugs (see Table 155.l): ethionamide, cycloserine, para-aminosalicylic acid (PAS), capreomycin, and kanamycin. Newer drugs, fluoroquinolones (gatifloxacin and moxifloxacin) and amikacin, are available but unproven. Finally, clofazimine and thiocetazone (not available in the United States) may be used but also are unproven. These second-line drugs are often rather toxic, and close monitoring is necessary. Monthly bacteriologic studies are necessary to monitor response to treatment.

Because of high failure and relapse rates in MDR-TB, surgical resection of the major diseased area of the lung is again becoming necessary after reasonable medical treatment has been given to reduce the bacterial load.

Preventive therapy for recent contacts with MDR-TB is controversial. However, two possible regimens are PZA plus EMB and PZA plus oxafloxacin for 12 to 24 months, during which periodic clinical, bacteriologic, and radiologic monitoring must be maintained.

The combination of RIF and PZA or rifabutin and PZA are suggested for shorter periods of time, but the regimens are highly toxic. Experts should be consulted prior to the use of the regimen.

TREATMENT REGIMENS FOR HIV-INFECTED PERSONS

In the United States the current 6-month treatment consisting of INH, RIF, PZA, and EMB or SM daily for 2 months, followed by INH and RIF daily or twice weekly for another 4 months, is not adequate in HIV-infected patients. The CDC recommends that therapy for patients with HIV infection be prolonged to 9 months or for at least 6 months following conversion of sputum cultures to negative (Table 155.3). Treatment-limiting side effects are frequent in HIV-infected patients, and they require innovative measures. Intermittent regimens (2 or 3 doses a week) are generally well tolerated in such situations.

Rifabutin may be used in place of RIF. However, the current recommendation is that HIV-infected patients with CD4 cell counts $<100/mm^3$ should receive therapy daily during the intensive phase and daily or thrice weekly during the continuation phase.

If adverse affects such as uveitis and cytopenia occur, medication must be discontinued at once.

SMEAR-NEGATIVE TUBERCULOSIS

Positive sputum smears indicate a large bacterial population and advanced disease, whereas negative smears generally suggest less advanced disease. We have treated a large number of patients having 3 initial specimens with negative smears but 1 or 2 positive cultures with INH and RIF for 6 months. Relapses are no more common than in smear-positive cases treated for 9 months. Occasionally a patient who is smear negative is also culture negative but is treated for TB on the basis of clinical and x-ray findings. Regimens for such patients have included 4 months of INH plus RIF. Another suggested regimen for smear-negative TB is INH, RIF, PZA, and EMB for 2 months, followed by INH and RIF for an additional 2 months (4 months total). However, HIV-infected patients should be treated for a minimum of 6 months.

EXTRAPULMONARY TUBERCULOSIS

The bacterial load in extrapulmonary TB usually is much smaller than in cavitary pulmonary TB. Thus, 6- to 9-month regimens (see Table 155.3) are adequate for treatment of extrapulmonary TB. Figure 155.3 indicates the steps in the diagnosis of pulmonary and extrapulmonary TB. We have successfully treated many patients with extrapulmonary TB with INH and RIF, but the increasing incidence of drug resistance necessitates additional drugs. It is generally recommended that the duration of therapy be prolonged in TB spondylitis (Pott's disease) and meminges to 9 to 12 months Corticosteroids may be added for patients with tuberculous pericarditis and tuberculous meningitis.

DIRECTLY OBSERVED THERAPY

The fact that most of the 6-month regimens may be given intermittently 2 or 3 times per week has led to the development of some innovative regimens. The Denver regimen consists of DOT administration of daily INH, RIF, PZA, and SM or EMB for 2 weeks, followed by twice-weekly doses for 6 weeks and then twice-weekly administration of INH or RIF for another 16 weeks. Another DOT regimen is INH, RIF, PZA, and EMB or SM 3 times a week for 6 months (Table 155.3, options 2 and 3).

To ensure completion of therapy, DOT is the preferred initial strategy and deserves special

Specific Organisms – Bacteria

emphasis. DOT can be provided daily or intermittently in the office, clinic, or in the field by trained personnel. Using DOT can only improve the outcome. Aggressive interventions may be initiated when the patient misses doses.

Therapy in Special Situations

PREGNANCY

Treatment with INH, RIF, and EMB is safe in pregnancy. Streptomycin should not be used because of toxicity to the eighth nerve of the fetus. Experience with PZA is limited in pregnancy, and at present it should be avoided if possible. If PZA is not included in the treatment regimen, the minimum duration of therapy is 9 months.

RENAL FAILURE

INH and RIF dosages need not be altered in renal failure because these drugs are excreted by the liver. Renal dialysis patients should receive the drugs after dialysis. EMB dosage must be reduced to 8 to 10 mg/kg in advanced renal failure. Streptomycin and aminoglycosides should be avoided in these patients, and the level should be monitored if they must be used in very unusual circumstances. PZA dosage should be reduced to 15 to 20 mg/kg.

LIVER DISEASE

Alcoholic liver disease does not preclude use of anti-TB drugs. However, monitoring for side effects must be careful and regular. In overt liver failure the therapy should consist of INH and EMB until liver function returns to normal. At that time RIF and/or PZA may be added to the regimen.

Combined Preparations

In the United States, two commercial preparations of combination drugs are available. It is advantageous to use combination preparations because they preclude the taking of only one bactericidal drug, which encourages drug resistance. Rifamate is a combination capsule of INH, 150 mg, and RIF, 300 mg, and 2 capsules are the recommended daily dose. Another preparation, Rifater, contains INH, 50 mg, RIF, 120 mg, and PZA, 300 mg, in each tablet; the recommended dose is 5 tablets daily. We strongly recommend the use of combination preparations for therapy as a safeguard against development of drug resistance and medication errors, particularly for patients not on DOT.

Corticosteroid Therapy

Corticosteroids are not routinely used in the treatment of TB. Prednisone, 20 to 30 mg/day, may improve the general sense of well-being, reduce fever, increase appetite, and improve nutrition of markedly toxic or severely debilitated patients. The drug should be tapered off gradually after 4 to 8 weeks. In disseminated TB associated with hypoxemia and respiratory failure, prednisone, 40 to 60 mg/day, may improve oxygenation. Steroids have been successfully used in AIDS patients with TB, but they may promote opportunistic infections. Most authorities believe that complicated tuberculous meningitis should be treated with prednisone, 60 to 80 mg/day, slowly tapered after 8 to 12 weeks. Some advise corticosteroid therapy for all cases of tuberculous pericarditis to prevent constrictive pericarditis.

MONITORING AND FOLLOW-UP OF PATIENTS

Intense bacteriologic monitoring is necessary during therapy of pulmonary TB. We recommend that 3 to 5 specimens of bronchial secretions (sputum) be examined initially by smear and culture, followed by drug susceptibility testing. During therapy, at least 1 specimen of sputum should be examined every 2 weeks until conversion to negative occurs. This permits early detection of noncompliance and impending failure. After completion of treatment, to detect early relapse, 1 specimen every 3 months 3 times should be examined before discharging the patient from the clinic.

Monitoring for side effects should be done monthly after explaining to the patient the symptoms of side effects for which to be alert (eg, nausea, vomiting, anorexia, dark urine, jaundice). Blood should be collected for baseline complete blood count and renal and hepatic function tests. We do not recommend routine monthly blood studies. Rather, the patients are advised to discontinue medication when symptomatic and to report for repeat hepatic function studies at that time. The drugs are then adjusted to the laboratory findings. Some clinicians, however, do recommend routine blood studies, either of all patients or only of those at risk for hepatotoxicity due to underlying liver disease, baseline abnormalities, and so on. For EMB, vision and color studies are performed monthly, and for SM or other aminoglycosisdes or capreomycin monthly examination for balance and hearing loss are performed.

PROPHYLAXIS

For prophylaxis, see Chapter 111, Nonsurgical Antimicrobial Prophylaxis.

SUGGESTED READING

American Thoracic Society, CDC, and Infectious Disease Society of America. Treatment of tuberculosis. *Am J Respir Crit Care Med.* 2003;167:603–662.

Dutt AK, Moers D, Stead WW. Short course chemotherapy for extrapulmonary tuberculosis. Nine years' experience. *Ann Intern Med.* 1986;104:771.

Furin J, Nardell EA. Multidrug-resistant tuberculosis: an update on the best regimens. *Infect Med.* 2006;23:493–504.

Goble M, Iseman MD, Madsen LA, et al. Treatment of 171 patients with pulmonary tuberculosis resistant to isoniazid and rifampin. *N Engl J Med.* 1993;328:527–532.

Iseman MD. Treatment of multidrug-resistant tuberculosis. *N Engl J Med.* 1993;329:784–791.

Nahid P, Pai M, Hopewell PC. Advances in the diagnosis and treatment of tuberculosis. *ProcAm Thoracic Soc.* 2006;3:103–110.

Sharme SK, Mohan A. Multidrug-resistant tuberculosis: a menace that threatens to destabilize tuberculosis control. *Chest.* 2006;130:261–272.

Weiss SE, Slocum PC, Blais FX, et al. The effect of directly observed therapy on the rates of drug resistance and relapse in tuberculosis. *N Engl J Med.* 1994;330:1179–1184.

Yew DD, Leung CC. Update in tuberculsis 2006. *Am J Respir Crit Care Med.* 2007;175:541–546.

156. Nontuberculous Mycobacteria

Timothy R. Aksamit and David E. Griffith

INTRODUCTION

The nontuberculous mycobacteria (NTM) are ubiquitous in the environment; so much so that some experts feel they should be referred to as "environmental mycobacteria." Although there are more than 120 identified NTM species, the most common NTM associated with human disease are *Mycobacterium avium* complex (MAC), *Mycobacterium kansasii*, *Mycobacterium fortuitum*, and *Mycobacterium abscessus*. Many other NTM species can cause human disease but are generally rarely encountered clinically, whereas a few NTM species, most notably *Mycobacterium gordonae*, are frequently isolated as specimen contaminants and almost never cause disease.

Infection is thought to occur from environmental exposure to the NTM with three potential portals of entry; the respiratory tract, the gastrointestinal tract, and direct inoculation of the skin and soft tissues. There are no documented occurrences of either human-to-human or animal-to-human transmission.

The most common clinical manifestation of NTM infection in the immunocompetent host is chronic pulmonary disease. Symptoms are usually insidious in onset and include cough, sputum production, fatigue, weight loss, weakness, hemoptysis, and night sweats. MAC is the most common respiratory pathogen. Patients with MAC lung disease are divided between two groups. The first are primarily female patients without a history of pre-existing lung disease who have noncavitary disease characterized by nodular densities and bronchiectasis, usually in the right middle lobe and lingua. The second group are primarily male patients with pre-existing lung disease, most often chronic obstructive lung disease, and cavitary abnormalities radiographically, similar to tuberculosis.

Lymphadenitis is the most common NTM disease manifestation in children and is usually due to MAC or, less commonly, *Mycobacterium scrofulaceum*. The most important differential diagnosis is tuberculosis lymphadenitis, although NTM account for approximately 90% of mycobacterial lymphadenitis in children (but only 10% in adults). Symptoms are usually minimal with unilateral involvement of submandibular, submaxillary, preauricular, or cervical lymph nodes most common. Skin and soft-tissue infections are usually due to *Mycobacterium marinum* or the "rapidly growing mycobacteria" (RGM), *Mycobacterium abscessus*, *M. fortuitum*, and *Mycobacterium chelonae* and are the result of direct inoculation either after trauma or surgery. Dissemination of NTM pathogens is most often associated with the severe immunosuppression of advanced acquired immunodeficiency syndrome (AIDS) and caused by MAC. Disseminated NTM infections can occur in other immunocompromised states, sometimes associated with indwelling foreign bodies such as venous catheters, dialysis catheters, or other prosthetic devices.

DIAGNOSTIC CRITERIA OF NONTUBERCULOUS MYCOBACTERIAL LUNG DISEASE

The diagnostic criteria for NTM lung disease include a compilation of clinical, radiographic, and microbiologic criteria. Although a diagnosis of NTM lung disease may be suspected by one or more of these three criteria, all must be present to establish a diagnosis. Clinical, radiographic, and microbiologic criteria are equally important. The minimum evaluation of a patient suspected of NTM lung disease should include (1) chest radiograph or, in the absence of cavitation, chest high resolution computed tomography (HRCT) scan, (2) 3 or more sputum specimens for acid-fast bacilli (AFB) analysis, and (3) exclusion of other disorders such as tuberculosis and lung malignancy.

The following criteria apply to symptomatic patients with radiographic infiltrates, nodular or cavitary, or an HRCT scan that shows multifocal bronchiectasis with multiple small nodules. These criteria fit best with MAC, *M. kansasii*, and *M. abscessus*. There is not enough known about most other NTM to be certain that these diagnostic criteria are universally applicable for all NTM respiratory pathogens. Expert consultation should be obtained when NTM are

Table 156.1 Treatment of Nontuberculous Mycobacterial Infections (see text for details)

NTM Species	Disease	Treatment	Comment
MAC	Pulmonary[a]	Clarithromycin 500 mg BID or azithromycin 250 mg/day plus ethambutol 15 mg/kg/day plus rifampin 600 mg/day Consider streptomycin or amikacin 10–15 mg/kg IM or IV for severe disease	Treat for 1 year if negative AFB cultures Rifabutin 150–300 mg daily may be substituted for rifampin
MAC	Disseminated	Clarithromycin 500 mg BID or Azithromycin 500 mg/day with Ethambutol 15 mg/kg/day ± Rifabutin 300 mg/day	Treatment lifetime or may be stopped with CD4+ T-cell count over 100 cells/μL for 12 months
MAC	Lymph node Involvement	Complete surgical excision of involved nodes usually curative	If adjunctive chemotherapy necessary, see drugs for pulmonary disease
M kansasii	Pulmonary	Rifampin 600 mg/d Isoniazid 300 mg/d Ethambutol 15 mg/kg/d	Treat for 1 year of negative AFB cultures; clarithromycin and Moxifloxacin also with excellent activity against M. kansasii
M. kansasii	Disseminated	Substitute rifabutin 150–300 mg/d for rifampin in HIV + MAC	Treatment duration as for disseminated
M. abscessus	Pulmonary	Clarithromycin, 500mg BID, plus amikacin, 10–15 mg/kg 3–5 times per wk	Consider second parenteral drug such as cefoxitin, imipenem or tigecylcine.
M. abscessus	Soft tissue	Clarithromycin, 500mg BID plus amikacin, 10–15 mg/kg 3–5 times per week for a minimum of 2 wks	Consider second parenteral drug for severe disease. Removal of foreign body and surgical debridement also important
M. marinum	Soft tissue	Clarithromycin, 500 mg BID, plus ethambutol, 15 mg/kg/day. Treat 1–2 months after resolution of symptoms (usually 3–4 mo total)	Susceptible to multiple agents. Surgical debridement may also be important.
M. fortuitum	Pulmonary	2 agents to which the organism is susceptible for 6 months. Consider parenteral med for severe disease.	Susceptible to multiple medications including quinolones, doxycycline, trimethoprim/sulfa, macrolides, amikacin.
M. fortuitum	Soft tissue	As above. Treatment 3–6 mo	
M. simiae, M. xenopi M. malmoense M. szulgai		Too little information to make standard or routine recommendation	Usually a macrolide-based regimen

[a] Consider 3× weekly therapy (TIW) with clarithromycin 1000 mg, ethambutol, 25 mg/kg/dose, and rifampin, 600 mg, for mild nodular/bronchiectatic (noncavitary) disease.

recovered that are either infrequently encountered or that usually represent environmental contamination.

Clinical criteria include respiratory or systemic symptoms attributed to NTM lung disease not attributable to other established diagnoses. Radiographic findings as noted above may vary, especially in the context of whether there is pre-existing lung disease. In the absence of radiographic changes related to pre-existing lung disease or of cavitary change, the most common findings include nodular infiltrates, cylindrical bronchiectasis, and consolidation. Pleural disease, prominent mediastinal/hilar adenopathy, air-fluid levels, and ground glass opacities on high resolution chest computed tomography are

Specific Organisms – Bacteria

not commonly seen in non–human immunodeficiency virus (HIV) patients with NTM lung disease. Microbiologic criteria also may vary. If three sputum results are available at least 2 AFB cultures should be positive, regardless of AFB smear results. In the absence of at least 2 positive cultures, consideration should be given to repeating 3 sputum specimens for AFB smear and culture or obtaining bronchoscopy with wash or lavage. If only one bronchial wash or lavage is available, 1 positive culture regardless of smear is necessary. If the sputum or bronchial wash results are nondiagnostic or another disease cannot be excluded, transbronchial or lung biopsy with mycobacterial histopathologic features (granulomatous inflammation or AFB) and yielding an NTM on culture or biopsy showing mycobacterial histopathologic features (granulomatous inflammation or AFB) and 1 or more sputums or bronchial washings that are culture positive for an NTM are required.

The preferred staining procedure is the fluorochrome method. Specimens should be cultured on both liquid and solid media. Species that require special growth conditions and/or lower incubation temperatures include *Mycobacterium haemophilum*, *Mycobacterium genavense* and *Mycobacterium conspicuum*. These species can cause cutaneous and lymph node disease. In general, NTM should be identified to the species level. Methods of rapid species identification include commercial DNA probes (MAC, *M. kansasii*, and *M. gordonae*) and high-performance liquid chromatography (HPLC). Routine susceptibility testing of MAC isolates is recommended for clarithromycin only. Routine susceptibility testing of *M. kansasii* isolates is recommended for rifampin only. Routine susceptibility testing, for both taxonomic identification and treatment of RGM (*M. fortuitum*, *M abscessus*, and *M. chelonae*), should be for amikacin, imipenem (*M. fortuitum* only), doxycycline, the fluorinated quinolones, a sulfonamide or trimethoprim–sulfamethoxazole, cefoxitin, clarithromycin, linezolid, and tobramycin (*M. chelonae* only).

DIAGNOSTIC CRITERIA OF NONTUBERCULOUS MYCOBACTERIAL EXTRAPULMONARY DISEASE

The diagnosis of extrapulmonary NTM disease also requires a compilation of clinical, microbiologic, and histopathologic test results in the context of lack of other diagnoses to explain symptoms and findings. Microbiology and histopathology results are generally of most value.

Specifically, AFB smear and culture of fluid or tissue is required. Specimens can be obtained by needle aspirate, core biopsy, or excisional biopsy. Tissue biopsy is generally the most sensitive means of obtaining a specimen for culture to establish extrapulmonary NTM disease. In some instances, histopathologic findings of granulomatous inflammation with or without AFB organisms present may be suggestive of NTM disease. However, prior to treatment for extrapulmonary NTM disease, definitive identification by culture is recommended.

GENERAL PRINCIPLES OF THERAPY FOR NONTUBERCULOUS MYCOBACTERIA (TABLE 156.1)

The greatest misunderstanding about treatment regimens for NTM pathogens is the result of the expectation that all NTM infections should respond in a predictable manner to antimicrobial therapy, in a manner similar to *M. tuberculosis*. That is, treatment regimens should be based on in vitro susceptibility testing, and the NTM pathogen should respond to antimicrobial agents based on in vitro susceptibility results. The most difficult and frustrating aspect of NTM therapy for most clinicians is the lack of a clear association between in vitro susceptibility results and clinical (in vivo) response for many NTM pathogens, including the most common one, MAC. For many NTM, including MAC, laboratory cutoffs for "susceptible" and "resistant" do not have a demonstrable clinical correlate and have not been confirmed to be clinically meaningful. The situation is complicated further because there is a spectrum of response by NTM pathogens based on in vitro susceptibilities. For instance, diseases caused by *M. kansasii*, *M. fortuitum*, and *M. marinum* respond predictably to treatment regimens based on in vitro susceptibilities. Response of disease caused by MAC correlates with in vitro susceptibility to macrolides (clarithromycin and azithromycin), but not other agents. Last, there are a number of NTM species (eg, *M. abscessus*, *Mycobacterium simiae*, *M. malomoense*, *Mycobacterium xenopi*) for which there is no established correlation between in vitro susceptibilities and in vivo response for any antimicrobial agents. The explanation(s) for the dichotomy between in vitro susceptibility results and in vivo response (clinical outcome) for many NTM is (are) currently not known. The clinician must use in vitro susceptibility data for many NTM with the awareness that, unlike tuberculosis, NTM disease may not be eradicated in a given patient with therapy based on in vitro susceptibility results.

RECOMMENDED DRUG TREATMENT FOR MAC LUNG DISEASE

As discussed in the general principals of NTM therapy, the macrolides (clarithromycin and azithromycin) are the only antimicrobial agents for which there is a demonstrated correlation between in vitro susceptibility and in vivo response for MAC lung disease. The cornerstones of MAC therapy, therefore, are the macrolides, clarithromycin, and azithromycin with the addition of ethambutol. These agents are then combined with companion drugs, usually a rifamycin and, possibly, an injectable aminoglycoside. It is necessary to include companion drugs with the macrolide to prevent the emergence of macrolide-resistant MAC isolates. The macrolides should *never* be used as monotherapy for treatment of MAC disease (pulmonary or disseminated).

An important illustration of how the dichotomy between in vitro susceptibility results and in vivo response in MAC disease can be detrimental is provided by the example of ethambutol. There has not been a demonstrated correlation between ethambutol in vitro susceptibility and clinical response in any previous study; however, the duration of ethambutol use is associated with improved microbiological response for patients receiving an intermittent clarithromycin-containing regimen, and the exclusion of ethambutol from treatment regimens is a major risk factor for the development of macrolide-resistant MAC. It would be potentially risky to the patient for a physician to exclude ethambutol from a multidrug MAC treatment regimen based on in vitro susceptibility results.

There is another difficult-to-explain phenomenon associated with MAC drug therapy. Patients who have failed prior MAC therapy, with or without a macrolide, have lower sputum conversion rates with macrolide-containing treatment regimens, even with macrolide-susceptible MAC isolates, than do patients with no prior therapy. Although the explanation for this observation is also not clear, it is evident that the best chance for treatment success in MAC lung disease is the first treatment effort.

The recommended treatment length for MAC pulmonary disease is a duration of therapy that includes 12 months of sputum culture negativity. This treatment goal dictates that patients should have sputum collected for acid-fast bacilli (AFB) analysis on a regular basis throughout the course of treatment.

For most patients with nodular/bronchiectatic disease, those with fibrocavitary disease who cannot tolerate daily therapy, or those patients for whom disease suppression is an appropriate goal, intermittent, 3 times weekly, therapy is recommended. Recommended intermittent drug dosages include (1) clarithromycin, 1000 mg, or azithromycin, 500 to 600 mg, (2) ethambutol, 25 mg/kg, and (3) rifampin, 600 mg, given 3 times weekly (TIW). Intermittent therapy is not recommended for patients with cavitary disease or patients who have received previous therapy for MAC.

The recommended regimen for patients with fibrocavitary disease or severe nodular/bronchiectatic disease, includes (1) clarithromycin, 1000 mg/day (or 500 mg twice daily), or azithromycin, 250 mg/day; (2) ethambutol, 15 mg/kg/day; and (3) rifampin, 10 mg/kg/day (maximum 600 mg/day). For some patients, the doses of clarithromycin may need to be split (eg, 500 mg twice daily) because of gastrointestinal intolerance, and for patients of small body mass (less than 50 kg) or age over 70 years, the clarithromycin dose may need to be reduced to 500 mg/day or 250 mg twice a day because of gastrointestinal intolerance.

A more aggressive and less well-tolerated treatment regimen for patients with severe and extensive (multilobar), especially fibrocavitary, disease consists of clarithromycin, 1000 mg/day (or 500 mg twice a day), or azithromycin, 250 mg/day, rifabutin, 150 to 300 mg/day, or rifampin, 10 mg/kg/day (maximum 600 mg/day), ethambutol, 15 mg/kg per day, and consideration of inclusion of either amikacin or streptomycin for the first 2 or 3 months of therapy (see dosage discussion below). Patients receiving clarithromycin and rifabutin should be carefully monitored for rifabutin-related toxicity, especially hematologic (leukopenia) and ocular (uveitis) toxicity.

Macrolide-resistant MAC lung disease is associated with a very poor prognosis. The two major risk factors for macrolide-resistant MAC disease are macrolide montherapy or treatment with macrolide and inadequate companion medications. The treatment strategy associated with the most success includes both the use of a multidrug regimen, including a parenteral aminoglycoside (streptomycin or amikacin) and surgical resection ("debulking") of disease. The optimal drug regimen for treating macrolide-resistant strains is unknown, but some experts recommend ethambutol, rifabutin, and an injectable agent. The role of other drugs, such as moxifloxacin or clofazimine, is not known.

Patients whose disease is predominantly localized to one lung and who can tolerate resectional surgery might also be considered for surgery if there is poor response to drug therapy, the development of macrolide-resistant MAC disease, or the presence of significant disease-related complications such as hemoptysis. Whenever possible, this surgery should be performed at centers with thoracic surgeons who have considerable experience with lung resectional surgery for mycobacterial disease, which is potentially associated with significant morbidity and mortality.

DISSEMINATED MAC DISEASE

Successful treatment of disseminated MAC in persons with AIDS is based on treatment of both the mycobacterial infection and the HIV infection. Clinicians must, therefore, be aware of the drug–drug interactions between the antimycobacterial and antiretroviral medications. Current guidelines for the use of antimycobacterial drugs with HIV therapies can be found at www.cdc.gov/nchstp/tb/TB_HIV_DRUGS/TOC.htm.

All patients should be treated with clarithromycin, 1000 mg/day or 500 mg twice daily, or, as an alternative, azithromycin at a dose of 500 mg daily and ethambutol at the dose of 15 mg/kg daily. Rifabutin, if added, should be used at a dose of 300 mg daily, with adjustments for interactions with antiretroviral drugs. As with macrolide-resistant MAC lung disease, patients with macrolide-resistant strains are far less likely to be successfully treated. Other drugs that should be considered for inclusion are amikacin and moxifloxicin. Clofazimine has been associated with excess mortality in the treatment of disseminated MAC disease and should not be used. Treatment of MAC in patients with AIDS should be considered lifelong, unless immune restoration is achieved by antiretroviral therapy. MAC treatment may be stopped for patients who are asymptomatic and have achieved a CD4+ T-cell count of over 100 cells/μL for at least 12 months.

Preventive therapy for disseminated MAC is recommended for all HIV-infected patients with less than 50 CD4+ T cells/μL. Based on efficacy and ease of use, azithromycin—given as 1200 mg once weekly—is the preferred agent. Clarithromycin is also effective; however, it is considered an alternative agent

because it must be given twice daily and the risk of breakthrough with macrolide-resistant strains is higher with daily clarithromycin than with weekly azithromycin. Rifabutin is also effective but should be used only when a macrolide cannot be tolerated. Primary MAC prophylaxis should be discontinued among adult and adolescent patients who have responded to antiretroviral therapy with an increase in CD4+ T-lymphocyte counts to more than 100 cells/μL for more than 3 months. Primary prophylaxis should be reintroduced if the CD4+ T-lymphocyte count decreases to less than 50 to 100 cells/μL.

MAC LYMPHADENOPATHY

The treatment of choice for MAC lymphadenopathy, as well as localized lymphadenopathy due to most NTM pathogens, is complete surgical resection of the involved lymph nodes. When complete surgical resection is not possible, due for instance to nerve impingement or encasement by the infected nodes, then chemotherapy with MAC treatment regimens similar to those for lung and disseminated disease would be necessary.

M. KANSASII PULMONARY DISEASE

The recommended regimen for treating pulmonary *M. kansasii* disease includes daily rifampin (600 mg/day), isoniazid (300 mg/day), and ethambutol (15 mg/kg/day) for a duration that includes 12 months of negative sputum cultures. Limited data suggest that intermittent therapy with rifampin, ethambutol, and clarithromycin for *M. kansasii* disease can also be successful. The recommended treatment duration, as with MAC lung disease, is a duration that includes 12 months of sputum AFB culture negativity.

Patients whose *M. kansasii* isolates have become resistant to rifampin as a result of previous therapy have been treated successfully with a regimen that consists of high-dose daily isoniazid (900 mg), high-dose ethambutol (25 mg/kg/day), sulfamethoxazole (1.0 g 3 times a day) combined with several months of streptomycin or amikacin. The excellent in vitro activity of clarithromycin and moxifloxacin against *M. kansasii* suggests that multidrug regimens containing these agents and at least 1 other agent based on in vitro susceptibilities, such as ethambutol or sulfamethoxazole, are likely to be even more effective for treatment of a patient with rifampin-resistant *M. kansasii* disease.

DISSEMINATED *M. KANSASII*

The treatment regimen for disseminated disease should be the same as for pulmonary disease. Because of the critically important role of rifamycins in the treatment of *M. kansasii* disease, it is important to construct *M. kansasii* and antiretroviral treatment regimens that are compatible (see Web site in disseminated MAC disease discussion above). An option for treating HIV-infected patients who receive an antiretroviral regimen not compatible with rifamycins is to substitute a macrolide or moxifloxacin for the rifamycin. There is no recommended prophylaxis regimen for disseminated *M. kansasii* disease.

M. ABSCESSUS DISEASE

Mycobacterium abscessus isolates are uniformly resistant to the standard antituberculous agents. *Mycobacterium abscessus* isolates generally have low or intermediate minimum inhibitory concentration (MIC), compared to achieveable drug levels, to clarithromycin, amikacin, and cefoxitin. Some isolates have low or intermediate MICs to linezolid and imipenem.

For serious skin, soft-tissue, and bone infections caused by *M. abscessus*, clarithromycin, 1000 mg/day, or azithromycin, 250 mg/day, should be combined with 1 or more of the parenteral medications (amikacin, cefoxitin, or imipenem). Intravenous amikacin is given at a dose of 10 to 15 mg/kg daily to adult patients with normal renal function to provide peak serum levels in the low 20 µg/mL range. The lower dose (10 mg/kg) should be used in patients over the age of 50 and/or in patients in whom long-term therapy (greater than 3 weeks) is anticipated. The amikacin combined with high-dose cefoxitin (up to 12 g/day given intravenously in divided doses) is recommended for initial therapy (minimum 2 weeks) until clinical improvement is evident. Limited cefoxitin availability may necessitate the choice of an alternative agent such as imipenem (500 mg 2 to 4 times daily), which is a reasonable alternative to cefoxitin. For serious disease, a minimum of 4 months of therapy is necessary to provide a high likelihood of cure. For bone infections, 6 months of therapy is recommended. Surgery is generally indicated with extensive disease, abscess formation, or where drug therapy is difficult. Removal of foreign bodies such as breast implants or percutaneous catheters is important and likely essential to recovery.

In contrast to the efficacy of medication regimens for nonpulmonary disease, no antibiotic regimens based on in vitro susceptibilities have been shown to produce long-term sputum conversion for patients with *M. abscessus* lung disease. The goal of 12 months of negative sputum cultures while on therapy may be optimal, but there is no medication strategy to reliably achieve this goal. Alternative goals of therapy such as symptomatic improvement, radiographic regression of infiltrates, or improvement in sputum culture positivity, short of conversion to negative cultures, are more realistic for *M. abscessus* lung disease. Combination therapy (as outlined above) with macrolide plus 1 or more parenteral agent (amikacin, cefoxitin, or imipenem for 2–4 months) usually produces clinical and microbiologic improvement, but cost and morbidity are significant impediments to a curative course of therapy. For some patients, symptoms can be controlled with intermittent periods of therapy with clarithromycin or azithromycin alone or in combination with one or more parenteral drugs. Curative therapy for *M. abscessus* lung disease is more likely to be obtained with limited disease and a combination of surgical resection of involved lung and chemotherapy. Drugs that show some potential but are not extensively tested include linezolid and tigecycline. Unfortunately, with current antibiotic options, *M. abscessus* is a chronic incurable infection for most patients.

M. MARINUM DISEASE

Mycobacterium marinum isolates are susceptible to rifampin, rifabutin, ethambutol, clarithromycin, sulfonamides, and trimethoprim–sulfamethoxazole; intermediately susceptible to streptomycin, doxycycline, and minocycline; and resistant to isoniazid and pyrazinamide.

For skin and soft-tissue infections due to *M. marinum* a reasonable approach is to treat with 2 active agents for 1 to 2 months after resolution of symptoms, typically 3 to 4 months in total. Some experts believe that minimal disease can be treated with a single agent. Excellent outcomes have also been reported for the combinations of clarithromycin and rifampin, clarithromycin and ethambutol, and the combination of ethambutol and rifampin. Clarithromycin and ethambutol are likely to provide the optimal balance of efficacy and tolerability for most patients, with the addition of rifampin in cases of osteomyelitis or other deep structure infection. Surgical debridement may also be indicated especially for disease involving the closed spaces of the hand and for disease that has failed to respond to standard therapy.

EMERGING AREAS OF NTM INFECTIONS

Increased numbers of published reports have highlighted several emerging areas of NTM infections since the mid-1990s. These newer and somewhat less common infections are worth noting and have linked growing numbers of individuals developing NTM infections to specific underlying disease conditions or specific home, work, or nosocomial environmental exposures, including cystic fibrosis (CF), hypersensitivity pneumonitislike lung disease (hot tub lung), and health care–associated NTM infections, respectively.

CYSTIC FIBROSIS-ASSOCIATED NTM DISEASE

A recent cross-sectional assessment from multiple CF centers across the United States found that approximately 13% of all surveyed CF patients, and 40% over the age of 40, had NTM isolated from sputum. Similar to non-CF NTM pulmonary disease, most NTM isolated were MAC (76%) or *M. abscessus* (18%). The explanation for this high prevalence of NTM in CF patients remains uncertain. Ambient exposure to NTM organisms from ubiquitous environmental water and soil sources coupled with abnormal host pulmonary factors such as altered mucociliary clearance and structural abnormalities accompanying advancing bronchiectasis may contribute to the development and phenotypic expression of NTM pulmonary disease commonly encountered in this group of patients. The diagnosis of NTM pulmonary disease in CF patients is similar to that of patients with non-CF NTM disease with the recognition that underlying bronchiectasis and other pathogens are present and may account for respiratory symptoms and radiographic abnormalities. The decision to treat NTM pulmonary infection in CF patients is complicated by a paucity of information about the effect of NTM infection on the natural history of CF, although CF patients with heavy *M. abscessus* growth from sputum appear to be at particular risk for more rapidly progressive disease and, in some instances, respiratory failure. Overall, treatment decisions require consideration of benefits weighed against risks and medication side effects for individual patients. Treatment regimens for CF patients with NTM lung disease are also similar to those of non-CF NTM pulmonary disease. Cystic fibrosis patients on azithromycin for noninfective purposes should have surveillance for NTM in sputum prior to and during treatment with macrolides to avoid macrolide monotherapy in a patient with occult or undiagnosed NTM disease.

HYPERSENSITIVITY PNEUMONITISLIKE NTM PULMONARY DISEASE

Several series of patients developing hypersensitivity pneumonitislike lung disease following NTM exposure have been reported since the mid-1990s. Most reports describe development of a typical pattern of hypersensitivity pneumonitislike lung disease in association with hot tub exposure. Some investigators have used the term *hot tub lung* to describe this presentation. In the cases of exposure to hot tubs, MAC has been the mycobacterial organism isolated from sputum, bronchoalveolar lavage, tissue, and hot tub water. Furthermore, comparison of MAC isolates from the hot tub water and lung specimens when assessed by genotyping methods has demonstrated identical matches. Controversy still exists, however, as to whether hot tub lung is an infectious process, inflammatory process, or combination of processes.

Hypersensitivity pneumonitislike lung disease patients tend to be young and without pre-existing lung disease. The clinical presentation varies widely from mild respiratory symptoms to respiratory failure requiring mechanical ventilatory support. Key elements to the diagnosis of MAC hypersensitivitylike lung include a compatible clinical history (subacute onset of respiratory symptoms, hot tub exposure), characteristic radiographic findings, and MAC isolates in sputum, bronchoalveolar lavage, tissue, and hot tub water (and compatible histopathology when available).

Patient prognosis is generally excellent independent of severity on presentation. The most benefit is gained by simply removing the patient from antigen exposure. In the case of hot tub lung, removal from antigen exposure generally involves drainage of hot tub water and complete avoidance of hot tub use. Whether continued exposure to ambient environmental MAC organisms can propagate the hypersensitivity pulmonary reaction is uncertain. For select patients with hypersensitivity pneumonitislike lung disease, use of systemic corticosteroids may be of benefit and hasten recovery of pulmonary symptoms, gas exchange abnormalities, and radiographic abnormalities. Likewise, antimycobacterial therapy with the same medications as standard pulmonary MAC lung disease may be required in some patients but with shorter durations of therapy, usually 3 to 6 months. Most patients can be expected to have complete or near complete resolution of respiratory symptoms as well as pulmonary function and radiographic abnormalities.

HEALTH CARE–ASSOCIATED NTM DISEASE

Transmission of NTM disease in the health care setting has most frequently been linked to tap (municipal) water exposure. Although various NTM species (including MAC, *M. kansasii*, *M. xenopi*, and *M. simiae*) have been isolated from municipal water supplies, *M. fortuitum* and *M. abscessus* have most often been implicated in health care–associated NTM disease. Even with use of potent disinfectants, including organomercurials, chlorine, bromine, 2% formaldehyde, and glutaraldehyde after tap water exposure, NTM organisms may persist on equipment or devices. The inability to eliminate these organisms underscores the importance of avoidance of tap water for preventing health care–associated NTM disease. Examples of health care–associated NTM infections include infections involving median sternotomy, plastic surgery procedures, liposuction, LASIK, dialysis-related outbreaks, long-term central intravenous catheters, tympanostomy tubes, and prosthetic devices such as heart valves, knee and hip joints, lens implants, and metal rod bone stabilizers. Pseudo-outbreaks have involved bronchoscopes contaminated with *M. abscessus* and *Mycobacterium immunogenum*. Documented outbreaks of hygiene-associated *M. fortuitum* and *Mycobacterium mageritense* furonculosis in association with use of contaminated whirlpool footbaths have been described in nail salons.

As a result of the increased understanding of environmental NTM reservoirs and reports linking the use of tap water to health care–associated NTM infections, it is recommended that tap water not be used in preparation of surgical procedures, prosthetics, and intravascular catheters, not be used in cleaning of fiberoptic endoscopes, and not be used to rinse the mouth out prior to collecting expectorated sputum samples. Moreover, recognition that alternative medicines or unapproved substances for injection may also be at risk of contamination by NTM warrants caution against use of these products as well.

SUGGESTED READING

Griffith DE, Aksamit T, Brown-Elliot BA, et al. An official ATS/IDSA statement: diagnosis, treatment, and prevention of nontuberculous mycobacterial diseases. *Am J Respir Crit Care Med*. 2007;175:367–416.

Griffith DE, Brown-Elliott BA, Langsjoen B, et al. Clinical and molecular analysis of macrolide resistance in *Mycobacterium avium* complex lung disease. *Am J Respir Crit Care Med*. 2006;174(8):928–934.

Hanak V, Kalra S, Aksamit TR, et al. Hot tub lung: presenting features and clinical course of 21 patients. *Respir Med*. 2006;100:610–615.

Mehta AC, Prakash UBS, Garland R, et al. American College of Chest Physicians and American Association for Bronchoscopy Consensus Statement: prevention of flexible bronchoscopy-associated infection. *Chest*. 2005;128:1742–1755.

Olivier KN, Weber DJ, Wallace RJ Jr, et al. Nontuberculous Mycobacteria in Cystic Fibrosis Study Group. Nontuberculous mycobacteria. I: Multicenter prevalence study in cystic fibrosis. *Am J Respir Crit Care Med*. 2003;167(6):828–834.

157. Vibrios

Duc J. Vugia

Vibrios are motile, rod-shaped, facultative-anaerobic, gram-negative bacteria that can cause gastroenteritis, wound infection, and septicemia in humans. They are naturally found in marine, estuarine, and brackish waters in the United States and in other parts of the world. In the United States, they are recovered from the environment most commonly in summer and fall, when the water is warm. Vibrios have also been isolated from a variety of fish and shellfish, including oysters, clams, mussels, crabs, and shrimp. Human cases of illness associated with *Vibrio* infection occur mostly in summer and fall, and usually follow ingestion of raw or undercooked shellfish, particularly oysters, or exposure of a wound to fish, shellfish, or seawater. In countries with endemic or epidemic cholera, infection with *Vibrio cholerae* may occur after ingestion of any contaminated food or water; in the United States, cholera is endemic along the Gulf Coast.

Analysis of 5S ribosomal ribonucleic acid sequence revealed 34 *Vibrio* spp., 12 of which have been isolated from human clinical specimens. The major clinical presentations associated with infection with these 12 species are shown in Table 157.1. Rarely, vibrios have also been recovered from bone, cerebrospinal fluid, ear, gallbladder, sputum, and urine.

GASTROENTERITIS AND CHOLERA

Clinical Presentation

Gastroenteritis is the most common clinical presentation of infection with most pathogenic vibrios. The disease ranges in severity from mild, self-limited diarrhea to frank, life-threatening cholera.

Cholera is a profuse, watery diarrhea mediated via an enterotoxin produced by epidemic strains of *V. cholerae* O1 and O139 and by some non-O1 strains. After attachment of toxigenic vibrios to intestinal epithelial cells, the cholera toxin, consisting of one A (activation) unit and five B (binding) units, is generated. It stimulates intracellular cyclic AMP, resulting in a secretory diarrhea. Other symptoms include nausea, vomiting, abdominal cramps, and muscle cramps of extremities; fever is typically not seen because the disease is toxin mediated and there is no invasion of the intestinal epithelium. Illness develops 4 hours to 5 days after ingestion of the bacteria and can rapidly lead to severe dehydration, electrolyte imbalance, acidosis, and death. Cholera usually lasts less than 7 days even without antibiotic therapy.

Gastroenteritis due to vibrios other than *V. cholerae* O1 and O139 may also be mediated via an enterotoxin, but the diarrhea is normally not so severe. However, bloody stool, low-grade fever, and elevated white blood cell count may be noted along with nausea, vomiting, and abdominal cramps. The median incubation period is 1 day, ranging from 4 hours to 5 days, and the duration of illness is typically less than 7 days, ranging from 1 to 15 days.

Therapy

For cholera, prompt replacement of fluid volume and electrolytes with an appropriate intravenous or oral solution is critical. If the patient has severe dehydration (loss of at least 10% of body weight) or cannot drink, intravenous fluid replacement with Ringer's lactate is recommended. Other intravenous solutions do not contain similar proportions of necessary electrolytes and are therefore not optimal. If the patient can drink, a solution containing glucose and adequate electrolyte replacement is recommended, such as those prepared with the oral rehydration salts (ORS) endorsed by the World Health Organization or commercially available ORS/electrolyte replacement solutions.

Treatment of cholera with antimicrobials is secondary to fluid and electrolyte replacement; appropriate antibiotics can decrease shedding of vibrios and duration of illness. Multidrug-resistant strains of *V. cholerae* O1 have been documented in Asia and in Africa, and antibiotic susceptibility testing should be performed on isolates from cholera patients. Recently, a single dose of azithromycin was found to be effective in the treatment of severe cholera in adults (1 g orally) and in children (20 mg/kg up

Vibrios

Table 157.1 Association of *Vibrio* with Major Clinical Presentations

Species	Gastroenteritis	Wound Infection	Septicemia
V. cholerae			
01	++	+	+
0139	++		+
Other non-01	++	+	+
V. alginolyticus	+	++	+
V. carchariae		+	
V. cincinnatiensis			+
V. damsela		+	+
V. fluvialis	++	+	+
V. furnisii	+		
V. hollisae	++	+	+
V. mimicus	++	+	+
V. metschnikovii	+	+	+
V. parahaemolyticus	++	++	+
V. vulnificus	+	++	++

++, Common; +, rare.

to a maximum of 1 g orally). Alternatively, for adults, ciprofloxacin either 1 g orally in a single dose or 500 mg orally twice daily for 3 days can be used. However, in a study in Bangladesh comparing azithromycin to ciprofloxacin for the treatment of cholera in adults, single-dose ciprofloxacin was found clinically and bacteriologically ineffective, and local strains of *V. cholerae* O1 had diminished in vitro susceptibility to ciprofloxacin. For adults with recent travel in the Americas where tetracycline resistance is not yet a problem, doxycycline 100 mg orally twice daily for 3 days or tetracycline 500 mg orally 4 times daily for 3 days can still be effective. As quinolones and macrolides are used more commonly, resistance to these classes of antibiotic may increase and, therefore, cholera patients treated with any antibiotic should have their isolates tested for susceptibility and the patients closely followed for appropriate clinical response.

For severe or prolonged gastroenteritis due to other vibrios, fluid and electrolyte replacement along with quinolone or doxycycline treatment is in order. However, mild or moderate gastroenteritis is usually self-limited and may not need therapy other than oral rehydration.

EXTRAINTESTINAL INFECTIONS
Clinical Presentations

For extraintestinal sites, wound infection and septicemia are the most common clinical presentations. Wound infection with vibrios occurs after exposure of a break in skin to seawater or after a skin injury from handling fish or shellfish. Wound infection may be mild and self-limited or severe and invasive. Septicemia, which may be primary following ingestion or secondary (eg, following wound infection), indicates severe disease.

Among vibrios causing extraintestinal infections, *Vibrio vulnificus* frequently causes two important clinical syndromes: primary septicemia and wound infections. Primary septicemia occurs predominantly in adults with liver disease, including cirrhosis and hemochromatosis, with alcoholism, with other chronic underlying diseases, including renal failure and diabetes, or with immune suppression, including cancer and human immunodeficiency virus (HIV) infection. In these susceptible persons, septicemia usually follows ingestion of raw shellfish, typically oysters. Between 7 and 48 hours after eating shellfish containing *V. vulnificus*, infected patients present with fever, chills, nausea, vomiting, abdominal pain, diarrhea, mental status changes, suggestive skin lesions (including bullae, cellulitis, and ecchymoses), and often hypotension or shock. Mortality for patients with *V. vulnificus* primary septicemia is greater than 50%, and it increases greatly with hypotension within 12 hours of hospitalization and when appropriate antibiotic therapy is delayed beyond 72 hours after onset of illness.

Vibrio vulnificus wound infection, however, results from injury to the skin from handling fish or shellfish or exposure of a fresh wound to seawater. Any healthy person may acquire this infection, but persons with the underlying diseases listed previously are at higher risk

for secondary septicemia and death. Infected persons develop inflammation of the wound, fever, and chills 4 hours to 4 days after exposure. Wound infections range from mild cellulitis to severe necrotizing fasciitis and myositis requiring extensive debridement or amputation. Secondary disseminated skin lesions such as bullae may be due to secondary septicemia (Figure 157.1).

Therapy

For invasive diseases of *Vibrio*, particularly *V. vulnificus*, prompt treatment with early antibiotic administration, appropriate wound management, and supportive care are crucial. Doxycycline, 100 mg, intravenously every 12 hours combined with a third-generation cephalosporin (eg, ceftazidime 2 g intravenously [IV] every 8 hours) should be given without delay. Alternatively, a fluoroquinolone such as ciprofloxacin, 400 mg IV every 12 hours, can also be used. The combination of ciprofloxacin and cefotaxime has been found synergistically active against *V. vulnificus* in vitro. The duration of treatment should be individualized to the

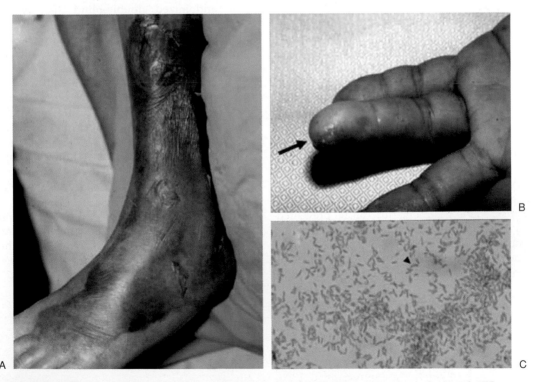

Figure 157.1 (A) Characteristic skin lesions associated with *Vibrio vulnificus* infection on the leg of a 75-year-old patient with liver cirrhosis in whom septic shock and bacteremia developed. **(B)** *Vibrio vulnificus* bacteremia developed 1 day after a fish bone injury on the fourth finger of the left hand (*arrow*) in a 45-year-old patient with uremia. **(C)** Gram-negative curved bacilli isolated from a blood sample of the 45-year-old patient with uremia. [Photos from Hsueh, et al. *Vibrio vulnificus* in Taiwan. *CDC Emerg Infect Dis*. 2004;10(8).]

presentation and clinical course but should be considered for at least 7 to 14 days. Necrotic tissue should be surgically debrided and, occasionally, amputation of an affected limb may be necessary.

LABORATORY DIAGNOSIS

For a patient with a gastrointestinal or cholera-like illness thought to be caused by *Vibrio*, physicians should specify culture for vibrios when ordering stool cultures. Ideally, specimens should be collected before treatment with antimicrobials. Vibrios are isolated by direct inoculation of stool onto a selective medium, such as thiosulfate-citrate-bile salts-sucrose agar.

Selective media are not necessary for extraintestinal infections because common media used to culture blood and wounds contain at least 0.5% sodium chloride, which is adequate to grow halophilic (salt-loving) vibrios.

For cholera patients already treated with antimicrobials and whose stool culture was either negative or not processed for vibrios, *V. cholerae* vibriocidal or antitoxin antibodies can be detected by serologic assays.

PREVENTION

Most *Vibrio* gastroenteritis, cholera, and primary *V. vulnificus* septicemia can be prevented. For prevention of cholera, travelers should be informed on whether cholera is endemic in the country or region being visited and take appropriate precautions with all foods and drinks. In general, well-cooked foods and hot or carbonated drinks are safe. There is no cholera vaccine available currently in the United States. And, although an oral cholera vaccine is commercially available in some other countries, it is not recommended for most travelers. In the United States, *Vibrio* gastroenteritis can be prevented by avoiding consumption of raw or undercooked shellfish. Patients with underlying liver and other chronic diseases or with immunosuppression, which puts them at increased risk of

V. vulnificus septicemia, should avoid raw oysters and other raw shellfish.

Wound infections are probably not preventable, because vibrios exist naturally in certain waters and on a variety of fish and shellfish. Nonetheless, an exposure history in a patient with an infected wound should raise clinical suspicion and prompt consideration of treatment for possible infection with a *Vibrio*.

SUGGESTED READING

Chiang S-R, Chuang Y-C. *Vibrio vulnificus* infection: clinical manifestations, pathogenesis, and antimicrobial therapy. *J Microbiol Immunol Infect*. 2003;36:81–88.

Hlady WG, Klontz KC. The epidemiology of *Vibrio* infections in Florida, 1981–1993. *J Infect Dis*. 1996;173:1176–1183.

Hoge CW, Watsky D, Peeler RN, Libonati JP, Israel E, Morris JG Jr. Epidemiology and spectrum of *Vibrio* infections in a Chesapeake Bay community. *J Infect Dis*. 1989;160:985–993.

Khan WA, Saha D, Rahman A, Salam MA, Bogaerts J, Bennish ML. Comparison of single-dose azithromycin and 12-dose, 3-day erythromycin for childhood cholera: a randomized, double-blind trial. *Lancet*. 2002;360:1722–1727.

Kim D-M, Lym Y, Jang SJ, et al. In vitro efficacy of the combination of ciprofloxacin and cefotaxime against *Vibrio vulnificus*. *Antimicrob Agents Chemother*. 2005;49:3489–3491.

Morris JG Jr. Cholera and other types of vibriosis: a story of human pandemics and oysters on the half shell. *Clin Infect Dis*. 2003;37:272–280.

Saha D, Karim MM, Khan WA, Ahmed S, Salam MA, Bennish ML. Single-dose azithromycin for the treatment of cholera in adults. *N Engl J Med*. 2006;354:2452–2462.

Steinberg EB, Greene KD, Bopp CA, Cameron DN, Wells JG, Mintz ED. Cholera in the United States, 1995-2000: trends at the end of the twentieth century. *J Infect Dis*. 2001;184:799–802.

158. Yersinia

Royce H. Johnson

INTRODUCTION

Yersinia genus includes several species. The most important for human disease are *Yersinia enterocolitica*, *Yersinia pseudotuberculosis*, and *Y. pseudotuberculosis* subspecies *pestis*. More commonly *Y. pseudotuberculosis* subspecies *pestis* is listed as *Yersinia pestis*. *Yersinia pseudotuberculosis* and *Y. pestis* are clearly closely related species by analysis of the genome. However, *Y. enterocolitica* and *Y. pseudotuberculosis* produce clinically similar disease and both are quite distinct from that produced by subspecies *Y. pestis*; hence, in this chapter the older terminology *Y. pestis* will be used, and *Y. enterocolitica* and *Y. pseudotuberculosis* discussed separately.

YERSINIA PESTIS

The well-known unfortunate events of September 11, 2001, have produced a resurgence in interest in an ancient organism. Additionally, *Y. pestis* has been classified as a re-emerging pathogen. *Yersinia pestis* was first identified by Alexander Yersin in 1894 during an outbreak in Hong Kong. *Yersinia pestis* is typically a zoonosis with human infection an incidental event. Domestic dogs and cats can also transmit the disease to humans. The disease is variably distributed throughout the world. Its distribution in the United States is largely limited to the west, particularly New Mexico, Arizona, and California.

Natural infection is most commonly from the bite of an infected flea. Inhalation of infected respiratory secretions or handling or ingestion of infected meat may result in infection. The majority of patients present with febrile lymphadenitis or bubonic disease. The incubation period is typically 2 to 6 days. Inguinal and femoral nodes are most frequently noted. Cervical and axillary node involvement is less common. Septicemic disease without lymphadenitis may present as undifferentiated gram-negative sepsis often with gastrointestinal symptoms. Plague pneumonia is the result of primary respiratory acquisition. This may occur from the respiratory secretions of animals or humans or from bioterrorism aerosols. Secondary pneumonic disease from bacteremia also occurs. Less common sites of infection include the eye, skin, and meninges. A careful epidemiologic history is essential in the evaluation of patients with lymphadenitis, sepsis, or pneumonia.

Specimens and cultures from patients with suspected *Y. pestis* must be handled with extreme caution. Smear and culture of lymph node aspirate, sputum, cerebrospinal fluid, buffy coat, or blood should be undertaken as directed by the clinical presentation. A gram stain or the preferred Wayson stain should be prepared. *Yersinia pestis* has the classic bipolar safety pin morphology on direct smear. *Yersinia pestis* is easily propagated on normal laboratory media aerobically or anaerobically. Identification can be undertaken with any of a number of systems appropriate for gram-negative organisms. Difficulty with an exact identification sometimes occurs. All suspected specimens should be referred to an appropriate public health reference laboratory for confirmation whether identification is clear or not.

Antigen detection by newer technology including microchip assay analysis is rapidly becoming available in many laboratories. If *Y. pestis* infections are suspected, expert advice regarding specimen handling and testing should be sought.

Therapy (Table 158.1)

Streptomycin has been used since 1948 with great success, although this drug may not be readily available in the United States, necessitating the use of alternative regimens. When streptomycin is available it should be used at a dosage of 15 to 30 mg/kg/day every 12 hours. Intramuscular (IM) treatment is recommended, but intravenous (IV) therapy can be used if required by the clinical circumstances. A 7- to 10-day course of streptomycin is recommended. Appropriate monitoring for renal, vestibular, and auditory toxicity is required. Because of the availability problems with streptomycin, gentamicin has been used. In vitro

Yersinia

Table 158.1 Therapy of Y*ersinia pestis*

Preferred Antibiotic	Classificatin for Use
Streptomycin, 15 mg/kg/d IM q12h (or IV if necessary)	If immediate availability is a problem, call direct to Pfizer Pharmaceuticals
Doxycycline, 100 mg PO or IV q12h	Not for use during pregnancy or in children ≤8 y
Chloramphenicol, 1 g (25 mg/kg) IV or PO q6h with dosage reduction as patient stabilizes to 500 mg (15 mg/kg) q6h	Predominantly for patients with meningitis and children in whom tetracycline is not indicated

data and retrospective review of human cases suggest similar efficacy. Gentamicin, 5 to 7 mg/kg/day in 3 divided doses given every 8 hours, is recommended. Monitoring for toxicity as with streptomycin is needed. Drug blood level assays are also desirable.

In children, pregnant women, and patients with meningitis, IV and oral chloramphenicol can be used as an alternative. As with streptomycin, availability may be a problem. Initial doses of 1 g (24 mg/kg) followed by 500 mg (15 mg/kg) every 6 hours can be used for a total course of 7 to 10 days. Trimethoprim–sulfamethoxazole, other aminoglycosides, and third-generation cephalosporins are likely to be effective. Some question has been raised regarding the efficacy of ciprofloxacin and other fluoroquinolones. No evaluable data exist regarding this issue.

There are also reports of natural drug resistance that is probably plasmid mediated and potentially multidrug resistant. Resistance to ampicillin, chloramphenicol, kanamycin, streptomycin, sulfonamides, and tetracyclines were found. This appeared to be based on a plasmid derived from enteric organisms. Multidrug-resistant bioterrorism constructs are also a possibility.

YERSINIA ENTEROCOLITICA AND YERSINIA PSEUDOTUBERCULOSIS

Yersinia enterocolitica is an increasingly well-recognized pathogen with protean manifestations. *Yersinia pseudotuberculosis*, a much rarer pathogen, causes gastrointestinal illness and rarely sepsis. *Yersinia enterocolitica* is widely distributed in nature and also has been identified in food, particularly pork, contaminated milk, and untreated water. Only certain serotypes of *Y. enterocolitica* typically produce gastrointestinal

disease. The O:3 serogroup is most commonly responsible for disease in the United States. This serogroup can be distinguished by its failure to ferment D-xylose.

Unlike many enteric pathogens, *Y. enterocolitica* is found most often in cool climates. The disease is reported most commonly from northern Europe, Japan, Canada, and the United States. The incubation period is 1 to 14 days, typically at the shorter end of this spectrum. Individuals with iron overload or receiving treatment with deferoxamine are at increased risk, as are individuals who are immunocompromised. Alkalinization of the stomach may also create an increased risk of infection.

The most common presentations of *Y. enterocolitica* are enteritis or enterocolitis. Children are the most frequently affected. The most typical illness is suggestive of shigellosis, with diarrhea (occasionally bloody), fever, abdominal pain, and vomiting. *Yersinia enterocolitica* may manifest as mesenteric lymphadenitis and present with abdominal pain that mimics appendicitis. The distinction from true appendicitis can often be made by careful ultrasound or computed tomography evaluation. *Yersinia enterocolitica* can also cause suppurative infections: pharyngitis with or without cervical lymphadenitis, hepatic abscess and pulmonary, genitourinary, and musculoskeletal infection. Bacteremia, endocarditis, pericarditis, and myocarditis have all been reported. Rare cutaneous infections have also been described.

Yersinia enterocolitica has also been shown to precipitate disease through immunopathologic mechanisms. Erythema nodosum, anterior uveitis, and reactive arthritis have all been reported. There is also a possible link to inflammatory bowel disease.

Therapy (Table 158.2)

Antipseudomonal penicillins and second-generation cephalosporins are not sufficiently active to be recommended on a routine basis. Only limited clinical information on aztreonam and imipenem–cilastatin is available; in vitro susceptibility testing suggests that these agents are active. Third-generation cephalosporins, especially ceftriaxone, have in vitro and clinical data to suggest significant utility, although there have been clinical failures. Similarly, aminoglycosides, chloramphenicol, trimethoprim–sulfamethoxazole, and doxycycline may be useful. Doxycycline may be particularly useful in less critically ill patients.

Table 158.2 Therapy of *Yersinia enterocolitica*

Preferred Agents for Serious Illness	Agents Likely to Be Effective	Agents Not Likely to Be Effective
Fluoroquinolones	Doxycycline	Penicillin
Ceftriaxone	Trimethoprim–sulfamethoxazole	Ampicillin
	Aminoglycosides	Amoxicillin–clavulanate
	Aztreonam	First-generation cephalosporins
	Imipenem	
	Chloramphenicol[a]	

[a] Not recommended in usual circumstances.

Probably the best information on in vitro sensitivity, animal models, and anecdotal human experience is for fluoroquinolones. These data suggest that these agents may be the drugs of choice for severe *Y. enterocolitica* infection.

Duration of treatment that has been shown to be effective has varied between 2 and 6 weeks. Initial therapy is most typically begun with an IV drug in severely ill individuals, with completion of therapy on an oral basis.

Yersinia pseudotuberculosis rarely requires therapy when presenting as mesenteric adenitis or gastrointestinal disease. Patients with sepsis may be treated with streptomycin or doxycycline; ampicillin can also be used.

SUGGESTED READING

Abdel-Haq NM, Papadopol R, Asmar BI, et al. Antibiotic susceptibilities of Yersinia enterocolitica recovered from children over a 12-year period. *Int J Antimicrob Agents.* 2006;27:449–452.

Centers for Disease Control and Prevention (CDC). Human plague—four states, 2006. *Morbid Mortal Weekly Rep.* 2006;55 (34):940–943.

Galimand M, Guiyoule A, Gerbaud G, et al. Multidrug resistance in Yersinia pestis mediated by a transferable plasmid. *N Engl J Med.* 1997;337(10):677–680.

Hadou T, Elfarra M, Alauzet C, et al. Abdominal aortic aneurysm infected by *Yersinia pseudotuberculosis. J Clin Microbiol.* 2006;44 (9):3457–3458.

Heijden I, Res PC, Wilbrink B, et al. Yersinia enterocolitica: a cause of chronic polyarthritis. *Clin Infect Dis.* 1997;25:831–837.

Jelloul L, Frémond B, Dyon JF, et al. Mesenteric adenitis caused by Yersinia pseudotuberculosis presenting as an abdominal mass. *Eur J Pediatr Surg.* 1997;7:180–183.

Klein EJ, Boster DR, Stapp JR, et al. Diarrhea etiology in a children's hospital emergency department: a prospective cohort study. *Clin Infect Dis.* 2006;43:807–813.

Olesen B, Neimann J, Böttiger B, et al. Etiology of diarrhea in young children in Denmark: a case-control study. *J Clin Microbiol.* 2005;43(8):3636–3641.

Perdikogianni C, Galanakis E, Michalakis M, et al. Yersinia enterocolitica infection mimicking surgical conditions. *Pediatr Surg Int.* 2006;22:589–592.

Stenseth NC, Samia NI, Viljugrein H, et al. Plague dynamics are driven by climate variation. *Proc Natl Acad Sci U S A.* 2006; 103:13110–13115.

159. Miscellaneous Gram-Positive Organisms

Sohail G. Haddad, Roberto Baun Corales, and Steven K. Schmitt

PEDIOCOCCUS SPECIES

Pediococci are gram-positive cocci that grow in pairs and tetrads. Normal inhabitants of the gastrointestinal tract, they are used extensively in industry to ferment cheese and other dairy products, soy products, and alcoholic beverages. Eight species of pediococci are recognized, but only the closely related *Pediococcus acidilactici* and *Pediococcus pentosaceus* have been identified as human pathogens. In recent years, these organisms have been increasingly recognized as a cause of bacteremia and pneumonitis in the immunocompromised host. These organisms have also been isolated from intra-abdominal infections such as peritonitis and hepatic abscesses. Risk factors for *Pediococcus* infections include prior antibiotic therapy, abdominal surgery, and gastric feeding.

Diagnosis is made by isolation and identification of the organism from cultures of blood or other body fluids. As one of the lactic acid bacteria associated with foods, *Pediococcus* species may be difficult to distinguish from enterococci and *Leuconostoc* species. Approximately 95% of clinical isolates will cross-react with group D streptococcal antisera. Tests that aid in distinguishing pediococci from other organisms include a negative pyrrolidonylarylamidase (PYRase) test and the absence of gas production from glucose. With newer application of molecular genetic techniques to determine relatedness of food-associated lactic acid bacteria, reorganization of the genus with novel morphologic or phenotypic differentiation of *Leuconostoc* species from *Pediococcus* species is being studied.

Pediococci are intrinsically highly resistant to vancomycin and other glycopeptides. Most strains are moderately susceptible to penicillin and ampicillin. Minimum inhibitory concentrations (MICs) are variable for cephalosporins. Imipenem appears active against all isolates, as does gentamicin. In vitro susceptibility to linezolid and daptomycin has been demonstrated. Resistance to quinupristin–dalfopristin, erythromycin, clindamycin, tetracycline, tobramycin, and amikacin has been described. If a serious *Pediococcus* infection is suspected (eg, on the

basis of the characteristic tetrad morphology on Gram stain), intravenous penicillin at a dosage of 12 million or more units daily or imipenem may be used as empiric therapy. Susceptibility testing, preferably by MIC rather than disk diffusion, should be performed to determine appropriate therapy (Table 159.1).

LEUCONOSTOC SPECIES

Leuconostoc species are gram-positive coccobacilli that recently have been increasingly recognized as human pathogens. These organisms are normally found in dairy products and vegetable matter and are used in the production of wine, dairy products, and dextrans. *Leuconostoc* species are not usually considered part of the normal human flora, but they have been isolated from the feces, vagina, and gastric fluid, primarily in hospitalized patients. Antibiotic therapy, particularly with vancomycin, to which leuconostocs are intrinsically resistant, may contribute to gastrointestinal colonization with these organisms.

Leuconostoc species may cause bacteremia in otherwise healthy neonates. Recent reports of other infections produced by these organisms include endocarditis caused by *Leuconostoc mesenteroides*; empyema and bacteremia caused by *Leuconostoc cremoris* in a burn patient; after liver transplantation; and from a thrombotized central venous catheter. Serious infections such as bacteremia and pneumonia almost always occur in immunocompromised patients, although a case of meningitis in a previously healthy teenager has been described. At least four *Leuconostoc* species (including *L. mesenteroides*, *Leuconostoc paramesenteroides*, *L. cremoris*, and *Leuconostoc citreum*) may cause human infections. Risk factors for *Leuconostoc* infection include lengthy hospitalization, intravascular catheters, prior antibiotic therapy, prematurity, short gut syndrome, and serious underlying disease.

Diagnosis is based on identification of the organism from cultures of blood or other sterile body fluids. On Gram stain the organisms appear as pairs or chains of slightly elongated gram-positive cocci that may appear rodlike.

Table 159.1 Recommended Drug of Choice for the Miscellaneous Gram-Positive Organisms

Organism	Antibiotic (Ab) (Alternative Ab)	Route	Dosage	Duration
Pediococcus	Penicillin G Imipenem (Cephalosporins) (Linezolid)	IV	12 million U	(10–14 d)[a]
Leuconostoc	Penicillin G Ampicillin (Clindamycin) (Erythromycin) (Daptomycin)	IV	≥12 million U	(10–14 d)[a] 4 to 6 wk for endocarditis
Lactobacillus	Penicillin G Penicillin G and gentamicin (Clindamycin) (Erythromycin) (Linezolid)	IV IV IV	12 million U daily 20–24 million U daily for endocarditis 1.0 mg/kg q8h	(10–14 d)[a] 6 wk
Oerskovia	Penicillin G, TMP–SMX (Vancomycin)	IV	(Moderate to high dosage)[a]	4–6 wk for endocarditis
Rothia	Penicillin G, (Vancomycin) (Cephalosporins) (Fluoroquinolones)	IV	20 million U daily for endocarditis	6 wk
Arcanobacterium	Erythromycin Penicillin V Penicillin G ± aminoglycosides (Clindamycin) (Tetracycline) (Linezolid)	PO/IV PO IV	40 mg/kg (4 divided doses) 250–500 mg QID 2 million U q4h (for endocarditis)	10 d Until clinical response 4–6 wk
Rhodococcus	Vancomycin (V) or imipenem plus rifampin (AIDS) or erythromycin (Sulfonamides) (Chloramphenicol) (Linezolid)	IV IV PO IV/PO	1 g q12h 500 mg q6h 600 mg/d 500 mg–1 g QID	2 wk 2–4 wk
Abiotrophia Granulicatella Gemella	Ampicillin or penicillin + gentamicin			

[a] Suggested by some authorities.
Abbreviations: TMP-SMX = trimethoprim–sulfamethoxazole; AIDS = acquired immunodeficiency syndrome

They may be difficult to distinguish from viridans streptococci, enterococci, lactobacilli, or pediococci. Helpful tests include the production of gas from glucose; a negative catalase, oxidase, and PYRase test; and the absence of arginine hydrolysis.

Leuconostoc isolates, like pediococci, are uniformly resistant to vancomycin and other glycopeptides. Most strains are susceptible to penicillin, clindamycin, and gentamicin. Susceptibility to the cephalosporins, quinolones,

and trimethoprim–sulfamethoxazole (TMP–SMX) is variable. Among newer agents directed against gram-positive organisms, daptomycin and linezolid show activity against *Leuconostoc* sp. Resistance to quinupristin/dalfopristin has been demonstrated. Penicillin, the drug of choice, should be given at relatively high dosages (≥12 million units daily). In the case of penicillin allergy or resistance, therapy should be based on results of susceptibility testing. Appropriate therapy may also include removal of potentially infected devices such as indwelling intravascular catheters.

LACTOBACILLUS SPECIES

Lactobacillus species are gram-positive rods that normally inhabit the human mouth, vagina, and gastrointestinal tract. More than 50 species of lactobacilli are recognized, many of which are used in the production of cheese, yogurt, pickles, and fermented beverages. Lactobacilli are widely considered to have low pathogenicity, and recent attention has focused on their possible roles as probiotic bacteria promoting beneficial health effects, as part of prevention and treatment protocols for pseudomembranous colitis, as vehicles for oral immunization, and as part of treatment policies called *ecoimmunonutrition*. Nevertheless, they have been reported to cause infections, including bacteremia, endocarditis, intra-abdominal and hepatic abscesses, meningitis, and pneumonia. Risk factors for serious infections caused by *Lactobacillus* species include underlying immunocompromised state (including human immunodeficiency virus [HIV] disease) and gastrointestinal surgery. Prior antibiotic therapy, particularly with vancomycin (to which most lactobacilli are resistant), has also been identified as a clinical risk factor. In patients with *Lactobacillus* bacteremia and endocarditis, a recent review identified cancer, recent surgery, and diabetes mellitus as underlying risk factors. In this series, *Lactobacillus* bacteremia was a marker for serious and rapidly fatal underlying illness. Additional history of dental infection or manipulation is common.

Diagnosis is based on identification of the organism from sterile body fluids. Lactobacilli are gram-positive rods, but they may appear coccoid if grown on solid media. Cultures grown in broth are more reliable for assessing morphology. Some *Lactobacillus* isolates may be difficult to distinguish from *Leuconostoc* species and streptococci. The combination of tests for gas production from glucose, arginine hydrolysis, PYRase, and carbohydrate fermentations should allow proper identification.

Intravenous penicillin (≥12 million units daily) is generally the drug of choice for serious infections. Endocarditis should be treated with penicillin 20 million to 24 million units daily plus gentamicin for 6 weeks. Lactobacilli are usually resistant to glycopeptides such as vancomycin. Susceptibility to cephalosporins and quinolones is variable, and most isolates are resistant to tetracycline and TMP–SMX. Most strains are susceptible in vitro to clindamycin, a possible alternative therapy in penicillin-allergic patients, but few clinical data are available. Lactobacilli are usually susceptible in vitro to linezolid but may be resistant to daptomycin and quinupristin/dalfopristin. Because of variable activity, susceptibility testing is critical in developing a treatment regimen. In the patient allergic to β-lactams who has endocarditis, penicillin desensitization should be considered.

OERSKOVIA AND CELLULOSIMICROBIUM SPECIES

Oerskovia species are yellow, gram-positive, non–acid-fast organisms with extensively branched filaments. They were first described by Orskov in 1938 as "motile *Nocardia*." Their usual habitat is soil, although they have also been isolated from decaying plant materials and grass cuttings. Two species of *Oerskovia* were originally recognized: *Oerskovia turbata* and *Oerskovia xanthineolytica*. Recently, *O. xanthineolytica* has been reclassified as *Cellulosimicrobium cellulans*, and *O. turbata* has been proposed for reclassification as a novel *Cellulosimicrobium* species. Both are rare causes of opportunistic infection in humans but should be considered as potential pathogens of low virulence, especially in the setting of indwelling devices. Reported infections caused by *Oerskovia* and *Cellulosimicrobium* species include native and prosthetic valve endocarditis, peritonitis, central venous catheter infections, bacteremia in immunocompromised hosts (including patients with acquired immunodeficiency syndrome [AIDS]), prosthetic joint infection, keratitis, and endophthalmitis due to a penetrating eye injury. Several reported cases have been associated with exposure to soil and bacterial contamination of hydrophilic contact lens solutions.

The diagnosis of *Oerskovia* and *Cellulosimicrobium* infections rests on laboratory identification from clinical specimens. Gram stain may reveal pleomorphic gram-positive nonmotile rods that can be mistaken for *Corynebacterium* spp. Culture reveals yellow colonies that are catalase positive when grown aerobically. They may be distinguished from other *Nocardia*-like organisms in that they are facultatively anaerobic and do not produce aerial mycelia. Identification is based on carbohydrate fermentation testing.

Successful treatment of *Oerskovia* infections generally requires removal of the contaminated foreign body in addition to appropriate antibiotic therapy, although some published cases report treatment without removal of infected vascular or peritoneal catheters. Antibiotics to which clinical isolates of *Oerskovia* and *Cellulosimicrobium* have been reported to be susceptible include penicillin (including extended-spectrum penicillins), vancomycin, TMP–SMX, cephalothin, and amikacin. Intermediate susceptibility or resistance has been described for ampicillin, ciprofloxacin, doxycycline, erythromycin, gentamicin, clindamycin, and the third-generation cephalosporins. Therapy should be based on susceptibility testing of the isolate. However, if culture results suggest *Oerskovia* infection, empiric parenteral penicillin or TMP–SMX therapy seems prudent while awaiting results of susceptibility testing.

ROTHIA SPECIES

Rothia dentocariosa is a small gram-positive pleomorphic rod. These organisms, common components of the normal oral microflora, were first isolated from carious dentine. The first description of human disease due to *Rothia* species was not reported until 1975, when the organism was recovered from a periappendiceal abscess. More recently, a number of case reports have described *Rothia* species as causing native and prosthetic valve endocarditis, aortic root abscess, and pneumonia. The patient often has a history of recent dental infection or dental manipulation; however, a recent report includes identification in throat cultures of healthy individuals. Complications, including mycotic aneurysm, cerebral abscess, and perivalvular abscess, are common. *Rothia* species may also cause bacteremia without endocarditis (particularly in immunocompromised patients), pneumonia, peritonitis, and infections of the head and neck. *Rothia dentocariosa* has been isolated in lymph nodes of patients with cat scratch disease (CSD), suggesting a possible role, together with *Bartonella henselae*, in the pathogenesis of CSD. Recent data show another species of this genus (*Rothia mucilaginosa*, formerly known as *Stomatococcus mucilaginosa*) to be a member of the normal oral flora. This species have been described as opportunistic agents of infection in cases of endocarditis, meningitis, peritonitis, and other infections.

Diagnosis of *Rothia* infections depends on identification of the organism from the cultures of blood or other body fluids. *Rothia* species are catalase positive, nonmotile, urease negative, and indole negative. The organisms may appear branched, resembling *Actinomyces* or *Nocardia* species. They are distinguished from these genera by carbohydrate fermentation testing. *Rothia mucilaginosa* forms cocci in clusters and displays variable catalase reactions ranging from negative to weakly positive to strongly positive. The inability to grow in 5% NaCl distinguishes *R. mucilaginosa* from members of *Staphylococcus* and *Micrococcus* genera.

Penicillin is the drug of choice for treatment of infections due to *Rothia* sp. Because rare isolates may be resistant to penicillin, susceptibility testing should be performed. For endocarditis due to penicillin-susceptible strains, intravenous penicillin at dosages of 20 million units per day for 6 weeks is recommended. In the case of penicillin resistance or drug allergy, vancomycin, netilmicin, or teicoplanin therapy may be effective. *Rothia* species may also be susceptible in vitro to ciprofloxacin, rifampin, cephalosporins, and gentamicin. Resistance to amikacin, kanamycin, ciprofloxacin, and TMP–SMX has been described. In endocarditis cases due to *Rothia* sp., cardiac surgery may be beneficial when antimicrobial therapy alone is unsuccessful. Dental evaluation should also be considered in patients with infections due to *Rothia* species because carious or infected teeth may be a source of recurrent infection.

ARCANOBACTERIUM SPECIES

Arcanobacterium haemolyticum (formerly known as *Corynebacterium haemolyticum*) are facultatively anaerobic gram-positive to gram-variable pleomorphic rods (slender at first, sometimes clubbed, or in angular arrangements) that are nonmotile and nonsporulating. They are considered commensals of human nasopharynx and skin and are transmitted person to person by the droplet route. *Arcanobacterium* species have been recognized as causes of pharyngitis and cervical lymphadenopathy (indistinguishable from the pharyngitis caused by *S. pyogenes*) with additional symptoms of fever, pruritus, nonproductive cough, scarlatiniform skin rash with mild desquamation, and occasional formation of peritonsillar abscesses. Cutaneous infections, including ulcers, wound infection, cellulitis, and paronychia, are marked in some cases by the elaboration of lipid-hydrolyzing enzyme (sphingomyelinase D), producing dermonecrosis. Sepsis syndrome has been seen, with intravenous drug abuse and diabetes identified as risk factors. Central nervous system (CNS) infections (brain abscess, cerebritis, meningitis), endocarditis, osteomyelitis, otitis media, sphenoidal sinusitis, empyema, and cavitary pneumonia have also been described.

Diagnosis is made by isolation and identification of the organism from cultures of blood, pharynx, skin lesions, or other clinical specimens (eg, CNS abscess, cerebrospinal fluid [CSF], aortic valve, bone). Isolates of *Archanobacterium* spp. are weakly acid fast, but this characteristic is typically not used for identification. On Loeffler's medium, the morphology closely resembles *Corynebacterium diphtheriae*. Tests that aid in diagnosis include fermentation of dextrose, lactose, and maltose but not mannitol or xylose. Colonies appear circular, discoid, opaque, and whitish, with a rough surface and friable consistency, a uniform feature at 48 hours of a black opaque dot at the center of each colony, and hemolysis at 24 to 48 hours incubation. Because *Archanobacterium* species may present as part of polymicrobic infections with typical respiratory pathogens, they are often overlooked. Diagnosis often occurs only after repeated isolation. Increased awareness in microbiology laboratories of this organism may allow further elucidation of its pathogenicity in soft-tissue infections.

Most isolates of *A. haemolyticum* are susceptible to erythromycin, gentamicin, clindamycin, and cephalosporins. New studies report susceptibility to linezolid as well. They are resistant to sulfonamides and nalidixic acid in vitro. The drug of choice is erythromycin, 40 mg/kg orally or intravenously in 4 divided doses per day (2 g maximum). Although there have been reports of treatment failure with penicillin attributed to tolerance and failure to penetrate the intracellular location of the pathogen, penicillins with or without aminoglycosides are also widely used antibiotics, in most cases with success. In cases of abscess or tissue necrosis, surgical drainage or debridement may be a necesssary adjunct to antibiotic therapy.

RHODOCOCCUS SPECIES

Rhodococcus equi (formerly known as *Corynebacterium equi*), readily found in soil contaminated with stool of horses and other animals, are nonfastidious, strict aerobic gram-positive bacteria displaying rod-to-coccus pleomorphism, with fragmenting and occasionally palisading forms. *Rhodococcus* are well-documented veterinary pathogens, causing granulomatous pneumonia in foals. They have been recognized as opportunistic pathogens found in immunocompromised patients, including transplant patients and HIV-infected persons. Documented clinical presentations include slowly progressive granulomatous pneumonia, with lobar infiltrates progressing to cavitating lesions on chest radiograph; abscesses of the central nervous system, pelvis, and subcutaneous tissue; and lymphadenitis. Vertebral osteomyelitis and pulmonary malakoplakia have also been reported. Mortality exceeds 50% among AIDS patients with documented *R. equi* pneumonia, which is associated with a high rate of relapse despite adequate treatment. A newly described species of *Rhodococcus*, *Rhodococcus tsukamurella*, may cause multiple lung cavitary lesions in immunosuppressed patients and patients with indwelling foreign bodies.

Rhodococcus equi forms salmon pink colonies on blood agar from clinical specimens after 2 to 3 days of incubation. Colonies can be mucoid and coalescing; growth on Lowenstein–Jensen medium allows earlier detection of pigment. Synergistic hemolysis (resembling the CAMP test), displayed by cross-streaking on sheep blood agar with any of a number of other bacteria, including *Arcanobacterium haemolyticum*, *Staphylococcus aureus,* and *Corynebacterium pseudotuberculosis*, has been helpful in the diagnosis. In addition, *Rhodococcus* isolates are nonreactive to catalase and urease and exhibit acid-fast staining. Some diagnostic laboratories use a commercial kit (API CORYNE strip; bioMerieux-Vitek, Hazelwood, MO) for identification. Prompt identification is necessary for optimal patient management.

Most strains are susceptible to inhibition by glycopeptide antibiotics, rifampin, and macrolides. Susceptibility to linezolid has been documented. Resistance to β-lactam antibiotics (except carbapenems) has been reported. The high relapse rate and attributable mortality rate, especially among AIDS patients, makes it difficult to recommend a standard treatment protocol. Repeat cultures are warranted during treatment to discover acquired resistance. A combination of at least two antibiotics parenterally (including a glycopeptide and rifampin) followed by oral maintenance therapy is recommended. Surgical lung resection has been used with some success, sometimes in combination with antimicrobial therapy. Antimicrobial prophylaxis may prove of benefit in AIDS patients. Recent data suggest treatment for *R. tsukamurella* infections to be combination of β-lactam and aminoglycoside, along with removal of affected medical devices.

ABIOTROPHIA AND *GRANULICATELLA* SPECIES

These two new genera were once considered nutritionally deficient mutants of viridans streptococci. They are members of normal oral cavity flora and have been documented as agents of endocarditis. They form gram-positive cocci in pairs and chains under optimal nutritional conditions (pyridoxal-supplemented media) but may display pleomorphic cellular morphology when growth conditions are suboptimal. Strains of these genera usually grow as small α-hemolytic colonies on chocolate agar but not on sheep blood agar unless the medium is supplemented or other bacteria are present to provide compounds needed for growth. Most strains exhibit positive PYR and LAP tests. They are susceptible to β-lactam agents, although elevated MICs for β-lactams have been observed for some strains. Hence, a combination of ampicillin and gentamicin is recommended for endovascular infections with these organisms.

GEMELLA SPECIES

This genus has recently grown to include a total of four species (*Gemella haemolysans*, *Gemella morbillorum*, *Gemella bergeriae*, and *Gemella sanguinis*). Most strains are PYR and LAP positive. They produce colonies on blood agar that resemble viridans streptococci. Although the cellular morphology of *G. morbillorum* resembles that of streptococci, *G. haemolysans* forms *Neisseria*-like diplococci that may also be arranged in tetrads and clusters and may appear to be gram variable. *Gemella haemolysans* is part of the normal flora of the oral cavity, and *G. morbillorum* is part of the normal flora of gastrointestinal tract. *Gemella* strains have been isolated from cases of endocarditis, meningitis, and other infections. It has been shown that these organisms are susceptible to vancomycin, penicillin G, and ampicillin. Synergy is seen between penicillin or vancomycin and gentamicin or streptomycin. Hence, penicillin and gentamicin are recommended for the treatment of *Gemella* endocarditis.

HELCOCOCCUS SPECIES

Helcococcus kunzii is currently the only species in this genus of PYR-positive, LAP-negative cluster-forming cocci that has been isolated from human clinical specimens. It forms small, nonhemolytic, slowly growing colonies on blood agar. This species has been described in recent reports as an agent of wound infection and bacteremia. They are susceptible to vancomycin and β-lactam agents.

LACTOCOCCUS SPECIES

The genus *Lactococcus* was created recently to accommodate non-β-hemolytic Lancefield group N streptococci normally isolated from dairy products. Members of this genus resemble either streptococci or enterococci in terms of phenotypic traits and are infrequently isolated opportunistic pathogens. Lactococci have been isolated from cases of endocarditis and a variety of other infections. They are susceptible to vancomycin and other β-lactam agents.

GLOBICATELLA SPECIES

The description of the species *Globicatella sanguinis* is α-hemolytic, PYR positive, LAP negative, and salt tolerant. They form cocci in chains. *Globicatella* sp. have been identified as a rare cause of shunt-associated meningitis and bacteremia. They are susceptible to vancomycin and β-lactam agents.

AEROCOCCUS GENUS

The most well-known species of this genus, *Aerococcus viridans*, forms clusters and has been noted as an infrequent cause of infection in compromised hosts. Another species, *Aerococcus urinae*, has been well documented as an agent of urinary tract infections and endocarditis in immunocompromised patients. Aerococci form α-hemolytic colonies on blood agar. *Aerococcus viridans* colonies are larger than those of *A. urinae*. These two species also differ in other phenotypic traits (*A. viridans* is PYR positive and LAP negative, whereas *A. urinae* is PYR negative and LAP positive). *Aerococcus urinae* is susceptible in vitro to a number of β-lactam agents and vancomycin; time-kill studies suggest a need for combination therapy, including an aminoglycoside for bactericidal therapy in endovascular infection.

SUGGESTED READING

Alcaide ML, Espinoza L, Abbo L. Cavitary pneumonia secondary to *Tsukamerella* in AIDS patient: first case and review of literature. *J Infect*. 2004;49:17–19.

Barton LL, Rider ED, Coen RW. Bacteremic infection with *Pediococcus*: vancomycin-resistant opportunist. *Pediatrics*. 2001; 107:775–776.

Boudewijns M, Magerman K, Verhaegen J, et al. *Rothia dentocariosa*, endocarditis and mycotic aneurysms: case report and review of literature. *Clin Microbiol Infect*. 2003;9:222–229.

Chow KM, Szeto CC, Chow VCY, et al. *Rhodococcus equi* peritonitis in continuous ambulatory peritoneal disease. *J Nephrol*. 2003;16:736–739.

Goyal R, Singh NP, Mathur M. Septic arthritis due to *Arcanobacterium haemolyticum*. *Ind J Med Microbiol*. 2005;23:63–65.

Handwerger S, Horwitz H, Coburn K, et al. Infection due to *Leuconostoc* species: six cases and review. *Rev Infect Dis*. 1990;12:602–610.

Husni RN, Gorden SM, Washington JA, et al. *Lactobacillus* bacteremia and endocarditis: review of 45 cases. *Clin Infect Dis*. 1997;25:1048–1055.

Niamut SML, van der Vorm ER, van Luyn-Wiegers CGL, Gokemeijer JDM. *Oerskovia xantheineolytica* bacteremia in an immunocompromised patient without foreign body. *Eur J Clin Microbiol Infect Dis*. 2003;22:274–275.

Ruoff KL. Miscellaneous catalase-negative, Gram-positive cocci: emerging opportunists. *J Clin Microbiol*. 2002;40:1129–1133.

Salvana EMT, Frank M. *Lactobacillus* endocarditis: case report and review of cases reported since 1992. *J Infect Dis*. 2006;53:5–10.

Tan TY, Ng SY, Thomas H, Chan BK. *Arcanobacterium haemolyticum* bacteraemia and soft-tissue infections: case report and review of literature. *J Infect*. 2006;53:69–74.

Urbina BY, Gohh R, Fischer SA. *Oerskovia xanthineolytica* endocarditis in a renal transplant patient: case report and review of literature. *Transplant Infect Dis*. 2003;5:195–198.

160. Miscellaneous Gram-Negative Organisms

Sampath Kumar and Kamaljit Singh

Most gram-negative infections are caused by organisms in the Enterobacteriaceae or Pseudomonadaceae families; however, a few are caused by a heterogeneous group of gram-negative organisms. These organisms do not fit conveniently into a single genera and have undergone frequent taxonomic changes, making understanding them even more difficult for clinicians. The clinical presentation varies widely, affecting different types of hosts and requiring a variety of antibiotics for therapy (Table 160.1). Varied predisposing environmental and host factors are outlined in Table 160.2.

ACINETOBACTER

Acinetobacter is a member of the family *Moraxellaceae*, with at least 25 genospecies and two commonly recognized clinical species, *Acinetobacter calcoaceticus* (formerly *A. calcoaceticus* var. *Iwoffii*) and *Acinetobacter baumannii* (formerly *A. calcoaceticus* var. *anitratus*). Because of problems in separating these two strains using phenotypic tests, some laboratories have chosen to report them as "*A. calcoaceticus-baumannii* complex." They are nonmotile, oxidase-negative, gram-negative coccobacilli often appearing as diplococci and thus are easily confused with *Neisseria* or *Haemophilus* spp. They differ from Enterobacteriaceae in that they do not grow anaerobically or reduce nitrates. They are distinguished from *Neisseria* and *Moraxella* by their negative oxidase reaction. Virulence factors include a polysaccharide capsule that may prevent phagocytosis and fimbriae that potentiate adherence to epithelial cells.

Acinetobacter spp. are widely distributed in the environment, found in food, soil, water, and sewage. *Acinetobacter* spp. may be found on inanimate surfaces, including hospital equipment such as ventilator tubing, resuscitation bags, humidifiers, sinks, mist tents, dialysis baths, angiography catheters, pressure transducers, and plasma protein solutions. They are found on the skin of many animal species and humans usually as commensal organisms. They are found as part of the normal oral flora and in the genitourinary and gastrointestinal tracts.

Acinetobacter baumannii is the most commonly found species in human clinical specimens followed by *Acinetobacter lwoffii*. *Acinetobacter baumannii* is increasingly recognized as one of the most important causes of nosocomial infections and is of particular concern because of its propensity for multidrug resistance. Most infections due to *A. baumannii* are nosocomial, occurring in severely debilitated patients who have been exposed to broad-spectrum antibiotics in the intensive care unit, mechanical ventilators, and invasive devices (eg, central venous catheters). In addition, *A. baumannii* is increasingly noted as a cause of serious infections among military personnel returning from the Middle East, often with carbapenem-resistant strains of *A. baumannii*. A wide variety of human infections due to *Acinetobacter baumannii* have been reported, including pneumonia (most often related to endotracheal tubes), septicemia, endocarditis, meningitis, urinary tract infections, wound infections, abscesses, peritonitis, osteomyelitis, and eye infections. The most common sites of isolation of *A. baumannii* are the respiratory and urinary tracts. The mortality can be as high as 40% to 60% in patients with septic shock and up to 30% in patients with ventilator-associated pneumonia, usually associated with underlying disease (eg, diabetes, malignancy, and renal failure). *Acinetobacter* spp. play a significant role in the colonization of hospitalized patients, making it difficult to differentiate true infection from colonization.

Acinetobacter baumannii is commonly multidrug resistant, and treatment is best guided by specific antibiotic testing and sensitivity patterns within each hospital. *Acinetobacter lwoffii* tends to be more susceptible than the other *Acinetobacter* spp. Most *A. baumannii* strains are resistant to penicillin, ampicillin, first-generation cephalosporins, gentamicin, and chloramphenicol and show variable susceptibility to second- and third-generation cephalosporins, trimethoprim–sulfamethoxazole, and tetracyclines. Ampicillin–sulbactam and sulbactam alone have intrinsic bactericidal activity and have been used with good success in susceptible strains. In recent years, many institutions have

Table 160.1 Antimicrobial Therapy of Miscellaneous Gram-Negative Bacilli

Organism	First-Line Therapy	Alternative Therapy
Acinetobacter	Ampicillin–sulbactam, piperacillin–tazobactam, imipenem–cilastin, meropenem, ceftazidime, amikacin	Fluroquinolones, trimethoprim–sulfamethoxazole, minocycline, tigecycline, colistin
Achromobacter	Imipenem–cilastin, meropenem	Piperacillin–tazobactam, ceftazidime, trimethoprim–sulfamethoxazole
Alcaligenes	Imipenem–cilastin, meropenem, trimethoprim–sulfamethoxazole	Amoxicillin–clavulanate, ceftazidime, piperacillin–tazobactam
Capnocytophaga canimorsus	Penicillin	Clindamycin, imipenem–cilastin, ampicillin–sulbactam, amoxicillin–clavulanate
Pseudomonas oryzihabitans/luteola	Fluoroquinolones, ceftazidime, piperacillin–tazobactam	Imipenem–cilastin, meropenem, aztreonam, aminoglycosides, trimethoprim–sulfamethoxazole
Chromobacterium	Imipenem–cilastin, ciprofloxacin	Tetracycline, trimethoprim–sulfamethoxazole, gentamicin
Chryseobacterium meningosepticum	Vancomycin	Fluroquinolones, minocycline, rifampin, trimethoprim–sulfamethoxazole
Ochrom-bactrum anthropi	Imipenem–cilastin	Trimethoprim–sulfamethoxazole, tetracyclines, aminoglycosides, fluoroquinolones

noted increasing resistance to aminoglycosides and carbapenems among *A. baumannii* strains. For pan-resistant strains of *A. baumannii,* colistin (or polymyxin B) and tigecycline may offer reasonable therapeutic alternatives.

ACHROMOBACTER

Achromobacter spp. are widely distributed in nature, including soil and water. They may be part of the normal flora of the lower gastrointestinal tract. *Achromobacter* spp. have been found as contaminants in disinfectants, diagnostic tracer solutions, intravenous computed tomography contrast solutions, hemodialysis solutions, ventilators, humidifiers, and pressure transducers.

The genus *Achromobacter* consists of a number of species of which two are of clinical relevance: *Achromobacter xylosoxidans* and *Achromobacter denitrificans* (previously *Alcaligenes denitrificans*). These are gram-negative rods that are oxidase positive and grow on MacConkey agar. They have been commonly reported as causative agents in a variety of nosocomial and community-acquired infections. *Achromobacter xylosoxidans* has been isolated from many types of specimens, including blood, cerebrospinal fluid (CSF), bronchial washings, urine, and wounds.

It represents an opportunistic pathogen and has been reported to cause meningitis and ventriculitis after neurosurgical manipulation, bacteremia, endocarditis, otitis, endophthalmitis, corneal ulcers, pharyngitis, pneumonia, wound infections, peritonitis and urinary tract infections, and abscesses. Mortality can approach 52% in patients with *A. xylosoxidans* bacteremia.

Achromobacter xylosoxidans colonizes the respiratory tract of cystic fibrosis patients and is associated with exacerbations of pulmonary symptoms. Antibiotic selection should be guided by susceptibility testing. Imipenem–cilastatin is the most consistently effective agent in vitro against *A. xylosoxidans*. Trimethoprim–sulfamethoxazole, piperacillin–tazobactam, ticarcillin–clavulanic acid, ceftazidime, and the quinolones may also be effective. For severe infections, combination therapy may be necessary; however, synergistic activity has not been established. Most strains are resistant to penicillin, ampicillin, first- and second-generation cephalosporins, and aminoglycosides.

Achromobacter denitrificans is reported to have been isolated from clinical specimens but its pathogenic role remains controversial. It has been reported to cause otitis externa and bacteremia associated with intravenous catheters.

Table 160.2 Environmental and Host Factors Predisposing to Infections with Miscellaneous Gram-Negative Bacilli

Organism	Environmental Factors	Host Factors	Infection
Acinetobacter	Ventilator tubing, resuscitation bags, humidifiers, sinks, mist tents, dialysis bags, angiography and IV catheters, pressure transducers, plasma protein solutions	Severely debilitated, recent surgery, instrumentation	Septicemia, endocarditis, meningitis, pneumonia, UTI, wound infections, abscesses, peritonitis, osteomyelitis, eye infections
Achromobacter	Contaminant in disinfectants, diagnostic tracers solution, IV CT contrast, hemodialysis solutions, ventilators, humidifiers, pressure transducers	Severely debilitated, recent neurosurgery	Community-acquired bacteremia, meningitis, chronic otitis media, hospital-acquired meningitis, bacteremia, ventriculitis, endocarditis, endophthalmitis, corneal ulcers, pharyngitis, pneumonia, wound infections, peritonitis, UTI, abscesses
Alcaligenes	Dairy products, rotten eggs, hospital equipment	Severely debilitated	Septicemia, native and prosthetic valve endocarditis, meningitis, meibomianitis, chronic purulent otitis, pyelonephritis, hepatitis, appendicitis, diarrhea
Capnocytophaga	Normal oral, gastrointestinal, respiratory, and vaginal flora of humans; *C. canimorsus* in canine oral flora	Severely immunocompromised, children with malignancies, neutropenia, mucositis, asplenia, alcohol abuse	Bacteremia, septicemia, keratitis, conjunctivitis, endophthalmitis, corneal ulcer, endocarditis, pericardial abscess, mediastinitis, lung and subphrenic abscess, empyema, peritonitis, abdominal abscess, septic arthritis, lymphadenitis, juvenile periodontitis
Chromobacterium	Enters through the skin or ingestion of contaminated food or water	Neutrophil defects (eg, chronic granulomatous disease)	Local cellulitis, lymphadenitis, septicemia, osteomyelitis, arthritis, meningitis, ocular infections, and pneumonia
Chryseobacterium	Soil, water, use of contaminated fluids in the hospital, nebulizers, flush solutions, pressure transducers, contaminated disinfectants and anesthetics, ice machines, peritoneal dialysis solutions	Neonates, premature infants, adult immunocompromised patients	Neonates: meningitis, hydrocephalus Adults: endocarditis, pneumonia, peritonitis, keratitis, wound infection, meningitis
Pseudomonas oryzihabitans/luteola	Soil, water, flushing solutions	Patients with indwelling foreign material, malignancies, immunosuppressive therapy, postsurgical state, history of IVDU, chronic renal failure, bone marrow transplant, cirrhosis	Septicemia, bacteremia, subdural empyema, pneumonia, peritonitis, biliary tract infection, abscesses, wound infection, empyema, line infections, prosthetic joint infections

Abbreviations: UTI = urinary tract infection; CT = computed tomography; IVDU = intravenous drug use.

ALCALIGENES

Alcaligenes consist of gram-negative rods or cocci that are oxidase positive and obligate aerobes. *Alcaligenes faecalis* (previously named *Alcaligenes odorans*) is the most commonly isolated species in the clinical laboratory. They produce a greenish color on blood agar plates and a characteristic fruity, apple odor. These organisms are found in soil and water as well as on normal human skin and in gastrointestinal tract flora. Dairy products and rotten eggs have been sources of *Alcaligenes*. These organisms have also been isolated from hospital equipment.

Clinically important infections are found in severely debilitated patients. Most infections are opportunistic and acquired from contaminated hospital equipment (eg, nebulizers, respirators, and lavage fluid). It is a rare cause of bacteremia, native and prosthetic valve endocarditis, meningitis, chronic purulent otitis, meibomianitis, pyelonephritis, hepatitis, appendicitis, and urinary tract infection. *Alcaligenes* isolated from the blood of patients with septicemia is thought to be associated with contaminated hospital equipment; however, blood isolates have also been obtained from patients without clinical evidence of sepsis. *Alcaligenes faecalis* isolation from the urine is often considered to be a contaminant and it is also found in diabetic ulcers with mixed flora, and its clinical significance is difficult to determine.

Alcaligenes faecalis is generally susceptible to trimethoprim–sulfamethoxazole and chloramphenicol. Sensitivity to the β-lactam drugs, quinolones, and aminoglycosides is variable. On the basis of in vitro studies, third-generation cephalosporins or the addition of clavulanic acid to amoxicillin or ticarcillin may be more consistently effective. Greater antibiotic resistance is seen in hospitals.

CAPNOCYTOPHAGA

Capnocytophaga encompasses a group of capnophilic (CO_2 requiring), microaerophilic gram-negative rods. The organisms are slow growing, thin, and often fusiform bacilli that display gliding motility on agar media. *Capnocytophaga* are classified in the family Flavobacteriaceae along with *Flavobacterium*, *Chrysobacterium*, and *Weeksella* species. There are five clinically relevant human species of *Capnocytophaga*: *Capnocytophaga ochracea*, *Capnocytophaga sputigena*, *Capnocytophaga haemolytica*, *Capnocyto phaga granulose*, and *Capnocytophaga gingivalis* (formerly Centers for Disease Control and Prevention dysgonic fermenter-1 or CDC DF-1). These species are oxidase, catalase, and indole negative. *Capnocytophaga canimorsus* (formerly DF-2) and *Capnocytophaga cynodegmi* (formerly DF-2-like organism) are part of the normal oral flora of domestic animals. These species are oxidase and catalase positive and indole negative, and they reduce nitrates.

Capnocytophaga are part of the normal flora of humans isolated from the oropharynx, vagina, and gastrointestinal tract. They are causative agents of localized juvenile periodontitis (together with *Actinobacillus actinomycetemcomitans*) and other periodontal disease. *Capnocytophaga* may also cause systemic disease in immunocompromised patients with hematologic malignancies and neutropenia, particularly with chemotherapy-associated oral lesions or mucositis. These patients usually present with bacteremia and septicemia. In immunocompetent patients, *Capnocytophaga* may be isolated from polymicrobial infections of the respiratory tract or contaminated wounds (eg, clenched fist injuries). It has also been reported to cause keratitis, conjunctivitis, endophthalmitis, corneal ulcers, endocarditis, pericardial abscess, mediastinitis, pulmonary abscesses, empyema, septic arthritis, cervical and inguinal lymphadenitis, sinusitis, thyroiditis, osteomyelitis, peritonitis, abdominal abscess, chorioamnionitis, and congenital bacteremia/neonatal sepsis.

Capnocytophaga species are generally susceptible to clindamycin, erythromycin, tetracycline, chloramphenicol, quinolones, and imipenem–cilastatin. Susceptibilities are variable for penicillin, expanded-spectrum cephalosporins, and metronidazole. In general, these organisms are resistant to aztreonam, aminoglycosides, vancomycin, trimethoprim, and colistin. β-Lactamase production has been reported in 2.5% to 32% of isolates (detected by the nitrocefin test). Clindamycin is thought to be the most active drug in vitro. In immunocompromised patients with bacteremia, antibiotics should be given for 10 to 14 days after documenting negative blood cultures. For immunocompetent patients, the duration of therapy should be dictated by the site and extent of infection and should be given in conjunction with adequate surgical drainage.

Capnocytophaga canimorsus and *C. cynodegmi* are part of the normal oral flora of dogs and cats. *Capnocytophaga canimorsus* is isolated more commonly and appears to be more virulent. It is generally associated with dog bites causing a wide spectrum of illness ranging from mild to fulminant infection, including sepsis and death. The case-fatality rate is approximately 25%. Predisposing factors to serious infection include underlying illness such as liver cirrhosis, alcohol abuse, and immunosuppression (steroids or hematologic malignancies). In predisposed persons, particularly asplenic patients, the infection tends to be fulminant, with shock, disseminated intravascular coagulation, hemorrhagic skin lesions mimicking meningococcemia, gangrene, renal failure, and death. More than 75% of cases report exposure to a dog, either through ownership or a bite. The most common clinical manifestations are septicemia and bacteremia, but *C. canimorsus* has been reported to cause meningitis, endocarditis, pneumonia, empyema, corneal ulcer, septic arthritis, cellulitis, and wound infections after a dog bite or cat scratch.

The diagnosis is established by blood cultures, although other specimens may also yield the organism (eg, wound cultures, CSF). In most reports, cultures become positive within 3 to 7 days. In asplenic patients, the organism may be demonstrated on a Gram stain of the buffy coat. In one alcoholic patient, the organisms were seen on a peripheral blood smear.

Routine susceptibility tests of *C. canimorsus* are difficult to perform because of slow growth. However, it is generally reported to be susceptible to most antibiotics, including penicillins, imipenem–cilastin, erythromycin, vancomycin, clindamycin, third-generation cephalosporins, chloramphenicol, rifampin, doxycycline, and quinolones. Susceptibility to aminoglycosides and trimethoprim is unclear and may depend on the method used. Penicillin is considered the drug of choice for *Capnocytophaga* infections.

CHROMOBACTERIUM

Chromobacterium violaceum is the species most commonly isolated in the clinical laboratory although it is seldom regarded as pathogenic. *Chromobacterium violaceum* is a slightly curved gram-negative rod that is facultatively anaerobic and produces a distinctive water-insoluble violet pigment on blood agar. The organism grows within 24 hours on conventional media. It is motile, with both polar and lateral flagellae that are antigenically distinct. Humans with neutrophil defects (eg, chronic granulomatous disease) may be particularly susceptible to infections with this organism.

Chromobacterium is generally found in the environment (soil, fresh water, and food). It grows optimally at 20°C to 37°C (68°F to 98.6°F); hence, most infections have been documented in tropical or subtropical climates. It is a rare infection, thought to enter the body through the skin, although ingestion of contaminated food or water may play a role. The most common clinical presentation is a local cellulitis and regional or diffuse lymphadenitis. Hematologic dissemination may occur, resulting in septicemia and multiorgan failure. Mortality is 60% to 70%, depending on the host

and accuracy of diagnosis. Other presentations have included fever, skin lesions, abdominal pain, osteomyelitis, arthritis, meningitis, ocular infections, and pneumonia.

Chromobacterium violaceum is generally very susceptible to chloramphenicol, gentamicin, and tetracycline. It is uniformly resistant to cephalosporins and generally resistant to most penicillins. It has variable sensitivity to some of the carboxypenicillins and ureidopenicillins. Trimethoprim–sulfamethoxazole has been used successfully as outpatient therapy after prolonged intravenous therapy with other agents.

CHRYSEOBACTERIUM

Chryseobacterium spp. (former *Flavobacterium* spp.) are long, thin, slightly curved, occasionally filamentous, oxidase-positive gram-negative rods. They are common inhabitants of soil and water. *Chryseobacterium meningosepticum* is the species most commonly associated with human infections, but *Chryseobacterium gleum*, *Chryseobacterium indologenes*, and other *Chrysobacterium* species have also been implicated in human disease. Members of *Chryseobacterium odorans* (*F. odorans*) have been renamed *Myroides odoratus* and *Myroides odoratimimus*.

Chryseobacterium meningosepticum are uncommon pathogens in adults and rarely cause infections in children beyond the newborn period. It is highly pathogenic for premature infants and has been associated with neonatal sepsis and meningitis. The development of meningitis may be insidious. The prognosis is extremely poor, with mortality >60%. Half of the survivors develop significant neurologic complications, including hydrocephalus. Although rarely encountered it is important to diagnose the disease accurately because epidemics may occur in nurseries. Meningitis has also been reported in adult immunocompromised patients. Other clinical presentations in adults include endocarditis, pneumonia, peritonitis, keratitis, and wound infections. Most of the described cases are nosocomial infections associated with the use of contaminated fluids in the hospital (nebulizers, flush solutions for arterial catheters, pressure transducers, ice machines, contaminated disinfectants, contaminated anesthetics, peritoneal dialysis). *Chryseobacterium indologenes*, although frequently isolated in clinical specimens, rarely has clinical significance. Bacteremia has been described with *C. indologenes* particularly in immunocompromised patients, but mortality appears low even when patients are pre-scribed antibiotics without activity against *C. indologenes.*

Antimicrobial selection is difficult as *Chryseobacterium* are inherently resistant to multiple antibiotics, and susceptibilities vary with the method used. Most *Chryseobacteria* produce β-lactamases and are resistant to β-lactam drugs, aminoglycosides, tetracyclines, and chloramphenicol but are susceptible to agents used for treating infections caused by gram-positive bacteria (eg, clindamycin, trimethoprim–sulfamethoxazole, rifampin, and vancomycin). Most reports have recommended vancomycin for treatment of serious infections due to *C. meningosepticum.* Erythromycin and rifampin have both been given concurrently intravenously and intrathecally with some success. Development of resistance on therapy has been demonstrated with erythromycin, rifampin, ciprofloxacin, and trimethoprim–sulfamethoxazole. Antimicrobial therapy should be continued for at least 2 weeks after sterilization of the CSF. Recovery is the rule in immunocompetent older patients infected with contaminated materials; however, the prognosis is poor in immunocompromised patients.

PSEUDOMONAS ORYZIHABITANS AND PSEUDOMONAS LUTEOLA (FORMERLY FLAVIMONAS ORYZIHABITANS AND CHRYSEOMONAS LUTEOLA)

Pseudomonas oryzihabitans and *Pseudomonas luteola* are oxidase negative, aerobic gram-negative rods with a distinct yellow pigment. After 48 hours of incubation, colonies are typically rough or wrinkled. They are found in water, soil, and other damp environments. Eighty-four percent of the reported cases have been associated with the presence of a foreign material, including intravascular catheters, dialysis catheters, or artificial grafts. Other associated host factors include malignancy, immunosuppressive therapy, postsurgical state, chronic renal failure, previous antibiotic therapy, intravenous drug use, long-term corticosteroid use, liver cirrhosis, and bone marrow transplantation. Infections associated with these organisms include sepsis, bacteremia, line infections, pneumonia, prosthetic joint infections, subdural empyema, peritonitis, biliary tract infections, surgical wound infections, abscesses, and empyema.

In many studies, resistance has been shown to the first- and second-generation cephalosporins, and most isolates are also resistant to ampicillin and tetracycline. They are sensitive to the ureidopenicillins, third-generation cephalosporins, carbapenems, aminoglycosides, and quinolones. There is a difference in susceptibility to trimethoprim–sulfamethoxazole: *P. luteola* is resistant and *P. oryzihabitans* is sensitive. Clinically, most patients have been treated with ciprofloxacin with a favorable outcome. The increase in number of reported cases is frequently related to the presence of intravascular catheters in immunocompromised patients and dialysis catheters in continuous ambulatory peritoneal dialysis.

OCHROBACTRUM

These are oxidase-positive, gram-negative coccobacilli formerly designated CDC group Vd-1 and Vd-2 and *Achromobacter* groups A, C, and D. Currently there are two designated *Ochrobactrum* species, *Ochrobactrum anthropi* and *Ochrobactrum intermedium*, although it is very difficult to differentiate the two species in the routine clinical microbiology laboratory. *Ochrobactrum anthropi* is an opportunistic pathogen affecting immunocompromised patients and is often associated with vascular device–related infections, hemodialysis, urinary and respiratory tract infections, continuous ambulatory peritoneal dialysis peritonitis, activation-induced cell death, and pacemaker infections. *Ochrobactrum anthropi* is usually susceptible to aminoglycosides, trimethoprim–sulfamethoxazole, tetracyclines, and imipenem–cilastin but is resistant to most semisynthetic penicillins and cephalosporins.

OLIGELLA, RHIZOBIUM, SHEWENELLA, SPHINGOMONAS, ROSEOMONAS, WEEKSELLA, AND BERGEYELLA

Oligella consist of two species, *Oligella urethralis* and *Oligella ureolytica*. Most isolates have been isolated from human urine often associated with indwelling Foley catheters and can rarely cause bacteremia, septic arthritis, and pyelonephritis. *Oligella* spp. are susceptible to most antibiotics.

Rhizobium spp. (former *Agrobacterium*) are occasionally isolated from clinical specimens but rarely linked with human infection. *Rhizobium* (*Agrobacterium*) *radiobacter* has been most commonly isolated from blood followed by peritoneal dialysate, mainly associated with infections of transcutaneous devices in immunocompromised patients. Antibiotic susceptibility is variable, and treatment should be guided by individual susceptibility testing. Most isolates are susceptible to cefepime, carbapenems, piperacillin–tazobactam, and quinolones.

Shewanella putrefaciens and *Shewanella algae* are the type species most commonly isolated from human clinical specimens. They are associated with skin and soft-tissue infections and bacteremia, especially in immunocompromised patients. They are usually susceptible to most antibiotics except for penicillin and cephalothin.

Sphingomonas paucimobilis is a yellow-pigmented, oxidase-positive, gram-negative rod that classically infects immunocompromised patients and is isolated from a variety of clinical specimens, including blood, CSF, urine, wounds, and the hospital environment. Most strains are susceptible to tetracycline, trimethoprim–sulfamethoxazole, aminoglycosides, and imipenem–cilastin with variable susceptibility to penicillins and quinolones.

Roseomonas are a pink-pigmented gram-negative coccobacilli. *Roseomonas* spp. are most commonly isolated from blood, usually due to device-associated bacteremia. They are also associated with intra-abdominal abscesses and urinary tract infections. Most infections have been treated with imipenem–cilastin, aminoglyosides, or tetracyclines, and *Roseomonas* spp. are usually resistant to penicillins and cephalosporins.

The genus *Weeksella* contained two species *Weeksella virosa* and *Weeksella zoohelcum*, now reclassified as *Bergeyella zoohelcum*. Both species are oxidase negative and susceptible to penicillin. *Bergeyella zoohelcum* is part of the normal oral flora of dogs and cats, and human isolates frequently result from dog or cat bites.

SUGGESTED READING

Bergogne-Berezin E, Towner KJ. Acinetobacter spp. as nosocomial pathogens: microbiological, clinical and epidemiologic features. *Clin Microbiol Rev*. 1996;9:148–165.

Hsueh P-R, Hsiue T-R, Wu J-J, et al. Flavobacterium indologenes bacteremia: clinical and microbiological characteristics. *Clin Infect Dis*. 1996;23:550–555.

Kern WV, Oethinger M, Kaufhold A, et al. Ochrobactrum anthropi bacteremia: report of four cases and short review. *Infection*. 1993;21:306–310.

Mandell WF, Garvey GJ, Neu HC. Achromobacter xylosoxidans bacteremia. *Rev Infect Dis*. 1987;9:1001–1005.

Nerad JL, Black S. Miscellaneous gram negative bacilli: acinetobacter, cardiobacterium, actinobacillus, chromobacterium, capnocytophaga, and others. In: Gorbach SL, Bartlett JG, Blacklow NR, eds. *Infectious Diseases*. 3rd ed. Philadelphia, PA: WB Saunders; 2003.

The nonfermentative gram-negative bacilli. In: Winn W Jr, Allen S, Janda W, et al., eds. *Koneman's Color Atlas and Textbook of Diagnostic Microbiology*. 6th ed. Baltimore, MD: Lippincott Williams & Wilkins; 2003.

Rahav G, Simhon A, Mattan Y, et al. Infections with Chryseomonas luteola (CDC Group Ve-1) and Flavimonas oryzihabitans (CDC Group Ve-2). *Medicine (Baltimore)*. 1995;74:83–88.

Schreckenberger PC, Daneshvar MI, Weyant RS, Hollis DG. Acinetobacter, achromobacter, chryseobacterium, moraxella and other nonfermentative gram-negative rods. In: Murray PR, Baron EJ, Jorgensen JH, Pfaller MA, Yolken RH, eds. *Manual of Clinical Microbiology*. 8th ed. Washington, DC: ASM Press; 2003.

Warren JS, Allen SD. Clinical, pathogenetic, and laboratory features of Capnocytophaga infections. *Am J Clin Pathol*. 1986;86:513–518.

PART XIX

Specific Organisms – Spirochetes

161. Syphilis and Other Treponematoses

Adaora A. Adimora

Treponemes are members of the family Spirochaetaceae, which also contains *Borrelia* and *Leptospira*. Although most treponemes do not cause disease in human beings, a few cause substantial morbidity. This chapter briefly reviews the clinical manifestations and treatment of syphilis in adults and the nonvenereal treponematoses, yaws, pinta, and bejel.

SYPHILIS
Clinical Manifestations

Like other treponemal diseases, the clinical manifestations of syphilis are divided into early and late stages. Early syphilis is further divided into primary, secondary, and early latent stages. During the latent syphilis stage, patients have positive serologic tests for syphilis but no other signs of disease. The Centers for Disease Control and Prevention (CDC) classifies patients in the latent stage as having early syphilis if they acquired infection during the preceding year. Otherwise, persons with latent disease are classified as having either late latent syphilis or latent syphilis of unknown duration. Although clinical staging is useful for diagnosis and treatment, it is also imprecise; overlap between stages is relatively common.

PRIMARY AND SECONDARY SYPHILIS
Treponema pallidum, the causative agent of syphilis, usually enters the body through breaks in the epithelium that occur during sexual contact. Some organisms persist at the site of entry, whereas others disseminate via the lymphatic system throughout the body, proliferating and stimulating an immune response. The incubation period of primary syphilis is usually about 21 days, although extremes of 10 to 90 days have been noted.

The first clinical manifestation is usually a chancre at the site of genital trauma. The chancre begins as a red macule that subsequently becomes papular and then ulcerates. The lesion is painless and has a well-defined margin and thickened, rubbery base. If untreated, the chancre persists for 3 to 6 weeks and then heals.

Nontender regional lymphadenopathy also develops.

In untreated individuals, *T. pallidum* disseminates throughout the body, and secondary syphilis develops about 3 to 6 weeks after the chancre's onset. Common symptoms include malaise, headaches, sore throat, fever, musculoskeletal pains, and weight loss. Physical examination reveals rash in 75% to 100%, regional or generalized lymphadenopathy in 50% to 85%, and mucosal ulceration in 5% to 30% of persons with secondary syphilis. The appearance of the rash can vary greatly, but lesions are often maculopapular or papulosquamous and often involve the entire body, including the palms and soles (Figure 161.1). Broad, flat lesions, known as *condylomata lata,* may develop in warm, moist areas, such as the scrotum, vulva, or perianal regions. Patchy alopecia and shallow painless mucosa ulcerations, called *mucous patches,* may also be seen. Like the chancre, these manifestations of secondary syphilis resolve spontaneously with or without therapy. A small proportion of patients develop complications, such as hepatitis, syphilitic glomerulonephritis with nephrotic syndrome, anterior uveitis, choroiditis, arthritis, bursitis, or osteitis. A wide variety of neurologic complications, including meningitis, cranial nerve palsies, transverse myelitis, nerve deafness, and cerebral artery thrombosis, can occur.

NEUROSYPHILIS
Treponema pallidum often invades the meninges during the course of secondary syphilis. Inadequately treated infection may spontaneously resolve or may result in either asymptomatic meningeal involvement or symptomatic acute meningitis. Further progression of infection causes persistent asymptomatic neurosyphilis or a variety of neurologic syndromes, such as meningovascular syphilis, tabes, or paresis.

Syphilitic meningitis most commonly occurs during the first year of infection. Most patients do not have a rash of secondary syphilis when they present with syphilitic meningitis, and meningitis is sometimes the first manifestation of syphilis. The clinical

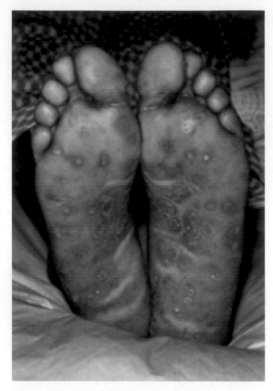

Figure 161.1 Secondary syphilis. Papulo-squamous lesions on soles. (Courtesy of David Schlossberg, MD.)

picture may suggest a viral aseptic meningitis, as patients may present with headache, fever, stiff neck, photophobia, and a mild cerebrospinal fluid (CSF) lymphocytic pleocytosis. Differential diagnosis includes meningitis caused by enteroviruses and other viruses, tuberculosis, cryptococcus, and Lyme disease. Cerebral involvement may result in seizures or hemiplegia. Cranial nerve palsies are especially common. Characteristic CSF findings include a lymphocytic pleocytosis, increased protein, and hypoglycorrhachia in slightly less than half of cases. Nontreponemal serologic testing is positive in blood and CSF. Penicillin yields a prompt response.

Meningovascular syphilis usually occurs about 5 to 12 years after infection in patients between the ages of 30 and 50 years and may involve the cerebrum, brainstem, or spinal cord. The pathophysiology involves chronic meningitis and infarction due to syphilitic endarteritis. In cerebrovascular syphilis, the middle cerebral artery is most commonly involved, and hemiparesis, aphasia, and seizures commonly occur. CSF usually reveals a lymphocytic pleocytosis with increased protein and a positive CSF Venereal Disease Research

Laboratory (VDRL) test. Spinal syphilis, a relatively uncommon entity, may present as meningomyelitis or transverse myelitis.

The major parenchymatous forms of neurosyphilis are general paresis and tabes dorsalis, which tend to occur 15 to 20 and 20 to 25 years, respectively, after initial infection. Both are now uncommon diseases.

General paresis is a chronic meningoencephalitis that results from direct invasion of the brain by *T. pallidum* and combines both psychiatric and neurologic manifestations. Early symptoms, such as irritability, memory loss, headache, and personality changes, may evolve into emotional lability, paranoia, and confusion. Pupillary abnormalities occur in more than half of patients with general paresis. Abnormal reflexes, slurred speech, and tremors are also common. In untreated patients, the interval between onset of symptoms and death can range from a few months to about 5 years.

Serum nontreponemal serologic tests are reactive in 95% to 100% of patients with generalized paresis. CSF VDRL is usually positive, but a negative result alone does not exclude the diagnosis. Differential diagnosis includes Alzheimer's disease, chronic alcoholism, and multiple sclerosis.

Tabes dorsalis is characterized by lightning pains and various combinations of other neurologic signs and symptoms, such as ataxia; bladder disturbances; pupillary abnormalities; absent ankle or knee reflexes; Romberg's sign; impaired vibratory and position sense; and development of extremely large, unstable, painless joints known as Charcot's joints. Lightning pains are paroxysms of severe stabbing pains, which usually occur in the legs. Although most patients have positive serum VDRL tests, 10% of patients with tabes have nonreactive serum VDRL serology. CSF may be normal or may reveal lymphocytic pleocytosis and elevated protein.

NONNEUROLOGIC MANIFESTATIONS OF TERTIARY SYPHILIS

Syphilitic heart disease, now an uncommon cause of cardiovascular disease, occurs 15 to 30 years after initial infection. During the early phases of infection, *T. pallidum* organisms disseminate to the heart and lodge in the aortic wall, where they may cause endarteritis of the vasa vasorum of the aorta with resultant scarring and destruction of the vessel's wall. Major cardiac manifestations include thoracic aneurysm, aortic regurgitation (without associated aortic stenosis), and coronary ostial stenosis.

Late benign syphilis is another now uncommon form of tertiary syphilis. It results from the chronic inflammatory response to *T. pallidum* and the formation of a granulomatous type of lesion called a *gumma*. Gummas may be ulcerative, nodular, or noduloulcerative and most commonly occur in the skin and bones but may also invade the viscera, muscles, and other structures.

Laboratory Tests

DIRECT MICROSCOPIC EXAMINATION

Direct microscopic examination can provide immediate diagnosis of primary and secondary syphilis. Dark-field microscopy must be used because *T. pallidum's* narrow width (0.15 μm) renders the organism below the level of resolution of light microscopy. Wet preparations can be made from the skin or mucous membrane lesions of primary or secondary syphilis; examination reveals tightly coiled organisms 6 to 14 μm long and 0.25 to 0.30 μm wide, with corkscrew motility. When examination of specimens must be delayed or oral lesions evaluated, direct fluorescent antibody testing can be useful. This test specifically detects *T. pallidum* and eliminates confusion with oral treponemal saprophytes the morphology of which is similar to that of *T. pallidum*.

SEROLOGIC TESTS

Serologic tests for syphilis measure either nonspecific nontreponemal antibody or specific treponemal antibody.

Nontreponemal antibody tests measure immunoglobulin G (IgG) and immunoglobulin M (IgM) antibodies formed by the host against lipid from *T. pallidum's* cell surfaces. These tests are used to screen for disease and disease activity; titers fall progressively over time and should decrease in response to therapy. The following nontreponemal tests are commonly used: VDRL test, rapid plasma reagin (RPR), automated reagin screen test (ART), unheated serum reagin test (USR), and the reagin screen test (RST). False-positive nontreponemal test results occur in 1% to 2% of the general population, but false-positive titers are usually less than 1:8. False-negative results may be seen in 10% to 20% of primary, latent, and late syphilis.

Specific treponemal antibody tests are usually used to confirm a current or past diagnosis of syphilis. These tests detect antibodies formed in response to treponemal antigens. Treponemal tests usually remain reactive after treatment, but

a small proportion of infected persons become seronegative. Commonly used treponemal tests include the fluorescent antibody absorption (FTA-ABS), microhemagglutination assay for antibodies to *T. pallidum* (MHA-TP), and the hemagglutination treponemal test for syphilis (HATTS).

CSF EVALUATION

CSF should be examined in all syphilis patients with neurologic signs or symptoms and in those with latent syphilis if any of the following are present: eye involvement, other evidence of active syphilis, human immunodeficiency virus (HIV) infection, or treatment failure. CSF of patients with latent syphilis should also be examined when duration of infection is known to be less than 1 year if nonpenicillin therapy is planned or the serum RPR or VDRL is greater than 1:32.

When CSF specimens are free of blood contamination, a positive CSF VDRL test almost always indicates neurosyphilis. Diagnosis is unclear, however, in patients with negative CSF serology, a positive blood serologic test, increased CSF protein levels, and slight pleocytosis. Although such patients may have asymptomatic neurosyphilis, other diagnoses should be considered.

Treatment and Follow-Up

Treatment and follow-up are outlined in Tables 161.1 and 161.2.

Syphilis in Persons with HIV Infection

Because syphilis and HIV infection share means of transmission and other risk factors, both infections often coexist. Moreover, syphilis, like other genital ulcer diseases, facilitates HIV transmission. Clinical observation and case reports suggest that HIV-infected patients may experience a more aggressive course of syphilis, with more frequent occurrence of neurosyphilis. Occasional unusual serologic reactions occur; false-positive nontreponemal tests and false-negative treponemal tests have been documented. Following treatment for syphilis, nontreponemal titers may fall more slowly in HIV-positive patients than in individuals who are HIV negative, although the clinical significance of this slower decline may be small. Nevertheless, available data suggest that HIV infection does not significantly change the presentation, clinical course, or response to treatment of syphilis.

Table 161.1 Management of Syphilis in Nonpregnant Adults without Known HIV Infection

Primary and Secondary Syphilis

Treatment

    Benzathine penicillin G, 2.4 million U IM once

    If penicillin allergy:

        Doxycycline, 100 mg PO BID for 2 wk or tetracycline, 500 mg PO QID for 2 wk

        Azithromycin 2 g PO once (but avoid this regimen in regions where resistance of *Treponema pallidum* to azithromycin has been noted)

        Ceftriaxone 1 g IM or IV for 8–10 days (caution: some patients with penicillin allergy are also allergic to ceftriaxone)

Management and follow-up

    HIV testing

    If evidence of neurologic or ophthalmic disease, evaluate for neurosyphilis and do slit-lamp examination

    Repeat serology and clinical examination at 6 and 12 mo

    If symptoms persist or recur, or if 4-fold increase in RPR or VDRL titer occurs, repeat HIV testing and re-treat

    If RPR or VDRL titers do not fall 4-fold within 6 mo of treatment, repeat HIV testing and consider LP

Latent Syphilis

Treatment

    Early latent syphilis (duration ≤1 y)

        Benzathine penicillin G, 2.4 million U IM once

        If penicillin allergy:

            Doxycycline, 100 mg PO BID for 2 wk *or* tetracycline, 500 mg PO QID for 2 wk

            Azithromycin 2 g PO once (but avoid this regimen in regions where resistance of *T. pallidum* to azithromycin has been noted)

            Ceftriaxone 1 g IM or IV for 8–10 days (caution: some patients with penicillin allergy are also allergic to ceftriaxone)

    Late latent syphilis or latent syphilis of unknown duration

        Benzathine penicillin G, 2.4 million U IM every wk, for 3 wk

        If penicillin allergy:

            Doxycycline, 100 mg PO BID for 4 wk or tetracycline, 500 mg PO QID for 4 wk

Management and follow-up

    HIV testing

    Examine accessible mucosal surfaces (e.g., mouth, perineum and perianal areas, etc.) to evaluate for internal mucosal lesions

    Clinical evaluation for evidence of tertiary disease (e.g., aortitis, neurosyphilis, gumma, iritis)

    Examine CSF before treatment if any of the following are present:

        Neurologic or ophthalmic signs or symptoms

        Evidence of active tertiary syphilis (eg, aortitis or gumma)

        Treatment failure

        HIV infection with late latent syphilis or syphilis of unknown duration

    Repeat quantitative VDRL or RPR at 6, 12, and 24 mo

        Patients with a normal CSF examination should be re-treated for latent syphilis if:

            Serologic titers increase 4-fold or

            An initially high titer (≥1:32) fails to fall at least 4-fold within 12–24 mo or

            Patient develops signs or symptoms consistent with syphilis

Tertiary Syphilis (Gumma or Cardiovascular Syphilis without Neurosyphilis)

Treatment

    Benzathine penicillin G, 2.4 million U IM weekly for 3 wk

    If penicillin allergy, use treatment for late latent syphilis

Management

    Examine CSF

Neurosyphilis

Treatment

    Aqueous crystalline penicillin G, 3 million to 4 million U IV q4h for 10–14 days; some experts follow with benzathine penicillin G, 2.4 million U IM weekly for 3 wks

    Alternative (if compliance is certain):

        Procaine penicillin, 2.4 million U IM every day for 14 d, plus probenecid, 500 mg PO QID for 14 days; some experts follow with benzathine penicillin G, 2.4 million U IM weekly for 3 wks

Management

    HIV testing

    Repeat CSF examination every 6 mo until CSF cell count is normal

    Consider re-treatment if cell count has not decreased after 6 mo or if CSF is not normal after 2 y

Abbreviations: HIV = human immunodeficiency virus; RPR = rapid plasma reagin; VDRL = Venereal Disease Research Laboratory test; LP = lumbar puncture; CSF = cerebrospinal fluid.

Table 161.2 Treatment of HIV-Positive Patients with Syphilis

Primary and Secondary Syphilis
Treatment
Benzathine penicillin G, 2.4 million U IM once
Alternative: benzathine penicillin G, 2.4 million U IM weekly × 3 wk
If penicillin allergy: manage according to recommendations for HIV-negative patients with primary and secondary syphilis
(see Table 161.1)
Management
Clinical and serologic evaluation 3, 6, 9, 12, and 24 mo after therapy
Examine CSF if RPR or VDRL titers fail to show a 4-fold decrease by 4 mo or there is other evidence of treatment failure
If CSF normal, re-treat with penicillin G, 2.4 million U IM weekly × 3 wk
If CSF suggests neurosyphilis, treat for neurosyphilis as in Table 161.1
Early Latent Syphilis
Manage and treat according to recommendations for HIV-negative patients with primary and secondary syphilis (see Table 161.1). Patients with penicillin allergy whose compliance with therapy or follow-up cannot be ensured should be desensitized and treated with penicillin
Late Latent Syphilis or Latent Syphilis of Unknown Duration
Treatment and management
Examine CSF
If CSF normal, give benzathine penicillin G, 2.4 million U IM weekly × 3 wk
If penicillin allergy: manage according to recommendations for HIV-negative patients with late latent syphilis or latent syphilis of unknown duration. However, patients with penicillin allergy whose compliance with therapy or follow-up cannot be ensured should be desensitized and treated with penicillin
If CSF suggests neurosyphilis, treat for neurosyphilis as in Table 161.1
Management
Clinical and serologic evaluation 6, 12, 18, and 24 mo after therapy
Examine CSF and re-treat accordingly if:
Clinical symptoms develop or RPR or VDRL titers rise 4-fold at any time or RPR or VDRL titer fails to fall 4-fold between
12 and 24 m
Neurosyphilis
Treatment and management as in Table 161.1
Abbreviations: CSF = cerebrospinal fluid; RPR = rapid plasma reagin; VDRL = Venereal Disease Research Laboratory test; HIV = human immunodeficiency virus.

Careful evaluation and follow-up of all HIV-positive patients with syphilis are essential. CSF should be evaluated to exclude central nervous system (CNS) involvement in all HIV-infected syphilis patients with latent syphilis or neurologic signs or symptoms. Vigilant follow-up is essential to document resolution of infection and allow prompt evaluation and retreatment if relapse, reinfection, or other complications occur. HIV-positive patients with syphilis should be treated with penicillin if at all possible; those with a history of hypersensitivity should undergo desensitization.

NONVENEREAL TREPONEMATOSES

Yaws, pinta, and bejel (endemic syphilis) are caused respectively by *T. pallidum* subspecies *pertenue; Treponema carateum;* and *T. pallidum* subspecies *endemicum.* These diseases, seen mainly in tropical and subtropical regions, are transmitted by direct contact with infected skin lesions and not primarily by sexual contact. Like venereal syphilis, these diseases have self-limited primary and secondary stages, a latent stage, and a late stage with destructive lesions. The causative agents are morphologically indistinguishable from *T. pallidum* subspecies *pallidum,* and the serologic responses they elicit are identical to those of venereal syphilis. Diagnosis can be made by dark-field examination of lesions or serologic testing. Long-acting penicillin G, the treatment of choice, has dramatically decreased the incidence of these diseases in endemic regions.

Yaws occurs in the tropical regions of Africa, southeast Asia, South America, and Oceania. About 3 to 5 weeks after infection, papules develop, which enlarge, erode, and then spontaneously heal. A generalized secondary eruption of similar lesions occurs weeks to months later, sometimes associated with osteitis or periostitis. In the late stage, infected persons may develop hyperkeratoses on the palms and soles; plaques, nodules, and ulcers of the skin; and gummatous bone lesions.

Pinta occurs in remote parts of Mexico, Central America, and Colombia. About 7 to 21 days after infection, small, red, pruritic papules develop, which enlarge, become squamous, and merge with other primary lesions. These lesions eventually heal, but residual hypopigmentation persists. Three to twelve months after the appearance of the primary lesions, small scaly papules known as *pintids* appear. These may eventually become brown, gray, or blue and may recur as long as 10 years after initial infection. Depigmented lesions develop in the late stage.

Bejel occurs in Africa and western Asia. Unlike yaws and pinta, bejel is spread not only by direct contact but also by eating and drinking utensils. Primary lesions are seldom seen. Secondary manifestations include mucous patches, condylomata lata, split papules at the angles of the mouth, and lymphadenopathy. Gummatous lesions of the skin, nasopharynx, and bones are common in the late stage.

SUGGESTED READING

Centers for Disease Control and Prevention. Azithromycin treatment failures in syphilis infections – San Francisco, California, 2002–2003. *MMWR Morb Mortal Wkly Rep.* 2004;53:197–198.

Centers for Disease Control and Prevention. 2006 Sexually transmitted disease treatment guidelines. *MMWR Morb Mortal Wkly Rep.* 2006;55(RR-11):22–30. UpToDate Online. www.uptodateonline.com

Chulay JD. *Treponema* species (yaws, pinta, bejel). In: Mandell GL, Bennett JE, Dolin R, eds. *Principles and Practice of Infectious Diseases.* 5th ed. New York, NY: Churchill Livingstone; 2000.

Gordon SM, Eaton ME, George R, et al. The response of symptomatic neurosyphilis to high-dose intravenous penicillin G in patients with human immunodeficiency virus infection. *N Engl J Med.* 1994;331:1469–1473.

Gourevitch MN, Selwyn PA, Davenny K, et al. Effects of HIV infection on the serologic manifestations and response to treatment of syphilis in intravenous drug users. *Ann Intern Med.* 1993;118:350–355.

Hook EW III, Marra C. Acquired syphilis in adults. *N Engl J Med.* 1992;326:1060–1069.

Musher DM. Early syphilis. In: Holmes KK, Mardh PA, et al., eds. *Sexually Transmitted Diseases.* 3rd ed. New York, NY: McGraw-Hill; 1999.

Swartz MN, Musher DM, Healy BP. Late syphilis. In: Holmes KK, Mardh PA, et al., eds. *Sexually Transmitted Diseases.* 3rd ed. New York, NY: McGraw-Hill; 1999.

Riedner G, Rusizoka M, Todd J, et al. Single-dose azithromycin versus penicillin G benzathine for the treatment of early syphilis. *N Engl J Med.* 2005;353: 1236–1244.

162. Lyme Disease

Janine Evans and Stephen E. Malawista

Lyme disease, a systemic illness caused by the spirochete *Borrelia burgdorferi*, is the most common tick-borne disease in the United States. In 2005, 45 states reported 23 305 cases of Lyme disease using the Council of State and Territorial Epidemiologists (CTSE)/Centers for Disease Control and Prevention (CDC) surveillance case definition. Since the original discovery of Lyme arthritis in the mid-1970s the clinical spectrum of Lyme disease has expanded to include a wide variety of organ systems, primarily the skin, joints, nervous system, and heart. Protean symptoms, uncertainty in diagnosis because of lack of definitive testing methods, and public fear of late sequelae of disease often lead to overdiagnosis and overtreatment. Although optimal therapy of some of the clinical features of Lyme disease is unclear, better understanding of its natural history, epidemiology, and pathogenesis helps in the often confusing and difficult decisions related to diagnosis and treatment.

Borrelia burgdorferi has been isolated from blood, skin, cerebrospinal fluid (CSF) specimens, and (rarely) other specimens from infected patients, although, with the exception of skin biopsy specimens, culture of *B. burgdorferi* from sites of infection is a low-yield procedure. *Borrelia burgdorferi* displays phenotypic and genotypic diversity and has been classified into 11 separate genospecies, 3 of which are pathogenic to humans: *Borrelia burgdorferi sensu stricto*, which includes all strains studied thus far from the United States and some European and Asian strains, and *Borrelia garinii* and *Borrelia afzelii*, which are found in Europe and Asia. *Borrelia afzelii* is primarily associated with a chronic skin lesion, *acrodermatitis chronica atrophicans,* rare in the United States, and *B. garinii* is predominant among CSF isolates.

Lyme disease occurs in three principal foci in the United States: the Northeast, the upper Midwest, and, to a lesser extent, the Pacific Coast. These areas correspond to the distribution of the predominant tick vectors of Lyme disease in the United States, *Ixodes scapularis* (please see Chapter 199, Human Babesiosis, Figure 199.2) in the East and Midwest and *Ixodes pacificus* in northern California. Lyme disease also occurs widely in Europe, where it is transmitted by the sheep tick, *Ixodes ricinus.* The largest number of reported cases in Europe are from Germany, Austria, Slovenia, and Sweden. *Ixodes scapularis* have a 3-stage, 2-year life cycle. Transovarial passage of *B. burgdorferi* is rare. Ticks become infected with spirochetes by feeding on spirochetemic animals, typically small mammals, during larval and nymphal stages. In highly endemic areas from 20% to, >60% of *I. scapularis* carry *B. burgdorferi.* Humans are only an incidental host of the tick; contact is typically made in areas of underbrush or high grasses but may occur in well-mown lawns in endemic areas. Lyme disease occurs most commonly during May through July when nymphal *I. scapularis* feed. Animal models show that transmission is unlikely to occur before a minimum of 36 hours of tick attachment and feeding.

CLINICAL MANIFESTATIONS

Clinical features of Lyme disease are typically divided into three general stages termed early localized, early disseminated, and late persistent infection. These stages may overlap, and most patients do not exhibit all stages. Direct invasion of the organism with a resultant vigorous inflammatory reaction has been demonstrated to be responsible for many of the clinical manifestations associated with Lyme disease, and the manifestations respond to antibiotic therapy. Some features, such as late neurologic deficits and chronic arthritis, may respond poorly to treatment. It is not clear that live organisms are responsible for these later symptoms. Seroconversion can occur in asymptomatic individuals but is rare with strict surveillance.

Early Localized Disease

Erythema migrans (EM), the hallmark of Lyme disease, begins at the site of a deer tick bite after 3 to 32 days (Figure 162.1). It is reported by 60% to 80% of patients, appearing as a centrifugally expanding erythematous macule or

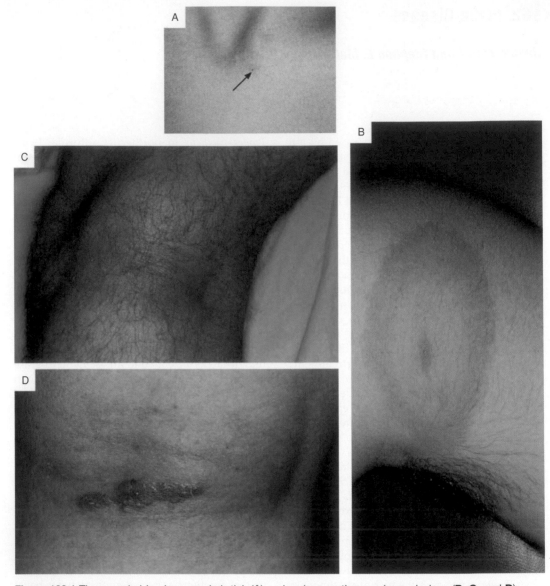

Figure 162.1 The nymphal *Ixodes scapularis* tick (**A**) and various erythema migrans lesions (**B**, **C**, and **D**). Lyme disease usually begins with a slowly expanding skin lesion, erythema migrans, which occurs at the site of a tick bite. **A:** Tiny (1 to 2 mm in diameter), nymphal *I. scapularis* tick (*arrow*) attached near the neck of a child. **B:** Shows a classic erythema migrans lesion (9 cm in diameter) near the axilla. The lesion has partial central clearing, a bright red outer border, and a target center. **C:** Pale, homogeneous erythema migrans lesion (12 cm in diameter) on the back of a knee. **D:** Erythema migrans lesion (10 cm in diameter) with a vesicular center on the back of a knee. In each instance, *Borrelia burgdorferi* was isolated from a skin-biopsy sample of the lesion. (Courtesy of Dr. Vijay Sikand, East Lyme, Connecticut, and the SmithKline Beecham Lyme Disease Vaccine Trial. Steere A. *N Engl J Med*. 2001;345:115–125.)

papule, often with central clearing. The thigh, groin, and axilla are common sites. The lesion may be warm, pruritic, and painful but is often asymptomatic and easily missed if out of sight. Occasionally, these lesions may develop blistering or scabbing in the center, remain an even, intense red without clearing, or develop a bluish discoloration. Spirochetes are present in the EM lesion and can be readily cultured from the expanding edge. Mild musculoskeletal flulike symptoms such as a low-grade fever, chills, malaise, headache, fatigue, arthralgias, and myalgias may accompany EM lesions. Theoretically such symptoms can occur without dissemination of the organism via local generation of cytokines. Untreated EM resolves within several weeks and treated lesions within several days.

Specific Organisms – Spirochetes

Early Disseminated Disease

In some patients the spirochete disseminates hematogenously to multiple sites causing characteristic clinical features. Secondary annular lesions, sites of metastatic foci of *Borrelia* in the skin, develop within days of onset of EM in about half of U.S. patients. They are similar in appearance to EM but are generally smaller, migrate less, and lack indurated centers. In addition to musculoskeletal flulike symptoms, mild hepatitis, splenomegaly, sore throat, nonproductive cough, testicular swelling, conjunctivitis, and regional and generalized lymphadenopathy may sometimes occur during early stages.

Diagnosis of early localized and early disseminated Lyme disease is based on clinical presentation, because serologic confirmation is often lacking and culture not readily available. Erythema migrans is diagnostic of Lyme disease although atypical lesions and rashes mimicking EM may be confusing. A history of a tick bite and residence or travel in an endemic area should be sought in patients presenting with rashes compatible with EM or a flulike illness in summer. Specific immunoglobulin M (IgM) antibody responses against *B. burgdorferi* develop 2 to 6 weeks after the onset of EM. Immunoglobulin G (IgG) antibody levels appear approximately 6 weeks after disease onset but may not peak until months or even years into the illness. The highest titers occur during arthritis. Antibodies are typically detected using indirect immunofluorescence, enyzme-linked immunosorbent assay (ELISA), and immunoblotting (Western blot). Antibody responses may persist for months to years after successful eradication of infection.

Late Disease

Late manifestations of Lyme disease typically occur months to years after the initial infection. In the United States, arthritis is the dominant feature of late Lyme disease, reported in approximately 60% of untreated individuals. Less often, individuals develop late chronic neurologic disease. Another late finding (years) associated with this infection is a chronic skin lesion, *acrodermatitis chronica atrophicans*, well known in Europe but rare in the United States. These late manifestations are discussed below.

Therapy

EARLY LYME DISEASE

The symptoms of early Lyme disease resolve spontaneously in most cases; therefore, the goals of therapy for early localized and mild early disseminated Lyme disease are to shorten the duration of symptoms and reduce the risk of developing serious late manifestations of infection. Treatment of these stages with oral antibiotics is adequate in the majority of patients (see Table 162.1). In patients with acute disseminated Lyme disease but without meningitis, oral doxycycline appears to be equally as effective as parenteral ceftriaxone in preventing the late manifestations of disease. Initial studies of treatment for early Lyme disease reported therapy with phenoxymethyl penicillin, erythromycin, and tetracycline, in doses of 250 mg 4 times a day for 10 to 20 days, shortened the duration of symptoms of early Lyme disease. Phenoxymethyl penicillin and tetracycline were superior to erythromycin in preventing late manifestations of disease. Subsequent clinical trials have proven amoxicillin and doxycycline to be equally efficacious. Amoxicillin has largely replaced penicillin because of greater in vitro activity against *B. burgdorferi*. It is the preferred antibiotic choice in children younger than 8 years. Concomitant use of probenecid has not been definitively shown to improve clinical outcome and is associated with a higher incidence of side effects. Doxycycline is usually selected over tetracycline because of its twice-daily dose schedule, increased gastrointestinal absorption and tolerability, and greater central nervous system (CNS) penetration. Doxycycline is effective in treating *Anaplasma phagocytophilum* (formerly known as *Ehrlichia phagocytophila*), an organism also transmitted by *Ixodes scapularis* ticks; amoxicillin is not. Cefuroxime axetil, an oral second-generation cephalosporin, has been shown to be about as effective as amoxicillin and doxycycline in treating early Lyme disease; azithromycin, an azilide analogue of erythromycin, somewhat less so. Macrolide antibiotics are not recommended as first-line therapy for early Lyme disease. Long-term follow-up of patients treated during early stages of Lyme disease support the current dosing regimens. Patients who received a 14- to 21-day course of a recommended antibiotic rarely developed late manifestations of illness. Recent studies have indicated that a 10-day course of doxycycline is adequate therapy for EM. Jarisch–Herxheimer-like reactions, an increased discomfort in skin lesions and temperature elevation occurring within hours after the start of antibiotic treatment, have been encountered in 14% of patients treated for early Lyme disease. They typically occur within 2 to 4

Table 162.1 Treatment Guidelines

Antibiotic Regimen	Comments
Erythema migrans	
Amoxicillin, 500 mg 3× daily for 14–21 d	Pediatric dose is 25–50 mg/kg/d 3× daily; also effective
Doxycycline (vibramycin), 100 mg 2× daily for 10–21 days	against *Anaplasma phagocytophilum*; not recommended for children under 8 years of age, pregnant or lactating women
Cefuroxime axetil (Ceftin), 500 mg 2× daily for 14–21 days	Pediatric dose 30 mg/kg/d 2× daily
Azithromycin (Zithromax), 500 mg daily for 7–10 days	Not recommended as first-line therapy; less effective than other regimens
Early disseminated disease (without neurologic, cardiac, or joint involvement)	
Initial treatment is the same as for erythema migrans except duration of treatment may be extended to 21–28 days	
Neuroborreliosis **Isolated seventh nerve palsy**	
Initial treatment is the same as for erythema migrans except duration of treatment is 21–28 days. The need for cerebrospinal fluid examination remains controversial	
All other neurologic manifestations (including meningitis, radiculoneuritis, peripheral neuropathy, encephalomyelitis, chronic encephalopathy)	
Ceftriaxone (Rocephin), 2 g daily for 14–30 days	30-day regimen associated with fewer relapses in patients with chronic encephalopathy
Penicillin G, 20 million units daily for 14–28 days	Pediatric dose 200 000–400 000 units/kg/d every 4 h
Cefotaxime sodium (Claforan), 2 g q8h	Pediatric dose 150–200 mg/kg/d in 3–4 divided doses for 14–28 d
Doxycycline, 100 mg 2× daily (oral or intravenous) for 14–28 days	No published experience in the United States
Carditis	
Doxycycline, 100 mg orally 2× daily for 21 d	For first degree heart block, PR interval ≤0.3 sec
Amoxicillin, 500 mg 3× daily for 21 d	For first degree heart block, PR interval ≤0.3 sec
Ceftriaxone, 2 g daily for 14–21 d	Optimal duration of therapy is unknown
Penicillin G, 20 million units daily for 14–30 d	Optimal duration of therapy is unknown, given in divided doses every 4 h
Arthritis	
Amoxicillin, 500 mg 4× daily for 30–60 d	Oral regimens should be limited to patients without evidence of neurologic involvement oral treatment may be extended for 60 days if no response to 30-d course
Doxycycline, 100 mg 2× daily for 30–60 d	
Cefuroxime axetil, 500 mg 2× daily for 30–60 d	For patients with doxycycline and penicillin allergy
Ceftriaxone, 2 g daily for 14–30 days	
Lyme disease in pregnancy	
Amoxicillin, 500 mg 3× daily for 21 d	For early localized disease only
Ceftriaxone, 2 g daily for 14–28 days	
Penicillin G, 20 million units daily for 14–28 d	Given in divided doses every 4 h
Asymptomatic tick bite	
No treatment or single dose of 200 mg doxycycline	For pregnant women, a 10-d course of amoxicillin may be considered
Asymptomatic seroconversion	No treatment necessary

hours of starting therapy, are more common in severe disease, and are presumably due to rapid killing of a large number of spirochetes.

Minor symptoms, including arthralgia, fatigue, headaches, and transient facial palsy, are common following treatment and generally resolve over a 6-month period. Patients with disseminated disease are most likely to experience persistent symptoms. These symptoms may be due to retained antigen rather than ongoing infection with *B. burgdorferi*, because longer courses of antibiotics have not been shown to shorten their duration. Prolonged courses of antibiotics should be reserved for those patients with evidence of persistent infection with *B. burgdorferi*.

Lyme Carditis

Cardiac involvement occurs in up to 10% of untreated patients. Transient and varying degrees of atrioventricular block several weeks to months after a tick bite are the most common manifestations. Other features are pericarditis, myocarditis, ventricular tachycardia, and, on rare occasions, a dilated cardiomyopathy; valvular disease is not seen. Carditis is typically mild and self-limited, although patients may present quite dramatically in complete heart block, and some require the insertion of a temporary pacemaker. In most cases, carditis resolves completely, even without treatment with antibiotics. Studies examining endomyocardial biopsy specimens from patients with Lyme carditis have indicated that direct invasion of *B. burgdorferi* into myocardium and an associated inflammatory reaction are responsible for the clinical events. Although optimal treatment of carditis is unknown, oral therapy for mild forms of cardiac involvement is usually sufficient. Intravenous antibiotics and cardiac monitoring are recommended for patients with varying high-degree heart block and more serious cardiac involvement. The benefit of concomitant use of aspirin or prednisone and antibiotics in treating patients with Lyme carditis is uncertain. Despite the generally benign course of Lyme carditis, several cases of permanent heart block have been reported, presumably caused by a vigorous inflammatory response. Short courses of prednisone may be considered in patients with prolonged dense heart block despite adequate antibiotic therapy.

Dilated cardiomyopathy is a rare complication of Lyme disease reported in Europe but not yet in the United States. The majority of the patients were from endemic areas for Lyme disease, had other clinical features of disease, and were seropositive for anti-*B. burgdorferi* antibodies. Their myopathy was cured by antibiotic treatment.

Early Neurologic Disease

Early neurologic involvement occurs in 15% to 20% of untreated patients and appears within 2 to 8 weeks after the onset of disease. Manifestations include cranial nerve palsies, meningitis or meningoencephalitis, and peripheral neuritis or radiculoneuritis, often appearing in combination. Unilateral or bilateral seventh nerve palsies are the most common neurologic abnormalities. Presenting symptoms depend on the area of the nervous system involved: Patients with meningitis present with fever, headache, and a stiff neck; those with Bannwarth's syndrome (primarily in Europe) develop severe and migrating radicular pain lasting weeks to several months; and those with encephalitis have concentration deficits, emotional lability, and fatigue. In patients with early CNS involvement, analysis of cerebrospinal fluid (CSF) typically reveals a lymphocytic pleocytosis. Specific antibodies against *B. burgdorferi* may also be present and concentrated in the CSF relative to the serum concentration; they are useful to confirm diagnoses.

Intravenous antibiotics are recommended for all cases of neuroborreliosis except isolated seventh nerve palsy. Patients presenting with a Bell-like palsy who have features that suggest possible CNS involvement, such as high fever, headache, or stiff neck, should undergo a lumber puncture looking for evidence of more extensive disease. The most experience in the treatment of CNS Lyme disease has been with aqueous penicillin and third-generation cephalosporins. Although optimal duration of therapy is unknown, it is recommended that patients be treated for 2 to 4 weeks. Ceftriaxone, in doses of 1 to 2 g per day, is the agent of choice because of better CNS penetration and ease of administration. Patients with persistent symptoms after recommended antibiotic therapy pose a particular management problem. It is often unclear whether these symptoms are due to resolving inflammation or ongoing infection. Meningitis and sensory symptoms usually resolve within days to weeks; other features may take months to improve. In most cases it is not necessary to continue antibiotic therapy until complete recovery.

Late Manifestations

ARTHRITIS

Arthritis is the dominant feature of late Lyme disease, occurring in up to 60% of untreated patients days to years after initial infection (mean of 6 months). The initial pattern of involvement may be migratory arthralgias (early) followed in 60% of patients by intermittent attacks of arthritis lasting from days to months. Large joints, particularly the knee, are most commonly involved. Swelling is often prominent, with large effusions and Baker cysts. Serologic testing in patients presenting with arthritis is positive in almost all cases.

Lyme arthritis has been treated successfully with oral and intravenous antibiotics. In early studies examining response to benzathine penicillin, 2.4 million units intramuscularly weekly for 3 weeks, 7 of 20 patients responded compared with 0 of 20 in the control group. Intravenous ceftriaxone, 2 to 4 g daily for 2 to 4 weeks, has been thought to be superior to benzathine penicillin. Oral regimens using doxycycline, 100 mg twice a day for 4 weeks, and amoxicillin plus probenecid, 500 mg of each orally 4 times a day for 4 weeks, have reported success in 18 of 20 patients and 16 of 18 patients, respectively. However, in 6 patients in each group, resolution of arthritis did not occur until 1 to 2 months after the 1-month treatment regimen (ie, resolution after sufficient treatment may be slow). Thus, a recommendation of an additional 4 weeks of oral antibiotics for those with persistent arthritis after the first month, is arguable. Some effusions take months to resolve completely.

A small subgroup of Lyme arthritis patients develop a chronic, potentially erosive arthritis unresponsive to antibiotics. These patients often have major histocompatability class II gene products, human leukocyte antigen death receptor 4 (HLA DR4) accompanied by strong serum IgG responses to *Borrelia* outer surface proteins A or B (OspA or OspB). Repeated courses of antibiotics have not been shown to improve clinical outcome. Treatment with anti-inflammatory medications and intra-articular steroid injections can be helpful in reducing joint swelling. Surgical synovectomy has cured a number of such patients. Resolution of the arthritis eventually occurs; in some patients it may take 3 to 5 years.

Late Neurologic Lyme Disease

Chronic neurologic syndromes, which are relatively uncommon, may occur months to years after initial infection. Cognitive dysfunction, affective changes, seizures, ataxia, peripheral neuropathies, and chronic fatigue have all been reported. The most common late-stage neurologic syndrome reported in the United States, called Lyme encephalopathy, is characterized by subtle cognitive impairment. Because these complaints are often nonspecific, and may be associated with post-Lyme syndromes, it is important to look for and document evidence of ongoing *B. burgdorferi* infection. Lymphocytic pleocytosis is uncommon in late neurologic disease, but increased intrathecal *B. burgdorferi*–specific antibodies may well be present. Careful evaluation with neuropsychological testing can help to distinguish cognitive abnormalities in Lyme disease from those associated with chronic fatigue states and depression. Chronic neurologic dysfunction usually improves with antibiotics but may not completely reverse. Late neurologic manifestations of Lyme disease are treated with intravenous antibiotics. Agents with demonstrated efficacy are aqueous penicillin and third-generation cephalosporins. Doxycyline, both oral and intravenous forms, have been reported to be successful in treating late CNS Lyme disease in Europe.

Ocular Disease

Ocular lesions in Lyme disease are rare but have involved every portion of the eye and vary depending on the stage of the disease. The most common ophthalmic presentations in early disease include conjunctivitis, photophobia, and neuro-ophthalmological manifestations due to cranial nerve palsies. The incidence of seventh nerve palsies are similar in Europe and the United States. The most severe ocular manifestations occur in late stages; they include episcleritis, symblepharon, keratitis, iritis, chorioditis, panuveitis, and retinal vasculitis. Serologic testing in these patients is typically positive.

Experience treating late ocular lesions in Lyme disease is scanty. The most success has been with the use of intravenous ceftriaxone in doses of 2 to 4 g daily for 10 to 14 days.

Pregnancy

Intrauterine transmission of *B. burgdorferi* is uncommon, usually occuring in cases of obvious disseminated infection during pregnancy. No uniform pattern of congenital anomaly has been reported. Prenatal exposure to Lyme disease has not been found to be associated with an increased risk of adverse pregnancy outcome. Optimal treatment of the pregnant patient with Lyme disease is unknown, but the recommended regimens have not been associated with adverse outcomes. Oral antibiotics for early localized disease is sufficient, and intravenous antibiotics are recommended for patients with symptoms suggesting disseminated disease.

Tick Bites

The risk of infection from a deer tick bite in a Lyme disease endemic area is low. In mice, infected ticks have been attached for over a 36-hour period before significant risk of developing Lyme disease occurred. In a controlled double-blind study in patients with tick bites, no patient asymptomatically seroconverted, no treated patient developed EM, and the 2 of 182 untreated patients who did develop EM were successfully treated with oral antibiotics. These results support marking and watching a tick bite, and should EM develop, treating it early, when antibiotics are most effective. A single dose of doxycycline has been shown to be effective in reducing the development of Lyme disease. The Infectious Diseases Society of America (IDSA) guidelines recommend offering the single-dose doxycycline if the attached tick can be reliably identified as an adult or nymphal *I. scapularis* tick, it is estimated to have been attached for >36 hours, prophylaxis can be started within 72 hours after tick attachment, and the local rate of infection of these ticks with *B. burgdorferi* is greater than 20%. Doxycycline prophylaxis for children under 8 years is not recommended.

Seropositive Patients with Nonspecific Symptoms

Patients with nonspecific symptoms such as myalgias, arthralgias, concentration difficulties, and fatigue are frequently tested for Lyme disease. Some patients, especially those from endemic areas, test positively and are treated for presumed Lyme disease, often without improvement in their symptoms. In several studies, over 50% of patients reporting to Lyme disease clinics did not have evidence of Lyme disease, and the reason for a lack of response to antibiotics was an incorrect diagnosis. Objective clinical evidence in support of the diagnosis of Lyme disease should be sought before initiating antibiotics, treatment should be given for the recommended duration and then discontinued, and the patient should be observed for resolution of symptoms.

Post-Lyme Disease Syndrome

Some patients continue to have subjective symptoms after completion of recommended courses of antibiotics for Lyme disease. Symptoms typically include arthalgias, myalgias, fatigue, and neurocognitive difficulties. A recent study of patients treated for EM reported that approximately 5% to 15% of patients experienced subjective symptoms when evaluated 6 to 12 months after treatment. Such symptoms may persist for 5 or more years after treatment. This syndrome does not appear to be related to persistent infection with *B. burgdorferi*. In a study of patients with post-Lyme disease syndrome there were no significant outcome differences between the groups who received intravenous ceftriaxone for 30 days followed by oral doxycycline for 60 days and those that received placebo. The IDSA guidelines do not recommend antibiotic therapy for patients with chronic (>6 months) subjective symptoms after recommended treatment regimens for Lyme disease.

Prevention of Lyme Disease

Recommended personal protective measures against tick bites include wearing light-colored clothing, long-sleeve shirts, and long pants; tucking pant legs into socks; using a tick repellent on clothing and exposed skin; and performing regular body checks for ticks–strategies that require significant self-motivation. Environmental strategies include the application of acaricides onto vegetation where the ticks live, acaricides delivered directly to tick hosts to kill ticks on the animals, and exclusion of deer from targeted areas. The last is not practical in most environments.

Public interest in human and veterinary vaccines prompted researchers to develop a safe and effective human vaccine for the prevention of Lyme disease. The results of two large safety and efficacy trials using recombinant OspA preparations reported the vaccines to be safe and effective in preventing Lyme disease in most people. LYMErix was approved by the Food and Drug Administration (FDA) in 1999 for use in individuals aged 15 and older. The vaccine manufacturer discontinued production in 2002, citing insufficient consumer demand. Protection provided by this vaccine diminishes over time. Individuals who received the Lyme disease vaccine prior to 2002 are probably no longer protected against Lyme disease.

Summary

Antibiotic regimens are recommended according to results of clinical trials and evolving clinical judgments and depend on the stage of infection and the organ system involved. Successful eradication of the infecting organism, *B. burgdorferi*, appears to occur in the large majority of patients with Lyme disease using these treatment guidelines. Patients with persistent symptoms following antibiotic therapy, particularly those with previous evidence of disseminated disease, pose a difficult management problem. Most persistent symptoms are likely due to retained antigens and not the result of persistent infection or to noninfectious sequelae such as fibromyalgia. In the former patients, resolution of symptoms occurs over the course of weeks to months and does not require prolonged courses of antibiotics; in the later, treatment is that of the associated syndrome. Rarely, persistent or recurrent symptoms are due to continued or recurrent infection and require additional courses of antibiotics. Such patients require careful diagnostic evaluation to determine the need for additional treatment.

SUGGESTED READING

Hayes EB, Piesman J. How can we prevent Lyme disease. *New Engl J Med*. 2003; 348:2424–2430.

Klempner MS, Hu LT, Evans J, et al. Two controlled trials of antibiotic treatment in patients with persistent symptoms and a history of Lyme disease. *New Engl J Med*. 2001;345:85–92.

Malawista SE. Resolution of Lyme arthritis, acute or prolonged: a new look. *Inflammation*. 2000;24:493–503.

Malawista SE. Lyme disease. In: Koopman WJ, Moreland LW, eds. *Arthritis and Allied Conditions*. 15th ed. Philadelphia, PA: Lippincott Williams & Wilkins; 2005: 2645–2664.

Piesman J, Gern L. Lyme borreliosis in Europe and North America. *Parasitiology*. 2004;129: S191–S220.

Rahn DW, Evans J, eds. *Lyme Disease*. Philadelphia, PA: American College of Physicians; 1998.

Steere AC, Angelis SM. Therapy for Lyme arthritis, strategies for the treatment of antibiotic-refractory arthritis. *Arth Rheum*. 2006;54:3079–3086.

Wormser, GP. Early Lyme disease. *New Engl J Med*. 2006;354:2794–2801.

Wormser GP, Dattwyler RJ, Shapiro ED, et al. The clinical assessment, treatment, and prevention of Lyme disease, human granulocytic anaplamosis, and babesiosis: clinical practice guidelines by the Infectious Diseases Society of America. *Clin Infect Dis*. 2006; 43:1089–1134.

163. Relapsing Fever

Joseph J. Burrascano

The relapsing fevers are a group of rapidly progressive and severe septic illnesses caused by a variety of species and strains of *Borrelia* spirochetes. Relapsing fever infections have been reported in all continents except Antarctica and Australia and in America in at least 15 states. This illness is becoming increasingly important, because with increasing travel and resurgence of infected disease vectors, disease incidence may now be on the rise.

Relapsing fever can be louse-borne or tick-borne, and these two types differ in geographic distribution and severity, with the former being the more severe. The soft ticks that are the vectors usually feed at night, with a painless bite and a duration of attachment of just 15 to 30 minutes. Thus, exposures often go unnoticed (see Figure 163.1).

It is difficult to separate *Borrelia* into individual serotypes, for they are able to shift phenotypes and thus express different surface antigens, which allows this organism to adapt to a variety of hosts. After the vector

bite the spirochetes enter the bloodstream and live persistently despite the development of specific antibodies. A characteristic of this infection is that the *Borrelia* undergo regular antigenic shifts, thus presenting the immune system with a different antigenic profile over time, resulting in immune evasion and recurrent, regular relapses.

The illness begins 3 to 12 days after exposure and is characterized by recurrent episodes of spirochetemia causing acute systemic symptoms and fever lasting on the average 1 week, separated by several days to weeks of asymptomatic or minimally symptomatic periods. Manifestations are multisystemic, and protean and tissue damage occurs primarily as the result of a vasculitic process often associated with disseminated intravascular coagulation (DIC) Fever, headache, photophobia, nausea, vomiting, myalgias, and arthralgias are associated with fleeting erythematous patches, hepatosplenomegaly with abnormal liver function tests, and various manifestations of

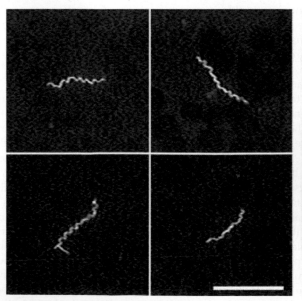
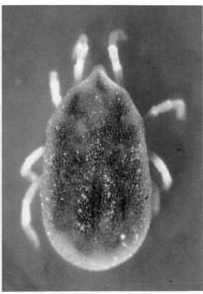

A   B

Figure 163.1 A: *Borrelia hermsii* in the blood of one patient stained with rabbit hyperimmune serum and antirabbit fluorescein isothiocyanate. Scale bar = 20 mm. **B:** An *Ornithodoros hermsi* nymph. The length of the tick is 3.0 μm, excluding the legs. (Courtesy of Dr. Tom Schwan, Rocky Mountain Lab of the National Institute of Allergy and Infectious Diseases.)

Table 163.1 Treatment of Relapsing Fever

Antibiotic	Adult Dose	Children's Dose
Preferred		
Doxycycline	100 mg BID	Not to be given to children
Tetracycline	500 mg QID	Not to be given to children
Alternative Choices		
Erythromycin	500 mg QID	40 mg/kg/d in 4 doses
Penicillin V	500 mg QID	50 mg/kg/d in 4 doses
Amoxicillin	500 mg TID	50 mg/kg/d in 3 doses
Chloramphenicol	500 mg QID	50 mg/kg/d in 4 doses
Parenteral Choices		
Ceftriaxone	2 g q24h	50–75 mg/kg/d given in 1 or 2 daily doses
Supportive Therapy as Needed		
Acetaminophen, tepid baths, analgesics Blood and volume replacement Vitamin K 30 mg IM B-complex tablets, 50 mg each, 1× daily, or B6 50 mg IM Specific treatment for DIC Bedrest the first 24 h		

Abbreviation: DIC = disseminated intravascular coagulation.

the bleeding diathesis. These periods end by crisis, with a rapid rise then fall of temperature, pulse rate, peripheral vascular resistance, and blood pressure. Acute myocardial insufficiency may result, and fatalities can occur especially in compromised hosts.

Borrelia are neurotropic, and cases of meningitis, encephalitis, and even uveitis have been reported. In addition, transplacental transmission can occur, resulting in intrauterine growth retardation, impaired fetal circulation, and septic newborns, as well as placental damage and inflammation and decreased maternal hemoglobin levels. Paradoxically, pregnancy has a relative protective effect on the mother, in whom symptoms are generally less severe than in matched, nonpregnant patients.

Acute episodes are terminated by a vigorous antibody response; relapses are caused by the organism's unique ability to undergo antigenic shifts that allow these changed strains to proliferate until a new antibody response can be mounted. Over time, relapses diminish in severity and eventually disappear. Recently, however, chronic forms of this illness with manifestations similar to those seen in late, disseminated Lyme disease have been reported, with recurrent symptoms and spirochetemia lasting for years despite repeated treatments.

Diagnosis is made by dark-field exam of peripheral blood smears during an acute episode or febrile period. Polymerase chain reaction assays of the peripheral blood during these times can be more sensitive than even blood smears, but this test may not be available in commercial labs. Convalescent specific antibody titers are often elevated, as are nonspecific febrile agglutinins.

TREATMENT

Treatment is 2-fold and includes antibiotics and supportive measures. Jarisch–Herxheimer (J-H) reactions are seen in 80%, occur within several hours after the onset of therapy, and confirm the diagnosis. Mediated by cytokines, J-H reactions can be particularly severe if antibiotics are initiated during an acute attack, especially in the louse-borne type. Clinically this resembles a typical crisis, with rigors, a rapid temperature spike, a rise in respiratory and pulse rate, and often a fall in blood pressure. Abdominal pain, nausea, and vomiting occur and are accompanied by leukopenia and thrombocytopenia. Supportive measures include aggressive correction of hypovolemia, control of pyrexia, and administration of vitamins K and B6. Pretreatment with aspirin, acetaminophen, or even corticosteroids does not ameliorate this reaction.

Antibiotics are given for 10 days minimum and are often repeated for recurrent flares. More prolonged courses are occasionally needed for late relapses and the chronic forms. Parenteral antibiotics can be given to the more acutely ill individual and to those unable to tolerate oral dosing. Prophylactic dosing of antibiotics after exposure is currently being studied. Although cell wall agents (the penicillins and cephalosporins) can be useful, treatment failures have been reported. Therefore, the tetracyclines and macrolides are the drugs of choice if not contraindicated (see Table 163.1).

Worldwide, relapsing fevers are most prevalent in areas of poor living conditions and especially after natural or other disasters when personal hygiene and adequate housing are lacking. Therefore, it is imperative that a search be made for concurrent illnesses and nutritional deficiencies likely to be present in this setting.

SUGGESTED READING

Felsenfeld O. *Borrelia*. St. Louis, MO: Warren H. Green, Inc.; 1971.

LaVoie PC. Borrelia hermseii, the inciting agent in a case of juvenile polyarthritis? Abstract presented at the IV International Conference on Lyme Borreliosis. June 18–21, 1990. W/Th-P-85.

Lim LL, Rosenbaum JT. Borrelia hermsii causing relapsing fever and uveitis. *Am J Ophthalmol*. 2006;142(2):348–349.

Negussie Y. Detection of plasma tumor necrosis factor, interleukins 6 and 8 during the Jarisch-Herxheimer reaction of relapsing fever. *J Exp Med*. 1992;175:1207.

Schwann TG. Analysis of relapsing fever spirochetes from the Western United States. *J Spirochetal and Tick Borne Diseases*. 1995;2(1):3–8.

164. Leptospirosis

Christopher D. Huston

Leptospirosis is an infection with spirochetes from the genus *Leptospira*. Infections are most commonly caused by *Leptospira interrogans*, of which more than 200 serovars infect humans. People become infected by exposure to animal urine or urine-contaminated surface water. *Leptospira* penetrate intact mucous membranes and abraded skin and disseminate widely via the bloodstream. Symptoms develop 7 to 12 days after exposure. Most patients have an abrupt onset of a self-limited, 4- to 7-day anicteric illness characterized by fever, headache, myalgias, chills, cough, chest pain, neck stiffness, and/or prostration (Table 164.1). An estimated 10% of patients will present with jaundice, hemorrhage, renal failure, and/or neurologic dysfunction (Weil's disease). The major clinical manifestations of disease result from infection of capillary endothelial cells leading to vasculitis (Table 164.2).

Classically, leptospirosis has been considered a biphasic illness. However, many patients with mild disease will not have symptoms of the secondary "immune" phase of illness, and patients with very severe disease will have a relentless progression from onset of illness to jaundice, renal failure, hemorrhage, hypotension, and coma. The illness is biphasic in about half of patients, with relapse occuring approximately 1 week after resolution of the initial febrile illness. A late complication is anterior uveitis, seen in up to 10% of patients months to years after convalescence. Leptospirosis in pregnancy is associated with spontaneous abortion but children with congenitally acquired leptospirosis have not been described to have congenital anomalies.

Case fatality rates for leptospirosis are less than 1%, and the illness is usually self-limited. Liver and renal dysfunction are reversible, with return to normal function over 1 to 2 months. The mortality rate for icteric disease has been reported in different studies to be 2.4% to 11.3%, with deaths resulting from renal failure, gastrointestinal and pulmonary hemorrhage, and the adult respiratory distress syndrome.

Table 164.1 Symptoms and Signs of Leptospirosis

Abrupt onset (70%–100%)
Fever, chills, rigors (98%)
Headache (93%–97%)
Myalgias, muscle tenderness (40%–80%)
Vomiting, diarrhea, abdominal pain (30%–95%)
Conjunctival suffusion (33%–100%)
Hepatomegaly (5%–22%; 80% of icteric cases)
Splenomegaly (5%–25%)
Meningeal signs (12%–44%)
Mental status changes (7%–21%)
Oliguria (10%)
Cough (10%–20%)
Chest pain (11%)
Skin rash (9%–18%)
Jaundice (1.5%–6%)

DIAGNOSIS

Leptospirosis most often manifests as a nonspecific flulike illness, so recognition of epidemiologic risk factors is essential (Table 164.3). Occupational exposure to animal urine (eg, veterinarians) has classically been considered the chief epidemiologic risk, but recent outbreaks highlight the importance of recreational water use (eg, reservoirs) and risks associated with adventure tourism. Epidemiologic risks should be sought in patients with a flulike illness, respiratory illness, aseptic meningitis, acute hepatitis, acute renal failure, pericarditis, atrioventricular block, or anterior uveitis. In some developing countries, leptospirosis is more common than hepatitis A as a cause of acute hepatitis. Useful means to distinguish icteric leptospirosis from acute viral hepatitis include the prominent myalgias, conjunctival

Table 164.2 Pathogenesis of Leptospirosis

Infectious vasculitis with damage to capillary endothelial cells resulting in the following:
Renal tubular dysfunction Hepatocellular dysfunction Pulmonary hemorrhage Muscle focal necrosis Coronary arteritis Extravascular fluid shifts

Table 164.3 Epidemiology of Leptospirosis

Leptospira are excreted in animal urine and survive in the environment for up to 6 mo
Disease is common in the tropics, especially in urban slums.
Incubation period ranges from days up to 4 wk after exposure (mean 10–12 d).
Recreational exposures include windsurfing, kayaking, swimming, and adventure tourism.

Occupational exposures:
    New Zealand dairy farmers (incidence of 1.1
        infections/10 person-years), Glasgow sewer
        workers (3.7/10 person-years), and U.S. Army
        soldiers undergoing jungle warfare training in
        Panama (4.1/10 person-years)
    Veterinarians, abbatoir workers, and others with
        exposure to rat urine/bites (homeless people,
        rodent control workers)

Outbreaks seen after floods

Table 164.4 Laboratory Findings of Leptospirosis

Renal failure – acute interstitial nephritis (15%–70%)
Jaundice with only 2- to 3- fold elevations in transaminases and alkaline phosphatases, conjugated bilirubinemia (2%–60%)
Myositis with elevated creatine phosphokinase (MM band) (20%–62%)
Thrombocytopenia (50%)
Cerebrospinal fluid pleiocytosis (80%–90%): ≤300 cells/mL, lymphocyte predominance .
Abnormal chest radiographs (20%–70%) Patchy alveolar pattern in lower lobes with or without interstitial/alveolar hemorrhage
Electrocardiogram abnormalities: sinus tachycardia, myocarditis, first-degree atrioventricular block
ELISA for IgM antibodies most sensitive test in first week of illness, but limited specificity
Microagglutination test MAT for leptospirosis antibodies positive within first 1–2 wk of illness

Table 164.5 Treatment of Leptospirosis

Outpatient treatment: Doxycycline, 100 mg PO BID for 7 days in adults
Severe infection requiring hospitalization: Penicillin, 6 million U IV qd or Ceftriaxone, 1 g IV/IM qd
Chemoprophylaxis: 200 mg doxycycline PO 1×/wk
Jarisch–Herxheimer reaction rare

suffusion, elevated serum creatine phosphokinase, and the relatively mild (2- to 3-fold) elevations in transaminases seen in leptospirosis (Table 164.4). It is possible in some cases to grow the organism from blood or cerebrospinal fluid collected during the first 7 to 10 days of illness or from urine collected during the second or third week. However, the diagnosis is usually made retrospectively by a 4-fold rise in antibody titer as measured by the microscopic agglutination test (MAT). Agglutinins characteristically appear within the first 1 to 2weeks of illness and peak at 3 to 4 weeks. Although not species or serovar specific, enzyme-linked immunsorbent assay (ELISA) kits to detect immunoglobulin M (IgM) antibodies enable diagnosis during the first week of illness.

THERAPY

Antibiotic treatment is most beneficial when started within 4 days of illness. Doxycycline, 100 mg orally twice daily for 7 days started within 48 hours of illness, decreased the duration of illness by 2 days in one study, and is recommended for mild illness. Penicillin at a dosage of 6 million units per day has been successful for early treatment of severe disease, and ceftriaxone (1 g daily) appears to be equally efficacious and has the benefits of simpler dosing schedules and potential intramuscular administration (Table 164.5). A benefit of antibiotic therapy given later in the disease course has not been uniformly seen. Jarish–Herxheimer reactions (fever, rigors, hypotension, and tachycardia) rarely occur on initiation of antibiotic therapy. Supportive care and treatment of the hypotension, renal failure (including dialysis), and hemorrhage that can complicate leptospirosis are crucial for a good outcome.

SUGGESTED READING

Centers for Disease Control and Prevention. Leptospirosis and unexplained acute febrile illness among athletes participating in triathlons—Illinois and Wisconsin, 1998. *MMWR Morb Mortal Wkly Rep.* 1998;47:673–676.

Centers for Disease Control and Prevention. Outbreak of acute febrile Illness among participants in EcoChallenge Sabah 2000—Malaysia, 2000. *MMWR Morb Mortal Wkly Rep.* 2000;49:816.

Lecour H, Miranda M, Magro C. Human leptospirosis—a review of 50 cases. *Infection.* 1989;17:8–12.

McClain JB, Ballou WR, Harrison SM, et al. Doxycycline therapy for leptospirosis. *Ann Intern Med.* 1984; 100:696–698.

Panaphut T, Domrongkitchaiporn S, Vibhagool A, et al. Ceftriaxone compared with sodium penicillin G for treatment of severe leptospirosis. *Clin Infect Dis.* 2003; 36:1507–1513.

Watt G, Padre LP, Tuazon ML, et al. Placebo-controlled trial of intravenous penicillin for severe and late leptospirosis. *Lancet.* 1988:1:433–435.

PART XX

Specific Organisms – Mycoplasma and Chlamydia

165. Mycoplasma

Ken B. Waites

Mycoplasmas are the smallest free-living organisms and are unique among prokaryotes in that they lack a cell wall, a feature that is largely responsible for their biologic properties and lack of susceptibility to many commonly prescribed antimicrobial agents. Mycoplasmas are usually mucosally associated, residing primarily in the respiratory and urogenital tracts and rarely penetrating the submucosa, except in the case of immunosuppression or instrumentation, when they may invade the bloodstream and disseminate to many different organs and tissues throughout the body. Intracellular localization occurs in some species and may contribute to chronicity that characterizes many mycoplasmal infections.

There are at least 17 species of mycoplasmas and ureaplasmas for which humans are believed to be the primary host, and numerous others of animal origin that have been detected occasionally, most often in the setting of immunosuppression. Several human mycoplasmal species are commensals in the upper respiratory or lower urogenital tracts. Five species are responsible for the majority of clinically significant infections that may come to the attention of the practicing physician. These species are *Mycoplasma pneumoniae*, *Mycoplasma hominis*, *Mycoplasma genitalium*, *Ureaplasma urealyticum*, and *Ureaplasma parvum*. *Mycoplasma fermentans* is another mycoplasma of human origin that may behave as an opportunist. *Mycoplasma fermentans* has been detected in throat cultures of children with pneumonia, in some cases when no other etiologic agent was identified, but the frequency of its occurrence in healthy children is not known. This mycoplasma has also been detected in adults with an acute influenzalike illness and in bronchoalveolar lavage specimens from patients with the acquired immunodeficiency syndrome and pneumonia. *Mycoplasma amphoriforme* is the newest human mycoplasma to be described. It has been detected in a small number of patients with recurrent bronchitis, but its true role as a human pathogen has not yet been established. Other mycoplasmas of animal origin occasionally cause zoonotic infections in humans.

MYCOPLASMA PNEUMONIAE RESPIRATORY DISEASE

Mycoplasma pneumoniae occurs endemically and occasionally epidemically in persons of all age groups, most commonly in school-age children, adolescents, and young adults. The common misconception that *M. pneumoniae* disease is rare among young children and older adults has sometimes led to failure of physicians to consider this organism in differential diagnoses of respiratory infections in these age groups. Failure to consider *M. pneumoniae* as an etiologic agent in cases of severe pneumonia may also lead to misdiagnosis because this organism can in fact cause severe respiratory disease that has caused death in a few cases. *Mycoplasma pneumoniae* is perhaps best known as the primary cause of "walking or atypical pneumonia," but the most frequent clinical syndrome is tracheobronchitis or bronchiolitis, often accompanied by upper respiratory tract manifestations. Typical complaints can persist for weeks to months and include hoarseness, fever, cough that is initially nonproductive but later may yield small to moderate amounts of nonbloody sputum, sore throat, headache, chills, coryza, and general malaise. The throat may be inflamed, but cervical adenopathy is uncommon. Bronchopneumonia, involving 1 or more lobes, develops in 3% to 10% of infected persons, accounting for 20% or more of community-acquired pneumonias overall. The incubation period is generally 1 to 3 weeks and spread throughout households often occurs. Recent epidemiologic studies have shown *M. pneumoniae* was second only to *Streptococcus pneumoniae* as an etiologic agent of pneumonia in adults requiring hospitalization. Hospital admission may be necessary in about 10% of children and adults, but recovery is usually complete without sequelae. Some people may experience extrapulmonary complications at variable time periods after onset of or even in the absence of respiratory illness. Such complications most commonly include skin rashes, pericarditis, hemolytic anemia, arthritis, meningoencephalitis, peripheral neuropathy, and pericarditis. Other nonspecific manifestations include nausea, vomiting, and diarrhea. Mycoplasmal infection may also be associated with exacerbations of chronic bronchitis and asthma. Whether the organism can act independently in the pathogenesis of asthma has not been firmly established, but the fact that it can induce a number of inflammatory mediators such as immunoglobulin E (IgE), substance P, and neurokinin 1 and that administration of macrolide antibiotics improves lung function of asthmatic persons with evidence of mycoplasmas in their airways suggests this possibility is worthy of further study.

Autoimmune reaction is thought to be responsible for many of the extrapulmonary complications associated with mycoplasmal infection. However, *M. pneumoniae* has been isolated from extrapulmonary sites such as synovial fluid, cerebrospinal fluid (CSF), pericardial fluid, and skin lesions and it has also been detected by polymerase chain reaction (PCR) assays in various extrapulmonary sites. Therefore, direct invasion must always be considered. The frequency of direct invasion of these sites is unknown because the organism is rarely sought.

The hemogram is often normal, but about one-fourth of patients may develop leukocytosis and one-third may demonstrate an elevated erythrocyte sedimentation rate. The cellular response of the sputum is mononuclear, with no bacteria visible by Gram stain. In about 50% of patients, a cold agglutinin titer of ≥1:32 may develop by the second week of illness, disappearing by 6 to 8 weeks. This is not a specific test for *M. pneumoniae*, because other microorganisms may induce similar reactions.

Lung involvement tends to be unilateral, but can be bilateral. Diffuse reticulonodular or interstitial infiltrates involving the lower lobes appearing as streaks radiating from the hilus to the base of the lung are the most common radiographic abnormalities. True lobar consolidation is uncommon, but pleural effusion may develop in about 25% of cases. Abnormalities on chest radiographs often appear more severe than the clinical condition of the patient would predict. Radiographic presentation of mycoplasmal pneumonia in a pediatric patient is shown in Figure 165.1.

Due to widespread lack of diagnostic services for confirmation of mycoplasmal infection, length of time until results can be obtained, impracticality of obtaining diagnostic specimens in patients who are not producing significant respiratory secretions, and similarity of clinical syndromes due to different microorganisms, clinicians often do not attempt to obtain a microbiologic diagnosis in mild to moderately ill outpatients suspected of having *M. pneumoniae* infection and elect to treat empirically. Several viruses, *Chlamydophilia pneumoniae*, *Streptococcus pneumoniae*, *Haemophilus influenzae*, *Moraxella catarrhalis*, *Legionella* species, and even some mycobacteria or fungi, can produce respiratory infections that are clinically indistinguishable and that may occur simultaneously with mycoplasmal infection. Thus, if the microbial etiology of community-acquired respiratory disease is to be known, appropriate laboratory tests for these other agents must be obtained. However, it is rarely practical to attempt to confirm laboratory

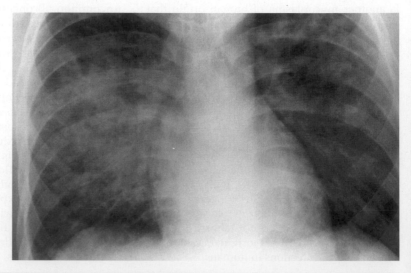

Figure 165.1 Chest radiograph from a pediatric patient with mycoplasmal pneumonia demonstrating severe interstitial disease bilaterally, with both patchy nodular areas and central alveolar areas of increased opacity on the right side. (Radiograph courtesy of Dr. Susan D. John, originally published in *Radiographics*. 2001;21:121–132 as Figure 4.b.)

diagnosis of specific respiratory viral infections, and laboratory testing for *C. pneumoniae*, like that for *M. pneumoniae*, is expensive and often is not widely available except in reference laboratories. However, if the illness is of sufficient severity to require hospitalization, search for a specific microbiological etiology is justified. If mycoplasmal respiratory infection is to be confirmed, culture, molecular-based, and/or serological tests are necessary. Clinical laboratories may offer culture service through a reference laboratory familiar with the complex cultivation requirements of mycoplasmas.

Respiratory tract specimens suitable for mycoplasmal culture include throat swabs, sputum, tracheal aspirates, bronchial lavage fluid, pleural fluid, or lung biopsy tissue according to the patient's clinical condition. Care should be taken in specimen collection, inoculation into a suitable transport medium (such as SP4 broth at bedside whenever possible), and not allowing desiccation. Freezing at −70°C is advised if specimens cannot be transported to the diagnostic laboratory immediately after collection. Growth in culture is slow, requiring ≥3 weeks in some cases. Growth of a glucose-fermenting mycoplasma in SP4 broth and development of microscopic spherical colonies approximately 100 μm in diameter on SP4 agar as shown in Figure 165.2 are presumptive evidence of *M. pneumoniae*. Because some of the upper respiratory commensal mycoplasmal species may also grow on this medium, it is advisable to confirm the identity of the organisms using the PCR assay. Due to the turnaround time, expense, and limited availability, culture is rarely used for routine diagnosis of *M. pneumoniae* infection.

Serology is most frequently used to confirm *M. pneumoniae* infection. Enzyme-linked immunosorbent assays are now preferred over the older, less-sensitive complement fixation assays or cold agglutinin titers. Because primary infection does not guarantee protective immunity against future infections and residual antibody may remain from earlier encounters with the organism, there has been a great impetus to develop sensitive and specific tests that can differentiate between acute and remote infection. Definitive diagnosis requires seroconversion documented by paired serum specimens obtained 2 to 4 weeks apart and assayed at the same time. Although single-titer qualitative and quantitative immunoglobulin M (IgM) assays purported to detect current infection have now become available, it is not clear how long IgM persists after acute infection, and as many as

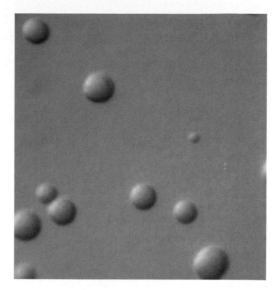

Figure 165.2 Spherical colonies of *Mycoplasma pneumoniae* approximately 100 μm in diameter growing on SP4 agar. Magnification: 126×.

50% of adults may not mount a detectable IgM response. Conversely, some children may not mount a measurable immunoglobulin G (IgG) response. Therefore, reliance on a single serological test can be clinically misleading, and paired assays for both IgM and IgG are recommended. Even then, the interpretation of serological results can sometimes be complex and inconclusive. Measurement of immunoglobulin A (IgA) may also be valuable to characterize acute infection, but very few commercial tests provide information on this immunoglobulin class.

Molecular-based systems for detection of *M. pneumoniae* utilizing the PCR assay have been developed for research purposes, and limited information is available describing the application of this methodology in a clinical setting. Presently there are currently no commercially available rapid diagnostic methods based on direct antigen detection or nucleic acid amplification for documenting the presence of *M. pneumoniae* in clinical specimens to assist the practicing physician on a routine basis. The rapid advances in molecular diagnostic techniques may one day result in the PCR assay becoming the test of choice for detection of slow-growing, fastidious organisms such as *M. pneumoniae*. The possibility of multiplex PCR tests to detect mycoplasmas simultaneously with other atypical etiologic agents of community-acquired pneumonias such as *Chlamydophila* and *Legionella* may eventually prove useful for screening purposes.

TREATMENT OF *MYCOPLASMA PNEUMONIAE* INFECTIONS

Formerly it was believed that mycoplasmal respiratory infections were entirely self-limited and no antimicrobial treatment was indicated. More recently it has been shown that appropriate antimicrobial therapy will shorten the symptomatic period and hasten radiological resolution of pneumonia and recovery, even though organisms may be shed for several weeks. In general, the clinical efficacy of antimicrobial therapy is correlated with severity of pneumonia and elapsed time of illness before treatment is begun. A summary of treatment alternatives for *M. pneumoniae* respiratory infections is provided in Table 165.1.

Mycoplasma pneumoniae is generally susceptible to macrolides, ketolides, tetracyclines, and fluoroquinolones such that in vitro susceptibility testing to guide therapy is not indicated at present. Susceptibility testing would also be impractical most of the time because clinical isolates are rarely available. Macrolide resistance in *M. pneumoniae* has been known to occur for many years, but there is little or no information on its prevalence or clinical significance. The recent emergence of macrolide-resistant *M. pneumoniae* in Japan that possesses ribosomal mutations and has diminished clinical response to macrolide therapy is worrisome. Oral erythromycin has long been a drug of choice for mycoplasmal respiratory infections, but its use has been reduced in recent years due to the availability of better-tolerated drugs in this class with improved pharmacokinetics and shorter treatment durations.

The newer macrolides clarithromycin, azithromycin, and dirithromycin and the ketolide telithromycin are broad-spectrum agents used primarily for treatment of community-acquired respiratory infections caused by a wide array of bacteria. These agents are very active in vitro against *M. pneumoniae* and inhibit its growth at comparable or lower minimum inhibitory concentrations (MICs) than those of erythromycin. All of these drugs have proven clinical efficacy and approved therapeutic indications for pneumonia caused by this organism. Care must be taken because of numerous potential drug interactions with these newer macrolides as well as telithromycin. Clarithromycin and azithromycin are available as pediatric oral suspensions and azithromycin is also available as an intravenous formulation in addition to the tablet or capsule formulations. Telithromycin is approved only for use

in adults with mild to moderate pneumonia. Tetracycline and its analogs are also effective in vivo and in vitro but should not be used in children due to potential bone and tooth toxicity. Clindamycin is effective in vitro, but limited reports suggest it may not be active in vivo and should not be considered a first-line treatment. None of the β-lactams, sulfonamides, or trimethoprim is effective in vitro or in vivo against *M. pneumoniae*.

The newer fluoroquinolones exhibit bactericidal antimycoplasmal activity, but are less potent in vitro than the macrolides against *M. pneumoniae*. Development of new quinolones with documented clinical efficacy and approved indications for treating *M. pneumoniae* such as levofloxacin, moxifloxacin, gemifloxacin, and sparfloxacin has been driven largely by the need for therapeutic alternatives for β-lactam and macrolide-resistant *Streptococcus pneumoniae* and the desire for agents that can be used as empiric monotherapy for respiratory infections due to other typical and atypical organisms. At the present time, quinolones are not approved for use in persons <18 years of age, but these drugs have achieved widespread use for treatment of respiratory infections in adults, mainly in the ambulatory setting. A potential disadvantage of fluoroquinolone usage is the effect these broad-spectrum agents can have on the gram-negative enteric flora. For this reason, tailored empiric therapy with a macrolide that has minimal effect on enteric organisms is preferred in most instances when disease is of mild to moderate severity.

Mycoplasmas are slow-growing organisms; thus one would logically expect respiratory infections to respond better to longer treatment courses than might be offered for other types of infections. Thus, a 14- or even 21-day course of oral therapy is appropriate for most drugs, but some of the newer agents have shown clinical efficacy against mycoplasmal pneumonias with shorter durations. For example, a 5-day course of oral azithromycin is approved for treatment of community-acquired pneumonia due to *M. pneumoniae*.

In addition to the administration of antimicrobials for management of *M. pneumoniae* infections, other measures such as cough suppressants, antipyretics, and analgesics should be given as needed to relieve the headaches and other systemic symptoms. Because most extrapulmonary manifestations are diagnosed late in the course of disease, the benefit of early treatment is unknown. If treatment of extrapulmonary mycoplasmal infections such

Table 165.1 Treatment Options for Respiratory Tract Infections Caused by *Mycoplasma pneumoniae*[a]

Drug	Route	Pediatric	Adult	Comments
		Dosage/24 h		
Doxycycline	PO	4 mg/kg loading dose d 1, then 2–4 mg/kg/d in 1–2 doses × 10–14 d	200 mg loading dose day 1, then 100 mg q12h × 9–13 d	Pregnancy category D Tetracyclines are contraindicated in children under 8 years of age unless there is no other alternative
	IV	Same as PO	Same as PO	
Tetracycline	PO	25–50 mg/kg/d in 4 doses × 10–14 d	250–500 mg q6h × 10–14 d 500 mg-1 gq6–12h × 10–14 d	Pregnancy category D Tetracyclines are contraindicated in children under 8 years of age unless there is no other alternative
	IV	10–20 mg/kg/d in 2–4 doses × 10–14 d		
Erythromycin	PO	20–50 mg/kg/d in 3–4 doses × 10–14 d	250–500 mg base/stearate q6h or 400–800 mg ethylsuccinate q6h × 10–14 d	Pregnancy category B
	IV	25–40 mg/kg/d in 4 doses × 10–14 d	Same as PO	
Dirithromycin	PO	Not recommended	500 mg qd × 14 d	Pregnancy category C Dirithromycin is not approved for use in persons under 12 years of age. No IV formulation is available.
Azithromycin	PO	10 mg/kg/d on day 1, then 5 mg/kg/d × 4 d; not to exceed 250 mg/d	500 mg d 1, then 250 mg q d × 4 d or 2 g given as a single dose	Pregnancy category B IV formulation is not approved for use in persons under 16 years of age
	IV	Not recommended	500 mg qd IV × 2 d, then 500 mg PO qd × 7–10 d	
Clarithromycin	PO	15 mg/kg/d in 2 doses × 7–14 d	250–500 mg q12h × 7–14 d (immediate release) or 1 g qd × 7 d (extended release)	Pregnancy category C No IV formulation is available
Levofloxacin	PO	Not recommended	750 mg qd × 5 d	Pregnancy category C Fluoroquinolones are not approved for use in persons under 18 years of age
	IV	Not recommended	Same as PO	
Sparfloxacin	PO	Not recommended	400 mg day 1, then 200 mg qd × 9 d	Pregnancy category C Fluoroquinolones are not approved for use in persons under 18 years of age. No IV formulation is available. Phototoxicity limits its usefulness
Moxifloxacin	PO	Not recommended	400 mg qd × 7–14 d	Pregnancy category C Fluoroquinolones are not approved for use in persons under 18 years of age
	IV	Not recommended	Same as PO	
Gemifloxacin	PO	Not recommended	320 mg qd × 7 d	Pregnancy category C Fluoroquinolones are not approved for use in persons under 18 years of age. No IV formulation is available
Telithromycin	PO	Not recommended	800 mg qd × 7–10 d	Pregnancy category C Not approved for use in persons under 18 years of age. No IV formulation is available

[a] Treatment recommendations are primarily for management of community-acquired pneumonia with antibiotics approved for treatment of this condition, although they are also appropriate for tracheobronchitis due to this organism. Choice of routes for administration are dependent on the severity of the clinical condition being treated. Most *M. pneumoniae* infections can be adequately treated with oral medication.

Specific Organisms – Mycoplasma and Chlamydia

as arthritis or pericarditis is necessary, and/or the patient is immunosuppressed, selection of an agent that exhibits bactericidal activity such as a fluoroquinolone may be most appropriate, and administration of the drugs for longer durations may be required.

Fortunately, the treatments of choice for *M. pneumoniae* are appropriate for many of the other microbial agents responsible for community-acquired respiratory infections. This is especially important in view of the fact that, in the major proportion of ambulatory patients seeking medical care, the identity of their infectious organism is never determined.

GENITAL *MYCOPLASMA* AND *UREAPLASMA* INFECTIONS

Ureaplasma spp. and *M. hominis* can be isolated from the lower genital tract in the majority of sexually active women; their occurrence is somewhat less frequent in men. The presence of genital mycoplasmas in so many asymptomatic persons has made it difficult to prove their pathogenic potential. For some conditions such as urethritis and urinary calculi for *Ureaplasma* spp. and pelvic inflammatory disease (PID) for *M. hominis*, evidence is sufficient to implicate these organisms as etiologic agents in a portion of clinical cases. For other conditions such as prostatitis and bacterial vaginosis the evidence is not as clear-cut. Only a subgroup of otherwise healthy adult men and women who are colonized will develop clinically significant genitourinary disease due to these organisms, but the risk factors are poorly understood. Table 165.2 summarizes diseases believed to be associated with or caused by genital mycoplasmas and ureaplasmas.

The ability of genital mycoplasmas to be transmitted vertically from mother to offspring in utero or at the time of delivery has led to considerable efforts to ascertain their role as perinatal pathogens. Isolation of *Ureaplasma* spp. from the chorioamnion of pregnant women has been consistently associated with histological chorioamnionitis and is inversely related to birth weight, even when adjusting for duration of labor, rupture of fetal membranes, and presence of other bacteria. *Ureaplasma* spp. can be isolated from endometrial tissue of healthy, nonpregnant women, indicating that they may be present at the time of implantation and might therefore be involved in early pregnancy losses. Numerous studies have shown that the presence of ureaplasmas alone or with other bacteria in the chorioamnion is independently associated with birth at ≤37 weeks of gestation, regardless of the duration of labor. The ability of ureaplasmas to invade the amniotic fluid early in gestation and initiate inflammation provides the setting through which they can also produce inflammation in the lower respiratory tract of the developing fetus and neonate. Over the past several years there has been increasing evidence that these organisms may cause congenital pneumonia and initiate events leading to chronic lung disease of prematurity or bronchopulmonary dysplasia.

Superficial mucosal colonization in the newborn period tends to be transient and without sequelae, but neonates, especially those born preterm, have been shown to be susceptible to development of a variety of systemic conditions due to either *M. hominis* or ureaplasmas, including bacteremia and meningitis.

For nearly 30 years *U. urealyticum* was the only species known to infect humans. However, this species was recently subdivided into two separate species, *U. urealyticum* and *U. parvum*, based on 16s ribosomal RNA (rRNA) sequences. *Ureaplasma parvum* is the more common species isolated from clinical specimens, but both species may occur simultaneously. Most clinical studies have not distinguished between the two species except in very recent years because sophisticated nucleic acid amplification tests are necessary to discriminate between them. Evidence is accumulating that suggests *U. urealyticum* may be more pathogenic in some conditions, but definitive data are still lacking. Extragenital infection with *M. hominis* and/or *Ureaplasma* spp. beyond the neonatal period is usually associated with some degree of immunocompromise, such as congenital hypogammaglobulinemia, iatrogenic immunosuppression following solid organ transplantation, or with invasive procedures such as instrumentation of the urinary tract. Ureaplasmas are the most common etiologic agents of septic arthritis in the setting of congenital antibody deficiencies and should be considered early when attempting to diagnose these conditions.

Mycoplasma genitalium was first isolated in 1980 from urethral specimens in men with urethritis. This mycoplasma occurs much less commonly in the lower urogenital tract than *M. hominis* or *Ureaplasma* spp. Appreciation of its role in human disease was initially hampered by its slow growth and fastidious cultivation requirements. However, availability

Table 165.2 Diseases Associated with or Caused by Genital Mycoplasmas

Disease	*Ureaplasma* spp.	*M. hominis*	*M. genitalium*
Male urethritis	+	−	+
Chronic prostatitis	±	−	±
Epididymitis	±	−	−
Urinary calculi	+	−	−
Cystitis/pyelonephritis	+	+	−
Bacterial vaginosis	±	±	−
Cervicitis	−	−	+
Pelvic inflammatory disease	−	+	+
Infertility	±	−	−
Chorioamnionitis	+	±	−
Spontaneous abortion	±	±	−
Prematurity/low birth weight	+	−	−
Intrauterine growth retardation	+	−	−
Postpartum/postabortal fever and endometritis	+	+	−
Neonatal pneumonia	+	+	−
Neonatal chronic lung disease	±	−	−
Neonatal bacteremia/ meningitis	+	+	−
Neonatal abscesses	+	+	−
Extragenital disease in adults[a]	+	+	−

[a]These include conditions such as septic arthritis, bloodstream invasion, abscesses, wound infections, lung infections, endocarditis, and osteomyelitis.
Key: − = no association or causal role demonstrated (in some conditions for *M. genitalium* this may reflect the fact that no studies using appropriate techniques to detect this organism have been performed); + = causal role; ± = significant association and/or strong suggestive evidence, but causal role not proven.

of the PCR assay as a research tool for its detection in clinical specimens has greatly enhanced understanding of the role of *M. genitalium* in human disease. Several clinical studies support a causal role for this mycoplasma in male urethritis, indicating it may be responsible for as many as 15% to 25% of all cases, as well as for female cervicitis and PID.

Both *M. hominis* and ureaplasmas grow rapidly and can be detected in cultures of appropriate specimens within 2 to 5 days. Proper handling and bedside inoculation of transport broth are recommended to enhance recovery of these organisms. Urethral or wound swabs, cervicovaginal or prostatic secretions, urine, respiratory specimens such as those described for *M. pneumoniae*, CSF, and blood or other body fluids or tissues are appropriate for culture, depending on the clinical setting. Cultures are available mainly

Specific Organisms – Mycoplasma and Chlamydia

through reference laboratories. *M. hominis* produces typical fried-egg colonies on agar and can be presumptively identified by rate of growth, colony morphology (Figure 165.3), and arginine hydrolysis. Definitive identification requires characterization by PCR. Ureaplasmas can be identified to genus level by typical colony morphology on A8 agar and urease activity (Figure 165.4). Speciation of ureaplasmas requires assay by PCR. Techniques for isolation of *M. genitalium* in culture have been described, but its extremely slow growth, sometimes requiring several weeks to form colonies, and difficult cultivation have essentially limited diagnostic measures to PCR assays performed mainly for research purposes.

Genitourinary or extragenital diseases known to be due to or associated with mycoplasmas warrant appropriate diagnostic tests when available and treatment if infection is confirmed. This is of particular importance if the organisms are recovered in the absence of other possible microbial etiologies and if the infection is present in a normally sterile site such as blood, synovial fluid, or CSF. Many of the conditions associated with a mycoplasmal etiology can also be due to a variety of microbial agents, and some conditions such as PID can be polymicrobial. Therefore, the selection of drugs must take into account multiple causes.

TREATMENT OF GENITAL *MYCOPLASMA* AND *UREAPLASMA* INFECTIONS

Oral tetracyclines have historically been the drugs of choice for use against urogenital infections due to *M. hominis*, but resistance now occurs in 20% to 40% of isolates. A recent survey of clinical isolates of *Ureaplasma* spp. from several states found that 45% possessed the *tetM* transposon conferring resistance to this class of drugs. The degree of resistance may vary according to geographical area, type of patient population, and previous exposure to antimicrobial agents. Recent reports of fluoroquinolone resistance in both *M. hominis* and *Ureaplasma* spp. in North America and Europe lend support to the recommendation that in vitro susceptibility testing is indicated when these organisms are recovered from a normally sterile body site, from immunocompromised hosts, and/or from persons who have not responded to an initial treatment. Susceptibility testing can be accomplished in 3 to 5 days by a reference laboratory once the organism is isolated. Treatment alterna-

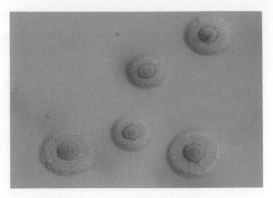

Figure 165.3 Fried egg–type colonies of *Mycoplasma hominis* up to 110 μm in diameter growing on A8 agar. Magnification: 132×.

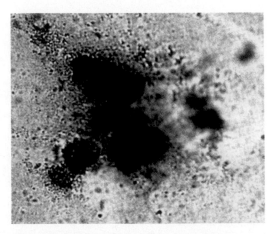

Figure 165.4 Granular brown urease-positive colonies of *Ureaplasma* species 15 to 60 μm in diameter growing from a vaginal specimen on A8 agar. Magnification: 200×.

tives for urogenital infections in adults and neonatal infections are provided in Tables 165.3 and 165.4, respectively.

Clindamycin is an alternative treatment for *M. hominis* and is effective against tetracycline-resistant strains, but it is much less active against *Ureaplasma* spp. In contrast, macrolides are generally active against ureaplasmas, whereas *M. hominis* is typically resistant. A single dose of azithromycin is approved for treatment of urethritis due to *Chlamydia trachomatis* and has been shown to work as well clinically as doxycycline in persons with urethritis due to *Ureaplasma* spp. Despite apparent in vitro susceptibility, tetracycline or erythromycin treatment of vaginal mycoplasmas in women is not always successful.

Clinical studies have encountered treatment failures with the tetracyclines for urethritis caused by *M. genitalium*, and it was initially

Table 165.3 Treatment Options for Urogenital and Systemic Infections in Adults Caused by *Mycoplasma hominis*, *Mycoplasma genitalium*, and *Ureaplasma* species[a]

Drug	Route	Dosage/24 h	Comments
Doxycycline	PO IV	200 mg loading dose d 1, then 100 mg q12h × 7 d Same as PO	Pregnancy category D. Activity may be inhibited in some strains of *M. hominis* and *Ureaplasma* spp. possessing *tetM*. Treatment failures have been described for *M. genitalium* urethritis
Tetracycline	PO IV	250–500 mg q6h × 7 d 125–500 mg q6–12h × 7 d	Pregnancy category D. Activity may be inhibited in some strains of *M. hominis* and *Ureaplasma* spp possessing *tetM*
Erythromycin	PO IV	250–500 mg q6h × 7 d Same as PO	Pregnancy category B. Macrolides are not active against *M. hominis*
Azithromycin	PO IV	500 mg × 1 d then 250 mg × 4 d; or 1 g single dose 500 mg/d × 2 d, then 500 mg PO qd	Pregnancy category B. Macrolides are not active against *M. hominis*. In vitro resistance and treatment failures have been described for *M. genitalium* urethritis.
Clindamycin	PO IV	150–450 mg q6h × 7 d 150–900 mg q6–8h × 7 d	Pregnancy category C. Clindamycin is not active against *Ureaplasma* spp.
Ofloxacin	PO IV	200–400 mg q12h × 7 d Same as PO	Pregnancy category C. Fluoroquinolones are not approved for use in persons under 18 years of age
Levofloxacin	PO IV	500 mg qd × 7–14 d Same as PO	Pregnancy category C. Fluoroquinolones are not approved for use in persons under 18 years of age
Moxifloxacin	PO IV	400 mg q12h × 10 d Same as PO	Pregnancy category C. Fluoroquinolones are not approved for use in persons under 18 years of age. Moxifloxacin does not have approved indications for treatment of urogenital infections, but it has been effective in men with *M. genitalium* urethritis who failed treatment with azithromycin.

[a] Treatment options are based on accepted regimens for urogenital infections involving other microorganisms that are expected to be suitable for infections caused by genital mycoplasmas based on in vitro susceptibility data in circumstances where there are no approved microbiological indications. Route and duration of treatment are dependent on the severity of the clinical condition being treated. For extragenital and/or systemic infections, particularly those involving immunocompromised persons, a longer duration of treatment may be necessary than those listed. Joint infections may require several weeks to months of antimicrobial administration.

believed that azithromycin would be a better option. However, recent reports of treatment failures with azithromycin and detection of *M. genitalium* isolates with elevated MICs to this drug indicate that it may not always be effective. Macrolide-resistant *M. genitalium* infections have been successfully treated with fluoroquinolones.

Fluoroquinolones have become useful alternatives for treatment of certain infections caused by *M. hominis*, *M. genitalium*, and *Ureaplasma* spp. within the urogenital tract and in some extragenital locations. Activity of fluoroquinolones is not affected by tetracycline or macrolide resistance. Ciprofloxacin and ofloxacin are generally less active in vitro against these organisms than are levofloxacin and moxifloxacin. Very few clinical antibiotic trials have included microbiologic data specific for genital mycoplasmas, and there have been no systematic comparative evaluations of treatment regimens for extragenital infections in adults or for neonatal infections. Thus, treatment recommendations in Tables 165.3 and 165.4, including dosages and duration, are based largely on in vitro susceptibility data, outcomes of treatment trials evaluating clinical response to syndromes such as PID and urethritis that may be due to genital mycoplasmas, and individual case reports. For infections such as urethritis that may be venereally transmitted, sexual contacts of the index case should also receive treatment.

Experience with mycoplasmal or ureaplasmal infections in immunocompromised patients, especially those with hypogammaglobulinemia who have been the best studied, demonstrate

Table 165.4 Treatment Options for Neonatal Infections with *Mycoplasma hominis* and *Ureaplasma* spp[a]

Drug	Route	Dosage/24 h	Comments
Doxycycline	PO	4 mg/kg loading dose d 1, then 2–4 mg/kg/d in 1–2 doses × 10–14 d	Tetracyclines are contraindicated in children ≤8 y of age unless no other alternative is available. Activity may be inhibited in some strains of *M. hominis* and *Ureaplasma* spp. possessing *tetM*. This drug has been used to successfully treat neonatal meningitis due to *M. hominis* and *Ureaplasma* spp., but treatment failure has been reported with *Ureaplasma* spp.
	IV	Same as PO	
Tetracycline	PO	25–50 mg/kg/d in 4 doses	Tetracyclines are contraindicated in children ≤8 y of age unless no other alternative is available. Activity may be inhibited in some strains of *M. hominis* and *Ureaplasma* spp. possessing *tetM*
	IV	10–20 mg/kg/d in 2–4 doses	
Chloramphenicol	PO	Not recommended	Chloramphenicol has been used successfully to treat neonatal meningitis due to *M. hominis* and *Ureaplasma* spp., but there has also been a report of treatment failure with *M. hominis*. Frequent monitoring of hematological parameters and blood levels of the antibiotic are necessary due to its potential toxicity
	IV	For neonates up to 2 weeks of age, use 25 mg/kg/d in 1 dose, thereafter 50 mg/kg/d in 1 dose	
Erythromycin	PO	20–50 mg/kg/d in 3–4 doses	Macrolides are not active against *M. hominis*. Despite poor CSF penetration, this drug has been used successfully to treat neonatal meningitis due to *Ureaplasma* spp., but treatment failure has also been reported
	IV	25–40 mg/kg/d in 4 doses	
	IV	Same as PO	
Clindamycin	PO	10–25 mg/kg/d in 3–4 doses × 10–14 d	Clindamycin is not active against *Ureaplasma* spp. This drug has been used to successfully treat neonatal infections due to *M. hominis*
	IV	10–40 mg/kg/d in 3–4 doses Do not exceed 15–20 mg/kg/d	

[a] No treatment guidelines for neonatal infections with genital mycoplasmas are available. Treatment options have been compiled based on in vitro susceptibility data and information described in published case reports. Dosages listed are based on data applicable to older infants and children when neonate-specific recommendations are unavailable.
Abbreviations: CSF = cerebrospinal fluid.

that, even though mycoplasmas are primarily noninvasive mucosal pathogens in the normal host, they have the capacity to produce destructive and progressive disease. Infections may be caused by resistant organisms refractory to antimicrobial therapy and require prolonged administration of a combination of intravenous antimicrobials, intravenous immunoglobulin, and/or antisera prepared specifically against the infecting species. Even with aggressive therapy, relapses are still likely to occur. Repeat cultures of affected sites may be necessary to monitor in vivo response to treatment.

Isolation of *M. hominis* or *Ureaplasma* spp. from CSF with pleocytosis, progressive hydrocephalus or other neurologic abnormality, pericardial fluid, pleural fluid, tracheal aspirate in association with respiratory disease, abscess material, or blood are justification for specific treatment in critically ill neonates when no other verifiable microbiologic etiologies of the clinical condition are apparent. Parenteral tetracyclines have been used most often to treat neonatal meningitis due to either *M. hominis* or

Ureaplasma spp. despite contraindications, but erythromycin for *Ureaplasma* spp., clindamycin for *M. hominis*, or chloramphenicol for either species are alternatives. No single drug has been successful in every instance in eradication of these organisms from CSF of neonates. Even though azithromycin has a number of advantages over erythromycin from the pharmacokinetic standpoint, there has been minimal clinical experience with this drug in treatment of neonatal ureaplasmal infections, and there are no guidelines for its use in this setting. Overall treatment guidelines for neonates are the same as for urogenital and systemic mycoplasmal infections in adults with appropriate dosage modifications based on weight, except that the intravenous route should be used for serious systemic infections when possible. Duration of treatment and drug dosages for neonatal mycoplasmal infections have not been critically evaluated, but a minimum of 10 to 14 days of therapy is suggested based on experience in individual cases where microbiologic follow-up has been assessed.

OTHER MYCOPLASMAL SPECIES

A variety of mycoplasmal species can be isolated from the upper respiratory or urogenital tract of humans. Some of them occur fairly commonly as commensals in healthy persons, whereas others are found less often. Some of these organisms have been implicated in case reports as agents of invasive disease, usually in immunosuppressed persons. No guidelines for their detection or treatment are possible due to the infrequency of isolation and lack of clinical isolates on which in vitro susceptibility tests have been performed. In the case of *M. fermentans*, its antimicrobial susceptibilities are generally similar to those of *M. hominis*, but scant information is available for other species. If a clinical isolate of one of these opportunistic mycoplasmal species is available, in vitro susceptibility tests should be determined to guide treatment, providing the organism will grow well enough in vitro to perform the test. Otherwise, empiric use of drugs shown to be effective against other mycoplasmal species should be considered, with the choice being based on the type of infection encountered and status of the host.

SUGGESTED READING

Bradshaw CS, Jensen JS, Tabrizi SN, et al. Azithromycin failure in *Mycoplasma genitalium* urethritis. *Emerg Infect Dis*. 2006;12: 1149–1152.

Kraft M, Cassell GH, Park J, et al. *Mycoplasma pneumoniae* and *Chlamydia pneumoniae* in asthma: effect of clarithromycin. *Chest*. 2002;121:1782–1788.

Marston BJ, Plouffe JF, File TM Jr, et al. Incidence of community-acquired pneumonia requiring hospitalization: results of a population-based active surveillance Study in Ohio. The Community-Based Pneumonia Incidence Study Group. *Arch Int Med*. 1997;156:1709–1718.

Schelonka R, Katz B, Waites KB, et al. A critical appraisal of the role of *Ureaplasma* in development of bronchopulmonary dysplasia using meta-analytic techniques. *Pediatr Infect Dis J*. 2005;24:1033–1039.

Suzuki S, Yamazaki T, Narita M, et al. Clinical evaluation of macrolide-resistant *Mycoplasma pneumoniae*. *Antimicrob Agents Chemother*. 2005;50:709–712.

Talkington DT, Waites KB, Schwartz S, et al. Emerging from obscurity: Understanding the pathogenesis, associated syndromes, and epidemiology of *Mycoplasma pneumoniae*. In: Scheld WM, Craig WA, Hughes JM, eds. *Emerging Infections*. 5th ed. Washington, DC: ASM Press; 2001:57–84.

Waites KB, Talkington DF. *Mycoplasma pneumoniae* as a human pathogen. *Clin Microbiol Rev*. 2004;17:697–728.

Waites KB, Talkington DF. New developments in human diseases caused by mycoplasmas. In: Blanchard A Browning G, eds. *Mycoplasmas: Pathogenesis, Molecular Biology, and Emerging Strategies for Control*. Norwich, UK: Horizon Scientific Press; 2005:289–354.

Waites KB, Katz B, Schelonka RL. Mycoplasmas and ureaplasmas as neonatal pathogens. *Clin Microbiol Rev*. 2005;18:757–789.

Yasuda M, Maeda S, Deguchi T. In vitro activity of fluoroquinolones against *Mycoplasma genitalium* and their bacteriological efficacy for treatment of *M. genitalium*-positive nongonococcal urethritis in men. *Clin Infect Dis*. 2005;41:1357–1359.

166. *Chlamydia Pneumoniae*

Margaret R. Hammerschlag

The first isolates of *Chlamydia* (*Chlamydophila*) *pneumoniae* were obtained serendipitously during trachoma studies in the 1960s. After the recovery of a similar isolate from the respiratory tract of a college student with pneumonia in Seattle, Grayston and colleagues applied the designation TWAR after their first two isolates, TW-183 and AR-39. *C. pneumoniae* appears to be a common human respiratory pathogen. The mode of transmission remains uncertain but probably involves infected respiratory tract secretions. Spread of *C. pneumoniae* within families and enclosed populations such as military recruits has been described. The proportion of community-acquired pneumonia in children and adults associated with *C. pneumoniae* infection has ranged from 0% to >44%, varying with geographic location, the age group examined, and the diagnostic methods used. Early studies that relied on serology suggested that infection in children younger than 5 years was rare; however, subsequent studies using culture and/or polymerase chain reaction (PCR) have found the prevalence of infection in children beyond early infancy to be similar to that found in adults.

Studies that have used culture have found a poor correlation with serology, especially in children. Although 7% to 13% of children 6 months to 16 years of age enrolled in two multicenter pneumonia treatment studies were culture positive and 7% to 18% met the serologic criteria for acute infection with the microimmunofluorecence (MIF) test, they were not the same patients. Only 1% to 3% of the culture-positive children met the serologic criteria, and approximately 70% were seronegative. By age 20, approximately 50% of persons will have detectable anti-*C. pneumoniae* immunoglobulin G (IgG). Seroprevalence may exceed 80% in some populations.

Prolonged culture positivity lasting from several weeks to several years after acute infection has been reported. Asymptomatic nasopharyngeal carriage also occurs in 2% to 5% of adults and children. The role that asymptomatic carriage plays in the epidemiology of *C. pneumoniae* is not known, but possibly these persons serve as a reservoir for spread of infection.

The spectrum of disease associated with *C. pneumoniae* is expanding. Most infections are probably mild or asymptomatic. Initial reports emphasized mild atypical pneumonia clinically resembling that associated with *Mycoplasma pneumoniae*. Generally, pneumonia associated with *C. pneumoniae* is not clinically indistinguishable from other pneumonias. Co-infection with other pathogens, especially *M. pneumoniae* and *Streptococcus pneumoniae*, can be a frequent occurrence. *C. pneumoniae* has been associated with severe illness and even death, although the role of pre-existing chronic conditions as contributing factors in many of these patients is difficult to assess. In some cases, however, *C. pneumoniae* clearly appears to be implicated as a serious pathogen, even in the absence of underlying disease. *C. pneumoniae* has been isolated from the empyema fluid in several patients with severe pneumonia.

The role of host factors in *C. pneumoniae* infection remains to be determined. *C. pneumoniae* appeared to be responsible for 14% to 19% of episodes of acute chest syndrome in children with sickle-cell disease. *C. pneumoniae* infection in these patients appeared to be associated with more severe hypoxia than infection with *M. pneumoniae*. *C. pneumoniae* may act as an inflammatory trigger for asthma.

The role of *C. pneumoniae* in upper respiratory infections is less well defined. *C. pneumoniae* has been isolated from the middle ear fluid of children and adults with otitis media and has also been implicated as a cause of pharyngitis. *C. pneumoniae* infection has been implicated in a wide variety of chronic diseases and conditions, including atherosclerosis, Alzheimer's disease, macular degeneration, and arthritis. However, many of these studies are hampered by the lack of standardized methods for the diagnosis of *C. pneumoniae* infection.

LABORATORY DIAGNOSIS

A specific laboratory diagnosis of *C. pneumoniae* infection can be made by isolation of the organism from nasopharyngeal or throat swabs, sputa, or pleural fluid, if present. The nasopharynx appears to be the optimal site for isolation of the organism. The relative yield from throat swabs and sputum is not known. Isolation of *C. pneumoniae* requires culture in tissue; the organism cannot be propagated in cell-free media. *C. pneumoniae* grows readily in cell lines derived from respiratory tract tissue, specifically, HEp-2 and HL cells. Culture with an initial inoculation and one passage should take 4 to 7 days.

Nasopharyngeal cultures can be obtained with Dacron-tipped, wire-shafted swabs. Each lot of swabs should be treated in a mock infection system to ensure that no inhibitory effects occur on either the viability of cells or recovery of chlamydiae. Specimens for culture should be placed in appropriate transport media, usually a sucrose phosphate buffer with antibiotics and fetal calf serum, and stored immediately at 4°C for no longer than 24 hours. Viability decreases if specimens are held at room temperature. If the specimen cannot be processed within 24 hours, it should be frozen at −70°C until culture can be performed. After 72 hours of incubation, culture confirmation can be performed by staining with either a *C. pneumoniae* spp.–specific or a *Chlamydia* genus–specific (antilipopolysaccharide [LPS]) fluorescein-conjugated monoclonal antibody.

Because isolation of *C. pneumoniae* was initially considered to be difficult and limited, emphasis was placed on serologic diagnosis. The MIF test is not standardized or U.S. Food and Drug Administration (FDA) approved. Although enzyme immunoassay (EIA) serology test kits offer the promise of standardized performance and objective end points, none have been evaluated adequately in comparison to culture or PCR. Most have been compared only with MIF. None have FDA clearance or approval for use in the United States. One commercial assay, the Medac rELISA, uses a recombinant LPS antigen; others are based on LPS-extracted EBs or synthetic peptides. These kits can measure IgG, immunoglobulin M (IgM), and immunoglobulin A (IgA) antibodies, but cutoffs vary from kit to kit, and the criteria for a positive result (acute infection, past infection) can be very complex. The Centers for Disease Control and Prevention (CDC) has proposed modifications of the serologic criteria for diagnosis of *C. pneumoniae* infection. Although the MIF test was considered to be the only serologic test currently acceptable, the criteria were made significantly more stringent. Acute infection as determined by MIF was defined as a 4-fold rise in IgG or an

IgM titer of 16 or greater, and the use of a single elevated IgG titer was discouraged. However, the use of paired sera also affords only a retrospective diagnosis, which is of little help in terms of deciding how to treat a patient. An IgG titer of 16 or greater was considered to indicate past exposure, but neither elevated IgA titer nor any other serologic marker was thought to be a validated indicator of persistent or chronic infection. The CDC did not recommend the use of any EIA for detection of antibody to *C. pneumoniae*.

PCR appears to be the most promising technology in the development of a rapid, non-culture method for detection of *C. pneumoniae*. More than 25 in-house PCR assays for detection of *C. pneumoniae* in clinical specimens have been reported in the literature. None of these assays is standardized or extensively validated in comparison to culture for detection of *C. pneumoniae* in respiratory specimens. None is commercially available or has FDA approval. Major variations in these methods include collecting and processing specimens, primer design, nucleic acid extraction, detection and identification of amplification products, and ways to prevent possible false-positive and inhibitory reactions. Recent studies suggest significant interlaboratory variation in performance of PCR for *C. pneumoniae*. Use of nested PCRs has been associated with a high risk of contamination due to amplicon carryover. Real-time PCR may be the method of choice, and several assays have been reported in the literature, but none have been adequately validated compared to culture in respiratory specimens.

THERAPY

Chlamydia pneumoniae is susceptible to tetracyclines, macrolides, and quinolones. Most of the treatment studies of pneumonia caused by *C. pneumoniae* published thus far have relied entirely on diagnosis by serology; consequently, microbiologic efficacy could not be assessed. Anecdotal reports have suggested that prolonged courses, up to 3 weeks, of either tetracyclines or erythromycin may be needed to eradicate *C. pneumoniae* from the nasopharynx of adults with flulike illness and pharyngitis. The results of two pediatric multicenter pneumonia treatment studies found that 10-day courses of erythromycin and clarithromycin and 5 days of azithromycin suspension were equally efficacious; they eradicated the organism in 79% to 86% of children. Quinolones, including levofloxacin and moxifloxacin, also

Table 166.1 Regimens for respiratory tract infection caused by *C. pneumoniae*

Adults	Children
Doxycycline, 100 mg 2 × a day for 14–21 d	Erythromycin suspension, 50 mg/kg/d for 10–14 days
Tetracycline, 250 mg 4 × a day for 14–21 d	Clarithromycin suspension, 15 mg/kg/d for 10 days
Azithromycin, 1.5 g over a period of 5 d	Azithromycin suspension, 10 mg/kg on day 1 followed by 5 mg/kg/d once daily on days 2 to 5
Levofloxacin, 500 mg/d orally or intravenously for 7–14 d	
Moxifloxacin, 400 mg/d orally for 10 d	

have been demonstrated to have 70% to 80% efficacy in eradicating *C. pneumoniae* from adults with community-acquired pneumonia. Most patients improved clinically despite persistence of the organism. Persistence does not appear to be secondary to the development of antibiotic resistance.

Based on these limited data, regimens for respiratory tract infection caused by *C. pneumoniae* are listed in Table 166.1. Some patients may require retreatment.

SUGGESTED READING

Dowell SF, Peeling RW, Boman J, et al. Standardizing *Chlamydia pneumoniae* assays: recommendations from the Centers for Disease Control and Prevention (USA) and the Laboratory Centre for Disease Control (Canada). *Clin Infect Dis.* 2001;33,492–503.

Hammerschlag MR. Advances in the management of *Chlamydia pneumoniae* infections. *Exp Rev Anti-Infect Ther.* 2003;1:493–504.

Kumar S, Hammerschlag MR. Acute respiratory infection due to *Chlamydia pneumoniae:* current status of diagnostic methods. *Clin Infect Dis.* 2007;44:568–576.

Rockey DD, Lenart J, Stephens RS. Genome sequencing and our understanding of chlamydiae. *Infect Immun.* 2000;68:5473–5479.

167. *Chlamydia Psittaci* (Psittacosis)

Alfred E. Bacon III

Chlamydophila psittaci was identified simultaneously by three investigators in 1930. It is one of four species within the genus *Chlamydia*. Based on RNA sequencing, it is currently considered distinct from *Chlamydophila pneumoniae* and *Chlamydia trachomatis,* despite phenotypic and physiologic similarities that have taxonomically bound them for many years. The organism is an obligate intracellular pathogen that contains both RNA and DNA but lacks a classic cell wall. These characteristics contribute to both the clinical manifestations as well as determine therapeutic options. *Chlamydophila psittaci* has a wide range of host species, including birds, humans, and lower mammals. *Chlamydophila pneumoniae*, however, is found only in humans, and *Chlamydia trachomatis* only in humans and mice.

The systemic illness associated with *C. psittaci* has been termed *psittacosis* because of its association with parrots and psittacine birds. Subsequently, many avian species have been found to harbor *C. psittaci* and to transmit the organism to humans, causing disease. The term *ornithosis* would be more appropriate; however, it is not traditional. The organism can be carried for years in birds, remaining latent causing disease many years after acquisition. Transmission to humans can occur even in the absence of disease in the bird. Excretion in the feces with aerosolization is the typical mode of transmission. Human-to-human transmission has been documented rarely and usually in the setting of severe disease. Health care workers have acquired the disease, but it is not felt warranted to isolate patients when hospitalized. Cases of mammal to human acquisition have been described in the setting of placental aeration at birth but these cases are likely caused by the now separate species *C. abortus.*

Individuals epidemiologically at risk for *C. psittaci* infection include abattoir and veterinary workers as well as those exposed to aviaries. Poultry breeders (particularly turkey farmers) are at significant risk, accounting for most outbreaks. A variable degree of illness exists in the birds infected with *C. psittaci*, ranging from asymptomatic to full-blown disease manifested by anorexia, dyspnea, and diarrhea. Birds may resolve the illness spontaneously, and a waxing and waning clinical course is not unusual. Therefore, a history of contact with birds is pertinent even if the bird is seemingly healthy. Up to 20% of patients may not recall bird exposure but contact as innocuous as mowing a lawn or being exposed to airborne feces is adequate exposure. It remains a distinctly unusual cause of pneumonia with only 813 cases reported to the Centers for Disease Control and Prevention (CDC) from 1988 to 1998. Underreporting in the setting of accepted clinical criteria may play a role in this lack of recognition.

CLINICAL SYNDROMES

Following inhalation in aerosol form, the organism travels to the alveoli and then disseminates to regional lymph nodes and the reticuloendothelial system. Dissemination does not always occur, limiting disease to the chest. The organism invades and even multiplies successfully in a wide range of host cells, including macrophages and neutrophils. Multiple organ involvement is not uncommon, and the systemic nature of this disease cannot be overstated.

The classic presentation is one of an atypical pneumonia, although systemic infections in the absence of pneumonia has been well described as a typhoidal disease, even with cutaneous manifestations such as Horder's spots. Cough is often a later clinical sign, preceded by fever, malaise, and often severe headache by a number of days. The presence of severe headache is felt to be a sentinel component of the disease. The incubation period ranges from 5 to 21 days, and in up to 20% of patients, no history of exposure to a bird can be elicited. Diarrhea is very common.

Neurologic involvement and encephalopathic features have been reported. Endocarditis, myocarditis, and septicemia can occur. Rash, panniculitis, and even joint disease seen as human leukocyte antigen (HLA)-B27 reactive arthritis occur rarely. Recently, a follicular conjunctivitis has been described caused by "nontrachoma" chlamydia, including *C. psittaci*. Anecdotal reports of vasculitis and cerebral vascular disease have been linked to *C. psittaci* but lack convincing clinical or diagnostic criteria.

Physical findings commonly include pulmonary consolidation and an altered mental status. As with other intracellular pathogens, a temperature–pulse dissociation is often reported. Laboratory data are rarely unique to *C. psittaci* infection; however, hepatocellular damage is present in almost 50% of patients. An abnormal chest x-ray film is evident in 80% of infected individuals, almost uniformly a lobar infiltrate as opposed to a diffuse pattern.

DIAGNOSIS

The diagnosis *C. psittaci* infection is based on serologic confirmation of exposure to the pathogen in the proper clinical setting. As with most cases of atypical pneumonia, a thorough history looking for exposures, systemic symptoms, and atypical features is crucial. Culturing the organism is difficult and hazardous in the laboratory. Two serologic assays are readily available. A complement fixation antibody assay with a 4-fold or greater change in titer between acute and convalescent phase era confirms the diagnosis. A random titer greater than 1:32 with a compatible illness is presumptively diagnostic. The complement fixation assay, however, does cross-react with *C. trachomatis* and *C. pneumoniae*. More recently used is a serum microimmunofluorescence assay. This assay has a higher specificity and can be successful diagnostically with demonstration of immunoglobulin M (IgM) antibody directed at *C. psittaci*. Evaluation of acute and convalescent sera is still recommended. However, it is important to note that the serologic response can be blunted when therapy is initiated early.

Rapid diagnostic testing has been utilized rarely in the diagnosis of *C. psittaci* infection: Immunohistochemical identification of *C. psittaci* antigen in clinical specimens has been successfully reported, and real-time polymerase chain reaction applied directly to both culture and clinical specimens has shown great specificity and sensitivity. Unfortunately, these techniques are not readily available in the clinical setting. In the acute setting, when therapy is initiated, the diagnosis of *C. psittaci* infection truly rests on clinical grounds, with an exposure history and a compatible clinical presentation.

THERAPY

The therapy of choice for *C. psittaci* infections, both systemic and limited, is a tetracycline. Doxycycline, 100 mg orally twice a day, is the preferred agent. The systemic nature of the infection and reports of relapsing disease require a prolonged course of therapy. The identification of relapsing disease has led most authors to suggest a course of at least 14 days, and most encourage 21 days total. In the seriously ill population requiring intravenous therapy the dosing is the same for doxycycline. In patients with endocarditis, a more prolonged course is necessary, and patients rarely have survived without valve replacement in addition to prolonged doxycycline therapy.

Traditionally, erythromycin, 500 mg orally four times a day, is the second-line drug for *C. psittaci* pneumonia. Because relapses and failures in therapy have been reported, a 21-day course of therapy is indicated. Newer macrolide agents, particularly azithromycin, have been studied in chlamydia infections, specifically *C. psittaci*. Azithromycin appears both in vitro and in vivo to be an excellent alternative to doxycycline. A 7-day course at 10 mg/kg of body weight has been effective in experimental models. This reflects the increased intracellular concentration of this agent as well as the prolonged half-life. There are fewer data to support the use of clarithromycin. This agent has been shown to be effective in the treatment of infections caused by other *Chlamydia* species.

In the treatment of conjunctivitis where *C. psittaci* is suspected, a 4- to 10-week course of either doxycycline or erythromycin is appropriate. More traditional agents have also shown efficacy, including chloramphenicol, 500 mg four times a day for 14 days. Patients failing this regimen have done well with the addition of rifampin.

There are growing data on the use of quinolones in the management of *C. psittaci* infections. These agents have shown excellent activity against other *Chlamydia* species. In vitro and animal model data have delineated activity of a broad range of quinolones against *C. psittaci*, most notably ofloxacin, ciprofloxacin, moxifloxacin, and sparfloxacin. Ofloxacin in a dose of 200 mg orally twice daily has shown efficacy in a small population of patients with confirmed infection with *C. psittaci*. The use of Levaquin at 500 mg daily for 21 days would likely be similarly supported.

Many reports in the literature demonstrate a prompt clinical response to doxycycline in patients infected with *C. psittaci*. A patient's failure to show symptomatic improvement within 48 hours should prompt a reevaluation of the diagnosis or a suspicion of deep-seated infection such as endocarditis.

SUGGESTED READING

Centers for Disease Control and Prevention. Compendium of measures to control Chlamydia psittaci infection among humans (psittacosis) and pet birds (avian chlamydia). *Mor-bid Mortal Weekly Rep.* 2000;49(RR08):1–17.

Donati M, et al. Comparative in-vitro activity of moxifloxacin, minocycline and azithromycin against Chlamydia spp. *J Antimicrob Chemother.* 1999;43:825–827.

Freidank H, et al. Evaluation of a new commercial microimmunofluorescence test for detection of antibodies to Chlamydia pneumoniae, Chlamydia trachomatis, and Chlamydia psittaci. *Eur J Clin Microbiol Infect Dis.* 1997;16:685–688.

Leitman T, et al. Chronic follicular conjunctivitis associated with Chlamydia psittaci or Chlamydia pneumoniae. *Clin Infect Dis.* 1998;26:1335–1340.

Leroy O, et al. Therapy of pneumonia due to Legionella, Mycoplasma, Chlamydia and Rickettsia with Ofloxacin. *Pathol Biol.* (Paris) 1989;10:1137–1140.

Miyashita N, et al. In vitro and in vivo activity of sitafloxacin against Chlamydia spp. *Antimicrob Agents Chemother.* 2001;45: 3270–3272.

Niki Y, et al. In vitro and in vivo activities of azithromycin, a new azalide antibiotic, against Chlamydia. *Antimicrob Agents Chemother.* 1994;38:2296–2299.

Schlossberg D. Chlamydia psittaci (psittacosis). In: Mandel GL, Bennett JE, Dolin R, eds. *Mandell, Douglas, and Bennett's Principles and Practice of Infectious Diseases.* 6th ed. New York, NY: Churchill Livingstone; 2005.

Schlossberg D, et al. An epidemic of avian and human psittacosis. *Arch Intern Med.* 1993;153:2594–2596.

Yang JM, et al. Development of a rapid real-time PCR assay for detection and quantification of four familiar species of Chlamydiaceae. *J Clin Virol.* 2006; 36:79–81.

Yung AP, Grayston ML. Psittacosis: a review of 135 cases. *Med J Aust.* 1988;148:228–233.

PART XXI

Specific Organisms – Rickettsia, Ehrlichia, and Anaplasma

168. Rickettsial Infections

Paul D. Holtom

The definition of the Rickettsiaceae family has changed since the mid-1980s on the basis of new genetic tools, allowing the discovery of new species and the reclassification of other species. The Rickettsiaceae are aerobic, small, gram-negative coccobacilli that are obligate intracellular parasites of eukaryotic cells. The Rickettsiales now consist of the genus *Rickettsia*, the new genus *Orientia*, and the *Ehrlichia* group. There are three groups of Rickettsiae based on clinical presentation: the spotted fever group, the typhus group, and scrub typhus. *Coxiella burnetii*, the agent that causes Q fever, is covered in this chapter but is now classified in the γ-proteobacteria group, together with *Legionella* and *Francisella tularensis*.

The pathogenesis of illness due to the Rickettsiae is vasculitis. The rickettsiae proliferate in the endothelial lining cells of the small arteries, capillaries, and veins. Erhlichiae invade and proliferate in their target cells of the hematopoietic and lymphoreticular systems, whereas in Q fever the organisms are inhaled and proliferate in the lungs, causing inflammation and bacteremic seeding of other organs, particularly the liver. All of the important rickettsial infections are vectorborne, whereas Q fever usually results from inhalation of dust contaminated by the birth fluids of domestic ungulates.

In any discussion of the treatment of rickettsioses it is important to stress that proper treatment cannot be given unless the diagnosis is suspected. Confirmation of the diagnosis is almost always delayed. The arthropodborne rickettsioses are diseases of the spring and summer in temperate climates. Q fever can occur at any season if exposure to aerosols of the organism occurs. Given an appropriate geographic, temporal, and/or occupational history, the triad of fever, headache, and rash should cause the physician to suspect a disease caused by the Rickettsiae. Fever, headache, and leukopenia or thrombocytopenia suggest ehrlichiosis. As early treatment is important in preventing fatalities, particularly in Rocky Mountain spotted fever (RMSF), therapy should be instituted when the diagnosis is suspected.

Confirmation of the diagnosis is almost always serologic and thus retrospective, because antibodies occur no earlier than the second week of illness in any of the rickettsioses. The Weil–Felix reaction, which depends on the development of agglutinating antibodies to the heterologous antigens of *Proteus* OX-2, OX-19, and OX-K, is not sensitive or specific enough to diagnose RMSF. Antibodies to specific rickettsial antigens can be detected by indirect immunofluorescence or enzyme immunoassay.

ROCKY MOUNTAIN SPOTTED FEVER

RMSF was first described in the late 1800s in the Bitterroot Valley of Idaho. Although originally recognized in the western United States, it now has a higher documented prevalence in the South Atlantic states and in the south-central region. The causative agent is *Rickettsia rickettsii*, a member of the spotted fever group of rickettsial infections.

Rickettsia rickettsii is transmitted to humans by the bite of an infected tick. Ticks are both the vectors and the main reservoirs of this agent; the specific tick responsible for transmission varies from region to region: In the eastern United States, the dog tick, *Dermacentor variabilis*, is the usual vector, whereas in the western United States it is the wood tick, *Dermacentor andersonii*. The adult tick transmits the disease to humans during feeding, releasing *R. rickettsii* from the salivary glands after feeding for 6 to 10 hours. Humans can also be infected by exposure to infected tick hemolymph, which may occur during the removal of ticks from persons or domestic animals, especially when the tick is crushed between the fingers.

The incubation of RMSF ranges from 2 to 14 days, with a median of 7 days. Virtually all patients have fever, usually above 38.9°C (102°F). The major diagnostic sign is the rash, seen in approximately 90% of the patients, which usually occurs within 3 to 5 days after the onset of fever. Fewer than half of the patients show the rash during the first 3 days of the illness. The rash typically starts around the wrists and ankles, but it may start on the trunk or be diffuse at onset. Although involvement of the palms is considered characteristic, this does not occur in all patients and often occurs late in the course of the disease (Figure 168.1). Other common symptoms include severe headache, myalgias, and gastrointestinal complaints such as nausea, vomiting, and severe abdominal pain.

Complications of RMSF include meningismus, meningitis, renal failure, pulmonary involvement, hepatic dysfunction with development of jaundice, splenomegaly, myocarditis, and thrombocytopenia. Although in the early reports the case fatality rate was greater than 20% in the absence of early therapy, in recent series of patients death occurs in 4% to 8% of the cases. In those with fulminant RMSF, death occurs 8 to 15 days after the onset of symptoms.

Diagnosis of RMSF is primarily based on a high clinical suspicion in the setting of a patient with fever, headache, and myalgias with exposure to ticks. Rash is found in only 14% of patients on the first day of illness and in 49% of patients during the first 3 days. Serological diagnosis is retrospective. A skin biopsy of a rash lesion (when present) can show *Rickettsia rickettsii* with immunohistochemistry or immunofluorescent staining. This has a specificity of 100% and a sensitivity of 70% but is useful only in patients who have developed a rash.

Treatment of RMSF requires the administration of an effective antibiotic for 7 days, continuing for 2 days after the patient has become afebrile. Early therapy is important, as the risk of death is 5 times greater in patients treated after day 5 of illness. The antibiotic of choice is oral doxycycline, 100 mg every 12 hours. Tetracycline, 25 to 50 mg/kg/day in 4 doses, is also effective. In patients with hypersensitivity to tetracyclines and in pregnant patients,

chloramphenicol, 50 to 75 mg/kg/day, is an alternative. Although tetracyclines are usually avoided in young children because they can cause staining of the teeth, doxycycline is recommended for children of all ages, both because RMSF is a life-threatening disease and because it is unlikely that a single course of doxycycline would cause staining of the teeth. Glucocorticosteriods have been given to severely ill patients in the past, but there is no documentation of their efficacy. No vaccine is currently available to prevent RMSF.

OTHER SPOTTED FEVER GROUP RICKETTSIA

There are 11 other members of the spotted fever group of *Rickettsia* that have been shown to cause infection in humans (listed in Table 168.1). Successful treatment for them has been reported using doxycycline (200 mg/day), tetracycline (25 mg/kg/day), chloramphenicol (2 g/day), or ciprofloxacin (1500 mg/day) for 5 to 7 days.

Rickettsia akari causes the nonfatal disease rickettsialpox, first reported in 1946 in New York but rarely diagnosed. The usual incidence in New York City is 5 cases per year, and it has been reported in eastern Europe, South Africa, and Korea. The reservoir for this infection is the house mouse, *Mus musculus*, and the vector for transmission to humans is the mouse mite *Allodermanyssus sanguineus*. A painless papule that ulcerates and forms an eschar occurs at the site of the mite bite some 3 to 7 days before the onset of symptoms in most cases. Manifestations include chills, fever, headache, myalgia, backache, and photophobia. Rigors and profuse diaphoresis may be seen. Within 2 to 3 days after onset, a generalized papulovesicular rash

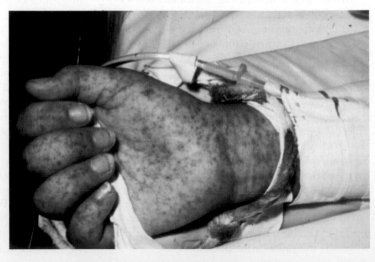

Figure 168.1 Petechial rash in Rocky Mountain spotted fever. (Courtesy of David Schlossberg, MD.)

Table 168.1 Diseases Caused by Rickettsia

Disease	Organism	Geographic Distribution	Vector
Spotted Fever Group			
Rocky Mountain spotted fever	*Rickettsia rickettsii*	Western Hemisphere	Tick
Boutonneuse	*Rickettsia conorii*	Africa, Mediterranean, India	Tick
Queensland tick typhus	*Rickettsia australis*	Australia	Tick
North Asian tick typhus	*Rickettsia sibirica*	Russia, Asia, Africa, France	Tick
Japanese spotted fever	*Rickettsia japonica*	Japan, China	Tick
Flinders Island spotted fever	*Rickettsia honei*	Australia, Thailand	Tick
African tick-bite fever	*Rickettsia africae*	Sub-Saharan Africa, West Indies	Tick
	Rickettsia parkeri	United States	Tick
	Rickettsia slovaca	Europe	Tick
	Rickettsia aeschlimannii	Africa	Tick
Fleaborne spotted fever	*Rickettsia felis*	Western Hemisphere, Europe	Flea
Rickettsialpox	*Rickettsia akari*	United States, Russia, Korea, Africa	Mite
Typhus Group			
Epidemic typhus	*Rickettsia prowazekii*	Western Hemisphere, Africa, Asia	Louse
Murine typhus	*Rickettsia typhi*	Worldwide	Flea
Scrub typhus	*Orientia tsutsugamushi*	Asia, Australia, South Pacific	Mite
Ehrlichia			
Human monocytotropic ehrlichiosis (HME)	*Ehrlichia chaffeensis*	North America, eastern Asia	Tick
Human granulocytotropic Anaplasmosis (HGA)	*Anaplasma phagocytophilum*	North America, Europe, Asia	Tick
Other			
Q fever	*Coxiella burnetii*	Worldwide	?Ticks

occurs. The rash begins as red papules 2 to 10 mm in diameter that vesiculate and heal by crusting. The disease is benign. Death and complications are very rare. Treatment is the same as the other *Rickettsia* with doxycycline, tetracycline, or chloramphenicol.

EPIDEMIC OR LOUSEBORNE TYPHUS

This classic plague of humanity is caused by *Rickettsia prowazekii* and transmitted by the human body louse *Pediculus humanus corporis*. The bacteria may remain latent in humans for many years after the initial infection and then relapse when persons are stressed by other disease or deprivations. Thus, during war and refugee exodus, when people are stressed and deprived and poor hygiene promotes the spread of lice, a rickettsemic person may initiate the cycle and cause an epidemic. This relapsing disease is generally milder than an initial attack, presumably because it occurs in a person with some established immunity. This recrudescent typhus is called Brill–Zinsser disease. An extrahuman reservoir has been identified in southern flying squirrels, *Glaucomys volans*, which are found throughout the eastern United

States. Humans are infected by flying squirrel fleas.

The characteristic incubation period is 8 to 16 days. The onset is usually abrupt, with intense headache, progressive fever, chills, and severe myalgia. Rash begins on about the fifth day of illness, usually on the axillary folds and upper trunk and spreads centrifugally. The rash begins as pink macules that fade on pressure but progresses to become maculopapular, darker, petechial, and nonfading on pressure. The rash may become confluent and involve the entire body, but the face, palms, and soles are spared. In the preantibiotic era, mortality was seen in 13%, occurring a median of 12.5 days after onset of the illness; survivors defervesced a median of 14 days after onset. Indigenously acquired typhus related to flying squirrel exposure is a similar but milder illness.

The established therapy for epidemic typhus is doxycycline (100 mg twice daily), tetracycline (25 to 50 mg/kg/day in 4 doses), or chloramphenicol (60 to 75 mg/kg/day in 4 doses) given for 7 to 10 days. In epidemic situations where the availability of doxycycline may be limited, a single dose of 200 mg of doxycycline may be effective, but a small proportion of patients may relapse. No vaccine is currently available for the prevention of typhus; the only prevention available is control of body lice by hygiene and insecticides such as permethrin.

MURINE TYPHUS

Murine typhus, caused by *Rickettsia typhi*, has worldwide distribution, especially in tropical and subtropical seaboard regions. Its most important reservoirs are *Rattus* spp., and the classic vector that spreads the organisms from rats to people is the flea *Xenopsylla cheopis*.

The disease is clinically less severe than epidemic typhus, with reported case fatality rates of 1% to 4%. Illness begins 1 to 2 weeks after a bite from an infected flea. At first it is nonspecific, with fever, headache, chills, myalgia, and nausea. Rash is seen in about 20% of patients at presentation and in about 50% sometime during the illness. The skin lesions are macular or maculopapular. The trunk is most often involved, but the extremities are involved in about half the patients who develop rash. The rash may also be seen on the palms and soles. The rash is frequently salmon colored and evanescent, but frank hemorrhagic vasculitic rash may develop. Occasionally, patients develop central nervous system (CNS) abnormalities, hepatic or renal failure, respiratory failure, or hematemesis.

Rickettsia typhi is treated with doxycycline, tetracycline, or chloramphenicol. Antimicrobial therapy should be continued for 2 to 3 days after defervescence.

SCRUB TYPHUS

Scrub typhus occurs when a larval stage trombiculid mite (chigger), infected with *Orientia tsutsugamushi*, bites a susceptible human host. The disease occurs from Korea and Japan to China, southeast Asia, India, and south to Australia.

Some 6 to 18 days after a chigger bite, the patient develops high fever, severe headache, mental changes, lymphadenopathy, and myalgia. An eschar may be found at the site of the bite. The severity of the signs and symptoms is widely variable, depending on the virulence of the responsible strain and the degree of susceptibility of the host. After about 5 days a macular rash, sometimes evanescent, may occur, beginning on the trunk and spreading to the extremities. Complications include

multiple organ system dysfunction and hemorrhage, pneumonia, heart failure, respiratory failure, and renal failure. Case fatality rates as high as 30% in untreated patients have been reported, but treatment shortens the duration of illness and essentially eliminates fatalities.

Doxycycline and chloramphenicol are the recommended treatments. Doxycycline can be given as a single dose of 200 mg or for a course of 3 to 7 days. Alternative drugs include rifampin (600–900 mg/day) and azithromycin (500 mg initial dose, then 250 mg daily).

Q FEVER

Q fever, an infection caused by *Coxiella burnetii*, can present as an acute infection with an influenzalike illness, including pulmonary and hepatic involvement, or it can develop into a chronic infection with endocarditis and chronic hepatitis.

Coxiella burnetii is an extremely infectious organism. In fact, a single inhaled organism is sufficient to initiate infection. It is endemic worldwide except in New Zealand. *Coxiella burnetii* infects many species of animals, and the infection usually results in long-lasting parasitism. Q fever in humans is usually caused by the inhalation of aerosolized particles from infected domestic animals; these particles can be airborne over long distances.

Infection with *C. burnetii* is often asymptomatic. Those with clinical illness most commonly have an acute febrile illness, which may be associated with pneumonia, hepatitis, or meningoencephalitis. Patients can go on to develop a chronic illness characterized by endocarditis and granulomatous hepatitis.

The incubation period for Q fever can be as short as 4 to 5 days, but it typically ranges from 9 to 39 days. Fever is the most common symptom, occurring in almost all patients, and the temperature often spikes to 40°C to 40.5°C (104°F to 105°F). Other signs and symptoms include chills, headache (often severe), retrobulbar pain, myalgias and arthralgias, neck pain and stiffness, pleuritic chest pain, cough, nausea and vomiting, diarrhea, jaundice, hepatomegaly, and splenomegaly. Unlike the rickettsial diseases, Q fever does not usually present with a rash, although a transient erythematous macular rash has been noted in about 4% of patients. The manifestations of Q fever usually resolve within 2 to 4 weeks, although some patients have had fever as long as 9 weeks. Case fatality rates from acute Q fever are very low (none in most series), but in hospitalized patients the case fatality rate has been reported as 2.4%.

Chronic Q fever is usually manifested by endocarditis, a rare, severe, and often fatal complication of *C. burnetii* infection. Most patients have pre-existing valvular heart disease, often a prosthetic valve. Other manifestations include chronic hepatitis, infections of vascular prostheses and aneurysms, osteomyelitis, and interstitial pulmonary fibrosis. The illness evolves slowly, manifesting any time from 1 to 20 years after the acute infection, and presents clinically as a culture-negative endocarditis, although fever is often absent in Q fever endocarditis.

The diagnosis of Q fever is based on clinical suspicion but can be confirmed by serological findings. Several tests are available to detect *C. burnetii*–specific antibodies in sera, including the complement fixation (CF) and the indirect fluorescent antibody (IFA) test. In acute Q fever, antibodies to the *C. burnetii* phase II antigen are produced, which become detectable 8 to 14 days after the onset of illness. Although a phase II CF titer of 1:8 or an IFA titer of greater than 1:50 is considered significant, confirmation of the diagnosis is made by a 4-fold rise in titer between acute and convalescent serum specimens. In chronic Q fever, the phase I antibody level becomes elevated. A phase I CF antibody titer greater than 1:200 or an immunoglobulin G IFA titer of 1:800 or greater is considered diagnostic for chronic Q fever.

Most acute Q fever infections resolve spontaneously, but because of the concern about the development of chronic Q fever and because some studies suggest that therapy shortens the duration of fever, we recommend specific antimicrobial therapy for acute Q fever. The treatment of choice is tetracycline or doxycycline for 2 weeks; other effective therapies include cotrimoxazole (trimethoprim–sulfamethoxazole), chloramphenicol, rifampin, and (in vitro) telithromycin.

The treatment of chronic Q fever has never been the subject of controlled studies. No antibiotics have been found to be bactericidal for *C. burnetii*, although several (including tetracycline, doxycycline, cotrimoxazole, rifampin, ciprofloxacin, and telithromycin) have been shown to be bacteriostatic. There are recommendations to use doxycycline in combination with a quinolone (such as ciprofloxacin), rifampin, or hydroxychloroquine, any of these regimens given for 2 years of treatment.

SUGGESTED READING

Bakken JS, Dumler JS. Human granulocytic ehrlichiosis. *Clin Infect Dis.* 2000; 31:554–560.

Bakken JS, Dumler JS. Clinical diagnosis and treatment of human granulocytotropic anaplasmosis. *Ann NY Acad Sci.* 2006;1078:236–247.

Holman RC, Paddock CD, Curns AT, et al. Analysis of risk factors for fatal Rocky Mountain spotted fever: evidence for superiority of tetracyclines for therapy. *J Infect Dis.* 2002;184:1437–1444.

Paddock CD, Zaki SR, Koss T, et al. Rickettsialpox in New York City: a persistent urban zoonosis. *Ann NY Acad Sci.* 2003;990:36–44.

Parker NR, Barralet JH, Bell AM. Q fever. *Lancet.* 2006;367(9511):679–688.

Reynolds MG, Krebs JS, Comer JA, et al. Flying squirrel-associated typhus, United States. *Emerg Infect Dis.* 2003;9:1341–1343.

169. Ehrlichiosis and Anaplasmosis

Johan S. Bakken and J. Stephen Dumler

Ehrlichiosis is the collective name for infections caused by obligate intracellular gram-negative bacteria in the genera *Ehrlichia* and *Anaplasma* that belong to the family Anaplasmataceae. Members of these two genera cycle in nature between invertebrate (arthropod) and vertebrate (mammalian) hosts, and some species occasionally cause zoonotic infections in humans. Three species are currently known to cause human tick-borne infection in the United States and Europe and include *Ehrlichia chaffeensis*, the agent of human monocytic ehrlichiosis (HME), *Ehrlichia ewingii*, the agent of human ewingii ehrlichiosis (HEE), and *Anaplasma phagocytophilum*, the agent of human granulocytic anaplasmosis (HGA).

In nature *Ehrlichia* and *Anaplasma* species reside in specific hard-body tick hosts, and the bacteria are passaged transstadially with each successive developmental tick stage. *Amblyomma americanum* (the Lone Star tick) is the tick vector for *E. chaffeensis* and *E. ewingii*, and the endemic range of the Lone Star tick is predominately in the south and southeastern United States from Maryland to Texas. In addition, all documented reports of human infections with these species have been limited to the North American continent. In contrast, *A. phagocytophilum* cycles within *Ixodes* species ticks, including *Ixodes scapularis* (the deer tick) in the eastern United States, *Ixodes pacificus* (the black-legged tick) in some regions of the U.S. Pacific coast (northern California, Oregon, and Washington), and *Ixodes ricinus* (the wood tick) and *Ixodes persulcatus* in Europe and Asia. *Ixodes* species ticks are also vectors for *Borrelia burgdorferi* (the agent of Lyme borreliosis), and most cases of HGA have been reported from the same areas where Lyme borreliosis occurs endemically. Thus far, HGA has been reported in 13 U.S. states and 11 countries in Europe, including Austria, the Czech Republic, France, Italy, Latvia, The Netherlands, Norway, Poland, Russia, Slovenia, Spain, and Sweden. Active surveillance studies in southeastern Missouri have identified HME incidence rates ranging as high as 414 cases per 100 000 population. Correspondingly, the incidence rate for HGA varied up to 58 cases per 100 000 in some regions of Connecticut and Wisconsin. Only a limited number of cases of HEE have been recognized in a few states in central United States, but it is anticipated to be common. Most cases of HME and HGA develop during the period between April and October, and as many as 75% of patients have noted 1 or more tick bites 1 to 2 weeks prior to the onset of symptoms. Male patients outnumber females by a factor of 3 to 2, and even though ehrlichiosis affects all age groups, symptomatic infection is less frequent in children. The assigned case fatality rate is 0.5% and 3.0% for HGA and HME, respectively. Table 169.1 summarizes some of the epidemiologic characteristics associated with HME, HEE, and HGA.

When the tick vector takes a blood meal from a mammal host bacteria become injected with the tick saliva into the mammal host. Once injected the bacteria preferentially infect specific circulating leukocytes and cause a nonspecific febrile illness. *Ehrlichia chaffeensis* typically infects monocytes and macrophages, whereas *E. ewingii* and *A. phagocytophilum* infect neutrophilic granulocytes. The bacteria adhere to specific leukocyte cell-membrane receptors and enter through the host cell cytoplasmic membrane by endocytosis. Once inside, the bacteria reside within cytoplasmic endosomes, where they multiply to form infectious aggregates called morulae (Latin), because of the resemblance to a mulberry. Through a combination of direct and indirect effects, the bacteria subvert the host cell, allowing it to tolerate their presence by altering intracellular signaling and the cell regulatory gene response (eg, the phagosome maturation process to develop into a lysosome vesicle becomes arrested, the host cell oxidative burst response is downregulated, and the timed onset of host cell apoptosis is delayed).

Even though they differ with respect to epidemiology and geographical distribution, HME, HEE, and HGA present as clinically similar illnesses with similar characteristic, albeit nonspecific alterations in routine hematologic and chemistry laboratory tests. The incubation

Table 169.1 Epidemiologic Characteristics, Incidence Rates and Reported Cases Associated with Human Monocytic Ehrlichiosis (HME), Human Ewingii Ehrlichiosis (HEE), and Human Granulocytic Anaplasmosis (HGA) in the United States (USA)

Bacterial Species	Ehrlichia Chaffeensis	Ehrlichia Ewingii	Anaplasma Phagocytophilum
Tick vector	*Amblyomma americanum*	*A. americanum*	*Ixodes ricinus* *Ixodes scapularis* *Ixodes pacificus*
Clinical illness	HME	HEE	HGA
Year first reported	1987	1999	1994
Known geographic distribution	Mid-Atlantic USA Southeast USA South Central USA	South Central USA	North and central Europe Upper Atlantic (USA) Upper Midwest (USA) Pacific coast (USA)
Target leukocyte	Monocyte Macrophage	Neutrophilic granulocyte	Neutrophilic granulocyte
Incidence rate (cases/10 000)	6	Unknown	14
Reported cases (*n*)*	2845	≤50	3505

period for HME, HEE, and HGA varies between 1 and 2 weeks following tick exposure or a recognized tick bite. The symptoms and signs of ehrlichiosis range from asymptomatic to fatal disease, and clinical severity varies proportionally with patient age and comorbid illnesses. HME, HEE, and HGA are clinical syndromes and are most commonly manifested by the abrupt onset of nonspecific fever, shaking chills, severe headache, and myalgias (Table 169.2), but diagnosis may be difficult because of the undifferentiated nature of the symptoms. Between one-third and one-half of patients who become symptomatic require hospitalization for up to 1 week or longer.

Laboratory test abnormalities observed with HME, HEE, and HGA are similar and nonspecific and include various permutations of leukopenia and thrombocytopenia with a differential leukocyte count that often reveals increased proportions of band neutrophils and a corresponding decrease in the lymphocyte concentrations. In addition, most patients manifest mild to moderate increases in serum hepatic transaminase concentrations suggesting hepatocellular injury. Albeit relatively insensitive, the diagnosis can be confirmed by blood smear examination, because morulae may be observed in peripheral blood leukocytes of 1% to 20% of patients with HME and as many as 60% of patients with HGA during the first week of infection (Figure 169.1). Polymerase chain reaction (PCR) is also an excellent tool for diagnosing HME, HEE, and HGA during

the early stage of infection, and sensitivity and specificity rates range from approximately 50% and >95%. However, the availability of PCR is currently limited to large commercial, academic medical, or public health reference laboratories. More than 95% of patients with HME and HGA form specific antibodies during the course of the infection, and serologic testing of acute and convalescent sera using the indirect fluorescent antibody (IFA) detection is currently the most sensitive method for laboratory confirmation of HME and HGA, even though the diagnosis can only be arrived at retrospectively. No specific serologic test exists for HEE.

Laboratory criteria for diagnosis of probable HME and HGA include a compatible exposure history and clinical illness combined with (a) the detection of morulae in peripheral blood, (b) a single positive IFA titer, or (c) positive PCR of acute phase blood. The criteria for a confirmed case of HME or HGA requires (a) demonstration of seroconversion (4-fold or greater change in serum antibody titer) with *E. chaffeensis* or *A. phagocytophilum*, (b) isolation of *E. chaffeensis* or *A. phagocytophilum* in culture from blood, or (c) a single elevated IFA titer combined with either detection of morulae in the peripheral blood smear *or* a positive PCR.

THERAPY

Ehrlichia and *Anaplasma* are uniformly susceptible to tetracycline, tetracycline derivatives, and rifampin. However, in vitro antibiotic

Table 169.2 Symptoms and Signs Observed in Patients with Human Monocytic Ehrlichiosis (HME) and Human Granulocytic Anaplasmosis (HGA)

Prevalence of Complaint	Symptom or Sign	HME (%) N = 155–633	HGA (%) N = 232–521
Common	Fever (T > 38.0°C)	97	94
	Malaise	82	97
	Headache	80	72
	Rigors	61	82
	Myalgias	57	86
Less common	Anorexia	66	48
	Nausea	64	39
	Arthralgias	41	40
Uncommon	Diarrhea	23	8
	Cough	26	21
	Confusion	19	14
	Rash	31	6

Abbreviation: T = temperature.

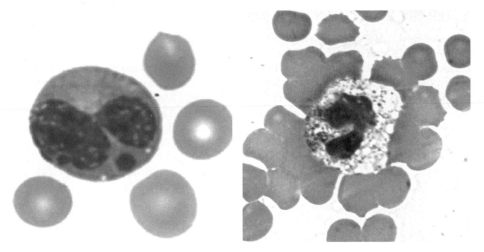

Figure 169.1 *Ehrlichia chaffeensis* morula (**left**) in a peripheral blood monocyte, and *Anaplasma phagocytophilum* morula (**right**) in a peripheral blood neutrophil (Wright stain; original magnifications: 360× and 400×, respectively).

susceptibility testing of obligate intracellular bacteria is complicated, and treatment recommendations have therefore been based on the experience from empirical antibiotic treatment of infected humans as well as animals. Even though HME and HGA can manifest as self-limited febrile illnesses that often resolve spontaneously without therapy, it is currently recommended that any patient who is diagnosed with acute infection should receive active antibiotic treatment. Doxycycline, 100 mg administered twice daily (oral or intravenous route), is the treatment of choice for adults. Doxycycline, 2 mg/kg, maximum dose 100 mg, given twice daily, is also the preferred treatment for children who are seriously ill. The

response to doxycycline therapy is rapid, and most patients become afebrile and resolve their symptoms within 24 to 36 hours. In fact, failure to respond to doxycycline therapy should prompt further clinical evaluation of the patient for an alternative diagnosis. The optimal duration of therapy with doxycycline has not been established. Serologic surveys have demonstrated that 15% to 20% of patients with active HGA also are seroreactive with *Borrelia burgdorferi*, the agent of Lyme borreliosis. Doxycycline therapy should therefore be administered for 10 to 14 days to ensure adequate coverage for potential co-incubating Lyme borreliosis.

Although no trials to show clinical efficacy have been conducted, treatment with rifampin may be considered for patients who have specific contraindications to tetracycline drugs, including pregnant women, patients who have known hypersensitivity to tetracycline class drugs, and children younger than 8 years who have a mild to moderate illness suitable for management in the outpatient setting. The dose of rifampin is 300 mg given twice daily for adults and 10 mg/kg (maximum dose 300 mg) twice daily for children for 5 to 7 days.

Human ehrlichiosis is for the most part a self-limited clinical illness that resolves spontaneously, even without active antibiotic therapy. Unlike Lyme borreliosis, HME, HEE, and HGA have not been reported to be associated with persistent infection. The long-term prognosis after resolved HME, HEE, and HGA appears favorable, and patients should expect to make a complete recovery.

SUGGESTED READING

Aguero-Rosenfeld ME, Horowitz HW, Wormser GP, et al. Human granulocytic ehrlichiosis: a case series from a medical center in New York State. *Ann Intern Med.* 1996;125:904–908.

Bakken JS, Dumler JS. Ehrlichiosis and anaplasmosis. *Infect Med.* 2004;21:433–451.

Bakken JS, Dumler JS. Clinical diagnosis and treatment of human granulocytotropic anaplasmosis. *Ann NY Acad Sci.* 2006; 1078:236–247.

Bakken JS, Dumler JS, Chen SM, Eckman MR, Van Etta LL, Walker DH. Human granulocytic ehrlichiosis in the upper Midwest United States. A new species emerging? *JAMA.* 1994;272:212–218.

Buller RS, Arens M, Hmiel SP, et al. Ehrlichia ewingii, a newly recognized agent of human ehrlichiosis. *N Engl J Med.* 1999; 341:148–155.

Chapman AS, Bakken JS, Folk SM, et al. Diagnosis and management of tickborne rickettsial diseases: Rocky Mountain spotted fever, ehrlichioses, and anaplasmosis—United States: a practical guide for physicians and other health-care and public health professionals. *MMWR Recomm Rep.* 2006;55:1–27.

Dumler JS. Anaplasma and Ehrlichia infection. *Ann NY Acad Sci.* 2005;1063:361–373.

Fishbein DB, Dawson JE, Robinson LE. Human ehrlichiosis in the United States, 1985 to 1990. *Ann Intern Med.* 1994; 120:736–743.

Maeda K, Markowitz N, Hawley RC, Ristic M, Cox D, McDade JE. Human infection with Ehrlichia canis, a leukocytic rickettsia. *N Engl J Med.* 1987;316:853–856.

Olano JP, Hogrefe W, Seaton B, Walker DH. Clinical manifestations, epidemiology, and laboratory diagnosis of human monocytotropic ehrlichiosis in a commercial laboratory setting. *Clin Diagn Lab Immunol.* 2003;10:891–896.

Specific Organisms – Fungi

Specific Organisms – Fungi

170. Candidiasis

Christopher F. Carpenter and Jorgelina de Sanctis

Candida species are common causes of disease ranging from superficial cutaneous and mucocutaneous infections to invasive infections such as candidemia and disseminated candidiasis. There are more than 150 species of *Candida*, but only 9 are frequent human pathogens. The most common isolate is *Candida albicans* (Figure 170.1); other encountered pathogens include *Candida tropicalis* (Figure 170.2), *Candida parapsilosis*, *Candida glabrata*, *Candida krusei* (Figure 170.3), *Candida kefyr*, *Candida lusitaniae*, *Candida dubliniensis*, and *Candida gulliermondii*. Less commonly isolated species with medical significance include *Candida lipolytica*, *Candida famata*, *Candida rugosa*, *Candida viswanathii*, *Candida haemulonii*, *Candida norvegensis*, *Candida catenulate*, *Candida ciferri*, *Candida intermedia*, *Candida utilis*, *Candida lambica*, *Candida pulcherrima*, and *Candida zeylanoides*. Most species are commensal organisms, colonizing the skin, gastrointestinal tract, and vagina, and they become opportunistic pathogens only when the host has compromised immunologic or mechanical defenses or when there are changes in the host's normal flora, such as those triggered by broad-spectrum antibiotic use.

Diagnosis of *Candida* infections continues to be primarily via culture, although the insensitivity, and at times protracted nature, of contemporary yeast culture methods have prompted the development of rapid and sensitive nonculture diagnostic methods, including polymerase chain reaction (PCR) and antigen detection assays. For example, an enzymatic assay (Fungitell, Associates of Cape Cod, Inc.) for β-1,3-D-glucan, a unique component of the cell wall in many fungi that is detectable in serum during invasive candidiasis, was recently approved for clinical use. New methods to reduce time to species identification are also now available, for example, the CHROMagar Candida (CHROMagar Microbiology) (Figure 170.4) and PNA FISH (AdvanDx) tests. Given that several *Candida* species have intrinsic or a high rate of acquired resistance to antifungal agents, these tests may prove to be cost-effective approaches for guiding early appropriate antifungal therapy in

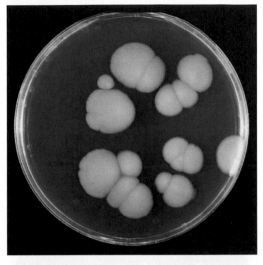

Figure 170.1 *Candida albicans*, SABHI agar plate. (Courtesy of Dr. William Kaplan, CDC Public Health Image Library.)

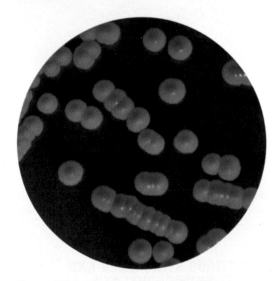

Figure 170.2 *Candida tropicalis*. CHROMagar. (Courtesy of Troy Biologicals, Inc.)

certain clinical settings. Furthermore, as with resistance in bacterial and viral pathogens, the level of acquired resistance for certain *Candida* species has risen, presumably in part due to an increased use of antifungal agents (Table 170.1). Fortunately, newer antifungal agents have

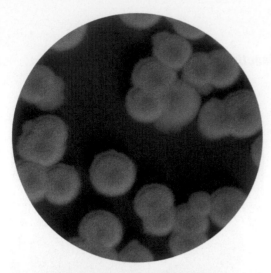

Figure 170.3 *Candida krusei*. CHROMagar. (Courtesy of Troy Biologicals, Inc.)

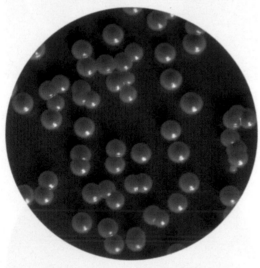

Figure 170.4 *Candida albicans*. CHROMagar (Courtesy of Troy Biologicals, Inc.)

become available for the treatment of *Candida* infections, including advance generation triazoles and the echinocandins (Table 170.2).

INFECTIOUS SYNDROMES AND TREATMENT/PROPHYLAXIS

Mucocutaneous Candida Syndromes

CUTANEOUS CANDIDIASIS

Primary cutaneous candidiasis is commonly seen in normal hosts manifesting as diaper dermatitis and intertriginous infections. Other manifestations include balanitis, vulvitis, paronychia, onychia, and folliculitis. Cutaneous candidiasis most commonly presents in skin areas that are moist and/or occluded, although other areas where altered local skin immunity has occurred, such as burn sites, are susceptible to infection. Patients who are systemically immunocompromised, including patients with diabetes mellitus, are also at increased risk. The diagnosis is usually made on clinical grounds. Findings may include an erythematous rash of intertriginous areas, such as the inguinal region, with satellite lesions, or the lesions may be papular, pustular, or ulcerated. Microscopic examination of skin scrapings revealing budding yeast cells and hyphae may be used to confirm the diagnosis. Positive cultures for *Candida* species may also assist with diagnosis; however, false-positive results may occur because of colonization or contamination and thus culture is generally not recommended. Bacterial superinfection may also occur with cutaneous candidiasis and necessitates concomitant antibacterial treatment. Nonantimicrobial methods are important in both prophylaxis and treatment of cutaneous candidiasis. These include maintenance of a dry skin surface, frequent diaper changes, and control of hyperglycemia in diabetics. Topical antifungals such as nystatin cream or an imidazole cream, applied twice daily, are the mainstay of treatment. Systemic therapy for paronychia or onychia with fluconazole, itraconazole, or terbinafine may be required.

CHRONIC MUCOCUTANEOUS CANDIDIASIS

Individuals with chronic mucocutaneous candidiasis suffer from persistent and recurrent *Candida* infections of the skin, nails, and mucous membranes. The disease is a complex disorder that may manifest as one of many different syndromes with variable severity. It can occur at any age but is most commonly recognized in children younger than 3 years. T-cell dysfunction is the primary immune abnormality associated with chronic mucocutaneous candidiasis, although deficits in humoral immunity, neutrophil function, and complement activity are also often found. The disorder may also be associated with abnormal function of the thyroid, parathyroid, and/or adrenal glands, as well as with diabetes mellitus, thymoma, and interstitial keratitis. Other opportunistic bacterial or viral infections may occur. Other than esophagitis, invasive infections are rarely encountered.

Therapy for mucosal infections is dominated by the triazole antifungal agents. These drugs may be used topically or systemically and are safe and efficacious. A significant problem with mucosal disease is its propensity for repeated

Table 170.1 *Candida* Species and Susceptibility Patterns

Species	Triazoles		Extended-Spectrum Triazoles	Polyenes	Echinocandins	Risk Factors
	Fluconazole	Itraconazole	Voriconazole Posaconazole	Amphotericin B	Caspofungin, Anidulafungin, and Micafungin	
C. albicans	S	S	S	S	S	HIV/AIDS, surgery
C. glabrata	S-DD to R	R	S-I	S-I	S	Hematologic malignancies, azole prophylaxis
C. parapsilosis	S	S-DD	S	S	S-I	Foreign bodies, azole prophylaxis, neonates
C. tropicalis	S	S	S	S	S	Neutropenia
C. krusei	R	R	S	S-I	S	Hematologic malignancies, azole prophylaxis
C. guillermondii	S	S	S	R	S	Azole prophylaxis, previous amphotericin treatment
C. lusitaniae	S	S	S	R	S	Previous amphotericin treatment

Abbreviations: HIV = human immunodeficiency virus; AIDS = acquired immunodeficiency syndrome; S = susceptible; S-DD = susceptible-dose dependent; S-I = intermediate; R = resistant.

Table 170.2 Antifungal Agents

Class	Antifungal
Polyene	Conventional amphotericin B Lipid formulations of amphotericin B (liposomal amphotericin B, amphotericin B lipid complex, and amphotericin B colloid dispersion)
Triazole	Fluconazole Itraconazole Voriconazole (extended spectrum) Posaconazole (extended spectrum)
Echinocandin	Caspofungin Anidulafungin Micafungin

relapses. This occurs in some special situations (immunocompromised hosts), therefore requiring long-term suppression, with the associated risk of resistance emergence.

OROPHARYNGEAL AND ESOPHAGEAL CANDIDIASIS

As normal members of the gastrointestinal tract flora, *Candida* species become pathogenic in the oropharynx and esophagus in patients with various risk factors, including impaired cell-mediated immunity (eg, human immunodeficiency virus [HIV] infection, chronic mucocutaneous candidiasis, stem cell and solid organ transplant recipients), diabetes mellitus, extremes of age, or esophageal achalasia or reflux or the use of progesterone, broad-spectrum antibiotics, or immunosuppressive medications such as corticosteroids.

Oral candidiasis most commonly presents as thrush: painless white pseudomembranous plaques on the surfaces of the oropharynx that can be removed by scraping with a tongue blade. It may also present in more symptomatic forms as erythematous mucosal patches without the pseudomembranous plaques (erythematous candidiasis), rough plaques that cannot be removed by scraping (*Candida* leukoplakia or hyperplastic candidiasis), and cracking and erythema at the corners of the lips (angular cheilitis). As with cutaneous candidiasis, the diagnosis is usually made clinically; however, microscopic examination of scrapings can confirm diagnosis (again, culture is not recommended because colonization commonly occurs). Empirical therapy with a topical antifungal should be considered for oral thrush unless it is associated with esophageal candidiasis, in which case systemic therapy is usually required. Nystatin suspension or clotrimazole troches are common first-line agents for oropharyngeal candidiasis; however, both require frequent administration. Systemic therapy with fluconazole and other azoles is also effective for thrush and may occasionally be required. Maintenance therapy in patients with chronic immunosuppression may be necessary, although this may lead to emergence of resistant *Candida* species and thus should be avoided if possible. In patients with HIV, antiretroviral therapy, via reconstitution of the immune system, routinely leads to a resolution of oral candidiasis. Angular cheilitis may be treated with topical imidazole creams or nystatin.

Esophageal candidiasis often presents as a sense of obstruction and/or pain (retrosternal, subxiphoid, or rarely cervical) on swallowing and can be mimicked by or coincide with cytomegalovirus esophagitis, herpes simplex virus esophagitis, esophageal aphthous ulcers, eosinophilic esophagitis, or pill esophagitis. The infection ranges from superficial to erosive, and patients also may be asymptomatic. Empirical therapy is frequently initiated with a systemic triazole antifungal (usually fluconazole); rarely in refractory esophageal infections, an echinocandin, extended-spectrum triazole, or low dose amphotericin B may be required, and in some patients long-term suppressive therapy might be needed. In refractory cases, esophagoscopy with mucosal brushings or biopsy may be necessary to confirm the diagnosis, test for antifungal resistance, and evaluate for other potential concomitant pathogens or disorders (Figures 170.5 and 170.6).

VULVOVAGINAL CANDIDIASIS

Vulvovaginal candidiasis (VVC) is a common infection in women of childbearing age and is the most common form of mucosal candidiasis. Although pregnancy, oral contraceptive use, antibiotic use, diabetes mellitus, HIV infection, intrauterine devices, and diaphragm use may be identified as predisposing host risk factors, often no precipitating factor can be found. Vaginal candidiasis often occurs in conjunction with vulvar candidiasis, and VVC may be classified as complicated or uncomplicated on the basis of clinical presentation, microbiology, host factors, and response to therapy (Table 170.3). The mechanism by which asymptomatic colonization transforms into symptomatic VVC

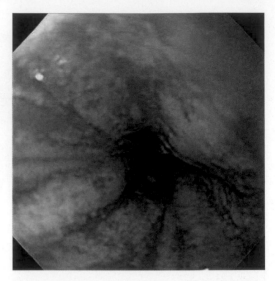

Figure 170.5 Endoscopic view, candida esophagitis.

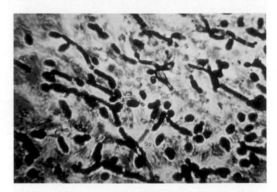

Figure 170.6 Photomicrograph of esophageal candidiasis (silver stain, ×100). (Courtesy of Sherry Brinkman, CDC Public Health Image Library.)

remains unclear. The clinical manifestations of VVC are primarily vulvar pruritus and vaginal discharge. Dyspareunia, dysuria, and vaginal irritation also may be present, although none of these symptoms are very sensitive or specific for VVC. Signs include erythema and edema of the vulva with erythema of the vagina. There may be no or minimal vaginal discharge of variable consistency. As with other forms of mucocutaneous candidiasis, the diagnosis is typically made clinically, but confirmation is easily obtained by observing budding yeast, with or without pseudohyphae, on a wet mount or 10% potassium hydroxide preparation of vaginal secretions; concurrent evaluation for other pathogens is also important.

Uncomplicated VVC may be effectively treated by short-course topical formulation (single dose and regimens of 1–3 days). Fluconazole as a single dose of 150 mg is

Table 170.3 Classification of Vulvovaginal Candidiasis (VVC)

Uncomplicated VVC	Complicated VVC
All of the following: • Sporadic and infrequent VVC • Mild to moderate VVC • Likely to be *Candida albicans* • Nonimmunocompromised women	At least one of the following: • Recurrent VVC • Severe VVC • Non-*albicans* VVC • Women with uncontrolled diabetes mellitus, debilitation, or immunosuppression, or women who are pregnant

Source: CDC, *Sexually Transmitted Diseases Treatment Guidelines.* MMWR. 2006; 55: RR-11.

commonly used. The topically applied imidazoles are more effective than nystatin. Treatment with azoles results in relief of symptoms and negative cultures in 80% to 90% of patients who complete therapy. Complicated VVC, including recurrent VVC (RVVC, usually defined as 4 or more episodes of symptomatic VVC in 1 year), affects a small percentage of women (≤5%). Vaginal cultures should be obtained to confirm the clinical diagnosis and to identify unusual species, including non-*albicans* species, particularly *Candida glabrata,* for which conventional antifungal therapies may not be as effective. Each individual episode of RVVC caused by *C. albicans* usually responds well to short-duration oral or topical azole therapy; however, some specialists recommend a longer duration of initial therapy (7–14 days). Suppressive antifungal therapy is effective in reducing RVVC. Unfortunately, 30% to 50% of women will have recurrent disease after suppressive therapy is discontinued. VVC in pregnancy should be managed with only topical imidazoles, and therapy in patients with HIV should not differ from that for seronegative women.

Candidemia and Disseminated Candidiasis

CANDIDEMIA

Candida species are the fourth most common cause of nosocomial bloodstream infection in the United States. Crude mortality rates of candidemia range from 30% to 61% with attributable mortality ranging as high as 49%. There are several reasons for the high mortality associated with candidemia, including the ability of *Candida* spp. to form biofilms on catheters and other surfaces, creating a difficult-to-eradicate nidus of infection. Despite an increased recognition of risk factors for invasive *Candida* infection, it remains very difficult to clinically predict which patients will develop infection.

For example, colonization with yeast remains a leading risk factor for infection in the intensive care unit (ICU). However, the prevalence of colonization in the ICU is high (50%–70% or more), which corresponds to a low predictive value given the relatively low rate of invasive infection. Nevertheless, colonization in ICU patients with unexplained fever, leukocytosis, and hypotension merits strong consideration of invasive candidiasis and candidemia as a potential cause. Candidemia is defined as the isolation, from at least 1 blood culture, of a pathogenic *Candida* species, and all patients with candidemia require treatment. It is often catheter related and when possible, all vascular devices should be removed. Furthermore, it is important to determine the extent of the infection to define both the prognosis as well as the treatment course. The susceptibility of the host is also important, as dissemination to areas such as the eye, liver, spleen, kidney, heart, skin and soft tissues, bone, central nervous system (CNS), and gastrointestinal tract may occur more commonly in those who are immunocompromised. These organs/systems often (approaching 50% of all deep infections) may also be infected without culture evidence of candidemia.

All patients with candidemia should be treated aggressively. In general, amphotericin B formulations, the triazoles, and the echinocandins play a role in treatment. *Candida albicans* is usually susceptible to most antifungals, including fluconazole, whereas other species are more likely to demonstrate reduced susceptibility or resistance to select antifungals. For example, *C. krusei* is intrinsically resistant to fluconazole and itraconazole but is usually susceptible to the extended-spectrum triazoles, echinocandins, and amphotericin B formulations. *Candida glabrata* has dose-dependant susceptibility to fluconazole and itraconazole, and it may be frankly resistant to these antifungals. It also typically shows some degree of cross-resistance to the newer triazoles, although both voriconazole and posaconazole offer significantly more activity. The echinocandins have activity against most *Candida* species, although *C. parapsilosis* typically has relatively higher minimum inhibitory concentrations to these antifungals; the clinical relevance of this finding is not clear.

For clinically stable nonneutropenic patients, potential antifungal choices include fluconazole (6 mg/kg/day), voriconazole (6 mg/kg every 12 hours on day 1 then 3–4 mg/kg every 12 hours), caspofungin (70 mg on day 1 followed by 50 mg/day), micafungin (100 mg/day), anidulafungin (200 mg on day 1 followed by 100 mg/day), amphotericin B (0.6–1.0 mg/kg/day), or a lipid-based amphotericin B formulation (generally dosed between 3 and 5 mg/kg/day). Higher doses and/or combination therapy may be required in patients with a suboptimal response or risk factors for a poor outcome. For patients who are neutropenic or who are deteriorating and unstable, initial treatment with amphotericin B or lipid-based amphotericin B formulation, an echinocandin, or combination therapy may be considered. All treatments should be extended for at least 2 weeks after the last positive blood culture and resolution of sepsis; for neutropenic patients resolution of neutropenia should also factor into the decision to stop therapy.

CHRONIC DISSEMINATED CANDIDIASIS

Chronic disseminated candidiasis (CDC, formerly hepatosplenic candidiasis) is an indolent process most commonly found in patients with severe persistent neutropenia (eg, in patients with acute leukemia or stem cell transplant recipients) that frequently becomes apparent when the neutrophil count is recovering. It typically involves the liver and/or spleen, although other organs such as the kidney or lung may be involved. Computed tomography (CT) or magnetic resonance imaging (MRI) studies are more than 90% sensitive, but only later in the disease course. Typically, multiple small hepatic and splenic abscesses are identified. Signs and symptoms of CDC include right upper quadrant tenderness, elevated transaminases and alkaline phosphatase concentrations, and hepatosplenomegaly; none are particularly sensitive or specific. Blood cultures are often negative, and biopsy may be required to confirm the diagnosis. Often, fluconazole is used in the initial management of nonneutropenic, stable patients. In neutropenic or unstable patients or in patients infected with a non-*albicans* species,

an amphotericin B formulation, extended-spectrum triazole, or an echinocandin should be considered for therapy. Therapy should be continued until calcification or resolution of lesions. Notably, in patients who receive repeated courses of antineoplastic therapy or who persistently remain immunosuppressed, prolonged suppression may be required (please see previous section, Candidemia, for recommended dosing).

Other Forms of Invasive Candidiasis

ENDOCARDITIS

Patients with *Candida* endocarditis and patients with bacterial endocarditis share both risk factors (intravenous drug use, cardiac surgery, prosthetic heart valves, abnormal native heart valves, and central venous catheters) and clinical presentation (fever, nonspecific signs and symptoms, cardiac murmur, and congestive heart failure). Mycotic emboli to major arteries are more common in *Candida* endocarditis, and blood cultures are often negative. The diagnosis should be considered in all patients with candidemia. Evidence of a valvular vegetation by transthoracic or the more sensitive transesophageal echocardiogram, establishes the diagnosis. Definitive treatment requires surgical resection of the infected valve (histopathologic examination and culture of the valvular material should be obtained for confirmation and susceptibility testing) and administration of an amphotericin B formulation plus flucytosine, 25 to 37.5 mg/kg orally 4 times a day, for 6 to 8 weeks after the surgery. There are several case reports of successful treatment of *Candida* endocarditis with caspofungin, and combination therapy may also be considered (eg, an azole with an echinocandin or amphotericin B), although evidence is lacking. Chronic suppression with fluconazole may be an alternative when the valve cannot be replaced. Patients should be monitored for a minimum of 1 year postoperatively due to the propensity for relapse (please see Candidemia section for recommended dosing).

CENTRAL NERVOUS SYSTEM INFECTIONS

Meningitis is the most common form of CNS candidiasis. Other forms of infection include mycotic aneurysms and cerebral abscesses. Low-birth-weight or premature infants and immunosuppressed hosts are at increased risk for *Candida* meningitis. Other risk factors include thermal burns, recent neurosurgery, and the presence of ventricular shunts and drains. Signs and symptoms are similar, yet often less severe, when compared with bacterial meningitis, and typically there is a more indolent and chronic course. Cerebrospinal fluid (CSF) analysis reveals a monocytic or neutrophilic pleocytosis, elevated protein, and either normal or depressed glucose. The diagnosis is difficult because the organism is present in low numbers in the CSF and the yield of standard CSF cultures is poor, thus repeated CSF cultures may be required. Combined therapy with amphotericin B (0.7–1.0 mg/kg/day) and 5-flucytosine (targeting serum levels of 40–60 µg/mL) is recommended as initial therapy; other antifungals may also be of benefit but are poorly studied. The antifungals should be continued for at least 4 weeks after resolution of signs and symptoms of infection. Removal of any ventricular shunt or drain is usually required to achieve eradication.

OCULAR INFECTIONS

Ocular candidiasis presents most commonly as chorioretinitis rather than endophthalmitis. Up to 15% of patients with candidemia have retinal lesions, often visible within 1 week of the onset of illness. The mortality rate in ICU patients with *Candida* endophthalmitis appears to be considerably higher than the mortality rate in patients with candidemia alone. Diagnosis requires a high degree of clinical suspicion. All patients with candidemia should be screened for sight-threatening endophthalmitis by an ophthalmologist; however, additional screening is advocated up to 2 weeks after negative findings on initial expert examination. Other manifestations may include iritis, choroidal neovascular membrane formation, and retinal detachment. Lesions may be sight threatening; diagnosis relies on characteristic ocular findings such as white lesions on the retina with ill-defined borders with possible vitreal extension. Vitreal aspiration may be required for diagnosis. The sensitivity of vitreous humor cultures remains low, ranging from 33% to 50%. PCR testing of vitreous samples may also play a role in ocular candidiasis. Symptoms may include bulbar pain, scotomas, and blurred vision. Recommended systemic therapy for endophthalmitis includes an amphotericin B formulation with or without flucytosine or fluconazole monotherapy at doses for candidemia. Fluconazole has superior vitreal penetration and less toxicity compared with amphotericin B. Voriconazole has also good ocular tissue penetration. Few data are available to support the use of echinocandins or newer triazoles. Typically, up to 6 to 12 weeks of therapy is anticipated for endophthalmitis. Vitrectomy with intravitreal amphotericin B should be considered for severe endophthalmitis, or evidence of progression or an absence of response (see also Chapter 15, Endophthalmitis).

GASTROINTESTINAL CANDIDIASIS

Candida peritonitis may develop in patients on peritoneal dialysis, after gastrointestinal surgery, as a complication of candidemia, or as an extension of local organ or tissue infection. In addition, gastric and duodenal mucosal infections may develop in patients with peptic ulcer disease or mucosal neoplasm. Other rare intra-abdominal manifestations of *Candida* infection include isolated pancreatic abscess, gangrenous cholecystitis, and obstruction of the common bile duct with a *Candida* fungus ball. *Candida albicans* is the predominant species isolated in intra-abdominal infections, but *C. glabrata* has assumed an increasing role in some centers. Diagnosis is made by paracentesis or by endoscopic, percutaneous, or open biopsy. Therapy with an amphotericin B formulation or fluconazole is reasonable for initial therapy; extended-spectrum triazoles and the echinocandins may also be considered, especially if non-*albicans* species are suspected or documented. Surgical exploration should be considered, and removal of any devices is also warranted.

BONE AND SOFT-TISSUE INFECTION

Bone and soft-tissue infections are rare complications of *Candida* dissemination or direct extension of a local *Candida* infection and are diagnosed by needle aspiration or via surgical debridement. They also may result from exogenous inoculation during trauma, intra-articular injection, a surgical procedure, or injection drug use. Treatment usually requires a combination of surgical debridement and often prolonged systemic antifungals, and either amphotericin B or high-dose fluconazole should be considered for initial therapy; extended-spectrum triazoles and echinocandins may have a role as well, but few data are available.

RESPIRATORY TRACT CANDIDIASIS

Pneumonia due to *Candida* sp. is very rare and poorly defined as a clinical entity because positive cultures cannot distinguish between true infection and either colonization or contamination of samples with oropharyngeal contents. This infection may be primary (eg, due to aspiration) or secondary (eg, due to hematogenous seeding). Without firm diagnostic criteria, the determination of appropriate antifungal therapy is difficult. In one review the only criterion found of documented primary *Candida* pneumonia was histologic demonstration of the fungus in lung tissue. Therapy with conventional amphotericin B is recommended, and triazoles and echinocandins may also have a role.

Patients with *Candida* empyema generally have an underlying predisposing condition such as malignancy. Most cases are nosocomially acquired, occurring frequently with concomitant bacterial infection. Diagnosis is made with isolation of a fungal species from an exudative pleural effusion in association with clinical signs of infection. Treatment via drainage and systemic antifungals with an amphotericin B formulation or fluconazole is appropriate. The newer triazoles and echinocandins also may be considered, but data are limited.

GENITOURINARY *CANDIDA* INFECTIONS

The isolation of *Candida* in the urine is common in hospitalized or nursing home patients, especially in those with indwelling urinary catheters. It is often difficult to distinguish patients with asymptomatic candiduria from those with true *Candida* urinary tract infections. Infections are more common and potentially more serious in patients who are taking broad-spectrum antibiotics or immunosuppressive agents, in patients with diabetes mellitus or who are otherwise immunosuppressed, and in patients with genitourinary abnormalities (including obstructive uropathy and renal transplant recipients). The diagnosis is problematic, as high colony count is not a strong indicator of infection, and pyuria in this setting is not always helpful. Frequently, the clinical suspicion combined with signs and symptoms of infection and culture results post removal of the catheter may be all that is available for the clinician. In most episodes of candiduria, catheter removal is often all that is required. *Candida* infection of the bladder also must be distinguished from infection of the kidney, although the two entities can coexist. Invasive infection of the kidney is unusual and is more difficult to treat. Other genitourinary syndromes (eg, epididymoorchitis) often require percutaneous culture for diagnosis.

Antifungal treatment for candiduria is recommended if symptoms of urinary tract infection are present, for patients with neutropenia, for low-birth-weight infants, for renal transplant recipients, or for patients undergoing urologic manipulation. Appropriate therapy includes either fluconazole, 200 mg/day for 7 to 14 days, or amphoB, 0.3 to 0.5 mg/kg/day for up to 1 week. Amphotericin B bladder irrigations are not routinely recommended, and other systemic antifungals (eg, the echinocandins, posaconazole, and voriconazole) do not achieve adequate urine levels to be considered optimal for treatment. *Candida* epididymoorchitis requires drainage and possibly orchiectomy along with systemic antifungals.

SUGGESTED READING

Centers for Disease Control and Prevention, Workowski KA, Berman SM. Sexually transmitted diseases treatment guidelines, 2006. *MMWR Recomm Rep.* 2006 Aug 4;55(RR-11):1–94.

Fridkin SK. The changing face of fungal infections in health care settings. *Clin Infect Dis.* 2005;41:1455–1460.

Krogh-Madsen M, Arendrup MC, Heslet L, Knudsen JD. Amphotericin B and caspofungin resistance in Candida glabrata isolates recovered from a critically ill patient. *Clin Infect Dis.* 2006;42:938–944.

Ostrosky-Zeichner L, Pappas PG. Invasive candidiasis in the intensive care unit. *Crit Care Med.* 2006;34:857–863.

Ostrosky-Zeichner L, Alexander BD, Kett DH, et al. Multicenter clinical evaluation of the (1,3) beta-D-glucan assay as an aid to diagnosis of fungal infections in humans. *Clin Infect Dis.* 2005;41:654–659.

Pappas PG. Invasive candidiasis. *Infect Dis Clin North Am.* 2006;20(3):485–506.

Pappas PG, Rex JH, Sobel JD, et al. Guidelines for the treatment of candidiasis. Infectious Diseases Society of America. *Clin Infect Dis.* 2004;38:161–189.

Tortorano AM, Kibbler C, Peman J, Bernhardt H, Klingspor L, Grillot R. Candidaemia in Europe: epidemiology and resistance. *Int J Am Ag.* 2006;27:359–366.

171. Aspergillosis

Sanjay Ram and Stuart M. Levitz

Aspergillus is readily isolated from samples of soil, decaying vegetation, water, and air worldwide. *Aspergillus fumigatus*, followed by *Aspergillus flavus, Aspergillus niger*, and *Aspergillus terreus*, are the most common species that cause human disease. Aspergillosis follows exposure of a susceptible host to the ubiquitous conidia (spores). Germinating conidia form hyphae, the invasive form of the fungus. *Aspergillus* hyphae average 2 to 4 μ in diameter and are septate, with dichotomous (Y-shaped) branching (Figure 171.1). The spectrum of diseases caused by the aspergilli is wide and profoundly influenced by the underlying immune status of the host.

CLINICAL MANIFESTATIONS AND DIAGNOSIS OF INVASIVE ASPERGILLOSIS

Although inhalation of conidia is common, invasive disease is relatively rare. The vast majority of affected patients are severely immunosuppressed. Major risk factors include profound, prolonged neutropenia due to cytotoxic chemotherapy and macrophage dysfunction due to high doses of corticosteroids. In patients who have undergone hematopoietic stem cell transplantation, additional risk factors are graft-versus-host disease and cytomegalovirus infection. Invasive aspergillosis also is particularly common in individuals with chronic granulomatous disease (CGD), a rare genetic disorder characterized by a defective phagocyte respiratory burst. Finally, recent studies have suggested that critically ill patients are at risk for invasive aspergillosis, even without aforementioned risk factors.

Invasive pulmonary aspergillosis, with or without dissemination, is the most common form of disease. Signs and symptoms of invasive aspergillosis are nonspecific. Fever is almost always present. Radiographic features include patchy densities or well-defined nodules that may be single or multifocal and can progress to cavitation or consolidation. High-resolution computed tomography (CT) scanning has greater sensitivity than plain films.

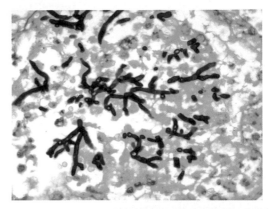

Figure 171.1 Photomicrograph demonstrating *Aspergillus* hyphae in a lung at autopsy in a liver transplant patient who died of systemic aspergillosis. The hyphae are stained with methenamine silver. (Courtesy of Dr. Barbara Banner, University of Massachusetts Medical School.)

Macronodules (nodules greater than 1 cm in diameter) are present in the vast majority of patients with invasive pulmonary aspergillosis. Nodules may be surrounded by a perimeter of ground-glass opacity, the so-called halo sign (Figure 171.2). Cavitation ("air-crescent sign") is less common and tends to occur as a later manifestation of disease. *Aspergillus* sinusitis is the second most common manifestation. Its clinical features include fever, localized pain, proptosis, and monocular blindness. Less common manifestations include cutaneous aspergillosis, which may be seen at intravenous catheter insertion sites in neutropenic patients, as invasive fungal dermatitis in premature neonates and children with acquired immunodeficiency syndrome (AIDS), or at sites of burn wounds in immunocompromised persons. Cerebral aspergillosis occurs in 10% to 20% of all cases of invasive aspergillosis. Involvement of the epiglottis, larynx, liver, cardiac valves, thyroid, kidneys, pericardium, and peritoneum has also been reported.

Invasive aspergillosis must be strongly suspected in any high-risk patient with fever unresponsive to broad-spectrum antibiotics, and empiric antifungal therapy should be considered. Although *Aspergillus* can be a laboratory

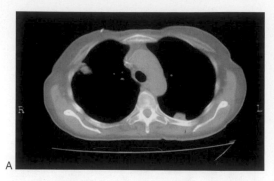 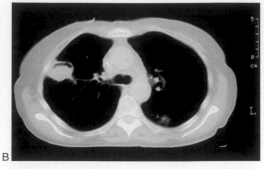

Figure 171.2 High-resolution computed tomography scans from patients with invasive pulmonary aspergillosis. **A:** Two pleural based nodules can be seen. The one on the right is surrounded by a gray area of low attenuation (halo sign). **B:** Air-crescent sign in a patient recovering from neutropenia. (Courtesy of the *Aspergillus*/ Aspergillosis Web site: www.aspergillus.org.uk. Copyright by the Fungal Research Trust. Used with permission.)

contaminant or a colonizer of the bronchial tree and sinuses, a positive culture for *Aspergillus* in a high-risk patient is predictive of invasive disease and should not be ignored. However, in patients with established disease, cultures and even biopsies are often negative.

In an effort to improve prognosis with earlier detection, nonculture methods to detect *Aspergillus* antigens and nucleic acids in clinical specimens of high-risk patients have been studied. Tests to detect two cell wall antigens released by growing *Aspergilli*, galactomannan and β-glucan, are clinically available. A meta-analysis concluded that the double-sandwich enzyme-linked immunsorbent assay (ELISA) for serum galactomannan has excellent specificity but only moderate sensitivity. The test performed better in patients with hematological malignancies than in those with solid organ transplants. False positives have been noted in patients receiving piperacillin–tazobactam and amoxicillin–clavulanate due to contamination of some lots of the antibiotic formulations with galactomannan. False negatives are considerably more common in patients receiving antifungal prophylaxis. A chromogenic assay to detect β-glucans in clinical specimens is commercially available and in preliminary studies has performed comparably to galactomannan testing. Tests to detect *Aspergillus* DNA and RNA in clinical samples remain investigational but show promise, particularly when used in combination with the galactomannan ELISA. It should be emphasized that these surrogate detection markers cannot definitively establish or exclude a diagnosis of aspergillosis and clinical correlation is required. Moreover, macronodules and air-crescent signs on chest CT scan may occur while antigen detection assays are still negative.

TREATMENT OF INVASIVE ASPERGILLOSIS

Licensed drugs with activity against *Aspergillus* include amphotericin B, itraconazole, voriconazole, posaconazole, caspofungin, micafungin, and anidulafungin. Fluconazole and ketoconazole do not inhibit *Aspergillus* at clinically obtainable concentrations and should not be used to treat aspergillosis. It is somewhat difficult to rank the active drugs in terms of relative efficacy because few randomized comparative trials have been performed. Studies based on comparisons to historical controls are problematic due to significant differences in the patient populations. A multicenter, randomized trial compared voriconazole with amphotericin B in 277 patients with definite or probable acute invasive aspergillosis. The voriconazole regimen demonstrated superior efficacy and a 22% relative survival benefit. Moreover, there were fewer treatment-related adverse events in the voriconazole group. This study has been criticized due to its unblinded design, the use of conventional (rather than lipid-based) amphotericin B preparations, and the allowance of a switch to other licensed antifungal medications. Nevertheless, the large survival benefit that was seen has firmly established voriconazole as the drug of choice for initial treatment of invasive aspergillosis. An important caveat though is voriconazole is not effective therapy against zygomycosis, which can present is a similar manner to aspergillosis.

In the above study, two doses of 6 mg/kg of intravenous voriconazole were administered on day 1, followed by 4 mg/kg/day. A switch to oral voriconazole at a dose of 200 mg twice a day was allowed after 1 week. Transient visual disturbances, including blurred vision, altered color perception, and photophobia, are common with voriconazole and tend to resolve without incident. Other side effects that have been observed include rash and liver function test abnormalities. Voriconazole interacts with many of the P450 isoenzymes; thus, interactions with other drugs are common. In patients with an estimated creatinine clearance <50 mL/min, accumulation of the intravenous vehicle occurs; these patients should be given oral voriconazole whenever possible.

In addition to voriconazole, other licensed triazoles with activity against *Aspergillus* are itraconazole and posaconazole. Itraconazole appears to have the least potent activity and is mainly used for the treatment of aspergillomas and allergic bronchopulmonary aspergillosis (see below). Posaconazole appears more promising and has the added advantage of having useful activity against zygomycetes, but clinical experience with its use for primary treatment of invasive aspergillosis is limited. Moreover, as of this writing, the drug was only available orally. Fluconazole and ketoconazole do not have any useful clinical activity against *Aspergillus*.

For patients who cannot take voriconazole because of contraindications or intolerance, amphotericin B is generally used for the treatment of invasive aspergillosis. (Amphotericin B should not be used to treat *A. terreus* due to intrinsic resistance.) However, controversy exists regarding the optimal daily dosage and formulation. For the conventional amphotericin B desoxycholate formulation, following a test dose of 1 mg, dosages ranging from 0.6 to 1.5 mg/kg/day have been recommended, with higher dosages reserved for those patients who are severely ill and/or profoundly immunosuppressed. Fevers, chills, and rigors, observed in a significant number of patients treated with amphotericin B, may be alleviated by premedication with acetaminophen, meperidine, 25 to 50 mg given intravenously, or the addition of 25 to 50 mg of hydrocortisone sodium succinate to the infusion solution. Amphotericin nephrotoxicity has been associated with sodium-depleted states and may be reduced by giving 1 L of normal saline a day to patients with no contraindications to volume expansion. As amphotericin B causes renal tubular losses of potassium and magnesium, their levels should be monitored closely and supplementation provided as needed. The dosage of amphotericin B must be individualized depending on factors such as the expected duration and degree of immunosuppression, and the extent of the disease.

In an effort to reduce the toxicity associated with the conventional amphotericin B preparation, lipid-associated formulations have been developed. Currently available formulations include amphotericin B lipid complex, amphotericin B colloidal dispersion, and a liposomal preparation. Comparisons between the different formulations of amphotericin B are difficult to make due to the lack of well-designed randomized trials. However, at the usual daily dosages recommended for the treatment of invasive aspergillosis (3 to 5 mg/kg/day), the lipid formulations appear to be as efficacious as amphotericin B deoxycholate. The lipid formulations are less nephrotoxic than the conventional preparation, but because of their considerably greater cost, we limit their use to patients who are at high risk for amphotericin B nephrotoxicity due to pre-existing renal disease, concomitant receipt of other nephrotoxic agents, or inability to tolerate saline loading. A recent clinical trial comparing 3 and 10 mg/kg/day of liposomal AmB as primary therapy for invasive aspergillosis found the lower dose was equally effective but less toxic.

Three members of the echinocandin class of antifungal drugs, caspofungin, micafungin, and anidulafungin, are licensed for use. All have modest activity against *Aspergillus* in vitro and in animal models, although none has been adequately studied in comparative clinical trials for primary treatment of invasive aspergillosis. In an open study of 83 patients with invasive aspergillosis who were refractory or intolerant to amphotericin B, a favorable response to caspofungin therapy was observed in 37 (45%) of the subjects. Due to poor oral absorption, the echinocandins must be administered intravenously. Although infusion-related reactions and liver function test elevations are relatively common, serious side effects of this class of drugs are rare.

Due to the high failure rate associated with monotherapy for invasive aspergillosis, combination regimens as initial and salvage therapy have been tried. Randomized studies have not been reported, and comparisons with historical controls must be interpreted cautiously. Due to the potential for antagonism between the azoles and amphotericin B, most studies have utilized caspofungin in combination with either amphotericin B or voriconazole. No firm conclusions can be drawn, and clearly randomized trials are needed. It is the authors' practice to treat most cases of invasive aspergillosis with voriconazole monotherapy, but to switch to combination therapy if progression results.

Regardless of whether monotherapy or combination therapy is utilized, the duration of treatment should be individualized depending on the extent of disease and degree of immunosuppression. Most patients will require several months of treatment. Surgery should be considered as an adjunct to treatment in instances where there is localized disease, particularly in cases where there is progression despite antifungal therapy or further courses of neutropenia-inducing chemotherapy are anticipated. Whenever possible, immunosuppression should be withdrawn or decreased. In neutropenic patients, recombinant granulocyte colony-stimulating factor (G-CSF) may improve outcome by decreasing the duration of neutropenia and increasing the functional activity of neutrophils.

PROPHYLAXIS AND PRE-EMPTIVE TREATMENT OF INVASIVE ASPERGILLOSIS

Given the high mortality associated with established disease, strategies for the prevention of invasive aspergillosis have been advocated and are summarized in Table 171.1. Numerous studies have examined empiric antifungal therapy in neutropenic patients with persistent or recurrent fevers despite empiric antibacterial therapy. This group is at high risk for invasive fungal infections, particularly aspergillosis and candidiasis, but also other opportunistic mycoses, including zygomycosis and fusariosis. Thus, ideal agents will have activity against a broad spectrum of opportunistic fungi. However, for those for whom the duration of neutropenia is expected to be short, candidiasis is the main concern, with aspergillosis and other mold infections being less common.

The earlier studies, published in the 1980s, established that amphotericin B deoxycholate could decrease the incidence of invasive fungal infections in patients with persistent neutropenic fevers. Subsequent noninferiority studies compared amphotericin B (either deoxycholate or lipid-based formulations) to fluconazole, itraconazole, voriconazole, and caspofungin. An important caveat in interpreting these studies is the variability in inclusion criteria and end points defining success. Most studies have used composite end points to assess success; this has the unfortunate consequence of counting failure due to death or a breakthrough invasive fungal infection the same as failure due to premature drug discontinuation.

Fluconazole has been successfully used in patient populations at low risk of invasive aspergillosis. Itraconazole and caspofungin have demonstrated noninferiority compared with amphotericin B. In a large study comparing voriconazole to liposomal amphotericin B, the criteria for noninferiority were just barely missed, mainly due to more patients in the voriconazole arm being prematurely removed from the study. As the study had an open-label design, investigator bias against the then-experimental drug likely contributed to these results. Importantly, there were fewer breakthrough fungal infections in the voriconazole group.

A recently reported study compared posaconazole (200 mg 3 times daily) with either fluconazole (400 mg/day) or itraconazole (200 mg/day) in 602 patients undergoing intensive chemotherapy for acute myelogenous leukemia or myelodysplastic syndrome. Patients received antifungal medications with each cycle of chemotherapy until complete remission or for up to 12 weeks. Remarkably, during the treatment phase of the study, only 2 cases of aspergillosis were seen in the posaconazole arm compared with 20 in the fluconazole–itraconazole arm. Moreover, there was a significant overall survival benefit in favor of posaconazole. Similarly, a significant reduction in cases of aspergillosis and in mortality was seen in a study comparing posaconazole with fluconazole for allogeneic hematopoietic stem cell transplant recipients with graft-versus-host disease. Posaconazole needs to be given with food for optimal absorption. It is an inhibitor of CYP3A4, thus dose adjustments must be made if patients are on other drugs, such as cyclosporine, sirolimus, and tacrolimus, that are metabolized by this enzyme.

ASPERGILLOSIS IN PATIENTS WITH AIDS

Patients with late-stage AIDS are predisposed to the development of invasive aspergillosis. Classical risk factors such as neutropenia and corticosteroid therapy are found in about half the cases. Atypical manifestations may be seen, including ulcerative or pseudomembranous tracheobronchitis aspergillosis, which may be only minimally invasive. Cough, fever, wheezing, hypoxemia, and hemoptysis are the main clinical features. Bronchoscopy helps confirm the diagnosis.

The incidence of invasive aspergillosis in the AIDS population has markedly declined due to the immune reconstitution associated with

Table 171.1 Prevention of Invasive Aspergillosis

Preventive Strategy	Comments

1. Avoidance of exposure to *Aspergillus* conidia
  a. Avoidance of environmental exposure
 	
  b. High-efficiency particulate air (HEPA) filters or laminar air flow (LAF)
	Heavily contaminated areas include compost heaps, grain silos, moldy hay, and marijuana
	Although expensive, HEPA and LAF may be considered for patients at very high risk of invasive aspergillosis, particularly if mold counts are high

2. Prophylaxis of high risk patients	Posaconazole should be considered in very high-risk groups[a]
3. Administration of colony-stimulating factors to neutropenic patients	Expensive. May be considered as part of an overall strategy to reduce infections in selected patients
4. Pre-emptive, empirical administration of antifungals to neutropenic patients with fevers despite broad-spectrum antibacterial agents	Strongly recommended[a]
5. Secondary prophylaxis (antifungal treatment to prevent recrudescence of invasive aspergillosis in patients who will become immunosuppressed)	Due to high relapse rates, voriconazole or amphotericin B should be given at the onset of chemotherapy or neutropenia. Consider surgical resection of localized disease[a]

[a] See text for details.

the administration of antiretroviral therapy. Although therapy for this group of patients is similar to that for patients without human immunodeficiency virus (HIV) infection, two points are worth emphasizing. First, long-term prognosis will be dramatically improved if immune reconstitution can be achieved with the administration of effective antiretroviral therapy. Second, the clinician must take into account potential drug interactions between antifungal and antiretroviral drugs. For example, the protease inhibitor, ritonavir, induces the metabolism of voriconazole.

ASPERGILLOMAS

Pulmonary aspergillomas are the result of saprophytic colonization of *Aspergillus*, usually within pre-existing lung cavities. The diagnosis is most often made by chest radiography, where a round to oval intracavitary mass partially surrounded by a radiolucent crescent of air is seen. Serum precipitins and sputum cultures for *Aspergillus* are positive in about 90% and 50% of cases, respectively. Hemoptysis is the most common symptom, and in most cases is mild and self-limited. Rarely, extrapulmonary aspergillomas can form, particularly in the sinuses.

Therapy for aspergillomas must be individualized according to the pulmonary and immunologic status of the host, but in most cases a conservative approach with close clinical follow-up is recommended. Resection generally is reserved for those with life-threatening hemoptysis. However, many patients are not surgical candidates due to poor baseline lung function. Bronchial artery embolization can be tried as a temporizing measure for massive hemoptysis in patients with a high operative risk. Other measures, including intracavitary instillation of amphotericin B, oral itraconazole, and oral voriconazole, have been associated with reduction in cavity size and severity of hemoptysis in case reports. In one series of 40 patients, all patients had short-term resolution of hemoptysis following instillation of a locally formulated paste consisting of amphotericin B, fatty acids, and emulsifying wax.

A subset of patients with aspergillomas tend to be chronically ill, with fever, weight loss, pulmonary symptoms, and leukocytosis. This entity, termed chronic necrotizing pulmonary aspergillosis or "semi-invasive" aspergillosis, is seen in patients with chronic pulmonary disorders and mild systemic immunocompromise like diabetes mellitus, alcoholism, low-dose corticosteroids, or malnutrition. Whenever possible, host defenses should be strengthened by diminishing factors responsible for immunosuppression. In some cases, dramatic clinical responses have been observed following a course of antifungal therapy. Resection may be considered in the small subset of patients with focal disease whose pulmonary function and underlying disease do not preclude surgery.

ALLERGIC MANIFESTATIONS OF *ASPERGILLUS*

Extrinsic allergic alveolitis occurs in nonatopic individuals who are exposed to *Aspergillus* conidia, as in "malt-workers lung" or "farmers lung," following their exposure to moldy grain or hay. Spontaneous recovery usually occurs over several weeks, without the need for corticosteroids. Exposure to *Aspergillus* in individuals with asthma can result in an exacerbation of their disease (extrinsic asthma).

Allergic bronchopulmonary aspergillosis (ABPA) is a syndrome characterized by asthma, proximal bronchiectasis, immediate cutaneous reactivity to *Aspergillus*, elevated serum immunoglobulin E (IgE) concentrations, and elevated serum immunoglobulin G (IgG) and IgE antibodies specific to *A. fumigatus*. Pulmonary infiltrates, peripheral eosinophilia, serum precipitins against *Aspergillus* antigens, and expectoration of fungus-laden mucus plugs may also be seen. Major predisposing factors are asthma and cystic fibrosis.

The goals of therapy are to reduce acute inflammation and minimize long-term lung damage. For patients with ABPA and pulmonary infiltrates, the primary treatment is prednisone in doses of 0.5 to 1.0 mg/kg/day for 1 to 2 weeks, followed by an alternating day regimen and then a gradual taper over a 3- to 6-month period. Total IgE levels in the serum directly correlate with disease activity and response to corticosteroids. A meta-analysis of data from two randomized trials comparing a 16-week course of itraconazole in doses of 200 mg twice daily with placebo concluded that itraconazole treatment was associated with fewer exacerbations and improved immunological parameters. However, improvements tended to be modest, and resistance of the fungus to itraconazole can emerge. Therefore, itraconazole should be considered as an adjuvant to corticosteroids rather than primary therapy. The role of voriconazole and posaconazole in the treatment of ABPA has not been adequately assessed, but these newer azoles would be predicted to have efficacy at least equal to that of itraconazole.

Currently, two oral formulations of itraconazole are available: capsules and an oral aqueous acidified solution in 5% hydroxypropyl-β-cyclodextrin. Absorption of the capsular form is best in an acidic environment, and in the presence of a meal. Histamine-2 blockers and antacids may interfere with absorption. In contrast, the oral aqueous hydroxypropyl-β-cyclodextrin solution should be taken without food. This preparation achieves peak serum concentrations about 60% higher than the capsules but is more expensive and is associated with a higher incidence of gastrointestinal side effects. Drugs that induce hepatic microsomal enzymes (eg, rifampin, isoniazid, phenytoin, phenobarbital, and carbamazepine) may significantly reduce serum itraconazole levels. Itraconazole itself slows hepatic drug metabolism and may increase the toxicity of phenytoin, oral hypoglycemics, digoxin, warfarin, and cyclosporine. Plasma concentrations of itraconazole can be measured in patients for whom absorption or drug metabolism problems are suspected, although therapeutic levels have not been established.

Allergic *Aspergillus* sinusitis usually responds to surgical debridement and drainage. Recurrences following surgery may be prevented by the use of intranasal steroid sprays or systemic corticosteroids in selected cases.

Saprophytic colonization of the paranasal sinuses and external auditory canal in immunocompetent patients must be distinguished from allergic and invasive forms of the disease. Surgical debridement and drainage of the sinuses and treatment of the chronic otitis is usually curative. Antifungal therapy in the absence of tissue invasion generally is not indicated.

SUGGESTED READING

Cornely OA, Maertens J, Winston DJ, et al. Posaconazole vs. fluconazole or itraconazole prophylaxis in patients with neutropenia. *N Engl J Med.* 2007;356(4):348–359.

Denning DW. Invasive aspergillosis. *Clin Infect Dis.* 1998;26(4):781–803.

Giron J, Poey C, Fajadet P, et al. CT-guided percutaneous treatment of inoperable pulmonary aspergillomas: a study of 40 cases. *Eur J Radiol.* 1998;28(3):235–242.

Herbrecht R, Denning DW, Patterson TF, et al. Voriconazole versus amphotericin B for primary therapy of invasive aspergillosis. *N Engl J Med.* 2002; 347(6):408–415.

Maertens J, Raad I, Petrikkson G, et al. Efficacy and safety of caspofungin for treatment of invasive aspergillosis in patients refractory to or intolerant of conventional antifungal therapy. *Clin Infect Dis.* 2004;39(11): 1563–1571.

Marr KA, Carter RA, Boeckh M, et al. Invasive aspergillosis in allogeneic stem cell transplant recipients: changes in epidemiology and risk factors. *Blood.* 2002;100(13):4358–4366.

Martino R, Viscoli C. Empirical antifungal therapy in patients with neutropenia and persistent or recurrent fever of unknown origin. *Br J Haematol*. 2006;132(2):138–154.

Pfeiffer CD, Fine JP, Safdar N. Diagnosis of invasive aspergillosis using a galactomannan assay: a meta-analysis. *Clin Infect Dis*. 2006;42(10):1417–1727.

Stevens DA, Kan VL, Judson MA, et al. Practice guidelines for diseases caused by Aspergillus. Infectious Diseases Society of America. *Clin Infect Dis*. 2000;30(4):696–709.

Stevens DA, Schwartz HJ, Lee JY, et al. A randomized trial of itraconazole in allergic bronchopulmonary aspergillosis. *N Engl J Med*. 2000;342(11): 756–762.

Wark PA, Gibson PG, Wilson AJ. Azoles for allergic bronchopulmonary aspergillosis associated with asthma. *Cochrane Database Syst Rev*. 2004;(3):CD001108.

172. Zygomycosis (Mucormycosis)

Scott F. Davies

The older term *mucormycosis* refers to a group of highly lethal fungal infections caused by the members of the order Mucorales, which include various species of the genera *Rhizopus*, *Absidia*, and *Mucor* (all from the family Mucoraceae). Most infections are caused by *Rhizopus* species. It is incorrect to use the term *mucormycosis* to refer only to infections caused by members of the genus *Mucor*, which are only a small minority of the total infections. An even broader term—*zygomycosis*—is increasingly preferred because it encompasses not only the entire order Mucorales (which includes infections due to *Cunninghamella* species) but also the order Entomophthorales, including *Conidiobolus* species, which have on rare occasions caused invasive pulmonary infections in profoundly immunosuppressed patients. Figure 172.1 gives an overview of the taxonomy of the causative organisms. For the remainder of this chapter the term *zygomycosis* will be used to refer to infections caused by any member of this expanded taxonomy. In common usage the two terms are virtually synonymous, but recent publications are trending in this direction, whereas legacy publications generally have used the older terminology.

The causative agents of zygomycosis are found throughout the world, associated with decaying organic matter. They grow as a mycelium (broad nonseptate hyphae with short stubby right-angle branches) in nature and in infected mammalian tissue.

PATHOGENESIS

Airborne spores of the fungi settle on the skin or are inhaled into the nose, the pharynx, and the lung. The organism has little chance of invading healthy tissue defended by neutrophils. *Rhizopus* organisms grow best at acid pH in a high-glucose environment. A specific enzyme, ketone reductase, plays an important role. Thus diabetic ketoacidosis provides a favorable opportunity for the fungus to locally invade tissues of the upper airway, resulting in the fulminant rhinocerebral form of zygomycosis. Once established, the fungus is angioinvasive, leading to infarction of tissues and wider areas of necrosis, in which the fungus thrives. The tissue response to the fungus includes pyogenic inflammation, but there is little tendency for granuloma formation. A second form of disease is pulmonary zygomycosis, in which infection occurs in the lung or, less commonly, in proximal airways. The disease resembles invasive pulmonary aspergillosis and occurs, although much less commonly, in the same substrate: patients with profound neutropenia and patients in whom phagocyte function is depressed by high-dose glucocorticoid therapy. Like *Aspergillus* species, agents of zygomycosis are angioinvasive in the lung, leading to tissue necrosis and eventually to pyemic spread to distant sites, including the skin, kidney, and brain. Rare forms of zygomycosis include a direct cutaneous infection that can complicate severe burns and the gastrointestinal form of the illness, associated with profound protein malnutrition (usually in infants), in which organisms directly invade the bowel wall, causing hemorrhage, bowel infarction, peritonitis, and death.

When uncontrolled diabetes is the main predisposing factor, rhinocerebral zygomycosis is more common. When hematological malignancy and organ transplantation are the predisposing factors, pulmonary zygomycosis is more common. Patients being treated for leukemia and bone marrow transplantation recipients appear to have an increasing risk of zygomycosis. The changing spectrum of antifungal agents being used for prophylaxis and empiric antifungal therapy in these patients may be playing a role. Early use of fluconazole for these indications reduced candida infections but likely shifted what was once a 50:50 split more heavily toward invasive *Aspergillus* infections. More recently, other triazoles highly active against *Aspergillus* (including itraconazole and now voriconazole) have been used, reducing *Aspergillus* infections but likely resulting in higher frequency of zygomycosis. There are several studies implicating itraconazole and voriconazole prophylaxis as independent risk factors for development of invasive zygomycosis.

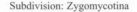

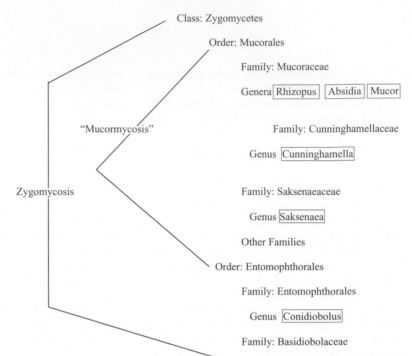

Figure 172.1 Taxonomy of organisms causing zygomycosis.

Kingdom: Fungi

Division: Zygomycota

Subdivision: Zygomycotina

Class: Zygomycetes

Order: Mucorales

Family: Mucoraceae

Genera | Rhizopus | Absidia | Mucor

"Mucormycosis"

Family: Cunninghamellaceae

Genus | Cunninghamella

Zygomycosis

Family: Saksenaeaceae

Genus | Saksenaea

Other Families

Order: Entomophthorales

Family: Entomophthorales

Genus | Conidiobolus

Family: Basidiobolaceae

Genus | Basidiobolus

CLINICAL MANIFESTATIONS

Rhinocerebral zygomycosis is an extremely fulminant infection. Infection begins in the nose, sometimes manifested by dark, blood-tinged discharge from one or both nostrils. Necrosis of the nasal septum and turbinates then follow, with spread to the paranasal sinuses. In sequence, the disease accelerates with ulceration and necrosis of sinus walls, periorbital cellulitis, and direct invasion of the orbit, eye, cavernous sinuses, and brain. Arterial thrombosis adds to the extent of tissue destruction. Early clinical findings include eye pain, decreased visual acuity, and cranial nerve palsies. A black eschar from ischemic necrosis, either in the nose or on the palate, is a strong signal of disease presence. Early symptoms and signs may be followed by seizures and progressive decrease in level of consciousness. Death may occur in 1 week.

Pulmonary zygomycosis is acquired by inhalation or possibly by micro-aspiration from colonized sinuses. The disease presents as an acute or subacute pneumonia, with fever, cough, and purulent sputum. Some patients have pleuritic pain and hemoptysis from superimposed pulmonary infarction caused by invasion of pulmonary vessels. The most characteristic finding on chest radiograph is a wedge-shaped area of dense infiltrate in the lung periphery. The spectrum of radiographic abnormalities also includes large masses (even to 6 to 10 cm in size), multiple nodules, and multiple peripheral infiltrates. Focal areas of consolidation often cavitate as the infection progresses. Metastatic abscesses may develop in the brain, liver, spleen, kidney, and skin. Metastatic skin lesions often show extensive necrosis (ecthyma gangrenosum) and offer easy diagnosis with a simple punch biopsy. Clinically, the illness cannot easily be distinguished from invasive aspergillosis. Most cases occur in patients with hematologic malignancy who have prolonged neutropenia. Cases of pulmonary zygomycosis also occur in organ transplant recipients, in patients receiving a long course of high-dose glucocorticoid therapy for malignant or nonmalignant disorders, and even in diabetic patients.

Desferoxamine therapy, used for chelation in some patients receiving long-term dialysis and in other iron-overloaded states, is also a risk factor for zygomycosis because it mobilizes iron from peripheral storage sites and makes it more available to the fungus as a growth factor.

Endobronchial zygomycosis is a rare form of pulmonary zygomycosis that has been reported mainly in patients with advanced acquired immunodeficiency syndrome (AIDS). Patients have irritative cough, purulent sputum, and often hemoptysis. Physical findings may include a localized wheeze. The chest radiograph may be normal or may show segmental or even lobar infiltrates with significant volume loss distal to the obstructed airway. Several other unusual forms of zygomycosis also have been reported in this population. Isolated renal zygomycosis has been described in AIDS patients who abuse drugs intravenously or have long-term intravascular access catheters for various therapeutics. Nodular skin lesions have also been reported in AIDS patients who abuse drugs intravenously. Intravenous drug abusers have been described with cerebral zygomycosis of the basal ganglia.

DIAGNOSIS

The diagnosis of rhinocerebral zygomycosis can often be strongly suspected based on the setting of diabetic ketoacidosis and the clinical features of the illness. High suspicion and early recognition are important. Specific diagnosis usually depends on histopathologic demonstration of characteristic broad nonseptate hyphae in biopsies of diseased tissue (Figure 172.2). Positive cultures are confirmatory and the only way to define the exact species causing the infection. Positive cultures for causative organisms of zygomycosis must be interpreted cautiously

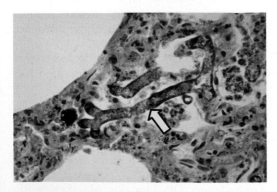

Figure 172.2 Mucormycosis: Hyphae (*arrow*) vary from 6 to 50 μm in diameter, are nonseptated, and typically branch at 90° angles. (Courtesy of www.doctorfungus.org © 2007).

and in clinical context because the organisms are ubiquitous in the environment and occasionally can be recovered from the skin, pharynx, and sputum of patients without disease. No useful skin tests or serologic tests are available.

The diagnosis of pulmonary zygomycosis is also highly dependent on the clinical setting, with leukemia and bone marrow transplantation most important predispositions, followed by organ transplantation. Prior use of itraconazole or voriconazole for prophylaxis or empiric antifungal therapy may also be a risk factor. The disease resembles invasive aspergillosis in similar hosts and can be distinguished only by histopathology or by culture.

TREATMENT

Rhinocerebral zygomycosis has a very high mortality, probably beyond 80% of all cases. Successful therapy is most likely if the diagnosis is made early and based entirely on clinical findings. There are three aspects to the treatment. First, the diabetic ketoacidosis must be controlled. Second, and most importantly, aggressive surgical debridement of all necrotic tissue must be done. Sometimes, a sequence of several procedures are needed as the limits of the diseased tissue become more apparent. Finally, full doses of amphotericin B (AMB) or one of its lipid derivatives must be given quickly. Amphotericin B likely contributes to successful outcome but is not sufficient in itself without metabolic control and surgical debridement.

Pulmonary zygomycosis is also highly lethal. Once there is spread to distant sites and particularly to the brain, fatal outcome is nearly certain. Localized pulmonary disease can sometimes be managed successfully. Again, a three-pronged approach is necessary. First, the predisposing causes must be reversed. This means return of neutrophils (either spontaneously or aided by marrow-stimulating biologicals) and/or rapid taper of glucocorticoid therapy to the extent it is possible. Second, amphotericin B or a lipid derivative should be started and escalated quickly to full dosages. Amphotericin B-deoxycholate doses of up to 1.0 to 1.5 mg/kg/day are recommended. That dosing usually worsens renal function is one reason for strong consideration of the more expensive lipid-based formulations. Third, if the patient stabilizes, strong consideration should be given to surgical resection of necrotic lung tissue, if the lung disease is localized and the risk of thoracotomy is reasonably low. The decision to operate must be appropriate in the context of the patient's underlying disease. There are anecdotal reports of successful treatment of pulmonary zygomycosis by surgical resection alone. In most cases, the preoperative diagnosis was uncertain, total excision of all involved lung was accomplished, the diagnosis was established by histopathology of the resected tissue, and the patient recovered fully without other therapy.

When possible, isolated renal zygomycosis in patients with AIDS should be treated with nephrectomy combined with amphotericin B. When nephrectomy is either not possible or is not a reasonable option given the overall condition of the patient, amphotericin B alone should be used. There are some anecdotal successes using amphotericin B without surgery.

Unfortunately, amphotericin B is not highly effective for zygomycosis. The high doses recommended are nephrotoxic, particularly in some of the patients most at risk, who often have underlying renal dysfunction and are frequently receiving other nephrotoxic drugs, including aminoglycosides and other antibacterial agents, antiviral agents such as ganciclovir, and immunosuppressives, including cyclosporin. Alternative lipid-based amphotericin preparations reduce renal toxicity greatly. Although less toxic, they are more expensive and are not proven to be more effective. The dosage is 5 mg/kg/day (or even higher in some cases) and is usually tolerated without renal embarrassment. One large series summarizing the compassionate use of amphotericin B lipid complex (ABLC) for all indications includes 24 cases of zygomycosis with 17 partial or complete responses. A similar publication summarizing compassionate use of liposomal AMB (AmBisome) for all indications (from the United Kingdom) includes only three cases of zygomycosis: two rhinocerebral cases that were successfully treated and one pulmonary case that died within 3 days of onset of treatment. There have also been a few anecdotal reports detailing the successful use of either ABLC or liposomal AMB for various forms of zygomycosis. In toto, these reports suggest some promise for the newer forms of AMB. Further experience will have to be gained before the exact role for these agents is determined.

As mentioned above, itraconazole and voriconazole are triazoles with activity against aspergillus. Wide use of these agents for prophylaxis and empiric antifungal therapy in patients with hematological malignancy likely has increased the incidence of zygomycosis. A possible real advance in treatment is the development of posaconazole, the first triazole compound with activity against the zygomycetes. Compassionate use in a large series of 91 patients with zygomycosis (69 proven disease, 22 probable) who had failed or were intolerant to prior antifungal treatment (usually a form of AMB) showed a success rate of 60% at 12 weeks. That exceeds historical success rates with prior standard therapy. Although posaconazole is not yet approved for use in zygomycoses, the prudent approach pending further data might be to start patients with proven disease on liposomal AMB plus posaconazole (not neglecting other aspects of therapy), continuing both until clinical response, and then extending the course of posaconazole to a total of 12 or more weeks. This recommendation is very fluid, and up-to-date information should be checked before considering a specific treatment regimen.

Finally, hyperbaric oxygen therapy has been proposed based on limited and anecdotal reports, as an adjunctive therapy for some patients with zygomycosis. Most published experience has been with the rhinocerebral form of the illness. Although successes have been reported, this therapy is not standard and does not reduce the need for early diagnosis, metabolic control, debridement of all necrotic tissue, and rapid escalation to full doses of either standard or newer lipid-based forms of AMB.

SUGGESTED READING

Boelaeret JR, van Roost GF, Vergauwe PL, et al. The role of desferoxamine in dialysis-associated mucormycosis: report of three cases and review of the literature. *Clin Nephrol*. 1988;29:261–266.

Chamilos G, Marom EM, Lewis RE, Lionakis MS, Kontoyiannis PD. Predictors of pulmonary zygomycosis versus invasive pulmonary aspergillosis in patients with cancer. *Clin Infect Dis*. 2005;41(1):60–66.

Couch L, Theilen F, Mader JT. Rhinocerebral mucormycosis with cerebral extension successfully treated with adjunctive hyperbaric oxygen therapy. *Arch Otolaryngol Head Neck Surg*. 1988;114;791–794.

Ferguson BJ, Mitchell TG, Moon R, et al. Adjunctive hyperbaric oxygen for treatment of rhinocerebral zygomycosis. *Rev Infect Dis*. 1988;10:551–559.

Kontoyiannis DP, Lionakis MS, Lewis RE, Zygomycosis in a tertiary-care cancer center in the era of Aspergillus-active antifungal therapy: a case-control observational study of 27 recent cases. *J Infect Dis*. 2005 Apr 15; 191(8): 1350-60. Epub 2005 Mar 16.

Kume H, Yamazaki T, Abe M, Tanuma H, Okudaira M, Okayasu I. Increase in aspergillosis and severe mycotic infection in patients with leukemia and MDS: comparison of the data from the Annual of the Pathological Autopsy Cases in Japan in 1989, 1993 and 1997. *Pathol Int*. 2003:53(11):744–750.

Ng TT, Denning DW. Liposomal amphotercin B (Ambisome) therapy in invasive fungal infections. Evaluation of United Kingdom compassionate use data. *Arch Intern Med*. 1995:155:1093–1098.

Rickerts V, Bohme A, Just-Nubling G. Risk factors for invasive zygomycosis in patients with hematologic malignancies. *Mycoses*. 2002;45(suppl 1):27–30.

Roden MM, Zaoutis TE, Buchanan WL, et al. Epidemiology and outcome of zygomycosis: a review of 929 reported cases. *Clin Infect Dis*. 2005;41(5):634–653.

Van Burik JA, Hare RS, Solomon HF, Corrado ML, Kontoyiannis DP. Posaconazole is effective as salvage therapy in zygomycosis: a retrospective summary of 91 cases. *Clin Infect Dis*. 2006;42(7):e61–e65.

Walsh TJ, Hiemenz JW, Seibel NL, et al. Amphotericin B lipid complex for invasive fungal infections: analysis of safety and efficacy in 556 cases. *Clin Infect Dis*. 1988;26;1383–1396.

173. Sporotrichosis

Ronald A. Greenfield

Sporotrichosis is a subacute or chronic fungal infection caused by *Sporothrix schenckii*. It occurs most commonly in cutaneous or lymphocutaneous forms resulting from direct inoculation of the pathogen but also occurs in a variety of extracutaneous forms. Among the extracutaneous forms, a primary sporotrichotic pneumonia, presumably acquired by inhalation, occurs rarely. More commonly, musculoskeletal or osteoarticular sporotrichosis occurs, either as a result of direct inoculation into tendons, bursae, and joints or as a result of hematogenous dissemination. Hematogenous dissemination may result in disseminated cutaneous sporotrichosis and/or infection of a variety of unusual sites, including the meninges.

EPIDEMIOLOGY

Sporothrix schenckii is widely distributed in nature; it grows on plant debris in soil, and on the bark of trees, shrubs, and garden plants. The fungus and the disease occur in much of the world, primarily in the tropical and temperate zones. The abundance of the organism and the reported incidence of the disease show great geographic variation, perhaps related to genotypic differences between organisms in different locales. The penetrating trauma that introduces the fungal conidia into the human host is most commonly accomplished by splinters, thorns, or woody fragments of plants, but any contact with plants or plant products (eg, sphagnum peat moss, mulch, hay, timber) accompanying minor skin trauma may initiate infection. Activities most frequently associated with acquisition of sporotrichosis include gardening (particularly rose gardening), landscaping, farming, berry-picking, horticulture, and carpentry. Skin test and serologic surveys demonstrate that most *S. schenckii* inoculations promote the development of immunity without clinically apparent infection. Zoonotic transmission also occurs from infected animals, particularly cats with extensive skin lesions, but may result from the scratch of any digging animal. Both pulmonary and disseminated sporotrichosis appear to occur more commonly in patients with a history of alcoholism.

Patients with immunosuppression due to human immunodeficiency virus (HIV) infection and acquired immunodeficiency syndrome (AIDS) appear to more frequently develop disseminated cutaneous sporotrichosis and hematogenously disseminated sporotrichosis, including sporotrichotic meningitis, than immunocompetent hosts. Although the incidence of HIV/AIDS-associated sporotrichosis is not precisely known, it is less than that of other endemic mycoses. Patients treated with immunosuppressive agents, including tumor necrosis factor-α antagonists, have also developed disseminated sporotrichosis.

LABORATORY DIAGNOSIS

Definitive diagnosis of sporotrichosis requires the isolation of *S. schenckii* in culture specimens from a normally sterile body site. Occasionally, the organism can be visualized in biopsied tissue specimens stained with periodic acid–Schiff, Gomori methenamine silver, or immunochemical stains (Figure 173.1). The organism can be recovered by fungal culture from sputum, pus, synovial fluid, bone drainage, and surgical specimens. Concentrations of organisms in joint fluid and particularly cerebrospinal fluid may be relatively low. Therefore repetitive large-volume cultures may be required for diagnosis. Serologic techniques for measurement of antibody are available but exhibit significant interlaboratory variability in sensitivity and specificity; they are best used to suggest the need for more aggressive attempts at definitive diagnosis.

CLINICAL MANIFESTATIONS
Cutaneous Sporotrichosis

The primary lesion develops at the site in the skin, 20 to 90 days after inoculation, most typically distally in the upper extremities. Over a few weeks, the initial small nodule enlarges, reddens, becomes pustular, and ulcerates,

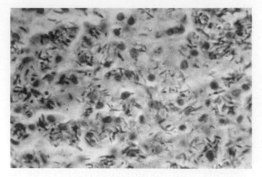

Figure 173.1 Histopathologic demonstration of the cigar-shaped yeasts of *Sporothrix schenckii* (CDC/Dr. Lucille K. Georg, CDC Public Health Image Library).

releasing purulent material from which the organism is readily cultured. Patients are typically afebrile and not systemically ill. In the lymphocutaneous form of the disease, an ascending chain of nodules develops along lymphatic channels of the skin, with the older distal lesions ulcerating and draining and the younger, more proximal lesions forming subcutaneous nodules that attach to the skin as they age and begin to ulcerate (Figure 173.2). The lesions are usually minimally painful, but extensive disease may result in functional impairment. Some patients exhibit no lymphangitic spread, and the disease presents as an indolent ulcerating plaque that persists for years if untreated (fixed cutaneous sporotrichosis). Patients often have received courses of antibacterial therapy without benefit before the process is recognized as sporotrichosis. The lymphocutaneous form of sporotrichosis can be mimicked by infection with *Nocardia*, *Mycobacterium marinum* and other mycobacteria other than tuberculosis, *Leishmania*, and *Francisella tularensis*.

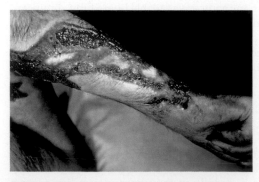

Figure 173.2 Lymphocutaneous sporotrichosis (CDC/Dr. Lucille K. Georg, CDC Public Health Image Library).

Pulmonary Sporotrichosis

Pulmonary sporotrichosis is a subacute or chronic pneumonitis with cavitation, usually in the upper lobes, clinically indistinguishable from mycobacterial infection or chronic pulmonary histoplasmosis. Almost all patients have underlying chronic obstructive pulmonary disease. They present with productive cough, sometimes with weight loss and increasing dyspnea, but rarely with fever, chills, or sweats. Diagnosis requires isolation of *S. schenckii* from sputum cultures or its histopathologic recognition in biopsy specimens.

Osteoarticular Sporotrichosis

Lesions of deeper tissues may occur in almost any organ, but there is a distinct predilection for the joints, particularly of the extremities, and the long bones adjacent to these joints. The resulting chronic arthritis is often confused with rheumatoid or other chronic inflammatory arthritis, not infrequently for 10 or more years, until destruction of adjacent bone or development of draining fistulae encourage efforts to establish the microbial etiology of the chronic osteomyelitis. Cutaneous or lymphocutaneous lesions are unusual in these patients. The process generally begins in a single joint, but additional joints may be involved successively. The patient usually has pain on motion, and the involved areas may be warm and red. Functional impairment resulting from osteoarticular sporotrichosis can become very severe.

Disseminated Sporotrichosis

Sporotrichotic lesions occur infrequently in many other organs such as the eye, the prostate, the oral mucosa, and the larynx, and the clinical manifestations in these patients depend on the organ involved. Involvement of the central nervous system (CNS) and meninges, which was distinctly rare in the pre-AIDS era, has become more common but is still rare in persons living with AIDS. Patients may present with subtle changes in mental status as the only symptom and are found to have chronic lymphocytic meningitis. Recovery of the fungus from extracutaneous lesions may be difficult, particularly in meningitis.

THERAPY

Spontaneous healing of the cutaneous forms of sporotrichosis has been reported, but without treatment, the lesions usually progress slowly with draining and scarring. In immunocompetent patients, the infection is not life threatening. Treatment options are presented in Table 173.1. Historically, cutaneous and lymphocutaneous sporotrichosis have been treated with saturated solution of potassium iodide (SSKI), although the mechanism of action and response rate have not been precisely determined. An initial dose of 5 to 10 drops diluted in liquid, preferably fruit juice, is given 3 times daily after meals, and increased dropwise to 120 drops per day or the maximum tolerated by the individual patient (frequently <60 drops per day). Although relatively inexpensive, this form of therapy is poorly accepted by many patients due to adverse effects, including increased lacrimation, increased salivation, metallic taste perversion, salivary gland swelling, gastrointestinal upset, and frequent rash.

Itraconazole is the treatment of choice for lymphocutaneous sporotrichosis; response rates of 89% to 100% have been demonstrated with itraconazole, 100 to 200 mg orally daily for 3 to 12 months, determined by continuing treatment for 1 month beyond resolution of all lesions. Itraconazole can be given either as capsules that must be taken with food and must not be coadministered with therapies that suppress gastric acidity and that have somewhat erratic absorption or as an itraconazole oral solution, which is less palatable and generally more expensive but avoids these drawbacks. In patients who do not respond to itraconazole initially, one can consider increasing the dosage of itraconazole to 400 mg/day. Alternative therapy includes terbinafine 500 mg orally twice daily, which has a reported cure rate of 87%. By historical comparison, treatment with fluconazole, 200 to 400 mg orally daily, was less effective (63%–71% response rate) than itraconazole. The effectiveness of higher doses of fluconazole is subject to speculation. Amphotericin B preparations should only be necessary as a treatment of last resort for patients with cutaneous or lymphocutaneous sporotrichosis. Because many strains of *S. schenckii* that cause fixed cutaneous sporotrichosis grow poorly in the laboratory at 37°C, local application of heat may be an effective adjunct to antifungal therapy.

Pulmonary sporotrichosis should be treated with either itraconazole, 200 mg orally twice daily, for patients with non–life-threatening infection or with an amphotericin B preparation (preferably a liposomal amphotericin B preparation because of better tolerability) in patients

Table 173.1 Treatment of Sporotrichosis

Form of Sporotrichosis	Preferred Treatment	Alternative Agents
Cutaneous or lymphocutaneous	Itraconazole	Terbinafine, SSKI, fluconazole, amphotericin B
Pulmonary	Itraconazole	Amphotericin B
Osteoarticular or musculoskeletal	Itraconazole	Amphotericin B
Disseminated	Amphotericin B	Amphotericin B plus flucytosine, itraconazole step-down therapy

Abbreviation: SSKI = saturated solution of potassium iodide.

with life-threatening or extensive pulmonary infection. For the latter patients who have the lung capacity to tolerate such a procedure, treatment with an amphotericin B preparation with subsequent surgical resection of involved lung areas may be the best therapy.

Itraconazole, 200 mg orally twice daily, should be initial therapy for patients with osteoarticular sporotrichosis. As with other joint and bone infections, drainage and debridement may be important surgical adjuncts to antimicrobial therapy. Conventional amphotericin B therapy appears to be approximately as effective as itraconazole but is less convenient and associated generally with more frequent adverse reactions; therefore, it is generally used only after failed itraconazole therapy. The role of liposomal amphotericin B preparations in osteoarticular sporotrichosis has not been defined. Fluconazole has been used with only modest success in osteoarticular sporotrichosis. Itraconazole treatment should generally be continued for 12 months, therapy with amphotericin B preparations for 6 to 10 weeks. Terbinafine therapy is not expected to be successful for osteoarticular sporotrichosis and should not be used. Voriconazole has poor activity in vitro against sporotrichosis and should not be used. Posaconazole has in vitro activity, but its role in vivo is undefined.

Sporotrichotic meningitis should be treated with amphotericin B, based on limited numbers of anecdotally reported cases; liposomal amphotericin B is preferred because of increased penetration into the cerebrospinal fluid. Based on possible in vitro synergy and anecdotal reports, the addition of flucytosine may be beneficial for patients with recalcitrant meningitis. Itraconazole may offer effective step-down therapy after clinical improvement.

Based on anecdotal experience, an amphotericin B preparation should be considered initial therapy for patients with disseminated sporotrichosis with or without AIDS. Itraconazole might be used for non–life-threatening infection and in cases in which meningitis has been actively excluded. Itraconazole may also play a role in lifelong suppressive therapy for patients with disseminated sporotrichosis and AIDS after initial induction therapy with an amphotericin B preparation.

SUGGESTED READING

Chapman SW, Pappas P, Kauffman C, et al. Comparative evaluation of the efficacy and safety of two doses of terbinafine (500 and 1000 mg per day) in the treatment of cutaneous or lymphocutaneous sporotrichosis. *Mycoses*. 2004;47:62–68.

Kauffman CA. Endemic mycoses: blastomycosis, histoplasmosis and sporotrichosis. *Infect Dis Clin N Am*. 2006;20:645–662.

Kauffman CA, Hajjeh R, Chapman SW. Practice guidelines for the management of patients with sporotrichosis. For the Mycoses Study Group. Infectious Diseases Society of America. *Clin Infect Dis*. 2000;30:684–687.

Kauffman CA, Pappas PG, McKinsey DS, et al. Treatment of lymphocutaneous and visceral sporotrichosis with fluconazole. *Clin Infect Dis*. 1996;22:46–50.

Kohli R, Hadley S. Fungal arthritis and osteomyelitis. *Infect Dis Clin N Am*. 2005;19:831–851.

Rocha MM, Dassin T, Lira R, et al. Sporotrichosis in patient with AIDS: report of a case and review. *Rev Iberoam Micol*. 2001;18:133–136.

Sharkey-Mathis PK, Kauffman CA, Graybill JR, et al. NIAID Mycoses Study Group. Treatment of sporotrichosis with itraconazole. *Am J Med*. 1993;95:279–285.

174. Cryptococcus

William G. Powderly

Infection with the yeast, *Cryptococcus neoformans*, is usually, although not always, a consequence of underlying immune compromise. Prior to the 1980s, infection was rare. Up to half of cases of cryptococcal disease were associated with lymphomas, and many other patients with cryptococcosis received corticosteroid therapy before the onset of the infection. Currently, the most common form of immunologic predisposition to cryptococcal infection is advanced infection with the human immunodeficiency virus (HIV) in patients with extremely low CD4+ lymphocyte counts. Since the beginning of the acquired immunodeficiency syndrome (AIDS) epidemic, cryptococcosis has emerged as a major cause of morbidity and mortality in persons infected, affecting between 5% and 10% of all AIDS patients in the United States at the peak of the epidemic in the mid-1990s. With the use of potent antiretroviral therapy (ART) for the treatment of HIV infection and the widespread use of the azole antifungals, the incidence of invasive cryptococcosis in the HIV-infected population has declined but has not disappeared. Indeed, in resource-poor settings cryptococcal meningitis is the second most common opportunistic infection in AIDS (after tuberculosis) and a leading cause of mortality.

PRESENTATION AND DIAGNOSIS

The most common manifestation of cryptococcal infection is meningitis. Most patients develop insidious features of a subacute meningitis or meningoencephalitis, with fever, malaise, and headache, and are generally symptomatic for at least 2 to 4 weeks before presentation. In patients with a more subacute or chronic course, mental status changes such as forgetfulness and coma can also be seen. Classic meningeal symptoms and signs such as stiff neck and photophobia occur in only about one-quarter to one-third of all patients and generally are less likely to occur in HIV-positive patients. The typical pattern in the cerebrospinal fluid (CSF) is chronic meningitis with a lymphocytic pleocytosis. However, the CSF may appear normal in HIV-positive patients with cryptococcal meningitis because the usual response to infection is usually markedly blunted. In fact, fewer than half of HIV-positive patients with cryptococcal meningitis have an elevated protein level, only about one-third have hypoglycorrhachia, and only about 20% have more than 20 white blood cells per cubic millimeter of CSF. The opening pressure is usually elevated in patients with cryptococcal meningitis (up to 70% of patients present with pressures greater than 20 cm H_2O) and is an important issue associated with therapy. India ink stain of the CSF is positive, showing encapsulated yeast, in about 75% of cases (Figure 174.1), and the cryptococcal antigen titer in the CSF is almost invariably positive with sensitivity of 93% to 100% and specificity of 93% to 98%. Serum cryptococcal antigen (sCRAG) is elevated in 95% of patients with meningitis. A positive sCRAG with titer above 1:8 suggests disseminated cryptococcosis. Such patients should be evaluated for possible meningeal involvement. False-positive sCRAG can happen secondary to infection with *Trichosporon beigelii* and secondary to residual disinfectant on laboratory test slides. Culture of *C. neoformans* from any body site should also be regarded as an indication for further evaluation and initiation of therapy. However, colonization of *Cryptococcus* can be found in the respiratory system. Patients with isolated positive respiratory cultures for *C. neoformans* should be carefully evaluated for disseminated infection; therapy might not be necessary in immunocompetent patients with no symptoms and negative sCRAG.

Cryptococcus neoformans can invade sites other than the meninges. Isolated pulmonary disease has been well described. It usually presents as a solitary nodule in the absence of other symptoms. Cryptococcus pneumonia has also been described (Figure 174.2). In immunocompromised patients, especially those with AIDS, disseminated disease is common. About half of HIV-positive patients with cryptococcal meningitis have evidence of pulmonary involvement at presentation, with clinical symptoms such as cough or dyspnea and abnormal chest radiographs. The chest radiographic finding is usually diffuse interstitial infiltrates in

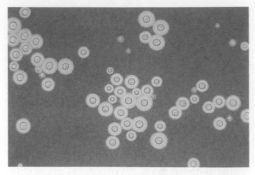

Figure 174.1 *Cryptococcus neoformans*. India ink stain, demonstrating capsules and budding. (Public Health Image Library, content provider: CDC, Dr. Leanor Haley.)

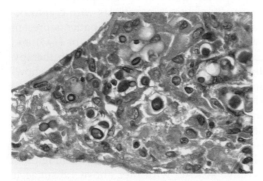

Figure 174.2 Cryptococcosis of lung in patient with AIDS. Mucicarmine stain. Histopathology of lung shows widened alveolar septum containing a few inflammatory cells and numerous yeasts of *C. neoformans*. The inner layer of the yeast capsule stains red with mucicarmine. (Public Health Image Library, content provider: CDC, Dr. Edwin P. Ewing, Jr.)

immunocompromised patients or focal lesions in immunocompetent patients. Concomitant opportunistic infections, especially with *Pneumocystis carinii*, occur in about 15% to 35% of patients. Cutaneous involvement is common and with this presentation suggests disseminated disease. The most common skin involvement resembles that of molluscum contagiosum. As many as three-quarters of patients with cryptococcal meningitis have positive blood cultures. Infection of bone, eye, adrenal glands, prostate, and urinary tract has also been described. The prostate gland represents a reservoir of infection and potential source of reinfection after completion of therapy.

THERAPY

Much of our current concepts regarding treatment for cryptococcal infection come from large controlled trials performed during the height of the AIDS era before the availability of effective antiretroviral therapy. Although these studies provide the basis of current treatment guidelines for cryptococcal meningitis, it is not clear how well they apply to patients without AIDS and in the current era.

Management of cryptococcal infection depends on the extent of disease and the patient's immune status. A solitary pulmonary nodule in a normal host may not need treatment, provided the patient has careful follow-up. The advent of relatively safe antifungals such as fluconazole permits a short course of therapy for most patients with localized disease. Extrapulmonary disease is generally managed in the same way as meningitis. A search for the underlying problems should be initiated in patients who are not known to be immunosuppressed, including an HIV antibody test and CD4 lymphocyte count, because cryptococcal infections have been described as one of the manifestations of so-called isolated CD4 T-cell lymphocytopenia. Drugs generally used in the treatment of cryptococcal infection are summarized in Table 174.1.

Cryptococcal Infection in Normal Hosts

Before the AIDS era, the standard treatment for cryptococcal meningitis had been the combination of amphotericin B and flucytosine (5-FC). The National Institute of Allergy and Infectious Diseases (NIAID)-sponsored Mycosis Study Group (MSG) showed that amphotericin B, 0.3 mg/kg, plus 5-FC for 6 weeks was effective and less nephrotoxic than amphotericin B, 0.4 mg/kg, given alone for 10 weeks. A subsequent study compared 4 weeks of combination therapy with a 6–week course and concluded that 4 weeks of combination therapy was acceptable for patients who did not have risk factors that correlated with a high frequency of relapse. The factors predicting relapse are shown in Table 174.2. The MSG investigators suggested that patients at risk of relapse were candidates for longer therapy. However, this regimen was not uniformly successful and had a mortality approaching 20%, so it is clear that a better approach is needed.

Untreated cryptococcal meningitis is uniformly fatal, so all patients with meningitis must be treated. Most of the available evidence suggests that amphotericin B–based therapy remains the gold standard and the combination of an amphotericin B preparation plus 5-FC should be regarded as the best initial treatment (Figure 174.3). Recent studies indicate that this combination is most likely to lead

Specific Organisms – Fungi

Table 174.1 Drugs Used in the Treatment of Cryptococcal Infection

Drugs	Dosage	Side Effects	Drug Interactions	Comments
Amphotericin B	0.7–1.0 mg/kg/day 3–6 mg/kg/day (liposomal) 5 mg/kg/day (lipid complex)	Immediate hypersensitivity reaction, fever, hypotension, nausea and vomiting during administration, hypokalemia, and nephrotoxicity	Nephrotoxic drugs (eg, aminoglycosides, pentamidine, foscarnet, cidofovir)	Liposomal or lipid complex formulation should be considered in patients with renal dysfunction
Flucytosine (5-FC)	25 mg/kg q6h	Gastrointestinal, bone marrow suppression	Nephrotoxic drugs	Dosage must be reduced in patients with renal dysfunction; drug level should be monitored
Fluconazole	400 mg/day (acute therapy), 200 mg/day (suppressive therapy)	Nausea, rash, and hepatitis	Rifabutin (increased rifabutin levels); rifampin (decreased fluconazole levels)	Dosage may need to be adjusted in renal dysfunction
Itraconazole	200–400 mg BID	Nausea, abdominal pain, rash, headache, edema, and hypokalemia	Rifamycins, ritonavir, phenobarbitol, phenytoin all decrease itraconazole levels The effect of nevirapine is unknown; the drug should not be used concomitantly with terfenadine or astemizole Antacids, histamine blockers decrease itraconazole absorption Itraconazole itself acts as a moderate inhibitor of cytochrome P450 system and can increase levels of indinavir, cyclosporin, digoxin, and phenytoin	Absorption of itraconazole is dependent on food and gastric acid and may be erratic; the newer solution is better absorbed

Table 174.2 Factors Predicting Relapse of Cryptococcal Meningitis

Immunosuppression
Presentation with neurologic abnormalities
CSF leukocyte count ≤20 cells/mm^3
CSF antigen titer >1:32
Positive India ink stain after 4 wk of treatment
CSF antigen titer greater than 1:8 after 4 wk of treatment
Abbreviation: CSF = cerebrospinal fluid.

to more effective and more rapid clearance of the fungus from the CSF, which is probably the best surrogate marker for ultimate successful therapy. This conceptual approach is consistent with clinical trial data in AIDS that amphotericin B–based therapy is superior to initial therapy with azoles. The different amphotericin B preparations have not been shown to have important differences in response rates of cryptococcal meningitis, although clearly the lipid-based formulations are less toxic than amphotericin B deoxycholate. The use of saline loading (ie, giving a bolus of 250 to 500 mL of normal saline before amphotericin B infusions) appears to minimize nephrotoxicity. Because some degree of nephroxicity is inevitable if amphotericin B deoxycholate is given for 4 to 6 weeks, my preference is to administer liposomal amphotericin at a dose of 5 mg/kg as treatment for cryptococcal meningitis in normal hosts. Although it is unclear whether 5-FC is necessary with higher dosages of amphotericin B, I recommend its use at a dosage of 37.5 mg/kg 4 times daily. Levels must be measured to minimize toxicity (especially bone marrow suppression), and dosages must be adjusted for renal insufficiency.

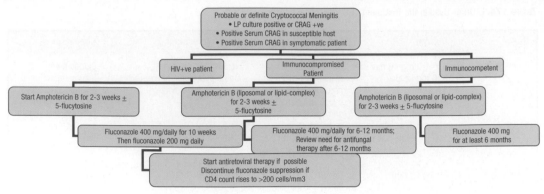

Figure 174.3 Treatment of cryptococcal meningitis.

It is clear that normal subjects with no evident risk factors for a poor outcome respond well to 4 weeks of combination therapy, and this is often curative. Azole therapy (ie, fluconazole, 400 mg orally daily) for 3 to 6 months is likely to be effective in such patients but has not been well studied. Pulmonary cryptococcosis without meningeal involvement can be treated initially with fluconazole. However, for meningitis, there is no controlled trial of fluconazole, especially comparing initial azole therapy with an amphotericin B–based regimen. With current available data, amphotericin B plus 5-FC is still recommended as standard therapy for cryptococcal meningitis. Fluconazole can be used to treat patients (or to complete a course of treatment) who cannot tolerate amphotericin B or patients without neural involvement. In many circumstances (need for intravenous access, difficulties with outpatient parenteral therapy, toxicity) a full course of parenteral amphotericin B is impractical or undesirable, and a switch to fluconazole is preferred. Timing of such a switch is uncertain. There is insufficient evidence to advocate using changes in cryptococcal antigen as a guide to making treatment decisions, but it is probably reasonable to consider using the clearance of yeast from CSF as an indicator for switching treatment from polyene to oral azole therapy. In most patients, this is likely to take 2 to 3 weeks to achieve, suggesting this is probably the minimum amount of amphotericin B therapy that should be used.

Once patients have been switched to fluconazole, the next question becomes how long to treat? Unfortunately, there are absolutely no well-controlled studies to answer this question. Given the potential severity of cryptococcal infection, the most prudent recommendation would be to treat with fluconazole for 6 to 12 months after clearance of CSF has been documented.

Cryptococcal Infection in AIDS

In early reports, the experience with treatment with amphotericin B and 5-FC regimens in patients with AIDS was not favorable, and the acute mortality was reported to be 10% to 25%. In addition, the regimen was thought to be too toxic for patients with AIDS. Multiple clinical factors have been identified in studies as predictors of a poor outcome, as summarized in Table 174.3. These initial poor outcomes led to a search for more effective treatment strategies.

The availability of the orally active antifungal triazoles fluconazole and itraconazole led to a number of controlled comparative trials. In each trial, the azole antifungals were effective in about 50% of patients. Similarly, in a study directly comparing fluconazole and itraconazole, fewer than 50% of patients responded to either drug. Thus at least 50% of patients treated initially with azole antifungals will fail to respond. Most studies of amphotericin B report response rates of 70% to 80% or more.

Given this experience, the NIAID/MSG and the AIDS Clinical Trials Group (ACTG) investigated a strategy of induction amphotericin B (for 2 weeks) followed by azole treatment. Patients with cryptococcal meningitis were randomized to receive 2 weeks of amphotericin B (0.7 mg/kg/day) with either 5-FC (25 mg/kg every 6 hours) or matching placebo. The study was designed to address two questions: (1) Does adding 5-FC to amphotericin B as induction therapy for cryptococcal meningitis improve 2- or 10-week survival compared with induction with amphotericin B alone and (2) is itraconazole as effective as fluconazole in suppressing relapse of cryptococcal meningitis

Specific Organisms – Fungi

Table 174.3 Factors at Baseline Predictive of a Poor
Outcome in AIDS Patients with Cryptococcal Meningitis

Decreased mental status at diagnosis
CSF leukocyte count ≤20 cells/mm^3
High titer of CSF cryptococcal antigen
Positive blood culture for *C. neoformans*
Age ≤35 y
Hyponatremia
Abbreviations: AIDS = acquired immunodeficiency syndrome; CSF = cerebrospinal fluid.

during the maintenance phrase of treatment? At
the end of 2 weeks, patients who were stable
or improved were again randomized to receive
either fluconazole, 400 mg per day, or itraconazole, 200 mg twice daily. The acute mortality
with this regimen was 6%. The addition of 5-FC
to amphotericin B did not improve the mortality and clinical course. However, 5-FC was well
tolerated. Furthermore, the use of 5-FC as initial
therapy has been associated with a decreased
risk of later relapse of cryptococcal meningitis.
There was no significant difference in clinical
symptoms, response rate, or mortality among
patients randomized to either fluconazole or
itraconazole. In light of these data, this approach
is recommended as a standard one for the treatment of acute cryptococcal meningitis in AIDS.

The availability of the alternative formulations of amphotericin B raises the issue of their
use in cryptococcal meningitis. Several studies
have shown that both liposomal amphotericin B
and amphotericin B lipid complex are effective
in AIDS-associated cryptococcal meningitis.
None show superiority to amphotericin B
deoxycholate, and most patients tolerate a
short course of amphotericin B deoxycholate
(10–14 days) without significant nephrotoxicity.
Thus the role of lipid preparations of amphotericin B in AIDS-associated cryptococcal meningitis remains uncertain, although they may be
useful in patients with impaired renal function.
There have been some studies looking at high
doses of fluconazole and at fluconazole–5-FC
combinations, but none are robust enough to
allow any recommendations.

An important aspect of management of acute
cryptococcal meningitis in AIDS is the recognition that clinical deterioration may be caused
by increased intracranial pressure (ICP), which
may not respond rapidly to antifungal therapy.
Analyses have shown a relationship between
baseline opening pressure and long-term

outcome, with the median survival in patients
with the highest pressures being significantly
less than those in patients whose pressures
were normal. I believe that all patients with
cryptococcal meningitis should have opening
pressure measured when a lumbar puncture is
performed, and strong consideration should be
given to reducing such pressure if the opening
pressure is high (>25 cm H$_2$O). Lumbar puncture
with removal of 30 mL of spinal fluid daily is
often effective. If elevated opening pressure
persists with neurologic symptoms despite serial lumbar puncture, lumbar drainage should
be considered. Some patients have required
placement of lumbar peritoneal shunts for
persistently elevated ICP despite successful
antifungal therapy. The role of corticosteroids in
this situation is not known, and I do not recommend their use.

The advent of ART has changed the natural
history of AIDS-related cryptococcal infection.
Prior to effective HIV therapy, lifelong maintenance therapy was required in AIDS patients
with cryptococcal infection to prevent relapse
of infection. Relapse rates of 50% to 60% and a
shorter life expectancy were reported in patients
who did not receive long-term suppressive
therapy. Fluconazole, 200 mg daily, is the drug
of choice. Routine monitoring by measurement
of sCRAG has not been shown to predict relapse,
although elevations of antigen in the CSF may
predict recurrence. However, it is now clear that
long-term suppressive treatment can be stopped
if the patient's immune system recovers with antiretroviral therapy (usually defined as the CD4+
T-cell count increasing to >200 cells/mm^3).

All HIV-positive patients with cryptococcal
meningitis should receive ART. Efavirenz-based
therapy has been shown to be well-tolerated in
patients receiving fluconazole for cryptococcal
meningitis. Timing of the initiation of ART is
uncertain. A potential complication of the restoration of the immune system is a more vigorous
inflammatory response to the underlying infection or immune reconstitution inflammatory
syndrome (IRIS). In the case of cryptococcal
meningitis, IRIS may manifest as an apparent
recurrence of meningitis, with all the features
of the initial meningitis presentation. Lumbar
puncture will typically show inflammation
but, by definition, will remain culture negative.
Rarely, the syndrome may present outside the
central nervous system (CNS) as pulmonary
infiltrates or hilar/mediastinal lymphadenitis
due to extra-CNS *Cryptococcus*. Typically IRIS
presents following an initial clinical improvement. The majority of cases of IRIS occur within

30 days of starting antiretroviral therapy, and the frequency of IRIS following initiation of antiretroviral therapy in cryptococcal meningitis has varied from 10% to 50% in different series. IRIS has been found more frequently in patients who are antiretroviral naïve before HAART therapy. It is also more commonly seen in those with a higher CSF cryptococcal antigen, probably due to increased antigen producing a greater inflammatory response. Starting HAART within 30 days of diagnosis of cryptococcal meningitis was also associated with a higher likelihood of IRIS, presumably due to a greater antigenic burden. The pathogenesis of IRS is unclear but thought to represent an overexuberant immunological response to a high antigen load in the context of an immune response that is recovering but not yet fully normal. Clinically there can be considerable morbidity and even mortality. If an immune reconstitution syndrome develops due to *C. neoformans*, patients should remain on antiviral therapy and continue antifungal treatment. Anti-inflammatory treatment may be needed for symptom management, and in some cases, immunosuppressive therapy such as corticosteroids has been used.

Cryptococcal Infection in Other Immunocompromised Hosts

Management of cryptococcal meningitis in the setting of organ transplantation or lymphoma is also uncertain. The MSG found patients with underlying immunosuppression to have poor outcomes when treated with amphotericin B and 5-FC and to be likely to relapse. Further more, amphotericin B nephrotoxocity complicates the use of immunosuppressives such as cyclosporin in such patients. However, there is very little published experience with the use of fluconazole, itraconazole, fluconazole plus 5-FC in this setting, and these agents are also associated with significant drug interactions. An approach similar to that used with AIDS patients (ie, an initial period of treatment with amphotericin B plus 5-FC followed by fluconazole) is recommended. Because nephrotoxicity

is an issue in many of these patients, liposomal amphotericin B is generally preferred, again for at least 2 to 3 weeks. An area of considerable uncertainty is the duration of fluconazole therapy after acute therapy. Suppressive antifungal therapy for at least 1 year after the completion of acute treatment is recommended. In some patients with persistent immunosuppression, such as solid organ transplant recipients, it may be necessary to continue treatment even further, although again there are very limited data on which to base a recommendation.

SUGGESTED READING

Brouwer AE, et al. Combination antifungal therapies for HIV-associated cryptococcal meningitis: a randomised trial. *Lancet*. 2004;363:1764–1767.

Dismukes WE, et al. Treatment of cryptococcal meningitis with combination of amphotericin B and flucytosine for 4 as compared with 6 weeks. *N Engl J Med*. 1987;317:334–341.

Mussini C, et al. Discontinuation of maintenance therapy for cryptococcal meningitis in patients with AIDS treated with highly active antiretroviral therapy: an international observational study. *Clin Infect Dis*. 2004;38:565–571.

Pappas PG, et al. Cryptococcosis in human immunodeficiency virus-negative patients in the era of effective azole therapy. *Clin Infect Dis*. 2001;33:690–699.

Powderly WG. Antifungal treatment for cryptococcal meningitis. *Intern Med J*. 2006;36: 404–405.

Saag MS, et al. Practice guidelines for the management of cryptococcal disease. *Clin Infect Dis*. 2000;30:710–718.

Saag MS, et al. Comparison of amphotericin B with fluconazole in the treatment of acute AIDS-associated cryptococcal meningitis. *N Engl J Med*. 1992;326:83–89.

van der Horst CM, et al. Treatment of cryptococcal meningitis associated with the acquired immunodeficiency syndrome. *N Engl J Med*. 1997;337:15–21.

175. Histoplasmosis

Alvaro Lapitz, Mitchell Goldman, and George A. Sarosi

INTRODUCTION

Histoplasma capsulatum is a thermal dimorphic fungus found most frequently in soil in the midwestern United States. Bird and bat excreta rich in organic nitrogen support the growth of the fungus. Sites associated with blackbird roosts are the most commonly identified sources of outbreaks nowadays, whereas domestic chicken coops were the source of the fungus in the past. When sites are disturbed the spores become airborne, producing the infective aerosol. The lung is considered the portal of entry in almost every case of histoplasmosis. The spores of *H. capsulatum* are inhaled, and once in the alveoli they convert to a yeast, which is the tissue invasive form. The now multiplying yeasts are phagocytosed by alveolar macrophages that are initially incapable of killing the fungus. The ingested yeasts multiply inside the macrophages and are spread throughout the body via the lymphatics during the preimmune phase of the illness to organs rich in reticulo-endothelial cells. Once adequate cell-mediated immunity (CMI) develops, the now "armed" macrophages can either kill or wall off the infecting organisms. When immunity is at a high level, as seen in normal individuals, necrosis occurs, which in time becomes calcified. These calcified granulomas are seen in the lung, hilar lymph nodes, liver, and spleen of individuals who successfully limited the infection.

Individuals infected with *H. capsulatum* develop adequate CMI. If CMI fails to develop, progressive dissemination will occur.

CLINICAL MANIFESTATIONS

Localized Pulmonary and Self-Limited Infections

Most *H. capsulatum* infections are asymptomatic. After low-level exposure, some patients develop a localized form of infection that manifests as fever, chills, headaches, myalgia, anorexia, cough, and chest pain. Erythema multiforme or erythema nodosum may develop in some instances. The incubation time following low-level, outdoor exposure is approximately 14 days. This form of acute localized pulmonary infection is self-limited; after 2 to 4 weeks, most immunocompetent patients will have recovered completely, and treatment is usually not necessary. Chest radiograph usually shows localized areas of pneumonitis, but it may be normal as well. Ipsilateral hilar lymph nodes are usually enlarged. Healing may be complete with normalization of the radiograph but frequently multiple cycles of central necrosis and peripheral calcification occur leaving the characteristic "coin" lesion as a proof of prior infection.

When the infective aerosol is unusually large, fulminant infection may occur, leading to severe hypoxemia and respiratory failure, requiring prompt and aggressive treatment. Patients who inhale large inocula may develop multiple nodular lesions of variable size. The radiologic appearance of an overwhelming infective dose leads to a diffuse micronodular infiltrate.

Patients with underlying emphysema may develop upper lobe infiltrates after exposure. The resultant infection may result in cavitation. The radiographic appearance of this infection mimics reactivation tuberculosis. Low-grade fever and anorexia with weight loss are common. Without treatment, most of these patients develop progressive and destructive disease. The clinical and radiologic similarities to tuberculosis make the diagnosis challenging.

Late complications of healed and calcified histoplasmosis are related to the location of the calcified lymph nodes, which may involve and compress various mediastinal structures. A rare late complication is the development of mediastinal fibrosis, which can lead to crippling complications, such as the superior vena cava syndrome.

Progressive Disseminated Histoplasmosis

During the preimmune phase of the infection it is believed that the fungus disseminates widely in all infected individuals. With the development of adequate CMI, the cells of the reticuloendothelium are responsible for limiting spread of the disease.

In the immunosuppressed patient or at extremes of age this dissemination becomes progressive. This form of the disease is known as progressive disseminated histoplasmosis (PDH), and prognosis is poor without treatment. Fever and weight loss are the most common symptoms, and hepatosplenomegaly is a frequent finding.

Dissemination to the oropharyngeal or gastrointestinal mucosa, the skin, and the adrenal glands may also occur (Figure 175.1). The patient may develop respiratory distress and hepatic or renal failure. Coagulopathy and shock may complicate severe cases. Central nervous system (CNS) involvement may also occur either as chronic meningitis or focal lesions. In PDH the mortality is close to 100% without treatment. In severely ill patients, mortality may still be high despite treatment.

Prior to the widespread use of cytotoxic agents and glucocorticoids, most patients with PDH had underlying lymphoreticular malignancies, most commonly Hodgkin's disease. Currently the most common underlying disease of patients with PDH is the acquired immunodeficiency syndrome (AIDS). Through the growing use of organ transplantation and newer immune modulating treatments such as the tumor necrosis factor (TNF) blocking agents for multiple disorders, an ever increasing number of individuals remain at risk for PDH.

DIAGNOSIS

The gold standard is the recovery of the organism from biologic material, but unfortu-nately this is very time consuming and may require up to 30 days for identification of the organism.

Sputum cultures are not very useful in the cases of suspected acute pulmonary infection because the inoculum is usually not high enough and only rarely do patients have productive cough. In patients with acute disseminated histoplasmosis and in those with chronic pulmonary or cavitary infections, sputum cultures are frequently positive. When bronchoscopy and bronchoalveolar lavage are employed with the appropriate stains, the sensitivity of obtaining respiratory secretions increases. Biopsy of accessible lesions (Figure 175.2) and bone marrow can be used in the cases of diffuse infection.

Detection of the histoplasma polysaccharide antigen offers high sensitivity and rapid diagnosis for patients with large inoculum acute pulmonary disease and for patients with PDH. Sensitivity for antigen detection is considerably higher in the urine than in serum, and the rare cases of antigenemia with no antigenuria are thought to represent false-positive results. This supports the initial testing of urine only as part of the initial evaluation. Antigenemia is useful, however, in anuric patients. Antigenuria is also useful when monitoring treatment because the levels decrease with successful therapy and increase with relapse of the disease.

Serologic tests like complement fixation and immunodiffusion are also helpful in some cases and may be the only means by which an infection can be diagnosed in immunocompetent individuals. In immunocompetent patients, it frequently takes 2 to 6 weeks for the development of detectable antibodies. The use of antibody for diagnosis of histoplasmosis is most helpful in the cases of chronic pulmonary

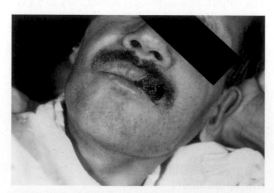

Figure 175.1 Upper lip lesion as manifestation of disseminated histoplasmosis. (Public Health Image Library, Centers for Disease Control and Prevention (CDC), Susan Lindsley, VD.)

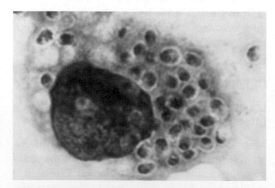

Figure 175.2 Histiocyte containing numerous yeast cells of *Histoplasma capsulatum*. Giemsa stain. (Public Health Image Library, Centers for Disease Control and Prevention (CDC), Dr. D. T. McClenan.)

Specific Organisms – Fungi

Table 175.1 Recommendations for Treatment of Patients with Histoplasmosis

Manifestation	Treatment
Acute pulmonary: moderately severe or severe when symptoms persist for 4 weeks or longer	Itraconazole, 200 mg 3× daily for 3 days, followed by itraconazole, 200–400 mg daily for 6–12 wk
Acute pulmonary with severe manifestations	Liposomal amphotericin, 3–5 mg/kg/d for up to 2 wk, followed by itraconazole, 200 mg 3× daily for 3 d, then itraconazole, 200 mg 2× daily for 12 additional wk Amphotericin deoxycholate, 0.7 mg/kg/d, is also effective and may be substituted for liposomal amphotericin in patient at low risk for renal damage
Chronic cavitary pulmonary	Itraconazole, 200 mg 3× daily for 3 days, followed by itraconazole, 200 mg 2× daily for at least a year. Itraconazole levels should be measured in patients where resolution is slow. Amphotericin B deoxycholate may also be used at the dose of 0.7 mg/kg/d for 12–16 wk
Progressive disseminated: moderately severe/severe, with or without HIV/AIDS	Liposomal amphotericin B, 3 mg/kg/d for 1–2 wk or until stability, followed by itraconazole, 200 mg 3× daily and then 200 mg 2× daily for at least 1 y; other lipid formulations may be used as well as the deoxycholate preparation if needed
Progressive disseminated mild to moderate	Oral itraconazole, 200 mg daily for 3 d followed by 200 mg 2× daily for at least a year
Central nervous system	Liposomal amphotericin B, 5 mg/kg/d for a total of 175 mg/kg, followed by itraconazole 200, mg 2–3× daily for at least 1 year

histoplasmosis and for those who have persistent symptoms following recent infection. Antibody tests have also provided an invaluable epidemiologic tool.

As in the case of antigen detection there is also clinical correlation between the severity of the disease and the antibody response. In the immunosuppressed patient the response may be weaker and in some cases it may not be demonstrated. Although there is an extensive literature for the histoplasma skin test, it is no longer available.

TREATMENT

The vast majorities of patients with acute histoplasmosis are asymptomatic or have a mild self-limited disease and do not require antifungal treatment. In the few patients where treatment is required, therapy (Table 175.1) depends on the clinical scenario.

Acute localized pulmonary infection resolves without therapy in the vast majority of cases, and treatment is indicated only when symptoms persist for more than 4 weeks. In these patients itraconazole, 200 mg 3 times daily for 3 days, followed by itraconazole, 200 to 400 mg daily for 6 to 12 weeks, is recommended if symptoms persist for 4 weeks or longer.

In the more severe cases of acute diffuse pulmonary histoplasmosis in the immunocompetent host that requires hospitalization, lipid formulation of amphotericin B in doses of 3 to 5 mg/kg/day is recommended for up to 2 weeks, followed by itraconazole, 200 mg 3 times daily for 3 days and then 200 mg twice daily for 12 additional weeks, is recommended. The parent compound, amphotericin B deoxycholate, is also effective, but the potential for nephrotoxicity limits its use. The usual dose is 0.7 mg/kg infused daily. Methylprednisolone, 0.5 to 1.0 mg/kg/day intravenously, may be used in severely ill, hypoxemic, or ventilated patients for up to 2 weeks.

The treatment of chronic pulmonary histoplasmosis is itraconazole, 200 mg 3 times daily for 3 days, followed by itraconazole, 200 to 400 mg/daily for at least a year, but therapy may be extended if resolution is slow. Itraconazole levels should be monitored, especially in patients where the resolution is slow. Amphotericin B is also effective when used for 12 to 16 weeks. Relapses after apparently successful treatment may occur, and close follow-up is indicated.

The treatment of severe PDH is liposomal amphotericin B at the dose of 3 mg/kg/day for 1 to 2 weeks or until clear-cut clinical improvement occurs. This is followed by oral itraconazole, 200 mg 3 times daily for 3 days followed by 200 mg twice daily for at least 12 months. Other lipid preparations may be substituted in appropriate doses. Amphotericin B deoxycholate is also effective in patients at low risk for renal failure. Mildly ill patients with PDH may be treated with oral itraconazole alone for at least 12 months. PDH in AIDS patients is treated in a similar fashion. Chronic suppressive therapy with itraconazole is recommended for patients who do not recover immune function. CNS histoplasmosis is treated with liposomal amphotericin B, 5 mg/kg/day, for a total of 175 mg/kg over 4 to 6 weeks, followed by itraconazole, 200 mg 2 to 3 times daily for at least 1 year.

In areas highly endemic for histoplasmosis, particularly during periods of time when high rates of histoplasmosis are observed, prophylaxis with 200 mg of itraconazole daily may be considered for patients with AIDS if the CD4 count is <150 cells/mm^3.

SUGGESTED READING

Dismukes WE, Bradsher RW, Cloud GC, et al. Itraconazole therapy for blastomycosis and histoplasmosis. NIAID Mycoses Study Group. *Am J Med*. 1992;93: 489–497.

Johnson PS, Wheat LJ, Cloud GC, et al. Safety and efficacy of liposomal amphotericin B compared with conventional amphotericin B for induction therapy of histoplasmosis in patients with AIDS. *Ann Intern Med*. 2002;137:105–109.

Wheat J, Hafner R, Korzun AH, et al. Itraconazole treatment of disseminated histoplasmosis in patients with the acquired immunodeficiency syndrome. AIDS Clinical Trial Group. *Am J Med*. 1995;98: 336–342.

Wheat J, Sarosi GA, McKinsey D, et al. Practice guidelines for the management of patients with histoplasmosis. *Clin Infect Dis*. 2000;30:688–695.

176. Blastomycosis

Peter G. Pappas

Blastomycosis is a systemic pyogranulomatous disease caused by the thermally dimorphic fungus *Blastomyces dermatitidis*. The disease is endemic to parts of the midwestern and south-central United States and Canada, although blastomycosis has been reported worldwide, including isolated reports from Africa and Central and South America. Within the United States and Canada, the disease is concentrated in areas along the Mississippi and Ohio River basins and the Great Lakes. In endemic areas, small point-source outbreaks of blastomycosis have been associated with recreational and occupational activities occurring in wooded areas along waterways. Current evidence indicates that *B. dermatitidis* exists in warm moist soil enriched by organic debris, including decaying vegetation and wood.

Most infections with *B. dermatitidis* occur through inhalation of aerosolized spores, although infection through direct inoculation has been reported rarely. Primary infections are usually asymptomatic or may result in a self-limited flulike illness. Hematogenous dissemination of organisms from the lung can result in extrapulmonary manifestations.

Blastomycosis is usually recognized as a chronic, indolent systemic fungal infection associated with various pulmonary and extrapulmonary manifestations. Pulmonary blastomycosis usually manifests as a chronic pneumonia syndrome characterized by productive cough, chest pain, hemoptysis, weight loss, and low-grade fever. There are no distinguishing radiologic features of pulmonary blastomycosis, although one or more fibronodular infiltrates or mass lesions with or without cavitation are common, often mimicking other granulomatous diseases or bronchogenic carcinoma. Hilar adenopathy and pleural effusions are uncommon. Rarely, diffuse pulmonary infiltrates consistent with adult respiratory distress syndrome may occur secondary to blastomycosis. The skin is involved in 40% to 80% of cases, and multiple organ involvement occurs in approximately 50% to 60% of cases. After lung and cutaneous disease, bone and joint disease is most common, followed by disease of the male genitourinary tract (especially the prostate and epididymis). Central nervous system (CNS) involvement is uncommon but may present as either granulomatous meningitis or an intracerebral mass lesion. *Blastomyces dermatitidis* is an uncommon opportunistic pathogen but may cause overwhelming disease in the immunocompromised host. Among patients with predisposing factors, chronic glucocorticosteroid use, solid organ transplant, and advanced human immunodeficiency virus (HIV) disease are the most common underlying conditions.

DIAGNOSIS

The definitive diagnosis of blastomycosis requires a positive culture for *B. dermatitidis* from clinical specimens. A presumptive diagnosis is based on the finding of broad-based budding yeasts with doubly refractile cell walls compatible with *B. dermatitidis* on histopathologic examination of clinical specimens (Figure 176.1). Ten percent potassium hydroxide (KOH) is used to prepare wet specimens for examination, whereas fixed specimens are usually stained with hematoxylin and eosin, periodic acid–Schiff (PAS), or Gomori's methenamine silver (GMS) reagents. Serologic assays are of limited value in the diagnosis of blastomycosis. The complement fixation assay for serum antibody is highly cross-reactive and of little diagnostic value. Recent studies suggest that immunodiffusion or enzyme immunoassay (EIA) tests for A antigen of *B. dermatitidis* or antibody to more purified antigens have potential as serologic markers of disease. A recently licensed *Blastomyces* EIA urine antigen assay is sensitive but nonspecific and gives false-positive results among patients with active histoplasmosis, paracoccidioidomycosis, and penicilliosis. The blastomycin skin test antigen lacks sufficient sensitivity and specificity and should not be used as a diagnostic test.

TREATMENT

Presently, three drugs are approved for the treatment of blastomycosis: amphotericin B,

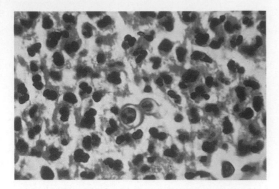

Figure 176.1 Histopathology of blastomycosis of skin. Cell of *Blastomyces dermatitidis* undergoing characteristic broad-based budding, surrounded by neutrophils. Multiple nuclei are visible. (Public Health Image Library, Centers for Disease Control and Prevention (CDC).)

itraconazole, and ketoconazole. Traditionally, amphotericin B has been the mainstay of therapy for all forms of blastomycosis, but studies and experience gained since the early 1990s indicate that ketoconazole, itraconazole, and fluconazole are highly effective alternative oral therapies, particularly in patients with chronic indolent disease without involvement of the CNS. Although no comparative trials have been performed, itraconazole appears to have greater efficacy and less toxicity than either fluconazole or ketoconazole and therefore is the oral agent of choice. In a recently published trial, 95% of patients with non–life-threatening, non-CNS blastomycosis were treated successfully with itraconazole, 200 to 400 mg daily for 2 to 6 months. This approximates the observed efficacy seen with amphotericin B. Clinical data regarding the use of ketoconazole and fluconazole suggest similar efficacy of these two agents, with at least 80% of patients responding to 400 to 800 mg daily for 6 months. Most patients with blastomycosis can be started on oral itraconazole, 200 mg daily and advanced by 100-mg increments at monthly intervals to a maximum of 400 mg daily in patients with persistent or progressive disease. In patients with more aggressive disease, an initial dose of 400 mg is appropriate. Ketoconazole and fluconazole are usually initiated at a dose of 400 mg daily and advanced by 200-mg increments monthly to 800 mg daily in patients with persistent or progressive disease. Therapy with any of the azoles should be given for a minimum of 6 months. Clinical experience with the expanded spectrum triazoles, including voriconazole and posaconazole, is very limited in all forms of blastomycosis; however, based on in vitro susceptibility data, one would anticipate excellent clinical activity of these compounds. Among the azoles, ketoconazole is the least well tolerated, but it is considerably less expensive than either itraconazole or fluconazole.

Amphotericin B should be reserved for patients with overwhelming life-threatening or CNS disease, patients who are immunocompromised, and those in whom oral therapy has failed. A total dose of 1.5 to 2.5 g is sufficient therapy for most patients. In selected patients, an induction dose of amphotericin B (totaling about 500 mg) for a rapid fungicidal effect to gain control of the disease may be useful, followed by oral therapy with itraconazole for at least 6 months. For patients with CNS involvement, several reports suggest that fluconazole and voriconazole, two azoles with significant CNS penetration, may have potential as therapeutic agents among individuals who have had an initial favorable response to amphotericin B. There is only limited clinical experience and are few published data concerning the use of the lipid formulations of amphotericin B in the treatment of blastomycosis, and there are no data to suggest superior efficacy of these agents compared with conventional (deoxycholate) amphotericin B. The use of the lipid formulations of amphotericin B to treat blastomycosis should probably be restricted to patients with pre-existing renal disease and in whom renal or other dose-limiting toxicities occur while receiving amphotericin B.

The treatment of acute pulmonary blastomycosis remains controversial. Many investigators suggest close observation without therapy in patients who are not immunocompromised; however, this nihilistic approach has become less common given the extensive safety and efficacy profile of the azole compounds. Available data suggest that most cases of acute pulmonary blastomycosis resolve spontaneously without therapy, although careful long-term evaluation of these untreated patients is important to monitor for evidence of active disease.

All patients with chronic blastomycosis should receive antifungal therapy. Cure rates of at least 90% should be expected, with relapse rates of less than 10%. A few patients, especially chronically immunocompromised individuals such as organ transplant recipients, patients receiving chronic glucocorticosteroid treatment, and patients with acquired immunodeficiency syndrome require long-term suppressive therapy to prevent relapse.

SUGGESTED READING

Bradsher RW, Chapman SW, Pappas PG. Blastomycosis. *Infect Dis Clin North Am.* 2003;17:21–40.

Chapman SW, Bradsher RW, Campbell GD Jr, et al. Practice guidelines for the management of patients with blastomycosis. *Clin Infect Dis.* 2000;30:679–683.

Treatment of blastomycosis and histoplasmosis with ketoconazole. Results of a prospective randomized clinical trial. National Institute of Allergy and Infectious Diseases Mycoses Study Group. *Ann Intern Med.* 1985;103:861–872.

Dismukes WE, Bradsher RW Jr, Cloud GC, et al. Itraconazole therapy for blastomycosis and histoplasmosis. *Am J Med.* 1992;93: 489–497.

Kauffman CA. Endemic mycoses: blastomycosis, histoplasmosis, and sporotrichosis. *Infect Dis Clin North Am.* 2006;20:645–662.

Lemos LB, Guo M, Baliga M. Blastomycosis: organ involvement and etiologic diagnosis: a review of 123 patients from Mississippi. *Ann Diag Pathol.* 2000;4:391–406.

Meyer KC, McManus EJ, Maki DG. Overwhelming pulmonary blastomycosis associated with the adult respiratory distress syndrome. *N Engl J Med.* 1993;329:1231–1236.

Pappas PG, Threlkeld MG, Bedsole GD, et al. Blastomycosis in immunocompromised patients. *Medicine* (Baltimore). 1993;72: 311–325.

Pappas PG, Bradsher RW, Kauffman CA, et al. Treatment of blastomycosis with higher doses of fluconazole. The National Institute of Allergy and Infectious Diseases Mycoses Study Group. *Clin Infect Dis.* 1997;25: 200–205.

Perfect JR, Marr KA, Walsh TJ, et al. Voriconazole treatment for less-common, emerging or refractory fungal infections. *Clin Infect Dis.* 2003;36:1122–1131.

177. Coccidioidomycosis

Laurence F. Mirels and Stanley C. Deresinski

BACKGROUND

Coccidioidomycosis, first described over a century ago by Alejandro Posadas, is a disease of protean manifestations endemic primarily to ecologic regions of the Western Hemisphere characterized as the Lower Sonoran Life Zone. This includes areas in the southwestern United States (California, Arizona, western Texas, and selected areas of New Mexico, Nevada, and Utah), northern Mexico, and scattered foci in Central and South America. Within these general endemic areas the incidence of coccidioidomycosis may vary significantly due to geographic pockets and climatic conditions particularly favorable for infection. The etiologic agent, classically known as *Coccidioides immitis*, is a dimorphic fungus that grows in its soil reservoir in the mycelial (mould) phase. Under appropriate conditions, infectious spores, dubbed arthroconidia, disarticulate from mycelia and are carried airborne and inhaled, reaching the alveoli of the host. There the organism converts to the parasitic spherule phase, which reproduces by a process characteristic of *Coccidioides* species known as endosporulation. Infection usually is controlled locally and confined to the site(s) of initial alveolar implantation. In some cases, such as if the infecting inoculum is large and/or the host is unable to mount an effective immune response, a chronic pulmonary infection may result or infection may go on to spread within the thorax or distantly, via the lymphatics and bloodstream. Disseminated (extrapulmonary) infection, especially when it involves the meninges, carries with it considerable potential for morbidity and mortality and therefore must always be treated.

Recent data from molecular genetic and genomic studies suggest that the genus *Coccidioides* actually consists of two largely geographically separated species: *Coccidioides immitis* (found primarily in California) and *Coccidioides posadasii* (found in Arizona, Texas, and outside the United States). There are no substantial phenotypic differences between the species and the differentiation of one from the other is not routinely performed in the clinical laboratory. Similarly, no specific diagnostic, therapeutic, or prognostic ramifications have been attributed to the two different species which therefore are referred to collectively as *Coccidioides* spp. Both species are highly infectious when cultured in the laboratory and have been considered as potential agents of biological warfare; as such, they are the only fungi listed as select agents by the Centers for Disease Control and Prevention and must be handled accordingly.

PRIMARY INFECTION

Approximately 60% of people infected with *Coccidioides* spp. develop either no symptoms whatsoever or perhaps a mild, nondescript illness. They become aware of their prior infection by virtue of the development of a positive skin test (the reagent necessary for such testing is not currently commercially available) or anticoccidioidal antibody. These individuals are generally immune to repeat primary infection. After an incubation period of 7 to 21 days, approximately 40% of acutely infected people develop appreciable "flu-like" symptoms, including fever, sweats, myalgia, arthralgia, anorexia, weight loss, and fatigue, the latter often being profound and, along with fever, frequently among the patient's major concerns. These constitutional symptoms are usually accompanied by a spectrum of respiratory complaints ranging from dry cough to symptoms such as pleuritic chest pain, tachypnea, and dyspnea. Reflecting this spectrum, the chest radiograph may be normal or may reveal scattered, patchy segmental infiltrates or dense lobar infiltrate(s) (Figure 177.1). Pleural effusion, often diminutive, is noted in about 20% of chest films. In more severe cases, as may be seen following particularly heavy exposures or in infections of the immunocompromised, the chest radiograph may demonstrate diffuse reticulonodular infiltrates, a miliary pattern, or a pattern consistent with acute respiratory distress syndrome (ARDS). In fulminant cases, hemodynamic changes, including septic shock, may be present. In the acute phase, some patients will develop a transient diffuse erythematous macular skin eruption, erythema

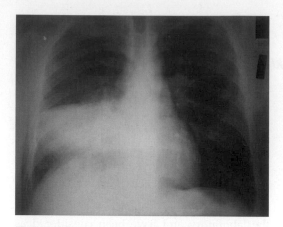

Figure 177.1 Primary pulmonary coccidio-idomycosis. This 18-year-old male Pacific Islander presented with community-acquired pneumonia, and the abovechest radiograph shows a dense right middle lobe infiltrate. Coccidioidomycosis was suspected as the patient had recently moved to California's Central Valley to attend college, demonstrating the importance of the travel history in such settings. He was treated with fluconazole for 6 months and recovered uneventfully.

nodosum, or, less commonly, erythema multiforme. These lesions are not the result of fungal dissemination but rather appear to represent immune reactions to the fungal infection, as does a self-limited arthritis ("desert rheumatism"), which may also occur. Development of erythema nodosum traditionally has been associated with subsequent successful resolution of disease, as if the immune processes resulting in this particular skin eruption reflect an underlying immune response favorable for the containment of coccidioidal infection.

Because the presentation of acute coccidioidomycosis resembles those of many other respiratory infections, a travel history placing the patient in an endemic area in the weeks prior to onset of illness can greatly expedite the diagnosis and emphasizes the importance of a detailed exposure history for all such patients, not only for consideration of coccidioidomycosis but for other endemic mycoses or even more exotic infections (eg, severe acute respiratory syndrome, avian influenza, hantavirus pulmonary syndrome). Although no findings are unique to acute coccidioidomycosis, those that tend to suggest this diagnosis include unexpectedly pronounced fever, fatigue, and weight loss and immune phenomena such as erythema nodosum. Eosinophils may be elevated on peripheral smear. Radiographic hints, when present, include thin-walled cavity or nodule formation at sites of infiltrates and pronounced hilar adenopathy. Such patients all

too frequently have been deemed ill enough to have been prescribed one or more courses of antibacterial antibiotics, with minimal effect, prior to consideration of the diagnosis of coccidioidomycosis or its serendipitous discovery via a positive sputum culture.

The vast majority of patients successfully overcome the acute infection without treatment. Symptoms, particularly fatigue, may take many months to resolve completely. These patients also develop a positive skin test, seroconvert, and are generally immune to subsequent primary infection. Persisting radiographic residua in the form of pulmonary nodules or cavities develop in approximately 10%. It is believed that viable organisms may remain latent for decades after resolution of the primary infection and apparent reactivation occurs occasionally, particularly in patients who become immunosuppressed later in life.

CHRONIC PULMONARY AND DISSEMINATED COCCIDIOIDOMYCOSIS

Development of chronic pulmonary infection or clinically important dissemination following primary infection is fortunately uncommon, occurring in approximately 1% of such people. Those who become ill with their primary infection appear to be at increased risk for progression to chronic pulmonary or disseminated infection (perhaps 10% of cases on average), possibly because severe symptoms during the acute phase are an early indication of an inability of the host to effectively control this infecting organism. In addition, certain characteristics define individuals or groups with a greatly increased risk of dissemination or progressive pneumonitis (Table 177.1) and, once these complications occur, tend to be more refractory to treatment. Included are those who are overtly immunocompromised due to underlying illness (eg, human immunodeficiency virus/acquired immunodeficiency virus [HIV/AIDS], lymphoma) or due to receipt of immunosuppressants (eg, patients who have undergone transplantation or treatment for rheumatological disorders). For reasons that remain unexplained, Filipinos and African Americans are clearly at increased risk as are Hispanics, to a somewhat lesser extent. Pregnant women (especially in the third trimester) or women in the immediate postpartum state are notorious for having great difficulty controlling their infections. Transmission to the fetus prior to or during birth is rare but does occur. Diabetes mellitus, particularly if poorly

Specific Organisms – Fungi

Table 177.1 Risk Factors for Dissemination

Ethnicity: Filipino > African American > Hispanic
Pregnancy and the postpartum period
Immunodeficiency states, including acquired immunodeficiency syndrome
Diabetes

controlled, has been repeatedly associated with chronic cavitary pulmonary disease and likely also leads to an increased risk of dissemination. Heavy exposures to infecting arthroconidia likely propel even healthy patients toward chronic or disseminated disease.

Following primary infection, approximately 1 in 200 individuals goes on to develop persistent infections that are confined to the lung. Such patients may display pulmonary cavities with more thickened walls (Figure 177.2) and chronic symptoms of dry to productive cough, chest pain, shortness of breath, and hemoptysis, each of which may wax and wane. A distinct subgroup will develop a destructive, progressive fibrocavitary pulmonary infection with fibrotic changes in the lung parenchyma and bronchiectasis. In addition to the symptoms mentioned earlier, these patients are often plagued with constitutional symptoms such as fever and weight loss, which may progress to cachexia. Antibody titers in this group tend to be high. Complications associated with cavities include bacterial superinfection (recurrent), fungus ball formation (due to *Coccidioides* spp. or other fungi), and rupture into the pleura with (hydro-)pneumothorax, empyema, and/or bronchopleural fistula. In the absence of profound immunocompromise, individuals with chronic pulmonary disease frequently do not have chronic extrapulmonary foci of infection and vice versa.

Disseminated disease usually becomes clinically evident within 6 months of the initiating infection. Evaluation of the patient may reveal involvement of only a single anatomic site or of a multitude of different sites and organ systems. Dissemination may occur in patients who were asymptomatic with their primary infection, and in those with symptomatic primary infections it is common for pulmonary symptoms and findings on chest radiograph to have resolved completely at the time of presentation. Both of these circumstances tend to obscure the diagnosis of coccidioidomycosis.

Skin lesions are the most frequently recognized manifestation of extrapulmonary

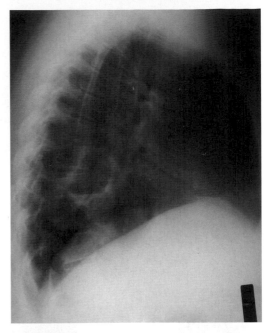

Figure 177.2 Chronic cavitary pulmonary coccidioidomycosis. Chest radiograph of a 21-year-old Hispanic woman with type II diabetes and known chronic cavitary coccidioidomycosis. She presented with 1 week of low-grade fever and increasing productive cough. Her lateral chest radiograph shows a chronic cavity with thickened walls and an air-fluid level consistent with bacterial superinfection. She responded to a 14-day course of amoxicillin–clavulanate and remained on fluconazole.

dissemination. Lesions may be single or numerous, range in size from several millimeters to many centimeters in diameter, and, even in the same patient, may take on a variety of forms, including smooth to verrucous papules, plaques, ulcers, or pustules (Figure 177.3A). Bone is a frequent site of dissemination with vertebrae, often numerous, being particularly favored. The cranium, pelvis, ribs, tibia, feet, and hands are other common targets. In some cases bone lesions are asymptomatic, whereas in other settings they cause the patient constant, gnawing pain. These lesions are usually lytic, may be highly destructive, and may be accompanied by extensive adjacent soft tissue involvement. Bone scans and magnetic resonance imaging (MRI) are particularly useful modalities for identifying bone lesions and for evaluating the extent of bone and neighboring soft-tissue involvement, respectively (Figure 177.4). Dissemination to joints is not infrequent and may be heralded by rapid or more insidious development of findings typical of septic arthritis. The knee is affected most frequently followed by joints of the ankle and foot, wrist, hands, and the elbow.

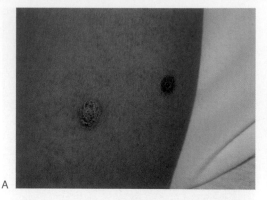

A

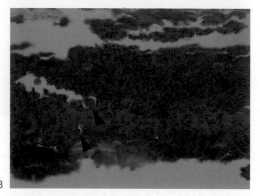

B

Figure 177.3 Disseminated coccidioidomycosis, skin lesions. **A:** This 26-year-old previously healthy Filipino man presented with coccidioidomycosis featuring numerous skin lesions of varying size and appearance. This photograph shows two suspicious lesions on the arm, each measuring ~5 mm in diameter. **B:** Photomicrograph of a punch biopsy of the skin which was taken from the margin of the verrucous lesion shown in the adjacent photograph. There is significant lymphocytic infiltration, and numerous spherules are evident (several of which are highlighted by arrowheads) thus making the diagnosis of disseminated coccidioidomycosis. (Original magnification, 400×, tissue stained with hematoxylin and eosin). This patient made a full recovery and continues on itraconazole.

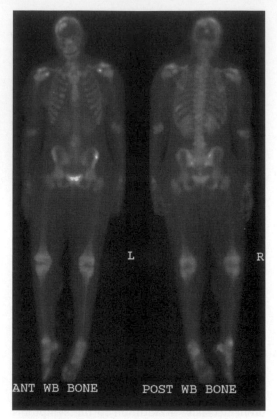

Figure 177.4 Disseminated coccidioidomycosis, bone lesions. This 14-year-old healthy African American adolescent presented with widely disseminated coccidioidomycosis. These delayed whole-body three-phase bone scan images demonstrate abnormal uptake indicative of a multitude of bone lesions that were subsequently verified by magnetic resonance imaging, computed tomography, or plain film: vertebral lesions are seen throughout the length of the spine; there are multiple lesions of the calvaria, lesions affecting the right sixth rib, the left tenth rib, both shoulders, the right ankle, and the right ischium are readily appreciated. Of note, only her shoulder and lower spine lesions were symptomatic. She was successfully treated medically with 1 month of intravenous amphotericin B, which was transitioned to itraconazole. She continues on itraconazole.

Pelvic joints may be involved, intervertebral disks are usually spared. Arthrocentesis may lead to the diagnosis; however, synovial biopsy offers a higher yield. Subcutaneous abscesses may represent primary sites of dissemination but often prove to have resulted from suppuration of a lymph node or extension of pus from a deeper (sometimes surprisingly distant) focus via fistula or erosion through tissue planes.

The central nervous system is a major site of dissemination. It is the manifestation most likely to result in permanent disability or death, as it can be difficult or impossible to control and complications occur with a disappointingly high frequency. *Coccidioides* spp. typically cause

a chronic granulomatous meningitis, most often involving the basilar meninges of the brain and those of the upper spinal cord (Figure 177.5). Central nervous system involvement generally occurs within months of the primary infection but occasionally is seen after much longer intervals. Symptoms may be abrupt or insidious in onset and progress inexorably at a tempo that varies from patient to patient. If the underlying disease remains untreated it virtually always will lead to death within 2 years. Patients complain primarily of headache with anorexia, nausea, vomiting, visual

Specific Organisms – Fungi

changes, generalized weakness, and ataxia as possible associated symptoms (often being secondary to the development of hydrocephalus). Progressive lassitude and altered mentation often are the dominant findings and result in a clinical picture quite distinct from that normally conjured up based on other commonly encountered causes of meningitis. Furthermore, patients may have surprisingly mild symptoms even in the face of impressive cerebrospinal fluid (CSF) findings, meningeal signs are often subtle if not absent entirely, and patients may be afebrile throughout their course. Therefore the threshold to evaluate patients by lumbar puncture and radiographic imaging must be low. Hydrocephalus develops commonly and can do so well into the course of appropriate, effective therapy. Vasculitis is a common consequence of central nervous system infection and may lead to a variety of complications such as stroke or seizures. Abscess formation, cranial nerve involvement, myelitis, arachnoiditis, and syrinx formation are also occasionally seen.

Other sites involved with some regularity in disseminated disease include lymph nodes, liver, spleen, male and female genitourinary tracts, peritoneum, pericardium, thyroid, and the eye.

DIAGNOSIS

The diagnosis of coccidioidomycosis is best made by direct examination of tissues or secretions for characteristic fungal forms (Figure 177.3B) and by culture, which usually requires 2 to 6 days for recovery of the organism. Skin testing with coccidioidal antigens is not diagnostically useful and, at any rate, reagents for this purpose are no longer commercially available. Serologic tests that identify anticoccidioidal immunoglobulin M (IgM) and immunoglobulin G (IgG) antibodies in body fluids, however, are both sensitive and specific. The magnitude of the complement-fixing (CF) antibody titer has the valuable property of correlating with the extent of disease so that most patients with dissemination will have serum titers of 1:16 or greater. Furthermore, the CF titer is useful for guiding therapy: A titer that falls over time is indicative of a successful therapeutic strategy, whereas a persistently rising titer suggests a need for change or intensification of therapy. Of note, false-negative IgM and IgG results may be seen early in the course of infection, therefore, repeating these tests at a later time in the undiagnosed patient with suspected coccidioidomycosis may be fruitful.

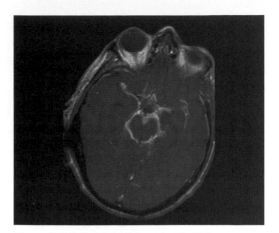

Figure 177.5 Coccidioidal meningitis. This 48-year-old Hispanic man with type II diabetes presented with headache and obtundation. This axial T1-weighted magnetic resonance image taken after the administration of contrast shows abnormal enhancement of the leptomeninges at the base of the brain. Hydrocephalus was treated by placement of a ventriculoperitoneal shunt, and a lumbar reservoir was placed to facilitate delivery of intrathecal amphotericin, which was given along with fluconazole. He made a full recovery and now continues on fluconazole alone.

False-negative results are also occasionally encountered in severely immunocompromised patients, such as those with advanced AIDS. There is no specific test for coccidioidal antigens in body fluids presently, but recent data suggest that certain *Histoplasma* antigen tests may cross-react, particularly early in the course of infection and in patients with widespread disease. If validated, such antigen tests could thus serve as excellent complements to the antibody-based diagnostic tests. Blood cultures are not part of the core work-up because they are usually negative outside of the setting of overwhelming disease. Similarly, urine cultures only occasionally yield the organism early in the course of infection or if the genitourinary tract is involved (eg, prostatitis). In patients with meningitis, analysis of the CSF demonstrates a predominantly mononuclear pleocytosis (usually 50 to 500 cells/µL, with the percentage of polymorphonuclear leukocytes present tending to decrease over time), elevated protein (usually 100 to 500 gm/dL, sometimes >1000 gm/dL), and low glucose—a picture that also suggests tuberculosis. Eosinophils, although not invariably present, are often found (usually at 1% to 10% of CSF white blood cells). In the patient with meningitis, CSF eosinophils, and an appropriate travel history, coccidioidomycosis should be strongly suspected. Culture or cytological evaluation of CSF in coccidioidal meningitis yields the organism in only a minority, but antibodies to the organism can be detected in the fluid in >90% of cases. Nucleic acid amplification-based tests for the detection of *Coccidioides* spp. in body fluids or tissue specimens may ultimately prove to be an important advance in the diagnosis of coccidioidomycosis, but they are not yet available for general use.

Patients with coccidioidomycosis are not contagious and need not be placed in isolation. Objects such as linens, bandages, and casting materials contaminated with body fluids containing the organism (eg, pus or sputum) are capable of supporting its conversion to the infectious mycelial form over a period of several days at room temperature. All such fomites should therefore be collected daily and sterilized using standard hospital practices for handling biological waste.

TREATMENT

Azoles have largely supplanted the use of amphotericin B in the treatment of coccidioidomycosis. Table 177.2 summarizes treatment recommendations. Many clinicians prefer amphotericin B as initial therapy in situations where immediate control is needed such as life-threatening, fulminant, or rapidly progressive infections, with transition to azole therapy after stabilization. Amphotericin B is also preferred during pregnancy due to the teratogenicity of the azoles. Intravenous lipid formulations of amphotericin B appear to be effective and can certainly be administered with fewer complications than amphotericin B deoxycholate; however, they have yet to be shown more effective than amphotericin B deoxycholate in clinical trials. Whether an azole is used from the outset or for later replacement of amphotericin B, either fluconazole or itraconazole may be safely chosen. Itraconazole was compared directly with fluconazole in the treatment of 191 patients with progressive, nonmeningeal coccidioidomycosis, including 70 with pulmonary, 71 with soft-tissue, and 50 with bone/joint infection. Clinical response (≥50% improvement at 8 months) overall was 50% in the fluconazole group and 63% for those assigned to itraconazole ($P = .07$). There was a trend toward statistical significance in those with bone/joint infection, with response rates of 26% in the fluconazole and 52% in the itraconazole group ($P = .06$), leading some clinicians to prefer itraconazole, at least, in these settings. The extended spectrum triazoles,

Table 177.2 Summary of Treatment Recommendations

Primary Pulmonary

No dissemination risk: No treatment or fluconazole, 400 mg daily, or itraconazole, 200 mg BID for approximately 3–6 mo or for 3 mo after complete resolution of clinical infection. All patients should be followed closely.

Dissemination risk or severe disease: fluconazole, ≥400 mg daily, or itraconazole, ≥200 mg BID for approximately 3–6 mo, including ≥3 mo after resolution of clinical infection.

Pulmonary Cavity (Uncomplicated) or Fibrocavitary Disease

Observation or fluconazole, 400 mg daily for ≥6–12 mo, and assess for response. Individualized management of complications. Surgical resection in selected cases.

Progressive Pulmonary or Disseminated (Nonmeningeal)

Immediately life threatening: amphotericin B deoxycholate, 0.6–1.0 mg/kg/d to approximate total of 2000 mg; or equivalent dose of lipid formulation of amphotericin B, 3.0–5.0 mg/kg/d; consideration given to transition to fluconazole or itraconazole when disease is controlled. Alternatively, fluconazole, ≥400 mg daily, or itraconazole, ≥200 mg BID. The duration of therapy is usually at least 2 yr; some patients may require lifelong therapy. Individualized management depending on site(s) of involvement

Slowly progressive or stable: fluconazole, ≥400 mg daily, or itraconazole, ≥200 mg BID. The duration of therapy is usually at least 2 years; some patients may require lifelong therapy. Individualized management depending on site(s) of involvement.

Meningitis

Fluconazole, ≥400 mg daily (many advocate starting dose of ≥800 mg), or itraconazole ≥200 mg BID (doses as high as 600 mg BID have been used, recommend checking serum levels).

or

Amphotericin B directly into cerebrospinal fluid (usually with an oral triazole dosed as above) transitioned to oral azole alone (usually dosed at no lower than 400 mg total daily). Patients must be evaluated frequently for the emergence of complications and serial CSF analyses must be performed to document response to therapy, particularly early in the course.

Due to the high relapse rate, patients with coccidioidal meningitis usually continue on antifungal therapy for life.

HIV-infected Patients

All HIV infected patients with CD4+ lymphocyte count ≤250 cells/μL with any form of coccidioidomycosis should receive antifungal therapy. If the infection is immediately life threatening, initial treatment with amphotericin B is preferred. With stabilization, fluconazole or itraconazole may be used, with careful attention to drug interactions with some antiretrovirals. Consider discontinuation if nonmeningeal disease, therapy has been prolonged and the CD4+ count is stably >250. For meningeal disease, lifelong antifungal treatment regardless of CD4+ count achieved.

Pregnant Patients

Amphotericin B, 0.6–1.0 mg/kg/d

Abbreviations: HIV = human immunodeficiency virus; CSF = cerebrospinal fluid.

voriconazole and posaconazole, clearly have activity against *Coccidioides* spp. Initial experience with posaconazole thus far has been very promising, and anecdotal data exist supporting the use of voriconazole in patients with coccidioidomycosis. Until further information becomes available, posaconazole and voriconazole will likely find use primarily in salvage settings. Similarly, echinocandins have been reported, either alone or in combination with other antifungals, to show activity in the treatment of coccidioidomycosis. Further study of the use of this class of compounds is needed before recommendations may be made.

There is a tendency to use increasingly higher dosages of azoles. To ensure adequate bioavailability, patients treated with orally administered itraconazole should have a determination of their serum levels of this drug and its active metabolite, hydroxyitraconazole. Based on similar interindividual variability in drug levels, it would appear advisable to measure serum concentrations of voriconazole and posaconazole if these agents are used. Determining serum azole levels over time has the additional benefits of allowing assessment of possible drug–drug interactions and patient adherence.

UNCOMPLICATED PRIMARY PULMONARY INFECTION

In the majority of cases, primary infection with *Coccidioides* is self-limited. No controlled studies evaluating the efficacy of treatment of patients with primary disease have been performed. For this reason, many clinicians do not treat such patients unless they fall into one of the known groups at higher risk of dissemination. Nonetheless, despite the lack of solid evidence that therapy shortens the duration of symptoms or prevents dissemination, it is reasonable to also consider treatment of at least some low-risk patients, especially those most acutely ill. The presence of a high complement-fixing antibody titer in a patient who otherwise appears to be at low risk for dissemination would add further weight favoring potential benefits of treatment.

The recommended antifungals for this purpose are fluconazole, 400 mg daily, or itraconazole, 200 mg twice a day. Pregnant patients requiring treatment should receive amphotericin B. The optimal duration of treatment of the primary infection is uncertain but should probably be a total of 3 to 6 months or continued until complete resolution of clinically apparent disease has occurred plus an addi-

tional 3 months. Patients in categories carrying a high risk of dissemination who also have high titers of CF antibody may benefit from even more prolonged therapy.

Whether patients are treated or not, it is imperative that they are followed regularly for at least 2 years to make certain that their infection resolves successfully or to detect complications related to infection as early as possible. Evaluations should include a complete review of systems, physical examination, serum CF antibody titer, and, as appropriate, repeat radiographic studies or cultures. For those on azoles, monitoring for side effects and periodically obtaining routine bloodwork (eg, liver function tests, electrolytes, complete blood count) and serum drug levels are advisable.

PROGRESSIVE PULMONARY OR NONMENINGEAL DISSEMINATED INFECTION

Although azoles are effective in most cases, some clinicians still consider amphotericin B to be the treatment of choice in those cases of progressive pulmonary or disseminated coccidioidomycosis that are immediately life threatening. Nonmeningeal coccidioidomycosis that is progressing at a more indolent pace, however, is generally treated with an orally administered azole.

Ketoconazole, at a dosage of 400 mg once daily, has proven effective but shows erratic bioavailability, possibly accounting for the relatively low response rates reported in some studies. This, at least in part, results from a requirement of gastric acid for its absorption from the gastrointestinal tract. Higher dosages of the drug do not appear to significantly improve response rates. Ketoconazole interferes with the biosynthesis of testosterone and cortisol and may result in decreased libido and gynecomastia in men and, rarely, in adrenal insufficiency. As with all the azoles, hepatotoxicity may occur. Although ketoconazole remains an option, questions surrounding its efficacy as well as its side-effect profile have led to a preference for fluconazole or itraconazole.

Itraconazole capsules, most commonly dosed at 200 mg twice daily with food, also require gastric acid for optimal absorption. An oral suspension of itraconazole, formulated with cyclodextrin, has improved bioavailability but may cause diarrhea at the doses typically used. Triazoles are metabolized extensively by the hepatic P450 enzyme system, and both ketoconazole and itraconazole participate in numerous significant pharmacokinetic interactions with other drugs. A partial list of medications with which these interactions occur includes diphenylhydantoin, carbamazepine, cyclosporine, tacrolimus, rifampin, isoniazid, antiretroviral protease inhibitors and nonnucleoside reverse transcriptase inhibitors, warfarin, vinca alkaloids, oral hypoglycemics, and statins. The concomitant use of proton pump inhibitors or H_2 blockers is to be avoided as they will lead to substantial decreases in the absorption of ketoconazole and itraconazole when given in pill form.

Fluconazole, at dosages of 400 mg or more daily, is also very effective. Some clinicians have used doses as high as 2000 mg daily. Its absorption, which does not depend on the presence of gastric acid, is more reliable than that of ketoconazole and itraconazole, and it does not affect human sterol synthesis to an important extent. Although it may interact with other drugs, such as those listed above for the other azoles, most such interactions tend to be more limited in magnitude. Recent evidence in patients with AIDS indicates that fluconazole interacts with clarithromycin and rifabutin.

Administration of a combination of an azole and amphotericin B is used by some clinicians in patients failing monotherapy, but there is only limited evidence to support this assertion. The role of the newer agents, voriconazole and posaconazole, is uncertain, but limited data suggest they may be useful as salvage agents in patients failing other therapies.

As a rule of thumb, treatment of nonmeningeal disseminated or progressive pulmonary coccidioidomycosis should continue for at least 2 years or for 1 year after the infection appears to have resolved completely, whichever is longer. Nonetheless, relapses frequently occur despite such prolonged treatment regimens using the currently available armamentarium, and many patients ultimately require significantly longer, potentially lifelong, courses of antifungal therapy. Furthermore, because relapse occurs frequently after the discontinuation of antifungal therapy in coccidioidomycosis, the need for continued, long-term, careful observation of such patients while off of therapy cannot be overemphasized. Patients with persisting immunosuppression or immunodeficiency should continue to be treated for at least as long as this state continues. Those with immunodeficiency secondary to AIDS should be maintained on therapy at least until such time as their CD4+ lymphocyte count remains reliably above 250 cells/μL.

MENINGITIS

A multicenter study demonstrated a response (defined as elimination of ≥40% of baseline abnormalities) of 79% with a daily dose of fluconazole of 400 mg given for a median duration of 37 months in the treatment of coccidioidal meningitis. Daily doses of fluconazole of 800 mg or more may be associated with an improved early response to therapy but also with a greater incidence of adverse reactions. Itraconazole, at total dosages of 400 mg or more daily, may be similarly effective. In either case, relapse after discontinuation of drug administration is extremely frequent, particularly if intrathecal amphotericin B has never been included in the treatment regimen, and lifelong suppressive therapy is to be expected. Patients undergoing treatment for meningitis should be followed closely, especially in the first months after diagnosis and the initiation of therapy to demonstrate that improvement is occurring. Evaluations should include a review of systems, physical examination, lumbar puncture to follow the opening pressure, cell count, protein, glucose and CF antibody titer, and, potentially, radiographic imaging. Evidence of disease progression necessitates immediate intensification of therapy (minimally a trial of an increased dose of the current therapy or conversion to an entirely different antifungal with intrathecal amphotericin favored in more severe cases). Similarly, evidence of complications, such as the development of hydrocephalus, requires immediate action. The treatment of coccidioidal meningitis is often complex and complicated and should probably be attempted only by, or in close collaboration with, clinicians experienced in its management.

Treatment of coccidioidal meningitis previously invariably involved the administration of amphotericin B directly into the CSF, and this method of therapy continues to be recommended for initial control of infection by some clinicians. Injection is usually accomplished via the lumbar, lateral cervical, or cisternal route by direct puncture or through the use of implanted devices such as the Ommaya reservoir. Amphotericin may also be administered into the lateral ventricles by use of such a device if needed. CSF flow patterns should be defined by radionuclide or dye studies when determining which route(s) is optimal for the delivery of amphotericin to the sites of central nervous system infection because the flow of CSF may be disrupted by blockages or loculations.

When administering intrathecal amphotericin by the lumbar route, some clinicians prefer using the "hyperbaric" technique, which allows delivery of the drug in high concentration to the basilar meninges, where the major burden of infection is ordinarily found. In addition, the rapid removal of drug from the lumbar area theoretically decreases the likelihood of some of the possible local complications induced by amphotericin, such as radiculitis, myelitis, arachnoiditis, and spinal artery thrombosis. In this method, amphotericin B is slowly delivered intrathecally in sterile, preservative-free 10% dextrose in water. Immediately after administration, the patient is placed in the Trendelenburg position for 30 to 45 minutes. Treatment is initiated at a dose of 0.01 to 0.05 mg and escalated, initially on a daily basis, until a maximum tolerated dose is reached (usually between 0.5 and 1.5 mg). Once clinical and laboratory improvement have been documented, the frequency of administration is gradually decreased. It has been suggested that a dosage of at least 0.75 mg 3 times weekly with rapid escalation to a cumulative dose of 20 mg is associated with better survival than less aggressive approaches.

Concomitant azole therapy is usually given to patients receiving intrathecal amphotericin in the hopes of decreasing the total amount of amphotericin B necessary to achieve a stable response to therapy.

The development of hydrocephalus, either communicating or noncommunicating, is a frequently encountered complication. This should be suspected when the patient's neurologic status deteriorates; nausea, vomiting, ataxia, or weakness develops; or if the CSF protein concentration increases to high levels. Hydrocephalus should be managed by the placement of a CSF shunting device. Central nervous system vasculitis may complicate coccidioidal meningitis. Although no comparative data exist, some clinicians suggest administration of corticosteroids along with maximal antifungal therapy in patients with this complication.

OTHER INFECTIONS

In the absence of immunosuppressive disease or therapy, antifungal treatment is not required in the case of a stable, solitary pulmonary nodule caused by Coccidioides spp. Coccidioidomycosis of the airways may be effectively treated with an azole.

Chronic pulmonary cavities respond poorly to antifungal therapy and, if asymptomatic,

may best be left untreated. Complications include bacterial superinfections, which are amenable to standard antibacterial therapy, and hemoptysis. On occasion, hemoptysis may be the result of the development of a fungus ball. Cavitation may be progressive despite chemotherapy. All of these complications are potential indications for surgical intervention. An alternative approach to the management of a pulmonary fungus ball in the patient who is a poor surgical candidate is intracavitary instillation of amphotericin B. Rarely, a coccidioidal cavity may rupture into the pleural space, resulting in pyopneumothorax. This complication should be managed surgically with concomitant administration of an antifungal agent.

Chronic fibrocavitary pneumonia requires prolonged antifungal therapy, usually with an azole; surgical resection of the affected tissues may be of value in some cases.

The musculoskeletal system is a common site of involvement in cases of disseminated infection. In addition to antifungal chemotherapy, surgical debridement may be warranted in some cases of osteomyelitis. The benefit of synovectomy in chronic coccidioidal arthritis remains unproved, but many believe it hastens the response to therapy and leads to improved functional outcomes.

PATIENTS WITH AIDS

All HIV-infected patients with a CD4+ lymphocyte count ≤250 cells/μL with any form of coccidioidomycosis should receive antifungal therapy. The reduced gastric acidity of many AIDS patients may lead to reduced bioavailability of orally administered itraconazole. In addition, attention must be paid to the possibility of pharmacokinetic interactions between some antiretrovirals and the azole antifungal agents. Discontinuation of therapy may be considered in nonmeningeal disease if the CD4+ lymphocyte count has stably exceeded 250 cells/μL. Patients with meningitis will likely require ongoing treatment for life.

SUGGESTED READING

Ampel NM. Coccidioidomycosis in persons infected with HIV type 1. Clin Infect Dis. 2005;41(8):1174–1178.

Blair JE, Logan JL. Coccidioidomycosis in solid organ transplantation. Clin Infect Dis. 2001;33(9):1536–1544.

Galgiani JN, Catanzaro A, Cloud GA, et al. Fluconazole therapy for coccidioidal meningitis. The NIAID-Mycoses Study Group. *Ann Intern Med*. 1993;119(1):28–35.

Galgiani JN, Catanzaro A, Cloud GA, et al. Comparison of oral fluconazole and itraconazole for progressive, nonmeningeal coccidioidomycosis: a randomized, double-blind trial. Mycoses Study Group. *Ann Intern Med*. 2000;133(9):676–686.

Galgiani JN, Ampel NM, Blair JE, et al. Coccidioidomycosis. *Clin Infect Dis*. 2005;41(9):1217–1223.

Johnson RH, Einstein HE. Coccidioidal meningitis. *Clin Infect Dis*. 2006;42(1):103–107.

Labadie EL, Hamilton RH. Survival improvement in coccidioidal meningitis by high-dose intrathecal amphotericin B. *Arch Intern Med*. 1986;146(10):2013–2018.

Pappagianis D. Serologic studies in coccidioidomycosis. *Semin Respir Infect*. 2001;16(4):242–250.

Stevens DA. Coccidioidomycosis. *N Engl J Med*. 1995;332(16):1077–1082.

Stevens DA, Shatsky SA. Intrathecal amphotericin in the management of coccidioidal meningitis. *Semin Respir Infect*. 2001;16(4):263–269.

178. *Pneumocystis* Pneumonia

Walter T. Hughes

The diffuse bilateral pneumonitis caused by *Pneumocystis jirovecii* (also called *Pneumocystis carinii*) occurs almost exclusively in immunocompromised patients with cancer, organ transplantation, congenital immunodeficiency disorders, and acquired immunodeficiency syndrome (AIDS). The organism is known to cause pneumonitis occasionally in patients without underlying immunodeficiency.

CLINICAL FEATURES

The clinical manifestations of *Pneumocystis* pneumonitis are fever, cough, tachypnea, and dyspnea progressing to cyanosis. The onset may be abrupt or subtle.

With an abrupt onset, fever, marked increase in respiratory rate, and severe dyspnea occur within 24 to 48 hours. The disease progresses rapidly with marked decrease in arterial oxygen tension (PaO$_2$) and increase in alveolar-arterial oxygen gradient. The chest radiograph shows bilateral diffuse alveolar disease with an air bronchogram. Without treatment, the disease worsens and within a month all patients will have died. Even in fatal cases and even in the most severely compromised host, the organism and the disease remain localized to the lung, with rare exception. When specific and supportive treatment is introduced early in the disease, the mortality rate can be reduced to around 10% in most medical centers. Abrupt onset tends to occur in patients with cancer, organ transplantation, and AIDS.

With a subtle onset, an increase in respiratory rate occurs, with or without fever. No abnormality may be found by chest radiograph early in the course, although computed tomography (CT) scans may show perihilar infiltrates. The disease slowly progresses over 1 to 2 weeks to the more severe and life-threatening disease described above for abrupt-onset presentation. The subtle pattern is seen in some AIDS patients, rarely in cancer and transplant patients, and usually in the infantile epidemic form of the pneumonitis. In the immunocompromised host, the subtle form progresses to a fatal outcome if untreated. However, during the outbreaks of infantile plasma cell pneumonitis caused by *Pneumocystis*, approximately half of the patients will eventually recover without treatment.

DIAGNOSIS

A definitive diagnosis of *Pneumocystis* pneumonitis requires the identification of the organism in tissue or secretions from the lung. Specimens are usually obtained by bronchoalveolar lavage (BAL). Induced sputum samples may contain the organism but less often than BAL. Open lung or transbronchial lung biopsy is the most sensitive source for diagnostic material. Specimens from BAL, induced sputum, and biopsy are processed with Gomori–Grocott methenamine silver, Giemsa, Papanicolaou, and fluorscein-labeled antibody (Merifluor; Meridian Bioscience, Inc., Cincinnati, OH) stains (Figure 178.1). No serologic method is of diagnostic value. The polymerase chain reaction (PCR) amplification of *P. jirovecii* DNA sequences from BAL, sputum, and oral wash specimens shows promise for diagnostic purposes, but lack of standardized and commercially available methods preclude its use in routine clinical practice.

THERAPY

Trimethoprim–sulfamethoxazole (TMP–SMX) is the drug of first choice for treatment. Moderately and severely ill patients should receive 15 mg of TMP and 75 mg of SMX/kg intravenously per day in 4 doses 6 hours apart. Patients with mild pneumonitis who can take oral medication may be treated with 20 mg of TMP and 100 mg of SMX/kg/day in 4 doses by mouth. The total daily dose should not exceed 400 mg of TMP plus 2000 mg of SMX. Usually, 14 to 21 days of therapy is required, and most patients who qualify for prophylaxis will continue taking the drug at one-fifth the therapeutic dose for life or until no longer at risk for recurrence or reinfection. Adverse reactions are uncommon in non-AIDS patients, but

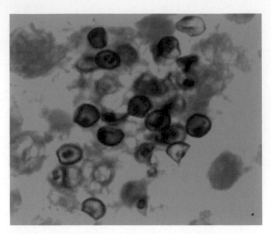

Figure 178.1 *Pneumocystis jirovecii* in lung biopsy. Gomori's methenamine silver stain. The thick-walled cysts are 4 to 7 µm in diameter. Collapsed cysts resemble crescents or cups. In some cysts, thickened areas of the inner cyst wall produce easily seen dense structures that may be single or paired. (Courtesy of David Schlossberg, MD.)

about 40% of those with AIDS have significant reactions to TMP–SMX. Rash, neutropenia, and fever are the most common treatment-limiting events. Some patients can tolerate mild reactions while TMP–SMX is continued. Rare but life-threatening reactions include Stevens–Johnson syndrome, hepatic necrosis, aplastic anemia, agranulocytosis, thrombocytopenia, and allergic reactions. Leucovorin is not used routinely with TMP–SMX therapy.

Patients who cannot tolerate or who fail to respond to TMP–SMX may be changed to other effective drugs. These include atovaquone, pentamidine isethionate, and trimetrexate with leucovorin, which have been approved by the Food and Drug Administration (FDA). Other effective drugs with proved efficacy, but not FDA approved, are dapsone–trimethoprim and clindamycin plus primaquine. The drug of second choice is usually pentamidine isethionate, but recent studies indicate that atovaquone is equally effective and less toxic. The production and sale of trimetrexate were terminated by the manufacturer in February 2007.

Pentamidine isethionate, 4 mg/kg/day as a single intravenous dose, may be used for *Pneumocystis* pneumonitis of any severity. This drug is similar in efficacy to TMP–SMX, but >50% of patients, including patients without AIDS, have significant adverse effects. These include nephrotoxicity, leukopenia, hypoglycemia, hyperglycemia, diabetes, pancreatitis, hyperkalemia, hypotension, thrombocytopenia,

hypocalcemia, and Stevens–Johnson syndrome. Pentamidine can be given intramuscularly, but serious injection site reactions are common. Aerosolized pentamidine has only limited therapeutic effect but is relatively safe. There is no oral preparation of pentamidine. Avoid the use of pentamidine with other nephrotoxic drugs such as amphotericin B, aminoglycosides, and cisplatin.

Atovaquone is available in only a suspension formulation (750 mg/5 mL). The adult dosage is 750 mg 3 times daily by mouth (total adult dose is 2250 mg/day). Children should be given 30 to 40 mg/kg/day in 3 doses. Infants aged 3 to 24 months require a dose of 45 mg/kg/day. It is important for each dose to be given after a meal high in fat to achieve maximal absorption. Clinical experience with atovaquone for the treatment of *Pneumocystis* pneumonitis has been limited to patients with mild and moderate disease, $AaDO_2$ of 45 mm Hg or less. No serious adverse effects or toxic dose have been reported. The most common adverse effects are diarrhea, headache, rash, and nausea.

Dapsone, 100 mg (total dose) per day, plus trimethoprim, 15 mg/kg/day in 3 doses, orally is efficacious. For children ≤13 years the dose of dapsone is 2 mg/kg/day. Adverse events include anemia, neutropenia, methemoglobinemia, and rash. About one-third of the patients intolerant to TMP–SMX may also be intolerant to dapsone–trimethoprim.

The combination of clindamycin, 600 mg every 6 hours intravenously for 10 days, and then 450 mg orally ever 6 hours to complete a 21-day course; plus primaquine, 30 mg of the base per day orally for 21 days, is another regimen shown to be efficacious in limited studies.

Supportive therapy for patients with a PaO_2 of 70 mm Hg or less, or arterial-alveolar gradient of 35 mm Hg or greater, includes the administration of a corticosteroid, such as prednisone, 40 mg twice a day on days 1 to 5, 40 mg once daily on days 6 to 10, and 20 mg/day on days 11 to 21.

PREVENTION

Pneumocystis pneumonitis can be effectively prevented with chemoprophylaxis. Indications for prophylaxis include the following:

- Human immunodeficiency virus (HIV)-infected adults and children 6 years of age and older, with CD4+ T-lymphocyte counts (%) of ≤200 cells/µL (15%); children 1 to 5 years with counts of ≤500 cells/µL (15%); and all HIV-infected infants and indeterminant infants of HIV-infected mothers 1 to 12 months of age (see Chapter 100, Prophylaxis of Opportunistic Infections in HIV Infection)

- Immunocompromised patients who have recovered from one or more episodes of *Pneumocystis* pneumonitis
- Certain high-risk patients with cancer, organ transplantation, and/or congenital immune deficiency disorders. Patients at especially high risk are those with lymphoproliferative malignancies, those on corticosteroid therapy, those who are bone marrow and/or certain solid organ transplant recipients, those with brain tumor on intensive chemotherapy, those with severe combined immunodeficiency syndrome, and those with persistent CD4+ T-lymphocyte counts <T200 cells/µL.

TMP–SMX is the preferred drug with any of the following schedules: 160 mg TMP+800 mg SMX once or twice a day to adults, either daily or 3 days a week. Some evidence suggests that 80 mg TMP+400 mg SMX is also effective in adults. Infants and children should receive 5 mg TMP+25 mg SMX per kilogram daily or 3 days a week, but not to exceed the adult doses.

For patients who cannot tolerate TMP–SMX the drugs atovaquone, dapsone, or aerosolized pentamidine may be used in the following dosages: atovaquone, 750 mg twice daily for adults and 30 mg/kg/day for infants and children 1 to 3 and >24 months and 45 mg/kg/day for infants 4 to 24 months of age, or dapsone, 100 mg as a single or divided dose daily, or dapsone, 2 mg /kg daily (maximum 100 mg/day) or 4 mg/kg (maximum 400 mg) weekly. Alternatively, aerosolized pentamidine, 300 mg delivered by nebulizer once a month, may be used.

Pneumocystis pneumonia prophylaxis can usually be safely discontinued in HIV-infected patients responding to highly active antiretroviral therapy (HAART) with a sustained level of CD4+ T lymphocytes >200 cells/µL in adults and proportionate levels in children.

SUGGESTED READING

Arcenas RC, Uhl JR, Buckwalter SP, et al. A real-time polymerase chain reaction assay for detection of *Pneumocystis* from bronchoalveolar lavage fluid. *Diag Microbiol Infect Dis*. 2006;54:169–175.

Centers for Disease Control and Prevention. Guidelines for preventing opportunistic infections among HIV-infected persons: 2002 Recommendations of the U.S. Public Health Service and Infectious Diseases Society of America. *Morbid Mortal Weekly Rep*. 2002;51(RR-8):4–5.

Centers for Disease Control and Prevention. Treating opportunistic infections among HIV-exposed and infected children: recommendations from CDC, The National Institutes of Health and Infectious Diseases Society of America. *Morbid Mortal Weekly Rep*. 2004;53(RR-14):4–6.

Huang L, Morris A, Limper AH, et al. An official ATS workshop summary: recent advances and future directions in *Pneumocystis* pneumonia. *Proc Am Thorac Soc*. 2006;3:655–664.

Hughes WT. Use of dapsone in the prevention and treatment of *Pneumocystis carinii* pneumonia: a review. *Clin Infect Dis*. 1998;27:191–204.

Hughes WT. Pneumocystis pneumonitis in non-HIV-infected patients: update. In: Walzer PD, Cushion MT, eds. *Pneumocystis Pneumonia*. 3rd ed. New York, NY: Marcel Dekker; 2005:407–434.

Nassar A, Zapata M, Little JV, Siddiqui MT. Utility of reflex Gomori methenamine silver staining for Pneumocystis jirovecii on bronchoalveolar lavage cytologic specimens: a review. *Diagn Cytopathol*. 2006;34:719–723.

Thomas CF Jr, Limper AH. Pneumocystis pneumonia. *N Engl J Med*. 2004;350:2487–2498.

Torres HA, Chemaly RF, Storey R, et al. Influence of type of cancer and hematopoietic stem cell transplantation on clinical presentation of *Pneumocystis jiroveci* pneumonia in cancer patients. *Eur J Clin Microbiol Dis*. 2006;25:382–388.

179. Miscellaneous Fungi and Algae

George A. Pankey and Donald L. Greer

Many species of fungi and algae may cause disease among the increasing population of individuals at risk. These microorganisms, loosely called *opportunistic agents*, cannot cause disease unless two major criteria are met: (1) the patient suffers from some predisposing factor that has mechanically (eg, trauma) or immunologically (eg, organ transplantation) decreased the capacity to resist infection and (2) the infecting agent can survive and multiply at body temperature (37°C [98.6°F]). At present, the number of these opportunistic agents reported to cause infection exceeds 200.

Although some opportunistic fungal infections are noteworthy for specific predisposing factors (eg, ketoacidosis, zygomycete infection), neutropenia or a defect in cell-mediated immunity is the usual predisposing factor. However, any trauma, disease state, or pharmacologic insult to host defenses increases the chance of fungal invasion, even from a patient's own normal flora.

The microorganisms considered in this chapter (Table 179.1) are ubiquitous but are uncommon causes of disease in humans. Therefore the diagnosis is usually made when a patient has an infectious disease that does not respond to antibacterial therapy, when the microbiology laboratory reports the isolation of one of these agents, or when the pathologist identifies a fungus or alga on histopathology.

A high degree of suspicion of an opportunistic agent is necessary for appropriate clinical specimens to be sent to the pathology department. Any material may be examined for fungi and algae, but the laboratory cannot guess the clinical diagnosis, and it is essential that the physician indicates the suspected pathogens and informs the laboratory. For example, to maximize the yield from blood cultures, a lysis centrifugation of cultured blood should be requested.

Many of the pathogens considered in this chapter require special media or conditions for culture. However, the challenge is not isolating the agent once it is suspected but the relevance of the isolate to the clinical picture. Mere isolation of a ubiquitous agent does not indicate

Table 179.1 Opportunistic Fungi and Algae

Hyalohyphomycoses
Long septate hyphae in tissue *Fusarium* species *Penicillium marneffei* *Scedosporium apiospermum (Pseudallescheria boydii)*
Phaeohyphomycoses (Dematiaceae)
Short septate hyphae, pseudohyphae, and/or yeast with melanin in cell walls identified by Fontana–Mason stain *Alternaria* *Bipolaris* *Cladosporium* *Curvularia* (see Figures 179.1 and 179.2) *Dactylaria (Ochroconis)* *Exophiala* *Exserohilum* *Phialophora* *Wangiella*
Opportunistic Yeast or Yeastlike Fungi
Hansenula species; only yeast in tissue *Malassezia (Pityrosporum) furfur:* Yeast only in deep tissue; "meatballs and spaghetti" in stratum corneum (tinea versicolor) *Rhodotorula:* "Red yeast" *Saccharomyces cerevisiae* *Trichosporon beigelii:* Yeast, pseudohyphae, arthroconidia, true hyphae
Protothecosis
Achlorophyllic unicellular algae produce spherical cells that multiply by cytoplasmic cleavage, forming a morula in tissue *Prototheca wickerhamii* *Prototheca zopfii*

pathogenesis. For causation to be proved, the culture must be confirmed either by tissue invasion as seen on biopsy or by repeatedly positive cultures from a usually sterile body fluid. The appearance of these agents in tissue is extremely variable (see Table 179.1). A culture is imperative for specific identification.

Virtually all of these species grow rapidly at 25°C to 30°C (77°F to 86°F). Most of the common contaminants, or opportunistic fungi, can be identified to genus in a clinical microbiology laboratory; however, a mycology expert is usually needed to identify the species. Fortunately, treatment of all species within the genus is typically the same. There are no reliable serologic tests, and direct microscopy using Gram, potassium hydroxide, India ink, and Papanicolaou preparations of lesion scrapings and sputum is often not helpful.

THERAPY

Therapy is often unsatisfactory without total surgical excision. This is a result both of the severity of the patient's underlying disease and the lack of effective drugs. It is unlikely that there will ever be enough cases to conduct double-blind therapeutic trials, even if the pharmaceutical industry develops new drugs. At present, these opportunistic agents are tested in vitro against antifungal agents developed primarily to treat fungi that more commonly produce disease in immunocompromised patients, such as *Candida* and *Cryptococcus.* Therefore only anecdotal case reports and small series are available in the literature. In addition, antifungal susceptibility testing in general is still in its infancy, with few laboratories even attempting it. Variations in susceptibility occur with these organisms, just as they do with bacteria, but the information is less readily available and not well standardized. Therefore, when these fungi are isolated, they should be sent to a reference laboratory for susceptibility testing, including synergy studies, with the hope of obtaining helpful information for a specific patient.

Failure of response to antifungal drugs occurs because: (1) the drug is fungistatic (most drugs) rather than fungicidal (amphotericin B, voriconazole), (2) combination therapy was not used, (3) the drug has no in vitro activity, (4) neutropenia was not reversed, (5) ketoconazole or itraconazole (oral) was given with antacid therapy, or (6) the dosage is too low. For example, very high dosages of fluconazole (up to 2 g/day) may be more effective than lower dosages, and liposomal formulations of amphotericin B clearly allow much higher dosages without increasing toxicity. The echinocandins are not active in vitro against these miscellaneous fungi and algae.

The initial therapeutic approach in adults for infection caused by these microorganisms reflects our personal experience and information from the literature. An infectious disease consultation should be obtained for all patients for advice regarding length and modifications of therapy. Optimal therapies with the agents discussed in this chapter (Table 179.2) remain controversial at best. Clearly, surgical excision of localized skin and subcutaneous lesions is

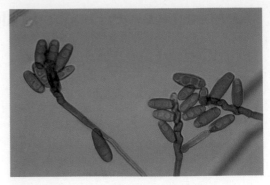

Figure 179.1 Conidiophores and conidia of the fungus *Curvularia harveyi.* (Centers for Disease Control and Prevention/Dr. William Kaplan – Public Health Image Library.)

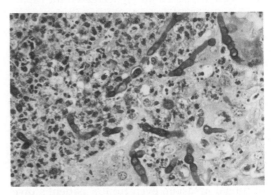

Figure 179.2 Phaeohyphomycosis of subcutaneous tissue due to the fungus *Curvularia harveyi.* Note characteristic pigmented hyphae that are septated and irregularly swollen, with yeastlike structures, as opposed to the septated but straight-walled hyphae of Aspergillus. (Centers for Disease Control and Prevention/Dr. William Kaplan.)

critical. Pharmaceutical companies evaluating antifungal agents may make them available for compassionate use for patients failing or intolerant to Food and Drug Administration (FDA)-approved agents.

Correction of the immunosuppression, if possible, is the major approach to the hospitalized patient with neutropenia or other immunosuppression. When this cannot be accomplished, prolonged antifungal therapy will be necessary, although the morbidity and mortality will remain high.

PREVENTION

It is important that immunocompromised patients are educated about the possibility of acquiring fungal infection from the environment. Prompt recognition by patient and physician of the possibility of these pathogens in

Table 179.2 Therapy of Infections by Opportunistic Fungi and Algae[a]

Pathogen	Characteristics	Therapy	Comments
Fusarium species	Blood culture positive in patient with fever and hematopoietical stem cell transplant; extensive burn; taking high-dose corticosteroids; or receiving cytotoxic chemotherapy. Multiple purpuric cutaneous nodules with central necrosis; keratitis	Correct neutropenia (G-CSF, GM-CSF) Liposomal amphotericin B, 5–7mg/kg/d, plus voriconazole	Little correlation between the clinical results and in vitro susceptibility to agents used. Reversal of neutropenia necessary for recovery.
Penicillium marneffei	Pneumonia; adenitis; skin lesions; osteomyelitis	Liposomal amphotericin B, 5–7 mg/kg/d, for 12 wk followed by itraconazole, 400 mg/d orally, for 10 wk	Fluconazole not effective. AIDS-defining opportunistic infection in southeast Asia
Scedosporium (*Pseudallescheria boydii*)	Mycetoma; sinusitis; pneumonia; endocarditis; meningitis; osteomyelitis; arthritis; brain abscess; keratitis	Surgical removal if possible; voriconazole	Amphotericin B not effective. Cannot be distinguished from *Aspergillus* by histopathology.
Dematiaceae (Phaeohyphomycosis): (chromoblastomycosis)	Skin and subcutaneous tissue; sinusitis; occasional dissemination.	Surgical removal if possible. Itraconazole or voriconazole orally for 6 months	Use better-absorbed cyclodextrin suspension formulation of itraconazole.
Trichosporon beigelii	Fungemia in neutropenic patients; nodular skin lesions containing the organism; pneumonia	Correct neutropenia Liposomal amphotericin B, 5–7 mg/kg/d Voriconazole for nonresponsive patients	False-positive reaction with cryptococcal latex agglutination.
Malassezia (*Pitysporum*)	Usually associated with lipid infusions, folliculitis in AIDS patients; tinea versicolor	Remove intravascular catheters Voriconazole if fungemia persists Topical selenium sulfide, ketoconazole or miconazole for folliculitis and tinea versicolor	Amphotericin B is not very active in vitro
Hansenula species	Fungemia	Remove intravascular catheters Liposomal amphotericin B, 5–7 mg/kg/d Voriconazole for nonresponsive patients	
Rhodotorula species	Fungemia; meningitis; peritonitis	Remove intravascular catheters Liposomal amphotericin B, 5–7 mg/kg/d	
Saccharomyces cerevisiae	Fungemia	Liposomal amphotericin B, 5–7 mg/kg/d	Probiotic use
Prototheca	Skin and soft tissue; occasional dissemination	Voriconazole (skin/soft-tissue) Liposomal amphotericin B, 5–7 mg/kg/d (disseminated)	

[a] Drug dose varies with age, weight, etc.
Abbreviations: AIDS = acquired immunodeficiency syndrome; G-CSF = granulocyte colony-stimulating factor; GM-CSF = granulocyte-macrophage colony-stimulating factor.

infected skin lesions following trauma is necessary to avoid surgery or dissemination. Proper intravascular catheter care and prevention of neutropenia are critical for the hospitalized patient.

SUGGESTED READING

Antachopoulos C, Papakonstantinou E, Dotis J, et al. Fungemia due to Trichosporon asahii in a neutropenic child refractory to amphotericin B: clearance with voriconazole. *J Pediatr Hematol Oncol.* 2005;27:283–285.

Bernal MD, Acharya NR, Lietman TM, et al. Outbreak of Fusarium keratitis in soft contact lens wearers in San Francisco. *Arch Ophthalmol.* 2006;124:1051–1053.

Bonifaz A, Saul A, Paredes-Solis V, Araiza J, Gierro-Arias L. Treatment of chromoblastomycosis with terbinafine: experience with four cases. *J Dermatolog Treat.* 2005;16:47–51.

Centers for Disease Control and Prevention (CDC). Update: Fusarlum keratitis–United States, 2005–2006 *MMWR Morb Mortal Wkly Rep.* 2006;55(20):563–564.

Crespo-Erchiga V, Florencio VD. Malassezia yeasts and pityriasis versicolor. *Curr Opin Infect Dis.* 2006;19:139–147.

Cuenca-Estrella M, Gomez-Lopez A, Mellado E, et al. Head-to-head comparison of the activities of currently available antifungal agents against 3,378 Spanish clinical isolates of yeasts and filamentous fungi. *Antimicrob Agents Chemother.* 2006;50:917–921.

Kane SL, Dasta JF, Cook CH. Amphotericin B lipid complex for Hansenula anomala pneumonia. *Ann Pharmacother.* 2002;36:59–62.

Lamaris GA, Chamilos G, Lewis RE, Safdar A, Raad II, Kontoyiannis DP. *Scedosporium* infection in a tertiary care cancer center: a review of 25 cases from 1989–2006. *Clin Infect Dis.* 2006;43:1580–1584.

Lionakis MS, Kontoyiannis DP. Fusarium infections in critically ill patients. *Semin Respir Crit Care Med.* 2004;25:159–169.

Mens H, Hojlyng N, Arendrup MC. Disseminated Penicillium marneffei sepsis in a HIV-positive Thai woman in Denmark. *Scand J Infect Dis.* 2004;36:507–509.

Muñoz P, Bouza E, Cuenca-Estrella MN, et al. Saccharomyces cerevisiae fungemia: an emerging infectious disease. *Clin Infect Dis.* 2005;40:1625–1634.

Perfect JR. Treatment of non-Aspergillus moulds in immunocompromised patients, with amphotericin B lipid complex. *Clin Infect Dis.* 2005;40(suppl 6):S401–S408.

Raad II, Hachem RY, Herbrecht R, et al. Posaconazole as salvage treatment for invasive fusariosis in patients with underlying hematologic malignancy and other conditions. *Clin Infect Dis.* 2006;42:1398–1403.

Torres HA, Bodey GP, Tarrand JJ, Kontoyiannis DP. Protothecosis in patients with cancer: case series and literature review. *Clin Microbiol Infect.* 2003;9:786–792.

PART XXIII

Specific Organisms – Viruses

180. Cytomegalovirus

Jeffery L. Meier

Cytomegalovirus (CMV), a human-restricted betaherpesvirus, infects nearly half the U.S. population. CMV prevalence differs widely according to age, socioeconomic status, sexual activity, and race/ethnicity. Over 90% of the overall U.S. population is infected by 80 years of age, and an estimated one-half million women of childbearing age are infected each year. Congenital CMV infection involves approximately 1% of all newborns and is the leading infectious cause of birth defects.

CMV infection is lifelong and usually asymptomatic, even as virus is shed into secretions. Primary CMV infection occasionally results in self-limiting acute illness (eg, heterophile-negative mononucleosis, viral syndrome, or hepatitis) and very rarely causes protracted or severe disease in otherwise healthy persons. Primary CMV infection of women during pregnancy increases risk of symptomatic congenital CMV infection. Approximately 8000 of the ~35 000 congenitally CMV-infected babies born each year in the United States have sequelea, including hearing loss, vision loss, mental retardation, or death. Persons with profound cellular immune deficiency, such as accompanies acquired immunodeficiency syndrome (AIDS) and hematopoietic stem cell or solid organ transplantation, are predisposed to debilitating or life-threatening CMV disease resulting from primary, reactivation, or recurrent infection. CMV causes a broad spectrum of disease, and the leading clinical manifestations vary among the different patient types but commonly include retinitis, gastrointestinal disease, hepatitis, pneumonitis, or encephalitis. Unrestrained CMV replication can directly damage a variety of organs and tissues and have immunomodulatory effects that are indirectly linked to sequelae of allograft dysfunction or rejection, superinfections with opportunistic pathogens, posttransplant lymphoproliferative disorder, and decrease in survival of human immunodeficiency virus (HIV)-positive persons living in the era of highly active antiretroviral therapy.

CMV is shed into saliva, urine, breast milk, semen, and cervical secretions. Infants and young children often shed CMV into urine, and sometimes saliva, for several weeks to months after a primary infection. Immunosuppression or concomitant illness may promote viral shedding at any time during infection. Close mucosal contact with infectious body fluids is the prime mode of CMV transmission. CMV persists in virtually all tissues, and its latent DNA genome is carried in monocytes, dendritic cells, and their precursors. For this reason, CMV-seronegative recipients of solid organs, bone marrow, or blood products obtained from CMV-seropositive donors are at increased risk of CMV infection.

DIAGNOSIS

The definitive diagnosis of CMV disease rests on the detection of active CMV infection in the tissue of a patient with a compatible illness. Detection of characteristic cytomegalic inclusions (Figure 180.1) in the involved tissue verifies the diagnosis. The diagnosis may also be confirmed by detection of CMV in tissue by viral culture, immunohistochemical analysis (CMV antigen), or in situ hybridization (CMV nucleic acid). A tissue-based diagnosis is not feasible for the diagnosis of CMV retinitis, which is mostly a disease of persons with advanced AIDS

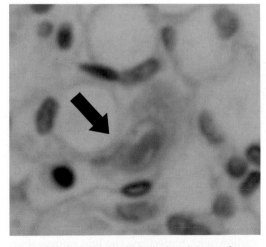

Figure 180.1 Cytomegalic inclusion disease. Arrow points to characteristic CMV infected cell, which is large and contains intranuclear and ground-glass cytoplasmic inclusions. H&E staining.

(CD4+ T lymphocyte count ≤50 cells/µL) and accounts for 85% of the CMV end-organ disease in these patients. CMV retinitis is diagnosed by recognition of characteristic retinal lesions that typically have perivascular infiltrate, atrophy, and hemorrhage. AIDS-associated CMV encephalitis, polyradiculopathy, and myelitis are diagnosed in persons having a positive cerebrospinal fluid (CSF) test for CMV DNA or viral culture and a compatible clinical presentation, including supportive radiographic and laboratory findings. The CMV syndrome that typically affects transplant recipients is diagnosed on the basis of specific clinical criteria plus evidence of CMV in blood by viral culture, viral antigen, or nucleic acid assay. Probable CMV disease in transplant recipients is defined as a compatible clinical illness plus evidence of CMV in blood, bronchoalveolar lavage (pneumonitis), or CSF (central nervous system disease).

Quantification of CMV antigen or nucleic acid load in blood improves ability to predict likelihood of CMV disease. However, the accuracy of this prediction and the alarm values vary among the different patient populations, conditions of immunosuppression, and specific methods of assay. In transplant recipients, the determination of CMV viremia level is useful for guiding pre-emptive therapy and monitoring effect of treatment for CMV disease. Neonatal CMV blood load correlates with risk of sequelea in congenitally infected newborns. Use of the methodology in persons living with AIDS has potential pitfalls: Although level of CMV blood load correlates with risk for CMV end-organ disease, substantial CMV viremia may occur in the absence of concomitant end-organ disease; CMV viremia is not uncommonly absent in patients with new or relapsing CMV retinitis; and the clinical value of using viremia-guided pre-emptive therapeutic strategies to prevent CMV end-organ disease is unclear.

Assessment of CMV antibody levels in immunocompromised persons is seldom helpful in establishing the diagnosis of CMV disease, but anti-CMV immunoglobulin G (IgG) serostatus is routinely determined to assess risk for CMV infection and disease. Interpretation of anti-CMV immunoglobulin M (IgM) antibody values from commercially available assays is confounded by high rates of false-positive and -negative results, and CMV-specific IgM is detected in settings of primary infection, reactivation, and reinfection. The IgM immunoblot assay is used to confirm a positive anti-CMV IgM screening test. A recent primary infection is serologically distinguished from reactivation or reinfection by presence of a low- to moderate-avidity anti-CMV IgG index. The laboratory diagnosis of CMV mononucleosis in the otherwise normal host is discussed in Chapter 183, Epstein–Barr Virus and Other Causes of the Infectious Mononucleosis Syndrome. Pregnant women with confirmed primary CMV infection (positive anti-CMV IgM immunoblot and low- to moderate-avidity anti-CMV IgG index) should have a detailed ultrasound examination and be considered for amniocentesis to test for CMV by polymerase chain reaction (PCR) if the diagnosis of congenital CMV infection is uncertain and requires confirmation.

THERAPY

Five antiviral agents (ganciclovir, valganciclovir, cidofovir, foscarnet, and fomivirsen) have been approved by the U.S. Food and Drug Administration (FDA) for therapy of CMV infection, although the FDA-approved indications for their use vary. Table 180.1 summarizes the recommended dosing schedules for these agents and of their use in clinical practice.

AIDS

Oral valganciclovir, the ganciclovir intraocular implant plus oral valganciclovir, and formulations of intravenous ganciclovir, foscarnet, and cidofovir are all effective initial therapeutic approaches for AIDS-associated CMV retinitis. Selection among the initial options is based on individualized patient characteristics (eg, location of retinal lesion; ability to absorb oral medication, adhere to treatment, and achieve immune recovery; feasibility of therapy administration; and concomitant medications and illness). Oral valganciclovir is often chosen as initial therapy. The ganciclovir intraocular implant plus oral valganciclovir is superior to intravenous ganciclovir in preventing relapse of CMV retinitis and may be the preferred initial therapy for patients with immediately sight-threatening retinitis or who are unlikely to achieve sufficient immune reconstitution from anti-HIV therapy. The implant requires replacement every 6 to 8 months in the absence of immune recovery. The management of CMV retinitis requires close monitoring by an experienced ophthalmologist and for potential adverse effects of the anti-CMV therapy. Optimization of antiretroviral therapy to achieve sufficient immune recovery (CD4+ T-lymphocyte count >100–150 cell/µL) is key for controlling CMV. After initial treatment

Table 180.1 Preventive and Treatment Regimens for CMV

Agent	Indications	Dosing Regimen	Toxicities	Monitoring	Comments
Intravenous					
Ganciclovir	Treatment of visceral or disseminated disease	Induction: 5 mg/kg q12h × 14–21d Maintenance: 5 mg/kg qd (modify dose in renal failure)	Catheter-related complications, neutropenia, thrombocytopenia	Induction: CBC 2×/wk, Cr weekly Maintenance: CBC qwk, Cr q1–3wk	If ANC 500–750, consider SQ G-CSF If ANC ≤500 or platelets ≤25 K, hold ganciclovir Increased toxicity of AZT or imipenem; increased level of didanosine (ddI) May cause infertility and may be teratogenic or embryotoxic. Adjust dosage for reduced renal function
	Prophylaxis or pre-emptive therapy in transplant recipients	5 mg/kg qd or BID (modify dose in renal failure)			
Foscarnet	Treatment of visceral or disseminated disease	Induction: 90 mg/kg q12h (or 60 mg/kg q8h) × 14–21d Maintenance: 90–120 mg/kg qd (modify dose in renal failure)	Catheter-related complications, nephrotoxicity, paresthesias, cation chelation, genital ulcerations, nausea	Induction: CBC, Cr, cations (K^+, Mg^{2+}, Ca^{2+}), and phosphate 2–3× qwk Maintenance: Cr, cations, and phosphate qwk, CBC q2wk	If Cr >2.8, hold foscarnet until Cr ≤2.1 mg/dL Adjust dosage for reduced renal function Hydration reduces renal toxicity
Cidofovir	Treatment of retinitis (limited experience with use for salvage therapy for CMV disease in other viscera)	Induction: 5 mg/kg/wk × 2; infuse over 1 h Maintenance: 5 mg/kg q2wk; infuse over 1 h (reduce dose to 3 mg/kg if Cr increase 0.3 mg/dL)	Nephrotoxicity, neutropenia, uveitis, ocular hypotony, probenecid rash Probenecid contraindicated in persons with severe sulfa allergy	Induction: Cr and UA every dose Maintenance: Same plus intraocular pressure qmo	1–2 L saline hydration, with 1 L given before cidofovir infusion; probenecid, given 3 h before (2 g) 3 h (1 g) and 8 h (1 g) after cidofovir infusion Do not use if Cr >1.5 mg/dL CrCl ≤55 mL/min, ≥2+ proteinuria or receiving other nephrotoxic agents
Intraocular					
Fomivirsen	Treatment of retinitis, if refractory or intolerant to other therapies	Induction: 330 mg intravitreal injection every other week × 2 Maintenance: 150–330 mg intravitreal injection qmo	Uveitis, increased intraocular pressure	Ophthalmologic follow-up, with intraocular pressure	Do not use in patients recently (2–4 wk) treated with cidofovir Topical steroids useful for management of uveitis
Ganciclovir implant	Treatment of retinitis	Surgical: Intraocular implantation via pars plana of (4.5 mg) implant; replacement q6–8mo Concomitant systemic therapy: see oral valganciclovir maintenance	Transient blurred vision, retinal detachment, hemorrhage, infection	Ophthalmologic follow-up	Requires addition of systemic therapy to reduce CMV disease risk in contralateral eye and other organs Implant releases 1 µg/h of ganciclovir

(continued)

Table 180.1 *(continued)*

Agent	Indications	Dosing Regimen	Toxicities	Monitoring	Comments
Oral					
Valganciclovir	Treatment of visceral or disseminated disease	Induction: 900 mg BID × 14–21d Maintenance: 900 mg qd (modify dose in renal failure	Neutropenia, thrombocytopenia	Induction: CBC 2x/wk, Cr weekly Maintenance: CBC qwk, Cr q1–3wk	If ANC 500–750, consider SQ G-CSF If ANC ≤500 or platelets ≤25 K, hold ganciclovir Increased toxicity of AZT or imipenem; increased level of ddI
	Prophylaxis or pre-emptive therapy in transplant	900 mg qd or BID, with food (modify dose in renal failure)			May cause infertility and may be teratogenic or embryotoxic. Adjust dosage for reduced renal function
Ganciclovir	Prophylaxis in transplant recipients	1 g TID, with food (modify dose in renal failure)	Neutropenia	CBC and Cr q2wk	
Valaciclovir	Prophylaxis in solid organ transplant recipients	2 g QID (modify dose in renal failure)	Hallucinations, confusion	CBC and Cr q2wk	Less effective than ganciclovir; therefore, use limited to low-risk patients
CMV Immunoglobulin					
CMV immunoglobulin intravenous (CytoGam)	Treatment of CMV pneumonitis in bone marrow transplant recipients Prophylaxis in solid organ transplant recipients	400 mg/kg days 1, 2, and 7 200 mg/kg day 14 plus IV ganciclovir (see IV ganciclovir) 50–150 mg/kg q2–4wk (various dosing regimens have been used)	Fever, myalgia, arthralgia, nausea, wheezing, hypotension, aseptic meningitis	Vital signs before, during, and after infusion	Derived from pooled adult human plasma containing high titers for antibody for CMV Increase infusion rate as tolerated, 15–60 mg/kg/h

Abbreviations: SQ = subcutaneous injection; CBC = complete blood count; Cr = serum creatinine; ANC = absolute neutrophil count; AZT = zidovudine; CMV = cytomegalovirus; UA = urine analysis; AIDS = acquired immunodeficiency syndrome; G-CSF = granulocyte colony-stimulating factor.

(induction therapy) for 14 to 21 days, secondary prophylaxis (maintenance therapy) is continued for at least 6 months after sufficient immune recovery has been achieved. Secondary prophylaxis is resumed if CD4+ T-lymphocyte count falls below 100 cells/μL. Systemic anti-CMV therapy should be a component of both initial treatment and secondary prophylaxis to provide protection to the contralateral eye and to other organs. Immune recovery uveitis is an inflammatory response to CMV that occasionally results from antiretroviral therapy–associated immune reconstitution and is treated with periocular or oral corticosteroids. An early first relapse (≤3 months) of CMV retinitis will often respond to reinstituting the same initial treatment regimen. Prior to 1996, the incidence of CMV resistance to antiviral drugs was approximately 25% to 30% by 1 year after diagnosis of retinitis, regardless of whether using ganciclovir, foscarnet, or cidofovir. In more recent years, the 2-year incidence of resistance to ganciclovir has been 9%, based on culturing of resistant CMV from blood. Low-level ganciclovir-resistant CMV may still respond to intravitreal injection of ganciclovir or the ganciclovir intraocular implant. A CMV with high-level ganciclovir resistance (median inhibition concentration [IC_{50}] >30 μM) requires treatment with an alternative anti-CMV drug, but is frequently cross-resistant to cidofovir and occasionally cross-resistant to foscarnet. Resistance testing by standard viral culture or molecular-based assays helps guide therapy. Intravitreous injection of fomivirsen is indicated for the treatment of CMV retinitis intolerant or resistant to the other anti-CMV therapies. The addition of CMV immunoglobulin is not beneficial.

Clinical studies indicate that either intravenous ganciclovir or foscarnet is effective therapy for AIDS-associated CMV esophagitis and colitis. Treatment duration is 21 to 28 days or until the illness has resolved, and secondary prophylaxis is not always needed. Oral valganciclovir is an option if oral absorption is not a problem. CMV pneumonitis may also respond to treatment with these agents. The combination of ganciclovir and foscarnet is recommended for initial treatment of CMV neurological disease. Unlike ganciclovir or foscarnet, cidofovir is not very effective at reducing AIDS-related CMV viremia.

Transplantation

The application of either antiviral prophylaxis or pre-emptive therapy in the early transplant period is an effective strategy for preventing CMV disease in recipients of hematopoietic stem cell and solid organ transplantation. Antiviral prophylaxis is given upfront to avert CMV replication, whereas pre-emptive therapy requires active viral surveillance and selective use of anti-CMV agent for early subclinical evidence of significant CMV replication. Although guidelines are published for the prevention and management of CMV infection and disease in recipients of hematopoietic stem cell and solid organ transplantation, there is considerable variability among centers in the exact regimens and protocols used. Oral valganciclovir, intravenous ganciclovir, or oral ganciclovir is effective prophylaxis. Pre-emptive therapy is usually initiated with full-treatment doses of oral valganciclovir or intravenous ganciclovir (induction phase) and is followed by suppressive therapy (maintenance phase) in certain types of transplant recipients. Intravenous foscarnet is also effective for prophylaxis and pre-emptive therapy, but is usually reserved for patients intolerant to or failing ganciclovir. Prophylaxis with high-dose acyclovir or valaciclovir decreases risk of CMV disease but is less effective than ganciclovir and is primarily reserved for use in low-risk renal transplant recipients. Late-onset CMV disease is increasingly recognized as a complication in both hematopoietic stem cell and solid organ transplant recipients. Use of high potency anti-CMV prophylaxis for extended duration may increase incidence of late-onset CMV disease in solid organ transplant recipients. Active CMV infection arising during or after lengthy exposure to ganciclovir heightens concern of possible ganciclovir resistance. Intravenous immunoglobulin is not recommended for prevention of CMV disease in hematopoietic stem cell, and is not generally used in solid organ transplant recipients.

Established CMV disease in transplant recipients is treated with intravenous ganciclovir, intravenous foscarnet, or oral valganciclovir. Limited clinical data, primarily obtained in hematopoietic stem cell transplant recipients, suggest that intravenous cidofovir may have a role as salvage therapy but poses a significant risk for renal damage. The combination of intravenous ganciclovir and foscarnet, each at half dose, is less effective than use of either drug alone at full dose in treatment of solid organ transplant recipients. The combination of intravenous ganciclovir and CMV hyperimmune globulin is the recommended therapy for CMV pneumonia in bone marrow transplant recipients.

Congenital Infection

Six weeks of intravenous ganciclovir therapy started in neonates with symptomatic congenital CMV infection appears to decrease risk for hearing impairment, but dose-limiting bone marrow toxicity is common and the long-term toxicity potential is unknown.

The Otherwise Normal Host

Symptomatic CMV illness in immunocompetent persons (eg, heterophile-negative mononucleosis, viral syndrome, or hepatitis) is usually self-limiting, although symptoms may resolve slowly over many weeks (mean duration of symptoms, ~8 weeks). Some patients experience relapsing symptoms before the illness abates. Use of valganciclovir or ganciclovir is reserved for severe protracted illness or evidence of tissue-invasive disease and should be carefully weighed against risks for potential adverse effects (ie, bone marrow and gonadal toxicities).

ANTIVIRAL AGENTS

Ganciclovir and Valganciclovir

Ganciclovir is a guanosine analog that requires initial phosphorylation by the CMV phosphotransferase (UL97 gene) for antiviral activity. The addition of two more phosphates by cellular enzyme produces ganciclovir triphosphate. This active metabolite inhibits the CMV DNA polymerase (UL54 gene) and is incorporated into replicating DNA to block chain elongation. The median effective inhibitory dose (median effective dose [ED_{50}]) of ganciclovir is ≤6 μM. The standard intravenous dose of 5 mg/kg provides serum peak and trough levels of 32.8 μM and 0.2 μM, respectively. The intracellular half-life of the active metabolite is 16.5 hours. Ganciclovir concentration in vitreous fluid and CSF is somewhat lower and more variable than that in serum, explaining some treatment failures in CMV disease involving the retina or central nervous system (CNS). Ganciclovir is eliminated by the kidneys, requiring dosage adjustments according to creatinine clearance. Oral ganciclovir has a bioavailability of only 6% to 9% and has been supplanted by valganciclovir. Valganciclovir is an orally administered prodrug of ganciclovir that attains levels approximating that produced by standard dosing of intravenous ganciclovir. Its tolerability profile is similar to that of intravenous ganciclovir. Ganciclovir also has activity against herpes simplex virus 1 (HSV-1), HSV-2, varicella-zoster virus (VZV), Epstein–Barr virus (EBV), human herpesvirus 6 (HHV-6), HHV-7, and herpes B virus.

Granulocytopenia is a frequent adverse effect of ganciclovir. Thus, use of other marrow-toxic agents should be avoided (eg, zidovudine) or minimized. Colony-stimulating factors can be used to ameliorate the problem. Thrombocytopenia, anemia, and CNS toxicity (eg, headache, seizures, and confusion) may also be observed. In animal studies, ganciclovir was teratogenic and carcinogenic and caused infertility. Ganciclovir given intravenously also introduces risk of catheter-related infection, whereas the intraocular implant may be complicated by endophthalmitis (0.3%).

Ganciclovir resistance mostly results from mutations in the CMV UL97 phosphotransferase gene and is less commonly due to mutations in the CMV UL54 DNA polymerase gene. CMV isolates having intermediate sensitivity to ganciclovir exhibit IC_{50} values between 6 and 12 μM, whereas ganciclovir-resistant isolates have IC_{50} values ≥12 μM. CMV isolates exhibiting high-level resistance (IC_{50} values ≥30 μM) often have mutations in both viral enzymes and are also likely to be cross-resistant to cidofovir. Alternative treatment for ganciclovir-resistant virus includes foscarnet, cidofovir, or fomivirsen.

Foscarnet

Foscarnet (phosphonoformic acid) directly inhibits viral DNA polymerase activity. The drug is cleared by the kidneys, so dosage adjustment according to creatinine clearance is required. The major toxicity is renal impairment, which may be reduced by hydration. Mineral and electrolyte abnormalities, such as hypocalcemia, hyperphosphatemia, hypophosphatemia, hypokalemia, and hypomagnesemia, are common. Although manageable, these abnormalities can precipitate seizures. Chelation of ionized calcium by foscarnet may result in numbness, tingling, and paresthesias, which may be prevented by slowing the infusion rate. Other notable adverse events include anemia, granulocytopenia, genital ulcers, and catheter-related sepsis. Foscarnet should not be used in persons receiving amphotericin B, aminoglycosides, intravenous pentamidine, or other nephrotoxic agents.

Cidofovir

The phosphorylation of cidofovir by cellular enzymes renders it active for inhibition of the viral DNA polymerase and termination of DNA chain elongation. The active metabolite has a long intracellular half-life (17 to 65 hours). Cidofovir is a nephrotoxic drug and is contraindicated in persons who have pre-existing renal insufficiency (Cr >1.5 mg/dL, CrCl ≤55 mL/min, or ≥2+ proteinuria) or are receiving other nephrotoxic agents. Intravenous prehydration and administration of probenecid is needed to minimize nephrotoxicity. Probenecid is contraindicated in those persons with history of a severe sulfa allergy. Neutropenia, ocular hypotony, and metabolic acidosis (Fanconi's syndrome) are other potential toxicities of the drug. Cidofovir was gonadotoxic, embryotoxic, and carcinogenic in animals.

Fomivirsen

Fomivirsen is a phosphorothioate antisense oligonucleotide that inhibits CMV replication by binding to and inactivating an essential viral messenger RNA (IE2). This drug is active against CMV strains that are resistant to ganciclovir, foscarnet, and/or cidofovir. Fomivirsen is given only by intravitreal injection and does not provide treatment of systemic CMV disease. Uveitis is a common complication of fomivirsen that can be alleviated with topical corticosteroid. Cidofovir may exacerbate uveitis and should not be used with fomivirsen.

Cytomegalovirus Immunoglobulin

Intravenous CMV immunoglobulin (CMVIG) is human immunoglobulin that is enriched

4-fold to 8-fold in anti-CMV antibody titer compared with standard preparations of intravenous immunoglobulin. CMVIG is used for passive immunoprophylaxis to prevent or attenuate CMV disease in certain high-risk solid organ transplant populations. It is also of clinical value when combined with intravenous ganciclovir for treatment of CMV pneumonia in bone marrow transplant recipients. CMVIG might have a role in the prevention and treatment of congenital CMV infection, but additional studies are needed.

PRIMARY PREVENTION

A vaccine for prevention of CMV infection and disease is a high-priority goal that has not yet been achieved. Uses of passive immunoprophylaxis and chemoprophylaxis in transplant recipients are addressed above. For CMV-seronegative persons at high risk of CMV disease or sequelea resulting from primary infection, measures are taken to prevent exposure to the virus. CMV seronegative or leukocyte-depleted blood products are used to prevent transfusion-transmitted CMV infection. Sexually active persons not in long-term monogamous relationships are advised to use condoms during sex. The risk of CMV transmission from changing diapers and wiping oral secretions of toddlers is reduced by attention to hand hygiene and avoidance of these activities.

SUGGESTED READING

Benson CA, Kaplan JE, Masur H, Pau A, Holmes KK. Treating opportunistic infections among HIV-infected adults and adolescents: recommendations from CDC, the National Institutes of Health, and the HIV Medicine Association/Infectious Diseases Society of America. *Morbid Mortal Weekly Rep*. 2004;53(RR15):1–112.

Biron KK. Antiviral drugs for cytomegalovirus disease. *Antiviral Res*. 2006;71:154–163.

Crumpacker CS, Wadhwa S. Cytomegalovirus. In: Mandell GL, Bennett JE, Dolin R, eds. *Mandell, Douglas, and Bennett's Principles and Practices of Infectious Diseases*. 6th ed. New York, NY: Elsevier Churchill Livingston; 2005.

Hodson EM, Jones CA, Webster AC, et al. Antiviral medications to prevent cytomegalovirus disease and early death in recipients of solid-organ transplants: a systematic review of randomized controlled trials. *Lancet*. 2005;365:2105–2115.

Sullivan KM, Dykewicz CA, Longworth DL, et al. Preventing opportunistic infections after hematopoietic stem cell transplantation: the Centers of Disease Control and Prevention, Infectious Diseases Society of America, and American Society for Blood and Marrow Transplantation Practice Guidelines and Beyond. *Hematology Am Soc Hematol Educ Program*. 2001:392–421.

181. Dengue and Dengue-Like Illness

Niranjan Kanesa-thasan and Charles H. Hoke, Jr.

Dengue virus, a mosquito-transmitted flavivirus, is the most common arbovirus infection of humans. Any of four dengue virus serotypes (1, 2, 3, and 4) may cause illness. Infection confers long-lasting protection against reinfection with the same dengue virus serotype but not against other serotypes. Hence, repeated dengue virus infections are possible if an individual is exposed sequentially to several serotypes. Infection with dengue virus may result in dengue fever or the more severe forms of disease known as dengue hemorrhagic fever (DHF) and dengue shock syndrome (DSS).

Classical dengue, or breakbone fever, is most commonly a self-limited, nonfatal acute viral illness in adults and children. An incubation period of 3 to 8 days precedes the sudden onset of fever to 39°C to 41°C (100.4°F to 102.2°F), frontal headache, muscle ache, and retroorbital pain. Prominent malaise and arthralgias may be accompanied by altered taste perception, nausea, and vomiting. Various rashes are often observed during illness, ranging from evanescent generalized maculopapular rashes to localized petechial rashes. Minor hemorrhagic manifestations such as epistaxis or gum bleeding may be present, but occasionally significant occult bleeding results from gastrointestinal ulcers. There is a characteristic transient depression of circulating neutrophil, lymphocyte, and platelet counts. Generally dengue fever resolves uneventfully, with defervescence in 7 days or less.

Occasionally, persons infected with dengue virus develop DHF at or near the time of defervescence, when systemic capillary leakage results in hemoconcentration (more than 20% rise in hematocrit) and thrombocytopenia (platelet count less than 100 000/mm^3). Manifestations of DHF may include a positive tourniquet test, ascites, pleural effusion, and spontaneous bleeding. Coagulopathies of varying intensities are present in most affected individuals. DHF may rapidly progress to DSS, with rapid or feeble pulse, narrow pulse pressure ($\leq$20 mm Hg), hypotension, and clammy extremities. DSS typically occurs on day 4 or 5 of illness. The World Health Organization's clinical grading scheme for DHF based on severity may be helpful in classification and management of patients (Table 181.1). In this scheme, DSS is classified as grade III or IV DHF. There is current debate about simpler and more sensitive case definitions for dengue disease.

The risk of DHF is highest in individuals who have been previously infected with another dengue serotype. DHF most often affects children in dengue-endemic areas (Figures 181.1A and 181.1B), where several serotypes may cocirculate. However, adults may be at risk for DHF if a dengue serotype is introduced to a region after another serotype was widespread. Varying epidemiological patterns in different countries suggest that more remains to be learned regarding the prognosis of dengue infection in specific groups.

DIAGNOSIS

Dengue should be included in the differential diagnosis of persons (civilian or military) returning to the United States from any endemic area (southeast Asia, the Indian subcontinent, Central and South America, the Pacific region, Africa, and the Middle East), but diagnosis on clinical grounds alone is not possible. Diagnosis is confirmed by isolation of virus from plasma or serum and/or demonstration of dengue-specific immunoglobulin M (IgM) antibody. A 4-fold rise in dengue hemagglutination-inhibiting antibody titer also provides evidence of recent infection. Serologic tests may be complicated by cross-reactive antibodies to other flaviviruses, such as Japanese encephalitis virus or yellow fever virus. Virus is best isolated from patients during their febrile period, and dengue-specific antibody is detected in specimens obtained following defervescence. Hence, paired specimens should be acquired when possible during the acute illness and again after convalescence, ideally with an interval exceeding 1 week. Sera for virus isolation should be stored at −70°C (−94°F) and shipped on dry ice to a state health laboratory; if such handling is not possible, storage and shipment at 4°C (39.2°F) is preferable to other procedures.

Table 181.1 Treatment and Classification of Dengue and Dengue Hemorrhagic Fever

Grade	Symptoms	Signs	Treatment

Dengue fever	Headache
	Retroorbital pain
	Myalgia
		Fever (39°–40°C [100.4°F–102.2°F]
		Rash (blanching, erythematous)
			Treat symptoms.
			  Use anti-inflammatory agents (not
			  aspirin).
			Monitor clinical status daily.
			Determine Hct and platelet count.

DHF grade I	Same as above	Hemoconcentration (>20% rise in Hct) Thrombocytopenia (≤100 000/mm³) Positive tourniquet test	Same as above, plus: Monitor vital signs q2h, then q6h. Determine Hct, platelet count. Provide oral hydration.
DHF grade II	Same as above	Hemoconcentration and thrombocytopenia Spontaneous bleeding	Same as above, plus: Type and cross-match. Determine PT and PTT.

DHF grade III	Restlessness
	Confusion
	Lethargy
		Hemoconcentration and
		  thrombocytopenia
		Rapid weak pulse
		Narrowed pulse pressure (≤20 mm Hg)
		Hypotension
		Cold clammy skin
			Same as above plus:
			Administer isotonic intravenous fluids
			  (rapid 20 mL/kg bolus).
			Obtain electrolytes; ALT/AST.
			Monitor vital signs more frequently
			  (≤q30 min).
			Follow urine output

DHF grade IV	Depressed sensorium
	Stupor
		Hemoconcentration and
		  thrombocytopenia
		Undetectable pulse and blood pressure
			Same as above, plus:
			Administer intravenous colloid or
			  plasma 10–20 mL/kg.
			Provide critical care support as needed.

Adapted from Technical Advisory Committee. *Dengue Hemorrhagic Fever: Diagnosis, Treatment and Control.* 2nd ed. Geneva: World Health Organization; 1997.
Abbreviations: Hct = hematocrit; PT = prothrombin time; PTT = partial thromboplastin time; ALT = alanine aminotransferase; AST = aspartate aminotransferase.

The reverse-transcriptase polymerase chain reaction has increasingly been used to detect circulating viral genome, and is more sensitive and faster than traditional viral culture.

Clinicians should suspect dengue fever in travelers with acute febrile syndromes within 2 weeks of return from tropical countries. The presence of rash accompanied by thrombocytopenia and neutropenia will help support, but not predict, the clinical diagnosis. Malaria is clinically indistinguishable from dengue and should be specifically sought, as malaria may be fatal without timely treatment. Other causes of acute fever and exanthem, such as scrub typhus, Rocky Mountain spotted fever, leptospirosis, measles, rubella, typhoid fever, and meningococcal disease, should be considered in the differential diagnosis. The hemorrhagic fever viruses (eg, Ebola and Junin) and other exotic viruses with similar initial clinical presentations must be kept in mind if a patient with suspected DHF has a history of travel to a tropical or remote location (see Chapter 192, Clinical Management of Viral Hemorrhagic Fevers).

THERAPY

Management of suspected dengue is challenging because diagnostic confirmation of infection is usually not available at the time of treatment. Furthermore, it is impossible to identify individuals at risk for severe dengue at the time of presentation. Treatment of uncomplicated dengue fever is supportive. Relief of symptoms may be achieved with nonsteroidal anti-inflammatory agents; aspirin is best avoided because of the risks of bleeding and of Reye's syndrome. Because of the nonspecific presentation and the risk of sudden and treatable vascular collapse and a differential diagnosis that includes potentially fatal, treatable conditions, all individuals suspected of having dengue should be hospitalized. Patients should be monitored frequently for sudden drop in blood pressure at the time of defervescence, onset of restlessness, confusion, or lethargy. Examination should focus particularly on evaluation of pulse or blood pressure (BP) changes, cool extremities, thrombocytopenia, and hematocrit. All cases of suspected or

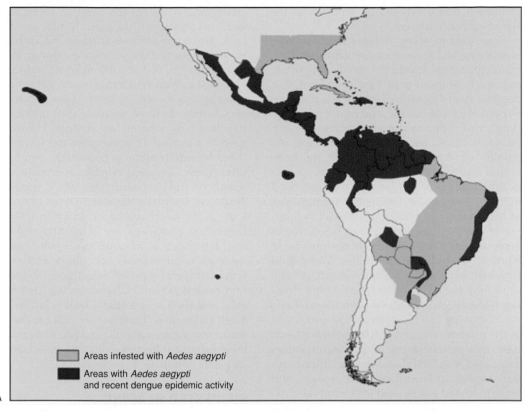

Figure 181.1A Dengue distribution, Western Hemisphere (Centers for Disease Control and Prevention).

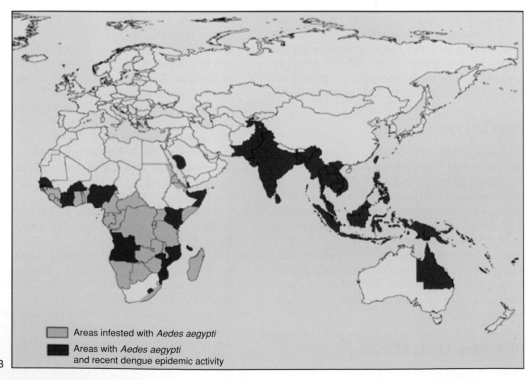

Figure 181.1B Dengue distribution, Eastern Hemisphere (Centers for Disease Control and Prevention).

confirmed dengue should be reported to the state health department.

Treatment of severe dengue requires close monitoring and support of circulatory and hematologic status. Relatively simple supportive measures, properly and timely applied, can decrease mortality to less than 1%. The phenomena of DHF are reversible, and recovery is often rapid after appropriate supportive therapy. Hence, judicious use of fluid resuscitation and monitoring of vital signs (pulse, BP) and urine output are required to avoid both hypovolemia in initial stages of disease and fluid overload in the recovery phase. Frequent determinations of hematocrit and platelet counts aid monitoring of plasma repletion through resolution of hemoconcentration and thrombocytopenia. In addition, a rapid drop in hematocrit after fluid replenishment without improvement in vital signs may suggest onset of spontaneous bleeding. If bleeding is present, it is advisable to obtain blood for type and cross-match. Determination of the prothrombin and partial thromboplastin times may indicate degree of the coagulopathies associated with DHF. Disseminated intravascular coagulation is distinctly uncommon, and heparin should not be used for treatment.

Treatment of DSS requires aggressive use of isotonic (Ringer's lactate or physiologic saline, 20 mg/kg intravenous [IV] bolus) and colloid fluids (plasma or dextran compound 10 to 20 mg/kg IV as needed). In cases of profound shock, critical care support, including ventilation, may be required. Intravenous steroids do not decrease mortality in DSS. Ribavirin did not prevent dengue virus replication in animal trials, and its use in DHF or DSS is unjustified.

PREVENTION

Cases of dengue infection are increasing with the unchecked spread of the primary mosquito vectors *Aedes aegypti* and *Aedes albopictus* (the tiger mosquito). Both species are well adapted to humans and widely dispersed in cities throughout the world, including many cities in the United States. The vectors are daytime feeders and feed repeatedly indoors. Travelers in dengue-endemic areas should avoid mosquitoes during the day if possible, particularly at dawn and dusk. Use of insect repellents is strongly recommended.

DENGUE-LIKE ILLNESSES

Other mosquito-borne viruses may also cause epidemics of self-limited dengue-like illnesses characterized by abrupt onset of fever, malaise, myalgias, arthralgias, headache, and rash. These arboviruses include the alphaviruses (chikungunya, O'nyong-nyong, Ross River, Mayaro, and Sindbis viruses) and flaviviruses (eg, West Nile virus fever). Recent chikungunya outbreaks in both Africa and India may, if they continue, increase the numbers of travelers with dengue-like disease. However, specific diagnosis of acute arboviral fevers on clinical grounds alone is impossible. Serologic or virologic diagnosis requires specialized research or public health laboratory support. Treatment is usually directed to relief of symptoms with anti-inflammatory agents and fluids. Prevention comprises use of insect repellents and avoidance of mosquitoes. Scrub typhus, meningococcal disease, and Rocky Mountain spotted fever may resemble dengue. Diagnosis may be delayed until laboratory data are available, and each is potentially fatal if not recognized and treated. Therefore an initial antibiotic treatment regimen should include therapy for these fulminant bacterial diseases until laboratory data eliminate their possibility.

SUGGESTED READING

Deen JL, Harris E, Wills B, et al. The WHO dengue classification and case definitions: time for a reassessment. *Lancet*. 2006;368:170–173.

Halstead SB. More dengue, more questions. *Emerg Infect Dis*. 2005;11:740–741.

Innis BL. Dengue and dengue hemorrhagic fever. In: Porterfield J, Tyrrell D, eds. *Handbook of Infectious Diseases: Exotic Viral Infections*. Vol. 3. London: Chapman & Hall; 1996.

Nimmannitya S. Dengue and dengue hemorrhagic fever. In: Cook GC, Zumla AI, eds. *Manson's Tropical Diseases*. 21st ed. Philadelphia, PA: WB Saunders; 2004.

Rigau-Perez JG, Clark GG, Gubler DJ, et al. Dengue and dengue hemorrhagic fever. *Lancet*. 1988;352:971–977.

Suh KN, Kozarsky PE, Keystone JS. Evaluation of fever in the returned traveler. *Med Clin North Am*. 1999;83:997–1017.

Technical Advisory Committee. Dengue Hemorrhagic Fever: Diagnosis, Treatment, Prevention, and Control. 2nd ed. Geneva: World Health Organization; 1997.

Wichmann O, Gascon J, Schunk M, et al. Severe dengue virus infection in travelers: risk factors and laboratory indicators. *J Infect Dis*. 2007;195: 1089–1096.

Wilder-Smith A, Schwartz E. Dengue in travelers. *N Engl J Med*. 2005;353:924–932.

182. Enteroviruses

Michael N. Oxman

Enteroviruses (EV), so named because most members infect the alimentary tract and are shed in the feces, cause a variety of diseases in humans and lower animals. They constitute 1 of the 6 major subgroups, or genera, of the family Picornaviridae [*pico*, "small"; *rna*, "ribonucleic acid"]. The other genera of Picornaviridae are the Rhinoviruses, Cardioviruses, Aphthoviruses, and 2 newly designated genera, Hepatovirus, the prototypic member of which is human hepatitis A virus; and Parechovirus, which contains 2 serotypes that were previously classified as *echoviruses* types 22 and 23. Three additional genera have been proposed: Erbovirus, Kobuvirus, and Teschovirus.

PHYSICAL AND BIOCHEMICAL PROPERTIES

Enteroviruses, like all members of the Picornavirus family, are small, spherical, non-enveloped viruses approximately 30 nm in diameter. Their genome consists of a linear, single-stranded, unsegmented molecule of RNA (approximately 7500 nucleotides) that has the same polarity as messenger RNA.

Enteroviruses are stable over a wide range of pH (pH 3 to 10) and retain infectivity for days at room temperature, weeks at refrigerator temperature, and indefinitely when frozen at –20°C or lower.

CLASSIFICATION OF ENTEROVIRUSES

Historically, human EV have been subclassified into polioviruses, group A and group B coxsackieviruses, and echoviruses on the basis of antigenic relationships, differences in host range, and types of disease produced (Table 182.1). By 1969, 67 species (serotypes) of human EV had been identified and classified according to these criteria, although reclassification and redundancy have reduced this number from 67 to 61.

PATHOGENESIS OF ENTEROVIRUS INFECTIONS

After ingestion of fecally contaminated material, virus implants in susceptible tissues of the pharynx and distal small intestine. Whereas some replication occurs in the pharynx, the primary site of infection is the distal small intestine; virus traverses the intestinal lining cells without causing detectable cytopathology and reaches Peyer's patches in the lamina propria, where significant replication occurs. Within 1 or 2 days, virus spreads to regional lymph nodes and, on about the 3rd day, small quantities escape into the bloodstream (the "minor viremia") and are disseminated throughout the reticuloendothelial system and to other receptor-bearing target tissues. In most cases, infection is contained at this stage by host defense mechanisms with no further progression, resulting in asymptomatic infection. In a minority of infected persons, replication continues in reticuloendothelial tissues producing, by about the 5th day, heavy sustained viremia (the "major viremia") that coincides with the "minor illness" of poliovirus infection and with the "nonspecific febrile illness" caused by other human EV.

The major viremia disseminates large amounts of virus to target organs, such as the spinal cord, brain, meninges, heart, and skin, where further virus replication results in inflammatory lesions and cell necrosis. In most such patients, host defense mechanisms quickly terminate the major viremia and halt virus replication in target organs; only rarely is virus replication in target organs extensive enough to be clinically manifest. Although other host defense mechanisms (eg, macrophages, natural killer [NK] cells, interferon production) are doubtless involved, neutralizing antibodies play a major role in terminating viremia and limiting EV multiplication in target tissues. Serotype-specific neutralizing antibodies may be detected in the serum within 4 or 5 days of infection, and they generally persist for life. Evidence for the critical role of antibodies in terminating infection is provided by the occurrence of chronic persistent EV infections in agammaglobulinemic children. Host defenses do not, however, terminate virus replication in the intestine, and fecal shedding continues for weeks after both symptomatic and asymptomatic EV infections. Reinfection (ie, virus excretion by a person with pre-existing homotypic antibodies) is

Table 182.1 Classification of Human Enteroviruses (EV)[a]

Enterovirus Group	Number of Serotypes	Numerical Designation	Growth in Primate Cell Culture	Pathogenicity for Suckling Mice	Pathogenicity fo Monkeys
Poliovirus	3	1–3	+	−	+
Coxsackievirus, group A	23	A1–22, A24[b]	+/−[c]	+	−[d]
Coxsackievirus, group B	6	B1–B6	+	+	−
Echovirus	29	1–9, 11–21, 24–27, 29–34[e]	+	−	−
Enterovirus	4	68–71[f] +	Variable[g]		Variable[h]

[a] Many EV strains have been isolated that do not conform to these criteria.
[b] Coxsackievirus A23 has been reclassified as echovirus 9.
[c] Except for a few serotypes (eg, A7, A9, A16), primary isolates of group A coxsackieviruses grow poorly or not at all in cell culture; virus isolation requires inoculation of suckling mice.
[d] Coxsackievirus A7 is neurovirulent in monkeys.
[e] Echovirus 10 has been reclassified as reovirus type 1; echovirus 28 has been reclassified as rhinovirus 1 A; echovirus 22 and echovirus 23 have been reclassified as parechovirus 1 and parechovirus 2, respectively, members of a new *Parechovirus* genus.
[f] Hepatitis A virus, formally classified as human EV 72, is now classified as a member of the *Hepatovirus* genus.
[g] EV-70 and- 71 are pathogenic for suckling mice.
[h] EV-70 and- 71 are neurovirulent in monkeys.

relatively uncommon. When it occurs, infection is confined to the alimentary tract and is not associated with illness, and the duration of virus shedding is markedly reduced.

EPIDEMIOLOGY

Human EVs are worldwide in distribution, and humans are their only known reservoir. The prevalence of EV infection varies markedly with season and climate, and with the age and socioeconomic status of the population studied. In tropical and semitropical regions, EV infections are frequent throughout the year. In temperate climates, the incidence of infection is markedly increased in the summer and early fall; within the United States, climatic and socioeconomic factors affect the prevalence of EV infections. Enterovirus isolation rates from young children are 2- to 3-fold higher in southern than in northern cities and 3- to 6-fold higher in lower than in middle and upper socioeconomic districts.

Transmission of human EV is chiefly by the fecal–oral route directly from person to person or through fomites; spread by respiratory secretions plays a lesser role. After infection by most serotypes, virus can be recovered from the oropharynx and intestine of both symptomatic and asymptomatic individuals, but virus is shed in greater amounts and for a longer period (a month or more) in the feces.

Young children have the highest rates of infection, and EVs are most efficiently disseminated by infected children younger than 2 years. Spread is from child to child, and then within family groups, and is facilitated by crowding and poor hygiene. Secondary attack rates of approximately 90% for polioviruses, 75% for coxsackieviruses, and 50% for echoviruses are observed in families.

Although the epidemiology of most EV is similar, patterns of infection with some serotypes are distinctive. EV-70 and coxsackievirus A24, etiologic agents of acute hemorrhagic conjunctivitis, are transmitted by direct inoculation of the conjunctivae by fingers and fomites contaminated with infected tears. Replication of these viruses in the alimentary tract, if it occurs at all, is limited. Coxsackievirus A21 is shed primarily from the upper respiratory tract, where it produces a rhinoviruslike illness. It is transmitted by respiratory secretions.

The incubation period for illnesses caused by EV may vary from less than 1 day to more than 3 weeks, but it is generally 2 to 7 days. It is shortest when symptoms are the direct result of virus replication at the portal of entry (eg, acute hemorrhagic conjunctivitis caused by EV-70 or coxsackievirus A24) and longest when they reflect tissue injury that involves immunopathology in target organs infected following viremia (eg, some forms of coxsackievirus myocarditis).

CLINICAL MANIFESTATIONS OF ENTEROVIRUS INFECTIONS

The majority of nonpolio EV infections (50% to 80%) are asymptomatic. Most symptomatic infections consist of *undifferentiated febrile illnesses* ("summer grippe"), often accompanied by upper respiratory symptoms. These are generally mild and last only a few days. This syndrome is totally nonspecific; it can be caused by virtually any EV serotype, as well as by members of a number of other virus families (eg, adenoviruses, paramyxoviruses, orthomyxoviruses). The so-called characteristic EV syndromes, such as aseptic meningitis, hand-foot-and-mouth disease (HFMD), and pleurodynia, are, in fact, unusual manifestations of EV infection. They represent the very small tip of a very large iceberg.

Some clinical syndromes are highly associated with certain EV serotypes or subgroups (Table 182.2), but even these associations are not specific. The same syndrome may also be caused by a number of other EV serotypes. Conversely, a single EV serotype may cause several different syndromes, even within the same outbreak. The more important syndromes are discussed below.

CENTRAL NERVOUS SYSTEM SYNDROMES

Aseptic Meningitis

Aseptic meningitis is the most common clinical syndrome caused by EV that results in medical attention, and EVs are responsible for more than 80% of the cases of aseptic meningitis in children and adults in developed countries in which an etiologic agent is identified. Almost every EV serotype has been implicated. Although attack rates are generally highest in children, cases also occur in adults, especially during larger outbreaks. Initial symptoms, which are typical of the *undifferentiated febrile illness* (eg, fever, headache, malaise, myalgias, and sore throat), are followed, usually within a day, by signs and symptoms of meningitis, including a more severe headache that is often retrobulbar, photophobia, meningismus, stiffness of the neck and back, and nausea and vomiting,

especially in children. The illness is sometimes biphasic-like poliomyelitis. The cerebrospinal fluid (CSF) is clear and under slightly increased pressure. The total cell count, which can vary from less than $10/mm^3$ to more than $3000/mm^3$, averages 50 to $500/mm^3$. Initially, neutrophils may predominate (although they rarely exceed 90%), but they are quickly replaced by mononuclear cells. The glucose concentration is usually normal, although levels less than 40 mg/dL are occasionally observed. The protein concentration is normal or slightly elevated but rarely exceeds 100 mg/dL. Fever and signs of meningeal inflammation subside in 3 to 7 days, although pleocytosis may persist for an additional week or more. The great majority of children and adults recover fully without sequelae. However, enteroviral meningitis during the first year of life may result in permanent neurologic damage, as evidenced by paresis, reduced head circumference, spasticity, and impaired intellectual function, in up to 10% of affected infants.

In some cases, especially those caused by echoviruses, coxsackieviruses A9 and A16, and EV-71, meningitis may be accompanied by a rash, which, if petechial, may raise the spectre of meningococcemia.

Paralytic Disease

Paralytic disease may occur in the course of many nonpolio EV infections. It is similar, but generally less severe, than that caused by polioviruses. Muscle weakness is far more common than frank paralysis, and recovery is usually complete, although occasional patients suffer cranial nerve palsies or severe, sometimes fatal, bulbar involvement. In contrast to paralytic poliomyelitis, which in the prevaccine era occurred in epidemics, cases of paralysis associated with nonpolio EV are generally sporadic. However, several nonpolio EVs produce paralytic disease with sufficient frequency to cause local outbreaks and epidemics. A variant of coxsackievirus A7, once thought to be a fourth serotype of poliovirus, has caused outbreaks, as well as numerous sporadic cases of paralytic disease. Paralytic disease resembling poliomyelitis, with a significant incidence of residual paralysis and muscle atrophy, has been observed in patients with acute hemorrhagic conjunctivitis caused by EV-70. EV-71 is a highly neurotropic virus associated with a variety of central nervous systems (CNS) syndromes, including aseptic meningitis, encephalitis, acute cerebellar ataxia, Bell's palsy, acute flaccid paralysis, and bulbar poliomyelitis.

Table 182.2 Clinical Manifestations of Nonpolio Enterovirus (EV) Infections[a]

Clinical Syndrome	Group A Coxsackieviruses[b]	Group B Coxsackieviruses	Echoviruses[c]	Enteroviruses
Asymptomatic infection	All serotypes	All serotypes	All serotypes	All serotypes
Undifferentiated febrile illness ("summer grippe") with or without respiratory symptoms	All serotypes	All serotypes	All serotypes	68, 70, 71
Aseptic meningitis (often associated with an exanthem)	1, 2, 3, 4, 5, 6, 7, 8, 9, 10, 11, 14, 16, 17, 18, 22, 24	1, 2, 3, 4, 5, 6	1, 2, 3, 4, 5, 6, 7, 8, 9, 10, 11, 12, 14, 16, 17, 18, 19, 20, 21, [22], [23], 25, 30, 31, 33	70, 71
Encephalitis	2, 4, 5, 6, 7, 9, 10, 16	1, 2, 3, 4, 5	2, 3, 4, 6, 7, 9, 11, 14, 17, 18, 19,[22], 25, 30, 33	70, 71
Paralytic disease (poliomyelitislike)	4, 5, 6, 7, 9, 10, 11, 14, 16, 21, 24	1, 2, 3, 4, 5, 6	1, 2, 4, 6, 7, 9, 11, 14, 16, 17, 18, 19, 30	70, 71
Myopericarditis	1, 2, 4, 5, 7, 8, 9, 14, 16	1, 2, 3, 4, 5, 6	1, 2, 3, 4, 6, 7, 8, 9, 11, 14, 16, 17, 19, [22], 25, 30	
Pleurodynia	1, 2, 4, 6, 9, 10, 16	1, 2, 3, 4, 5, 6	1, 2, 3, 6, 7, 8, 9, 11, 12, 14, 16, 19, [23], 25, 30	
Herpangina	1, 2, 3, 4, 5, 6, 7, 8, 9, 10, 16, 22	1, 2, 3, 4, 5	6, 9, 11, 16, 17, [22], 25	71
Hand–foot–and–mouth disease	4, 5, 7, 9, 10, 16	2, 5	7	71
Exanthems	2, 4, 5, 6, 7, 9, 10, 16	1, 2, 3, 4, 5	2, 4, 5, 6, 9, 11, 16, 18, 25	71
Common cold	2, 10, 21, 24	1, 2, 3, 4, 5	2, 4, 8, 9, 11, 20, 25	
Lower respiratory tract infections (broncheolitis, pneumonia)	7, 9, 16	1, 2, 3, 4, 5	4, 8, 9, 11, 12, 14, 19, 20, 21, 25, 30	68, 71
Acute hemorrhagic conjunctivitis[d]	24			70
Generalized disease of the newborn	3, 9, 16	1, 2, 3, 4, 5	3, 4, 6, 7, 9, 11, 12, 14, 17, 18, 19, 20, 21, [22], 30	

[a] A great many EV serotypes have been implicated in most of these syndromes, at least in sporadic cases. The serotypes listed are those that have been clearly and/or frequently implicated. Serotypes with the strongest association are underlined.
[b] Because isolation of many of the group A coxsackieviruses requires suckling mouse inoculation, they are likely to be underreported as causes of illness.
[c] Echovirus types [22] and [23] were found to differ substantially in nucleotide and amino acid sequence from other EV and to have 3, rather than 4, capsid proteins. Consequently, they have been reclassified as parechoviruses 1 and 2, the first members of a new Picornavirus genus, *Parechovirus*. Epidemiologic and clinical features of these viruses are similar to those of the echoviruses.
[d] Conjunctivitis without hemorrhage is frequently seen in association with other manifestations in patients infected with many group A and group B coxsackieviruses and echoviruses, especially coxsackieviruses A9, A16, and B1-B5 and echoviruses 2, 7, 9, 11, 16, and 30.

Specific Organisms – Viruses

Encephalitis

Encephalitis is a well-recognized but uncommon manifestation of EV infection. Enteroviruses account for only 10% to 20% of the cases of encephalitis in the United States of proven viral etiology. In most cases, encephalitis complicates the course of aseptic meningitis; parenchymal involvement is indicated by the onset of confusion, coma, abnormalities of motor function, hemiparesis, vasomotor instability, cranial nerve palsies, cerebellar ataxia, and focal or generalized seizures, singly or in various combinations. Cerebral involvement is usually generalized, but focal encephalitis does occur and may be clinically indistinguishable from herpes simplex encephalitis. Recovery from enteroviral encephalitis is usually complete, although neurologic sequelae and deaths do occur, especially in young infants and during EV-71 epidemics. The large epidemics of EV-71 HFMD in the Asia-Pacific region that began in 1997 have been associated with a syndrome of brainstem encephalitis and rapidly fatal pulmonary edema and hemorrhage that was previously described in only one case of EV-71 infection in 1995.

OTHER REPORTED NEUROLOGIC COMPLICATIONS

Enteroviruses, particularly coxsackie A viruses, appear to be an important cause of febrile seizures in children during EV season. Other neurologic syndromes, including Guillain–Barré syndrome, transverse myelitis, and Reye's syndrome, have been reported in patients with a number of different EV infections.

Epidemic Pleurodynia (Bornholm Disease)

Epidemic pleurodynia is an acute febrile viral illness characterized by the sudden onset of intense paroxysmal lower thoracic or abdominal pain. Synonyms include Bornholm disease, devil's grip, epidemic myalgia, epidemic benign dry pleurisy, and Sylvest disease. The name *pleurodynia* (*pleura*, "side"; *odyne*, "pain") reflects the characteristic intercostal location of the pain and does not connote disease of the pleura. Pleurodynia is usually an epidemic disease, but sporadic cases do occur.

Pleurodynia is characterized by the abrupt onset of fever and sharp, paroxysmal pain over the lower ribs or upper abdomen. In about 25% of patients, this is preceded by a 1- or 2-day prodrome of headache, malaise, anorexia, sore throat, and diffuse myalgia. The pain varies in intensity, but is often severe. It is accentuated, sometimes elicited, by deep breathing, coughing, and movement. In adults, the pain is primarily in muscles of the thorax, especially the intercostals. In children, abdominal muscles are more often involved. Occasionally it may involve muscles in the neck or limbs.

Multiple paroxysms of pain occur, each lasting from a few minutes to several hours. The initial paroxysm is usually the most severe, and patients frequently appear relatively well between paroxysms. The acute illness generally lasts for 2 to 6 days, with a range of 12 hours to 3 weeks. The disease is often biphasic; the initial pain and fever resolve and the patient is asymptomatic for a day or more, and then the pain and fever recur, frequently at the same site. Rarely, patients will have several recurrences over a period of several weeks or will have a late recurrence after being symptom free for a month or more. Group B Coxsackieviruses, especially B3 and B5, are the principal cause. Transmission is primarily from person to person, and multiple family members may be attacked almost simultaneously or in rapid succession at intervals of 2 to 5 days.

Pleurodynia is a disease of skeletal muscle, not of the pleura or peritoneum. As in most enteroviral diseases, infection is initiated in the alimentary tract. Pleurodynia may be confused with any of a number of more serious diseases. When the pain is thoracic, these include pneumonia, pulmonary infarction, rib fracture, costochondritis, and myocardial infarction. When the pain is abdominal, it can be difficult to differentiate pleurodynia from serious causes of acute abdominal pain, such as peritonitis, cholecystitis, appendicitis, perforated peptic ulcer, and acute intestinal obstruction. Pleurodynia may also be confused with the pain of pre-eruptive herpes zoster, herniated intervertebral disk, and renal colic.

Treatment of pleurodynia is symptomatic. Heat applied to affected muscles may also be useful. Despite the tendency of the disease to relapse, patients with epidemic pleurodynia eventually recover completely.

MYOCARDITIS AND PERICARDITIS CAUSED BY ENTEROVIRUSES

Enteroviruses have emerged as the major recognized infectious cause of myocarditis and pericarditis in North America and western Europe. Neonatal infections frequently result in severe myocarditis, widespread involvement of other organs, and high mortality whereas, in older children and adults, pericarditis often predominates and the disease is generally benign and self-limited. In fact, it appears that the clinical manifestations are generally so subtle that cardiac involvement during enteroviral infections is often unrecognized. However, idiopathic dilated cardiomyopathy may, in many cases, be a late sequela of both recognized and unrecognized enteroviral myocarditis.

Increasing use of endomyocardial biopsy and the application of in situ hybridization and, especially, reverse transcription–polymerase chain reaction (RT–PCR) for detection and amplification of enteroviral nucleic acid has substantially improved our ability to establish the etiology in cases of myocarditis and pericarditis. The group B coxsackieviruses are the most common etiologic agents of myocarditis and pericarditis. They appear to account for approximately 50% of sporadic cases of acute myocarditis and for virtually all cases that have occurred in epidemics. Group B coxsackieviruses also appear to account for 30% or more of sporadic cases of acute nonbacterial pericarditis.

At least two-thirds of the cases occur in males, but in females the risk of cardiac involvement also appears to be increased during pregnancy and immediately postpartum.

Idiopathic dilated cardiomyopathy may in many instances represent the end stage of an immunologically mediated disease initiated by an episode of enteroviral myocarditis. This notion is supported by the development of chronic cardiomyopathy in approximately 10% of patients observed long term after group B coxsackievirus myocarditis and by the demonstration of progressive fibrosis in such patients by serial endomyocardial biopsies.

Treatment of enteroviral myopericarditis is primarily supportive. It should include control of pain with analgesics; careful monitoring for arrhythmias, heart failure, and hemodynamic compromise; and prompt treatment of these complications if they arise. Bed rest is an important component of therapy because of clear evidence in mice with coxsackievirus B3 myocarditis that exercise markedly increases the extent of myocardial necrosis and mortality during the acute phase of the disease. Adequate oxygenation should be assured and fluid overload avoided and promptly treated if it develops. In severe cases cardiac assist devices may be lifesaving. Corticosteroids should not be administered to patients with suspected enteroviral myocarditis or pericarditis. Their use during the acute phase of viral myocarditis has been associated with rapid clinical deterioration.

The majority of children and adults with enteroviral myopericarditis recover without obvious sequelae. Acute mortality is low (0% to 5%), and deaths occur as a result of arrhythmias or congestive heart failure in patients with myocarditis; cardiac tamponade is extremely rare in enteroviral pericarditis.

Approximately 20% of patients experience one or more episodes of recurrent myopericarditis within 1 year of their initial illness, and persistent electrocardiographic (ECG) abnormalities are observed in 10% to 20% of patients. Cardiomegaly persists in 5% to 10% of patients, and long-term follow-up suggests that 10% or more may develop chronic cardiomyopathy. Constrictive pericarditis rarely occurs following enteroviral pericarditis.

INSULIN-DEPENDENT DIABETES MELLITUS

Epidemiologic evidence suggests a role for EV, especially group B coxsackieviruses, in the etiology of insulin-dependent diabetes mellitus (IDDM). A number of serologic studies have found evidence of a higher frequency of coxsackievirus B infection in children with new-onset IDDM than in matched controls, and maternal EV infections during pregnancy have been associated with the subsequent development of IDDM in offspring during early childhood. Moreover, enteroviral RNA has been identified by RT–PCR in children with new-onset IDDM at a higher frequency than in matched controls.

MUCOCUTANEOUS SYNDROMES CAUSED BY ENTEROVIRUSES

Enteroviruses are the leading cause of exanthematous disease in the United States and most other developed countries. Almost all EVs can cause maculopapular eruptions, and most serotypes are occasionally responsible for petechial or papulovesicular exanthems and enanthems, as well. Moreover, a given EV may cause more than one pattern of mucocutaneous disease, even within a single infected household. Consequently, except for HFMD, which is usually caused by coxsackievirus A16 or EV-71, there are no clinical or epidemiologic characteristics of any given enteroviral rash that point to a specific EV as its cause.

The epidemiology of enteroviral exanthems and enanthems is the epidemiology of enteroviral infections in general. The vast majority occur during the summer and early fall. The incidence of enanthems and exanthems in infected persons varies among different EVs and even among different strains of the same EV. For example, enanthems and exanthems are often seen in >50% of infected children during outbreaks of infection caused by echovirus 9 or coxsackievirus A16 but are rare during outbreaks caused by echovirus 6 or coxsackievirus A7. Host factors, especially age, are also important; infants and young children are more likely to develop mucocutaneous lesions, whereas other manifestations of EV infection, such as aseptic meningitis, are more likely to develop in older children and adults. Thus, during outbreaks of echovirus 9 infection, rash is often seen in the majority of infected children younger than 5 years of age, but in less than 5% of infected adults, and it is not uncommon when evaluating an adult with aseptic meningitis and no rash to find that a child in the same household is convalescing from an illness characterized by a maculopapular rash. Enteroviral exanthems and enanthems occur in outbreaks and as sporadic cases.

Enteroviral lesions in the oropharyngeal mucosa and skin are manifestations of a systemic virus infection and in contrast to the pathogenesis of the lesions of acute herpetic gingivostomatitis, human papillomavirus infections (warts), and acute hemorrhagic conjunctivitis, which are the direct result of exogenous virus infection and replication in epithelial cells at the portal of entry.

The obligatory occurrence of alimentary tract replication and viremia before mucocutaneous lesions develop explains the 3- to 10-day incubation period and the frequent occurrence of prodromal signs and symptoms. Moreover, the simultaneous dissemination of virus to a number of target organs explains the concurrent appearance of other manifestations of EV infection, such as aseptic meningitis and myopericarditis.

Enanthems

The oropharyngeal mucosa is involved to some degree during most symptomatic enteroviral infections. This is usually manifest by mild pharyngitis and mucosal erythema, but it may also result in a variety of enanthems. These may consist of macules, papules, vesicles, petechiae, or ulcers, and they may occur alone or in association with exanthems and other manifestations of systemic enteroviral infection. They are often transient and frequently unrecognized, but they occasionally lead to diagnostic confusion, for example, when they resemble Koplik's

spots and accompany a morbilliform exanthem in a child infected by echovirus 9. Two enanthems are sufficiently unique to warrant separate description.

HERPANGINA

Herpangina (*herpes*, "vesicular eruption"; *angina*, "inflammation of the throat") is a syndrome characterized by sudden onset of fever, sore throat, pain on swallowing, and a vesicular enanthem of the posterior pharynx. It is seen primarily in children between ages 3 and 10. The disease begins abruptly, after a 3- to 10-day incubation period, with temperature ranging from 38°C to 41°C, sore throat, and pain on swallowing. There may also be anorexia, vomiting, and abdominal pain. Fever tends to be greater in younger children, who may suffer febrile convulsions; older children and adults frequently complain of headache and myalgia. On examination there is pharyngeal erythema but little or no tonsillar exudate. The characteristic lesions are discrete 1- to 2-mm vesicles and ulcers surrounded by 1- to 5-mm zones of erythema. Lesions are few, averaging 4 to 5 per patient, with a range of 1 or 2 to 20. They occur most frequently on the anterior tonsillar pillars, the posterior edge of the soft palate, and the uvula, and less frequently on the tonsils, the posterior pharyngeal wall, and the posterior buccal mucosa. They begin as small papules, progress to vesicles, and ulcerate within 24 hours. The shallow ulcers, which are moderately painful, may enlarge over the next 1 or 2 days to a diameter of 3 to 4 mm. Symptoms generally disappear in 3 or 4 days, but the ulcers may persist for up to a week. Most cases are mild and resolve without complications, but herpangina is occasionally associated with exanthems, aseptic meningitis, or other serious manifestations of systemic EV infection.

Outbreaks of herpangina are common during the summer, and sporadic cases are also observed. Group A coxsackieviruses account for the majority of outbreaks.

ACUTE LYMPHONODULAR PHARYNGITIS

Acute lymphonodular pharyngitis is a variant of herpangina that has been described in children infected with coxsackievirus A10. The lesions have the same distribution as typical cases of herpangina, but instead of evolving into vesicles and ulcers, they remain papular and are infiltrated with lymphocytes to form 2- to 3-mm gray-white nodules surrounded by narrow zones of erythema. The disease is otherwise indistinguishable from herpangina.

HAND-FOOT-AND-MOUTH DISEASE

HFMD (vesicular stomatitis with exanthem) is a mild enteroviral disease characterized by a vesicular eruption in the mouth and over the extremities. It occurs most frequently in children younger than 5 years. After an incubation period of 3 to 6 days, the disease begins with mild fever ranging from 38°C to 39°C, anorexia, malaise, and, often, a sore mouth. Within 1 or 2 days vesicular lesions appear in the oral cavity, most frequently on the anterior buccal mucosa and the tongue, but also on the labial mucosa, gingivae, and hard palate. In the majority of preschool children, but in only about 10% of infected adults, the oral lesions are accompanied by vesicular skin lesions, most often on the dorsal or lateral surfaces of the hands and feet and on the fingers and toes but not infrequently on the palms and soles. Less often, lesions occur on the buttocks or more proximally on the extremities and, rarely, on the genitalia. They are generally 3 to 7 mm in diameter and surrounded by a narrow zone of erythema. They range from 2 or 3 to 30 or more; consist of subepidermal vesicles containing a mixed inflammatory infiltrate of lymphocytes, monocytes, and neutrophils; and are accompanied by acantholysis and cellular degeneration in the overlying epidermis. HFMD is caused most frequently by coxsackievirus A16; less frequently by EV-71 and coxsackieviruses A5, A9, and A10; and occasionally by coxsackieviruses A4, A7, B2, and B5. Outbreaks and sporadic cases occur primarily in the summer and early fall. It may be accompanied by more serious manifestations, especially when caused by EV-71.

Exanthems

Enterovirus exanthems themselves are benign, but they are clinically important for at least three reasons: (1) They constitute direct evidence of EV dissemination and thus provide a clue to the presence and the etiology of coexistent disease referable to other infected target organs, such as the heart and the CNS; (2) they represent the "tip of the iceberg" of EV infection in the community; and (3) they are often confused with other infectious exanthems, some of which have more serious consequences, require specific control measures, or are amenable to specific anti-infective therapy. Misdiagnosis of EV rashes assumes added significance as we prepare to deal with the threat of bioterrorism involving the use of smallpox.

The most common cutaneous manifestation of EV infection is an erythematous maculopapular rash that appears together with fever and other manifestations of systemic infection. This is also a common manifestation of infection by a variety of other organisms, but it is more often caused by EV. Only certain EVs (eg, echovirus 9) cause this syndrome with high frequency, but almost all can produce it at least occasionally. The rash begins on the face and quickly spreads to the neck, trunk, and extremities. It consists of 1- to 3-mm erythematous macules and papules that may be discrete (*rubelliform*, resembling rubella) or confluent (*morbilliform*, resembling measles). It usually lasts for 2 to 5 days and does not itch or desquamate. Enteroviral exanthems are generally not accompanied by significant posterior cervical, suboccipital, or postauricular lymphadenopathy, but there are many exceptions. For example, posterior cervical and suboccipital lymphadenopathy similar to that seen in rubella has been observed in many children with exanthems caused by coxsackievirus A9.

Enteroviral rashes are sometimes petechial and occasionally purpuric. Although this pattern is seen most frequently in echovirus 9 and coxsackievirus A9 infections, it is observed occasionally with many other EV serotypes.

Vesicular exanthems are most often seen as a component of HFMD (see earlier), but several EVs, including echovirus 11, coxsackievirus A9, and EV-71, may cause vesicular exanthems without an associated enanthem. The lesions resemble those caused by varicella-zoster and herpes simplex viruses. In contrast to varicella, however, vesicular rashes caused by EV are usually peripheral in distribution and consist of relatively few lesions that heal without crusting. When they are not associated with HFMD, vesicular lesions caused by EV are often confused with insect bites or poison ivy. Echovirus 11 and several coxsackievirus serotypes have been associated with skin lesions resembling papular urticaria, lesions that usually result from insect bites.

Enteroviral rashes are generally accompanied by fever; they develop at or within 1 or 2 days of its onset. In some cases, however, the rash does not develop until the fever subsides, a pattern resembling that of *roseola infantum* (exanthem subitem), a benign sporadic disease of infants aged 6 to 24 months now known to be caused by human herpesvirus 6.

Herpangina is most often confused with bacterial pharyngitis, tonsillitis, or pharyngitis caused by other viruses. Other considerations include HFMD, primary herpes simplex virus infections, particularly acute herpetic pharyngotonsillitis, and herpes zoster involving the palate.

The vesicular lesions of HFMD resemble those caused by herpes simplex and varicella-zoster viruses. Patients with primary herpetic gingivostomatitis usually have more toxicity, cervical lymphadenopathy, and more prominent gingivitis. Their cutaneous lesions are usually perioral but may occasionally involve a finger that has been in the mouth. Recurrent herpes simplex (herpes labialis) usually involves the vermilion border of the lip or the adjacent skin, is rarely accompanied by lesions on the hands or feet, often has a neuralgic prodrome, and frequently has a history of recurrent episodes. The cutaneous lesions of varicella are generally more extensive and are centrally distributed, sparing the palms and soles. Oral lesions are far less prominent in varicella, and its prevalence in winter and spring further distinguish it from HFMD. Like vesicular lesions caused by herpes simplex and varicella-zoster virus, EV vesicles are generally more superficial and evolve more rapidly than those caused by variola and vaccinia viruses.

Aphthous stomatitis is distinguished from HFMD by the absence of fever and other signs of systemic illness, the absence of cutaneous lesions, and often by a history of recurrence. Maculopapular exanthems caused by EV are distinguished from measles and rubella by their summertime occurrence; the usual absence of posterior cervical, suboccipital, and postauricular lymphadenopathy; and their relatively short incubation period. The absence of significant coryza and conjunctivitis further distinguishes the typical enteroviral exanthems from measles. In addition, the probability of measles and rubella is markedly reduced in persons with a well-documented history of adequate immunization.

When enteroviral rashes are maculopapular they may be confused with drug reactions; when they are petechial they may be confused with bacterial or rickettsial rashes. When enteroviral rashes are petechial or purpuric it is impossible to rule out meningococcemia on clinical grounds alone, and when the rash is associated with aseptic meningitis (as is often the case in echovirus 9 and coxsackievirus A9 infections), it is clinically indistinguishable from meningococcal meningitis. Laboratory investigation is required, even during proven outbreaks of enteroviral disease, because concurrent enteroviral and meningococcal infections can occur.

Enteroviral enanthems and exanthems are generally benign self-limited illnesses that require only symptomatic therapy for headache and sore throat. When illness mimics meningococcemia or meningococcal meningitis, antimicrobial chemotherapy should be initiated until bacterial infection is ruled out by appropriate cultures and antigen-detection assays.

RESPIRATORY TRACT DISEASE CAUSED BY ENTEROVIRUSES

A number of EVs have been associated with mild upper respiratory tract illness in children and adults, especially coxsackieviruses A21, A24, and B1 through B5 and echoviruses 9 and 11. Many of the EVs, most notably coxsackievirus A21, produce illnesses that resemble the common cold, except for a higher incidence of fever. In contrast to most other EVs, coxsackievirus A21 is shed primarily from the upper respiratory tract rather than in feces. Enteroviruses have also been associated with lower respiratory tract illnesses in infants and children, although rarely in adults. These include tracheitis, bronchitis, croup, bronchiolitis, and pneumonia. Surveillance data indicate that EVs account for 2% to 10% of viral respiratory disease and that 10% to 15% of symptomatic EV infections are associated with respiratory symptoms. The respiratory illnesses caused by EVs are clinically indistinguishable from similar illnesses caused by viruses more commonly considered to be respiratory tract pathogens, such as rhinoviruses, influenza viruses, parainfluenza viruses, respiratory syncytial virus, and adenoviruses. However, infections with these viruses occur most frequently during the winter, whereas EV infections occur primarily in the summer and early fall.

ACUTE HEMORRHAGIC CONJUNCTIVITIS

Acute hemorrhagic conjunctivitis (AHC) is an acute, highly contagious, self-limited disease of the eye characterized by sudden onset of pain, photophobia, conjunctivitis, swelling of the eyelids, and prominent subconjunctival hemorrhages. Since its first appearance in 1969, AHC has occurred in explosive epidemics throughout the world.

AHC is a highly contagious disease. In contrast to most enteroviral infections, it is transmitted by direct inoculation of the conjunctivae with virus-contaminated fingers or fomites (ie, transmission is eye to finger or fomite to eye). EVs-70 and the coxsackievirus A24 variant are both naturally occurring temperature-sensitive viruses that replicate optimally at 33°C to 35°C, the temperature of the conjunctivae. There appears to be little or no virus replication in the alimentary tract. Virus is abundant in the conjunctivae and in the ocular exudate, from which it can be readily isolated early in infection. During epidemics, all age groups are affected.

AHC begins with the sudden onset of eye pain and foreign body sensation, lacrimation, photophobia, blurred vision, and bulbar conjunctivitis. Signs and symptoms rapidly increase in severity with the development of palpebral conjunctivitis, conjunctival edema, swelling of the eyelids, subconjunctival hemorrhages in the bulbar conjunctivae, and a serous or seromucoid ocular discharge containing large numbers of polymorphonuclear leukocytes. The subconjunctival hemorrhages, which are the hallmark of the disease, range from discrete petechiae to confluent hemorrhages that occupy virtually the entire bulbar conjunctiva. AHC often begins unilaterally, but it rapidly spreads to the other eye. Signs and symptoms peak within 24 to 36 hours of onset, by which time most patients have also developed hypertrophy of palpebral follicles and papillae, preauricular lymphadenopathy, and punctate epithelial keratitis with tiny corneal erosions that are often seen only by slit-lamp examination after fluorescein staining. Clinical improvement usually begins by the 2nd or 3rd day, and recovery is generally complete without sequelae within 7 to 10 days. Constitutional symptoms, including headache, low-grade fever, and malaise, occur in a minority of patients.

Poliomyelitislike motor paralysis occurs as a rare complication of AHC caused by EV-70, but not in AHC caused by coxsackievirus A24. It occurs predominantly in adult males. The neurologic disease generally does not begin until 2 to 5 weeks after AHC (range of 5 to 60 days or more), thus its relationship to the conjunctivitis is often overlooked by physicians as well as by the patients themselves.

AHC almost always resolves spontaneously without sequelae, and treatment is symptomatic. Topical application of antihistamine/decongestant eye drops and cold compresses may be used to reduce discomfort. Corticosteroids, a component of many topical ophthalmic preparations, are contraindicated. Transmission of AHC can be prevented by careful handwashing, avoidance of contaminated washcloths and towels, and sterilization of all ophthalmologic instruments. These practices should be routine in eye clinics.

DIAGNOSIS

The enteroviral etiology of a disease may be suspected on clinical and epidemiologic grounds, but the multiplicity of agents capable of causing most clinical syndromes associated with EV infections makes it impossible to establish a specific etiologic diagnosis on the basis of such information alone. Virus isolation from the site of pathology (eg, CSF in aseptic meningitis, brain biopsy in encephalitis, myocardial tissue and pericardial fluid in myopericarditis) has been the "gold standard" of enteroviral diagnosis. Isolation of an EV from the nasopharynx or feces is less definitive, because isolation of an EV from these sites may be due to an intercurrent asymptomatic EV infection or prolonged virus shedding from an earlier EV infection and be etiologically unrelated to the observed illness.

The recent development and commercialization of methods for the detection and identification of EV RNA that employ RT–PCR make it possible to provide an accurate diagnosis of EV infection within a few hours, with a sensitivity substantial greater than virus isolation and a specificity of 100%. Serologic testing has a very limited role in the diagnosis of enteroviral infections because of the great diversity of serotypes and the lack of a common antigen.

TREATMENT AND PREVENTION

Specific antiviral chemotherapeutic and chemoprophylactic agents are not yet available for EV infections. Thus treatment is symptomatic and, in severe disease, supportive. Corticosteroids, which have a deleterious effect on coxsackievirus-infected mice, should not be administered during acute EV infections. Strenuous exercise and intramuscular injections, both of which may precipitate paralysis of the involved muscles during EV viremia, should also be avoided during the acute, presumably viremic, phase of symptomatic EV infections. Intravenous immunoglobulin (IVIG), which contains high titers of neutralizing antibodies to many EVs, appears to have been useful in some agammaglobulinemic patients with chronic enteroviral meningoencephalitis. IVIG may also have a role in the treatment of enteroviral infections in other patients with severely compromised B lymphocyte function. Infants with generalized neonatal EV infections are unlikely to have received transplacental antibodies to the causative virus from their mothers. Consequently it seems reasonable to administer IVIG to such infants in an attempt to terminate their viremia and limit virus replication in infected tissues. Prophylactic IVIG should also be considered for patients with compromised B lymphocyte function, including bone marrow transplant recipients. Several promising inhibitors of EV replication belong to a class of anti-EV drugs known as capsid binding inhibitors or (WIN) compounds that bind within a hydrophobic pocket under the floor of the receptor-binding canyon in the EV capsid. This binding inhibits EV replication by blocking receptor attachment and/or virus uncoating. One of these compounds, pleconaril, has broad and potent anti-EV activity, excellent bioavailability, and a very favorable safety profile. Clinical trials have demonstrated benefit in children and adults with EV meningitis and in adults with respiratory infections caused by EV and rhinoviruses. However, the drug is not currently available. Live attenuated and inactivated poliovirus vaccines have been remarkably successful in preventing paralytic poliomyelitis.

Pre-exposure administration of immune serum globulin reduces the risk of paralytic poliomyelitis. Because immune serum globulin also contains neutralizing antibodies to many nonpolio EVs, it would probably prevent many nonpolio EV diseases as well. This approach probably reduces the frequency of severe enteroviral infections in agammaglobulinemic patients receiving replacement therapy. However, the benign nature of most EV infections, the fact that exposures are rarely recognized (most result from contact with an asymptomatically infected person), and the relatively short half-life of exogenous immune serum globulin make this approach to prevention impractical in most situations. Nursery outbreaks of severe enteroviral disease provide an exception. The administration of IVIG to all infants in the nursery offers protection to those infants without transplacentally acquired neutralizing antibody who have not yet been infected.

SUGGESTED READING

Graves PM, Norris JM, Pallansch MA, et al. The role of enteroviral infections in the development of IDDM. *Diabetes*. 1997;46:161–168.

Ho M. Enterovirus 71: the virus, its infections and outbreaks. *J Microbiol Immunol Infect*. 2000;33:205–216.

Modlin JF. Coxsackieviruses, echoviruses, and newer enteroviruses. In: Mandell GL, et al., eds. *Principles and Practice of Infectious Diseases*. 5th ed. New York, NY: Churchill Livingstone; 1999.

Modlin JF. Coxsackieviruses, echoviruses, and newer enteroviruses. In: Mandell GL, et al., eds. *Principles and Practice of Infectious Diseases*. 6th ed. New York, NY: Churchill Livingstone; 2005:2148--2161.

Pallansch MA, Roos RR. Enteroviruses: polioviruses, coxsackieviruses, echoviruses and newer enteroviruses. In: Knipe DM, Howley PM, eds. *Fields Virology*. 4th ed. Philadelphia, PA: Lippincott Williams & Wilkins; 2001:723–775.

Pevear DC, Tull TM, Seipel ME. Activity of pleconaril against enteroviruses. *Antimicrob Agents Chemother*. 1999;43:2109–2115.

Rotbart HA. Enteroviruses. In: Richman DD, Whitley RJ, Hayden FG, eds. *Clinical Virology*. 2nd ed. Washington DC: ASM Press; 2002:971–994.

183. Epstein–Barr Virus and Other Causes of the Mononucleosis Syndrome

Jeffery L. Meier

Epstein–Barr virus (EBV) infects nearly all persons in the world at some time. The virus persists indefinitely in their B lymphocytes and is shed intermittently from oropharyngeal tissue into oral secretions. Transmission of EBV occurs when susceptible individuals come in close oral contact with infectious saliva. Casual contact is generally insufficient to transmit infection, and spread of EBV among susceptible household contacts is infrequent. Occasionally, the virus is transmitted by blood products or donor tissues. About 95% of all persons will have acquired EBV by the end of their 3rd decade of life. Persons living with low standards of hygiene, such as occurs in developing countries or low socioeconomic conditions, often acquire EBV in childhood, and nearly everyone becomes infected by adulthood. In contrast, persons adhering to a high standard of hygiene often have EBV infection delayed until adolescence or early adulthood, when sexual intimacy becomes a factor in transmission.

INFECTIOUS MONONUCLEOSIS

Presentation

Most EBV infections do not produce illness. When EBV does cause disease, the spectrum of illness is varied (Table 183.1). Infectious mononucleosis (IM) is the paradigmatic illness associated with EBV infection. The IM syndrome is largely the product of an exuberant immunologic response to a newly acquired EBV infection, and in healthy persons IM does not arise from EBV reactivation. This illness commonly occurs among adolescents and young adults (15 to 25 years) and seldom appears in persons of other ages. This is because most infants and children do not overtly exhibit findings of acute infection and most older adults are no longer susceptible to EBV, although they do retain the capacity to develop IM. Approximately 25% to 50% of young adults experiencing primary EBV infection will develop IM.

The diagnosis of IM is based on a characteristic clinical and laboratory presentation (Table 183.2). A primary EBV infection (IM) is

Table 183.1 EBV-Related Illness

Acute
Infectious mononucleosis (IM)
Atypical presentations or complications of IM

Chronic
Chronic active infection (extremely rare)
Oral hairy leukoplakia

Lymphoproliferative Disorders
Consequence of congenital or acquired immunosuppression
X-linked (Duncan disease)

Other Disorders
African Burkitt's lymphoma
Nonkeratinizing nasopharyngeal carcinoma
Primary central nervous system lymphoma in AIDS
Some smooth muscle cell tumors and thymomas
Hodgkin's disease (EBV DNA in 40%–65% of tumors)

Abbreviations: EBV = Epstein–Barr virus; AIDS = acquired immunodeficiency syndrome.

exceedingly likely in persons presenting with the following: classic clinical triad of fever, pharyngitis, and cervical lymphadenopathy; absolute peripheral lymphocytosis; atypical lymphocytosis that is >10% of the differential; and heterophile antibodies. As these criteria are relaxed, the probability of EBV causing the mononucleosis (mono)-like syndrome decreases accordingly. Conversely, the absence of any of these criteria does not rule out EBV. For example, as many as 5% to 10% of EBV mono episodes will remain heterophile negative. In addition, some of the characteristic features of IM may not be evident until later in the illness. Atypical lymphocytosis, for instance, may not be impressive until the second week of illness. Unusual clinical presentations of primary EBV infection are more likely to occur in infants, young children, older adults, and immunosuppressed persons.

Malaise and fatigue are often prominent symptoms of IM, and their resolution is generally more gradual than other symptoms. Approximately 10% of patients report fatigue and impaired functional status at 6 months after the acute illness. This delay in recovery is not the

Table 183.2 Clinical and Laboratory Findings in Uncomplicated Infectious Mononucleosis

Percentage of Patients	>50%	10%–50%	≤10%
Symptoms	Sore throat, malaise, fatigue, headache, sweats	Anorexia, myalgia, chills, nausea	Cough, arthralgias, abdominal discomfort
Signs	Lymphadenopathy, fever, pharyngitis	Splenomegaly, hepatomegaly, palatal petechiae, periorbital edema	Rash, jaundice
Labs	>50% mononuclear cells >10% atypical lymphocytes Heterophile antibodies Mild LFT increase Mild thrombocytopenia Cold agglutinins	Mild neutropenia Antinuclear antibodies Rheumatoid factor	Bilirubinemia >3 mg/100 mL Hematuria Pyuria Proteinuria

Abbreviation: LFT = liver function test.

result of ongoing EBV activity and is not distinguished by physical examination, serologic, or laboratory findings. Mild retroorbital headache is also common but short lived. Fever is typically in the range of 38°C to 39.5°C (100°F to 103.1°F) and subsides in 1 to 2 weeks, although it occasionally persists up to 4 weeks. Concomitant sweats and chills also occur. Fever above 40°C (104°F) is rare and should prompt a search for a superimposed bacterial infection (eg, bacterial pharyngitis or peritonsillar abscess). Exudative tonsillopharyngitis occurs in one-third of uncomplicated IM cases; this usually resolves in the first 2 weeks of illness. Petechiae located on the uvula and at the junction of soft and hard palates suggest EBV but may be seen in other viral infections such as rubella. Symmetric posterior cervical lymphadenopathy is a common characteristic of IM. Anterior cervical lymph node enlargement is common as well. Lymphadenopathy may take several weeks to resolve; rarely, it persists for months. Hepatitis is present in approximately 90% of IM cases and is usually mild, although transaminases above 500 IU/L and clinical jaundice are possible. Splenomegaly occurs in nearly one-half of IM cases. Severe abdominal discomfort is unusual and should raise a concern of splenic rupture. Rash is infrequent in the absence of antibiotics and, if present, often takes the form of a faint morbilliform eruption. The peripheral blood lymphocytosis often peaks during the second or third week of illness, and mild neutropenia and thrombocytopenia are common.

In elderly persons, the acute EBV illness is less likely to present with pharyngitis, lymphadenopathy, and splenomegaly. A prolonged febrile course or jaundice occurs with greater frequency. Atypical lymphocytosis may be delayed and of lesser magnitude. Infants and young children with EBV mono are more likely to be heterophile negative and have coryza, exudative pharyngitis, rash, and hepatosplenomegaly.

Complications

Most episodes of IM are uneventful. However, any one of a wide range of complications may occur (Table 183.3). These complications may at times either greatly overshadow or develop in the absence of typical IM features. Most complications of IM resolve without sequelae, but rare fatalities do occur, largely as the result of encephalitis, splenic rupture, hepatic failure, myocarditis, or bacterial infection related to neutropenia. Airway obstruction can result from excessive lymphoid hyperplasia in tonsillar tissue. Enlarged spleens are susceptible to traumatic rupture; spontaneous rupture is rare. Autoantibodies may arise to produce hemolytic anemia, thrombocytopenia, or neutropenia.

Infectious mononucleosis may evolve into a life-threatening lymphoproliferative disorder in persons with profound acquired or congenital cellular immunodeficiency. In a rare inherited disease, the X-linked lymphoproliferative disorder, young males develop a fulminant mononucleosis after acquiring EBV. Many die of hemorrhage and infection; survivors have aplastic anemia, dysgammaglobulinemia, and lymphoma. EBV can also rarely cause chronic active infection (chronic IM), which results in interstitial pneumonitis, massive lymphadenopathy, hepatosplenomegaly, marrow failure, dysgammaglobulinemia, Guillain–Barré

Table 183.3 Complications of Infectious Mononucleosis

Neurologic

Encephalitis, meningitis, Guillain–Barré syndrome, Bell's palsy, optic neuritis, psychosis, transverse myelitis, Reye's syndrome

Splenic

Rupture of enlarged spleen (traumatic or spontaneous rupture)

Respiratory

Upper airway obstruction from hypertrophy of lymphoid tissue, interstitial pneumonitis (especially, in children with HIV)

Hematologic

Autoimmune hemolytic anemia, critical thrombocytopenia, agranulocytosis, aplastic anemia, hemophagocytic syndrome

Hepatic

Fulminant hepatitis, hepatic necrosis

Cardiac

Myocarditis, pericarditis

Immunologic

Anergy, lymphoproliferative syndromes, hypogammaglobulinemia

Dermatologic

Cold-mediated urticaria, leukocytoclastic vasculitis, ampicillin-associated rash, erythema multiforme, erythema nodosum

Abbreviation: HIV = human immunodeficiency virus.

syndrome, and uveitis. The diagnosis is substantiated by demonstrating high levels of EBV in blood or tissues; EBV-specific antibodies also reach very high titers. Chronic fatigue syndrome is heterogeneous in form or etiology, is infrequently triggered by EBV-induced IM, and is not maintained by persistent EBV activity.

Serology

Heterophile antibodies are a long-established marker of EBV-induced IM and are rarely produced outside of this setting. They are uncommonly observed in viral hepatitis, primary human immunodeficiency virus (HIV) infection, malaria, and lymphoma. Rapid latex slide tests and solid-phase immunoassays have supplanted traditional methods, such as the Paul–Bunnell–Davidsohn test, for detection of heterophile antibodies. Heterophile antibodies are defined based on their ability to recognize specific animal erythrocytes (eg, causing agglutination of sheep, horse, and cow erythrocytes) and to not react with guinea pig kidney cells. They do not recognize EBV antigens, and their titers do not correlate with severity of illness. Heterophile antibodies are sometimes not detected until the second or third week of the illness, resolve in 3 to 6 months, and do not reappear.

EBV-specific serologies are useful to ascertain the role of EBV in illness not fulfilling the classical criteria of IM. Antibodies against viral capsid antigen (anti-VCA) are demonstrable in virtually all episodes of IM. Anti-VCA immunoglobulin M (IgM) evolves quickly during primary EBV infection, is usually detectable when patients first present, and may linger for weeks to months. A comparison of paired acute and convalescent anti-VCA immunoglobulin G (IgG) titers is less helpful for the diagnosis of primary infection because the titer is often near its peak when patients first present. This antibody titer falls slowly and persists lifelong, ranging from 1:40 to 1:2560, as determined by the immunofluorescence assay (IFA). Antibodies to EBV early antigens (anti-EA) of the diffuse and restricted types develop in most IM cases and wane with time. The persistence of these antibodies in low titers is of no clinical significance. Antibodies to EBV nuclear antigens (anti-EBNA) are usually not detected by IFA in the acute symptomatic phase of IM but do appear in convalescence and persist for life; some enzyme-linked assays are more likely to detect these antibodies during the acute illness.

Caution should be used when interpreting EBV-specific antibody titers. Comparison of results acquired at different times, in different places, or by different methods may be misleading.

OTHER CAUSES OF MONO SYNDROME

Primary infections with cytomegalovirus (CMV), toxoplasma, HIV, rubella, and viral hepatitis (eg, hepatitis A, B, and C), as well as bacterial pharyngitis, are often considered as other possible causes of mono syndrome, particularly when heterophile antibodies are absent. Although each of these other causes of mono syndrome may exhibit distinctive clinical and general laboratory features (Table 183.4), the definitive diagnosis usually relies on the outcome of specific laboratory tests (Table 183.5). EBV should also be kept in the differential diagnosis of heterophile-negative mono syndrome.

CMV accounts for the majority of heterophile-negative mono episodes. CMV mono may closely resemble IM because both

Table 183.4 Differential Diagnosis of Mononucleosislike Syndrome

Variables	EBV	CMV	Toxoplasma	HIV	Bacterial Pharyngitis[a]	Rubella	HAV, HBV, HCV
Fever	++	++	+	++	++	+	++
Sore throat	++	+	+	++	++ abrupt	+/– coryza	–
Exudative pharyngitis	+	+/–	–	+/– aphthous ulcers	+	–	–
Anterior cervical LN	++	+	++	++	++	+	+/–
Posterior cervical LN	++	+	++	++	+/– mild	++	+/–
Rash	+/– but common with ampicillin	+	+/–	++	+/– scarlatiniform	++	+/–
Hepatitis	++	++	+/–	+	–	+/–	++
Jaundice	+/–	+/–	–	–	–	–	++
Splenomegaly	++	+	+/–	+/–	–	+/–	+
Atypical lymphs	++	++	+ ≤10% of cells	+/– ≤10% of cells	–	+/– ≤10% of cells	+ ≤10% of cells
Heterophile antibodies	++ absent in 5%–10%	–	–	–	–	–	–

Key: ++ = present in >50% of cases; + = present in 10% to 50% of cases; +/– = present in 10% of cases; – = absent or rare;
Abbreviations: EBV = Epstein–Barr virus; CMV = cytomegalovirus (glandular fever); HIV = human immunodeficiency virus (acute retroviral syndrome); HAV = hepatitis A virus; HBV = hepatitis B virus; HCV = hepatitis C virus; LN = lymphadenopathy; lymphs = peripheral lymphocytes.
[a] Primarily β-hemolytic streptococci; consider diphtheria, *Arcanobacterium hemolyticum*, *Neisseria gonorrhoeae*, mycoplasma, and Vincent's angina.

often produce fever, hepatitis, and atypical lymphocytosis. However, cervical lymphadenopathy and pharyngitis tend to be milder in CMV mono. The diagnosis of acute CMV infection in the immunocompetent patient is confirmed by serological evidence of a positive anti-CMV IgM plus low- to moderate-avidity anti-CMV IgG index or CMV IgG seroconversion. Detection of CMV antigen or DNA in peripheral blood also supports the diagnosis. Absence of CMV in urine by viral culture makes the diagnosis less likely, but a positive urine culture lacks specificity.

Acute HIV infection is frequently accompanied by a mono syndrome. In acute retroviral syndrome, unlike IM, a rash is common, exudative pharyngitis is infrequent, tonsillar hypertrophy is minimal, and oral or genital ulcers are sometimes observed. A transient peripheral lymphopenia is followed 2 to 3 weeks later by lymphocytosis in which a small proportion of cells may be reactive. A diagnosis is made during the acute illness by detection of HIV RNA or p24 antigen in blood despite the negative or indeterminate result of HIV antibody testing.

Streptococcal pharyngitis may be distinguished from IM on the basis of its abrupt onset and absence of any associated posterior cervical lymphadenopathy, hepatosplenomegaly, and atypical lymphocytosis. Toxoplasmosis, which is an uncommon cause of mono syndrome in the United States, does not produce exudative pharyngitis or a peripheral atypical lymphocytosis that exceeds 10% of the differential. Rubella may present with fever and lymphadenopathy, but the rash, coryza, arthralgias, and minimal atypical lymphocytosis distinguish it from IM. The diagnosis of viral hepatitis is suggested by prominent hepatic involvement in the absence of pharyngitis or marked lymphadenopathy.

Other conditions or agents that uncommonly produce an acute monolike illness include

Specific Organisms – Viruses

Table 183.5 Diagnostic Studies in Mononucleosislike Syndrome

Variables	EBV	CMV	Toxoplasma	HIV	Bacterial Pharyngitis[a]	Rubella	HAV, HBV, HCV
Antibody response: acute[b]	+ Heterophile + IgM VCA +/− anti-EA (IFA) − anti-EBNA (IFA)	+ IgM CMV, low- to moderate-avidity CMV IgG	+ IgM Toxo, low- to moderate-avidity Toxo IgG	−HIV Ab	None	+ IgM rubella	+ IgM HAV, + IgM HBc, − HCV Ab
Convalescent	+/− 4-fold increase IgG VCA +/− anti-EA (IFA) + anti-EBNA (IFA)	+ 4-fold increase IgG CMV	+ IgG Toxo serocon/version (several test-types available)	+ HIVAb +Confirmatory immunoblot	+ Elevated or rising ASO or anti-DNase B	+ 4-fold increase IgG rubella	+ IgG HAV, + or − anti-HBs + IgG HBc, + HCV Ab
Nucleic acid or antigen detection	None	+/− CMV antigen or DNA in blood WBC or DNA in plasma	None	+ plasma HIV RNA PCR +/− p24 Ag	+ Rapid Strept test	None	+ HBs Ag + plasma HCV RNA PCR
Culture	Impractical	+ Urine, saliva	Impractical	Impractical	+ Throat swab, blood agar	Impractical	None

Key: + = typically present; +/− = sometimes present; − = usually absent.

Abbreviations: EBV = Epstein–Barr virus; CMV = cytomegalovirus; Toxo = toxoplasma; HIV = human immunodeficiency virus; HAV = hepatitis A virus; HBV = hepatitis B virus; HCV = hepatitis C virus; VCA = EBV viral capsid antigens; EA = EBV early antigens; IFA = immunofluorescence assay; EBNA = EBV nuclear antigens; EIA = enzyme-linked immunoassay; HBc = HBV capsid antigens; HBs = HBV surface antigen; p24 = HIV core protein; PCR = polymerase chain reaction.

[a] Applies primarily to group A streptococcus; special media required to culture *Corynebacterium diphtheriae*, *Neisseria gonorrhoeae*, and *Arcanobacterium haemolyticum*.

[b] IgM and heterophile status determined with acute serum. Paired acute and convalescent sera should be analyzed simultaneously to accurately determine change in antibody titer.

human herpesvirus 6 (HHV-6), parvovirus B19, hematologic disorders, and drug reactions.

MANAGEMENT

Epstein–Barr Virus

The management of primary EBV infection (Table 183.6) rarely demands more than general supportive care, which includes adequate rest, hydration, antipyretics, and analgesics. Complications of IM may require additional supportive measures (eg, maintenance of airway during obstructive tonsillar enlargement or encephalitis, transfusions for severe hemolytic anemia or thrombocytopenia, splenectomy for splenic rupture). Activity should be restricted in proportion to the degree of symptoms and any splenomegaly. Most students can return to school in less than 2 to 3 weeks. Contact sports should be avoided for 1 month or until absence of splenomegaly is verified. This recommendation aims to decrease risk of traumatic splenic rupture that involves enlarged spleens and occurs within the first month of infection, during either the acute symptomatic or early convalescent phase of the illness. Ultrasonography can detect splenomegaly that is not appreciated on physical examination, and this nonpalpable splenomegaly also resolves in 1 month. For the athlete with resolving IM who wants to participate in contact sports during the first month of illness, ultrasonography can be used to exclude nonpalpable splenomegaly.

The virally induced exudative tonsillopharyngitis that accompanies IM commonly leads to a search for β-hemolytic streptococci. Anywhere from 3% to 30% of throat cultures obtained randomly during IM will grow group A streptococci, reflecting differences in the age of patients and in prevalence of streptococcal carriage in the community. Although streptococcal infection and colonization are clinically indistinguishable in persons with EBV pharyngitis, as many as 30% of individuals harboring this bacterium will eventually show serologic evidence of infection. For this reason, treatment for 10 days with penicillin or erythromycin is advised, particularly to prevent poststreptococcal sequelae. Ampicillin should not be used because it causes rash in more than 85% of cases; amoxicillin also appears to cause rash frequently. The empiric use of antibiotics in uncomplicated IM is not recommended, as most studies of this approach have not shown efficacy.

Table 183.6 Management of Acute Infectious Mononucleosis

Uncomplicated Cases

Supportive care: hydration, rest, antipyretic, analgesic (eg, acetaminophen or nonsteroidal antiinflammatory agent)

Activity restriction: restrict in proportion to degree of symptoms and splenomegaly; avoid contact and collision sports for 1 mo or until absence of splenomegaly verified

If throat culture contains β-hemolytic streptococci, treat with 10 d of penicillin or erythromycin

Avoid ampicillin- and amoxicillin-containing regimens

Corticosteroid use is not indicated

Complicated Cases

Additional supportive care: maintenance of airway during obstruction or encephalitis; splenectomy for splenic rupture; transfusions for critical anemia or thrombocytopenia

Corticosteroids are useful in selected situations[a]: impending airway obstruction from tonsillar enlargement; persistent severe illness; autoimmune hemolytic anemia or thrombocytopenia; aplastic anemia; considered in encephalitis, myocarditis, or pericarditis

[a] Sixty-mg dose equivalent of prednisone per day for 2 to 3 d and then tapered over 1 to 2 wk.

Antiviral agents such as acyclovir, ganciclovir, and foscarnet inhibit EBV replication during lytic (productive) infection but do not inhibit amplification of latent EBV genomes in proliferating B cells. Valaciclovir, an orally administered prodrug of acyclovir, and formulations of intravenous and high-dose oral acyclovir greatly inhibit oropharyngeal shedding of EBV in persons with IM. This inhibition occurs even if corticosteroid is administered and ceases after discontinuation of the antiviral agent. However, combined evidence from several controlled trials indicates that acyclovir is not clinically efficacious in acute IM, and the proportion of circulating B cells containing EBV is not consistently reduced.

EBV-associated oral hairy leukoplakia usually resolves with immune reconstitution resulting from treatment of HIV but may respond to high-dose oral acyclovir (800 mg 5 times per day). Acyclovir or ganciclovir is used for treatment of posttransplant lymphoproliferative disorders, although the therapeutic efficacy is unclear. Acyclovir may be useful in some cases of chronic IM.

The routine use of a corticosteroid as therapy for uncomplicated IM is not recommended. Although some clinicians use corticosteroids to quickly relieve symptoms of uncomplicated IM, several small controlled trials varying in design have not consistently found this practice to be clinically effective and have not fully addressed the potential for short- and long-term adverse effects. Of the studies showing benefit, a modest reduction in the duration of fever and tonsillopharyngeal symptoms is noted. In a double-blind, placebo-controlled study, the combination of prednisolone and acyclovir did not significantly decrease duration of IM symptoms. Corticosteroids have not been shown to decrease lymphadenopathy or hepatosplenic involvement. Corticosteroids have been associated with rare reports of encephalitis, myocarditis, and peritonsillar abscess and with theoretical concerns of producing adverse effects on long-term immunity or number of latently infected cells with malignancy potential.

Corticosteroids are clinically useful in the management of certain complications of IM (Table 183.6). Such therapy may quickly ameliorate impending airway obstruction from tonsillar enlargement. A short course of a corticosteroid is worth consideration in exceptional situations of severe protracted IM (ie, fever, prostration, weight loss). Corticosteroids may also reduce the severity of autoimmune thrombocytopenia and hemolytic anemia, and their use can be considered for intractable or desperate cases of encephalitis, myocarditis, and pericarditis. When required, corticosteroid therapy is initiated with 60 mg of predisone equivalent per day given orally (or intravenously) for 2 to 3 days, and then tapered over a period of 1 to 2 weeks.

Therapy of Other Causes of Mono Syndrome

The mono syndrome associated with CMV, toxoplasma, HIV, rubella, or the hepatitis viruses is usually self-limiting and, like IM, is primarily managed with supportive care. However, HIV, pregnancy, and underlying cellular immunosuppression are circumstances in which additional therapeutic interventions may be required. For instance, specific antimicrobial therapy is warranted in persons with profound cellular immune deficiency who develop CMV mono or acute toxoplasmosis (see Chapter 99, Differential Diagnosis and Management of Opportunistic Infections Complicating HIV Infection). Because primary CMV, toxoplasma, and rubella infections in pregnancy pose a risk for congenital infection and disease, an obstetrician with expertise in this area should be consulted. Primary toxoplasmosis of pregnancy necessitates antimicrobial therapy (see Chapter 197, Toxoplasma). Antiretroviral therapy given during pregnancy can substantially reduce perinatal HIV transmission, but its use requires knowledge of the attendant toxicities and risks (see Chapter 93, Pregnancy and the Puerperium: Infectious Risks). Immediate antiretroviral therapy should be considered in persons with acute HIV infection (see Chapter 97, HIV-1 Infection: Antiretroviral Therapy).

PREVENTION

There is not a vaccine for prevention of EBV infection or disease. Hospitalized patients with IM need not be isolated. Transmissibility of EBV during asymptomatic viral shedding remains possible long after the acute illness. Restricting intimate contact can decrease transmission of EBV but is generally neither practical nor feasible. Avoidance of intimate contact is reasonable when the complications of EBV infection could be devastating.

SUGGESTED READING

Candy B, Hotopf M. Steroids for symptom control in infectious mononucleosis (review). *Cochrane Database Syst Rev.* 2006;19;3: CD004402.

Chervenick PA. Infectious mononucleosis: the classic clinical syndrome. In Schlossberg D, ed. *Infectious Mononucleosis.* 2nd ed. New York, NY: Springer-Verlag; 1989.

Johannsen EC, Kaye KM, Schooley RT. Epstein-Barr virus (infectious mononucleosis). In: Mandell GL, Bennett JE, Dolin R, eds. *Mandell, Douglas, and Bennett's Principles and Practices of Infectious Diseases.* 6th ed. New York, NY: Elsevier Churchill Livingstone; 2005.

Straus SE, Cohen JI, Tosato G, Meier J, NIH conference. Epstein-Barr virus infections: biology, pathogenesis, and management. *Ann Intern Med.* 1993;188:45–58.

Torre D, Tambini R. Acyclovir for treatment of infectious mononucleosis: a meta-analysis. *Scand J Infect Dis.* 1999;31:543–547.

Epstein–Barr Virus and Other Causes of the Mononucleosis Syndrome

184. Hantavirus Cardiopulmonary Syndrome in the Americas

Gregory Mertz and Michelle J. Iandiorio

INTRODUCTION

Hantavirus cardiopulmonary syndrome (HCPS) is a viral zoonosis that may result in cardiogenic shock and respiratory failure with significant associated mortality. Hantavirus infection has been identified throughout much of North, Central, and South America. In the United States 453 cases of HCPS have been reported through September 2006 with a case fatality rate of 35%. The majority of these cases have been from the southwest. The incidence is even greater in South America, particularly in Argentina, Brazil, Chile, and Paraguay. In Chile 495 cases have been reported through 2006, with a case fatality rate of 37%.

VIROLOGY

HCPS is caused by an infection with a hantavirus. There have been approximately 20 New World hantaviruses identified since their discovery in 1993. The New World hantaviruses differ from the Old World hantaviruses that cause hemorrhagic fever with renal syndrome (HFRS) and are found primarily in Asia and Europe. The most common hantavirus causing HCPS in Canada and the United States is *sin nombre* virus (SNV). Other hantaviruses that cause significant disease in Central and South America include Andes virus (ANDV) in Chile and Argentina, Choclo virus in Panama, and Laguna Negra virus in Paraguay. The hantaviruses are small single-stranded negative-sense RNA viruses that belong to the family Bunyaviridae, a family known to include other viruses that cause significant zoonotic illnesses.

EPIDEMIOLOGY

Hantavirus infection is spread to humans by a rodent reservoir. The primary rodent responsible for human transmission in North America is the deer mouse, *Peromyscus maniculatus*. These asymptomatic rodent hosts shed the virus in urine, feces, and saliva. Humans are thought to be infected when the aerosolized excreta are inhaled. People are exposed most often when they are cleaning enclosed areas where dried excreta are disturbed. Exposure through rodent bite has also been identified. Human-to-human transmission has only been documented with ANDV infections in Chile and southern Argentina. In both Chile and southern Argentina, approximately one-third of cases occur in household clusters, and most secondary cases in these clusters result from person-to-person transmission. In a recent prospective study of household contacts of patients with HCPS in Chile, Ferrés et al. reported a significantly higher risk of the development of HCPS in sex partners and other close household contacts as compared to members of the household who slept in different rooms and denied sexual contact.

CLINICAL SYNDROME

Most cases involve an individual with a prolonged exposure history, so it is often difficult to determine the exact incubation period. In a small series from Chile where individuals had brief periods of exposure to high-risk areas, the median incubation period between exposure and onset of clinical disease was 18 days, with a range of 11 to 32 days. Clinical disease begins with a febrile prodrome consisting of 2 days to a week of fevers and myalgias, often with associated headache, backache, abdominal pain, nausea, and diarrhea. After several days with nonspecific prodromal symptoms, the cardiopulmonary phase starts abruptly with cough and dyspnea. This stage of disease may be mild, requiring only supplemental oxygen, or severe, causing rapid pulmonary edema and respiratory failure requiring mechanical ventilation. Severe disease is also characterized by cardiogenic shock, hemoconcentration, and lactic acidosis that may result in profound shock, cardiac arrhythmias, and death. The cardiopulmonary phase usually lasts 2 to 4 days. If the patient survives the cardiopulmonary phase, the patient will proceed into the diuretic phase with subsequent resolution of the pulmonary edema. Convalescence is prolonged and may include weakness, fatigue, and impaired exercise tolerance with abnormal diffusion capacity.

DIAGNOSIS

Early presumptive diagnosis is critical because patients often progress to shock and death before definitive diagnosis can be made. The appropriate exposure history is helpful but not always present. Clinical diagnosis during the prodrome is difficult as there may be no cough, a normal chest radiograph, and no lab abnormalities except for thrombocytopenia.

A definitive diagnosis of HCPS is based on serological testing for hantavirus-specific immunoglobulin G (IgG) and immunoglobulin M (IgM) antibodies. These antibodies become positive during the febrile prodrome, but the clinician must have a high degree of suspicion to order the tests. In addition, the serologic test results are usually not available for at least 8 to 24 hours.

The serologic tests available in the United States are the enzyme-linked immunosorbent assay (ELISA), which is available at many state health departments via the Centers for Disease Control and Prevention (CDC), and a strip immunoblot assay (SIA). An acute infection is characterized by a positive IgM and negative IgG or a 4-fold rise in IgG titers. Nested reverse transcription–polymerase chain reaction (RT–PCR) can detect hantavirus RNA in peripheral mononuclear cells and in serum but is limited to research laboratories. Hantavirus RNA has been detected in peripheral blood cells up to 2 weeks before the onset of symptoms or detection of antihantavirus antibodies.

A presumptive diagnosis can generally be made at the onset of the cardiopulmonary phase on the basis of the clinical presentation, radiologic findings, and a review of the peripheral blood smear. Characteristic hemodynamic findings may also be helpful in establishing a diagnosis. The chest radiograph will show findings consistent with pulmonary edema, including bilateral pulmonary infiltrates, Kerley B lines, indistinct hilar borders, and peribronchial cuffing, which progress rapidly over the next 12 hours. A peripheral blood smear should be evaluated by an experienced pathologist. Clues to the diagnosis include the following: thrombocytopenia (platelet count ≤150), left-shift (presence of myeloblasts), a lack of toxic granulation in neutrophils, hemoconcentration (hematocrit >50 in men and >48 in women), and >10% immunoblasts among lymphocytes. When evaluating a patient in whom there is a high clinical suspicion of HCPS, 4 of 5 of these peripheral blood criteria have a sensitivity of 96% and a specificity of 99%. Unfortunately, these criteria apply only once the patient is already in the cardiopulmonary phase and therefore cannot be used for diagnosis in the prodromal stage. Other clinical findings in this later stage include a low cardiac index associated with a high systemic vascular resistance, in contrast to parameters found in septic shock. Occasionally, hyponatremia and/or transaminitis may be found.

TREATMENT

When there is clinical suspicion of HCPS, the patient should be transported to a facility in which cardiovascular and ventilatory support is available. Volume resuscitation should be avoided, as this can exacerbate the pulmonary edema. Supplemental oxygen should be provided, including ventilatory support if necessary. A pulmonary artery catheter should be placed for the monitoring of cardiac index and systemic vascular resistance. Early use of pressors should be utilized when appropriate. Dobutamine is preferred because this ionotrope allows for afterload reduction. High-dose norepinephrine or dopamine can be used in addition to dobutamine, if necessary.

If extracorporeal membrane oxygenation (ECMO) is available, the patient should be evaluated by the critical care and ECMO team, including cardiothoracic or vascular surgery, as soon as a presumptive diagnosis is made. In patients who are continuing to deteriorate despite full ventilatory and pressor support, ECMO should be considered. The University of New Mexico Hospital (UNMH) in Albuquerque, New Mexico, has the most experience with the use of ECMO for this condition. The criteria for the use of ECMO at this institution include a cardiac index less than 2.3 L/min/m^2, PaO_2/FiO_2 of less than 50, and a lack of response to conventional support. Exclusion criteria include age over 70 years, severe pre-existing comorbid disease, and neurologic impairment. Of the 35 patients treated with ECMO at UNMH through February 2006, 23 survived to discharge.

There is no antiviral therapy approved for the treatment of HCPS, and intravenous ribavirin did not show any survival benefit in a placebo-controlled trial in North America. There is currently an ongoing controlled trial of methylprednisolone treatment, but the results of this trial are not yet available.

SUGGESTED READING

Crowley MR, Katz RW, Kessler R, et al. Successful treatment of adults with severe Hantavirus pulmonary syndrome with extracorporeal membrane oxygenation. *Crit Care Med*. 1998;26:409–414.

Ferres M, Vial P, Marco C, et al. Prospective evaluation of household contacts of persons with hantavirus cardiopulmonary syndrome in Chile. *J Infect Dis*. 2007;195:1563–1571.

Koster F, Foucar K, Hjelle B, et al. Presumptive diagnosis of hantavirus cardiopulmonary syndrome by routine complete blood count and blood smear review. *Am J Clin Pathol*. 2001;116:665–672.

Lázaro ME, Cantoni GE, Calanni LM, et al. Clusters of hantavirus infection, southern Argentina. *Emerg Infect Dis*. 2007;13:104–110.

Mertz GJ, Hjelle B, Crowley M, Iwamoto G, Tomicic V, Vial PA. Diagnosis and treatment of new world hantavirus infections. *Curr Opin Infect Dis*. 2006;19:437–442.

Mertz GJ, Miedzinski L, Goade D, et al. Placebo-controlled, double-blind trial of intravenous ribavirin for hantavirus cardiopulmonary syndrome in North America. *Clin Infect Dis*. 2004; 39:1307–1313.

Vial PA, Valdivieso F, Mertz G, et al. Incubation period of hantavirus cardiopulmonary syndrome. *Emerg Infect Dis*. 2006;12: 1271–1273.

185. Herpes Simplex Viruses 1 and 2

David W. Kimberlin and Richard J. Whitley

THE VIRUS

Herpesviruses are generally defined as large enveloped virions with an icosapentahedral nucleocapsid consisting invariably of 162 capsomeres arranged around a double-stranded DNA core. The two antigenically distinct types of herpes simplex virus (HSV) are HSV-1 and HSV-2. Considerable homology exists between the HSV-1 and HSV-2 genomes, with most of the polypeptides specified by one viral type being antigenically related to polypeptides of the other viral type. Although this results in considerable cross-reactivity between the HSV-1 and HSV-2 glycoproteins (g), unique antigenic determinants allow for differentiation between these two viruses (eg, gG-1 and gG-2). Surrounding the viral genome and nucleocapsid is a tightly adherent membrane known as the *tegument*. A lipid envelope containing the viral glycoproteins loosely surrounds the tegument.

PATHOLOGY AND PATHOGENESIS

Cutaneous HSV infection causes ballooning of infected epithelial cells, with nuclear degeneration, loss of intact cellular membranes, and the formation of multinucleated giant cells. Ultimately, cells lyse and release clear fluid containing large quantities of virus, with subsequent accumulation of cellular debris and inflammatory cells between the epidermal and dermal layers. Multinucleated giant cells are usually present at the base of the vesicle. An intense inflammatory response extends from the base of the vesicle into the dermis, producing the erythema that classically surrounds a cluster of HSV vesicles. As the lesions heal, vesicular fluid becomes purulent as more inflammatory cells are recruited to the site of infection. Scab formation then follows. Scarring is uncommon.

When infection involves mucous membranes, shallow ulcers are more common than vesicles because of rapid rupture of the very thin cornified epithelium present at mucosal sites. Nevertheless, the histopathologic findings of mucosal lesions are similar to those of skin lesions.

EPIDEMIOLOGY

Although HSV-1 is found most commonly in the oropharynx, it is an increasingly common cause of first episode genital herpes and can infect any organ system. Factors that influence the frequency of primary HSV-1 infection include geographic location, socioeconomic status, and age. Throughout childhood and adolescence, African Americans maintain approximately twice the prevalence of HSV-1 antibodies as white children, with 40% of African American children being seropositive for HSV-1 by 5 years of age. By the age of 60 years, however, both African Americans and whites have a similarly high prevalence of HSV-1 antibody (up to 90%).

Recurrences of herpes labialis have been associated with physical or emotional stress, fever, exposure to ultraviolet light, tissue damage, and immune suppression. As with primary infections, recurrent disease may occur in the absence of clinical symptoms. At any given time, 1% of normal children and 1% to 5% of normal adults asymptomatically excrete HSV-1, as demonstrated by viral culture. Recent studies employing polymerase chain reaction (PCR) suggest that these numbers may be at least 3-fold higher.

HSV-2 causes 75% to 80% of the cases of recurrent genital HSV infections in the United States. As would be expected, antibodies to this virus are rarely found before the onset of sexual activity. Among adolescents and adults, factors that correlate with seroprevalence for HSV-2 include sex (higher for women than for men), race (higher for African Americans than for whites), marital status (higher for persons previously married than for single or married persons), number of sexual partners (increasing likelihood with increasing number of partners), and income level (higher probability for those persons earning lesser amounts of money).

The propensity for recurrence of genital HSV infection depends on a variety of factors, including sex (more common in men), viral type (more common with HSV-2), and the presence and titer of neutralizing antibodies (more common in the presence of high neutralizing antibody titers). Overall, 60% to 90% of patients with primary genital HSV-2 infection will experience clinically apparent recurrence of infection.

CLINICAL MANIFESTATIONS
Oropharyngeal HSV Infection

Primary oropharyngeal infection with HSV-1 occurs most commonly in young children between 1 and 3 years of age. It is usually asymptomatic. The incubation period ranges from 2 to 12 days, with an average of 4 days. Symptomatic disease is characterized by fever to 104°F, oral lesions, sore throat, fetor oris, anorexia, cervical adenopathy, and mucosal edema. Oral lesions initially are vesicular but rapidly rupture, leaving 1- to 3-mm shallow gray-white ulcers on erythematous bases. These lesions are distributed on the hard palate, the anterior portion of the tongue, along the gingiva, and around the lips (Figure 185.1). In addition, the lesions may extend down the chin and neck due to drooling. Total duration of illness is 10 to 21 days.

Primary infection in young adults has been associated with pharyngitis and often a mononucleosislike syndrome. In such patients, ulcerative lesions on erythematous bases frequently are apparent on the tonsils.

Primary gingivostomatitis results in viral shedding in oral secretions for an average of 7 to 10 days. Virus can be isolated from the saliva of asymptomatic children and adults as well. Virus is also shed in the stool.

Recurrent orolabial HSV lesions are often preceded by a prodrome of pain, burning, tingling, or itching. These symptoms generally last for less than 6 hours, followed within 24 to 48 hours by the appearance of painful vesicles, typically at the vermillion border of the lip (Figure 185.2). Lesions usually crust within 3 to 4 days, and healing is complete within 8 to 10 days. Recurrences occur only rarely in the mouth or on facial skin of immunocompetent patients.

Genital HSV Infection

Genital HSV disease (Figure 185.3) is usually acquired by sexual contact with an infected partner. Historically, virtually all cases of genital herpes were caused by HSV-2 but, with changing sexual behavior, as many as 50% of cases today are the consequence of HSV-1. The incubation period of primary disease ranges from 2 to 12 days. Lesions persist for an average of 21 days. In 70% of patients, primary infections are associated with fever, malaise, myalgias, inguinal adenopathy, and other signs and symptoms of systemic illness. Complications include extragenital lesions, aseptic meningitis, and sacral autonomic nervous system dysfunction with associated urinary retention. Women tend to experience more severe primary infections and are more likely to develop complications.

In males, primary genital HSV infection usually manifests as a cluster of vesicular lesions on erythematous bases on the glans or shaft of the penis. In females, primary genital HSV lesions usually involve the vulva bilaterally. Concomitant HSV cervicitis occurs in 90% of women with primary HSV-2 infection of the external genitalia. In women, the lesions rapidly ulcerate and become covered with a gray-white exudate. Lesions may be exquisitely painful.

Recurrent genital HSV-2 infection can be either symptomatic or asymptomatic. A prodrome

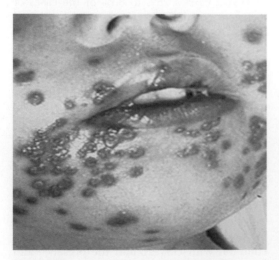

Figure 185.1 Herpes simplex gingivostomatitis.

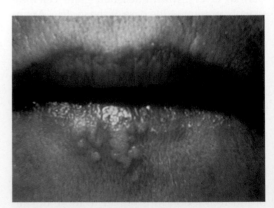

Figure 185.2 Recurrent herpes simplex labialis.

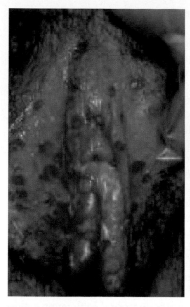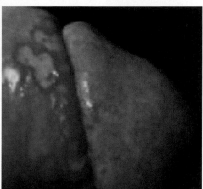

Figure 185.3 Genital HSV infection in woman (primary infection) and man (recurrence).

of itching, burning, tingling, or tenderness may be noted several hours before a recurrence. The duration of disease is shorter during recurrent infection (7 to 10 days), and fewer lesions are present. In men, lesions usually appear on the glans, or shaft, of the penis. In women, lesions occur most commonly on the labia minora, labia majora, and perineum. Cervical excretion of HSV occurs in 10% of women with recurrent genital lesions. Systemic symptoms are uncommon in recurrent genital HSV disease. Genital HSV-1 infections are much less likely to recur.

Transmission usually occurs in the absence of clinical symptoms, and occurs more often from men to women. Importantly, HSV-2 seropostive but asymptomatic individuals are just as likely to transmit infection as those who are symptomatic.

Other Primary HSV Skin Infections

Alteration in the barrier properties of skin, as occurs in atopic dermatitis, can result in localized HSV skin infection (eczema herpeticum). Most cases resolve over a 7- to 9-day period without specific therapy. Localized cutaneous HSV infection after trauma is known as herpes gladitorium (wrestler's herpes or traumatic herpes).

HSV infection of the digits results in herpetic whitlow. Such lesions may be the result of autoinoculation, as in the case of infants, or exogenous exposure, as occurs among medical and dental personnel.

Ocular HSV Infection

Herpetic infection of the eye usually presents as either a blepharitis or a follicular conjunctivitis. As disease progresses, branching dendritic lesions develop. Symptoms include severe photophobia, tearing, chemosis, blurred vision, and preauricular lymphadenopathy. An ophthalmologist should always be involved in the care of such patients.

Central Nervous System HSV Infection

Central nervous system (CNS) signs and symptoms of HSV disease can begin suddenly or can follow a 1- to 7-day period of nonspecific influenzalike symptoms. Prominent CNS features include headache, fever, altered consciousness, and focal neurologic findings such as focal seizures. Clinical signs and symptoms may reflect the characteristic frontal and temporal lobe localization, such as memory loss, anosmia, olefactory hallucinations, speech disorders, and behavioral disturbances, often accompanied pathologically by focal necrosis (Figure 185.4).

Neonatal HSV Infections

Neonatal HSV infection can be classified as (1) disease localized to the skin, eye, and/or mouth (SEM) (45% of cases); (2) encephalitis, with or without SEM involvement (30% of cases); and (3) disseminated infection that

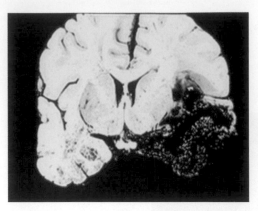

Figure 185.4 Brain with temporal lobe necrosis.

involves multiple organs, including the CNS, lung, gastrointestinal tract, liver, adrenals, skin, eye, and/or mouth (25% of cases). Infants with disseminated and SEM disease usually present for medical attention within the first 2 weeks of life, whereas infants with disease localized to the CNS usually present between the second and third weeks of life. Presenting signs and symptoms can include any combination of irritability, seizures (both focal and generalized), lethargy, tremors, poor feeding, temperature instability, bulging fontanelle, respiratory distress, jaundice, disseminated intravascular coagulopathy, shock, and cutaneous vesicles. It is important to note that >40% of infants with disseminated disease and >30% of infants with encephalitis will never have skin vesicles during the course of illness. Even in cases of SEM disease, almost 20% of neonates do not have skin lesions.

HSV in the Immunocompromised Host

Patients compromised by immunosuppressive therapy, underlying disease, or malnutrition are at increased risk for severe HSV infection. Disseminated disease may occur with widespread dermal, mucosal, and visceral involvement. Alternatively, disease may remain localized but persist for much longer periods of time than would be seen in immunocompetent hosts.

DIAGNOSIS

Type-specific serologic tests allow the distinction between HSV-1 and HSV-2. These tests can be utilizied to determine those people at risk for infection or those previously infected but who remain unaware of their status. The diagnosis of HSV is best achieved by either the isolation of HSV by culture or the detection of viral DNA by PCR. If skin lesions are present, a scraping of the vesicles should be transferred in appropriate viral transport medium on ice to a diagnostic virology laboratory. Other sites from which virus may be isolated include the cerebrospinal fluid (CSF), urine, throat, nasopharynx, conjunctivae, and duodenum. The presence of intranuclear inclusions and multinucleated giant cells on a Tzanck prep are indicative of, but not diagnostic for, HSV infection. The application of PCR to lesion scrapings is becoming increasingly valuable for proof of HSV, especially late in the course of vesicular evolution.

In HSV encephalitis, CSF findings are variable but often include a moderate pleocytosis with a predominance of mononuclear cells, elevated protein level, and normal or slightly decreased glucose. The electroencephalogram (EEG) generally localizes spike and slow wave activity to the temporal lobe, even when obtained very early in the disease course. Computed tomography (CT) of the brain may initially be normal or reveal only edema, but as the disease progresses can demonstrate temporal lobe involvement as well. Detection of HSV DNA in the CSF by PCR has become the diagnostic method of choice; however, it must be performed only by a reliable laboratory.

TREATMENT

Herpes Labialis

The treatments of choice for herpes labialis are acyclovir, valacyclovir, or famciclovir. Orally administered acyclovir at a dosage of 400 mg 5 times daily for 5 days reduces the duration of pain and time to the loss of crusts by about one-third, but only if treatment is started during the prodromal or erythematous stage of recurrent infection. Similar benefit is achieved with valaciclovir (2 g twice daily for 1 day, taken about 12 hours apart). Clinical benefit is achieved only if therapy is initiated very early after recurrence. Recently, 1-day therapy with famciclovir was approved by the Food and Drug Administration. When administered during prodrome, 1500 mg administered once accelerates healing.

Topical therapies provide little benefit in the management of herpes labialis. Although these therapies are licensed, these authors do not recommend their use. Similarly, data do not support the use of long-term suppressive treatment with acyclovir for the prevention of herpes labialis.

Table 185.1 Antiviral Therapy in Herpes Simplex Virus (HSV) Infections

Type of Infection	Drug	Route and Dosage[a]	Comments
Genital HSV			
Initial episode	Acyclovir	200 mg PO 5×/d ×10 d	Preferred route in normal host
		5 mg/kg IV q8h ×5 d	
	Valaciclovir	1 g PO BID ×10 d	Reserved for severe cases
	Famciclovir	250 mg PO TID ×10 d	
Recurrent episode	Acyclovir	200 mg PO 5×/d ×5 d	
	Valaciclovir	500 mg PO BID × 3 d	
	Famciclovir	1 g PO BID x 1 d	
Suppresion	Acyclovir	400 mg PO BID	
	Valaciclovir	500 mg or 1 g PO qd	
	Famciclovir	250 mg PO BID	
Herpes labialis	Acyclovir	400 mg PO 5×/d x 5 d	
	Valaciclovir	2 g PO BID for 1 d, taken about 12 h apart	
	Famciclovir	1500 mg administered once	
Mucocutaneous HSV in immunocompromised patient	Acyclovir	200–400 mg PO 5×/d ×10 d	
		5–10 mg/kg IV q8h ×7–10 d	
	Valaciclovir	500 mg BID PO	
	Famciclovir	500 mg TID PO	
HSV encephalitis	Acyclovir	10–15 mg/kg IV q8h ×14–21 d	
Neonatal HSV	Acyclovir	20 mg/kg IV q8h ×14–21 d	
Herpetic conjunctivitis	Trifluridine	1 drop q2h while awake ×7–14 d	Alternative: vidarabine ointment

Adapted from Whitley R, Gnann J. *N Engl J Med.* 1992;327:782.
[a] The dosages are for adults with normal renal function unless otherwise noted.

Genital Herpes

The treatments of choice include acyclovir (oral or intravenous), valacyclovir (oral), or famciclovir (oral). Although topical acyclovir is approved for treatment of genital herpes, it is not recommended. Treatment of primary genital herpes in the normal host decreases the duration of symptoms, viral shedding, and time to healing of lesions (Table 185.1). However, neither systemic nor topical treatment of primary HSV lesions reduces the frequency or severity of recurrences. Episodic administration of oral or topical acyclovir for the treatment of recurrent genital HSV lesions provides only a modest benefit, with duration of lesions being shortened at most by 1 to 2 days. However, daily administration of oral acyclovir, valacyclovir, or famciclovir can effectively suppress recurrences of genital herpes in 60% to 90% of patients. Importantly, suppressive therapy does not totally prevent reactivation; thus, transmission can occur, albeit less frequently. Treatment should be interrupted approximately yearly to reassess the need for continued suppression.

Both valaciclovir and famciclovir are now licensed for the treatment and suppression of genital HSV. There is a pharmacokinetic advantage with these medications. For recurrent infection, valaciclovir is administered at 500 mg twice daily for 3 days, and famciclovir is administered at 1 g twice daily for 1 day.

The transmission of genital HSV infection can be decreased by administration of valacyclovir (500 mg once daily) to the infected partner.

Mucocutaneous HSV Infections in Immunocompromised Patients

In immunocompromised patients, the three aforementioned antiviral drugs all diminish the duration of viral shedding, as well as substantially accelerate the time to cessation of pain and to total healing of HSV lesions. In addition, prophylactic administration of these drugs to such patients significantly reduces the incidence of symptomatic HSV infection (see Table 185.1).

Herpes Simplex Keratoconjunctivitis

Idoxuridine (Stoxil), trifluridine (Viroptic), and vidarabine ophthalmic drops all are effective and licensed for treatment of HSV keratitis. Trifluridine is the most efficacious and the easiest to administer, and as such is the drug of choice for HSV ocular disease (see Table 185.1).

Herpes Simplex Encephalitis

In patients with HSV encephalitis, acyclovir administration greatly reduces mortality and has a modest impact on morbidity. Dosage and length of therapy are shown in Table 185.1. Outcome is more favorable when therapy is instituted early in the disease course.

Neonatal HSV Infections

Intravenous acyclovir is the drug of choice in the treatment of neonatal HSV infection (see Table 185.1). Therapy is most efficacious if instituted early in the course of illness. Because of the exceptional safety profile of acyclovir, an intravenous dosage of 60 mg/kg/day divided every 8 hours should be given. Duration of therapy is 14 to 21 days.

Infants with ocular involvement caused by HSV should receive topical antiviral medication in addition to parenteral therapy. Trifluridine is the treatment of choice for ocular HSV infection in the neonate (see Table 185.1).

SUGGESTED READING

Kimberlin DW. Neonatal herpes simplex infection. *Clin Microbiol Rev.* 2004;17(1):1–13.

Kimberlin DW, Rouse DJ. Genital herpes. *N Engl J Med.* 2004;350:1970–1977.

Wald A, Corey L, Cone R, Hobson A, Davis G, Zeh J. Frequent genital herpes simplex virus 2 shedding in immunocompetent women: effect of acyclovir treatment. *J Clin Invest.* 1997;99:1092–1097.

Whitley RJ, Cobbs CG, Alford CA Jr, et al. Diseases that mimic herpes simplex encephalitis: diagnosis, presentation, and outcome. *JAMA.* 1989;262:234–239.

Whitley RJ, Kimberlin DW, Roizman B. Herpes simplex viruses. *Clin Infect Dis.* 1998;26:541–555.

Xu F, Sternberg MR, Kottiri BJ, et al. Trends in herpes simplex virus type 1 and type 2 seroprevalence in the United States. *JAMA.* 2006;296:964–973.

Ruth M. Greenblatt

Human herpesviruses 6, 7, and 8 (HHV-6, HHV-7, and HHV-8) are DNA viruses enclosed in a capsid that produce lytic and latent infection of lymphocytes and other cell types. Latent infection has been implicated in the etiology of several malignancies, although causation of malignancy has been established only for HHV-8 at this time. Reactivation of latent infection occurs intermittently, with replication of virus in various tissues and secretions. HHV-6, -7, and -8 constitute a diverse group in terms of their biology and pathogenesis and the diseases they produce; HHV-6 and -7 are able to infect a broader array of cell types than HHV-8. Clinical presentation ranges from asymptomatic infection or mild illnesses, such as exanthem subitum in the case of HHV-6, extending to life-threatening disease in the immune compromised host, such as HHV-8–associated Kaposi's sarcoma or HHV-6 encephalitis. Selected clinical and virologic characteristics are summarized in Table 186.1, and limited antiviral treatment information is presented in Table 186.2.

HUMAN HERPESVIRUS 6

HHV-6 is a member of the *Betaherpesvirinae* group, of which cytomegalovirus was the previously recognized human pathogen, and is placed in the genus *Roseolovirus*. HHV-6 consists of two related variants, HHV-6A and HHV-6B, that have 90% DNA homology and cannot be distinguished by serologic tests, but have distinctive molecular, cell culture, and clinical features. Seventy to 100% of adults have serologic evidence of HHV-6 infection with both variants worldwide. Infection follows a 2-week incubation period and most often occurs between the ages of 6 and 15 months.

Shedding and Tissue Tropism

HHV-6B is shed in saliva, which is an important vehicle of transmission (perhaps most often from mother to child). The virus is not found in breast milk. After primary infection, viral replication occurs in salivary glands and recurs during periodic episodes of reactivation and shedding, which decrease in frequency over time. Both variants primarily infect CD4+ T cells; the A variant also infects CD8 cells. HHV-6 infection of fibrolasts, other lymphocytes, hepatocytes, epithelial and endothelial cells, astrocytes, oligodendrocytes, and microglia can be demonstrated in vitro. The virus is highly neurotropic with a central nervous system (CNS) site of latency. HHV-6 is unique among human herpesviruses in that its DNA integrates into specific locations on chromosomes 1, 17, and 22. HHV-6 DNA integration into germ cells can result in inheritance of HHV-6 genetic elements and is associated with persistent high-level viremia. Congenital transmission does not result in clinical sequelae, which further distinguishes HHV-6 from cytomegalovirus (CMV). HHV-6A is proportionately associated with more congenital infections than acquired infections. High-level viremia suggestive of chromosomal integration is uncommon but not rare (reported in 3% of blood donors in a recent British study but the prevalence may vary significantly with location).

Infection in Immunocompetent Hosts

The clinical presentation of HHV-6A is not well characterized. Primary infection with HHV-6B is associated with fever, ≥40°C, that lasts 3 to 7 days and then suddenly declines. Fever is followed by a maculopapular rash (exanthema subitum [ES] or roseola infantum or sixth disease) on the trunk, face, and neck in a subset of patients, apparently more often in Japan. Malaise, otitis media, and gastrointestinal (GI) and respiratory symptoms are also common. It is estimated that HHV-6 may account for 20% to 25% of all emergency room visits for children 6 to 12 months of age. Approximately one-third of all febrile seizures in children younger than 2 years appear to be related to HHV-6 in the United States; other viruses are more frequently implicated in other parts of the world, particularly Asia. Febrile seizures occur in roughly 20% of children with ES. Encephalomeningitis is a rare complication, and both variants can be recovered from cerebrospinal fluid (CSF); the A variant may be more persistent at this site.

Table 186.1 Clinical Features of Human Herpesviruses (HHV) 6, 7, and 8

Virus	Age of First Infection	Sites of Shedding	Unique Attribute	Clinical Features of Primary Infection	Clinical Features of Infection in Compromised Hosts
HHV-6A	Most before 2 years	Serum, CSF	Chromosomal integration and germ cell transmission occurs	Not known	? pneumonitis, ?disseminated infections
HHV-6B	Most before 2 years, congenital and perinatal transmission is possible	Saliva, cervical secretions, stool, serum	Chromosomal integration and germ cell transmission occurs and is associated with persistent high-grade viremia	Pityriasis rosea, exanthem subitum, fever, febrile seizures, respiratory and GI symptoms	Pneumonitis, hepatitis, hemorrhagic cystitis, colitis, bronchiolitis obliterans, encephalitis, allograft rejection, suppression of bone marrow engraftment, retinitis, role in GVHD, optic neuritis, hemophagocytosis, dissemination, rash
HHV-7	Early childhood	Saliva, breast milk		Less frequent cause of exanthem subitum and other exanthems	Unknown
HHV-8	Most commonly after puberty, occasionally in childhood	Saliva, semen	Cancer-producing virus	None to febrile illness of infancy	Kaposi's sarcoma, multicentric Castleman's disease, primary effusion lymphoma, and others

Abbreviations: CSF = cerebrospinal fluid; GI = gastrointestinal; GVHD = graft-versus-host disease.

As in many other viral illnesses, the severe complications are more common in adults with primary infection, but mononucleosislike syndrome, hepatitis, hemophagocytosis, thrombocytopenia, encephalitis and/or fatal dissemination can occur in adult primary infections. HHV-6 has been implicated, controversially, as an etiologic agent of multiple sclerosis; a bystander role is difficult to exclude. The somewhat beneficial effects of high-dose herpes antiviral drugs in some forms of multiple sclerosis (MS) recently provided more evidence that a herpesvirus, including HHV-6, may be involved in this disease. Shedding of HHV-6, along with several other human herpesviruses, has been noted in drug-induced hypersensitivity syndromes; current evidence indicates that reactivation of viral replication commonly follows the onset of drug hypersensitivities, continues after discontinuation of the offending drug, and could underlie the association between drug hypersensitivity and subsequent graft-versus-host disease.

Infection in Immunocompromised Hosts

Active HHV-6B infection is frequently detected in immunocompromised hosts, such as bone marrow and solid organ transplant recipients; serious HHV-6 infections can occur, including pneumonitis, colitis, hemorrhagic cystitis, encephalitis (most often involving the temporal lobe), hepatitis, and acute graft-versus-host disease. HHV-6 infection may contribute to rejection of transplanted allografts. Fatalities have been reported, including after primary infection in a transplant recipient. Fever, rash, and encephalitis are most frequently reported. Most infections occur 2 to 4 weeks posttransplantation. HHV-6 replication is associated with bronchiolitis obliterans among lung transplant recipients, which is associated with eventual graft failure. Active HHV-6 infections may occur concurrently with CMV or HHV-7, making distinction of the clinical manifestations due to each virus difficult. HHV-6 also produces chronic infection in human immunodeficiency virus (HIV)-infected persons, with manifestations that include encephalitis, pneumonitis, and retinitis. HHV-6 can also suppress production of key inflammatory mediators and lymphocyte proliferative responses, producing defects in cell-mediated immunity. Like some other herpesviruses, HHV-6 increases susceptibility of CD4 cells to HIV and may facilitate

Table 186.2 Summary of in Vivo and in Vitro Information Regarding Antiviral Treatment of HHV-6, HHV-7, and HHV-8

Virus	Treatment Indication	Drug	Comment
HHV-6B	Evidence of disseminated infection in solid organ or stem cell transplant recipient	Ganciclovir, foscarnet, cidofovir	Limited clinical trial data, CMV dosing presumed to be required
	Some efficacy of CMV prophylaxis in prevention	Acyclovir prophylaxis	
HHV-7	None known	None known	
HHV-8	KS, MCD, PEL in AIDS patient	1. HAART regimen	Potent antiretroviral combination treatment
		2. Cidofovir, or ganciclovir, or foscarnet	CMV dosing, duration not known Proven efficacy
		3. Chemo- and radiotherapies as needed.	
	PEL, MCD, HIV and non-HIV	Interferon-α	Efficacy with responses in some patients. Can be combined with antiviral agents
	KS in solid organ transplant recipient	1. Withdraw as much immunosuppressive therapy as possible	Presumed CMV dosing, no clinical data, theoretical efficacy at best
		2. Ganciclovir or foscarnet	

Abbreviations: HHV = human herpesvirus; CMV = cytomegalovirus; KS = Kaposi's sarcoma; AIDS = acquired immunodeficiency syndrome; MCD = multicentric Castleman's disease; PEL = primary effusion lymphoma; HAART = highly active antiretroviral therapy.

HIV-disease progression. As is the case for CMV, combination antiretroviral therapy appears to have reduced the incidence of serious HHV-6 infections in acquired immunodeficiency syndrome (AIDS).

Detection of Infection

The very high prevalence of infection, the course of intermittent reactivation, and the occurrence of chromosomal integration must be considered in the interpretation of diagnostic tests for HHV-6; detection of virus does not necessarily indicate disease or reactivation. Viral culture of peripheral blood mononuclear cells is the gold standard for viral detection and can be accomplished using standard cell culture or shell viral techniques. Detection of HHV-6 DNA in either cellular or acellular specimens using polymerase chain reaction (PCR) is also suggestive of active HHV-6 replication and is positive in children with ES and a variety of immunocompromised individuals. Immunohistochemistry can detect cells with active infection in biopsy or cytologic specimens. Serologic tests include indirect immunofluorescence assay (IFA), anticomplement immunofluorescence assay, competitive radioimmune assay, neutralization, and enzyme immunoassays (EIA). The EIA tests are more easily quantified and are less subjective. Primary infection can be demonstrated serologically by seroconversion of immunoglobulin G (IgG) from

negative to positive in children and adults or the presence of immunoglobulin M (IgM) in children. The presence of IgM in adults may indicate either primary infection or reactivation from latency. A 4-fold increase in serum IgG by IFA or a 1.6-fold increase by EIA suggests recent infection. In classic ES, etiologic diagnosis is seldom necessary. Culture or PCR testing of blood, CSF, urine, and other body fluids has been employed to identify HHV-6 infections. Culture and PCR methods can distinguish between the A and B variants; serology cannot.

Treatment of HHV-6 Infection

In culture, ganciclovir, cidofovir, and foscarnet have much better activity against both HHV-6 variants than does acyclovir. Case reports describe clinical responses to gancyclovir, cidofovir, or foscarnet in transplant recipients with encephalitis, although treatment failures are also reported. CMV prophylaxis may reduce salivary shedding of HHV-6 in allograft recipients, but it does not fully prevent viral replication and viremia. Viral resistance in the setting of CMV prophylaxis has not been reported. Treatment is recommended for virologically confirmed infection in the setting of posttransplant bone marrow suppression, encephalitis, or pneumonitis. Analogous to CMV, bone marrow transplant recipients who receive high-dose acyclovir, despite lack of efficacy in vitro, appear to have fewer HHV-6 infections.

Human Herpesvirus 7

HHV-7 is similar in terms of morphology and genome sequence to HHV-6, the viruses resembling each other more than CMV. The virus is also a member of the Betaherpesvirinae group, genus *Roseolovirus* (along with HHV-6); it infects CD4-positive T lymphocytes, and latent infection occurs. Primary infection occurs during childhood and is probably most often asymptomatic. Cross-reactivity between HHV-6 and HHV-7 in some assay systems may have complicated early studies of the viruses, and HHV-6 and HHV-7 may reactivate each other. Infection is very common; serum antibodies can be identified in >85% of adults. Salivary shedding occurs even more frequently than in the case of HHV-6 (can be found in saliva from 75% of adults), and exposure to oral secretions is likely the major mode of transmission. The virus can be detected in breast milk, CSF, cervical tissue, and peripheral blood lymphocytes. Congenital infection is rare, if it occurs at all.

HHV-7 infrequently causes ES, far less commonly than HHV-6B. Other febrile illnesses of childhood have been reported in association with development of serum antibodies. The detection of HHV-7 DNA in blood from transplant recipients is common and occurs even among patients who receive CMV prophylaxis with ganciclovir. HHV-7 can also be detected in urine. T cells that respond to HHV-6 antigens may also respond to HHV-7, perhaps providing some level of partial immunity. There is currently no published information on the treatment of apparent HHV-7 infections.

Human Herpesvirus 8

HHV-8 is a member of the Gammaherpesvirinae group, of which Epstein–Barr virus (EBV) was the only previously recognized human pathogen. Relatively little is known about primary HHV-8 infection. In central Africa, a region in which Kaposi's sarcoma (KS) was common before the HIV epidemic, HHV-8 infection appears to be a relatively common cause of the first febrile illness in infants and may be associated with respiratory symptoms in some cases. In these areas an increasing incidence of HHV-8 infection occurs with age; prevalence of infection reaches 39% in early and 48% by late adolescence. HHV-8 viremia usually precedes the onset of associated lymphoproliferative conditions and cancers.

KAPOSI'S SARCOMA

Moritz Kaposi first described classic KS in 1872 as a rare skin tumor seen primarily in elderly men of Mediterranean or Ashkenazi Jewish origin. The clinical characteristics of conditions associated with HHV-8 infection are summarized in Table 186.3; KS is the most common of these. Because several types of cells (many of which are inflammatory) are present in KS lesions, and not of a single clone or specific pattern of cytogenetic mutations, as seen in most cancers, some researchers question whether KS is a true malignancy. The endemic or African form of KS was recognized in the early part of this century and is confined to equatorial areas where, until the AIDS era, it accounted for up to 10% of all malignancies. The iatrogenic form primarily occurs in solid organ transplant recipients and tends to be an aggressive illness with rapid dissemination, unless immune suppressive therapies are discontinued, and occurs most often in the first 2 years following transplantation. It is likely that most cases are associated with pretransplant infection in the graft recipient. Kaposi's sarcoma in the setting of solid organ transplantation can mimic PTLD and involve the donor organ. AIDS KS has a variable course, which can range from isolated skin lesions to more aggressive disease with rapid dissemination. For AIDS KS, prognosis is best in persons with no other AIDS defining conditions, relatively higher CD4 cell counts, and age less than 50 years.

In a 1990 study, the risk of KS was at least 20 000 times greater among AIDS patients than the general population and 300 times greater among AIDS patients than other immunosuppressed groups. AIDS KS is most prevalent among men who have sex with men, regardless of intravenous drug use, than in other HIV exposure groups (such as injection drug users). Overall, epidemiological evidence supports the notion that AIDS KS is caused by a sexually transmissible agent. Early KS lesions appear as faint red-violet or brown macules that can be mistaken for more benign skin conditions. Lymphedema is common and can occur out of proportion to the extent of skin and lymphatic involvement, perhaps due to the release of inflammatory mediators.

MULTICENTRIC CASTLEMAN'S DISEASE (MCD AND MCD-ASSOCIATED PLASMABLASTIC LYMPHOMA)

MCD is a rare lymphoproliferative condition characterized by angiofollicular hyperplasia associated with fever, adenopathy, and splenomegaly; several clinical variations exist. It

Table 186.3 Clinical Characteristics of Conditions Associated with HHV-8 Infection

Condition	Setting	Clinical Characteristics
Classic KS	A rare condition seen among elderly men of Mediterranean or Ashkenazi Jewish descent. No known environmental etiologic precipitator	Often involves lower extremities, slowly progressive, primarily cutaneous, often not cause of death
Endemic KS	A relatively common cause of cancer (or a cancerlike condition) in children and adults residing in central Africa. No known environmental etiologic precipitator	Variable from mild (like classic) to locally aggressive disease
Iatrogenic KS	Seen in solid organ transplant recipients and other recipients of medication-induced immunologic suppression	Aggressive condition that often improves or resolves with withdrawal of immunosuppressive therapy, and may recur with reinstitution
AIDS KS	AIDS-defining illness in HIV-infected patients, most often homosexual men (in developed countries). One of the most common HIV-associated malignancies, the incidence is falling	Often aggressive condition that progressively includes metastatic mucosal or cutaneous foci (often the mouth, face, and genitalia), and then may extend to lymphatic, pulmonary, and GI tract disease. Often responds to potent antiretroviral combination therapy
Multicentric Castleman's disease	HHV-8 DNA present in virtually all HIV-associated cases, approximately half of cases in HIV-uninfected persons	Associated with fever
Primary effusion lymphoma	Most common in AIDS patients, most cases reported in men, but occurs in women. Has been reported in recipients of solid organ transplants	Aggressive lymphoma which typically presents with ascites or pleural effusion
Germinotrophic lymphoproliferative disorder	A rare, recently recognized condition reported in HIV-uninfected adults	HHV-8–expressing plasmablasts within the germinal centers of lyphoid B-cell follicles possible with immunoglobulin gene rearrangements. Presents with lymphadenopathy and has been treated with chemotherapy

occurs most commonly, but not exclusively, in AIDS patients with KS. HHV-8 DNA sequences have been detected in mononuclear cells and lesional tissue from most MCD patients when optimal methods are used. Survival is variable, and clinical recurrences are common. Chemo- and radiotherapies can be effective, the efficacy of immune modulation therapy is under investigation, and some responses have been reported with antiviral agents that inhibit HHV-8 (see section Treatment of HHV-8 Infection).

PRIMARY EFFUSION LYMPHOMAS

Primary effusion lymphoma (PEL) is a rare malignancy of relatively mature B cells occurring as a subset of AIDS-related non-Hodgkin lymphomas, although rare cases have been reported in the absence of HIV infection. PEL presents as a neoplastic effusion of the pleural, pericardial, and peritoneal cavities in the absence of a solid tumor mass. PEL diagnoses require typical body cavity malignant

effusions and the presence of HHV-8; no other lymphomatous effusion expresses HHV-8. Solid lymphomas have been reported prior and subsequent to PEL. Recently extracavitary solid lymphoma that expresses HHV-8 has been reported in both HIV-infected and -uninfected persons. These nodal and non-nodal tumors have large cell lymphoblastic or immunoblastic morphology, resemble PEL cells, and express a group of proteins that were previously recognized as characteristic of PEL. PEL tend to occur in the setting of advanced HIV-associated immunodepletion, whereas the HHV-8–positive solid tumors tend to occur with less severe immunodepletion.

GERMINOTROPIC LYMPHOPROLIFERATIVE DISORDER

Recently several cases of a lymphoproliferative disorder characterized by the presence of plasmablasts within the germinal centers of lymphoid follicles have been reported. The plasmablasts express HHV-8 and demonstrate rearrangements of immunoglobulin genes. This condition is responsive to chemo- and radiotherapies.

PATHOGENESIS

HHV-8 genes have been found to code for viral products that resemble cellular cytokines and other regulators of local immune response and tissue growth. These findings may provide insight into the mechanism by which the virus promotes development of KS, BCBL, and MCD. Elevated blood levels of some of these viral inflammatory products are known to precede the onset of KS. HIV proteins may augment this inflammatory process, explaining the synergistic effect that dual HIV/HHV-8 infection appears to have on the development of KS.

DETECTION OF INFECTION

Standardized methods for detection of HHV-8 infections have not yet been established. Prevalence rates depend on testing method as well as the population being evaluated. DNA detection techniques such as PCR may be of limited value in studying the epidemiology of HHV-8 because infected tissue must be directly sampled and the technique is cumbersome and sensitive to laboratory error. Indirect immunofluorescence and enzyme immunoassays have been developed for the detection of antibodies to lytic and latent HHV-8 antigens. Antibody assays have ranged from 80% to 98% sensitivity in KS patients (when compared with PCR). In general, the prevalence of antibody to lytic antigens is higher than antibody to latent antigens. Higher levels of serum antibodies to HHV-8 antigens have been identified in KS patients than in persons without KS.

EPIDEMIOLOGY AND MODES OF TRANSMISSION

HHV-8 antibodies are highly prevalent among patients with KS and in homosexual men. The prevalence of serological reactivity is also relatively high in areas where KS was endemic prior to the AIDS epidemic as summarized in Table 186.4. Outside of geographic regions in which HHV-8 infection is prevalent, such as sub-Saharan Africa, HHV-8 infection is most prevalent among men who have sex with men, increasing with the total number of lifetime sexual partners. In heterosexual populations, a history of prior sexually transmitted disease is a relatively consistent risk factor for

Table 186.4 Estimated Prevalence of HHV-8 Infection in Various Populations

Population	% Prevalence
Sub-Saharan Africa, general population	30–60
Mediterranean countries, general population	4–35
Developed countries, general population	5–10
Developed countries, men who have sex with men	21–67
Developed countries, injection drug users	5–50
U.S. women with HIV infection	4–15
Abbreviations: HHV = human herpesvirus; HIV = human immunodeficiency virus.	

HHV-8 serum antibody. An increased prevalence of HHV-8 infection has been reported in some groups of injection drug users, but because these populations also tend to have a high prevalence of risky sexual behaviors and sexually transmitted diseases, it is not clear that injection drug use is an independent risk factor. In addition, increased prevalence rates of HHV-8 infection have been identified among adolescents who report same-sex sexual partners, history of certain sexually transmitted infections, and various other factors. Early childhood infection appears to be common in high prevalence areas, although in utero transmission is uncommon.

Most studies show that the detection of HHV-8 DNA in semen and genital tissues is limited to the high-risk populations of homosexual men, residents of central Africa, and persons with KS. HHV-8 DNA sequences have also been identified in saliva and oral tissues of patients with KS and in HIV-infected patients without KS. These studies indicate that HHV-8 is present in the oropharynx and could be transmitted via saliva contact in a manner analogous to EBV. Curiously, HHV-8 has a far lower prevalence rate and later age of infection than HHV-6, HHV-7, and EBV, infections in which saliva is more clearly a key vehicle for transmission. HHV-8 can be transmitted via blood products, which is a relatively common occurrence in high prevalence areas. In the U.S. transplant setting, the prevalence of HHV-8 increases from an average of approximately 5% preoperatively to 15% after surgery, probably the result of blood product and donor organ transmission.

TRANSMISSION VIA ALLOGRAFTS AND BLOOD PRODUCTS

Kaposi's sarcoma is a relatively common cancer among solid organ transplant recipients and it is associated with HHV-8 infection. BCBL has also been reported in allograft recipients. HHV-8 can be transmitted via renal allografts, and screening of donated tissue has been recommended. Although KS can occur among patients who were infected with HHV-8 prior to receiving an allograft, it is unclear if the risk is greater among persons who were HHV-8 infected or uninfected prior to transplantation. Because HHV-8 can be identified in blood from healthy donors, parenteral transmission of the pathogen is possible but does not appear to occur commonly.

TREATMENT OF HHV-8 INFECTION

HHV-8 DNA includes two sequences that indicate potential susceptibility to thymidine kinase and phosphotransferase inhibitors, drugs that are active against other human herpesviruses. HHV-8 shares only limited DNA homology with these other viruses; it is most similar to EBV. In general, in vitro drug susceptibility tests have limited utility for this pathogen; however, ganciclovir, foscarnet, and cidofovir have demonstrated the most consistent inhibition. Systemic administration of cidofovir, foscarnet, ganciclovir, and interferon-α have been reported to induce response or remission in patients with AIDS KS, often in conjunction with antiretroviral therapy and/or chemotherapy. The clinical course of AIDS KS has improved greatly in the years since the introduction of highly active antiretroviral therapy (HAART) regimens; antiretroviral protease inhibitors may have direct inhibitory effects on KS in addition to facilitating improvement in immune functions. Foscarnet and ganciclovir were shown to be effective in preventing KS among HIV-infected men during the pre-HAART era, although this approach has been largely displaced by antiretroviral therapies. Dosage of the antiviral therapies is based on anticytomegalovirus therapy; specific dosing recommendations for HHV-8 are not available. Traditional treatment for KS, MCD, and PEL includes reduction or elimination of any immunosuppressive treatment, chemotherapy, and/or radiation therapy. Case reports indicate that the use of ganciclovir or cidofovir can result in treatment responses or resolution in PEL and MCD but not in KS. Valganciclovir has been used successfully to prevent recurrence of PEL. Interferon-α has been effective in the treatment of HIV-associated PEL, MCD, and non-HIV MCD but does not eliminate HHV-8 viremia. Interferon-α combined with HAART has been shown to be effective in the treatment of about 5 of 13 HIV-KS patients in a phase one clinical trial.

SUGGESTED READING

Carbone A. AIDS-related non-Hodgkin's lymphomas: from pathology and molecular pathogenesis to treatment. *Hum Pathol.* 2002;33(4):392–404.

Casper C. The aetiology and management of Castleman disease at 50 years: translating pathophysiology to patient care. *Br J Haematol.* 2005;129(1):3–17.

Casper C, Meier AS, Wald A, Morrow RA, Corey L, Moscicki AB. Human herpesvirus 8 infection among adolescents in the REACH cohort. *Arch Pediatr Adolesc Med.* 2006;160(9):937–942.

De Bolle L, Naesens L, De Clercq E. Update on human herpesvirus 6 biology, clinical features, and therapy. *Clin Microbiol Rev.* 2005;18(1):217–245.

Du MQ, Diss TC, Liu H, et al. KSHV- and EBV-associated germinotropic lymphoproliferative disorder. *Blood.* 2002;100(9):3415–3418.

Hall CB, Caserta MT, Schnabel KC, et al. Congenital infections with human herpesvirus 6 (HHV6) and human herpesvirus 7 (HHV7). *J Pediatr.* 2004;145(4):472–477.

Henke-Gendo C, Schulz TF. Transmission and disease association of Kaposi's sarcoma-associated herpesvirus: recent developments. *Curr Opin Infect Dis.* 2004;17(1):53–57.

Hladik W, Dollard SC, Mermin J, et al. Transmission of human herpesvirus 8 by blood transfusion. *N Engl J Med.* 2006;355(13):1331–1338.

Humar A. Reactivation of viruses in solid organ transplant patients receiving cytomegalovirus prophylaxis. *Transplantation.* 2006;82(suppl 2):S9–S14.

Leong HN, Tuke PW, Tedder RS, et al. The prevalence of chromosomally integrated human herpesvirus 6 genomes in the blood of UK blood donors. *J Med Virol.* 2007;79(1):45–51.

Stebbing J, Sanitt A, Nelson M, Powles T, Gazzard B, Bower M. A prognostic index for AIDS-associated Kaposi's sarcoma in the era of highly active antiretroviral therapy. *Lancet.* 2006;367(9521):1495–1502.

Zerr DM. Human herpesvirus 6: a clinical update. *Herpes.* 2006;13(1):20–24.

187. Influenza

Leanne Gasink, Neil Fishman, and Harvey M. Friedman

Influenza is an important epidemic viral infection that has caused significant morbidity and mortality throughout history. The first worldwide pandemic was documented in 1580, and 31 pandemics have been described since then. The most severe occurred in 1918–1919, when at least 20 million deaths were recorded worldwide, including approximately 550 000 in the United States. The last pandemic was in 1968, but milder epidemics continue to occur every 1 to 3 years. The Centers for Disease Control and Prevention (CDC) document 10 000 to 40 000 excess deaths in the United States during most epidemics. Recently, the possibility of a worldwide pandemic due to a highly pathogenic avian influenza has become of great concern. Significant resources worldwide have been dedicated to the detection and containment of avian influenza outbreaks and the development of response plans to influenza epidemics at international, national, and local levels.

INFLUENZA VIRAL STRUCTURE AND PATHOPHYSIOLOGY

Influenza viruses are medium-sized enveloped RNA viruses belonging to the family Orthomyxoviridae. Three genera, influenza virus types A, B, and C, have been described. Influenza A and B viruses are important causes of human disease, whereas influenza C virus causes only sporadic upper respiratory infections.

The morphologic characteristics of all influenza virus types are similar. The envelope is composed of a lipid bilayer, with a layer of matrix protein on the inner surface and spike-like surface projections of glycoproteins on the outer surface. These glycoproteins have either hemagglutinin or neuraminidase activity and are responsible for the attachment of the virus to human cells, for the release of virus from infected cells, and for the stimulation of the host immune response. Hemagglutinins initiate the infectious process by binding to sialic acid residues on surface receptors of respiratory epithelial cells. After proteolytic cleavage, the hemagglutinins fuse with the host cell membrane. The neuraminidase cleaves sialic acid that is present on the host cell surface and promotes release of viral particles from infected cells. Within the envelope of influenza A and B viruses are eight segmented pieces of nucleocapsid composed of a nucleoprotein and segmented single-stranded RNA, whereas influenza C virus contains seven fragments.

EPIDEMIOLOGY

One of the most remarkable features of influenza virus is the frequency of change in antigenicity. Antigenic variation is annual with influenza A virus but less common with influenza B virus. Therefore, immunity to the influenza viruses is partial and temporary. This phenomenon explains why influenza remains a major epidemic disease of humans. Two types of antigenic variation have been described, principally involving the two external glycoproteins of the virus, hemagglutinin and neuraminidase. The more dramatic but less common alteration, antigenic shift, results from genetic reassortments, frequently between human and other animal strains of the virus. Shifts that produce immunologically novel strains of the influenza A virus herald the larger epidemics and worldwide pandemics and tend to occur sporadically. Since World War I, antigenic shifts have generally occurred approximately every 10 to 15 years, although the most recent shift occurred in 1977. The second and more common change, antigenic drift, is produced by single point mutations in the hemagglutinin or neuraminidase genes that result in changes of one or a few amino acids. Antigenic shift is seen only with influenza A virus. Although antigenic drift affects both influenza A and B viruses, changes in the latter occur less frequently. Three subtypes of hemagglutinin, H1 (variants H0, H1, Hsw1), H2, and H3, and two subtypes of neuraminidase, N1 and N2, are recognized among human influenza A viruses. Recently, however, cases of human infection with subtypes of hemagglutinin and neuraminidase previously known only to cause influenza oubreaks among birds have been documented, most notably H5N1, but cases of other strains have also occurred. Only a few strains of either influenza A or B virus tend to dominate during each annual influenza season.

Most influenza infections are acquired through human-to-human transmission of small-particle aerosols. Localized epidemics begin rather abruptly, usually in children, reach a sharp peak in 2 to 3 weeks, and last 5 to 6 weeks. Attack rates during such outbreaks can approach 10% to 40%. Although influenza is virtually always active somewhere in the world, infection is most common during the winter. The peak influenza season extends from December through April in the Northern Hemisphere. Influenza season is defined by viral isolation, whereas an epidemic is defined by a rise in pneumonia and influenza deaths above the epidemic threshold in the CDC's 121-city mortality surveillance system. Although influenza affects all segments of the population, severe infections and major complications are most common in patients who are young, elderly, or debilitated.

H5N1 strain is one of only a few avian influenza viruses to cross the species barrier and infect humans. Endemic in many wild bird populations, H5N1 has resulted in the death of hundreds of millions of birds since first appearing in Asia. Since 1997 several hundred cases of laboratory-confirmed human H5N1 have been reported. Isolated cases have resulted from human-to-human transmission of the virus, but close contact with infected poultry has been the primary source for human infection. The H5N1 virus is known to mutate rapidly and has become progressively more pathogenic in poultry, is increasingly stable in the environment, and is expanding its mammalian host range. Humans have little or no existing immunity to H5N1; therefore, if the virus adapts such that efficient and sustained human-to-human transmission is possible, a worldwide pandemic is likely to occur. The World Health Organization (WHO) is leading a global effort to detect outbreaks and respond to human cases, monitoring the threat of an H5N1 pandemic.

CLINICAL MANIFESTATIONS

Uncomplicated Influenza

Classic influenza is characterized by abrupt onset of symptoms after an incubation period of 1 to 2 days. Many patients can pinpoint the hour of onset. Systemic signs and symptoms predominate initially. They include fever, chills or rigors, headaches, myalgias, malaise, and anorexia. Myalgias and headache are the most troublesome symptoms, with severity related to the height of the febrile response. Severe pain of the intraocular muscles often can be elicited on lateral gaze. Myalgias in the calf muscles may be particularly prominent in children. The systemic symptoms usually persist for approximately 1 week. Respiratory symptoms, such as dry cough and nasal discharge, also present at the onset of illness and begin to dominate the clinical presentation as fever resolves. Cough is the most common and troublesome of these later complaints and can take 2 weeks or more to resolve completely.

Complications of Influenza

The complications of influenza can be classified as pulmonary or nonpulmonary and result either from progression of the viral process itself or from secondary bacterial infections. Two manifestations of pneumonia are associated with influenza, primary influenza viral pneumonia, and secondary bacterial pneumonia (Table 187.1). Extrapulmonary complications of influenza occur less often and are most prevalent during larger, more severe outbreaks. These include myositis (more common with influenza B infection), myocarditis, pericarditis, transverse myelitis, encephalitis, and Guillain–Barré syndrome. A toxic shocklike syndrome has occurred in previously healthy children and adults during outbreaks of influenza A or B. This syndrome has been attributed to the effects of the viral infection on the colonization and replication characteristics of toxin-producing staphylococcus. Reye's syndrome has also been described in children treated with aspirin during influenza outbreaks. The major causes of death are pneumonia and exacerbation of chronic cardiopulmonary conditions. Of those who die, 80% to 90% are aged 65 years or older.

H5N1 Infection

Most cases of H5N1 have occurred in healthy young adults, approximately 2 to 4 days after exposure to infected birds. Initial symptoms include high fever and an influenzalike illness. In contrast to infection with human influenza viruses, lower respiratory tract involvement and clinically apparent pneumonia are almost universal. Watery diarrhea may be present before the development of respiratory symptoms. Progression to multiorgan failure, including

Table 187.1 Pulmonary Complications of Influenza

Feature	Primary Viral Pneumonia	Secondary Bacterial Pneumonia
Setting	Cardiovascular disease Pregnancy Young adults (in large outbreaks)	Age >65 years Chronic pulmonary, cardiac, or metabolic disease
History	Rapid progression after typical onset	Biphasic illness, with worsening after clinical improvement
Physical examination	Diffuse crackles	Consolidation
Sputum culture	Normal oral flora	*Streptococcus pneumoniae* *Staphylococcus aureus* *Haemophilus influenzae*
Isolation of influenza virus	Yes	No
Chest radiograph	Diffuse bilateral interstitial disease	Consolidation
Response to antibiotics	No	Yes
Mortality	Variable, high during some pandemics	Variable, generally low

respiratory failure, renal dysfunction, and cardiac compromise, is common. Atypical presentations, such as encephalopathy, gastroenteritis, and mild respiratory disease, have been reported, but frequencies of such presentations are unknown. Among laboratory-confirmed cases reported to the WHO, the fatality rate has been 60%. Death occurs on average 9 to 10 days after the onset of illness. Asymptomatic infection likely occurs as well, as indicated by seropositivity in populations at risk. However, the incidence is unknown.

DIAGNOSIS

Isolation of virus and detection of viral antigen in respiratory secretions offer the greatest utility for diagnosis in the setting of acute illness. Rapid diagnostic tests employing immunological and molecular techniques are becoming increasingly available and can be performed quickly, although some assays require considerable laboratory expertise. Serologic tests such as hemagglutinin inhibition antibody titers that compare acute and convalescent sera are sensitive and specific but do not yield results in time to affect clinical decisions. Generally, the diagnosis is established on epidemiologic grounds. A clinical presentation with fever, headache, myalgias, and cough is usually sufficient to diagnose influenza during a winter outbreak.

Studies have documented the accuracy of clinical diagnosis during an influenza outbreak to be 60% to 85%.

THERAPY

Two classes of antiviral drugs are available for treatment of influenza. The neuraminidase inhibitors zanamivir (Relenza) and oseltamivir (Tamiflu) are available for treatment of both influenza A and B infection. Neuraminidase is a viral enzyme that cleaves sialic acid residues, promoting the release of influenza virus from infected cells. The antiviral drugs inhibit neuraminidase activity and alter virus release. Zanamivir has poor oral bioavailability and is formulated as a dry powder for oral inhalation using a disk inhaler. Oseltamivir is the ethyl ester prodrug of the active compound and is well absorbed orally. When given within 2 days after the onset of symptoms, both drugs decrease the duration of symptoms by about 1 day. Data regarding the ability of neuraminidases to decrease influenza-related complications and/or severity of illness are limited. However, current data suggest that oseltamivir decreases the severity of disease, the incidence of secondary complications, and the use of antibiotics. Both drugs are generally well tolerated, although zanamivir can cause bronchospasm and respiratory compromise in patients with chronic respiratory diseases.

Oseltamivir causes nausea and vomiting, but this rarely results in discontinuation of therapy. Resistance can develop while the patient is receiving therapy, although this is uncommon. Neuraminidase inhibitors appear to be useful in treating patients infected with H5N1; however, resistance has been reported and clinical effectiveness has not been demonstrated.

An older class of drugs, the M2 inhibitors, amantadine and rimantadine, are approved in the United States for the treatment of influenza A, but are not effective against influenza B. The M2 inhibitors prevent viral replication by blocking the M2 protein ion channel, thus preventing fusion of the virus and host cell membranes. Both drugs have been shown to reduce the duration of symptoms of clinical influenza and decrease the severity of fever and other symptoms in randomized trials. However, compared to neuraminidase inhibitors they have several disadvantages. Amantadine causes several minor reversible central nervous system (CNS) toxicities, including insomnia, dizziness, nervousness, and difficulty concentrating, especially in the elderly, that can result in the early discontinuation of therapy. Rimantadine has fewer CNS side effects. The use of M2 inhibitors is becoming limited by increasing resistance among influenza A isolates, and use has not been recommended during recent influenza seasons. The utility of these drugs for the treatment of influenza in the future is unknown, and they should not be used for the treatment of influenza until efficacy is re-established.

PREVENTION

Vaccine

Vaccination is the mainstay of influenza prevention. Because influenza viruses undergo frequent antigenic alterations, a new vaccine containing antigens expected to predominate in the upcoming winter epidemic is prepared each year. The CDC, in conjunction with the WHO, tracks influenza activity throughout the world to predict the components of the annual influenza vaccine. In general, vaccines contain two types of influenza A and one influenza B virus. In the United States, two forms of influenza vaccine have been approved, a trivalent inactivated vaccine for intramuscular administration and a trivalent live-attenuated, cold-adapted influenza vaccine for intranasal administration. The latter has the potential to produce mild signs and symptoms of influenza infection because it contains live virus. The protective efficacy of influenza vaccination depends on the similarity between the viruses used in the vaccine and those in circulation, as well as an indvidual's age and immune status. In healthy adults younger than 65 years, a well-matched vaccine prevents influenza illness among 70% to 90% of adults and results in decreased work absenteeism. During poorly matched seasons, efficacy is closer to 50% among healthy persons and 40% among those at high risk. In older populations, the efficacy against influenza respiratory illness may be less, but vaccination is most effective at decreasing hospitalization, secondary complications, and death due to influenza. Influenza vaccination produces protective antibody titers in human immunodeficiency virus (HIV)-infected persons with high CD4+ T-lymphocyte cell counts, but there has not been a consistent antibody response in individuals with advanced HIV disease (HIV-1 RNA levels >100 000 copies/ mL) and low CD4 counts (≤200/mL). Regardless, all HIV-infected patients should be vaccinated because influenza may result in considerable morbidity and mortality and vaccination could result in the production of protective antibody.

Adults with acute febrile illnesses usually should not be vaccinated until their symptoms have abated. However, minor illnesses with or without fever are not a contraindication. Both the intramuscular and intranasal vaccines are initially grown in embryonated hen eggs and are contraindicated in persons with egg allergies. The live, attenuated intranasal vaccine is approved only for healthy individuals between ages 5 and 49 years. It should not be given to persons with chronic cardiovascular, pulmonary, renal, or metabolic diseases, immunodeficient persons, children or adolescents taking chronic aspirin, persons with a history of Guillian–Barré syndrome, and pregnant women. The optimal time for organized vaccination campaigns for persons in high-risk groups is usually mid-October through mid-November. Recommendations for the use of influenza vaccine are listed in Table 187.2.

Chemoprophylaxis

Chemoprophylaxis is an important adjunct to vaccination. Persons can still be vaccinated after an outbreak of influenza has begun; however, development of antibiodies takes 2 weeks, thus chemoprophylaxis may be considered in high-risk individuals until immunity develops. Chemoprophylaxis may also be effective at controlling outbreaks in settings such as nursing homes and long-term care facilities. Even in

Table 187.2 Recommended Recipients of Annual Influenza Vaccine

Groups at Increased Risk for Influenza-Related Complications and Severe Disease
Persons ≥50 years of age
Children aged 6–59 months
Women who will be pregnant during influenza season
Children and adolescents (aged 6 months–18 years) who are receiving long-term aspirin therapy and, therefore, might be at risk for experiencing Reye's syndrome
Adults and children who have chronic disorders of the pulmonary or cardiovascular systems (not hypertension)
Adults and children with chronic diseases such as chronic metabolic diseases, renal dysfunction, hemoglobinopathies, or immunodeficiency
Adults or children with any condition that compromises respiratory function
Persons Who Live with or Care for Persons at High Risk
Residents of nursing homes and other chronic-care facilities that house persons of any age who have chronic medical conditions
Persons who live with or care for persons at high risk for influenza-related complications, including healthy household contacts and caregivers of children aged 0–59 months, elderly persons, and persons with chronic medical illness
Health care workers

Adapted from Recommendations of the Advisory Committee on Immunization Practices, Centers for Disease Control and Prevention, 2006.

settings with high vaccination rates, chemoprophylaxis may be necessary because vaccination is not completely protective. Chemoprophylaxis may also be considered as a supplement to vaccination in patients who may be expected to have a poor antibody response.

The neuraminidase inhibitors, oseltamivir and zanamivir, are approved for prophylaxis of influenza A and B. When given to healthy adult volunteers, both zanamivir, at a dosage of 10 mg/day over a 4-week period, and oseltamivir, at 75 mg/day over a 6-week period, have been shown to reduce laboratory-confirmed cases by 82% and 84%, respectively. Both drugs are also effective at decreasing secondary spread of influenza. Lower rates of influenza among household contacts of suspected cases of influenza were documented in patients who took zanamivir at a dosage of 10 mg/day for 10 days or oseltamivir, 75 mg/day for 7 days, compared to placebo.

Amantadine and rimantadine are approved for use as prophylactic agents against influenza A virus. Their level of efficacy is about 50% to 80%, and protection may be additive to that of the vaccine. However, high rates of drug resistance in the United States make M2 inhibitors a poor choice for chemoprophylaxis unless the epidemic strain is known to be susceptible to these agents.

PANDEMIC PREPAREDNESS

The emergence of the avian influenza virus, H5N1, has raised awareness of the possibility of a severe, worldwide influenza pandemic. In the event of an influenza pandemic it is expected that global spread will occur and that all countries will be susceptible. During a pandemic, an estimated 30% or more of individuals may become ill. The health care system will likely become overwhelmed, supplies (eg, vaccine, antivirals, antibiotics, ventilators, personal protective equipment) will be in short supply, and there will not be adequate hospital beds to meet health care needs. Public health measures, including school closings, travel bans, and individual quarantine, may cause significant social disruption. Absenteeism could likely exceed 40% and have profound effects on commerce, the economy, and the supply of goods and services.

The effects of a pandemic could be lessened by proper planning for such an event. Preparedness on federal, state, and local levels is important, but business and health care sectors as well as individuals must also plan and prepare. Hospitals, clinics, and long-term care facilities should develop pandemic preparedness plans that include the development of surveillance systems for identifying potential outbreaks, plans for communication (eg, with public officials, employees, and patients), strategies for dealing with surges in patient volume (including triage, admissions, cohorting, and facility access), and protocols for dealing with sick and exposed employees and the reassignment of worker duties. Other important issues include developing guidelines for the distribution of antivirals, vaccine, and medical supplies that may be limited. Health care workers should also encourage patients to develop their own pandemic preparedness plans with their families.

The CDC provides checklists, guidelines, and suggestions for pandemic planning in health care, family, school, business, and community, state, and local government settings. Given the almost guaranteed limited availability of vaccine and antiviral medication during the initial waves of a pandemic, the CDC is also promoting nonpharmacologic interventions to limit transmission of the virus. This strategy has been termed *targeted layered containment* and includes isolation of ill persons and voluntary quarantine of household contacts, social distancing measures (eg, school closure, increased use of telecommuting in the workplace), cancellation of public events and public gatherings (including closure of houses of worship), and individual infection control measures (such as hand hygiene and cough etiquette) (www.pandemicflu.gov).

SUGGESTED READING

Cooper NJ, Sutton AJ, Abrams KR, et al. Effectiveness of neuraminidase inhibitors in treatment and prevention of influenza A and B: systematic review and meta-analysis of randomised controlled trials. *BMJ*. 2003;326:1235.

Stiver G. the treatment of influenza with antiviral drugs. *CMAJ*. 2003;168:49–56.

The Writing Committee of the World Heath Organization (WHO). Consultation on human influenza A/H5: avian influenza A (H5N1) infection in humans. *N Engl J Med*. 2005;353:1374.

Treanor, JJ. Influenza virus. In: Mandell GL, Bennett JE, Dolin R, eds. *Mandell, Douglas and Bennett's Principles and Practices of Infectious Diseases*. 6th ed. New York: Churchill Livingstone; 2005;2062–2085.

Recommendations and Reports: Prevention and control of influenza: recommendations of the advisory committee on immunization practices. *Morbid Mortal Weekly Rep*. 2006;55(RR-10).

188. Papillomavirus

Lawrence J. Eron

Human papillomaviruses (HPV) cause 10 000 cases of cancer of the cervix each year, as well as 3700 deaths annually. In addition, they are the cause of the most common sexually transmitted disease, genital warts, with an annual incidence of 6.2 million and a prevalence of 20 million infections (Figure 188.1). Because they produce persistent infection that in most cases is subclinical and because they are easily transmitted via intercourse, they infect more than 75% of sexually active people during their lifetime.

Of the more than 100 different DNA types of HPV, distinguished on the basis of relatedness of their genomes, 40 infect the genital area. These 40 genital types fall into two groups, distinguished on the basis of the types of disease that they produce. The first group, which includes the two most common HPV types, 6 and 11, causes exophytic condylomata, referred to as genital warts (Figure 188.2), as well as low-grade dysplasia of the vulva, vagina, and cervix. The second group, typified by types 16 and 18, causes high-grade dysplasia of the cervix, vagina, and vulva, which appears as white areas after the application of acetic acid (Figure 188.3). Low-grade dysplasia is referred to as squamous intraepithelial lesions (SIL) grade I, moderate dysplasia as SIL grade II, and severe dysplasia as SIL grade III. Both groups of HPV viruses may produce asymptomatic infection, subclinical disease, or clinically apparent disease (Figure 188.4).

HPV may also infect the perianal region and the distal rectum above the dentate line. In people infected with human immunodeficiency virus (HIV), HPV may produce small, innocent-appearing ulcers that on biopsy are shown to be squamous cell carcinomas. HIV infection, as well as other immunodeficiency states, increases the likelihood that dysplastic lesions of the cervix may evolve into invasive carcinomas. Recurrent or refractory genital warts may be surrogate markers for concomitant infection by HIV, and it is important to test for HIV in patients with HPV infection, as with any other sexually transmitted disease.

PRINCIPLES OF THERAPY

There are certain principles that should be emphasized regarding the treatment of HPV infection. When HPV types 6 and 11 cause external genital warts or mild dysplasia of the cervix, vulva, or vagina, afflicted individuals may experience depression and a sense of social isolation. Nonetheless, as many infections are asymptomatic, an alternative for some patients with genital warts or mild dysplasia is no treatment.

Second, in up to 30% of cases, infection by these low-grade HPV types may be transient (Figure 188.5). Persistence of HPV types 6 and 11, when it does occur, will not evolve into a malignant state. Therefore, treatment directed at lesions showing mild dysplasia should be no worse than the disease itself.

Third, when HPV types 16 and 18 produce moderate or severe dysplasia of the cervix, it may be a premalignant or malignant condition. Although moderate or severe dysplasia may remit without treatment, patients with this condition should be followed closely to detect the development of carcinoma in situ.

Fourth, treatments that extirpate clinically evident disease usually do not eliminate the underlying HPV infection. Because the virus can be shed asymptomatically from apparently normal tissue adjacent to the treated areas, removal of a wart or dysplastic tissue has not been shown to decrease transmissibility of HPV infection. Because many external genital warts resolve spontaneously and there is no likelihood that the viral reservoir can be eliminated by treatment, the primary goal of treatment of external genital warts is to ameliorate symptoms.

TOPICAL TREATMENTS

Topical treatments may be categorized as either cytotoxic or immune. These treatments are recommended for exophytic condylomata and for low-grade dysplasia. Cytotoxic treatments may be further subdivided into patient-applied and provider-applied formulations. Podophyllotoxin and imiquimod

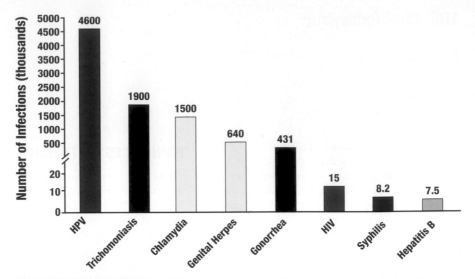

Figure 188.1 Human papillomaviruses (HPV) are the cause of the most common sexually transmitted disease, genital warts, with an annual incidence of 6.2 million and a prevalence of 20 million infections. HIV = human immunodeficiency virus.

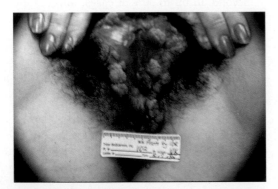

Figure 188.2 Exophytic condylomata also referred to as genital warts.

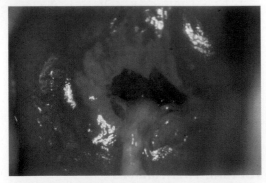

Figure 188.3 High-grade dysplasia of the cervix, vagina, and vulva, appears as white areas after the application of acetic acid.

are two patient-applied treatments, whereas trichloro- and bichloroacetic acid (TCA and BCA, respectively), 5-fluorouracil, and cidofovir are examples of provider-applied treatments.

Guidelines for treatment suggest that clinicians become familiar with and prescribe one patient-applied treatment and one provider-applied treatment. It is recommended to begin with a patient-applied treatment first where reliability and compliance can be assured.

Podophyllotoxin (Condylox) is the active ingredient of podophyllin and is applied to external genital warts twice daily, 3 days per week, repeated weekly for up to 5 weeks. Efficacy rates up to 60% have been reported, but recurrences following treatment are in excess of 33%. It may cause local irritation and discomfort and should not be used in pregnant patients.

Imiquimod cream (Aldara) is a potent inducer of interferon and other cytokines and induces an immune response against genital warts. When topically applied thrice weekly for 8 weeks, clearance rates of 56% have been reported in women and lesser rates in men. Recurrences occur up to 19% of the time. Like podophyllotoxin, it may cause local irritation and discomfort and should not be used in pregnant women.

TCA and BCA may be formulated in 50% to 85% solutions, applied twice daily, 3 days per week, and repeated weekly. Unlike the two previous therapies, they can be used in pregnant women. When applied to external warts or vaginal warts, they produce a white slough that peels away in a few days. Their efficacy rate is comparable to the other topical therapies and is less effective on highly keratinized squamous epithelium, such as the penile shaft, scrotum, and labia majora. As with the previous therapies, they are irritating and may cause discomfort.

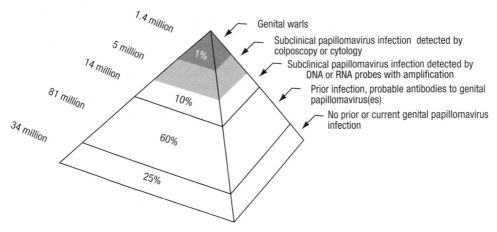

Figure 188.4 Human papillomaviruses may produce asymptomatic infection, subclinical disease, or clinically apparent disease.

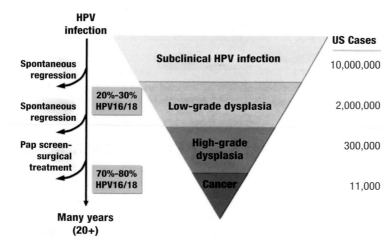

Figure 188.5 Infection by low-grade human papillomavirus (HPV) types may be transient.

Two other topical preparations are available for use in the treatment of genital warts: 5-fluorouracil (Effudex) and cidofovir. The former can be applied topically but is intensely irritating. Cidofovir is an acyclic nucleoside analog with broad-spectrum antiviral activity against DNA viruses. It has been used as a topical formulation to treat external genital warts with clearance rates up to 33%.

CYTODESTRUCTIVE TREATMENTS

Because topical treatments are plagued by low eradication rates and high recurrence rates, it is recommended that patients with persistent or recurrent HPV infection be referred to a specialist for consideration of cytodestructive treatment. This is especially true for cases involving moderate to severe dysplasia of the cervix,

vagina, and vulva, as well as the penis. The simplest and most cost-effective cytodestructive procedures are surgical excision and cryotherapy. Cryotherapy utilizes a nitrous oxide probe or liquid nitrogen applied via cotton-tip applicator as two 1-minute freeze–thaw cycles. It is somewhat more efficacious than topical treatments, with clearance rates up to 80% and recurrence rates of 25%. Cryotherapy is less painful than surgical excision, and usually does not require any type of anesthesia. However, it involves repeated treatments (usually at least three) administered at weekly intervals. Cryotherapy may cause considerable swelling and discomfort following treatments and should not be used on the urethral meatus.

Surgical excision is as effective as cryotherapy with similar relapse rates, but it requires local anesthesia with painful, intradermal injection of lidocaine. As with other surgical procedures, it may be complicated by postoperative pain and occasionally infection.

Electrocoagulation of genital warts and loop electrical excisional procedure of dysplastic tissue of the cervix are reported to be more effective than surgical excision or cryotherapy, with clearance rates up to 94% but with relapse rates of 22%. Like surgical excision, they require local anesthesia with lidocaine and may be complicated by postoperative pain. The smoke plume generated during treatment must be captured by an exhaust apparatus, as it contains infectious HPV DNA.

Laser ablation, used extensively in the treatment of HPV infection of the cervix, offers precise control of the depth of tissue destruction, unlike electrocoagulation and cryotherapy. It requires local and sometimes general anesthesia and is more expensive than any other treatment. Efficacy rates as high as 90% have been reported with relapse rates similar to all other cytodestructive treatments. As with electrocoagulation, the smoke plume must be captured by an exhaust apparatus.

IMMUNITY TO HPV INFECTION

Although the prevalence of HPV infection is high in young women, only a minority (≤5%) of infected women develop persistent infection and SIL. In most cases of HPV type 16 infection, it may be transient if the individual develops a sufficient immune response to the virus. The median duration of an HPV type 16 infection is 11 months. For types 6 and 11 infection, it is even shorter. In those with persistent infection by types 16 or 18, it may take decades for infection to progress to squamous cell carcinoma of the cervix (SCCC).

Viral, environmental, and host factors, in association with HPV types 16 and 18 infection, are undoubtedly involved in the development of the evolution of highly dysplastic SIL to SCCC. Polymorphisms among HPV type 16 variants are associated with more aggressive infection. These HPV type 16 variants exhibit an increased risk of the development of high-grade SIL and SCCC than the prototype virus. In addition to viral factors and host immunity, numerous environmental factors that are associated with progression of SIL to SCCC have been identified, including smoking, long-term oral contraceptive use, high parity, and other STDs.

In addition to these factors, susceptibility to SCCC has been attributed to genetic polymorphisms in the major histocompatibility complex (MHC) genes. Higher risk for SCCC is associated with certain MHC alleles. These human leukocyte antigen (HLA) polymorphisms point directly to a role of the immune response in the control of HPV infection.

Modulating the immune response to decrease persistent infection and recurrence rates following treatment is the "holy grail" of HPV treatment. By increasing helper CD4 and cytotoxic CD8 lymphocyte activity, patients with recurrent or recalcitrant disease that fails to respond to cytotoxic and cytodestructive measures may be salvaged. Interferon and other cytokines have the potential to stimulate an immune response that might not only remove the wart but might also eradicate the viral reservoir. Unfortunately, neither intralesional injection with various α interferons (Intron-A, Roferon, Alferon) nor topical administration of an interferon inducer (Aldara) has produced higher efficacy rates than far less expensive topical and cytodestructive therapies. Parenteral (ie, intramuscular) administration of interferon, despite considerable success in the treatment of other viral diseases such as hepatitis B and C, has not proven effective in the treatment of genital warts.

HPV GENOME AND CARCINOGENESIS

HPV contains a circular, double-stranded DNA genome, consisting of 8 structural genes in 2 distinct regions (Figure 188.6). The early region is composed of 6 early genes (E1-2 and E4-E7) that control viral replication, transcription, and cell transformation. The late region is composed of 2 late genes (L1 and L2) that encode the viral coat proteins. The "long control region" regulates the expression of the other 8 genes. In productive infection, as is the case for types 6 and 11, both early and late regions of the virus are transcribed into messenger RNA (mRNA), which codes for proteins essential for viral DNA replication and for coat proteins. Many copies of HPV DNA are produced in each infected cell as circular, extrachromosomal plasmids. The net result is mature infectious virions.

In contrast to productive infection, when type 16 or 18 infects a cell, late genes are not transcribed, and viral coat proteins are not synthesized. No mature virions are produced. Instead the circular HPV genome inserts itself into the host chromosome disrupting the E2 gene, resulting in the loss of E1 and E2 gene function (Figure 188.6). Normally E1 and E2 downregulate E6 and E7 expression, but with the loss of E1 and

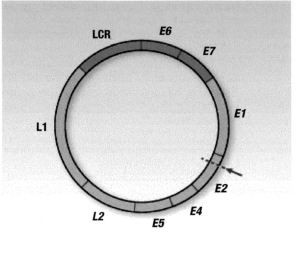

Figure 188.6 Human papillomavirus contains a circular, double-stranded DNA genome, consisting of 8 structural genes in 2 distinct regions.

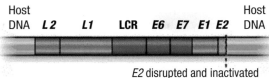

E2 control, E6 and E7 functions are upregulated. The E6 and E7 gene products then inactivate host antioncogenes that normally control cell growth and differentiation. Two examples of antioncogenes are p53 and pRB (retinoblastoma tumor suppressor protein), which in the normal state arrest host cell division in the G1 phase. This allows the cell time to repair damaged DNA before progressing to the S (DNA replication) phase. The loss of this repair mechanism results in cell transformation, which renders the host genome susceptible to other carcinogens, such as smoking. The time between initial HPV infection and the development of SCCC is between 10 to >20 years.

HPV PREVENTION

Because the viral genome is highly conserved and because HPV uses cellular enzymes to replicate (and thus cannot easily develop resistance in contrast to HIV for example), a vaccine has been developed from viruslike particles derived from the viral coat protein L1 that contains no infectious DNA (and therefore is not infectious). This vaccine produces neutralizing antibodies that protect against viral infection. Although it may be difficult for vaccines to produce high-titer neutralizing antibodies at mucosal surfaces, cytotoxic CD8 lymphocytes eliminate nascently HPV-infected cells undergoing productive infection at the basal layer of the skin. The vaccine is >95% effective in the prevention of infection by HPV types 6, 11, 16, and 18. Types 16 and 18, however, represent only 70% of cancer-causing types. Vaccine administration is recommended for females, age 9 to 26, the earlier the better to induce immunity prior to the female sexual debut, which in 77% occurs by age 19. Once sexual activity begins, the incidence of HPV infection rises to 40% within 2 years and to >50% within 4 years. The vaccine is a 3-dose series administered over 6 months and remains effective for at least 5 years.

Because the HPV genome contains two oncogenes, E6 and E7, that are involved in the production of SCCC, vaccines against the products of these oncogenes could be used therapeutically in the treatment of cervical cancer. In animals, such a vaccine can protect against challenge with tumors expressing E6 and E7 antigens. Vaccine-induced tumor rejection occurs when CD8 lymphocytes encounter these antigens in the context of MHC-restricted loci. The possibility of vaccinating women with preinvasive, but high-grade, SILs is being pursued, although such a vaccine has not yet been shown to be useful in humans.

In patients with SCCC, a downregulation of MHC molecules may induce an immunotolerant state, seemingly precluding a robust immune response to a therapeutic vaccine. Nonetheless, the possibility of utilizing this vaccine to treat SCCC would be of enormous benefit in the developing world, where it is the leading cause of cancer-related deaths in women.

In addition to vaccines, the most cost-effective strategy for reducing HPV infection is the consistent use of condoms. Until recently, no study has shown conclusive efficacy of condom use. However, in a well-designed and executed study, condoms reduced the incidence of genital HPV infection from 89.3 per 100 patient-years to 37.8. In those women whose partners used condoms 100% of the time, there were no cervical SILs observed in 32.1 patient-years, whereas 14 were detected in 96.8 patient-years among women whose partners used condoms less than 100% of the time.

SUGGESTED READING

Aho J, Hankins C, Tremblay C, et al. Genomic polymorphism of human papillomavirus type 52 predisposes toward persistent infection in sexually active women. *J Infect Dis*. 2004;190:46–52.

Beutner KR, Wiley DJ, Douglas JM, et al. Genital warts and their treatment. *Clin Infect Dis*. 1999;28(suppl 1):S37–S56.

Bosch FX. *Progress in Preventing Cervical Cancer*. New York, NY: Academy for Healthcare Education, Inc.; 2005:5–8.

Eron LJ. Papillomavirus. In: Schlossberg D, ed. *Current Therapy of Infectious Disease*. 2nd ed. St. Louis, MO: Mosby; 2001: 613–615.

Eron LJ. Human papillomaviruses and anogenital disease. In: Gorbach SL, Bartlett JG, Blacklow NR, eds. *Infectious Diseases*. 3rd ed. Philadelphia, PA: Lippincott Williams & Wilkins; 2004.

Frazer IH, Cox JT, Mayeaux EJ, et al. Advances in prevention of cervical cancer and other human papillomavirus-related diseases. *Pediatr Infect Dis J*. 2006;25:S61–S81.

Koutsky L. Epidemiology of genital human papillomavirus infection. *Am J Med*. 1997;102:3–8.

Maciag PC, Schlecht NF, Souza PSA. Polymorphisms of the human leukocyte antigen DRB1 and DZB1 genes and the natural history of human papillomavirus infection. *J Infect Dis*. 2002;186:164–172.

Stoler MH. A brief synopsis of the role of human papillomaviruses in cervical carcinogenesis. *Am J Obstet Gynecol*. 1996;175:1091–1098.

Wiley DJ, Douglas J, Beutner K, et al. External genital warts: diagnosis, treatment, and prevention. *Clin Infect Dis*. 2002;35(suppl 2): S210–S224.

Winer RL, Hughes JP, Feng Q. Condom use and the risk of genital human papillomavirus infection in young women. *N Engl J Med*. 2006;354:2645–2654.

189. Acute and Chronic Parvovirus Infection

Neal S. Young

B19 parvovirus is the only member of the *Parvoviridae* family known to cause diseases in humans. Parvoviruses are small viruses with unenveloped icosahedral capsids that contain a single-stranded DNA genome. These physical properties contribute to viral resistance to heat, solvents, and extreme chemical conditions. Because of their limited genome, parvoviral propagation depends on infection of mitotically active cells. In the taxonomy of the parvovirus family, B19 and closely related simian parvoviruses constitute the *Erythrovirus* genus, separated from autonomous animal parvoviruses, dependoviruses (which require coinfection with a second virus for efficient propagation in cell culture), and insect parvoviruses called densoviruses.

B19 parvovirus has extreme tropism for human erythroid progenitor cells, which are responsible for the generation of circulating erythrocytes. In tissue culture, B19 has been propagated only in bone marrow, fetal liver, peripheral blood, and rather inefficiently in a few leukemic cell lines. B19 replication in patients has been detected in blood and marrow. Specificity for erythroid cells follows from the cellular receptor for the virus, globoside or P antigen, a tetrohexoseceramide present on erythroid cells, megakaryocytes, endothelial cells, and some placental cell types, as well as fetal liver and heart. Parvovirus infection is terminated by host production of neutralizing antibodies. Failure to produce neutralizing antibodies can result in persistent infection. Recently, cellular immune responses to parvoviruses have been measured and some CD4 and CD8 T-cell epitopes defined.

B19 DISEASES

Serologic studies have shown that more than half of the adult population has antibodies to B19 parvovirus; although most infection occurs during childhood, the seropositivity rate continues to rise with age. Probably the majority of infections are asymptomatic. Reliable diagnostic assays are now widely available. The presence of immunoglobulin G (IgG) to virus only signifies past infection. Immunoglobulin M (IgM) or virus DNA detected by direct hybridization testing indicates recent infection. The interpretation of a positive DNA study obtained by gene amplification (polymerase chain reaction) is more problematic, as individuals may not clear small amounts of virus for many months after an acute infection, and laboratory contamination can produce false-positives.

Fifth Disease

This common childhood exanthem is caused by acute parvovirus infection. The slapped-cheek rash and the evanescent maculopapular eruption over the trunk and proximal extremities are typical (Figure 189.1). Children may be febrile but usually have few symptoms. Meningitis and encephalitis have been reported as very rare complications. The blood of children with fifth disease contains IgM antibody to B19 but little if any virus; because the syndrome is due to immune complex formation between virus and antibodies, affected individuals are not considered infectious. Reassurance and antipyretics as needed are sufficient for this self-limited illness.

In adults, acute parvovirus infection may be more serious. Adults have more rheumatic complaints than do children, and there may be frank joint inflammation and a pattern of distribution and chronicity mimicking rheumatoid arthritis; occasionally rheumatoid factor will be present. However, in most cases, symptoms resolve within a few days or weeks, and parvovirus is not a cause of rheumatoid arthritis. The basis of chronic joint complaints in some patients is not understood, but symptoms usually can be addressed with conventional anti-inflammatory drug therapy.

Transient Aplastic Crisis and Other Hematologic Syndromes

Transient aplastic crisis is caused by parvovirus infection in patients with hemolytic anemia, compensated hemolysis (as in many cases of hereditary spherocytosis), or increased demand for red cell production (iron deficiency,

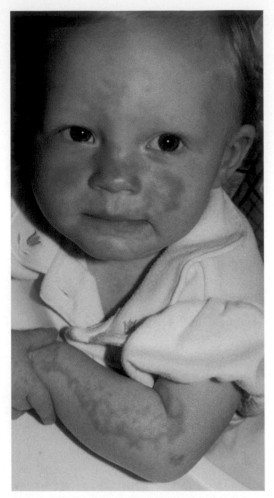

Figure 189.1 Fifth disease; note characteristic maculopapular rash with "slapped cheek" appearance.

acute hemorrhage). B19 briefly interrupts erythropoiesis in most persons infected but without consequence because of the long survival of circulating red blood cells. Transient aplastic crisis is manifested by anemia, reticulocytopenia, and red cell aplasia in the marrow. There may be moderate thrombocytopenia and neutropenia in addition to the severe anemia, especially in patients with functioning spleens. The syndrome may be accompanied by marrow necrosis and may be fatal, especially in young children. As the anemia is self-limited, transfusion is adequate therapy. Specific antibody production terminates the episode and likely prevents recurrence.

Hydrops Fetalis and Congenital Infection

Parvovirus infection of the pregnant woman may be transmitted to the fetus. Midtrimester

events have been best characterized; first trimester infection may result in abortion, and third trimester infection has not been associated with adverse outcomes. Infection of the fetus is predominantly in the liver, the site of red cell production; the heart may also be affected (fetal myocardial cells express P antigen). Untreated, the fetus develops severe anemia and heart failure leading to the massive edema of hydrops and death at birth or shortly afterward (Figure 189.2). In utero blood transfusions have apparently been successful in a few instances; however, untreated fetal infection need not result in mortality or morbidity. As ultrasound diagnosis may not be definitive, a conservative recommendation is to document progressive hydrops on serial testing before intervention.

Congenital parvovirus infection after transfusion treatment of hydrops can produce chronic anemia from birth. Only a few infants have been described: In all, virus was localized to the marrow and did not circulate, and gene amplification was required to detect the low levels of B19 DNA. The pathology of the marrow was erythroid hypoplasia (Diamond–Blackfan anemia) or erythroid dysplasia resembling congenital dyserythropoietic states. There may

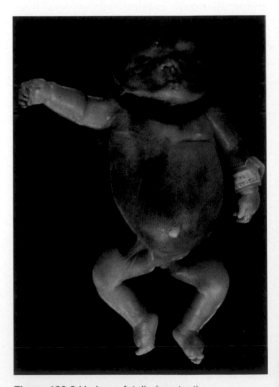

Figure 189.2 Hydrops fetalis (see text).

be associated immunodeficiency; one infant died of overwhelming bacterial infection from a catheter source. Transfusions can maintain the hemoglobin, but immunoglobulin therapy has not been effective.

Persistent Infection

In the absence of an appropriate immune response, B19 infection can become chronic. Persistent infection has been observed in congenital immunodeficiency (Nezelof syndrome), acquired immunodeficiency syndrome (AIDS) secondary to human immunodeficiency virus (HIV) 1 infection, and during therapy with cytotoxic or immunosuppressive drugs. The deficit in the immune response may be subtle; B19 infection may be the only evidence of a congenital syndrome and the first sign of AIDS. Clinically, the patients have typical pure red cell aplasia with severe anemia, absent reticulocytes in the blood, and a paucity of red cell precursors in the marrow. Scattered giant pronormoblasts, the mark of B19 infection, may signal the diagnosis, which is established by DNA hybridization studies of serum.

Persistent infection results from inability to mount an effective humoral immune response, measured either as neutralizing antibodies in functional tissue culture experiments or by immunoblot binding of viral capsid proteins. Most AIDS patients lack any antibodies to B19; some congenital cases may have circulating IgM to B19 suggestive of a class-switch abnormality. Fortunately, commercial immunoglobulin preparations are a good source of effective antibodies to parvovirus. Administration of IgG 0.4 g/kg/day intravenously for 5 to 10 days terminates infection. The reticulocyte count dramatically increases after the first week, the marrow shows healthy normoblastic erythroid proliferation, and the hemoglobin rises to a level appropriate for the patient. Treatment can be curative, and the virus may no longer be detectable in some patients who have congenital immunodeficiency or whose immunosuppressive therapy is discontinued. In contrast, AIDS patients have intense chronic parvoviremia, and IgG treatment appears to reduce but not eliminate the virus (Figure 189.3). Although relapse after some months is common, recurrent anemia responds to a second course of IgG. Monthly maintenance injections of IgG have been used in a few patients.

OTHER POSSIBLE ASSOCIATIONS

The associations of B19 parvovirus with other clinical syndromes is less secure. Apparent links to childhood neutropenia, idiopathic thrombocytopenic purpura, vasculitis, and juvenile rheumatoid arthritis have not been reproducible. A major technical problem has been the

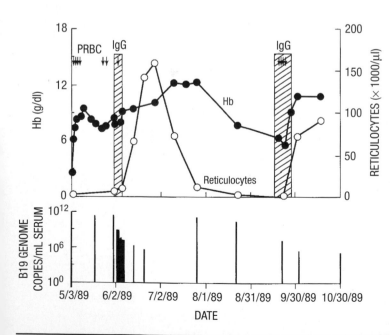

Figure 189.3 Immunoglobulin G (IgG) treatment of B19 persistence in acquired immunodeficiency syndrome (AIDS), illustrating recurrence predicted by molecular studies and the effectiveness of repeated treatment.

use of gene amplification methods, which not only are susceptible to false-positive results but also are positive in a high proportion of normal individuals: Viral DNA has been found in almost half of knee joints biopsied for trauma and in 20% of normal bone marrows using this sensitive method. Polymerase chain reaction–derived data that are reported without other clinical or serologic evidence of recent infection should be especially suspect. Nevertheless, B19 parvovirus may be linked to some types of hepatitis. In addition, paroxysmal cold hemoglobinuria, a severe childhood hemolytic anemia that usually follows a viral illness, is a good candidate as a B19 parvovirus syndrome because of the presence of the pathogenic Donath–Landsteiner antibody, directed against erythrocyte P antigen, the virus's cellular receptor. Fetal and childhood myocarditis might also follow parvovirus infection, because the P antigen receptor is present on maturing heart cells.

VACCINE DEVELOPMENT

Effective vaccines to prevent parvovirus infection in animals have been produced by tissue culture modification of virus. For B19, which resists conventional cell culture, recombinant empty capsids have been produced in a baculovirus system by expression of a portion of the parvovirus genome; they contain no viral DNA. Capsids enriched for the highly immunogenic VP1 protein elicit strong neutralizing antibody responses in test animals and, with the appropriate adjuvant, in normal volunteers.

SUGGESTED READING

Brown KE. Detection and quantitation of parvovirus B19. *J Clin Virol*. 2004;31:1–4.

De Jong EP, de Haan TR, Kroes AC, et al. Parvovirus B19 infection in pregnancy. *J Clin Virol*. 2006;36:1–7.

Ergaz Z, Ornoy A, et al. Parvovirus B19 in pregnancy. *Reprod Toxicol* 2006;21:421–435.

Frickhofen N, Abkowitz JL, Safford M. Persistent parvovirus infection in patients infected with human immunodeficiency virus type 1 (HIV-1): a treatable cause of anemia in AIDS. *Ann Intern Med*. 1990;113:926–933.

Kurtzman G, Cohen BJ, Field AM, et al. The immune response to B19 parvovirus infection and an antibody defect in persistent viral infection. *J Clin Invest*. 1989;84:1114–1123.

Lindner J, Barabas S, Saar K, CD4+ T-cell responses against the VP1-unique region in individuals with recent and persistent parvovirus B19 infection. *J Vet Med*. 2005;52:351–361.

Mouthon L, Guillevin L, Tellier Z. Intravenous immunoglobulins in autoimmune- or parvovirus B19-mediated pure red cell aplasia. *Autoimmun Rev*. 2005;4:264–269.

Serjeant GR, Serjeant BE, Thomas PW, Anderson MJ, Patou G, Pattison JR, et al. Human parvovirus infection in homozygous sickle cell disease. *Lancet*. 1993; 341:1237–1240.

Sokal EM, Melchior M, Cornu C, et al. Acute parvovirus B19 infection associated with fulminant hepatitis of favourable prognosis in young children. *Lancet*. 1998;352:1739–1741.

Young NS, Brown KE. Parvovirus B19. *N Engl J Med*. 2004;350:586–597.

190. Rabies

Anita Venkataramana, Nicoline Schiess,
Anita Mahadevan, Susarla K. Shankar, and Avindra Nath

HISTORY

The first clear recognizable reference to rabies was from writings by Aristotle in circa 380 BC in which he described the symptoms and transmission of rabies in dogs. Despite centuries of observations on the transmission, symptoms, and a myriad of unsuccessful remedies, the disease remained invariably fatal until approximately 1885 when Louis Pasteur developed the first rabies vaccine in Paris. Unable to identify the intangible virus—indeed unaware at that time of even the difference between bacteria and viruses—he cultured it in the spinal cords of rabbits and, ultimately, injected it into Joseph Meister, a young boy severely attacked by a rabid dog on his way home from school. Given the severity of his wounds on his face, hands, and legs he undoubtedly would have died; however, he received a series of 13 injections, survived, and subsequently spent his life working as a guard at the Pasteur Institute.

EPIDEMIOLOGY

In 2001, the Centers for Disease Control and Prevention (CDC) reported that there were 7473 cases of rabies in animals in the United States but no human rabies infection. Hawaii has been the only state kept free of rabies infection in humans and animals. Ninety-three percent of cases were in wild animals. In the United States the largest reservoirs remain in raccoons followed by skunks, bats, foxes, and coyotes. Raccoon and fox reservoirs are mainly from the eastern states; bat and skunk cases were also found in parts of the south, Pacific Northwest, and California. Domestic animals only accounted for about 6.8% of rabies. Interestingly, cats are found to be infected with rabies almost double the infections of dogs. The cases of rabid cats have risen by 8.4%, whereas the cases in other animals have declined. This paradox may be due to administration of vaccines in certain animals, especially dogs. Cats, however, are viewed as not being a potential threat, which would certainly allow infection to go unnoticed.

In Europe, rabies reservoir is mainly the fox; whereas the bat is the main reservoir in Australia, Mexico, and parts of South America. Worldwide, death from rabies is usually from a rabid dog. It is found on all continents except Antarctica. The highest prevalence of rabies worldwide is still in the developing countries, with India being in the lead followed by China, Nepal, and Myanmar. In Europe, Lithuania had the highest rate of cases followed by Ukraine. According to the World Health Organization (WHO) *Rabies Bulletin—Europe* (2006), 17 countries in total reported the rabies virus. High-risk groups include veterinarians or unprotected rural workers, especially in endemic areas that should be sought out and appropriate where intervention be offered.

PATHOGENESIS AND PATHOLOGY

The virus replicates at the wound site for a period of days and then, via retrograde axoplasmic flow, moves up the peripheral nerves to the anterior horn cells in the spinal cord. Both sensory and motor nerves can propagate the infection. Once the central nervous system (CNS) is seeded with the virus, it then centrifugally spreads back to the periphery. This process involves infection of nonneural tissues, especially with infection of the salivary glands, where the virus is transmitted.

Postmortem examination of the brain shows perivascular inflammation of the gray matter, neuronal degeneration, and the characteristic cytoplasmic inclusions called the Negri bodies (Figure 190.1A). Renal tubular necrosis has also been demonstrated at autopsy. In 2005, a few cases of rabies were also reported from organ recipients. Some of the neuropathological features in the latter study showed Duret hemorrhages, widespread neuronal loss, perivascular lymphocytic infiltration, and extensive spinal cord pathology.

CLINICAL SYMPTOMS

The clinical course in humans is acute, usually progressing from initial symptoms to death within 2 to 3 weeks, even with intensive supportive

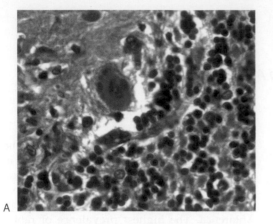

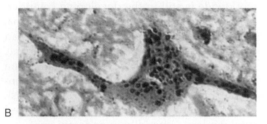

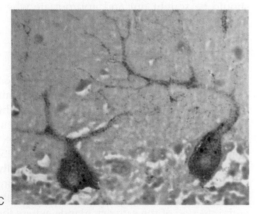

Figure 190.1 Histopathology of human rabies encephalitis. **A:** Eosinophilic Negri bodies in a Purkinje cell. **B:** Anterior horn cell immunostaining for rabies virus. **C:** Purkinje cells immunostaining for rabies virus antigen.

care. The incubation period of rabies can vary from a few days to several years. The length of the incubation period varies with the infecting strain and is thought to be inversely related to the size of the inoculum and the proximity of the bite to the CNS. Approximately half of the patients develop pain or paresthesias at the wound site. A diagnosis of rabies should not always depend on a history of an animal bite. Often the exposure is not obvious. The prodrome includes low-grade fevers, loss of appetite, and anxiety. Most patients have "furious rabies" characterized by marked hyperactivity, disorientation,

hallucination, or bizarre behavior, which lead to an initial psychiatric evaluation. This hyperactivity later becomes intermittent and may be spontaneous or precipitated by tactile, auditory, or visual stimuli. Hydrophobia (spasm of the pharynx and larynx provoked by drinking or the sight of water) and aerophobia (similar effect produced by blowing air on the face of the patient) are considered hallmarks of the disease. The inability to swallow from paralysis of bulbar muscles may also result in hypersalivation. Seizures, which are more common in children, may also occur during this stage, as can dysfunction of the autonomic nervous system. Rarely, there may be respiratory distress with medullary involvement. A few patients die during this stage, but most go on to develop progressive paralysis and eventually coma. In some patients, the paralytic state dominates the entire clinical picture; hence, it is termed *paralytic rabies*. Paralysis or paresis involves the proximal muscles and can be accompanied by constipation, urinary retention, and respiratory failure. Alternatively, inflammation and demyelination of the peripheral nerve causes an ascending lower motor neuron weakness without anterior horn cell involvement. Physical exam shows a motor weakness involving the respiratory muscles and loss of deep tendon reflexes with maintained consciousness. This lack of involvement of spinal cord motor neurons and brainstem is called an "escape phenomenon." In some patients, however, the clinical manifestations can be nonspecific; hence, in all patients with unknown cause of progressive encephalitis, the possibility of rabies should be considered. In patients receiving intensive supportive care, the average duration of illness between onset of paralysis and death is 7 days. Once neurologic symptoms have developed, survival is rare.

DIAGNOSIS

Prior to available accurate lab tests, a potentially infected animal was placed in isolation for observation. If it died a characteristic rabies death, the diagnosis was established. With the advent of the microscope in 1903, intracytoplasmic inclusion bodies were discovered in infected brain tissue by Aldelchi Negri, who at the time was an assistant of Camillo Golgi. These structures were subsequently called Negri bodies. In the 1980s the direct fluorescent antibody (DFA) test was formed, which remains to this day the diagnostic gold standard (Figure 190.1). For postmortem diagnosis in animals, fresh unfixed brain tissue is necessary for DFA testing as fixed tissue with agents such as formalin may yield inaccurate results. Brain tissue is the only sample tissue type for diagnosis as saliva and salivary gland excretion of the virus can be intermittent. The predictive value of a negative brain DFA test is 100%.

Routine laboratory tests and diagnostic studies are of little value in the diagnosis of rabies. Examination of the cerebrospinal fluid (CSF) may show leukocytosis, but protein and glucose assays are often normal. Antibodies to the virus in an unvaccinated patient with encephalitis confirms the diagnosis. In addition, saliva samples can be cultured and then tested for viral nucleic acid. A tissue diagnosis can be made in premortem humans using the DFA test on a skin sample from the back of the neck. Polymerase chain reaction (PCR) can also be used in diagnosis, but DFA is still considered the gold standard as PCR is hampered by obtaining universal *Lyssavirus* primers. Although real-time PCR is a more sensitive method than conventional PCR, DFA remains a reliable, cost-effective, and efficient way to establish a diagnosis.

In 2006, the CDC reported an interesting case of encephalitis in a 15-year-old girl from Wisconsin who was bitten by a bat. Antibody titers to rabies virus were found in CSF and serum to suggest the diagnosis. She survived the infection. Another young boy developed encephalitis of undetermined etiology that progressed rapidly. He developed rabies-specific immunoglobulin G antibodies in increasing titers, which brought about the diagnosis. Rabies virus could not be detected in the CSF by PCR; however, antibodies to the rabies virus were present.

Magnetic resonance imaging (MRI) changes most likely occur in the early stages of the infection. More extensive involvement of various regions of the brain has been shown in advanced stages on serial imaging. There are no specific features that are attributable to the rabies virus. Patients with acute rabies encephalitis have been shown to have T2 hyperintense lesions in the brainstem, thalami, hippocampus, and subcortical white matter. Mild signal changes can also be seen in the brain stem and spinal cord of some patients. Enhancement with gadolinium contrast is not present until the patient is comatose.

TREATMENT

Treatment efforts are concentrated on preventing and treating complications of established infection and protecting those who come in contact with the patient from virus exposure. Neither vaccine nor rabies immunoglobulin increases survival in symptomatic patients and should be avoided. Steroids should also be avoided in the treatment of cerebral edema if it develops. Universal precautions should be followed by hospital staff, and respiratory precautions are recommended for suctioning. Postexposure prophylaxis is recommended for contacts who were bitten or had clear contamination of mucous membranes to the patient's saliva, urine, or other body tissue.

Postexposure Prophylaxis

Once an individual is bitten by an animal presumed to have rabies, it is vital to immediately begin the immunization. Raccoons, skunks, foxes, and coyotes are the wild animals most often infected with the rabies virus. Patients exposed to these animals should receive postexposure prophylaxis as soon as possible. Transmission of rabies virus can occur from minor, even unrecognized, bites from bats. Therefore, rabies postexposure prophylaxis is recommended for all persons with bite, scratch, or mucous membrane exposure to a bat and should be considered if the history indicates that a bat was physically present, even if the person is unable to reliably report contact that could have resulted in a bite. An unprovoked attack by a domestic animal is more likely than a provoked attack to indicate that the animal is rabid. If the animal has been vaccinated, it is unlikely to be infected; if not vaccinated but otherwise healthy, the animal should be confined and observed for 10 days. Any illness during this time should be evaluated by a veterinarian and the public health department. Vaccination can be withheld if the animal remains healthy during this time. Small rodents (eg, squirrels, hamsters, guinea pigs, gerbils, chipmunks, rats, mice) and lagomorphs (including rabbits and hares) are almost never infected with the rabies virus and have not been known to transmit rabies to humans. Large rodents such as woodchucks are sometimes found to be infected. Therefore, in cases involving rodent exposure, the state or local health department should be consulted before initiating prophylaxis. Postexposure therapy for rabies is highly effective, and no failures have been recorded in patients who have received all three arms of treatment. Failures have occurred only on deviation from the recommended protocol.

Local Wound Care

The abraded skin after a bite must be cleaned by soap and water or povidone-iodine solution.

Even scratches or contaminated skin from saliva should be cleaned the same way. It has been found that cleaning the wound would help reduce the chances of developing rabies. There are no areas that are deemed more susceptible after a bite. All bites in any area should be treated with the same level of care. Tetanus prophylaxis and antibiotics may be necessary to prevent secondary infection.

Vaccination

Postexposure therapy is given by both passive immunoglobulin with Rabies Immune Globulin (RIG) and the vaccine in those who have not been vaccinated by the rabies vaccine previously. The RIG is administered as a one-time dose at the beginning and at the same time as the vaccine itself. The RIG should be given within the first 7 days of the vaccine because after this time period the vaccine production of antibody is thought to have occurred. The recommended dose of RIG is 20 IU/kg body weight and it is the dose for any age group. It is typically administered around the bite wound. The RIG and vaccine should not be given at the same site.

In the United States, there are currently three Food and Drug Administration (FDA)-approved vaccines. The human diploid cell vaccine (HDCV), under the trade name Imovax, can be administered intramuscularly (IM) and intradermally (ID). The rabies vaccine adsorbed (RVA) and the purified chick embryo cell vaccine (PCEC), trade name RabAvert, are the other vaccines, and these are given only by the intramuscular route. Vaccine is given as 1.0 mL IM in the deltoid area (the outer thigh may be used in younger children, but vaccine should not be given in the gluteal area) on days 0, 3, 7, 14, and 28. All of these vaccines are used for both pre-exposure and postexposure prophylaxis. The only exception when postexposure vaccination is not given would be when an individual is actually found to have the infection. The infection itself would serve as the antigen load. The older vaccine, Semple vaccine, is still used in developing countries and has been associated with severe and life-threatening complications. The newer vaccines are quite safe with rare occurrence of vaccine-related neurological deficits.

Pre-exposure Vaccination

Pre-exposure prophylaxis should be offered to persons at high risk for exposure to rabies. Persons who work with rabies virus in research laboratories or vaccine-production facilities are at highest risk for exposure and should have rabies antibody titers checked every 6 months. Other laboratory workers (eg, those performing rabies diagnostic testing), spelunkers, veterinarians and staff, and animal-control and wildlife officers in areas where animal rabies is enzootic should also have antibody measurements done every 2 years. Booster doses (IM or ID) of vaccine should be administered to maintain an adequate serum titer. The immunization practices advisory committee (ACIP) recommends three pre-exposure doses of the HDCV given IM or ID at 0, 7, and 21 or 28 days. This ensures both seroconversion and adequate duration of protective antibody. Routine serologic testing after vaccination is not needed as seroconversion has been uniform. Patients who are immunosuppressed or taking medications such as chloroquine, which may interfere with antibody response to the vaccine, should postpone pre-exposure vaccinations and consider avoiding activities for which rabies pre-exposure prophylaxis is indicated. When this is not possible, they should be vaccinated and their antibody titers checked.

EDUCATION

Prevention is the best cure. Knowledge is extremely vital in this disease. People should be informed of preventative measures if they are considered to be a high-risk group. The CDC has immensely resourceful web-based information for individuals who have concerns or common questions related to a dog bite. They have recommendations for people who would like to have a dog as a household pet. Casual handshaking or standing next to someone who may be infected are not considered to be risks of acquiring the infection. Changing bed linen from an infected individual does not pose a threat, either. Certain risks seen in the domestic setting, barring animal bites, would also be from sexual activity, sharing utensils or cigarettes, and saliva contact from an infected source (CDC). A healthy person undergoing post-exposure prophylaxis (PEP) does not constitute a potential threat for infecting others. If a person is found to be infected, the local health department should be notified once the infection is documented. In an unknown case of encephalitis, especially in children, a history must be ascertained about recent animal bites. Patients may not recognize that certain animals can be a threat for a rabies virus infection.

As there is currently no cure for rabies infection once it has reached the CNS, determining a definitive, positive diagnosis does not aid the patient directly. However, it is an important part of the work-up and differential for an acute encephalitis in that a negative result points toward a different cause for the encephalitis. Alternatively, a positive result is important from a public health perspective and garners patient isolation a necessity. It also aids in establishing a more detailed history for possible exposure in other family members.

SUGGESTED READING

Burton EC, Burns DK, Opatowsky MJ, et al. Rabies encephalomyelitis: clinical, neuroradiological and pathological findings in 4 transplant recipients. *Arch Neurol.* 2005; 62:873–882.

Centers for Disease Control and Prevention. Human rabies prevention—United States, 1999: recommendations of the Advisory Committee on Immunization Practices (ACIP). MMWR 1999;48(No. RR-1):1-41.

Fisher DJ. Resurgence of rabies: a historical perspective on rabies in children. *Arch Pediatr Adolesc Med.* 1995;149:306–312.

Hemachudha T, Wacharapluesadee S, Laothamatas J, Wilde H. Rabies. *Curr Neurol Neurosci Rep.* 2006;6:460–468.

Laothamatas J, Hemachudha T, Mitrabhakdi E, Wannakrairot P, Tulayadaechanont S. MR imaging in human rabies. *Am J Neuroradiol.* 2003;24:1102–1109.

Mitrabhakdi E, Shuangshoti S, Wannakrairot P, et al. Difference in neuropathogenetic mechanisms in human furious and paralytic rabies. *J Neurol Sci.* 2005;238:3–10.

Wilkinson L. The development of the virus concept as reflected in corpora of studies on individual pathogens. *Med Hist.* 1977; 21:15–31.

191. Varicella-Zoster Virus

John A. Zaia

Varicella-zoster virus (VZV) is one of the 8 herpesviruses of humans and is the cause of chickenpox (varicella) and shingles (zoster). Chickenpox, the exanthem caused by primary infection with VZV, usually occurs in children. Shingles, the clinical syndrome of segmental, unilateral, exanthem, and neuralgic pain due to reactivation of latent VZV infection, usually occurs many years after the primary infection. In the immunodeficient person, both primary and reactivated VZV infection can lead to severe generalized virus dissemination, the life-threatening form of VZV infection. The availability of antiviral agents for management of VZV infection has raised the importance of recognizing this infection in high-risk groups. Prior to the introduction of the VZV vaccine in the United States in 1995, approximately 4 million cases of chickenpox occurred each year, 83% in children younger than 9 years. There are an estimated 1 million cases of herpes zoster in the United States per year, with the annualized incidence of 1.5 to 3.0 cases per 1000 persons, and the incidence and severity of disease increases with age. A VZV vaccine was approved in 2006 for prevention of shingles in persons older than 60 years.

CLINICAL PRESENTATION
Chickenpox

In healthy unvaccinated children, VZV infection manifests as a vesicular exanthem often associated with prodromal malaise, pharyngitis, rhinitis, and abdominal pain. At the median, the rash appears 15 days after VZV exposure; the range is 10 to 21 days. The vesicular eruption emerges in successive crops over the first 3 to 4 days of illness, usually with concomitant enanthem. Each skin vesicle appears on an erythematous base, resulting in the descriptive image of a dewdrop on a rose petal. This stage of infection may be missed because of rupture of the vesicle, which then quickly undergoes inflammatory changes and crusting. The exanthem usually begins on the head and quickly progresses to the trunk, arms, and, finally, the legs. It is common to see all stages

of the exanthem, including macules, vesicles, papules, and crusts, in the same region of the skin, and this should be looked for in the examination of the patient (Figure 191.1). Fever can be expected for the first 3 to 4 days of the exanthem, and much of the morbidity is associated with the extent of the cutaneous rash. In addition, primary VZV infection invades the mucosal surfaces of respiratory, alimentary, and genitourinary systems, and the patient with chickenpox can have severe laryngitis, laryngotracheobronchitis, vaginitis, urethritis, pancreatitis, and enteritis. Severe abdominal pain or back pain is a hallmark of progressive VZV infection in the immunocompromised individual.

Since the introduction of VZV vaccine, the age-unadjusted incidence of chickenpox has been approximately 3 cases per 1000 population, and the hospitalization rate for complications of chickenpox has decreased dramatically. Complications of chickenpox remain highest in persons younger than 1 year and older than 15 years and consist of bacterial superinfection of skin, dehydration, pneumonia, encephalitis, and hepatitis. Bacterial skin infections and bacterial pneumonias occur in the youngest groups, and before the antibiotic era severe bacterial infections, including osteomyelitis,

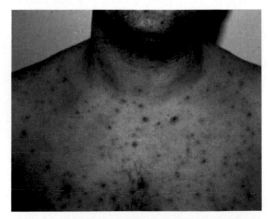

Figure 191.1 Varicella. Note various stages of lesions in each area of eruption. (Courtesy of David Schlossberg, MD.)

were not uncommon complications of chick-enpox. The rate of encephalitis, previously ~1 per 11000 cases in the age group 5 to 14 years, and of VZV-associated Reye's syndrome have been virtually eliminated, first with the recommendation against aspirin use in VZV infection and then with the VZV vaccine. With the availability of the vaccine, hospitalizations for chickenpox have significantly decreased and VZV-associated mortality is at an all-time low of less than 0.1 per million population.

Shingles

Shingles occurs when VZV infection reacti-vates in cranial or spinal nerve ganglia and then spreads to the cutaneous nerves. The in-cidence of disease in those older than 75 years is approximately 10 per 1000 person-years, and this can be significantly reduced with the zoster vaccine. The incidence is also increased in immunosuppressed patients. The clinical presentation and major complications of this disease derive from the neural origin of the virus infection. The most common area of in-volvement is the trunk, presumably because this is the area of greatest primary VZV in-fection, followed by cranial dermatomes and then by cervical and lumbar dermatomes. Thus, shingles presents with pain and with a vesicular eruption in a unilateral cutaneous distribution. Rarely, a pain syndrome, called *zoster sine herpete*, can be the only symptom of this disease. The pain of herpes zoster that persists for 30 days after the healing of skin le-sions is termed postherpetic neuralgia (PHN). PHN increases in frequency with age and is a major problem in patients with shingles after age 50 years. Virus reactivation in the spinal or cranial nerve ganglia causes intense inflam-mation with hemorrhagic necrosis of nerve cells, eventual destruction of portions of the ganglion, poliomyelitis of posterior spinal columns, and leptomeningitis. This intense inflammation results in nerve dysfunction manifested clinically by symptoms of men-ingitis and myelitis, with or without hyper-esthesia (in which nonnoxious stimuli can be painful) or even paresis at sites of involved nerves. Thus, in severe cases, in addition to allodynia, there may be weakness or paraly-sis of limbs, of facial muscles, and of muscles within abdominal viscera. In addition, intense inflammation of the cutaneous site of infection results in scarring of the involved epidermis. This is a particular concern when the cornea or other ophthalmic structures are involved.

DIAGNOSIS

The history and physical examination remain the primary methods for diagnosing chicken-pox and shingles. In chickenpox, look for le-sions in all stages of development, including macules, vesicles, pustules, and crusted le-sions. The rash of chickenpox can be mistaken for a diverse array of entities, such as rashes due to herpes simplex virus, coxsackie and other enteroviruses, mycoplasma, streptococ-cal impetigo, rickettsialpox, insect bites, and delayed-type hypersensitivity reactions such as poison ivy. Zosteriform herpes simplex occurs in approximately 4% of suspected shingles cases. For laboratory confirmation of diagno-sis, for both chickenpox and zoster, the most accurate method is DNA polymerase chain re-action (PCR) assay but the most rapid is the di-rect immunofluorescent stain of a skin scraping for VZV antigen using a commercially available kit. The Tzanck prep, a method to demonstrate multinucleated giant cells in skin scrapings stained with Wright–Giemsa, and virus isola-tion by tissue culture have been superseded by these assays. Conventional methods of culture of VZV or serology for VZV antibody can also be used to confirm the diagnosis, but the results of these tests will not be available as rapidly and therefore are less useful.

DETECTION OF SUSCEPTIBILITY TO VZV

For purposes of immunization, the revised definition of likely VZV immunity includes written documentation of age-appropriate immunization, history of chickenpox from a reliable source, laboratory evidence of immu-nity or infection, or birth in the United States before 1966. In adults, the simplest method of reliably ruling out susceptibility to chick-enpox is to obtain a history of chickenpox or of having cared for children with chickenpox, because a positive history from adults has a 97% to 99% correlation with serologic confir-mation. A negative history from an adult fails to conform to a negative serologic status in 72% to 93%. Therefore, serologic tests are nec-essary to determine whether a person with a negative history of chickenpox, who has not been vaccinated, has been infected with VZV. Commercial assays, fluorescent or enzyme-linked immunoassays, and a very rapid latex agglutination assay are useful except in per-sons who have received blood products and have acquired passive antibody.

PREVENTION AND THERAPY
VZV Vaccine

The live, attenuated VZV vaccine (Varivax) was approved in the United States in 1995 and is recommended for persons older than 12 months. Every person in the United States who does not have indicators for VZV immunity (see text immediately above) should have 2 doses of varicella vaccine. Specifically, infants older than 12 months and toddlers should have 2 doses in childhood, with the first given at approximately 1 year of age, usually as the measles, mumps, and rubella (MMR)-V vaccination, and the second given at some later time such as at the 5- to 6-year routine visit. Those 13 years of age and older should receive 2 doses of vaccine separated by an interval of at least 4 weeks. Each dose, for infants and adults, is 0.5 mL administered subcutaneously.

In addition to normal children, VZV vaccine use is particularly encouraged in eligible health care and day-care workers, college students, prisoners, military recruits, nonpregnant women of childbearing age, and international travelers. Protection from chickenpox can be expected in 90% to 95% depending on age. The vaccine is not recommended for infants <1 year old, for immunosuppressed persons, for those on salicylate therapy, for pregnant women, or those allergic to components of the vaccine, including neomycin, gelatin, and monosodium glutamate.

Chickenpox

OVERALL ASSESSMENT

The goal in management is to treat the symptoms of primary VZV infection and to prevent complications if possible. The three stages of management are (1) establishing the likelihood of the diagnosis, (2) determining whether antiviral therapy is indicated, and (3) ruling out secondary bacterial infection, other complications, and failure of previous antiviral treatment. In children, chickenpox usually requires minimal medical attention, but if there is an atypical course or severe skin involvement, the patient should have a physical examination to assess the level of hydration, the need for temperature control, the baseline mental status, and other physical findings that suggest complications. This is particularly true if any risk factors for severe disease are present, such as concomitant immunosuppressive therapy and age above 18 years.

SYMPTOMATIC THERAPY

Itching is the major symptom of chickenpox, and antipyretic management is important. Warm baths containing baking soda (1/3 cup per bathtub) or emulsified oatmeal (Aveno) can temporarily relieve pruritus. This can be combined with the oral administration of either diphenhydramine (Benadryl) 1.25 mg/kg every 6 hours or hydroxyzine (Atarax, Vistaril) 0.5 mg/kg every 6 hours. In older children, cold pramoxine HCl 1% lotion with calamine 8% (Caladryl) can be used, but this should be avoided in infants because of the risk of excessive surface exposure and absorption of drug or vehicle (alcohol 2.2%). Fever should be controlled with acetaminophen, but salicylates should not be used because administration of certain salicylates to children with chickenpox increases the risk of subsequent Reye's syndrome. For severe dysuria, a cold compress on the genital area during urination will ease the pain and minimize the likelihood of a functional bladder obstruction.

ANTIVIRAL THERAPY

Acyclovir (Zovirax) is the only agent licensed in the United States for the treatment of chickenpox. It is indicated for treatment of chickenpox in certain normal persons, for disseminated VZV infection in immunosuppressed persons, and for treatment of shingles. Oral acyclovir should be used in otherwise healthy persons with chickenpox who are at risk for moderate to severe disease, such as those older than 12 years, those with chronic cutaneous or pulmonary disorders, those receiving chronic salicylate therapy, and those receiving short, intermittent, or aerosolized courses of corticosteroids or aerosolized corticosteroids (Table 191.1). The American Academy of Pediatrics (AAP) does not recommend that otherwise normal children younger than 12 years receive oral acyclovir for chickenpox. In immunocompetent persons, virus replication ceases at approximately 72 hours after onset of rash, and it is likely that there is only a small period of time when such treatment would be useful. However, studies have shown that treatment of chickenpox within 24 hours of the onset of rash reduces the duration and magnitude of fever and the number and duration of skin lesions. Therefore, some experts recommend using oral acyclovir in secondary household cases because disease is usually more severe in these children. The data are insufficient regarding the safety and efficacy of acyclovir therapy for

Table 191.1 Antiviral Treatment of Varicella-Zoster Virus (VZV) Infection[a]

Agent	Indication	Creatinine Clearance (mL/min/1.73 M^2)	Dose	Dosing Interval	Duration (days)
Oral acyclovir	Chickenpox >age 12 y	>25	20 mg/kg up to 800 mg	4 times/d	5
		10–25	Same	q8h	5
		0–10[b]		q12h	5
	Shingles	>25	20 mg/kg up to 800 mg	5 times/d	5–7
		10–25	Same	q8h	5–7
		0–10[b]	Same	q12h	5–7
IV acyclovir	Life-threatening VZV infection	>50	500 mg/M^2 or 10 mg/kg[c,d]	q8h	7
		25–50	Same	q12h	7
		10–25	Same	q24h	7
		0–10[b]	250 mg/M^2	q24h	7
Famciclovir	Shingles >age 18 y	>60	500 mg	q8h	7
		40–59	500 mg	q12h	7
		20–39	500 mg	q24h	7
		≤20	250 mg	q24h	7
Valacyclovir	Shingles >age 18 y	>50	1000 mg	q8h	7
		30–49	1000 mg	q12h	7
		10–29	1000 mg	q24h	7
		≤10	500 mg	q24h	7
Foscarnet	Acyclovir-resistant VZV[e]	>100[f]	60 mg/kg	q8h	7–10

[a] See package insert for recommended dose adjustment of all drugs.
[b] An additional dose is recommended after each hemodialysis treatment.
[c] To minimize renal toxicity an adequate urine output is required. This can be assured if the acyclovir is infused at a concentration of approximately 4 mg/mL over 1 hour and the same volume of fluid is given over the next hour.
[d] Use ideal body weight for height to calculate dose in obese person: M^2, square meter of body surface area.
[e] Foscarnet is recommended by experts for treatment of life-threatening acyclovir-resistant VZV infection, but this is not an U.S. Food and Drug Administration (FDA)-approved indication for foscarnet use. Appropriate informed consent should be obtained before such use.
[f] Foscarnet is nephrotoxic, and dosage should be based on creatinine clearance. Guidelines for dosage adjustment are listed in the package information.

infants younger than 12 months, and it is not recommended.

All adults with chickenpox should receive oral acyclovir, and those with rapidly progressive infection should be treated with intravenous acyclovir. Valacyclovir (Valtrex) and famciclovir (Famvir), both of which are approved for treatment of shingles, are not approved in the United States for treatment of chickenpox. All immunosuppressed persons with chickenpox should be treated with intravenous acyclovir until the course of infection is defined. However, as noted by the AAP, some experts have used oral acyclovir in highly selected immunocompromised persons who are at relatively low risk for developing complications and in whom follow-up is assured. Case-by-case evaluation of risks versus benefits is necessary, but for many groups the risk of disseminating infection is sufficiently high and so unpredictable that intravenous treatment should be recommended in nearly all cases.

Intravenous acyclovir should be used for the pregnant patient with serious complications of varicella, but, if acyclovir is used routinely for the pregnant woman with uncomplicated chickenpox, it should be recognized that the risk and benefits to the fetus and mother are mostly unknown. Varicella-zoster immune-globulin (VZIG) is licensed for use in high-risk individuals at the time of exposure to VZV infection but is not recommended for treatment of chickenpox.

BACTERIAL INFECTIONS

Pyoderma is the most frequently observed bacterial complication of varicella. It can be minimized by attention to good hygiene, including daily bathing with bacteriostatic soap, trimming of children's fingernails to minimize excoriation of itchy skin, and early recognition of superinfection. Streptococcal and staphylococcal bacterial infections can be associated with bacteremia and subsequent osteomyelitis, with scarlet fever, and with bacterial synergetic gangrene. Therefore, aggressive management of bacterial infection is warranted.

RESPIRATORY TRACT INFECTION

In addition to the occasional laryngitis and laryngotracheobronchitis that can occur during chickenpox, bacterial superinfection can affect the lower respiratory tract, producing pneumonia and bronchitis. Pneumonia is most often due to the usual respiratory pathogens, including *Streptococcus pneumoniae*, *Haemophilus influenzae*, and *Staphylococcus aureus*. Viral pneumonia is more likely to be a problem in older persons with chickenpox, and pulmonary status should be monitored during treatment.

GASTROINTESTINAL COMPLICATIONS

When death occurs during VZV infection, the gastrointestinal tract is invariably involved. Specific attention must be given to bleeding, particularly in the immunosuppressed person. Vomiting is not a usual part of the clinical course of this infection, and it should alert the physician to look for abdominal or central nervous system complications. Also, surgical emergencies such as appendicitis and intussusception can occur during varicella. Mild hepatitis is seen in a majority of children with chickenpox, usually asymptomatic elevation of hepatic enzymes for which no treatment is necessary. However, elevation of serum or urinary amylase indicates pancreatitis, which may require supportive treatment. As noted, the concomitant use of aspirin in the child with chickenpox has been associated with an increased incidence of Reye's syndrome. Although this is rare today, Reye's syndrome and other metabolic diseases must be excluded in any child with varicella in whom there is vomiting and changes in mental status.

ENCEPHALITIS

Cerebral complications may be either cerebral or cerebellar abnormalities; the latter is a more benign disease. Cerebellar ataxia, the most common syndrome associated with varicella encephalitis, is generally a benign entity thought to be due to postinfectious demyelination. There is no evidence that acyclovir treatment is necessary in postchickenpox cerebellitis, but it is prudent to include antiviral therapy in any cerebral presentation of VZV infection, especially if it may be associated with continued viral replication such as in acquired immunodeficiency syndrome (AIDS) or other immunosuppressive states.

BLEEDING DISORDERS

Bleeding disorders during or just after chickenpox are due to disseminated intravascular coagulation, vasculitis, or idiopathic thrombocytopenic purpura (ITP), which can occur during active infection or convalescence. These should be managed according to conventional treatment, and there is no VZV-specific management regimen.

IMMUNOSUPPRESSED PATIENTS

As noted, acyclovir is the only indicated drug for the treatment of VZV infections in the immunosuppressed patient, whether disseminated chickenpox, disseminated shingles, or localized shingles. Three other commercial antiviral drugs, valacyclovir, famciclovir, and foscarnet (Foscavir), have activity against VZV. Valacyclovir and famciclovir are indicated for the treatment of shingles as described below (see Table 191.1). Foscarnet is recommended for the treatment of acyclovir-resistant VZV.

Shingles

OVERALL ASSESSMENT

The major complication of shingles is postherpetic pain. For this reason effective analgesic medication must be a principal part of treatment, and the initial assessment should be directed to a determination of general medical status and tolerance for narcotic-based therapy. In addition, there is increasing evidence that, early antiviral therapy can lessen late neuralgia; therefore, institution of specific anti-VZV agents is important in certain patients.

SYMPTOMATIC THERAPY

A hallmark of shingles is intense inflammation, and the cutaneous site of disease can take weeks to heal. The patient or caretaker should be instructed to have daily soaks with salt solutions and dressing changes to minimize bacterial infection and speed healing. If the eye is involved, an ophthalmologist should be consulted for use of topical anti-inflammatory or antiviral medication and for long-term evaluation. Management of pain will vary from patient to patient, but it usually begins with acetaminophen–codeine combinations and increases to more potent analgesia if indicated. In severe postherpetic neuralgia, if there is no response to conventional pain management, a specialist in pain management should be consulted, and in this setting gabapentin, tricyclic antidepressant medications, and other methods of pain control can be tried. Local nerve block has been used for refractory pain. Topical pain medications are not recommended, because the source of pain stimulation is central.

Use of corticosteroids in the acute phase of disease remains controversial, but studies combining corticosteroids and antiviral therapy have shown improvement in the acute processes, including pain, but these have not shown a decrease in PHN. There were more side effects with steroid use, and these should not be used on patients with certain obvious risk factors such as diabetes mellitus or gastritis. Corticosteroids for shingles should never be prescribed without concomitant antiviral medications. Because early treatment with antivirals alone can significantly reduce late postherpetic pain, this must be the focus of initial therapy.

ANTIVIRAL THERAPY

Acyclovir, valacyclovir, and famciclovir are licensed in the United States for the treatment of shingles in otherwise normal persons (see Table 191.1). Acyclovir is the agent of choice for immunocompromised persons and is the only intravenous agent available for treatment of shingles. Valacyclovir is the prodrug of acyclovir and, because of better bioavailability, is preferred over acyclovir for oral therapy of shingles. Famciclovir is an oral prodrug of the antiviral agent penciclovir, which has potent activity against VZV, and famciclovir undergoes rapid biotransformation to the active antiviral compound. Safety and efficacy in children has not been established for either valacyclovir or famciclovir. Also, because of the potential for tumorigenicity in rats, famciclovir should not be given to pregnant or nursing mothers unless nursing is discontinued.

Valacyclovir and famciclovir are the agents of choice for outpatient management of shingles and should be used in those older than 50 years because of their established efficacy in decreasing PHN. The decision to treat adults younger than 50 years with antiviral agents should be made on individual assessment.

Involvement of the first branch of the trigeminal nerve can result in severe pain syndromes and involvement of the eye that can be sight-threatening. Therefore, ophthalmic zoster should be managed in consultation with an ophthalmologist.

MANAGEMENT OF EXPOSURE TO VZV

The spread of infectious VZV from a person with chickenpox is by air droplets from naso-pharyngeal secretions, which usually requires face-to-face exposure indoors for an hour but can also be via air currents to susceptible individuals without direct contact. The period of respiratory infectivity is generally considered to begin 48 hours prior to the onset of exanthem and to continue for 4 days after onset. In addition, the vesicular fluid can spread the virus by direct contact, so infectivity by contact with skin lesions is possible until they are crusted. Shingles can also spread by direct contact or by exposure to airborne infectious material. The incubation period for chickenpox following exposure to shingles is the same as for exposure to chickenpox—15 days with a range of 10 to 21 days. The varicella attack rate in susceptible children on household exposure to chickenpox is approximately 90% and is 25% on exposure to household shingles.

IMMUNOCOMPROMISED HOST EXPOSED TO VZV

Until the VZV vaccine became available in the United States, the only protection from VZV infection was passive immunization at the time of exposure. Families and school personnel must continue to be aware of exposure to VZV in high-risk persons so that VZIG can be administered within 96 hours. Any susceptible person at risk for complications of VZV (Table 191.2) should receive passive immunization if exposure was adequate to communicate disease and occurred within approximately 4 days. Adequacy of exposure is defined as indoor face-to-face exposure for 1 hour with a person during the infectious phase. VZIG should not be used in any person with a history of chickenpox except persons who have undergone bone marrow transplantation. Immunosuppressive therapy should be stopped during the incubation period, although this precaution is waived if the underlying disease requires continued treatment, such as initial therapy for acute leukemia. Although not approved for such use, especially in children ≤12 years, valacyclovir, given at a dose of 1000 mg orally 3 times daily or 500 mg in those weighing less than 40 kg, can be effective in settings of acute exposure to VZV to prevent the development of chickenpox. Because VZIG has a significant failure rate and may not be as readily available, this method of prevention of chickenpox in at-risk immunosuppressed patients deserves consideration.

NORMAL ADULTS EXPOSED TO VZV

More than 90% of adults have had VZV, and although reinfection occurs after exposure

Table 191.2 Groups at Risk for Complications of VZV Infection[a]

Susceptible persons on immunosuppressive therapy[b]
Persons with congenital cellular immunodeficiency
Person with an acquired immunodeficiency, including AIDS
Persons older than 20 years
Newborn infants exposed to onset of maternal varicella less than 5 days before or 2 to 7 days after birth
Premature infants weighing <1 kilogram[c]

[a] Susceptible (antibody negative) persons exposed to VZV by indoor face-to-face contact with an infected person less than 2 days before or anytime during vesiculopustular stage of chickenpox are at highest risk and should receive VZIG.
[b] All cytoreductive chemotherapy and radiotherapy is considered immunosuppressive. The immunosuppressive dose of prednisone equivalent can vary in individual cases but is in the range of 1 to 2 mg/kg/d
[c] The risk of complications of VZV infection in this group, which is poorly defined, is based on the likelihood of protective maternal antibody versus gestational age at birth.
Abbreviations: VZV = varicella-zoster virus; AIDS = acquired immunodeficiency syndrome; VZIG = varicella-zoster immune-globulin.

to chickenpox, these persons do not usually develop disease, although some cutaneous lesions can occur. Susceptible adults are at risk for life-threatening chickenpox, and they are the source of unexpected epidemics. One adult population known to have a high rate of susceptibility to chickenpox is immigrants from subtropical climates. Serologic tests of susceptibility should be considered in any such immigrants working in a health care setting with subsequent immunization in the seronegatives. The decision to use VZIG in susceptible healthy adults following close exposure to VZV should be made on an individual basis, taking into consideration the person's health, the type of exposure, and the likelihood of previous chickenpox. Valacyclovir prophylaxis, as described above, is an unapproved alternative in this setting.

NOSOCOMIAL VZV

Control of nosocomial infections requires three actions: (1) routine continuous surveillance of VZV susceptibility among hospital staff, with VZV vaccination as indicated; (2) adequate isolation of contagious VZV infections; and (3) rapid evaluation of and response to exposure. Hospitals that care for immunodeficient children should screen staff

at the time of employment for susceptibility. This can be done efficiently by performing antibody tests on those who have a negative or unknown history of chickenpox. Susceptible employees should be vaccinated and excluded from care of patients with VZV infection until approximately 1 month after the second dose of vaccine. Exposed susceptible health care workers should be furloughed from the eighth day after initial exposure until 21 days after the last exposure.

If the VZV exposure is from a patient, he or she should be discharged if possible. If not possible, the patient should be placed in isolation designed to prevent spread of infection by both air and direct contact. Optimally this consists of a private room with negative air pressure relative to the corridor, with gown and glove precaution guidelines posted on the door and restricted entry for susceptible persons. Isolation should remain in effect until skin lesions are crusted.

After control of the source of infection comes quick assessment of 3 types of information: (1) the nature of the exposure and whether it is likely to result in secondary infections, (2) the susceptibility to VZV of the exposed patients or staff, and (3) the risk for complications in these exposed patients. Thus, the initial step is to define the hospital areas in which a definitive VZV exposure has occurred and then to focus on which patients in these areas are at risk for infection. Once susceptibility or positive history of varicella is determined and serologic evaluation of those with ambiguous or negative history is done, all susceptible patients who are exposed should be discharged if possible. Those remaining in the hospital should be placed in respiratory isolation between days 8 and 21 postexposure or for 8 to 28 days for those receiving VZIG. Those remaining in the hospital without exposure should be placed in a cohort that protects them from exposures.

MANAGEMENT OF THE PREGNANT WOMAN

A syndrome of congenital varicella consisting of low birth weight, cutaneous scarring, limb hypoplasia, microcephaly, and other brain and eye abnormalities can occur in the baby of a pregnant woman who has chickenpox. Teratogenic damage results only from first- and second-trimester infection, and clinically apparent disease occurs only in approximately 2% of infants born after maternal varicella in early pregnancy. For this reason, experts advise that maternal chickenpox is not a medical indication for abortion. There is no reliable diagnostic method, including amniocentesis and ultrasound, for determining teratogenic intrauterine infection. It is recommended that, after exposure in pregnancy, susceptibility be determined and that the susceptible person be given VZIG. With regard to antiviral therapy in the setting of pregnancy, acyclovir, valacyclovir, and famciclovir are category B drugs, meaning that, if there is a clinical need for the drug, it is considered safe to use it. However, it is generally recommended that these agents be used only if the benefit to the pregnant woman clearly exceeds the potential risk to the fetus.

SUGGESTED READING

Centers for Disease Control and Prevention. Prevention of varicella: updated recommendations of the Advisory Committee on Immunization Practices (ACIP). *Morbid Mortal Weekly Rep*. 1999;48(RR-6):1–5.

Enders G, Miller E, Cradock-Watson J, et al. Consequences of varicella and herpes zoster in pregnancy: prospective study of 1739 cases. *Lancet*. 1994;343: 1548–1551.

Gnann JW Jr, Whitley RJ. Clinical practice: herpes zoster. *N Engl J Med*. 2002;347(5): 340–346.

Nguyen HQ, Jumaan AO, Seward JF. Decline in mortality due to varicella after implementation of varicella vaccination in the United States. *N Engl J Med*. 2005;352(5):450–458.

Oxman MN, Levin MJ, Johnson GR, et al. A vaccine to prevent herpes zoster and postherpetic neuralgia in older adults. *N Engl J Med*. 2005;352(22): 2271–2284.

Preblud SR. Age-specific risks of varicella complications. *Pediatrics*. 1981;68:14–17.

Zaia JA, Grose C. Varicella and herpes zoster. In: Gorbach S, Bartlett J, Blacklow N, eds. *Infectious Diseases*. 2nd ed. Philadelphia, PA: W. B. Saunders; 1998:2081.

192. Viral Hemorrhagic Fevers

Daniel G. Bausch

INTRODUCTION

The term *viral hemorrhagic fever* (VHF) refers to an acute systemic illness classically involving fever, a constellation of initially nonspecific signs and symptoms, and a propensity for bleeding and shock. VHFs are caused by small, single-stranded, lipid-enveloped RNA viruses from four families (Table 192.1). Although VHFs collectively exist worldwide, the distribution of any given virus is generally restricted by the distribution of its natural reservoir and/or arthropod vector. Depending on the specific disease, virus may be transmitted to humans through direct exposure to contaminated blood or excreta of the animal reservoir or through the bite of an arthropod. Secondary human-to-human transmission also occurs with Ebola, Marburg, Crimean Congo hemorrhagic fever (CCHF), and the arenaviruses, especially Lassa (Table 192.1).

PATHOLOGY AND PATHOGENESIS

Consideration of the underlying pathogenesis helps guide treatment. Although the pathophysiology of the VHFs varies with the specific virus, certain common hallmarks can be identified, namely microvascular instability and impaired hemostasis. Contrary to popular thought, mortality in VHF usually results not directly from exsanguination, but rather from a process akin to septic shock, with insufficient effective circulating intravascular volume leading to cellular dysfunction and multiorgan system failure. In fact, external bleeding is seen in a minority of cases.

After inoculation, virus typically replicates in local tissues and regional lymph nodes and is then subsequently disseminated through the lymph and blood monocytes to a broad number of tissues and organs, including the liver, spleen, lymph node, adrenal gland, lung, and endothelium. Migration of tissue macrophages ensues, with secondary infection of permissive parenchymal cells. The particular organs most affected vary with the VHF. Inflammatory cell infiltrates are usually mild, consisting of a mix of mononuclear cells and neutrophils. The interaction of virus with immune cells, especially macrophages and endothelial cells, either directly or indirectly via soluble mediators, results in cell activation and the unleashing of an inflammatory and vasoactive process consistent with the systemic inflammatory response syndrome. Impaired hemostasis may entail endothelial cell, platelet, and/or coagulation factor dysfunction. Disseminated intravascular coagulation (DIC) is frequently noted in some VHFs. Tissue damage may ultimately be mediated through direct necrosis of infected cells or indirectly through apoptosis of immune cells and induced perturbations of normal organ homeostasis. Data from animal models suggest that cardiac inotropy may be directly or indirectly inhibited in some VHFs, further impairing organ perfusion. Adrenal or pituitary gland necrosis with consequent vascular collapse has been postulated but not specifically demonstrated. Virus is cleared rapidly in survivors, with the exception of a few immunologically protected sites, such as the chambers of the eye and gonads, resulting in sexual transmission months after recovery from acute disease (best documented for Ebola, Marburg, and Lassa viruses).

The pathogenesis of most VHFs appears to be related to unchecked viremia due to virus-induced impairment of cellular immunity. One exception is hemorrhagic fever with renal syndrome (HFRS), where virus is usually cleared prior to the most severe phase of the disease and the host immune response may play a detrimental role. The unique process of antibody-mediated enhancement may facilitate the development of dengue hemorrhagic fever.

CLINICAL PRESENTATION

Although the clinical presentation may differ for each VHF as it progresses, in most cases the limited data do not permit clear distinctions, especially in the early phases of disease. At presentation, most patients show nonspecific signs

Table 192.1 Principal Viruses Causing Hemorrhagic Fevers

Virus	Disease	Geographic Distribution
Filoviridae		
Ebola	Ebola hemorrhagic fever	Sub-Saharan Africa, Philippines?
Marburg	Marburg hemorrhagic fever	Sub-Saharan Africa
Arenaviridae[b]		
Lassa	Lassa fever	West Africa
Junin	Argentine hemorrhagic fever	Argentine pampas
Machupo	Bolivian hemorrhagic fever	Beni department, Bolivia
Guanarito	Venezuelan hemorrhagic fever	Portuguesa state, Venezuela
Sabiá[c]	Proposed name: Brazilian hemorrhagic fever	Rural area near Sao Paulo, Brazil?
Flexal[d]	Proposed name: None	Brazilian Amazon
Bunyaviridae		
Hantaan, Seoul, Puumala, Dobrava, others (see also Chapter 184, Hantavirus Cardiopulmonary Syndrome in the Americas)	Hemorrhagic fever with renal syndrome	Hantaan: northeast Asia; Seoul: urban areas worldwide; Puumala and Dobrava: Europe
Rift Valley fever	Rift Valley fever	Sub-Saharan Africa
Crimean-Congo hemorrhagic fever	Crimean-Congo hemorrhagic fever	Africa, Middle East, Balkans, southern Russia, western China
Flaviviridae		
Yellow fever	Yellow fever	Africa, South America
Dengue	Dengue fever and dengue hemorrhagic fever	Tropics and subtropics worldwide
Omsk hemorrhagic fever	Omsk hemorrhagic fever	Western Siberia
Kyasanur Forest disease	Kyasanur Forest disease	Karnataka state, India
Alkhumra hemorrhagic fever[f]	Proposed name: Alkhumra hemorrhagic fever	Saudi Arabia

[a] Although some endemic transmission of the filoviruses (Ebola > Marburg) and Rift Valley fever virus occurs, these viruses have <200. Filovirus epidemics have been recognized with increasing frequency during the period 1994–2006.
[b] Although evidence of infection with the North American arenavirus Whitewater Arroyo has been noted in sick persons, its role
[c] First discovered in 1990. Only 3 cases (1 fatal) of Sabiá virus infection have been noted, 2 of them related to laboratory infection.
[d] A single case of human infection (nonfatal) with Flexal virus has been reported from a presumed laboratory exposure in Belem,
[e] Based on estimates from the World Health Organization. Significant underreporting occurs. Incidence may fluctuate widely
[f] Alkhumra is considered by some to be a variant of Kyasanur Forest disease virus. Controversy exists over the proper spelling

Principal Reservoir/Vector	Annual Cases	Case:Infection Ratio	Human-to-Human Transmissibility
Unknown	—[a]	1:1	High
Unknown	—[a]	1:1	High
Rodent (the "multimammate rat" or *Mastomys natalensis*)	100 000–300 000	1:5–10	Moderate
Rodent (the "corn mouse" or *Calomys musculinus*)	~100	1:1.5	Low
Rodent (the "large vesper mouse" or *Calomys callosus*)	≤50	1:1.5	Low
Rodent (the "cane mouse" or *Zygodontomys brevicauda*)	≤50	1:1.5	Low
Unknown (Rodent?)	—[c]	1:1.5	Low?
Rodent (*Oryzomys* species)	—[d]	Unknown	Unknown
Rodent (Hantaan: the "striped field mouse" or *Apodemus agrarius*; Seoul: the "Norway rat" or *Rattus norvegicus*; Puumala: the "bank vole" or *Clethrionomys glareolus*; Dobrava: the "yellow-necked field mouse" or *Apodemus flavicollis*)	50 000–150 000	Hantaan: 1:1.5 Others: 1:20	No
Domestic livestock/mosquitoes (*Aedes* and others)	100–100 000[a]	1:100	No
Wild and domestic vertebrates/tick (*Hyalomma* spp.)	~500	1:1–2	High
Monkey/mosquito (*Aedes aegypti*, other *Aedes* and *Haemagogus* spp.)	5000–200 000[e]	1:2–20	No
Human/mosquito (*Aedes aegypti*)	Dengue fever: 100 million, Dengue hemorrhagic fever: 100 000–200 000[e]	1:10–100 depending on age, previous infection, genetic background, and infecting serotype	No
Rodent/tick (*Ixodes*), maintenance cycle incompletely understood	100–200	Unknown	Not reported
Vertebrate (rodents, bats, birds, monkeys, others)/tick (*Ixodes*)	400–500	Unknown	Not reported, but laboratory infections have occurred
Ticks?	≤50	Unknown	Not reported

most often been associated with epidemics. Ebola hemorrhagic fever epidemics typically involve <500 people and Marburg

as a pathogen has not been clearly established.
Disease from this virus is presumed to be similar to the other South American arenavirus hemorrhagic fevers.
Brazil, in 1978.
depending on epidemic activity.
of the virus, written as "Alkhurma" in some publications.

Table 192.2 Clinical Aspects of the Viral Hemorrhagic Fevers

Disease	Incubation Period (days)	Onset	Bleeding	Rash	Jaundice
Filoviridae					
Ebola hemorrhagic fever	3–21	Abrupt	++	+++	+
Marburg hemorrhagic fever	3–21	Abrupt	++	+++	+
Arenaviridae					
Lassa fever	5–16	Gradual	+	++	0
South American hemorrhagic fevers[a]	7–14	Gradual	+++	0	0
Bunyaviridae					
Hemorrhagic fever with renal syndrome	9–35	Abrupt	+++	0	0
Rift Valley fever[b]	2–5	Abrupt	+++	+	++
Crimean-Congo hemorrhagic fever	3–12	Abrupt	+++	0	++
Flaviviridae					
Yellow fever	3–6	Abrupt	+++	0	+++
Dengue hemorrhagic fever	3–15	Abrupt	++	+++	+
Omsk hemorrhagic fever	3–8	Abrupt	++	0	0
Kyasanur forest disease	3–8	Abrupt	++	0	0
Alkhumra hemorrhagic fever[c]	3–8	Abrupt	++	+	+

[a] Data are insufficient to distinguish between Argentine, Bolivian, Venezuelan, and Brazilian hemorrhagic fevers. They are thus
[b] Hemorrhagic fever, encephalitis, and retinitis may be seen in Rift Valley fever independently of each other.
[c] Based on preliminary observations. Fewer than 100 cases have been reported.
Key: 0 = sign not typically noted/organ not typically affected, + = sign occasionally noted/organ occasionally affected, ++ = sign

and symptoms difficult to distinguish from a host of other febrile illnesses (Table 192.2). Illness typically begins with fever and constitutional symptoms, including general malaise, anorexia, headache, chest or retrosternal pain, sore throat, myalgia, arthralgia, lumbosacral pain, and dizziness. The pharynx may be erythemic or, less frequently, exudative, especially in Lassa fever, incorrectly leading to a diagnosis of streptococcal pharyngitis (Figure 192.1A). Gastrointestinal signs and symptoms readily ensue, including nausea and vomiting, epigastric and abdominal pain and tenderness (especially in the right upper quadrant in Ebola hemorrhagic fever), and diarrhea. VHF has sometimes been mistaken for acute appendicitis or other abdominal emerg-

encies. Hepatosplenomegaly is frequently seen, but it is unknown whether this is specific to the VHF or simply represents the high underlying prevalence of hepatosplenomegaly in populations in sub-Saharan Africa where most clinical observations have been made. A dry cough, sometimes accompanied by a few scattered rales on auscultation, is frequently noted, but prominent pulmonary symptoms or the presence of productive sputum early in the course of disease are uncommon. Conjunctival injection or hemorrhage is seen in about a third of the patients but is *not* typically accompanied by itching, discharge, or rhinitis (Figures 192.1B and C). Various forms of skin rash, including morbilliform, maculopapular, petechial, and

Specific Organisms – Viruses

Heart	Lung	Kidney	Central Nervous System	Eye	Case Fatality Ratio	Clinical Management
++?	+	+	+	+	50%–90%	Supportive
++?	+	+	+	+	35%–80%	Supportive
++	+	0	+	0	2%–20%	Ribavirin
++	+	0	+++	0	15%–30%	Convalescent plasma, ribavirin
++	+	+++	+	0	Hantaan: 5–15% Seoul: ≤ 1% Puumala: ≤ 1%	Ribavirin
+?	0	+	++	++	50%	Ribavirin?
+?	+	0	+	0	15%–30%	Ribavirin
++	+	++	++	0	20%–50%	Supportive
++	+	0	+	0	Untreated: 10–15% Treated: ≤1%	Supportive
+	++	0	+++	+	1%–3%	Supportive
+	++	0	+++	+	3%–5%	Supportive
+	+	0	++	+	20%–25%	Supportive

frequently grouped as the "South American hemorrhagic fevers."

commonly noted/organ commonly affected, +++ = sign characteristic/organ involvement severe.

ecchymotic, may be seen, depending on the specific VHF (Figure 192.1D).

In severe cases, patients progress to vascular instability and hemorrhage. Evidence of vascular instability may include conjunctival injection/hemorrhage, facial flushing, edema, bleeding, hypotension, shock, and proteinuria (Figures 192.1B, C, E–H). The likelihood of clinically discernible hemorrhage varies with the infecting virus and may be manifested as hematemesis, melena, hematochezia, metrorrhagia, petechiae, purpura, epistaxis, and bleeding from the gums and venupuncture sites (Figures 192.1E–G). Hemoptysis and hematuria are infrequently seen. Hemorrhage is almost never present in the first 48 hours of illness. Central nervous system manifestations, including disorientation, gait anomalies, convulsions, and hiccups may be noted in end-stage disease. Renal insufficiency or failure may occur, especially in HFRS, as the name implies. Pregnant women often present with spontaneous abortion and vaginal bleeding. With the exception of yellow fever, jaundice is not typical of the VHFs. Radiographic and electrocardiogram (EKG) findings generally correlate with the physical exam.

The clinical course of VHF usually unfolds quite rapidly, with death in fatal cases 7 to 10 days after symptom onset. Distinct phases of disease and recovery are classically described for HFRS, yellow fever, and dengue hemorrhagic fever, although they are not seen in all

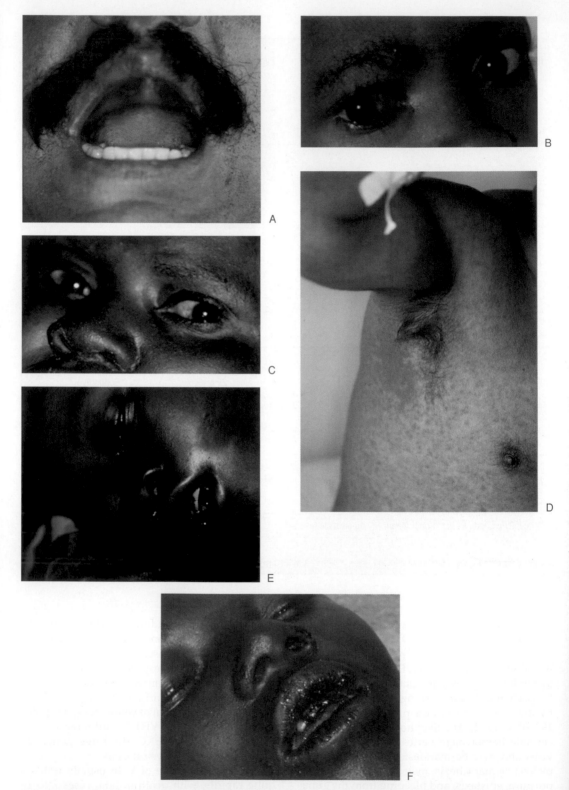

Figure 192.1 Clinical manifestations of viral hemorrhagic fever. **(A)** Soft and hard palate erythema in Lassa fever. **(B)** Subconjunctival hemorrhage in Lassa fever. **(C)** Subconjunctival hemorrhage in Ebola hemorrhagic fever. **(D)** Maculopapular skin rash in Lassa fever. **(E)** Severe oral and nasal mucosal bleeding in Ebola hemorrhagic fever. **(F)** Mild oral and nasal mucosal bleeding in Lassa fever. **(G)** Rectal bleeding in Ebola hemorrhagic fever. **(H)** Facial edema in Lassa fever.

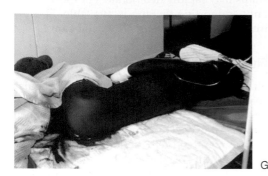 G

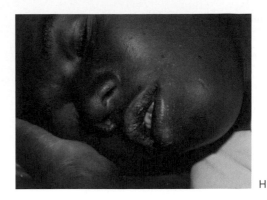 H

Figure 192.1 (continued)

cases. Common indicators of a poor prognosis include shock, bleeding, neurological manifestations, high viremia (or surrogate measurements of antigen or genome copies), and elevated levels of aspartate aminotransferase (>150 IU/L). Maternal and fetal mortality are elevated in pregnancy, especially during the third trimester. However, mild and even asymptomatic cases have been reported even for what are considered the most virulent VHFs. Reasons for the heterogeneity in severity are largely unknown, although differences in route and dose of infection, underlying comorbid illness, and genetic predisposition have been postulated. An association between certain major histocompatibility markers and severity of disease has been reported for HFRS.

DIFFERENTIAL DIAGNOSIS

The early nonspecific clinical presentation of VHF makes it extremely difficult to diagnose clinically, especially outside of the setting of a recognized outbreak. The differential diagnosis includes a broad array of febrile illnesses that may vary by geographic region (Table 192.3). A diagnosis of VHF should be considered in patients with a clinically compatible syndrome who, within 3 weeks prior to disease onset, (1) traveled in areas where a VHF is known or suspected to be endemic, (2) had potential direct contact with blood or bodily fluids of a person or animal with VHF during their acute illness (this group most often is composed of health care workers), (3) had contact with live or recently killed wild animals (especially nonhuman primates) in or recently arriving from an area where a VHF is endemic, (4) worked in a laboratory or animal facility where hemorrhagic fever viruses are handled, or (5) had sexual relations with someone recovering from a VHF in the last

3 months. Acts of bioterrorism must be considered if VHF is strongly suspected in a patient without any of the above criteria, especially if clusters of cases are seen. It should be remembered that most VHFs are rare even in persons possessing one of the above risk factors, so alternative diagnoses, especially malaria and typhoid fever, should always be aggressively sought.

LABORATORY DIAGNOSIS

Prompt laboratory confirmation is imperative, although testing is presently available only in a few specialized laboratories. In the United States, testing can be arranged through the Centers for Disease Control and Prevention (404-639-1115). Assays commonly used in the diagnosis of the VHFs include the enzyme-linked immunosorbent assays (ELISAs) for viral antigen and specific immunoglobulin M (IgM) and immunoglobulin G (IgG) antibodies, polymerase chain reaction, virus culture, and immunohistochemistry on postmortem tissues. Immunofluorescent antibody assays, which are more subjective and often lack specificity, have been largely supplanted by ELISA. A variety of new diagnostic approaches are currently being researched.

CLINICAL MANAGEMENT

The rarity of most VHFs and their typical occurrence in remote and resource-poor settings make controlled studies on clinical management difficult. Most recommendations represent the informal consensus of experienced clinicians and investigators. Because of their associated severity, risk of secondary spread, high degree of public scrutiny, and unfamiliarity on the part of most physicians, consultation with infectious disease specialists or other clinicians with experience treating patients with VHFs should be

Table 192.3 Differential Diagnosis of the Viral Hemorrhagic Fevers

Parasites
Malaria
Amebiasis
Giardiasis
African trypanosomiasis (acute phase)

Bacteria
Typhoid fever
Bacillary dysentery (including shigellosis, campylobacteriosis, salmonellosis, and enterohemorrhagic *Escherichia coli*)
Meningococcemia
Staphylococcemia
Septicemic plague
Streptococcal pharyngitis (may mimic the exudative pharyngitis sometimes seen in Lassa fever)
Tularemia
Acute abdominal emergencies (appendicitis and peritonitis)
Pyelonephritis and poststreptococcal glomerulonephritis (may mimic hemorrhagic fever with renal syndrome)
Anthrax (inhalation or gastrointestinal)
Psittacosis

Viruses
Influenza
Arbovirus infection (including dengue, yellow fever, and West Nile fever)
Viral hepatitis (including hepatitis A, B, and E, Epstein-Barr, and cytomegalovirus)
Measles
Rubella
Hemorrhagic or flat smallpox
Alphavirus infection (including chikungunya and o'nyong-nyong)
Other viral hemorrhagic fevers (see Table 192.1)

Spirochetes, Rickettsia, Ehrlichia, and Coxiella
Relapsing fever
Leptospirosis
Spotted fever group rickettsia (including Rocky Mountain spotted fever, Boutonneuse fever, African tick bite fever)
Typhus group rickettsia (including murine- and louse-borne typhus)
Q fever
Ehrlichiosis

Noninfectious Etiologies
Thrombotic thrombocytopenic purpura
Acute glaucoma (may mimic the acute ocular manifestations of Rift Valley fever)
Leukemia (may resemble the leukemoid reaction occasionally seen in hemorrhagic fever with renal syndrome)

sought as soon as the diagnosis is considered. Furthermore, all suspected cases of VHF should be reported immediately to local, state, and federal health authorities. Patients should be placed in isolation (see Infection Control below) and, if possible, in an intensive care unit, as the clinical status may rapidly deteriorate. For most VHFs, only supportive therapy is available. Specific treatment guidelines are provided below.

Fluid Management

Fluid management in VHF poses a particular challenge. Severe microvascular instability often dictates aggressive fluid replacement, which may also prevent DIC. However, overaggressive and unmonitored rehydration may lead to significant third-spacing and pulmonary edema, especially given the impaired cardiac function present in some VHFs. Although invasive hemodynamic monitoring through the placement of a Swan–Ganz catheter would seem to be in order, with the exception of peripheral intravenous lines, indwelling vascular devices should probably be considered contraindicated due to the risk of bleeding at the site, although they have been occasionally placed without reported complications. The decision whether to place an indwelling catheter or reply on blood pressure cuff values should probably be made on a case-by-case basis.

Because the pathogenesis of most advanced and severe cases of VHF is consistent with septic shock, it is reasonable to implement proven management strategies for this condition. Early goal-directed therapies have been shown to mitigate both mortality and organ dysfunction. Crystalloids (normal saline or Ringers lactate) and, if necessary, vasopressors should be infused to maintain central venous pressure between 8 and 12 mm Hg or mean arterial blood pressure above 65 mm Hg. Although the matter remains a subject of debate, dopamine and norepinephrine are presently the vasopressor regimen of choice. Dobutamine should be added if the above measures, along with blood transfusion (see below), fail to maintain the target blood pressure and adequate organ perfusion, based on clinical grounds. Peritoneal and hemodialysis have been employed extensively in patients with HFRS without frequent complications, although there is little published experience with the other VHFs. Low-dose dopamine and sodium bicarbonate have not been shown to be efficacious in septic shock and are not recommended. Similarly, routine use of vasopressin or intensive insulin therapy is not recommended.

Blood Products and Management of DIC

Bleeding may be profuse in some VHFs, especially CCHF and Ebola and Marburg hemorrhagic fevers. Significant internal bleeding from the gastrointestinal tract may occur even in the absence of external hemorrhage. Nevertheless, blood products should not be given empirically, but rather to meet defined clinical and laboratory parameters in the face of clinically significant hemorrhage. Extrapolating from data on septic shock, packed red blood cells should be transfused to maintain a hematocrit over 30%, with the usual attention to the risk of volume overload. Whole blood may be a reasonable substitute in developing world sites where packed cells are not available.

The possibility of DIC should be specifically assessed and treatment implemented when a patient manifests consistent laboratory parameters (see Clinical Laboratory Testing below) *and* active bleeding. Treatment should not be based on laboratory results alone except in preparation for an invasive procedure or when platelet levels fall to dangerously low levels. Replacement therapy with various blood products is the mainstay. Transfusion of platelet concentrate (1–2 U/10 kg) should be considered when the platelet count is <50 000/μL in a bleeding patient or <10 000/μL without bleeding. The platelet count should generally rise by at least 2000/μL per unit of platelets transfused, although a lesser response may occur if there is ongoing DIC and platelet consumption. Platelet aggregation may be impaired in some VHFs, especially Lassa fever, promoting hemorrhage even when platelet counts are not drastically low.

Transfusion of fresh frozen plasma (FFP) (15–20 mL/kg) should be considered when bleeding is present and fibrinogen levels are <100 mg/dL. Fibrinogen concentrates (total dose 2–3 g) or cryoprecipitates (1 U/10 kg) may be administered in place of FFP, although FFP has the theoretical advantage of containing all coagulation factors and inhibitors deficient in DIC and no activated coagulation factors. Vitamin K (10 mg on 2 consecutive days) may be given to patients with DIC to replenish stores of vitamin K–dependent coagulation enzymes, especially if underlying malnutrition or liver disease is suspected. Folic acid has also sometimes been added in DIC to prevent the detrimental effect of acute folate deficiency on platelet production.

Oxygenation and Ventilation

Impaired gas exchange is not typically a prominent feature of VHF, especially in the early phases of disease and in the absence of iatrogenic pulmonary edema. Due to the risk of bleeding, arteriopuncture for blood gas determination should be kept to a minimum, relying when possible on the respiratory rate and pulse oximetry. Oxygen should be administered by nasal cannula or face mask to patients with unfavorable parameters. Mechanical ventilation has rarely been available or employed in the treatment of VHF and should probably be avoided unless absolutely necessary due to the risk of barotrauma and consequent pleuropulmonary hemorrhage. When required, low tidal volumes (ie, lung-protective ventilation) would be best.

Antiviral Drugs

The only currently available specific antiviral therapy for the VHFs is the guanosine analog ribavirin (Table 192.2). The best data are for Lassa fever, for which intravenous ribavirin has been shown to decrease mortality in severe disease from 55% to 5% when begun within the first 6 days of illness. Based on limited data, the drug appears also to be efficacious in other arenavirus hemorrhagic fevers as well. Ribavirin has been shown to reduce mortality in HFRS if administered within 4 days of onset. The Chinese drug chongcao shenkang has also been reported to be efficacious in HFRS. Numerous observational studies and anecdotal reports support the use of ribavirin in CCHF, although randomized prospective studies have not been performed. In vitro and animal data show activity of ribavirin against Rift Valley fever virus, but a prospective trial in humans in Saudi Arabia in 2000 was stopped after an increase in encephalitis was noted in the ribavirin group. However, retrospective analysis showed some significant baseline discrepancies between the treatment and control groups, making definitive conclusions difficult. In vitro data also generally show activity of ribavirin against dengue and yellow fever viruses, but clinical studies have not been performed. The drug is not efficacious and should not be used for Ebola or Marburg hemorrhagic fevers.

Pharmacokinetic and sensitivity testing for ribavirin has not been extensively performed for each VHF. The intravenous dose used is derived from that found efficacious in Lassa fever: 30 mg/kg loading dose, followed by 15 mg/kg every 6 hours for 4 days, followed by 7.5 mg/kg every 8 hours for 6 days (total course 10 days). The drug should be diluted in 150 mL of 0.9% saline and slowly infused. The main side effects of intravenous ribavirin are a mild-to-moderate anemia, which infrequently necessitates transfusion and disappears with cessation of treatment, and rigors when the drug is infused too rapidly. Oral ribavirin has also been reported to be efficacious in many VHFs, especially CCHF, but few controlled data are available.

Convalescent Plasma

The most data on the use of convalescent plasma are for arenavirus infections. Transfusion of appropriately titered convalescent plasma within the first 8 days of illness reduces the case fatality of Argentine hemorrhagic fever (AHF) from 15% to 30% to <1%. However, this therapy has been associated with a convalescent-phase neurologic syndrome characterized by fever, cerebellar signs, and cranial nerve palsies in 10% of those treated. The syndrome occurs after a period of 7 to 80 days (mean 20 days) free of symptoms and differs from the neurologic manifestations seen in the acute disease. Given this complication and the potential transmission of concomitant viruses, such as human immunodeficiency virus (HIV) and hepatitis viruses, with convalescent plasma, substitution of ribavirin for plasma in the treatment of AHF should be considered, although direct comparisons of the two have yet to be conducted.

Animal studies show convalescent plasma to be efficacious in Lassa fever as well, but only if it contains a high titer of neutralizing antibody (which cannot uniformly be assumed) and there is a close antigenic match between the infecting viruses of the donor and recipient. Given these major constraints, ribavirin is a better choice. The efficacy of convalescent plasma has not been extensively investigated in other VHFs, with the exception of Ebola hemorrhagic fever, in which data from animal models and a limited number of observations in human do not show efficacy.

Coagulation Modulators

A growing body of literature suggests that disturbances in the procoagulant–anticoagulant balance play an important role in the mediation of septic shock. Although a number of the anticoagulant therapies for septic shock have been investigated, including heparin sulfate, antithrombin III, and tissue-factor pathway inhibitor, only activated protein C has shown clinical efficacy (24 µg/kg/hour constant infusion) and been U.S. Food and Drug Administration (FDA) approved. However, recent studies have cast some doubt on these findings. Furthermore, serious bleeding, including intracranial hemorrhage, was noted as an adverse effect of ac-

tivated protein C, a finding that would seem to contraindicate its use in VHF. However, the mechanism of activated protein C may not, in fact, be via direct anticoagulation but rather through modulation of inflammation. Conceivably, early use could mitigate the pathogenic processes in VHF that ultimately result in hemorrhage, with no additional risk of bleeding due to the drug itself.

A small study of Ebola-infected monkeys treated with activated protein C as postexposure prophylaxis showed a small survival benefit (18%). A slightly higher benefit (33%) was seen in monkeys treated with a recombinant inhibitor of tissue factor–initiated blood coagulation (rNAPc2), but efficacy trials have not been conducted in humans. Until the issue is more systematically explored, use of activated protein C should be made on a case-by-case basis. The use of heparin in septic shock and DIC is controversial and should be considered contraindicated until more data on its safety and efficacy are available, although lower mortality was recently noted in heparin-treated patients with severe sepsis in a phase III clinical trial.

Immune Modulators

Recognition that overactive immune responses, both innate and adaptive, may play deleterious roles in the pathogenesis of septic shock has prompted trials of various immune modulators, including ibuprofen, corticosteroids, anti-tumor necrosis factor-alpha (TNF-α), nitric oxide inhibitors, and various interleukins, but none have shown conclusive benefit. A few clinical trials of corticosteroids in HFRS have provided conflicting results. A small study of recombinant interleukin-2 showed that the drug reduces the degree of acute renal insufficiency in HFRS, but further studies are needed before this can be considered the standard of care.

There has been renewed interest in the use of corticosteroids for possible adrenal insufficiency in septic shock. Interestingly, viral infection of the adrenal cortex as well as adrenal gland necrosis have been reported in humans and animals with various VHFs. Results of trials of corticosteroid replacement in shock have been mixed. The matter is further complicated by controversy over the best way to assess adrenal insufficiency. Measurement of free cortisol in response to adrenocorticotropin stimulation is probably best but not always technically feasible. Furthermore, the use of corticosteroids might exacerbate the immunosuppression that is a common component of some VHFs. Until more conclusive studies are conducted, corticosteroids should probably not be administered unless adrenal insufficiency is specifically and unequivocally demonstrated, the target blood pressure is not maintained despite adequate fluid repletion and vasopressors, or in conjunction with mannitol if cerebral edema is suspected. If necessitated, physiological doses should be used (hydrocortisone 200–300 mg/day in 3 or 4 doses administered by continuous infusion for 7 days).

Antibiotics and Secondary Infection

Patients should be covered with appropriate antibacterial and/or antiparasitic therapy (especially for malaria if traveling in the tropics) until a diagnosis of VHF can be confirmed or when secondary infection is suspected. These drugs should be stopped once the diagnosis of VHF is established.

Pain Control

Oral acetaminophen, tramadol, opiates, or other analgesics should be used as needed for pain control. Intramuscular and subcutaneous injections and the use of salicylates or nonsteroidal anti-inflammatory drugs should be avoided because of the risk of hematoma. Antiemetics, such as the phenothiazines, are frequently warranted. Prophylactic therapy for stress ulcers with H_2 receptor antagonists or proton pump inhibitors is appropriate, although the efficacy of the latter has not been specifically demonstrated.

Management of Seizures and Other Central Nervous System Manifestations

Seizures sometimes occur in late-stage VHF but can usually be managed with benzodiazepines or phenytoin. The use of sedatives and neuromuscular blocking agents should also be minimized as much as possible due to potential exacerbation of the encephalopathy, polyneuropathy, and myopathy associated with sepsis. When necessary, low dose, short-acting psychoactive drugs, such as haloperidol or the benzodiazepines, may be used, with careful attention to potential vasodilation and hypotension.

Clinical Laboratory Testing

A broad range of clinical laboratory parameters should be monitored in patients with VHF (Table 192.4). Third spacing, vomiting, diarrhea, decreased fluid intake, and the administration of intravenous fluids may result in significant electrolyte imbalance. Laboratory tests for DIC should be specifically assessed in each patient and, if present, D-dimer levels monitored in response to therapeutic measures. Although hyperglycemia has not been reported to be a frequent problem in VHF, glucose should be monitored and levels kept <150 mg/dL via the use of intravenous insulin because strict glucose control has been shown to reduce morbidity and mortality in patients with septic shock and an intensive care unit (ICU) stay of >5 days.

Nutrition

Attention should be given to adequate nutrition, especially if the patient's course is prolonged or the patient is malnourished. Gut feeding is preferable to parenteral alimentation. Nasogastric tubes may be theoretically indicated for patients unable to eat, but there is little practical experience with their use in the VHFs. Exacerbation of gastrointestinal bleeding and heightened risk of transmission to health care workers during tube placement are concerns.

Management of Pregnancy

Uterine evacuation appears to lower maternal mortality in VHF and should be considered because it may be lifesaving for the mother, and fetal loss and neonatal mortality often approach 100% anyway. Although technically contraindicated in pregnancy, ribavirin should similarly be considered as a lifesaving measure for the mother in severe cases of the VHFs for which the drug is efficacious.

Postexposure Prophylaxis

Contrary to popular belief, secondary attack rates in most VHFs are low (15%–20%). Thus, postexposure prophylaxis should be considered only in persons with distinct high-risk exposures, usually either a needle stick or other direct and specific unprotected contact with blood or body fluids of a patient during their acute illness. As persons with VHF are not infectious before the onset of symptoms, prophylaxis should never be given when the only exposure was during the incubation period.

Postexposure prophylaxis with oral ribavirin has been recommended for some VHFs, especially Lassa fever, although no systematically collected data on its efficacy are available.

Table 192.4 Indicated Laboratory Tests and Characteristic Findings in the Viral Hemorrhagic Fevers

Test	Characteristic Findings and Comments
Leukocyte count	Early: moderate leukopenia, sometimes with atypical lymphocytes; Later: leukocytosis with left shift
Hemoglobin and hematocrit	Hemoconcentration
Platelet count	Mild-to-moderate thrombocytopenia
Electrolytes	Sodium, potassium, and acid-base perturbations, depending upon fluid balance and stage of disease
BUN/creatinine	Renal failure may occur late in disease
AST, ALT, amylase	Increased, usually AST > ALT
Coagulation studies (PT, PTT, fibrinogen, fibrin split products, platelets, D-dimer)	DIC common
Urinalysis	Proteinuria common
Blood culture	Used to exclude VHF or may indicate secondary infection
Stool culture	Used to exclude bacillary dysentery
Thick and thin smears for malaria (or other molecular-based assay)	Negative in VHF unless coinfection with malaria
Febrile agglutinins or other assay for *Salmonella typhi*	Negative in VHF unless coinfection with *S. typhi*

Abbreviations: ALT = alanine aminotransferase; AST = aspartate aminotransferase; DIC = disseminated intravascular coagulation; VHF = viral hemorrhagic fever; BUN = blood urea nitrogen; PT = prothrombin time; PTT = partial thromboplastin time.

Convalescent plasma is also routinely given as postexposure prophylaxis for AHF, including for nursing children of an infected mother, because Junin virus can be found in breast milk. Recombinant-based vaccines for Ebola and Marburg viruses have recently been shown to be efficacious as postexposure prophylaxis in animal models but are not yet approved for use in humans.

Vaccines

Vaccines for the VHFs are at various stages of development. The 17D live-attenuated yellow fever vaccine has an excellent protection and safety profile, despite recent recognition of rare serious adverse events in elderly persons. Confirmed previous vaccination with 17D should essentially rule out yellow fever. A highly efficacious live-attenuated vaccine, Candid 1, also exists for AHF, although it is only licensed in Argentina. Candid 1 may also be effective in Bolivian hemorrhagic fever but does not protect against other arenavirus infec-

tions. Vaccines for HFRS, Rift Valley fever, and Kyasanur Forest disease exist and appear to be efficacious, although most have not been widely tested and are not widely available. A number of vaccine candidates have recently been shown to be efficacious in animal models of Ebola, Marburg, and Lassa virus infection. None are yet approved for use in humans, although a recombinant vaccine for Ebola hemorrhagic fever has been shown to be safe and immunogenic in Phase I studies.

CONVALESCENCE AND SEQUELAE

Persons who survive VHF usually suffer no obvious long-term sequelae. Notable exceptions include deafness in Lassa fever and optic retinopathy with vision loss in Rift Valley fever, both of which appear during early convalescence and may persist, to some degree, for life. Convalescence may be prolonged, especially for Ebola and Marburg viruses, with the potential for persistent myalgia, arthralgia, anorexia and weight loss, alopecia, pancreatitis, uveitis, and orchitis up to a year after infection. The psychological effects of VHF may also be significant, with some patients experiencing depression or posttraumatic stress. Clinical management during convalescence includes the use of warm packs, acetaminophen, nonsteroidal anti-inflammatory drugs, cosmetics, hairgrowth stimulants, anxiolytics, antidepressants, nutritional supplements, and nutritional and psychological counseling as indicated. Uveitis in patients recovering from Ebola virus infection responds to topical steroids and atropine. Because of the risk of sexual transmission during convalescence, abstinence or condom use is recommended for 3 months after acute illness. Similarly, it is prudent to avoid breast-feeding during convalescence unless there is no other way to support the baby.

INFECTION CONTROL

Established isolation measures should be implemented as soon as the diagnosis of VHF is considered. Although normal barrier nursing precautions to prevent parenteral and droplet exposure to blood and bodily fluids probably suffice in most instances, these are usually upgraded to "VHF precautions" once the diagnosis is entertained, which include the use of surgical masks, face shields, double gloves, gowns, and head and shoe covers. Disinfection of items coming into direct contact with the patient with bleach, including chemical or heat inactivation of human waste, is advised. Although there is little evidence for aerosol transmission between humans, it is prudent to place the patient in a negative airflow room if available. Small-particle aerosol precautions, such as the use of high-efficiency particulate air filter masks, should be employed when performing procedures which may generate aerosols, such as endotracheal intubation. The hospital laboratory should be alerted to the possible diagnosis of VHF before sending any specimens so that appropriate precautions can be implemented. When possible, the use of point-of-care diagnostic assays performed by the treatment team can further limit exposure. Patients with arboviral hemorrhagic fevers should be cared for in mosquito-protected rooms or a mosquito net placed over the bed.

Contact tracing should be initiated once a case of person-to-person transmissible VHF is confirmed. Patients with VHF are generally contagious only when symptomatic and especially toward the later and most serious stages of illness. VHF has not been reported in persons whose contact with an infected person occurred only during the incubation period. Given the low secondary attack rates, especially outside of caretakers, widespread contact tracing, laboratory testing, or postexposure prophylaxis are not indicated for casual contacts. Virus can be found in a wide variety of bodily fluids during the acute illness, including blood, saliva, stool, and breast milk. Potentially exposed persons should be monitored with twice-daily temperature checks for the duration of the incubation period of the VHF in question and immediately placed in isolation if fever or other suggestive signs and symptoms develop.

FUTURE DIRECTIONS

To date, most recommended therapeutic interventions for the VHFs are based on uncontrolled observations. Thus, the true impact of these measures in decreasing morbidity and mortality remains to be proven. Since the mid-1990s, concern about the use of hemorrhagic fever viruses as bioweapons has driven research on various experimental therapies and vaccines, with the promise of expanded options in the future. Nevertheless, the first priority is to optimize supportive care. One step forward would be the development of formal and detailed consensus treatment guidelines, including standard forms for clinical record-keeping during outbreaks. These guidelines would then serve as a benchmark to implement, monitor, reevaluate, and improve the various therapeutic measures. A concerted effort must be made to insure that appropriate care is made available both in industrialized countries and in the developing world where most VHFs are endemic. This will be a challenging task, necessitating a broad array of partners and resources, but the fundamental knowledge and technology to provide such care are available if the political will is there.

ACKNOWLEDGEMENTS

The author thanks Mike Bray, Delia Enria, Onder Ergonul, Tom Geisbert, Frederique Jacquerioz, Benjamin Jeffs, Sheik Humarr Khan, A.G. Sprecher, and Ellen Yang for thoughtful review of the manuscript and Corrie West for assistance with its preparation.

SUGGESTED READING

Bausch DG. Marburg and Ebola viruses. PIER: *The Physicians' Information and Education*

Resource. American College of Physicians, electronic publication: http://pier.acponline.org/physicians/diseases/d891/d891.html. Accessed March 12, 2007.

Bausch DG, Ksiazek TG. Viral hemorrhagic fevers including hantavirus pulmonary syndrome in the Americas. *Clin Lab Med*. 2002;22(4):981–1020, viii.

Bernard GR, Vincent JL, Laterre PF, et al. Efficacy and safety of recombinant human activated protein C for severe sepsis. *N Engl J Med*. 2001;344(10):699–709.

Centers for Disease Control and Prevention. *Infection Control for Viral Haemorrhagic Fevers in the African Health Care Setting*. Atlanta, GA: Centers for Disease Control and Prevention; 1998.

Enria DA, Mills JN, Flick R, et al. Arenavirus infections. In: Guerrant RL, Walker DH, PF Weller, eds. *Tropical Infectious Diseases: Principles, Pathogens and Practice*. 2nd ed. Philadelphia, PA: Elsevier Churchill Livingstone; 2006:734–755.

Jeffs B. A clinical guide to viral haemorrhagic fevers: Ebola, Marburg and Lassa. *Trop Doct*. 2006;36(1):1–4.

Mahanty S, Bray M. Pathogenesis of filoviral haemorrhagic fevers. *Lancet Infect Dis*. 2004;4(8):487–498.

McCormick JB, King IJ, Webb PA, et al. Lassa fever. Effective therapy with ribavirin. *N Engl J Med*. 1986 Jan;314(1):20–26.

Peters CJ, Zaki SR. Overview of viral hemorrhagic fevers. In: Guerrant RL, Walker DH, Weller PF, eds. *Tropical Infectious Diseases: Principles, Pathogens, and Practice*. Philadelphia, PA: Churchill Livingstone; 2006:726–733.

Russell JA. Management of sepsis. *N Engl J Med*. 2006;355(16):1699–1713.

193. Intestinal Roundworms

Kathryn N. Suh and Jay S. Keystone

Nematodes (roundworms) are the most common parasites infecting humans worldwide. Of almost half a million species of roundworms, approximately 60 are known to be pathogenic to humans. Among the most prevalent human infections are those due to the intestinal (lumen-dwelling) nematodes. *Ascaris lumbricoides* and *Trichuris trichiura* each infect over 1 billion people worldwide; hookworm (*Ancylostoma duodenale* and *Necator americanus*) infects almost the same number. Other important nematodes of humans include *Strongyloides stercoralis* and *Enterobius vermicularis*. Co-infection, in particular with *A. lumbricoides* and *T. trichiura*, is common.

Ascaris lumbricoides, hookworm, and *T. trichiura*, collectively referred to as geohelminths (or soil-transmitted helminths), share the requirement for eggs or larvae to mature in soil in order to be infective to humans. The majority of infections caused by these species are asymptomatic and associated with low worm burdens, whereas the minority (15%–35%) of infected individuals harbor the majority of the worm burden and suffer from more intense symptoms. The natural history of geohelminthic infections is usually one of decreasing worm burden over time. Due to the obligate soil stage of maturation, these parasites cannot be transmitted from person to person. In contrast, *S. strongyloides* is able to complete its entire life cycle within the human host, and like *E. vermicularis*, both person-to-person transmission and autoinfection can occur.

The prevalence and intensity of helminthic infections, and in particular geohelminthic infections, are related to poverty, educational and agricultural standards, population density, and sanitary (public health) conditions, all of which have a far greater impact on the burden of disease than do ecologic factors.

ASCARIASIS

Ascariasis is among the earliest recorded and most prevalent helminthic infections of humans. Disease is caused by *A. lumbricoides*; infection due to the closely related porcine ascarid *Ascaris suum*

has been reported following accidental ingestion of ova. Ascariasis is widely distributed throughout the world, with the highest prevalence in Asia and in young children. Complications of infection are generally related to a high worm burden, and thus only a minority of infected individuals is at risk of serious morbidity. The prevalence of ascariasis is attributable in part to the prodigious output of eggs by each adult female and the ability of these eggs to survive in a diverse range of environmental conditions.

The life cycle of *Ascaris* is shown in Figure 193.1. Fertilized eggs are excreted in stool, embryonate, and become infective after a period of weeks to months in soil, depending on environmental conditions. One to 2 days after infective eggs are ingested, larvae are released in the small bowel, penetrate the intestinal wall, travel to the pulmonary circulation, and enter the lungs, where they ascend the trachea and are swallowed. Larvae mature into adults in the small intestine, where they live for up to 18 months. Egg production occurs 3 to 4 months after initial ingestion; females can produce more than 200 000 eggs per day.

Most *Ascaris* infections are asymptomatic. Adult worms may be seen in emesis or stool and are occasionally coughed up or extruded through the nose. Loeffler's syndrome, characterized by migratory pulmonary infiltrates and peripheral eosinophilia, results from larval migration through the pulmonary parenchyma and may be seen within 2 weeks of ingestion. Clinical manifestations include fever, dyspnea, wheezing, and dry cough. Gastrointestinal complications are generally due to a heavy adult worm burden (eg, intestinal obstruction from worm masses) or to migration of a single adult worm into the bile or pancreatic duct or the appendix. Complications from worms in other organs are rare.

Ascariasis is diagnosed by the demonstration of ova, larvae, or adult worms. Eggs are readily demonstrated in stool. Barium studies occasionally demonstrate adult worms, either by outlining them with barium or by visualizing ingested barium within the gut of the worm. Eosinophilia is not a feature of adult

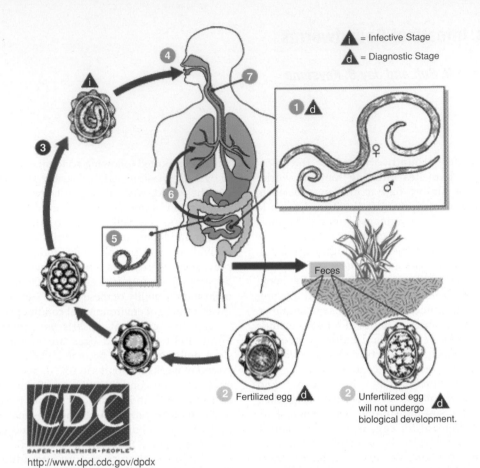

i = Infective Stage

d = Diagnostic Stage

Feces

2 Fertilized egg d

2 Unfertilized egg
will not undergo
biological development. d

CDC
SAFER·HEALTHIER·PEOPLE™

http://www.dpd.cdc.gov/dpdx

Figure 193.1 Life cycle of *Ascaris lumbricoides*. Adult worms ❶ live in the lumen of the small intestine. A female may produce approximately 200 000 eggs per day, which are passed with the feces. ❷ Unfertilized eggs may be ingested but are not infective. Fertile eggs embryonate and become infective after 18 days to several weeks ❸, depending on the environmental conditions (optimum: moist, warm, shaded soil). After infective eggs are swallowed ❹, the larvae hatch ❺, invade the intestinal mucosa, and are carried via the portal, then systemic circulation to the lungs ❻. The larvae mature further in the lungs (10 to 14 days), penetrate the alveolar walls, ascend the bronchial tree to the throat, and are swallowed ❼. On reaching the small intestine, they develop into adult worms ❶. Between 2 and 3 months are required from ingestion of the infective eggs to oviposition by the adult female. Adult worms can live 1 to 2 years. Source: Division of Parasitic Diseases, National Center for Infectious Diseases, Centers for Disease Control and Prevention, Atlanta, GA. http://www.dpd.cdc.gov/DPDx/HTML/Ascariasis.htm, accessed 3 December 2006.

ascariasis but is a common finding during the migration phase.

Because of the potential for worm migration, all infections, whether symptomatic or not, should be treated. When mixed helminthic infections are being treated, *Ascaris* should always be treated first, because medications may stimulate worms to migrate. Mebendazole or albendazole are appropriate first-line therapies (Table 193.1).

TRICHURIASIS

Like ascariasis, trichuriasis is a widely distributed disease. Humans are the only hosts

of *Trichuris trichiura* (whipworm, so named for the characteristic morphology of adult worms). It is most common in tropical climates, with the highest prevalence in children. Human disease may rarely be caused by related species of porcine (*Trichuris suis*) and canine (*Trichuris vulpis*) whipworm.

Eggs passed in stool embryonate after 2 to 4 weeks of maturation in soil. There is no tissue (pulmonary) phase; eggs are deposited directly in the cecum, where larvae hatch and mature into adults over several days. Adult worms survive for up to 8 years in the cecum, where they remain attached to the intestinal mucosa. Eggs production begins 2 to 3 months after

Table 193.1 Treatment of Intestinal Roundworm Infections

Disease	Drug	Adult and Pediatric Dose
Ascariasis	Albendazole or	400 mg 1×
	Mebendazole or	100 mg BID × 3d or 500 mg 1×
	Pyrantel pamoate or	11 mg/kg (max 1g) daily × 3 d
	Ivermectin	150–200 µg/kg 1×
Trichuriasis	Albendazole or	400 mg daily × 3 d
	Mebendazole or	100 mg BID × 3 d or 500 mg 1×
	Ivermectin	200 µg/kg daily × 3 d
Hookworm	Albendazole or	400 mg once
	Mebendazole or	100 mg BID × 3d or 500 mg 1×
	Pyrantel pamoate	11 mg/kg (max 1 g) daily × 3 d
Strongyloidiasis Immunocompetent	Ivermectin or	200 µg/kg daily × 2 d
	Albendazole	400 mg BID × 7 d
Immunosuppressed	Ivermectin plus	200 µg/kg daily ×2 d[a]
	Albendazole	400 mg BID × 7 d[a]
Pinworm[b]	Albendazole or	400 mg 1×
	Mebendazole or	100 mg 1×
	Pyrantel pamoate	11 mg/kg (max 1 g) 1×
Trichostrongyliasis	Ivermectin or	200 µg/kg 1×
	Pyrantel pamoate or	11 mg/kg (max 1 g) 1×
	Albendazole or	400 mg 1×
	Mebendazole	100 mg BID × 3 d

[a] In disseminated strongyloidiasis, therapy should be continued until parasite has cleared.
[b] Regardless of the agent used, therapy must be repeated 2 to 4 weeks after the first course.

initial infection, with females releasing up to 20 000 eggs per day.

Most infected individuals are asymptomatic. Moderate worm burdens may cause nonspecific gastrointestinal symptoms, including abdominal pain or distension or diarrhea. Heavy worm burdens more often affect children and may lead to profuse bloody diarrhea or rectal prolapse, the hallmark of trichuriasis in endemic areas. Iron deficiency anemia may also be present, but eosinophilia is uncommon.

The diagnosis of *T. trichiura* infection rests on demonstration of eggs or adult worms. Endoscopy may reveal colitis and the presence of visible worms hanging within the intestinal lumen. Treatment with mebendazole or albendazole is curative (Table 193.1).

HOOKWORM INFECTION

Hookworm infection affects approximately 740 million individuals, with most cases in Asia and sub-Saharan Africa. Disease due to *Necator americanus* is most common and is found predominantly in tropical climates, whereas *Ancylostoma duodenale* infection is more geographically restricted, occurring in northern India, North Africa, the Middle East, and the southeastern United States. Prevalence increases throughout early childhood and then plateaus in early adulthood, with worm burden remaining essentially constant (or declining modestly) throughout the life of the infected host. Other hookworm species, including *Ancylostoma ceylanicum* and *Ancylostoma caninum*, rarely cause enteritis, whereas *Ancylostoma braziliense* infection typically causes cutaneous larva migrans.

The life cycle of hookworm resembles that of *Ascaris*. Eggs are excreted in stool and hatch in soil, and within 7 days larvae become infective. Following penetration of intact skin, larvae migrate through lymphatics to enter the bloodstream and travel to the lungs, ascend the trachea, and are swallowed. *Ancylostoma duodenale* larvae may also cause infection by the oral route. Within the small intestine, larvae mature into adults and attach themselves to the intestinal mucosa. *Ancylostoma duodenale* adults survive for up to 1 year, and *N. americanus* for up to 9 years. Egg production begins 1.5 to 2 months after infection. Females release 5 to 30 thousand eggs per day, depending on the infecting species.

An intensely pruritic erythematous maculopapular eruption, "ground itch," may develop at entry points of filariform larvae. Dermatitis is more likely with repeated exposure and can be complicated by secondary infection. Loeffler's syndrome may occur 10 to 14 days after infection. Nausea, epigastic pain, or abdominal tenderness may be present early in the course of disease and with heavy worm burdens. Infection by the oral route may lead to pharyngeal irritation, hoarseness, cough, and nausea (Wakana disease). The hallmark of hookworm infection is chronic iron deficiency anemia, which results from local blood loss at the site of attachment of the adult worms as well as from their ingestion of blood. The occurrence and severity of anemia depend on the infecting species of hookworm, the intensity of infection, the iron reserves of the host, and the availability of iron in the diet; therefore, hookworm anemia is mostly seen in the Third World, where a hemoglobin of 3 to 8 g/dL is not unusual. Complications of severe anemia, including weakness, fatigue, and high-output cardiac failure, are common.

In addition to laboratory findings of iron deficiency anemia, eosinophilia is common. Hypoalbuminemia may result from protein-losing enteropathy. The diagnosis is made by identification of hookworm ova in the stool; fecal concentration techniques are not usually required. Occasionally, rhabditiform larvae may be present in stool and must be differentiated morphologically from those of *Strongyloides*. Mebendazole and albendazole are drugs of choice for treatment (Table 193.1).

STRONGYLOIDIASIS

Human strongyloidiasis is caused primarily by *S. stercoralis*, which is endemic to Africa, Asia, southeast Asia, and Central and South America. Disease is also found in the Caribbean and, to a much lesser extent, in Europe, Japan, Australia, and parts of the southern United States. Infection caused by *Strongyloides fuelleborni*, found sporadically in Africa and Papua, New Guinea, is relatively rare. Strongyloidiasis affects between 30 and 100 million individuals worldwide.

The life cycle of *S. stercoralis* is complex (Figure 193.2). Rhabditiform larvae released in the stool of infected hosts mature into infective (filariform) stages in soil. Infection usually results from the penetration of intact skin by filariform larvae. These travel via the circulatory system to the lungs where they penetrate the alveoli, ascend the trachea, are swallowed, and then mature into adult worms in the small intestine. Although sexual reproduction does take place within the intestine, adult females are also parthenogenetic (capable of reproduction without males). Eggs are deposited in the intestinal mucosa, hatch, and release rhabditiform larvae, which are excreted in the stool to begin another cycle. Additionally, however, rhabditiform larvae may transform directly into filariform larvae and lead to either autoinfection or, in the appropriate clinical setting (ie, immunosuppression), to disseminated disease (hyperinfection syndrome). Rhabditiform larvae have the capacity to develop into adults in soil where they reproduce sexually (heterogonic development) and give rise to infective filariform larvae (Figure 193.2).

Most infected persons have low worm burdens and are persistently infected for life, often with minimal or no symptoms. If symptoms are present they are generally intermittent, with long asymptomatic periods between episodes. Acute infection may be apparent with very rapid (1–2 cm/hour) migratory serpiginous skin lesions (larva currens) or urticaria at the sites of larval penetration; cutaneous larva migrans from dog or cat hookworms may produce a similar picture, but with much slower migration in skin (1–2 cm/day). Larva currens in the perianal area is pathognomonic of chronic strongyloidiasis. Urticarial rashes may occur over many years during chronic infection. Pulmonary manifestations of disease are unusual due to the

Specific Organisms – Parasites

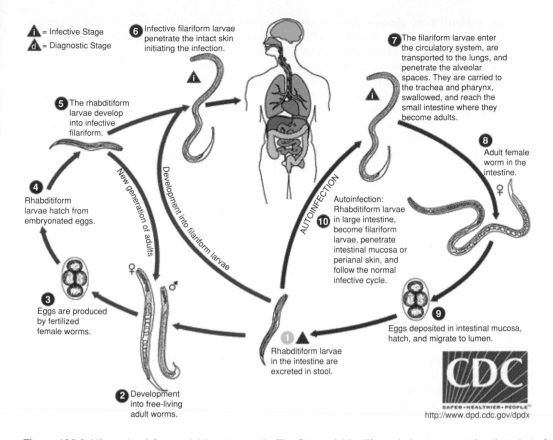

Figure 193.2 Life cycle of *Strongyloides stercoralis*. The *Strongyloides* life cycle is more complex than that of most nematodes with its alternation between free-living and parasitic cycles and its potential for autoinfection and multiplication within the host. In the free-living cycle, rhabditiform larvae passed in the stool ➊ can either molt twice and become infective filariform larvae (direct development) ➏ or molt 4 times and become free-living adult males and females ➋ that mate and produce eggs ➌ from which rhabditiform larvae hatch ➍. The latter in turn can develop ➎ either into a new generation of free-living adults (as represented in ➋) or into infective filariform larvae ➏. The filariform larvae penetrate the human host skin to initiate the parasitic cycle ➏. In the parasitic cycle, filariform larvae in contaminated soil penetrate the human skin ➏ and are transported to the lungs where they penetrate the alveolar spaces; they are carried through the bronchial tree to the pharynx, are swallowed, and then reach the small intestine ➐. In the small intestine they molt twice and become adult female worms ➑. The females live threaded in the epithelium of the small intestine and by parthenogenesis produce eggs ➒, which yield rhabditiform larvae. The rhabditiform larvae can either be passed in the stool ➊ (see "free-living cycle" above) or can cause autoinfection ➓. In autoinfection, the rhabditiform larvae become infective filariform larvae, which can penetrate either the intestinal mucosa (internal autoinfection) or the skin of the perianal area (external autoinfection); in either case, the filariform larvae may follow the previously described route, being carried successively to the lungs, the bronchial tree, the pharynx, and the small intestine where they mature into adults; or they may disseminate widely in the body. To date, occurrence of autoinfection in humans with helminthic infections is recognized only in *S. stercoralis* and *Capillaria philippinensis* infections. In the case of *Strongyloides*, autoinfection may explain the possibility of persistent infections for many years in persons who have not been in an endemic area and of hyperinfections in immunodepressed individuals. Source: Division of Parasitic Diseases, National Center for Infectious Diseases, Centers for Disease Control and Prevention, Atlanta, GA. http://www.dpd.cdc.gov/DPDx/HTML/Strongyloidiasis.htm, accessed 3 December 2006.

small numbers of larvae passing through the lungs, except at the onset of a heavy infection or, more commonly, when disseminated disease is present (see below). Epigastric pain mimicking peptic ulcer disease and persistent abdominal pain, diarrhea, and anorexia are common manifestations of symptomatic chronic infection. Abdominal bloating, distention, and intestinal malabsorption can also occur.

Hyperinfection syndrome most often occurs in the presence of impaired cellular immunity, typically due to the use of systemic steroids. Other chemotherapeutic agents, hematologic malignancies (notably lymphoma), organ transplants, malnutrition, chronic alcoholism, and co-infection with human T-lymphotrophic virus 1 (HTLV-1) are also predisposing factors. Interestingly, human immunodeficiency virus infection is not associated with an increased risk of disseminated disease. Insidious gastrointestinal symptoms may be present. Pulmonary disease is the most common extraintestinal manifestation of hyperinfection syndrome and is characterized by diffuse pulmonary infiltrates with dyspnea, cough, wheezing, or hemoptysis. In uncontrolled hyperinfection, filariform larvae also penetrate organs not normally involved in the life cycle, including the urinary tract, liver, and brain. Gram-negative bacillary infections, including bacteremia, peritonitis, meningitis, and sepsis, may result from the concurrent migration of bacteria and larvae across the bowel wall. The triad of hemorrhagic pneumonitis, enteritis, and gram-negative bacteremia in an immigrant who is immunocompromised should lead to consideration of disseminated strongyloidiasis. The mortality rate for disseminated disease is approximately 50%.

The diagnosis of chronic strongyloidiasis is difficult due to the nonspecific symptoms of the disease and the minimal, irregular larval output in stool. Demonstration of larvae in clinical specimens (eg, stool, bronchial washings in disseminated infection) is diagnostic but insensitive. In gastrointestinal infection, a single stool specimen may fail to detect larvae in up to 70% of cases, although sensitivity approaches 100% with 7 consecutive stool samples. Specialized laboratory techniques (eg, Baermann concentration; Harada–Mori filter paper test) and duodenal aspirates are more sensitive than single stool examinations but are impractical to perform. The agar plate method, in which stool is plated on solid medium and incubated for up to 72 hours, is highly sensitive (96%) but has a slow turnaround time. Agar plate specimens containing S. stercoralis larvae will, after incubation, reveal linear tracks formed by bacteria that have been carried by motile larvae. Peripheral eosinophilia is present in up to 80% of patients with intestinal disease and can be a clue to diagnosis, but it is rarely a feature of disseminated infection (although pulmonary eosinophilia may be noted in the latter). Strongyloides serology is available and has a reported sensitivity of 88% to 95% and specificity of 39% to 99%. Its use is limited by cross-reactivity with other helminthic infections (in particular filariasis, ascariasis, and acute schistosomiasis), and the inability of a positive result to distinguish between treated or ongoing infection, because antibodies may

persist for years following effective treatment. However, because several studies have shown that antibody levels drop significantly over the first year following successful therapy, serology may be used to determine test of cure.

Treatment of strongyloidiasis in asymptomatic individuals is often successful, whereas those with disseminated disease may require prolonged or repeated courses of therapy. Currently, ivermectin is considered the treatment of choice. If possible, immunosuppressant therapy should be discontinued in those with hyperinfection. Recommended regimens are summarized in Table 193.1.

ENTEROBIASIS

In contrast to other gastrointestinal helminthic infections, Enterobius vermicularis infection (pinworm, threadworm) does not respect socioeconomic boundaries. Enterobius vermicularis is ubiquitous, found in both urban and rural settings worldwide. Enterobiasis is the most common helminthic infection in North America and is among the most prevalent throughout the world. Humans are the only hosts, with infection occurring most commonly in young children.

Eggs are ingested, either by the fecal–oral route or by exposure to contaminated fomites. There is no tissue phase of infection. Larvae hatch in the upper gastrointestinal tract and mature into adults. Adult worms mate in the small intestine before migrating to the appendix and cecum, where they survive for up to 13 weeks. Gravid females migrate to the perianal area, where they release over 10 000 eggs daily, beginning 3 to 7 weeks after infection.

Symptoms are rarely serious, but may be problematic. Nocturnal pruritis ani is the most common symptom and can lead to insomnia and irritability. Local bacterial infection as a result of scratching can occur. Gastrointestinal and other attributable symptoms appear to be infrequent. Abdominal pain or diarrhea should prompt a search for Dientamoeba fragilis, because the co-infection rate with E. vermicularis may be as high as 50%. There is no evidence of an association between pinworm infection and behaviors such as tooth grinding, nail biting, or enuresis.

Eosinophilia is not a feature of enterobiasis. The diagnosis is established by identifying adult worms or eggs. The most reliable approach is the cellulose tape test using transparent adhesive tape to demonstrate eggs on perianal skin. A wooden tongue depressor draped with tape with the sticky side out is firmly pressed against the perianal skin immediately on waking in the morning, before defecation or bathing. The tape is removed, placed sticky side down on a slide, and examined under a microscope. Ninety percent of infections can be detected with three slides obtained on consecutive mornings, and seven tests detect 100% of infections. In contrast, routine stool examination for ova and parasites is positive in only 10% to 15% of infected persons.

The treatment of enterobiasis is summarized in Table 193.1. In the absence of reinfection or autoinfection, a primary infection will clear without treatment in 30 to 45 days. Because intrafamilial transmission is common, treatment of the entire family is usually recommended. A second course of therapy administered 2 to 4 weeks after the first is recommended to treat possible autoinfection or reinfection, because medications are relatively ineffective against developing larvae and newly ingested eggs. Specific personal hygiene measures such as good hand hygiene, daily bathing in the morning, the use of underwear and pyjamas for sleeping at night, daily change of underwear, and regular laundering of bedclothes are also important for eradication of infection. Recurring infections should be treated at least 4 times at 2-week intervals.

TRICHOSTRONGYLIASIS

Trichostrongylus species are parasites of herbivores such as sheep, cattle, and goats, primarily in the Middle East and Asia; humans are accidental hosts. Ova released in the feces of infected animals hatch in soil within 1 to 2 days, and pass through three free-living stages before becoming infective. Human infection typically results from ingestion of larvae in contaminated food or water, although larvae can also penetrate skin. There is no tissue phase, and adults reside embedded in the duodenal or upper jejunal mucosa. Little is known about the pathology of human trichostrongyliasis.

Most human infections are mild and asymptomatic, but diarrhea, flatulence, and epigastric pain may occur. Peripheral eosinophilia may be marked but is more commonly absent. Diagnosis depends on identification in stool of ova, which are often difficult to differentiate from hookworm ova. Ivermectin is recommended for treatment (Table 193.1).

ANISAKIASIS

Anisakiasis (herring worm or codworm disease), caused by infection with the third-stage larvae of *Anisakis simplex* or *Pseudoterranova decipiens*, is most prevalent in Japan and less frequent in Hawaii and the coastal areas of North America and northern Europe. It is acquired by consumption of raw or inadequately cooked marine fish or squid, as found in sushi or ceviche, for example. The primary hosts of anisakids are sea mammals, including dolphins, porpoises, whales, seals, sea lions, and walruses. Eggs released in feces mature in seawater. Free-swimming second-stage larvae are ingested by small marine crustacea and develop into third-stage (infective) larvae in squid and predatory fish. Herring, salmon, mackerel, cod, and squid, among others, are important sources of infection for humans. Larvae ingested by consumption of raw or inadequately cooked fish invade the submucosa of the stomach or intestine but cannot mature into adult worms in the human host. The larvae cause local inflammation and hemorrhage that generally last about 10 days.

Anisakiasis is categorized into gastric, intestinal, or extraintestinal disease. Gastric anisakiasis usually presents acutely after ingestion of infected food and presents with severe epigastric pain, nausea, and vomiting. Acute symptoms subside in a few days, but intermittent nausea, vomiting, and vague abdominal pain may persist for weeks to months. Symptoms of intestinal anisakiasis develop 1 to 5 days after the infecting meal and are due to invasion of the distal ileum. Abdominal pain, nausea, vomiting, and mild leukocytosis occur. Extraintestinal complications include peritonitis and pleurisy caused by larval perforation of the intestinal wall. Hypersensitivity reactions, including anaphylaxis, have also been associated with anisakiasis.

With the appropriate history and presenting symptoms, the diagnosis of gastric anisakiasis can be most easily confirmed by endoscopy. An ulcerated lesion and the protruding larva may be visualized. Intestinal and extraintestinal anisakiasis are difficult to differentiate from other causes of acute abdomen, and patients often undergo laparotomy. Serologic diagnosis may be helpful but is not readily available. Peripheral eosinophilia is common. Treatment includes removal of the parasite and supportive care, although even untreated infection subsides in a few days. Antihelminthic therapy for human anisakiasis is not well established.

SUGGESTED READING

Bethony J, Brooker S, Aobonico M, et al. Soil-transmitted helminth infections: ascariasis, trichuriasis, and hookworm. *Lancet.* 2006;367:1521–1532.

Concha R, Harrington W Jr., Rogers AI. Intestinal strongyloidiasis. Recognition, management, and determinants of outcome. *J Clin Gastroenterol*. 2005;39:203–211.

Crompton DWT. Ascaris and ascariasis. *Adv Parasitol*. 2001;48:285–375.

Elston DM. What's eating you? Enterobius vermicularis (pinworms, threadworms). *Cutis*. 2003;71:268–270.

Hotez PJ, Brooker S, Bethony JM, et al. Hookworm infection. *N Engl J Med*. 2004;351:799–807.

Johnson EH, Windsor JJ, Clark CG. Emerging from obscurity: biological, clinical, and diagnostic aspects of Dientamoeba fragilis. *Clin Microbiol Rev*. 2004;17:553–570.

Khuroo MS. Ascariasis. *Gastroenterol Clin North Am*. 1997;25:553–577.

Lim S, Katz K, Krajden S, et al. Complicated and fatal Strongyloides infection in Canadians: risk factors, diagnosis, and management. *Can Med Assoc J*. 2004;171:479–484.

Ralph A, O'Sullivan MVN, Sangster NC, et al. Abdominal pain and eosinophilia in suburban goat keepers – trichostrongyliasis. *Med J Aust*. 2006;184:467–469.

194. Tissue Nematodes

Thomas A. Moore

Tissue-dwelling helminths include a large number of nematodes, cestodes, and trematodes that cause a wide variety of clinical manifestations. Immunoglobulin E (IgE) elevations tend to accompany eosinophilia due to helminth infections, but a normal level does not eliminate parasitic disease. The diagnostic considerations can be narrowed through an understanding of the various parasites, specifically the geographic distribution, the likelihood of exposure in endemic areas, incubation period, and knowledge of the common manifestations of infection. Serologic tests are sometimes helpful, but panels of helminth serologic tests are most likely to be unrewarding if not confusing. Treatment strategies must be tailored to the individual parasitic disease.

TRICHINOSIS

Trichinosis develops when raw or inadequately cooked meat containing the encysted larvae of *Trichinella* species is eaten. The larvae are released from the cysts and attach to the mucosa of the small intestinal villi, where they develop into male and female adult worms. The infective newborn larvae invade striated muscle, where they encyst within individual muscle fibers.

Trichinosis has a worldwide distribution, occurring in temperate and tropical climates. In the United States, trichinosis has historically been associated with eating *Trichinella*-infected pork from domesticated sources. Improved observance of standards and regulations in the U.S. commercial pork industry has resulted in a steady reduction of *Trichinella* prevalence among swine. The number of reported cases related to eating nonpork products has remained constant, however, and now for the first time exceeds the number of reported cases related to eating pork.

In the 5-year period from 1997 through 2001, 72 cases of trichinosis were reported to the Centers for Disease Control and Prevention (CDC). Of these, 31 cases (43%) were associated with eating wild game: 29 with bear meat, 1 with cougar meat, and 1 with wild boar meat. In comparison, only 12 cases (17%) were associated with eating commercial pork products, including 4 cases traced to a foreign source. Nine cases (13%) were associated with eating noncommercial pork from home-raised or direct-from-farm swine where U.S. commercial pork production industry standards and regulations do not apply.

Among U.S. travelers, most cases of trichinosis have been associated with consumption of wild pigs, especially the bush pig and warthog. Meat from other sources can result in trichinosis as well, and outbreaks of the disease have been associated with consumption of meat from bears, walruses, and horses. Most reported travel-related infections have been associated with visits to Mexico, southeast Asia, and sub-Saharan Africa.

The severity of symptoms depends on the absolute number of ingested larvae. Because most infections result from ingestion of a small number of larvae, most infected persons are asymptomatic. The adult worm in the small intestine may cause gastrointestinal symptoms within a week of infection. Symptoms include abdominal discomfort, vomiting, and diarrhea, which may evolve into fulminant enteritis in unusually heavy infections. However, most clinical manifestations are related to systemic invasion by larvae, and they usually begin in the second week after infection, peak over a week's time, and then slowly subside. These symptoms include fever and myositis with pain, swelling, and weakness. Myositis usually begins in the extraocular muscles and progresses to involve the masseters, neck muscles, and limb flexors. Other symptoms include headache, cough, and dysphagia. Occasionally subconjunctival or subungual splinter hemorrhages develop. A petechial or macular rash is sometimes seen. In fulminant infection myocarditis, pneumonia, and encephalitis occasionally lead to death.

Fever and eosinophilia associated with periorbital edema and myositis are the cardinal features of trichinosis. Eosinophilia begins about 10 days after infection and may be quite high. The erythrocyte sedimentation rate is usually normal. Elevated creatine phosphokinase and lactate dehydrogenase levels reflect extensive muscle involvement.

Serologic testing is available from the CDC, but antibodies are not detectable until at least 3 weeks after infection. Although muscle biopsy may confirm the diagnosis, it is usually unnecessary.

THERAPY

The goal of treatment in early infection is to limit muscle invasion by larvae; when this has already occurred, the goal is to reduce muscle damage, which is responsible for the major clinical manifestations. Specific treatment with mebendazole, 400 mg twice daily for 10 days, or albendazole, 400 mg twice daily for 10 days, has been shown to be effective for intestinal and muscle stages. Thiabendazole is no longer used because of its side effects. The mainstays of symptomatic treatment remain bed rest and salicylates. Glucocorticoids (prednisone, 60 mg/day for 7 days with a subsequent taper over 7 days) are effective for severe symptoms not relieved by salicylates. Persons who are known to have recently eaten trichinous meat should be given a 7-day course of albendazole 400 mg orally twice daily to eliminate the intestinal infection.

FILARIASIS

Of the eight filarial species capable of infecting humans, the four that cause the most disease worldwide are *Brugia malayi*, *Wuchereria bancrofti*, *Onchocerca volvulus*, and *Loa loa*. Because only a small proportion of insect bites is infective, the disease generally occurs only after long exposure in an endemic area. The clinical manifestations of filariasis depend in part on the immune response of the host. Generally the response to the parasite in endemic populations is dampened, and a large parasite burden is common. In contrast, individuals who have grown up outside of endemic regions and who move or travel to these regions and become infected manifest prominent signs and symptoms of inflammatory reactions to the parasites and usually have a low parasite burden.

Lymphatic Filariasis

Lymphatic filariasis is caused by infection with one of the lymph-dwelling filariae; specifically, *W. bancrofti*, *B. malayi*, or *B. timori*. The bite of an infected mosquito deposits larvae in the subcutaneous tissue. Over time, they mature into adult worms. These threadlike adults reside in afferent lymphatic channels or sinuses of lymph nodes.

Wuchereria bancrofti, found in tropical and subtropical regions throughout the world, is the most widely distributed of the human filariae. In most of the world the parasite is nocturnally periodic, meaning that microfilariae are scarce in peripheral blood during the day but increase at night. In the Pacific Islands, however, the microfilariae are subperiodic; microfilaremia is seen throughout the day, reaching maximal levels in the afternoon. Brugian filariasis occurs throughout Asia and the Far East, including India and the Philippines. This form of filariasis is nocturnally periodic, except in forested areas, where it is subperiodic.

Among endemic populations, the common manifestations of lymphatic filariasis include asymptomatic microfilaremia, filarial fevers, and lymphatic obstruction. Most infected individuals are clinically well and have an asymptomatic condition associated with microfilaremia. More than half of these patients have hematuria, proteinuria, or both. Filarial fevers are acute episodes of high fever and chills accompanied by signs of lymphatic inflammation (lymphangitis and lymphadenitis) and transient lymphedema. The episodes spontaneously abate after a week to 10 days but can recur. Importantly, the lymphangitis develops in a descending fashion, opposite the direction seen in cellulitis. Regional lymphadenopathy is often present and thrombophlebitis can also develop. Both upper and lower extremities may be involved, but genital involvement, which may manifest as epididymitis, funiculitis, and scrotal pain and tenderness, is found exclusively with *W. bancrofti*.

Damage to the lymphatics, which may result in obstruction or lymphatic dysfunction, manifests early as pitting edema. The edema may progress with time, eventually resulting in the characteristic features of elephantiasis, which include thickening of subcutaneous tissues, hyperkeratosis, and fissuring of the skin. Lymphedema alone renders the patient susceptible to recurrent bacterial and fungal infections. Hydrocele formation is the most common manifestation of lymphatic filariasis, and scrotal lymphedema may also develop (Figure 194.1). If the retroperitoneal lymphatics are obstructed, chyluria develops.

Persons new to endemic areas (expatriates, transmigrants) who acquire lymphatic filariasis usually develop symptoms and signs of acute lymphatic inflammation such as lymphangitis,

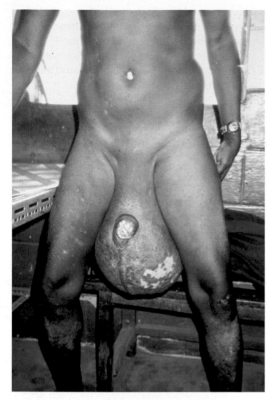

Figure 194.1 Massive scrotal swelling in lymphatic filariasis.

lymphadenitis, and, in the case of *W. bancrofti*, genital pain, but they may also develop allergy-like problems such as hives, urticaria, and eosinophilia.

Lymphatic filariasis is diagnosed by a combination of an appropriate epidemiologic history, physical findings, and laboratory tests. However, a definitive diagnosis can be made only by detecting the parasite. Adult worms in lymphatics are generally inaccessible, and excisional biopsies are unhelpful; however, ultrasonographic examination of the scrotum or breast in females using a high-frequency (7.5–10 MHz) transducer with Doppler may demonstrate motile adult worms within dilated lymphatics (the so-called filarial dance sign). Additional supportive data can be obtained with the use of lymphoscintigraphy, which (in early infections) will demonstrate a paradoxically brisk lymphatic flow on the affected side.

Microfilariae can be detected in blood and occasionally in other body fluids. Detection of microfilariae in the blood is most efficiently performed by filtering 1 mL or more of blood through a polycarbonate filter with 3-μm pores or examining the sediment from a Knott's prep (1 mL of blood with 10 mL of 2% formalin). The

timing of blood collection is critical and should be based on the periodicity of the microfilariae in the endemic region in question. Filtration of blood for nocturnally periodic microfilariae must be performed between 10 PM and 4 AM. It is important to note that a 10- to 14-day period is required for microfilarial periodicity to adjust to the local time zone.

Assays that detect circulating antigens of *W. bancrofti* (but not *Brugia* spp.) are commercially available and permit the diagnosis of filariasis in patients without microfilaremia. Polymerase chain reaction (PCR)-based assays that detect DNA of *W. bancrofti* and *B. malayi* have been developed but are not commercially available.

Data supporting filarial infection include eosinophilia, elevated serum IgE levels, and antifilarial antibodies in the serum. Serologic studies have greater diagnostic value in persons new to endemic areas. A negative or low antibody level effectively rules out active infection in this population. However, interpretation of serologic findings may be problematic because of cross-reactivity between filarial antigens and antigens of other helminths, such as *Strongyloides stercoralis*.

THERAPY

The mainstay of treatment for lymphatic filariasis remains diethylcarbamazine (DEC) 6 to 8 mg/kg/day in either single or divided doses for 14 days. DEC, an orphan drug, can be obtained from the CDC drug service (telephone 404–639–3670). Although extended treatment is usually necessary to kill the adults, the drug rapidly kills microfilariae. The severity of adverse reactions correlates with the pretreatment level of microfilaremia. Usually the reactions, which include fevers, headache, lethargy, arthralgias, and myalgias, can be easily managed with antipyretics and analgesics. Side effects of treatment can be minimized by pretreating with glucocorticoids (0.5-1.0 mg/kg/d) then initiating treatment with a small dose of DEC (e.g., a single 50 mg tablet).

A note of caution: The geographic distribution of onchocerciasis and loiasis overlap with lymphatic filariasis, and coinfection occurs. Because treatment of onchocerciasis and loiasis with DEC can result in severe adverse effects, it is imperative that the clinician excludes the possibility of coinfection with these organisms prior to giving DEC to patients with lymphatic filariasis.

Because adult worms may survive the initial treatment, symptoms can recur within a few months after therapy, and retreatment is recommended for such patients. Some individuals have suggested treating such patients with DEC at the standard dose of 6 to 8 mg/kg/day for 1 week each month for 6 to 12 months. Combination therapy with DEC and either albendazole or ivermectin has been tried in populations for mass chemotherapy of filariasis and other helminths, with good success; however, the use of these combination regimens to treat individual patients cannot be recommended at this time.

The optimal treatment of acute lymphatic inflammation is unknown, and these attacks usually resolve in 5 to 7 days without therapy. Treatment of chronic lymphatic obstruction is problematic. If the infection is recognized early, some signs of lymphatic obstruction can be reversed. In severely damaged lymphatics, however, only supportive measures may be helpful. These include elevation of the infected limb, use of elastic stockings, and good foot care with use of antifungal topical ointments and antibacterial antiseptics containing iodine. Prophylactic antibiotics should be considered for prevention of recurrent bacteremia and cellulitis. Hydroceles can be managed surgically, and surgical decompression with a nodovenous shunt may provide relief for severely affected limbs. No treatment has proved satisfactory for chyluria. DEC is useful for prophylaxis, but the optimal dose and frequency have not been established.

Tropical Pulmonary Eosinophilia

Tropical pulmonary eosinophilia (TPE) is a distinct syndrome caused by immunologic hyperresponsiveness to *W. bancrofti* or *B. malayi*. The syndrome affects men 4 times as commonly as women, often in the third decade of life. Most cases have been reported from Pakistan, India, Sri Lanka, southeast Asia, and Brazil.

It has been hypothesized that the symptoms and signs of TPE are due to trapping of microfilariae in the pulmonary vasculature, where they incite intense eosinophilic alveolitis. The clinical entity is characterized by paroxysmal cough and wheezing that is usually nocturnal and probably related to the nocturnal periodicity of the microfilariae, anorexia, and low-grade fever. Extreme eosinophilia (>3000/μL), high IgE levels, marked elevations of specific antifilarial antibodies, and a therapeutic response to DEC are required for the diagnosis.

THERAPY

DEC is recommended at 4 to 6 mg/kg/day for 14 days. Symptoms usually dramatically resolve within the first week of therapy. Most patients with this syndrome are already being treated with corticosteroids, and these can be readily tapered as the clinical situation warrants. Relapse occurs in 12% to 25% of treated patients and requires retreatment.

Loiasis

Also known as "African eyeworm," loiasis results from infection with *Loa loa* acquired in the rain forests of West and Central Africa. After the bite of an infected tabanid (horse) fly, the parasites are inoculated into the subcutaneous tissue, where they mature and mate. Although the adults reside in the subcutaneous tissue, they migrate widely over the body. The microfilariae released into the blood by the adult female exhibit diurnal periodicity.

Clinical manifestations, mostly due to the host's response to the migrating adult worm, differ between natives to endemic areas and newcomers. In the indigenous population, microfilaremia is generally asymptomatic, remaining subclinical until the adult migrates through the subconjunctival tissues of the eye or causes Calabar swellings, which are angioedematous lesions that develop in response to proteins excreted by the migrating adult worm and are most often noted in the extremities (Figure 194.2). The swelling develops after the adult has migrated through the tissue, so biopsy of the lesion is fruitless. Nephropathy, encephalopathy, and cardiomyopathy are rare. In nonresidents, allergic or hypersensitivity responses are predominant, microfilaremia is rare, but Calabar swellings occur more frequently and are more debilitating. Peripheral blood eosinophilia, parasite-specific immunoglobulin G (IgG), and vigorous lymphocyte proliferation to parasite antigens are typical.

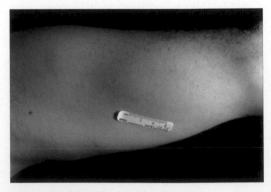

Figure 194.2 Calabar swelling of loiasis.

Definitive diagnosis requires the identification of either microfilariae in peripheral blood or isolation of the adult worm. The microfilariae can be identified with the technique described for lymphatic filariasis. However, because the microfilariae of *Loa loa* exhibit diurnal periodicity, blood must be filtered between noon and 4 PM after the patient has been in the local time zone for 10 to 14 days. The adult worm is difficult to find unless it crawls across the eye. The worm is not found in Calabar swellings, and biopsy of these lesions is not indicated. In amicrofilaremic patients the diagnosis must be based on a characteristic history and clinical presentation, blood eosinophilia, and elevated levels of antifilarial antibodies.

THERAPY

The drug of choice to treat loiasis is DEC, which is effective against both the adult worm and microfilariae. It is dosed as 8 to 10 mg/kg/day (in 3 doses) for 21 days. A single course of therapy is curative in the majority of patients with loiasis, although multiple courses of therapy may be required, and clinical relapses may occur up to 8 years following apparently successful treatment. It is not unusual for treated patients to develop localized inflammatory reactions such as subcutaneous papules or vermiform hives. These reactions, which are distinct from Calabar swellings, are a response to dying adult worms. The adult worms can be surgically extracted from these lesions, but removal is usually unnecessary.

Greater caution is warranted in patients who have microfilaremia. Treatment of such individuals with standard dosages of DEC has resulted in severe neurologic complications and even death caused by microfilariae in the central nervous system (CNS). To reduce the risk of developing treatment-induced encephalopathy, some experts have tried to reduce the microfilarial burden by performing apheresis of the blood before initiating treatment with DEC. In addition, gradual institution and escalation of DEC doses has been tried with apparent success. In this regimen, DEC should be gradually instituted, giving 0.5 mg/kg for the first dose then doubling every 8 hours until the full dose of 8 to 10 mg/kg/day (in 3 doses) is achieved. Prednisone (1 mg/kg/day) should be used during the first 3 to 6 days of treatment, and the first dose of prednisone should be given at least 6 hours before the first dose of DEC.

Because onchocerciasis occurs in the same geographic areas as loiasis and treatment of onchocerciasis with DEC can result in severe adverse effects, the clinician must rule out co-infection with onchocerciasis.

Other side effects of treatment are pruritus, fever, anorexia, lightheadedness, and hypertension. These symptoms usually resolve after the first few doses. A single course of DEC cures roughly half of those treated, and additional courses are frequently necessary to achieve cure. The decision to repeat treatment must be made on clinical grounds, because no objective laboratory data can predict treatment failures. Albendazole is an attractive treatment option for patients with very high levels of microfilaremia. Treatment at a dose of 200 mg twice daily for 3 weeks results in a gradual decline in microfilaremia over several months.

Once an individual has developed loiasis, serious consideration should be given to providing prophylaxis if that person is planning on returning to an endemic area. Although once-weekly treatment with DEC has been shown to be effective prophylaxis, the drug is difficult to come by in tropical countries because it is now manufactured only in the United States. Instead, albendazole 400 mg/day once weekly is an acceptable alternative, although the efficacy of this regimen is not clearly established.

Onchocerciasis

Infection with *Onchocerca volvulus* is the second leading infectious cause of blindness worldwide. Onchocerciasis occurs mainly in sub-Saharan Africa (where about 98% of the infected individuals live) and is found in savanna and rain forest. It is also found in Yemen and is scattered throughout Central and South America (Brazil, Colombia, Ecuador, Guatemala, Mexico, and Venezuela). Areas of transmission are focal because the *Simulium* blackfly vector flies only within a few kilometers of the streams where it breeds.

After the bite of an infected blackfly, larvae penetrate the skin and migrate into the subcutaneous tissue, where they mature into adults. About 7 to 36 months after infection, the gravid female releases microfilariae, which migrate throughout the skin and concentrate in the dermis. There they can be ingested by female blackflies during their feeding to complete the life cycle. Most of the symptoms of onchocerciasis result from microfilariae migrating through host tissues, primarily the skin, lymph nodes, and eyes. As with the other filariases, clinical presentations differ between individuals from endemic and nonendemic areas. However, pruritus is the most frequent manifestation of onchocerciasis in all individuals. An itchy, erythematous, papular rash prominent early in the infection is also seen (Figure 194.3). With chronic infection there is epidermal atrophy, loss of elasticity with exaggerated wrinkling, and loose, redundant skin. The pigmentary changes have led to the term "leopard skin." Lymph node involvement, usually found in persons from endemic areas, presents as inguinal and femoral lymphadenopathy that may lead to enlargement of lymph nodes, which hang down (so-called hanging groin).

The most serious result of infection is blindness. It usually affects only individuals from endemic areas with moderate to heavy infections. Ocular complications occur more frequently with savanna strains, and the endosymbiont *Wolbachia*—found in some strains—appears to play an important role. Lesions may be found anywhere in the eye, and the most common early finding is conjunctivitis with photophobia. In the cornea, microfilariae in the anterior chamber of the eye elicit an inflammatory reaction resulting in punctate keratitis with "snowflake" opacities. In Africa, sclerosing keratitis, which may develop later, is the most common cause of blindness. Anterior uveitis and iridocyclitis occur in about 5% of infected Africans. In the Americas, secondary glaucoma may result from damage to the anterior uveal tract. Chorioretinal lesions, constriction of the visual fields, and frank optic atrophy may also develop.

Laboratory findings differ between persons from endemic and nonendemic areas. Eosinophilia and elevated IgE are prominent findings in infected individuals. Eosinophilia

and IgE levels are greater in natives of endemic areas, a finding that is contrary to the findings in the other filariases.

Like the other filariases, definitive diagnosis rests on the detection of an adult worm in an excised nodule or, more commonly, microfilariae in a skin snip. Skin snips are easily and bloodlessly obtained by sampling the most superficial skin layers using a corneoscleral punch. However, a 25-gauge needle may also be used to carefully tent up the skin, while a scalpel is used to excise the most superficial layers of skin. The sample is incubated in saline or tissue culture medium on a glass slide or in a flat-bottomed microtiter plate at 37°C (98.6°F) for at least 2 hours.

THERAPY

Ivermectin (Stromectol, Mectizan) is the drug of choice for treating onchocerciasis. Given as a single dose of 150 µg/kg on an empty stomach, it is available in 3 and 6-mg tablets. It is generally available to most pharmacies in the United States. Treatment with this agent is contraindicated in children younger than 5 years, pregnant or breast-feeding women, and patients with CNS disorders that may increase the penetration of ivermectin into the CNS. Because ivermectin does not kill adult worms, the effect of the drug lasts 6 to 12 months. Retreatment is generally required either yearly or semiannually.

Reactions to treatment are usually mild, occur within 3 days following treatment, and include a transient exacerbation of pruritus, dizziness, headache, arthralgias, rash, or edema. More serious reactions are exceptionally rare and have only been reported in patients who were coinfected with *Loa loa*.

In contrast to ivermectin, treatment with doxycycline, 100 mg/day for 6 weeks, leads to death of the endosymbiont *Wolbachia*, resulting in complete cessation of early embryogenesis of *O. volvulus* microfilariae for at least 18 months.

Nodulectomy has been advocated as a way to decrease the parasitic load; however, approximately two-thirds of the nodules are located very deeply in the body, making this approach infeasible. Priority should be given to removing nodules located on the head, because they are associated with a major risk of ocular complications.

Other Filarial Infections

Humans can harbor infections with other filariae, most notably *Mansonella* species: *Mansonella streptocerca*, *Mansonella perstans*, and *Mansonella*

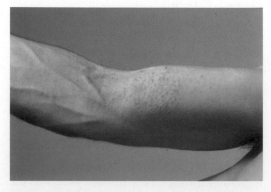

Figure 194.3 Papular eruption in onchocerciasis.

Specific Organisms – Parasites

ozzardi. Most of these organisms are discovered incidentally, but occasionally, infected persons develop clinical manifestations of illness.

Mansonella streptocerca, found in central Africa, is transmitted by biting midges. The major clinical manifestations, which are limited to the skin, are analogous to onchocerciasis, with pruritus, papular rashes, pigmentation changes, and occasionally inguinal adenopathy. The diagnosis is made by finding the characteristic unsheathed microfilariae in skin snips. DEC 6 mg/kg/day (in 3 doses) for 21 days is the recommended therapy.

Mansonella perstans, also transmitted by biting midges, is found in both central Africa and South America. The clinical manifestations, which are poorly defined, may resemble loiasis, with pruritus and transient angioedema, fever, headache, and arthralgias. Occasionally pericarditis and hepatitis occur. The diagnosis is established by the demonstration of typical microfilariae in blood or serosal effusion. As with other filariases, eosinophilia and antifilarial antibodies are often seen. Although no therapy is conclusively effective, DEC 8 to 10 mg/kg/day for 21 days is recommended.

Mansonella ozzardi is found only in Central and South America and the Caribbean. No clear picture of infection with this organism has been established. Diagnosis relies on finding the microfilariae, which circulate in the peripheral blood without periodicity. Although a single case report describes successful treatment with ivermectin, no broader studies of efficacy have been performed.

Humans are accidental hosts for a variety of filariae that primarily infect small mammals. The parasite never completely develops, and the worms are usually found incidentally. The canine heartworm *Dirofilaria immitis* occurs mainly in the southeastern United States. The bite of an infected mosquito deposits the parasite, which develops in the subcutaneous tissues, and then migrates to the pulmonary vasculature, where it is trapped and dies. It usually presents as a solitary pulmonary nodule that cannot be easily differentiated from other nonparasitic causes of pulmonary nodules. Eosinophilia is seen in fewer than 15% of infected persons and is only seen in the early stages of the lesion. Other *Dirofilaria* can cause discrete subcutaneous nodules. *Brugia* of small mammals can cause isolated lymph node enlargement in humans, but eosinophilia and antifilarial antibodies are uncommon. These zoonotic infections are diagnosed and cured by excisional biopsy.

DRACUNCULIASIS

Dracunculiasis is an uncommon infection distributed unevenly throughout the tropics, usually in arid regions where populations bathe or wade in water used for drinking such as step wells. The infection develops after the consumption of water contaminated with water fleas infested with *Dracunculus medinensis* larvae. The larvae are released in the stomach, pass into the small intestine, and penetrate the mucosa, ultimately reaching the retroperitoneum, where they mature and mate. The infection remains largely asymptomatic until about a year later, when the female worm migrates to the subcutaneous tissues, usually in the legs. A tender papule forms and is occasionally associated with a generalized reaction that may include urticaria, dyspnea, nausea, and vomiting. The lesion develops into a vesicle that eventually ruptures and ulcerates, exposing a portion of the gravid worm. On contact with water, large numbers of larvae are released and then ingested by crustaceans to complete the life cycle.

THERAPY

Metronidazole (750 mg/day in 3 doses for 10 days) it is recommended, although it exerts no direct antiparasitic activity.

The effects of these agents are similar, with symptomatic pain relief, reduced incidence of secondary infections, and improved healing of ulcers, allowing removal of the worm over the course of a week by progressively winding it around a small stick by a few centimeters a day. Topical applications of hydrocortisone and tetracycline ointments have the same effect.

UNUSUAL TISSUE HELMINTH INFECTIONS

Toxocariasis

Infections with *Toxocara canis* from dogs and, less commonly, *Toxocara cati* from cats may produce the syndromes of visceral or ocular larva migrans. Because these nematodes are normally parasitic for other host species, the larvae do not develop into adult worms and elicit eosinophilic inflammation as they migrate through host tissues. Visceral larva migrans is seen mainly among preschool children, but most infections remain subclinical.

Humans acquire toxocariasis mainly by eating soil contaminated with the infective eggs shed in the stool of the host animal.

Specific Organisms – Parasites 1349

Tissue Nematodes

Visceral larva migrans (VLM) is also usually asymptomatic, but those who seek medical attention present with fever, malaise, anorexia, weight loss, cough, wheezing, and rashes. Eosinophilia, the hallmark feature of VLM, may be strikingly elevated. Hepatomegaly is typical, but splenomegaly is seen in only a minority of those infected. Neurologic involvement is uncommon, and death, which is even rarer, is due to severe brain, lung, or heart involvement. Serum antibodies to *Toxocara* larvae are a useful adjunct in establishing the diagnosis, but elevated titers are also found in patients without VLM.

Ocular larva migrans (OLM) is occasionally associated with clinically recognized VLM but is usually unaccompanied by systemic symptoms or signs. The typical patient is an older child who presents with unilateral visual deficits, ocular pain, leukocoria, or strabismus. In the early stages, the lesion is raised above the level of the retina and closely mimics retinoblastoma. After the acute phase has subsided, the lesion remains a well-defined circumscribed area of retinal degeneration. Serum antibodies to *Toxocara* larvae may be present, but because many patients with OLM have low or negative titers, they are unhelpful unless compared with titers in vitreous and aqueous humor, which are generally higher in affected patients.

Patients with serologic evidence of toxocariasis who have mild or no symptoms fall into the category of "covert" toxocariasis. Children with hepatomegaly, cough, sleep disturbance, abdominal pain, and headache are more likely to have elevated toxocaral antibody titers. Eosinophilia, when present, is often mild. Recurrent abdominal pain is often the sole presenting complaint. Adults can be affected as well, demonstrating nonspecific symptoms of weakness, pruritus, rash, difficulty breathing, and abdominal pain.

As with other tissue nematodes, the diagnosis of toxocariasis is made initially on clinical grounds, with confirmatory testing playing a secondary role.

THERAPY

The majority of patients with toxocariasis do not require treatment. Although generalized treatment recommendations are limited by a paucity of controlled clinical data, treatment is generally reserved for patients with severe disease. Albendazole, 400 mg twice daily for 5 days, is the currently recommended therapy for acute VLM. Alternatively, a 21-day course of mebendazole, 20–25 mg/kg/day, has also been shown to be effective.

Albendazole has been found to be effective in OLM, but higher doses (adults, 800 mg twice a day; children, 400 mg twice a day) have been used in these clinical studies. Treatment should extend 4 weeks, with concomitant glucocorticoids, 0.5–1.0 mg/kg/day, for 2 to 4 weeks.

Cutaneous Larva Migrans ("Creeping Eruption")

Cutaneous larva migrans (CLM), also known as "creeping eruption," is a zoonosis caused by animal hookworms, most often those of the dog (*Ancylostoma caninum*) or cat (*Ancylostoma braziliense*). As with human hookworms, the infection starts when the worm enters the skin from contaminated soil that is protected from desiccation and temperature extremes, such as on beaches and under houses. As in toxocariasis, the worm cannot complete the infective cycle, so it continues to burrow through the subcutaneous tissues, resulting in the characteristic serpiginous, erythematous, elevated, and pruritic skin lesion (Figure 194.4). The pruritus is sometimes incapacitating. The infection is often seen in travelers who have walked barefoot on beaches frequented by roaming cats and dogs. Systemic symptoms and eosinophilia are rare.

THERAPY

Without treatment the lesions resolve spontaneously over 4 weeks, although the patients are often miserable with pruritus. Treatment with a single dose of ivermectin (150 to 200 µg/kg on an empty stomach) or a 3-day course of albendazole (400 mg daily) has been shown to resolve the infection within 1 week, although retreatment is sometimes necessary.

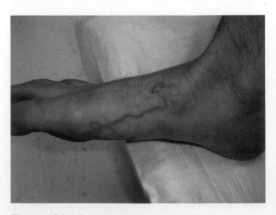

Figure 194.4 Cutaneous larva migrans.

Eosinophilic Meningitis Due to Helminths

Eosinophilic meningitis due to infection with helminths is most often caused by the rat lungworm *Angiostrongylus cantonensis*, followed by the nematode *Gnathostoma spinigerum* and the raccoon ascarid *Baylisascaris procyonis*. However, the condition has been reported to be a consequence of infection with other helminths, specifically *Schistosoma japonicum*, *Paragonimus* species, and *Taenia solium* cysticerci. Eosinophilic meningitis occurs widely throughout southeast Asia and the Pacific, including Hawaii, but is focally distributed in many other tropical areas worldwide.

Humans acquire angiostrongyliasis incidentally by eating raw infected mollusks, vegetables contaminated with mollusk slime, or marine fauna that have eaten the infected mollusks themselves, such as crabs and freshwater shrimp. Although nausea, vomiting, and abdominal discomfort may occur soon after eating the larvae, most patients have no symptoms until after an incubation period that ranges from 2 to 30 days (average about 2 weeks). At that time, patients develop an intermittent excruciating headache that may either be insidious or abrupt. Peripheral blood eosinophilia is prominent and lasts for about 3 months. Typical cerebrospinal fluid (CSF) findings consist of an elevated initial pressure, turbid fluid showing a pleocytosis with at least 10% eosinophilia, and elevated protein content but normal glucose. Diagnosis is based on the clinical findings, as recovery of the larvae from CSF or ocular fluids is rare. Treatment is mostly supportive. The headache responds poorly to analgesics and sedatives, but removal of CSF affords symptomatic relief and may be repeated as necessary. Corticosteroids have been tried in severe cases with some benefit. Because clinical deterioration and death can result from the inflammatory reaction to dying worms, antihelminthic therapy is likely contraindicated.

Infection with the raccoon ascarid *Baylisascaris procyonis* uncommonly causes a severe form of VLM usually associated with severe brain involvement and/or characteristic eye findings termed *diffuse unilateral subacute neuroretinitis* (DUSN). The developing worm can sometimes be found in the retina and killed by laser treatment. Albendazole treatment may be tried in persons with systemic disease or if the larval worm cannot be found.

Gnathostoma spinigerum, an intestinal parasite of dogs and cats, has been found to cause

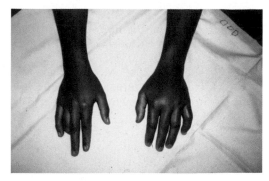

Figure 194.5 Angioedema of left hand in gnathostomiasis.

human infections most commonly in southeast Asia, although other foci of gnathostomiasis have recently been reported in Mexico and East Africa. Humans usually acquire the parasite by eating undercooked freshwater fish that harbor the encysted larvae. Gnathostomiasis is always associated with leukocytosis and hypereosinophilia. Intermittent subcutaneous swelling associated with edema and pruritus is the most common manifestation (Figure 194.5), mimicking the Calabar swelling of loiasis. However, the most feared complication of gnathostomiasis is eosinophilic myeloencephalitis, which can be fatal. This neurologic condition begins as intense radicular pain and is followed by paralysis of the lower extremities and urinary retention. Sudden onset of severe headache followed by coma and death may occur. The diagnosis of gnathostomiasis is usually established clinically. The only serologic test available is performed in Bangkok, Thailand, and samples can be sent via the CDC. Albendazole (400 mg twice daily for 28 days) is the mainstay of treatment. Occasionally, the worm will erupt from the skin shortly after treatment is initiated. Removal of the worm is both diagnostic and curative. Adjunctive treatment should include corticosteroids and adequate analgesia when indicated.

SUGGESTED READING

Ament CS, Young LH. Ocular manifestations of helminthic infections: onchocerciasis, cysticercosis, toxocariasis, and diffuse unilateral subacute neuroretinitis. *Int Ophthalmol Clin*. 2006;46(2):1–10.

Caumes E. Treatment of cutaneous larva migrans. *Clin Infect Dis*. 2000;30(5):811–814.

Despommier D. Toxocariasis: clinical aspects, epidemiology, medical ecology, and molecular aspects. *Clin Microbiol Rev*. 2003;16(2): 265–272.

Dupouy-Camet J, Kociecka W, Bruschi F, et al. Opinion on the diagnosis and treatment of human trichinellosis. *Expert Opin Pharmacother.* 2002;3:1117–1130.

Keiser PB, Reynolds SM, Awadzi K, Ottesen EA, Taylor MJ, Nutman TB. Wolbachia in posttreatment reactions. *J Infect Dis.* 2002;185:805–811.

McCarthy J, Moore TA. Emerging helminth zoonoses. *Int J Parasitol.* 2000; 30(12–13):1351–1360.

Moore TA, Reynolds JC, Kenney RT, et al. Diethylcarbamazine-induced reversal of early lymphatic dysfunction in a patient with bancroftian filariasis: assessment with use of lymphoscintigraphy. *Clin Infect Dis.* 1996;23:1007–.

Ong RK, Doyle RL. Tropical pulmonary eosinophilia. *Chest.* 1998;113:1673–1679.

Rajan TV. Natural course of lymphatic filariasis: insights from epidemiology, experimental human infections, and clinical observations. *Am J Trop Med Hyg.* 2005;73(6):995–998.

Ruiz-Tiben E, Hopkins DR. Dracunculiasis (Guinea worm disease) eradication. *Adv Parasitol.* 2006;61:275–309.

Slom TJ, Cortese MM, Gerber SI, et al. An outbreak of eosinophilic meningitis caused by *Angiostrongylus cantonensis* in travelers returning from the Caribbean. *N Engl J Med.* 2002; 346:668–675.

Twum-Danso NA. Serious adverse events following treatment with ivermectin for onchocerciasis control: a review of reported cases. *Filaria J.* 2003;2(Suppl 1):S3.

Udall DN. Recent updates on onchocerciasis: diagnosis and treatment. *Clin Infect Dis.* 2007;44(1):53–60.

195. Schistosomes and Other Trematodes

James H. Maguire

The trematode flatworms that infect human beings include the schistosomes, which live in venules of the gastrointestinal or genitourinary tract, and other flukes that inhabit the bile ducts, intestines, or bronchi. The geographic distribution of each species of trematode parallels the distribution of the specific freshwater snail that serves as its intermediate host (Table 195.1). Schistosomes infect as many as 200 million persons worldwide; infections caused by the other flukes are more limited in distribution and number. Trematode infections last for years; most are subclinical, and in general only the small proportion of persons who have heavy worm burdens develop severe disease.

SCHISTOSOMIASIS

Clinical Presentation

A history of contact with possibly infested freshwater in an endemic area should prompt an evaluation for schistosomiasis, even in the absence of symptoms (Figure 195.1). Clinical manifestations that suggest the diagnosis vary according to the stage of infection. Some persons complain of intense pruritus or rash shortly after the infective cercariae penetrate the skin. Previously uninfected visitors to endemic areas may develop acute schistosomiasis, or Katayama fever, 2 to 10 weeks after exposure, as the immune system begins to respond to maturing worms and eggs. Symptoms range from mild malaise to a serum sicknesslike syndrome that lasts for weeks and may be life threatening. Common features include fever, headache, abdominal pain, myalgia, dry cough, diarrhea, hepatosplenomegaly, lymphadenopathy, urticaria, and marked eosinophilia.

Chronic infections with schistosomes usually are asymptomatic and often are accompanied by a slight or moderate eosinophilia. Long-term residents of endemic areas may harbor heavy infections for long periods and thus are more likely than transient visitors to have symptoms. Disease is the consequence of egg deposition in tissues and the ensuing inflammatory and fibrotic response (Figure 195.2).

In infections due to *Schistosoma mansoni*, *Schistosoma japonicum*, *Schistosoma mekongi*, and *Schistosoma intercalatum*, involvement of the bowel leads to mucosal inflammation and microulcerations, diarrhea, bleeding, polyps, and strictures. Embolization of eggs to the liver results in hepatosplenomegaly, periportal fibrosis, portal hypertension, and esophageal varices. Hematuria and dysuria are the first symptoms of chronic infection by *Schistosoma haematobium*; later, fibrosis and calcification of the bladder and lower ureters results in hydroureter and hydronephrosis (Figure 195.3), and squamous cell carcinoma of the bladder may develop. Ectopic deposition of eggs in the skin, genitalia, and other organs occurs during both the acute and chronic stages of infection with all species of schistosomes. Transverse myelitis, seizures, and other serious sequelae result from egg deposition in the central nervous system. In endemic areas, chronic infections of even moderate intensity have been associated with anemia, poor nutritional status, and cognitive impairment.

Diagnosis

The most direct method of diagnosis is microscopic examination of stool or urine for schistosome eggs (Figure 195.4). Because egg output is low in light infections, concentration techniques and examination of several specimens obtained on different days should be routine. Egg should be counted to estimate the intensity of infection and to monitor the response to therapy. Counts above 400 eggs per gram of feces or 10 mL of urine are considered heavy and are associated with an increased risk of complications. Microscopic examination of snips of rectal mucosa obtained at proctoscopy may reveal eggs when stool examination is negative.

Serologic tests for antibodies to schistosomes are available at several commercial laboratories in the United States and at the Centers for Disease Control and Prevention (CDC) in Atlanta. The CDC uses a sensitive and specific Falcon assay screening test/enzyme-linked

Table 195.1 Geographic Distribution of Important Trematodes[a,b]

Schistostomes	
Schistosoma mansoni	South America, Caribbean, Middle East, Africa
Schistosoma japonicum	China, Philippines, Indonesia, Thailand
Schistosoma mekongi	Cambodia, Laos
Schistosoma intercalatum	West and Central Africa
Schistosoma haematobium	Africa, Middle East
Biliary and Liver Flukes	
Clonorchis sinensis	China, Taiwan, Korea, Japan, Vietnam
Opisthorchis viverrini	Thailand, Laos, Cambodia
Opisthorchis felineus	Eastern Europe, former Soviet Union
Fasciola hepatica	Europe, North Africa, Asia, western Pacific, Latin America
Fasciola gigantica	Africa, western Pacific, Hawaii
Lung Flukes	
Paragonimus westermani and other species	Far East, South Asia, Philippines, Central and South America, West Africa
Intestinal Flukes	
Fasciolopsis buski	Far East
Heterophyes heterophyes	Far East, Egypt, Middle East
Metagonimus yokogawai	Far East
Nanophyetus salmincola	Pacific Northwest

[a] Parasites may be limited to certain countries in the regions listed and certain foci within these countries.
[b] Many less common trematodes that infect human beings are not listed here.

immunosorbent assay (FAST-ELISA) for screening and a highly specific immunoblot for confirmation and species determination. These tests cannot distinguish active from past infections but are useful for the diagnosis of acute schistosomiasis before eggs are shed in the stool. Serologic tests may be used to screen previously unexposed travelers and expatriates to determine whether stool or urine examination is necessary. In such persons a positive serologic test is presumptive evidence of infection when microscopy is negative.

Persons with confirmed schistosomiasis should be evaluated for evidence of disease. Evaluation of infections due to the intestinal schistosomes includes measurement of liver function tests and tests for chronic hepatitis B and C to rule out concomitant hepatocellular disease. Heavy infection or evidence of liver disease should prompt an ultrasound to document periportal fibrosis and signs of portal hypertension (Figure 195.5). Esophageal varices are visualized by barium swallow or endoscopy. Urinalysis, urine culture, and serum creatinine determination are indicated for persons with *S. haematobium* infection. Ultrasonography or other imaging studies detect complications such as hydronephrosis, polyps, stones, and carcinoma of the bladder.

THERAPY

All persons with schistosomiasis should receive treatment. Eradication of infection is desirable because even a single pair of worms may deposit eggs in the central nervous system. In endemic areas where reinfection is inevitable, the goal is to reduce worm burdens to levels that are unlikely to produce disease. Successful treatment not only prevents complications but also may cause regression of polyps and fibrotic lesions. Fortunately, available drugs are safe and highly effective after one or a few oral doses.

The drug of choice for treating all species of schistosomes is praziquantel (Table 195.2). Praziquantel causes an influx of calcium ions across the tegument of the adult worm, leading to a tetanic contraction and vacuolization of the tegument that makes the parasite susceptible to immune destruction. Cure rates range from 65% to 90%, and in persons not cured, egg excretion is reduced by >95%. A few reports suggest that resistance to praziquantel may be developing. Adverse effects,

Specific Organisms – Parasites

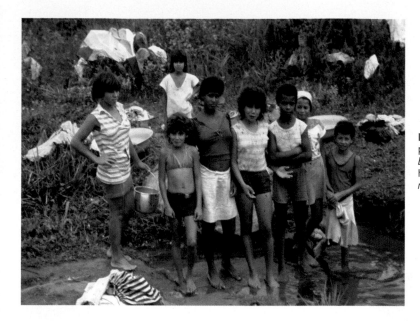

Figure 195.1 Shallow pond infested with *Biomphalaria*, the snail host of *Schistosoma mansoni* in Brazil.

which are usually mild and last less than 24 hours, may be caused by reactions to dying worms rather than drug toxicity. Patients occasionally report malaise, headache, dizziness, or abdominal discomfort. Nausea, vomiting, diarrhea, bloody stools, fever, and urticaria are uncommon. The World Health Organization has judged praziquantel safe for pregnant or lactating women. Persons with known or suspected cysticercosis should remain under observation during therapy because of the risk of seizures or other neurologic consequences of dying cysticerci. Praziquantel is metabolized in the liver, and the dosage need not be reduced because of renal insufficiency.

Oxamniquine, 15 mg/kg/day in 1 dose, is an alternative treatment for *S. mansoni* infections. It is used mainly in Brazil, where it is as effective as praziquantel. Drug resistance has been documented. Side effects include transient dizziness, drowsiness, headache, and, in persons with a history of epilepsy, seizures. Metrifonate, an inhibitor of acetylcholinesterase that is effective only against urinary schistosomes, is no longer available.

Severely ill persons with acute schistosomiasis should receive corticosteroids as well as antischistosomal drugs. Treatment of acute infection should not be delayed, but because maturing schistosomes are less susceptible to praziquantel than are adult worms, patients should receive a second dose 4 to 6 weeks after the first. Artemisinin derivatives have activity against immature parasites and may be useful for preventing or curing acute schistosomiasis.

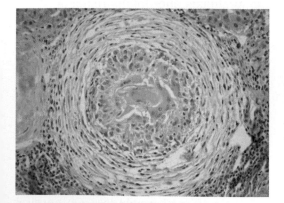

Figure 195.2 Granuloma around egg of *Schistosoma mansoni* that embolized to the liver and was trapped in a small branch of the portal vein.

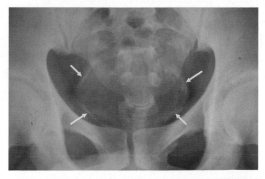

Figure 195.3 Plain radiograph of the pelvis showing calcification of the wall of the bladder and lower ureters (*arrows*).

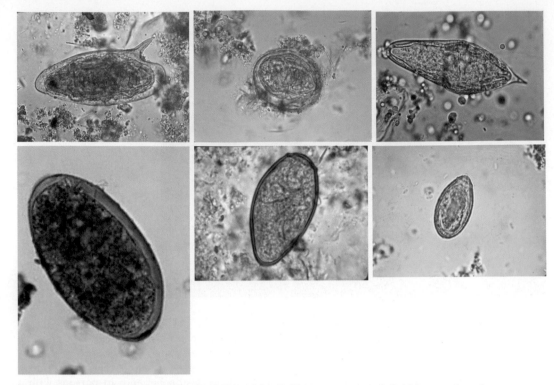

Figure 195.4 Trematode eggs. **Top row, left to right:** *Schistosoma mansoni*, *Schistosoma japonicum*, *Schistosoma haematobium*. **Bottom row, left to right:** *Fasciola hepatica*, *Paragonimus westermani*, *Clonorchis sinensis*.

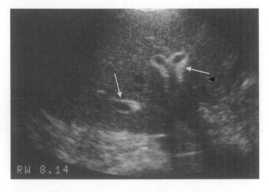

Figure 195.5 Ultrasound of the liver showing periportal fibrosis. Two portal tracts (one of the tracks is bifurcated) are surrounded with an area of increased echo (*arrows*).

Because antischistosomal drugs may temporarily inhibit egg laying by adult worms, stool and urine should be examined 3 and 6 months after completion of therapy. Eosinophilia, hematuria, and other symptoms that persist beyond this time should prompt repeat parasitologic studies and evaluation for causes other than schistosomiasis. Serologic tests may remain positive for years after successful treatment and are of limited utility for the assessment of cure.

OTHER TREMATODE INFECTIONS

More than 65 species of trematodes other than schistosomes infect 40 million or more persons worldwide. Most are parasites of wild and domestic animals. Human beings become infected by ingestion of metacercariae encysted in freshwater fish, crustacea, and plants, the second intermediate hosts.

Clonorchiasis and Opisthorchiasis

The oriental liver flukes *Clonorchis sinensis*, *Opisthorchis viverrini*, and *Opisthorchis felineus* inhabit the biliary tree of persons who ingest infected carp and other freshwater fish without proper cooking. Most patients are asymptomatic, but eosinophilia is possible. An acute illness resembling Katayama fever occasionally occurs 2 to 3 weeks after initial exposure. Persons with heavy infections for many years develop symptoms due to irritation and inflammation of biliary epithelium. Patients complain of right upper quadrant discomfort, anorexia, and weight loss. On physical examination the liver is palpable and firm. Cholangitis, pancreatitis, and cholangiocarcinoma are infrequent.

Table 195.2 Treatment of Trematode Infections

Parasite	Drug of Choice	Dosage
Schistosoma mansoni, S. haematobium, S. intercalatum[a]	Praziquantel	40 mg/kg/d in 2 doses ×1 d
Schistosoma japonicum, S. mekongi	Praziquantel	60 mg/kg/d in 2 or 3 doses ×1 d
Clonorchis sinensis, Opisthorchis spp.	Praziquantel	75 mg/kg/d in 3 doses ×1 d
Fasciola hepatica, F. gigantica	Triclabendazole	10 mg/kg ×1 or 10 mg/kg x 2 doses 6 h apart
Paragonimus spp.	Praziquantel	75 mg/kg/d in 3 doses ×2 d
Fasciolopsis buski, Heterophyes heterophyes, Metagonimus yokogawai	Praziquantel	75 mg/kg/d in 3 doses ×1 d
Nanophyetus salmincola	Praziquantel	60 mg/kg/d in 3 doses ×1 d

[a] To increase the likelihood of a complete cure, praziquantel 60 mg/kg/day in 2 or 3 split doses can be given to persons with schistosomiasis who have left an endemic area. Many experts suggest that persons who acquired *S. mansoni* infection in Africa should also receive 60 mg/kg/day in 2 or 3 split doses.

Diagnosis is made by finding eggs in the stool (Figure 195.4) or identifying adult worms during endoscopic retrograde cholangiopancreatography (ERCP) or surgery for complications. Ultrasonography or computed tomography (CT) is useful in symptomatic cases for demonstrating dilation and stricture of bile ducts, thickening of the gallbladder wall, and stones. A single course of praziquantel eradicates infection in more than 85% of cases (Table 195.2). A 7-day course of albendazole is an alternative therapy.

Fascioliasis

Infection with the sheep liver fluke *Fasciola hepatica* and the closely related *Fasciola gigantica* results from ingestion of uncooked watercress or other fresh aquatic vegetation from sheep- and cattle-raising parts of the world. After excysting in the duodenum, immature worms pass through the bowel wall and peritoneal cavity to invade the liver and burrow through the parenchyma to the bile ducts. This migration provokes an acute syndrome of fever, nausea, tender hepatomegaly, eosinophilia, and urticaria that lasts for weeks to months. Aberrant migration may produce nodules in the skin, painful inflammation of the intestinal wall, pleural effusion, or lesions in the lungs, brain, or elsewhere. Chronic fascioliasis is usually subclinical, but some persons have symptoms due to inflammation and obstruction of bile ducts.

The definitive diagnosis is made by demonstrating eggs in samples of stool, bile, or duodenal aspirates (Figure 195.4) or by recovering worms at surgery. Serologic tests are useful during acute infection because symptoms develop 1 to 2 months before eggs are detectable in the stool. Ultrasonography and ERCP may demonstrate adult worms and biliary pathology, and CT or magnetic resonance (MR) shows migratory hypodense lesions in the liver corresponding to necrosis along the path of larval migration.

Treatment of fascioliasis is with 1 or 2 doses of the veterinary drug triclabendazole which is available from Victoria Pharmacy in Zurich, Switzerland (Table 195.2). If given with food, treatment is successful in around 80% of cases, and a repeat course will cure most of the remaining cases. The alternative drug, bithionol, is poorly tolerated. Unlike infections with other flukes, fascioliasis responds poorly to praziquantel.

Paragonimiasis

Infection with *Paragonimus westermani*, the oriental lung fluke, and, less commonly, other species of *Paragonimus*, follows ingestion of raw or poorly cooked freshwater crabs or crayfish. An acute phase with fever, abdominal and chest pain, cough, and eosinophilia corresponds to migration of immature parasites through the bowel wall, diaphragm, and pleura en route to the lungs. The inflammatory reaction to adults encapsulated in the lungs and the shedding of eggs into the bronchial tree are responsible for chronic symptoms. Patients complain of cough, rusty or golden sputum, hemoptysis, vague chest pains, and dyspnea on exertion. Radiographs of the chest show poorly defined infiltrates, cysts, nodules, cavities, calcified lesions, and pleural effusions that on aspiration are seen to contain eosinophils. The findings may suggest tuberculosis. Bronchiectasis, bacterial pneumonia, or empyema complicates heavy infections. Extrapulmonary migration of flukes is common, and it gives rise to migratory subcutaneous nodules, involvement of abdominal viscera, or focal lesions of the central nervous system. Cerebral paragonimiasis is characterized by headache, seizures, focal neurologic deficits, cerebrospinal fluid eosinophilia, and cystic lesions on radiographs and scans.

The diagnosis of paragonimiasis is established by identifying expectorated eggs in the sputum, swallowed eggs in the feces, or worms and eggs in biopsy specimens (Figure 195.4). Several examinations of stool and sputum may be necessary. Serologic tests, such as the immunoblot offered by the CDC, are useful for diagnosis of light infections and extrapulmonary infections.

The treatment of choice for paragonimiasis is praziquantel (Table 195.2). Alternatives include triclabendazole and bithionol. Because an inflammatory reaction to dying worms may precipitate seizures or other neurologic complications, corticosteroids should be used simultaneously with praziquantel for cerebral paragonimiasis.

Intestinal Fluke Infections

Adult intestinal flukes live attached to the mucosa of the duodenum and jejunum, where they cause local inflammation and ulceration. Of the dozens of species that infect human beings, *Fasciolopsis buski*, the giant intestinal fluke, is the best known. Infection is acquired by eating uncooked aquatic plants, such as water caltrop, water chestnut, and watercress. Heavily infected persons develop hunger pains that suggest peptic ulcer disease, diarrhea with mucus, and in extremes cases, malabsorption, ascites, anasarca, and intestinal obstruction. Eosinophilia is common.

Other important intestinal flukes include *Heterophyes heterophyes* and *Metagonimus yokogawai*, both of which are acquired by ingestion of raw or undercooked freshwater fish. Symptoms caused by these parasites resemble those produced by *Fasciolopsis*, but embolization of eggs that enter the circulation may cause severe myocarditis or cerebral hemorrhage. The source of infection with *Nanophyetus salmincola* is raw or poorly cooked salmon or trout. Manifestations include abdominal pain, watery diarrhea, and eosinophilia.

The diagnosis of all intestinal fluke infections is made by demonstrating eggs in the feces. Because the number of eggs excreted may be low, concentration techniques and repeated examinations are recommended. Praziquantel is the drug of choice (Table 195.2). Alternatives include triclabendazole and, for *Fasciolopsis* and *Heterophes* infections, niclosamide.

SUGGESTED READING

Blair D, Xu ZB, Agatsuma T. Paragonimiasis and the genus, *Paragonimus*. *Adv Parasitol*. 1998;42:113–222.

Gryseels B, Polman K, Clerinx J, LucKestens L. Human schistosomiasis. *Lancet*. 2006;368: 1106–1118.

Keiser J, Engels D, Buscher G, Utzinger J. Triclabendazole for the treatment of fascioliasis and paragonimiasis. *Expert Opin Investig Drugs*. 2005;14:1513–1526.

Keiser J, Utzinger J. Emerging foodborne trematodiasis. *Emerg Infect Dis*. 2005;11: 1507–1514.

King S, Scholz T. Trematodes of the family Opisthorchiidae: a minireview. *Korean J Parasitol*. 2001;39:209–221.

Lun ZR, Gasser RB, Lai DH, et al. Clonorchiasis: a key foodborne zoonosis in China. *Lancet Infect Dis*. 2005;5:31–41.

MacLean JD, Cross J, Siddhartha M. Liver, lung, and intestinal fluke infections. In: Guerrant RL, Walker DH, Weller PF, eds. *Tropical Infectious Diseases: Principles, Pathogens, and Practice*. 2nd ed. Philadelphia, PA: Elsevier, 2006;1349–1369.

Meltzer E, Artom G, Marva E, Assous MV, Rahav G, Schwartz E. Schistosomiasis among travelers: new aspects of an old disease. *Emerg Infect Dis*. 2006;12:1696–1700.

Ross AG, Vickers D, Olds GR, Shah SM, McManus DP. Katayama syndrome. *Lancet Infect Dis*. 2007;7:218–224.

World Health Organization. Report of the WHO informal consultation on the use of praziquantel during pregnancy/lactation and albendazole/mebendazole in children under 24 months (WHO/CDS/CPE/PVC/2002.4). Geneva: World Health Organization; 2002.

196. Tapeworms (Cestodes)

Zbigniew S. Pawlowski

Cestodes cause intestinal (eg, taeniasis, hymenolepiasis) and/or tissue parasitoses (eg, cysticercosis, echinococcosis). Most of intestinal tapeworm infections are meat-borne zoonoses, whereas tissue infections with larval cestodes are fecal-borne, acquired mainly through ingestion of the tapeworm eggs from human, dog, or fox faeces.

TAENIA SAGINATA AND *TAENIA ASIATICA* TAENIASIS

Taenia saginata, the beef tapeworm, sometimes >5 m long, may live up to 30 years in the small intestine of humans, who are its only natural host. Humans are infected by ingestion of the cysticercus, a bladder worm <1 cm in diameter, present in raw or undercooked beef.

Taenia saginata infections can spread easily because of a high fecundity of the tapeworm (>500 000 eggs produced daily for years), wide and long-term contamination of the environment with eggs, bovine cysticercosis that may escape routine meat inspection when of a low intensity, and, finally, common consumption of raw beef. More than 10% of nomads are infected in East Africa; in Europe the annual incidence in urban populations is <0.1%; in the United States and Canada, *T. saginata* taeniasis is uncommon and observed mainly among migrants from Latin America.

Taenia saginata infection occurs mainly in well-nourished middle-aged individuals who are raw beef eaters. Complaints include vague abdominal pains, nausea, weight loss or gain, and some perianal discomfort caused by gravid proglottids (about 6 per day) crawling actively out of the anus. Sometimes, the patient passes a longer part of tapeworm strobila; in that case the expulsion of proglottids may stop for some weeks. The diagnosis is set up by questioning and macroscopic examination of expulsed tapeworm proglottids. *Taenia* eggs are found more often on anal swabs than in feces. Tests detecting parasite antigen in feces are highly sensitive and specific and may detect the infections even when proglottids or eggs are not expelled.

Treatment of *T. saginata* taeniasis with praziquantel or niclosamid is safe and effective in 95% and 80% of cases, respectively. Praziquantel is given orally in a single dose of 5 to 10 mg/kg an hour after a light breakfast. Niclosamid is preferred for children younger than 4 years and for pregnant women. Niclosamid (use only the original products, recently manufactured) should be chewed thoroughly on an empty stomach in a single dose of 2 g for adults, 1 g for children who weigh 10 to 35 kg, and 0.5 g for smaller children. For both drugs adverse effects, such as abdominal discomfort, headache, and dizziness, are rare and transient. Tapeworm is usually expelled in fragments within a few hours; the scolex, indicating elimination of the entire worm, is often difficult to find. Therefore, successful therapy can be confirmed only when no proglottids reappear within 4 months after treatment.

Taenia asiatica, described recently in several Asian countries, is a sister species of *T. saginata*, similar morphologically but a distinct species when examined by molecular techniques. Its life cycle is different; small cysticerci develop in liver and viscera of pigs and a range of wild animals. Humans become infected by eating raw viscera, especially liver, of the infected animals. The diagnosis and treatment are similar to *T. saginata*. *Taenia asiatica* as well as *T. saginata* do not produce cysticercosis in humans.

TAENIA SOLIUM TAENIASIS AND CYSTICERCOSIS

Taenia solium (pork tapeworm) infection is common in Latin American countries, Central and South Africa, India, Indonesia, and China. Intestinal infection is acquired by eating undercooked pork containing cysticerci. Cysticercosis, a cystic larval form developing in the tissues, is acquired by ingesting *T. solium* eggs present in contaminated food or water or on hands spoiled with feces (autoinfections or family infections are not uncommon). Human cysticercosis may be common in endemic countries; sporadic cases of cysticercosis are diagnosed in humans in the United States and in Europe, having been acquired abroad or from immigrants infected with *T. solium* tapeworm.

The pork tapeworm is smaller than *T. saginata*, and its proglottids are usually expelled with feces, starting 2 months after ingestion of infected pork. Clinical symptoms and signs of taeniasis are not characteristic and similar to *T. saginata* infection. The diagnosis is made by examination of the expelled proglottids or detecting the specific coproantigens. Finding *Taenia* eggs in feces can only confirm the diagnosis of taeniasis (*T. solium* eggs are morphologically indistinguishable from those of *T. saginata*). Proglottids and feces should be handled with care because *T. solium* eggs are infective for humans.

Treatment of *T. solium* taeniasis is mandatory as soon as possible, in both confirmed and suspected cases, due to a danger of spreading eggs causing cysticercosis in humans and/or pigs. Treatment of intestinal infection is the same as for *T. saginata* taeniasis; on rare occasions, praziquantel may provoke symptoms in concomitant asymptomatic cysticercosis. Evaluation of treatment is by frequent fecal examination for *Taenia* eggs during the second and third months after the anthelmintic therapy.

In cysticercosis, *T. solium* cysticerci may be localized in muscle and subcutaneous tissues (Figure 196.1A) without much symptomatology; the clinically important are mainly the cases of neurocysticercosis, ocular cysticercosis, and heart cysticercosis. Neurocysticercosis is suspected when epileptiform seizures (70% to 90% of the cases), intercranial hypertension, or psychiatric disturbances occur, especially in adolescents or adults living in endemic areas or having contact with a *T. solium* carrier (autoinfection is common). The most malignant forms of cysticercosis are at ventricular and basal cisternal parasite localizations. In case the subcutaneous nodules are present (which is uncommon, except in India), the final diagnosis can be made by biopsy demonstrating a scolex or typical structures of cysticercus wall. Most often, cysticerci are diagnosed by finding cysticercuslike structure(s) in the brain, spine, eye, or heart by computed axial tomography (CAT) or magnetic resonance imaging (MRI) scans (Figure 196.1B). In some cases the inflammatory reaction or edema and ventricular dilatation are present. In ocular cysticercosis the diagnosis can be made by ophthalmoscopy. Less often cysticercosis is suspected on the basis of ultrasound scanning and/or x-ray examination, particularly if calcifications are present (Figure 191.1C). Positive serological tests, especially enzyme immunoassay (EIA) and (EITB) assays,

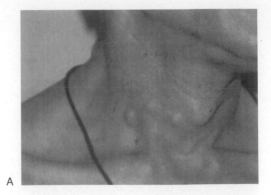

A

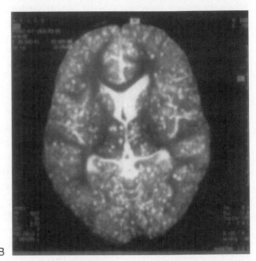

B

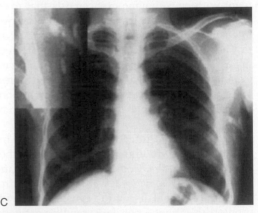

C

Figure 196.1 Cysticerci in subcutaneous location **(A)**, on brain computed tomographe (CT) showing innumerable cysticerci (starry-night appearance) **(B)**, and in soft tissues **(C)**, (Courtesy Dr. S.K. Gaekwad.) Bradley. *Neurology in Clinical Practice.* 4th ed. Butterworth-Heineman; 2004.

support the clinical diagnosis but cannot differentiate between active and passed infections.

Neurocysticercosis is often asymptomatic; in such cases, indications for treatment must be considered carefully. Symptomatic cases, which can be active or inactive (calcified). Therapy can be via specific anthelmintic treatment, surgery, corticosteroids, or symptomatic treatment. The choice of treatment has to be individually tailored. Anthelmintic therapy with praziquantel or albendazole is indicated in active cysticercosis with several parenchymal cysts or with clinical signs of vasculitis, encephalitis, and arachnoiditis. Traditionally, praziquantel is given orally in a daily dose of 50 mg/kg for 14 days, but a shorter regimen with a higher dose has been recently proposed. Albendazole is given orally in a daily dose of 15 mg/kg for 8 days. For parenchymal brain cysticerci, the efficacy is about 60% for praziquantel and 85% for albendazole. Damage to cysticerci, caused by both drugs, may result in a local inflammatory reaction and edema, which necessitates a concomitant additional corticosteroid or antihistamine drug therapy.

Surgical extirpation is indicated for single parenchymal, intraventricular, spinal, and ocular cysticerci and with focal symptoms (eg, cranial nerve dysfunction). A ventricular shunt is indicated in hydrocephalus. Corticosteroids and immunosuppressants may control vasculitis and encephalitis. Antiepileptic drugs are used mainly in inactive cysticercosis with granulomatous or calcified lesions. The global disability and mortality from neurocysticercosis are still considerable but its control measures are introduced only locally.

HYMENOLEPIS NANA INFECTIONS

Hymenolepis nana, the dwarf tapeworm, 15 to 40 mm long, lives only up to 3 months in human small intestine. Some of the tapeworm eggs are expelled with feces and constitute a source of autoinfection or infection for other people. The other eggs hatch in the human intestine and develop within a month into cysticercoids in intestinal villi and later into the next generation of adult tapeworms in the same host.

Such a cycle facilitates spread of infection in close communities (day-care centers, schools, psychiatric institutions) as well as permits intensive infections of thousands of tapeworms, especially in malnourished or immunodeficient individuals. Usually a specific immunity develops and regulates the intensity and duration of infection, which occurs mainly in children and often clears spontaneously in adolescence. Hymenolepiasis is very common in regions with a hot, dry climate; it is rare in countries with appropriate sanitation.

Intensive infections may cause diarrhea, abdominal pains, and general symptoms such as weight loss, pallor, and weakness. Diagnosis is made by finding characteristic *H. nana* eggs in feces. Treatment with a single dose of praziquantel, 15 to 25 mg/kg, is highly effective; in intensive infections treatment must be repeated after 3 weeks. Niclosamid is much less effective and requires repeated courses of 7 days with the same daily doses as for *T. saginata* taeniasis. Successful treatment has to be confirmed by negative fecal examination every 2 weeks for 2 months after therapy.

Other Intestinal Cestodes

Diphyllobothriasis, caused by *Diphyllobothrium latum* and *D. pacificum*, still occurs around unpolluted large lakes in moderate climates (the Great Lakes in the United States and Canada and lakes in Finland and Switzerland) and along the Pacific Coast in South America, respectively. An uncommon clinical complication of diphyllobothriasis is vitamin B12 deficiency. Diagnosis is made by finding characteristic eggs during fecal examination. Treatment is a single dose of praziquantel, 15 to 25 mg/kg. Evaluation of successful therapy is by repeated fecal examination some months after.

Hymenolepis diminuta (rat tapeworm) and *Dipylidium caninum* (dog tapeworm) infections occur accidentally in humans and are usually nonintensive and asymptomatic. They are diagnosed by fecal examination and can be easily treated by a single dose of praziquantel, 15 mg/kg.

Spirometra spp., a tapeworm parasitizing a broad spectrum of amphibian hosts, reptiles, birds, and mammals, may be a sporadic but worldwide cause of sparganosis, larval worms infection, mainly in the subcutaneous tissue or in an orbit.

Cystic Echinococcosis (Hydatid Disease)

Echinococcus granulosus is a tiny tapeworm living in the small intestine of some carnivores, mainly dogs. *Echinococcus granulosus* eggs, which are excreted in dog feces and contaminate an environment, are the source of cystic echinococcosis in various animals, mainly sheep or pigs, and sporadically in humans. Echinococcosis is still common in sheep-breeding regions in South America, Mediterranean countries, Middle East, Central Asia, and China. Small enzootic foci are found in

Alaska, California, southern Utah, northern Arizona, and New Mexico. In Europe, sporadic cases of cystic echinococcosis are frequently caused by an *E. granulosus* strain, originating from pigs.

Echinococcus cysts develop mainly in the liver (about 65%) or lungs (25%), but they can invade any tissue, including the brain, kidney, spleen, heart, and bone. Clinical manifestations are diverse, depending on location, size, and number of the cysts as well as the complications resulting from cyst's rupture and communication with biliary or bronchial systems or with adjacent body cavities. Bacterial infection of the cysts and secondary peritoneal echinococcosis are not uncommon. Clinical diagnosis is confirmed mainly by imaging techniques (sonography, CT, MRI, positive-emission tomography [PET], and/or x-ray examination. Classification of cystic echinococcosis in sonography is based on cyst morphology, considering also fertility and the content of the cyst; one can differentiate a cystic lesion (CL) stage, similarly to nonparasitic cysts, and C1 to C5 stages from young active cysts to old inactive cysts. Diagnosis can be confirmed by the serologic tests (sensitive enzyme-linked immunosorbent assay [ELISA], followed by more specific immunodiffusion or immunoblot tests). In some cases the clinical picture, imaging, and serology are not conclusive, and the final diagnosis is made by finding parasite hooks, protoscolices, or cyst wall fragments in sputum or in biopsy, surgical, or necropsy samples. In some specialized centers, cyst puncture with a fine needle guided by sonography and performed under the cover of albendazole is becoming widely used. Most commonly the differential diagnosis considers liver simple nonparasitic cysts.

The echinococcus cysts may be sterile or fertile (with protoscolices), simple or multiple, small or large (up to 20 cm in diameter), asymptomatic or symptomatic, active or inactive, complicated or noncomplicated. The choices of management are surgery, chemotherapy, PAIR (puncture, aspiration, injection of a cysticidal substance, and reaspiration), or observation without any intervention. Major indication for surgery are large, active, superficially located, and easy-to-rupture liver cysts and most of the brain, spinal, heart, and bone cysts. Surgery can be radical (removal of the whole intact cyst) or conservative (cystectomy and removal of the parasite but not the host pericyst). Surgery brings a risk of complications, such as anaphylactic shock or secondary echinococcosis and death (0.5% to 4%).

Chemotherapy is used more widely, mainly but not exclusively in inoperable cases. An important indication for chemotherapy before surgery or a puncture is prevention of secondary echinococcosis due to unintentional spillage of a cyst's contents. The drugs used are mebendazole, 40–50 mg/kg daily for at least 3 months, or albendazole, 10–15 mg/kg daily for at least 1 month. Sometimes repeated courses of treatment are necessary. Chemotherapy with both drugs brings a risk of embryotoxicity in early pregnancy. Careful clinical monitoring can prevent hepatotoxicity, neutropenia, and thrombocytopenia but not alopecia, which may occur.

PAIR is used rather in endemic regions with poor health care facilities. Unfortunately, no protoscolicide is both effective and safe; widely used now are 75% to 95% ethanol, 20% hypertonic sodium chloride solution, and 0.5% cetrimide. Formalin solution should no longer be used, as it can provoke sclerotic cholangitis.

Alveolar and Polycystic Echinococcosis

Echinococcus multilocularis tapeworms develop in the intestine of some carnivores, mainly foxes, but also dogs; the intermediate hosts are rodents such as voles, lemurs, and mice. Large natural enzoonotic foci of alveolar echinococcosis are in the region of the Alps (France, Switzerland, Germany, Austria), Siberia, northern Japan, Alaska, and northwest Canada. Humans are infected accidentally by *E. multilocularis* eggs present in fecally polluted natural environments (water, soil, berries) or on fox's skin or dog's hair.

Echinococcus multilocularis lesions, composed of clusters of tiny vesicles, usually begin in the liver, grow slowly in a tumorlike pattern, and metastasize to lungs and brain. Modern (PNM) classification of alveolar echinococcosis lesions in liver is based on the size of parasitic mass, involvement of the neighboring tissues, and distant metastases. The early clinical manifestations are usually vague; the advanced disease is invariably symptomatic due to liver lesions or lung or brain metastases. Diagnosis is based on imaging techniques and serological tests; the latter (eg, Em2+ and/or Em18) are highly specific. The differential diagnosis is mainly with neoplasma conditions. Treatment is by radical surgical resection of liver lesions followed by

Specific Organisms – Parasites

at least 2 years of chemotherapy. Recurrent or nonresectable lesions require lifelong chemotherapy with mebendazole or albendazole, which are parasitostatic rather than parasitocidal. Nitrazoxanide and amphotericin B are now suggested as potential alternative additional or combined drugs. The treatment has to be performed in specialized centers because of various and frequently severe complications, which may need another surgery or in rare cases a liver transplantation.

Polycystic echinococcosis occurs in humans in Central and South America and is caused by *Echinococcus vogeli* and *Echinococcus oligartrus,* the parasites of wild mammals. The numerous small cystic lesions can be found in the liver, lungs, abdominal cavity, stomach, heart, and orbit. The clinical course is similar to alveolar echinococcosis. Polycystic echinococcosis frequently requires surgery and responds well to albendazole.

SUGGESTED READING

Ammann RW, Eckert J. Cestodes. Echinococcus: parasitic diseases of the liver and intestines. *Gastroenterol Clin North Am.* 1996;25:655–689.

Eckert J, Gemmell MA, Meslin F.-X, Pawlowski ZS, eds. WHO/OIE manual on echinococcosis in humans and animals: a public health problem of global concern. Paris: WHO/OIE; 2001;1–265.

Ito A, Craig PS, Schantz PM, eds. Taeniasis/ cysticercosis and echinococcosis with focus on Asia and the Pacific. *Parasitol Int.* 2006;55(suppl):S1–S308.

Murrell KD, ed. *Guidelines on Taeniasis/ Cysticercosis.* Geneva: WHO/OIF/FAO; 2005:1–99.

Singh G, Prabhakar S, eds. Taenia solium cysticercosis: from basic to clinical science. Wallingford, Oxon, UK: CABI Publishing; 2002:1–457.

197. Toxoplasma

Roderick Go and Benjamin J. Luft

Toxoplasmosis, caused by the obligate intracellular parasite *Toxoplasma gondii*, is responsible for significant morbidity and mortality throughout the world. Although it has long been recognized as a serious congenital disease, it is only with the advent of acquired immunodeficiency syndrome (AIDS) and the increased use of immunosuppressive therapy that toxoplasmosis has reached epidemic proportions.

Humans are incidental hosts in the life cycle of *T. gondii*. Acute infection occurs via ingestion of meats or beverages contaminated with tissue cysts or tachyzoites or by handling cats, the definitive host. Once the human host develops an adequate immune response, tissue cysts are formed and a chronic or latent infection ensues. Antibodies against *T. gondii* will be present in serum for life. When a chronically infected person becomes immunocompromised, particularly with defects in cell-mediated immunity, devastating reactivation of the latent infection may occur.

CLINICAL MANIFESTATIONS AND DIAGNOSIS

Toxoplasmosis in the AIDS patient is most commonly manifested by toxoplasmic encephalitis (TE), usually alone but sometimes as part of a multiorgan infection. Isolated organ involvement without central nervous system (CNS) disease is uncommon. In most cases, TE develops when the CD4 lymphocyte count falls below $100/mm^3$, although the risk of developing overt infection begins when CD4 counts fall below $200/mm^3$. The clinical manifestations of TE are protean, including signs and symptoms of focal or generalized neurologic dysfunction or more commonly both, depending on the number, size, and location of the lesions. Cerebral edema, vasculitis, and hemorrhage, which can accompany active infection, also contribute to the disease process. Toxoplasmic encephalitis most commonly presents with a subacute onset of focal neurologic deficits with or without evidence of generalized cerebral dysfunction. Less often, seizures are the initial manifestation. Occasionally, signs and symptoms of generalized cerebral dysfunction dominate the presentation, and patients develop focal deficits as the infection progresses. The clinical presentation varies from an insidious process evolving over several weeks to a more acute or even fulminant course. Headaches may be focal or generalized and unremitting.

Serologic tests for diagnosis of toxoplasmosis in AIDS patients are useful only to identify human immunodeficiency virus (HIV)-infected individuals at risk for development of TE and as support for the diagnosis in AIDS patients with focal brain lesions. The Sabin–Feldman dye test is the accepted standard for measurement of immunoglobulin G (IgG) antibodies, which have been shown to be higher in AIDS patients with TE than in those without TE. The immunofluorescence assay (IFA), which is more commonly used, measures the same IgG antibodies as the dye test. Almost all AIDS patients with TE have detectable IgG. The absence of these antibodies strongly suggests another cause of the neurologic signs and symptoms.

The standard of care allows for the treatment of TE to be initiated on presumptive diagnosis when a typical neuroradiographic abnormality is noted on computed tomography (CT) or magnetic resonance imaging (MRI). MRI is more sensitive than CT in the demonstration of focal CNS lesions. The clinical diagnosis is a result of clinical and radiographic response to specific therapy because patients may have similar symptoms resulting from lesions of other causes, such as CNS lymphoma, progressive multifocal leukoencephalopathy, brain abscess, and focal lesions caused by other organisms, including *Cryptococcus neoformans*, *Aspergillus* spp., *Mycobacterium tuberculosis*, and *Nocardia* spp. The practice of presumptive therapy for patients who have not been receiving effective prophylaxis for *Toxoplasma* with a characteristic finding on CT or MRI and positive serology for *Toxoplasma* is widely accepted. With the use of these criteria, the predictive value has been estimated at 80%. However, for patients such as intravenous drug abusers in whom other CNS processes are more prevalent, the predictive value of a positive serology for *Toxoplasma* is reduced, and the widespread use of prophylaxis may further reduce it. Toxoplasmic encephalitis is predominantly intra-axial, so significant meningeal involvement is uncommon. Examination of cerebrospinal fluid (CSF) is used to exclude other diseases. However, detection of *T. gondii* DNA by polymerase chain reaction (PCR) in CSF has shown to be a promising tool in the definitive diagnosis of TE in AIDS patients with focal lesions.

The lungs are the second most common site of infection in AIDS patients and in recipients of bone marrow transplants. The clinical manifestations of toxoplasma pneumonia are nonspecific, similar to those seen with *Pneumocystis jirovecii* (formerly *Pneumocystis carinii*) pneumonia (PCP). Most patients have fever, a nonproductive cough, dyspnea, and occasionally hemoptysis. However, the onset of disease tends to be faster than with PCP. The chest roentgenogram typically reveals bilateral interstitial infiltrates, although multiple nodular infiltrates, single nodules, isolated cavitary disease, lobar infiltrates, pleural effusions, and hilar adenopathy may occur. Pneumothorax complicating toxoplasmic pneumonia has been reported, as well as adult respiratory distress syndrome (ARDS). The diagnosis relies on a high index of suspicion and the demonstration of *T. gondii* from bronchoalveolar lavage (BAL) fluid or biopsy specimens, given the nonspecific nature of both clinical and radiologic manifestations in most cases.

After cytomegalovirus (CMV) retinitis, ocular toxoplasmosis is the most common retinal infection in patients with AIDS. It is rarely reported, and the exact incidence of ocular toxoplasmosis is unknown. Patients usually present with decreased visual acuity and, less often, eye pain. Ocular toxoplasmosis may be the sole manifestation of infection or may accompany TE or disseminated disease. At times, ocular toxoplasmosis is a harbinger of TE. A CT scan of the head should be obtained to assess presence of concomitant TE. Funduscopic findings are consistent with a necrotizing chorioretinitis. The lesions, which may be single or multiple and bilateral and are usually nonhemorrhagic, are yellow-white areas of retinal necrosis with ill-defined fluffy borders. They occur at the posterior pole and may be associated with a moderate to severe inflammatory response in the vitreous and anterior chamber. These characteristics help in the differential diagnosis with CMV retinitis. Fluorescein angiography may also be helpful. Dye leakage tends to occur along the edge of the lesions in toxoplasmosis and to be more prominent in the center of lesions in CMV retinitis. Ocular toxoplasmosis should be suspected if the AIDS patient is seropositive for *T. gondii* and has changes in visual acuity with accompanying funduscopic changes. A prompt response to specific therapy should also be expected. Definitive diagnosis has been made by demonstrating the organism in retinal biopsy specimens or isolation of *T. gondii* from vitreal fluid.

THERAPY

Immunocompetent Host

Most infections in immunocompetent hosts are asymptomatic and do not require therapy. Lymphadenopathy, the most common manifestation, is self-limited and usually resolves within 1 to 3 weeks. Treatment should be considered only if systemic symptoms are severe or long lasting or in the rare event of visceral involvement (encephalitis, myocarditis, pneumonitis). Acute infection as a result of laboratory accidents or transfusions may be severe and should be treated. The treatment regimen of choice consists of a combination of pyrimethamine (Daraprim) and sulfadiazine or trisulfapyrimidine (a mixture of equal parts of sulfamethazine, sulfamerazine, and sulfadiazine) given for 2 to 4 weeks with folinic acid (leucovorin) (Table 197.1). In the event of pyrimethamine-induced hematologic toxicity, the dosage of folinic acid can be increased to 20 to 50 mg/day. For patients allergic to sulfa, clindamycin in combination with pyrimethamine and folinic acid has been used successfully (see Table 197.1).

For ocular toxoplasmosis, the drugs of choice are pyrimethamine and sulfadiazine or trisulfapyrimidine with folinic acid in the same dosages as described earlier. Therapy is given for 4 weeks and repeated as needed. Treatment is required to prevent relapse with the risk of progressive vision loss and other complications such as glaucoma. Adjunctive therapy with systemic corticosteroids (prednisone, 80 to 120 mg/day, or an equivalent) is indicated if the macula, optic nerve, or papillomacular bundle is involved.

Immunocompromised Host

For TE, the combination of pyrimethamine, 200 mg loading dose in 2 divided doses followed by 50 to 75 mg/day orally, plus sulfadiazine, 4 to 6 g/day orally in 4 doses, remains the mainstay of treatment (see Table 197.1). Oral folinic acid is added to preclude the hematologic toxicities

Table 197.1 Drugs for Treatment of Toxoplasmic Encephalitis and Extraneural Toxoplasmosis

Antimicrobial	Mode of Action	Metabolism	Adverse Effects	Recommended Dosage (Immunocompromised)	Recommended Dosage (Immunocompetent)
Pyrimethamine (Daraprim) oral	Inhibits folic acid synthesis	Readily absorbed by gut; hepatic metabolism, lipid soluble	Cytopenias, rash, GI intolerance	Acute: loading dose 200 mg then 50–75 mg daily; with oral folinic acid (leucovorin) 10–20 mg/d Maintenance: 25–50 mg/day with oral folinic acid 10–25 mg/d	Loading dose 200 mg daily for 2 d, then 50–75 mg daily for 2–4 wk; with oral folinic acid 10–20 mg/d
plus					
Sulfadiazine[a] oral	Inhibits folic acid synthesis; acts synergistically and sequentially with pyrimethamine	Readily absorbed by the gut; penetrates blood–brain barrier; some hepatic metabolism	GI intolerance, rash (Stevens–Johnson syndrome), cytopenias, nephrolithiasis, crystalluria, interstitial nephritis, encephalopathy	Acute: 1–1.5 g q6h Maintenance: 500–1000 mg/day QID	1–1.5 g q6h, 2–4 wk
or					
Clindamycin[a] oral and IV	Unknown; possibly inhibition of plastid and/or mitochondrial protein synthesis	Readily absorbed by gut; excellent tissue penetration	GI intolerance, rash, pseudomembranous colitis	Acute: 600 mg q6h (up to IV 1200 mg q6h) Maintenance: 300-450 mg PO q6–8h	300 mg q6h, 4 wk, repeat as needed

Abbreviation: GI = gastrointestinal.
[a] Used in combination with pyrimethamine
Adapted from Mofenson et al. MMWR Recomm Rep. 2004;53(RR–14):1.

associated with antifolate agents. Acute therapy is recommended for at least 6 weeks. Longer treatment durations may be needed if there is extensive clinical and radiographic disease or the response is incomplete at 6 weeks. Patients who cannot tolerate sulfas can be given clindamycin in combination with pyrimethamine as described. Prophylactic use of anticonvulsants is not recommended. Corticosteroids should not be used routinely but are indicated it there is evidence of increased intracranial pressure. In one study, 70% of AIDS patients treated for TE had a quantifiable clinical improvement by day 7 of therapy. Conversely, patients not responding to empiric therapy had evidence of progressive disease within the first 10 days. Ninety percent of patients had improvement on neuroradiographic studies within 6 weeks of starting therapy.

In immunocompromised hosts, maintenance therapy (secondary prophylaxis) should be initiated. The regimen is usually the same as that used for primary treatment but at half dose. Maintenance therapy should be continued for the life of the patient or until the underlying immunosuppression has resolved. In patients with AIDS, secondary prophylaxis can be discontinued if they have sustained CD4 counts greater than 200 cells/mm^3 for longer than 6 months.

The same chemotherapeutic regimens are used for extraneural toxoplasmosis; however, there are limited data available on the optimal length and outcome of treatment. As a rule, ocular toxoplasmosis responds favorably to therapy, and treatment of pulmonary infection has been reported to be successful in 50% to 77% of patients.

Intravenous trimethoprim–sulfamethoxazole (TMP–SMX, Bactrim, Septra), at 5 mg/kg/day trimethoprim component, has been used when oral therapy is contraindicated. Although TMP–SMX is available for oral use, response rates have been lower than standard regimens. Recently, trials have shown higher initial response rates

Table 197.2 Alternative Treatments of Toxoplasmosis in Immunocompromised Patients[a]

Antimicrobial	Mode of Action	Metabolism	Adverse Effects	Recommended Dosages
Atovaquone (Mepron)[a] oral	Uncoupling electron biosynthesis; inhibition of de novo pyrimidine biosynthesis	Suspension has better bioavailability than old tablet formulation; improved absorption if taken with food, particularly fatty foods	Rash, elevated liver function tests	Acute: suspension 1500 mg q12h Maintenance: suspension 750 mg q6–12h
Azithromycin (Zithromax)[a] oral	Unknown; possibly inhibition of plastid and/or mitochondrial protein synthesis	Readily absorbed by gut; high intracellular levels	GI intolerance	Acute: 900–1200 mg/d Maintenance: same
Trimethoprim–sulfamethoxazole (TMP–SMX)[b] (Bactrim, Septra) oral or IV	Inhibits folic acid synthesis	Renal metabolism	Rash, Stevens–Johnson syndrome, bone marrow suppression, hepatotoxicity, increased serum creatinine	Acute: 5 mg/kg TMP and 25 mg/kg SMX IV or oral BID

Abbreviations: GI = gastrointestinal.
[a] Used in combination with pyrimethamine or sulfadiazine.
[b] Used in combination with pyrimethamine.

when the dose was increased (trimethoprim, 6.6 to 10 mg/kg body weight per day).

The drugs described thus far are active only against the tachyzoite form of *T. gondii*. Surviving tissue cysts can reinitiate TE and other manifestations of reactivated latent disease if treatment is discontinued. Therefore it is necessary to give long-term suppressive therapy. Pyrimethamine, 25 to 50 mg/day, and sulfadiazine, 2 to 4 g/day orally in 4 doses, with 10 mg/day of oral folinic acid is recommended because of the low relapse rate associated with this combination. Clindamycin is used in cases of sulfa allergy. Atovaquone monotherapy at 750 mg 2 to 4 times a day may be considered in patients who are unable to tolerate pyrimethamine; however, this regimen has a 1-year relapse rate of 26%.

Primary chemoprophylaxis is a very attractive therapeutic option for patients known to be at risk for toxoplasmosis (ie, those with CD4 counts less than 100 cells/mm^3 and seropositive for anti-*T. gondii* antibodies). Retrospective data suggest that TMP–SMX, 1 double-strength tablet per day orally, is efficacious. Neither dapsone nor pyrimethamine, when used as a single agent, is consistently effective. However, the combination of pyrimethamine, 50 mg/week, plus dapsone, 50 mg/day, plus folinic acid has been a useful alternative. In patients with a sulfa allergy, desensitization is also an option.

Primary prophylaxis can be safely discontinued when the patient has sustained immune reconstitution with a CD4 count greater than 200 cells/mm^3 for 3 months.

Drug regimens being studied for their usefulness as initial and maintenance therapy (Table 197.2) include atovaquone (Mepron). A recent AIDS Clinical Trials Group (ACTG) trial evaluating the efficacy of atovaquone-containing regimens (either in combination with pyrimethamine or sulfadiazine) shows encouraging results, with greater than 80% initial response to therapy (unpublished data). As salvage therapy, atovaquone alone induced initial clinical response in 50% of study patients. The response to therapy with atovaquone has been directly correlated with serum drug levels achieved. The newest formulation of atovaquone is administered as an oral suspension 1.5 g twice daily with food, preferably fatty foods, to increase the bioavailability. The new macrolide antibiotics azithromycin (Zithromax) and clarithromycin (Biaxin) in combination with pyrimethamine have limited utility as alternative agents.

Pregnancy

Women who acquire toxoplasmosis (primary infection) during pregnancy expose their fetuses to risk of infection. Infection of the fetus

Table 197.3 Drugs Used in Treatment of Toxoplasmosis in Pregnant Women

In pregnant women infected during gestation	Medication	Dosage	Duration of Therapy
First 18 wk of gestation or until term if fetus found not to be infected by amniocentesis at 18 wk	Spiramycin[a]	1 g every 8 h without food	Until fetal infection is documented or until it is excluded at 18 wk of gestation
If fetal infection confirmed after wk 18 of gestation and in all women infected after wk 24	Pyrimethamine[b] plus	Loading dose: 50 mg each 12 h for 2 d; then beginning on day 3, 50 mg/d	Until term
	Sulfadiazine plus	Loading dose: 75 mg/kg; then beginning 50 mg/kg each 12 h (maximum 4 g/d)	Until term
	Leucovorin (folinic acid)	10–20 mg daily	During and for 1 wk after pyrimethamine therapy

From Remington JS, McLeod R, Thulliez P, Desmonts G. Toxoplasmosis. In: Remington JS, Klein JO, Wilson CB, Baker CJ, eds. *Infectious Diseases of the Fetus and Newborn Infant.* 6th ed. Philadelphia, PA: Elsevier; 2006.
[a] Spiramycin is not commercially available. Available only on request from the U.S. Food and Drug Administration (telephone number: 301-443-5680), and then with approval by physician's request to Sanofi–Aventis (908-231-3365).
[b] Adjusted for megaloblastic anemia, granulocytopenia, or thrombocytopenia.

may result in stillbirth, spontaneous abortion, or birth of a symptomatic or an asymptomatic infant. Rarely, transmission has been reported in cases where the mother contracts acute toxoplasmosis 6 to 8 weeks before conception. Fetal infection is less common when the mother is treated during pregnancy. Early diagnosis, through serology, amniotic sampling, and fetal ultrasonography, is important in further management (antibiotics or therapeutic abortion).

Pyrimethamine plus a sulfonamide or spiramycin, a macrolide antibiotic available in western Europe, Mexico, and Canada and through the Food and Drug Administration of the United States (301-443-9553), appears to decrease the incidence of congenital toxoplasmic infection when given to women who acquire *T. gondii* during pregnancy (Table 197.3). Pyrimethamine is teratogenic and should not be used until after the first trimester. There is no optimal medical therapy in the United States for treatment of women who become infected during the first trimester. However, sulfadiazine or trisulfapyrimidines should be used during the first trimester because sulfonamides alone have been shown to be effective in acute toxoplasmosis in animal models. If spiramycin can be obtained, pregnant women acutely infected in the first trimester may be treated until term with 30 to 50 mg/kg/day in 3 doses until fetal infection is confirmed or excluded. Treatment with spiramycin alone decreases the incidence of transmission but not the severity of established congenital infection. If fetal infection is suspected or confirmed after the first trimester, pyrimethamine and sulfadiazine plus folinic acid should be used to treat the maternal infection.

Pregnant women or women who are trying to become pregnant should be advised about risk factors for primary infection with toxoplasmosis. Education has been shown to be effective in decreasing the seroconversion rate during pregnancy. Women with cats should have someone else changing the litter box daily. They should avoid consuming undercooked meats, raw eggs, unpasteurized milk, or unfiltered water. All uncooked fruits and vegetables should be washed. Gloves should be used if they are working with soil, if they are preparing raw meat, or if they must change the cat litter box themselves. Proper hand hygiene should be practiced after working with soil, after handling the cat or the litter box, or after touching raw or undercooked meat.

SUGGESTED READING

Kravetz JD, Federman DG. Toxoplasmosis in pregnancy. *Am J Med.* 2005;118:212–216.

Luft BJ, Hafner R, Korzun AH, et al. Toxoplasmic encephalitis in patients with the acquired immunodeficiency syndrome. *N Engl J Med.* 1993;324:995–1000.

Mariuz P, Bosler EM, Luft BJ. Toxoplamosis in individuals with AIDS. *Infect Dis Clin North Am.* 1994;8:365–381.

Montoya JG, Liesenfeld O. Toxoplasmosis. *Lancet.* 2004;363:1965–1976.

Novati R, Castagna A, Morsica G, et al. Polymerase chain reaction for toxoplasma gondii DNA in the cerebrospinal fluid of AIDS patients with focal brain lesions. *AIDS*. 1994;8:1691–1694.

Pomeroy C, Filice GA. Pulmonary toxoplasmosis: a review. *Clin Infect Dis*. 1992;14: 863–870.

Porter SB, Sande MA. Toxoplasmosis of the central nervous system in the acquired immunodeficiency syndrome. *N Engl J Med*. 1992;327:1643–1648.

Remington JS, et al. Toxoplasmosis. In: Remington JS, Klein JO, Wilson CB, Baker CJ, eds. *Infectious Diseases of the Fetus and Newborn Infant*. 6th ed. Philadelphia, PA: Elsevier; 2006.

Torre D, Casari S, Speranza F, et al. Randomized trial of trimethoprim-sulfamethoxazole vs. pyrimethamine-sulfadiazine for therapy of toxoplasmic encephalitis in patients with AIDS. *Antimicrob Agents Chemother*. 1998;42:1346–1349.

Torres RA, Weinberg W, Stansell J, et al. Atovaquone for salvage treatment and suppression of toxoplasmic encephalitis in patients with AIDS. Atovaguone/Toxoplasmic Encephalitis Study Group. *Clin Infect Dis*. 1997;24:422–429.

198. Malaria: Treatment and Prophylaxis

Phyllis E. Kozarsky, Deborah J. Nicolls, and Jay S. Keystone

Malaria is the most important parasitic infection that causes disease in humans. More than a million persons, mostly children, die each year from malaria. It is also one of the most common causes of fever in returned travelers and recent immigrants from malaria-endemic areas.

Malaria is primarily caused by infection with 1 of 4 *Plasmodium* species: *Plasmodium falciparum*, *Plasmodium vivax*, *Plasmodium ovale*, and *Plasmodium malariae*. Occasionally human infection with a monkey malaria parasite, such as *P. knowlesi*, occurs. Treating malaria appropriately requires knowledge of the infecting species, the likely location in which the infection was acquired, and the geographic patterns of drug resistance. Figure 198.1 shows the worldwide distribution of malaria. When there is any doubt about the infecting species, the clinician should treat for the worst-case scenario, chloroquine-resistant *P. falciparum* (CRPF) malaria. Malaria caused by *P. vivax* and *P. ovale* may leave dormant forms, hypnozoites, in the liver after the blood phase has been eradicated. Thus, treatment of these two infections requires eradication of the erythrocytic phase followed by a second drug to eradicate the liver phase (terminal prophylaxis).

CLINICAL ASPECTS

Because death from malaria can occur within several days of the onset of symptoms, it is necessary to consider a febrile illness in a patient from a malarious endemic area to be a medical emergency. This is particularly so when symptoms begin within the first 2 months of arrival because more than 90% of those with malaria caused by *P. falciparum* present within this time. However, persons may develop symptoms of malaria 6 months to 1 year after departing a malarious region, particularly those infected with *P. vivax* or *P. ovale* or, in rare cases, *P. falciparum* in semi-immunes (usually from sub-Saharan Africa). The use of chemoprophylaxis may also modify the symptoms or delay the onset of malaria. For these reasons, anyone who develops fever within a year of travel to a malaria-risk area should have blood films performed to rule out malaria.

Infection with *Plasmodium* spp. occurs through the bite of a female *Anopheles* mosquito. The sporozoite is released into the human bloodstream and quickly travels to the liver, where it matures. Infected persons are asymptomatic at this stage of infection. Symptoms begin only after the parasites are released from the liver back into the bloodstream where they infect erythrocytes. The severity of symptoms depends on the proportion of erythrocytes infected by the *Plasmodium* spp. and the presence of partial immunity to *Plasmodium* infection due to prior exposure.

Initial symptoms typically do not occur until after 1 week to 10 days following a bite. They are nonspecific and include fever, chills, malaise, anorexia, headaches, and myalgias. Cough, abdominal pain, and diarrhea may also be present. Severe infection with *P. falciparum* is a multiorgan system disease, causing severe anemia, thrombocytopenia, metabolic acidosis, hypoglycemia, pulmonary edema, respiratory failure, renal failure, and coma. Even with treatment, severe malaria has an overall mortality of 15% to 20%; it is higher in the older population.

DIAGNOSIS

Prompt and accurate diagnosis is crucial to the effective management of malaria. The standard approach to diagnosing malaria is the examination of stained thick and thin blood films, but many laboratories do not have the expertise to examine the former. Thick films are 5 to 6 times as sensitive as thin films, allowing for the detection of low parasitemia levels; at low parasitemia levels, thin films may be negative. Thin films are better for determining the species of malaria. If the expertise to examine thick films is not available, as is usually the case in the middle of the night, thin blood films are better than none at all. Although the diagnosis may be missed on a thin blood film, a negative result will rule out a life-threatening infection, which is always associated with high parasitemia. If the initial blood films are negative, they should be repeated 2 or 3 times at 12-hour intervals.

A number of rapid diagnostic tests (RDTs) have been developed in recent years to assist with the diagnosis of malaria in areas where blood films are not readily available. These tests rely on the detection of various *Plasmodium* spp. antigens, including histidine-rich protein 2 (HRP2) and parasite lactate dehydrogenase (pLDH). They have a high degree of sensitivity and specificity for falciparum malaria and are probably equivalent to thick and thin films when performed by trained technicians. These tests tend to be more expensive than microscopy and are vulnerable to high temperatures and humidity; however, in areas where microscopy is not feasible, RDTs are important in the management of malaria. Also, RDTs may be valuable for office-based clinicians and emergency room personnel who do not have access to immediate laboratory support.

Polymerase chain reaction (PCR) may be used to confirm the diagnosis of malaria and is an important tool in identifying mixed infections. PCR is also more sensitive than thick films in detecting a low parasitemia; however, it is not a rapid technique and is not used in the routine diagnosis of malaria. It is often available in laboratory reference centers or as a research tool.

THERAPY

Increasingly, the treatment of malaria has been complicated in recent years by the rapid spread

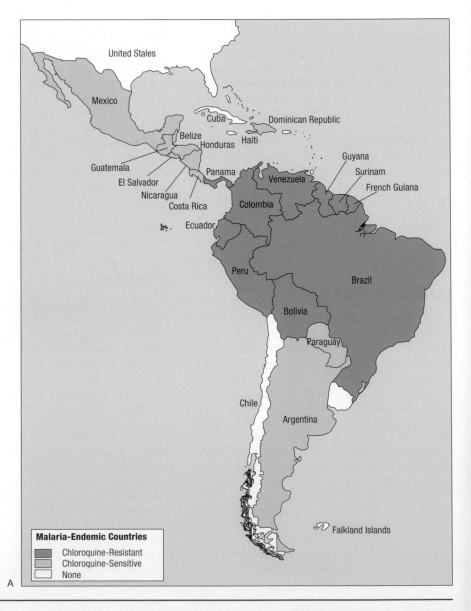

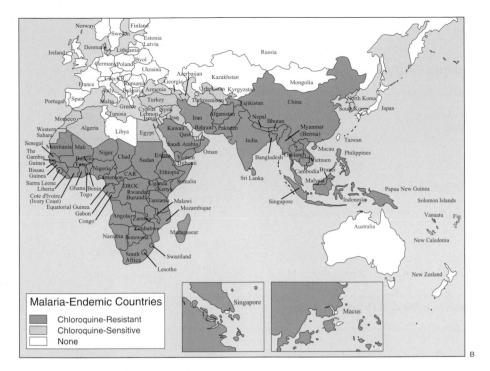

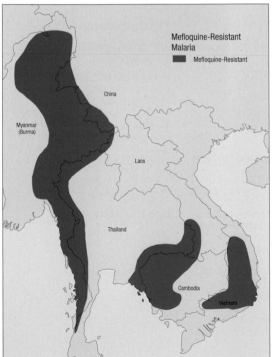

Figure 198.1 A and B: Distribution of malaria and chloroquine-resistant *Plasmodium falciparum* in the Western and Eastern Hemispheres, 2006. **C:** Distribution of mefloquine-resistant *Plasmodium falciparum*, 2006. (Courtesy of the Centers for Disease Control and Prevention.)

of drug-resistant strains. No longer do clinicians have to be concerned only with CRPF malaria but also with chloroquine-resistant and primaquine-resistant *P. vivax* malaria. Drug resistance has not been established in *P. ovale* or *P. malariae*. Drug regimens for treatment are provided in Table 198.1.

Plasmodium vivax Malaria

Plasmodium vivax malaria has very low mortality, but considerable morbidity in the developing world. The erythrocytic phase of *P. vivax* malaria is usually effectively treated with chloroquine; primaquine is then used to eradicate

Table 198.1 Treatment of Malaria

Drug	Adult Dosage	Pediatric Dosage
Chloroquine-Sensitive Malaria (All Species)		
Chloroquine 1 tablet (150 mg base = 250 mg salt) Plus in *Plasmodium vivax* and *Plasmodium ovale* only:	600 mg base immediately, followed by 300 mg base in 6, 24, and 48 h	10 mg base/kg (maximum 600 mg) immediately, followed by 5 mg base/kg in 6, 24, and 48 h
Primaquine	30 mg base/d × 14 d	0.5 mg base/kg/d × 14 d
Mefloquine	1.5 g (base) in single or divided dose over 12 h	15 mg salt/kg in individual dose over 12 h
Quinine sulfate plus one of the following:	650 mg salt TID × 3–7 d	10 mg salt/kg TID × 3–7 d
Doxycycline	100 mg BID × 7 d	4 mg/kg in 2 doses × 7 d
Clindamycin	900 mg TID × 3 d	20 mg/kg/d in 3 doses × 7 d
Tetracycline	250 mg QID × 7 d	25 mg/kg/d in 4 doses × 7 d
Primaquine (following both quinine and mefloquine)	30 mg base/d × 14 d	0.5 mg base/kg/d × 14 d
Uncomplicated Chloroquine-Resistant *Plasmodium falciparum*		
Quinine sulfate plus one of the following:	650 mg salt TID × 3–7 d	10 mg salt/kg TID × 3–7 d
Doxycycline	100 mg BID × 7 d	4 mg/kg in 2 doses × 7 d
Clindamycin	900 mg TID × 3 d	20 mg/kg/d in 3 doses × 7 d
Tetracycline	250 mg QID × 7 d	25 mg/kg/d in 4 doses × 7 d
Atovaquone–proguanil	250 mg atovaquone/100 mg proguanil = 1 adult tablet	62.5 mg atovaquone/25 mg proguanil = 1 pediatric tablet
	4 adult tablets daily × 3 d	5–8 kg: 2 ped tabs daily × 3 d 9–10 kg: 3 ped tabs daily × 3 d 11–20 kg: 1 adult tab daily × 3 d 21–30 kg: 2 adult tabs daily × 3 d 31–40 kg: 3 adult tabs daily × 3 d >40 kg: 4 adult tabs daily × 3 d
Mefloquine	1.5 g (base) in a single or divided dose over 12 h	15 mg/kg in a single or divided dose over 12 h
Treatment of Severe Illness; Parental Dose for All Species		
Quinine loading	20 mg/kg (salt) (1 mg salt = 0.83 mg base) in 300 mL of normal saline IV over 2–4 h Maintenance, 10 mg/kg q8h	Same as for adults
Quinidine loading	24 mg/kg (salt) in 300 mL of normal saline IV over 2–4 h Maintenance: 12 mg/kg q8h or 10 mg/kg (salt) IV over 1–2 h, then constant infusion of 0.02 mg/kg/min by infusion pump	Same as for adults
Plus one of the following:	If unable to tolerate orally:	
Doxycycline	100 mg IV q12h	If ≤45 kg: 4 mg/kg q12h If ≥45 kg: use same dose as adults
Clindamycin	10 mg/kg IV loading dose, then 5 mg/kg q8h	10 mg/kg IV loading dose, then 5 mg/kg q8h
Tetracycline	As above	As above

hepatic hypnozoites. Because primaquine is one of the most potent oxidizing agents known, a glucose-6-phosphate dehydrogenase (G6PD) level must be determined before primaquine therapy is initiated to prevent severe hemolysis in those with G6PD deficiency.

Chloroquine-resistant *P. vivax* malaria was first described in Indonesia in 1989. Since then, it has been shown to be highly endemic in Oceania and the Amazon basin of Peru, Brazil, Colombia, and Guyana. Malaria caused by chloroquine-resistant *P. vivax* should be suspected when the illness recurs within 28 days after a patient has received standard therapy with chloroquine and primaquine. Although studies from Indonesia suggested that a standard course of chloroquine combined with high-dose primaquine (2.5 mg/kg over 48 hours) would be effective therapy for drug-resistant *P. vivax* malaria, the regimen was not effective in strains from Guyana. Both mefloquine and halofantrine are effective, although the latter is not available in North America and should not be used routinely because of its adverse event profile.

When a relapse of *P. vivax* occurs more than 28 days after treatment with chloroquine and primaquine, primaquine resistance should be considered. Primaquine-resistant *P. vivax* malaria is often reported from Papua, New Guinea, Irian Jaya, other parts of southeast Asia and Somalia, and, less commonly, Colombia. Patients who fail the usual course of primaquine should receive 2 times the standard dose over 14 days, or a total dose of 6 mg/kg, to prevent further relapses.

Plasmodium ovale Malaria

Malaria caused by *P. ovale*, found mostly in Africa, is managed in the same way as chloroquine-sensitive *P. vivax*. No drug-resistant strains of *P. ovale* have been documented.

Plasmodium malariae and Uncomplicated Chloroquine-Sensitive *P. falciparum* Malaria

Chloroquine-sensitive *P. falciparum* malaria is confined to Central America north of Panama, Haiti, the Dominican Republic, parts of North Africa, and the Middle East. Outbreaks can occur in nonendemic areas, such as Jamaica or the southern United States, that may be located near another highly endemic area. Chloroquine in standard doses should be used to treat *P. falciparum* from these areas and *P. malariae* infections from any part of the world. Chloroquine does not eradicate the gametocytes of *P. falciparum* malaria that circulate harmlessly for several months after the other erythrocytic forms of the parasite have been eradicated.

Uncomplicated Chloroquine-Resistant *P. falciparum* Malaria

With the exception of the regions where chloroquine-sensitive *P. falciparum* malaria remains, malaria caused by *P. falciparum* should be considered chloroquine resistant. Artemisinin-based combination therapies (ACTs) are rapidly becoming the treatment of choice for *P. falciparum* malaria. Artemisinin and its derivatives are well tolerated and lead to a rapid reduction in parasitemia and fever; however, monotherapy is associated with a high rate of recrudescence. The combination of a second agent is necessary to ensure cure of the infection. ACTs currently recommended by the World Health Organization (WHO) include artemether-lumefantrine, artesunate plus amodiaquine, artesunate plus mefloquine, and artesunate plus sulfadoxine–pyrimethamine. Artesunate is available in parenteral, oral, and suppository forms. Atovaquone–proguanil has also been shown to be effective in ACTs but is very costly.

Unfortunately, artemisinin-based regimens are not available in the United States. Atovaquone–proguanil has recently become the drug combination of choice for the treatment of uncomplicated *P. falciparum* malaria infections, even for those who have acquired multidrug-resistant infection in areas of Thailand. The 3-day course of therapy is generally well tolerated, with a small percentage of individuals suffering from gastrointestinal upset. Dividing the dose twice daily and giving it with food may reduce this problem.

Quinine sulfate in combination with tetracycline, doxycycline, or clindamycin remains a very good regimen for the treatment of CRPF but is longer and less well tolerated than is atovaquone–proguanil. Clindamycin is usually reserved for pregnant women and for young children, in whom no tetracycline derivative is generally used. Because these second agents tend to be slower acting, it is important to institute quinine therapy as soon as the diagnosis is confirmed. Virtually everyone who takes quinine will suffer from cinchonism, and complaints of tinnitus, dizziness, headache, and possibly temporary hearing loss are common. If the parasitemia is 1% or greater, strong consideration should be given to the use of a loading dose of quinine (doubling the initial dose) and if oral medication is not tolerated, intravenous quinidine (quinine in Canada) is the drug of choice. This remains quite problematic as this agent tends not to be readily available in U.S. hospitals.

Mefloquine is also a very effective therapy for uncomplicated CRPF malaria, but it is not recommended for patients who acquired their infection in certain rural areas of southeast Asia, particularly along the Thai–Myanmar (Burma) or Thai–Cambodian borders, because of multi-drug resistance. Moreover, there is evidence for increasing drug resistance in these regions (see Figure 198.1). Studies confirm the development of cross-resistance among mefloquine, halo-fantrine, and quinine because of their chemical relatedness. Major concerns about the use of me-floquine for treatment of malaria are the severe neuropsychiatric adverse reactions (psychosis, convulsions), which occur 10 to 60 times as often as when the drug is used for prophylaxis; these complications are estimated to occur in 1:215 to 1:1700 of those treated for malaria. In an attempt to decrease the gastrointestinal side effects of mefloquine, the dose may be split and administered over 12 hours.

Due to the spread of drug resistance through southeast Asia, Africa, and the Amazon ba-sin, the use of pyrimethamine–sulfadoxine (Fansidar) is no longer recommended for the treatment of malaria, except when resistance patterns are known.

Halofantrine is widely used in malarious areas throughout the world; however, in stan-dard doses, it has limited effectiveness against malaria acquired along the borders of Thailand. Studies have documented cardiotoxicity with halofantrine, particularly in those who have taken the drug with food, as drug absorption increases 6-fold with a fatty meal. Halofantrine should be taken on an empty stomach. It is contraindicated in those with a family history of prolonged QT interval or conduction distur-bances or when any other QT-prolonging agent such as mefloquine or quinine has been admin-istered. An electrocardiogram is recommended before halofantrine administration.

Complicated *P. falciparum* Malaria

Severe malaria is a medical emergency. Management comprises four main areas: clinical assessment, specific antimalarial treat-ment, adjunctive therapy, and supportive care. When *P. falciparum* parasitemia reaches 5% or more, complications such as cerebral malaria,

renal failure, adult respiratory distress syn-drome (ARDS), and massive hemolysis may occur. It is not uncommon for ARDS to occur on the third to fourth day of treatment while the parasitemia is dropping. The mortality of even appropriately treated severe *P. falciparum* malaria ranges from 15% to 20%. Patients with complicated malaria, and those who can-not tolerate oral quinine because of vomiting, require parenteral therapy with quinine or quinidine. Because parenteral quinine prepara-tions are not readily available in most centers, quinidine should be used. However, because of its potential for cardiotoxicity, continuous electrocardiographic monitoring should be un-dertaken. Because both quinine and quinidine cause insulin to be released from the pancreas, it is important to monitor for hypoglycemia (use 10% dextrose in intravenous fluids), a common complication of severe malaria, espe-cially in pregnant women and children. Fluid balance should be corrected judiciously with the aim of avoiding fluid overload because of the risk of ARDS. Lactic acidosis, a common complication of severe malaria, indicates a poor prognosis. For parasitemias above 10%, particularly when other complications are pres-ent, exchange transfusion with at least 4 units of blood or red cell pheresis may be lifesaving. When patients present with severe *P. falciparum* malaria, it is prudent to rule out other concom-itant infections such as meningitis in those who are comatose and septicemia in those who are hypotensive.

PROPHYLAXIS

The primary goal of prophylaxis is to pre-vent *P. falciparum* infection in nonimmune travelers because almost all fatal cases are as-sociated with illness caused by this species. For decades, chloroquine was widely effective in the prevention and treatment of all species of malaria, and it remains the drug of choice for travel to areas in which chloroquine resistance is low or not yet described. However, with the spread of chloroquine resistance to much of Africa, Asia, and tropical South America, recom-mendations for antimalarial chemoprophylaxis have become more complicated. Figure 198.2 is an algorithm for determining an appropriate antimalarial chemoprophylactic regimen.

Areas within a country may differ with respect to risk. For example, travel in most areas in Kenya places travelers at risk for acquisition of CRPF. The risk is highest near Lake Victoria, intermediate on the coast, and

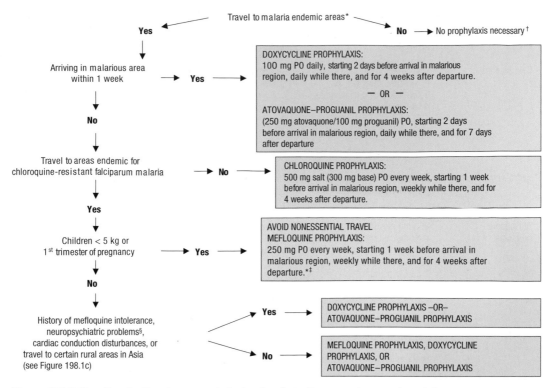

Figure 198.2 Algorithm for the chemoprophylaxis of malaria. Dosages given are for adults.
* Dosage recommendations are for adults. See Table 198.2 for pediatric dosages.
† Malaria in many coutries is confined to rural areas or regions not on usual tourist itineraries.
‡ Data collected suggest there is no significant increase in spontaneous abortions or congenital malformations when mefloquine is given during the first trimester; inadvertent use not a reason for termination of pregnancy.
§ Seizures, psychoses, depression, anxiety reactions.

lowest in the game parks. However, if the traveler will be staying only in Nairobi, the capital, where there is no malaria, prophylaxis is not necessary.

For travel in areas with CRPF infections, 1 of 3 chemoprophylaxis regimens is recommended: doxycycline, mefloquine, and atovaquone–proguanil (Table 198.2). All 3 regimens have comparable efficacy, except in areas with multidrug-resistant *P. falciparum*, particularly in certain rural areas of Asia where mefloquine resistance has been identified (see Figure 198.1). The decision about which regimen to use should be based on the presence of any contraindications to the use of a particular antimalarial drug and client preference; the latter is often determined by side-effect profile, convenience, and cost. Mefloquine has been associated with disabling neuropsychiatric side effects (anxiety, depression, headaches, nightmares, and irritability), which occur in approximately 1 in 200 users and more often in women. Dividing the dose twice weekly may reduce these effects. Severe reactions, including seizures and

psychosis, have been documented to occur in approximately 1:10,000 users, most often in those with underlying contraindications to the drug. Because the majority of adverse reactions to mefloquine occur with the first 3 doses, if possible, it would be advisable to commence the drug 4 weeks prior to departure to ascertain drug tolerance. Moreover, from a medical legal perspective, mefloquine should not be prescribed unless the traveler is fully informed about the drug's potential side effects and alternative prophylactic agents. Unlike mefloquine, atovaquone–proguanil and doxycycline can be started within 1 to 2 days of arriving in a malaria-risk area. Both drugs are usually well tolerated but are contraindicated in pregnancy, whereas mefloquine is not.

Long-term travel poses an additional challenge in the prevention of malaria. Long-term travelers have a higher risk of malaria than short-term travelers, and they frequently underuse personal protective measures and adhere poorly to continuous chemoprophylaxis regimens. Medications that are administered

Table 198.2 Malaria Chemoprophylaxis Regimens

Drug	Adult Dose	Pediatric Dose	Adverse Effects
Chloroquine	500 mg salt (300 mg base) PO weekly, starting 1 wk before travel and continue for 4 wk after travel	8.3 mg/kg salt (5 mg/kg base) PO 1×/wk	Bitter taste, headache, pruritus, rash, blurry vision, reversible corneal opacity, partial alopecia. Rare: retinopathy, blood dyscrasias, nail discoloration, nerve deafness, myopathy. May exacerbate psoriasis
Hydroxychloroquine	400 mg salt (310 mg base) PO weekly, as for chloroquine	6.5 mg/kg salt (5 mg/kg base) PO weekly (maximum 310 mg base)	As for chloroquine
Atovaquone–proguanil	250 mg atovaquone and 100 mg proguanil (1 adult tablet) PO daily, starting 1–2 d before travel and continue for 7 d after travel	Body weight 5–8 kg: ½ pediatric tab po daily (1 ped tab=: 62.5 atovaquone and 25 mg proguanil) 9–10 kg: ¾ ped tab PO daily 11–20 kg: 1 ped tab PO daily 21–30 kg: 2 ped tab PO daily 31–40 kg: 3 ped tab PO daily >40 kg: 1 adult tab PO daily	Nausea, abdominal pain, headache. May transiently increase transaminases. Rare: rash. Take with food. Do not use if creatinine clearance ≤30 mL/min
Doxycycline	100 mg PO daily, starting 1–2 d before travel and continue for 4 wk after travel	≥8 years old: 2 mg/kg PO daily (maximum dose 100 mg/d)	Esophageal irritation, GI upset, photosensitivity, vaginitis. Stains teeth of children aged ≤8 years and fetuses. Do not use in pregnancy
Mefloquine	250 mg salt (1 tablet) PO weekly, starting 1 wk before travel and continue for 4 wk after travel	Body weight ≤9 kg: 5 mg/kg salt weekly; body weight 10–19 kg: ¼ tablet weekly; body weight 20–30 kg: ½ tablet weekly; body weight 31–45 kg: ¾ tablet weekly; body weight >45 kg: 1 tablet weekly	Dizziness, nausea, diarrhea, headache, nightmares, altered dreams, insomnia, mood changes. Rare: seizure, psychosis. Do not use if history of psychosis, active depression, seizure disorder, or cardiac conduction abnormality
Primaquine Terminal prophylaxis	30 mg base PO daily for 14 d	0.5 mg/kg base PO daily for 14 d	GI upset. Take with food. CHECK G6PD LEVEL. Hemolysis with G6PD deficiency. Do not use in pregnancy
Primary prophylaxis	30 mg base daily, starting 1–2 d before travel and continue for 7 d after travel	0.5 mg/kg base PO daily, starting 1–2 d before travel and continue for 7 d after travel	

Abbreviations: GI = gastrointestinal; G6PD = glucose-6-phosphate dehydrogenase.

weekly may be easier to comply with compared with daily regimens.

Prolonged exposure to malaria in areas intensely endemic for *P. vivax* (for example, Central America, northwest Africa, South Asia, Oceania) warrants terminal malaria prophylaxis with primaquine phosphate to eradicate the hepatic hypnozoites and prevent relapsing malaria. As noted, G6PD levels should be checked before prescribing this drug, and it is contraindicated during pregnancy. Primaquine is usually taken after completing chloroquine, mefloquine, or doxycycline therapy. The adult dose is 30 mg base/day for 14 days. Primaquine

has also been used successfully as primary prophylaxis in partially immune residents of malaria-endemic areas and nonimmune travelers to malaria-endemic areas.

Because no antimalarial regimen is 100% effective, all travelers to malarious regions need to be meticulous about personal protection measures. Between dusk and dawn, when the *Anopheles* mosquitoes bite, travelers should wear permethrin-impregnated protective clothing (long sleeves, pants), use mosquito repellents, and sleep under permethrin-impregnated netting or in screened or air-conditioned rooms. Insect repellents that contain 35% or more

Specific Organisms – Parasites

diethyltoluamide (DEET) are very effective. Recently, the American Academy of Pediatrics and the United States Environmental Protection Agency have indicated that 30% DEET is safe for individuals as young as 2 months of age. Picaridin is a newly available insect repellent that appears to be quite efficacious, particularly in its 15% formulation that is available in Europe but not in North America. Travelers should always read and follow instructions on the containers so that the products are used safely and are reapplied at the best time intervals. Knock-down sprays should be used indoors and in infected areas before bedtime.

Because there is no worldwide consensus concerning malaria chemoprophylaxis, travelers should be advised to listen with great caution to antimalarial advice received from fellow travelers and overseas health care providers. Also, travelers should be advised to seek medical attention immediately in the event of fever during or soon after travel. They should tell their health care provider to test them for malaria and have blood films repeated 2 more times if the first one is negative. Also, it is important for travelers to know that malaria is often overdiagnosed in developing countries; therefore, they should be advised to continue their prophylaxis regimen even if they are diagnosed with malaria while abroad.

Physicians who are responsible for preventing and treating malaria will have to keep abreast of the global spread of drug resistance and the new agents being developed to combat this problem. Assistance may be sought from the Centers for Disease Control and Prevention by calling toll free 877-FYI-TRIP (394–8747) or through their Web site (www.cdc.gov/travel).

SUGGESTED READING

Baird JK, Hoffman SL. Primaquine therapy for malaria. *Clin Infect Dis.* 2004;39:1336–1345.

Baird JK. Effectiveness of antimalarial drugs. *N Engl J Med.* 2005;352:1565–1577.

Centers for Disease Control and Prevention. *Health Information for International Travel 2007–2008.* Philadelphia, PA: Mosby; 2007.

Chen LH, Keystone JS. New strategies for the prevention of malaria in travelers. *Infect Dis Clin North Am.* 2005;19:185–210.

Chen LE, Wilson ME, Schlagenhauf P. Prevention of malaria in long-term travelers. *JAMA.* 2006;296:2234–2244.

Franco-Paredes C, Santos-Preciado JL. Problem pathogens: prevention of malaria in travellers. *Lancet Infect Dis.* 2006;6:139–149.

Hill DR, Ericsson CD, Pearson RD, et al. The practice of Travel Medicine: guidelines by the Infectious Diseases Society of America. *Clin Infect Dis.* 2006;43:1499–1539.

Ochola LB, Vounatsou P, Smith T, Mabaso ML, Newton CR. The reliability of diagnostic techniques in the diagnosis and management of malaria in the absence of a gold standard. *Lancet Infect Dis.* 2006;6:582–588.

Schwartz E, Parise M, Kozarsky P, Cetron M. Delayed onset of malaria—implications for chemoprophylaxis in travelers. *N Engl J Med.* 2003;349:1510–1516.

World Health Organization. *Guidelines for the Treatment of Malaria.* Geneva, Switzerland: WHO Press; 2006.

199. Human Babesiosis

Tempe K. Chen and Peter J. Krause

Babesiosis is an emerging zoonotic disease caused by intraerythrocytic protozoa and transmitted by ticks. The first well-documented case of human babesial infection was reported in 1957 in a splenectomized resident of Yugoslavia, who died after an acute illness marked by anemia, fever, hemoglobinuria, and renal failure. Intraerythrocytic parasites were noted and tentatively identified as *Babesia bovis*. Since then, six *Babesia* species have been found to cause disease in humans: *Babesia microti*, *Babesia duncani* (formerly known as WA1), and MO1 in North America; *Babesia divergens* and EU1 in Europe; and TW1 in Taiwan. The clustering of cases of human *B. microti* infection in the United States contrasts with the sporadic occurrence of the disease in Europe, Africa, and Asia. Rarely, babesiosis may be transmitted through blood transfusion or perinatally.

EPIDEMIOLOGY

More than 90 species in the genus *Babesia* infect a wide variety of wild and domestic animals. Humans are an uncommon and terminal host for *Babesia* species, which depend on other species for survival. The most common cause for human babesiosis is *B. microti*, a babesia of rodents. The primary reservoir for *B. microti* in eastern North America is the white-footed mouse (*Peromyscus leucopus*). As many as two-thirds of *P. leucopus* have been found to be parasitemic in endemic areas. *Babesia* species are transmitted by hard-bodied (ixodid) ticks. The primary vector in eastern North America is *Ixodes scapularis* (also known as *Ixodes dammini*), which is the same tick that transmits *Borrelia burgdorferi*, the etiologic agent of Lyme disease, and *Anaplasma phagocytophilum*, the agent of human granulocytic anaplasmosis. Thus, simultaneous human infection with two or more of these pathogens may occur.

Each of the three active stages in the life cycle of *I. scapularis* (larva, nymph, and adult) takes a blood meal from a vertebrate host to mature to the next stage (Figure 199.1). The *Babesia* species ingested by one tick stage are transmitted to the next stage. The tick transmission cycle begins in late summer when newly hatched larvae ingest the parasite with a blood meal from an infected rodent and maintain the parasite to the nymphal stage. Nymphs transmit the *Babesia* species to rodents in late spring and summer of the following year. Larvae, nymphs, and adults can feed on humans, but the nymph is the primary vector (Figure 199.2). All active tick stages also feed on the white-tailed deer (*Odocoileus virginianus*), which is an important host for the tick but is not a reservoir for *B. microti*. An increase in the deer population over the past few decades is thought to be a major factor in the spread of *I. scapularis* and in the resulting increase in human cases.

Beginning in the 1980s, human babesiosis has been described with increasing frequency at sites in the northeastern and northern midwestern United States. Recent studies suggest that the endemic range continues to expand. In certain sites during years of high transmission, babesiosis may constitute a significant public health burden. For example, in one study of a highly endemic area in Rhode Island, approximately 9% of the population had evidence of previous *B. microti* infection compared with 11% of previous Lyme disease. Most human cases of babesiosis occur in the summer and in areas where the vector tick, rodents, and deer are in close proximity to humans. Rarely, babesiosis is acquired through transfusion of blood products. Whole blood, packed red cells, cryopreserved red cells, and platelets have been implicated. Transplacental/perinatal transmission of babesiosis also has been described.

PATHOGENESIS

Our understanding of the pathogenesis of human babesiosis is incomplete and is primarily based on studies done in animals. Cytoadherence of infected erythrocytes to vascular epithelium may diminish access of host immune factors to babesia, including prevention of transit of infected erythrocytes through the spleen where they would be destroyed, allowing babesia to complete their life cycle

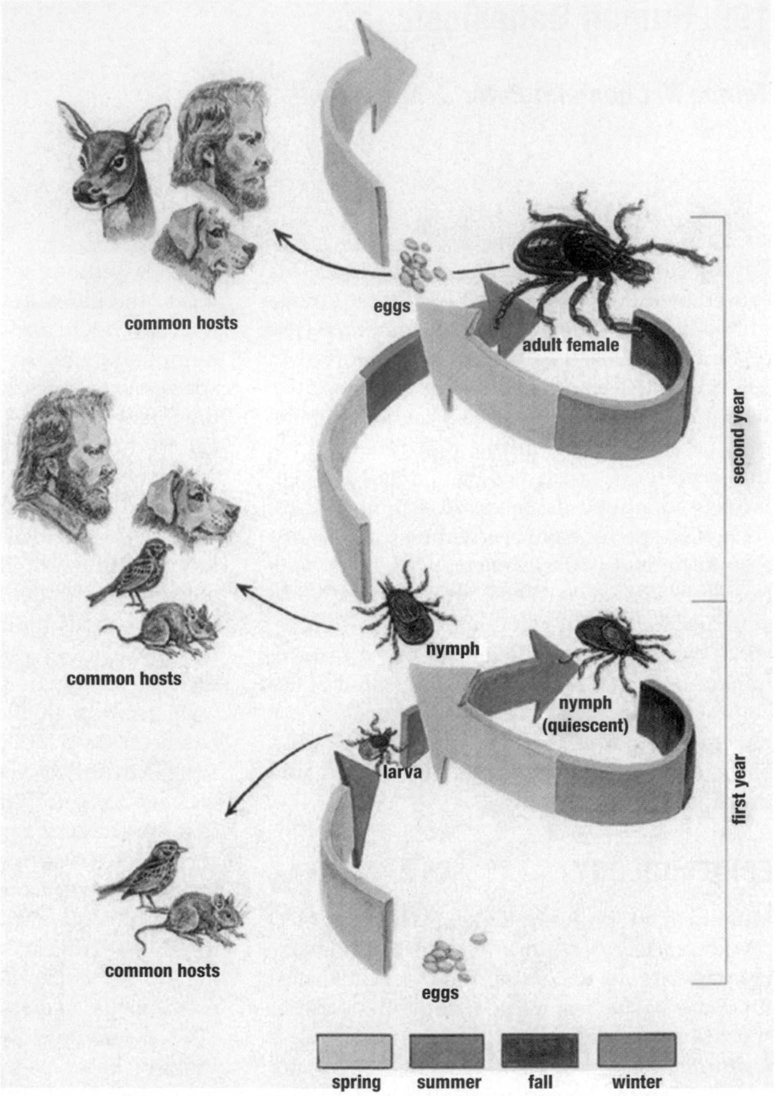

Figure 199.1 Life cycle of *Babesia microti.* (Reproduced with permission from D. W. Miller.)

and invade other erythrocytes. Excessive cytoadherence may lead to erythrocyte sequestration and obstruction of microvasculature with subsequent tissue anoxia, as has been demonstrated in cattle infected by *Babesia bovis.* Similarly, production of host proinflammatory cytokines such as tumor necrosis factor (TNF) and interleukin (IL)-1 help to destroy intracellular babesia; however, excessive cytokine production associated with moderate to severe disease probably accounts for the majority of clinical manifestations and complications of the disease. T and B cells macrophages, polymorphonuclear leukocytes, antibody, and complement also are important in clearing parasitemia and may contribute to disease pathogenesis.

CLINICAL MANIFESTATIONS

The clinical severity of babesiosis ranges from subclinical infection to fulminating disease resulting in death. In clinically apparent cases, symptoms of babesiosis begin after an incubation period of 1 to 9 weeks from the beginning of tick feeding or 6 to 9 weeks after transfusion. In most cases, there is a gradual onset of malaise, anorexia, and fatigue followed by intermittent temperatures as high as 40°C (104°F) and one or more of the following symptoms: chills, sweats, myalgia, arthralgia, nausea, and vomiting. Less commonly noted are emotional lability, hyperesthesia, headache, sore throat, abdominal pain, conjunctival injection, photophobia, weight loss, and nonproductive

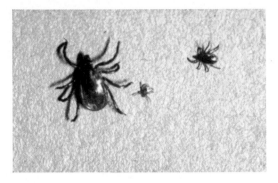

Figure 199.2 *Ixodes scapularis* (also known as *Ixodes dammini*) ticks showing larval, nymphal, and adult stages.

cough. The findings on physical examination generally are minimal, often consisting only of fever. Mild splenomegaly, hepatomegaly, or both are noted occasionally. Slight pharyngeal erythema, jaundice, retinopathy with splinter hemorrhages, and retinal infarcts also have been reported. Rash is seldom noted although ecchymoses and petechiae have been described in severe disease.

Symptoms usually persist for a few weeks to several months, with prolonged recovery of up to 18 months in severe cases. Parasitemia may continue even after a person feels well and may persist for >2 years with subsequent relapse of illness. Although prolonged symptomatic disease unresponsive to antimicrobial therapy or death may occur in immunocompromised hosts, complete recovery with or without therapy is the rule.

Patients at increased risk for more severe babesial disease include those who suffer from malignancy, have concomitant human immunodeficiency virus (HIV) infection, are asplenic, are older than age 50 years, are taking immunosuppressive medications, or are infected with *B. divergens* or *B. duncani*. Concurrent babesiosis and Lyme disease infection occurs in about 3% to 15% of patients experiencing Lyme disease in parts of southern New England and results in more severe illness than with either disease alone. Moderate to severe babesiosis may occur in children, but infection often results in mild disease and is generally less severe than in adults. Several cases of neonatal babesiosis have been described, usually following transfusion with infected blood, and sometimes resulting in severe illness. Symptoms and signs include lethargy, tachypnea, pallor, poor feeding, splenomegaly, hepatomegaly, jaundice, and generalized macular rash.

COMPLICATIONS

A severe form of babesiosis has been noted in some patients, consisting of fulminant illness lasting about a week and ending in death or a prolonged convalescence. Although more common in immunocompromised hosts or those experiencing *B. divergens* or *B. duncani* infection, severe babesiosis can occur in otherwise healthy individuals who are infected with *B. microti*. In a retrospective study of 136 patients with *B. microti* infection from Long Island, New York, 7 patients (5%) died. The patients with fatal illness ranged in age from 60 to 82 years, and only 1 was known to be immunocompromised. Signs and symptoms in severe cases include high fever, severe hemolytic anemia, hemoglobinemia and hemoglobinuria, jaundice, ecchymoses, petechiae, congestive heart failure, pulmonary edema, renal failure, adult respiratory distress syndrome, and coma. Patients with malignancy or HIV infection also may experience a chronic form of babesiosis that is unresponsive to multiple courses of standard antibabesial therapy.

DIAGNOSIS

Babesiosis should be suspected in any patient with unexplained febrile illness who has recently lived or traveled in endemic regions during the months of May through September, with or without a history of tick bite. There is often no recollection of a tick bite, because the unengorged *I. scapularis* nymph is about 2 mm in length.

Laboratory findings reflect the invasion and subsequent lysis of erythrocytes by the parasite and the immune response to infection. They include moderate to severe hemolytic anemia, an elevated reticulocyte count, thrombocytopenia, an elevated erythrocyte sedimentation rate, elevated serum bilirubin and liver enzyme concentrations, elevated serum blood urea nitrogen and creatinine concentrations, and proteinuria. The leukocyte count is normal to slightly decreased, with a "left shift." Atypical lymphocytes also may be noted on manual differential blood smear examination.

Specific diagnosis of babesiosis is made by microscopic demonstration of the organism using Giemsa-stained thin blood smears. *Babesia* species are round, oval, or pear shaped and have a blue cytoplasm with a red chromatin membrane (Figure 199.3). Multiple blood smears should be examined because only a few erythrocytes are infected in the early stage of the illness when most people seek medical attention. Fewer than 1% of erythrocytes

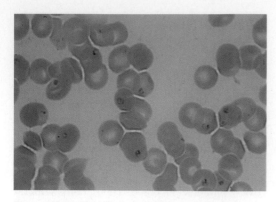

Figure 199.3 Ring forms of *Babesia microti* in human blood film (1000×).

may be parasitized initially and may escape detection. Maximum erythrocyte infection is approximately 10% in normal hosts but up to 85% in people who are immunocompromised. Thick blood smears may be examined, but the organisms appear as simple chromatin dots that may be mistaken for stain precipitate or iron inclusion bodies. Accordingly, only someone with extensive experience in interpreting thick smears should perform this method. The ring form is most common and is very similar to the rings of *Plasmodium falciparum*. Although the presence of tetrad forms ("Maltese cross") is said to be diagnostic, such elements are rarely encountered. Similarly, the absence of hemozoin (malarial pigment) is often considered to be generally diagnostic for the piroplasms, but early ring stages of the plasmodia also lack pigment. Diagnosis is thus made by a combination of criteria and, in severe cases, includes the presence of intense parasitemias, erythrocytes infected by multiple parasites, and basket-shaped merozoites that are often extracellular.

Physicians can further confirm babesial infection by use of serologic testing, small animal inoculation, and polymerase chain reaction (PCR). Both immunoglobulin G and immunoglobulin M immunofluorescent assay antibodies can be detected using the indirect IFA. The IFA is sensitive and specific and may quickly confirm a diagnosis of babesiosis when parasites are scarce or not detectable. During the acute phase of the illness, titers usually exceed 1:1024 but decline to 1:64 or less within 8 to 12 months. Thus, a babesial IFA titer of 1:1024 or greater usually signifies active or recent infection. A serological cutoff point of 1:64 generally is considered to be diagnostic. Although cross-reactions occur to different *Babesia* species and *Plasmodium* species with the IFA test, these titers are almost always low (1:16 or less). Where laboratory expertise exists, blood from the patient can be injected by the intravenous (IV) or intraperitoneal route into small laboratory animals such as hamsters or gerbils. If present in the patient, *B. microti* usually appears in the blood of the inoculated animal within 2 to 4 weeks. The PCR is a sensitive and specific test for detection of *Babesia* DNA. Proper technique must be used to prevent false-positive results. The diagnosis of babesiosis is suspect in symptomatic patients whose serum contains antibody to babesia, but whose blood lacks identifiable babesial parasites on smear or babesial DNA by PCR.

For *B. divergens* babesiosis, specific antibodies do not become detectable until at least 1 week after onset of illness. Because this infection is rapidly fulminating, serological diagnosis is not practical in the diagnosis of acute infection, but serological conversion serves as an aid in retrospective diagnosis in survivors. The high parasitemias that are present are easily detected by blood smear in the acute phase of infection. Infection by *B. duncani* may readily be detected by blood smear or by demonstrating specific antibody by IFA. This babesia may be cultivated *in vitro*. Unlike the IFA for *B. microti*, a higher cutoff value (>1:160) is required to impart specificity, for unknown reasons. In humans and in rodent models, tetrad forms are frequently seen in blood smears, but otherwise this agent is difficult to distinguish from *B. microti*.

Co-infection with the agents of Lyme disease (*B. burgdorferi*), human granulocytic anaplasmosis (*A. phagocytophilum*), or both may occur in patients experiencing babesiosis in geographic areas where these pathogens are endemic. Co-infection should be considered in patients who present with rash or more severe initial symptoms than are commonly observed with babesiosis alone.

TREATMENT

Early efforts to treat patients with babesiosis were unsuccessful, including use of the antimalarial drug chloroquine. The combination of clindamycin and quinine was the first effective antimicrobial therapy and remains the combination of choice for severe babesiosis. Clindamycin is given to adults 300–600 mg IV every 6 hours or 600 mg orally every 8 hours and to children in a 7–10 mg/kg/dose, up to a maximum dose of 600 mg, given IV or orally every 6–8 hours. Quinine is given as 650 mg orally every 6–8 hours in adults and 8 mg/kg/dose up to a maximum dose of 650 mg, given

Table 199.1 Treatment of Babesiosis

| Medication | Dose of Antibabesial Drug (All drugs given for 7 to 10 days or longer) | | Comment |
	Adults	Children	
Clindamycin plus	300–600 mg IV q/6h or 600 mg PO q/8h	7–10 mg/kg/dose IV or PO q6–8h (maximum 600 mg/dose)	This combination is the treatment of choice for severe babesiosis. Exchange transfusion or partial exchange transfusion should be considered in such patients
Quinine	650 mg PO q6–8h	8 mg/kg/dose PO q8h (maximum 650 mg/dose)	
Atovaquone plus	750 mg PO q12h	20 mg/kg/dose PO q12h (maximum 750 mg/dose)	This combination is the treatment of choice for mild to moderate babesiosis. A dose of 600–1000 mg/q24h may be used for immunocompromised adult patients
Azithromycin	500–1000 mg PO on d 1, then 250 mg PO/q24h	10 mg/kg as a single dose PO on d 1 (maximum 500 mg/dose), then 5 mg/kg PO q24h (maximum 250 mg/dose	

orally every 6 hours in children. Clindamycin and quinine generally is administered for 7 to 10 days. This combination frequently produces untoward reactions, such as tinnitus, vertigo, and gastrointestinal upset, and treatment failures have been reported in patients with splenectomy, HIV-infected patients, and those receiving concurrent corticosteroid therapy (Table 199.1).

The successful use of atovaquone and azithromycin for treatment of malaria and for treating babesiosis in a hamster model of infection suggested that this combination might also be useful against human babesiosis. In the first prospective, randomized trial of antibabesial therapy in humans, the combination of atovaquone and azithromycin was compared with that of clindamycin and quinine for treatment of adults with *B. microti* infection. The atovaquone and azithromycin combination was found to be as effective in clearing parasitemia and resolving symptoms as the clindamycin and quinine combination. Both drug combinations were given by mouth over 7 days. After 3 months, there was no evidence of piroplasms or amplifiable *B. microti* DNA in either group. Significantly fewer adverse effects were associated with the atovaquone and azithromycin combination. Three-fourths of patients receiving clindamycin and quinine experienced adverse drug reactions, and one-third were forced to decrease the dose or to discontinue the medication. Adverse effects of therapy included hearing loss, tinnitus, syncope, hypotension, and gastrointestinal (GI) symptoms (anorexia, vomiting, and diarrhea). By contrast, only 18% in the azithromycin and atovaquone group experienced symptoms consistent with adverse

drug reaction, and none required a decrease in dosage or discontinuation of medication. The conclusions of this study were (1) antibabesial therapy based on the atovaquone and azithromycin drug combination generally is superior to those based on clindamycin and quinine, mainly because the atovaquone and azithromycin regimen is well tolerated, whereas the clindamycin and quinine regimen frequently is not, and (2) physicians should consider the use of atovaquone and azithromycin in adult patients experiencing mild or moderate babesial symptoms and in others who cannot tolerate clindamycin and quinine. The currently recommended dose for atovaquone is 750 mg orally every 12 hours in adults or 20 mg/kg/ dose up to a maximum dose of 750 mg, given orally every 12 hours in children, whereas that for azithromycin is 500–1000 mg on day 1 and then 250 mg per day thereafter in adults or 10 mg/kg/day as a single dose (up to a maximum dose of 500 mg) given orally on day 1, and 5 mg/kg/dose (up to a maximum dose of 250 mg) given orally once per day thereafter in children. Higher doses of 600–1000 mg per day may be used for immunocompromised patients experiencing babesiosis.

The combination of pentamidine (240 mg IV/day) and trimethoprim–sulfamethoxazole (3 g/day) was found to be moderately effective in clearing parasitemia and symptoms due to *B. divergens*. Potential adverse reactions to pentamidine that include pain at the site of injection, formation of sterile abscess, and nephrotoxicity limit the use of this combination.

Clindamycin (administered intravenously) and quinine should be given for patients experiencing babesiosis who are more severely ill with high parasitemia (>10%), significant hemolysis, or renal or pulmonary compromise. In addition, exchange transfusion should be considered in such patients. Partial exchange transfusion (red blood cell) or complete exchange (whole blood exchange) as well as plasmapheresis are rapid and reliable methods of decreasing parasitemia by removing parasite-infected red blood cells from the circulation. They also help remove vasoactive elements such as cytokines and thromboplastic substances that may contribute to renal failure and disseminated intravascular coagulation. Due to the risks associated with multiple blood exposures, these techniques should not be considered as routine therapy but only used for those severely ill with babesiosis, such as patients with a high parasitemia and coma, hypotension, congestive heart failure, pulmonary edema, or renal failure. In combination with clindamycin and quinine, exchange transfusion is the treatment of choice for all cases of *B. divergens* babesiosis.

Patients with babesiosis should be monitored closely during therapy. In most cases, improvement will occur within 1 or 2 days after antiprotozoal therapy is begun. Symptoms generally resolve within 1 or 2 months after clindamycin and quinine or atovaquone and azithromycin therapy is completed. In severely ill patients (especially those with asplenia or HIV), the hematocrit and percentage of erythrocytes parasitized should be monitored daily or every other day until the patient has improved and the parasitemia has decreased to less than 5%. Blood smears should be examined every 4 hours following the first dose of clindamycin and quinine, and alternative therapy should be considered if parasitemia does not appear to appreciably decline within 24 hours. Some patients may have persistence of low-grade parasitemia for months following antibiotic therapy. Because low-grade parasitemia may be difficult to detect on thin blood smear, the more sensitive PCR for amplifying parasite DNA should also be considered. We suggest retreatment of patients with antibabesial therapy if patients show evidence of parasitemia in their blood for more than 3 months after initial therapy.

Physicians also should consider the possibility of co-infection with Lyme disease, human granulocytic anaplasmosis, or both in patients who experience especially severe or persistent symptoms despite appropriate antibabesial therapy. Such patients may benefit from the addition of doxycycline therapy because neither clindamycin and quinine nor atovaquone and azithromycin have been shown to be effective for the treatment of Lyme disease or human granulocytic anaplasmosis.

PREVENTION

Prevention of babesiosis can be accomplished by avoiding areas from May through September where ticks, deer, and mice are known to thrive. It is especially important for those at increased risk in endemic areas, such as asplenic individuals, to avoid tall grass and brush where ticks may abound. Use of clothing that covers the lower part of the body and that is sprayed or impregnated with diethyltoluamide (DEET), dimethyl phthalate, or permethrin (Permanone) is recommended for those who travel in the foliage of endemic areas. DEET has been shown to be more effective than other repellents against ticks, but the risk of adverse effects is greater. Topically applied DEET is absorbed into the systemic circulation and as much as 10% to 15% of each dose can be found in the urine. Dermatological effects such as bullous eruptions and urticaria have been documented. Systemic effects such as toxic encephalopathy, anaphylaxis, and grand mal seizures have been noted with higher DEET concentrations. Finally, DEET ingestion may be fatal to both children and adults. Thus, although DEET can help to prevent tick bites, care must be taken with repeated use of high concentration products.

A search for ticks on people and pets should be carried out and the ticks removed using tweezers to grasp the mouthparts without squeezing the body of the tick. Prophylactic antibiotics after a tick bite to prevent babesiosis is not indicated. Attempts to reduce the tick, mouse, or deer populations in endemic areas generally have not been effective. The American Red Cross excludes prospective blood donors with a history of babesiosis to prevent transfusion-related cases. Effective vaccines have been developed to prevent *B. divergens* and *B. bovis* infections in cattle, but no vaccines are currently available for the prevention of human babesiosis.

SUGGESTED READING

Hatcher JC, Greenberg PD, Antique J, et al. Severe babesiosis in Long Island: review of 34 cases and their complications. *Clin Infect Dis.* 2001;32:1117–1125.

Krause PJ, Telford SR, Spielman A, et al. Concurrent Lyme disease and babesiosis: evidence for increased severity and duration of illness. *JAMA.* 1996;275:1657–1660.

Krause PJ, Spielman A, Telford S, et al. Persistent parasitemia after acute babesiosis. *N Engl J Med*. 1998;339:160–165.

Krause PJ, Lepore T, Sikand VJ, et al. Atovaquone and azithromycin for the treatment of human babesiosis. *N Engl J Med*. 2000;343:1454–1458.

Krause PJ, Telford SR, Spielman A, et al. Comparison of PCR with blood smear and inoculation of small animals for diagnosis of *Babesia microti* parasitemia. *J Clin Microbiol*. 1996;34:2791–2794.

McQuiston JH, Childs JE, Chamberland ME, et al. Transmission of tickborne agents by blood transfusions: a review of known and potential risks in the United States. *Transfusion*. 2000;40:274–284.

Meldrum SC, Birkhead GS, White DJ, et al. Human babesiosis in New York state: an epidemiological description of 136 cases. *Clin Infect Dis*. 1992;15:1019–1023.

Persing DH, Herwaldt BL, Glaser C, et al. Infection with a Babesia-like organism in northern California. *N Engl J Med*. 1995;332:298–303.

Spielman A, Clifford CM, Piesman J, et al. Human babesiosis on Nantucket Island, U.S.A.: description of the vector, *Ixodes* (Ixodes) *dammini,* n. sp. (Acarina: Ixodidae). *J Med Entomol*. 1979;15:218–234.

Wittner M, Rowin KS, Tanowitz HB, et al. Successful chemotherapy of transfusion babesiosis. *Ann Intern Med*. 1982;96:601–604.

Wormser GP, Dattwyler RJ, Shapiro ED, et al. The clinical assessment, treatment, and prevention of Lyme disease, human granulocytic anaplasmosis, and babesiosis: clinical practice guidelines by the Infectious Diseases Society of America. *Clin Infect Dis*. 2006;43: 1089–1134.

200. Trypanosomiases and Leishmaniases

Anastácio de Queiroz Sousa, Selma M. B. Jeronimo,
and Richard D. Pearson

American trypanosomiasis (Chagas disease), human African trypanosomiasis (HAT, sleeping sickness), and leishmaniasis are caused by related protozoa of the family Trypanosomatidae, order Kinetoplastida (see Table 200.1). They have a unique mitochondrial structure, the kinetoplast, are transmitted in nature by insect vectors, and exist in multiple morphologic forms in their human hosts and insect vectors. They are important causes of morbidity and mortality in endemic areas of the world: Chagas disease in South and Central America, sleeping sickness in sub-Saharan Africa, and leishmaniasis in scattered areas on every continent except Antarctica. Although uncommon in industrial countries in North America and Europe, these diseases have been the source of increased attention in recent years. Infection with *Trypanosoma cruzi*, the cause of Chagas disease, is well documented among a subset of Latin American immigrants to the United States and Canada and poses a risk to them and to recipients of contaminated blood or transplanted organs. Cutaneous leishmaniasis is seen among tourists returning from endemic areas in Latin America and the Middle East as well as in military personnel serving in Iraq and Afghanistan. Canine visceral leishmaniasis has been reported in the United States among foxhounds and other dogs, but to date, humans have not been infected.

Despite several important recent advances, the treatment of Chagas disease, African trypanosomiasis, and leishmaniasis leaves much to be desired. Many of the drugs (Table 200.2) used for them are associated with frequent and potentially severe untoward effects, some require parenteral administration, and many must be administered over prolonged periods of time. Liposomal amphotericin B is the only one approved for use by the U.S. Food and Drug Administration. The others are considered investigational and can be obtained from the Centers for Disease Control and Prevention (CDC) Drug Service (Atlanta, Georgia) along with detailed information about their administration and side effects. The high cost of some of these drugs and lack of availability of others are important determinants in therapeutic decisions in impoverished endemic areas. The development of new drugs and vaccines has been slowed by the lack of financial incentive for pharmaceutical companies. Hopefully, more effective, less toxic approaches to chemotherapy and/or protective vaccines will become available in the future.

AMERICAN TRYPANOSOMIASIS (CHAGAS DISEASE)

Chagas disease, which is caused by *T. cruzi,* is transmitted by triatomine (reduviid or kissing) bugs that reside in adobe buildings in rural areas of Latin America. *Trypanosoma cruzi* infects a large number of animal species as well as humans. The parasite develops in the intestine of the triatomine bug and is passed in feces when it takes a blood meal. The bite causes itching, and parasites may enter the skin through the imperceptible bite site when the person scratches. They may also be transferred to the conjunctiva where they can enter in the absence of a lesion.

The invasion that follows can elicit a local inflammatory nodule or chagoma. When parasites invade through the conjunctiva, unilateral, painless, periorbital edema (Romaña's sign) may develop. After a period of local multiplication, trypomastigotes disseminate through the bloodstream producing acute Chagas disease with fever, other constitutional symptoms, carditis, and, rarely, meningoencephalitis. Death can result, but the acute phase can also be mild or asymptomatic. Symptoms usually resolve over 4 to 8 weeks as host immune responses develop. The indeterminate phase of infection follows in which persons are entirely asymptomatic but continue to harbor the parasite. Years later, 20% to 30% of infected individuals progress to chronic Chagas with cardiac, esophageal, or large intestinal involvement. Progressive, disseminated Chagas disease with carditis and/or brain abscesses has been reported in

Table 200.1 Diseases Caused by Protozoa of the Family Trypanosomatidae

Disease	Causative Agent	Geographic Distribution	Vector	Reservoir
American trypanosomiasis (Chagas disease)	*Trypanosoma cruzi*	Americas	Triatomine (Reduviid) bugs	Multiple species of animals
African trypanosomiasis (sleeping sickness)	*Trypanosoma brucei gambiense* *Trypanosoma brucei rhodesiense*	West and Central Africa East Africa	Tsetse flies (*Glossina* species)	Humans, domestic animals (minor role) Large game animals
Leishmaniasis (visceral, cutaneous, mucosal)	*Leishmania* species	Worldwide	Sand flies (*Phlebotomus* species and *Lutzomyia* species)	Rodents, canines (dogs, foxes), or humans

a limited number of persons with acquired immunodeficiency syndrome (AIDS), following transplants or associated with other immunocompromising conditions.

Trypanosoma cruzi is present in the bloodstream and organs of persons throughout the period of infection. Transmission can occur through transfusion of contaminated blood or transplantation of contaminated organs. This has posed ongoing problems in endemic areas in Latin America and is of increasing concern in North America related to immigration. Congenital transmission and accidental laboratory infections are also well documented.

The diagnosis of acute Chagas disease is frequently made by identifying the parasite in blood or body tissues (Figure 200.1). Several serological assays have been developed to detect antitrypanosomal antibodies in persons with indeterminate phase or chronic Chagas disease. The tests differ in their sensitivity and specificity. A screening test for anti–*T. cruzi* immunoglobulin G antibodies has recently been approved by the U.S. Food and Drug Administration to detect infected blood and organ donors in the United States. In addition to protecting potential recipients, screening will bring to medical attention a number of infected immigrants now living in the United States and Canada.

The drugs of choice are benznidazole or nifurtimox. Benznidazole has been the mainstay of therapy in Latin American countries. Nifurtimox has been used in the United States (available under an Investigational New Drug protocol from the CDC Drug Service). Untoward effects are common with both drugs and may necessitate premature discontinuation of therapy. Nifurtimox (Bayer 2502, Lampit; Bayer) is typically given for 90 to 120 days

(see Table 200.2 for dosage). The drug is better tolerated in children and adolescents than in adults; higher doses per kilogram of body weight are used in younger patients. Neurological and gastrointestinal side effects are common. They include sleep disturbances, restlessness, tremor, memory loss, paresthesias, weakness, polyneuritis, and, rarely, seizures, as well as anorexia, nausea, vomiting, abdominal pain, and weight loss. Other, rare side effects include fever, pulmonary infiltrates, and effusions.

Benznidazole (Rochagan, Roche) is usually administered for a period of 60 days. Higher doses are used in children. Side effects are frequent and include gastrointestinal disturbances, psychiatric manifestations, dose-dependent neuropathy, and cutaneous hypersensitivity reactions. On rare occasions hepatitis or neutropenia develops.

Treatment for Chagas disease is effective in the acute symptomatic stage of infection. The efficacy of treatment in preventing late complications in persons with indeterminate infection is uncertain. Many experts recommend treatment, particularly in children and young adults. Once the cardiac, esophageal, or large intestinal manifestations of chronic Chagas disease develop, neither drug appears to alter the outcome. Supportive therapy includes cardiotropic drugs for congestive heart failure and arrhythmias, pacemaker placement for heart block, and palliative endoscopic or surgical procedures for esophageal and intestinal megadisease. Nifurtimox has been used to prevent disseminated infection in a relatively small number of persons who have undergone cardiac transplantation for chagasic cardiomyopathy in the United States.

Table 200.2 Treatment of Trypanosomiasis and Leishmaniasis

Drug of Choice	Adult Dosage	Pediatric Dosage
American Trypanosomiasis/Chagas Disease (*Trypanosoma cruzi*)		
Nifurtimox[a,b] or Benznidazole	8–10 mg/kg/d in 3–4 doses × 90–120d 5–7 mg/kg/d in 2 divided doses × 30–90d	1–10 yrs : 15–20 mg/kg/d in 4 doses × 90–120d ≤12 yrs: 10 mg/kg/d in 2 doses × 30–90d 11–16 yrs: 12.5–15 mg/kg/d in 4 doses × 90d–120d
East African Sleeping Sickness (*Trypanosoma brucei rhodesiense*)		
Hemolymphatic stage Suramin[a]	100–200 mg (test dose) IV, then 1 g IV on days 1,3,7,14 and 21	20 mg/kg on days 1,3,7,14 and 21
Late stage with central nervous system involvement Melarsoprol[c]	2–3–6 mg/kg/d × 3d; after 7d 3.6 mg/kg/d × 3d; repeat again after 7d	2–3.6 mg/kg/d × 3d; after 7d 3.6 mg/kg/d × 3d; repeat again after 7d
West African Sleeping Sickness (*Trypanosoma brucei gambiense*)		
Hemolymphatic Stage Pentamidine[d,e]	4 mg/kg/d IM × 7d	4 mg/kg/d IM × 7d
Alternative: Suramin[a]	100–200 mg (test dose) IV, then 1g IV on days 1,3,7,14 and 21	20 mg/kg/d on days 1,3,7,14 and 21
Late stage with central nervous system involvement Melarsoprof[c] or Eflornithine[a,f]	2.2 mg/kg/d IV × 10d 400 mg/kg/d IV in 4 doses × 14d	2.2 mg/kg/d IV × 10d 400 mg/kg/d IV in 4 doses × 14d
Leishmaniasis (*Leishmania* species)[g]		
Visceral Liposomal amphotericin B[i] or Sodium stibo- gluconate[a] or Meglumine antimonate[a]	3 mg/kg IV (d 1-5) and 3 mg/kg/d d 14 and 21[j] 20 mg Sb/kg/d IV or IM × 28d[h] 20 mg Sb/kg/d IV or IM × 28d[h]	3 mg/kg IV (d 1-5) and 3 mg/kg/d d 14 and 21[j] 20 mg Sb/kg/d IV or IM × 28d[h] 20 mg Sb/kg/d IV or IM × 28d[h]
Alternative Miltefosine[k] or Amphotericin B[d]	2.5 mg/kg/d PO (max 150mg/d)× 28d 1 mg/kg IV daily or every second day for up to 8 wks	2.5 mg/kg/d PO (max 150mg/d)× 28d 1 mg/kg IV daily or every second day for up to 8 wks
Cutaneous[l] Sodium stibogluconate[a] or Meglumine antimonate[a]	20 mg Sb/kg/d IV or IM × 20d[h] 20 mg Sb/kg/d IV or IM × 20d[h]	20 mg Sb/kg/d IV or IM × 20d[h] 20 mg Sb/kg/d IV or IM × 20d[h]
Alternative[m] Pentamidine[d] or Paramomycin[d,o]	2-3 mg/kg IV or daily or every second day × 4-7 doses[n] Topically 2×/d × 10-20 d	2-3 mg/kg IV or daily or every second day × 4-7 doses[n] Topically 2×/d × 10-20 d
Mucosal[p] Sodium stibogluconate[a] or Meglumine antimonate[a] or Amphotericin B[d]	20 mg Sb/kg/d IV or IM × 28 d[h] 20 mg Sb/kg/d IV or IM × 28 d[h] 0.5-1 mg/kg IV daily or every second day for up to 8 wks	20 mg Sb/kg/d IV or IM × 28 d[h] 20 mg Sb/kg/d IV or IM × 28 d[h] 0.5-1 mg/kg IV daily or every second day for up to 8 wks

Reprinted with permission from The Medical Letter on Drugs and Therapeutics, Drugs for parasitic infections, August 2004, with modifications base on Drugs for Parasitic Infections, The Medical Letter, 2007:5:e1-e15 (http://www.medletter.org) and other resources.

[a] Available under an Investigational New Drug (IND) protocol from the CDC Drug Service, Centers for Disease Control and Prevention, Atlanta, GA 30333; 404-639-3670 (evenings, weekends, or holidays: 404-639-2888).

(continued)

Table 200.2 *(continued)*

[b] The addition of gamma interferon to nifurtimox for 20d in experimental animals and in a limited number of patients appears to shorten the acute phase of Chagas disease (McCabe RE, et al. *J Infect Dis.* 1991;163:912).

[c] In frail patients, begin with as little as 18 mg and increase the dose progressively. Pretreatment with suramin has been advocated for debilitated patients. Corticosteroids have been used to prevent arsenical encephalopathy (Pepin J, et al. *Trans R Soc Trop Med Hyg.* 1995;89:92). Up to 20% of patients with *T. b. gambiense* fail to respond to melarsoprol (Barrett MP. *Lancet* 1999;353:1113).

[d] An approved drug, but considered investigational for this condition by the FDA.

[e] For treatment of *T. b. gambiense*, pentamidine and suramin have equal efficacy, but pentamidine is better tolerated.

[f] Eflornithine is highly effective in *T. b. gambiense* but not against *T. b. rhodesiense* infections. It is available in limited supply only from the World Health Organization (WHO) and the CDC.

[g] Visceral infection is most commonly due to the Old World species *L. donovani* (kala-azar) and *L. infantum* and the New World species *L. chagasi*. Treatment duration may vary based on symptoms, host immune status, species, and area of the world where infection was acquired.

[h] May be repeated or continued; a longer duration may be needed for some patients (Herwaldt BL. *Lancet* 1999;354:1191).

[i] Three lipid formulations of amphotericin B have been used for treatment of visceral leishmaniasis. Largely based on clinical trials in patients infected with *L. infantum*, the FDA-approved liposomal amphotericin B (AmBisome) for treatment of visceral leishmaniasis (Meyerhoff A. *Clin Infect Dis.* 1999;28:42). Amphotericin B lipid complex (Abelcet) and amphotericin B cholesteryl sulfate (Amphotec) have also been used with good results but are considered investigational for this condition by the FDA.

[j] The FDA-approved dosage regimen for immunocompromised patients (e.g., HIV infected) is 4 mg/kg/d (d 1–5) and 4 mg/kg/d on d 10, 17, 24, 31, and 38. The relapse rate is high; maintenance therapy may be indicated, but there is no consensus as to dosage or duration.

[k] For treatment of kala-azar in adults in India, oral miltefosine 100 mg/d (~2.5 g/kg/d) for 3–4 wk was 97% effective after 6 mo (Jha TK, et al. *N Engl J Med.* 1999;341:1795; Sangraula H, et al, *J Assoc Physicians India.* 2003;51:686). Gastrointestinal adverse effects are common, and the drug is contraindicated in pregnancy. Resistance has been reported. The dose of miltefosine in an open-label trial in children in India was 2.5 mg/kg/d x 28d (Bhattacharya SK et al, *Clin Infect Dis.* 2004; 38:217). Miltefosine (Impavido) is available from the manufacturer (Zentaris, Frankfurt, Germany at info@zentoris.com).

[l] Cutaneous infection is most commonly due to the Old World species *L. major* and *L. tropica* and the New World species *L. mexicana, L. (Viannia) braziliensis,* and others. Treatment duration may vary based on symptoms, host immune status, species, and area of the world where infection was acquired.

[m] In a placebo-controlled trial in patients ≥12 years old, oral miltefosine was effective for the treatment of cutaneous leishmaniasis due to *L. (V.) panamensis* in Colombia but not *L. (V.) braziliensis* in Guatemala at a dosage of about 2.5 mg/kg/d for 28d. "Motion sickness," nausea, headache, and increased creatinine were the most frequent adverse effects (Soto J, et al. *Clin Infect Dis.* 2004;38:1266). See footnote j regarding miltefosine availability. For treatment of *L. major* cutaneous lesions, a study in Saudi Arabia found that oral fluconazole, 200 mg once/d x 6wk, appeared to speed healing (Alrajhi AA, et al. *N Engl J Med.* 2002;346:891).

[n] At this dosage pentamidine has been effective against leishmaniasis in Colombia where the likely organism was *L. (V.) panamensis* (Soto-Mancipe J et al. *Clin Infect Dis.* 1993;16:417; Soto J et al. *Am J Trop Med Hyg.* 1994;50:107); its effect against other species is not well established.

[o] Topical paromomycin should be used only in geographic regions where cutaneous leishmaniasis species have low potential for mucosal spread. A formulation of 15% paromomycin/12% methylbenzethonium chloride (Leshcutan) in soft white paraffin for topical use has been reported to be partially effective against cutaneous leishmaniasis due to *L. major* in Israel and against *L. mexicana* and *L. (V.) braziliensis* in Guatemala, where mucosal spread is very rare (Arana BA, et al. *Am J Trop Med Hyg.* 2001; 65:466). The methylbenzethonium is irritating to the skin; lesions may worsen before they improve.

[p] Mucosal infection is most commonly due to the New World species *L. (V.) braziliensis, L. (V.) panamensis,* or *L. (V.) guyanensis.* Treatment duration may vary based on symptoms, host immune status, species, and area of the world where infection was acquired.

Abbreviations: IV = intravenously; IM = intramuscularly; sb =

AFRICAN TRYPANOSOMIASIS (SLEEPING SICKNESS)

Human African trypanosomiasis is caused by *T. brucei gambiense*, which is endemic in West and Central Africa, and *T. brucei rhodesiense* in East Africa. Uganda is the only country where both exist. The African trypanosomes are transmitted by tsetse flies, which are found only in sub-Saharan Africa. Humans are the primary reservoir of *T. b. gambiense*, whereas *T. b. rhodesiense* is found primarily in large game animals. There are an estimated 50 000 to 70 000 new cases yearly although reporting is poor. Transplacental transmission and transmission through contaminated blood or transplanted organs can occur but are uncommon. *Trypanosoma b. gambiense* (West African trypanosomiasis) accounts for approximately 90% of all cases worldwide, but it is rarely encountered in the United States and in industrialized areas. There have been 36 reported cases of *T. b. rhodesiense* (East African trypanosomiasis) in the United States since 1967.

An indurated chancre may develop at the site of parasite inoculation. In *T. b. gambiense* infection, the early (hemolymphatic) stage is characterized by recurrent bouts of fever, rash, headaches, edema of the face, myalgias, arthralgias, other constitutional symptoms, and lymphadenopathy. Swollen posterior

Specific Organisms – Parasites

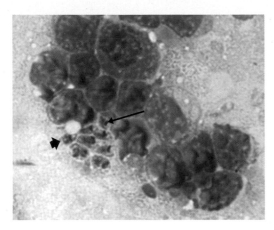

Figure 200.1 An imprint from a lymph node biopsy of a child with acute Chagas disease showing amastigotes (*arrowhead*), with large kinetoplast (*arrow*). Culture in LIT from the node and from whole blood grew *Trypanosoma cruzi*.

cervical nodes are known as Winterbottom sign. Trypanosomes are found in blood and lymph nodes. After a period of several weeks to months they invade the central nervous system, producing meningoencephalitis. Symptoms and findings include headaches, which may be severe, loss of concentration, personality changes, memory loss, seizures, difficulty walking, increased sleeping, and eventually obtundation, coma, wasting, and death.

In *T. b. rhodesiense* infection, systemic symptoms develop a few days to several weeks after the tsetse fly bites. A chancre may be present. Fever, headache, severe fatigue, irritability, lymphadenopathy, myalgias, and arthralgias follow. Death can occur within several weeks or months if treatment is not initiated. The courses may be indistinguishable, but *T. b. rhodesiense* infection is usually more acute and severe, and lymphadenopathy is not as prominent as it is with *T. b. gambiense* infection.

All cases of human African sleeping sickness must be treated. Given the complexity of the treatment regimens and toxicity of the drugs, consultation with experts at the CDC or elsewhere is recommended. Eflornithine, which has been called the "resurrection drug," is highly effective for hemolymphatic and central nervous system disease caused by *T. b. gambiense* and, when available, is the treatment of choice for West African sleeping sickness. Unfortunately, it is expensive and logistically difficult to administer in rural, endemic areas of Africa, and supplies are very limited. A 14-day course administered intravenously (IV) is recommended for late stage disease

(Table 200.2). Eflornithine is not active against *T. b. rhodesiense*.

Persons with hemolymphatic disease due to *T. b. gambiense* when eflornithine is not available are treated with either pentamidine isethionate, a 7-day course administered parenterally, or suramin. Pentamidine and suramin are of comparable efficacy for *T. b. gambiense*, but pentamidine is less toxic. Suramin sodium is used for *T. b. rhodesiense* under an investigational New Drug Protocol from the CDC Drug Service.

Toxicity is frequent with suramin and includes gastrointestinal disturbances such as nausea and vomiting; neurological side effects such as photophobia, hyperesthesias, and peripheral neuropathy; and urticaria and pruritus. Administration of the drug is occasionally associated with shock, renal toxicity, optic atrophy, or blood dyscrasias. A test dose of suramin is given IV prior to the administration of treatment doses.

Pentamidine isethionate is administered daily, intramuscularly (IM) or IV. If infused too rapidly, IV pentamidine can produce hypotension and shock. Gastrointestinal disturbances, pain at the injection site when the drug is given IM, liver enzyme abnormalities, and nephrotoxicity are other side effects. Some patients develop life-threatening hypoglycemia due to pancreatic beta cell injury and insulin release; insulin-dependent diabetes may follow. Rare side effects include acute pancreatitis, hyperkalemia, anaphylaxis, and ventricular arrhythmias.

Melarsoprol (*Arsobal*, Rhone-Poulenc Rorer) is used to treat persons with central nervous system involvement with *T. b. gambiense* in sites where eflornithine is not available, and it is the recommended drug for persons with *T. b. rhodesiense* and central nervous system infection. Melarsoprol is administered IV (see Table 200.2). Untoward effects are common with melarsoprol. In addition to encephalopathy, which occurs in as many as 18% of recipients and is fatal in 3% to 10%, treatment is frequently associated with nausea, vomiting, abdominal pain, peripheral neuropathy, hypertension, allergic reactions, and, rarely, shock. Administration of prednisolone, 1–2 mg/kg/day, appears to reduce the severity of arsenical encephalopathy and the risk of death by approximately half. A number of dosage regimens have been studied. Reduced doses of melarsoprol have been used in cachectic patients. A recent study found that a combination of low-dose melarsoprol plus nifurtimox (see Chagas disease above) was more effective than the standard melarsoprol regimen.

LEISHMANIASIS (CUTANEOUS, MUCOSAL, AND VISCERAL)

Leishmaniasis refers to the spectrum of disease caused by more than 20 *Leishmania* spp. that infect humans. The major clinical syndromes include cutaneous, mucosal, and visceral leishmaniasis, but a variety of other presentations, including post kala-azar dermal leishmaniasis, diffuse cutaneous leishmaniasis, disseminated cutaneous leishmaniasis, and viscerotropic leishmaniasis, have been described. *Leishmania* spp. are transmitted by sandflies in nature. In many areas of the world, leishmaniasis is a zoonosis with dogs, other canines, or rodents serving as reservoirs, and humans becoming infected when they venture into endemic habitats. An outbreak of canine visceral leishmaniasis has been reported in the United Kingdom among foxhounds and some other dogs. Infection seemed to have occurred by dog-to-dog transmission. There have been no human cases. In some sites such as India, humans are the only reservoir of visceral leishmaniasis. The manifestations of disease depend on complex and only partially understood interactions between the virulence characteristics of the infecting *Leishmania* sp. and the genetically determined cell-mediated immune responses of its human host (Figures 200.2–200.9).

In persons with cutaneous leishmaniasis, parasites multiply in macrophages at the site of inoculation in the skin. The morphology of the resulting lesion is variable. Often, a nodule develops, expands, and then ulcerates over a course of weeks. Lesions may be single or multiple. Some have a "pizzalike" appearance with a raised, erythematous, outer border, a central area of red granulation tissue, and a yellowish or brown overlying crust. Others are volcano-like or flat and plaquelike. They can persist for months to years but eventually heal leaving a burnlike scar as evidence of disease. In mucosal leishmaniasis due to *Leishmania (Viannia) braziliensis* and related species in Latin America, mucosal lesions of the nose, oral pharynx, and occasionally other sites develop months to years after the initial skin lesion has healed.

The majority of persons infected with *Leishmania donovani, Leishmania infantum Leishmania chagasi*, or other *Leishmania* species associated with visceral leishmaniasis are asymptomatic and have spontaneously resolving infections. In the subset of persons who develop progressive visceral leishmaniasis, known as kala-azar, parasites disseminate throughout the reticuloendothelial system. They are found within macrophages in the liver, spleen, bone marrow, and occasionally other organs. Patients typically present with massive splenomegaly, hepatomegaly, fever, weight loss, constitutional symptoms, and hypergammaglobulinemia. Visceral leishmaniasis has emerged in Spain, southern France, Italy, and elsewhere in southern Europe as an opportunistic infection in persons with AIDS and others with compromised cell-mediated immunity. Persons with concurrent visceral leishmaniasis and AIDS may present in the classical manner, but atypical presentations are common. Splenomegaly may be absent, and gastrointestinal and pleuro-pulmonary involvement are often seen.

The diagnosis of cutaneous or visceral leishmaniasis is suggested by a history of exposure in an endemic region and the clinical findings. It is confirmed by identifying leishmania amastigotes in blood, bone marrow, splenic aspirates, or tissue from patients with visceral leishmaniasis or in biopsies of skin lesions from those with cutaneous leishmaniasis. Antileishmanial antibodies are typically present at high titer in persons with visceral leishmaniasis, but they may be absent in persons with AIDS. Several assays are available; an enzyme-linked immunosorbent assay using a recombinant 39-kd kinesinlike antigen appears to be the most sensitive and specific for visceral leishmaniasis. Serological assays are of no diagnostic value in cutaneous leishmaniasis, as antileishmanial antibodies are variably present and at low titer. The leishmanin (Montenegro) skin test (Figure 200.10) is not available in the United States. It is negative in patients with visceral leishmaniasis, but it becomes positive after successful treatment. The test is typically positive in persons with cutaneous and mucosal leishmaniasis.

All patients with clinically apparent visceral leishmaniasis should be treated. Liposomal amphotericin B (AmBisome, Fugisawa) is the only drug licensed in the United States for this indication. It is as highly effective, as is amphotericin B deoxycholate, but it is less toxic. Although it is the drug of choice in industrialized countries, its cost and availability have limited its use in impoverished endemic areas.

Sodium sibogluconate (Pentostam) and meglumine antimonate (Glucantime), both pentavalent antimony compounds, have been used for decades to treat leishmaniasis. Pentostam is available through the CDC Drug

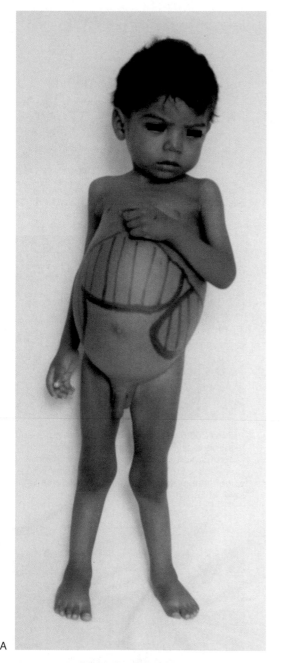
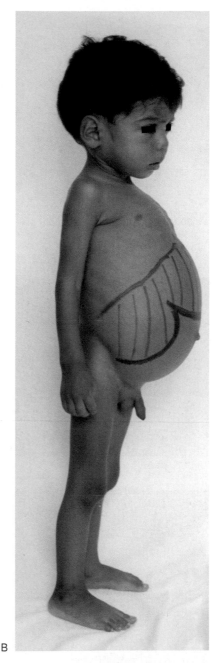

Figure 200.2 A and B: Brazilian child with advanced visceral leishmaniasis and massive heptosplenomegaly.

Service in the United States. These drugs are dosed on the basis of their pentavalent antimony content; Pentostam contains 100 mg of pentavalent antimony/mL and Glucantime contains 85 mg/mL. They remain the treatment of choice for visceral leishmaniasis in some areas of the world, but antimony resistance and treatment failures are now common in the Indian subcontinent. In South America, the Sudan, and other areas where pentavalent

antimony failures are infrequent, either Glucantime or Pentostam is given at a dose of 20 mg of pentavalent antimony/kg body weight/day IV or IM for 28 days.

When relapses occur in persons treated with pentavalent antimony, they are usually observed within the first 6 months. They can be treated with a second course of antimony or an alternative therapeutic regimen. Relapses are particularly common following therapy

Specific Organisms – Parasites

1395

Trypanosomiases and Leishmaniases

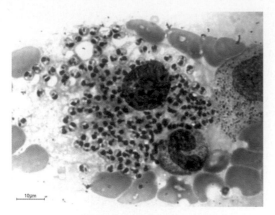

Figure 200.3 A macrophage with more than 100 amastigotes from a bone marrow aspirate of an AIDS patient with kala-azar.

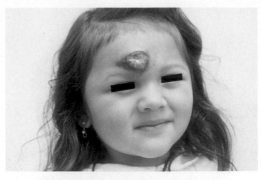

Figure 200.5 Brazilian child with cutaneous leishmaniasis due to *Leishmania Viannia braziliensis*.

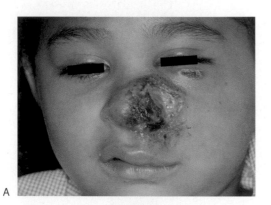

A

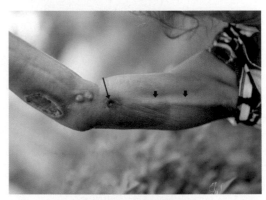

Figure 200.6 A Brazilian woman with cutaneous leishmaniasis, with lymphatic involvement (sporotricoid type) due to *Leishmania Viannia braziliensis*. Lymphatic (*arrowheads*) and where a punch biopsy was taken (*arrow*). Leishmania were seen in imprint and grown in NNN culture.

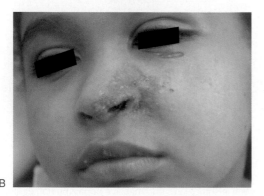

B

Figure 200.4 **A and B:** A child with cutaneous leishmaniasis with involvement of the nose, due to *Leishmania Viannia braziliensis*. Before and after treatment.

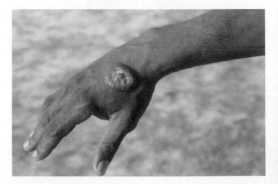

Figure 200.7 Patient with cutaneous leishmaniasis, due to *Leishmania Viannia braziliensis*. Hand involvement.

with pentavalent antimony in persons with AIDS. Treatment with liposomal amphotericin B is the treatment of choice. Suppressive antileishmanial therapy is advisable in that setting, but there have been no controlled trials to suggest the optimal drug or regimen. Many persons with visceral leishmaniasis in the developing world are severely wasted when they present and die from secondary bacterial or viral infections. Attention should focus on addressing their nutritional needs and treating secondary bacterial infections with appropriate antibiotics.

Specific Organisms – Parasites

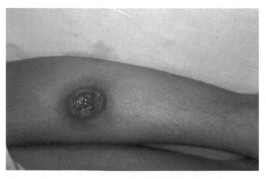

Figure 200.8 Patient with cutaneous leishmaniasis, due to *Leishmania Viannia braziliensis*. Leg involvement.

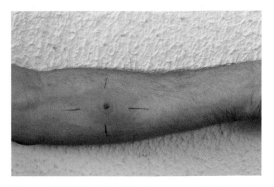

Figure 200.10 Positive Montenegro test (leishmanin skin test), 50 mm, with central necrosis, of a patient with mucosal leishmaniasis.

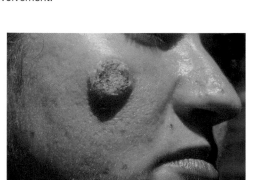

A

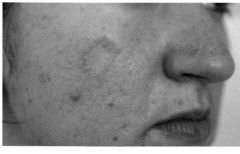

B

Figure 200.9 A and B: Cutaneous leishmaniasis due to *Leishmania Viannia braziliensis* before and after treatment.

The emergence of pentavalent antimony resistance in India and some other areas has stimulated the search for new drugs. Two new therapeutic approaches have been reported. Miltefosine, a phosphocholine analog that is administered orally, has been shown to be effective for the treatment of visceral leishmaniasis and post kala-azar dermal leishmaniasis in India. Gastrointestinal effects are a problem but have not prevented the completion of therapy in most study patients. The drug is embryotoxic and contraindicated in pregnancy. Resistance has been reported in India. Studies

now underway should determine its role in the treatment of visceral leishmaniasis in Latin America and elsewhere. The aminoglycoside paromomycin (aminosidin) has also been used parenterally in India to treat patients with pentavalant antimony-resistant *L. donovani*. Neither miltefosine nor parenteral paromomycin have been approved by the U.S. Food and Drug Administration.

Cutaneous leishmaniasis typically has a self-resolving course. If lesions are small, cosmetically inconsequential, show evidence of healing, and are not caused by *Leishmania* species associated with mucosal disease, treatment may not be necessary. For lesions that are large, cosmetically significant, or caused by *L. (V.) braziliensis* or related species associated with mucosal leishmaniasis, treatment is advisable. In many situations either Pentostam or Glucantime, 20 mg of pentavalent antimony/kg/day, for 20 days is used. Cutaneous leishmaniasis responds slowly, and lesions are often only partially healed at the completion of therapy.

Oral fluconazole, itraconazole, and ketoconazole are variably effective, depending on the infecting *Leishmania* species. For example, fluconazole, 200 mg/day for 6 weeks, resulted in a response rate of 90% in American troops with cutaneous leishmaniasis due to *Leishmania major*. Unfortunately, studies in the Americas have demonstrated high failure rates with imidazoles in persons infected with *L. braziliensis*. Topical administration of paromomycin (15%) and methylbenzethonium chloride (12%) in white paraffin has been used in persons with localized disease caused by *L. (Leishmania) major*. Amphotericin B deoxycholate is an effective but toxic alternative.

Persons with mucosal leishmaniasis are often treated initially with Pentostam or

Glucantime, 20 mg of pentavalent antimony/kg/day for 28 days; failures and relapses are common. Alternatives include amphotericin B, pentamidine isethionate, or granulocyte macrophage–colony-stimulating factor (GM-CSF) or interferon-γ administered concurrently with a pentavalent antimony. Liposomal amphotericin B has not been systematically assessed in the treatment for mucosal or cutaneous leishmaniasis. Plastic surgical repairs in persons with mucosal lesions should be delayed for 12 months after clinical cure because grafts may be lost if a relapse follows surgery.

SUGGESTED READING

Barrett M, Burchmore R, Stich A, et al. The trypanosomiases. *Lancet*. 2003;362: 1469–1480.

Bern C, Montgomery SP, Herwaldt BL, et al. Evaluation and treatment of Chagas disease in the United States: a systematic review. *JAMA* 2007;298:2171–2181.

The Medical Letter on Drugs and Therapeutics. Drugs for parasitic infections. http://www.medicalletter.org. 2007;5(Suppl):e1–e15.

Murray HW, Berman JD, Davies CR, Saravia NG. Advances in leishmaniasis. *Lancet*. 2005;366:1561–1577.

201. Intestinal Protozoa

Paul Kelly and Michael J. G. Farthing

Intestinal protozoal infection produces substantial morbidity and mortality in people of all ages, particularly in tropical and subtropical parts of the world. Amebiasis, giardiasis, cryptosporidiosis, and those infections associated with acquired immunodeficiency syndrome (AIDS) are important problems for health in many parts of the world, but some protozoa found in the human digestive system do not cause disease. Vaccines are not yet available for protection against these infections, and many are difficult to treat. The intestinal protozoa that produce important human infections are summarized in Table 201.1.

ENTAMEBA HISTOLYTICA

Entameba histolytica causes dysentery, chronic colonic amebiasis, and hepatic amebiasis. The last topic is dealt with in Chapter 202, Extraintestinal Amebic Infection. Amebic dysentery is a syndrome of bloody diarrhea caused by invasion of the colonic wall by trophozoites of *E. histolytica*. It is common in many parts of the world, especially West and southern Africa, Central America, and south Asia. In the United States, 3000 to 4000 cases are reported each year. There is now consensus that the species formerly recognized as *E. histolytica* in fact comprises two species: *E. histolytica* and *E. dispar.* The first is the pathogenic protozoan long associated with human invasive disease and with hepatic amebiasis, and the latter is a morphologically identical nonpathogenic protozoan first recognized as the nonpathogenic zymodeme of *E. histolytica.* The latter does not require treatment, but it cannot be differentiated from *E. histolytica* morphologically. Diagnosis of invasive amebiasis is achieved by the identification of hematophagous trophozoites in very fresh stool smears (Figure 201.1) or in colonic biopsies; the latter may also show typical flask-shaped ulcerations (Figure 201.2). Serologic testing using an immunofluorescent antibody test is now an important contribution to the diagnosis of a seriously ill patient, particularly in distinguishing colonic dilation resulting from amebiasis from that caused by ulcerative colitis.

Table 201.1 Intestinal Protozoa

The sarcodina (amebae)	Pathogenic Nonpathogenic	*Entameba histolytica* *Entameba dispar* *Entameba moshkovskii* *Entameba chattoni* *Endolimax nana* *Iodameba butschlii* *Dientameba fragilis*
The mastigophora (flagellates)	Pathogenic Nonpathogenic	*Giardia intestinalis* *Trichomonas hominis* *Chilomastix mesnili* *Embadomonas intestinalis* *Enteromonas hominis*
The ciliophora		*Balantidium coli*
The coccidia		*Cryptosporidium parvum* *Isospora belli* *Sarcocystis* species *Cyclospora cayetanensis*
The microspora		*Enterocytozoon bieneusi* *Encephalitozoon intestinalis*
Uncertain classification, uncertain pathogenicity		*Blastocystis hominis*

Treatment of invasive amebiasis is shown in Table 201.2. Treatment can be divided into two stages: (1) eradication of tissue forms with metronidazole, tinidazole, or nitazoxanide and (2) eradication of luminal carriage with diloxanide furoate. Dehydroemetine and iodoquinol, used formerly for the treatment of amebiasis, are toxic and no longer used.

Intestinal amebiasis may be complicated by acute toxic colitis, presenting in a similar manner to the dilation of acute severe ulcerative colitis. The patient will be febrile and unwell, sometimes with signs of peritoneal irritation, and a plain abdominal radiograph will indicate

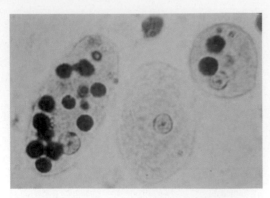

Figure 201.1 Trophozoites of *Entameba histolytica* with ingested erythrocytes (trichrome stain). Ingested erythrocytes appear as dark inclusions. Erythrophagocytosis is the only characteristic that can be used to differentiate morphologically *E. histolytica* from the nonpathogenic *E. dispar*. In these specimens, the parasite nuclei have the typical small, centrally located karyosome, and thin, uniform peripheral chromatin.
(Source: http://www.dpd.cdc.gov/dpdx/HTML/ ImageLibrary/Amebiasis.)

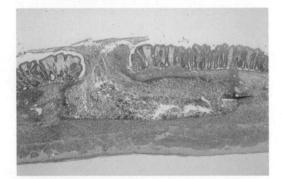

Figure 201.2 Histopathology of a typical flask-shaped ulcer of intestinal amebiasis.
(Source: Public Health Image Library, CDC/Dr. Mae Melvin).

dilation. Intravenous fluids must be given, the patient starved, and metronidazole and a third-generation cephalosporin given intravenously. Worsening dilation of the colon or perforation will necessitate surgery, but in the event of perforation, the outcome is poor. If treatment with metronidazole is started early in patients with severe amebic colitis, medical management should nearly always suffice, but surgery should not be delayed if perforation is impending.

Chronic amebiasis may be difficult to distinguish from intestinal tuberculosis or Crohn's disease but responds to metronidazole and diloxanide as above. Surgery is sometimes necessary because stricturing may persist.

GIARDIA INTESTINALIS

Giardia intestinalis infection, first recognized by Van Leeuwenhoek in 1681, is a cause of acute and persistent diarrhea and possibly malnutrition in children in many tropical and subtropical countries. It is also a well-recognized cause of traveler's diarrhea. In many cases it is self-limiting, but the course may be prolonged in immunoglobulin deficiencies. Asymptomatic infection is common. Diagnosis is by stool microscopy, although when this is negative and the clinical suspicion is strong, trophozoites may be detected in small intestinal fluid and mucosal biopsy specimens obtained by endoscopy. Fecal *Giardia* antigen enzyme-linked immunosorbent assays are now commercially available and increasingly used in many routine diagnostic laboratories.

A variety of drugs are now available for the treatment of giardiasis but none are regarded as safe in pregnancy, and treatment failures are not uncommon, requiring a second and sometimes a third course of therapy. Five classes of chemotherapy are available (Table 201.3): nitroimidazoles (metronidazole and tinidazole), benzimidazoles, particularly albendazole, nitazoxanide, nitrofurans (furazolidone), and paromomycin, which is the treatment of choice in pregnancy. If single agents fail repeatedly, combination therapy may be tried, but there are few controlled data to guide drug choice, dose, or duration.

BALANTIDIUM COLI

Balantidium coli infection manifests as a severe, sometimes life-threatening, colitis indistinguishable from amebic dysentery. It is uncommon but occurs in Central and South America, Iran, Papua, New Guinea, and the Philippines, usually in communities that live in close proximity to pigs, which are an important reservoir. Diagnosis is made by identification of the large trophozoites in feces or in rectal biopsies. Treatment is with tetracycline, 500 mg 4 times daily for 10 days (Table 201.4). Metronidazole and paromomycin are alternatives.

CRYPTOSPORIDIOSIS

Infection with *Cryptosporidium parvum* is likely to present as acute, self-limiting watery diarrhea in children or in travelers or as a waterborne epidemic. Most episodes require no specific therapy, but attention to fluid and electrolyte balance is important. Cryptosporidiosis is

Table 201.2 Drug Treatment of Amebiasis

		Adult Dosage	Child Dosage
Tissue Infection			
First choice	Metronidazole[a]	750 mg TID for 10 d	50 mg/kg/d for 10 d[b]
	Tinidazole[a]	2 g/d for 3 d	60 mg/kg/d for 3 d
Second choice	Nitazoxanide	500 mg BID for 3 d	Age 2–3 years:100 mg BID; age 4–11 years 200 mg BID for 3 d
	Paromomycin	30 mg/kg/d for 10 d[b]	30 mg/kg/d for 10 d[b]
Luminal Carriage			
First choice	Diloxanide furoate	500 mg TID for 10 d	20 mg/kg/d for 10 d[b]
Second choice	Paromomycin	30 mg/kg/d for 10 d[b]	30 mg/kg/d for 10 d[b]

[a] Must be followed by eradication of luminal carriage.
[b] In 3 doses.

Table 201.3 Drug Treatment of Giardiasis

Drug	Adult Dosage	Child Dosage	Efficacy
Metronidazole	2 g daily for 3 d	15 mg/kg/d for 10 d (maximum 750 mg daily)	>90%
Tinidazole	2 g single dose	75 mg/kg single dose	>90%
Albendazole	400 mg daily for 5 d		>85%
Nitazoxanide	100–200 mg 2× daily		85%
Furazolidone	100 mg QID for 10 d	2 mg/kg TID for 10 d	>80%
Paromomycin	500 mg 3× daily for 5–10 d		

associated with persistent diarrhea, even in apparently immunocompetent children, and in human immunodeficiency virus (HIV)-infected individuals often persists until death. Cryptosporidiosis is common in malnourished children in the tropics. In patients with HIV-related diarrhea, cryptosporidiosis can be found in 10% to 30% of cases in industrialized countries and 10% to 40% of cases in tropical populations. However, since the introduction of highly active antiretroviral therapy with multidrug regimens, this infection is much less frequent in those regions where these drugs are freely available. It remains a significant clinical challenge in patients in the tropics, where patients often present with advanced AIDS or compliance is often poor. Diagnosis is usually made by microscopy of fecal smears using a modified Ziehl–Neelsen stain, which reveals the red-staining 5-μm oocysts (Figure 201.3).

Although many drugs have been tried, only two have been shown to have any value in controlled trials: paromomycin and nitazoxanide. Hyperimmune bovine colostrum is a form of passive immunotherapy but is not in clinical use. Paromomycin (30 mg/kg/day in 3 doses) has been found to be of very limited efficacy. Nitazoxanide (1 g twice daily for 14 days) has been demonstrated to be effective in children and adults with and without AIDS-related diarrhea in randomized controlled trials. Recent uncontrolled data from the U.S. compassionate use program indicate that prolonged courses of 500–1500 mg nitazoxanide twice daily can be useful.

ISOSPORA BELLI

Isospora belli is uncommon in industrialized countries but may be found in up to 40% of patients with HIV-related diarrhea in Africa. In HIV-infected individuals it causes a clinical syndrome of persistent diarrhea and wasting, which is indistinguishable from that attributed to other intracellular enteropathogenic protozoa (*C. parvum*, microsporidia). There were reports

Table 201.4 Treatment of Ciliophora, Coccidia, and Microsporidia

Organism	Drug Regimen
Ciliophora	
Balantidium coli	Tetracycline, 500 mg QID for 10 d
Coccidia	
Cryptosporidium parvum	Nitazoxanide, 500 mg 2× daily for 3 d
Isospora belli	Trimethoprim–sulfamethoxazole, 1 DS tab PO QID for 10 d; Prophylaxis: 1 DS tab 3x/week
Sarcocystis species	As for *I. belli*
Cyclospora cayetanensis	Trimethoprim–sulfamethoxazole, 1 DS tab PO BID for 7 d
Microsporidia	
Enterocytozoon bieneusi	Fumagillin, 60 mg daily for 14 d
Encephalitozoon intestinalis	Fumagillin, 60 mg daily for 14 d
Blastocystis Hominis	
	The status of this organism as a pathogen is still the subject of controversy, so it is uncertain whether it requires treatment. It is our practice to attempt eradication with metronidazole, 750 mg TID for 10 days, when there are gastrointestinal symptoms and no other cause is apparent.

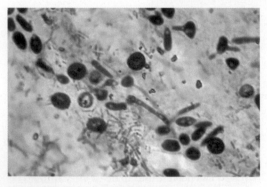

Figure 201.3 *Cryptosporidium* sp. micrograph of a direct fecal smear, using a modified Kinyoun stain; oil immersion; the *Cryptosporidium* sp. oocysts stain red. Source: Public Health Image Library, #5242; CDC/ *J Infect Dis*. 1983;137(5):824–828.

of isosporiasis before HIV infection appeared. Diagnosis rests on the identification in fecal smears of elongated, large sporocysts, which appear red with the modified Ziehl–Neelsen stain.

Trimethoprim–sulfamethoxazole (TMP–SMX) has been reported to be effective at a dosage of 160/800 mg 4 times daily for 10 days. In patients with AIDS, this needs to be followed with the same drug in a dose of 160/800 mg 3 times weekly indefinitely as prophylaxis against recurrence. Otherwise, recurrence is seen in 50% of patients with HIV infection at 2 months. An alternative drug is sulfadoxine–pyrimethamine (500/25 mg weekly) as secondary prophylaxis. Patients intolerant of sulfonamides could be given diclazuril, but only anecdotal evidence of its efficacy is available. It does not appear to respond to nitazoxanide.

SARCOCYSTIS SPECIES

Sarcocystis infection, which may give rise to a persistent diarrhea, is treated in the same way as *I. belli*. This infection is uncommon.

DIENTAMEBA FRAGILIS

Most infections with *Dientameba fragilis* are asymptomatic and do not require treatment. When required, treatment is as for amebiasis.

CYCLOSPORA CAYETANENSIS

Cyclospora cayetanensis is a newly recognized enteropathogen that causes traveler's diarrhea (especially in travelers to South America and Nepal) and foodborne outbreaks. In fecal smears, the oocysts resemble those of *C. parvum* in taking up carbol fuchsin in the modified Ziehl–Neelsen stain, but the oocysts are larger than *C. parvum* at 8–10 μm and they autofluoresce. Eradication is achieved using

TMP–SMX (160/800 mg twice daily) for 7 days. If infection persists, then TMP–SMX should be continued for a further 3–5 days. In patients who are intolerant to TMP–SMX, ciprofloxacin can be used but it is less effective.

MICROSPORIDIA

Two microsporidia are pathogenic in the human gastrointestinal tract: *Enterocytozoon bieneusi* and *Encephalitozoon intestinalis* (formerly known as *Septata intestinalis*). These organisms have only recently been described and are representatives of a phylum of primitive protozoa. They are intracellular parasites, which generally infect severely immunocompromised individuals. The most common manifestation is a persistent diarrhea associated with weight loss, but a syndrome of sclerosing cholangitis is also described. Diagnosis relies on detection of the parasite in duodenal biopsies obtained at endoscopy or on the finding of the spores in the feces using a variety of stains. *Encephalitozoon intestinalis* may cause a disseminated infection with renal spore excretion.

Treatment of *E. intestinalis* infection is with albendazole, 400 mg twice daily for 1 month, but maintenance treatment may be needed if relapse occurs following the cessation of therapy, although eradication may be achieved in some patients. Albendazole in this dose often leads to temporary suppression of *E. bieneusi* infection, but fumagillin, 60 mg daily for 14 days, results in symptomatic improvement and parasite clearance in some patients.

SUGGESTED READING

Amadi B, Mwiya M, Musuku J, et al. Effect of nitazoxanide on morbidity and mortality in Zambian children with cryptosporidiosis: a randomized controlled trial. *Lancet.* 2002;360:1375–1380.

Farthing MJG. Clinical aspects of human cryptosporidiosis. In: Petry F, ed. *Cryptosporidiosis and Microsporidiosis.* Basel: Karger; 2000:50–74.

Farthing MJG. Treatment options for the treatment of intestinal protozoa. *Nature Clin Gastroenterol Hepatol.* 2006:436–445.

Farthing MJG, Cevallos AM, Kelly P. Intestinal protozoa. In: Cook GC, ed. *Manson's Tropical Diseases.* 7th ed. London: WB Saunders; 2005.

Hoge CW, Shlim DR, Ghimire M, et al. Placebo-controlled trial of cotrimoxazole for *Cyclospora* infections among travellers and foreign residents in Nepal. *Lancet.* 1995;345:691–693.

Molina JM, Tourneur M, Chevret S, et al. Fumagillin treatment of intestinal microsporidiosis. *N Engl J Med.* 2002;346:1963–1969.

Rossignol JF, Ayoub A, Ayers MS. Treatment of diarrhea caused by Giardia intestinalis and Entamoeba histolytica or E. dispar: a randomized, double-blind, placebo-controlled study of nitazoxanide. *J Infect Dis.* 2002;184:381–384.

Tannich E. Entamoeba histolytica and E. dispar: comparison of molecules considered important for host tissue destruction. *Trans Roy Soc Trop Med Hyg.* 1998;92:593.

Zaat JO, Mank T, Assendelft WJ. Drugs for treating giardiasis. *Cochrane Database of Systematic Reviews.* (2): CD000217, 2000.

Zulu I, Kelly P, Njobvu L, et al. Nitazoxanide for persistent diarrhea in Zambian acquired immune deficiency syndrome patients: a randomized-controlled trial. *Aliment Pharmacol Ther.* 2005;21:757–763.

202. Extraintestinal Amebic Infection

Robert Huang and Sharon Reed

Extraintestinal manifestations of invasive amebic disease, although far less common than amebic colitis, are still a significant cause of morbidity and mortality worldwide, accounting for approximately 50000 deaths annually. The most common presentation, amebic liver abscess, can be diagnosed clinically by its characteristic presentation in conjugation with appropriate epidemiologic risks and supported by several serologic or antigen-based detection tests. Without treatment, amebic liver abscess is almost always fatal, but with prompt and appropriate treatment, the chance of a cure is nearly universal. Other, more rare, manifestations of invasive amebiasis also occur and will be discussed as well. The foundation of successful invasive amebiasis treatment has been metronidazole and the related nitroimidazole, tinidazole, which recently gained U.S. Food and Drug Administration (FDA) approval.

AMEBIC LIVER ABSCESS

In addition to amebic colitis and its complications, extraintestinal manifestations of invasive *Entameba histolytica* infections can occur, led in frequency by amebic liver abscesses. An estimated 10% of the worldwide 40 to 50 million symptomatic amebic infections will either present as or be complicated by amebic liver abscess. Adult men are 7 to 10 times more likely to have amebic liver abscess than women, but there is no difference between the sexes in children. It has been suggested that the different gender rates in adults may have to do with protective effects of estrogen in women and the role of alcohol in men with hepatocellular damage setting up a nidus for infection during portal drainage from an infected colon. As with other invasive amebic infections, amebic liver abscesses occur predominantly in the developing world with endemic disease seen in Central and South America, Africa, and Asia. Travelers to countries with endemic disease are at risk for developing amebiasis and liver disease. Longer stays are associated with increased risk; however, liver abscesses have been

reported in visitors with exposure as short as 4 days. Another population at risk in developed countries includes homosexual men who have an increased risk of intestinal amebiasis compared to the general population. Finally, those with cell-mediated immune defects including chronic steroid users, pregnant women, alcoholics, the malnourished, and those with malignancy may also be at increased risk of invasive *Entameba histolytica* infection and subsequent liver abscess.

The clinical presentation of amebic liver abscesses has been well described in several large reviews. Fever and right upper quadrant pain are the most frequent complaints and also the most consistent findings on examination (Table 202.1). The duration of disease influences the symptoms, as patients with symptoms for more than 2 weeks tend to be afebrile and have weight loss and more focal abdominal pain. The classic finding of point tenderness in the right upper quadrant or intercostal tenderness has been frequently noted in earlier literature but is likely neither sensitive nor specific. At most, only about one-third of patients have concomitant diarrhea or dysentery within the few weeks prior to their symptoms.

Approximately 80% of the liver abscesses are found in the right lobe of the liver, thus explaining the location of pain. The pain may also be located in the epigastrium, right lower chest, or the right shoulder tip (referred pain). Left-sided abdominal pain, corresponding to an abscess in the left lobe of the liver, is less common. Localized swelling or generalized hepatomegaly may be noted on exam depending on the size and location of the abscess or abscesses. Abscesses high in the right lobe of the liver may not result in hepatomegaly but, if of significant size, can lead to elevation of the right hemidiaphragm, which is evident on a chest radiograph.

Laboratory findings in a patient with amebic liver disease include leukocytosis (white blood cell (WBC) count >12000/µL), an elevated alkaline phosphatase, and, occasionally, elevated transaminases. It is uncommon to see an elevated bilirubin, and thus jaundice in a febrile

Table 202.1 Clinical Findings for Patients with Amebic Liver Abscess

Clinical Findings	%
Fever	85%–90%
Right upper quadrant pain	84%–90%
Hepatomegaly	30%–50%
Weight loss	33%–50%
Diarrhea	20%–33%
Cough	10%–30%
WBC count >12 000/µL	80%
Elevated level of alkaline phosphatase	70%

From Petri and Singh. *Clin Infect Dis.* 1999;29:1117–1125.
Abbreviation: WBC = white blood cell.

patient with right upper quadrant pain should point the clinician toward another diagnosis. A mild degree of anemia (anemia of chronic disease) is present in many cases, particularly with symptoms for more than 2 weeks.

Diagnosis

The definitive diagnosis of amebic liver abscess is made by finding invasive trophozoites on microscopic exam from tissue or pus obtained from the abscess or culturing the organism in vitro. However, due to the low yield and relative contraindications to needle aspiration of a suspected amebic liver abscess, other means of making the diagnosis represent the practical standard. Serologic testing for antibodies to *E. histolytica* is >80% sensitive in disease more than 1 week old, and nearly 99% sensitive in recovering patients. A negative test essentially rules out the diagnosis except in early infection (≤1 week). It is important to use an enzyme immunoassay (EIA) or agar gel dilution to test serology as an indirect hemagglutination often remains positive for years at high titer, and residents of an endemic region may have positive antibodies to *E. histolytica* that do not represent acute disease. Serum antigen detection tests to the *E. histolytica* Gal/GalNAc lectin are new and gave a positive result in >95% of patients with amebic liver abscess in a study in Bangladeshi patients prior to treatment, comparing favorably to currently available serum antibody tests. Importantly, after treatment

with metronidazole, circulating antigen levels were rarely detected (15%), making the test potentially useful for the diagnosis of acute disease in endemic countries. Molecular diagnosis using polymerase chain reaction (PCR) assays are highly sensitive and specific but require time, skill, and lab resources, all of which may be lacking in the resource-poor settings where amebiasis is common and thus will likely remain a research tool for the near future.

A number of imaging modalities are useful in supporting the diagnosis of amebic liver abscess. Chest radiographs in approximately 50% of patients with liver abscesses demonstrate an elevated right hemidiaphragm or other abnormality such as discoid atelectasis. Ultrasonography, computer tomography (CT) scanning, and magnetic resonance imaging (MRI) are all quite sensitive; however, the availability of these studies in amebiasis endemic areas is often limited. In the majority of cases, imaging demonstrates a single round or oval, homogeneous, hypoechoic lesion. Low attenuation lesions with septations or an observable fluid level or debris also may be seen (see Figures 202.1 and 202.2). Unfortunately, although gallbladder and ductal abnormalities

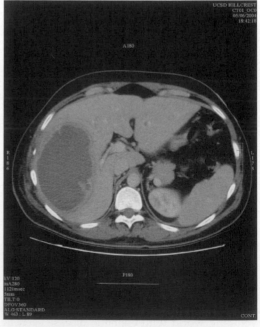

Figure 202.1 Contrast computed tomography (CT) scan image of an amebic liver abscess. The abscess appears as a hypoattenuating mass within the right lobe of the liver with an irregular, multiseptated rim with a thin rim of surrounding edema.

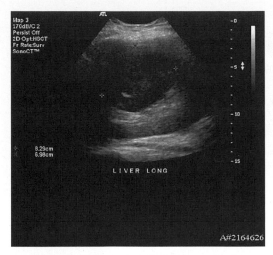

Figure 202.2 Ultrasound of the same amebic liver abscess as Figure 202.1.

are seen more often in pyogenic liver abscess, there are really no specific radiographic features distinguishing pyogenic from amebic liver abscesses; therefore, imaging only serves as an aid to confirming the clinical suspicion of an intrahepatic process. Amebic liver abscesses are reportedly "cold" on gallium scan, possibly with a bright rim, whereas pyogenic liver abscesses are "hot"; however, these studies are almost never necessary or available in most situations.

Aspiration of a liver abscess for the purpose of diagnosis is not generally recommended except in cases where immediate exclusion of a pyogenic abscess is clinically warranted. The classic gastronomic description of amebic pus as "anchovy paste" or "chocolate sauce" refers to the thick, acellular, proteinaceous debris consisting of necrotic hepatocytes and few polymorphonuclear cells obtained by successful aspiration. Amebic trophozoites are magenta colored by periodic acid–Schiff staining, making them easy to visualize, but finding trophozoites in an aspirate only occurs in 20% to 30% of cases, with a higher yield from the edge of the abscess.

The differential diagnosis of amebic liver abscesses includes pyogenic abscess, hepatocellular carcinoma, especially with necrosis, and echinococcal cyst. On imaging, the differential can often be narrowed to pyogenic abscess versus amebic liver abscess, with the clinical and radiographic findings being largely indistinguishable. Some epidemiologic differences may help to increase the likelihood of pyogenic liver abscess: age >50 years old, no sex predominance, underlying diabetes

mellitus, biliary disease, and lack of travel to an endemic country. Nevertheless, these clues do not rule out amebic liver abscess, especially in a patient living in a country where the disease is endemic.

Treatment

The treatment of amebic liver abscess has been based for the past several decades on the effective tissue amebicide metronidazole. Metronidazole, a nitroimidazole compound, has been demonstrated in a number of trials to be effective in a dose of 750 mg 3 times daily for 7–10 days for adults and 35–50 mg/kg/day in 3 doses for 7–10 days for children (Table 202.2). Lower doses and shorter courses may be effective for mild to moderate cases of amebic colitis but are not recommended for liver abscesses. Metronidazole is generally well tolerated but the disulfiramlike reaction to alcohol is important to mention to patients, especially because those developing amebic liver abscesses often have a history of alcohol use/abuse. Minor side effects such as nausea, vomiting, anorexia, and a metallic taste occur more frequently than rare neurologic adverse effects such as vertigo, seizures, and encephalopathy. The drug should be discontinued if these latter effects or, rarely, neutropenia occurs. Long-term use of metronidazole is also known to cause peripheral neuropathy, but the duration of therapy for invasive amebic disease should not approach that at which this adverse event occurs.

The related imidazole compound, tinidazole, has been reported as effective as a single 2-g dose for treatment of liver abscess in South Africa. Tinidazole was recently approved by the FDA after its use for years in other countries. The recommended dose for amebic liver abscess is 2 g/day for 3–5 days in adults and 50 mg/kg/day for 3–5 days in children. It is generally better tolerated than metronidazole and offers a shorter course; however, it is more expensive and less well studied.

The imidazoles are more than 90% effective in the treatment of amebic liver abscess.

Although clinical cases of resistance have been demonstrated in the related protozoa, *Giardia lamblia*, and resistance can be demonstrated in vitro, no clinical cases of metronidazole-resistant amebiasis have been documented. Treatment with these agents typically results in defervescence, decreased abdominal pain, and normalization of the WBC count within 3 days.

Table 202.2 Drug Treatment of Amebic Liver Abscess[a]

Drug of Choice	Adult Dose	Pediatric Dose	Side Effects
Metronidazole	750 mg IV/PO TID x 7–10 d	35–50 mg/kg/d in 3 doses ×7–10 d	Common: nausea, vomiting. metallic taste
			Occasional: peripheral neuropathy, vertigo, seizures, encephalopathy
			Disulfiram effect: nausea, vomiting with alcohol ingestion
Tinidazole[tt]	2 g IV/PO qd ×5 d	60 mg/kg/d (maximum 2 g) ×5 d	Similar side effect profile as metronidazole: better tolerated with less nausea and vomiting

[a] All treatments should be followed by luminal amebicidal agent, described in text and detailed in Chapter 201, Intestinal Protozoa.
[b] Used only as alternative to metronidazole.

Therapeutic aspiration of amebic liver abscesses is now typically reserved for several specific circumstances. Disease not responding to 3–5 days of medical therapy with persistent fever or pain, imminent rupture of an abscess >15 cm, or a left lobe abscess that may rupture into the pericardium have all been cited as reasons to drain abscesses. Blind needling of the liver for the purposes of diagnosis or treatment is dangerous and ultrasonographic or CT-guided aspiration is recommended in all instances when available.

All treatment regimens with a tissue amebicide should be followed by treatment with a luminal amebicide to eliminate intestinal carriage of the organism that could lead to relapse if not treated. Paromomycin, a non-absorbed aminoglycoside, taken for 7 days is the preferred luminal amebicide in the United States. It is safe in pregnancy, has minimal gastrointestinal side effects, and ototoxicity and nephrotoxicity rarely occur. Diloxanide furoate is also effective and well tolerated and has few side effects but is not commercially available in the United States. Iodoquinol is likewise effective but has some serious side effects such as optic neuritis and peripheral neuropathy, and requires a 20-day course. Nitazoxanide, a 5-nitrothiazolyl derivative, is active against a range of protozoa and is approved by the FDA for the treatment of diarrhea caused by *Cryptosporidium parvum* and *Giardia lamblia* in children. Its activity against *E. histolytica* has been demonstrated in vitro, and one double blind, placebo-controlled trial

suggested efficacy as well; however, it has not been directly compared to the standard luminal amebicides already mentioned.

The usual response to medical therapy of an amebic liver abscess is rapid resolution of fever and pain. There is no reason to get a follow-up ultrasound early in the course, as lesions may actually enlarge acutely, but they ultimately completely resolve within a year. Serology by EIA typically reverts to negative within 6 months.

AMEBIC PLEUROPULMONARY DISEASE

The most common pulmonary manifestation of invasive amebiasis is development of a serous, sympathetic effusion in the right pleural cavity due to a right-sided liver abscess. Rupture of a liver abscess into the chest cavity can lead to empyema, producing signs such as cough, dyspnea, and pleuritic chest pain. Thoracentesis will reveal the classic anchovy paste fluid described above. Classically, patients who develop bronchopleural fistula will expectorate the contents of the liver abscess. Although unpleasant, prior to amebicidal agents this occurrence was deemed a good prognostic sign, as it was an effective means of draining the abscess. In addition, hematogenous spread of amebic trophozoites can rarely cause disease in the lung parenchyma leading to consolidation and sometimes lung abscess. Treatment of pleuropulmonary disease involves the use of a tissue amebicide, such as metronidazole, and, in the case of empyema, drainage with a chest tube. Amebic pneumonia and lung abscesses from hematogenous spread are successfully treated with metronidazole alone.

AMEBIC PERICARDITIS

The most serious complication of a left-lobe amebic liver abscess is rupture into the pericardium leading to pericarditis and, potentially, cardiac tamponade. In one large series, the incidence of pericardial rupture was approximately 1% of all liver abscess cases. A left-lobe liver abscess threatening the pericardial sac may cause irritation and a serous effusion. According to one group of authors, this pericardial effusion should be referred to as the "presuppurative phase," rather than simply a sympathetic or reactive effusion because it heralds an impending rupture. The rapidity of leakage of amebic pus into the pericardial sac determines both the signs and symptoms that develop. A slow leak gives more insidious symptoms of gradually increasing shortness of breath, unmitigated fever, and patient deterioration, whereas a rapid rupture into the pericardium may cause cardiac tamponade and the associated chest pain, tachypnea, pulsus paradoxus, elevated neck veins, and hypotension.

The evaluation of amebic pericarditis begins with establishing the diagnosis of an invasive amebic infection with positive serologic testing in a patient with left-lobe liver abscess and a compatible epidemiologic history. An electrocardiogram will show evidence of pericarditis, and chest radiography demonstrates an elevated and immobile left diaphragm. Confirming the diagnosis is only definitively accomplished by aspiration of the pericardium, which, along with effective tissue amebicides, is the treatment of choice. A concomitant large liver abscess should also be aspirated and repeat aspirations performed if needed to eliminate the risk of further pericardial accumulation. Fibrous constriction is unusual after the above treatment, and surgical treatment is unnecessary in most cases.

AMEBIC PERITONITIS

In about 2% of amebic liver abscesses, intraperitoneal abscess and peritonitis complicate the case. The associated physical exam findings of an acute abdomen are usually present. Compared to amebic peritonitis due to perforation of the colon from amebic colitis, patients with ruptured liver abscesses and peritonitis have better outcomes because there is not concomitant colonic bacterial flora contaminating the peritoneum. Treatment of amebic peritonitis due to liver abscess rupture is with metronidazole plus therapeutic paracentesis to drain infected collections.

OTHER MANIFESTATIONS OF INVASIVE AMEBIC DISEASE

Although very rare, amebic brain abscesses can occur by hematogenous seeding of trophozoites and may present with altered mental status, headache, and focal neurologic signs in a patient with known amebiasis. Computed tomography scanning of the head reveals often multiple space-occupying lesions, which, early in the course of disease, may be low-attenuation circumscribed areas without a clear rim or enhancement. Treatment involves an extended course of metronidazole, which has good central nervous system penetration, and possible surgical drainage depending on the size of the lesion(s) and severity of the symptoms.

Amebic splenic abscesses, also resulting from hematogenous spread of amebic trophozoites, can be visualized with ultrasound or CT scan and is treated medically with metronidazole. Splenectomy is occasionally required.

Urinary tract amebiasis, manifesting as perinephric abscesses, are again due to hematogenous spread of amebic trophozoites and treated with metronidazole. Genital amebiasis is more common in women than men, with vaginitis, vulvovaginal amebiasis, cervicitis, and salpingitis all having been reported. These cases may be sexually transmitted; consequently, ulcerative penile lesions in a sexual partner should be evaluated for possible amebiasis. Invasive carcinoma of the penis and carcinoma of the cervix are often initially suspected as the clinical appearance of the amebic ulcerative lesions mimics that of these malignancies. An epidemiologic study in Japan found a link between genital amebiasis and homosexuals engaging in anal sex with partners with amebic colitis. The treatment for these manifestations of the disease is again with metronidazole, and sexual partners should always be treated as well.

SUGGESTED READING

Adams EB, MacLeod IN. Invasive amoebiasis II: ameobic liver abscess and its complications. *Medicine*. 1977;56:325.

Ayeh-Kumi PF, Petri WA Jr. Diagnosis and management of amebiasis. *Infect Med*. 2006, 23:301–310.

Katzenstein D, Rickerson V, Braude A. New concepts of amebic liver abscess derived from hepatic imaging, serodiagnosis, and hepatic enzymes in 67 consecutive cases in San Diego. *Medicine*. 1982;61:237.

Reed SL. Amoebiasis: an update. *Clin Infect Dis*. 1992;14:385–393.

Stanley SL Jr. Amoebiasis. *Lancet*. 2003; 361:1035.

PART XXV

Antimicrobial Therapy – General Considerations

203. Principles of Antibiotic Therapy

Richard A. Gleckman[†] and John S. Czachor

Since the mid-1990s, there has been the recognition of a very disturbing trend of antibiotic resistance among a wide variety of pathogens that are causing serious disease in patients residing in the community, in long-term care facilities, and in hospitals. A partial list consists of the following bacteria: *Streptococcus pneumoniae*, resistant to penicillin, first- and second-generation cephalosporins, macrolides/azilides, tetracyclines, trimethoprim–sulfamethoxazole (TMP–SFX), and fluoroquinolones; *Staphylococcus aureus*, resistant to oxacillin, cephalosporins, clindamycin, fluoroquinolones, and, very rarely, vancomycin; ampicillin and vancomycin-resistant *Enterococcus* spp.; extended-spectrum β-lactamase–producing *Escherichia coli* and *Klebsiella pneumoniae* resistant to broad-spectrum cephalosporins; *Salmonella* spp., resistant to ampicillin, chloramphenicol, TMP–SFX, fluoroquinolones, and third-generation cephalosporins; *Campylobacter* spp., resistant to fluoroquinolones; *Helicobacter pylori*, resistant to clarithromycin; *Vibrio cholerae*, resistant to ciprofloxacin; aminoglycoside and fluoroquinolone-resistant *Pseudomonas aeruginosa*, *Stenotrophomonas maltophilia*, and *Acinetobacter* spp.; clindamycin-resistant *Bacteroides fragilis*; and *Mycobacterium tuberculosis* organisms resistant to all available drugs.

The pharmaceutical companies have responded to this grave concern and have developed several new agents (quinupristin–dalfopristin, linezolid, daptomycin, and dalbavancin) that inhibit the growth of gram-positive bacteria, and a new compound, tigecycline, that possesses inhibitory activity for a wide range of gram-positive, gram-negative, and anaerobic bacteria. Although some data are available, it is premature to precisely establish the indications for these new antibiotics, their potential to cause toxicities and drug–drug interactions, and to identify *the* preferred agent for a specific infection.

Another event that has merited attention is the continuously evolving novel indications for antibiotics for both infectious and noninfectious disorders. Recent studies have suggested a role for telithromycin in the treatment of the acute exacerbation of asthma, and doxycycline to treat lymphangioleiomyomatosis, and to prevent tick-borne relapsing fever.

When selecting an antibiotic, the clinician must reflect on a number of issues. Some of the more common factors that merit consideration include the patient's drug allergy history; the relative safety of the medication; the potential of the antibiotic to cause a significant drug–drug interaction; the mechanism of the drug's elimination from the body; the agent's historical "track record" in the therapy of the specific infection being treated; the route of administration of the antibiotic; and the cost of the medication. For the oral administration of antibiotics there are the additional concerns of patient compliance and adequate drug absorption.

PHARMACOKINETICS AND PHARMACODYNAMICS

Pharmacokinetics refers to the disposition of an antibiotic throughout the human body. This encompasses such principles as absorption, bioavailability, distribution, protein binding, metabolism, and elimination. Pharmacodynamics refines the concept of pharmacokinetics by describing the interaction between the concentration of the antibiotic at the site of the infection over time and its subsequent effect on the infection itself. Pharmacodynamics is useful for establishing optimum dosing regimens. The absorption of most oral antibiotics occurs by passive diffusion in the small intestine. Some antibiotics, including vancomycin, aminoglycosides, and aztreonam, are not adequately absorbed when given orally. On occasion, this can be advantageous. Oral neomycin can be prescribed as a preoperative preparation prior to large bowel surgery or the treatment of hepatic encephalopathy, whereas oral vancomycin has been an effective treatment for the therapy of *Clostridium difficile*–related colitis. Other drugs, such as cefpodoxime proxetel and cefuroxime axetil, are administered as prodrugs to facilitate absorption. Food interferes with the absorption of some antimicrobials; for example, penicillin, ampicillin, cephalexin, tetracycline, and azithromycin.

A fundamental tenet of antimicrobial activity is that it must achieve therapeutic concentrations at the tissue source of the infection. Multiple factors influence the distribution of antibiotics from plasma to these sites: the nature of the capillary bed (those fenestrated by small pores versus those unfenestrated capillaries of the brain, leptomeninges, and vitreous humor), the lipid solubility, the degree of protein binding (as only unbound drug is antibacterially active and capable of diffusing across capillaries), and the presence of active transport pumps (located in the choroids plexus of the brain, retina, kidneys, and biliary ducts).

Antibacterial agents are eliminated from the body through hepatic and biliary excretion (ceftriaxone and piperacillin), hepatic metabolism (clindamycin, chloramphenicol, metronidazole, erythromycin, sulfonamides, some tetracyclines, isoniazid, rifampin), and predominantly renal excretion (most penicillins and cephalosporins, imipenem, aminoglycosides, nitrofurantoin, most tetracyclines, ofloxacin, vancomycin, TMP–SFX). It is essential that the clinician be aware of renal compromise from congestive heart failure, hypertension, diabetes, medication, and physiologic alteration with age, because this will mandate a dosage reduction for those compounds predominantly eliminated by renal excretion. The estimated glomerular filtration rate (using the Cockcroft–Gault equation or the Modification of Diet in Renal Disease [MDRD] equation) has traditionally been used to help determine appropriate drug doses for antimicrobials eliminated primarily by renal excretion when the measured creatinine clearance is not available.

Concentration-dependent antimicrobial agents function such that optimal bacterial killing occurs while the concentration of the antibiotic is above the minimum inhibitory concentration (MIC) of the organism. The aminoglycosides are one example of this type and are usually administered as once-daily dosing (unless prescribed for synergistic purposes), taking advantage of the observation that the ratio of the maximum peak drug concentration to organism MIC (8 to 12) correlates with clinical response. Other concentration-dependent antimicrobials include fluoroquinolones, daptomycin, and metronidazole. Alternatively, those compounds that are concentration independent or time dependent measure their success by the percentage of time the drug concentration exceeds the MIC of an organism. Drugs in this class include vancomycin, clindamycin, the macrolides, and the β-lactam group. There may be some benefit for continuous intravenous administration of the β-lactam antibiotics, thereby maintaining sustained drug levels above the MIC of the pathogen, particularly in the severely ill or immunocompromised patient.

The postantibiotic effect (PAE) is another pharmacodynamic concept that may impact antimicrobial choice. This refers to the persistent suppression of bacterial regrowth following limited exposure to an antibiotic and can be considered the time it takes for the organism to recover from this exposure. Classically, drugs that affect protein synthesis or nucleic acid synthesis, such as the fluoroquinolones, aminoglycosides, tetracyclines, macrolides, chloramphenicol, and rifampin, have significant PAEs against gram-negative organisms, although the only β-lactam antibiotics that share this property are the carbapenems.

SELECTION OF THERAPY

Table 203.1 delineates some of the more important host and drug features that influence antibiotic selection. Additional concerns relate to adherence to the therapeutic regimen and cost of the medication. Antibiotics that can be administered infrequently lend themselves to out-of-hospital administration. Daptomycin, ertapenem, and ceftriaxone can usually be infused as infrequently as once a day. The development of new oral antimicrobial agents that can be given as infrequently as once or twice per day achieves enhanced compliance. Compounds such as the fluoroquinolones, metronidazole, and linezolid have excellent absorption, resulting in high serum levels without the need for intravenous administration. Some medications, although still available, including chloramphenicol and erythromycin estolate, are infrequently prescribed, having fallen out of favor due to adverse effects, unfavorable pharmacokinetics and/or pharmacodynamics, or a limited spectrum of activity.

Antibiotic combinations are used to manage selected infections (Table 203.2). There are potential disadvantages, however, to the administration of antibiotic combinations such as increased untoward events, heightened costs, and suprainfection.

With few exceptions, the optimal duration of antibacterial treatment has not been defined by rigorous controlled trials. Recommended duration of antibacterial therapy has predominantly evolved from clinical experience. Treatment duration is influenced by a number of factors, including the immune competence of the host,

Table 203:1 Selection of Therapy

Host Factor	Special Antibiotic Concern
Drug allergy	Safety record
Site of infection	Success record
Pregnancy	Most likely organism(s) and susceptibility
Epidemiologic information	Bactericidal/bacteriostatic
Renal function	Penetration into privileged sites (CNS,
Recent antibiotic exposure	endocardium)
Infection acquisition (community/ECF/	Potential to cause major untoward event
hospital)	
Concomitant medication	

Abbreviations: CNS = central nervous system; ECF = extended care facility.

Table 203.2 Combination Therapy

Tuberculosis
Disseminated *Mycobacterium avium* complex
Helicobacter pylori
Endocarditis (α-hemolytic streptococcus, enterococcus)
Life-threatening infection caused by *Pseudomonas aeruginosa*
Empiric treatment -Pneumococcal meningitis until susceptibility confirmed -Febrile, severely neutropenic host -Polymicrobic infection -Life-threatening infection with inapparent source

the nature of the organism(s), and the site(s) of infection. As a general statement, patients with cellulitis, an exacerbation of chronic bronchitis, community-acquired sinusitis/pharyngitis, and uncomplicated urinary tract infections are candidates for a treatment course of approximately 10 days. Newer, more potent, and highly active therapies have begun to reduce the length of treatment for selected diseases. Treatment courses of 3 days are standard for uncomplicated cystitis, and respiratory infections, such as community-acquired pneumonia in selective hosts, have been shortened to 5 days with the use of fluoroquinolones. Alternatively, patients with bacterial osteomyelitis, chronic bacterial prostatitis, endocarditis, and *Legionella* pneumonia require antibacterial treatment for 3 weeks to 3 months.

SPECIAL POPULATIONS
The Pregnant Patient

Physiologic changes in the urinary tract and complications of parturition predispose the pregnant woman to urinary tract infections, as well as chorioamnionitis and endometritis. Antibiotic selection for the pregnant woman must take into consideration the potential for drug-induced toxicities for both the woman and her developing fetus. Animal studies and epidemiologic data (generated from pregnant women who were exposed to antibacterial agents because of clinical need) suggest that penicillins, including those in combination with a β-lactamase inhibitor, cephalosporins, aztreonam, erythromycin, azithromycin, clindamycin, and metronidazole, have not demonstrated human fetal risk. Sulfonamides should be avoided late in pregnancy because of the potential to develop neonatal kernicterus. Chloramphenicol should not be administered to the mother near term as the newborn does not possess the appropriate liver enzyme to metabolize this drug, and hence the "gray baby" syndrome can result. The aminoglycosides gentamicin, tobramycin, and amikacin, should not be administered to pregnant women, especially ecclamptic women, unless there is a compelling reason. If they must be prescribed, serum concentrations must be monitored carefully.

The fluoroquinolones are not recommended for use in pregnancy because of their adverse effects on developing cartilage seen in animal studies. Tetracyclines are contraindicated in pregnant women because these compounds can interfere with normal development of teeth and bones in the fetus and have caused hepatorenal failure and death, particularly when administered intravenously to treat pyelonephritis, in pregnant women.

The Elderly Patient

There are a number of factors that distinguish the administration of antibiotics in elderly patients: concern about compliance with the

Table 203.3 Adverse Drug Reaction

Drug	Untoward Event
Aminoglycoside	Nephrotoxicity, ototoxicity
Amoxicillin–clavulanic acid (chronic administration)	Hepatotoxicity
TMP–SFX	Blood dyscrasias, hyperkalemia
Fluoroquinolone	Seizure
Doxycycline	Esophageal stricture/ulcer
Nitrofurantoin (chronic administration)	Pulmonary fibrosis, hepatitis, agranulocytosis
Abbreviation: TMP–SFX = trimethoprim–sulfamethoxazole.	

medication, because of poor memory, impaired vision, diminished hearing, or difficulty in opening child-resistant containers; the decrease of renal function with normal aging, and the need to make appropriate dosage adjustment of medications to prevent antibiotic-related toxicities; the potential for drug–drug interactions, as many geriatric patients take numerous medications daily; and the presence of concomitant medical disorders, such as congestive heart failure and atherosclerotic vascular disease, that can adversely influence antibiotic distribution and penetration. Elderly patients appear to experience adverse drug reactions from antibacterial compounds more frequently than younger patients do (Table 203.3).

ANTIBIOTIC USE IN CONTINUOUS RENAL REPLACEMENT THERAPY

For critically ill patients with infection, acute renal insufficiency often develops. Acute renal failure is associated with increased morbidity and mortality in patients with sepsis. Continuous renal replacement therapies (CRRT), an alternative to traditional hemodialysis and better tolerated by hemodynamically unstable patients, decreases the incidence of adverse biomarkers. Appropriate dosing of antimicrobial agents for patients receiving CRRT remains poorly defined, as the pharmacokinetics of drug removal in critically ill patients undergoing CRRT is complex. Those antibiotics with low protein binding capacity and/or poor tissue penetration have enhanced removal. Mechanical or operational factors associated with CRRT play a role in antibiotic therapy in these patients as well, and increasing the blood flow or dialysate flow rate of CRRT may increase drug clearance. Tables 203.4 and 203.5

list antibiotic dose alterations for patients with CRRT. Loading doses are necessary for vancomycin and levofloxacin.

ROUTE OF ADMINISTRATION

Antibiotics are administered intravenously when the patient has systemic perfusion issues (septic shock, hypotension), has bacterial infection at a unique or protected site (eg, leptomeninges, endocardium, a deep neck infection, epiglottitis, endophthalmitis, myopercarditis, mediastinitis, septic thrombophlebitis), has an infection that is imminently life endangering (eg, meningococcemia, Rocky Mountain spotted fever, plague, bacteremia), has an infection that precludes oral administration because of nausea/vomiting or impaired function of the gastrointestinal tract (peritonitis, appendicitis, ascending cholangitis, pancreatic abscess), or has an infection that cannot be managed with an oral compound. Traditionally, physicians have prescribed an intravenous antibiotic simply because a patient was admitted to the hospital. However, the decision to hospitalize a patient does not automatically dictate that the antibacterial therapy must be administered intravenously. Unless one of the indications previously listed is present, some serious infections can be successfully managed by oral antibiotics: uncomplicated pyelonephritis, uncomplicated community-acquired pneumonia, and traditional cellulitis (cellulitis not precipitated by a unique exposure).

Adverse Reactions

Antibiotic-induced untoward events are a concern not only because they result in host injury but also because these adverse events interrupt

Table 203.4 Drugs Not Requiring Dosage Alteration During Continuous Renal Replacement Therapies

Aztreonam	Linezolid
Azithromycin	Meropenem
Cefepime	Metronidazole
Ceftriaxone	Moxifloxacin
Clindamycin	Oxacillin
Doxycycline	Quinupristin–dalfopristin
Gatifloxacin	Rifampin
Imipenem	

Table 203.5 Drugs Requiring Dosage Alteration During CRRT[a]

Amikacin	Penicillin
Ampicillin/sulbactam	Piperacillin
Cefazolin	Piperacillin–tazobactam
Ciprofloxacin	Ticarcillin–clavulanic acid
Daptomycin	Tobramycin
Gentamicin	TMP–SFX
Levofloxacin	Vancomycin

[a] Dose reduction as compared to normal renal function.
Abbreviations: CRRT = continuous renal replacement therapies; TMP–SFX = trimethoprim–sulfamethoxazole.

and complicate treatment, thereby requiring the administration of alternative and often more expensive and potentially toxic medication. Antibiotic-induced untoward events can also serve as a source of medical litigation.

Adverse events attributed to antibiotics are usually caused by three mechanisms: exaggerated response to the known pharmacologic effects of the drug, immunologic reactions to the drug or its metabolites, and toxic effects of the medication or its metabolites. Many of the antibiotic-related adverse events are initiated by an extension of the drug's normal pharmacology, and these events are often avoided by appropriate dosage adjustment.

In addition to the direct influence of the antibiotic, host factors such as genetic constitution, integrity of drug elimination mechanisms, and concomitant medical disorders can affect the frequency and severity of antibiotic-induced untoward events. Human immunodeficiency virus (HIV)-infected patients are predisposed to oxacillin-induced hepatitis and cutaneous reactions attributed to TMP–SFX and aminopenicillins. TMP–SFX causes more non–dose-related gastrointestinal intolerance, fever,

and altered liver function in patients with the acquired immunodeficiency syndrome. Ampicillin-induced rash is more common in patients with infectious mononucleosis.

The penicillin family of drugs is usually well tolerated, but on occasion they can cause hypersensitivity events, including fever, rash (maculopapular and urticarial), anaphylaxis, exfoliative dermatitis, erythema multiforme, serum sickness, and hemolytic anemia. When administered intravenously in high doses, particularly to patients with renal impairment, they have the potential to cause central nervous system toxicity, manifested by myoclonic jerks, seizures, and coma. Table 203.6 lists selective penicillins, carbapenems (imipenem, meropenem, ertapenem), and cephalosporins and the unique adverse drug reactions attributed to these compounds.

The most notorious side effects of clindamycin are diarrhea and *C. difficile*–related colitis. This drug has rarely caused drug fever, blood dyscrasias, and hepatotoxicity. Doxycycline has caused diarrhea and, on occasion, photosensitivity, rash, hepatitis, and, particularly in elderly patients, esophageal ulcerations and strictures.

Uncommon adverse events attributed to vancomycin include rash, fever, nephrotoxicity, ototoxicity, and reversible, transient hematopoietic toxicity. The most dramatic side effect is the red man syndrome, a nonimmunologically mediated reaction consisting of pruritis and erythema with or without hypotension, which appears to be dependent on dose, frequency of administration, and rate of infusion. With regard to the newer antibiotics designed to manage gram-positive infections caused by vancomycin-resistant organisms, quinupristin–dalfopristin can cause severe arthralgias and myalgias; chronic administration of linezolid has produced myelosuppression, optic neuropathy, and peripheral neuropathy; infusion of daptomycin has elicited myopathy and paresthesias/dysesthesias; and tigecycline has been associated with nausea, vomiting, and headache. Gastrointestinal symptoms are the most common untoward events attributed to the administration of the new semisynthetic lipoglycopeptide dalbavancin.

Rash, fever, and gastrointestinal adverse events are the most common side effects produced by TMP–SFX. Additional rare untoward events include nephrotoxicity, hyperkalemia, hematologic derangements (neutropenia, thrombocytopenia, agranulocytosis, aplastic anemia, megaloblastic anemia), hepatitis,

Table 203.6 Penicillin-Family, Carbapenem, and Cephalosporin Adverse Events

Ampicillin	*C. difficile* colitis, interstitial nephritis
Amoxicillin–clavulanic acid (chronic administration)	Hepatotoxicity
Nafcillin	Neutropenia
Ticarcillin, carbenicillin	Hypokalemia, fluid overload, platelet-mediated bleeding
Imipenem–cilastatin	Seizures
Ceftriaxone	Diarrhea, hemolytic anemia, biliary sludge
Cefotetan	Hemolytic anemia
Cefoperazone diarrhea	Hypoprothrombinemic bleeding
Ceftazidime	Alteration of hepatic function
Cefditoren	Diarrhea

pancreatitis, pseudomembranous colitis, and central nervous system events, including headache, insomnia, vertigo, ataxia, and aseptic meningitis.

Adverse events attributed to the macrolides have included nausea, vomiting, abdominal pain, diarrhea, and rarely antibiotic-associated colitis, pancreatitis, cholestatic jaundice, acute hepatitis, and reversible ototoxicity. Telithromycin, a ketolide, has the potential to cause gastrointestinal disturbances, headache, and dizziness. The major adverse event related to the administration of telithromycin is severe hepatotoxicity.

The most common adverse events associated with the administration of the fluoroquinolones are gastrointestinal symptoms, nervous system toxicity (headache, dizziness, insomnia, agitation, hallucinations), and allergic reactions, including pruritis and rash. Rare adverse events attributed to the quinolones include seizures, elevation of liver enzymes, and tendinopathy. Administration of the fluoroquinolones, particularly gatifloxacin, is associated with an increased risk of dysglycemia.

There has been renewed interest in the old antibiotic, polymyxin E (colistimethate sodium), as therapy for patients with life-endangering infections caused by drug-resistant *Pseudomonas aeruginosa* and *Acinetobacter baumannii*. This agent has the potential to elicit both neurotoxic side effects and nephrotoxicity.

Antibiotic Allergy

Antibiotic-induced allergic reactions are immunologically mediated and most commonly involve the skin as pruritus, a maculopapular eruption, or urticaria. More significant antibiotic-induced allergic reactions include erythema multiforme (Stevens–Johnson syndrome), toxic epidermal necrolysis, exfoliative dermatitis, angioedema, and anaphylaxis. Antibiotic-induced allergic reactions are not confined to the skin: Amoxicillin–clavulanic acid and macrolides have caused cholestatic liver injury, and high-dose administration of penicillins and cephalosporins have caused hemolysis and cytopenias. Patients with infectious mononucleosis, cystic fibrosis, and HIV infection appear to be particularly predisposed to antimicrobial-induced allergic reactions.

Among the most feared allergic reactions to penicillins and cephalosporins are angioedema and anaphylaxis. These events are usually attributed to drug-specific immunoglobulin E (IgE) antibodies from prior drug administration, but these serious untoward events can also result from direct release of mast-cell mediators following the first dose of antibiotic. Vancomycin and fluoroquinolones can also cause direct mast cell release in the absence of drug-specific IgE antibodies. Skin testing has been very accurate for identifying penicillin-related IgE antibodies and for determining the risk for patients experiencing an immediate reaction (see Chapter 206, Hypersensitivity to Antibiotics).

There appears to be an increased risk of cephalosporin-induced reactions among patients with positive results on penicillin skin tests. If a patient has a history of a presumed IgE-mediated reaction to a penicillin (angioedema, anaphylaxis), it is best to avoid a cephalosprin, particularly because skin testing material is not currently available for cephalosporins, and drug desensitization can be complicated by severe allergic reactions. Although structurally similar to the β-lactam antibiotics, aztreonam can be safely administered to patients who have experienced an anaphylactic reaction following the administration of a member of the penicillin family. It is considered potentially harmful to administer imipenem to patients with a history of immediate hypersensitivity to penicillins; however, recent investigation suggests that those patients with negative skin testing to imipenem–cilastatin can safely be offered this antibiotic.

Drug–Drug Interactions

Drug–drug interactions can be subtle or life-endangering, and they occur when one drug modifies the pharmacokinetics (absorption, distribution, metabolism, or excretion) or pharmacodynamics of another drug. Magnesium antacid reduces the absorption of nitrofurantoin, food diminishes the absorption of azithromycin, and antacids, sucralfate, ferrous sulfate, and zinc alter the bioavailability of oral tetracyclines and quinolones. Oral antacids lower the plasma concentrations of cefditoren. The angiotensin-converting enzyme inhibitor quinapril has a high concentration of magnesium, and it impedes the absorption of the quinolones. Suppression by oral tetracyclines, erythromycin, or TMP–SFX of upper intestinal bacteria that inactivate digoxin can result in digoxin-induced toxicity. Administration of doxycyline has been associated with failure of oral contraceptive preparations. Alcohol ingestion in patients receiving metronidazole can result in a disulfiram reaction, and caution should be used when prescribing metronidazole to patients receiving zalcitabine, didanosine, or stavudine, as there is the potential for additive peripheral neuropathy.

Drug–drug interactions have not been a major concern for patients receiving the penicillins, carbapenems, aztreonam, and the cephalosporins. Theophylline and cyclosporine can reduce the threshold for seizures in patients receiving imipenem, and meropenem decreases the serum concentrations of valproic acid to subtherapeutic levels in patients with seizure disorders. There is the potential for enhanced aminoglycoside-induced nephrotoxicity and/or ototoxicity when patients receive vancomycin, amphotericin B, cyclosporine, cisplatin, and ethacrynic acid.

Ciprofloxacin has the potential to inhibit the metabolism of theophylline through its effect on the enzymes of the cytochrome P450 system and produce theophylline toxicity. Ciprofloxacin can also alter cyclophosphamide pharmacokinetics in patients with non-Hodgkin's lymphoma. There is a potential concern when fluoroquinolones are used to treat patients taking medications (antipsychotics, tricyclic antidepressants, and antiarrhythmics) that predispose to the development of torsades de pointes. Levofloxacin and moxifloxacin have been associated with enhancement of the effect of warfarin. Gatifloxacin administration to patients receiving oral hypoglycemic agents can produce severe and resistant hypoglycemia.

Erythromycin is extensively metabolized by cytochrome P450 3A isozymes (CYP3A), and when this antibiotic is coadministered with medications that are strong inhibitors of CYP3A, such as azole antifungal drugs, diltiazem, verapamil, and protease inhibitors, sudden cardiac death can occur. Coadministration of sirolimus and erythromycin in transplant recipients increase the blood concentrations of the immunosuppressant. Clarithromycin is oxidized by the cytochrome P450 system, and this compound results in decreased clearance of those other agents given concurrently that are metabolized by the same enzyme system. Administration of clarithromycin to a patient taking a statin (3-hydroxy-3-methylglutaryl coenzyme A reductase inhibitor) other than pravastatin can result in rhabdomyolysis. Coadministration of digoxin and clarithromycin can result in digitalis intoxication. The ketolide telithromycin is an inhibitor of the cytochrome P450 3A4 (CYP-3A4) enzyme and should not be prescribed to patients receiving cisapride, pimozide, simvastatin, lovastatin, atorvastatin, and class IA and class III antiarrhythmic agents.

Serotonin toxicity (fever, agitation, mental status changes, myoclonus, and tremors) has been associated with the coadministration of linezolid and medications that increase concentrations of serotonin in the central nervous system, such as the selective serotonin reuptake inhibitors. If the patient's infection requires linezolid therapy, such as for treatment of a life-endangering infection caused by *Enterococ-cus faecium* or methicillin-resistant *Staphylococcus aureus,* the selective serotonin reuptake inhibitor should be discontinued, and the patient monitored for the serotonin syndrome. Coadministration of TMP–SFX with phenytoin, glipizide, methotrexate, and thiazide diuretics has caused phenytoin toxicity, enhanced hypoglycemia, bone marrow suppression, and severe hyponatremia, respectively. TMP–SFX can enhance warfarin-induced anticoagulation and ganciclovir-induced bone marrow suppression, and it can diminish cyclosporine concentrations, resulting in a transplant rejection. Neutropenia and thrombocytopenia can occur in renal allograft recipients who receive azathioprine and more than 3 weeks of treatment with TMP–SFX. TMP–SFX has caused hyperkalemia when prescribed to patients receiving a potassium-sparing diuretic.

Quinupristin–dalfopristin is a potent inhibitor of CYP3A4, and it should be used with caution when patients are receiving drugs that are substrates of 3A4, such as cyclosporine, nifedipine, protease inhibitors, and statins.

DRUG MONITORING

Monitoring the adequacy of antibiotic treatment involves the physician critically assessing the patient's response on a regular basis, as determined by the resolution of both the systemic and local inflammatory response and, in part, measured by results obtained from laboratory studies, microbiology data, and radiologic exams. In general, antibiotic concentrations in blood are not routinely measured. Aminoglycoside antibiotics are an exception, however, because serum concentrations of these compounds are performed to ostensibly reduce the risk of nephrotoxicity and ototoxicity and to ensure appropriate therapeutic levels. Better outcomes for treating patients with gram-negative bacteremia are noted if peak levels of gentamicin and tobramycin exceed 5 μg/mL and peak amikacin concentrations exceed 20 μg/mL. Avoiding elevated aminoglycoside levels may result in decreased ototoxic and nephrotoxic effects. Serial audiometric testing to assess ototoxicity should be considered for those patients receiving long-term administration of aminoglycosides and vancomycin. Some practitioners also measure vancomycin troughs to assist their choice of dosage interval and drug amount, and appropriate levels may reduce the incidence of ototoxicity. The serum bactericidal test has been used to predict clinical cure for patients with osteomyelitis and gram-negative bacillary bacteremia. Peak serum bactericidal titers of ≥1:8 are recommended to treat bacterial endocarditis but do not predict the clinical outcome for these patients. Titers greater than or equal to 1:16 have been suggested for chronic osteomyelitis therapy.

Outpatient Parenteral Antibiotic Therapy

Outpatient parenteral antibiotic therapy is designed to either avoid hospitalization or to continue treatment initiated in the hospital and to provide therapy that is therapeutically equivalent to the inpatient setting, while enhancing the patient's quality of life and achieving significant cost savings. The decision to initiate outpatient parenteral antibiotic therapy is influenced by the following factors: availability of an adequate oral treatment; the patient's clinical status and acceptance of this form of treatment; the home environment and support systems; the potential for treatment plan compliance; the availability of competent, professional follow-up; and the reimbursement status. Outpatient parenteral antibiotic therapy has been a safe and effective form of treatment for patients with a wide array of infectious diseases, such as pneumonia, complicated urinary tract infections, pelvic inflammatory disease, endocarditis, Lyme disease, visceral abscesses, and, most commonly, skin infections and osteomyelitis. Antibiotics such as ceftriaxone, vancomycin, daptomycin, ertapenem, and aminoglycosides lend themselves to outpatient parenteral antibiotic therapy because these compounds can be administered infrequently. Some of these agents (eg, ertapenem) can treat polymicrobic infections, thus avoiding administration of multiple agents, whereas others (eg, vancomycin, daptomycin) manage infections caused by drug-resistant pathogens. Those patients who are to receive an aminoglycoside should be informed of the risks of developing hearing impairment and vestibular toxicity and advised to immediately report the development of dizziness and reduced hearing. Consideration should be given to performing serial measurements of serum creatinine and aminoglycoside concentrations, as well as serial audiograms, particularly for patients with renal insufficiency. In addition to antibiotic-related adverse events, outpatient intravenous antibiotic infusion poses the risk of access-related complications.

Switch (Step-Down) Therapy

The availability of numerous safe and effective oral antimicrobials (cephalosporins, penicillins, sulfonamides, tetracyclines, macrolides, azalides, fluoroquinolones, and, more recently, ketolides and oxazolidinones) that are well absorbed and can be administered infrequently provides the opportunity for switch or step-down therapy. This approach, available to the patient who has stabilized and appears to be "turning the corner," as manifested by resolution of fever with improved appetite and strength, has been successfully used to treat patients with the most common community-acquired infections necessitating hospitalization and parenteral therapy, namely pneumonia, exacerbation of chronic bronchitis, pyelonephritis, and cellulitis. Switch therapy frees the patient from the inconvenience, discomfort, and risks of intravenous access, results in considerable cost savings, and permits earlier hospital discharge. Switch therapy requires patient compliance with the medication and adequate intestinal absorption of the antimicrobial.

ANTIBACTERIAL PROPHYLAXIS

Appropriately administered antibiotic prophylaxis is the standard of care for patients who undergo selective surgical procedures. The ideal prescribed agent should cause minimal untoward events, should not select for virulent organisms, achieves adequate local tissue levels, is relatively inexpensive, demonstrates inhibitory activity for the bacteria anticipated to cause postoperative infection, and should be infused (usually 30–60 minutes before the surgery begins) so that therapeutic concentrations are present prior to the initial operative incision (see Chapter 112, Surgical Prophylaxis).

In addition to their indication for the prevention of postoperative infections, antibacterial agents have been effective for the prevention (primary/secondary) of a number of nonsurgical disorders, including rheumatic fever, syphilis, travelers' diarrhea, tuberculosis, invasive meningococcal disease, pertussis, diphtheria, plague, and recurrent cystitis in women. Although no definite studies have confirmed that antibiotic prophylaxis provides protection against the development of endocarditis during bacteremia-producing procedures, it is currently recommended that patients with moderate- to high-risk cardiac conditions receive antibiotic prophylaxis when subjected to selective dental, respiratory tract, gastrointestinal tract, and genitourinary tract bacteremia-producing procedures (see Chapter 111, Nonsurgical Antimicrobial Prophylaxis).

Antimicrobial Failure

When a patient is not responding to antimicrobial therapy, there is a temptation to administer an alternative compound with an extended spectrum of activity. This approach is often valid, particularly for the seriously ill patient. It is essential, however, for the clinician to establish an accurate diagnosis, because noninfectious disorders often masquerade as infection. For example, hypersensitivity to an insect bite, acute gout, a fixed drug reaction, Lyme disease, necrotizing fasciitis, and anaerobic myonecrosis can initially resemble traditional bacterial cellulitis; Charcot joint in the diabetic simulates osteomyelitis; pulmonary infarction, lung cancer, adult respiratory distress syndrome, aspiration of gastric contents, drug-induced pneumonitis, and congestive heart failure can imitate an infectious pneumonia; and vasculitis can resemble endocarditis. There should be consideration given to those factors that have the potential to impede successful antibiotic treatment (obstruction, necrotic tissue, undrained abscess, or an infected prosthetic device), the possibility of a polymicrobic infection, the development of drug resistance or a superinfection, or infection in a "privileged site," such as meningitis, endocarditis, or chronic bacterial prostatitis, disorders that require antimicrobials with unique penetration properties.

The clinician should also consider drug compliance and adequacy of drug dosage and recognize that selective infections, such as bacterial endocarditis, bacterial meningitis, and life-threatening infections in granulocytopenic hosts, require a bactericidal antibiotic.

An additional factor that can impact antibiotic treatment for patients is the recognition that numerous patients self-prescribe antibiotics prior to their first encounter with physicians. This practice can alter the anticipated microbiological cause, the manifestations of the infection, and the clinical response of the infection.

In addition to antibiotics, survival of seriously ill, infected patients often requires early institution of adjunctive treatments. Therapies that merit consideration include vigorous fluid administration (goal-directed therapy), cardiovascular support with a vasopressor or an inotropic agent, oxygen delivery via lung-protective ventilation, continuous renal replacement therapy, administration of dexamethasone specifically for the patient with pneumococcal or tuberculous meningitis, and infusion of activated protein C for those adult patients, without a likelihood of bleeding, who have sepsis and an Acute Physiology and Chronic Health Enquiry (APACHE II) score >25.

Inappropriate Administration

There are no convincing scientific data to support the administration of antibiotics to otherwise healthy patients who experience rhinitis and nonbacterial pharyngitis, laryngitis, acute bronchitis, or acute sinusitis. These infections are predominantly self-limited viral disorders. Antibiotic administration to these patients will serve only to add to health care–related costs, promote the spread of antibiotic-resistant organisms, and place patients at risk of adverse drug reactions. Additional disorders for which antibiotics are not indicated include witnessed aspiration pneumonia, colonized noninfected wounds, and asymptomatic bacteriuria, unless the latter condition is identified in a pregnant woman.

Antibiotic therapy is not appropriate treatment for the patient with persistent unexplained fever. These patients merit a thorough evaluation, consisting of a comprehensive medical history and physical examination, complemented with the judicious application of laboratory and radiographic studies. Empiric administration of an antibiotic to the patient with protracted fever may serve to obscure and/or delay the correct diagnosis and result in untoward drug-induced events.

When making decisions regarding the administration of antibiotics, clinicians should be guided by accurate susceptibility data for those clinically significant isolates recovered from appropriately collected specimens, as well as expert consultation, and evidence based medicine as published in the practice guidelines of the Infectious Diseases Society of America.

SUGGESTED READING

Clay KD, Hanson JS, Pope SD, et al. Brief communication: severe hepatotoxicity of telithromycin: three case reports and literature review. *Ann Intern Med*. 2006;144:415–420.

Craig WA. Pharmacokinetic/pharmacodynamic parameters: rationale for antibacterial dosing of mice and men. *Clin Infect Dis*. 1998;26:1–12.

Estes L. Review of pharmacokinetics and pharmacodynamics of antibacterial agents. *Mayo Clin Proc*. 1998;78:1114–1122.

Noskin GA. Tigecycline: a new glycylcycline for treatment of serious infections. *Clin Infect Dis*. 2005;41:S303–S314.

Park-Wyllie LY, Juurlink DN, Kopp A, et al. Outpatient gatifloxacin therapy and dysglycemia in older adults. *N Engl J Med*. 2006;354:1413–1415.

Romano A, Viola M, Guéant-Rodriguez RM, et al. Imipenem in patients with immediate hypersensitivity to penicillins. *N Engl J Med*. 2006;354:2835–2837.

Stein GE. Safety of newer parenteral antibiotics. *Clin Infect Dis*. 2005:41(suppl 5):S293–S302.

Trotman RL, Williamson JC, Shoemaker M, Salzer WL. Antibiotic dosing in critically ill patients receiving continuous renal replacement therapy. *Clin Infect Dis*. 2005; 41:1159–1166.

Zinner SH. The search for new antimicrobials: why we need new options. *Expert Rev Anti Infect Ther*. 2005;3:907–913.

204. Antifungal Therapy

Nathan P. Wiederhold and Thomas F. Patterson

This chapter focuses on the use of drugs that treat systemic mycoses (Table 204.1). Treatment of cutaneous fungal infections is discussed in Chapter 25, Superficial Fungal Infection of the Hair, Skin, and Nails.

AMPHOTERICIN B

Amphotericin B is a polyene antifungal synthesized by *Streptomyces nodosus*. Its chemical structure confers it with amphoteric properties that are essential for the drug's ability to form channels through the cytoplasmatic membrane. The pores formed from preferential binding of amphotericin B to ergosterol, the primary fungal cell sterol, result in an increase in membrane permeability, leading to a loss of essential elements such as potassium and other molecules that impairs fungal viability. Amphotericin B binds with less affinity to cholesterol, the primary cell sterol of mammalian cells, which are therefore less affected by amphotericin B than is the fungal target.

Amphotericin B is commercially available as a complex with sodium deoxycholate: commercial vials contain amphotericin B, 50 mg, sodium deoxycholate, 41 mg, and a sodium phosphate buffer, 25.2 mg. The clinical pharmacology of amphotericin B is characterized by extensive binding to plasma proteins (>90%) and wide distribution to the peripheral compartment with preferential accumulation in liver and spleen, with lesser amounts in kidney and lung. Intravenous administration of therapeutic doses results in peak plasma levels of 1.0 to 1.5 µg/mL falling to 0.5 to 1.0 µg/mL 24 hours later. At therapeutic doses, less than 5% of the drug each dose is excreted in the urine. The elimination of the amphotericin B is not altered in patients with renal or liver dysfunction and does not require dose adjustment in patients who are anephric or undergoing hemodialysis. Cerebrospinal fluid (CSF) levels are low, although higher concentrations occur in brain tissue. Amphotericin B also diffuses poorly into other body fluids such as saliva, amniotic fluid, aqueous humor, and vitreous humor. However, drug concentrations in inflamed pleura, peritoneum, aqueous humor,

and joint spaces are roughly two-thirds of the trough plasma concentration.

For clinical administration, amphotericin B is diluted in 5% dextrose (at a concentration of ≤0.1 mg of amphotericin B per milliliter of diluent) and infused intravenously over 2 to 4 hours at dosages of 0.5 to 1.5 mg/kg/day. The most common side effects of amphotericin B treatment are acute infusion-related reaction and nephrotoxicity. The acute infusion-related reaction consists of a syndrome of chills, fever, and tachypnea that typically occurs 30 to 45 minutes after beginning the first infusion and may last for 2 to 4 hours. Premedication with acetaminophen (650 mg given orally or rectally), hydrocortisone (25 to 50 mg given intravenously or mixed with the amphotericin B infusion solution), and diphenhydramine (50 mg given orally or rectally) can diminish the frequency and severity of these reactions. Chills may be terminated by the administration of meperidine (50 mg given intravenously). The acute symptoms associated with amphotericin B infusion can be serious. The occurrence of severe infusion reactions is considered an indications for use of lipid-associated amphotericin B preparations, which are usually significantly better tolerated (see below).

The other major side effect of amphotericin B is the development of nephrotoxicity, which occurs through a decrease in the glomerular filtration, rate as a result of a direct vasoconstrictive effect on afferent renal arterioles, reducing glomerular and renal tubular blood flow. The nephrotoxicity may be exacerbated by other nephrotoxic agents (Table 204.2). There is evidence that renal vasoconstriction is partially reversible by salt loading with 500 to 1000 mL of normal saline before each infusion. Other renal effects include potassium and bicarbonate wasting and decreased erythropoietin production. Permanent loss of renal function can occur if the drug is continued in the setting of worsening renal function. Other chronic toxicities include nausea and vomiting, anorexia, normocytic normochronic anemia (with the hematocrit rarely falling below 20% to 25%), and, rarely, thrombocytopenia, leukopenia, and peripheral vein phlebitis.

Table 204.1 Antifungal Agents: Therapeutic Options

Disease	Therapy	
	Primary	**Alternative**
Aspergillosis: Invasive	Voriconazole 6 mg/kg IV q12h for 2 doses then 4 mg/kg or 200 mg PO q12h	Liposomal formulations of AmB (see Table 204.3 for dosage) Caspofungin 70 mg IV × 1 dose, then 50 mg IV/d AmB, 1.0–1.5 mg/kg/d IV Posaconazole 800 mg/d in 2 to 4 doses Itraconazole 400 mg/d PO (oral solution preferred)
Blastomycosis	Itraconazole, 200–400 mg/d PO for 6 mo; or AmB, 0.5 mg/kg/d to a total dose of ≥1.5 g for critically ill patients	Fluconazole, 400–800 mg/d for at least 6 mo
Candidiasis		
Candidemia	Fluconazole, 400 mg/d IV ×7 d then PO for 7+ d to complete 14-d course after last positive blood culture, or anidulafungin, 200 mg IV × 1 dose then 100 mg IV/d, or caspofungin, 70 mg IV × 1 dose then 50 mg IV/d, or micafungin, 100 or 150 mg IV/d, or AmB, 0.5–0.6 mg/kg/day IV for 14-d course If neutropenic, AmB, 0.6–1.0 mg/kg/day, or anidulafungin, 200 mg IV × 1 dose then 100 mg IV/day, or caspofungin, 70 mg IV × 1 dose then 50 mg IV/day, or micafungin, 100 or 150 mg IV/day, or fluconazole, 400–800 mg/d ×7 day IV then PO (if no prior azole therapy) until neutropenia resolved	Fluconazole 800 mg/d IV for 5–8 d then PO plus AmB 0.5–0.7 mg/kg (for 5–8 d) In patients who fail to respond or deteriorate, higher dosages may be used (AmB, 0.8–1.0 mg/kg/d IV, or fluconazole, 800 mg/d PO) Avoid fluconazole in patients with recent azole exposure, or if Candida *krusei* likely
Hepatosplenic candidiasis	AmB, 0.8–1.0 mg/kg/d IV ± 5-FC, 37.5 mg/kg PO q6h, or Fluconazole, 800 mg/d IV	AmB lipid complex (ABLC), 5 mg/kg/d
Coccidiomycosis		
Nonmeningeal (AIDS and non-AIDS)	Fluconazole, 400–800 mg/d PO for 12–18 mo	Itraconazole, 200 mg BID PO × 12–18 mo, or AmB, 0.6–1.0 kg/d IV; total dose, ≥2.5 g In AIDS patients, lifetime suppressive treatment with fluconazole, 200–400 mg/d PO, or itraconazole, 200–400 mg/d PO Posaconazole, voriconazole investigational
Meningeal (AIDS and non-AIDS)	Fluconazole, 400–600 mg/d PO indefinitely	AmB IV as for nonmeningeal Posaconazole, voriconazole investigational
Cryptococcosis		
Nonmeningeal	AmB, 0.7 mg/kg/d IV ± 5-FC 25 mg/kg PO q6h until response, then fluconazole, 400 mg/d PO for 8–10 wk, or Lipid AmB 3–5 mg/kg/d IV ± 5-FC as above	Fluconazole 400–800 mg/d IV Posaconazole, voriconazole investigational

Disease	Therapy	
	Primary	Alternative
Meningeal	AmB, 0.7 mg/kg/d IV ± 5-FC, 25 mg/kg PO q6h for 2 wk, then fluconazole, 400 mg/d PO for 8–10 wk, *or* Fluconazole, 400 mg/d PO ×8–10 wk (for less severely ill patients)	Fluconazole, 400 mg/d PO ×6–10 wk, then suppressive treatment, or lipid AmB 3–5 mg/kg/d IV, ×2 wk, followed by fluconazole, 400 mg/d PO ×8–10 wk
Histoplasmosis		
Non-AIDS	Itraconazole, 200 mg/d PO for 9 mo; if life threatening, AmB, 0.7–1.0 mg/kg/d or lipid AmB 3–5 mg/kg/d IV ×14 d, followed by itraconazole, 400 mg/d × 8–10 wk if clinical response	
Disseminated AIDS	AmB, 0.7–1.0 mg/kg/d IV or lipid AmB 3–5 mg/kg/d ×14 days, followed by itraconazole, 400 mg/day ×8–10 wk, then begin suppressive treatment with itraconazole 200 mg/d PO	Itraconazole, 300 mg BID PO ×3 d, then 200 mg BID PO ×12 wk, or 400 mg/d ×12 wk, then 200 mg/d PO
Zygomycosis	Surgery plus AmB, 0.8–1.5 mg/kg/d IV or lipid AmB 5–7.5 mg/kg/d IV	Liposomal formulations of AmB (see Table 204.3 for dosage) Posaconazole, 200 mg PO 4× daily followed by 400 mg PO 2× daily
Sporotrichosis		
Lymphocutaneous	Itraconazole, 200 mg/d PO ×6 mo	Potassium iodide solution (SSKI), 10–15 gtt TID ×6–12 wk
Extracutaneous	AmB, 1.5–3.0 g total course (may require adjunctive intraarticular therapy or surgery)	Itraconazole, 200–300 mg PO BID ×6 mo, then 200 mg PO BID long term

Note: Dosages and duration of therapy given are approximations based on clinical response and underlying condition in the host. Individual responses and therapeutic requirements may vary.
Abbreviations: AmB = amphotericin B; 5-FC = flucytosine; AIDS = acquired immunodeficiency syndrome.

Amphotericin B is active against most fungal pathogens that cause systemic or deep-seated infections. Despite its significant dose-limiting toxicities, amphotericin B remains an option for many mycoses because of its broad spectrum of activity and fungicidal activity, although the availability of better tolerated and effective alternative agents (including lipid formulations of amphotericin B, the extended-spectrum azoles, or the echinocandins) have limited indications for the use of amphotericin B deoxycholate. Recommendations for appropriate dosages of amphotericin B and for duration of therapy remain poorly defined for most infections. In the past, total doses of 1 to 2 g for serious infections (which is approximately 15 to 30 mg/kg over a 6-week period) were usually recommended. However, the dosage and duration of amphotericin B depend largely on response of infection to therapy and resolution of underlying host immunodeficiency (eg, resolution of neutropenia). Increasingly, a therapeutic approach that includes aggressive "induction" courses of amphotericin B followed by "consolidation" therapy with an azole, which can be administered orally, is used. This strategy has been evaluated most thoroughly in cryptococcal meningitis, but clinical reports have documented success of sequential amphotericin B to azole therapy in candidemia (using oral fluconazole), invasive aspergillosis (with an oral anti-*Aspergillus* azole such as voriconazole or itraconazole), and endemic fungi (coccidioidomycosis and histoplasmosis with fluconazole and itraconazole, respectively). Generally, a 2-week (or until signs of infection have resolved or significantly improved) course of amphotericin B can be followed by azole therapy.

Local instillation is rarely indicated due to the advances in alternative agents. Historically, itrathecal amphotericin B was a mainstay of therapy for coccidioidal meningitis, but the use of intrathecal amphotericin B is associated

Table 204.2 Antifungal Drug–Drug Interaction

Antifungal Agent	Other Drug	Effect
Amphotericin B/amphotericin B lipid formulations	Antineoplastic drugs	↑ Nephrotoxicity risk
	Foscarnet	↑ Nephrotoxicity risk
	Corticosteroids and adrenocorticotropic hormone	May potentiate hypokalemia
	Digitalis	↑ Toxicity of Digitalis if K$^+$ ↓
	Flucytosine	Possible ↑ toxicity of flucytosine due to decreased clearance
	Nephrotoxic drugs: aminoglycosides, cidofovir, cyclosporin, foscarnet, pentamidine	↑ Nephrotoxicity of Amphotericin

Azoles

FLU	ITZ	VOR	POS		
	+			Isoniazid	Decreased itraconazole concentrations
+	+	+	+	Rifampin/rifabutin	↑ Levels of rifampin/rifabutin, ↓ serum levels of FLU, ITZ, VOR, POS
+				Theophyllines	↑ Levels of theophylline with toxicity
+	+	+	+	Phenytoin	↑ Levels of phenytoin, ↓ serum levels of FLU, ITZ, VOR, POS
+				Zidovudine	↓ Levels of zidovudine
	+			Didanosine	↓ Absorption of ITZ
	+			Indinavir	↑ Levels of indinavir
	+	+		Nelfinavir	↑ Levels of nelfinavir, ↑ serum levels of ITZ, VOR
	+	+		Saquinavir	↑ Levels of saquinavir, ↑ serum levels of ITZ, VOR
+	+	+	+	Cyclosporin, tacrolimus, sirolimus	↑ Levels of cyclosporin, tacrolimus, sirolimus
+	+	+	+	Antihistamines (e.g., terfenadine, astemizole)	↑ Levels of terfenadine (cardiac arrhythmias)
	+			Proton pump inhibitors	↑ Absorption of ITZ
	+		+	H$_2$-blockers, antacids, sucralfate	↑ Absorption of ITZ, POS
+	+	+	+	Cisapride	↑ Levels of cisapride (arrhythmias, ↑ QT interval)
+	+	+	+	Midazolam/triazolam	↑ Levels of benzodiazepines
+	+	+	+	Amytriptyline	↑ Levels of amytriptyline
	+			Methadone	↑ Levels of methadone
	+	+		Carbamazepine	↓ Levels of ITZ, VOR

Antifungal Agent				Other Drug	Effect
+	+	+	+	Oral anticoagulants	↑ Levels of anticoagulants
+	+	+		Oral hypoglycemics	↑ Levels of oral hypoglycemics
+	+	+	+	Lovastatin/simvastatin	↑ Levels of statins; rhabdomyolysis reported
Echinocandins					
Anidulafungin					
Caspofungin				Cyclosporine	↑ Levels of caspofungin
				Tacrolimus	↓ Levels of tacrolimus
				Rifamin, phenytoin, efavirenz, nevirapine	↓ Levels of caspofungin
Micafungin				Nifedipine	↑ Levels of nifedipine
				Sirolimus	↑ Levels of sirolimus

Data from Gilbert DN, Moellering RC Jr, Sande MA, eds. *The Sanford Guide to Antimicrobial Therapy.* 36th ed. Hyde Park, VT: Antimicrobial Therapy; 2006, and Kwon-Chung KJ, Bennett JE. *Medical Mycology.* Philadelphia, PA: Lea & Febiger; 1992.
Abbreviations: FLU = fluconazole; ITZ = itraconzole; VOR = voriconazole; POS = posaconzole

with substantial toxicity; consequently, that approach is now usually reserved for patients in whom systemic therapy, including high dosages of an azole, fails. In other cases, local instillation of amphotericin B into the bladder via a Foley catheter has been used for urinary tract candidiasis, but systemic azole therapy, usually with fluconazole, is well tolerated and effective for that indication.

New lipid preparations of amphotericin B have been developed in an attempt to reduce the nephrotoxicity of the conventional form of amphotericin B deoxycholate. The administration of such liposomal forms modifies the pharmacologic and toxicologic properties of amphotericin B. Characteristics of the commercially available lipid amphotericin B preparations, amphotericin B lipid complex (ABLC, Abelcet), amphotericin B colloidal dispersion (ABCD, Amphotec), and liposomal amphotericin B (L-AMB, AmBisome) are shown in Table 204.3. Serum levels of L-AMB are higher than those achieved with standard amphotericin B, but serum levels of ABLC and ABCD are similar to those of amphotericin B deoxycholate. The advantage of the administration of amphotericin B in lipid complexes or in liposomes is the reduced rate of nephrotoxicity, allowing the delivery of larger amounts of the drug. Although few direct comparisons of the preparations have been performed, the fewest infusion reactions appear to occur with L-AMB with slightly more reactions, including chills and fevers, associated with ABLC. The highest incidence of infusion-related toxicities, including hypoxia, have been reported with ABCD.

The lipid amphotericin B formulations have shown efficacy in many indications, including their use as salvage therapy for patients who fail amphotericin B deoxycholate or who are intolerant to it. In addition, L-AMB was shown to have fewer adverse events and to reduce proved emergent fungal infections when used as empiric therapy for persistent fever in febrile neutropenic patients, although no change in overall outcome was noted. However, despite the improved therapeutic index of these amphotericin B formulations as compared with amphotericin B deoxycholate, they have not been shown superior in efficacy. The use of these preparations in patients with severe fungal infection who have baseline renal insufficiency or who are at very high risk for nephrotoxicity (eg, allogenic bone marrow transplant recipients receiving nephrotoxic medications) is justified. In addition, in patients who have infections that respond poorly to amphotericin B, including infections caused by Zygomycetes, *Fusarium,* and other invasive molds such as *Aspergillus,* it is possible that high doses of lipid formulations of amphotericin B will improve outcome. Although increases in the doses of lipid formulations are also associated with increased toxicity, their increased therapeutic index has largely resulted in replacement of amphotericin B deoxycholate for invasive fungal infections.

Table 204.3 Amphotericin B Lipid Formulations

Amphotericin B Lipid Formulations	Structure	Indications	Dosages
Amphotericin B lipid complex (ABLC) (Abelcet)	Ribbonlike structures of a bilayered membrane formed by combining a 7:3 mixture of dimyristoyl-phosphatidylcholine and dimyristoylphosphatidylglycerol with amphotericin B (drug/lipid ratio of 1:1)	Invasive fungal infections in patients refractory or intolerant to amphotericin B deoxycholate	5 mg/kg/d as single infusion
Amphotericin B cholesteryl sulfate complex colloidal dispersion (ABCD), (Amphotec)	Disklike structures of cholesterol sulfate complexed with amphotericin B in equimolar concentration	Treatment of patients who either failed or are intolerant to amphotericin B deoxycholate; increased toxicity noted	3–4 mg/kg/d (up to 6 mg/kg/d)
Liposomal amphotericin B (Ambisome)	Small unilamellar liposomes about 55–75 nm in diameter made up of a bilayer membrane of hydrogenated soy phosphatidylcholine and distearoylphosphatidylglycerol stabilized by cholesterol and combined with amphotericin B in a 2:0.8:1:0.4 ratio	Empirical treatment for presumed fungal infection in febrile neutropenic patients; treatment of patients with *Aspergillus* species, *Candida* species, and/or *Cryptococcus* species infection refractory to amphotericin B deoxycholate, or in patients in whom renal impairment or toxicity precludes the use of amphotericin B deoxycholate	3–5 mg/kg/d as single infusion

Data from Hiemenz JW, Walsh TJ. Lipid formulations of amphotericin B: recent progress and future directions. *Clin Infect Dis*. 1996;22(suppl 2):5133.

AZOLES

Similar to the polyenes, azole antifungal agents also target ergosterol albeit through a alternative mechanism of action. By binding to lanosterol 14-α-demethylase, these agents inhibit ergosterol biosysnthesis resulting in disruption of the fungal cell membrane. The primary members of this class used in the treatment of invasive mycosis are fluconazole, itraconazole, voriconazole, and posaconazole.

Fluconazole is commercially available in both an oral and an intravenous preparation. Following oral administration, fluconazole is nearly completely absorbed with a bioavailability >90% and is widely distributed into the tissues, including the CSF (concentrations in CSF and urine concentrations are 70% to 90% those found in the plasma). The half-life of fluconazole is approximately 30 hours, and the majority of this primary route of elimination is as unchanged drug in the urine. Doses may need to be adjusted in renal failure.

Itraconazole is available in both oral (capsule and solution) and intravenous formulations. Unlike fluconazole, itraconazole capsules have low and erratic bioavailability due to poor water solubility, which may be influenced by

gastric pH. An oral solution and intravenous itraconazole formulation are available, both of which utilize hydroxy-propyl-β-cyclodextrin as an excipient to overcome the insolubility of itraconazole in aqueous solution. The oral solution has improved the bioavailability and consistency of plasma levels of itraconazole. Due to its high lipophilicity itraconazole is extensively distributed to the tissues. Itraconazole is highly protein bound (>99%) and is extensively metabolized by cytochrome P450 3A4, with less than 1% of drug found unchanged in the urine. The half-life of itraconazole is 24 hours. Due to the extensive hepatic metabolism, the oral formulations do not require dose adjustments in renal failure. However, accumulation of the cyclodextrin component may occur following intravenous administration due to extensive elimination in the urine.

Similar to both fluconazole and itraconazole, voriconazole is also available as an oral and intravenous preparation. Following oral administration, the bioavailability of voriconazole is approximately 90%. Voriconazole undergoes extensive hepatic metabolism primarily by cytochrome P450 2C19 and, to a lesser extent, 2C9 and 3A4 isoenzymes. The bioavailability of voriconazole may be influenced by polymorphisms in 2C19, with homozygous poor metabolizers having peak plasma concentrations and overall exposures, as measured by the plasma area under the curve, 4-fold higher than those of homozygous extensive metabolizers. Compared to the other azoles, the half-life of voriconazole is relatively short, approximately 6 hours. However, at higher doses voriconazole demonstrates nonlinear kinetics in adults due to saturable metabolism and is distributed extensively to the tissues. Similar to itraconazole, the intravenous formulation contains a cyclodextrin excipient (sulfobutyl ether β-cyclodextrin), which may accumulate with decreased renal function.

Currently, posaconazole is available only as a suspension for oral administration. The bioavailability of this agent is greatly enhanced when coadministered with a high-fat meal. Posaconazole has a large volume of distribution, suggesting extensive tissue distribution, and is extensively protein bound (99%). Unlike itraconazole and voriconazole, posaconazole does not undergo phase I metabolism (mediated by cytochrome P450 enzymes) but instead is metabolized via glucuronidation (phase II metabolism). The half-life of posaconazole is 25 hours, and the majority of elimination occurs in the feces as unchanged drug.

The azole antifungals are generally well tolerated with a mild side-effect profile consisting of nausea, vomiting, headache, dizziness, rash, pruritus, and anorexia. These effects occur in fewer than 5% of patients and are often dose related. Notably, itraconazole oral solution may be associated with significant gastrointestinal adverse effects, including nausea, vomiting, and osmotic diarrhea, due to the cyclodextrin component. In addition, administration of itraconazole at doses greater than 400 mg/day can cause hypokalemia, hypertension, and pedal edema. Voriconazole has been associated with visual disturbances and cutaneous phototoxicity. Visual disturbances, which may manifest as photophobia or abnormal vision, are transient, have not resulted in long-term toxicity, and abate with continued treatment.

Each member of this class can cause hepatotoxicity (estimates of toxicity range from 1 in every 10000 to 50000 patients after a mean of 4 weeks of therapy). Typically, the liver dysfunction is characterized by asymptomatic elevation of transaminases in the range of 2 to 3 times the upper limit of normal. Mild, asymptomatic transaminase elevations can be managed without drug discontinuation and close follow-up. Symptomatic liver dys-

function, however, requires discontinuation of treatment. Enzyme elevations are reversible but may take months to normalize. However, cases of fatal hepatotoxicity have been reported with itraconazole, voriconazole, and posaconazole, although the latter appears to be associated with less hepatotoxicity due to its lack of hepatic metabolism.

Due to similarities between ergosterol and cholesterol biosynthesis, drug interaction can occur via inhibition of cytochrome P450 enzymes by azole antifungals. In addition, itraconazole, voriconazole, and, to a lesser extent, fluconazole are also substrates of cytochrome P450 enzymes. Although posaconazole does not undergo phase I metabolism, it is an inhibitor of cytochrome P450 3A4. In addition, posaconazole is a substrate for P-glycoprotein efflux. Thus, coadministration of azoles with drugs that are substrates, inhibitors, or inducers of these enzymes may result in significant drug interactions (Table 204.2). Therefore, careful consideration is required prior to the addition or removal of an azole to or from an existing drug regimen. Monitoring patients for signs and symptoms of toxicity or subtherapeutic effects, and when possible measuring concentrations of coadministered drugs, may also be necessary.

Fluconazole has been used extensively in the treatment of systemic yeast infections, including primary therapy for candidemia, particularly that caused by *Candida albicans* but also other yeasts, including *Candida tropicalis*, *Candida parapsilosis*, and *Candida glabrata*. Only *Candida krusei* is inherently resistant to fluconazole, although resistance may develop to fluconazole and other azoles in *C. glabrata*. Fluconazole is also effective in the therapy of cryptococcal infections, including meningitis, with most use for consolidation therapy after initial therapy with amphotericin B and for long-term suppressive therapy in immunosuppressed patients, including those with acquired immunodeficiency syndrome (AIDS). Fluconazole is an alternative, when appropriate, to amphotericin B in the management of *Coccidioides immitis* meningitis. In addition, fluconazole is indicated for the prophylaxis of yeast infection in patients with chemotherapy-induced neutropenia.

Itraconazole is indicated for the therapy of endemic mycoses, including histoplasmosis, blastomycosis, and sporotrichosis, usually used after amphotericin B in severely ill patients or as primary therapy in patients with less extensive infection. It may be used for sequential therapy

following initial amphotericin B in invasive aspergillosis, as primary therapy in less immunosuppressed patients with less extensive infection, and as prophylaxis in patients with chemotherapy-induced neutropenia and in allogeneic stem cell transplant recipients with graft-versus-host disease receiving corticosteroids. In addition, itraconazole is effective in cutaneous and systemic infection resulting from dematiaceous fungi, including *Exophiala* species and *Bipolaris* species.

Voriconazole has a broad spectrum of activity against *Aspergillus* species, including *Aspergillus terreus*, *Candida* species, including those resistant to fluconazole (*C. krusei*), *Scedosporium apiospermum*, and *Fusarium* species. In vitro activity has also been demonstrated against *Cryptococcus neoformans*, *Blastomyces dermatitidis*, *C. immitis*, and *Histoplasma capsulatum*. Voriconazole has become the drug of choice for the primary treatment of invasive aspergillosis and infections caused by *S. apiospermum* and *Fusarium* species. It is also indicated for invasive candidiasis and esophageal candidiasis, including fluconazole-resistant species, although cross-resistance (particularly in *C. glabrata*) can occur as it can with posaconazole and the other azoles. Voriconazole has also been shown to be effective as early or pre-emptive therapy for presumed *Aspergillus* infections.

Posaconazole has been shown to be effective for the salvage treatment of invasive aspergillosis and invasive candidiasis, although it is only licensed in Europe for the former and has a limited role in serious *Candida* infections due to the lack of an intravenous formulation. Similar to voriconazole, posaconazole has a broad spectrum of activity against a wide range of both yeast and filamentous fungi, including *Aspergillus* and *Candida* species, the dimorphic fungi *C. immitis*, *H. capsulatum*, and *B. dermatitidis*, and *C. neoformans*. However, unlike voriconazole, posaconazole also has in vitro and in vivo activity against Zygomycetes. Studies have also demonstrated the potential utility of this agent in the treatment of invasive infections caused by *Fusarium* species. Excellent efficacy of posaconazole has also been demonstrated as antifungal prophylaxis both in neutropenic patients and in allogeneic stem cell transplant recipients postengraftment with graft-versus-host disease.

ECHINOCANDINS

The echinocandins anidulafungin, caspofungin, and micafungin are large, cyclic, semisynthetic lipopeptides. Through noncompetitive inhibition of glucan synthase, these agents deplete β-1,3-glucan, a primary component of the cell wall of many pathogenic fungi, including *Aspergillus* and *Candida* species.

Due to their high molecular weight and poor bioavailability, each member of this class is available only for intravenous administration. Each echinocandin contains a hexapeptide nucleus. However, differences in the *N*-acyl side chain are responsible for variability in the physiochemical properties among these agents. Anidulafungin is insoluble in water and must be reconstituted with 20% weight/weight dehydrated alcohol prior to further dilution in 5% dextrose or physiologic saline. Anidulafungin is not metabolized but rather undergoes spontaneous chemical degradation to an open-ring peptide following intravenous administration. This echinocandin is also extensively protein bound (>99%). The majority of the plasma concentration–time profile is characterized by a half-life of approximately 26 hours, followed by a long terminal half-life (52 hours). Caspofungin does undergo phase I metabolism (hydrolysis and *N*-acetylation) as well as some spontaneous chemical degradation to an open-ring peptide. However, distribution to the tissues, not excretion or metabolism, is the primary determinant of plasma clearance. Similar to anidulafungin, a half-life between 9 and 11 hours characterizes the majority of the plasma concentration–time profile, followed by a long terminal half-life of 40 to 50 hours. Caspofungin is also extensively protein bound (97%). Micafungin does undergo limited phase I metabolism. However, the primary route of elimination is as unchanged drug in the feces. Similar to anidulafungin and caspofungin, micafungin is also extensively protein bound (99.5%), with an elimination half-life between 13 and 15 hours.

Due to their inhibition of glucan synthase, a fungal specific target without a mammalian homolog, the echinocandins are very well tolerated with few clinically significant drug interactions. The primary adverse effects reported in clinical trials are generally mild to moderate in severity and include rash, headache, nausea, vomiting, diarrhea, and infusion-related reactions. Mild elevations in transaminases and alkaline phosphate have also been reported. None of the members of this class act as inhibitors or inducers of cytochrome P450 isoenzymes, nor do they undergo extensive metabolism by these enzymes. Table 204.2 lists potential drug–drug interactions associated with the echinocandins.

Therapeutic Uses

The echinocandins have a broad spectrum of activity against *Candida*, including non-*albicans* species and isolates resistant to fluconazole and *Aspergillus* species. However, these agents lack activity against *C. neoformans*, *Fusarium* species, and Zygomycetes. Each member of this class has been shown to be effective in the treatment of candidemia, invasive candidiasis, and esophageal candidiasis. In addition, caspofungin and micafungin have also been shown to be effective in the treatment of invasive aspergillosis, including in patients with refractory infections, although only caspofungin is licensed for that indication. Caspofungin has also been shown to be effective in the setting of febrile neutropenia, whereas micafungin is efficacious as prophylaxis in patients with neutropenia.

FLUCYTOSINE

The clinical usefulness of flucytosine (5-FC) is limited by its narrow spectrum of activity, frequent emergence of resistance, and toxicity. Flucytosine is usually administered at a dosage of 150 mg/ kg/day in 4 divided doses, although 100 mg/kg/day in 4 divided doses may be used in combination with amphotericin B for cryptococcal meningitis. More than 90% of the drug is excreted unchanged in the urine, and patients with renal insufficiency require dosage reduction. As an approximation, the total daily dose should be reduced to 75 mg/kg with a creatinine clearance of 26 to 50 mL/min and to 37 mg/kg when the creatinine clearance is 13 to 25 mL/ min. In azotemic patients, blood levels should be measured and dosage should be adjusted so that serum levels do not exceed 50 to 100 µg/mL. The drug readily diffuses to the CSF and achieves concentrations of about 74% of serum. Flucytosine is usually well tolerated and results in minor and uncommon adverse effects, such as rash, diarrhea, and mild hypertransaminasemia. The presence of azotemia or the concomitant use of amphotericin B might exacerbate the toxicity, resulting in severe leukopenia, thrombocytopenia, and enterocolitis. These complications seem to occur in many, but not all, patients with blood levels exceeding 100 µg/mL.

Flucytosine has been used extensively to treat chromomycosis. It is not used alone because of the rapid development of resistance and the availability of other less toxic agents, although it has activity in candidiasis and cryptococcosis. Importantly, 5-FC has been shown to have synergistic effects in combination with amphotericin B against most isolates of *Candida*, *Cryptococcus neoformans*, and possibly *Aspergillus*. The combination of amphotericin B and 5-FC has been proved useful in the treatment of cryptococcal meningitis in terms of more rapid sterilization of CSF and possibly in reducing rate of relapse. Flucytosine has been used with amphotericin B for invasive *Aspergillus* infections as well as in the therapy of refractory candidemia, although its benefit in these infections has not been shown in controlled trials. Flucytosine has also been used in combination with fluconazole in both cryptococcal infections and against *Candida*.

NEW THERAPIES

Investigational Azoles

New azoles are in various stages of development, including ravuconazole (BMS-207,147) and isovuconazole (BAL4815 and the oral prodrug BAL8557). Ravuconazole has been shown to have a broad spectrum of activity against *Candida* species, *C. neoformans*, *Aspergillus* species, and other opportunistic molds and yeasts. A similar broad spectrum of activity has been demonstrated for isovuconazole, including Zygomycetes.

Other Agents

The pradimicins are antifungal compounds that bind to cell wall mannoproteins in a calcium-dependent manner that causes osmotic-sensitive lysis, causing leakage of intracellular potassium. They are active against *Aspergillus* species, *Candida* species, and *C. neoformans*. Although this class of agent is not currently in active clinical development because of toxicities of the prototype compounds, they represent an important new antifungal target. Nikkomycins compounds are potent chitin-synthase inhibitors, which are necessary for cell wall synthesis. Nikkomycin Z has shown activity against *C. immitis* and *B. dermatitidis* alone and against *Candida* species, *C. neoformans*, and *Aspergillus fumigatus* in combination with azoles. Sordarins are a new class of antifungals in early development that inhibit protein synthesis through the binding to elongation factor 2. These compounds have shown to have activity against a wide range of fungi, including *Candida* species, *C. neoformans*, *Pneumocystis jirovecii* (formerly *Pneumocystis carinii*), and some filamentous fungi as well as emerging invasive fungal pathogens.

FUTURE DIRECTIONS

Despite the increasing number of antifungal agents, treatment of fungal diseases still remains unsatisfactory. In many cases, host factors such as neutropenia associated with cytotoxic chemotherapy or other causes of underlying immunosuppression play a pivotal role as important risk factors for the acquisition of fungal infections as well as for response to therapy. Future research efforts should be aimed at reducing risk of acquiring fungal infections as well as improving host defenses against these opportunistic pathogens. The use of recombinant hematopoietic growth factors, such as recombinant cytokine granulocyte–colony-stimulating factor and granulocyte macrophage–colony-stimulating factor has been demonstrated to shorten the duration of neutropenia in patients undergoing cyototoxic chemotherapy. These growth factors may be useful in reducing risk for opportunistic mycoses as well as improving host responses in these infections.

Another approach has been the development of monoclonal antibodies against the fungal pathogen. Efungumab is a monoclonal antibody fragment against a conserved heat shock protein 90 (Hsp90) that has activity against *Candida*, *Aspergillus*, and *Cryptococcosis* that was synergistic with liposomal amphotericin B in candidemia. Combination therapy, particularly with antifungal agents and/or biologicals that target distinct fungal targets, may be a means for improving overall outcomes in these difficult-to-treat infections. Future research efforts are essential in improving clinical responses of antifungal agents in the therapy of systemic mycoses in severely immunosuppressed hosts.

SUGGESTED READING

Dodds ES, et al. Pharmacology of systemic antifungal agents. *Clin Infect Dis*. 2006; 43(suppl 1):S28.

Gallis HA, Drew RH, Pickard WW. Amphotericin B: 30 years of clinical experience. *Rev Infect Dis*. 1990;12:308–329.

Gilbert DN, Moellering RC Jr, Eliopoulos GM, Sande MA, eds. *The Sanford Guide to Antimicrobial Therapy*. 37th ed. Sperryville, VA: Antimicrobial Therapy; 2007.

Groll AH, Piscitelli SC, Walsh TJ. Clinical pharmacology of systemic antifungal agents: a comprehensive review of agents in clinical use, current investigational compounds, and putative targets for antifungal drug development. *Adv Pharmacol*. 1998;44:343–500.

Hiemenz JW, Walsh TJ. Lipid formulations of amphotericin B: recent progress and future directions. *Clin Infect Dis*. 1996;22(suppl 2): S133–S144.

Kauffman CA. Clinical efficacy of new antifungal agents. *Curr Opin Microbiol*. 2006;9:483–488.

Ostrosky-Zeichner L, Marr KA, Rex JH, Cohen SH. Amphotericin B: time for a new "gold standard." *Clin Infect Dis*. 2003;37:415-425.

Pappas PG, Rex JH, Sobel JD, et al. Guidelines for treatment of candidiasis. *Clin Infect Dis*. 2004;38:161–189.

Patterson TF. Advances and challenges in the management of invasive mycoses. *Lancet*. 2005;366:1013–1025.

Wiederhold NP, Lewis RE. The echinocandin antifungals: an overview of the pharmacology, spectrum and clinical efficacy. *Exp Opin Investig Drugs*. 2003;12:1313–1333.

205. Antiviral Therapy

Frank L. Tomaka and Roger J. Pomerantz

Successful antiviral therapy continues to be one of the most difficult challenges facing the physician today. The reasons stem from some intrinsic characteristics of the major human viral pathogens. Because all viruses parasitize host cell enzymes and structures to varying degrees, designing or discovering drugs that specifically target the virus without toxicity is difficult. Additionally, many viruses establish a latent infection in the host, during which they are essentially quiescent. Elimination of such latent viruses from the host has so far remained an elusive goal. Some of the most serious viral infections today stem from the reactivation of latent viruses during periods of impaired cell-mediated immunity.

Most of the currently available antiviral agents target the virus by exploiting differences in viral and host replication processes. Many viruses have their own specific DNA polymerases, which are more susceptible to inhibition by specific drugs than the cellular DNA replication enzymes. Thus many antiviral agents are nucleoside analogs. In addition, some of these compounds accumulate preferentially in virus-infected cells or are activated by virus-encoded enzymes, increasing their specificity. Nevertheless, unlike many antibacterial agents, most antiviral agents remain far from being "magic bullets" and can have considerable dose-related toxicities.

This chapter describes the Food and Drug Administration (FDA)-approved antiviral drugs, their primary uses, their pharmacokinetics and potential interactions, and the major toxicities associated with their administration. Since 2001, there have been dramatic changes in the approach to the therapy of human immunodeficiency virus type 1 (HIV-1). These changes and the available antiretroviral drugs are discussed in Chapter 97, HIV-1 Infection: Antiretroviral Therapy. There have also been additions to the armamentarium against other viruses and some new uses discovered for old drugs. New viral diseases and syndromes continue to emerge and promise to remain a major challenge to all practicing physicians, emphasizing the need for continued research aimed at developing new and effective antiviral agents.

ACYCLOVIR

Acyclovir (9-[2-hydroxy-ethoxy)methyl] guanine sodium), a guanine derivative, has in vitro activity against herpes simplex virus (HSV) types 1 and 2, varicella-zoster virus (VZV), Epstein–Barr virus (EBV), and cytomegalovirus (CMV), but it is used primarily in HSV and VZV infections. Acyclovir is preferentially taken up by HSV-infected cells and is phosphorylated by HSV thymidine kinase, which is necessary for conversion to the active triphosphate form. It inhibits viral DNA polymerase and causes DNA chain termination when incorporated into replicating DNA.

Acyclovir may be used in primary episodes of genital herpes to reduce the time of viral shedding and time to healing at a dose of 200 mg orally 5 times per day for 10 days. Acyclovir can be used as chronic suppressive therapy to decrease the incidence of recurrent genital herpes at 400 mg orally twice daily. Therapy should be evaluated periodically to reassess the need for chronic suppression. In some patients, pre-emptive therapy with 200 mg 5 times a day for 5 days at the first sign of a recurrence is enough to prevent its development. An ointment is available for primary herpes genitalis, but its impact on the natural course of the infection is marginal. Many physicians use acyclovir for the treatment of herpes labialis in a fashion similar to the treatment of genital herpes.

Acyclovir reduces mortality in HSV encephalitis and should be used at high dosages (10 mg/kg intravenously [IV] every 8 hours). Severe mucosal and cutaneous infections in immunocompromised patients may require IV therapy (5 mg/kg every 8 hours). HIV-1–infected patients often require oral suppression to prevent recurrences. Refractoriness to therapy in such patients may indicate the development of acyclovir resistance.

Acyclovir is also active against VZV, but treatment of VZV infections requires higher dosages than treatment of uncomplicated HSV infections. Acyclovir, 800 mg 5 times daily for 7–10 days, should be used in immunocompromised patients with herpes zoster (shingles) to prevent dissemination and in an attempt to shorten the time to healing. Such treatment does not convincingly alter the subsequent development of postherpetic neuralgia, however. Ophthalmic zoster, involving the first branch of the trigeminal nerve, warrants evaluation by an ophthalmologist and immediate therapy, which may be given orally. VZV has also been associated with the syndrome of acute retinal necrosis, which should be treated as a medical emergency.

Acyclovir is effective in the treatment of primary varicella or chickenpox, shortening the duration and severity of illness when begun within 24 hours after the onset of rash. Whether such treatment of children affects long-term immunity or the subsequent incidence of zoster remains to be demonstrated. Chickenpox in pregnant women may be life threatening, particularly when varicella pneumonia develops. It is our practice to treat all adults with clinical varicella pneumonia with IV acyclovir. Acyclovir treatment of neonates with VZV or HSV infection is also indicated.

Oral acyclovir, 400 mg 5 times a day, or IV therapy is effective in preventing mucocutaneous HSV infections in both solid organ and bone marrow transplant patients. It may be given longer term (6 months) to decrease the incidence of VZV infections in bone marrow transplant recipients.

Acyclovir may be of some benefit in EBV-induced lymphoproliferative disease in immunocompromised patients, but it is not clinically useful in EBV disease such as mononucleosis. Incidentally, acyclovir is of no utility in the treatment of chronic fatigue immune dysfunction syndrome (CFIDS) because this syndrome has no causal association with EBV infection. Acyclovir is active and has been clinically useful against *Herpesvirus simiae*, or B virus, an endemic herpesvirus of certain primate species, which, when transmitted to humans has resulted in severe neurologic disease and death.

Pharmacokinetics

Acyclovir has good tissue distribution. It is excreted renally. The serum half-life is 2.5 to 3 hours. Dose adjustment is necessary in patients with impaired renal function.

Major Toxicities

Central nervous system (CNS) effects range from confusion to seizures and coma, especially in the settings of renal insufficiency, underlying altered mental status, and old age. Renal failure may occur from precipitation in the renal tubules. When administering high IV doses, it is important to ensure adequate hydration of the patient. Acyclovir is potentially teratogenic, but inadvertent or therapeutic administration during pregnancy has occurred without obvious adverse effects.

ADEFOVIR

Adefovir dipivoxil (9-[2-[bis[(pivaloyloxy) methoxy]ethyl]adenine]) is a nucleotide analog that inhibits reverse transcriptase. It is indicated for the treatment of chronic hepatitis B infection with active viral replication and either elevated serum aminotransferases (alanine aminotransferase [ALT] or aspartate aminotransferase [AST]) or histologically active disease. Adefovir competitively inhibits hepatitis B virus (HBV) DNA polymerase, causing DNA chain termination. The recommended dose of adefovir is 10 mg daily. It had previously been in the advanced development stages for the treatment of HIV infection at significantly higher doses. The development for this indication was discontinued due to renal toxicity.

Pharmacokinetics

Following oral intake, adefovir dipivoxil is readily converted to adefovir. It is renally excreted by both glomerular filtration and tubular secretion. The dosing interval should be adjusted in patients with renal impairment.

Major Toxicities

Associated adverse events include asthenia, headache, abdominal pain, gastrointestinal (GI) upset, pruritus, lactic acidosis, hepatomegaly with steatosis, and nephrotoxicity with prolonged use. An exacerbation of hepatitis can occur when treatment is discontinued.

Drug Interactions

Adefovir may potentiate or be potentiated by drugs that decrease renal function or compete for active tubular secretion.

AMANTADINE

Amantadine hydrochloride (1-adamantanamine hydrochloride) is used to treat Parkinson's disease and as an antiviral agent that prevents uncoating of influenza A virus after host cell entry. It is indicated for the prophylaxis of unimmunized high-risk patients in the presence of a documented outbreak of influenza A. It is also useful in those high-risk patients who have had an anaphylactic reaction to egg proteins or prior influenza vaccination. Amantadine does not impair antibody response and so may be used concurrently with the influenza vaccine to provide protection until the development of immunity. Treatment of influenza A with amantadine may be useful if instituted early in disease (≤48 hours after onset). Dosage is 200 mg/day, which may be given as two 100-mg doses. Prophylaxis should be given for at least 10 days after exposure. It may be used for 90 days when the vaccine is contraindicated. Drug-resistant strains develop rapidly and may limit its usage in children, who shed virus for prolonged periods of time.

Pharmacokinetics, Major Toxicities, and Drug Interactions

Amantadine is excreted renally. Its more frequent toxicities are related to the central nervous system (CNS): dizziness, insomnia, confusion, and seizures. Anticholinergic drugs and amantadine used concurrently may lead to unacceptable atropinelike effects. Hydrochlorothiazide and triamterene used with amantadine have led to increased amantadine levels.

CIDOFOVIR

Cidofovir is an acyclic nucleoside derivative with antiviral activity. Cidofovir was designed to minimize the resistance that develops in response to nucleoside analogs that require phosphorylation by viral enzymes, such as acyclovir and ganciclovir. Although cidofovir must be diphosphorylated to become active, it does not require phosphorylation by viral kinases. Rather, cidofovir is activated by cellular enzymes. Cidofovir is more active against herpesvirus DNA polymerases than cellular DNA polymerases and thus has selective antiviral activity.

Cidofovir is primarily used for the treatment of CMV retinitis in acquired immunodeficiency syndrome (AIDS) patients and has been FDA approved for this indication in adults. Its use in other CMV infections and in other immunocompromised patients has not been adequately evaluated. Cidofovir has been effective in delaying the progression of CMV retinitis in AIDS patients, including those who have failed ganciclovir or foscarnet therapy. Ganciclovir-resistant strains of CMV, which carry mutations in the UL97 phosphokinase gene, generally remain susceptible to cidofovir. However, other ganciclovir-resistant mutants, especially those carrying mutations in the DNA polymerase gene may be cross-resistant to cidofovir. CMV strains resistant to ganciclovir, foscarnet, and cidofovir have also been described.

Intravenous cidofovir is administered with probenecid to prevent rapid secretion of the drug by the renal tubules. Creatinine clearance should be estimated by calculation or directly measured before initiating therapy with cidofovir. The nephrotoxic potential of cidofovir is such that a creatinine clearance less than 55 mL/ min, a serum creatinine greater than 1.5 mg/dL, or 2+ proteinuria is a contraindication to its use. Induction therapy with cidofovir is initiated at a dosage of 5 mg/kg once weekly for 2 weeks, followed by the same dose once every 2 weeks as maintenance therapy. Intravenous saline prehydration with 1 L of normal saline immediately before cidofovir infusion is mandatory to prevent nephrotoxicity. If possible, an additional liter of saline should be administered with and after cidofovir over a 1- to 3-hour period. In addition, great care should be taken to monitoring renal function with both urine and serum measurements, and the importance of taking the probenecid should be emphasized. Probenecid is administered as follows: 2 g 3 hours before infusion and 1 g at 2 and 8 hours after infusion.

Pharmacokinetics

Approximately 70% of cidofovir is eliminated unchanged by the kidneys. Its plasma half-life is approximately 2.5 hours, but it has a long-lasting antiviral effect. The latter is the result of the intracellular persistence of its active phosphorylated metabolite.

Major Toxicities

As described, the major toxicity of cidofovir is its nephrotoxicity. Neutropenia has occurred in approximately 20% of cidofovir recipients in clinical trials.

Drug Interactions

The most important drug interactions are those leading to additional nephrotoxicity. Additive or synergistic nephrotoxic effects with other drugs known to result in nephrotoxicity, such as aminoglycosides or amphotericin B, have not been studied. In addition, the potential for probenecid effects on the metabolism and disposition of other drugs must be considered.

ENTECAVIR

Entecavir (2-amino-1,9-dihydro-9-[hydroxy-3-(hydroxymethyl)-2-methylenecyclopentyl]-6H-purin-6-one, monohydrate) is a nucleoside analog that works by inhibiting HBV polymerase. It is indicated for the treatment of chronic hepatitis B infection in adults with evidence of active viral replication and either persistently elevated serum aminotransferases (ALT or AST) or histologically active disease. For the treatment of chronic hepatitis B infection in adults and adolescents (16 years old or older) who are nucleoside treatment naïve, the dosing is 0.5 mg daily. For patients with hepatitis B viremia also being treated with lamivudine or who have lamivudine resistance, the dose is 1 mg daily. Dose adjustment is necessary for patients with decreased renal function.

Pharmacokinetics

Entecavir has a bioavailability of 100% following oral administration when the patient is fasting. It is predominantly eliminated by the kidney predominately as unchanged drug. It undergoes both glomerular filtration and tubular secretion.

Major Toxicities

Commonly reported side effects include headaches, fatigue, dizziness, and (GI) upset. Severe acute exacerbations of hepatitis have occurred when treatment has been discontinued.

Drug Interactions/Precautions

Entecavir may potentiate or be potentiated by drugs that decrease renal function or compete for active tubular secretion.

FAMCICLOVIR

Famciclovir, a diacetyl 6-deoxy analog of penciclovir (9-[4-hydroxy-3-hydroxymethylbut-1-yl] guanine), is a nucleoside analog that has a spectrum of activity similar to that of acyclovir. Famciclovir is an inactive prodrug of penciclovir. After oral administration, famciclovir is rapidly metabolized to active penciclovir, which is phosphorylated by viral thymidine kinase and has a mechanism of action similar to acyclovir. Famciclovir is more bioavailable than acyclovir and has a prolonged intracellular half-life, which permits thrice-daily dosing. Famciclovir is approved for treatment of herpes zoster (500 mg 3 times daily for 7 days) and is similar to acyclovir in ameliorating the course of the acute attack. It is also claimed, on the basis of two studies, that famciclovir shortens the duration of postherpetic neuralgia. It is also indicated for the treatment and suppression of recurrent genital HSV (treatment: 1000 mg every 12 hours for 1 day; suppression: 250 mg every 12 hours for up to 1 year) and recurrent herpes labialis in immunocompetent patients (1500 mg as a single dose). For the treatment of orolabial or genital herpes in HIV-infected patients, it is recommended that famciclovir 500 mg be given every 12 hours for 7 days.

Pharmacokinetics

Famciclovir is excreted renally. The serum half-life is 2.5 to 3 hours, but the intracellular half-life is 10 to 20 times longer. Dose adjustment is necessary in patients with reduced renal function.

Major Toxicities

In clinical trials, no major adverse effects have been reported to date. No adverse effects were observed on embryo-fetal development in animal testing. However, no adequate and well-controlled studies have been conducted in pregnant women. Testicular toxicity was observed in animal models, and decreased fertility was observed in male rats after 10 weeks of administration at 1.9 times the human dosage.

Drug Interactions

Probenecid may lead to increased famciclovir levels. Famciclovir may lead to increased digoxin levels.

FOMIVIRSEN

Fomivirsen, a novel agent active against CMV, is a prototype of an "antisense" approach to antiviral therapy. Fomivirsen has engendered much excitement as a possible forerunner of a class of agents targeted against specific molecular targets in the genome of bacterial and viral pathogens. Fomivirsen consists of a synthetic oligonucleotide with a DNA sequence complementary to the messenger RNA (mRNA) of the immediate early transcriptional unit IE2 of human CMV. Its presumed mechanism of action is to bind to and inactivate CMV messenger RNA. Interestingly, however, fomivirsen-resistant mutant strains of CMV derived in the laboratory carry mutations outside of the gene targeted by fomivirsen, leaving open the possibility that its mechanism of action may be unrelated to its ability to bind to its intended RNA target. Fomivirsen is administered by intravitreal injection. Fomivirsen injection may be considered in situations in which conventional therapy, including systemic or intravitreal ganciclovir, foscarnet, or cidofovir, has failed or is contraindicated. Induction therapy consists of 330 µg by intravitreal injection every other week for 2 doses, followed by maintenance therapy once every 4 weeks. Response is usually observed within days, with a reported median time to response of 8 days. Intravitreal injection of fomivirsen, as might be expected, does not provide any systemic anti-CMV treatment.

Pharmacokinetics

Systemic absorption after intravitreal injection is thought to be minimal. Metabolism is via exonucleases and catabolism of the resultant mononucleotides.

Major Toxicities

Transient increases in intraocular pressure and inflammation have been reported. Retinal toxicity has been noted with injection of amounts above the recommended dosage. Systemic toxicity or interactions with other drugs have not been reported.

FOSCARNET

Foscarnet (phosphonoformic acid) binds to pyrophosphate binding sites on viral DNA polymerases and reverse transcriptases. This compound does not bind to cellular DNA polymerases at virus-inhibitory concentrations. Foscarnet is active against all herpesviruses and has some direct activity in vitro against HIV-1. Foscarnet is used in AIDS patients with CMV retinitis who cannot tolerate or worsen on ganciclovir. Foscarnet is not curative but delays progression to greater than 3 months versus less than 1 month without therapy. Induction treatment is given at 60 mg/kg IV every 8 hours for 2 to 3 weeks, followed by maintenance therapy at 90 mg/kg once daily. Foscarnet is also used in resistant VZV and HSV infections in AIDS patients.

Pharmacokinetics

Foscarnet is excreted renally. Its half-life is variable and highly dependent on renal function, which is invariably impaired by foscarnet. Thus, close monitoring of renal function with dosage adjustment is mandatory in all patients.

Major Toxicities

The major toxicity of foscarnet is impairment of renal function. In addition, hypocalcemia, hypophosphatemia, hyperphosphatemia, hypomagnesemia, and hypokalemia may occur.

Drug Interactions

Foscarnet may interact with pentamidine, increasing the risk of fatal hypocalcemia and may have additive effects on anemia due to zidovudine.

GANCICLOVIR

Ganciclovir (9-(1,3-dihydroxy-2-propoxymethyl) guanine, a guanine derivative) is a major antiviral agent used against CMV. Ganciclovir is phosphorylated by viral and then cellular kinases and preferentially accumulates in CMV-infected cells. It competitively inhibits viral DNA polymerase and is incorporated into DNA, acting as a chain terminator. Ganciclovir is used primarily in AIDS-associated CMV retinitis, colitis, pneumonitis, and disseminated disease. Efficacy in AIDS is clearly established only for retinitis, in which it slows progression and is not curative. Retinitis is treated with an induction phase (5 mg/kg every 12 hours for 14 to 21 days) followed by maintenance at the same dose once a day. Rarely maintenance may also be given orally as 1000 mg 3 times daily with food. Patients who fail while receiving maintenance therapy may be "reinduced" or changed to foscarnet. Ganciclovir tablets can also be used for the prevention of CMV disease in patients with advanced HIV infection. The recommended dose for this indication is 1000 mg 3 times a day with food.

Recently, an intravitreal ganciclovir implant for the treatment of CMV retinitis has become available. Because such local therapy does not prevent the development of CMV disease elsewhere, most importantly in the contra-lateral eye (see also the section Fomivirsen), combination therapy with systemic ganciclovir has been studied. A recently completed large-scale study demonstrated that oral ganciclovir, albeit at a dosage of 4.5 g/day, prevented the development of retinitis in the unaffected eye almost as well as did IV ganciclovir. CMV retinitis is much less common since the advent of highly active antiretroviral therapy (HAART), and prophylaxis may be unneces-sary in those patients achieving immune recon-stitution. However, CMV retinitis often occurs in patients in whom antiretroviral therapy has already failed. The role of intravitreal and pro-phylactic ganciclovir in the setting of HAART and earlier antiretroviral therapy for HIV-1 will thus undoubtedly be further defined in the future.

Ganciclovir prevents CMV disease in high-risk transplant patients when given for 7 to 14 days at the same dosages as for induction therapy. The duration of maintenance therapy depends on the intensity of immunosuppres-sion and should be given for at least 100 days after the transplant in the case of bone marrow transplant patients. Treatment of established CMV pneumonia in bone marrow transplant patients is effective when combined with IV immunoglobulin.

Pharmacokinetics, Major Toxicities, and Drug Interactions

Ganciclovir is excreted renally. Dose reduc-tions based on creatinine clearance are neces-sary in patients with impaired renal function. The major toxicity of ganciclovir is hemato-logic, often causing anemia, neutropenia, and thrombocytopenia. All cytotoxic drugs that inhibit cell replication have the potential to significantly increase the marrow toxicity of ganciclovir. These include chemotherapeu-tic agents, trimethoprim–sulfamethoxaszole, dapsone, zidovudine, and other nucleoside analogs. Other adverse events associated with ganciclovir use include renal insufficiency, fever, diarrhea, anorexia, vomiting, and sweat-ing. Cyclosporin, amphotericin B, and other nephrotoxic agents should be used with caution because of the increased risk of combined neph-rotoxicity. Probenecid may lead to increased ganciclovir levels.

Ganciclovir has demonstrated teratogenic and carcinogenic effects in animal studies.

IMIQUIMOD

Imiquimod (1-(2-methylpropyl)-1H-imidazo [4,5-c]quinolin-4-amine) is a topical agent that may be used for the treatment of condyloma acuminata. It can also be used to treat actinic keratosis and superficial basal cell carcinoma. Its mode of action is unknown but it ap-pears to act as an immune response modifier. Imiquimod induces mRNA encoding cytokines, including interferon-α at the application site. Human papillomavirus (HPV) L1 mRNA and HPV DNA levels decrease significantly follow-ing treatment. It has no direct antiviral activity. Systemic absorption appears to be minimal, and local reactions appear to be the major toxicity. However, its long-term effects and safety have not been evaluated.

INTERFERONS

Interferons are naturally occurring glycopro-teins with antiviral, antitumor (antiprolif-erative), and immunomodulatory activities. They are induced by viral infection, especially double-stranded RNA viruses. Interferon-α is primarily synthesized by B lymphocytes and interferon-β by fibroblasts and other cells. Interferon-α and interferon-β are closely re-lated. Interferon-α is actually a heterogeneous family of proteins encoded by multiple simi-lar genes. Interferon-γ is produced by T lym-phocytes and is induced by mitogenic stimuli, such as antigen-presenting cells and antigen. Interferon-γ also has macrophage-activating functions and other interleukin activities, modulating the function of other lymphocytes. Recently, a form of interferon termed *interferon alfacon-1* was introduced. Interferon alfacon-1 is not found in nature, but its structure was derived by combining the sequences of various naturally occurring interferons and produced by recombinant DNA technology.

The mechanism(s) of action of interfer-ons is varied. Their antiviral effect is partly mediated by inducing cellular enzymes that lead to a shutdown of protein synthesis in virus-infected cells, as well as activating RNA degradation.

Route of Administration and Major Toxicities

Administration is subcutaneous, intramus-cular (IM), or intralesional. Major toxicities commonly observed are flulike symptoms, fe-ver (in almost all patients treated), myalgias, fatigue, and alopecia. Exacerbation of some autoimmune diseases and psoriasis with interferon has been observed. Depression has been associated with administration of some interferons. Ophthalmologic side effects such as retinal hemorrhages have been rarely reported concomitantly with interferon therapy.

Interferon-α2a

Interferon-α2a (recombinant human protein made in *Escherichia coli*) may be used in the treatment of the following conditions: (1) AIDS-associated Kaposi's sarcoma (the response correlates with extent of HIV-1 progression more than the severity of Kaposi's sarcoma) and (2) chronic hepatitis C (see the following section).

Interferon-α2b

Interferon-α2b (recombinant human protein made in *E. coli*) is used in the treatment of the following conditions:

- Condyloma acuminata: Interferon-α2a is injected intralesionally for the treatment of condyloma acuminata. Injection of 1 million units per lesion is performed with a tuberculin syringe on alternate days, 3 times a week for 3 weeks. The product literature should be consulted for other details regarding administration and dosage.
- AIDS-associated Kaposi's sarcoma: The dosage is 30 million units/m^2 3 times a week, administered IM or subcutaneously. If tolerated, treatment may be continued until resolution of tumors.
- Chronic hepatitis C: Interferon treatment decreases transaminase levels and may lead to sustained virologic response. The benefit extends beyond period of therapy. Relapse may be treated with combination ribavirin and interferon therapy. Interferon-naive patients may also be treated with combination therapy. The dosage is 3 million units subcutaneously 3 times weekly. The optimal duration of therapy in different situations remains to be defined.
- Chronic hepatitis B: A virologic response with loss of eAg (and sAg in some patients) and improved transaminases may occur. Lasting remission may also be occasionally obtained. Interferon-α2b has been administered as 5 million units daily or 10 million units 3 times a week for this indication.

Interferon-α3n

Interferon-α3n is a purified natural human leukocyte interferon. It is produced by infecting human leukocytes with Sendai virus and then purifying the induced interferon. It is used intralesionally for condyloma acuminata.

Interferon Alfacon-1

Interferon alfacon-1 is used in the treatment of chronic hepatitis C. A dose of 9 μg is administered subcutaneously 3 times a week for 24 weeks.

Peginterferon-α2a

Peginterferon-α2a is a covalent conjugate of interferon-α2a and a PEG (polyethylene glycol) moiety. Pegylation lowers the systemic clearance of interferon-α2a 100-fold, thereby increasing the mean terminal half-life after subcutaneous dosing from 5.1 hours to 80 hours. Peginterferon-α2a is indicated as monotherapy and in combination with ribavirin for the treatment of chronic hepatitis C infection in patients with compensated liver disease. Efficacy, defined by achieving sustained virologic response, is greater with the use of peginterferon-α2a compared to interferon-α2a. This has been demonstrated in both monotherapy trials and in combination therapy (with ribavirin) trials. The recommended dose for the treatment of chronic hepatitis C in monotherapy and in combination therapy with ribavirin is 180 μg subcutaneously weekly. The side-effect profile is similar to that of interferon-α2a. However, there is a higher incidence of injection site reactions with the use of peginterferon-α2a.

Peginterferon-α2b

Peginterferon-α2b is a covalent conjugate of interferon-α2b and monomethoxypolyethylene glycol (PEG). Its use is indicated for the treatment of chronic hepatitis C, as monotherapy and in combination with ribavirin in patients with compensated liver disease. Virologic response rates are superior with the use of peginterferon-α2b compared to interferon-α2b in patients with hepatitis C genotype 1. The superiority is less clear in the treatment of other hepatitis C genotypes. When used as monotherapy, the recommended dose is 1.0 μg/kg/week, subcutaneously. When used in combination with ribavirin, peginterferon-α2b is dosed 1.5 μg/kg/week. The side-effect profile is similar to that of interferon-α2b with the exception of a higher incidence of injection site reactions/inflammation with the pegylated agent.

LAMIVUDINE

Lamivudine (2R,cis)-4-amino-1-(2-hydroxymethyl-1,3-oxathiolan-5-yl)-(1H)-pyrimidin-2-one) is a pyrimidine analog most commonly used as part of combination regimens for treatment of HIV-1 infection. Lamivudine also inhibits hepatitis B DNA polymerase and may be used as treatment for chronic hepatitis B infection. Treatment with 100 mg daily has been shown to result in serologic conversion, virologic response, and histologic improvement. Treatment has been associated with the development of lamivudine-resistant mutants. Treatment of HIV-1–positive patients with lamivudine alone is not recommended because it is likely to result in rapid appearance of lamivudine-resistant HIV–1 strains. Lactic acidosis with severe hepatomegaly and steatosis are rare side effects of lamivudine. The majority of lamivudine is excreted unchanged in the urine.

Pharmacokinetics

Lamivudine is rapidly absorbed after oral intake. It is phosphorylated intracellularly. The incorporation of monophosphorylated lamivudine into viral DNA by HBV polymerase causes chain termination. The majority of lamivudine is eliminated unchanged in the urine. The mean elimination half-life is between 5 and 7 hours. Dose adjustment is necessary in patients with impaired renal function.

Adverse Events

Serious adverse events reported with the use of lamivudine in patients with chronic hepatitis B infection include lactic acidosis, hepatic steatosis, pancreatitis, and post-treatment exacerbation of hepatitis B.

Drug Interactions

As lamivudine is mainly eliminated by active organic catonic secretion into the urine, the possibility exists of interactions with other drugs eliminated by a similar mechanism. However, no clinically relevant interactions are known that would require dose adjustments.

OSELTAMIVIR

Oseltamivir phosphate [(3R,4R,5S)-4-acetyl-amino-5-amino-3(1-ethylpropoxy)-1-cyclohex-ene-1-carboxylic acid, ethyl ester, phosphate (1:1)] is a neuraminidase inhibitor. It is indicated for the treatment of uncomplicated influenza in patients at least 1 year old. It is also indicated for the prophylaxis of influenza in this same population. By inhibiting influenza virus neuraminidase, it is believed to alter viral particle aggregation and release. For the treatment of influenza in adults and adolescents, oseltamivir is dosed 75 mg twice daily for 5 days. Treatment should be started within the first 2 days of the commencement of symptoms. For prophylaxis of influenza, oseltamivir should be prescribed 75 mg once daily for a minimum of 7 days. The treatment should be started within 2 days of exposure.

Pharmacokinetics

Oseltamivir is absorbed by the GI tract and is converted to the carboxylate salt by hepatic esterases. Oseltamivir carboxylate is eliminated in the urine by both glomerular filtration and tubular secretion. The product package insert should be reviewed for information regarding plasma concentrations following various dosing schedules in renally impaired patients.

Drug Interactions

Clinically significant drug interactions are unlikely to occur.

Common Toxicities

Associated adverse events include GI upset, bronchitis, abdominal pain, dizziness, headache, insomnia, and fatigue.

PALIVIZUMAB

Palivizumab is a monoclonal antibody directed against the F protein of respiratory syncytial virus (RSV). It is used for the prevention of RSV infection in high-risk pediatric patients by passive immunization. Palivizumab is a "humanized" monoclonal antibody. It is produced in vitro and was developed using recombinant technology. It is genetically composed of 95% human and 5% murine sequences. It is administered as an IM injection at a dose of 15 mg/kg of body weight. Its efficacy has been demonstrated in children with bronchopulmonary dysplasia (BPD) and premature infants born at less than 35 weeks' gestation. Use of the monoclonal antibody resulted in a 55% decrease in the rate of hospitalization due to RSV infections. However, the severity of infection occurring despite prophylaxis did not appear to be significantly affected.

Pharmacokinetics and Major Toxicities

The mean half-life in pediatric patients was 20 days. Although no major toxicities have been observed, the potential for local and anaphylactic reactions may exist with this preparation, as with all protein injections.

PENCICLOVIR

Penciclovir is a nucleoside analog similar to ganciclovir in structure. It has activity similar to that of acyclovir and is available only as a topical preparation for recurrent herpes labialis. In clinical trials, it shortened the duration of symptoms by half a day, if applied within 1 hour of the beginning of symptoms and again every 2 hours while awake. Thus, its unimpressive performance is similar to that of all topical preparations available for the treatment of herpes infections, other than in the eye.

RIBAVIRIN

Ribavirin (1-β-D-ribofuranosyl-1H-1,2,4-triazole-3-carboxamide) is a synthetic nucleoside that interferes with viral RNA transcription, but its complete mechanism of action may be more complex. Ribavirin has a broad spectrum of activity against RNA viruses, including RSV, hepatitis C, measles virus, Lassa fever virus, and hantaviruses.

A major use for ribavirin is as combination therapy with interferon-α against chronic hepatitis C. Oral ribavirin combined with injected interferon-α (see below) has been shown to produce a sustained virologic response when used either as initial therapy or after relapse in patients previously treated with interferon-α alone. Oral dosage is based on the patient's body weight and is 400 mg in the morning and 600 mg in the evening daily for those weighing less than 75 kg. For those weighing more than 75 kg, the dosage is 600 mg twice a day. For previously untreated patients, treatment should be administered for 24 to 48 weeks. Discontinuation of therapy should be considered in those who have not responded by 24 weeks. For patients who have relapsed after interferon therapy, the recommended duration is 24 weeks. There are no safety and efficacy data beyond this period, but these recommendations may change based on future studies. The combination of ribavirin and interferon-α may be effective in interferon nonresponders, but its utility in this setting or in liver transplantation has not been established. It is commonly necessary to adjust the dosage based on adverse effects in individual patients. The need for close monitoring and dosage modification based on parameters, such as white blood cell count and hemoglobin, is emphasized.

Ribavirin is administered as an aerosol for confirmed, severe, lower respiratory (RSV) infection in infants or the immunosuppressed adult host. Because ribavirin has in vitro activity against Lassa fever virus and hantaviruses, it has been used intravenously in Lassa fever cases, in hemorrhagic fevers, and in the recent hantavirus pulmonary syndrome outbreak in the United States. Management of these rare and often fatal infections mandates contact with the Centers for Disease Control and Prevention (Atlanta, Georgia).

Pharmacokinetics

Ribavirin is rapidly absorbed after oral administration and undergoes first pass metabolism. The elimination half-life of ribavirin is more than 300 hours after multiple dosing. Ribavirin thus accumulates over the long term in vivo. Aerosolized ribavirin is absorbed systemically with a plasma half-life greater than 9 hours.

Major Toxicities

Ribavirin is potentially mutagenic, teratogenic, and embryotoxic. Documentation that a female patient is not pregnant and two methods of contraception while receiving therapy and for 6 months after treatment is therefore recommended. It is also recommended that similar precautions be observed if the male partner is being treated. Hematologic side effects, principally hemolytic anemia, are common, and the recommendations for dosage adjustment and discontinuation vary depending on whether the patient has known cardiac disease. Ribavirin by the aerosol route may lead to respiratory failure in chronic obstructive pulmonary disease (COPD) and asthma. Of note, the drug may precipitate in the mechanical ventilator and lead to an inability to ventilate the patient.

Drug Interactions

It is not recommended to coadminister didanosine with ribavirin due to increased exposure to didanosine.

RIMANTADINE

Rimantadine hydrochloride (α-methyltricyclo-[3.3.1.1/3.7]decane-1-methanamine hydrochloride) is a structural analog of amantidine. It has essentially the same indications as amantadine, and the dosage is the same. It is associated with fewer CNS side effects, however. Unlike amantadine, rimantadine undergoes extensive metabolism, and the dosage may need to be adjusted in those with either hepatic or renal insufficiency.

Drug Interactions

Aspirin and acetaminophen reduce plasma levels of rimantadine slightly, whereas cimetidine may lead to increased levels.

TELBIVUDINE

Telbivudine (1-[(2S,4R,5S)-4-hydroxy-5-hydroxy-methyltetrahydrofuran-2-yl]-5-methyl-1H-pyrimidine-2,4-dione) is a nucleoside analog with activity against HBV DNA polymerase. It is indicated for the treatment of chronic hepatitis B infection in adult patients with evidence of viral replication and either persistently elevated aminotransaminases or histologically active disease. The recommended dosage is 600 mg once daily. The optimal duration of treatment has not yet been determined.

Pharmacokinetics

Telbivudine is phosphorylated by cellular kinases to the active triphosphate form (telbivudine 5'-triphosphate), which competes with thymidine 5'-triphosphate. When telbivudine 5'-triphosphate is incorporated by the viral DNA, it causes chain termination. Telbivudine is primarily eliminated by renal excretion as unchanged drug. Patients with moderate to severe renal impairment require modification of the dosing interval.

Adverse Events

In clinical studies, telbivudine was well tolerated. However, lactic acidosis and severe hepatomegaly with steatosis have been reported. Severe exacerbations of hepatitis can occur after discontinuing therapy with telbivudine. No teratogenic toxicity has been seen in animal studies.

Drug Interactions

No clinically remarkable drug–drug interactions are known.

TRIFLURIDINE

Trifluridine (trifluorothymidine) is a fluorinated pyrimidine analog that interferes with DNA synthesis and is used topically for the treatment of HSV keratitis. Trifluridine may cause local irritation and palpebral edema.

VALACYCLOVIR

Valacyclovir (L-valine,2-[(2-amino-1,6-dihydro-6-oxo-9H-purin-9-yl)methoxy]ethyl ester, monohydrochloride) is a valyl ester of acyclovir that is metabolized to acyclovir after oral administration, resulting in plasma levels of acyclovir similar to those achieved with IV acyclovir. However, such higher bioavailability is expected to be dependent on factors such as GI absorption and hepatic function. Valacyclovir given at a dosage of 1 g 3 times daily has been shown to reduce time to healing and postherpetic neuralgia in herpes zoster and to do so more effectively than acyclovir. Valacyclovir may also be used in primary (1 g twice daily for 10 days) and recurrent (500 mg 3 times per day) genital herpes. In patients with normal immune function, valacyclovir 1 g daily can be used as suppressive therapy of recurrent genital herpes. Herpes labialis can be treated with valacyclovir 2 g every 12 hours for 1 day. In most respects, valacyclovir is appropriate when oral acyclovir is used and may be a potential substitute for IV acyclovir. However, the exact situations in which oral valacyclovir may be safely substituted for IV acyclovir, especially in the immunosuppressed patient, remain to be defined.

Pharmacokinetics

Valacyclovir is readily absorbed from the GI tract after oral intake and is almost completely converted to acyclovir and L-valine via first-pass intestinal and/or hepatic metabolism. Acyclovir is primarily excreted in the urine.

Major Toxicities

The major toxicities are similar to those of acyclovir.

Drug Interactions

There are no known clinically significant drug–drug interactions. Probenicid coadministration does result in an increase of the acyclovir Cmax and area under the curve but are of doubtful clinical relevance.

VALGANCICLOVIR

Valganciclovir hydrochloride (L-valine, 2-[(2-amino-1,6-dihydro-6-oxo-9H-purin-9-yl)methoxy]-3-hydroxypropyl ester, monohydrochloride) is a nucleoside analog and is the prodrug of ganciclovir. After oral administration, valganciclovir is rapidly converted to ganciclovir by hepatic and intestinal esterases. The active metabolite, ganciclovir triphosphate, is formed by phosphorylation by both viral and cellular kinases. Ganciclovir triphosphate is virustatic, by inhibiting viral DNA synthesis.

Valganciclovir is indicated for the treatment of AIDS-related CMV retinitis and for the prevention of CMV disease in high-risk recipients of kidney, heart, and kidney–pancreas transplants. It is commonly used for the prevention of CMV disease in HIV-1–infected patients who are felt to be at high risk for CMV disease because of a severely impaired immune system (most often determined by a very low CD4 lymphocyte count. It has significant advantages over ganciclovir, as it is administered orally thereby avoiding the need for indwelling catheters. For treatment of active CMV retinitis, it is recommended to induce the patient with 900 mg twice daily for 21 days, followed by maintenance with 900 mg daily. Valganciclovir should be dosed with food. To prevent CMV disease in patients who have received a kidney, heart, or kidney–pancreas transplant, valganciclovir, 900 mg, should be dosed daily (with food) within 10 days of transplant until 100 days post-transplantation.

Pharmacokinetics

Valganciclovir is well absorbed from the GI tract and is rapidly hydrolyzed to ganciclovir in the intestinal wall and in the liver. The major route of elimination is by renal excretion through glomerular filtration and active tubular secretion. The terminal half-life following oral administration of valganciclovir is 4.08 hours in healthy or HIV/CMV-positive patients. The terminal half-life in transplant patients is 6.48 hours. Dose adjustment is necessary in patients with renal impairment.

Major Toxicities

As for ganciclovir, the major toxicity of valganciclovir is hematologic, often causing anemia, neutropenia, and thrombocytopenia. Additional adverse effects associated with its use include GI upset, fever, headache, peripheral neuropathy, paresthesias, tremors, renal insufficiency, and infections. Valganciclovir may be teratogenic or embryotoxic in humans.

Drug Interactions/Precautions

The clinician should avoid coadministering other drugs with the potential to suppress the bone marrow. Caution should also be exercised when considering the coadministration of other agents with nephrotoxic potential. Probenicid causes increased levels of valganciclovir. An increased incidence of seizures has been noted with the concomitant use of imipenem and cisplatin.

VIDARABINE

Vidarabine (Ara-A, adenine arabinoside) is a purine analog made from *Streptomyces antibioticus* that inhibits viral DNA polymerases. It has been supplanted by acyclovir because of the greater efficacy and lower toxicity of acyclovir in HSV and VZV infections. It was the first agent used against HSV encephalitis but has been made almost obsolete by acyclovir. Acyclovir-resistant strains of HSV and VZV are currently treated with foscarnet. Vidarabine is currently only used as an ointment for the treatment of herpetic keratitis caused by HSV-1 and HSV-2.

ZANAMIVIR

Zanamivir (5-(acetylamino)-4-[(aminoiminomethyl)-amino]-2,6-anhydro-3,4,5-trideoxy-D-glycero-D-galacto-non-2-enonic acid) is a neuraminidase inhibitor that is indicated for the treatment of influenza A and influenza B in patients aged ≥7 years who have been symptomatic for no longer than 2 days. It is also indicated for the prophylaxis of influenza in patients who are at least 5 years old. It is not recommended for patients with underlying airway disease such as chronic obstructive pulmonary disease (COPD) or asthma. It is administered to the respiratory tract by oral inhalation. It has been proposed that the mechanism of action of zanamivir is through inhibition of influenza virus neuroaminidase with possible alteration of viral particle aggregation and release.

Zanamivir is dosed as two inhalations every 12 hours for 5 days for the treatment of influenza.

Pharmacokinetics

Between 4% and 17% of oral inhaled zanamivir is systemically absorbed. It is renally excreted unchanged. Unabsorbed drug is excreted fecally. The serum half-life is between 2.5 and 5.1 hours.

Common Toxicities

The use of zanamivir can precipitate bronchospasm and decline in pulmonary function. Many of theses cases have occurred in patients with underlying airway disease, such as asthma or COPD. Other common adverse events associated with its use are GI upset, sinusitis, dizziness, headache, bronchitis, cough, and allergic reactions (including oropharyngeal edema and rash).

Drug Interactions

There are no clinically relevant known pharmacokinetic drug interactions.

SUGGESTED READING

Keeffe EB, Marcellin P. New and emerging treatment of chronic hepatitis B. *Clin Gastroenterol Hepatol.* 2007 Mar;5(3):285–294.

Knipe D, Howley P, Griffin D, Lamb R, Martin M, Straus S, eds. *Fields Virology.* Philadelphia, PA: Lippincott, Williams, & Wilkins; 2006.

Sethi A. Approach to the management of patients with chronic hepatitis C who failed to achieve sustained virologic response. *Infect Dis Clin North Am.* 2006;20(1):115–135.

Gulfem E. Celik and N. Franklin Adkinson, Jr.

Adverse drug reactions (ADRs) are usefully separated into type A reactions (predictable from known pharmacologic properties and largely dose related) and type B reactions (unpredictable and restricted to a vulnerable subpopulation). Type B reactions comprise 10% to 15% of all ADRs and include *immunologic drug reactions, drug intolerance* (eg, tinnitus after single aspirin tablet), and *idiosyncratic reactions*, some of which are pseudoallergic (eg, aspirin-induced reactions).

Immune mechanisms are thought to be involved in 6% to 10% of all ADRs. Allergenic drugs can induce the entire spectrum of immunopathologic reactions, which are clinically indistinguishable from reactions elicited by foreign macromolecules (Table 206.1). Gell and Coombs' type I reactions are caused by drug/antigen-specific immunoglobulin E (IgE) that binds to high-affinity Fc-IgE receptors on mast cells and basophils. Cross-linking these receptors leads to the release of vasoactive mediators such as histamine and cysteinyl leukotrienes. Typical syndromes include urticaria, anaphylaxis, rhinitis, and bronchoconstriction, which can occur immediately in a previously sensitized individual. Type II cytolytic reactions are generally confined to rapidly haptenating drugs such as penicillins and are based on immunoglobulin G (IgG)-mediated cytotoxic mechanisms, resulting mainly in blood cell cytopenias. Type III reactions are immune complex mediated and may involve complement activation and stimulation of Fc-α receptor–activated inflammatory cells. Drug-specific immune complexes result from high-dose, prolonged therapy and may produce drug fever, a classic serum sickness syndrome, and various forms of cutaneous vasculitis. Type IV reactions are mediated by T lymphocytes and cause "delayed hypersensitivity reactions," the most typical examples being delayed maculopapular exanthem and contact dermatitis from topically applied drugs. Many drug-induced hypersensitivity reactions such as bullous, pustular, and some morbilliform skin eruptions that are presumed to have an immune etiology did not seem to fit into the older Gell and Coombs classification.

Recent studies of T-cell subsets and functions in the pathogenesis of delayed-onset immune reactions have suggested subcategories of type IV reactions as shown in Table 206.1.

However, some drug reactions resemble allergic syndromes but are not immunologic in origin. These nonimmune hypersensitivity reactions are also known as "pseudoallergic reactions." Most pseudoallergic reactions mimic type 1 IgE-mediated reactions such as urticaria, angioedema, bronchospasm, and anaphylaxis. In such cases basophils and mast cells are activated by nonimmune mechanisms, and vasoactive mediators are released.

In this chapter, we review type B ADRs to antibiotics with a focus on current concepts in the diagnosis and management of allergies to β-lactam antibiotics, the prototype of immunologic drug allergies. We also address the management of multiple antibiotic sensitivity syndromes.

EPIDEMIOLOGY OF ANTIBIOTIC ALLERGY

β-Lactams and sulfonamides are the most prevalent causes of antibiotic hypersensitivity. In a cross-sectional survey of a general population from Porto, Portugal, history of hypersensitivity to penicillin and other β-lactam antibiotics was found in 4.5% of adults. History of hypersensitivity to sulfonamides has been reported to occur in 2% to 4% of populations, but is increased among acquired immunodeficiency syndrome (AIDS) patients to 40% to 80%. Immunologic reactions to the newer classes of antibiotics are often rare and poorly documented. The perceived relative risk of immunologic drug reactions with commonly used antibiotics is given in Table 206.2.

BURDEN OF ANTIBIOTIC ALLERGY

β-Lactams are among the most commonly prescribed antibiotics for treatment of many types of bacterial infections. However, recent data show a significant decrease in β-lactam prescriptions, in part due to a rising prevalence

Table 206.1 Features of Immunopathologic Reactions to Antibiotics and Management Strategies

Reaction Category	Clinical Manifestation	Common Examples for Antibiotics	Timing for Sensitization with the First Use of the Drug
Type I (IgE)	Urticaria, angioedema, rhinitis, bronchospasm, anaphylaxis	β-lactam antibiotics Sulfamethoxazole	Required: 1 to 2 wk
Type II (IgG and complement)	Hemolytic anemia, drug-induced nephritis, thrombocytopenia, neutropenia	Penicillins Cephalosporins Sulfonamides	Required: 1 to 2 wk
Type III (IgG immune complexes)	Serum sickness, fever, vasculitis	Penicillins Cephalosporins Sulfonamides Streptomycin	Required: 10–21 d
Type IVa (Th1 lymphocytes)	Allergic contact dermatitis	Penicillins Neomycin Bactrim	Required: 1 to 3 wk
Type IVb (Th2 lymphocytes)	Maculopapular eruptions	Penicilillins, especially diaminopenicillins like amoxicillin and ampicillin Sulfonamides	Required: 4–14 d
Type IVc cytotoxic lymph. [perforin/granzyme B]	Contact dermatitis, Maculopapular and bullous exanthema, hepatitis, SJS, TEN	Sulfonamides Penicillins Macrolides	Required: 1–2 wk
Nonimmunologic	Urticaria, angioedema, rhinitis, erythema bronchospasm	Vancomycin (red man syndrome)	Not required Reaction may occur with first dose

Abbreviations: DPT = drug provocation tests; ESR = erythrocyte sedimentation rate; CRP = C-reactive protein,
[a] Only validated for penicillin skin testing which has high negative predictive value. Positivity may be helpful with certain
[b] Clinically false positivity may occur.
According to Gell and Combs, as modified.

of histories of allergy, which can exceed 30% in intensive care environments. Emergence of bacterial resistance as well as introduction of newer antibiotics have also contributed to this trend. Prescriptions of quinolones and macrolides as alternative antibiotics for common infections have been increasing as has the use of vancomycin in patients with histories of penicillin allergy, yet only 10% to 20% of the subjects with a history of penicillin reactions have positive type I skin tests. Unevaluated histories of antibiotic allergies lead to the substitution of often less effective or more toxic, and almost always more expensive, alternative drugs, resulting in high medical and economic burdens on medical care. In a retrospective study of hospital practice, penicillin-allergic patients had higher antibiotic costs and were more likely to receive a broader spectrum antibiotic such as cephalosporins, macrolides, and

quinolones. At the Mayo Clinic, prophylactic vancomycin use in patients with a history of penicillin or cephalosporin allergy undergoing elective orthopedic surgery was substantially reduced by targeted allergy consultation and penicillin allergy skin testing. Similar benefits are likely to occur in patients with histories of other antibiotic allergies who are appropriately evaluated before alternative antibiotics are selected.

CLINICAL FEATURES

The presentation of antibiotic allergies is similar to known hypersensitivity reactions, and the clinical features are variable depending on the type and severity of the reaction and the organ systems affected (Table 206.1). Many factors such as the immunologic profile of the antibiotic; treatment factors, including dosage,

Onset after Re-exposure to the Drug	Skin Tests	In Vitro Tests	Readministration of the Drug (DPT/Desensitization)
Usually within 1 h (rarely after hours)	Immediate (wheal/flare)[a] Intradermal tests	RAST (serum IgE) Serum mast cell tryptase level Basophil activation	Desensitization if skin test +
Many days or weeks	None	Complete blood count Coombs tests	Cautious DPT
Usually days to weeks	None	ESR CRP Immune complex Serum complement levels	Cautious DPT
8–120 h	Patch tests Intradermal tests (delayed response at 48–72 h)	Lymphocyte transformation tests	Likely contraindicated
	Patch tests Intradermal tests (delayed response at 48–72 h)	Lymphocyte transformation tests[b]	DPT useful
	Patch tests Intradermal tests (delayed response at 48–72 h)	Lymphocyte transformation tests[b]	Contraindicated (for bullous exanthem and SJS/TEN)
Within minutes, Infusion rate dependent	None	None	Slow infusion Use premedication

RAST = radioallergosorbent test; IgE = immunoglobulin E; IgG = immunoglobulin G; SJS = Stevens–Johnson syndrome; TEN = toxic epidermal necrolysis.
antibiotics; however, negative skin tests do not exclude the diagnosis for many immediate reactions to antibiotics.

administration route, and frequency; host factors such as immune status and comorbidities; and the inflammatory milieu in which antibiotics are used can influence the frequency and of characteristics of hypersensitivity reactions.

The skin is the most common organ involved in antibiotic reactions. Maculopapular eruptions (MPEs), urticaria, and pruritus are the most common presentations that typically occur after hours, days, or even weeks of antibiotic exposure but can also be part of an acute allergic reaction. Immunologic drug reactions require a sensitization period, whereas a nonimmunological mast cell release can occur on first exposure in susceptible patients. Antibiotics can also cause severe but rare exfoliative skin syndromes such as toxic epidermal necrolysis (TEN) and Stevens–Johnson syndrome (SJS). Other targeted organ manifestations such as interstitial pneumonitis and immune cytopenias are rare. Life-threatening reactions such as anaphylaxis are also rare. Although β-lactams are the most common antibiotic class inducing anaphylaxis, IgE antibody responses have also been documented for sulfonamides; those now in use are given in Table 206.3.

CLINICAL ASSESSMENT

Drug allergy syndromes are recognized by the constellation of signs and symptoms identified with a particular mechanism of immunopathology (Table 206.1). Appropriate diagnosis of these cases depends largely on careful history taking, with attention to prior drug experience and the chronology of the reaction, supplemented by compatible physical and laboratory findings, and knowledge of drug allergenicity profiles. For atypical or discordant reactions, skepticism

Table 206.2 Relative Risks of Immunologic Reactions to Commonly Used Antibiotics

Risk of Inducing an Immunologic Reaction[a]	Antibiotic (or its class)
Common (>2%)	Penicillins Antimicrobial sulfonamides Nitrofurantoin
Intermediate (0.1%–2%)	Bacitracin Cephalosporins Penems Itraconazol Quinolones Minocycline
Rare (0.1%)	Monobactam (aztreonam) Aminoglycosides Amphotericin B Chloramphenicol Clindamycin Flucanozole Griseofulvin Ketaconazole Macrolide antibiotics Vancomycin Tetracyclines Polymyxin Metronidazole

[a] Among patients receiving multiple courses of therapy.

is appropriate to avoid labeling the patient as "drug allergic" incorrectly.

Step 1: Initial Evaluation

HISTORY TAKING

A detailed history is essential for the initial evaluation of patients with suspected drug allergies. The history guides a decision about performing further diagnostic testing and other evaluation strategies. It is also possible to make a reasonable decision about risks of reintroduction of the suspected drug by using historical detail. Medical records that describe previous reactions and treatment can be very helpful, especially in patients with vague histories or clouded consciousness. Occasionally, information provided by a relative or friend who witnessed the event can also be very helpful in differential diagnosis.

The clinical history of suspected drug allergy should be focused on both medication-related and patient-related factors. The medication(s) implicated, clinical features of the reaction(s), and the previous exposure and reaction to each drug and related compounds as well as comorbid disorders of the patients should be recorded. For example, patients with chronic urticaria often attribute cutaneous reactions to drugs and foods. Similarly symptoms of chest tightness or pain, dyspnea, and tachycardia after use of a drug can be a sign of underlying cardiovascular disease. Other patient comorbidities include the high frequency of amoxicillin-induced morbilliform rashes in patients with mononucleosis, and frequent trimethoprim–sulfamethoxazole reactions in AIDS patients. Another example is that patients with cystic fibrosis have a higher risk for immune reactions to antibiotics, probably because of frequent re-exposure.

History taking provides information helpful in assessing the likelihood of immune mediation. Immunologic reactions require a sensitization period, so putatively allergic patients should have a history of prior use of the either the drug itself or a structurally related compound. For first drug exposure, an immunologic reaction may be seen after 3 to 10 days, which can be sufficient for primary sensitization. Nonimmunologic reactions do not require sensitization, and reactions may be seen even after the first dose. Pseudoallergic reactions can often be distinguished from IgE-mediated reactions with similar clinical manifestations by reliable histories of previous drug use. Based on clinical features and the chronology of the reaction, conclusions can often be drawn about whether a reaction is immunologically mediated (Table 206.1).

PHYSICAL EXAMINATION

Direct observation of patients undergoing presumed drug reactions can be useful for both differential diagnosis and objective assessment of severity, which can often be exaggerated in retrospective patient accounts. A complete physical examination is desirable as many organ systems have the potential for involvement. For skin reactions occuring with drug use, a detailed dermatologic examination is often helpful. Viral exanthems are easily confused with maculopapular drug eruptions. Fever and coryza or pharyngitis can help to identify the former.

Step 2: Decision about Application of Further Diagnostic Testing

History alone is often not sufficient for establishing current drug sensitivity. Only 10% to 20% of subjects with a convincing history of IgE-dependent penicillin allergy will be positive by validated skin testing, indicating a very low diagnostic accuracy of history alone for current sensitivity. Data with other drugs are similar,

Table 206.3 Clinical Features of Hypersensitivity Reactions

Antibiotic	Common	Less Common/Rare
β-lactams	Urticaria, MPE	Exfoliative dermatitis, TEN, SJS, serum sickness syndrome, vasculitis, cytopenias, anaphylaxis, nephritis
Sulfonamide	Fixed drug eruption HIV(+): Delayed MPE+fever, urticaria, angioedema	Erythema multiforme, SJS, TEN Anaphylactic reactions
Quinolones	Urticaria, FDE, photoallergic reactions	Acute interstitial nephritis, acute hepatitis, serum sickness, SJS, TEN, MPE, acute pancreatitis, anemia; thrombocytopenia
Macrolides	Urticaria, angioedema, FDE, and MPE	TEN, vasculitis
Vancomycin	"red man syndrome," lineary IgA bullous dermatosis	MPE, FDE, vasculitis, thrombocytopenia, erythema multiforme, and urticaria anaphylaxis

Abbreviations: FDE = fixed drug eruptions; MPE = maculopapular eruption; TEN = toxic epidermal necrolysis; SJS = Stevens–Johnson syndrome; IgA = immunoglobulin A; HIV = human immunodeficiency virus.

suggesting that sensitivity may wane with time. Drug provocation tests that are the gold standard for the diagnosis of current drug allergy have a similarly low positivity rate in patients with history of drug allergy. All of this indicates that diagnosis of current sensitivity based on history alone is often not advisable. Further diagnostic tests for definite diagnosis may be needed.

Unfortunately, many *in vivo* and *in vitro* diagnostic tests for allergy have shown limited value in the diagnosis of allergy to haptenic (small molecular weight) drugs.

Although skin testing provides valuable information for the diagnosis of immediate reactions to penicillins and in some cases to other β-lactams, the validity of skin tests with other antibiotics is limited as the antigenic determinants are not adequately known. *In vitro* tests for drug-specific IgE to antibiotics is of limited value because they are less sensitive than intradermal tests. A positive result, however, is usually reliable and corresponds to skin test results. If there is no contraindication, drug provocation testing with the offending drug is the most reliable test for diagnosis of current antibiotic hypersensitivity for many haptenic drug allergies. Because such testing carries some risk for the patient, its use is usually restricted to cases where alternative antibiotics are unacceptable or there are multiple antibiotic sensitivities. A stepwise approach to the diagnosis of antibiotic allergy is given in Figure 206.1. Diagnostic testing can be pursued based on likely immunopathology as given in Table 206.1.

EVALUATION OF IMMEDIATE-TYPE SENSITIVITIES
Skin Testing for β-Lactam Antibiotics

Intradermal skin testing with a 15- to 20-minute readout of wheal and flare has been validated for detecting drug-specific IgE antibodies to penicillins and other β-lactam antibiotics. A major determinant analog (*penicilloyl-polylysine*) and minor determinants (*benzylpenicilloate, benzylpenilloate,* and *benzylpenicillin* isomers of penicillin) are used for skin test evaluation for IgE-dependent penicillin allergy. IgE antibodies to minor determinants are clinically associated with anaphylactic reactions and can predict the risk of more severe reactions. IgE antibodies to the major penicilloyl determinant correlate loosely with risk for urticarial reactions.

Testing is undertaken with two or more reagents, usually penicilloyl-polylysine (Pre-Pen) antigen and either penicillin alone (10 000 IU/mL) or a mixture of minor antigens, including at least benzylpenicillin and benzylpenicilloate (10 mM each). Of these minor determinants, only benzylpenicillin is available commercially in the United States. Academic allergy centers may have made their own skin testing materials for experimental use. Skin prick testing

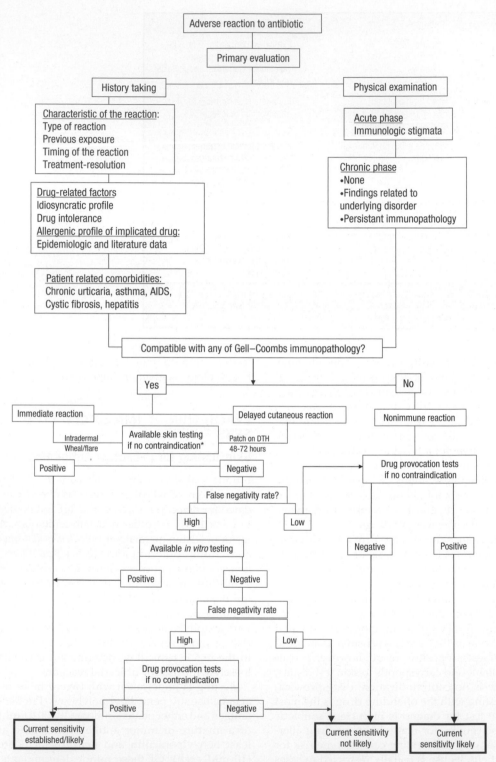

Figure 206.1 A diagnostic algorithm for evaluation of putative immunologic reactions to antibiotics.

*Contraindication for skin immunoglobulin E testing are extensive skin lesion, recent antihistamine use, and history of serious immediate systemic reaction with allergen exposure. AIDS = acquired immunodeficiency syndrome; DTH = ;

with full-strength reagents is done first, and if these tests are negative at 15 minutes, they are followed by intracutaneous testing, raising an initial bleb of 2 to 3 mm. A wheal diameter of at least 3 mm greater than negative control is considered positive. In some centers, elective testing is followed by the administration of 1 to 3 doses of oral penicillin and a period of observation to confirm that the drug is tolerated. For hospitalized patients with serious infection, a rapid dose escalation of the intravenous antibiotic of choice is judiciously employed.

Falsely negative penicillin skin testing is rare, and all reports are of mild, self-limited, and/or transient reactions. About 75% to 90% of history-positive patients will have negative penicillin testing, allowing a large majority of such patients to be re-treated safely. Despite this substantial diagnostic power, it has been difficult to maintain persistant commercial sources for these reagents in the United States and Europe. Some academic centers have produced the reagents for their own use, but concerns persist about access to these orphan drug products.

Recent studies show promising results with cephalosporin skin tests. Concentrations of 2 to 3 mg/mL of a parenteral cephalosporin preparation are reported to be usually nonirritating, but each cephalosporin requires concurrent evaluation for its irritant potential in nonallergic subjects. Although a positive cephalosporin skin test implies the presence of drug-specific IgE antibodies, a negative test does not exclude immediate hypersensitivity.

Commercial cephalosporin skin test reagents are not currently available in the United States. Positive intradermal skin tests have been reported for imipenem and other β-lactams, but validated skin testing protocols have not been developed.

In Vivo Tests

Solid-phase immunoassays (radioallergosorbent test [RAST] and enzyme-linked immunosorbent assay) have been established for a wide variety of immediate-type drug allergies. Only with penicillin allergy have *in vitro* test results been systematically compared with skin tests. The consistent finding has been diagnostic sensitivity for penicilloyl–IgE by RAST of 65% to 85% compared with penicilloyl–polylysine skin tests and 32% to 50% compared with a combination of skin testing and challenge. Minor determinant penicillin IgE antibodies are not reliably detected by available immunoassays. In recent years, flow cytometry has been increasingly used in the diagnosis of allergy. Assessment of basophil activation by means of increase in surface markers such as CD63 has been investigated in penicillin allergy. In one study from Europe, sensitivity was ≤30% compared with a diagnosis confirmed by skin testing. As with unvalidated skin tests, a clearly positive result is of greater clinical value than a negative result, thus in vitro basophil activation tests remain investigational.

EVALUATION OF NONIMMEDIATE REACTIONS

Skin Testing

European studies suggest that both patch tests and intradermal tests with delayed cutaneous readouts (at 48 and 72 hours) are useful in evaluating nonimmediate reactions to aminopenicillins and certain β-lactams and that both can reliably predict the results of rechallenge. Additional studies are required to confirm and extend these results to other drug allergies and to define more precisely the clinical correlation and predictive value for re-treatment.

Other Tests

Drug-specific T lymphocytes, which are involved in some cutaneous hypersensitivity reactions, may be detected with the use of in vitro lymphocyte transformation tests, which are utilized in Europe but not approved for diagnostic use in the United States. However, sensitization may be found after recent treatment even in the absence of any clinical reactivity, and positive test results have been demonstrated after both immediate and delayed antibiotic-induced reactions caused by β-lactam antibiotics, sulfonamides, and quinolones.

USE OF DRUG PROVOCATION TESTS

Definitive diagnosis of drug allergy involves provocation testing as the last step, during which gradually increasing doses of the offending drug are given. Provocation testing may be necessary to accurately identify the responsible agent when multiple drugs are given simultaneously and a reaction occurs. It is particularly important not to incorrectly label a patient allergic to an antibiotic because it may severely restrict antibiotic choices for life.

Studies indicate that only a small minority of history-positive subjects have positive drug challenges. Drug provocation tests should be considered only after evaluating the risk–benefit ratio for an individual patient, and should be performed by experienced personnel in an appropriate environment. Informed consent of the patient should be obtained prior to the procedure.

MANAGEMENT OF ANTIBIOTIC ALLERGY

Alternatives for Drug-Allergic Patients

Three alternative approaches are available to provide acceptable pharmacotherapy for infection in antibiotic-allergic patients (Figure 206.2). The physician may choose to use an unrelated antibiotic, or potentially cross-reactive alternative, or to readminister the implicated antibiotic after desensitization. A structurally unrelated antibiotic is usually chosen if the trade-offs of safety, efficacy, and cost are acceptable. This often obtains in the treatment of uncomplicated outpatient infections. If there is no acceptable alternative to the offending drug class, a potentially cross-reacting member of the same antibiotic family may be administered using rapid dose escalation under careful observation. If a reaction occurs during graded challenge,

then a desensitization protocol is warranted. Classical desensitization is applied only for IgE-dependent allergy in patients with demonstrable or presumed IgE antibody responses. The procedure aims to induce a temporary state of drug tolerance.

Desensitization procedures usually start at 1/10 000 of the full dose with a 2- to 3-fold dose increment every 30 to 60 minutes. The procedure entails risk of acute allergic reactions, which occur in mild form in 30% to 80% of penicillin-allergic patients undergoing desensitization. Reactions are generally confined to local and mild systemic reactions during the desensitization procedure and, occasionally, late-occurring reactions during therapy, including urticaria or serum sickness and hemolytic anemia if prolonged high-dose therapy is used. Desensitization should usually be performed in a hospital setting where experienced personnel and emergency treatment are available. Desensitization is an active and reversible process dependent on the continuous presence of the drug. After drug discontinuation, the desensitized state dissipates over days to weeks, and repeat desensitization is usually required for subsequent treatment courses. Both oral and parenteral routes can be used to initiate desensitization therapy, and both appear equally

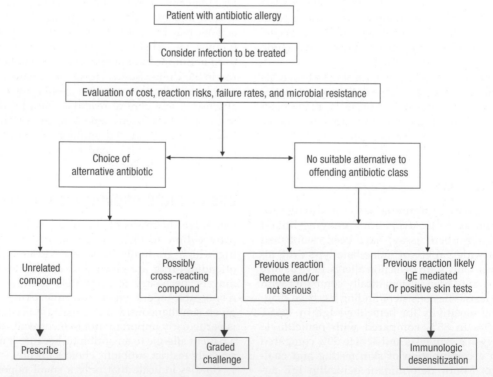

Figure 206.2. An approach to treating patients with antibiotic allergy.

Table 206.4 Oral Densensitization Protocol

Step[a]	Phenoxymethyl Penicillin (U/mL)	Amount (mL)	Dose (U)	Cumulative Dosage (U)
1	1 000	0.1	100	100
2	1 000	0.2	200	300
3	1 000	0.4	400	700
4	1 000	0.8	800	1 500
5	1 000	1.6	1 600	3 100
6	1 000	3.2	3 200	6 300
7	1 000	6.4	6 400	12 700
8	10 000	1.2	12 000	24 700
9	10 000	2.4	24 000	48 700
10	10 000	4.8	48 000	96 700
11	80 000	1.0	80 000	176 000
12	80 000	2.0	160 000	336 700
13	80 000	4.0	320 000	656 700
14	80 000	8.0	640 000	1 296 700
Observe patient for 30 minutes Changes to benzylpenicillin G IV (slow IV drip over 15 minutes)				
15	500 000	0.25	125 000	
16	500 000	0.50	250 000	
17	500 000	1.00	500 000	
18	500 000	2.25	1 125 000	

[a] 15-minute interval between steps.
Adapted from Sullivan TJ. Penicillin allergy. In: Lichtenstein LM, Fauci AS, eds. *Current therapy in allergy, immunology, and rheumatology*, Toronto: BC Decker; 1985:57.
Abbreviation: IV = intravenous.

effective in inducing clinical tolerance. The oral approach is arguably safer, although not always feasible.

A variety of desensitization protocols have been used succesfully for reintroducing β-lactams, trimethoprim–sulfamethoxazole, vancomycin, and other antimicrobials. Tables 206.4 and 206.5 show illustrative published protocols for penicillin.

Management of β-Lactam Allergy

β-Lactam antibiotics are the most commonly prescribed class of antibiotics and the most frequent cause of antibiotic allergy. It is the only group of antibiotics for which skin tests have been validated. This group includes penicillins, cephalosporins, carbapenems, and monobactams, all of which share a β-lactam ring but otherwise vary in nuclear structure and side chains.

If skin testing reagents are available, then therapy may be dispensed according to the result of skin tests. When reagents or consultants are not available, an approach is outlined in Figure 206.3. Patients with histories of a reaction to a β-lactam class other than penicillin should first be skin tested with the benzylpenicillin reagents and, if negative, with the diluted β-lactam chosen for use.

Cross-Reactivity among β-Lactam Antibiotics

Cross-reactivity within the penicillin class is virtually complete. A patient who is allergic to any penicillin is likely to react to all

Table 206.5 Parenteral Desensitization Protocol

Infection Number	Benzylpenicillin Concentration (U/mL)	Volume/Route (mL)
1	100	0.1 ID
2	100	0.2 SC
3	100	0.4 SC
4	100	0.8 SC
5	1 000	0.1 ID
6	1 000	0.3 SC
7	1 000	0.6 SC
8	10 000	0.1 ID
9	10 000	0.2 SC
10	10 000	0.4 SC
11	10 000	0.8 SC
12	100 000	0.1 ID
13	100 000	0.3 SC
14	100 000	0.6 SC
15	1 000 000	0.1 ID
16	1 000 000	0.2 SC
17	1 000 000	0.2 IM
18	1 000 000	0.4 IM
19	Continuous IV infusion (1 000 000 U/h)	

Doses are administered at 20-minute intervals. Observe skin wheal and flare response to intradermal doses.
ID = intradermal; SC = subcutaneous; IM = intramuscular; IV = intravenous.
Adapted from Wesis ME, Adkinson NF. Immediate hypersensitivity reactions to penicillin and related anitibiotics. *Clinical Allergy*. 1988;18:515–540.

penicillins. Immunologic cross-reactivity between cephalosporins and penicillins is readily demonstrated in vitro and by skin testing, yet multiple studies have shown that most patients with penicillin IgE responses can be safely treated with cephalosporins, especially those of third and fourth generation. Still, penicillin allergy conveys a relative risk of 4.4 to 10 for acute cephalosporin reactions, and in one series a majority of cases of fatal anaphylactic reactions to cephalosporins involved penicillin-allergic patients. Because of this, administration of cephalosporins to penicillin-allergic patients should be undertaken cautiously, especially for patients with previous life-threatening reactions to β-lactam antibiotics of any class.

Penicillin-allergic patients can be given the monobactam aztreonam with little risk because clinically significant cross-reactivity between penicillin and monobactams has not been demonstrated. In contrast, cross-reactions between aztreonam and ceftazidime have been reported, presumably due to identical side chains. The carbapenem antibiotics (imipenem, meropenem, and ertapenem) will induce positive skin tests in about half of penicillin-allergic patients. However, a recent clinical report from Europe found that 100% of 110 patients with positive penicillin skin tests tolerated imipenem. Cautious cross-treatment may be reasonably attempted.

Sulfonamide antimicrobials (sulfamethoxazole, sulfadiazine, sulfisoxazole, and sulfacetamide) are extensively cross-reactive and also cross-react with dapsone. Sulfonamide antimicrobial agents differ from other sulfonamide-containing medications by having an aromatic amine group at the N4 position and a substituted ring at the N1 position that are not found in nonantibiotic sulfonamide-containing drugs. Patients allergic to sulfonamide antibiotics generally tolerate thiazide diuretics, oral hypoglycemic agents, and other SO_2-containing drugs and vice versa.

Other Antibiotics

Immunologic reactions to quinolones and macrolides are very rare. These antibiotics mostly evoke maculopapular eruptions and occasionally urticaria and angioedema (Table 206.3). As there are no validated skin or in vitro tests, drug provocation tests are the only available diagnostic methods for these classes of antibiotics.

Vancomycin is associated with two main types of hypersensitivity reactions, namely an anaphylactoid reaction known as "red man syndrome" and anaphylaxis. Skin testing with vancomycin at ≤100 mg/mL is diagnostic for the presence of IgE antibodies that can be elicted by multiple courses of therapy. Limited efforts with skin testing have not been found useful.

Topical antibiotics such as bacitracin and neomycin usually cause delayed-type skin reactions. Although immediate-type reactions are rarely reported, repeated usage of bacitracin has been associated with near fatal anaphylaxis in a few cases. Hypersensitivity reactions to metronidazole are infrequently reported. Fixed drug eruptions and delayed-type

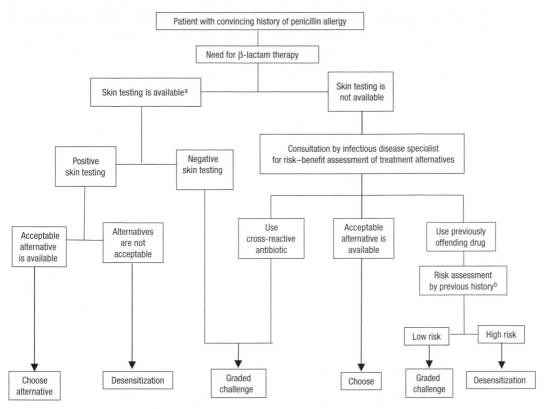

Figure 206.3 Diagnostic evaluation of patients with histories of penicillin allergy.

[a] Intradermal skin tests should include penicilloyl–polylysine (Pre-Pen) as a major determinant analog, plus one or more minor determinants (especially benzylpenicillin, benzylpenicilloate), the previously offending antibiotic if known and/or the currently desired antibiotic choice may be usefully included, especially in evaluating non–penicillin β-lactams.

[b] Risk assessment by previous history: High risk: Histories of bronchospasm, angioedema, hypotension, shock that occurred within 30 minutes of penicillin administration in the last year Low risk: History of isolated urticaria or maculopapular rash occurring after days of treatment remotely >5 years in the past.

skin reactions are the most common clinical presentations.

The general approach to antibiotic allergy as depicted in Figure 206.1 is also useful for management of adverse reactions to non–β-lactam antibiotics.

Multiple Antibiotic Allergy Syndromes

Some patients show a marked propensity to react to several chemically unrelated antibiotics and sometimes nonantibiotic drugs. This condition has been termed the multiple drug allergy syndrome (MDAS). In most cases, MDAS presents clinically as acute urticaria, angioedema on ingestion of offending drugs, but different rashes, including SJS, anaphylaxis, serum sicknesslike reactions, and immune cytopenias, have also been described. Mechanisms underlying multiple drug reactivity are still unclear. Published studies have suggested a high propensity to MDAS among patients with a history of allergy to β-lactams or any other

antimicrobial drug. Whether MDAS results from a facilitated ability to make immune responses to drug haptens or an increased vulnerability to drug-induced immunopathology has yet to be determined. Some cases of MDAS are "pseudoallergic" and reflect classically conditioned responses that can readily be misinterpreted as anaphylaxis.

Clinical management of MDAS is similar to that of patients with single antibiotic allergy. Avoidance of unnecessary use of drugs should be the first step. Preferential use of low-risk antibiotics such as macrolides and quinolones may be helpful. If validated skin or in vitro tests are available, they can be helpful in permitting re-administration of previously implicated drugs, especially β-lactams.

CONCLUSION

Patients relating a history of immune or nonimmune reactions to antibiotics are not rare in medical practice. As history alone has low diagnostic value, it is desirable that the history-positive patients should be evaluated by diagnostic tests when validated or by drug provocation tests when the index of suspicion is low. Although alternative antimicrobials can often be identified, they can have higher costs and treatment failures or greater toxicity to deal with. For the truly drug-allergic patient, management approaches include cautious administration of cross-reactive antimicrobials from the same class or drug desensitization. When approached systematically, almost all antibiotic-sensitive patients can be safely and effectively treated.

SELECTED READINGS

Adkinson NF Jr. Drug allergy. In: *Middleton`s Allergy: Priciples and Practice*. 6th ed. 2003;1 679–1691.Philadelphia, PA: Mosby.

Adkinson NF Jr, Essayan D, Gruchalla R, et al. Health and Environmental Sciences Institute Task Force. Task Force Report: future research needs for the prevention and management of immune-mediated drug hypersensitivity reactions. *J Allergy Clin Immunol.* 2002;109:S461–S478.

Gomes ER, Demoly P. Epidemiology of hypersensitivity reactions. *Curr Opin Allergy Clin Immunol.* 2005;5:309–316.

Greenberger PA. Drug allergies. *J Allergy Clin Immunol.* 2006;117:S464–S470.

Gruchalla RS, Pirmohamed M. Antibiotic allergy. *N Engl J Med.* 2006;354:601–609.

Hemstreet BA, Page RL. Sulfonamide allergies and outcomes related to use of potentially cross-reactive drugs in hospitalized patients. *Pharmacotherapy.* 2006;26:551–557.

Pichichero ME. A review of evidence supporting the American Academy of Pediatrics recommendation for prescribing cephalosporin antibiotics for penicillin allergic patient. *Pediatrics.* 2005;115:1048–1057.

Pichler JW. Immune mechanism of drug hypersensitivity. *Immunol Allergy Clin North Am.* 2004;24:373–397.

Romano A, Blanca M, Torres MJ, et al. Diagnosis of nonimmediate reactions to β-lactam antibiotics. *Allergy.* 2004;59:1153–1160.

Romano A, Viola M, Gueant-Rodriguez RM, Gaeta F, Pettinato R, Gueant JL. Imipenem in patients with immediate hypersensitivity to penicillins. *N Engl J Med.* 2006;354:2835–2837.

Solensky R. Drug hypersensitivity. *Med Clin North Am.* 2006;90:233–260.

Tilles AS, Slatore CG. Hypersensitivity reactions to non beta-lactam antibiotics. *Clin Rev Allergy Immunol.* 2003;24:221–228.

Verdel BM, Souverein PC, Egberts AC, Leufkens HG. Difference in risks of allergic reaction to sulfonamide drugs based on chemical structure. *Ann Pharmacother.* 2006;40: 1040–1046.

Wolcheck GW. Clinical evaluation and management of drug hypersensitivity. *Immunol Allergy Clin North Am.* 2004;24:357–371.

207. Antimicrobial Agent Tables

Divya Sareen, Michael Kessler, Rosalie Pepe, and David Schlossberg

INTRODUCTION

The following tables of antimicrobial agents are organized as follows:

The listings are alphabetical by generic name, with the corresponding brand name provided; available data are included for dosage, cost, change in absorption with food, pregnancy class, dosage adjustment for renal failure and dialysis, and major toxicities. Suggested Reading at the end of the tables indicate resources for references and for additional data.

Table 207.1 Antibacterial Agents

Name		Usual Dose			Change in Absorption with Food
Generic	Brand	Adult	Child	Cost (per Day)*	
Amikacin[c]	Amikin	15 mg/kg/d; divide q8–12h IV 10–40 mg IT q24h	15 mg/kg/d; divide q8–12h	$130.00	n/a
Amoxicillin	Amoxil	0.25–0.5 g PO q8h or 875 mg PO q12h or 1000 mg PO q12h (*Helicobacter pylori*)	6.6–13.3 mg/kg PO q8h (Neonate: 0–7 d, 25 mg/kg q12h; 1–4 wk 25 mg/kg q8h)	250 mg, 500 mg capsule: $0.75 875 mg: $3.48	Decreased
Amoxicillin–clavulanate	Augmentin	0.25–0.5 g PO q8h 875 mg PO q12h 2000 mg PO q12h XR tablets	6.6–13.3 mg/kg PO q8h	250 mg tab: $7.70 500 mg tab: $5.76 875 mg tab: $15.14 XR 100 mg tab: $14.24	Decreased
Ampicillin	Ampen, Omnipen	0.5–1 g PO q8h; 1–2 g IV q4–6h	12.5–25 mg/kg PO q8h 6.25–25 mg/kg IV q8h	$0.69–$1.20 PO $35.00 IV	Decreased
Ampicillin–sulbactam	Unasyn	1.5–3 g IV q6h	25–50 mg/kg IV q6h	$44.00 1.5 g $78.10 3 g	n/a
Azithromycin	Zithromax	5 g day 1; 0.25 g days 2–5 PO	—[b]	PO: $7.78 IV: $25.16	Decreased
Azlocillin	Azlin	2–4 g IV q4–6h	75 mg/kg IV q6h	Data not available	n/a
Aztreonam	Azactam	1–2 g IV q6–8h	30–50 mg/kg q6–12h (n.a.)	1 g: $125.00 2 g: $250.00	n/a
Bacampicillin	Spectrobid	0.4–0.8 g PO q12h	12.5–25 mg/kg PO q12h	$4.77–$9.55	None
Carbenicillin indanyl sodium	Geocillin	1–2 0.382-g tabs PO q6h	7.5–12.5 mg/kg PO q6h	$11.75	Increased
Carbenicillin	Geopen	5–6.5 g IV q4–6h	25–100 mg/kg IV q4–6h	Data not available	n/a
Cefaclor	Ceclor	0.25–0.5 PO q8h	20–40 mg/kg/d; divide q8h PO	250 mg $7.96 500 mg $15.56	Decreased
Cefadroxil	Duricef	0.5–1 g PO q12–24h	30 mg/kg/d; divide q12h PO	$8.91	Decreased

Pregnancy Class[a]	Dose Interval Adjustment for Reduced CrCl			Supplemental Dose in Dialysis		Major Toxicity
	>50	10–50	≤10	HD	PD	
D	q8–12h	q12–48h	>48h	2.5–3.75 mg/kg pHD	2.5 mg/kg/d IV or 3–4 mg/ 2 L dialysate removed	Renal toxicity, vestibular or auditory toxicity, CNS reactions, neuromuscular blockade (rare)
B	q8h	q8–12h	q16–24h	0.25–0.5 g	0.25 g q12h	Allergic reactions (rare: anaphylactic), rash, diarrhea, nausea, vomiting
B	q8h	q12h	q12–24h	0.25 g PO	—[b]	Allergic reactions (rare: anaphylactic), diarrhea, nausea, vomiting, cholestatic hepatitis
B	q4–6h	q8h	q12–24h	0.5–2 g	0.25 g PO q12h or 1–4 g IV q24h	Allergic reactions (rare: anaphylactic), diarrhea, nausea, vomiting
B	q6–8h	q8–12h	q24h	2 g ampicillin pHD	—[b]	Allergic reactions (rare: anaphylactic), diarrhea, nausea, vomiting
B	Usual	Usual	Usual	—[b]	—[b]	GI disturbance, headache
B	q4–6h	q8h	q12h	3 g pHD	—[b]	Allergic reactions (rare: anaphylactic), diarrhea, nausea, vomiting
B	q6–8h	q12–18h	q24h	⅛ first dose (60–250 mg) pHD	Usual dose (1–2 g) then usual dose at usual intervals	Rash, diarrhea, nausea, vomiting, elevated AST/ALT
B	q12h	q12h	—[b]	—[b]	—[b]	Allergic reactions (rare: anaphylactic), diarrhea, nausea, vomiting
B	—[b]	—[b]	—[b]	—[b]	—[b]	Allergic reactions (rare: anaphylactic), diarrhea, nausea, vomiting
B	q4h	2–3 g q6h	N.R.	0.75–2 g pHD	2 g q6–12h	Allergic reactions (rare: anaphylactic), diarrhea, nausea, vomiting
B	q8h	q8h	q8h	0.25–0.5 g	—[b]	Allergic reactions, GI disturbance, arthritis, serum sickness
B	q12–24h	0.5 g q12–24h	0.5 g q36h	0.5–1 g	—[b]	Allergic reactions, GI disturbance

(continued)

Table 207.1 *(continued)*

Name		Usual Dose		Cost (per Day)*	Change in Absorption with Food
Generic	Brand	Adult	Child		
Cefamandole	Mandol	0.5–2 g IV q4–8h	50–150 mg/kg/d; divide q4–8h IV	$36.25 (1 g q6h)	n/a
Cefazolin	Ancef, Kefzol	0.5–2 g IV q8h	25–100 mg/kg/d; divide q6–8h IV	$13.83 (1 g q8h)	n/a
Cefdinir	Omnicef	300 mg PO q12h	14 mg/kg/d PO qd divide q12–24h	$11.37	Minimal decrease
Cefditoren	Spectracef	400 mg PO BID	400 mg PO BID	$8.31	Increased
Cefepime	Maxipime	0.5–2 g IV q12h	50 mg/kg IV q8h (n.a.)	$45.20–$89.68	n/a
Cefixime	Suprax	0.4 g PO q24h	8 mg/kg/d; divide PO q24h	$8.00	Decreased
Cefmetazole	Zefazone	2 g IV q6–12h	—[b]	Data not available	n/a
Cefonicid	Monocid	0.5–2 g IV q24h	—[b]	Data not available	n/a
Cefoperazone	Cefobid	1–2 g IV q6–12h	25–100 mg/kg IV q12h (n.a.)	$36.00–$72.46	n/a
Cefotaxime	Claforan	0.5–2 g IV q8–12h; 3 g q6h for CNS	50–200 mg/kg/d; divide IV q4–8h (neonate: 0–7 d – 50 mg/kg q12h; 1–4 wk: 50 mg/kg q6–8h)	$136.80 2 g q6h	n/a
Cefotetan	Cefotan	1–2 g IV q12h	40–60 mg/kg/d; divide IV q12h (n.a.)	$29.26–$58.50	n/a
Cefoxitin	Mefoxin	1–2 g IV q6–8h	80–160 mg/kg/d; divide IV q4–8h	$33.75–$67.50	n/a
Cefpodoxime	Vantin	0.1–0.4 g PO q12h	5 mg/kg PO q12h	$10.90–$28.84	Increased
Cefprozil	Cefzil	0.25–0.5 g PO q12–24h	15 mg/kg PO q12h	$9.74–$19.82	No effect

Pregnancy Class[a]	Dose Interval Adjustment for Reduced CrCl			Supplemental Dose in Dialysis		Major Toxicity
	>50	10–50	≤10	HD	PD	
B	q4–8h	q8h	0.5–1 g q12h	0.5–1 g	—[b]	Thrombophlebitis with IV infusion, allergic reactions, GI disturbance
B	q8h	0.5–1 g q8–12h	0.5–1 g q24h	0.25–0.5 g	—[b]	Allergic reactions, GI disturbance, diarrhea
B	Usual	300 mg q24h	300 mg q24h	Not defined	Not defined	Anaphylaxis, toxic epidermal necrolysis, erythema multiforme, neutropenia
B	400 mg PO BID	200 mg PO BID	200 mg PO qd	None	—[b]	Anaphylaxis, leukopenia, neutropenia, thrombocytopenia
B	0.5–2 g IV q12h	q24h	0.25–0.5 g q24h	Dose pHD	0.5–2 g q48h	Nausea, diarrhea, vomiting, rash, phlebitis
B	q24h	0.3 g q24h	q48h	None	—[b]	Thrombophlebitis, allergic reactions, GI disturbance
B	q6–12h	q16–24h	q48h	—[b]	—[b]	Thrombophlebitis, allergic reactions, GI disturbance
B	q24h	4–15 mg/kg q24–48h	3–15 mg/kg q3–5 days	None	—[b]	Allergic reactions, GI disturbance, hypoprothrombinemia or hemorrhage
B	q6–12h	q6–12h	q6–12h	Dose after HD	—[b]	Thrombophlebitis, allergic reactions, GI disturbance
B	q8–12h	q12–24h	0.5 g q24–48h	0.5–2 g	—[b]	Thrombophlebitis, allergic reactions, GI disturbance
B	q12h	q24h	q48h	25% dose nonHD days, 50% HD	—[b]	Thrombophlebitis, allergic reactions, GI disturbance, hypoprothrombinemia, hemorrhage
B	q6–8h	q12–24h	0.5–1 g q12–24h	1–2 g	—[b]	Thrombophlebitis, allergic reactions, GI disturbance
B	q12h	q24h	q24h	Dose 3 × wk	—[b]	Allergic reactions, GI disturbance
B	q12–24h	50% dose q12–24h	50% dose q12–24h	—[b]	—[b]	Allergic reactions, GI disturbance

(continued)

Table 207.1 (continued)

| Name | | Usual Dose | | | Change in |
Generic	Brand	Adult	Child	Cost (per Day)*	Absorption with Food
Ceftazidime	Fortaz, Tazicef, Tazidime	1–2 g IV q8–12h	25–50 mg/kg IV q8h	$59.91 2 g q8h	n/a
Ceftibuten	Cedax	400 mg PO q12h	3–6 mg/kg PO q8h	$8.54	Increased
Ceftizoxime	Cefizox	1–3 g IV q6–8h	33–50 mg/kg IV q6–8h	$35.58–$66.09	n/a
Ceftriaxone	Rocephin	0.5–2 g IV q12–24h (neonate: 0–7 d, 50 mg/kg q24h; 1–4 wk, 50–75 mg/kg q24h)	50–100 mg/kg/d; divide IV q12–24h	$12.50 2 g q24h	n/a
Cefuroxime	Zinacef, Kefurox	0.75–1.5 g IV q8h	50–100 mg/kg/d divide IV q6–8h	$19.20–$40.32	n/a
Cefuroxime axetil	Ceftin	0.125–0.5 g PO q12h	0.125–0.25 g PO q12h	$4.86–$30.24	Decreased
Cephalexin	Keflex, Biocef, Keftab	0.25–1 g PO q6h	25–100 mg/kg/d; divide PO q6h	$2.76–$5.48	Unchanged
Cephalothin	Keflin	0.5–2 g IV q4–6h	80–160 mg/kg/d; divide IV q6h	$57.20	n/a
Cephapirin	Cefadyl	0.5–2 g IV q4–6h	40–80 mg/kg/d divide IV q6h	Data not available	n/a
Cephradine	Velosef	0.25–1 g PO q6h 0.5–2 g IV q4–6h	25–100 mg/kg/d; divide PO q6–12h 50–100 mg/kg divide IV q6h	$3.96–$7.76 PO IV: not available	Decreased
Chloramphenicol	Chloromycetin	0.25–0.75 g PO q6h 0.25–1 g IV q6h	50–100 mg/kg/d; divide q6h PO, IV	PO: Data not available IV: $10.00	Vitamins may increase absorption
Cinoxacin	Cinobac	0.25 g q6h, 0.5 g PO q12h	N.R.	$5.96	Delayed absorption and lower mean peak serum levels
Ciprofloxacin	Cipro	0.25–0.75 g PO q12h 0.2–0.4 g IV q12h	N.R.	$9.18–$11.64 PO $32.50–$62.50 IV	Decreased

Pregnancy Class[a]	Dose Interval Adjustment for Reduced CrCl			Supplemental Dose in Dialysis		Major Toxicity
	>50	10–50	≤10	HD	PD	
B	q8–12h	q12–24h	q24–48h	1 g load then 1 g pHD	0.5 g IV q24h or 250 mg/2 L dialysate	Thrombophlebitis, allergic reactions, GI disturbance
B	for CrCl 30: 400 mg q12–24h PO 12 For CrCl 5: 29–200 mg PO qd	for CrCl 30: 400 mg q24h PO 12 For CrCl 5: 29–200 mg PO qd	100 mg q24h	400 mg pHD		Seizures, anaphylaxis, TEN. Stevens–Johnson syndrome, erythema multiforme
B	q6–8h	0.25–1 g q12h	0.5 g q24h	Dose pHD	3 g q48h	Thrombophlebitis, allergic reactions, GI disturbance
B	q12–24h	q12–24h	q12–24h	None	—[b]	Thrombophlebitis, allergic reactions, GI disturbance, cholelithiasis
B	q8h	q8–12h	0.75 g q24h	0.75 g pHD	15 mg/kg pPD	Thrombophlebitis, allergic reactions, GI disturbance
B	q12h	q12h	0.25 g q24h	—[b]	—[b]	Allergic reactions, GI disturbance
B	q6h	q8–12h	q24–48h	0.25–1 g	—[b]	Allergic reactions, GI disturbance
B	q4–6h	1–1.5 g q6h	0.5 g q8h	0.5–2 g	Add up to 6 mg/kg to dialysate	Thrombophlebitis with IV infusion, allergic reactions, GI disturbance
B	q4–6h	q8h	q12h	7.5–15 mg/kg pHD then q12h	—[b]	Thrombophlebitis, allergic reactions, GI disturbance
B	q6h	0.5 g q6h	0.25 g q12h	0.25 g before HD, then 12, 36, and 48 h pHD	0.5 g q6h	Allergic reactions, GI disturbance
C	Usual	Usual	Usual	Dose pHD	Usual	Blood dyscrasias, gray baby syndrome, GI disturbance
C	q6h	0.25 g q12–24h	N.R.	—[b]	—[b]	Nausea, vomiting, dizziness, headache, tremors, confusion
C	q12h	0.25–0.5 g PO q12h, IV q12–24h	0.25–0.5 g PO q18h, IV q18–24h	0.25–0.5 g q24h, pHD on HD days	0.25–0.5 g q24h	Nausea, vomiting, dizziness, headache, tremors, confusion

(continued)

Table 207.1 *(continued)*

| Name | | Usual Dose | | Cost (per Day)* | Change in Absorption with Food |
Generic	Brand	Adult	Child		
Clarithromycin	Biaxin	0.25–0.5 g PO q12h	7.5 mg/kg q12h (n.a.)	$9.04	Increased or unchanged
Clindamycin	Cleocin	0.15–0.3 g PO q6h 0.3–0.9 g IV q6–8h	8–25 mg/kg/d; divide PO q6–8h 15–40 mg/kg/d; divide IV q6–8h (newborn: 0–7 d: 15 mg/kg/d q6–8h; 1–4 wk: 15–20 mg/kg/d q6–8h)	$4.76–$15.04 PO $26.24–$46.44 IV	Unchanged
Cloxacillin	Tegopen	0.5–1 g PO q6h	12.5–25 mg/kg PO q6h	$3.03	Decreased
Colistin		5–15 mg/kg/d PO q8h 2.5–5 mg/kg/d IV q6–12h	5–15 mg/kg/d; divide PO q8h 2.5–5 mg/kg/d; divide IV q6–12h	$4.00 IV	Not significantly absorbed orally
Dapsone		0.05–0.1 g PO q24h	1–2 mg/kg/d; divide q24h	$0.40	No effect
Daptomycin	Cubicin	4–6 mg/kg IV q24h	Not defined	$214.90	n/a
Dicloxacillin	Dynapen	0.25–0.5 g PO q6h	3.125–6.25 mg/kg PO q6h	$2.64–$4.80	Decreased
Doxycycline	Vibramycin	0.1 g PO, IV q12h	2.2 mg/kg PO, IV q12–24h	$1.04–$2.22 PO $29.50 IV	Decreased with milk, antacids
Enoxacin	Penetrex	0.4 g PO, IV q12h	N.R.	$3.58 PO	Decreased
Ertapenem	Invanz	1 g IM/IV qd	30 mg/kg/d IM/IV BID	$62.30	n/a
Erythromycin base	EryC, PCE, Emycin, Erytab	0.25–0.5 g PO q6h	30–50 mg/kg/d; divide q6h	$2.32 PO	Decreased

Pregnancy Class[a]	Dose Interval Adjustment for Reduced CrCl			Supplemental Dose in Dialysis		Major Toxicity
	>50	10–50	≤10	HD	PD	
B	q12h	q12–24h	q24h	—[b]	—[b]	GI disturbance, abnormal taste, headache
B	Usual	Usual	Usual	Usual	Usual	Diarrhea, including pseudomembranous colitis, allergic reactions
B	q6h	q6h	q6h	Usual	Usual	Allergic reactions (rare: anaphylactic), diarrhea, nausea, vomiting
Not established	q6–12h	2.5 mg/kg/d q12–24h	1.5 mg/kg q36h	—[b]	—[b]	Nephrotoxicity, CNS side effects including confusion, coma, seizures
C	q24h	q24h	q24h	—[b]	—[b]	Rash, headache, GI irritation, infectious monolike syndrome
B	4–6 mg/kg q24h	4–6 mg/kg q48h	4–6 mg/kg q48h	4–6 mg/kg q48h. Administer after dialysis session on dialysis days	4–6 mg/kg q48h	Arrhythmias, hypersensitivity rxn, anaphlyaxis, thrombocytopenia, myopathy
Not established	q6h	q6h	q6h	Usual	Usual	Allergic reactions (rare: anaphylactic), diarrhea, nausea, vomiting
D	q12h	q12h	q12h	Usual	Usual	GI disturbance, photosensitivity reactions, hepatic toxicity, esophageal ulcers
C	q12h	0.1–0.2 g q12h	0.1–0.2 g q12h	—[b]	—[b]	Nausea, vomiting, dizziness, headache, tremors, confusion
B	1 g IM/IV qd	CrCl ≤30: 500 mg qd	CrCl ≤30: 500 mg qd	30% of daily dose should be supplemented pHD	—[b]	Thrombocytopenia, increased LFTs, diarrhea, allergic reactions
B	q6h	q6h	q6h	Usual	Usual	GI disturbance; rare: allergic reactions, hepatic dysfunction, hearing loss

(continued)

Table 207.1 *(continued)*

| Name | | Usual Dose | | Cost (per Day)* | Change in Absorption with Food |
Generic	Brand	Adult	Child		
Erythromycin estolate	Ilosone	0.25–0.5 g PO q6h	3–50 mg/kg/d; divide q6h	$2.28	Decreased
Erythromycin ethyl succinate	EES, eryPed	0.4 g PO q8h	30–50 mg/kg/d divide PO q8h	$1.20	Increased
Erythromycin lactobionate	Erythrocin	0.5–1 g IV q6h	15–20 mg/kg/d; divide IV q6h	$14.80–$30.60 IV	n/a
Gentamicin[c]	Garamycin	3–5 mg/kg/d; divide IV q8h 4–8 mg/d IT	3–7.5 mg/kg/d; divide IV q8h (newborn: 0–7 d: 2.5 mg/kg q12h; 1–4 wk: 7.5 mg/kg/d q8h)	$5.18	n/a
Imipenem	Primaxin	0.5–1 g IV q6h	15–25 mg/kg IV q6h (n.a.) (neonate: 0–7 d: 25 mg/kg q12h; 1–4 wk 25 mg/kg q8h)	$83.40–$156.98	n/a
Kanamycin[c]	Kantrex	15 mg/kg/d; divide IV q8–12h	15 mg/kg/d; divide IV q8–12h (newborn: 0–7 d: 15–20 mg/kg/d q12h; 1–4 wk: 15 mg/kg/d q8–12h)	$1.31	n/a
Levofloxacin	Levaquin	0.25–0.75 g/d PO or IV	—[b]	$11.13–$23.90 PO $22.83–$60.59 IV	Unchanged
Lincomycin	Lincocin	0.5 g PO q6–8h 0.6–1 g IV q8–12h	30–60 mg/kg/d; divide PO q6–8h 10–20 mg/kg/d; divide IV q6h	$8.04 PO $36.57–$60.96 IV	Decreased
Linezolid	Zyvox	600 mg PO/IV q12h	>12 y 600 mg PO q12 0–11: 30 mg/kg PO/IV q8h	$154.68: PO $198.20 IV	Unchanged
Lomefloxacin	Maxaquin	0.4 g PO q24h	N.R.	$7.58	Decrease
Loracarbef	Lorabid	0.2–0.4 g PO q12–24h	15–30 mg/kg/d; q12h	$4.20–$6.38	Decreased
Meropenem	Merrem	0.5–1 g IV q8h	20–40 mg/kg IV q8h	$106.47–$212.94	n/a

Antimicrobial Therapy – General Considerations

Pregnancy Class[a]	Dose Interval Adjustment for Reduced CrCl			Supplemental Dose in Dialysis		Major Toxicity
	>50	10–50	≤10	HD	PD	
B	Usual	Usual	Usual	No change	No change	Cholestatic hepatitis, hearing loss or tinnitus, GI disturbance, hypersensitivity reactions
B	Usual	Usual	Usual	Usual	Usual	GI disturbance; rare: allergic reactions, hepatic dysfunction
B	Usual	Usual	Usual	Usual	Usual	GI disturbance; rare: allergic reactions, hepatic dysfunction, hearing loss
C	q8–12h	q12–48h	>48 h	1–1.7 mg/kg pHD	1 mg/2 L dialysate removed	Renal toxicity, vestibular and auditory toxicity, CNS reactions, neuromuscular blockade (rare)
C	q6h	0.5 g q8–12h	0.25–0.5 g q12h	0.25–0.5 pHD then q12h	—[b]	Fever, rash, nausea, vomiting, diarrhea, seizures (rare)
D	q8–12h	q12–48h	>48 h	4–5 mg/kg pHD	3.75 mg/kg/d	Cranial nerve VIII and renal damage
C	Usual	0.25 g q24–48h	0.25 g q48h	0.25 g q48h	0.25 g q48h	Diarrhea, nausea, headache
Not established	Usual	Usual	Usual	—[b]	—[b]	Diarrhea, including pseudomembranous colitis, allergic reactions
C	Usual	Usual	Usual	200 mg	—[b]	Leukopenia, pancytopenia, lactic acidosis, peripheral neuropathy, optic neuropathy
C	q24h	0.2 g q24h	0.2 g q24h	0.4 g load, then 0.2 g q24h	—[b]	Nausea, vomiting, dizziness, headache, tremors, confusion, photosensitivity
B	q12–24h	q24–48h	q3–5d	Dose pHD	—[b]	Allergic reactions, GI disturbance
B	0.5–1 g IV q8h	q12h	0.25–0.5 q24h	—[b]	—[b]	Nausea, diarrhea, vomiting, rash

(continued)

Table 207.1 *(continued)*

| Name | | Usual Dose | | Cost (per Day)* | Change in Absorption with Food |
Generic	Brand	Adult	Child		
Metronidazole	Flagyl	0.25–0.5 g PO q6–12h 0.5 g IV q6–8h	15 mg/kg/d; divide TID (n.a.)	$2.58–$2.92 PO $67.32 IV	Unchanged
Mezlocillin	Mezlin	3–4 g IV q4–6h	50 mg/kg IV q4–6h	$71.80 (4 g q6h)	n/a
Minocycline	Minocin, Dynacin	0.1 g PO, IV q12h	2 mg/kg PO, IV q12h	$6.80 PO $95.88 IV	Decreased with milk, antacids
Moxifloxacin	Avelox	400 mg PO/IV q24h	Not defined	$12.74 PO $43.75 IV	Absorption delayed
Nafcillin	Nallpen, Unipen	0.5–2 g IV q4–6h	150 mg/kg/d; divide IV q4–6h (neonate: 0–7 d; 25 mg/kg q8–12h; 1–4 wk: 25 mg/kg q6–8h)	$73.36 2 g q6h	Decreased (PO)
Neomycin	Neo-tabs	50 mg/kg/d; divide PO q6h	—[b]	$1.05 PO	Neomycin not significantly absorbed PO
Netilmycin[c]	Netromycin	4–6.5 mg/kg/d; divide IV q8–12h	3–7.5 mg/kg/d; divide IV q8–12h (newborn: 0–4 wk: 4–6.5 mg/kg/d q12h)	Data not available	n/a
Nitrofurantoin	Macrodantin, Macrobid	0.05–0.1 g PO q6h	5–7 mg/kg/d; divide q6h	$4.36–$7.44	Increased
Norfloxacin	Noroxin	0.4 g PO q12h	N.R.	$6.78	Decreased
Ofloxacin	Floxin	0.2–0.4 g PO, IV q12h	N.R.	$9.56–$12.00 PO $27.60–$55.20 IV	Decreased
Oxacillin	Bactocil	0.5–1 g IV q4–6h	37.5–50 mg/kg IV q6h (neonate: 0–7 d, 25 mg/kg q8–12h; 1–4 wk: 25 mg/kg q6–8h)	$2.10 PO $31.40 IV	Decreased

Pregnancy Class[a]	Dose Interval Adjustment for Reduced CrCl			Supplemental Dose in Dialysis		Major Toxicity
	>50	10–50	≤10	HD	PD	
B	Usual	Usual	Usual	Usual	Usual	Nausea, headache, metallic taste
B	q4–6h	q8h	q8h	2–3 g then 3–4 g q12h	3 g q12h	Allergic reactions (rare: anaphylactic), diarrhea, nausea, vomiting
D	q12h	q12h	q12h	Usual	Usual	GI disturbance, photosensitivity, hepatic toxicity, esophageal ulcers, vestibular toxicity; tooth discoloration
C	Usual	Usual	Usual	No change	No change	Anaphylaxis, phototoxicity, increased ICP, toxic psychosis
B	q4–6h	q4–6h	q4–6h	Usual	Usual	Allergic reactions (rare: anaphylactic), diarrhea, nausea, vomiting; platelet dysfunction with high doses
Not established	—[b]	—[b]	—[b]	—[b]	—[b]	Cranial nerve VIII and renal damage
D	q8–12h	q12–48h	>48 h	2 mg/kg pHD	—[b]	Renal toxicity, vestibular and auditory toxicity, CNS reactions, neuromuscular blockade (rare)
B	Usual	Avoid	Avoid	Avoid	Avoid	Rash, nausea/vomiting, pancreatitis, anemia, leukopenia, LFT elevation, neuropathy, urine discoloration
C	q12h	q24h	q24h	—[b]	—[b]	Nausea, vomiting, dizziness, headache, tremors, confusion
C	q12h	q24h	0.1–0.2 g q24h	0.2 g load; then 0.1 g q24h	—[b]	Nausea, vomiting, dizziness, headache, tremors, confusion
B	q4–6h	q4–6h	q4–6h	Usual	Usual	Allergic reactions (rare: anaphylactic), diarrhea, nausea, vomiting

(continued)

Table 207.1 *(continued)*

Name		Usual Dose			Change in Absorption with Food
Generic	Brand	Adult	Child	Cost (per Day)*	
Penicillin V	Pen–VeeK, Pen–V	0.25–0.5 g PO q6h	6.25–12.5 mg/kg PO q6h	$0.88–$1.48	Decreased
Penicillin G benzathine	Bicillin	600,000–2,400,000 U IM ×1	600,000 U IM ×1 (neonate: 1–4 wk: 50,000 U/kg IM ×1)	$101.76 2.4 million U	n/a
Penicillin G		0.5–1 g PO q6h 1–4 million U IV q4–6h	25,000–90,000 U/kg/d; divide q4–8h PO 25,000–400,000 U/kg/d; divide IV q4–6h (neonate: 0–7 d: 50,000–150,000 U/kg/d q8–12h; 1–4 wk: 75,000–200,000 U/kg/d q6–8h)	Data not available PO: $84.18 IV	Decreased
Piperacillin	Pipracil	3–4 g IV q4–6h	50 mg/kg IV q4–6h (n.a.)	$69.60 4 g q6h	n/a
Piperacillin–tazobactam	Zosyn	3.375 g IV q6–8h	90–112.5 mg/kg IV q8h	$78.60`	n/a
Polymyxin B	Aerosporin, Neosporin	15,000–25,000 U/kg/d IV q12h	15,000–25,000 U/kg/d IV q12h	$28.80	n/a
Procaine penicillin G	Wycillin	0.6–1.2 million U IM q12h	25,000–50,000 U/kg IM q12–24h	$39.58	n/a
Quinupristin–dalfopristin	Synercid	7.5 mg/kg IV q8h	—[b]	$453.75	n/a
Rifaximin	Xifaxan	200 mg PO TID	—[b]	$10.29	Unchanged
Sparfloxacin	Zagam	0.4 g PO ×1 d then 0.2 g/d	—[b]	$6.68	Unchanged
Spectinomycin	Trobicin	2 g IM qd	—[b]	$35.48	n/a
Streptomycin		0.5–1 g IV or IM q12h	20–40 mg/kg/d; divide IV or IM q6–12h	$18.20	n/a

Pregnancy Class[a]	Dose Interval Adjustment for Reduced CrCl			Supplemental Dose in Dialysis		Major Toxicity
	>50	10–50	≤10	HD	PD	
B	q6h	q6h	q6h	250 mg	—[b]	Allergic reactions (rare: anaphylactic), diarrhea, nausea, vomiting
B	Usual	Usual	Usual	Usual	Usual	Allergic reactions (rare: anaphylactic), diarrhea, nausea, vomiting
B	q4–6h	q4–6h	25%–50% of standard dose q4–6h	500,000 U	—[b]	Allergic reactions (rare: anaphylactic), diarrhea, nausea, vomiting
B	q4–6h	q6–8h	q8–12h	1 g pHD, then 2 g IV q8h	—[b]	Allergic reactions (rare: anaphylactic), diarrhea, nausea, vomiting; platelet dysfunction with high doses
B	q6–8h	2.25 g q6h	2.25 g q8h	—[b]	—[b]	Allergic reactions (rare: anaphylactic), diarrhea, nausea, vomiting
Not established	q12h	q12h	2250–3750 U/kg/d; divide q12h	—[b]	—[b]	Nephrotoxicity, flushing; CNS effects: confusion, seizures; allergic reactions
B	q12h	q12h	q12h	—[b]	—[b]	Allergic reactions (rare: anaphylactic), diarrhea, nausea, vomiting
—[b]	Usual	Usual	Usual	—[b]	—[b]	Pain at infusion site Thrombophlebitis, arthralgia, myalgia
C	—[b]	—[b]	—[b]	—[b]	—[b]	Headache, constipation, vomiting
C	Usual	0.2 g q48h	0.2 g q48h	—[b]	—[b]	Photosensitivity, diarrhea, nausea, headaches, cardiac arrhythmias in patients taking antiarrhythmic drugs
B	q24h	q24h	q24h	—[b]	—[b]	Pain at injection site, nausea, allergic reactions
D	q12h	7.5 mg/kg q24h	7.5 mg/kg q72–96h	0.5 g pHD	—[b]	Cranial nerve VIII damage, paresthesias, rash, fever, renal toxicity, neuromuscular blockade, optic neuritis

(continued)

Table 207.1 *(continued)*

Name		Usual Dose			Change in Absorption with Food
Generic	Brand	Adult	Child	Cost (per Day)*	
Sulfadiazine	Microsulfon	2–4 g/d; PO q4–8h	120–150 mg/kg/d; divide PO q4–6h	$12.64	Decreased
Sulfamethoxazole	Gantanol, Urobac	1 g PO q8–12h	50–60 mg/kg/d; divide PO q12h	$3.18	Decreased
Sulfisoxazole	Gantrisin	0.5–1 g PO q6h 25 mg/kg IV q6h	120–150 mg/kg/d; divide PO q4–6h	$4.16 PO	Decreased
Teichoplanin		0.2–0.4 g IV q24h	10 mg/kg IV q24h	Data not available	n/a
Telithromycin	Ketek	800 mg PO qd	—[b]	$9.38	Unchanged
Tetracycline	Achromycin	0.25–0.5 g PO q6h	25–50 mg/kg/d; divide q6–12h	$0.32–$0.48	Decreased with milk, antacids
Ticarcillin	Ticar	3 g q4–6h	50 mg/kg q4–6h (neonate: 0–7 d: 75 mg/kg q8–12h; 1–4 wk: 75 mg/kg q8h if <2 kg; 100 mg/kg q8h if >2 kg)	$77.28	n/a
Ticarcillin–clavulanate	Timentin	3.1 IV q4–8h	50 mg/kg IV q4–6h	$99.96	n/a
Tigecycline	Tygacil	100 mg IV ×1 then 50 mg IV q12h	—[b]	$118.76	n/a
Tobramycin[c]	Nebcin	3–5 mg/kg/d; divide IV q8h 4–8 IT mg/d	3–6 mg/kg/d; divide IV q8h (newborn: 0–7 d: ≤4 mg/kg/d q12h; 1–4 wk: 3–5 mg/kg/d q8h)	$27.30	n/a
Trimethoprim–sulfamethoxazole	Bactrim, Septra	0.16–0.8 g PO q12–24h 3–5 mg/kg IV q6–8h trimethoprim	6–12 mg/kg/d; divide q6–12h PO/IV	$1.32 PO $66.08 IV	Decreased
Trimethoprim	Proloprim	0.1 g PO q12h	4 mg/kg/d; divide PO q12h	$1.36	Decreased

Pregnancy Class[a]	Dose Interval Adjustment for Reduced CrCl			Supplemental Dose in Dialysis		Major Toxicity
	>50	10–50	≤10	HD	PD	
C	—[b]	—[b]	—[b]	—[b]	—[b]	Rash, photosensitivity, drug fever
C	—[b]	—[b]	—[b]	—[b]	—[b]	Rash, photosensitivity, drug fever
C	q6h	q8–12h	q12–24h	—[b]	—[b]	Rash, photosensitivity, drug fever
Not established	q24h	q48h	q72h	—[b]	—[b]	Ototoxicity
C	Usual	Usual	600 mg PO qd	Dose pHD	—[b]	QT prolongation, arrythmias, hepatotoxicity, visual disturbances
D	q6h	Use doxycycline	Use doxycycline	500 mg pHD	—[b]	GI disturbance, photosensitivity, hepatic toxicity, esophageal ulcers
B	q4–6h	q6–8h	2 g q12h	3 g pHD; then 2 g q12h	3 g q12h	Allergic reactions (rare: anaphylactic), diarrhea, nausea, vomiting
B	q4–6h	q6–8h	2 g IV q12h	3.1 g	3.1 g q12h	Allergic reactions (rare: anaphylactic), diarrhea, nausea, vomiting
D	Usual	Usual	Usual	Usual	—[b]	Tooth discoloration, pancreatitis, photosensitivity
D	q8–12h	q12–48h	>48 h	1 mg/kg pHD	1 mg/2 L dialysate removed	Renal toxicity, vestibular and auditory toxicity, CNS reactions, neuromuscular blockade (rare)
C	q6–12h	q24h	Avoid	4–5 mg/kg pHD	0.16–0.8 g q48h	Rash, nausea, vomiting
C	q12h	q18–24h	Avoid	—[b]	—[b]	Nausea, vomiting

(continued)

Table 207.1 *(continued)*

| Name | | Usual Dose | | Cost (per Day)* | Change in Absorption with Food |
Generic	Brand	Adult	Child		
Trovafloxacin	Trovan	0.2–0.2 g/d PO 0.2–0.3 g/d IV	—[b]	$6.39 PO $60.45 IV	Unchanged
Vancomycin	Vancocin	0.5–2 g PO q6–8h 1 g IV q12h 5–10 mg IT: q48–72h	40 mg/kg/d; divide PO q6–8h 40 mg/kg/d; divide IV q6–12h (newborn: 0–7 d: 15 mg/kg load, then 10 mg/kg q12h; 1–4 wk: 10 mg/kg q8h	$32.50 IV $38.56 oral solution $130.87 pulvules	Not absorbed

Abbreviations: CrCl = creatinine clearance (mL/min); HD = hemodialysis; PD = peritoneal dialysis; CNS = central nervous aminotransferase; N.R. = not recommended; IT = intrathecal; TEN = toxic epidermal necrolysis; RXN = reaction; P = post;
[a] Food and Drug Administration pregnancy categories: A = adequate studies in pregnant women, no risk; B = animal studies inadequate but benefit may exceed risk; D = evidence of human risk, benefit may outweigh risk; X = fetal
[b] Insufficient information available to make a recommendation.
[c] Aminoglycoside dosing may be modified after obtaining serum levels. The generally desired peak and trough concentrations trough ≤2 µg/mL; for amikacin and kanamycin, peak 15–30 µg/mL, trough ≤5–10 µg/mL. With once-daily administration amikacin, kanamycin and streptomycin, and desired serum levels are as follows: for gentamicin and tobramycin, peak streptomycin, peak 56–64 µg/mL, trough ≤1 µg/mL. The dose is infused over 60 minutes to avoid neuromuscular blockade.
* Fleming, T. 2007 Red Book, 2007.

Pregnancy Class[a]	Dose Interval Adjustment for Reduced CrCl			Supplemental Dose in Dialysis		Major Toxicity
	>50	10–50	≤10	HD	PD	
C	Usual	Usual	Usual	—[b]	—[b]	Hepatotoxicity, including severe liver failure, dizziness, nausea, headache
B	Levels vary; use serum assays and manufacturer's nomogram to guide dosage	Levels vary; use serum assays and manufacturer's nomogram to guide dosage	Levels vary; use serum assays and manufacturer's nomogram to guide dosage	None needed	None needed	Thrombophlebitis, fever, Chills, rash, cranial nerve VIII toxicity

system; GI = gastrointestinal; pHD = posthemodialysis; n/a = not approved; AST = aspartate aminotransferase; ALT = alanine LFT = liver function tests.

studies no risk, human studies inadequate, or animal toxicity, human studies no risk; C = animal studies show toxicity, human abnormalities in humans, risk exceeds benefit.

are as follows: for gentamicin and tobramycin, peak 6–12 μg/mL and trough ≤2 μg/mL; for netilmicin, peak 6–10 μg/mL, of aminoglycosides, doses are 5–7 mg/kg q24h for gentamicin and tobramycin, 6.5 mg/kg for netilmycin and 15 mg/kg q24h for 16–24 μg/mL, trough ≤1 μg/mL; for netilmicin, peak 22–30 μg/mL, trough ≤1 μg/mL; for amikacin and kanamycin and

Table 207.2 Antimycobacterial Agents

Name		Usual Dose		Cost (per Day)*	Change in Absorption with Food
Generic	Brand	Adult	Child		
Capreomycin	Capastat	1 g IM q24h	10–20 mg/kg q24h (n.a.)	$26.60	Unknown
Clofazimine	Lamprene	0.1 g PO q24h	—[b]	$0.42	Increased
Cycloserine	Seromycin	0.25–0.5 g PO q12h	10–20 mg/kg q12h (n.a.)	$8.38–$16.76	Decreased
Ethambutol	Myambutol	15–25 mg/kg PO q24h	10–15 mg/kg q24h (N.R.)	$4.76–$8.34	Unchanged
Ethionamide	Trecator	0.25–0.5 g PO q12h	15–20 mg/kg q24h (n.a.)	$7.10–$14.20	No data
INH + RIF + PZA	Rifater	6 tabs/d		$15.18	Decreased
INH + RIF	Rifamate	2 tabs/d		$6.84	Decreased
Isoniazid		0.3 g PO, IM q24h	10–20 mg/kg/d; divide PO, IM q12–24h	$0.14 PO $74.70 IM	Decreased
Paraamino salicylic acid	PAS	150 mg/kg q6–12h	150–360 mg/kg/d; divide q6–8h	Data not available	Decreased but advised
Pyrazinamide	15–30 mg/kg PO q24h	30 mg/kg/d; divide q12–24h (n.a.)		$2.26–$4.52	No data
Rifabutin (ansamycin)	Mycobutin	0.3 g PO q24h	—[b]	$16.65	Unchanged
Rifampin	Rifadin, Rimactane	0.6 g PO, IV q24h	10–20 mg/kg/d; divide PO, IV q12–24h	$3.86 PO $114.91 IV	Decreased
Rifapentine	Priftin	4 tabs 2×/wk	—[b]	$4.23	Increased
Streptomycin		1 g IM q24h	20–40 mg/kg IM q24h	$9.10	n/a

Abbreviations: CrCl = Creatinine clearance mL/min; HD = hemodialysis; PD = peritoneal dialysis; CNS = central nervous INH = isoniazid; PZA = Pyrazinamide; RIF = rifampin; pHD = post hemodialysis; pPD = post peritoneal dialysis.
[a] Food and Drug Administration pregnancy categories: A = adequate studies in pregnant women, no risk; B = animal studies studies inadequate but benefit may exceed risk; D, evidence of human risk, benefit may outweigh risk; X = fetal
[b] Insufficient information available to make a recommendation.
* Fleming, T. 2007 Red Book, 2007.

Pregnancy Class[a]	Dose Interval Adjustment for Reduced CrCl			Supplemental Dose in Dialysis		Major Toxicity
	>50	10–50	≤10	HD	PD	
C	q24h	7.5 mg/kg q24–48h	7.5 mg/kg 2×/wk	—[b]	—[b]	Renal and cranial nerve VIII toxicity, hypokalemia, sterile abscesses at injection site
C	q24h	q24h	q24h	—[b]	—[b]	Hyperpigmentation, ichthyosis, dry eyes, GI disturbance
C	q12h	q24h	0.25 g q24h	—[b]	—[b]	Anxiety, depression, confusion, hallucinations, headache, peripheral neuropathy
B	q24h	q24–36h	q48h	15 mg/kg/d pHD	15 mg/kg/d	Optic neuritis, allergic reactions, GI disturbance, acute gout
C	q12h	q12h	5 mg/kg q24h	—[b]	—[b]	GI disturbance, liver toxicity, CNS disturbance
As with individual drugs	q24h	q24h	Avoid	—[b]	—[b]	As with individual drugs
As with individual drugs	q24h	q24h	Avoid	—[b]	—[b]	As with individual drugs
C	q24h	q24h	½ dose in slow acetylators	5 mg/kg pHD	Daily dose pPD	Peripheral neuropathy, liver toxicity (possibly fatal), glossitis, GI disturbance, fever
C	—[b]	—[b]	—[b]	—[b]	—[b]	GI disturbance
C	q24h	q24h	12–20 mg/kg q24h	—[b]	—[b]	Arthralgia, hyperuricemia, liver toxicity, GI disturbance, rash
C	—[b]	—[b]	—[b]	—[b]	—[b]	Uveitis, orange discoloration of urine, sweat, tears; liver toxicity, GI disturbance
B	q24h	q24h	q24h	—[b]	—[b]	Orange discoloration of urine, sweat, tears; liver toxicity, GI disturbance, flulike syndrome
C	—[b]	—[b]	—[b]	—[b]	—[b]	Similar to rifampin
D	q24h	q24–72h	q72–96h	0.5 g pHD	—[b]	Vestibular nerve damage, paresthesias, rash, fever, pruritus, renal toxicity

system; GI = gastrointestinal; pHD = posthemodialysis; n.a. = not approved; N.R. = not recommended; IT = intrathecal;

no risk, human studies inadequate, or animal toxicity, human studies no risk; C = animal studies show toxicity, human abnormalities in humans, risk exceeds benefit.

Table 207.3 Antifungal Agents

| Name | | Usual Dose | | | Change in |
Generic	Brand	Adult	Child	Cost (per Day)*	Absorption with Food
Amphotericin B	Fungizone	0.25–1 mg/kg IV q24h	0.25–1 mg/kg IV q24–48h	$27.30	n/a
Amphotericin B lipid complex	Abelcet	5 mg/kg IV q24h	5 mg/kg IV q24h	$854.66	n/a
Amphotericin B liposomal	AmBisome	3–5 g/kg IV q24h	3–5 g/kg IV q24h	$1373.75	n/a
Amphotericin B cholesteryl sulfate complex	Amphotec	3–4 g/kg q24h	3–4 g/kg q24h	$480.00	n/a
Anidulafungin	Eraxis	100 mg IV q24h	No data	$225.00	n/a
Caspofungin	Cancidas	50 mg IV q12h	No data	$411.84	n/a
Clotrimazole	Mycelex	10 mg PO 5×/d	—[b]	$7.30	Not absorbed
Fluconazole	Diflucan	0.05–0.4 g PO, IV q24h	3–6 mg/kg qd (n.a.)	$5.62–$28.80 PO $31.86–$186.26 IV	Unchanged
Flucytosine	Ancobon	50–150 mg/kg/d; divide PO q6h	50–150 mg/kg/d; divide PO q6h	$81.06–$243.18	Decreased
Griseofulvin	Grisactin, Grifulvin, Fulvicin	0.5–1 g PO q24h	15 mg/kg/d PO q24h	$3.20	Increased
Itraconazole	Sporanox	0.2–0.4 g PO q24h 0.2 g PO q12h	—[b]	$18.56–$37.12 PO $498.60 IV	Increased

Pregnancy Class[a]	Dose Interval Adjustment for Reduced CrCl			Supplemental Dose in Dialysis		Major Toxicity
	>50	10–50	≤10	HD	PD	
B	q24h	q24h	q24h	Usual	Usual	Fever, chills, nausea with infusion; renal insufficiency, anemia
B	—[b]	—[b]	—[b]	—[b]	—[b]	Fever, chills, renal insufficiency (less than non-liposomal amphotericin)
B	—[b]	—[b]	—[b]	—[b]	—[b]	Fever, chills, renal insufficiency (less than non-liposomal amphotericin)
B	—[b]	—[b]	—[b]	—[b]	—[b]	Fever, chills, renal insufficiency (less than nonliposomal amphotericin)
C	No adjustment	No adjustment	No adjustment	—[b]	—[b]	Diarrhea, infusion site reaction, hypokalemia
C	No adjustment	No adjustment	No adjustment	No adjustment	No adjustment	Infusion site reaction, headache, nausea
C	—[b]	—[b]	—[b]	—[b]	—[b]	Contact dermatitis, erythema, burning, stinging, pruritius, urticaria, edema
C	q24h	50% dose q24h	25% dose q24h	—[b]	—[b]	Nausea, vomiting, rash, elevated liver enzymes
C	q6h	q12–24h	15–25 mg/kg q24h	20–37.5 mg/kg pHD	—[b]	Leukopenia
C	q24h	q24h	q24h	—[b]	—[b]	GI disturbance, allergic and photosensitivity reactions, blood dyscrasias, liver toxicity, exacerbation of SLE and leprosy
C	q12–24h	—[b]	—[b]	—[b]	—[b]	Nausea, rash, headache, edema, hypokalemia, hepatotoxicity

(continued)

Table 207.3 (continued)

| Name | | Usual Dose | | | Change in Absorption with |
Generic	Brand	Adult	Child	Cost (per Day)*	Food
Ketoconazole	Nizoral	0.2–0.4 g PO q12–24h	5–10 mg/kg/d; divide PO q12–24h	$3.14–$12.56	Increased
Micafungin	Mycamine	50 mg IV qd	No data	$116.88	n/a
Miconazole	Monistat	0.4–1.2 g IV q8h	20–40 mg/kg/d; divide IV q8h	Data not available (IV)	n/a
Nystatin	Mycostatin	400,000–1,000,000 U PO q8h	400,000–600,000 U PO q6h	$6.68 (20 mL)	Not absorbed
Posaconazole	Noxafil	200 mg PO TID	200 mg PO TID	$75.00	Increased
Voriconazole	Vfend	4 mg/kg IV q12h	4 mg/kg IV q12h 200 mg PO q12h	$380.10 IV $81.23 PO	n/a (IV) Decreased (PO)

Abbreviations: CrCl = Creatinine clearance mL/min; HD = hemodialysis; PD = peritoneal dialysis; CNS = central nervous
[a] Food and Drug Administration pregnancy categories: A = adequate studies in pregnant women, no risk; B = animal studies inadequate but benefit may exceed risk; D = evidence of human risk, benefit may outweigh risk; X = fetal abnormalities
[b] Insufficient information available to make a recommendation.
* Fleming T. 2007 Red Book, 2007.

Pregnancy Class[a]	Dose Interval Adjustment for Reduced CrCl			Supplemental Dose in Dialysis		Major Toxicity
	>50	10–50	≤10	HD	PD	
C	q12–24h	Usual	Usual	Usual	Usual	Nausea, vomiting, gynecomastia, decreased testosterone synthesis, rash, hepatotoxicity, adrenal insufficiency
C	q24h	No adjustment	No adjustment	—[b]	—[b]	Thrombophlebitis, rash, headache, leukopenia
C	q8h	q8h	q8h	—[b]	—[b]	Phlebitis, thrombocytosis, pruritus, rash, blurred vision, anaphylaxis (rare)
C	q8h	q8h	q8h	—[b]	—[b]	GI disturbance, allergic reactions
C	TID	No adjustment	No adjustment	—[b]	—[b]	Fever, nausea, vomiting, diarrhea, QT prolongation, hyperbilirubinemia (rare)
D	q12h	IV: Avoid use PO: No adjustment	IV: Avoid use PO: No adjustment	—[b]	—[b]	Abnormal vision, rash, torsades de pointes (rare)

system; GI = gastrointestinal; pHD = posthemodialysis; n.a. = not approved; SLE = systemic lupus erythematosus.
studies no risk, human studies inadequate, or animal toxicity, human studies no risk; C = animal studies show toxicity, human
in humans, risk exceeds benefit.

Table 207.4 Antiviral Agents

Name		Usual Dose		Cost (per Day)*	Change in Absorption with Food
Generic	Brand	Adult	Child		
Abacavir	Ziagen	0.3 g PO q12h	8 mg/kg PO q12h	$20.74	Unchanged
Acyclovir	Zovirax	0.2–0.8 g PO 2–5×/d 5–12 mg/kg IV q8h	0.2 g 5×/d (HSV) PO 20 mg/kg PO q6h, max 800 mg q6h (VZV) 25–50 mg/kg/d IV q8h	$4.90 PO (200 mg) $18.35 (800 mg) $14.00 IV (10 mg/kg/dose)	Unchanged
Amantadine	Symmetrel	0.1 g PO q12h	2.2–4.4 mg/kg PO q12h	$0.62	No data
Amprenavir	Agenerase	1.2 g PO q12h	—b	$25.76	Decreased with high-fat meal
Atazanavir	Reyataz	100–400 mg PO qd	—b	$9.65	Increased.
Cidofovir	Vistide	5 mg/kg IV q wk ×2 wk, then 5 mg/kg q2wk	—b	$126.86	n/a
Darunavir	Prezista	600 mg PO BID with 100 mg PO Ritonavir	—b	$32.50	Increased
Didanosine	Videx	0.167–0.2 g PO q12h	0.143–0.248 mg/m² divided PO q12h	$12.84	Decreased
Efavirenz	Sustiva	0.6 g PO qhs	—b	$18.44	Unchanged
Emtricitabine	Emtriva	200 mg PO qd	6 mg/kg PO sol qd (3 mo–17 y)	$12.81	Unchanged
Enfuvirtide	Fuzeon	90 mg SC BID	2 mg/kg SC BID	$85.09	n/a
Entecavir	Baraclude	0.5–1 mg PO qd	>16 y 0.5–1 mg PO qd	$26.68–$53.36	Decreased
Famciclovir	Famvir	0.125 g PO q12h (HSV) 0.5 g PO q8h (VZV)	—b	$6.76 HSV $33.79 VZV	Unchanged
Fosamprenavir	Lexiva	700–1400 mg PO BID	—b	$24.42–$48.44	Unchanged
Foscarnet	Foscavir	60 mg/kg IV q8h ×14–21 d; then 90 mg/kg/d	—b	$2228.94	n/a
Ganciclovir	Cytovene	5 mg/kg IV q12h ×14–21 d; then 5 mg/kg/d	5 mg/kg IV q12h	$87.01 IV	IV: n/a

Pregnancy Class[a]	Dose Interval Adjustment for Reduced CrCl			Supplemental Dose in Dialysis		Major Toxicity
	>50	10–50	≤10	HD	PD	
—[b]	—[b]	—[b]	—[b]	—[b]	—[b]	Nausea, hypersensitivity reaction with myalgias, fever, rash; anaphylaxis
C	2–5×/d PO IV q8h	2–5×/d PO IV q12–24h	0.2–0.8 g PO q24h 2.5–6 mg/kg IV q24h	0.5 g PO pHD	2–5 mg/kg/d	Headache, rash, renal toxicity, CNS symptoms (rare)
C	q12h	0.1–0.2 g 2–3×/wk	0.1–0.2 g qwk	—[b]	—[b]	Livedo reticularis, edema, insomnia, dizziness, lethargy
—[b]	Usual	Usual	Usual	Usual	Usual	Nausea, diarrhea, rash
B	—[b]	—[b]	—[b]	—[b]	—[b]	Hyperbilirubinemia, rash
C	Check prescribing information	Check prescribing information	Check prescribing information	—[b]	—[b]	Proteinuria, renal insufficiency, neutropenia
B	Usual	Usual	Usual	No supplement	No supplement	Erythema multiforme, neutropenia
B	q12h	q12–24h	100 mg PO q24h	Dose pHD	—[b]	Diarrhea, nausea, vomiting, pancreatitis, peripheral neuropathy
C	Usual	Usual	Usual	Usual	Usual	Drowsiness, CNS side effects, rash
B	Usual	q48–72h	q96h	Give dose after dialysis session on HD days	—[b]	Lactic acidosis, hepatotoxicity, neutropenia
B	Usual	Usual	—[b]	—[b]	—[b]	Injection site reactions, hypersensitivity rxn
C	Usual	0.25 mg–0.15 mg PO qd	0.05 mg PO qd	0.05 mg pHD	0.05 mg P capd	Lactic acidosis, elevated transaminases
B	0.5 g q8h 0.125 g q12h	0.5 g q12–24h; 0.125 g q12–24h	0.25 g q48h 0.125 g q48h	Dose pHD	ND	Headache, nausea
C	—[b]	—[b]	—[b]	—[b]	—[b]	Diarrhea, rash, nausea, hemolytic anemia (rare)
C	63–90 mg/kg/d maintenance	78–63 mg/kg/d maintenance	—[b]	—[b]	—[b]	Renal dysfunction, anemia, nausea, disturbances of calcium, magnesium, phosphorus, potassium metabolism
C	q12h	2.5 mg/kg q24h	1.25 mg/kg q24h	1.25 mg/kg pHD	—[b]	Neutropenia, thrombocytopenia

(continued)

Table 207.4 *(continued)*

Name		Usual Dose		Cost (per Day)*	Change in Absorption with Food
Generic	**Brand**	**Adult**	**Child**		
Indinavir	Crixivan	800 mg PO q8h	—[b]	$16.50	Decreased
Lamivudine	Epivir	150 mg PO q12h	4 mg/kg PO q12h	$12.86	Unchanged
Lopinavir/ ritonavir	Kaletra	400/100 mg PO BID	12 mg/3 mg/kg PO BID 6 mo–12 yr	$27.60	Increased
Nelfinavir	Viracept	0.75 g PO TID or 1.25 g PO q12h	0.2–0.3 mg/kg q8h	$7.57–$25.24	Increased
Nevirapine	Viramune	200 mg PO q24h ×14 d, then 200 mg PO q12h	—[b]	$12.02	Unchanged
Oseltamivir	Tamiflu	75 mg PO BID ×5 d	—[b]	$16.84	—[b]
Ribavirin	Copegus, Rebetol, Virazole	12–18 h/d ×3 d via aerosol, 0.4–0.6 g PO q12h, IV investigational	12–22 h/d × 6 d via aerosol	$34.88–$52.32 PO	—[b]
Rimantadine	Flumadine	0.1 g PO q12h	—[b]	$5.46	Unchanged
Ritonavir	Norvir	600 mg PO q12h	—[b]	$128.64	Unchanged
Saquinavir hard gel	Invirase	1.0 g PO q12h with 0.2 g PO ritonavir		$12.16	Increased
Saquinavir soft gel	Fortovase	1.2 g PO TID		$26.34	Increased
Stavudine	Zerit	0.04 g PO q12h	—[b]	$14.25	Unchanged
Telbivudine	Tyzeka	600 mg PO qd	>16 yr 600 mg PO qd	$20.29	Unchanged
Tenofovir	Viread	300 mg PO qd	—[b]	$20.10	Increased
Tipranavir	Aptivus	500 mg PO BID with 200 mg PO Ritonavir	—[b]	$37.25	Unchanged
Valacyclovir	Valtrex	1 g PO TID (VZV); 0.5 g PO BID (HSV)	Unchanged	$34.86 VZV $12.64 HSV	No effect

Pregnancy Class[a]	Dose Interval Adjustment for Reduced CrCl			Supplemental Dose in Dialysis		Major Toxicity
	>50	10-50	≤10	HD	PD	
C	—[b]	—[b]	—[b]	—[b]	—[b]	Nephrolithiasis, nausea, headache
C	150 mg PO q12h	100–150 g PO qd	25–50 mg PO qd	—[b]	—[b]	Headache, nausea, neutropenia, increased AST, and ALT
C	—[b]	—[b]	—[b]	—[b]	—[b]	Diarrhea, dyslipidemia, LFT elevation
B	Usual	Usual	Usual	Usual	Usual	Diarrhea, nausea
B	—[b]	—[b]	—[b]	—[b]	—[b]	Rash, including Stevens–Johnson syndrome; hepatotoxicity
—[b]	—[b]	—[b]	—[b]	—[b]	—[b]	Nausea, vomiting, headache
X	—[b]	—[b]	—[b]	—[b]	—[b]	Anemia, headache, hyperbilirubinemia, bronchospasm
C	q12h	q12h	q12h	—[b]	—[b]	Fewer CNS side effects than amantadine
B	Usual	Usual	Usual	Usual	Usual	Nausea, vomiting, diarrhea
B	Usual	Usual	Usual	Usual	Usual	Diarrhea, nausea
B	Usual	Usual	Usual	Usual	Usual	Diarrhea, nausea, headache
C	—[b]	—[b]	—[b]	—[b]	—[b]	Peripheral neuropathy, liver toxicity
B	Usual	q48h	q72h	q96h: give after the end of the dialysis session on dialysis days	—[b]	Lactic acidosis, myopathy, elevated CPK, elevated LFTs
B	Usual	q48h	Twice weekly	—[b]	pHD q 7d	Lactic acidosis, nephrotoxicity
C	Usual	Usual	Usual	Usual	—[b]	Diarrhea, hepatotoxicity, Hyperlipidemia, bleeding
B	Usual	12–24h	0.5 g q24h	0.5 g q24h	0.5 g q24h	Nausea, headache; thrombotic thrombocytopenic purpura in immunocompromised patients.

(continued)

Table 207.4 *(continued)*

Name		Usual Dose		Cost (per Day)*	Change in Absorption with Food
Generic	Brand	Adult	Child		
Valganciclovir	Valcyte	900 mg PO q12h × 21 d, then 900 mg PO q24h	—[b]	$160.17	Increased
Vidarabine	Vira-A	10–15 mg/kg/d IV over 12 h	10–15 mg/kg/day IV over 12 h	$3.86	n/a
Zalcitabine	Hivid	0.375–0.75 g PO q8h	0.75 g PO q8h (children >13 y)	$6.81–$8.53	Decreased
Zanamivir	Relenza	10 mg BID in half ×50	—[b]	$13.44	—[b]
Zidovudine	Retrovir	0.1 g PO q4h or 0.2 g PO q8h 1–2 mg/kg IV q4h	180 mg/m² PO q6h	$12.12 PO $27.10 IV	Decreased

Abbreviations: CrCl = Creatinine clearance mL/min; HD = hemodialysis; PD = peritoneal dialysis; CNS = central nervous aminotransferase; N.R. = not recommended; HSV = herpes simplex virus; VZV = varicella-zoster virus; LFT = liver function test;
[a] Food and Drug Administration pregnancy categories: A = adequate studies in pregnant women, no risk; B = animal studies inadequate but benefit may exceed risk; D = evidence of human risk, benefit may outweigh risk; X = fetal abnormalities
[b] Insufficient information available to make a recommendation.
* Fleming T. The Red Book, 2007.

Pregnancy Class[a]	Dose Interval Adjustment for Reduced CrCl			Supplemental Dose in Dialysis		Major Toxicity
	>50	10-50	≤10	HD	PD	
C	Usual	0.45 g q12–48h	N.R.	N.R.	N.R.	Neutropenia, thrombocytopenia
Not established	Usual	Usual	10 mg/kg/d over 12 h	Usual dose pHD	—[b]	GI disturbance, nausea, vomiting, thrombophlebitis
C	q8h	q12h	q24h	—[b]	—[b]	Peripheral neuropathy, stomatitis, esophageal ulcers, pancreatitis
—[b]	—[b]	—[b]	—[b]	—[b]	—[b]	Nasal and throat discomfort, headache and cough
C	q4h	q6h	q6–12h	100 mg pHD	100 mg q6–12h	Anemia, granulocytopenia, headache, nausea, insomnia, nail pigment changes

system; GI = gastrointestinal; pHD = posthemodialysis; n.a. = not approved; AST = aspartate aminotransferase; ALT = alanine rxn = reaction; capd = continuous ambulatory peritoneal dialysis; CPK = creatine phosphokinase.
studies no risk, human studies inadequate, or animal toxicity, human studies no risk; C = animal studies show toxicity, human in humans, risk exceeds benefit.

Table 207.5 Antiparasitic Agents

Name		Usual Dose		Cost (per Day)*	Change in Absorption with Food
Generic	Brand	Adult	Child		
Albendazole	Albenza	15 mg/kg/d PO	—[b]	$8.23	Increased
Artemisinin[e]		10 mg/kg/d ×5d	Same as adult	Data not available	—[b]
Atovoquone	Mepron	750 mg PO BID	—[b]	$40.90	Increased
Benznidazole[e]		5 mg/kg PO BID 1–4 mo	—[b]	Data not available	—[b]
Bithionol[d]	Bitin	30–50 mg/kg on alternate days ×10–15 d	Same as adult	Data not available	—[b]
Chloroquine HCL	Aralen HCL	300 mg PO qwk (prophylaxis) 600 mg PO, then 300 mg after 6, 24, 48 h 200 mg IM q6h (treatment)	5 mg/kg qwk PO (for prophylaxis) 10 mg/kg, then 5 mg/kg, same intervals as adult (treatment) IM treatment not recommended	$82.88 IM	Increased
Chloroquine phosphate	Aralen phosphate	500 mg PO qwk (prophylaxis) 1 g, then 500 mg after 6, 24, 48 h (treatment)	8.3 mg/kg qwk PO (prophylaxis)	$7.47 PO	Increased
Dehydroemetine[d]		1–1.5 mg/kg/d IM (maximum dose 90 mg)	1–1.5 mg/kg IM qd, divided in 2 doses	Data not available	—[b]
Diethyl carbamazine[d]	Hetrazan	Day 1: 50 mg PO Day 2: 50 mg TID Day 3: 50 mg TID Days 4–21: 6 mg/kg/d divided TID	Day 1: 1 mg/kg PO Day 2: 1 mg/kg TID Day 3: 1–2 mg/kg TID Days 4–21: 6 mg/kg/d divided TID	Available from manufacturer without charge for compassionate use only	—[b]
Diloxanide furoate[e]	Furamide	500 mg TID × 10d	20 mg/kg/d divided TID × 10 d	Data not available	—[b]
Eflornithine[e]	Ornidyl	400 mg/kg/d IV divided QID × 14 d then 300 mg/kg/d PO ×3–4 wk	—[b]	Data not available	—[b]

Pregnancy Class[a]	Dose Interval Adjustment for Reduced CrCl			Supplemental Dose in Dialysis		Major Toxicity
	>50	10–50	≤10	HD	PD	
Not established	—[b]	—[b]	—[b]	—[b]	—[b]	Diarrhea, abdominal discomfort, elevated AST, ALT and bone marrow suppression, alopecia with high dose
Not established	—[b]	—[b]	—[b]	—[b]	—[b]	Transient heart block, elevated AST and ALT, neutropenia, decreased reticulocyte count, abdominal pain, diarrhea, fever
C	—[b]	—[b]	—[b]	—[b]	—[b]	Rash, GI disturbance, fever, headache
Not established	—[b]	—[b]	—[b]	—[b]	—[b]	Peripheral neuropathy, rash, bone marrow suppression
Not established	—[b]	—[b]	—[b]	—[b]	—[b]	Hypotension, wheezing, angioedema, rash, hyperthermia, diarrhea, anorexia, nausea, vomiting, dizziness, headache
C	—[b]	—[b]	—[b]	—[b]	—[b]	Blurred vision (retinopathy with prolonged use), GI effects, pruritus, hemolysis in patients with G6PD deficiency
C	—[b]	—[b]	—[b]	—[b]	—[b]	Blurred vision (retinopathy with prolonged use), GI effects, pruritus, hemolysis in patients with G6PD deficiency
Not established	—[b]	—[b]	—[b]	—[b]	—[b]	Diarrhea, nausea, vomiting, cardiac arrhythmias, tachycardia
Not established	—[b]	—[b]	—[b]	—[b]	—[b]	Headache, malaise, arthralgia, nausea, vomiting, anorexia, pruritus, fever, hypotension, lymphadenitis, encephalopathy
Not established	—[b]	—[b]	—[b]	—[b]	—[b]	Flatulence
Not established	—[b]	—[b]	—[b]	—[b]	—[b]	Anemia, thrombocytopenia, leukopenia, nausea, vomiting, diarrhea, transient hearing loss

(continued)

Table 207.5 (continued)

| Name | | Usual Dose | | | Change in |
Generic	Brand	Adult	Child	Cost (per Day)*	Absorption with Food
Furazolidone	Furoxone	100 mg PO q6h	25–50 mg PO q6h	$10.32	—[b]
Halofantrine	Halfan	500 mg PO q6h ×3, repeat in 1 wk	8 mg/kg PO q6h ×3 (patient ≤40 kg), repeat in 1 wk	Data not available	Increased
Hydroxy-chloroquine	Plaquenil	400 mg PO qwk (prophylaxis) 800 mg, then 400 mg after 6, 24, 48 h (treatment)	5 mg/kg PO qwk (prophylaxis) 10 mg/kg, then 5 mg/kg at same intervals as adult (treatment)	$9.36 (2–day treatment course)	—[b]
Iodoquinol	Yodoxin, Diquinol	650 mg PO TID	30–40 mg/kg/d; divide PO TID	$3.63	Minimally absorbed
Ivermectin	Stromectol	200 μg/kg	—[b]	$27.20	Decreased
Mebendazole	Vermox	100 mg PO BID depending on infection being treated	Same as adults	$10.64	Minimally absorbed
Mefloquine	Lariam	250 mg/wk (prophylaxis) 1250 mg ×1 (treatment)	25 mg/kg PO qwk (prophylaxis)	$12.93 prophylaxis $64.66 treatment	Increased
Meglumine antimonate[e]	Glucantine	20 mg/kg IV ×2 d (850 mg/d limit)	—[b]	Data not available	n/a
Melarsoprol B[d]	Mel B, Arsobal	1.2 mg/kg IV TID × 3 d; repeat qwk ×2 wk	—[b]	Data not available	n/a
Niclosamide	Niclocide	2 g PO qd	0.5–1.5 g/d PO	Data not available	Not absorbed
Nifurtimox[d]	Lampit	3 mg/kg PO TID ×3 mo	—[b]	Data not available	—[b]
Niridazole[e]	Ambilhar	—[b]	—[b]	Data not available	—[b]

Pregnancy Class[a]	Dose Interval Adjustment for Reduced CrCl			Supplemental Dose in Dialysis		Major Toxicity
	>50	10–50	≤10	HD	PD	
Not established	—[b]	—[b]	—[b]	—[b]	—[b]	Nausea, vomiting, rash, fever, headache, hemolysis in patients with G6PD deficiency
Not established	—[b]	—[b]	—[b]	—[b]	—[b]	Abdominal pain, vomiting, diarrhea, headache, pruritus, rash
C	—[b]	—[b]	—[b]	—[b]	—[b]	Blurred vision, GI effects, pruritus; rare: cardiomyopathy
Not established	—[b]	—[b]	—[b]	—[b]	—[b]	Optic neuritis, peripheral neuropathy, anorexia, nausea, vomiting, diarrhea, skin reactions
Not established	—[b]	—[b]	—[b]	—[b]	—[b]	Fever, pruritus, headache, edema
B	—[b]	—[b]	—[b]	—[b]	—[b]	Diarrhea, nausea, vomiting, abdominal pain, fever, headache, neutropenia, thrombocytopenia
C	—[b]	—[b]	—[b]	—[b]	—[b]	Nausea, dizziness, seizures, bradycardia, rash
Not established	—[b]	—[b]	—[b]	—[b]	—[b]	Bradycardia, hypotension, rashes, facial edema, injection site pain, pancreatitis, leukopenia, nephrotoxicity
Not established	—[b]	—[b]	—[b]	—[b]	—[b]	Fever, hypertension, abdominal pain, vomiting, arthralgia, encephalopathy, rash, hemolysis in patients with G6PD deficiency
B	—[b]	—[b]	—[b]	—[b]	—[b]	Nausea, abdominal discomfort, diarrhea, drowsiness, dizziness, headache
Not established	—[b]	—[b]	—[b]	—[b]	—[b]	Nausea, vomiting, abdominal pain, anorexia, weight loss, restlessness, insomnia, paresthesias, seizures, rash, neutropenia
Not established	—[b]	—[b]	—[b]	—[b]	—[b]	Seizures, hallucinations

(continued)

Table 207.5 *(continued)*

| Name | | Usual Dose | | | Change in |
Generic	Brand	Adult	Child	Cost (per Day)*	Absorption with Food
Oxamniquine[e]	Vansil	12–60 mg/kg qd or divide BID	20–60 mg/kg divided BID	Data not available	Decreased
Paromomycin	Humatin	25–35 mg/kg PO divided TID 2–3 g qd divided QID in AIDS	—[b]	$30.33	Not absorbed
Pentamidine	Pentam, Nebupent	3–4 mg/kg/d IV 300 mg aerosolized q mo	3–4 mg/kg/d IV	$98.75 IV $98.75 aerosol	n/a
Piperazine citrate[e]	Antepar	2–3.5 g/d PO	65–75 mg/kg PO qd	Data not available	—[b]
Praziquantel	Biltricide	5–25 mg/kg ×1 (intestinal cestodiasis) 50–75 mg/kg/d, divided TID (other infections)	Not shown to be safe for children <4 y	$41.28	Increased
Primaquine phosphate		26.3 mg/d PO ×14 d 29 mg PO qwk × 8 wk	0.5 mg/kg/d PO 1.5 mg/kg PO q wk	$1.23	—[b]
Proguanil HCl and atovaquone	Malarone	400/1000 PO qd (treatment) 100/250 PO daily 1–2 d before entering endemic area, during stay, and for 7 d after return (prophylaxis)	50/125–1000/400 PO qd (depending on weight) (treatment) 25/62.5–100/250 PO qd (depending on weight) (prophylaxis)	$24.52 (treatment) $6.13 (prophylaxis)	Increased
Pyrantel pamoate	Antiminth, Pin-X	11 mg/kg (max 1 g/d) PO	11 mg/kg/d PO; not recommended for children ≤2 y	$7.23	—[b]

Pregnancy Class[a]	Dose Interval Adjustment for Reduced CrCl			Supplemental Dose in Dialysis		Major Toxicity
	>50	10–50	≤10	HD	PD	
Not established	—[b]	—[b]	—[b]	—[b]	—[b]	Dizziness, drowsiness, headache, nausea, vomiting, abdominal pain, orange-red discoloration of urine
Not established	—[b]	—[b]	—[b]	—[b]	—[b]	Anorexia, nausea, vomiting, abdominal pain, diarrhea, malabsorption
C	—[b]	—[b]	—[b]	—[b]	—[b]	Nephrotoxicity, hypotension, sterile abscess with IM injection, hypoglycemia or hyperglycemia, nausea, vomiting, abdominal pain, pancreatitis, hypocalcemia, cough and bronchospasm with inhalation
Not established	—[b]	—[b]	—[b]	—[b]	—[b]	Nausea, vomiting, diarrhea, abdominal cramps, headache, dizziness, rash, hemolytic anemia, ataxia
B	Usual dose	N.R.	N.R.	—[b]	—[b]	Transient dizziness, headache, drowsiness, fatigue, seizures, CSF reaction syndrome with treatment of neurocysticercosis, abdominal pain, nausea, rash
Not established	—[b]	—[b]	—[b]	—[b]	—[b]	Hemolytic anemia in patients with G6PD deficiency, nausea, vomiting, abdominal cramps, headache, pruritus
C	Usual	N.R. in patients with CrCl ≤ 30 mL/min	N.R. in patients with CrCl ≤ 30 mL/min	N.R. in patients with CrCl ≤ 30 ml/min	N.R. in patients with CrCl ≤ 30 ml/min	Rare hematologic toxicity
C	—[b]	—[b]	—[b]	—[b]	—[b]	Nausea, vomiting, cramps, dizziness, drowsiness, headache

(continued)

Table 207.5 *(continued)*

Name		Usual Dose		Cost (per Day)*	Change in Absorption with Food
Generic	Brand	Adult	Child		
Pyrimethamine	Daraprim	25–75 mg/d PO	0.5–2 mg/kg PO, divide BID Contraindicated for children ≤2 y	$0.61–$1.83	—[b]
Pyrimethamine + sulfadiazine	Fansidar	1 tab PO q wk (prophylaxis) 3 tabs PO ×1 (treatment)	½ tab PO 5–10 kg 1 tab 10–20 kg 1½ tab 21–30 kg 2 tabs 31–40 kg For children >2 y	$4.31/wk (prophylaxis) $12.93 (treatment course)	—[b]
Quinacrine HCl[e]	Atabrine	100 mg TID PC ×5 d	6 mg/kg TID PC ×5 d (≤50 kg)	Data not available	—[b]
Quinidine		10 mg/kg load over 1–2 h, then 0.02 mg/kg/min ×72 h	Same as adult	$89.84	Increased
Quinine	Legatrin Quinamm	325–650 g PO BID-TID	25–30 mg/kg/d PO; divide TID	$2.34–$4.68	—[b]
Spiramycine[e]	Rovamycine	3 g/d PO	50–100 mg/kg once or 2× daily (depending on infection being treated)	Data not available	No effect
Stibogluconate[d]	Pentostam	20 mg/kg IV qd × 20 d (not to exceed 850 mg)	—[b]	Data not available	n/a

Pregnancy Class	Dose Interval Adjustment for Reduced CrCl			Supplemental Dose in Dialysis		Major Toxicity
	>50	10–50	≤10	HD	PD	
C	—[b]	—[b]	—[b]	—[b]	—[b]	Bone marrow suppression with high doses, pulmonary eosinophilia, photosensitivity
C	—[b]	—[b]	—[b]	—[b]	—[b]	Leukopenia, hemolysis in patients with G6PD deficiency, rash and hypersensitivity reactions including Stevens–Johnson syndrome, hepatitis, pulmonary hypersensitivity reactions
C	—[b]	—[b]	—[b]	—[b]	—[b]	Nausea, vomiting, headache, dizziness, yellow discoloration of skin and urine, rash, fever, psychosis
C	—[b]	—[b]	—[b]	—[b]	—[b]	Diarrhea, abdominal pain, hypersensitivity reactions, systemic lupus erythematosuslike syndrome, elevated AST, elevated ALT, jaundice, cardiac arrhythmias
X	—[b]	—[b]	—[b]	—[b]	—[b]	Flushing, pruritus, rash, fever, tinnitus, headache, nausea, thrombocytopenia, hemolysis in patients with G6PD deficiency, hypoglycemia
—[b]	—[b]	—[b]	—[b]	—[b]	—[b]	QT interval prolongation, vasculitis, rash, diarrhea, increasad LFTs
Not established	—[b]	—[b]	—[b]	—[b]	—[b]	Abdominal pain, nausea, vomiting, malaise, headache, elevated AST and ALT, nephrotoxicity, myalgia, arthralgia, fever, rash, cough

(continued)

Table 207.5 *(continued)*

| Name | | Usual Dose | | | Change in |
Generic	Brand	Adult	Child	Cost (per Day)*	Absorption with Food
Suramin[d]	Germanin	1 g IV q wk ×5 wk (100-mg test dose)	—[b]	Data not available	n/a
Thiabendazole	Mintezol	25 mg/kg PO BID (maximum 3 g/d)	22 mg/kg PO BID	$7.56	—[b]
Trimetrexate	Neutrexin	45 mg/m²/d with leucovorin 20 mg/m² q6h; continue leucovorin at least 72 h after last dose	—[b]	$1412.40 (trimetrexate) + $68.00 (leucovorin)	n/a

Abbreviations: CrCl = Creatinine clearance mL/min; HD = hemodialysis; PD = peritoneal dialysis; AST = aspartate AIDS = acquired immunodeficiency syndrome; N.R. = not recommended; PC = after meals; CSF = cerebrospinal fluid.

[a] Food and Drug Administration pregnancy categories: A = adequate studies in pregnant women, no risk; B = animal studies no inadequate but benefit may exceed risk; D = evidence of human risk, benefit may outweigh risk; X = fetal abnormalities in

[b] Insufficient information available to make a recommendation.

[c] Available in the United States only from the manufacturer.

[d] Available from the Centers for Disease Control and Prevention drug service.

[e] Not available in the United States.

* Fleming T. The Red Book, 2007.

Pregnancy Class	Dose Interval Adjustment for Reduced CrCl			Supplemental Dose in Dialysis		Major Toxicity
	>50	10–50	≤10	HD	PD	
Fetal risk can not be ruled out	—[b]	—[b]	—[b]	—[b]	—[b]	Nausea, vomiting, shock, loss of consciousness, death during administration; fever, rash, exfoliative dermatitis, paresthesia, photophobia, renal insufficiency, diarrhea
C	—[b]	—[b]	—[b]	—[b]	—[b]	Anorexia, nausea, vomiting, dizziness
D	—[b]	—[b]	—[b]	—[b]	—[b]	Neutropenia (must be given with leucovorin); rash; elevated AST and ALT; reversible peripheral neuropathy

aminotransferase; ALT = alanine aminotransferase; GI = gastrointestinal; G6PD = glucose-6-phosphate dehydrogenase; n.a. = not approved; LFT = liver function test.
risk, human studies inadequate, or animal toxicity, human studies no risk; C = animal studies show toxicity, human studies humans, risk exceeds benefit.

SUGGESTED READING

Cunha BA. *Antibiotic Essentials*. Royal Oak, MI: Physicians' Press; 2006.

Fleming T. 2007 *Red Book: Pharmacy's Fundamental Reference*. Thomson Publishers; 2007.

Gilbert DN, Moellering RC, Eliopoulos GM, et al. *The Sanford Guide to Antimicrobial Therapy*. 36th ed. Sperryville, VA: Antimicrobial Therapy, Inc.; 2006.

Mandell GL, Bennett JE, Dolin R. *Principles and Practice of Infectious Diseases*. 6th ed. Philadelphia, PA: Elsevier; 2005.

Index

Chryseomonas luteola; see
Pseudomonas luteola
Ciclopirox, 174, 180, 177t
Cidofovir, 1435–1436, 1482t
  cytomegalovirus, 1244, 1241t
  cytomegalovirus retinitis, 105,
    104t
  esophageal infection, 345, 346t
  human herpesvirus, 1283t
  human papillomaviruses, 1297
  pregnancy, 725t
  progressive multifocal
    leukoencephalopathy, 573
Ciguatera, 362t, 364t
Cinchonism, 1375–1376
Cinoxacin, 1458t
Ciprofloxacin, 1458t
  acute cholangitis, 322f
  anthrax, 899–900
  bacterial meningitis, 512
  bronchitis, chronic, 201, 203,
    203, 202t
  Campylobacter infection, 927t
  chancroid, 437–438, 985t
  conjunctivitis, 82t
  diverticulitis, 384t, 384t
  donovanosis, 439
  drug–drug interactions, 1419
  endocarditis, 262t, 631
  gastroenteritis and cholera,
    1095–1096
  gonorrhea, 980t, 980t, 980t
  HACEK organisms, 966, 967t
  iritis, 98
  joint infection, 472
  Legionnaires' disease, 992t
  lung abscess, 243
  meningococcal infection,
    1000t, 1004t
  nosocomial pneumonia,
    230–231, 231t
  osteomyelitis, 480, 481t
  otitis media, 51
  peritoneal dialysis infection,
    667t
  peritonitis, 398
  pregnancy, 725t
  prostatitis, 443–444, 444t
  pyoderma, 148, 146t
  pyogenic liver abscess, 329t
  rat-bite fevers, 1041
  Shigella infection, 373, 1070,
    1071t, 1071t
  surgical prophylaxis, 800t
  trauma-related infections, 777t
  travelers' diarrhea, 861t
  urethritis, 412–413, 412t
  urinary tract infection, 453t,
    454t, 455t
Citrobacter freundii nosocomial
    pneumonia, 229, 230t, 230t
Citrobacter spp., 761

Clarithromycin, 1458t
  animal bites, 163t
  atypical pneumonia, 217t
  bronchitis, chronic, 202–203,
    202t
  C. pneumoniae, 1159t
  community-acquired
    pneumonia, 225, 225t,
    225t, 1026, 1026t
  drug–drug interactions, 1419
  H. pylori treatment, 974t
  impetigo, 145
  Legionnaires' disease, 991,
    992t
  M. avium complex in HIV
    patients, 714t
  M. pneumoniae, 1149t
  MAC lung disease, 1090–1091,
    1088t
  otitis media, 49t
  pregnancy, 725t
  rat-bite fevers, 1041
Clenched fist bites, 164–165
Clindamycin, 1458t
  actinomycosis, 883t
  acute supraglottitis, 208
  adverse reactions to, 1417,
    1416t
  animal bites, 163t
  aspiration pneumonia,
    237–238
  babesiosis, 1384–1385, 1385t
  bursitis, 476–477, 476f
  cellulitis, 153, 154t
  cytolytic vaginitis or
    vaginosis, 424
  deep neck infections, 74t
  dental infections, 62
  desquamative vaginitis, 425
  diabetic foot infection, 629
  diverticulitis, 384t
  Erysipelothrix spp., 962–963t
  gas gangrene, 159, 933
  impetigo, 145
  lung abscess, 242, 243t, 244t
  M. hominis, 1152, 1153t, 1154t
  M. hominis and Ureaplasma
    spp., 1153t, 1154t
  malaria, 1374t
  mediastinitis, 283
  ocular toxoplasmosis, 106
  osteomyelitis, 481t
  otitis media, 49t
  pelvic inflammatory disease,
    446t
  peritonitis, 400–401
  pharyngotonsillitis
  acute, 37
  chronic and recurrent, 37–38,
    36t
  pneumocystis pneumonia,
    1230

pregnancy, 725t
  psoas abscess, 500t
  pyoderma, 148, 146t
  sinusitis, 57
  spinal epidural abscess, 544
  surgical prophylaxis, 800t
  toxic shock syndrome, 132
  toxoplasmosis, 1367t
Clofazimine, 1476t
  chronic uveitis, 100
  leprosy, 995, 995t
  tuberculosis, 1084, 1080t
Clonazepam, 582–583
Clonorchiasis and
    opisthorchiasis, 1356–1357,
    1356f, 1357t
Clostridia, 929–934
  bacteremia, 934
  botulism, 929–931
    foodborne, 929–930
    infant, 931
    inhalation, 931
    pathogenesis, 929
    wound infection, 930–931
  C. difficile colitis, 367–369
  C. perfringens food poisoning,
    934
  gas gangrene, 933
  tetanus, 931–933
    cephalic, 932
    generalized, 931–932
    local, 932
    neonatal, 932
    vaccine, 932–933, 933t
Clostridial myonecrosis; see Gas
    gangrene
Clostridial spp., 159
Clostridium botulinum,
    361, 364t
  food poisoning, 360t, 364t,
    929–930
  infant, 931
  inhalation, 931
  laboratory tests for, 870
  neuropathy, 556–558
  pathogenesis, 929
  treatment, 876
  wound infection, 930–931
Clostridium difficile, 13
  diarrhea, 367–369
    diagnosis, 367
    implications, 368–369
    treatment, 367–368, 368t,
      368t
  gastroenteritis, 356t
  lung abscess, 243
  NAP1 strain, 368
  neutropenic patients, 594
Clostridium perfringens food
    poisoning, 360t, 364t, 934
  gas gangrene, 933
Clostridium spp.

IG; see Immunoglobulin (IG)

Iliopsoas abscess; see Psoas abscess

Imidazoles
dermatophyte infections, 176, 177t
esophageal infection (*Candida*). see Esophageal infections
fungal endocarditis, 261
leishmaniasis, 1397
liver abscess, amebic, 1407
vulvovaginal candidiasis, 1182–1183

Imipenem, 1458t
acute cholangitis, 322f
lung abscess, 243t
neutropenic patients, 598t
Nocardia infection, 1015t
nosocomial pneumonia, 230–231, 231t
pancreatitis, 334–336
pyelonephritis, 655–656
pyoderma, 148, 146t
pyogenic liver abscess, 329t
urinary catheter-related infections, 764t
Y. enterocolitica, 1101t

Imiquimod cream, 1296, 1438

Immune reconstitution inflammatory syndrome (IRIS), 699–706
history and definitions, 700, 700t, 700t
immune recovery with HAART, 699
microbiology, 702t
pathology, 700–704, 702t, 699f, 701f
C. neoformans-related, 701–702, 703f
cytomegalovirus-related, 702–703
hepatitis B and C, 704, 700t
herpes and varicella zoster viruses, 703
human herpesvirus-8, 704
JC virus, 704
M. avium complex-related, 700–701, 701f
M. tuberculosis related, 701, 703f
predisposing factors, 704–705, 702t, 705t
treatment, 705

Immunization Action Coalition (IAC), 807

Immunizations, 807–821
for adults, 812, 818t
anthrax, 899–900
for children, 807–812, 811t, 815t

combination, 812, 815t
F. tularensis, 1074
hepatitis A virus, 299, 820–821, 829
hepatitis B virus, 303, 741, 819, 827
hepatitis C virus, 304
HIV infected patients, 686–687, 687t
for influenza, 45–46, 208, 985, 985t, 1292, 1293t
Lyme disease, 1133
measles (rubeola), 137, 137t, 813–815
meningococcal infection, 1001–1002
mumps, 68, 429, 813–815
parvovirus infection, 1304
PCV7 and otitis media, 45–46, 51
pneumococcal, 819, 1029
polio, 819, 826
post-splenectomy infection, 677, 676t
preseptal cellulitis, 118
rabies, 829, 1308
routine, 812–821
rubella, 137, 138t, 813–815
special considerations, 821
supraglottitis prevention, 209
tetanus, 162, 559, 932–933, 933t
for travelers, 825–830, 828t
typhoid, 828–829
varicella-zoster virus, 815–819, 1313
viral hemorrhagic fever, 1330
viral influenza, 819–820
yellow fever, 827–828

Immunocompromised patients; see also Alcoholic patients; Elderly patients; HIV infection and AIDS
abdominal abscess, 388
actinomycosis treatment in, 884
acute cholecystitis, 322
alcoholics, 637t, 638t
aseptic meningitis syndrome, 520
bites, human and animal, 162t
blastomycosis, 1216
brain abscess, 532, 534–535, 535t
cat scratch disease, 907, 909–910, 909f, 909f, 910f
chronic hepatitis C, 314
corticosteroid use, 605–606
cryptococcus, 1210
cytomegalovirus retinitis, 103–105

deep neck infection treatment, 74t
Epstein-Barr virus, 306
erysipelas, 151
esophageal infection, 342, 343, 343–344, 344–345
esophageal infection (*Candida*), 339
hepatitis, 302–303
herpes simplex virus, 1278, 1279, 1279t
human herpesvirus-6, 1282–1283
L. monocytogenes. see Listeria
M. hominis and *Ureaplasma* spp., 1153–1154
mycetoma, 182
onychomycosis, 176
pericarditis, 265
pneumocystis pneumonia, 1230–1231
psoas abscess, 499t
pyogenic liver abscess, 328
Rhodococcus spp., 1107
rubeola, 137
septic emboli, 125
skin lesions, 141
splenic abscess, 392–393, 395
toxoplasmosis, 1366–1368, 1367t, 1368t
urethritis, 409, 409t
varicella-zoster virus, 1316, 1317t

Immunodeficiency
evaluation of, 587–591
approach to, 587, 591
B cell function, 588t, 587–588, 604
complement system, 591t, 590–591
IL-12/23 and interferon gamma pathways, 589
innate immune signaling (TLRs), 589
natural killer cell function, 589
neutrophil function, 589–590, 590t, 601–603
T cell function, 588–589, 589t
intravenous drug abusers, 633–634

Immunoglobulin (IG); see also Intravenous immunoglobulin (IVIG)
antibiotic hypersensitivity, 1446t
hepatitis A virus, 829, 828t
measles (rubeola), 137
parvovirus infection, 1303f
rubella, 138

Immunosuppression

adjunctive, 91–93
administration, 89–90
empiric, 90, 89f
Ketoconazole, 1478t
blastomycosis, 1215–1216
coccidioidomycosis, 1225–1226
dermatophyte infections, 177t
leishmaniasis, 1397
mycetoma, 185
otitis externa, 53
pityriasis versicolor, 180
pregnancy, 725t
Ketolides, *M. pneumoniae*,
1148–1150, 1149t
Kingella spp., 966t
Klebsiella pneumoniae
lung abscess, 241, 241–242
pancreatitis, 334t
urinary catheter-related
infections, 761
Klebsiella spp.
abdominal abscess, 388–389
acute cholecystitis, 322
CSF shunt infections, 575
metastatic endophthalmitis,
99
neutropenic patients, 593
nosocomial pneumonia, 229
penile implant infection, 780
pericarditis, 266t
pneumonia in neoplastic
patients, 602t
prostatitis, 443t
renal corticomedullary
abscess, 462
splenic abscess, 394t
Kuru; *see* Prion diseases
Kuttner's tumor (KT), 68

L

Laboratory Risk Indicator for
NECrotising fasciitis
[LRINEC], 157
Labyrinthitis, 52
Lacrimal gland infections, 69–70,
70t, 117
canaliculitis, 69, 117
dacryoadenitis, 70, 117
dacryocystitis, 69–70, 117
Lactobacillus crispatus, 415–416,
416t; *see also* Vaginitis and
cervicitis
Lactobacillus spp., 779–780, 1105,
1104t
Lactococcus spp., 1108, 1104t
Lamivudine, 1440, 1482t
for chronic hepatitis B, 313t,
313t
hepatitis B virus, 303
HIV infection, 691–692, 693t

Lancefield, Rebecca, 1055
Laryngitis, 209–210
Laryngotracheobronchitis,
205–207, 206t, 207t, 207f
Lateral pharyngeal space
infection, 74, 74t, 74t, 75t,
76f
Legionella pneumophila, atypical
pneumonia, 211, 213,
217–218, 216t
Legionella spp.
community-acquired
pneumonia, 223, 223t,
225t, 225t, 226t
lung abscess, 241
polymyositis, 492–493, 492t
Legionellosis, 987–992
diagnosis, 990–991
epidemiology, 987–988
etiology, 987, 987t
infectious syndromes, 989–990
nosocomial, 990, 991t
pneumonia, 989–990, 991t
Pontiac fever, 990
Legionnaires' disease, 213
in travelers, 835
water exposure, 857
pathogenesis, 988–989
Pontiac fever, 990
treatment, 991–992, 992t
Legionnaires' disease; *see*
Legionellosis
Leibovitz, E., 47
Leishmaniasis, 1394–1398, 1395f,
1396f
clinical presentation, 1396f,
1396f, 1396f, 1396f, 1397f,
1397f, 1397f
microbiology, 1389, 1398t
skin ulcers, 143t
in travelers, 835
treatment, 1391t
Lemierre's syndrome, 75–76, 76t,
285
Leprosy, 993–996
chronic uveitis, 100
classification and clinical
presentation, 993–994, 994f
diagnosis, 994–995
epidemiology, 993
neuropathy, 554
pathophysiology, 993
treatment (general), 995–996,
995t
treatment of reversal
reactions, 996, 996t
Leptospirosis, 1139–1148
clinical presentation, 1139,
1139t
diagnosis, 1139–1148, 1140t
epidemiology, 1140t
pathogenesis, 1140t

in travelers, 835
treatment, 1148, 1140t
water exposure, 856, 851t
Leuconostoc spp., 1103–1105,
1104t
Leukopenia, 6
Levofloxacin, 1458t
atypical pneumonia, 217–218,
217t, 217t
bronchitis, chronic, 201, 202t
C. pneumoniae, 1159t
community-acquired
pneumonia, 225t
diabetic foot infection, 629
gonorrhea, 980t, 980t, 980t
joint infection, 472
Legionnaires' disease, 991,
992t
lung abscess, 243
M. hominis and *Ureaplasma*
spp., 1153t
osteomyelitis, 480, 481t
pelvic inflammatory disease,
446t, 446t
pneumonia, 1026–1027, 1026t
prostatitis, 443–444, 444t
spinal epidural abscess, 544
trichomoniasis, 422, 422–423
urinary tract infection, 453t,
454t
Lincomycin, 1458t
pharyngotonsillitis
acute, 37
chronic and recurrent,
37–38, 36t
Lincosamide for cellulitis, 154t
Linezolid, 1458t
bursitis, 476–477, 476f
cellulitis, 155, 155t
community-acquired
pneumonia, 225–226
defibrillator and pacemaker
infections, 294–295, 295t
dental infections, 62
diabetic foot infection, 629
endocarditis, 257–258
mycetoma, 184
necrotizing fasciitis, 158–159,
158t
spinal epidural abscess, 544
Lipid A, 9, 10, 11
Liposomal amphotericin B, 1394,
1427, 1428t, 1478t
Listeria, 1005–1011
clinical presentation,
1007–1010
bacteremia, 1008
bacterial meningitis, 505,
511, 507t, 509t
brain abscess, 532, 532t
brain stem encephalitis,
1008

cerebritis and brain
abscess, 1009, 1009f
endocarditis, 1009
febrile gastroenteritis,
1009–1010
localized infection, 1009
meningitis, 1008, 1009t
in neonates, 1008
pericarditis, 266t
in pregnancy, 1007
diagnosis, 1010
epidemiology, 1005–1006
immunity, 1007
L. monocytogenes
bacterial meningitis, 505,
511, 507t, 509t
brain abscess, 532, 532t
pathogenesis, 1006–1007
pericarditis, 266t
treatment, 1010–1011,
1010t
L. spp. (other), 1005
microbiology, 1005
pathogenesis, 1006–1007
prevention, 1011, 1011t
treatment, 1010–1011, 1010t
Little, Paul, 47
Liver failure and hepatitis A
virus, 299
Liver transplantation
chronic hepatitis, 305
mushroom poisoning, 365
Loa loa, 1346–1347, 1346f
Loiasis, 1346–1347, 1346f
Lomefloxacin, 1458t
Loperamide, 354–355, 355t,
860–861, 861t
Lopinavir, 692–693, 694t, 1482t
Loracarbef, 1458t
Louse infestations, 167–169, 171t,
168f, 168f
Ludwig's angina, 1061–1063
deep neck infections, 74, 74t,
74t, 75t, 76f
dental infection, 59, 61, 61t
Lung abscess, 241–244
definition, 241
diagnosis, 241–242, 242t, 242f,
242f
imaging, 241
lower-airway specimen
techniques, 241
vs. necrotizing pneumonia,
241
treatment, 241–242
drainage, 244
duration, 243, 244t
empiric, 242–243, 243t
Lyme disease, 1127–1134
clinical presentation,
1127–1129, 1128f
early disseminated, 1129

early localized disease,
1127–1128
late disease, 1129
iritis, 98
myocarditis, 271, 272t
polyarthritis, 486
prevention and prophylaxis,
792t, 1133
in travelers, 835, 838–841,
839t, 846t
treatment, 1130t
arthritis, 1131–1132
carditis, 1131
early Lyme disease,
1129–1131
early neurologic disease,
1131
late neurologic Lyme
disease, 1132
ocular disease, 1132
post-Lyme syndrome,
1133
pregnancy and, 1132
seropositive patients with
nonspecific symptoms,
1133
tick bites, 1132–1133
Lymphadenopathy, 187–193
adenopathy and HIV
infection, 191–193, 193f
diagnosis, 192–193
anatomy and differential
diagnosis, 188t
clinical approach, 187
generalized, 191
localized, 189f, 190f, 190f,
191f, 188–191
Lymphatic filariasis, 1344–1345,
1345f
Lymphocytopenia, 6
Lymphocytosis, 6
Lymphogranuloma venereum,
434, 438–439
clinical presentation, 435t
diagnosis, 436t
prevalence, 434t
treatment, 438t

M
Macrolides; *see also specific
macrolides*
adverse reactions to, 1418,
1416t, 1454, 1449t
atypical pneumonia, 215–217
bronchitis, chronic, 202–203,
202t
Campylobacter infection,
926–927, 927t
cellulitis, 154t
community-acquired
pneumonia, 223–225,

225–226, 224t, 225t, 225t,
1026, 1026t
gastroenteritis, 355–356, 356t
Legionnaires' disease, 992t
M. pneumoniae, 1148, 1149t
MAC lung disease, 1090–1091,
1088t
otitis media, 49–50, 1028–1029
pertussis, 914, 915t
pharyngotonsillitis, 37, 36t,
35t
relapsing fever, 1136–1137,
1136t
sinusitis, 57
Macular edema, 97
Madura foot, 181–185
clinical presentation, 181–182,
182f, 183f, 183f
diagnosis, 182–184
differential diagnosis, 184
epidemiology, 181
microbiology, 181, 182t, 182t
pathogenesis, 181
treatment, 184–185
actinomycetoma, 184–185,
182t
eumycetoma, 185, 182t
Mafenide acetate, 784, 785
Malaria, 1371–1379
clinical presentation, 1371
diagnosis, 1371–1372
etiology and epidemiology,
1371, 1373f
pregnancy, 657
prophylaxis, 1376–1379,
1377f
in returning travelers, 833
treatment, 1372–1376, 1374t,
1378t
chloroquine-resistant *P.
falciparum* malaria,
1375–1376, 1373f
complicated *P. falciparum*
malaria, 1376
P. malariae and uncomplicated
chloroquine-sensitive *P.
falciparum* malaria, 1375
P. ovale malaria, 1375
P. vivax malaria, 1373–1375
Malassezia furfur, 179–180
Malathion, 167–168, 171t
Malignancy and fever of
unknown origin, 4
Mansonella spp., 1348–1349
Marginal blepharitis, 117
Marshall, Barry, 969
Mastitis, 660
Mastoiditis, 52
Meares-Stamey prostatitis
localization protocol, 441
Measles; *see* Rubeola
Mebendazole, 1488t

diagnosis
extrapulmonary disease, 1089
lung disease, 1087–1094
emerging areas of infection, 1093–1094
cystic fibrosis associated disease, 1093
healthcare associated disease, 1094
hypersensitivity pneumonitis-like lung disease, 1093–1094
treatment, 1088t
disseminated disease, 1091
M. abscessus disease, 1092
M. kansasii pulmonary disease, 1091–1092
M. marinum disease, 1092
MAC lung disease, 1090–1091
MAC lymphadenopathy, 1091
principles of, 1089–1090
Nontuberculosis mycobacterial keratitis, 90
Nontypeable *H. influenzae* (NTHi) and otitis media, 45, 46, 47, 48–50, 51–52
Nonvenereal treponematoses, 1125–1126
Norepinephrine, hantavirus cardiopulmonary syndrome, 1272
Norfloxacin, 1458t
pancreatitis, 334–336
peritonitis, 398
Norovirus
food poisoning, 359, 360t, 364t
gastroenteritis, 351
water exposure, 858, 858f
Norwalk virus; *see Norovirus*
Nosocomial infections, 733–737
A. baumannii, 1111–1112, 1112t, 1113t
Achromobacter spp., 1112, 1112t, 1113t
C. difficile-associated enteritis, 367–368
candiduria, 457
catheter-related infections. *see* Catheter-related infections
in diabetic patients, 630
endocarditis, 254–255
endophthalmitis, 109
gram-positive organisms causing, 954t
hospital-acquired fever, 745–747
infectious causes, 745t
noninfectious causes, 746t
impact of, 733–734, 733t
investigation of outbreak, 734t

Legionnaires' disease, 990, 991t, 992t
measures and programs, 735–737, 736t
in neonates, 647
new and continuing problems, 734–735, 734t
percutaneous injury. *see* Percutaneous injury
pneumonia. *see* Nosocomial pneumonia
post-transplantation, 611–612, 613t
sepsis and septic shock, 13t, 15t
transfusion-related infection, 749–753
clinical management, 752, 752f
contamination sources, 751–752
plasma and plasma-derived products, 751
platelets, 750–751, 751t
prevention, 752–753, 753t
risk associated with, 749–750, 749t
whole blood and erythrocytes, 750, 750t, 751t
urinary tract infection, 449
varicella-zoster virus, 1317
Nosocomial pneumonia, 229–232
diagnosis, 229–230
empiric monotherapy, 230–231, 231t
and HSV-1, 231–232, 232t
and Legionnaires' disease, 990, 991t
multidrug resistant therapy, 231, 230t
vs. respiratory secretion colonization, 229, 230t, 230t
types, 229
ventilator-associated, 229, 616, 733, 745t, 1037–1038
Nucleoside therapy for chronic hepatitis B, 311–312, 313t, 313t
progressive multifocal leukoencephalopathy, 572–573
Nucleoside/nucleotide reverse transcriptase inhibitors (NRTIs), 691–692, 689t, 690t, 693t, 742–744, 742t
Nucleotide analog therapy (chronic hepatitis B), 312–313, 313t, 313t, 313t, 5552.210f
Nystatin, 1478t

candidiasis, 421
chronic fatigue syndrome, 27

O

Obstructive sialadenitis, 68, 66t
Ochrobactrum spp., 1116, 1112t, 1113t
Octreotide, 355t
Ocular disease
candidiasis, 1185
conjunctivitis. *see* Conjunctivitis
endophthalmitis. *see* endophthalmitis
iritis. *see* Iritis
keratitis. *see* Keratitis
in Lyme disease, 1132
periocular infections, 117–120, 119t
definition, 117
eyelid, 117
periorbital, 118–120
retinitis, 103–107
acute retinal necrosis, 106–107, 106f
cytomegalovirus, 103–105, 103f, 103f, 1241t, 1435, 1443
in HIV infected patients, 716–718, 717t
ocular toxoplasmosis, 105–106, 105f, 1366
treatment, 104t, 1241t, 1443
Ocular larva migrans (OLM), 1350
Ocular medicamentosa, 84–85
Ocular toxoplasmosis, 105–106, 104t, 105f
Odontogenic infections; *see* Dental infections
Oerskovia spp., 1105–1106, 1104t
Ofloxacin, 1458t
bronchitis, chronic, 201, 202t
conjunctivitis, 82t
epididymitis, 430
gonorrhea, 980t, 980t, 980t
leprosy, 995, 995t
M. hominis and *Ureaplasma* spp., 1153t
meningococcal infection, 1004t
otitis media, 51
pelvic inflammatory disease, 446t, 446t
pregnancy, 725t
urinary tract infection, 453t
Ohnemilz; *see* Overwhelming postsplenectomy infection (OPSI)
Oligella spp., 1116
Oligoarthritis; *see* Polyarthritis and fever

renal papillary necrosis, 465, 462t, 465t
Renal papillary necrosis, 465, 462t, 465t
Reoviridae, 528, 522t
Respiratory syncytial virus (RSV), 215
    atypical pneumonia, 219, 214t, 216t
    community-acquired pneumonia, 226–227
    pharyngotonsillitis, 34
    treatment, 1441
Retinitis, 103–107
    acute retinal necrosis, 106–107, 106f
    cytomegalovirus, 103–105, 103f, 103f, 1241t, 1435, 1443
    in HIV infected patients, 716–718, 717t
    ocular toxoplasmosis, 105–106, 105f, 1366
    treatment, 104t, 1241t, 1443
Retropharyngeal space infection, 74–75, 74t, 74t, 75t, 76t
Reye's syndrome, 563–566
    in adults, 565
    clinical presentation, 563–564, 564t
    definition, 563
    pathology, 564
    pathophysiology, 564
    prognosis, 565
    vs. Reye's-like-syndrome, 565, 565t, 566t
    treatment, 564–565
Reynolds' pentad, 324
Rhabdomyolysis from polymyositis, 491
Rhabdoviridae, 523t
Rheumatic diseases
    acute rheumatic fever, 1065–1067, 1066t, 1066t
    fever of unknown origin, 4, 7
    prophylaxis, 794t
Rheumatic fever
    acute, 1065–1067, 1066t, 1066t
    incidence, 25
    myocarditis, 272t
    penicillin, 1055
    pericarditis, 266t
    postinfectious polyarthritis, 487–488, 485t
    prophylaxis, 794t
    toxic shocklike syndrome, 124–125
    treatment, 37
Rheumatoid factor, 6
Rhinosinusitis, 55–56; see also Sinusitis
Rhinoviruses, 209, 226–227

Rhizobium spp., 1116–1117
Rhodococcus equi, 1107, 1104t
    HIV infected patients, 714t, 717t
Rhombencephalitis, 1008
Ribavirin, 226–227, 1441–1442, 1482t
    for chronic hepatitis B, 316t, 317t, 316t
    for chronic hepatitis C, 314–317, 317t
    encephalitis, 528
    for viral hemorrhagic fever, 877
Rickettsia rickettsii, 1167–1168
Rickettsial infection, 834, 1167–1168, 1167–1171
    diseases caused by, 1169t
    murine typhus, 1170
    Q fever, 1170–1171
    Rocky Mountain spotted fever. *see* Rocky Mountain spotted fever
    scrub typhus, 1170
    spotted fever group Rickettsia, 1168–1169, 1169t
    typhus, epidemic or louseborne, 1169–1170
Rifabutin, 1476t
    nontuberculosis mycobacteria (MAC), 1088t
    pregnancy, 725t
Rifampicin for chronic uveitis, 100, 100
Rifampin, 1476t
    acute supraglottitis, 209
    bacterial meningitis, 512
    bartonellosis, 904f, 904t
    brucellosis, 835, 922–923, 923–924
    CSF shunt infections, 577t
    in diabetic patients, 628
    ehrlichiosis and anaplasmosis, 1174–1176
    endocarditis, 260–261, 631
    joint infection, 472, 471t
    Legionnaires' disease, 991, 992t
    leprosy, 995, 995t
    mediastinitis, 283
    meningococcal infection, 1004t, 1028t
    nontuberculosis mycobacteria (MAC), 1088t
    osteomyelitis, 480, 481t
    peritoneal dialysis infection, 667t
    pregnancy, 725t
    sinusitis, 57
    toxic shock syndrome, 132–133
    tuberculosis, 1080t

Rifapentine, 1476t
Rifaximin, 860, 861, 861t, 1458t
Rimantadine, 1442, 1482t
Ringer's lactate
    acute appendicitis, 378
    dengue, 1248–1250, 1248t
    food poisoning, 362
Ritonavir, 692, 694t, 1482t
Rocky Mountain spotted fever, 124, 125t, 838, 839t, 845, 846t, 1167–1168
    clinical presentation, 1168t
    treatment, 1168
Roseola, 138–139
    diagnosis, 138–139
    treatment and prevention, 139
Roseomonas spp., 1117
Rotaviruses, 351
Rothia dentocariosa, 1106, 1104t
Rothia spp., 1106, 1104t
Roundworms, intestinal, 1335–1341, 1337t
    anisakiasis, 1341
    ascariasis, 1335–1336, 1336f
    enterobiasis, 1340–1341
    hookworm, 1337–1338
    strongyloidiasis, 1338–1340, 1339f
    trichostrongyliasis, 1341
    trichuriasis, 1336–1337
Rubella, 135–137, 136t
    diagnosis, 137–138
    vs. infectious mononucleosis, 1266t, 1267t
    polyarthritis, 487
    treatment and prevention, 138
    vaccine, 137, 138t, 813–815, 826–827
Rubeola, 135–137, 136t
    diagnosis, 135–136
    pericarditis, 266t
    treatment and prevention, 136–137
    vaccine, 137t, 813–815, 826–827

S
Salicylic acid; *see* Acetylsalicylic acid
Salivary gland infections, 65–69
    acute bacterial sialadenitis, 65–67, 66f, 67t
    chronic bacterial sialadenitis, 67–68
    chronic sclerosing sialadenitis, 68
    granulomatous sialadenitis, 69
    obstructive sialadenitis, 68
    viral sialadenitis, 68–69
Salmonella spp., 1040–1048